—American Society of Superintendents of Training Schools for Nurses (renamed the National League of Nursing Education [NLNE] in 1912) became the first organized nursing group in the United States and Canada.

1897 Nurses' Associated Alumnae of United States and Canada organized. Renamed the American Nurses' Association (ANA) in 1911.

—Victorian Order of Nurses established in Canada by Lady Aberdeen. It conducted practically all public health nursing.

1899 International Council of Nurses (ICN) established by Mrs. Bedford Fenwick of Great Britain. United States and Canadian nurses were among its founders, and their national associations were among the first admitted to membership.

1900 *American Journal of Nursing*, first nursing journal in the United States to be owned, operated, and published by nurses, launched. Its publisher, incorporated in 1902, now also publishes *Nursing Research*, established in 1952; *Nursing Outlook*, 1953; *International Nursing Index*, 1966; *MCN: American Journal of Maternal-Child Nursing*, 1976; and *Geriatric Nursing: American Journal of Care for the Aging*, 1980.

1901 United States Army Nurse Corps formally established by act of Congress.

1903 First nurse practice acts passed in North Carolina, New Jersey, Virginia, and New York.

1905 *Canadian Nurse* journal inaugurated. By 1959 it was published in both English and French.

1908 Canadian National Association of Trained Nurses (CNATN) established. It later became the Canadian Nurses' Association (CNA).

—National Association of Colored Graduate Nurses (NACGN) established.

—United States Navy Nurse Corps formed.

1912 National Organization for Public Health Nursing (NOPHN) established.

—United States Children's Bureau created by Congress as part of the Department of Commerce and Labor.

1916 Criteria for a profession, set forth by Abraham Flexner in "Is social work a profession?" (published in *School and society*, volume 1), became yardsticks for nursing and continue to serve this function.

1917 NLNE published its first *Standard curriculum for schools of nursing*; revised editions, under slightly different titles, appeared in 1927 and 1937.

1919 Ethyl Johns established the first baccalaureate degree program in nursing in the British Empire at the University of British Columbia, Vancouver.

1922 Sigma Theta Tau, national honor society of nursing in the United States, founded by six nursing students at Indiana Training School for Nurses.

1923 Publication of *Nursing and nursing education in the United States*, better known as the Goldmark (or Winslow-Goldmark) Report. Originally intended to study education for public health nursing, the study committee extended its work to include all of nursing education, criticizing the low standards, inadequate financing, and lack of separation of education from service.

—Yale University (New Haven, Connecticut) and Western Reserve University (Cleveland, Ohio), each with the aid of endowments, established independent schools of nursing. In 1934, both started requiring a baccalaureate degree for admission to the schools and granted masters of nursing degrees.

1928 Publication of *Nurses, patients, and pocketbooks*, first report of the Committee on Grading of Nursing Schools appointed two years earlier. The report indicated that there was an oversupply of nurses in general but an undersupply of adequately prepared ones.

1929 American Association of Nurse-Midwives formed. It merged in 1969 with the American College of Nurse-Midwifery to become the American College of Nurse-Midwives.

1931 Weir Report in Canada recommended integration of nursing education into the provincial education system.

1932 Association of Collegiate Schools of Nursing (ACSN) established to promote nursing education on a professional and collegiate level and to encourage research.

1933 ANA launched campaign for hospitals to employ graduate nurses instead of relying heavily on nursing students for patient care.

1934 Publication of *Nursing schools today and tomorrow*, final report of the Grading Committee (which never did grade schools publicly). It confirmed the

(Continued on inside back cover)

Fundamentals of Nursing

Fundamentals of Nursing

Second Edition

Concepts and Procedures

Barbara Kozier, BA, BSN, RN, MN

Glenora Erb, BSN, RN

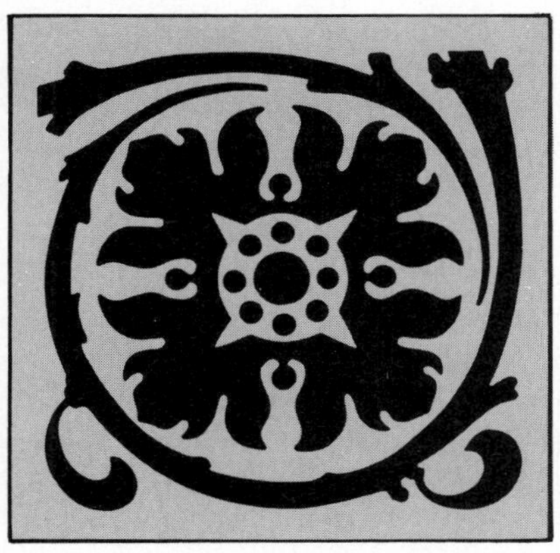

Addison-Wesley Publishing Company
Nursing Division, Menlo Park, California
Reading, Massachusetts • London • Amsterdam • Don Mills, Ontario • Sydney

Library of Congress Cataloging in Publication Data

Kozier, Barbara Blackwood.
Fundamentals of nursing.

Includes bibliographies and index.
1. Nursing. I. Erb, Glenora Lea, 1937– .
II. Title. [DNLM: 1. Nursing care. WY 100 K88fa]
RT41.K72 1983 610.73 82-22707
ISBN 0-201-11711-8

GHIJ-MU-898765

Addison-Wesley Publishing Company
Nursing Division
2725 Sand Hill Road
Menlo Park, California 94025

Sponsoring Editor: Nancy Evans
Production Editor: Zipporah W. Collins, assisted by Antonio Padial and Loralee Windsor
Copyeditors: Zipporah W. Collins, Antonio Padial
Book Design: Janet Bollow
Cover Design: Michael A. Rogondino
Illustrations: Jack P. Tandy
Photographs: William Thompson, RN, of Limited Horizons; George B. Fry III
Proofreaders: Nancy Cooney, Katherine L. Kaiser-Schwartz
Indexer: Elinor Lindheimer

"Significant Events in Nursing History" on the front and back endsheets was compiled by Edith P. Lewis, MN, FAAN

The authors and publishers have exerted every effort to ensure that drug selections and dosages set forth in this text are in accord with current recommendations and practice at the time of publication. However, in view of ongoing research, changes in government regulations, and the constant flow of information relating to drug therapy and drug reactions, the reader is urged to check the package insert for each drug for any change in indications of dosage and for added warnings and precautions. This is particularly important where the recommended agent is a new and/or infrequently employed drug.

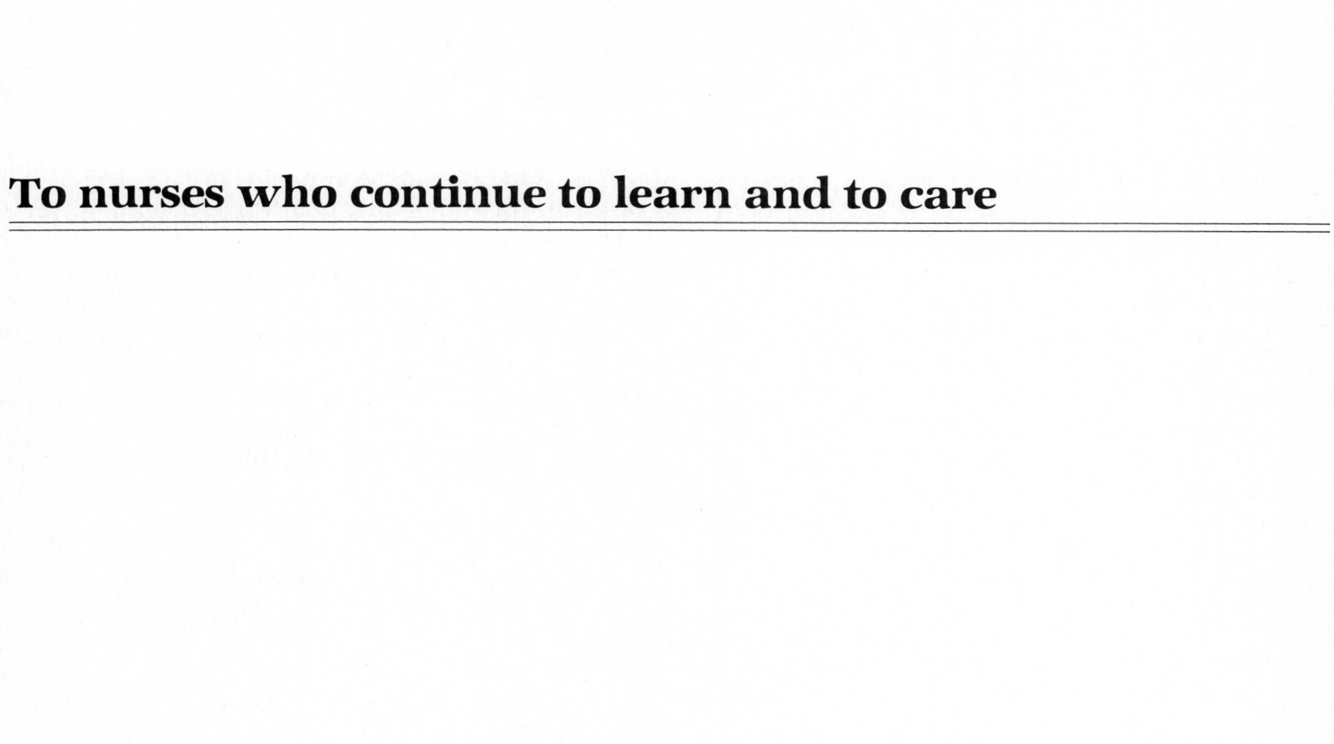

To nurses who continue to learn and to care

Preface

Look to the essence of a thing,
whether it be a point of doctrine, of practice,
or of interpretation.

MARCUS AURELIUS

What is the essence of nursing? Answers vary. Since the Nightingale era, experts have tried to define nursing, realizing that nursing continually redefines itself in response to the needs of a dynamic world. Although total consensus eludes the definers, many would agree that the essence of nursing embraces skilled, sensitive, personalized care for individuals, families, and communities.

Such care demands not only concern and commitment but also the understanding that springs from wide-ranging knowledge and the skills that grow from applying that knowledge in practice. This text provides a foundation on which the student can build such understanding, skills, and values. It integrates essential knowledge from the physical and behavioral sciences with clinical nursing procedures, presented against a background of nursing theory, history, trends, and issues.

Revised, Updated, and Expanded Throughout

Though unchanged in approach and purpose, this second edition has been redesigned in an inviting, streamlined format and incorporates both major and minor changes throughout. These changes reflect new ideas, new technology, changing attitudes, and valuable comments and suggestions from instructors using the first edition. New features include:

- Major focus on description and application of the five-step nursing process, particularly nursing diagnosis
- Expanded content on nursing as a profession, its history, theories, and philosophy, current issues, and emerging trends
- A chronology of significant events in nursing history on the inside covers
- Increased emphasis on psychologic aspects of care and life span implications
- Thorough revision and updating of every chapter
- New tables, charts, photographs, and drawings
- Revised objectives at the beginning of each chapter
- Lists of relevant terms, which are defined in the chapter and in the glossary
- Updated lists of suggested activities, suggested readings, and selected references at the end of each chapter
- Expanded glossary at the end of the text

Reorganized in Eight Units

The text has been reorganized into eight units plus appendices, glossary, and index. A needs approach has been retained, but the steps of the nursing process have been emphasized as a major organizational element throughout.

Unit I, Nursing and Health, orients the student to the nursing profession and its role within the health care system. Much new material has been added on conceptual models for nursing, contemporary nursing history, standards of nursing practice, education for professional nurses, roles of the nurse, professionalism, patient advocacy, resolving ethical problems, and alternative health care delivery systems.

Unit II, The Nursing Process, is almost totally new. It defines terms and activities associated with the nursing process, compares the nursing process with the medical process, and presents selected frameworks used for assessment. Chapter 6 clearly defines nursing diagnosis, shows how it differs from medical diagnosis, describes its components and its advantages, explains how to develop a nursing diagnosis, presents three major diagnostic processes, and cites factors affecting diagnostic ability.

Unit III, Concepts Basic to the Nursing Process, introduces the student to homeostasis, human needs, stress and adaptation, human values and culture. Revised throughout, this unit reflects major changes in the chapter on human values and culture. Two chapters present growth and development across the life span.

The developmental concepts introduced here are amplified in subsequent chapters that apply nursing assessment and intervention to clients of all ages.

Unit IV, Skills Basic to the Nursing Process, begins with assessment of vital signs, general assessment skills, and effective communication. A new Chapter 16 discusses functioning in groups. Revised chapters on teaching and learning and on recording and reporting complete the unit. All of these skills are considered essential to effective implementation of the nursing process.

Unit V, Protective Measures Related to Nursing Practice, discusses medical and surgical aseptic practices essential to safe nursing intervention.

Unit VI, Physiologic Needs of Patients, is comprised of 11 chapters that comprehensively cover these needs. The chapter on nutrition has been greatly expanded. Two unusually complete chapters on fluid, electrolyte, and acid-base balance and imbalance offer a thorough discussion of these important topics.

Unit VII, Psychosocial Needs of Patients, includes almost totally rewritten chapters on a healthy self-concept, sexuality, spiritual preference, stimulation, and accepting loss and death. Each of these chapters also applies the five-step nursing process.

Unit VIII, Special Nursing Measures, discusses medications, special procedures (tests and treatments), perioperative care, and wound care. All chapters reflect thorough revision, with major updates in the content on medications and special procedures.

Revised In-Text Learning Aids

Hundreds of illustrations supplement the clear, to-the-point text material, and accessibility of information continues to be a primary feature of the book's design. Selected step-by-step procedures demonstrate psychomotor skills, giving rationales for specific actions. Each chapter opens with all new behavioral objectives and a list of relevant terms that are defined within the chapter and in the glossary at the end of the text.

The general objectives are stated as broad learning outcomes, while the specific objectives clarify what is meant by each general objective. The specific objectives are stated as behavioral outcomes and form the basis for evaluation of the broad general objective. Students may find it helpful to add the words "by being able to" after each *general* objective.

Suggested readings and activities plus updated references conclude each chapter.

New Teaching-Learning Package

To help instructors and students gain maximum usefulness from this new edition, three new supplements are offered: a modular workbook, an instructor's manual, and an overhead transparency set.

1. *Modular Workbook for Nursing Fundamentals*, by Carol Marcus, RN, MS, and Kathleen Wilson, RN, MA, is a totally new supplement, carefully coordinated with the second edition of the text. Each module includes an introduction, directions to the student, objectives, learning experiences, summary, and post-test.
2. *Instructors' Manual,* by Margot Joan Fromer, BS, MA, M Ed, includes brief chapter summaries, suggested activities for helping students meet each major objective, and a bibliography of books, articles, films, and other resources.
3. *Overhead transparency set* includes more than 100 illustrations from the new edition and from *Techniques in Clinical Nursing.*

Present and future nurses likely will experience new dimensions of practice as patterns of health and disease change, the population ages, and attitudes and values about health care alter. These developments foster a growing opportunity for nurses to function with increased competence, accountability, and personal and professional satisfaction.

Yet, no matter how nursing roles, functions, and practice settings change, the essence endures. We have tried, in this text, to offer students a clear look at this essence and thus to open a new window on a world of caring. Just as nursing is shaped from within and without, this book's development will be shaped both by our experience as educators and practitioners and by comments from instructors and students who use it. We are gratified by the acceptance of the first edition and welcome suggestions for ways in which this second edition might make teaching and learning even more effective and enjoyable.

Barbara Kozier
Glenora Erb

Acknowledgments

We would like to extend our warmest appreciation and heartfelt thanks to:

• Our typist and friend, A. Goldie, Vancouver, British Columbia, who spent endless hours making this manuscript presentable for publication. Words cannot describe the support she provided to help us meet our writing deadlines.

• The illustrator, Jack Tandy, St. Louis, Missouri, whose explicit line drawings confirm the saying that one picture is worth a thousand words.

• The photographer, William Thompson, Palo Alto, California, whose realistic pictures and creative talents are evidenced throughout the book.

• The staff and patients of Stanford University Hospital, Stanford, California; Children's Hospital at Stanford, Palo Alto, California; the Visiting Nurse Association of San Mateo County, California; Casa Olga Intermediate Care, Palo Alto, California; and Planned Parenthood Association, Mountain View, California, who generously gave of their time for the photographs for this text; and Yolanda Wuth, Foto-Graphics, Mountain View, California, who developed much of the film.

• The sponsoring editor, Nancy Evans, whose experience as a nursing editor has provided valuable guidance to us during this revision. Her willingness to help in many ways has been greatly appreciated.

• The copy and production editor, Zipporah Collins, Berkeley, California, who offered meticulous editing, constant support and encouragement, optimism, and high standards; her associate, Antonio Padial, whose work and humor we have also enjoyed; the proofreader, Nancy Cooney, her assistant, Katherine Kaiser-Schwartz, and the indexer, Elinor Lindheimer, who made valuable contributions to the finished book.

• The page designer, Janet Bollow, San Anselmo, California, who has created a fresh, eye-appealing book for readers.

• Edith P. Lewis, former editor of *Nursing Outlook*, for her contribution of the Significant Events in Nursing History on the inside front and back covers.

• Carol Ren Kneisl, Associate Professor, Graduate Program, Mental Health/Psychiatric Nursing, State University of New York at Buffalo, for her contribution of the process recording in Chapter 15 and other helpful comments.

• The staff at Addison-Wesley Publishing Company, Medical/Nursing Division, whose behind-the-scenes activities in coordinating the efforts of all involved in this project have been helpful: Pat Waldo, Deborah Gale, Deb Collins-Stephens, Allan Wylde, Nick Keefe, and Wayne Oler.

• The many people at hospitals who provided sample clinical records for inclusion in the book:

Joyce Campbell, Director of Nursing, Lions Gate Hospital, North Vancouver, British Columbia.

Shirley Gemmel, Associate Director of Nursing, The Hospital for Sick Children, Toronto, Ontario.

Thelma Kleckner, Clinical Specialist, Quality Assurance and Research, Department of Nursing, and Edward J. Kowalewski, President, Medical Staff, at University of Maryland Hospital, Baltimore, Maryland.

Margaret Loh, Associate Vice-President for Nursing Service, Michael Reese Hospital and Medical Center, Chicago, Illinois.

B. Ratsoy, Director of Nursing at St. Paul's Hospital, Nursing Department, Vancouver, British Columbia.

Diana Ritchie, Director of Nursing, and Rosemary Weber, Public Relations, Mount St. Joseph Hospital, Vancouver, British Columbia.

Margaret Suttie, Coordinator, Inservice Education, The Montreal General Hospital, Montreal, Quebec.

F. Trout, Director of Special Projects at Vancouver General Hospital, Vancouver, British Columbia.

• The persons who reviewed portions of the manuscript and whose time, thought, and constructive comments were very helpful: Margaret M. Basteyns, Frances Best, Sister Kathleen Black, Betty L. Chang, Barbara J. Cohen, Mattie Collins, Patricia R. Cook, Mary Dowe, Margot Joan Fromer, Joanne Kovach, Norman Leslie, Edith P. Lewis, Norma R. Lipscomb, Mary H. Mayers, Robin Meize-Grochowski, Alma A. Miles, Sharon D. Moscatello, Joyce Johnson Neaves, Wilfred Parsons, Martha Primeaux, Judy Ribak, Brenda Rowe, Alice R. Roye, Betsy Todd, Edythe Tuchfarber, and Patricia A. Wagner.

• The many students and patients who have taught us both so much and in that way contributed greatly to this book.

• Our families and friends for their interest and encouragement.

Contents in Brief

Contents in Detail

Unit I Nursing and Health 1

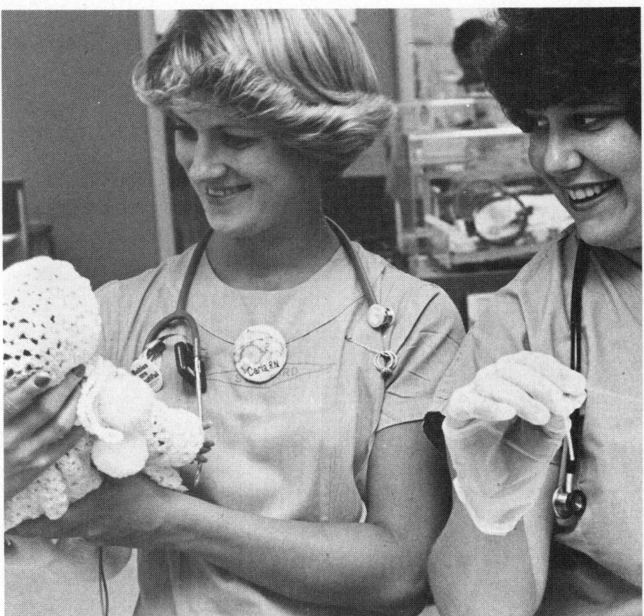

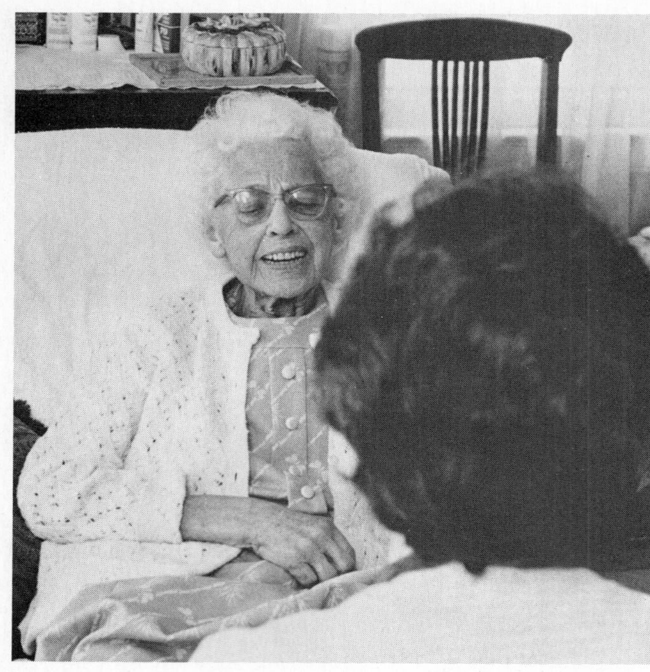

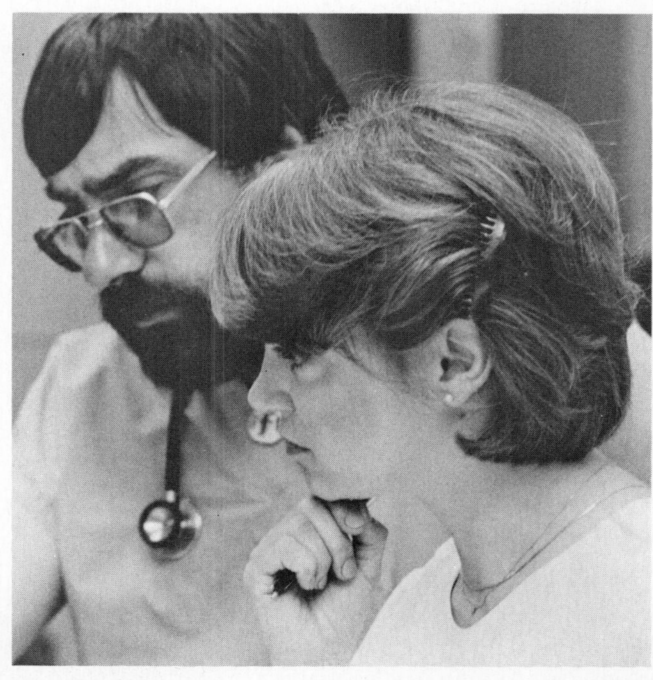

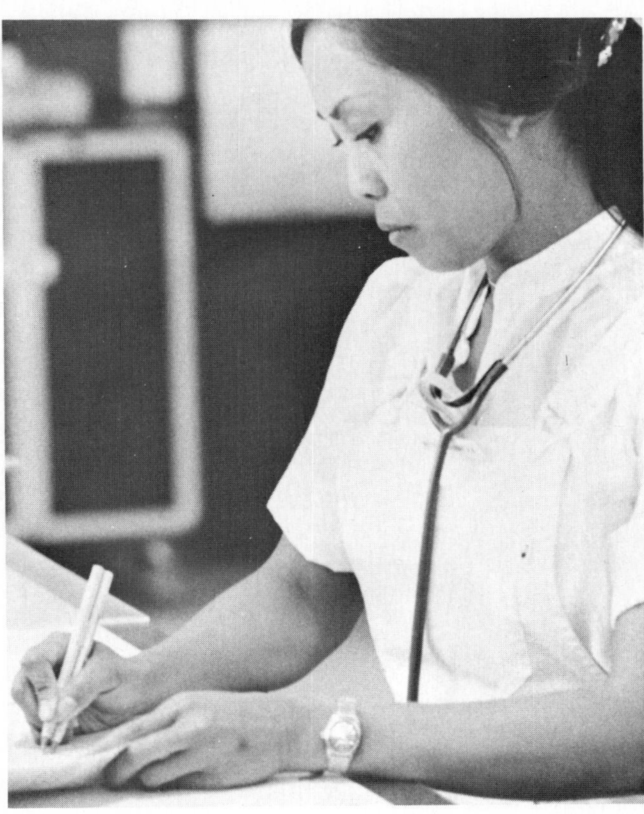

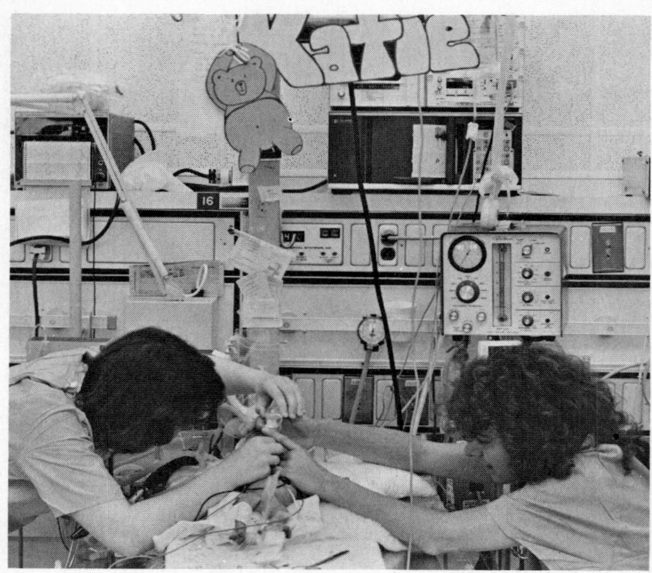

Chapter 6 Nursing Diagnosis and Planning 134

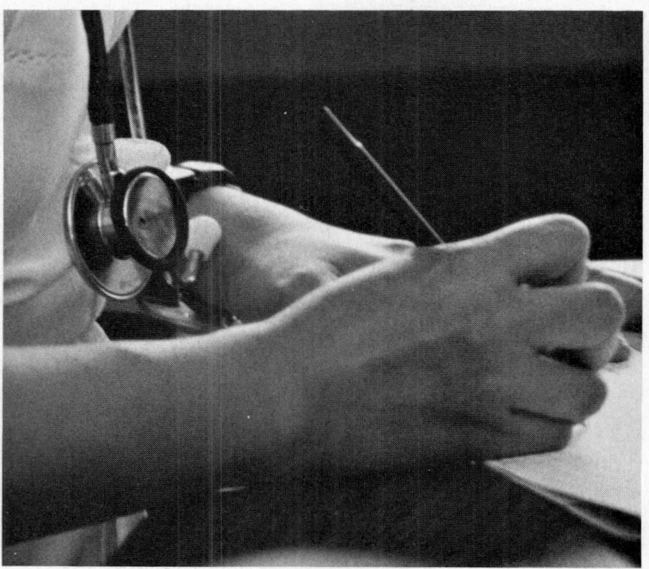

Chapter 7 Intervention and Evaluation 152

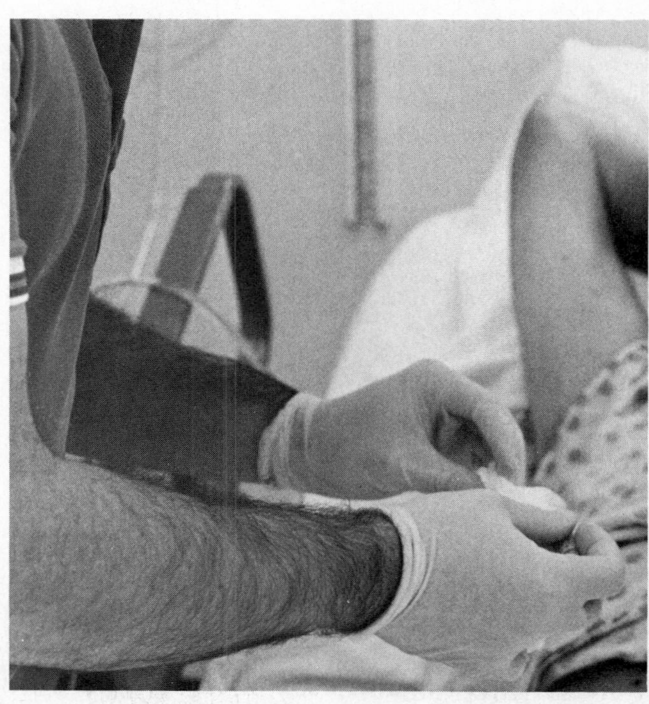

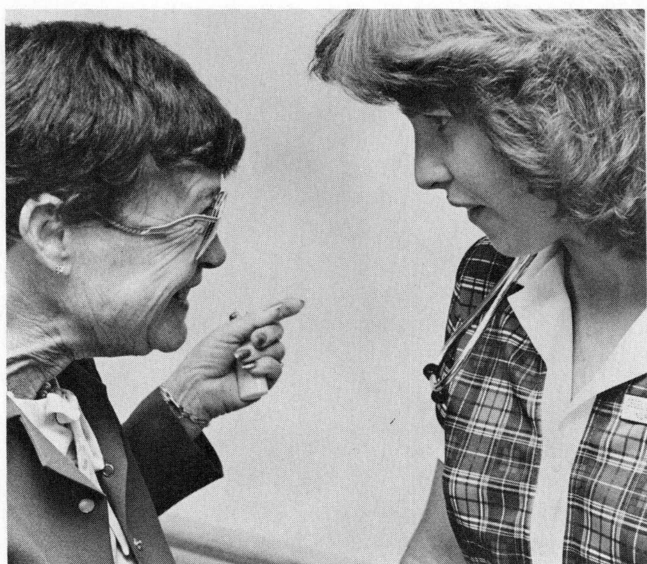

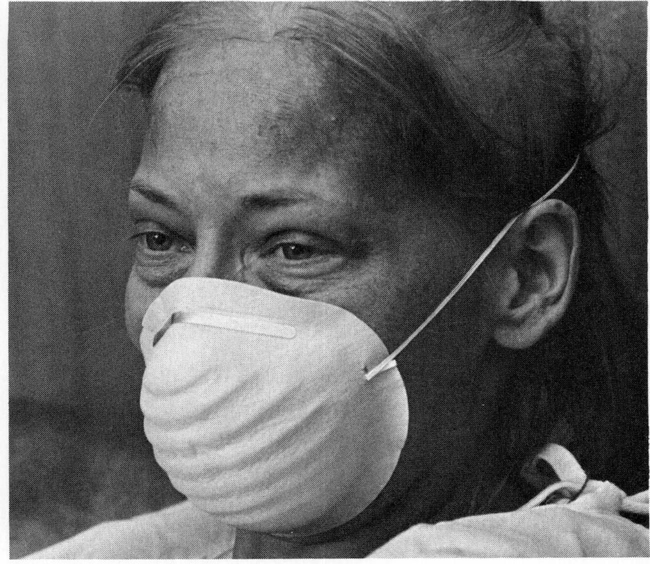

Unit III Concepts Basic to the Nursing Process 161

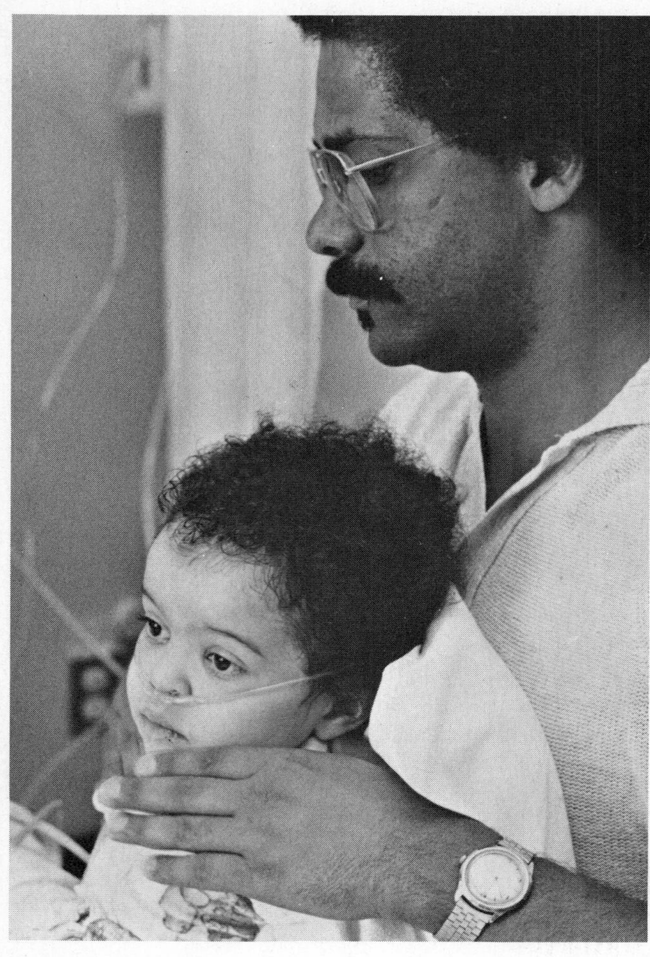

Chapter 11 Early Growth and Development 231

Chapter 12 Development from Adolescence to Late Adulthood 259

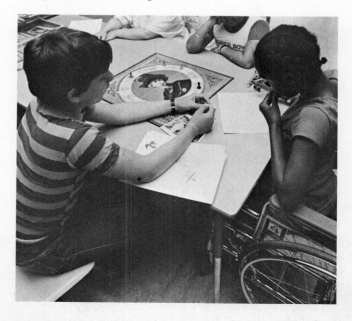

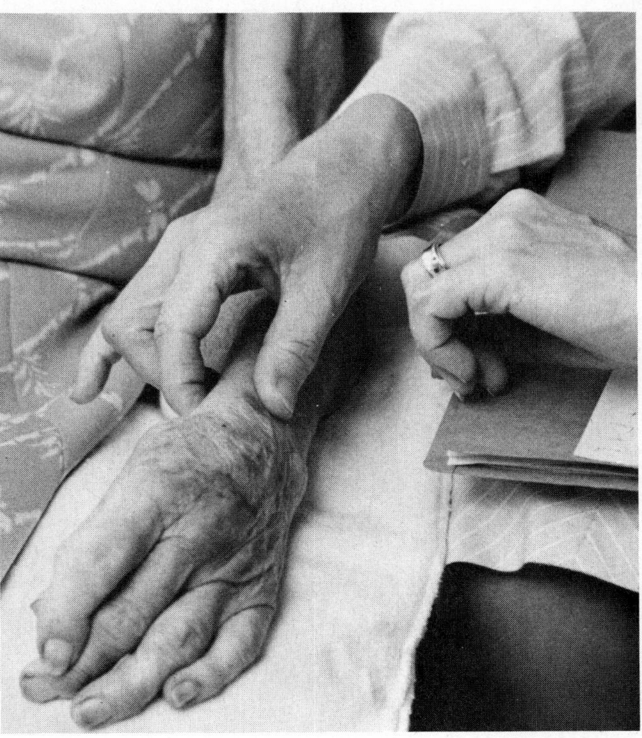

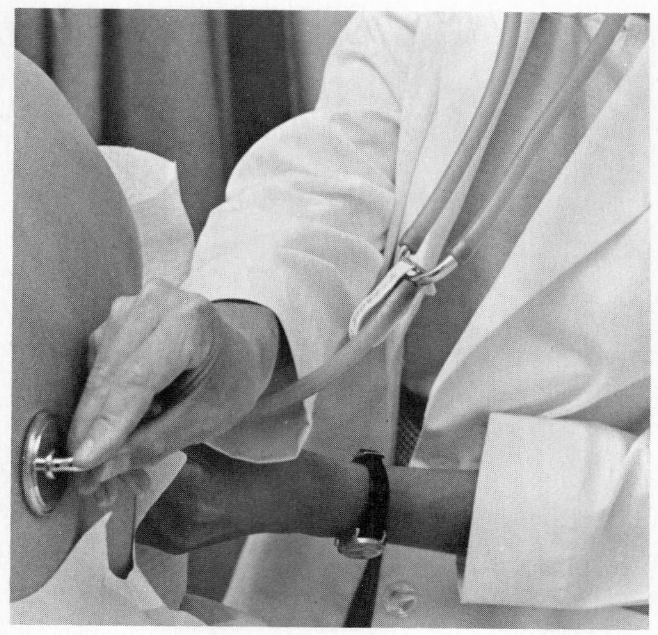

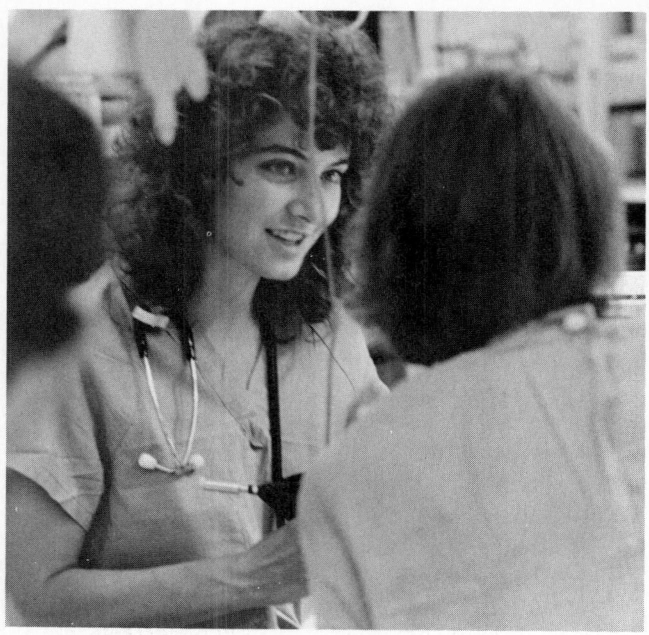

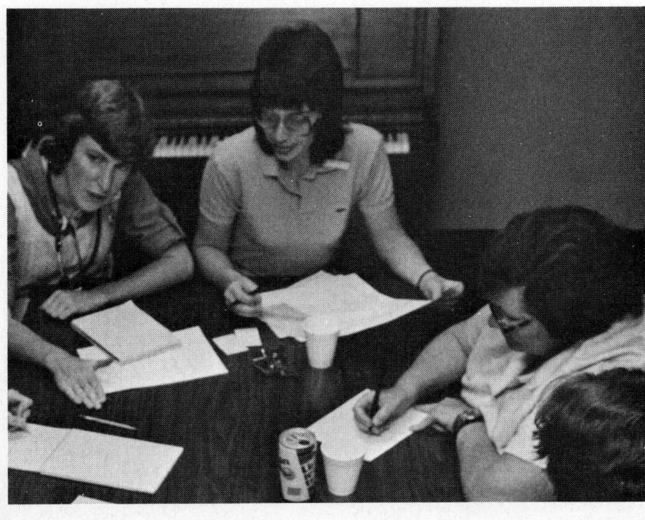

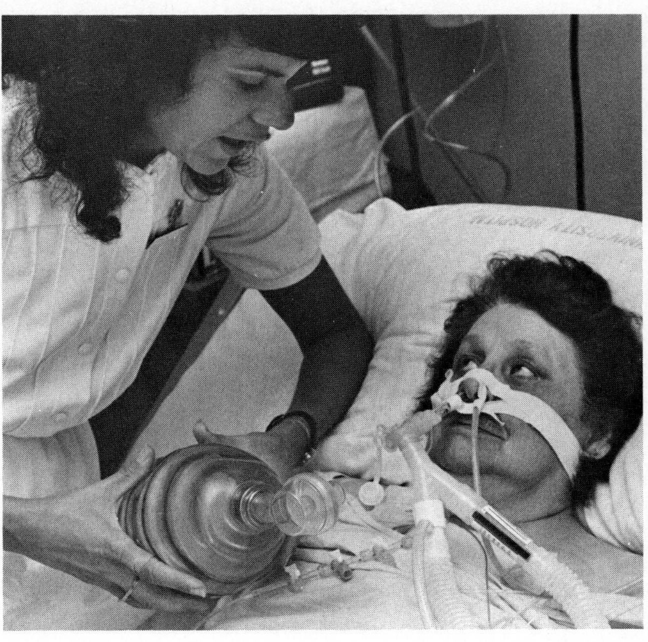

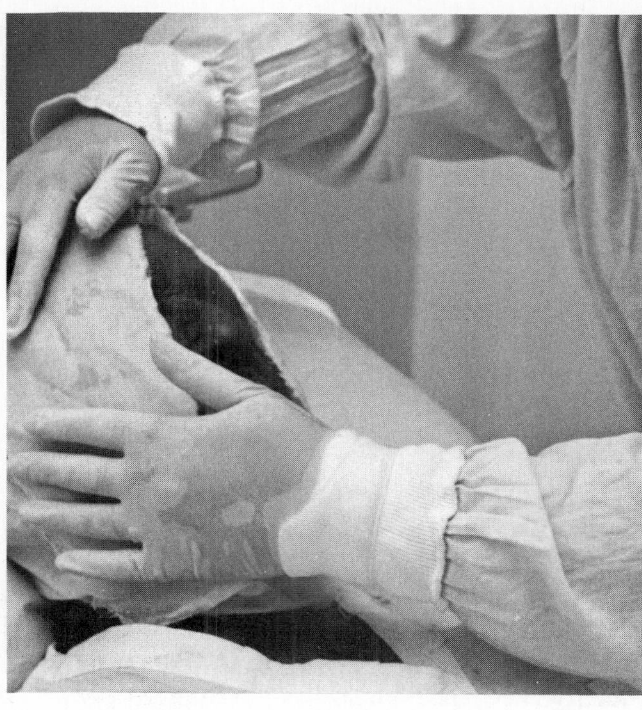

Unit V Protective Measures Related to Nursing Practice 441

Chapter 19 Medical Asepsis: Infection Control 443

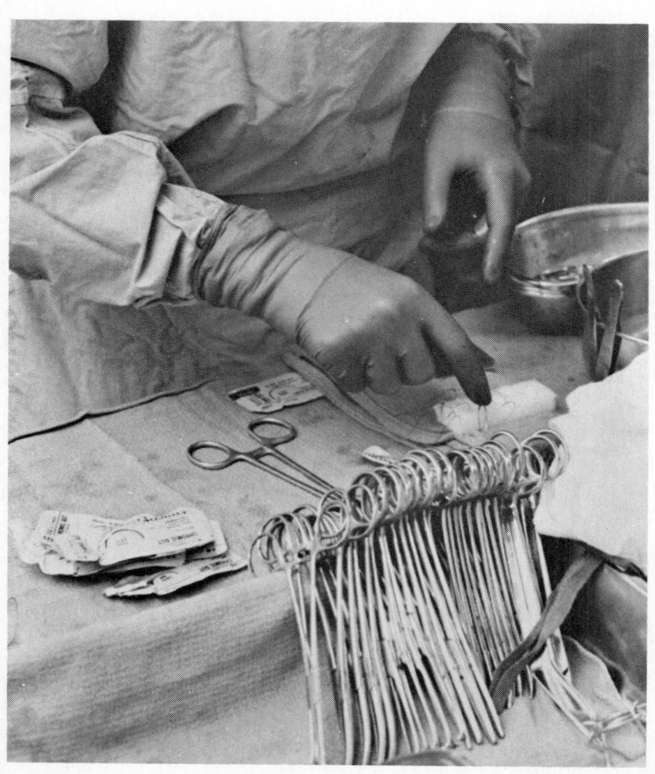

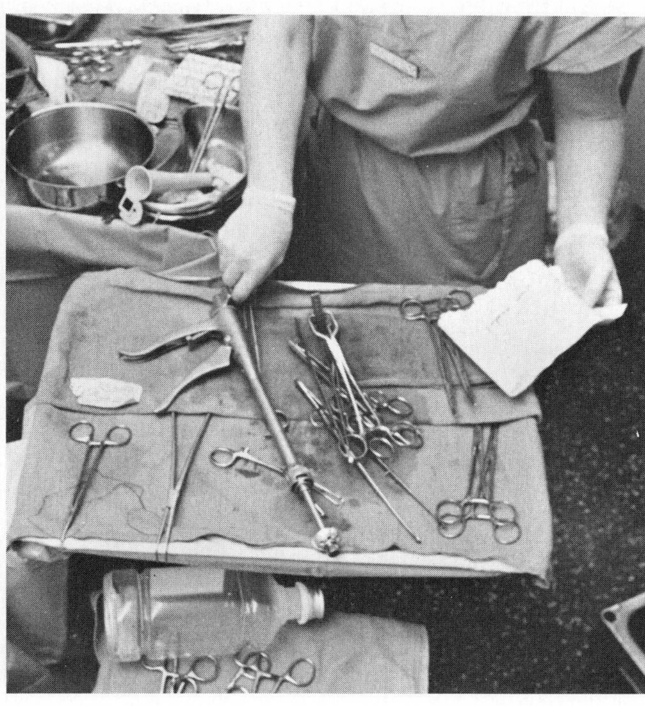

Chapter 20 Surgical Asepsis 466

Unit VI Physiologic Needs of Patients 481

Chapter 21 Personal Hygiene 483

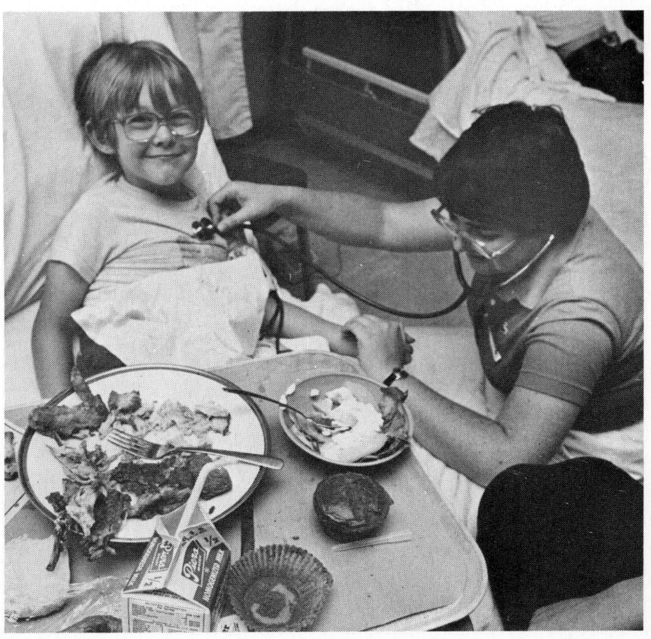

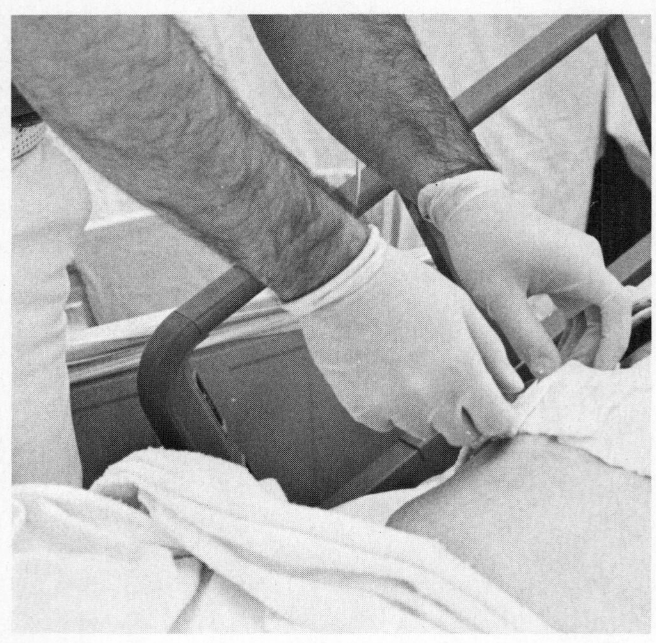

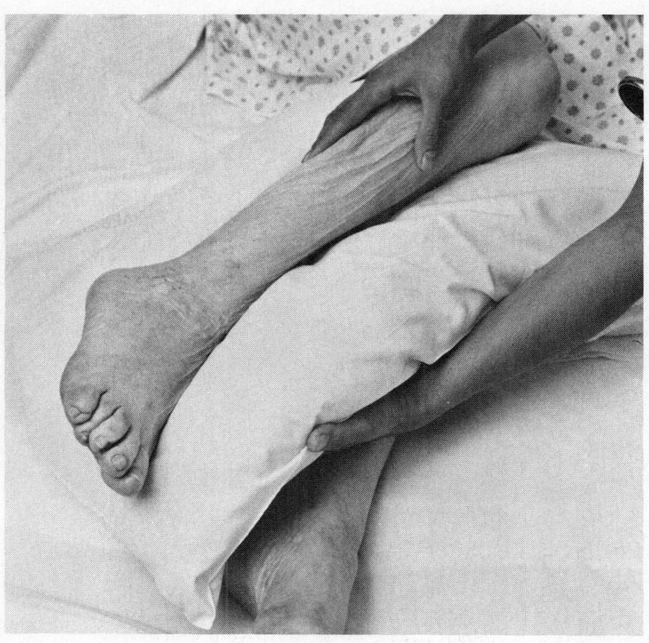

Chapter 22 Protection 530

Chapter 23 Body Alignment 551

Chapter 24 Exercise and Ambulation 581

Chapter 25 Rest, Sleep, and Relief from Pain 618

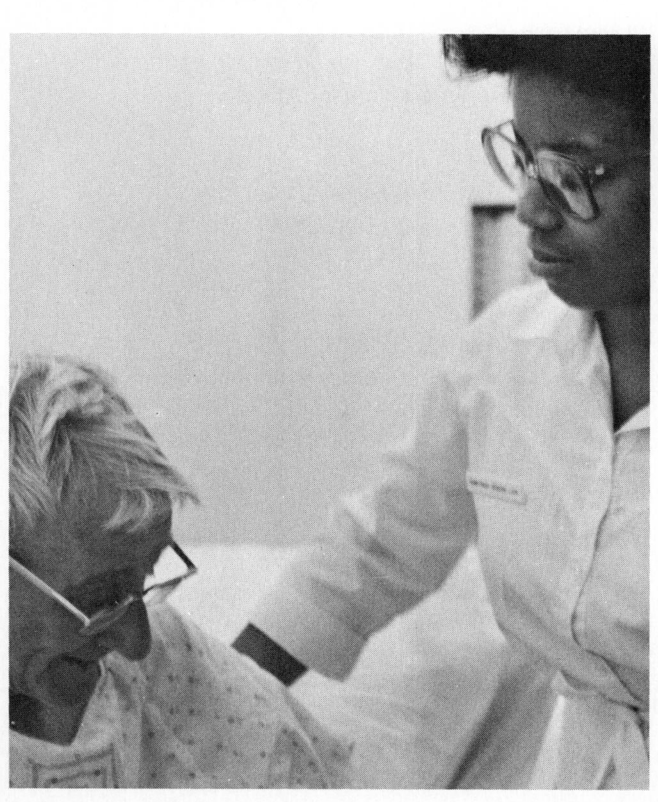

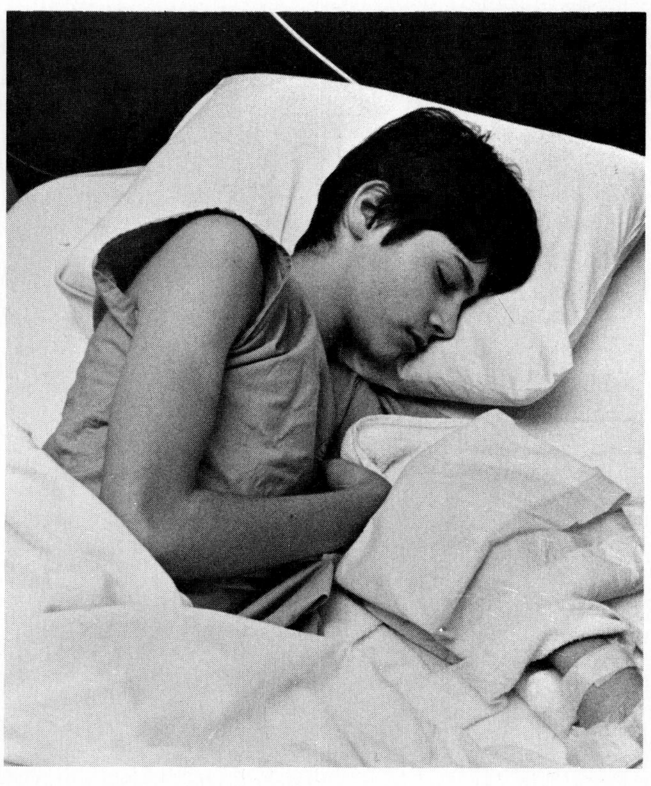

Chapter 26 Nutrition 650

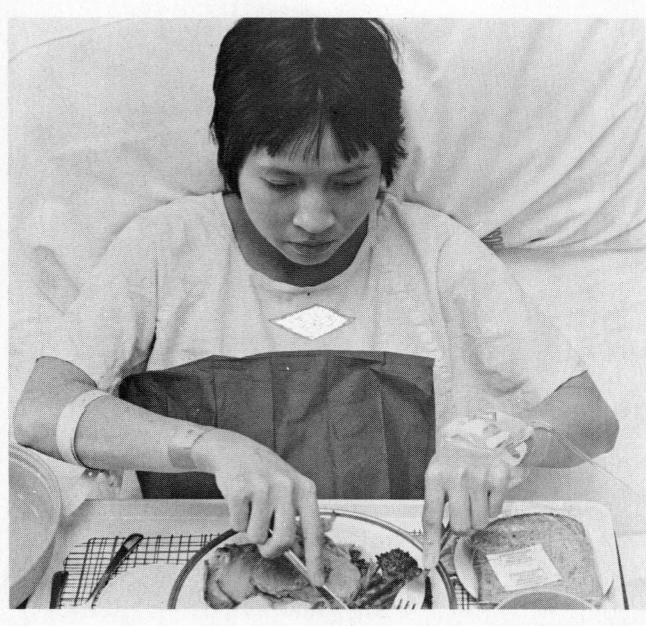

Chapter 27 Fecal Elimination 682

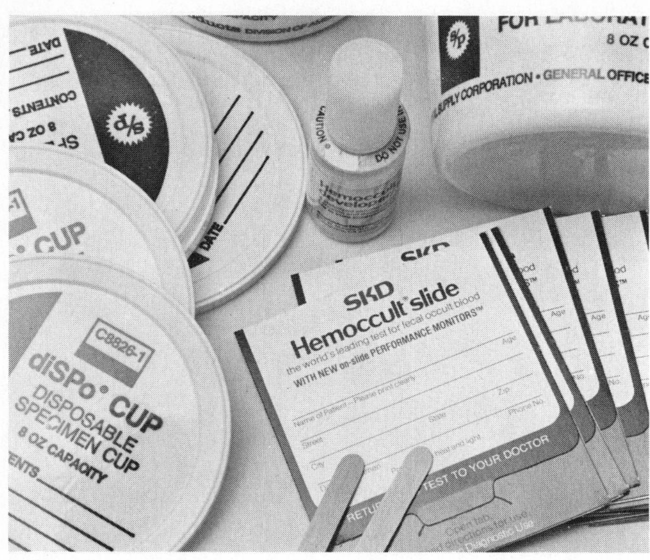
SKD
Hemoccult slide
WITH NEW on-slide PERFORMANCE MONITORS™
C8826-1
diSPo CUP
DISPOSABLE
SPECIMEN CUP
8 OZ CAPACITY
TEST TO YOUR DOCTOR

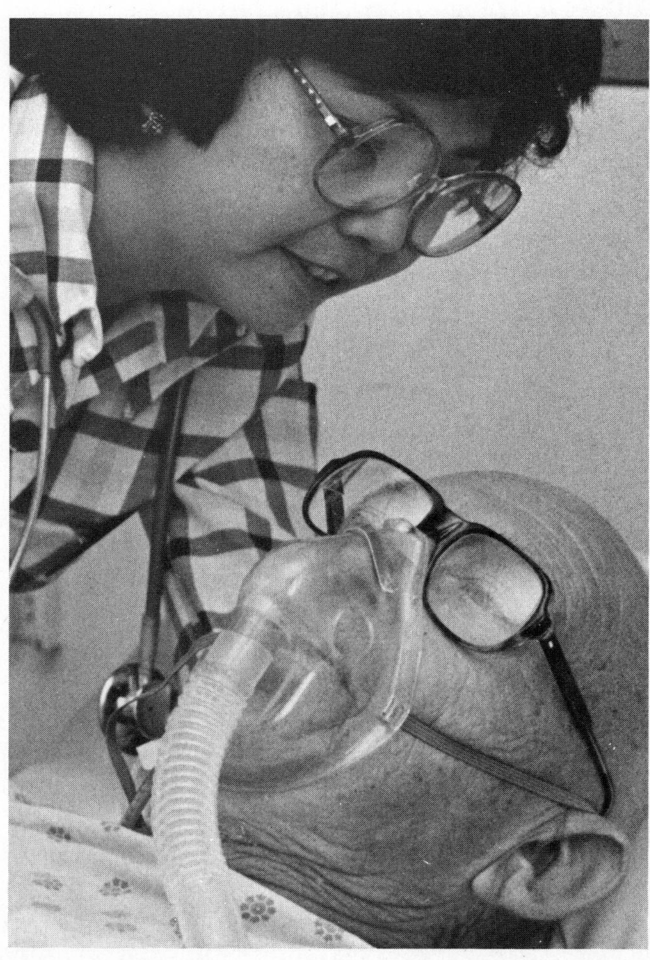

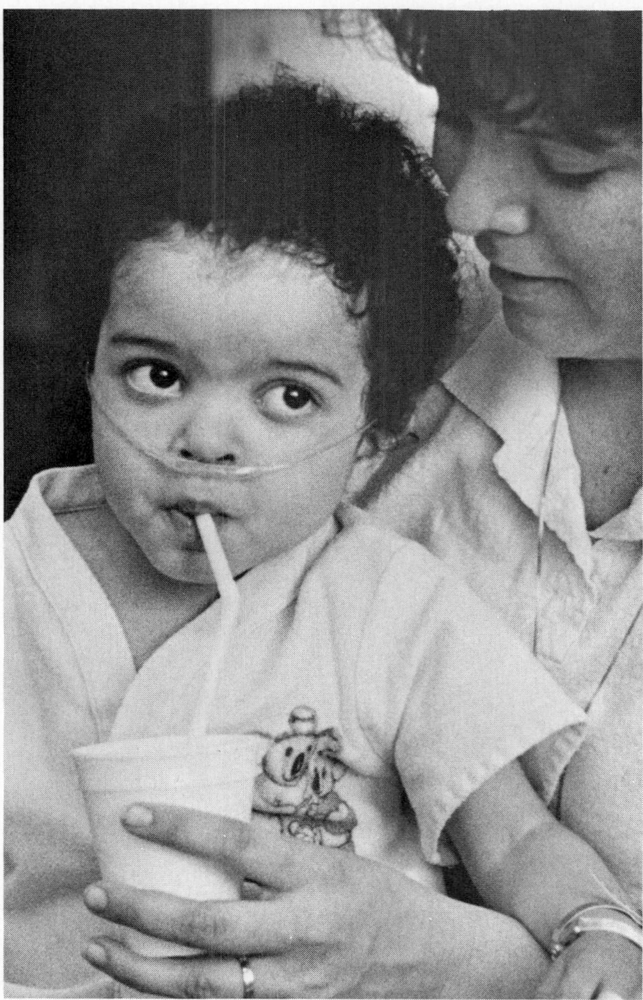

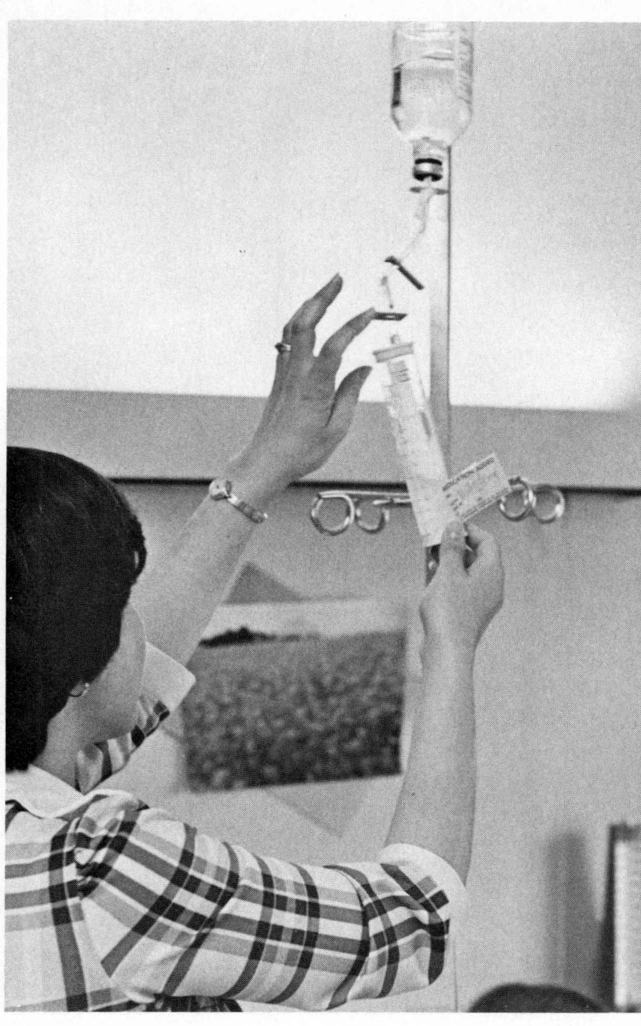

Unit VII Psychosocial Needs of Patients 833

Chapter 32 Healthy Self-Concept 835

Chapter 33 Sexuality 855

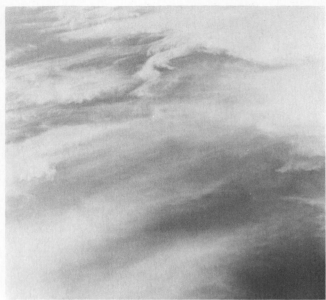

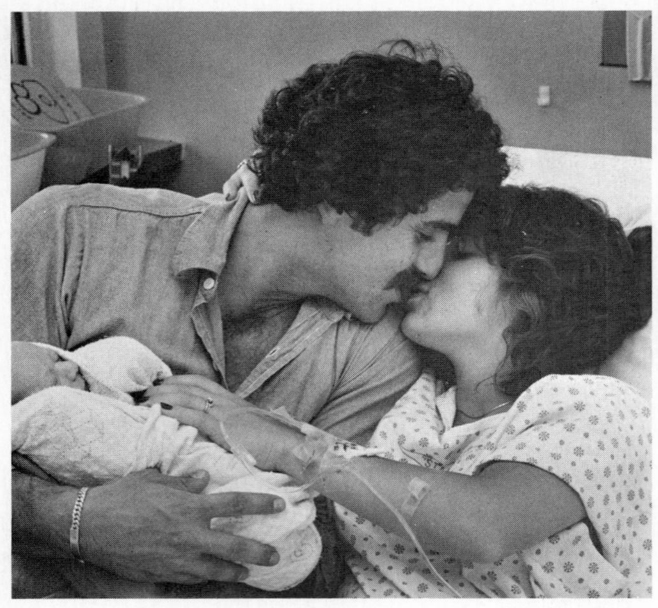

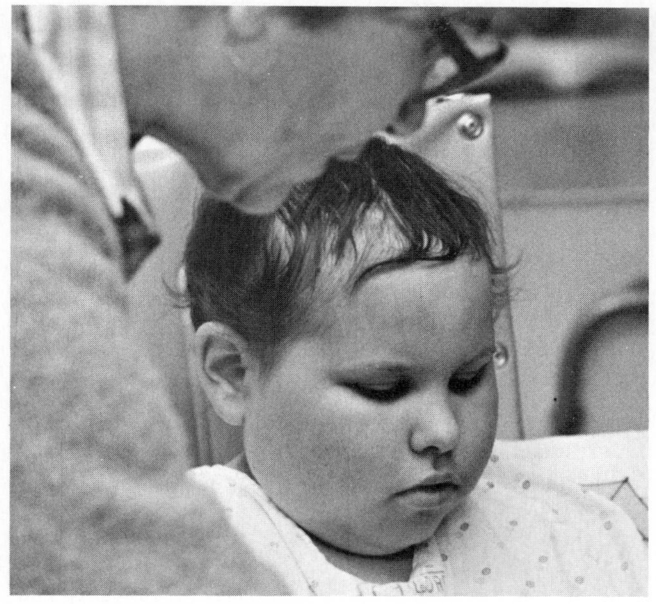

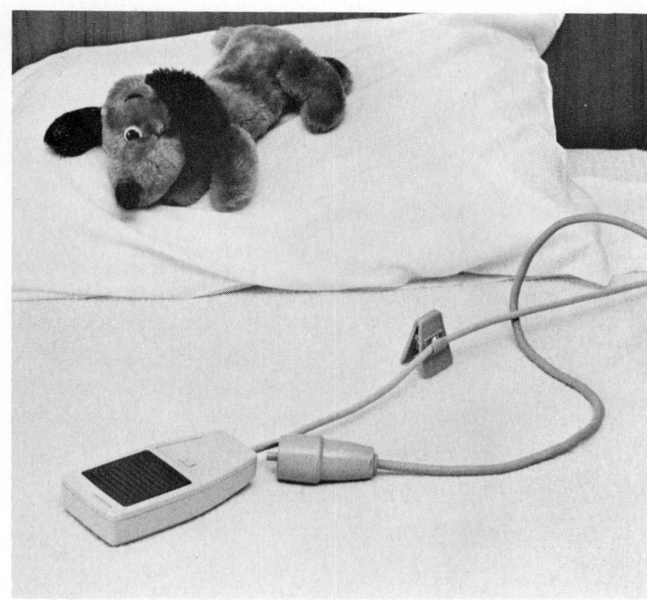

Chapter 36 Accepting Loss and Death 912

Unit VIII Special Nursing Measures 931

Chapter 37 Medications 933

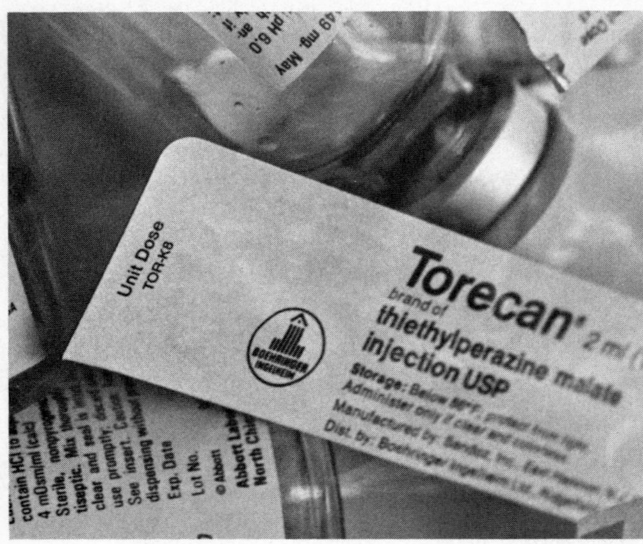
Unit Dose
Torecan
brand of
thiethylperazine maleate
injection USP

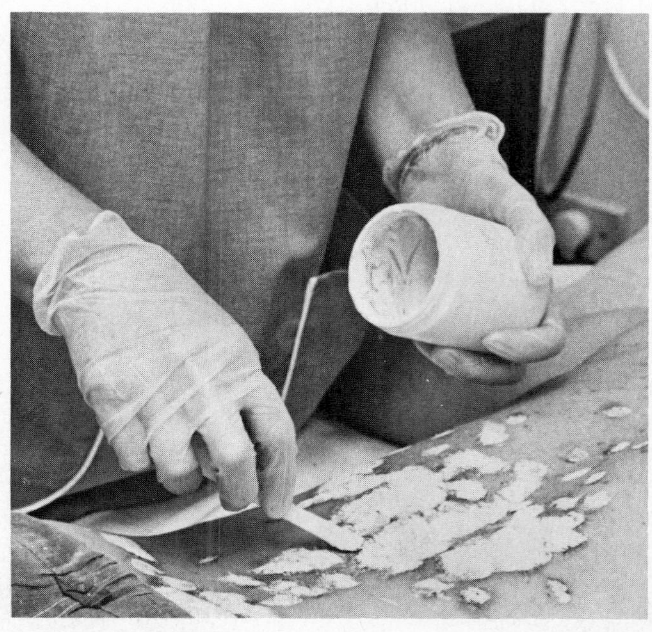

Chapter 39 Perioperative Care 1001

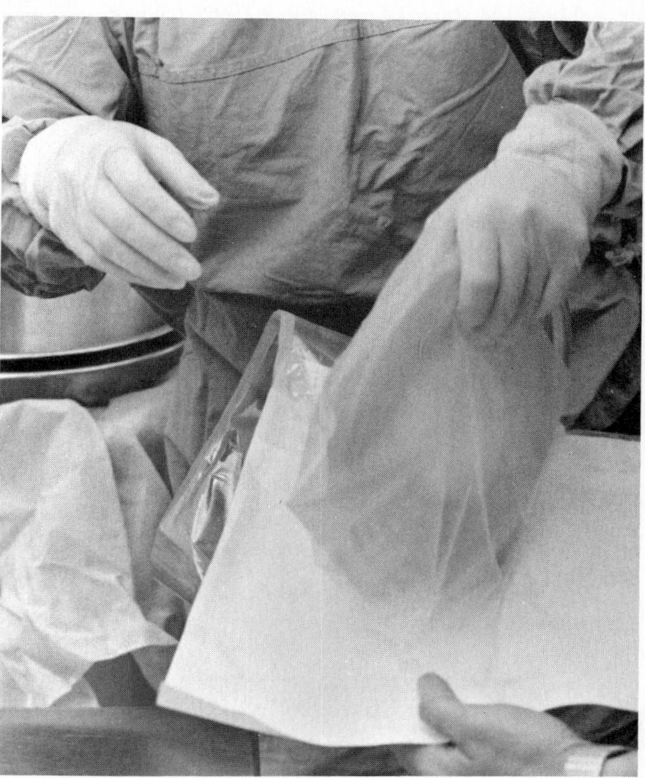

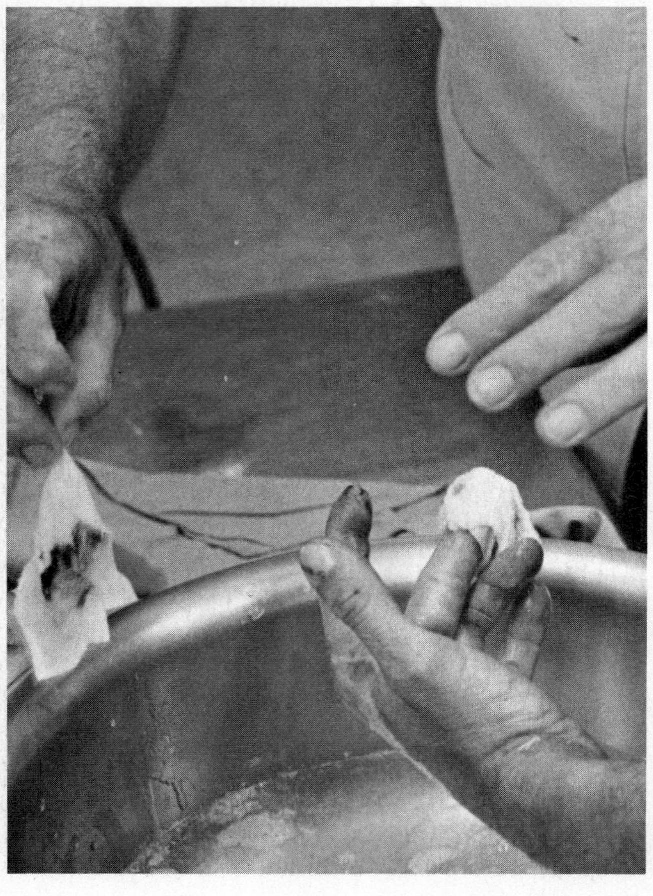

Fundamentals of Nursing

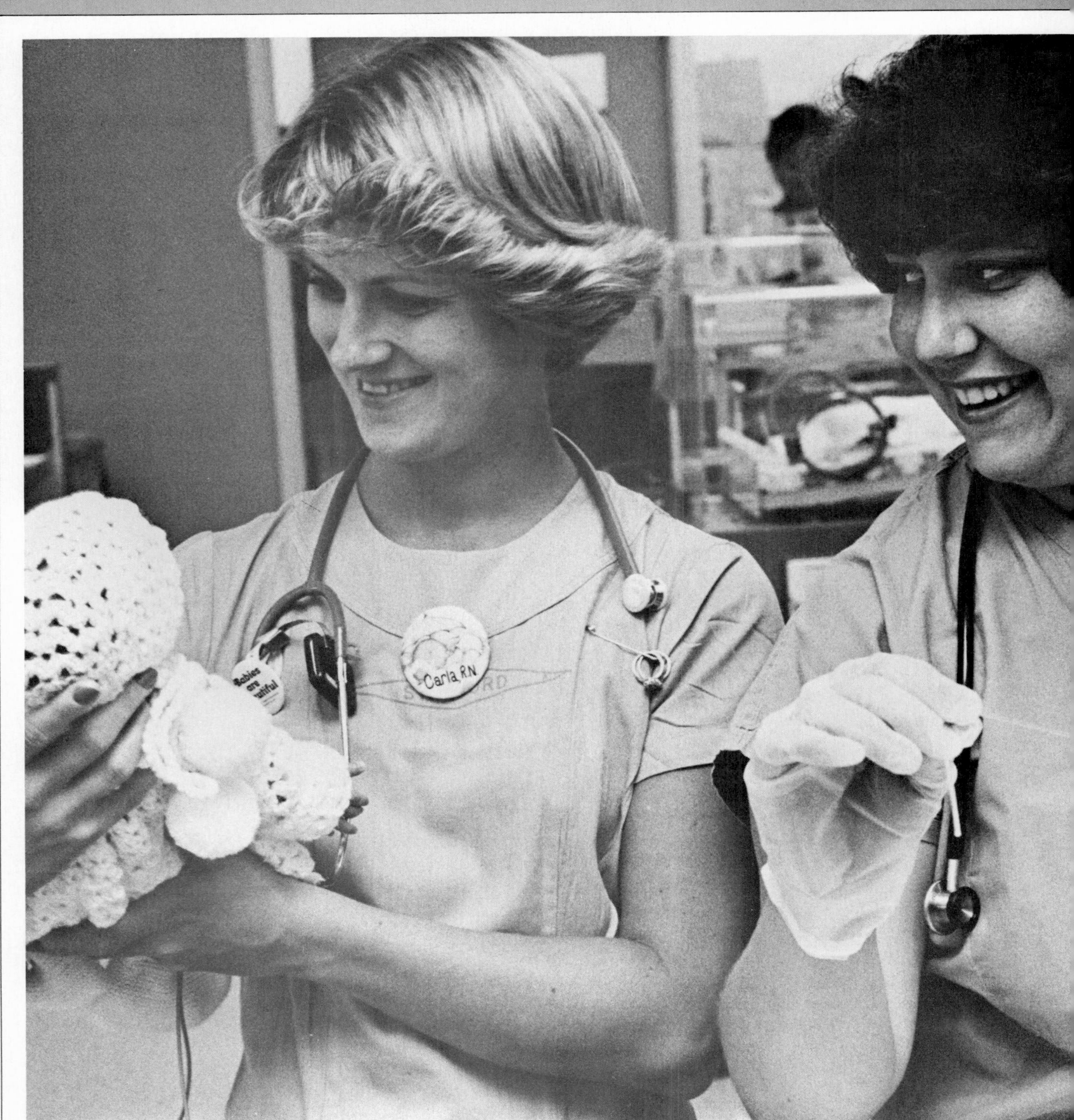
Carla, R.N

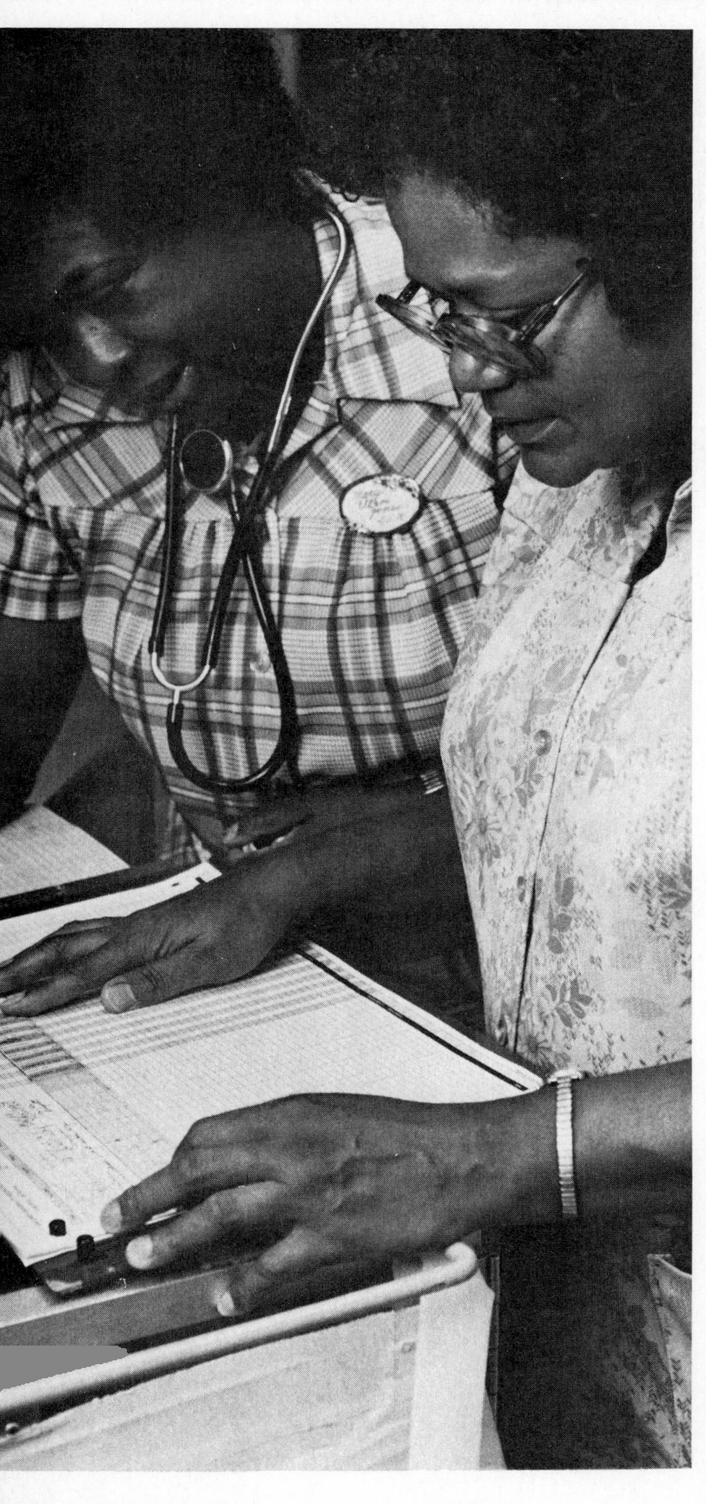

Unit I

Nursing and Health

CONTENTS

Chapter 1

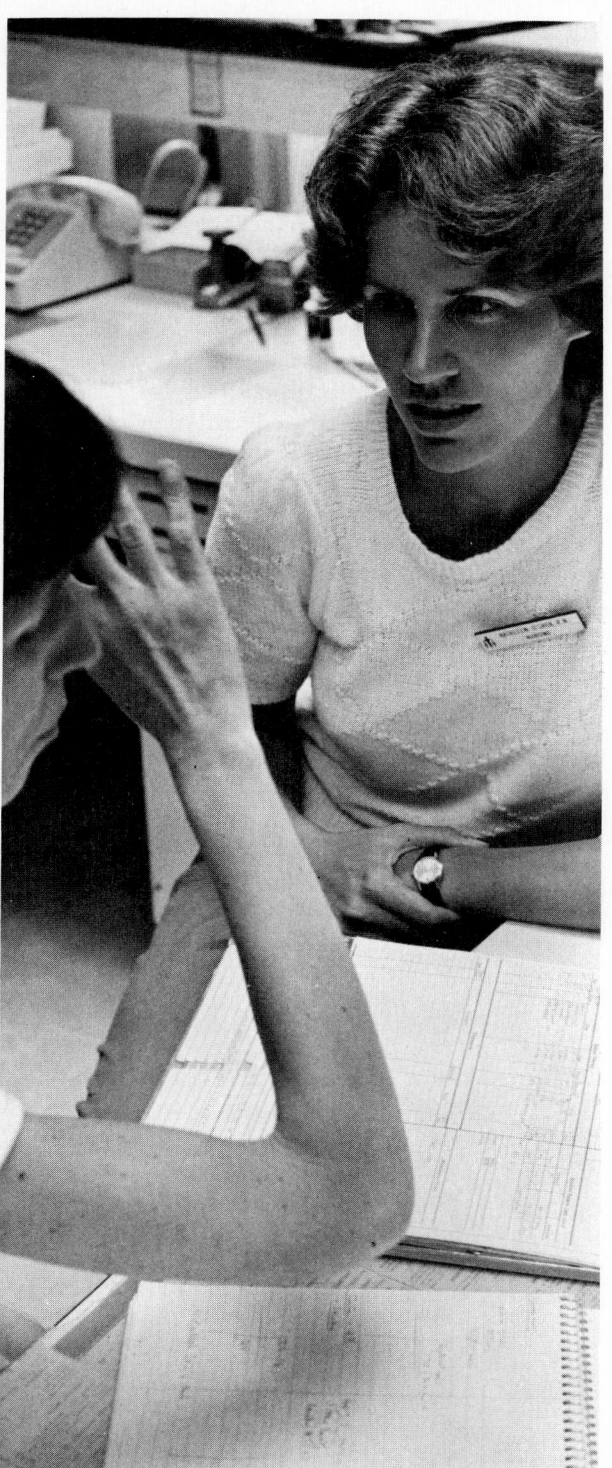

Nursing and the Nurse

CONTENTS

(Continued on next page)

Objectives

1. Know essential facts about nursing
   1.1 Define selected terms
   1.2 Identify essential aspects of nursing derived from nursing definitions cited in this chapter
   1.3 Identify Flaherty's characteristics of professionalism
   1.4 Outline four levels of nursing practice
   1.5 Identify three essential components of a conceptual model for nursing
   1.6 Identify seven major units of a conceptual model for nursing
   1.7 Identify the steps of the nursing process used to operationalize conceptual models for nursing
   1.8 Identify differences in the nurse's role in various settings for nursing practice
   1.9 Identify the major roles of the nurse
2. Understand past, present, and future factors influencing nursing practice
   2.1 Identify the significance of selected historic aspects of nursing
   2.2 Explain the significance of current factors influencing nursing practice
   2.3 Identify the significance of selected trends in nursing practice
3. Know facts about nursing education programs and organizations
   3.1 Describe some differences among various types of nursing education programs
   3.2 Identify some competencies for graduates of various types of nursing education programs
   3.3 Describe the ladder concept in nursing education
   3.4 Identify the functions of selected nursing and health organizations
4. Understand essential facts about the role of the nurse as a provider of health care
   4.1 Identify nine roles of the nurse related to the care of patients and families
   4.2 Explain Orem's five methods of assisting patients and families
   4.3 Identify six essential attributes required by nurses in a changing health care delivery system
   4.4 Identify three areas of learning basic to socialization into the nursing role
   4.5 Explain essential components of accountability and responsibility

Terms

accountability
concept
conceptual model
demography
dependent nursing function
empirical
framework
independent nurse practitioner
independent nursing function
model
morbidity
mortality
nurse clinician
nursing process
primary care
primary nursing
responsibility
socialization

What Is Nursing?

Nursing practice combines the science of health and the art of care, a humanistic blend of scientific knowledge, nursing philosophy, clinical practice, communication, and social sciences. Thus, today's nursing student must master an astounding number of professional concepts and skills. The purpose of this book is to help students meet that challenge by providing a comprehensive framework for holistic and humanistic nursing practice.

The book first examines the past, present, and future of nursing by viewing roles and functions of the nurse, components of nursing, and trends in nursing practice as these elements are influenced by various sociologic factors. In later chapters, these theories serve as the structure within which to apply principles of clinical practice. By integrating concepts with skills, today's nurse becomes a realistic practitioner of both the art and the science of this profession.

An Emerging Definition

Just as nursing today is different from the nursing practiced 50 years ago, it takes a vivid imagination to think about the nursing profession in the next 50 years. Ours is an ever-changing world. To comprehend present-day nursing and at the same time prepare for nursing in tomorrow's world, it is important to understand not only past events but contemporary nursing practice and the sociologic factors affecting it.

Various professional groups have set forth definitions of nursing. Nursing was defined by the International Council of Nurses (ICN) in 1973 as follows:

> The unique function of the nurse is to assist the individual, sick or well, in the performance of those activities contributing to health or its recovery (or to peaceful death) that he would perform unaided if he had the necessary strength, will or knowledge.

A further development in defining nursing was made by the American Nurses' Association (ANA) in 1973 in its Standards of Nursing Practice. This official definition states: "Nursing practice is a direct service, goal oriented, and adaptable to the needs of the individual, the family and community during health and illness."

In both definitions certain ideas and goals are emphasized. Drawing from these, and expanding on the elements involved we have created the following statements about nursing:

1. Nursing is nurturing, caring for, and caring about people.
2. Nursing is a service to patients, their families, and communities. Examples of community nursing practice are found in well-baby clinics, mental health day-care centers, and parenthood classes. See Figure 1–1.
3. Nursing can be either preventive or therapeutic. For example, a well child may need protection against poliomyelitis, requiring nursing services for immunization. A child ill with pneumonia may need nursing services in bed at home to treat the disease.
4. Nursing is a direct service, that is, one of direct contact between nurse and patient or nurse and family.
5. Nursing is adapted to the individual needs of the patient. Because each patient has unique characteristics and attributes, nursing must consider these in meeting patients' health needs.

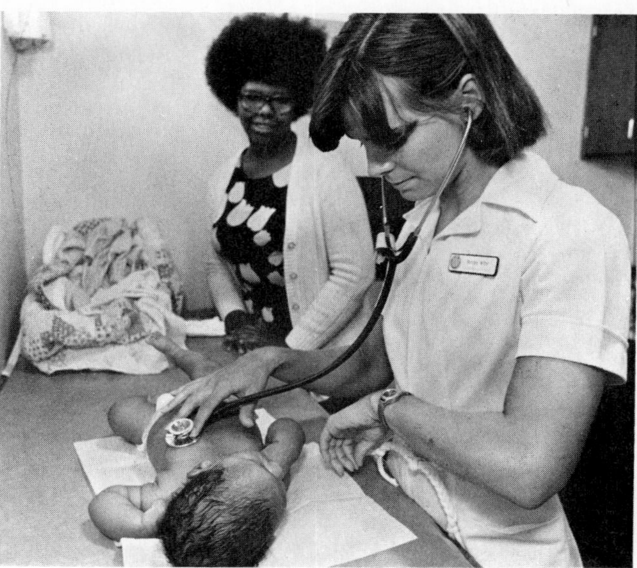

Figure 1–1 A nurse in a community clinic assesses an infant's health and offers a mother assistance with care.

Many other definitions of nursing have emerged over past decades. These definitions vary among nursing practice laws, practice settings, and geographic areas. They also vary in accordance with the types and functions of nurses and the beliefs of the person or group devising the definition.

Current definitions of nursing tend to include beliefs about (a) human beings as holistic responsible persons, (b) health and illness, (c) specific needs for nursing service, (d) the unique role of the nurse, and (e) the goals and consequences of nursing actions. For example, Dorothea Orem (1980:6, 7) defines nursing as:

> a service, a mode of helping human beings, and not a tangible commodity. Nursing's form or structure is derived from actions deliberately selected and performed by nurses to help individuals or groups under their care to maintain or change conditions in themselves or their environments. . . . Nursing has as its special concern the individual's need for self-care action and the provision and management of it on a continuous basis in order to sustain life and health, recover from disease or injury, and cope with their effects.

In this definition nursing is viewed as a helping service provided to individuals and groups. The individual is considered responsible for his or her own health in terms of performing self-care activities that maintain life, health, and well-being. When individuals have difficulty maintaining or meeting their self-care requirements, nurses provide assistance directed toward changing the individual's ability to perform self-care or adjusting the environment so that self-care needs are met.

The Canadian Nurses' Association (1980:6) has developed the following philosophical statement about nursing:

> The nursing profession exists in response to a need of society and holds ideals related to man's health throughout his life span. Nurses direct their energies toward the promotion, maintenance, and restoration of health, the prevention of illness, the alleviation of suffering and the ensuring of a peaceful death when life can no longer be sustained. Nurses value a holistic view of man and regard him as a biopsychosocial being who has the capacity to set goals and make decisions and who has the right and responsibility to make informed choices congruent with his own beliefs and values. Nursing, a dynamic and supportive profession guided by its code of ethics, is rooted in caring, a concept evident throughout its four fields of activity: practice, education, administration and research.

One of the major problems confronting the nursing profession today is the need to devise a definition of nursing that can be used nationally and internationally, that identifies the scope of nursing practice, and that clearly differentiates the role of the nurse from other health disciplines. The Professional Services Committee (PSC) of the International Council of Nurses (ICN) is currently examining this matter (ICN 1974).

An Evolving Profession

The history of nursing is one of constant evolution. The nursing profession owes much to the influence of Florence Nightingale (1820–1910), a woman with a vision. Emerging into this field in an age when nursing was regarded with vehement contempt, Nightingale crusaded to change the world's view of the nurse. No longer is nursing held in disrepute as it was in the 19th century. Nightingale's belief in education, her development of theories of nursing practice and hygiene techniques, and her campaign to emphasize prevention in health care are important facets of the nursing spectrum today.

In the early 20th century, however, some of Nightingale's ideals were temporarily misplaced. Medicine, in its zeal to control disease, frequently emphasized cure rather than prevention. Nurses were trained rather than educated, frequently working long hours performing hospital chores rather than spending time and energy with patients. Nurses all too often were allowed only to follow orders, not to make independent decisions about patient care. Nightingale's intentions for the nursing profession were ignored but fortunately not forgotten. Her vision was shared by nursing pioneers in the years that followed, and this vision is the motivating force behind the campaign today for similar aims. Our changing society, advances in medicine, current goals for human rights, and Nightingale's vision continue to spur change in the nursing profession.

Today one of the issues before nursing is the degree of professionalism it has attained. The traditional nursing role was one of humanistic caring, nurturing, comforting, and supporting. To these must be added specific characteristics for true professionalism, including education, a code of ethics, mastery of a craft, an informed membership involved in the organized profession, and accountability for actions (Flaherty 1979:61). Other criteria also indicate professionalism. Any of these provides a framework against which to measure the degree to which nursing is a profession.

Education

Historically nurses were educated through apprenticeship; however, increasingly nurses are obtaining baccalaureate degrees (see the discussion of baccalaureate education later in this chapter). As a profession, nursing needs to have a well-defined body of knowledge and expertise based on that unique body of knowledge. A number of nursing conceptual models (discussed later in this chapter) have been developed that contribute to the knowledge base of nursing education and to the direction for nursing research. However, this knowledge must be accepted by other professionals and by society for nursing to achieve full professionalism.

Code of ethics

Nurses generally place a high value on the worth and dignity of others. The nursing profession requires integrity of its members; that is, a member is expected to do what is considered right regardless of the personal cost. Nurses must respect the professional judgment of others and must develop nursing standards and establish mechanisms for identifying and dealing with unethical behavior.

Ethical codes must be subject to change as the needs and values of society change. Nursing has developed its own codes of ethics and in most instances has set up means to monitor the professional behavior of its members. See Chapter 3 for additional information on ethics.

Mastery of the craft

In a true profession, members have mastery of the knowledge and skills of the craft. Nurses are expected to have a depth of knowledge and skills that others without similar education do not have. They are also expected to make independent decisions using this body of knowledge, not merely to function as another professional directs. See the discussion of planning interventions later in this chapter.

Professional organization

A true profession has an informed membership that is involved in the professional organization. For example, nurses need to be aware of the issues confronting nursing and the trends in nursing practice.

Accountability

In the professional sense, nurses must ensure accountability for their own actions. This concept is discussed fully later in this chapter. The nurse participates in making decisions and learns to live with these decisions. See Chapter 3 for further information.

Levels of Care

Nursing involves an interrelationship of many people in different settings concerned with different ideas, techniques, and functions. Nursing is comprised of a combination of elements, but emphasis frequently is placed on only one aspect of being a nurse. For example, a nurse may have excellent communication and patient care skills, but may be sadly deficient in procedures such as monitoring a patient's vital signs.

Today there is an emphasis on the whole person. People are not merely physical beings but also social, moral, psychologic, and spiritual beings. The nurse applies a network of skills to the practice of nursing a whole patient. The nurse is concerned also with the family and the community and is aware of the effects of these groups on the patient's well-being in addition to the well-being of the groups themselves.

The nurse needs a knowledge of the theory and philosophy of nursing, the science of the human body and health, and procedures of nursing care.

Nurses practice nursing on four different levels:

1. *Promotion of health:* assisting people who are either healthy, disabled, or ill to increase their level of wellness (see the discussion of the health-illness continuum in Chapter 2). An example is the dietary advice a nurse gives to an obese person.
2. *Prevention of disease or injury:* assisting people who are either healthy or ill to prevent disease, for example, providing immunizations against smallpox.
3. *Restoration of health:* assisting a patient to return to health after illness, for example, teaching a patient to protect an incision and to change the surgical dressing or assisting a handicapped individual to attain the fullest physical, mental, social, and economic usefulness of which he or she is capable.
4. *Consolation of the dying:* assisting terminally ill patients of all ages to a peaceful death.

Even the nurse practicing in a highly specialized setting such as an intensive care unit or an elementary school employs these four levels of care. All levels are equally important in the total health picture of patient, family, and community.

Conceptual Models for Nursing

A conceptual model or framework is a way of looking at (conceptualizing) a discipline (e.g., nursing and what it is) in clear, explicit terms that can be communicated to others. Although most nurses have a clear idea of what nursing is, its uniqueness needs to be clearly stated to others, e.g., other health professionals and the public. The need for conceptual models for nursing has arisen in association with professionalism and a desire for collegial status with other health professionals. If nurses are to be considered health professionals, they have to communicate exactly what they do that makes their place in the interdisciplinary team unique and important.

Before discussing conceptual models, clarification of terms is necessary. A *concept* is a complex of ideas united to portray a large general idea (Wandelt 1970:313); a *model* is a pattern of something to be made; and a *framework* is a basic structure supporting anything. A *conceptual model*, therefore, can be defined as a basic structure in which a complex of ideas is united to portray a large general idea.

There are concepts of all kinds in nursing—about human beings, health, helping relationships, and communication. A conceptual model gives clear and explicit direction to the three areas of nursing: practice, education, and research. (Some nurses add a fourth field of nursing, administration; however, many consider administration a component of each of the three areas.) All conceptual models are frames of reference (conceptual and theoretic) but not all frames of reference are models, in that some are not specific enough to give clear direction for all aspects of that discipline in terms of practice, education, and research.

Because there is no consensus among nurses about the nature and structure of nursing, a number of models have been and are being developed. Each model bears the name of the person or group who developed it and reflects the beliefs of that developer. Some commonly known models since 1960 are those developed by Virginia Henderson (1966), Dorothy E. Johnson (1968), Dorothea E. Orem (1971), and Sister Callista Roy (1976). In 1980 the Canadian Nurses' Association (1980) Testing

Service (CNATS) also developed a model. See Components of Nursing Models next and Table 1-1 on page 10 for additional information.

Components of Nursing Models

There are three components of conceptual models: assumptions, a value system, and major units.

Assumptions

Assumptions are statements of facts (premises) or suppositions that people accept as the underlying theoretic foundation for the way nursing is conceptualized. Assumptions are derived from scientific theory or practice or both and either have been or can be verified. Some nursing models have drawn assumptions from adaptation theories; others from general systems theories (see Chapter 2, page 56). Most models also draw assumptions from practice.

Assumptions differ greatly from model to model since they are drawn from different premises. For example, assumptions about human beings (the client) vary considerably: Henderson views the client as a being with fourteen fundamental needs, Roy as a being with four modes of adaptation; Johnson as a being with eight behavioral subsystems; and Orem as an agent with six universal self-care requisites.

Values system

The values system is the beliefs that underlie the profession. Generally these beliefs are similar from model to model. Some of them are:

1. Nurses have a unique function even though they share certain functions with other health professionals.
2. Nursing is a service directed toward meeting the needs of well or ill persons or groups (families and communities) rather than directed toward specific aspects of disease or illness.
3. Nursing uses a systematic process (see Chapter 5) to operationalize its conceptual model.
4. Nursing involves a series of interpersonal relationships. The nurse-patient relationship (helping relationship) is of major importance. See Chapter 15.

Margretta Styles believes that nursing as a profession must have and hold a common ideology just as nations have their pledges of allegiance, societies their oaths and religions their creeds. Styles proposes the following (1982:61):

Declaration of Belief about the Nature and Purpose of Nursing*

I. I believe in nursing as an *occupational force for social good*, a force that, in the *totality of its concern* for all human health states and for mankind's responses to health and environment, provides a distinct, unique, and vital perspective, value orientation, and service.
II. I believe in nursing as a *professional discipline*, requiring a sound education and research base grounded in its own science and in the variety of academic and professional disciplines with which it relates.
III. I believe in nursing as a *clinical practice*, employing particular physiological, psychosocial, physical, and technological means for human amelioration, sustenance, and comfort.
IV. I believe in nursing as a *humanistic field*, in which the fullness, self-respect, self-determination, and humanity of the nurse engage the fullness, self-respect, self-determination, and humanity of the client.
V. I believe that nursing's *maximum contribution* for social betterment is dependent on:
  A. The well-developed *expertise* of the nurse;
  B. The *understanding, appreciation*, and *acknowledgment* of that expertise by the public;
  C. The organizational, legal, economic, and political *arrangements* that enable the full and proper expression of nursing values and expertise;
  D. The ability of the profession to maintain *unity* within diversity.
VI. I believe in *myself* and in my nursing *colleagues:*
  A. In our *responsibility* to develop and dedicate our minds, bodies, and souls to the profession that we esteem and the people whom we serve;
  B. In our *right* to be fulfilled, to be recognized, and to be rewarded as highly valued members of society.

Major units

Seven major units of the model are constructed from the assumptions and values:

1. Goal of nursing
2. Client (patient)
3. Role of the nurse
4. Source of difficulty of the client
5. Intervention focus
6. Modes of intervention
7. Consequences of nursing activity

A summary of these units in the major conceptual models is given in Table 1-1.

Goal of nursing The goal is the end or aim of nursing, what nursing is trying to achieve. This goal has to agree with the goals common to all health profes-

*From Styles, Margretta M.: *On nursing: Toward a new endowment*, St. Louis, 1982, The C. V. Mosby Company.

sionals—to improve health, to maintain health, to prevent health problems, to restore health, etc. However, each health discipline has a goal distinct enough to justify that discipline's presence on the health team. Specific nursing goals vary from model to model, depending on the assumptions stated about people. Goals need to be broad enough (a) to indicate what end the nursing profession is working toward, (b) to indicate what to teach future practitioners, and (c) to apply to nursing practice in all practice settings (community, hospital, home, health center, etc.). Before the 20th century, Florence Nightingale believed the goal of nursing was to make the patient as comfortable as possible and to put the patient in the best possible condition for nature to act and for the physician's treatment to take effect. For current goals of nursing, see Table 1–1.

Client The client unit refers not only to the person toward whom nursing service is directed but also to conceptions about that person. Most models indicate that the client is a biopsychosocial being, but they differ in exactly how he or she is conceptualized as such. Henderson views the client as a whole, complete, independent being who has fourteen fundamental needs, while Johnson views the client as a behavioral system composed of eight subsystems. See Table 1–1 for further information.

Role of the nurse The role of the nurse must be wanted, needed, and accepted by society just as the physician's curative role or the lawyer's defending role is wanted and accepted. Many nurses consider their role to be one of "caring"; however, caring is difficult to operationalize and needs to be clarified. In Orem's self-care model, the role of the nurse is to provide assistance to influence the client's development in achieving an optimal level of self-care; in Roy's adaptation model, the nurse's role is to promote the client's adaptive behaviors by manipulating stimuli. See Table 1–1 for additional information.

Source of difficulty The source of difficulty is that of the client, not that of the nurse. In other words it indicates the probable origin or cause of the client's problems that fall within the sphere of nursing competence. Clients in health care agencies have health problems that may be subcategorized as medical, psychologic, dietary, nursing, etc. The physician deals with medical problems, the psychologist or psychiatrist with psychologic problems, the dietician with dietary problems, and the nurse with nursing problems. The source of difficulty unit states more explicitly what a nursing problem is. For example, in Henderson's model the origin of the patient's problem is lack of strength, will, or knowledge; in Johnson's model it is functional or structural stress.

Intervention focus Another unit of each model indicates the target or focus of nursing intervention. The universally accepted intervention focus for the physician is the client's pathology. In Orem's self-care model the intervention focus for nurses is a deficit in the client's ability to maintain self-care; in Roy's adaptation model it is the stimuli the client is having difficulty adapting to. See Table 1–1 for additional information.

Modes of intervention The modes of intervention unit clarifies the means at the nurse's disposal when intervening. It is closely allied to the intervention focus and spells out specific ways in which the nurse helps the client. For example, in Roy's adaptation model the intervention focus is stimuli and the mode of intervention is manipulation of the stimuli. In contrast, Florence Nightingale believed the mode of intervention was manipulation of the environment. This was done by providing warmth, fresh air, light, food, and sanitation. See Table 1–1 for other intervention modes.

Consequences The last unit states the consequences that nursing expects to achieve. It reflects the nursing goal and the concept of the client. See Table 1–1 for the consequences of specific models.

One versus Several Models

Many nurses believe that there are advantages to having a single, universal model for nursing:

1. It would facilitate the development of nursing as a profession.
2. It would give all nurses a common framework, enhancing communication and research.
3. It would promote understanding about the nurse's role in nontraditional nursing settings, such as independent nurse practitioner practice, self-help clinics, and health maintenance organizations (HMOs), since many people believe nurses provide care for only sick persons.

In contrast, many nurses believe that use of one model alone may decrease creativity and overlook development of emerging roles in nursing. It is likely that this issue will not be resolved for many years. In the 21st century it is possible that many more models for nursing will be developed or existing ones refined in accordance with societal needs and with their tested usefulness.

Table 1–1 Summary of Major Units from Selected Conceptual Models for Nursing

Major units of model	*CNATS: developmental-adaptation model*	*Henderson: complementary-supplementary model*	*Johnson: behavioral system model*	*Orem: self-care model*	*Roy: adaptation model*
	Conceptual model for nursing*				
Goal of nursing	To help human beings achieve and sustain their optimal level of functioning	Independence in the satisfaction of human beings' 14 fundamental needs	Behavioral system equilibrium and dynamic stability	Achievement of optimal client self-care so that clients can achieve and maintain an optimal health state	Adaptation in each of the four adaptive modes in situations of health and illness
Client	A unique biopsychosocial being who functions as an integrated whole and whose modes of adaptation (patterns of responses to environmental and organismic stimuli) are both inborn and acquired	A whole, complete, and independent being who has fourteen fundamental needs: to breathe, eat and drink, eliminate, move and maintain posture, sleep and rest, dress and undress, maintain body temperature, keep clean, avoid danger, communicate, worship, work, play, and learn	A behavioral system composed of eight subsystems: affiliative, achievement, dependence, aggressive, eliminative, ingestive, restorative, and sexual	A unity who can be viewed as functioning biologically, symbolically, and socially and who initiates and performs self-care activities on his or her own behalf in maintaining life, health and well-being; self-care activities deal with: air, water, food, elimination, activity and rest, solitude and social interaction, hazards to life and well-being, and being normal	A biopsychosocial being who is in constant interaction with the environment and who has four modes of adaptation, based on: physiologic needs, self-concept, role function, and interdependence
Role of the nurse	To care for clients at critical periods of life in such a way that they may develop and use those modes of adaptation (motor, physiologic, social, affective, cognitive) that enable them to achieve the optimal level of functioning	A complementary-supplementary role to maintain or restore independence in the satisfaction of clients' fourteen fundamental needs	A regulator and controller of behavioral system stability and equilibrium	To provide assistance to influence clients' development in achieving an optimal level of self-care	To promote clients' adaptive behaviors by manipulating the focal, contextual, and residual stimuli

Table 1–1 continued

Major units of model	Conceptual model for nursing*				
	CNATS: developmental-adaptation model	*Henderson: complementary-supplementary model*	*Johnson: behavioral system model*	*Orem: self-care model*	*Roy: adaptation model*
Source of client difficulty	Actual or anticipated changes in stimulation, occurring at critical periods, which have the capacity to disrupt the optimal level of functioning	Lack of strength, will, or knowledge	Functional or structural stress	Any interference with self-care, by a person, object, condition, event, circumstance, or any combination of interferences	Coping activity that is inadequate to maintain integrity in the face of a need deficit or excess
Intervention focus	Modes of adaptation that require reinforcement (appropriate modes) or alteration (inappropriate modes) to sustain or restore the optimal level of functioning	The deficit that is the source of client difficulty	**1.** The mechanisms of control and regulation **2.** The functional imperatives	Inability to maintain self-care (a deficit in the self-care agency)	The focal, contextual, and residual stimuli
Modes of intervention	Manipulation of stimuli through the introduction of new ones, removal of existing ones, or modification of existing ones	Actions to replace, complete, substitute, add, reinforce, or increase strength, will, or knowledge	Actions to facilitate, inhibit, defend, or restrain the client in the face of functional or structural stress	Five general ways of assisting: acting for or doing for, guiding, supporting, providing a developmental environment, and teaching	Manipulation of the stimuli by increasing, decreasing, and/or maintaining them
Consequences of nursing activity	Sustained optimal level of functioning	**1.** Increased independence in satisfaction of the client's fourteen fundamental needs, or **2.** Peaceful death	Efficient and effective client behavior	Achievement of the client's optimal level of self-care	Adaptive responses to stimuli by the client

*The models are listed in alphabetical order.

CNATS model from Canadian Nurses' Association, *A definition of nursing practice: Standards for nursing practice* (Ottawa: Canadian Nurses' Association, 1980), reprinted by permission of the Canadian Nurses' Association Testing Service, Ottawa; Henderson's model from Virginia Henderson, *The nature of nursing* (New York: Macmillan Co., 1966); Johnson's model from Joan P. Riehl and Callista Roy, *Conceptual models for nursing practice*, 2nd ed. (New York: Appleton-Century-Crofts, 1980); Orem's model from Dorothea E. Orem, *Nursing: Concepts of practice*, 2nd ed. (New York: McGraw-Hill Book Co., 1980); Roy's model from Callista Roy, *Introduction to nursing: An adaptation model* (Englewood Cliffs, N.J.: Prenctice-Hall, 1976).

The Nursing Process

The conceptual model for nursing is an abstraction that is operationalized or brought to reality by the use of a process called the *nursing process*. See Chapter 5 for detailed information. This systematic process, not unique to nursing and similar to the scientific or problem-solving process, consist of five steps:

1. Collecting data (assessment)
2. Interpreting the data (nursing diagnosis)
3. Planning an intervention
4. Implementing the intervention
5. Evaluating the effectiveness of the other four steps

Assessment

Florence Nightingale wrote in *Notes on Nursing*, published in 1859:

> The most important practical lesson that can be given to nurses is to teach them what to observe—how to observe—what symptoms indicate improvement—what the reverse—which are of importance—which are none—which are the evidence of neglect—and of what kind of neglect.

The importance of observation has not diminished. This first step of the nursing process relies heavily on observation but has expanded over the years to encompass all data collected about a patient by various means: observation, physical examination, interviewing, laboratory tests, etc. The specific data that the nurse collects are directly associated with the second unit of the conceptual model for nursing: the client. For example, if the patient (client) is seen as a being with 14 fundamental needs, data are collected about these 14 needs. See Chapters 5, 13, and 14 for additional information regarding assessment.

Nursing Diagnosis

In the second step, the patient's problems are outlined in accordance with the nursing model used. In the past decade considerable attention has been given to the identification, development, and standardization of nursing diagnoses. These diagnoses describe a combination of signs and symptoms indicating actual or potential health problems that nurses are licensed to treat. See Chapter 6 for further information.

Planning Interventions

Planning nursing interventions is also directly related to the conceptual nursing model. Interventions are planned in accordance with the modes of nursing intervention outlined in the conceptual model (see page 9).

Nursing interventions can be described as either dependent or independent functions. *Dependent nursing functions* are those activities carried out at the request or with the guidance of the physician, for example, giving an antibiotic by injection to a patient every 4 hours. This dependent part of nursing practice cannot be minimized. Historically and legally nurses have an obligation to carry out physicians' orders. However, there is much more to nursing than the dependent part of practice. The independent part of nursing evolves from the conceptual model for nursing. *Independent nursing functions* are those activities carried out in the nurse's judgment, autonomously, without the physician's direct order. Examples are:

1. Assisting the patient with basic needs
2. Observing the patient's response and adaptation to illness
3. Observing the patient's response and adaptation to treatment
4. Teaching the patient self-care
5. Counseling the patient on health matters
6. Supervising or guiding the patient in rehabilitative activities related to daily living
7. Planning with the patient in a manner that develops the patient's sense of trust, self-worth, and, ultimately, self-realization

In addition to the dependent and independent functions of nursing, some nurses believe there is an interdependent part of nursing. It is obvious that all nursing activities are interdependent with the activities of other members of the health team to achieve a common goal for the patient. However, until the independent part of nursing is clarified, it is difficult to specify what is interdependent.

When planning interventions, nurses need to consider coordination of the patient's care, direction of the care provided by others, and plans for continuity of care.

Coordination of care

Coordination of total patient care involves helping all participants in a patient's care to work together as one unit toward a common goal. See also Chapter 2, page 49. The nurse works with patient and family as well as other members of the health team. Because the nurse is with the patient more than other health professionals are, and because of the nurse's relationship with the patient, this coordinating function is most effectively carried out by nurses. For example, if the nurse coordinates the time of laboratory and radiology tests that both require the patient to fast, the patient can be subjected to a delayed breakfast for only one morning instead of two. In another situation, the physician's orders may allow a patient to sit in a chair only three times a day for a brief period. The nurse and patient may plan this activity in conjunction with meal hours. This offers the patient the enjoyment of sitting up for meals and can also conserve the patient's energies.

Direction of care provided by others

The registered nurse is generally the member of the nursing team who delegates functions to other nursing personnel or to the family or the patient's other support persons. This delegation is done considering the particular needs of the patient and the skills of the nursing personnel or the support persons. After delegating these activities, nurses need to be available in case their assistance is required.

Primary nursing has been adopted in some hospitals. In this system, a patient is assigned to one nurse upon admission. This nurse is totally responsible for the care of three or four patients 24 hours of the day during their hospital stay. The primary nurse establishes the nursing care plan for the patient, and the plan is carried out by other nursing personnel when that nurse is off duty. For patients, the primary nursing concept in a hospital means there is one nurse in particular who is responsible for communication and care during their entire hospital stay. For nurses, this method of organization fosters independent nursing action and greater responsibility and accountability for patient care.

Plans for continuity of care

The patient does not cease to require care just because his or her physical presence is no longer directly in the nurse's view. The nurse plans for continuity of care to assist the patient to good health. Appropriate planning permits the patient to change physical settings, for example, from a hospital to home and family or from one hospital unit to another, with minimal disturbance to the patient and no disruption in care. Continuity is especially important when a patient requires care over a prolonged period. In this instance, many health personnel may be involved from time to time, making continuity planning a necessity. A systematic method of communication must be practiced; otherwise gaps may occur in patient care. For example, a patient may have a nursing order to increase activity as tolerated. Unless a plan is communicated, one nurse may interpret this to mean sitting in a chair for ten minutes twice a day, while another may expect the patient to walk to and from the bathroom. In a psychiatric nursing setting, it is essential that a consistent approach be provided by all health workers. For example, if a patient has difficulty making decisions, each nurse, occupational therapist, recreational therapist, and other health worker involved in this patient's care needs to encourage and help the patient to make decisions.

Implementing Interventions

Implementing the planned interventions draws on scientific knowledge that is not part of the nursing model. The nursing model instructs the nurse *what* to do and directly influences what nursing interventions are planned, but it does not tell the nurse *how* to do it. For example, a planned intervention may be to teach a patient and his wife how to give insulin. What to do is evident, but how to do it is not. To implement this plan effectively the nurse needs further knowledge about communication, helping relationships, learning, teaching strategies, techniques for giving injections, etc. This knowledge is drawn from sources other than the nursing model.

Evaluation of Care

Evaluating is a continuous nursing function. How is the patient adjusting and reacting? What does the patient see as needs? How does the patient see these needs changing? Has the patient achieved the desired consequences? The answers to these questions assist the nurse to evaluate the effectiveness of the total nursing process and the nursing model. The nursing process therefore needs to be flexible and responsive to the needs of the patient and support persons. For example, the nurse and a diabetic patient may decide to increase the patient's level of independence once the patient's severity of illness lessens. Rather than have the nurse test the patient's urine and administer the insulin, the nurse may begin to teach the patient, so that these activities can be carried out independently.

Settings for Nursing Practice

Settings for nursing practice can be grouped broadly into (a) hospitals, (b) community agencies, and (c) physicians' offices. In addition, other settings of practice are becoming available to the nurse. See Table 1–2.

In different settings there are differences in the degree of autonomy of the nurse, the nursing tasks required, and the relationships to physicians and other health workers. Today nurses have a variety of career choices and can pursue several of their personal and professional goals.

Table 1–2 Areas of Registered Nurse Employment

Practice setting	United States (1977–78)	Canada (1977)
Hospitals	65.0%	79.0%
Nursing homes, homes for aged	7.6%	5.6%
Physicians' and dentists' offices, family practice units	6.2%	1.5%
Community health agencies, schools, home care, public health agencies	9.0%	6.9%
Teaching institutions	3.4%	2.7%
Occupational health settings	2.2%	0.8%
Other (e.g., self-employed, private duty nursing)	6.6%	3.5%

From American Nurses' Association, *Facts about nursing 80–81* (New York: American Journal of Nursing Co., 1981), p. 3, and Statistics Canada, *Nursing in Canada* (Ottawa: Statistics Canada, 1978), p. 28.

Hospitals

Hospitals are health institutions that vary in size and in the services they provide. General hospitals treat patients with different health problems and different socioeconomic backgrounds. They range in size from the small hospital in a rural setting to the large metropolitan hospital of perhaps 2000 beds. A specialized hospital may be of any size, but it restricts its services to defined areas, such as obstetrics, pediatrics, or psychiatry. Nurses who are employed in hospitals generally have limited autonomy in their functions, although nurses in psychiatric settings may have more autonomy than nurses in many other areas of a hospital. Recently, however, nurses in specialty areas, such as intensive care units, have been functioning with increasing autonomy and with highly advanced skills.

Hospitals are bureaucratic organizations with regulations and policies that largely govern the activities of the employees. This is most obvious in large hospitals. Smaller institutions tend to be less formal and have fewer, more flexible policies. Nurses in hospitals are expected to fit into the system of the institution and to share its values as an organization. This expectation can conflict with the judgment of the nurse when assisting patients. For example, a patient who is accustomed to bathing in the evening may wish to continue this practice in the hospital as a relaxing measure to assist in sleep. The hospital, on the other hand, may not have a sufficient nursing staff working in the evening to provide the patient with the assistance required for a bath.

In hospital settings, nurses interact with a number of physicians and other health personnel. They perform a variety of nursing tasks, often at the direction of physicians. These tasks, such as giving medications, are usually dependent, cure-related activities, and as such they frequently take precedence over independent activities prescribed and initiated by nurses themselves. However, as patterns of nursing education change, as hospital policies change, and indeed as state and provincial legislative regulations change, the independent functions of the nurse are changing as well. Today's nurse is growing in responsibility and autonomy.

Community Agencies

Nurses are employed by community agencies for a wide range of nursing activities. A community can be a particular geographic area or a group of people brought together because of common interests. For example, a community might be a town or the teachers, students, and families associated with a specific school.

Community agencies include community clinics, public health agencies, industrial clinics, schools, and home nursing services. In these settings, nurses tend to function more independently than in hospitals. Their contact with physicians is episodic. In rural areas, contact with a physician may occur only when the nurse judges that a physician's advice or intervention is required.

Depending upon the purpose of the community agency, nurses' activities may include a mixture of care, cure, and coordination. Generally, nurses use more independent judgment in these settings, and the activities tend to be less related to the physician's cure regimen, than in hospitals.

Physicians' Offices

In physicians' offices, nurses have a minimum amount of independent function. The physician is generally there when the patients are present, and many of the nurse's activities are done in response to the physician's request. The nurse's function is related mainly to the physician's therapy.

Other Career Settings

More and more career possibilities are available for today's nurse. Besides nursing education or administration, there are career opportunities in nursing research and in various clinical specialties. See page 20. As physicians and other health professionals develop group practices (e.g., family practice clinics), nurses are joining the health team along with others (e.g., social workers and technologists) as a vital part of groups devoted to a broad range of services and holistic health.

In more and more states, nurses are being employed as independent nurse practitioners (described on page 20) in: (a) hospital practice settings such as inpatient and emergency areas; (b) ambulatory care settings such as private practice, hospital outpatient clinics, and community-based clinics; (c) institutions such as schools for the mentally and physically handicapped, public schools, and college health programs; and (d) community settings such as health departments and social service agencies. The vast majority (90%) of independent nurse practitioners are employed in settings (b)–(d) (Levine 1977:1800).

Career Patterns

A nursing career is flexible and open to personal and educational growth and expansion. Two differing but related career patterns, which include a broad range of nursing practice possibilities, are available to the nurse. One career pattern (episodic) emphasizes nursing practice that is essentially curative and restorative, generally acute or chronic in nature, and most frequently provided in hospital and inpatient facilities. The second career pattern (distributive) emphasizes nursing practice designed essentially for health maintenance and disease prevention, generally continuous in nature, seldom acute, and frequently operative in the community or in newly developing institutional settings.

The increasing complexity of nursing practice in a wide variety of settings and recognition that it is difficult for a nurse to function effectively in every setting are seen in the summary report and recommendations by the National Commission for the Study of Nursing and Nursing Education (1974:23).

Factors Influencing Nursing Practice

To understand nursing as it is practiced today and as it will be practiced tomorrow requires not only a historic perspective of nursing's evolution but also an understanding of some of the social forces presently influencing this profession. These forces usually affect the entire health care system, and nursing, as a major component of that system, cannot avoid the effects.

Historic Development

Nursing as an activity that provides help to the ill, to children, and to babies has existed since the earliest times. Before the early Christian period (1–500 A.D.), caring for the sick was chiefly done by women in their homes. Later, monastic orders provided nursing functions as part of their activities. The first nursing order, the Augustinian Sisters, was established in the Middle Ages. This was probably the first organized group to provide purely nursing services to people.

Prior to the Protestant Reformation in the 16th century, hospital facilities were organized chiefly by the Roman Catholic Church. With the Reformation, beginning in 1517, came a decline in people's interest in and support of the church and religion. This change resulted in an era in nursing history known as the "dark period." Hospitals were unsanitary places, dark and foreboding. Nursing was provided by women who were frequently described as drunk, heartless, and immoral. They were expected to carry out the housework of the hospital, wash the laundry, and do all the cleaning for very little reward. Nurses were not required to have any training, and it was not unusual for a nurse to work anywhere from 12 to 40 consecutive hours. This period of decline lasted until the middle of the 19th century.

The era of reform in nursing is marked by the work of the British nurse, Florence Nightingale, during the Crimean War (1854–56). Nightingale's efforts made nursing once again a respectable vocation. However, Nightingale's reform activities did not stop at respectability. Besides crusading for cleanliness and comfort in hospitals, Nightingale also worked toward educating the populace regarding health measures, in an effort to stave off the widespread diseases resulting from poor conditions in the cities. Nightingale believed in prevention and in nursing the whole person, calling upon her fellow nurses to make sure that patients always had fresh air, good water, proper medication, quiet, mobility, and knowledge of how to care for themselves in the future. Many of Nightingale's ideas are now standards of patient care. Education of nurses was a major goal of this reformer. Among her many other accomplishments was the establishment of the Nightingale School of Nurses at St. Thomas' Hospital, London, in 1860. This school is credited with providing the first planned educational program for nurses. She also assisted in establishing the first organized home nursing services.

In North America, establishment of nursing and health services was slow prior to the American Revolution (1775–83). One notable organization was the Nurse Society of Philadelphia, which gave women minimal instruction in obstetrics to enable them to provide maternity nursing services in home settings.

The late 1800s was a time of rapid reform of nursing services in the United States and Canada. Schools of nursing with planned educational programs were started. From these schools a number of nurses graduated who became the early leaders in the profession.

Isabel Hampton Robb had been a young schoolteacher in Canada. She decided to change her profession and entered the Bellevue Hospital Training School in New York. After graduation she nursed in Rome for two years and then she became superintendent of the Illinois Training School at 26 years of age. Three years later she went to Baltimore to organize a new school in connection with Johns Hopkins Hospital. Among her many accomplishments was a nursing textbook, which was recognized as a standard text for nursing schools in America.

Mary Adelaide Nutting, also from Canada, was in the first class at Johns Hopkins. After graduation she established a course of training for students prior to ward experience at Johns Hopkins. Later she reduced the nursing students' hours from 12 to 8 and lengthened the nurses' training to three years.

Mary Agnes Snively graduated from Bellevue and returned to Canada to take charge of the nurses' training at Toronto General Hospital. She is credited largely with the direction of Canadian nursing education and was the first president of the Canadian Nurses' Association.

Two American graduates from the New York Hospital, Lillian D. Wald and Mary Brewster, were the first to offer trained nursing services to the poor in the New York slums. What began as their home among the poor on the upper floor of a tenement is now famous as a center of public health nursing (the Henry Street Settlement). Soon after, school nursing was established as an adjunct to visiting nursing. Again Wald was involved, along with Lina L. Rogers.

Linda Richards, who graduated in 1873 from the New England Hospital for Women and Childen Training School for Nurses in Boston, is cited by many historians as America's first trained nurse (Jamieson, Sewall, and Suhrie 1966:224). She is credited with nursing reform in 12 major hospitals, some of which were specialized mental hospitals. She initiated training schools for students in mental health nursing, and included a period of training in general hospitals in their programs. She also founded the first training school for nurses in Japan.

Some, however, dispute that Richards was the first trained nurse. In a series of reports of Women's Hospital of Philadelphia there is evidence suggesting that Harriet Newton Phillips was the first trained nurse to receive a certificate from that hospital in 1864 (Large 1976:50). Phillips is also considered the first trained nurse in America to do community nursing, to do missionary service, and to take postgraduate training.

America's first trained black nurse was Mary Mahoney. She trained at the same hospital as Linda Richards and graduated in 1879 (Notter and Spalding 1976:15).

During the late 1800s the need for concerted actions by nurses was felt (in England first). In 1894 the Matrons' Council of Great Britain and Ireland was organized, followed by the American Society of Superintendents of Training Schools for Nurses of the United States and Canada. Alumnae associations also came together and formed the Nurses' Associated Alumnae of the United States and Canada in 1897. In 1908 the National Association of Colored Graduate Nurses was formed by a group of nurses who felt such an association could more readily further not only the nursing cause but their own special interests. From these organizations current national groups were founded. The Society of Superintendents divided nationally and ultimately became the Canadian National Association of Trained Nurses in 1908 (now the Canadian Nurses' Association) and the National League of Nursing Education in 1912. The Nurses' Associated Alumnae became the American Nurses' Association in 1911. See the section on nursing organizations later in this chapter.

After World War I, the Frontier Nursing Service (FNS) was established by a notable pioneer nurse, Mary Breckinridge. In 1918 she worked with the American Committee for Devastated France, distributing food, clothing, and supplies to rural villages in France and taking care of sick children. In 1921 Breckinridge returned to the United States with plans to provide health care to the people of rural America. She initially prepared herself by taking courses at Teachers College in New York (where she met Mary Adelaide Nutting and gained her approval) and midwifery training in London, and by developing prominent social contacts for fundraising. In 1925 Breckinridge and two other nurses began the FNS in Leslie County, Kentucky. Within this organization, Breckinridge began one of the first midwifery training schools in the United States.

The general trend from the beginning of formal organization of nursing in the late 1800s to the end of World War I was rapid expansion in the establishment of hospitals, with nursing schools dependent upon them for support. Hospitals in turn depended on the schools to carry the chief nursing load. During the war, greater numbers of young women were accepted for entrance and less consideration was given to selection requirements. Most schools by this time had been increased to three-year programs, but the 8-hour day originally proposed with those programs was less quickly adopted.

By 1920 the apprenticeship system of educating nurses was increasingly being criticized. In addition, the effectiveness of the nurse as a teacher of nurses was being questioned. Thus, a special postbasic course was offered at Teachers College, Columbia University, New York, to prepare nurses as teachers. Preparations for a postbasic public health nursing program were also made, in response to an influenza epidemic and the development of broader aims by the medical profession, which now included teaching the principles of healthful living to individuals, families, and community groups.

During the early 1920s, the Rockefeller Survey (Committee for the Study of Nursing Education) recommended that nursing schools be independent of hospitals and on a college level. As a result, two university schools of nursing were set up, one at Yale University, New Haven, Connecticut, the other at Western Reserve University, Cleveland, Ohio. The purpose of these experimental schools was to prove the feasibility of planning both classroom instruction and ward practice in accordance with the educational needs of the students. Emphasis was placed on the social welfare and health aspects of nursing. Both schools demonstrated the value of university standards in the nursing field.

Another far-reaching result of the Rockefeller Survey was a proposal by the National League of Nursing Education to undertake a comprehensive study of nursing education (1926–34) that would lead to the grading of nursing schools. It was believed that grading would establish standards for education in these schools. This was the beginning of the accreditation function that the National League for Nursing now carries out. See the section on nursing organizations later in this chapter.

During this period the concept of the clinical nurse specialist arose. In 1933, the need for "experts in the nursing art and specialists in the clinical branches they represent" was recognized (Stewart 1933:363). This concept, currently seen by many as a new role in nursing, was discussed by nursing leaders in the 1930s and '40s. In the early '40s it was thought that more emphasis needed to be placed on the clinical specialties in the advanced professional curricula of colleges and universities. Most advanced nursing curricula were preparing specialists in nursing school administration, teaching, and supervision, in public health, and in hospital administration and were not emphasizing the clinical specialties component. This component gained prominence with the needs of postwar society. Nurses returning from overseas were required to work in clinical areas not familiar to them, such as psychiatric nursing, which were needed to assist individuals to readjust to civilian life. By 1946 many nursing programs in the United States were providing more clinical content. Today the nurse clinician is a graduate of a master's or doctoral program in nursing with a major in a clinical specialty. This nurse is reponsible for increasing her or his own clinical knowledge and competence and for enhancing the quality of nursing care and the quality of the organizational climate for learning and research (McPhail 1971:16–18).

From its early days to the present, nursing has undergone change in every area. Rapid strides have been made in nursing education programs and in a wide variety of hospital and community nursing services. Throughout these changes, nursing has continued to provide a stable helping service to people.

Current Influences

It is difficult to escape the influences of society, science, and technology. Nursing, as a profession deeply involved with people, certainly cannot escape. Many factors influence the individual nurse, nursing practice, and, of course, patients. To function effectively amid media bombardment, rapid systems of communication, and advances in research, the nurse must develop in response to outside influences. The current major influences can be grouped into nine broad areas: (a) consumer demands and participation, (b) changing family structure, (c) economics, (d) science and technology, (e) legislation, (f) demography, (g) the nursing profession, (h) the women's movement, and (i) unionization.

Consumer demands

Consumers of nursing services (the public) have become an increasingly effective force in changing nursing practice. On the whole, people have become better educated and have more knowledge about health and illness than in the past. This is in no small measure because of television and the news media. Consumers also have become more aware of the needs of others for care. The ethical and moral issues raised by poverty and neglect have caused people to be more vocal about the needs of minority groups and the poor.

The public's concepts of health and nursing have also changed. People now believe that health is a right of all people, not just a privilege of the rich. People are bombarded by the media with the message that individuals must assume responsibility for their own health by obtaining a physical examination regularly, checking for the seven danger signals of cancer, and maintaining their mental well-being by balancing work and recreation. Interest in health and nursing services is therefore greater than ever. Furthermore, many people now want more than freedom from disease—they want energy, vitality, and a feeling of wellness.

Increasingly, the consumer has become an active participant in making decisions about health and nursing care. Planning committees concerned with providing nursing services to a community have active consumer membership. More and more state and provincial nursing associations have representatives of the community on their governing boards.

Family structure

The need for and provision of nursing services are being influenced by new family structures. An increasing number of people are living in structures other than the extended family and the nuclear family, and the family breadwinner is no longer necessarily the husband. An extended family consists of parents, children, grandparents, and sometimes aunts and uncles; a nuclear family consists only of parents and their children.

There are now many single men and women raising children and many two-parent families in which both parents work. It is also common for young parents to live at great distances from their parents. These families need support services such as day-care centers. Many families do not have grandparents or other relatives readily available to help in times of illness or to offer advice about childbearing and child health. The advice these parents get about their children usually comes from physicians and nurses as well as others.

Similarly, grandparents, who now may live alone and far from other members of the family, require homemaker and visiting nurse services when they are ill, to replace the care formerly provided by younger members of the family.

Economics

Another factor that has increased the demand and need for nursing services is the greater financial support provided through health insurance programs in the United States and Canada. Medicare, Medicaid, and other government programs as well as other public and private financing agencies have increased the demand for broad nursing services. Thus, health services such as new eyeglasses, hospitalization, and annual medical examinations are increasingly being used by people who could not afford these in the past. Federal governments recognized this need and markedly increased their budgets for health care in the past ten years.

This increase in expenditure is accompanied by an increase in the number of people who provide health services. In nursing alone, the number of practicing nurses in the United States grew from 750,000 in 1971 to 1,119,100 in 1980, an increase of 32.9% (American Nurses' Association [ANA] 1981:6). In Canada, the number of practicing nurses also increased during this period. Unfortunately, the current economic trend is a retrenchment in health care funding by governments, resulting in decreases in hospital beds and staff cuts.

Science and technology

Discoveries in science and related technologies, such as means to control many infectious diseases, have affected nursing. The vaccine for poliomyelitis has made largely obsolete the nursing skills required in the 1950s to assist the acutely ill patient with poliomyelitis. Advances in science also have an indirect effect on nursing. For example, as physicians acquire new knowledge and skills in cardiac surgery, nurses must acquire complementary knowledge and skills.

In some settings, technologic advances have required that nurses become highly specialized. Nurses frequently have to use sophisticated equipment for patient monitoring or treatment. As technologies change, nursing education changes, and some nurses require advanced education to perform effectively as members of the health team.

Development of new pharmaceuticals affects nursing practice. The discovery that lithium carbonate can be used to control the manic state of manic-depressive illness is an example. It has changed the role of the nurse from one of psychologically assisting the patient with behavior to one of counseling the patient about effective use of the medication.

New facts are being discovered in every field associated directly or indirectly with nursing. The social sciences offer a better understanding of human behavior and are building a knowledge of how the mind and the body are interrelated. Advances in technology are exemplified by the many machines now used to help patients maintain life. There seems to be no end to the discoveries and the knowledge explosion of the 20th century.

With this knowledge explosion, unfortunately, has come the charge by many that medical services—and some health professionals—have become dehumanized. Yet an increasing understanding of the psychologic, emotional, and spiritual aspects of care has developed to balance the technologic advances. As science and technology create methods of treating disease, it is the responsibility of all health professionals to remember that patients are human beings requiring warmth, care, and acknowledgment of self-worth. Often equipment is frightening to patients and their support persons. Medical vocabularly appears mysterious and is frequently misunderstood. The nurse dealing daily with patients is in an ideal situation to humanize technology as much as is possible. Explanations by nurses and their communications of support and recognition of the patients' needs to understand and to be supported help to humanize highly technical care.

Scientific developments have led to other changes in the nursing profession by indirectly affecting human health. For example, some industries have proven hazardous to employees because of the dangerous equipment used or because of harmful chemical residues. Trauma (injury) and disease are frequently the direct result of advanced technology; the classic example is automobile accidents, which are among the top five causes of death in North America. In addition, our advanced society frequently produces high levels of stress and diminished mental health. These problems created by technologic change present new challenges to the health team.

Legislation

Legislation about nursing practice and in relation to health matters affects both the public and nursing. Legislation governing nursing is discussed in Chapter 4. However, changes in legislation affecting health also affect nursing. For example, the laws governing abortions have recently been broadened in some states and in Canada. This change has lowered the birth rate significantly and has increased the need for nursing intervention associated with abortions.

Demography

Demography is the study of population statistics. It includes the distribution of the population by age and place of residence, *mortality* (death), and *morbidity* (incidence of disease) statistics. From demographic data, needs of the population for nursing services can be assessed. For example:

1. The total populations in both the United States and Canada have increased since 1900. The proportion of elderly people has also increased in both populations, creating an increased need for nursing services for this group. For further information on population, see Chapter 2, page 52.
2. Another study of the population indicates a shift of the primary residence of people from rural (country) to urban (city) settings. Concomitant with this are increased needs for nursing related to problems caused by pollution and by the effects on the environment of concentrations of people. Thus, most nursing services are now provided in urban settings.
3. Mortality rates in the United States have reflected a steady decrease, adding years to the average life span at the time of birth. Much of this decrease can be attributed to the control of infectious diseases such as smallpox and diphtheria. For additional mortality statistics, see Chapter 2.
4. Morbidity studies indicate (a) higher incidence of long-term illness; (b) increases in venereal disease, alcoholism, and drug addiction; (c) increases in lung cancer and heart disease; (d) an increase in automobile accidents; (e) an increase in homicide, especially among nonwhite men; and (f) high infant mortality (Somers 1971:18–20).

The nursing profession

Members of the nursing profession actively influence nursing services. Increasingly they have assumed more responsibility and accountability for nursing activities. They also have established functions for nurses outside of hospitals, such as in community clinics and home nursing. Recently the American Nurses' Association published a list of nursing standards in an attempt to determine the quality of nursing care provided to the public (see the section on trends in nursing practice later in this chapter). Beyond these activities, some members of the nursing profession are involved in health politics. Many are working with legislative committees to develop licensing standards for new branches of the nursing profession, such as nurse practitioners or nurse midwives. Others are developing programs in continuing education or specialized areas of nursing.

Accreditation of nursing education programs by the National League for Nursing has also influenced nursing. Many programs have steadily improved to meet the standards for accreditation over the years. As a result, graduates are better prepared to meet the demands of society as nurses. See page 33 for further information about the NLN.

The women's movement

The women's movement has brought public attention to women's rights, minority rights, and all human rights. Persons are seeking equality in all areas, particularly educational, political, economic, and social equality. Because the majority of nurses are women, this trend has altered the perspectives of nurses about economic and educational needs. As a result, nurses are increasingly asserting themselves as professional people who have a right to equality with men in health professions. They are demanding more responsibility in patient care and are becoming equal members of the health team.

Unionization

More and more nurses are using collective bargaining to deal with their concerns. The ANA has participated in collective bargaining for years on behalf of nurses. Today some nurses are joining other labor organizations that represent them at the bargaining table. There are instances in both the United States and Canada of nurses striking to support their demands and concerns. Often these concerns go beyond economic reward to issues about safe care for patients. Increasingly nurses are becoming aware of the strength they have through organized large numbers.

Trends in Nursing Practice

Some trends in nursing practice are subtle and slow to emerge, while others are obvious and seem to surface quickly. Not all the trends complement each other; some are divergent, if not in conflict. Over time, some aspects of nursing practice will emerge as prevailing trends; others may be modified by social forces. As nursing responds to societal conditions, some of these trends in nursing practice will gain emphasis.

Broadened Focus of Care

The focus of nursing care has broadened from care of the ill to care of people in both sickness and health, and from the patient to both patient and family or support persons or significant others. In the past, the nurse's role was chiefly to care for people who were ill. Nursing care was disease- and illness-oriented. More emphasis is now being placed on promoting health and preventing disease. It has been predicted that one day all diseases, including heart disease and cancer, will be conquered. At that time the nurse will be chiefly concerned with helping people to attain their optimum level of health.

Nursing care is also broadening to include a family focus. Assistance for a family might be directly related to the needs of the patient or it might be concerned with totally different health problems. For example, the family may need assistance in providing economical but nutritious meals to growing teenagers.

Modern nursing care also includes a holistic focus. Today's nurse deals with patients as emotional and social as well as physical beings. Care is provided not just for a particular disease or wound but also for the health of the whole person. The broadened focus of care requires an integration of skills and concepts.

Another aspect of the broader nursing focus is the movement of nursing practice to the community. At one time nurses worked only in institutions; now nursing services are provided in the community, often in homes and in clinics. These nursing activities not only assist those who are ill but also help those who are healthy to maintain wellness. This is one of the major areas of growth in the nursing services.

Increasing Scientific Basis

In the past, nursing was largely intuitive or *empirical* (relying on experience or observation, rather than on research). Through trial and error the nurse sensed the measures that would assist the patient, and many nurses became highly skilled in providing care through experience. Now much nursing has a scientific base, either from nursing research or from research in the biologic, physical, and social sciences. Some nursing practice today is still intuitive, but, as a theoretic base for nursing is developed, the scientific basis of the field will increase.

At one time nursing care was chiefly "ministering to the patient, wiping the fevered brow." Increasingly, nursing intervention, particularly in hospitals, necessitates using highly complex machines such as cardiac monitors, respirators, and computers. The patient and support persons remain the focus of nursing, but technologic advances affect the methods used to provide care.

Increased Independence

Nursing practice increasingly uses the independent judgment of nurses. At one time nursing was entirely dependent, that is, it was a result of a physician's order. Although these activities are still a part of nursing, more and more the nurse is functioning in areas that require independent judgment, such as teaching dietary practices to pregnant women or providing these women with primary prenatal care.

New Roles

The emergence of new roles for the nurse is a fourth trend. Many hospitals today employ *nurse clinicians*—nurses with advanced skills in a particular area of nursing practice, for example, psychiatric nursing. The clinician serves as a consultant to other nursing staff members and assists them with particular problems in identifying or meeting patient needs.

Another new role for the nurse is the expanded role of *independent nurse practitioner* in *primary care* (the first contact a patient has with the health care system). This nurse usually has an office in the community and functions independently, that is, patients come to the office for nursing. Some nurses, as independent practitioners, work closely with a group of physicians. In the past, the first person a patient met was usually the physician. Today, the primary care nurse takes medical histories and carries out physical examinations that traditionally were functions of the physician.

Development of Nursing Standards

One of the most recent trends in nursing is the establishment of standards for nursing practice. These standards provide patients and nurses with exact criteria against which care can be evaluated for effectiveness and excellence. Basic to the development of these standards are:

Table 1–3 American Nurses' Association Standards of Nursing Practice

Standard	Rationale
1. The collection of data about the health status of the client/patient is systematic and continuous. The data are accessible, communicated, and recorded.	Comprehensive care requires complete and ongoing collection of data about the client/patient to determine the nursing care and needs of the client/patient. All health status data about the client/patient must be available for all members of the health care team.
2. Nursing diagnoses are derived from health status data.	The health status of the client/patient is the basis for determining the nursing care needs. The data are analyzed and compared to norms when possible.
3. The plan of nursing care includes goals derived from the nursing diagnoses.	The determination of the results to be achieved is an essential part of planning care.
4. The plan of nursing care includes priorities and the prescribed nursing approaches or measures to achieve the goals derived from the nursing diagnoses.	Nursing actions are planned to promote, maintain, and restore the client/patient's well-being.
5. Nursing actions provide for client/patient participation in health promotion, maintenance, and restoration.	The client/patient and family are continually involved in nursing care.
6. The nursing actions assist the client/patient to maximize his health capabilities.	Nursing actions are designed to promote, maintain, and restore health.
7. The client/patient's progress or lack of progress toward goal achievement is determined by the client/patient and the nurse.	The quality of nursing care depends upon comprehensive and intelligent determination of nursing's impact upon the health status of the client/patient. The client/patient is an essential part of this determination.
8. The client/patient's progress or lack of progress toward goal achievement directs reassessment, reordering of priorities, new goal setting, and revision of the plan of nursing care.	The nursing process remains the same, but the input of new information may dictate new or revised approaches.

From American Nurses' Association, *Standards of nursing practice* (Kansas City, Mo.: American Nurses' Association, 1973). Reprinted with permission.

1. The needs of patients and support persons to have the assurance that they are receiving a safe and good standard of care.

2. The need of patients and health administrators to know that the standard of care is efficiently provided at an acceptable level. Both the consumer and the health administrator have become increasingly concerned about the costs of health care.

3. The need of nursing personnel to have precise standards against which they can measure the nursing they provide, thus protecting themselves and patients.

Nursing standards clearly reflect the specific functions and activities that nurses provide, as opposed to the functions of other health workers. The ANA's Standards of Nursing Practice are set forth in Table 1–3, and those of the CNA are summarized in Table 1–4.

The Nurse as a Provider of Health Care

Roles of the Nurse

Nursing is a system of interrelated people, skills, and concepts, and the roles of the nurse are interwoven in the system. The nurse has nine main roles in relation to the care of patients and their families or support persons. The emphasis of each role varies with the situation. The nurse adapts skills and methods of care to these interrelated roles as needs arise.

Table 1–4 Summary of Canadian Nurses' Association Standards for Nursing Practice

Standard	Elements	Standard	Elements
I. Nursing practice requires that a conceptual model for nursing be the basis for the independent part of that practice	1. Nurses are required to have a clear idea or conception of the distinct goal of nursing 2. Nurses are required to have a clear idea or conception of the client 3. Nurses are required to have a clear idea or conception of their role in response to the health needs of society 4. Nurses are required to have a clear idea or conception of the source of client difficulty 5. Nurses are required to have a clear idea or conception of the focus and modes of nursing intervention 6. Nurses are required to have a clear idea or conception of the expected consequences of nursing activities	II. Nursing practice requires the effective use of the nursing process as the method for carrying out the independent, interdependent, and dependent functions of nursing practice	1. Nurses are required to collect data in accordance with their conception of the client and consistent with their interdependent and dependent functions 2. Nurses are required to analyze data collected in accordance with their conception of the goal of nursing, their role, and the source of client difficulty, and consistent with their interdependent and dependent functions 3. Nurses are required to plan their nursing actions based upon the identified actual and potential client problems, in accordance with their conception of the focus and modes of intervention and consistent with their interdependent and dependent functions

Healing (therapeutic) role

The nurse has a healing or curative role. Nurses use techniques that help the natural processes of healing, such as changing a sterile dressing and administering medications. This role is illustrated most vividly by nurses employed by hospitals in acute settings, e.g., coronary care units. Here the patients are acutely ill and many of the nurses' activities are oriented to promoting the restorative processes of the body.

Caring (comforting) role

The caring role is difficult to define specifically. It is the role of human relations. The chief goal of the nurse in this role is to provide support; this should not be thought of as establishing dependence. The nurse supports the patient by attitudes and actions that show concern for patient welfare and acceptance of the patient as a person, not merely a chart.

The caring role has also been described as a comforting or soothing role. Nurses who comfort patients act to relieve anxiety, diminish pain, and restore a sense of well-being. The nurse recognizes that people have different backgrounds and ideas, many of which may be counter to the nurse's views. Nevertheless, the nurse provides care and maintains a harmonious environment to assist the patient's recovery. These activities maintain the patient's motivational equilibrium, facilitating the therapeutic function. It is important that the nurse's caring functions also support the therapeutic goals of the patient. For example, if one of the objectives for the patient is to regain independence in activities, then the caring functions must not foster dependence under the guise of support. Nurses are also careful not to make decisions for the patient but to encourage the

Table 1–4 continued

Standard	Elements
	4. Nurses are required to perform nursing actions that implement the plan **5.** Nurses are required to evaluate all steps of the nursing process in accordance with their conceptual model for nursing and consistent with their interdependent and dependent functions
III. Nursing practice requires that the helping relationship be the nature of the client-nurse interaction	**1.** Nurses are required to increase the likelihood that the client will perceive the health service experience as understandable, manageable, and meaningful at the outset **2.** Nurses are required to set mutually agreed upon expectations as a means of increasing the likelihood that the client will perceive the health service experience as understandable, manageable, and meaningful **3.** Nurses are required to ensure a successful termination of the helping relationship
IV. Nursing practice requires nurses to fulfill professional responsibilities in their independent, interdependent, and dependent functions	**1.** Nurses are required to respect statutes and policies relevant to the profession and the practice setting **2.** Nurses are required to comply with the Code of Ethics of their profession **3.** Nurses are required to function as members of a health team

Adapted from Canadian Nurses' Association, *A blueprint for a comprehensive examination for nurse registration/licensure* (Ottawa: Canadian Nurses' Association, May 1977), p. 2. Reprinted with permission.

patient and support persons to participate in planning care. Nurses carry out these caring functions with the welfare of the patient in mind.

The caring role is magnified in dealing with people who have long-term illnesses. These patients and their families have time to develop a relationship with nurses and often require supportive, caring functions more than therapeutic functions. Caring activities include those that preserve the dignity of the individual and those often referred to as the "mothering actions" in nursing.

Communicating role

Actions of communication include collecting information, conveying information to others, and influencing others. Nurses communicate with patients, their support persons, other nurses, and other members of the health team. The quality of a nurse's communication often affects the patient's return to health. For example, a nurse who communicates abruptly or incompletely to a patient may produce feelings of anxiety or worry in the patient that can delay recovery.

Teaching role

Nurses frequently act as teachers, imparting information and reinforcing changes in behavior. For effective learning to take place, a nurse must establish an environment in which patients can learn, determine with the patient the need to learn and readiness to learn, and design teaching strategies for the learning. The teaching role may be a formal one, in which the teaching is planned, or it may be more casual, for example, encouraging a patient to wash his feet daily during a bed bath.

Planning role

Planning by nurses occurs during all phases of the nursing process, including assessment, intervention, and evaluation. Planning is carried out so that anticipated goals can be met. Nurses plan with patients, their support persons, other nurses, and other health professionals.

Coordinating role

The nurse has a coordinating role involving patients, support persons, other nurses, and other health professionals. Coordinating can be described as pulling together or producing equilibrium. In coordinating, the nurse considers such matters as the time and sequence of activities, energies, and needs of others.

Protecting role

Nursing activities that are considered protecting include those that protect the patient from injury or complications. The nurse checks the functioning of a suction machine, the temperature of bath water, and the sterility of supplies, for example, to prevent patient injury. Activities that are protective are often called *preventive.*

Rehabilitating role

Rehabilitating activities are those that maximize a patient's capabilities and minimize limitations. These activities often help patients to change and to gain new skills, such as walking with crutches.

Socializing role

The socializing role of the nurse is one that is often forgotten. For patients who are separated from their support persons and normal activities, socializing offers a distraction and respite from the focus on illness. Patients do not always want a therapeutic conversation; sometimes they just want news of another world and conversation they can enjoy. This is particularly true of patients with long-term illnesses.

Methods of Nursing Assistance

For the nurse, providing assistance is a matter of course. Helping is fundamental to the nursing profession. Some methods of assisting are more effective than others, and some patients are more willing to receive assistance than others. People have different wants and needs, and the nurse must be flexible enough to adapt to them. Assistance must be given in a manner that does not destroy the patient's sense of self-worth.

Nursing practice involves helping the patient and/or support persons either directly or indirectly. *Direct activities* are those carried out in the presence of the patient or support persons. *Indirect activities* are carried out on the patient's behalf but not in the patient's presence, for example, a meeting between nurse and physician to discuss a change in medication for the patient. As the member of the health team closest to the patient, the nurse assumes the role of patient advocate, acquainting the physician with the patient's physical and emotional responses to treatment.

The choice of method of assistance to be used by a nurse depends on the particular situation. In providing care, the nurse needs to be sensitive to the patient on many levels and must be aware of change, selecting a method of help according to the requirements of the situation. Five methods of assisting identified by Dorothea Orem (1980:61) are:

1. Acting for or doing for another
2. Guiding another
3. Supporting another (physically or psychologically)
4. Providing an environment that promotes development of another's ability to meet present or future demands for action
5. Teaching another

Acting for or doing for another

The nurse's own abilities (physical and mental) may be used so that the patient's needs are met. When a patient is unconscious, the care plan is carried out using the nurse's judgment and without the patient's participation. For a nurse to act for a patient who is conscious, however, the patient must legally agree. In most situations, patients can assist in planning their care even if they cannot physically participate in it.

Doing for the patient occurs in a number of situations when it is not possible for the patient to care for himself or herself. Patients requiring this care include those who (a) have certain physical illnesses, (b) are incompetent, and (c) are very young or old.

Guiding another

The nurse may guide a patient either verbally or by action. The patient must be willing to accept the guidance or the instruction, and the nurse must be able to provide it. An example would be suggesting to a patient who was sitting in her chair for the first time after surgery that she return to bed for a rest before becoming too tired. In this situation the nurse is guiding the patient using knowledge of the patient's health and strength.

Supporting another

A person may be supported either physically or emotionally by a nurse. Often both types of support are given at the same time. For example, when a patient who has had a fractured hip gets out of bed for the first time, he may need physical support because of weakness and encouragement and emotional support to allay his fear of falling. Support may often be the first step in helping a patient to regain independent functioning.

Providing a developmental environment

Nurses may provide an environment that helps a patient set and meet appropriate goals. For example, a patient who has had an operation and is recovering well may be introduced to a patient who is anticipating the same type of surgery. A child may be taken to a playroom and provided with toys that will help him to exercise his arms. A severely depressed person may require surroundings that are sunny, cheerful, and attractively decorated as well as an atmosphere that is safe, simple, and unconfusing.

Teaching another

Nurses can assist patients by teaching them skills and knowledge. For learning to take place, the patient needs to be ready to learn and want to learn.

Appropriate activities need to be arranged for effective learning. For example, for a pregnant woman to learn prenatal exercises, she usually needs an opportunity to carry out the exercises while the nurse is present to assist her.

Accountability

Accountability means being answerable. Nurses have to be answerable for all their professional activities. They must be able to explain their professional actions and accept responsibility for them. Three questions naturally arise.

First, to whom is the nurse accountable? As a health care professional, the nurse is accountable to the patient; as an employee, the nurse is accountable to the employer; as a professional, the nurse is accountable to the professional association; and, as a member of the health team, the nurse is accountable to the patient's physician. Often, if nurses can determine to whom they are responsible, they can decide which direction to follow. For example, a nurse provides medications to a patient, the medications were ordered by a physician, the nurse lists them for the billing office of the hospital, and the nurse supports the patient in taking the medications and responds to his or her concerns regarding the illness. In these actions the nurse is accountable to the patient, to the physician, to the hospital, and to the patient, respectively. The nurse's chief accountability is to the patient.

Second, for what are nurses accountable? Nurses are accountable for all their professional nursing activities. Some of these are readily measured or observed; others remain elusive.

Third, by what criteria is accountability measured? The nurse's actions are evaluated against standards that are objective, realistic, and desirable. One measure might be the charting done by the nurse; another could be the plan of nursing interventions.

Two of the ways in which nursing practice is monitored are: comparing practice to a predetermined standard (nursing audit) and evaluation of nursing practice by peers (peer review). See Chapter 7 for further information.

Responsibility

Responsibility means reliability and trustworthiness. This attribute indicates that the professional nurse carries out required nursing activities conscientiously and that the nurse's actions are honestly reported.

When the patient becomes aware that the nurse is a responsible person with appropriate knowledge and skills, a sense of trust develops in the patient, relieving the anxiety that occurs when patients are unsure about the nurse's integrity and competence.

There are several ways in which the nurse can communicate this quality of responsibility:

1. By conveying a sincere interest in the patient.
2. By always following through with activities. If the nurse is delayed in doing something the patient expects, the nurse needs to provide an explanation about the delay.
3. By addressing the patient in a manner that conveys respect.
4. By talking with the patient about subjects the patient desires, rather than the nurse's own interests.
5. By not discussing other patients in a derogatory manner or conveying confidential information about them.
6. By accepting criticism from the patient and trying to see the patient's point of view.

Socialization into the Nursing Role

Socialization is a process by which individuals learn the knowledge, skills, and dispositions of a given group or society. Socialization into nursing is a complex process, because the role of the nurse is a complex one (see the section on roles of the nurse earlier in this chapter) and continues to undergo change (see the section on trends earlier). It is recognized that nurses must be able to assess, diagnose, plan, implement, and evaluate nursing care. To provide nursing in a changing health care delivery system, P. J. Estok (1977:11) notes that nurses must:

1. Utilize knowledge from the humanities and the physical, behavioral, and nursing sciences when making nursing practice decisions.
2. Have the psychomotor skills necessary to carry out nursing functions.
3. Accept an obligation to become involved with the changes required to improve the health care delivery system.
4. Make independent decisions and be accountable for their actions.
5. Be able to collaborate, coordinate, and consult effectively with clients and others in the health care delivery system.
6. Value learning and recognize the need for lifelong learning.

Socialization to the role of the nurse is, to a great extent, guided by the educational institution at which a nurse is trained. The ANA Code of Ethics (see Table 3–10 on page 88) also provides descriptions to guide nurses in the practice of nursing. The three areas of learning (knowledge, skills, and dispositions) described in the definition of socialization serve as a basis for considering nursing education:

1. Knowledge is the cognitive base of nursing practice, derived from the humanities and the physical, behavioral, and nursing sciences.
2. Psychomotor skills are the techniques of implementing nursing practice, e.g., administering an enema, changing a dressing, or maintaining the sterility of supplies.
3. Dispositions constitute a large area that includes attributes of professional commitment and values (such as accountability, responsibility, and caring). Values are discussed further in Chapter 3. Accountability and responsibility were discussed earlier in this chapter.

Education for Nurses

The nurse's function today is so complex that a nursing student requires knowledge in the biologic, physical, and social sciences. It is no longer possible for a nurse to acquire a safe level of skill through empirical means alone. Specific knowledge and skills are required that can be gained only through an organized nursing curriculum.

The traditional orientation of nursing education has been toward learning the skills required in hospitals. However, considerable evidence exists that the need for community and home services is increasing and that some negative aspects of hospitalization, such as separation from a family, should be avoided in many situations. As a result, nursing curricula are now focused more broadly on health as well as illness needs, and community as well as hospital needs, in addition to appropriate knowledge from the biologic, social, and physical sciences.

State laws in the United States and provincial laws in Canada recognize two types of nurses: the licensed practical (vocational) nurse (LPN or LVN) and the registered nurse (RN).

Registered Nursing Education

Basic education for registered nurses is provided in three types of programs: baccalaureate, associate degree, and diploma in the United States; and baccalaureate, two-year diploma, and three-year (or more) diploma in Canada.

Baccalaureate degree

Although baccalaureate nursing education programs were established in universities in both the United States and Canada in the early 1900s, it was not until the 1960s that the number of students enrolled in these programs increased markedly. In 1965, the ANA "position paper" on nursing education presented the position: "Education for those who work in nursing should take place within the general education system" (ANA 1965:107). This paper provided considerable impetus to move nursing education out of hospitals and into the general education system. It was followed by a study conducted by the National Commission for the Study of Nursing and Nursing Education. The commission's first report in 1970 reinforced the ANA recommendation. In the years since 1965, a number of diploma nursing schools have closed, while the number of baccalaureate programs has increased. By 1977–78, 31.1% of all nursing graduates were from baccalaureate programs, in contrast to 19.9% in 1968–69 (ANA 1981:133). A similar but less striking movement took place in Canada: In 1976, 9.5% of all nursing graduates (10,041) were from baccalaureate programs, compared to 3.8% in 1968. See Figure 1–2.

Most baccalaureate programs also admit registered nurses who have diplomas or associate degrees. Some programs have special curricula to meet the needs of these students, often in two-year programs. Some universities also offer nursing students the opportunity to pursue a self-paced or independent study program. Many accept transfer credits from other accredited colleges and universities and the opportunity to take challenge examinations when the student believes she or he already has the knowledge or skills taught in a course.

Another impetus toward baccalaureate education for all nurses was a resolution of the ANA, passed in 1978, stating that the minimum educational preparation for entry into professional nursing practice by 1985 should be a baccalaureate degree. However, the 1978 delegates also endorsed a resolution that diploma and associate degree graduates who are licensed to practice before 1985 will not be affected. Although most nurses recognize the move toward a baccalaureate degree as entry into professional nursing practice, the issue of licensure has yet to be resolved by individual state legislation.

In 1978, the Council of Baccalaureate and Higher Degree Programs approved the following statement* about baccalaureate education, identifying 11 characteristics descriptive of the graduate's abilities:

> The baccalaureate program in nursing, which is offered by a senior college or university, provides students with an opportunity to acquire: (1) knowledge of the theory[1] and practice in nursing; (2) competency in selecting, synthesizing, and applying relevant information from various disciplines; (3) ability to assess client needs and provide nursing interventions; (4) ability to provide care for groups of clients; (5) ability to work with and through others; (6) ability to evaluate current practices and try new approaches; (7) competency in collaborating with members of other health disciplines and with consumers; (8) an understanding of the research process and its contribution to nursing practice; (9) knowledge of the broad function the nursing profession is expected to perform in society; and (10) a foundation for graduate study in nursing.
>
> Nurses are prepared as generalists at the baccalaureate level to provide within the health care system[2] a comprehensive service of assessing, promoting, and maintaining the health of individuals and groups. These nurses are prepared to: (1) be accountable for their own nursing practice; (2) accept responsibility for the provision of nursing care through others; (3) accept the advocacy role in relation to clients; and (4) develop methods of working collaboratively with other health professionals. They will practice in a variety of health care settings—hospital, home, and community—and emphasize comprehensive health care, including prevention, health promotion, and rehabilitation services; health counseling and education; and care in acute and long-term illness.
>
> Baccalaureate nursing programs are conceptually organized to be consistent with the stated philosophy and objectives of the parent institution and the unit in nursing. These programs provide the general and professional education essential for understanding and respecting people, various cultures, and environments; for acquiring and utilizing nursing theory upon which nursing practice is based; and for promoting self-understanding, personal fulfillment, and motivation for continued learning. The structure of the baccalaureate degree program in nursing follows the same pattern as that of baccalaureate education in general. It is characterized by a liberal education at the lower division level, on which is built the upper division major. In baccalaureate nursing education, the lower division consists of foundational courses drawn primarily from the scientific and humanistic disciplines inherent in liberal learning. The major in nursing is built upon this lower division general

[1]Throughout this statement, theory is used in the universal sense as it applies to all disciplines.

[2]The health care system includes social, cultural, economic, and political components. It can be conceptualized from an individual perspective of nurse and client/family to the broad, national health care scene. For the most part, the graduates of baccalaureate programs in nursing work within the local health care system although fully aware of the regional and national health care scenes. The master's graduates in nursing are proficient in working within the local health care system and have learned to extend their influence and effectiveness to and through the regional and national levels.

*National League for Nursing, *Characteristics of Baccalaureate Education in Nursing* (New York: The League, 1979), pp. 1–3. Used with permission.

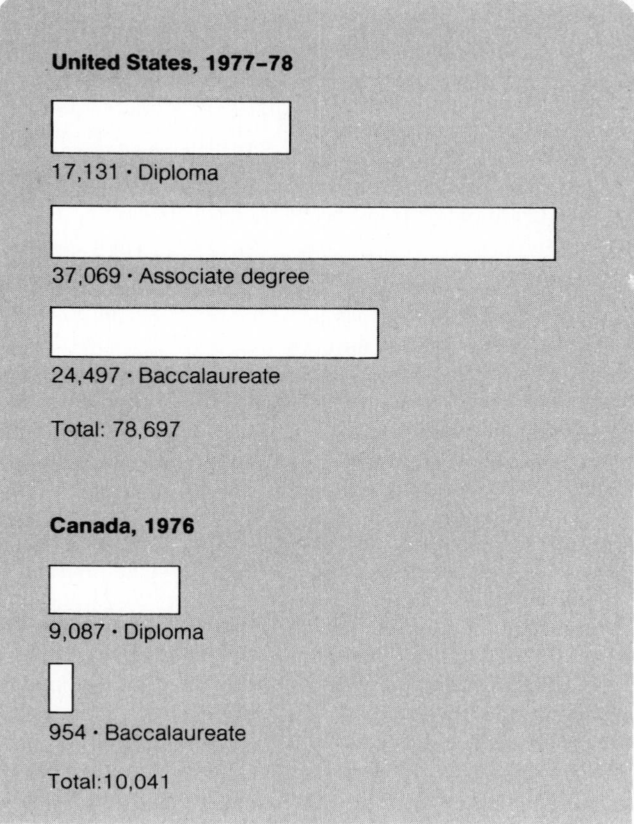

Figure 1–2 The number of graduates from nursing education programs in the United States and Canada. (From American Nurses' Association, *Facts about nursing 80–81* [New York: American Journal of Nursing Co., 1981], p. 133; and Statistics Canada, *Nursing in Canada* [Ottawa: Statistics Canada, 1980], p. 70.)

education base and is concentrated at the upper division level. Upper division studies include courses that complement the nursing component or increase the depth of general education.

Consistent with the foregoing characteristics and directly related to the Criteria for the Appraisal of Baccalaureate and Higher Degree Programs in Nursing, the graduate of the baccalaureate program in nursing is able to:

- Utilize nursing theory in making decisions on nursing practice.
- Use nursing practice as a means of gathering data for refining and extending that practice.
- Synthesize theoretical and empirical knowledge from the physical and behavioral sciences and humanities with nursing theory and practice.
- Assess health status and health potential; plan, implement, and evaluate nursing care of individuals, families, and communities.
- Improve service to the client by continually evaluating the effectiveness of nursing intervention and revising it accordingly.
- Accept individual responsibility and accountability for the choice of nursing intervention and its outcome.
- Evaluate research for the applicability of its findings to nursing actions.
- Utilize leadership skills through involvement with others in meeting health needs and nursing goals.
- Collaborate with colleagues and citizens on the interdisciplinary health team to promote the health and welfare of people.
- Participate in identifying and effecting needed change to improve delivery within specific health care systems.
- Participate in identifying community and societal health needs and in designing nursing roles to meet these needs.

These characteristics were developed by the professional nurse membership of the Council of Baccalaureate and Higher Degree Programs and are an expression of professional accountability to the consumer, both student and client.

Associate degree

Associate degree programs in nursing were blueprinted by Mildred L. Montag (1980) in 1951. It was proposed that a "nursing technician" be prepared whose education would be less extensive than that of the professional nurse. Montag intended that the technical nurse would carry out nursing responsibilities under the supervision of a professional nurse and that she or he would not carry out administrative responsibilities. The program of studies was designed to be terminal; that is, it was not considered the first two years of a baccalaureate program.

Associate degree programs are offered in the United States in junior and senior colleges and universities. Upon graduation from the program, the graduate receives an associate degree (AD) in nursing. In Canada, associate degrees are not offered, but similar educational programs confer a diploma upon graduation.

The number of graduates from associate degree programs in the United States has steadily increased. In 1977–78, 37,069 students graduated from these programs, accounting for 47.1% of graduates in nursing. This is a marked increase from 20.6% in 1968–69 (ANA 1981:133). In Canada, the first diploma nursing program was established within the general education system at the Ryerson Institute of Technology in Toronto in 1964. By 1973, 9001 students were in similar nursing programs across Canada (LaSor and Elliott 1977:161).

In 1977 and 1978, the Council of Associate Degree Programs, National League for Nursing, developed and approved the following statement* of competencies for graduates of associate degree programs in nursing:

Assumptions Basic to the Scope of Practice

The practice of graduates of associate degree nursing programs:

- Is directed toward clients who need information or support to maintain health.
- Is directed toward clients who are in need of medical diagnostic evaluation and/or are experiencing acute or chronic illness.
- Is directed toward clients' responses to common, well-defined health problems.
- Includes the formulation of a nursing diagnosis.
- Consists of nursing interventions selected from established nursing protocols where probable outcomes are predictable.
- Is concerned with individual clients and is given with consideration of the person's relationship within a family, group, and community.
- Includes the safe performance of nursing skills that require cognitive, psychomotor, and affective capabilities.
- May be in any structured care setting but primarily occurs within acute- and extended-care facilities.
- Is guided directly or indirectly by a more experienced registered nurse.
- Includes the direction of peers or other workers in nursing in selected aspects of care within the scope of practice of associate degree nursing.
- Involves an understanding of the roles and responsibilities of self and other workers within the employment setting.

Roles of Practice

Five interrelated roles have been defined for graduates of the associate degree nursing program based upon the above assumptions underlying the scope of practice. These roles are: provider of care, client teacher, communicator, manager of client care, and member within the profession of

*National League for Nursing, *Competencies of the Associate Degree Nurse on Entry into Practice* (New York: The League, 1978), pp. 3–11. Used with permission.

nursing. In each of these roles, decisions and practice are determined on the basis of knowledge and skills, the nursing process, and established protocols of the setting.

Role as a Provider of Care As a provider of nursing care, the associate degree nursing graduate uses the nursing process to formulate and maintain individualized nursing care plans by:

Assessing

- Collects and contributes to a data base (physiological, emotional, sociological, cultural, psychological, and spiritual needs) from available resources (e.g., client, family, medical records, and other health team members).
- Identifies and documents changes in health status which interfere with the client's ability to meet basic needs (e.g., oxygen, nutrition, elimination, activity, safety, rest and sleep, and psychosocial well-being).
- Establishes a nursing diagnosis based on client needs.

Planning

- Develops individualized nursing care plans based upon the nursing diagnosis and plans intervention that follows established nursing protocols.
- Identifies needs and establishes priorities for care with recognition of client's level of development and needs, and with consideration of client's relationship with a family, group, and community.
- Participates with clients, families, significant others, and members of the nursing team to establish long- and short-range client goals.
- Identifies criteria for evaluation of individualized nursing care plans.

Implementing

- Carries out individualized plans of care according to priority of needs and established nursing protocols.
- Participates in the prescribed medical regime by preparing, assisting, and providing follow-up care to clients undergoing diagnostic and/or therapeutic procedures.
- Uses nursing knowledge and skills and protocols to assure an environment conducive to optimum restoration and maintenance of the client's normal abilities to meet basic needs.
  —Maintains and promotes respiratory function (e.g., oxygen therapy, positioning, etc.).
  —Maintains and promotes nutritional status (e.g., dietary regimes, supplemental therapy, intravenous infusions, etc.).
  —Maintains and promotes elimination (e.g., bowel and bladder regimes, forcing fluids, enemas, etc.).
  —Maintains and promotes a balance of activity, rest, and sleep (e.g., planned activities of daily living, environmental adjustment, exercises, sensory stimuli, assistive devices, etc.).
  —Maintains an environment which supports physiological functioning, comfort, and relief of pain.
  —Maintains and promotes all aspects of hygiene.
  —Maintains and promotes physical safety (e.g., implementation of medical and surgical aseptic techniques, etc.).
  —Maintains and promotes psychological safety through consideration of each individual's worth and dignity and applies nursing measures which assist in reducing common developmental and situational stress.
  —Measures basic physiological functioning and reports significant findings (e.g., vital signs, fluid intake and output).
  —Administers prescribed medications safely.
- Intervenes in situations where:
  —Basic life support systems are threatened (e.g., cardiopulmonary resuscitation, obstructive airway maneuver).
  —Untoward physiological or psychological reactions are probable.
  —Changes in normal behavior patterns have occurred.
- Participates in established institutional emergency plans.

Evaluating

- Uses established criteria for evaluation of individualized nursing care.
- Participates with clients, families, significant others, and members of the nursing team in the evaluation of established long- and short-range client goals.
- Identifies alternate methods of meeting client's needs, modifies plans of care as necessary, and documents changes.

Role as a Communicator As a communicator, the associate degree nursing graduate:

- Assesses verbal and non-verbal communication of clients, families, and significant others based upon knowledge and techniques of interpersonal communication.
- Uses lines of authority and communication within the work setting.
- Uses communication skills as a method of data collection, nursing intervention, and evaluation of care.
- Communicates and records assessments, nursing care plans, interventions, and evaluations accurately and promptly.
- Establishes and maintains effective communication with clients, families, significant others, and health team members.
- Communicates client's needs through the appropriate use of referrals.
- Evaluates effectiveness of one's own communication with clients, colleagues, and others.

Role as a Client Teacher As a teacher of clients who need information or support to maintain health, the associate degree nursing graduate:

- Assesses situations in which clients need information or support to maintain health.
- Develops short-range teaching plans based upon long- and short-range goals for individual clients.
- Implements teaching plans that are specific to the client's level of development and knowledge.
- Supports and reinforces the teaching plans of other health professionals.
- Evaluates the effectiveness of client's learning.

Role as a Manager of Client Care As a manager of nursing care for a group of clients with common, well-defined health problems in structured settings, the associate degree nursing graduate:

- Assesses and sets nursing care priorities.
- With guidance, provides client care utilizing resources and other nursing personnel commensurate with their educational preparation and experience.
- Seeks guidance to assist other nursing personnel to develop skills in giving nursing care.

Role as a Member within the Profession of Nursing As a member within the profession of nursing, the associate degree nursing graduate:

- Is accountable for his or her nursing practice.
- Practices within the profession's ethical and legal framework.
- Assumes responsibility for self-development and uses resources for continued learning.
- Consults with a more experienced registered nurse when client's problems are not within the scope of practice.
- Participates within a structured role in research (e.g., data collection).
- Works within the policies of the employer or employing institution.
- Recognizes policies and nursing protocols that may impede client care and works within the organizational framework to initiate change.

Diploma

Nursing education originated in hospital-based programs. First developed by Florence Nightingale (circa 1860), these programs were operated by hospitals as training schools for nurses. Today diploma nursing programs continue to be hospital-based, may be two or three years in length, and often are associated with colleges or universities. A significant number of nurses practicing today are graduates of diploma programs. The impetus to close diploma nursing programs came from the ANA resolution discussed on page 26. In addition, hospitals found that the costs of operating educational programs were increasing, making them less viable financially. In 1969, there were 695 diploma nursing programs in the United States, while by 1981 there were only 311 (ANA 1981:152). Graduates of diploma nursing programs accounted for 18.9% of the total number of graduates in 1978–1979 (ibid., p. 133). Canada has moved rapidly from hospital-based programs to those based in educational institutions. Of the 172 diploma nursing programs in 1964, all but one (admitting 21 students) were hospital based, whereas in 1973, 78.5% of nursing students were in programs within the general educational system.

In 1978 the National League for Nursing approved the following statement* describing the roles and competencies of graduates of diploma nursing programs:

> The graduate of the diploma program in nursing is eligible to seek licensure as a registered nurse and to function as a beginning practitioner in acute, intermediate, long-term, and ambulatory health care facilities. In order to fulfill such roles, graduates should demonstrate the following competencies.[1]
>
> Assessment
> - Establishes a data base through a nursing history including a psychosocial and physical assessment.
> - Utilizes knowledge of the etiology, pathophysiology, usual course, and prognosis for the prevalent illnesses and health problems.
> - Establishes priorities when providing nursing care for one or more patients.
> - Recognizes the significance of non-verbal communication.
>
> Planning
> - Formulates a written plan of nursing care based on the assessment of patient needs.
> - Includes in the nursing care plan the effects of the family or significant others, life experiences, and social-cultural background.
> - Involves the patient, family, and significant others in the development of the nursing plan of care.
> - Incorporates the learning needs of the patient and family into an individualized plan of care.
> - Applies principles of organization and management in utilizing the knowledge and skills of other nursing personnel.
>
> Implementation
> - Meets the health needs of individuals and families.
> - Utilizes concepts, scientific facts, and principles when providing nursing care.
> - Performs technical nursing procedures.
> - Initiates appropriate intervention when environmental and safety hazards exist.
> - Initiates preventive, habilitative, and rehabilitative nursing measures according to the needs demonstrated by patients and families.
> - Performs independent nursing measures and/or seeks assistance from other members of the health team in response to the changing needs of patients.
> - Collaborates with physicians and members of other disciplines to provide health care.
> - Documents nursing interventions and patient responses.
> - Utilizes effective verbal and written communication.
>
> [1]Competency, as used in this document, is the ability to apply in practice situations the essential principles and techniques of nursing and to apply those concepts, skills, and attitudes required of all nurses to fulfill their role, regardless of specific position or responsibility.

*National League for Nursing, *Roles and Competencies of Graduates of Diploma Programs in Nursing* (New York: The League, 1978). Used with permission.

- Communicates pertinent information related to the patient through established channels.
- Assists the physician in implementing the medical plan of care.
- Applies knowledge of individual and group behavior in establishing interpersonal relationships.
- Teaches individuals and groups to achieve and maintain an optimum level of wellness.
- Utilizes the services of community agencies for continuity of patient care.
- Protects the rights of patients and families.

Evaluation
- Evaluates the effectiveness of nursing care and takes appropriate action.
- Initiates and cooperates in efforts to improve nursing practice.

Professionalism
- Recognizes the legal limits of nursing practice.
- Demonstrates ethical behavior in the performance of nursing.
- Practices nursing in a nondiscriminatory and nonjudgmental manner.
- Respects the rights of others to have their own value systems.
- Accepts responsibility and accountability for professional practice.
- Demonstrates flexibility in functioning in a changing society.
- Adjusts with minimal difficulty to the role of employee.

This revised statement by the Council of Diploma Programs in Nursing, National League for Nursing, was approved at the Council's April 1978 meeting.

Licensed Practical Nursing Education

Approved practical nursing programs are provided by community colleges, vocational schools, hospitals, and a variety of health agencies. These courses are usually a year in length and provide both classroom and clinical experiences. At the end of the program the graduate takes examinations to obtain a license as a practical nurse. In some states and provinces, applicants for licensure are assessed on the basis of their nursing experience rather than their formal education in an approved school. Licensed practical nurses are employed in hospitals and in community services such as home nursing. Their skills are basically those required for bedside nursing under the guidance of a registered nurse, who has the knowledge and skills to make more accurate nursing judgments.

Education for Expanded Nursing Roles

Expanded roles of nurses such as the nurse clinician and nurse practitioner are briefly discussed earlier in this chapter. Over 100 courses are available at American universities to prepare nurses for the independent nurse practitioner role. These courses provide preparation in primary care skills (e.g., history taking), physical examination, ordering laboratory tests, and assuming responsibility for management of selected patients with emphasis on primary care. Programs differ in length but all require that students be registered nurses. Certificate programs are about 5 months in length; master's programs are about 15 months (Levine 1977:1800).

Courses to prepare the nurse clinician are offered in many universities at the master's and doctoral levels. In these programs, nurses obtain skills and knowledge in a selected nursing area. There are also courses to enable the nurse to become a clinical specialist (Oda 1977:374).

Issues in Nursing Education

Technical and professional nurse

The 1965 resolution of the ANA discussed on page 26 delineated two kinds of nursing practice: technical and professional. The technical nurse is a graduate of an associate degree program, while the professional nurse has a baccalaureate degree. There is still considerable discussion about differentiating the two groups functionally. At present, both technical and professional nurses according to the above description are licensed as registered nurses.

Ladder programs in nursing

The ladder concept fosters progression of an individual from one educational level to another. The nurse who wishes to progress "up the ladder" can often obtain credit for experience and/or courses at an earlier level. Although associate degree programs were originally designed to be terminal programs, some universities now give academic credit toward a baccalaureate degree for these years.

Some universities, such as Villanova, permit students to transfer or take challenge examinations for up to 50% of all credits in the baccalaureate program (Nayer 1981:2057). Others admit nurses as prenursing students. Often emphasis is placed on independent learning and self-pacing for the baccalaureate nursing student.

An increasing number of master's and doctoral programs are being offered to students in nursing. Some master's courses prepare nurses in specialty areas, such as gerontologic nursing, care of the premature newborn, or adolescent psychiatric nursing, as well as in general nursing practice. Doctoral education can be obtained in areas such as nursing research, administration, nursing practice, and theory development.

Continuing education

Continuing education programs are conducted by a variety of educational institutions and health agencies. They are usually designed to meet one or more of the following purposes:

1. To keep nurses abreast of new techniques and knowledge
2. To assist nurses to attain expertise in a specialized area, such as intensive care nursing
3. To provide nurses with information essential to nursing practice, for example, knowledge about the legal aspects of nursing

Some state laws now require a nurse to obtain a certain number of continuing education credits in order to renew her or his license. Increasing numbers of continuing education courses are being offered.

Nursing Organizations

Nursing (and other health) organizations bring together health practitioners with the intention of improving the health and nursing services of people within their jurisdictions. Nursing organizations are established at the international, national, and local levels.

International Council of Nurses (ICN)

Illness and trauma do not stop at the boundaries of countries. Although different areas of the world and different countries have their own health problems, it is often in their mutual interest to cooperate in health and nursing matters. Because of the ease with which people can now travel around the world, problems in India, for example, can quickly become problems in North America. People traveling abroad frequently return home only to be stricken by an illness rarely seen in their own country. As the world grows closer through technologic advances, and people travel more, nurses must become increasingly concerned and involved with health matters of people all over the world. In 1973 the International Council of Nurses (ICN) stated in its Code for Nurses:

> The need for nursing is universal. Inherent in nursing is respect for life, dignity and rights of man. It is unrestricted by considerations of nationality, race, creed, color, age, sex, politics or social status.

The ICN was established in 1899. Nurses from both the United States and Canada were among the founding members. The council is a federation of national nurses' associations such as the American Nurses' Association and the Canadian Nurses' Association. In 1981, 95 national associations from different countries were affiliated with the ICN.

The purpose of the ICN is to provide a medium through which national nursing associations can work together and share common interests. By membership in the national association, a nurse is automatically a member of the ICN. The functions of the ICN are:

1. To promote the organization of national nurses' associations and advise them in their continued development.
2. To assist national nurses' associations to play their part in developing and improving (a) health service for the public, (b) the practice of nursing, and (c) the social and economic welfare of nurses.
3. To provide means of communication among nurses throughout the world for mutual understanding and cooperation.
4. To establish and maintain liaison and cooperation with other international organizations and to serve as representatives and spokespeople of nurses at the international level.
5. To receive and manage funds and trusts that contribute to the advancement of nursing or for the benefit of nurses.
6. To do any other things incidental or conclusive to the attainment of the objective of the ICN (ICN 1973b).

World Health Organization (WHO)

WHO is one of the special agencies of the United Nations. It is an intergovernmental agency, formed in 1948, whose primary aim is to bring all people in the world to the highest possible level of health. As of 1974, 143 countries were members of WHO. Its major activities are to provide assistance to countries in terms of improving health standards, education, and training, fighting disease, combatting water pollution, etc.

Nursing makes an essential contribution to the activities of WHO. American and Canadian nurses are frequently asked to go to countries that require assistance in nursing education and public health. About 300 nurses are at present working for WHO in countries other than their own.

American Nurses' Association (ANA)

The ANA is the national professional organization for nursing in the United States. It was founded in 1896 and was a charter member of the ICN along with Great Britain and Germany in 1899. The membership is open only to registered nurses. The purposes of the ANA are to foster high standards of nursing practice and to promote the educational and professional advancement of nurses so that all people may have better nursing care. The ANA is composed of the nurses' associations from the 50 states, Guam, the Virgin Islands, Puerto Rico, and the District of Columbia. These state associations are in turn divided into regional and local chapters.

In 1966 the ANA made provision for an Academy of Nursing, to recognize individuals for professional achievement and excellence in nursing. That year 36 charter members were named to the academy. In 1974 the political arm of the ANA, N-CAP (Nurses' Coalition for Action in Politics), was officially organized to work for the legislative objectives of the ANA.

Two significant actions of the ANA in recent years were its 1965 position paper on nursing education in the general educational system and its position on the educational preparation necessary for professional nursing (see the section on education for nurses earlier in this chapter). The ANA has also developed nursing standards for specific areas of nursing practice.

National League for Nursing (NLN)

The National League for Nursing, formed in 1952, is an organization of both individuals and agencies. Its objective is to foster the development and improvement of all nursing services and nursing education. People who are not nurses but have an interest in nursing services, for example, hospital administrators, can be members of the league.

The league has a broad range of activities, including provision of educational services such as workshops and recruitment assistance for nursing programs. It also conducts the state board examinations for licensure for registered nurses and licensed practical nurses.

One of the league's major functions is to accredit nursing programs, thus improving the standards of nursing education. Accreditation by the NLN is voluntary. As of January 1, 1979, 69.7% of all nursing programs in the United States were NLN accredited (ANA 1981:151).

Canadian Nurses' Association (CNA)

The CNA is the national nursing association in Canada. Its membership numbers 104,000 of the 170,000 registered nurses in Canada. The CNA has provincial organizations, which in turn have local chapters.

A significant function of the CNA is administration of the National Testing Service, which prepares examinations for graduate nurses seeking registration. These examinations are available to all provinces and territories and provide a nationwide standard for admission to practice nursing. The CNA has also been active in moving nursing education into the general education system and in establishing quality control through licensing and registering.

Nursing Student Organizations

In the United States the National Student Nurses' Association (NSNA) is the official preprofessional organization for students of nursing. It functions under the aegis of the ANA and NLN; however, it is autonomous in that it is financed and run by nursing students.

The purpose of NSNA is "to aid in the development of the individual student and to urge all students of nursing, as future health professionals, to be aware of, and contribute to, improving the health care of all people" (NSNA 1972:3).

The NSNA speaks for students of nursing when necessary and undertakes activities such as the recruitment of minority groups into nursing and participation in programs related to student suicide and the use of drugs on campus. Members of NSNA also attend ANA and ICN meetings to discuss issues with nursing students from other states and countries.

In Canada, nursing students have a similar organization, the Canadian Student Nurses' Association (CSNA), and the students attend provincial, national, and international meetings. The provincial student nurses' associations also have programs related to the needs of nursing students and concerns within the health field in general.

Other Organizations

Most nursing schools have alumni associations to which graduates can belong. These associations generally have programs of particular concern to the graduates and often have fundraising activities to support nursing students.

Sigma Theta Tau is the national honor society of nursing. It has chapters on many university campuses. Its purposes include recognizing achievement in scholarship in nursing studies.

Other organizations, such as the Red Cross, the National Black Nurses' Association, the Association of Operating Room Nurses, and the American Association of Nurse Anesthetists, serve particular segments of the nursing community. For the nurse who qualifies for membership, these organizations offer services and programs.

Nursing in Transition

We live in a world of cultural borrowing. Our ideas, philosophies, and technologies are blends of concepts from all over the globe. Professions have had to evolve with the developing world and recognize that everything is part of one vast earth—which is only one part of an even greater universe.

Humanity is a part of nature, and the practice of nursing is a part of humanity. As Florence Nightingale asked many times, "Can there be any greater work than this?" Indeed, were she alive today, she might add, "Can there be any greater time to do this work?" Nursing has come a long way. No longer disreputable, no longer a position of servitude, nursing is now an important career choice for many men and women who are vitally interested in preserving health. Its genuine emphasis on such goals as wellness, prevention, and humanism addresses the needs and rights of all persons.

It is the purpose of this book to present concepts important for nurses, basic physiology, and fundamental nursing skills, and to offer a means to integrate these three types of knowledge. The book will discuss legal problems, rights of patients, and rights of nurses as well as culture, values, and basic human needs. The differences that occur in people at various ages and various stages of development will be discussed in both physiologic and psychologic terms. Nursing techniques will be presented in the text and will also be summarized in Procedures. No one technique or idea makes a nurse. This book analyzes and synthesizes these concepts, integrating one with another to give a framework for a holistic, humanistic professional—today's nurse.

As science and civilization continue to develop, the role of the nurse will change. An even greater emphasis will be placed on disease prevention and health maintenance. Some branches of nursing will achieve greater autonomy and will provide more direct services in patient care. At all times and whatever complex changes occur, however, the most important aspect of nursing will be very simple: people.

Summary

The nurse in today's world faces the challenge of blending technology with humanity. As a constantly evolving profession, nursing has combined some of the reform concepts of Florence Nightingale with scientific advances of the past few decades. Therefore, a definition of nursing requires input from many sources on many levels. Contemporary definitions describe the nurturing (caring) function of the nurse as well as the helping functions, which require knowledge and skills on the part of the nurse. The goal of nursing is to assist individuals who are healthy or ill to achieve their optimal levels of functioning. Nursing is a service that involves direct contact, considers the individual differences of people, and serves individuals, families, and communities.

Many interrelated elements comprise the practice of nursing. The nurse integrates concepts with skills, to nurse patients as complete human beings. The nurse practices on four different levels: promotion of health, prevention of disease or injury, restoration of health, and consolation of the dying.

Conceptual models in nursing have been and are being developed to clarify the unique functions of the nurse. They have three components: assumptions, values, and major units. The major units of an effective nursing model include the goals of nursing, the client, the role of the nurse, the source of difficulty of the client, and the intervention focus, modes, and consequences.

Nursing practice involves the five steps of the nursing process: collecting data (assessment), interpreting data (diagnosis), and planning, implementing, and evaluating interventions. Within this context, the nurse assesses patients' needs, administers medications and therapies, and teaches patients self-care. Some of these activities are dependent functions; others are independent functions. The nurse also coordinates the care given by other health professionals, plans for continuity of care, evaluates care, and directs others in giving nursing care.

Four broad settings for nursing practice are hospitals, community agencies, local clinics, and physicians' offices. The degree of autonomy of the nurse, the nursing activities performed, and the relationships the nurse has with other health workers vary within these settings. The nurse may function more independently and may require more judgment skills in some settings than in others. New practice settings are becoming available to the nursing professional, including private practice and nursing research.

Vast changes have taken place in nursing in the past 50 years. Many factors have influenced these changes. The consumer of nursing services is increasingly active in exerting pressure for health care rather than disease cure. Changes from large extended families to small nuclear families or single-parent families have increased the need for homemaker and day-care services. Decreases in morbidity and mortality, changes in government legislation, and advances in technology all affect needs for nursing services.

Future trends in nursing practice are predictable to some degree by current social and economic forces. Nurses need to have increasing knowledge that is scientifically based and that deals with preventive health care. New roles are emerging and old roles changing to meet the demands for service and to maintain a high standard of care. Some of these are the expanded role of nurses in primary care, the new role of the nurse clinician, and the new role of the independent nurse practitioner.

Nine main roles of the nurse are: healing, caring, communicating, teaching, planning, coordinating, protecting, rehabilitating, and socializing. In the former two roles particularly, the nurse needs to select specific methods of helping patients and families. If the patient is dependent, the nurse must act for or do for the patient. For those who are less dependent but lacking in judgment, knowledge, or energy, the nurse needs to guide or support the patient. Provision of a developmental environment is also essential to the safety, growth, and security needs of patients. Finally, teaching is necessary to help patients acquire the knowledge to achieve or maintain their health. It is the nurse's responsibility to be sensitive and attuned to the method of helping that is warranted in a given situation.

Nurses need knowledge in the biologic, physical, and social sciences. Well-planned curricula in nursing education must include these as well as consider the future health and illness needs of consumers. At present, two types of licensed nurses are recognized in the state and provincial laws of the United States and Canada: the LPN and the RN. Nurses need to participate actively in continuing education programs and in their professional nursing associations to keep abreast of changes and to ensure provision of the best standards of nursing care to people.

In the years to come, nursing will continue to evolve. The modern nurse will continue to integrate concepts with skills, concentrating on humanistic care for the whole person.

Suggested Activities

1. In a clinical setting, observe the activities of a licensed practical nurse, an orderly, and a registered nurse. List the functions you observed. In a group discussion, compare these observations with those of other students, and prepare a composite list for each role.

2. In an appropriate clinical setting, observe a head nurse, a community nurse, and a clinical nurse specialist. List the functions you observed, and discuss these functions as they relate to the five components of nursing practice discussed in this chapter.

Suggested Readings

Greiner, P. A. December 1981. What has become of the traditional nurse? *Nursing Outlook* 29:720–21.

This article briefly describes the changes that have taken place since the "traditional nurse" ceased to be a reality. The author explains how the contemporary nurse's function differs from the image many people have of nursing.

Kellams, S. E. June 1977. Ideals of a profession: The case of nursing. *Image* 9:30–31.

The author discusses the goals toward which professions strive and relates these to the nursing profession. Two key professional goals are: (a) to develop and disseminate knowledge unique to the profession of nursing, and (b) to provide services in the interest of the public.

Smith, D. W. 1970. Change: How shall we respond to it? *Nursing Forum* 9(4):391–99.

This author discusses pressures from society, from other professional groups, and from within the nursing profession itself.

Watson, J. August 1981. Professional identity crisis—is nursing finally growing up? *American Journal of Nursing* 81:1488–90.

The author examines some of the personal and professional problems facing nursing and the internal and external forces affecting the profession. She also analyzes six existential criteria as they apply to mature professional status.

Selected References

American Nurses' Association. December 1965. American Nurses' Association first position on education for nursing. *American Journal of Nursing* 65:106–11.

———. 1973. *Standards of nursing practice.* Kansas City, Mo.: American Nurses' Association.

———. 1981. *Facts about nursing 80–81.* New York: American Journal of Nursing Co.

Anderson, N. D. June 1981. Ethel Fenwick's legacy to nursing and women. *Image* 13:32–33.

Barritt, E. R. 1973. Florence Nightingale's values and modern nursing education. *Nursing Forum* 12(1):6–47.

Bayer, M., and Brandner, P. January 1977. Nurse/patient peer practice. *American Journal of Nursing* 77:86–90.

Becktell, P. June 1981. Of women and walls. *Image* 13:34–36.

Bower, F. L., and Bevis, E. O. 1979. *Fundamentals of nursing practice: Concepts, roles, and functions.* St. Louis: C. V. Mosby Co.

Bullough, B. 1980. *The law and the expanding nursing role.* 2nd ed. New York: Appleton-Century-Crofts.

Canadian Nurses' Association. 1980. *A definition of nursing practice: Standards for nursing practice.* Ottawa: Canadian Nurses' Association.

Chamings, P. A., and Teevan, J. February 1979. Comparison of expected competencies of baccalaureate- and associate-degree graduates in nursing. *Image* 11:16–21.

Chaska, N. L. 1978. *The nursing profession: Views through the mist.* New York: McGraw-Hill Book Co.

Cohen, H. A. 1981. *The nurse's quest for a professional identity.* Menlo Park, Calif.: Addison-Wesley Publishing Co.

Estok, P. J. February 1977. Socialization theory and entry into the practice of nursing. *Image* 9:8–14.

Fagin, C. April 1971. Accountability. *Nursing Outlook* 19: 249–51.

———. January 1982. Nursing as an alternative to high cost care. *American Journal of Nursing* 82:56–60.

Fasano, M. A. April 1976. From LVN to RN in one year. *Nursing Outlook* 24:251–53.

Fawcett, J. 1980. On research and the professionalization of nursing. *Nursing Forum* 19(3):310–18.

Flaherty, M. J. 1979. The characteristics and scope of professional nursing. *Journal for Nursing Leadership and Management* 1:61, 63, 69.

Grissum, M., and Spengler, C. 1976. *Womanpower and health care.* Boston: Little, Brown and Co.

Hale, S. L., and Boyd, B. T. September 1981. Accommodating RN students in baccalaureate nursing programs. *Nursing Outlook* 29:535–40.

Henderson, V. 1966. *The nature of nursing.* New York: Macmillan Co.

———. October 1969. Excellence in nursing. *American Journal of Nursing* 69:2133–37.

———. 1972. *ICN basic principles of nursing care.* Geneva: International Council of Nurses.

Hull, R. T. December 1981. Responsibility and accountability, analyzed. *Nursing Outlook* 29:707–12.

International Council of Nurses. 1973a. *Code for nurses.* Geneva: International Council of Nurses.

———. 1973b. *Constitution and regulations.* Geneva: International Council of Nurses.

———. May/August 1974. Definition of 'nurse' will get further study. *International Nursing Review* 21:125.

Jamieson, E. M.; Sewall, M. F.; and Suhrie, E. B. 1966. *Trends in nursing history.* 6th ed. Philadelphia: W. B. Saunders Co.

Johnson, D. 1968. One conceptual model of nursing. Paper presented at Vanderbilt University, Nashville, Tenn., April 25, 1968.

Kalisch, B. J. January 1978. The promise of power. *Nursing Outlook* 26:42–46.

King, I. M. 1971. *Toward a theory for nursing: General concepts of human behavior.* New York: John Wiley and Sons.

Kluge, E. H. February 1982. Nursing: Vocation or profession? *Canadian Nurse* 78:34–36.

Large, J. T. October 1976. Harriet Newton Phillips, the first trained nurse in America. *Image* 8:49–51.

LaSor, B., and Elliott, M. R. 1977. *Issues in Canadian nursing.* Scarborough, Ont.: Prentice-Hall of Canada.

Lenburg, C. B. July 1976. The external degree in nursing: The promise fulfilled. *Nursing Outlook* 24:422–29.

Levine, E. November 1977. What do we know about nurse practitioners? *American Journal of Nursing* 77: 1799–803.

Lewis, E. P. May 1972. Accountability: How, for what, and to whom? (Editorial.) *Nursing Outlook* 20:315.

McPhail, J. October 1971. Reasonable expectations for the nurse clinician. *Journal of Nursing Administration* 1:16–18.

Marram, G.; Barrett, M. W.; and Bevis, E. O. 1979. *Primary nursing: A model for individualized care.* 2nd ed. St. Louis: C. V. Mosby Co.

Michelmore, E. August 1977. Distinguishing between AD and BS education. *Nursing Outlook* 25:506–10.

Millis, J. S. July 1977. Primary care: Definition of, and access to . . . . *Nursing Outlook* 25:443–45.

Montag, M. L. April 1980. Looking back: Associate degree education in perspective. *Nursing Outlook* 28:248–50.

National Commission for the Study of Nursing and Nursing Education. 1974. Summary report and recommendations. In Lysaught, Jerome P. *Action in nursing: Progress in professional purpose.* New York: McGraw-Hill Book Co.

National League for Nursing. 1976. *Accountability: Accepting the challenge.* Publication no. 16-1621. New York: National League for Nursing.

National Student Nurses' Association. 1972. *Bylaws.* New York: National Student Nurses' Association.

Nayer, D. D. November 1981. BSN doors are opening for RN students. *American Journal of Nursing* 81:2056–57, 2062–64.

Nightingale, F. 1860. *Notes on nursing: What it is, and what it is not.* London: Harrison. Reprinted in Bishop, F. L. A., and Goldie, S. 1962. *A bio-bibliography of Florence Nightingale.* London: Dawsons of Pall Mall.

Notter, L. E., and Spalding, E. K. 1976. *Professional nursing: Foundations, perspectives, and relationships.* 9th ed. New York: J. B. Lippincott Co.

Oda, D. June 1977. Specialized role development: A three-phase process. *Nursing Outlook* 25:374–77.

Orem, D. E. 1971. *Nursing: Concepts of practice.* New York: McGraw-Hill Book Co.

———. 1980. *Nursing: Concepts of practice.* 2nd ed. New York: McGraw-Hill Book Co.

Palmer, I. S. June 1981. Florence Nightingale and international origins of modern nursing. *Image* 8:28–31.

Pletsch, P. K. December 1981. Mary Breckinridge: A pioneer who made her mark. *American Journal of Nursing* 81:2188–90.

Riehl, J. P., and Roy, C. 1980. *Conceptual models for nursing practice.* 2nd ed. New York: Appleton-Century-Crofts.

Roy, C. 1976. *Introduction to nursing: An adaptation model.* Englewood Cliffs, N.J.: Prentice-Hall.

Sheahan, D., Sr. January 1978. Scanning the seventies. *Nursing Outlook* 26:33–37.

Sims, E. February 1977. Preparation for independent practice. *Nursing Outlook* 25:114–18.

Smoyak, S. A. November 1976. Specialization in nursing: From then to now. *Nursing Outlook* 24:676–81.

Somers, A. R. 1971. *Health care in transition: Directions for the future.* Chicago: Hospital Research and Educational Trust.

Statistics Canada. 1980. *Nursing in Canada: Canadian nursing statistics.* Ottawa: Statistics Canada.

Stewart, I. April 1933. Post graduate education–new and old. *American Journal of Nursing* 33:363.

Stuart, G. W. February 1981. How professionalized is nursing? *Image* 13:18–23.

Styles, M. M. January 1978. Dialogue across the decades. *Nursing Outlook* 26:28–32.

———. 1982. *On nursing: Toward a new endowment.* St. Louis: C. V. Mosby Co.

Wandelt, M. 1970. *Guide for the beginning researcher.* New York: Appleton-Century-Crofts.

Whitman, M. January 1982. Toward a new psychology for nurses. *Nursing Outlook* 30:48–52.

Williams, C. A. April 1977. Community health nursing—what is it? *Nursing Outlook* 25:250–54.

Chapter 2

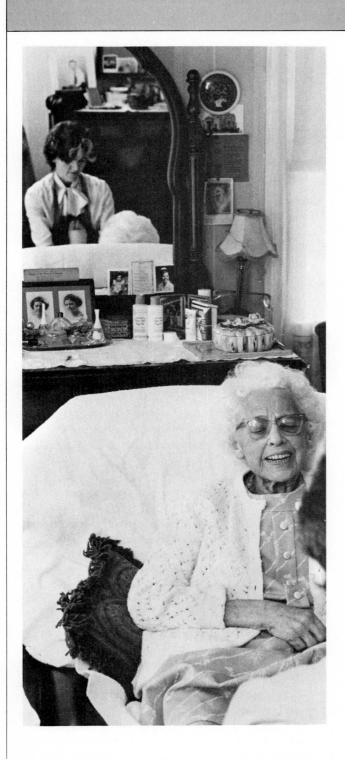

Health-Illness Continuum

CONTENTS

(Continued on next page)

Objectives

1. Understand essential facts about health, illness, the health-illness continuum, and hospitalization

- **1.1** Compare definitions of health outlined in this chapter
- **1.2** Explain Dunn's concept of the health-illness continuum
- **1.3** Identify factors influencing an individual's personal definition of health
- **1.4** Differentiate health state, health beliefs, and health practices
- **1.5** Contrast some definitions of illness and disease; identify three criteria individuals apply to judge whether they are ill
- **1.6** Identify factors affecting illness behavior
- **1.7** Identify five stages of illness and the significance of each
- **1.8** Identify effects of hospitalization on patients
- **1.9** Identify four aspects of the sick role
- **1.10** Identify common behavior changes in sick persons
- **1.11** Identify the effects of illness on family roles and functions

2. Understand current patterns and trends in health and illness

- **2.1** Identify factors responsible for the improving health of North Americans
- **2.2** Identify four major risk factors responsible for illness and mortality
- **2.3** Explain the health field concept
- **2.4** Relate some demographic statistics to problems, trends, and needs in the health-illness care system

3. Know essential facts about systems theory and models used by health professionals

- **3.1** Describe various models used by health professionals
- **3.2** Identify four characteristics of systems

4. Know essential facts about health care delivery systems

- **4.1** Identify four essential areas of a comprehensive health and illness care system
- **4.2** Describe various health care agencies
- **4.3** Identify specific problems in the current health-illness care delivery system
- **4.4** Identify five general ways of financing health-illness care
- **4.5** Identify aspects of alternative delivery systems

5. Understand the nurse's role in maintaining, promoting, and restoring health and in relating to other health professionals

- **5.1** Identify the nurse's role in primary, secondary, and tertiary prevention
- **5.2** Identify the nurse's role in supporting ill persons
- **5.3** Identify the roles of various health care providers
- **5.4** Differentiate the roles of various members of the nursing team

Terms

autonomy
boundary (systems theory)
closed system
coping mechanism
ecology
egocentricity
feedback
health
health belief
health-illness continuum
health practice
health state
health team
hospice
illness
input
model
morbidity
mortality
open system
output
palliative
physiatrist
privacy
psychosomatic
rehabilitation
role
somatic
system
theory
throughput

Health or wellness is a much sought-after state, yet for some an elusive state. Health means being of sound body, mind, and soul; yet this description does not really explain what health is, much less how to attain it. To identify illness, nurses need to know more explicitly just what a healthy body and a healthy mind are. Nurses also have specific responsibilities for promoting health. An understanding of health must include an understanding of the differences among individuals as well as the process of continually changing health as described in the health-illness continuum.

Illness is a universal phenomenon. Everyone at one time or another has experienced some illness, even if only a common cold. Illness has many connotations; thus different factors can affect both a nurse's and a patient's perspective of illness. Just as patients' beliefs are influenced by cultural and social backgrounds, so are nurses'. To really assist and understand patients, it is important for nurses to be aware of their own perspectives and beliefs, particularly those that may differ from patients' perspectives and beliefs.

The sick person assumes a role. A *role* is defined as "a pattern of behavior corresponding to a system of rights and duties and . . . associated with a particular position in a social group" (Wilson and Kolb 1949:208). A person in the sick role in North America has certain rights and responsibilities that are acknowledged by society. The sick person experiences certain emotions about illness; these may affect behavior. Therefore, caring for an ill person requires an understanding of how that person and his or her family react to illness.

The health team provides a wide range of assistance, to both the healthy and the ill or injured. Care of the healthy is receiving increasing emphasis in today's health care systems. Most members of the health team function under the supervision of an agency. Agencies vary in emphases and functions.

People use health services in various ways. To a large degree, how agencies are used and how much they are used are the measures of their effectiveness. Sometimes health services do not meet the needs of the people in the community. The nurse may see unmet needs and wonder why; knowledge of the enormous cost of health services, to the taxpayer and the patient, yields some measure of understanding. Failure to meet patients' needs, however, is difficult to condone, no matter what the reason.

Patterns and trends in health problems reveal how far health services have come and how far they have yet to go in preventing disease. An understanding of health trends will assist nurses to prepare for their future roles in the health care system and to understand contemporary change.

A complete health care system has four parts: health promotion, disease prevention, diagnosis and therapy, and rehabilitation. Nurses function in all these areas and need to be aware of health problems, whether obvious or hidden.

Definitions of Health

Health is a highly individual perception. Some people define health as the ability to carry out their normal daily tasks: A healthy woman is able to go to work and accomplishes her usual tasks; a healthy youngster can go to school and play baseball at noon. Other people consider themselves healthy only when they have vitality in their daily living and a feeling of wellness. However, definitions of vitality and wellness also vary. One person may consider herself well only when she functions at a high energy level. Another person may never have that amount of energy, yet consider himself well.

Meanings and descriptions of health vary with geography and culture. Health in a highly industrialized nation such as the United States is quite different from health in some deprived nations. In the latter, skin lesions may be considered normal and not a sign of ill health; indeed, the absence of lesions may be considered uncommon.

In summary, there is no absolute definition of health. There is no certain knowledge of how to attain the ultimate level of health, nor can health itself be measured.

In 1947 the World Health Organization (WHO) proposed a broad definition of health: "Health is a state of complete physical, mental, and social well-being, and not merely the absence of disease or infirmity" (WHO 1947:1). At that time, some considered this definition impractical; some view it as a possible goal for all people, while others consider complete well-being unobtainable. See the discussion of Dubos (1978) later in this section.

In 1953, in the United States, the President's Commission on Health Needs of the Nation stated: "Health is not a condition; it is an adjustment. It is not a state but a process. The process adapts the individual not only to our physical, but also our social environment" (President's Commission 1953:4). Dunn (1961) points out that an individual has different levels of wellness and that he or she responds to the environment as an integrated whole. Dunn calls optimum health "high-level wellness," which he defines as an integrated method of functioning that maximizes individuals' potential within their environments (ibid., p. 4).

Dunn also describes wellness in terms of a *health-illness continuum.* Wellness and illness are on opposite ends of the continuum. From high-level wellness on one side, a person's condition can move through good health, normal health, poor health, to extremely poor health and eventually to death on the other side. See Figure 2–1. Persons move back and forth within this continuum day by day. There is no distinct boundary across which people move from health to illness or from illness back to health. How persons perceive themselves and how others see them also affect their placement on the continuum. There is a considerable range in which people can be considered healthy or ill.

One's state of health is never constant; it is always changing. For example, a man may wake up in the morning with a headache; by noon he feels better, and by evening he feels quite well.

Health has also been defined as "the state of optimum capacity of an individual for the effective performance of his roles and tasks" (Parsons 1972:107). An emphasis in this definition is the capacity of the individual rather than a commitment to roles and tasks. By this definition, a person who does not wish to go to work is not necessarily unhealthy, yet people with diabetes, epilepsy, or paraplegia are healthy if they can perform roles and tasks effectively within their capacity.

Dubos (1978) views health as a creative process. Individuals are actively and continually adapting to their environments. In Dubos's view, the individual must have sufficient knowledge to make informed choices about his or her health and also the income and resources to act on choices. Dubos believes that complete well-being is unobtainable, thus contradicting the 1947 definition by the World Health Organization.

Rogers (1961) and Jahoda (1958) also describe health. Rogers refers to the "fully functioning person" and Jahoda suggests specific criteria by which to gauge mental health. For additional information see Chapter 8, page 177.

Factors Influencing Personal Definitions of Health

An individual's definition of health is often a personal one. It is frequently related to a number of factors or experiences, and it may or may not be in agreement with definitions of health professionals. The following factors influence an individual's definition of health:

1. *Developmental status.* The idea of health is frequently related to a person's level of development. The ability to conceptualize a state of health and the ability to respond to changes in health are related directly to age. An infant can be aware of pain but unable to verbalize it or take measures to seek help to relieve it. The nurse's knowledge of an individual's developmental status can facilitate assessment of the appropriateness of the person's behavior and help anticipate future behaviors.

Figure 2–1 The health-illness continuum from high-level wellness to death. (Adapted from H. L. Dunn, *Positive wellness in the human national posture* [Washington, D.C.: Government Printing Office], Developmental Note no. 58-DAP-7).

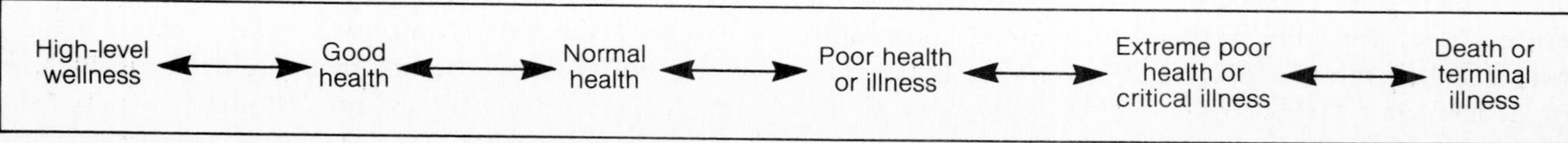

2. *Social and cultural influences.* Culture and social interactions also influence a person's notion of health. Each culture has ideas about health, and often these are transmitted from parents to children. For example, in some traditional Chinese families health is defined as a flow of energy (yin and yang). Yin is dark, cold, wet, negative, and female; yang is light, warm, dry, positive, and male. An imbalance of yin and yang results in disease.

Socioeconomic influences affect definitions of health. For example, people who do not have the money for health care might consider themselves healthy even when they have colds, whereas people with resources seek assistance for the same problem.

Another important influence is the reaction of a person's significant others (family and friends) to a health problem. If a man, for example, is told by significant others that a certain pain is normal, then he may consider the pain normal and himself healthy.

3. *Previous experiences.* Experiences with health and illness also affect people's perceptions of health. Some people may consider a pain or dysfunction normal because they have felt it before or often before. In addition, knowledge gained from these experiences helps determine people's definitions of health.

4. *Expectations of self.* Some people expect to be functioning at a high level physically and psychosocially all the time when they are healthy. They perceive any change in that level of functioning, therefore, as illness. Others expect variations in their level of functioning, and their definitions of health accommodate those variations.

Another factor related to self is how the individual perceives himself or herself generally. These perceptions relate to such aspects of self as esteem, body image, needs, roles, and abilities. When there is any threat or perceived threat to these views of self, the individual usually feels some anxiety. Often the individual needs to reassess his or her health and to redefine health. For example a 60-year-old man who can no longer play tennis as he was accustomed to do may need to examine and redefine his concept of health in view of his age and abilities.

Health Beliefs and Practices

The *health state* of an individual is the health of that person at a given time. In its general meaning, the term may refer to anxiety, depression, acute illness, etc., and thus describes the individual as a whole; *health state* also can describe such specifics as pulse rate and body temperature. *Health beliefs* of an individual are the concepts about health that an individual believes true. They may or may not be founded on fact. *Health practices* are activities that individuals carry out as a result of their health beliefs and definitions of health. These practices may or may not be those recommended by health care professionals. For example, an individual who believes that drinking a case of beer each day keeps the intestines free of infection may refuse to accept advice against this practice even in life-threatening situations. It is therefore important for nurses assessing an individual's state of health to be aware of that person's health beliefs and health practices. Nurses preparing a plan of care for an individual need to consider the person's health beliefs before they attempt to change health practices. Otherwise, the individual may reject the suggestions from nurses and become angry because of intrusion into his or her personal habits.

Nurses' Responsibilities for Health

Nurses play a major role in promoting health in people of all ages. Although individuals are in part responsible for their own health, the nurse has responsibilities and opportunities to promote health in individuals, families, and communities. Prevention can be a framework for presenting and interpreting health care requirements and their implications in nursing situations (Orem 1980:132). Leavell and others (1965) describe prevention as having three levels: primary, secondary, and tertiary.

Primary Prevention

Primary prevention includes health maintenance, health promotion, and disease prevention. Often the informed adult in a community can assume much of the responsibility at this level, for example by regularly flossing and brushing the teeth (see Chapter 21 for further information) or seeking appropriate immunizations. The role of the nurse at this level is to provide health education and such services as immunization.

Nurses can practice primary health promotion in a variety of settings: homes, schools, industry, and hospitals. Nurses can direct primary prevention to individuals, to groups, or more broadly to whole communities, for example, by working to change environmental control laws. Primary prevention activities should be incorporated into an individual's daily life. Often it may be necessary for a nurse to identify populations at risk in a community and to intervene before the health of those individuals is affected. An example of a group at risk is pregnant teenagers who eat junk food rather than a balanced diet.

Secondary Prevention

Secondary prevention includes interventions that prevent complications from disease processes. At this level, health promotion by the nurse involves an awareness of complications that could develop and intervention to prevent these complications. For example, nurses change the position of immobilized patients and provide skin care regularly to prevent decubitus ulcers. See Chapters 21 and 23 for additional information. Another example is maintaining an intravenous infusion accurately so that the patient receives the correct fluids and electrolytes. Supporting the patient and significant others is an important part of secondary prevention. The nurse promotes health by reducing the anxiety and fear that attend most illnesses.

Tertiary Prevention

Tertiary prevention includes assessing the abilities and disabilities of patients and intervening to help them overcome disabilities and adjust their functioning. This level of prevention is frequently called *rehabilitation*. Nursing at this level may be temporary or permanent. The patient or support persons may be able to learn the skills necessary to promote health, and the nurse's role may be teaching these skills. An example is teaching a female patient with a paralyzed limb to walk and then to function in her own house. See the section on rehabilitation later in this chapter for further information.

Definitions of Illness

Differentiation from Disease

Illness has been defined in a number of ways; it has been described as sickness or as a deviation from a healthy stage. More recently, sociologists have differentiated illness from disease. Illness in this context is considered a highly personal state in which the person feels ill; for example, the person feels pain or nausea and as a result tends to modify behavior in some way. Illness can be defined as "a state of disturbance in the normal functioning of the total human individual, including both the state of the organism as a biological system, and of his person and social adjustments" (Parsons 1972:107). This definition includes illness of organic or somatic origin (biologic disturbances) and illness of psychologic origin (personal and/or social changes).

Disease, by contrast, is solely a biologic entity; it is something that alters the function of the body in some way, such as an obstruction in a blood vessel or a tumor in the liver. With reference to these definitions, it is apparent that a person may feel ill without the presence of a disease. Also, a disease might be present, but the person may or may not feel ill. Generally speaking, illness can be any condition that causes a person to seek advice from a health professional. Illness behavior, then, is the behavior in this context.

Bauman (1965:206) found that people have three distinct criteria by which they consider themselves ill:

1. The presence of symptoms such as elevated temperature or pain
2. Their perceptions of how they feel; for example, good, bad, sick
3. Their ability to carry out daily activities, such as a job or schoolwork

Factors Influencing Illness Behavior

The illness behavior of a person is a culturally and socially learned response. Cultures differ widely in their responses to illness. Subcultures in the United States demonstrate these differences. For example, Jewish and Italian patients often respond to pain in emotionally expressive ways and tend to exaggerate the pain experienced, while Anglo-Americans tend to be stoic and less expressive. The Irish tend to deny the existence of the pain (Mechanic 1972:120).

These cultural responses are learned in early childhood. For example, if a hurt child cries and as a result receives help and comfort, the child learns that crying brings help and comfort. At the other extreme, a crying child who is repeatedly ignored learns crying does not bring comfort, but perhaps other types of behavior do.

This child may learn that stoicism elicits comfort and support from the family, who sees this behavior as admirable.

Social conditioning also affects illness behavior. For example, older children are usually more stoical than younger children; boys are socialized to react less to hurt or pain than girls. These sterotypical socialization patterns are changing, however. Although generalizations can be made about culturally learned behavior, there are wide variations within a culture that mitigate against predictive behavior assessment.

Even within the same culture there can be a wide variety of responses to the same illness. One person might dismiss a condition and not let it alter his or her life, while another with the same illness may show considerable change socially and emotionally. Often the way persons react is related to other stresses, problems, or coping difficulties that they have at that time rather than to the illness itself. Illness is stressful, and the total number of stresses a person has influences illness behavior. The nurse should be aware that even a minor complaint about illness may be a patient's way of seeking help for another problem.

Illness behavior can obtain some advantages for the patient. For example, a person who lives alone in a cold room and who falls ill and is admitted to a hospital receives the advantages of food, warmth, being cared for, escape from worry, and relief from maintaining life in a difficult environment. This is an extreme example of the secondary advantages of illness. More commonly nurses encounter simpler mechanisms. For example, a person develops a severe headache just before a dental appointment, thus avoiding a dreaded visit. Sometimes such a reaction is a symptom of an underlying problem, which manifests itself in illness behavior.

Stages of Illness

Suchman (1972:145) describes five stages of illness:

1. Symptom experience stage
2. Assumption of the sick role
3. Medical care contact stage
4. Dependent patient role stage
5. Recovery or rehabilitation stage

Symptom Experience Stage

The first stage of illness is the transition stage during which patients come to believe something is wrong. Either a significant person mentions that they look unwell, or patients experience some symptoms, which can appear insidiously. Initially, persons often go through a phase of denial and continue to function as if they felt well. During this period, they may not want to bother the family or physician with something that seems trivial. This behavior delays treatment, which is an unwise practice.

There are three aspects of the symptom experience stage: the physical experience of symptoms such as pain or high temperature; the cognitive aspect, that is, interpretation of the symptoms in terms that have some meaning to the person; and the emotional response of fear or anxiety.

During this stage unwell persons usually consult persons close to them about their symptoms or feelings. People validate with their spouses or partners, for example, that the symptoms are real and obtain support to seek a physician's advice. At this stage, sick persons sometimes try home remedies such as laxatives or cough medicines.

Assumption of the Sick Role

The second stage signals acceptance of the illness. At this time individuals decide that their symptoms or concerns are sufficiently severe to suggest that they are sick. They seek confirmation of the illness from family and friends and then assume the sick role, discussed later in this chapter. Some people seek professional help quickly; others continue self-treatment, often following the suggestions of family and friends.

In this stage, sick persons are usually afraid, but they now accept that they are ill even though they may not be able to accept the possible reasons. In conferring with people close to them, sick persons seek not only advice but also support for the decision to give up some activities and, for example, stay home from work.

At the end of this stage, sick persons experience one of two outcomes. They may find that the symptoms have changed and that they feel better. Still, they seek confirmation of improvement from the family; if family members support the patients' perceptions, they are no longer considered or consider themselves sick. Then the recovered persons resume normal obligations, such as returning to work or attending a school concert. If, however, the symptoms persist or increase and if lack of improvement is validated by the family or significant others, then sick persons know they should seek a physician's advice.

Medical Care Contact Stage

Sick persons seek the advice of a physician either on their own initiative or at the urging of significant others. When people go for medical advice, they are really asking for three types of information:

1. Validation of real illness
2. Explanation of the symptoms in understandable terms
3. Reassurance that they will be all right or prediction of what the outcome will be

If the physician does not validate illness, persons have two recourses: to return to normal activities or to seek another physician's advice. If the symptoms disappear, persons perceive that they really are not ill. If symptoms continue, persons return to the physician or go to a second physician for medical care. People who are repeatedly told that they are not ill may seek out quasi-practitioners as a last resort to alleviate the perceived symptoms. Some people will go from physician to physician until they find someone who provides a diagnosis that fits their own perceptions.

Most people also want an understandable explanation of their symptoms. When symptoms are not explained, patients may assume the physician does not believe them or perhaps that they are imagining the symptoms. Overly technical explanations, however, often confuse and frighten people.

People experience anxiety about seeking medical help. Even minor symptoms can be construed as serious. Therefore, the patient needs reassurance that he or she will be cured. Even when this reassurance cannot be given, most people want to know the likely outcome.

Dependent Patient Role Stage

When the physician has validated that the person is ill, the individual becomes a patient, dependent on the physician for help. During this stage sick persons may or may not be reluctant to accept a physician's recommendations. They may vacillate about what is best for them and alternately accept and reject the physician's suggestions. People vary greatly in the degree of ease with which they can give up their independence, particularly in relation to life and death. Role obligations—such as those of wage earner, father, or mother or of student, baseball team member, or choir member—complicate the decision to give up independence. It is also common for patient and physician to hold different notions of the nature of the illness, unless complete and open communication exists. During this stage, a nurse can often give the patient information that may allay some fears and/or provide data that support the physician's diagnosis. Misconceptions can result from limited information, which patients interpret in the light of their experiences. For example, a patient may be told by the physician that there is a small encapsulated growth in the right groin and that surgical removal is advised. If the patient's mother died after being told she had a growth in her breast, the patient may assume that he or she also will die.

Most patients accept their dependence on the physician, although people retain varying degrees of control over their own lives. For example, some patients request precise information about their diseases, their treatment, and the cost of treatment, and they delay the decision to accept treatment until they have all this information. Other patients prefer that the physician proceed with treatment and do not request additional information.

During this period, sick persons gradually become more passive and accepting. They require a predictable environment in which people are genuinely concerned about them. In addition to being concerned about themselves, some sick persons regress to an earlier behavioral stage in their development. As a result, patients may have fewer *coping mechanisms* (physical and emotional adaptive or defensive abilities). Frequently patients' reactions are related to previous experiences and to misconceptions about what will happen.

Children are accustomed to being dependent for some of their needs, although dependence varies with age and home situation. Since 1-year-old children are accustomed to being bathed and fed, this assistance is not a major adjustment when they are ill. Adults, however, are usually unaccustomed to this assistance, and they may find it difficult to relinquish independence and accept such help even if it is necessary. People have varying dependence needs. For some, illness may meet dependence needs that have never been met and thus provide satisfaction to the patient. Other people have minimal dependence needs and do everything possible to return to independent functioning. A few may even try to maintain independence to the detriment of their recovery.

Nurses need to assess the dependence needs of their patients and relate these to needs normally appropriate for their developmental stages. See Chapters 11 and 12. Patient behaviors that support independent functioning need to be encouraged once the patient is ready. Thus, nurses can assist patients to develop new ways of coping and decrease unhealthy dependence on others.

Recovery or Rehabilitation Stage

During the fifth stage, the patient learns to give up the sick role and return to former roles and functions. For patients with acute illnesses, the time as a patient is generally short, and recovery is usually rapid. Thus they find it relatively easy to return to their former life-styles. People who have long-term illnesses and who have to make adjustments in life-style find recovery more difficult. Recovery is particularly difficult for people who have to relearn skills such as walking or talking.

During this stage, readiness for social functioning lags behind physical functioning. Patients may be physically able to go out to dinner but find that functioning socially is still too stressful.

Nurses can assist patients to function with increasing independence by planning with patients those functions they can accomplish by themselves and those with which they need assistance. It is also important that the nurse convey an attitude of hope and support. Each person, even an infant, needs this to return to health.

Effects of Hospitalization

Normal patterns of behavior generally change with illness; with hospitalization, the change can be even greater. Hospitalization usually disrupts a person's privacy, autonomy, life-style, roles, and economics.

Privacy

When a patient enters a hospital the loss of privacy is instantly obvious. *Privacy* has been described as a comfortable feeling reflecting a deserved degree of social retreat. Its dimensions and duration are controlled by the individual seeking the privacy. It is a personal, internal state that cannot be imposed from without (Schuster 1976:245).

People need varying degrees of privacy and establish boundaries for privacy; when these boundaries are crossed, they feel invaded. Hospital personnel sometimes show little concern for patients' privacy. Patients are asked to provide information that often they consider private; they may share a room with strangers; and their health is frequently discussed with many health professionals, often in the hearing of others.

The boundaries for privacy are highly individual. The adult who lives alone may be used to privacy while eating, sleeping, and reading. A child from a large family may be accustomed to sharing these activities with others. It is important for nurses to ascertain what privacy means to the individual and try to support accustomed practices whenever possible.

Autonomy

Autonomy is the state of being independent and self-directed without outside control. People vary in their sense of autonomy; some are accustomed to functioning independently in most of their life activities while others are more accustomed to direction from others. An example of the former is a writer who lives alone and works independently. By contrast, a wife in a patriarchal home may be accustomed to having decisions made by her husband and receiving direction from him.

Hospitalized patients frequently give up much of their autonomy. Decisions about meals, hygienic practices, and sleeping are frequently made for them. This loss of individuality is often difficult to accept, and the patient may feel dehumanized into "just a piece of machinery."

Nurses have been trying to humanize care in recent years by learning about the patient as a person and by individualizing nursing care plans.

Life-Style

Hospitalization marks a change in life-style. Many hospitals determine when patients wake up and when they sleep. The woman who normally rises at 8:00 A.M. and the man who usually works until 11:00 P.M. must change their habits. Food in a hospital is mass produced, and individual differences in taste are rarely accommodated. Occasionally hospitals have relatively large populations from a particular culture and make special food arrangements, for example, a Chinese menu for traditional Chinese patients or Kosher foods for traditional Jewish patients. However, individual preferences are often not met.

Nurses can help patients adapt to life in a hospital by:

1. Making arrangements wherever possible to accommodate the patient's life-style, such as providing a bath in the evening rather than in the morning
2. Providing explanations about hospital routines
3. Encouraging other health professionals to become aware of the patient's life-style and to support healthy aspects of that life-style
4. Reinforcing desirable changes in practices with a view to making them a permanent part of the patient's life-style

Roles

People's life roles frequently change when they are hospitalized. A man or woman may no longer be the wage earner; parents may be unable to fulfill normal parental responsibilities. See the sections on the dependent patient role stage and the sick role in this chapter.

Economics

Hospitalization often places a genuine financial burden on patients and their families. Even though many people have health insurance, it may not reimburse all costs; in addition, many lose wages while they are hospitalized.

Nurses can be aware of these costs and provide care that is as economical as is safely possible; for instance, they can use only the minimum supplies necessary for safe care. Nurses also can support activities that promote health and that return patients to their normal activities as soon as possible.

The Sick Role

Characteristics of the Role

People assume the sick role when they accept illness and when that illness has been validated by a physician. The sick role describes the typical patient's behavior, but cannot, of course, describe every patient's behavior. Parsons (1964:436–37) describes four aspects of the sick role:

1. Patients are not held responsible for their condition.
2. Patients are excused from certain social roles and tasks.
3. Patients are obliged to try to get well as quickly as possible.
4. Patients or their families are obliged to seek competent help.

The patient in North American society is not held responsible for incurring an illness. Illness, though undesirable, is seen as beyond a person's control. Some subcultures view illness as punishment from God, and therefore consider the infirm responsible for their illnesses, because of their sins. This folk belief persists to some degree in American society. Often a patient will say, "What have I done to deserve this?" This remark reflects a sense of illness as punishment. Today, people are being held increasingly responsible for some illnesses, for example, the cardiac patient who smokes or the overweight person who develops diabetes.

Nurses can help patients assume the sick role by providing factual information and not judging the patient responsible for his or her illness. It is important not to reinforce behaviors that exacerbate or may have helped bring about an illness and to encourage behaviors that promote health.

The sick person is also excused from some normal duties. This is true whether the person has a cold or requires surgery. Social pressures on the sick and expectations of them by others usually depend on the prognosis and the severity of the illness. People who are severely ill and whose prognosis is poor or uncertain are permitted to be dependent and are so treated. People who are not seriously ill and whose prognosis is good are more likely to be encouraged to fulfill personal and social responsibilities. The person with a cold may still be expected to give a scheduled speech or to take an examination. People who are chronically ill may be permanently exempted from some duties or activities; for example, the father confined to bed is not expected to attend his daughter's field hockey games. In this situation, arrangements are usually made within the family for another person to fulfill the father's role while he is unable to do so.

Some patients may express feelings of guilt because they are unable to fulfill their normal responsibilities. Nurses can express support to patients who cannot fulfill their perceived roles and help them substitute other appropriate activities, when desirable. For example, a young father who cannot play ball with his son can help the son build a model airplane, thereby fulfilling the father's role in another way.

A third aspect of the sick role is the obligation of the person to get well as quickly as possible. The sick role is a dependent one, at least in some respects. The person who fears dependence may be threatened by assuming a sick role and having to seek help. This person might ignore advice despite the most serious consequences. Some people, however, find dependence gratifying. Some patients find dependence so satisfying that they perpetuate the sick role and do not try to get well or continue to complain of symptoms even after they are physically well. Some people in the dependent stage also find it satisfying to control others through excessive demands. With exceptions, people usually try to get well as quickly as possible.

Nurses can help patients assume a dependence appropriate to their developmental status and health. Part of the nurse's job is to reinforce both dependence and increasing independence at the appropriate times. For example, a man who is acutely ill may have to be shaved by the nurse; however, once he is stronger the nurse can assist him by providing shaving supplies and later complimenting him on his appearance.

The fourth aspect of the sick role is seeking competent help. This presupposes that competent help is available to the patient. It should also be recognized that the patient's notion of competent help may be different from the general population's. For example, a man with a whiplash injury may become dissatisfied with his physician's treatment because of his slow recovery and may go to a healer who uses hypnotism. Or a young woman may have a manner others find unpleasant—she talks a great deal and is domineering. She cannot keep a job for more than 2 months. Someone suggests that she see a physician or therapist. She decides instead to join a cult of young people, considering the members of the cult competent help.

Occasionally nurses need to encourage people to obtain competent help from health professionals. Nurses who are aware of the health facilities available in a community can assist people to obtain care. People may require considerable support before seeking assistance because, for example, they fear the health problem might be serious or they believe competent help might not be available. A nurse's function in these instances is to provide accurate information about available health facilities while recognizing patients' beliefs and their right to hold those views.

Behavior Changes of Sick Persons

Fearfulness

A person usually becomes fearful after assuming the sick role. Generally, the person is afraid of reduced functioning, changed social relationships, or death. The person worries about the outcome of the illness, particularly when the diagnosis is uncertain. The individual also worries about the effects of reduced functioning: "Will this illness mean a lower family income?" These changes often mean that patients must change their concept of themselves, e.g., from capable wage earner to part-time employee. Persons also worry about possible changes in social relationships. For example, if the wife becomes the major wage earner, how will the husband-wife relationship change? Nurses can assist patients by listening to their concerns and supporting realistic behavior and realistic plans for the future.

Regression

Persons threatened by illness feel anxious. In order to cope with anxiety they may regress to behavior more appropriate to an earlier stage of maturation. For example, 8-year-olds may wet the bed or suck their thumbs; adults may seek attention by constant demands. As a part of this regression, the patient may show a number of kinds of behavior: egocentricity, an exaggerated concern over small matters, narrowed interests, emotional overreaction, and some changes in the perception of people in the environment. Nurses should support behavior that is appropriate to the patient's age and should not reinforce regressive behavior but recognize that it is normally temporary.

Egocentricity

Egocentricity is excessive concern about oneself. When patients become egocentric, they are preoccupied with themselves and their illness. They usually do not want to hear about someone else's operation; they want to talk about their own operations or their own pains. Egocentricity is often more apparent when patients are in a hospital. In this setting, isolated from their families and their activities, patients have more time to think about themselves and their illnesses.

Concern over small matters

As patients become preoccupied with themselves, they show an exaggerated concern over small matters. They may fret about a wrinkle in a bedspread or be intolerant of delays. Most patients, however, are realistic and considerate of others most of the time. Nurses need to encourage expression of the exaggerated concerns of patients and understand that most of these are related to the sick role.

Narrowed interests

Patients' interests narrow chiefly when they are hospitalized or ill for a long time. This narrowing of interests may be due in part to stress, which reduces patients' perceptions of the world around them, or to a lack of energy, because weakened patients use all their energy to get well. Contributing to this problem is the fact that patients have been relieved of many of their responsibilities because of the illness. For these reasons, ill people are not necessarily interested in everything that interests them when they are well.

Sometimes, however, patients in hospitals become interested in something that normally does not interest them. For instance, a patient who usually takes no interest in baseball may follow the World Series avidly. This change in behavior usually has two causes: the fellowship of sharing the experience with other patients and the distraction it offers for a short time without demanding intense emotional involvement.

Emotional overreactions

Emotional overreactions are common in people who are ill; they cry more easily, become angry quickly, and have an increased need for affection and attention from others. The patient who has family and/or support persons generally gets this attention from them; but the patient who does not have visitors is supported emotionally chiefly by nurses. This is the caring aspect of nursing, the genuine concern frequently referred to as TLC (tender loving care). Children especially need the support and care usually provided by parents. Adults, too, need care and affection, but this need is not as pronounced as in children.

Changed perceptions of others

Hospitalized people often experience shifts in their perceptions of the people around them. The physician may become all powerful in the patient's eyes. The nurse may be seen in a mothering role, that is, comforting, supporting, and providing security. These perceptions may be unconscious or conscious.

Sometimes these new perceptions of others frustrate the patient. For example, if the nurse directs attention to other patients the patient may display anger or jealousy. This may be obvious in the children's units of a hospital, where a child who does not receive the nurse's attention all the time often expresses frustration in an angry outburst.

Effects of Illness on Family Members

When any person is ill, there is some effect on the family or significant others. The kind of effect and its extent are chiefly dependent on three factors: which member of the family is ill, how serious and long the illness is, and what cultural and social customs that family holds.

The changes that can occur within a family include:

1. Role changes
2. Task reassignments
3. Increased stress due to anxiety about the outcome of the illness for the patient and conflict about unaccustomed responsibilities
4. Financial problems
5. Loneliness as a result of separation and pending loss
6. Change in social customs

Each member of the family is affected differently depending on whether a grandmother, the father of a nuclear family, or a teenager is ill. Each of these people has a different role in the family, and each supports the family in different ways. Parents of young children, for example, have greater family responsibilities than parents of grown children.

The degree of change that family members experience is often related to their dependence on the sick person. For example, when a child is ill, there are few changes other than added responsibilities directly related to the child's illness. When the mother is ill, however, many changes are often necessary in the lives of the family members because others must assume her functions.

Sick Elderly Persons

When an elderly person is ill, a son or daughter often assumes the role of parent to the elderly person. Sons or daughters may find it necessary to provide housing, meals, and assistance with daily needs over a prolonged time. In other words, the parent-child roles are frequently reversed. This role reversal may be only temporary and may end when the illness ends, or it may become permanent. Since elderly people generally have few responsibilities, task reassignment is usually restricted to direct care for the sick person. Stress and concern about the outcome of the illness is present for all the family, in particular for the spouse of the sick person. Younger persons in the family often deal with serious illness in an elderly person by stating, "He has led a good life" or "She had so much pain the past years." In this way, the young prepare themselves for that person's death. This same reasoning is rarely applied to a child or younger adult who is ill.

When an elderly person is ill, adult sons and daughters may face conflicting responsibilities. A daughter who lives some distance away needs to maintain her job and look after her own family, but at the same time her parents need her in another city. How often should she visit? How should she fulfill her responsibilities? These questions pose problems for a family separated by miles.

The financial problems of the sick elderly can be a major problem for a family as well as a community. Because illness in this age group tends to be chronic, the costs of illness tend to be considerable.

Loneliness as a result of separation from or pending loss of an elderly person is usually felt most by that person's spouse. When a marriage has lasted for 50 or 60 years, elderly people find it difficult to envisage what life will be like without a husband or wife. Older people generally recognize that they are at the end of their lives, but separation and loneliness are prominent concerns. Grandchildren also experience anxiety about the outcome of a grandparent's illness, particularly if they have had long and pleasant ties and experiences. Primary ties are generally in the nuclear family (parents and children), however, and often the elderly person lives apart or in another city. When an elderly person is ill or hospitalized, the family life-style generally has minimal disruption. The greatest change in life-style is that it now must accommodate hospital visits to the elderly relative.

Sick Parents

When the sick person is a parent, the degree to which the family experiences change is related to the kinds of responsibilities the individual has and the number and age of dependents in the person's care. For example, when a father is ill for a long time, his roles are usually taken over by other members of the family, frequently the mother. Tasks such as doing chores in the house or attending a child's basketball games, for example, are either reassigned or not performed at all. Anxiety of family members about the outcome of a parent's illness is usually high, especially if the parent is the wage earner. The implications to the family of prolonged illness or death are great in almost all areas of living because of the needs of the dependents.

Prolonged illness of the mother can have equally serious consequences and be particularly disruptive if an outsider is employed to perform tasks formerly carried out by the mother. Children, especially young ones, in this situation suffer a loss in affection and feel insecure when their mother is away or too ill to function as usual. Often a lack of understanding about why their mother is in the hospital coupled with feelings of loneliness and not being wanted present problems. Sometimes the mother's functions are taken over by grandparents or by aunts and uncles as well as by the father. When a young mother has a serious illness of unknown outcome, the father and family face worrisome problems of how to manage over a long period of time. Most arrangements have financial implications and involve role changes for the father and children. In this situation, the father must become both father and mother and give up many of his normal social activities. The children may also need to assume more housekeeping functions.

Sick Children

Because a child is dependent on parents for so many daily needs, both sick children and their families need to make fewer role adjustments than sick adults and their families. Task reassignments are also generally minimal. Sometimes a younger sibling takes over a paper route for a sick brother or sister, and other members of the family share the sick child's chores.

Anxiety is experienced by all members of the family if the outcome of the illness is in doubt. A permanent disability has implications for schooling, earning a living, and future needs. Financial responsibility for chronic illness or a disability often can be a serious problem for young parents. Other children may feel neglected if an unusual amount of attention is given to the ill child. Husband and wife may also expend most of their energies visiting the hospital and have little time for each other. If extended, this situation can place great stress on a marriage.

When a child is admitted to the hospital, parents and siblings may experience some sense of loss; however, children usually continue with their daily activities, and there is minimal disruption in the home.

Health Team

The *health team* consists of a group of people from different disciplines who coordinate their skills to assist a patient and/or family. The choice of personnel for a particular team depends on the needs of the patient. In the present system of health care in North America, health teams commonly include physicians, nurses, dietitians, physiotherapists, social workers, occupational therapists, paramedical technologists, pharmacists, and inhalation therapists.

Physician

A physician is a person who is licensed to practice medicine in a particular jurisdiction. The physician has successfully completed a course of medical studies. In a hospital setting, the physician is responsible for medical diagnosis and for determining the therapy required by a person who is ill or injured. In a community setting, the physician may be involved in diagnosis and therapy or play a consulting role. An example of the latter is the physician who specializes in public health and who serves as a consultant to the school nurse.

Nurse

The role of the nurse was discussed in Chapter 1. Nursing skills can be described as psychomotor, affective, or cognitive. Psychomotor skills are the traditional skills of nurses. The use of the hands, whether to manipulate equipment or reposition a patient, for example, is a psychomotor skill. With increasing technology, psychomotor skills necessary for nursing are increasing steadily. Affective skills include the ability to incorporate cultural, attitudinal, and emotional elements into nursing. The nurse uses affective skills to individualize care. Caring and communicating roles (see Chapter 1) require affective skills. Cognitive skills include the ability to think, recall knowledge, apply knowledge, and evaluate. Cognitive skills are required in all aspects of the nursing process.

A number of nursing personnel may be involved in the health team and may have their own nursing team. Sometimes nurses find it necessary to provide some of the services normally given by other members of the team. This often happens in settings where all the health services required by a patient are not available. For example, a nurse might assist a patient who has had a cerebrovascular accident (stroke) by giving remedial exercises to restore function of the left arm. In an urban hospital these exercises would generally be taught by a physiotherapist; however, in a rural setting a physiotherapist's services often are not available, so the nurse frequently provides this assistance.

Dietitian or Nutritionist

When dietary and nutritional services are required, the dietitian or nutritionist may be a member of a health team. Dietitians in hospitals design special diets—for example, for a child who has diabetes mellitus—and they supervise the preparation of the meals according to the diet. The nutritionist in a community setting recommends healthy diets and gives broad advisory services about the purchase and preparation of foods.

Hospital dietitians are generally concerned with therapeutic diets. The community nutritionist often functions at the preventive level. Such dietitians promote health and prevent disease, for example, by advising families about balanced diets for growing children and pregnant women.

Physiotherapist

The physiotherapist (physical therapist) assists patients with musculoskeletal problems. The physiotherapist's functions are:

1. Assessing mobility and strength
2. Providing therapeutic measures, for example, exercises and heat applications to improve mobility and strength
3. Teaching patients new skills, for example, how to walk with an artificial leg
4. Teaching patients measures to prevent illness, for example, teaching deep breathing to a patient before surgery as a preventive measure against postoperative pneumonia

Most physiotherapists provide their services in hospitals; however, independent practitioners are establishing offices in communities and serving patients either at the office or in the patient's home.

Social Worker

The social worker counsels the patient and family about such problems as finances, marital difficulties, and adoption of children. It is not unusual for health problems to produce problems in living. For example, an elderly woman who lives alone and has a stroke resulting in impaired walking may find it impossible to continue to live in her third-floor apartment.

Occupational Therapist

The occupational therapist assists patients with some impairment of function to gain the skills they need to perform the activities of daily living. For example, a man with severe arthritis in his arms and hands might be taught how to adjust his kitchen utensils so that he can continue to cook. The therapist also teaches skills that are therapeutic and at the same time provide some satisfaction. For example, weaving is a recreational activity but also exercises the arthritic man's arms and hands. Occupational therapists coordinate their activities closely with those of other members of the health team.

Paramedical Technologist

Laboratory technologists, radiologic technologists, and nuclear medicine technologists are just three kinds of paramedical technologists in an expanding field of medical technology. *Paramedical* means having some connection with medicine. Laboratory technologists examine specimens such as urine, feces, blood, and discharges from wounds to provide the physician with exact information that facilitates the medical diagnosis and the prescription of a therapeutic regimen. The radiologic technologist assists with a wide variety of x-ray film procedures, from simple chest radiography to more complex fluoroscopy and radiography of the patient's stomach using a contrast medium. The nuclear medicine technologist, a more recent member of the technology group, uses radioactive substances to provide diagnostic information, for example, about a patient's liver and can administer therapeutic doses of radioactive materials as part of a therapeutic regimen. These technologists have highly specialized skills and knowledge important to patient care.

Pharmacist

The pharmacist prepares and dispenses pharmaceuticals in hospital and community settings. The role of the pharmacist in monitoring and evaluating the actions and effects of medications on patients is becoming increasingly prominent. Pharmacists are also actively involved in preparing individual dosages for patients in hospitals that employ the unit dose system. In some settings, pharmacists prepare medications for intravenous therapy.

Inhalation Therapist

The inhalation therapist or respiratory technologist is skilled in therapeutic measures used in the care of patients with respiratory problems. These therapists are knowledgeable about oxygen therapy devices, intermittent positive pressure breathing respirators, artificial mechanical ventilators, and accessory devices used in inhalation therapy. Frequently they are involved in diagnostic procedures such as pulmonary function tests. Programs in inhalation therapy are offered in postsecondary educational institutions. Students complete such programs in 2 or 3 years.

Health and Illness: Patterns and Trends

The health of North Americans is steadily improving. Probable reasons for this improvement are:

1. Earlier preventive efforts based on new knowledge obtained through research.
2. Improvements in sanitation, housing, nutrition, and immunization essential to disease prevention.
3. Individual measures to promote health and prevent disease. For example, increasing attention is being paid to exercise, nutrition, environmental health, and occupational health.

Evidence of gains in health status is cited in the Surgeon General's Report on Health Promotion and Disease Prevention (U.S. DHEW 1979:3):

1. In 1977, a record low of 14 infant deaths per 1000 live births was reported.
2. Between 1960 and 1975, the difference in infant mortality rates for nonwhites and whites was cut in half.
3. Between 1950 and 1977, the mortality rate for children aged 1 to 14 was halved.
4. A baby born in the United States today can be expected to live more than 73 years on average, while a baby born in 1900 could be expected to live only 47 years.
5. Deaths due to heart disease decreased in the United States by 22% between 1968 and 1977.
6. During the past decade the expected life span for Americans has increased by 2.7 years. In the previous decade it increased by only 1 year.

Four of the major risk factors responsible for illness and premature deaths cited by the surgeon general (U.S. DHEW 1979:7–8) are:

1. *Cigarette smoking.* This is clearly identified as a cause of most cases of lung cancer and a major factor increasing the risk of heart attacks.
2. *Alcohol and drug abuse.* Consumption of alcohol and drugs, even among youths, has grown substantially since the 1960s and accounts for significant illness, disability, and death.
3. *Injuries.* The highest death rate from accidents occurs among the elderly, but it is also substantial among those aged 15 to 24. Injuries from accidents may be caused by motor vehicles, firearms, falls, burns, poisons, recreational activities, and adverse drug reactions.
4. *Occupational risks.* Certain occupational hazards, such as exposure to asbestos, rubber, and plastic, are now being identified as potential cancer risks.

All of these risks present challenges to health care workers, especially nurses, in terms of prevention. Measures to enhance health include elimination of cigarette smoking; moderation of alcohol consumption; safety measures, such as using seat belts, to prevent accidents and injuries; and periodic screening for such health problems as cancer.

Health Field Concept

In 1974 Lalonde, Canadian minister of national health and welfare, introduced the health field concept, which views all causes of death and disease as having four contributing elements: (a) human biologic factors, such as genetic makeup and age; (b) behavioral factors or unhealthy life-styles; (c) environmental hazards; and (d) inadequacies in the health care system (Canada Department of National Health and Welfare 1974:31–34). Using these four elements as a framework, a group of United States experts devised a method to assess the relative contributions of each of these elements to the ten leading causes of death in 1976. The results indicated that approximately 50% of deaths were due to unhealthy behavior or life-style; 20% to human biologic factors; 20% to environmental factors; and 10% to inadequacies in health care (U.S. DHEW 1979:9). These results have implications for nursing; the most important is that a substantial number of deaths could be avoided by efforts directed at health promotion.

Demographics

Demographic statistics, such as age distribution, mortality, and morbidity also reflect trends and needs in the health and illness care system.

Population

Statistics reflect an increase in the total population and indicate the need for increased health and illness services. In both the United States and Canada there has been tremendous population growth, particularly since 1945. See Figure 2–2. A breakdown of the population reflects an increase in the number of elderly in both populations. In 1979, it was estimated that the total number of people in the United States over age 65 was 24 million, comprising 11% of the population (U.S. DHEW 1979:71). By the year 2030 it is estimated that there will be an increase to 50 million, or 17% of the population (U.S. DHEW 1979:71). In Canada a similar increase in the number of older people is anticipated: from 1.9 million in 1976 (Statistics Canada 1980:10) to 3.2 million by the year 2000.

Figure 2–2 Increases in population in the United States, 1900–1980, and Canada, 1901–1981. (From U.S. Department of Commerce, Bureau of the Census, *Population profile of the United States: 1980*, Series P, no. 363 [Washington, D.C.: Government Printing Office, June 1981], p. 9, and Statistics Canada, *Census of Canada* [Ottawa: Minister of Supplies and Services, 1981], p. 6.)

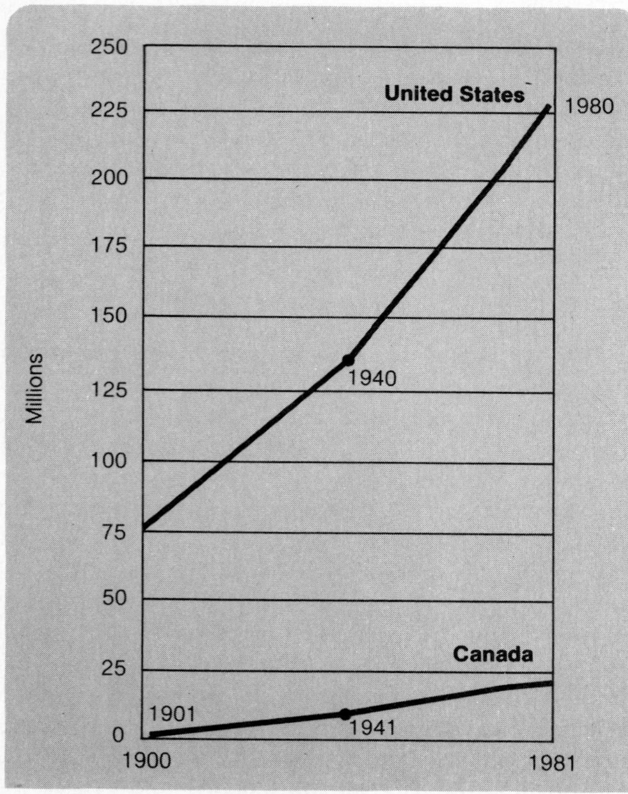

Increased life expectancy is largely due to the success with which many acute diseases are treated today. Reasons for the longer life span of women are multiple. Authorities believe that females have a biologic advantage, which requires more research to explain. Other factors contributing to increased relative longevity for women are the lower maternal death rate and the higher rate of cardiovascular-renal diseases in men. Two other factors affecting the male-to-female population balance are higher accident rates among males and the successful detection and treatment programs for breast and uterine cancer in women. Programs for lung cancer in men have been less successful. Although chronic diseases (those persisting over a long time) can affect people in all age groups, the elderly show the highest incidence of these conditions. Eighty percent of older people have one or more chronic conditions (DHEW 1979:71). Together with their dependence needs, the elderly require financial, housing, and health care assistance in ever-increasing numbers. Within this elderly group, the ratio in the United States is 100 women to 76 men in the over-65 age group (Somers 1971:16). In Canada in 1980 the life expectancy at birth for males was 76 years and for females 78 years, compared to 69.5 years for males and 77.1 years for females in 1974 (Canada Department of National Health and Welfare 1980:100, 1976:58).

In both the United States and Canada the very young require the most health services after the elderly. The very young make up a sizable proportion of the population. In the United States in 1973, there were about 52 million children under the age of 15, or nearly 24.4% of the population (DHEW, 1978:2). In Canada in 1975, there were about 6 million (25% of the population) under the age of 15 (United Nations 1976), a drop from 34% in 1961 (Statistics Canada 1980:10).

Mortality

Mortality means death, and mortality statistics are stated as a ratio of the population. The mortality rate of North American infants is falling, but the rate is still high for industrialized countries. In the United States in 1977, 14 of every 1000 babies died within the first 6 days of life (U.S. DHEW 1979:3). In Sweden the infant mortality rate is 9 per 1000.

The major causes of death in infants during the first 6 days of life are immaturity (low birth weights) and birth-associated events, such as lack of oxygen. Among infants 1 year and younger, the four most important causes of death are congenital malformations, sudden infant deaths, influenza and pneumonia, and accidents. Accidents cause most deaths among children 1 to 4 years of age. Among children 4 to 14 years of age, deaths are rare. However, the death rate increases again in people 15 to 24, with accidents and homicides as the major causes of death. In people older than 24 years, cardiovascular-renal disease and malignant neoplasms are the major causes of death. The major causes of death in the general population are shown in Table 2–1.

In Canada, diseases of the circulatory system and neoplasms together accounted for 117,893 deaths, or 70% of the total mortality in 1977. See Table 2–2.

Morbidity

Morbidity means illness; the morbidity rate is the ratio of sick to well people in a population. Morbidity statistics are more difficult to obtain than mortality statistics. One source of morbidity data is the number of days patients spend in hospitals. Of course, these data are not definitive because the majority of sick people do not require hospitalization. Public health agencies are another source of morbidity statistics, but these too are incomplete because only certain contagious diseases are reported to the agencies.

Morbidity statistics derived from patient hospital-days in Canada reflect the following disease distribu-

Table 2–1 Leading Causes of Death in the United States by Age Groups, 1976

Age	Cause	Approximate numbers
0–1 year	Immaturity-associated	11 per 1,000
	Birth-associated	7 per 1,000
	Congenital birth defects	4 per 1,000
	Sudden infant deaths	3 per 1,000
	Influenza and pneumonia	2 per 1,000
1–14 years	Accidents other than motor vehicle	25 per 100,000
	Motor vehicle accidents	19 per 100,000
	Cancer	9 per 100,000
	Birth defects	9 per 100,000
	Influenza and pneumonia	4 per 100,000
	Homicide	4 per 100,000
15–24 years	Motor vehicle accidents	69 per 100,000
	Homicide	50 per 100,000
	Accidents other than motor vehicle	40 per 100,000
	Suicide	24 per 100,000
	Cancer	11 per 100,000
	Heart disease	6 per 100,000
25–64 years	Heart disease	380 per 100,000
	Cancer	320 per 100,000
	Stroke	80 per 100,000
	Cirrhosis of liver	60 per 100,000
	Homicide	60 per 100,000
	Accidents other than motor vehicle	55 per 100,000
	Motor vehicle accidents	50 per 100,000
65 years and over	Heart disease	4,500 per 100,000
	Cancer	2,000 per 100,000
	Stroke	1,500 per 100,000
	Influenza and pneumonia	400 per 100,000
	Diabetes mellitus	250 per 100,000
	Arteriosclerosis	200 per 100,000

From U.S. Department of Health, Education, and Welfare, Public Health Service, Office of the Assistant Secretary for Health and Surgeon General, *Healthy people: The surgeon general's report on health promotion and disease prevention* (DHEW (PHS) Publication no. 79-55071) (Washington, D.C.: Government Printing Office, 1979).

Table 2–2 Major Causes of Death in Canada, All Ages, 1977

Cause of death	Total
Diseases of the circulatory system	81,474
Neoplasms	36,419
Accidents, poisonings, and violence	16,001
Diseases of the respiratory system	10,833
Diseases of the digestive system	6,130
Endocrine, nutritional, and metabolic diseases	3,719
Symptoms and ill-defined conditions	2,201
Diseases of the genitourinary system	1,976
Certain causes of perinatal mortality	1,956
Diseases of the nervous system and sense organs	1,809
Congenital anomalies	1,585
Other causes	3,395
Total, all causes	167,498

From Statistics Canada, Causes of death, in *Perspectives in Canada III* (Catalogue no. 84–203) (Ottawa: Minister of Supplies and Services, 1980), p. 68.

tion: Heart disease accounted for 9.2% of all causes of hospitalization; accidents, 7.8%; respiratory diseases, 7.4%; cerebrovascular disease, 7.2%; and mental disorders, 6.9%. Some major causes of morbidity in Canada, however, are not reflected in hospital-day statistics. Among these causes are alcoholism, sexually transmitted disease, dental disease, and psychologic disorders (Statistics Canada 1980:62). See Table 2–3.

Morbidity statistics do not reveal health problems related to age and development that the nurse needs to consider. These problems are discussed in Chapters 11 and 12. For example, children face developmental problems such as learning difficulties, behavioral disturbances, speech problems, and vision problems. Common problems of the adolescent include premarital pregnancy, abuse of alcohol and drugs, sexually transmitted disease, and mental illness.

Trends and Needs

It is possible to assess health statistics and to summarize some significant health trends and needs in the United States and Canada.

Trends

1. A high infant mortality rate, especially among nonwhite babies. In the United States, the black infant mortality rate is twice as high as the white rate, and the overall mortality rate is higher than in Sweden and Japan (U.S. DHEW 1979:23).
2. A high accident mortality rate among children ages 1 to 14. The United States rate is higher than the rates in Sweden and England.
3. A decline in the incidence of acute contagious disease.
4. An increase in mortality rates of teenagers due to homicides, motor vehicle accidents, and suicide.
5. An increase in use of alcohol and drugs.
6. A recent increase in premarital pregnancies and sexually transmitted disease among adolescents.
7. An increase in the death rate from chronic diseases, such as heart disease.
8. An increase in the death rate from lung cancer.

Needs

1. Improvement of maternal prenatal care to reduce factors contributing to low birth weight, such as inadequate nutrition, smoking, and alcohol consumption.
2. Early identification of problems that cause lack of oxygen to the fetus during labor and delivery, or prompt management of such problems when they do occur.
3. Early detection of developmental disorders in infants and children.
4. Prevention of childhood accidents and injuries.
5. Maintenance of immunization programs to prevent infectious diseases.
6. Promotion of measures to ensure optimal childhood development.
7. Improvement in the health, the physical, psychologic, and social attitudes, and the health habits of adolescents and young adults to prevent their later susceptibility to chronic diseases.
8. Education to help youths acquire skills and information needed to prevent pregnancy, alcohol and drug abuse, and sexually transmitted disease.
9. Improvement in life-styles of individuals to help them avoid major risk factors responsible for disease.
10. Improved screening programs to assist in the early identification of disease.

Models Used in the Health Professions

A *model* is "a symbolic depiction in logical terms of an idealized relatively simple situation showing the structure of the original system" (Hazzard and Kergin 1971:392). It is a conceptual representation of reality (Riehl and Roy 1980:6). A model, then, is not reality, just as a model airplane is not a real airplane but

Table 2–3 Patient-Days by Major Causes of Illness in Canada, 1976

Disease	Total days	Percentage of total, all causes
Heart disease	3,647,913	9.2
Accidents	3,081,365	7.8
Cerebrovascular disease	2,870,542	7.2
Respiratory diseases	2,932,022	7.4
Mental disorders	2,722,346	6.9
All deliveries	2,097,018	5.3
Diseases of the nervous system	1,977,629	5.0
Diseases of the musculoskeletal system	1,795,955	4.5
Arteriosclerotic diseases	1,145,382	2.9
Symptoms, senility, and ill-defined conditions	1,075,411	2.7
Other diseases of breast and female genitalia	909,239	2.3
Infections of kidney and urinary system	851,413	2.1
Infectious diseases	849,217	2.1
Diabetes	761,218	1.9
Other causes	12,902,630	32.6
Total, all causes	36,619,300	100.0

From Statistics Canada, *Perspectives in Canada III* (Ottawa: Minister of Supplies and Services, 1980), p. 62.

represents many aspects of an airplane. Many disciplines have models, which identify the essential concepts of the particular field. Models are based on assumptions and values of the discipline.

Nursing practice has traditionally borrowed and used models from other disciplines. It is only within the last 15 years that nurses have started to develop their own models of nursing, using nursing theory rather than theory from other disciplines. Nurses, however, do work with personnel from other disciplines. To work effectively with other professionals, nurses should understand other models as well as nursing models.

Medical Model

The medical model used by physicians views health and illness as organic phenomena. Emphasis is placed on disorders in the structure and function of the body (Phillips 1977:5). This is a disease-oriented approach to the patient; it is concerned with pathophysiology, biochemistry, and so on. Mental disorders are also considered illnesses.

Psychologic Model

The model used by psychologists represents normal growth and development and the defects that occur during the maturation process. Emphasis is placed on disruptions in the individual's development. Certain feelings and conduct are considered undesirable. The psychologic model does not deal with the relationship between humans and the environment.

Ecologic (Public Health) Model

In the ecologic, or public health, model, disease is considered to be caused by multiple factors both inside and outside the individual. (*Ecology* is the study of people's relationship to the environment.) The ecologic model is the basis of the concept of prevention.

Social Model

The social model is based on the assumption that social behavior is primarily the consequence of cultural variables that impinge on individuals (Phillips 1977:6).

Nursing Models

There are a number of nursing models accepted for use in nursing today. Some of these (Peplau Developmental Model, Systems-in-Change Model) are based on theories of growth. Others—such as the Betty Newman Health Care System Model, the Roy Adaptation Model, the Johnson Behavioral System Model, Orem's Self-Care Concept, and the Rogers Conceptual System for Unitary Man and Environment—are based on systems models. See the section on systems theory next in this chapter. There are also interaction models, such as the Riehl Interaction Model. See Chapter 1 for additional information on nursing models.

Systems Theory

Systems theory is being used increasingly by nurses as a way of understanding not only the systems within a person's body but families, communities, and nursing and health care. General systems theory provides a way of examining interrelationships and deriving principles. A *system* is a set of identifiable parts or components. The *boundary* of a system is the line that differentiates the parts of the system from parts external to the system. A *theory* is a scientifically acceptable general principle that governs practice or is proposed to explain observed facts. Four characteristics of all systems are:

1. *All components of a system are interrelated.* All components work together. If health care is the system, then nursing and medicine are components. The work of all health professions must be viewed as a unit, just as the body (a system) is seen as a whole and not a collection of disparate organs.

2. *A system responds as a whole (holistically) to changes of one of its parts.* When one aspect of a system changes, the entire system is affected. When nursing—a component of the health care delivery system—is changed, then the entire health care delivery system is affected. Similarly, when a person has a tumor of the liver, the individual as a whole is affected, that is, he or she may be nauseated, tired, anxious, etc.

3. *Each system is part of a larger system.* In the health care delivery system, nursing, medicine, etc., are subsystems. An individual is a subsystem of a larger system, the family. The larger system, immediately above the focal system, is called the *suprasystem.* If health care delivery on a state level is the focal system, then health care delivery on a federal level is the suprasystem.

4. *Because systems are interrelated the boundaries between systems are set as of a given time and may be set differently at another time.* The boundaries are set according to the purposes of the people working in the system at a particular time. At one particular time, a health care delivery system could include nursing, medicine, social work, and clients and their families. At another time, for instance, during a research study, the same system might include only medicine and nursing. During surgery, a physician and a nurse may view the kidney as a system even though in a larger context the kidney is a subsystem of the urinary system.

There are two general types of systems: closed and open. A *closed system* does not exchange energy or matter with its environment. Conventional physics and chemistry are limited to processes in a closed system. Therefore a closed system is in a static or steady state. The components of the system always remain in the system. An *open system* exchanges matter, energy, and information with the environment. All living systems, such as individuals, families, and communities, are open systems.

An open system depends on the quality and quantity of its input, output, and feedback for its functioning. *Input* consists of information, material, or energy that enters the system. After the input is absorbed by the system, it is processed in a way useful to the system. This process of transformation is called *throughput.* For example, in the digestive system, food is input; it is digested (throughput) so that it can be used by the body.

Output from a system is energy, matter, or information disposed of by the system as a result of its processes. Output from the digestive system is feces and caloric energy.

Feedback is a process that enables a system to regulate itself. Feedback gives the system the ability to control its input and output. For example, if a thirsty person drinks a glass of juice, feedback should indicate that the thirst was satisfied or unsatisfied. Feedback, which can be thought of in the context of outcome, is used to increase or decrease the system's equilibrium. With feedback, output from the system returns to the system, thus forming a feedback loop. Two types of feedback are positive and negative. Positive feedback signals change within the system, while negative feedback signals equilibrium or steadiness in the system. In this context, these two terms signify the opposite of their ordinary meanings. An example of positive feedback is pain and pallor in a postoperative patient following a position change. This feedback enables the nurse to reevaluate the appropriateness of the position, perhaps change the position, and report the feedback so the physician can relate it to the surgery and the patient's diagnosis.

For information on adaptation theory, see Chapter 9; for developmental theory, see Chapters 11 and 12; and for interaction theory, see Chapter 15.

Health Care Delivery System

Restorative and Preventive Care

The health care delivery system in North America provides two general types of services: illness care services (restorative) and health care services (preventive). Illness care services help the ill or injured. Health care services promote better health and help prevent disease and accidents. Although most facilities within the system—for example, hospitals, clinics, and physicians' offices—provide both types of services, illness care services predominate. In recent years, however, there has been increased awareness of the need to promote health and to prevent disease. Considerable emphasis has been placed on the role of the nurse in prevention. Often the community nurse's major thrust is to promote wellness and prevent illness, for example, through parent and child counseling.

In the past, health care facilities have been influenced largely by the needs of the people providing the service. For example, hospitals have developed in relation to medical and technologic advances and generally reflect the needs of physicians. Also, the public viewed health care facilities as sources of help primarily for the ill or injured. As a result, preventive health care facilities have been slow to develop. This delay can be attributed in great part to three factors:

1. Physicians are largely oriented to illness in their practice.
2. Consumers are more aware of treatment of illness than of prevention and health promotion.
3. The nurse's role as the chief provider of preventive health care has been slow to evolve, and frequently the treatment of illness takes precedence over preventive health care activities.

However, the cost of hospitalization and the disruption it causes in the lives of patients have given impetus to health promotion programs. For additional information, see the section on nurses' responsibilities for health in this chapter.

Comprehensive Health and Illness Care

Comprehensive health and illness care services encompass four areas: health promotion, prevention of disease and injury, diagnosis and treatment of disease and injury, and rehabilitation. None of these services is necessarily independent of the others; frequently they operate at the same time and overlap in their effects. For example, a patient receiving a diagnostic test, such as a chest radiograph for tuberculosis, might also be acquiring knowledge that will help him or her prevent disease; or a patient who is receiving iron pills to restore the blood's hemoglobin level may at the same time learn to prevent the problem through proper diet.

The concept of total health includes both physical and mental health. *Physical* (*somatic*) health refers to the body, whereas *mental* health refers to the mind as distinct from the body. *Psychosomatic*, also referred to as *somatopsychophysiologic*, refers to the interrelationship of mind and body; for example, emotional problems can be the cause of physical symptoms such as a headache.

Health promotion

Health promotion is one of the fastest growing areas of the health care system. As people become increasingly aware of good health and as diseases are conquered, more and more emphasis will be placed on this area. At present, health promotion is the major function of community nurses and community health workers generally. Programs in health promotion are directed toward five major areas: (a) maternal and child health, (b) mental health, (c) environmental health (physical fitness), (d) nutrition, and (e) dental health.

Prevention of disease and injury

Prevention of infectious disease has long been emphasized. It is a major nursing function. The longer life expectancy and lowered mortality figures of the 19th and early 20th centuries can be almost completely attributed to effective preventive programs against diphtheria, smallpox, typhus, typhoid fever, and tuberculosis. More recently there have been effective preventive programs against poliomyelitis.

Prevention is moving beyond its traditional focus on infectious diseases. Research is underway to prevent long-term diseases such as cardiovascular diseases. On national, state (provincial), and local levels, prevention programs in recent years have been aimed at combating and publicizing, through the news media, the dangers of tobacco, alcohol, and drug use.

Today, there are four major kinds of prevention programs:

1. Crisis programs to prevent mental health problems on an individual and family basis
2. Early detection programs for such chronic diseases as cardiovascular diseases
3. Safety programs aimed at preventing industrial and automobile accidents
4. Environmental programs to prevent pollution and destruction of the environment (water, air, forests, natural life)

Preventive health programs are often carried out by nurses and are generally oriented to the family and the community. The individual approach, typified by immunization programs to control infectious diseases, is still used and is still essential; however, the broader approach is being utilized increasingly to assist more people to prevent disease and injury.

The World Health Organization describes an increased-risk stage as the time when preventive measures can be taken to protect an individual who for some reason is particularly susceptible to disease. An example is the administration of tetanus antitoxin to a person who has a contaminated wound.

Diagnosis and treatment of disease and injury

The diagnosis and treatment of disease and injury have long occupied the leading position in health care service. Essentially, this area is the prerogative of the physician, and patients usually seek help at their own initiative. See the description of the medical model in this chapter.

In addition, there are diagnosis and treatment programs on a broad basis. Communitywide programs are now conducted to detect tuberculosis, sexually transmitted disease, cancer, hypertension, glaucoma, sickle cell anemia, and diabetes. Advertising stresses what symptoms to look for and the importance of consulting a physician. Mobile units visit local communities and offer several services, usually free of charge. Early detection is emphasized together with appropriate treatment.

During the early detection stage, the initial symptoms of disease appear. At this stage, detection and appropriate treatment can often prevent more serious problems; for example, early diagnosis and treatment of a breast growth is usually successful.

Rehabilitation

The concept of rehabilitation has gained considerable acceptance during the past 20 years. Before that time it was generally associated with vocational help and social guidance for people who had physical injuries, often as a result of accidents at work. Today, the concept is applied to all illness (physical and mental) and to injury. Rehabilitation affects every age group and segment of society. A contemporary definition of *rehabilitation* is "the restoration through personal health services of handicapped individuals to the fullest physical, mental and social and economic usefulness of which they are capable, including ordinary treatments and treatments in special rehabilitation centres" (Krusen 1964:1). Rehabilitation, then, is a process of restoring people to their previous level of health—that is, to their previous capabilities—or to the level that is possible for them. Rehabilitation, as distinct from maintenance, is an active concept and can be considered largely an educational function. Patients must actively participate in the process if it is to be effective.

The rehabilitation process involves the patient and a team of health personnel who have various specialized skills. A physician, often a specialist in rehabilitation medicine, usually heads the team; this physician is referred to as a *physiatrist.* A nurse, a social worker, an occupational therapist, a physical therapist, and sometimes a psychiatrist and a speech therapist form part of the rehabilitation team. These people, together with the patient and often the family and support persons, plan a program to help the patient achieve maximum use of capabilities.

Rehabilitation programs usually take place in independent centers in the community or in special units in hospitals. However, rehabilitation really starts the moment a patient enters the health care system. Thus, nurses are involved in rehabilitation whether they are employed on pediatric, psychiatric, or surgical units of hospitals or in the community. A rehabilitation process usually has four broad objectives:

1. To return affected abilities to the highest possible level of function
2. To prevent further disability
3. To protect the patient's present abilities
4. To assist the patient to use abilities

Rehabilitation is frequently a long process, and the need for programs and facilities is steadily increasing. The growing incidence of chronic disease and disability and the increasingly large groups of elderly persons in North American society mean an increased need for rehabilitation.

The success of any rehabilitation program depends largely on the individual's motivation to learn, his or her life-style before and after the illness, and the support of significant others. It is important that the disabled person be viewed as a total person, and not just in relation to the disability. The number of specialized health team members required varies from patient to patient. It is important for the success of any rehabilitation plan that the patient be able to see his or her own progress. Usually a plan of therapy and a record of progress are available, so the patient is encouraged to be an active, motivated participant in the planning and the program.

The nurse's function in a rehabilitation program is primarily (a) to prevent complications as a result of the deficit, (b) to limit the deficit as much as possible, and (c) to plan and implement the rehabilitation program. Specific nursing interventions that may be included in a rehabilitation program are bowel and bladder training, bathing and skin care, training in walking with special supports, and providing special fluid and diet requirements. These are discussed in subsequent chapters.

Often rehabilitation programs extend from a hospital or special rehabilitation setting into the home. Nurses from community agencies may help the patient and family continue a program and make the initial adjustments to living at home. Sometimes patients and their families join support groups of others with similar problems. There are organizations for people who have had strokes, "ostomies," emotional problems, and diseases such as multiple sclerosis. Peer support and social interaction through such groups help people learn new skills and adjust to handicaps.

Health Care Agencies

A wide variety of facilities and agencies provide illness and health care in the average community. Some of these are:

1. Physician's offices
2. Hospitals
3. Day-care centers
4. Nursing homes (personal care homes)
5. Residential institutions
6. Home care programs
7. Rehabilitation centers
8. Community health clinics
9. Health maintenance organizations and community health centers
10. Government agencies
11. Voluntary agencies
12. Special programs
13. Hospice services

Physicians' offices

The physician's office is one of the major sources of illness care in North America. The majority of physicians either have their own offices or work with several other physicians in a group practice. People usually go to a physician because they consider themselves ill, because a relative thinks the patient is ill, or because the patient feels the need of medical advice.

The physician with an office practice is oriented chiefly to illness. The average time the physician spends with a patient in an office visit is very short—6.1 minutes according to one study (Somers 1971:9). In this time the physician is concerned mainly with the diagnosis and therapy pertaining to the patient's immediate illness or injury.

Hospitals

Hospitals are the institutions through which restorative care to the ill and injured traditionally has been provided. They vary in size from the 12-bed rural hospital to the 1500-bed metropolitan hospital with a 50-bed day surgery center. Hospitals can be classified according to their ownership or control as governmental (public) and nongovernmental (private). Governmental hospitals are either federal, state, city, or county hospitals in the United States and federal or provincial hospitals in Canada. In both countries governments have traditionally provided hospital facilities for veterans, merchant mariners, and individuals with long-term illness. The United States government provides approximately 70% of the hospital beds in the country. Nongovernmental or private hospitals are generally owned or controlled by churches, industry, private groups of physicians or citizens, or fraternal orders.

Hospitals also are classified by the services they provide. General hospitals admit patients requiring a variety of facilities, including medical, surgical, obstetric, pediatric, and psychiatric services. Other hospitals offer only specialty services such as psychiatric or pediatric care.

Although hospitals are chiefly viewed as institutions that provide care, they have other functions, such as providing resources for health-related research and teaching. Hospital personnel may conduct research and educational programs, or they may provide resources for such personnel as university teachers to carry out research and teaching responsibilities.

Hospitals can be further described as acute or chronic. An acute hospital provides assistance to patients who are acutely ill or whose illness and need for hospitalization are relatively short-term, for example, a 1-day to perhaps 1-month stay. Long-term hospitals provide health services for longer periods, sometimes for years or the remainder of the patient's life.

The traditional organization within a hospital has been departmental. Departments such as medical, nursing, dietary, laboratory, maintenance, pharmacy, and purchasing carry out their functions, which may be directly or indirectly related to patient care. One of the limitations of this organizational pattern is the isolation of each department and subsequent discrepancies in personnel utilization and efficiency.

A more recent organizational structure for hospitals is the arrangement of the departments into systems and programs, each of which has a common characteristic. The systems provide a commonality among diverse functions; for example, the business system includes the functions of the business office, the accounting office, and the payroll office. Some or all of these might be separate departments in more traditional hospitals. The programs are the means of coordinating the resources of the various systems into care, teaching, and research functions. For example, in an ambulatory care program for patients, assistance is received from the four systems of business, quality control, patient care, and professional services in this manner:

1. The business system collects fees.
2. The quality control system establishes medical records.
3. The patient care system supplies nursing personnel and social services.
4. The professional service system provides physicians' services.

With the expansion of knowledge and skills in the health field, and with increasing costs, flexible organizational patterns are seen as a means of providing a diversity of services efficiently and effectively.

Day-care centers

Day-care centers either are attached to hospitals or operate independently to provide health services during daytime hours. Often these agencies provide a specific service. For example, the community mental health center cares for patients who have emotional problems but who do not require hospitalization, and day surgery centers provide surgical services for patients who do not require overnight hospitalization. The latter admit children or adults who require minor surgery (often in a hospital) in the morning. After the surgery, the patient returns to the center where members of the family often assist with care. The patient returns home the same day. These centers have two advantages: They permit the patient to continue to live at home while obtaining needed health care, and they free costly hospital beds for seriously ill patients.

Figure 2–3 Home nursing services provide assistance to an individual who is learning to use a walker.

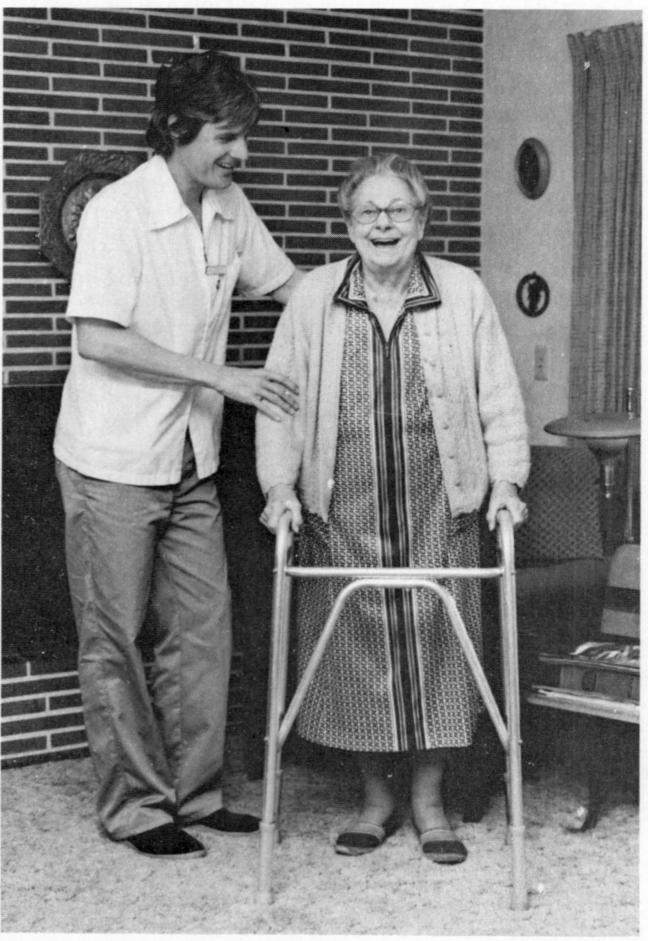

Nursing homes (personal care homes)

Many nursing homes are owned privately by individuals or groups of individuals, for example, physicians or ethnic groups, but some are publicly owned. A wide variety of institutions can be called nursing homes, and they offer a considerable variety of services. Generally, they provide long-term care, in contrast to the community hospital. Because long-term illness occurs most often in the elderly, many nursing homes have programs that are oriented to the needs of this age group.

Nursing homes are intended for people who require not only personal services (such as assistance in bathing and dressing, and meal preparation) but also some regular nursing care and occasional medical attention. However, the type of care provided to the patients varies considerably. Some homes admit and retain only residents who can dress themselves and are ambulatory. Other homes provide bed care for patients who are more incapacitated. Nursing homes can, in effect, become the patients' home, and consequently the people who live there are frequently referred to as residents rather than patients.

Residential institutions

A variety of other residential institutions provide primarily personal care services but also nursing services in varying degrees. Homes for the aged (rest homes, senior citizens' lodges) provide some nursing services in addition to personal care services. Other institutions provide rehabilitative services for persons with particular health problems, such as the mentally retarded, deaf, blind, and pregnant teenagers. Other facilities, usually called halfway houses and boarding homes, provide therapies for patients with specific problems, such as alcoholism or mental illness. These facilities allow individuals to receive treatment yet live in the community rather than in large institutions.

Home care programs

Home care programs operate out of hospitals and community agencies. In both instances a variety of nursing services can be provided to patients and to families. See Figure 2–3. Some of these services are well-baby visits to new parents to assist with initial care of the baby; bedside nursing for the chronically ill; administration of medications, for example, insulin to diabetics; and mental health assistance for patients and families who have emotional problems.

Some hospital-organized home care programs provide the services of a variety of health workers: physicians, nurses, social workers, therapists, and nutritionists. In addition, it is often necessary to provide services that enable people to maintain themselves at home. For example, the Meals-on-Wheels program provides prepared meals as required, and homemaker programs assist with household management.

As a complement to these home care programs, there are now laboratory visiting services in some metropolitan areas. Through this service, patients who are confined to their homes can have specimens taken and submitted to a laboratory for analysis.

Rehabilitation centers

Rehabilitation centers often exist as departments within hospitals and provide services to patients admitted to the hospital and to patients who come to the center on an appointment basis. Some rehabilitation centers also exist as separate health agencies with inpatient, outpatient, and home visiting services. These centers often combine the services of physical therapists, occupational therapists, social workers, and nursing personnel. Specialists such as speech and recreational therapists and vocational counselors may also be on the staff of a center. See the section on rehabilitation in this chapter.

Community health clinics

Many community agencies provide medical, dental, nursing, counseling, legal, and other social services. Some of these clinics are staffed by volunteers and tend to be relatively informal. They often provide services to students, transient youths, and minority and low-income groups. Usually services are available free of charge or for a minimal fee.

Other, more formal clinics are staffed by a physician and other health care workers—nurses, nutritionists, dentists, dental hygienists, public health inspectors, and physiotherapists. Nurses provide such services as immunization, screening (e.g., testing for hearing and vision defects), and home or school visits to provide counseling and health education.

Health maintenance organizations and community health centers

The term *health maintenance organization* (HMO) became popular in the United States in the early 1970s. It is not used in Canada, but in the early 1970s Canadians also expressed interest in establishing a network of community health centers (CHCs). Both organizations are designed to provide continuous primary health care—including preventive, diagnostic, curative, and rehabilitation services—to individuals and families. Their goals are to provide quality health care economically and to prevent illness. See the discussion of health maintenance organizations on page 65.

Government agencies

Government agencies are established at the local, state (provincial), and federal levels. Local health departments (county, bicounty, or tricounty) traditionally have responsibility for (a) developing programs that are responsive to the health needs of the people, (b) providing the necessary staff and facilities to carry out these programs, and (c) continually evaluating the effectiveness of the programs and monitoring changing needs. State health organizations (approximately 60 different organizations) are responsible for assisting the local health departments. In some remote areas, state departments also provide direct services to people.

The Public Health Service (PHS) of the United States Department of Health and Human Services is an official agency at the federal level. Its functions include:

1. Research and training in the health field
2. Assistance to communities in planning and developing health facilities
3. Assistance to states and local communities through financing and provision of trained personnel

The federal governments in both the United States and Canada maintain responsibility for the health of seamen and for health matters related to interstate and interprovincial transportation. Otherwise, health legislation is generally the responsibility of states in the United States and of the provinces in Canada.

Voluntary agencies

Voluntary health service agencies are supported by the people in a community. Examples are the National Heart Associations and Visiting Nurse Services (Associations). They are nonprofit organizations that rely on donations and, in some cases, on government grants for support. They are usually formed by volunteers in response to a specific recognized need, such as day care for the mentally retarded. Often they supplement official agencies' functions. Some voluntary agencies are oriented to the care of special groups in the community, others to special programs, such as pollution control.

Once a voluntary agency has pointed out a need in a community, an official agency may take over some of the voluntary agency's functions. For example, the American Cancer Society originally funded treatment for cancer, but its treatment functions were taken over by official government agencies, such as hospitals, and the cancer society retained its nontreatment functions, such as fund raising.

Special programs

Several special programs deal with particular health problems. These programs are operated and financed by various agencies, including governments. Examples are alcohol and drug abuse programs and cancer programs.

Hospice services

A *hospice*, traditionally, was a place where travelers could rest. Recently, the term has come to mean a health care facility for the dying. The *hospice movement* subsumes a variety of services given to the terminally ill, their families, and support persons. The movement sprang initially from dissatisfaction with the preoccupation of health personnel with technologic care and insufficient emphasis on caring and psychologic support. In the 1970s, the movement gained momentum. It derived impetus from new attitudes toward death and from the work of such people as Elisabeth Kübler-Ross, whose books challenged prevailing attitudes, and Cicely Saunders, founder of St. Christopher's Hospice in London. Saunders believed that the physical and social environments of dying people are as important as medical interventions on their behalf.

Currently there are five forms of hospice services (Wald 1980:174):

1. Home care services
2. Hospice teams in hospitals
3. Palliative care units in hospitals
4. Hospices with hospital affiliations
5. Autonomous hospices

Hospices are a haven for the dying because they emphasize the needs of the individual and help patients and their families plan for death. The central concept of the hospice movement, as distinct from the acute care model, is not saving life but improving or maintaining the quality of life until death. Important in this care are *palliative* measures, measures whose aim is relief rather than cure. Comfort and relief from pain are frequently the most important needs of the dying. Hospice care addresses the needs of the mind and the spirit as well: It is truly holistic.

Problems in the Delivery System

Currently there are a number of problems in the health-illness care system in North America. Many of the problems stem, at least partially, from the enormous changes in health-illness care during the past 30 years. Major advances in medicine and technology have meant better care for many. With this improved care, however, have come such problems as fragmentation of care, high costs of health-illness service, and outdated knowledge and skills of some practitioners in the health field.

Other problems have always existed with health-illness delivery systems and are present today. Some of these are unmet needs of the poor for care; unmet needs of minority groups for particular assistance; unmet needs of the illiterate, semiliterate, and poorly educated for information and knowledge; and unmet needs of the elderly. Another problem is uneven national distribution of health-illness services, so that limited resources are available in rural and inner-city areas, while more services are available in urban and suburban areas. The consumer is becoming more aware of these problems and is exerting increasing pressure to have them corrected, but corrections are gradual and must accommodate to economic and political realities.

Fragmentation of Care

Highly specialized techniques and new knowledge emerging during the past 30 years of research mean that an increasing number of health workers provide specialized services. They may be highly specialized technicians or technologists who have relatively narrow but exacting jobs, such as respiratory technologists, biomedical electronic technologists, and nuclear medicine technologists. Increased specialization is evident also among physicians. The number of physicians practicing primary care dropped from 56,852 in 1968 to 51,029 in 1974 (DHEW 1978:28). All this specialization means fragmentation of care and sometimes less than desirable total care. To patients, it may mean receiving care from 5 to 30 people during their hospital experience. This seemingly endless stream of personnel is often confusing and frightening. The patient feels like a cog in the wheel and asks, "Who really cares about me?" and "Who is really responsible?" The increasing number of health workers creates problems with the smooth flow of information and plans to help the patient. Again, the patient wonders, "Will someone forget to order my medication?" "Will someone help me get my meals when I return home from the hospital?" The concept of total care is more difficult to implement when so many people are involved.

Increased Cost of Services

The problem of financing health-illness services is increasingly severe. There are six major reasons for increased costs:

1. Existing equipment and facilities are continually becoming obsolete as research uncovers new and better methods in health-illness care.
2. Additional space and sophisticated equipment are required to provide the newest diagnostic and treatment methods.
3. Inflation increases all costs.
4. The total population has grown, and the demand for services has increased.
5. People increasingly recognize that health is a right of *all* people, hence larger numbers of people are seeking assistance in health matters.
6. The relative number of people who provide health-illness services has increased.

Health care costs have increased greatly in recent years. The cost of care for people who cannot afford health care, e.g., the poor and the aged, increased substantially from 1965 to 1978 (Enthoven 1980:15). In 1976, it was estimated that 92 to 95% of the population had some type of health insurance (ibid., p. 17); 5 to 8% had no insurance (ibid., p. xvi). See the section on financing health and illness services later in this chapter.

Outdated Knowledge and Skills

With the many discoveries in the health field, graduates rapidly become out of date in their skills unless they follow continuing education programs. Many professional groups are aware of this problem and are taking steps to require that practitioners be current and show evidence of updating their skills as a condition of licensing. In some states (e.g., Florida), continuing education units (CEUs) are mandatory for nursing licensure.

Needs of Ethnic and Poverty Groups

There is a cultural lag in the provision of health-illness services to ethnic groups within the community. The more sophisticated and impersonal health services become, the further they are removed from groups who are inwardly oriented and have a strong family tradition. These groups tend to rely on the private physician. They prefer the personalized care of someone who understands them and their families. Many such people look on the modern health care system with distrust.

Some people in the United States have no health insurance coverage. For the very wealthy, health insurance is no problem, but most people without insurance require assistance to maintain their health. Poverty is frequently accompanied by fear and ignorance: fear of what might happen if help were requested and ignorance about how and when to obtain health care. Quasi practitioners are sometimes sought by these groups in lieu of scientifically oriented health practitioners. Quasi practitioners are nonmedical healers who use a wide variety of methods that are not validated by scientific means. Among them are the faith healers, the magical healers, and the practitioners of folk medicine. Examples of the latter are the Hispanic *medicastro* (quack) and *curandero* (healer, medicine man) of the southwestern United States. There is little question that these groups meet some needs of people; however, the danger is that while people are being treated by them, diseases that could possibly be cured by medical and nursing care will become incurable. The emotional appeal of quasi practitioners is not restricted to the lower socioeconomic groups. Their appeal is broad, but they are less accepted by people who have some scientific education.

Special Needs of the Elderly

Because people over 65 are becoming an increasingly large group in the population, their health needs deserve special concern. Long-term illnesses are most prevalent in this group, and with these illnesses frequently come special needs for housing, treatment services, and financial support. The elderly need to feel they are still part of a community even though they are approaching the end of their lives. Feelings of being useful, wanted, and productive citizens are essential to their health. Special programs are being designed in communities so that many of the talents and skills of this group will be used and not lost to society. These programs—for example, partial employment—are designed especially for the elderly person.

Uneven Distribution of Health Services

Serious problems exist in the distribution in health services in both the United States and Canada. Two facets of this problem are (a) uneven distribution of physicians and (b) increased specialization. Uneven distribution is evidenced by the relatively high ratio of physicians to population in Washington, D.C., (318 per 100,000) and the relatively low ratio in Mississippi (69 per 100,000). Some rural areas in fact have no physicians. The increase in the number of specialists compared to the number of primary practice physicians means fewer primary services. The same problems exist for other health care workers, such as nurses and physiotherapists (Somers 1971:7).

Use of Health and Illness Services

In the United States and Canada more and more people are seeking help for health problems. In 1963, in the United States alone, approximately 65% of the population saw a physician at least once. Of this group over 8% were admitted to hospitals, and half of them had some surgical procedure (Anderson and Andersen 1972:387).

The hospital is the fastest growing part of health services. The admission rate increased from 59 per 1000 population in 1935 to 130 per 1000 population in 1971. Increased use has meant increased cost. With the advent of hospital insurance, more people are now admitted to hospitals; however, the average hospital stay is shorter than before. The shortening of the hospital stay can be explained by the change in the medical concept of care, which encourages early ambulation of patients, as well as by the increase in the number of patients admitted to hospitals with minor conditions. An additional factor in shortening hospital stays is the use of utilization review committees that adhere to criteria for average lengths of stay for patients with various conditions.

Physicians' services are also being called on increasingly. Young people tend to go to the physician because of acute diseases such as upper respiratory infections, and the elderly because of long-term and chronic conditions. The elderly use physicians' services more than any other group.

Preventive health services in the community can be categorized as follows:

1. Primary services, which prevent disease—for example, immunization against diphtheria
2. Secondary services, which check the development of a disease—for example, treatment of a middle ear infection
3. Tertiary services, which manage a disease that is neither curable nor preventable—for example, treatment for diabetes mellitus

An annual physical examination by the physician can be considered a preventive health service. In 1964 a survey indicated that approximately half of the population had had a physical examination within the year. People sought examinations for three major reasons, none of which predominated: The person was experiencing illness symptoms; the examination was required, for example, for a job; and the annual physical was a preventive measure (Anderson and Andersen 1972:396–397).

Financing Health and Illness Services

Health has been described as the fastest growing industry in the United States. The federal governments in both the United States and Canada have increased their budget allocations for health services substantially in recent years.

There are five general types of financing of health illness care:

1. *Voluntary insurance.* Health-illness care costs are covered by private insurance plans. The costs of these insurance plans, such as Blue Shield and Blue Cross, are borne by the individual or shared by the employer and the employee. One type of voluntary health insurance is the prepaid group plan sometimes referred to as a health maintenance organization (HMO). In these plans, participants pay for the services of physicians who participate in the plan and the facilities arranged for in the plan. An example is the Kaiser Permanente Medical Care Program in California and other states. Prepaid group plans provide for services required by the participants 24 hours a day. By advance payment, the individual takes out insurance against any health requirements in the future. These plans place heavy emphasis on promotion of health and prevention of disease and injury among participants.
2. *Social insurance.* Social insurance includes programs, such as Medicare, that provide for the costs of hospitalization; related care is financed through payroll taxes and general taxes. Social insurance covers most people who are over 65. Medicaid, by contrast, provides for the payment of physicians' services and certain health services. Participation in Medicaid is voluntary, and it is primarily designed for the elderly, although, since 1976, people under 65 who are disabled can also

participate. The monthly fee is divided between the person participating and the government. In Canada the government has financed hospital care through taxes since 1957, and physicians' services since 1968.

3. *Industry.* In many settings, industry provides for hospital and/or medical care and related services for employees and families. The rationale is that healthy workers are more productive workers. In North America, industry sometimes provides financial support to hospitals, especially in isolated mining and lumbering centers. When there are hospitals, workers and their families are more likely to be attracted to these centers and to stay there.

4. *Personal payment.* Sometimes patients bear the full expense of health care. Until the last 15 years, this was the major method of payment of hospitalization costs in the United States, and it is still used by some people. At present, personal payment is the major method for financing dental care, medicines, and ambulatory care.

5. *Charitable resources.* Charitable resources for medical payments are supported by donations from individuals or groups and by bequests. Charitable donations are still made by some philanthropic organizations to assist the poor and to support innovations. On the whole, however, charitable donations as a means of paying for health care are declining in importance.

Alternative Health Care Delivery Systems

Concerns about the fragmentation of health care services, lack of accessibility of services, and in particular rising costs have led to proposals about alternative health care delivery systems, often referred to as health maintenance organizations (HMOs) in the United States and community health centers (CHCs) in Canada.

Health Maintenance Organizations

The basic idea of the HMO arose in the 1930s when prepaid health care experiments were sponsored by unions, cooperatives, corporations, municipalities, and other organized groups. HMOs did not become popular, however, until the early 1970s when the Health Maintenance Organization Act was passed in 1973. The act was a response to a proposal made in 1970 by a group near Minneapolis, Paul M. Ellwood and his associates, calling for a national "health maintenance strategy" based on *competing private* comprehensive health care organizations, which they called health maintenance organizations. After the concept was accepted by government, the term *HMO* was broadened to "alternative health care financing and delivery systems" or "alternative delivery systems."

To be federally qualified, an HMO company must meet certain requirements: It must offer physicians' services, hospital and outpatient services, emergency services, short-term mental health services, treatment and referral for drug and alcohol problems, laboratory and radiologic services, preventive dental services for children under 12, and preventive health services.

Principles of alternative delivery systems

There are four major principles defining an alternative delivery system (Enthoven 1980:56–57):

1. *Premiums are paid to an organization that accepts responsibility for providing or arranging comprehensive services.* Premiums, set in advance on the basis of a fixed amount per person per month, must cover all or nearly all of the cost of services provided. Therefore the provider organization has a fixed budget within which it must operate. In comparison, the traditional insured fee-for-service system is organized so that premiums are paid to a financial intermediary, which pays providers of care *after* care has been given and the costs are incurred. In this system, physicians charge separately for each service performed. If more services are given, more costs are incurred. It is thought, therefore, that the traditional system provides incentives for physicians to provide more services (e.g., laboratory tests, x-ray films, technologic procedures) even when such services are of negligible benefit to the patient. The result is more costly care, because neither the providers of care nor the consumers assume responsibility for the cost of services.

2. *The patient accepts a limited choice of doctors that includes only those participating in the system.* In the traditional fee-for-service system, the patient has theoretically "free choice of physicians." However, in reality the patient's choice is limited by many factors, such as the willingness of the physician to accept the patient and the patient's limited knowledge about other physicians. In the alternative delivery system, the patient may choose a physician from those within the organization and can choose to join an HMO in which a favored doctor participates. What is more significant to patients than so-called free choice is that the HMO system is a cost-conscious provider of health care services because such systems are economically competitive.

3. *The provider organization is responsible for a voluntary enrolled population.* This means that the HMO can plan the availability of resources to meet the specific needs of its enrollees. For example, HMOs can emphasize prevention and less costly ways of treating problems. In comparison, the traditional insured fee-for-service system offers no incentive to physicians for effective prevention of medical problems or for treating them in less costly ways. Neither is there a defined or enrolled population to whom the physician gives care. Physicians are responsible only to those they willingly accept as patients.

4. *The provider organization organizes, provides, or arranges for health services in varying degrees.* Thus the organization can exercise management controls over quality of care, costs, location, and other aspects of the delivery of services. In the insured fee-for-service system the intermediary, which pays the bills after the fact, does not organize or manage the services.

The idea of alternative health care delivery systems is therefore based on economic competition: They provide health care at a lower cost. Concern with cost does not remove the responsibility to provide quality service. If one HMO fails to provide quality service, members of the plan can drop it and enroll in another.

Types of alternative delivery systems

There are three types of HMOs: prepared group practices (PGPs), individual practice associations (IPAs), and primary care networks (PCNs). They differ in the way their physicians are organized.

Prepared group practices Prepared group practices are the oldest type of HMO. The PGP contracts with a group of doctors in multiple specialties who work together out of a common facility. The physicians agree to provide comprehensive health care services for a certain fee, fixed in advance, to a defined population of voluntarily enrolled members. Variations exist among PGPs. Physicians may pool their income and distribute it as salaries or on the basis of a per capita payment plus a share of the program's net income. Some PGPs own their own hospitals. Some of the physicians' groups include a broad range of specialists; others are composed of general practitioners, pediatricians, and general internists who emphasize primary care. In the latter, patients are referred to outside specialists, when necessary, at no additional cost.

Many PGPs are sponsored by industrial companies, consumer cooperatives, labor unions, physician partnerships, insurance companies, and universities. The largest PGP system is Kaiser-Permanente Medical Care Program, which had 3.5 million members in seven states in 1978 (Enthoven 1980:58). Other leading PGPs include Ross-Loos in southern California, Group Health Association of Washington, D.C., Group Health Plan of St. Paul, Minnesota, and Group Health Plan of Puget Sound, Seattle, Washington. All of these have operated for more than 30 years.

There is growing evidence that PGPs are effective in reducing the total per capita costs of medical care compared to traditional insured fee-for-service systems. Other advantages of this system include ease of consultation for the consumers (because of the pool of specialty physicians available) and a professional climate that provides for mutual support and the lively exchange of ideas among physicians.

Individual practice associations Individual practice associations are the next most common type of HMO. The IPA consists of a central administrative core that contracts with individual or small groups of physicians to provide service to the HMO's subscribers. The IPA physicians maintain their existing practices in their own offices and are generally reimbursed on a fee-for-service basis. Thus the IPA is often described as a fee-for-service HMO. Generally, a significant majority of a community's physicians participate in an IPA; thus a wide choice of physicians is available to the HMO members. IPA physicians agree on a maximum fee schedule for providing health benefits such as hospital care, laboratory tests, and roentgenography. When the service is rendered to a member of the association, the association, not the member, is billed. The association is also responsible for hospital costs. It either pays hospital costs directly or teams up with an insurance carrier that offers a hospital insurance policy.

Examples of the IPA health delivery system are the San Joaquin Foundation for Medical Care in California, the Physicians Association of Clackamas County in Oregon, Comprecare in Colorado, and Physicians' Health Plan in Minnesota. A major criticism of the IPA plans is that, since the physicians are paid on a fee-for-service basis, they have no knowledge of or incentive to control total per capita costs of services for enrollees.

Primary care networks Primary care networks are comparatively new and small. The PCN is based on the primary care physician, who is a generalist and the "doctor of first contact." Primary care physicians usually include general and family practitioners, general internists, and pediatricians, who can treat most medical problems and direct the patient to appropriate specialists as required. Some plans, however, include specialists.

There is substantial variation among PCN plans. Generally the participating primary care physicians agree to provide all primary care services, arrange referrals, and supervise all other care (by specialists or hospitals) for each enrolled member. With the exception of emergency services, services not ordered by this physician are not covered. The physicians are either paid a negotiated fixed amount (capitation payment) per patient, which varies according to the age and sex of the patient, since medical needs vary by age and sex, or paid on a fee-for-service basis.

To control costs, an account is set up for each participating physician from which all referral service bills are paid. The physician must see and approve every bill prior to payment. Generally, if there is a surplus in the account at the year's end, the physician receives 50%; if there is a deficit the physician pays back 50% within defined limits. In addition, a medical director assisted by a board of participating physicians monitors the use of services, particularly hospitalization.

Examples of PCNs are the Wisconsin Physicians' Service Health Maintenance Program, SAFECO Life Insurance Company of Seattle in California and Washington, the Group Health Plan of Northeast Ohio, and Pennsylvania Blue Shield's Comprehensive Health Care Program. Advantages of PCNs are numerous. For example, the primary care physician (a) is accountable for total health services costs, (b) has an incentive to increase productivity, e.g., by employing nurse practitioners, (c) has an incentive to emphasize prevention of illness, and (d) is the "general manager" of the patient's total medical care.

Community Health Centers

In the early 1970s, considerable interest was expressed in Canada about development of community health centers to facilitate access to health services and reduce health costs. Recommendations in the 1972 Hastings report and by other provincial commissions on health services all suggested establishment of a network of community health centers or local community service centers (LCSC). Common principles of these proposals include (Soderstrom 1978:35):

1. Continuous primary health care that includes preventive, diagnostic, curative, and rehabilitative services should be available to individuals and families.
2. Health teams that include family physicians, dentists, clinical and public health nurses, and social workers should be used to provide coordinated health and social services.
3. Centers should be formally integrated into the rest of the health and social services systems by regionalization schemes, which divide a province into regions that have boards (councils) with financial powers and responsibility for planning and coordinating health services within the region. The board membership should include consumers, health service providers, and representatives of the provincial government.
4. Fee-for-service methods should not be used to reimburse centers for medical services provided.
5. General policies for the centers should be established by a governing board representing consumers, center staff, and government.

Despite the interest in CHCs, few are currently operating. Two widely known CHCs are at St. Catherines and Sault Ste. Marie in Ontario; the province of Quebec has the largest number of centers. The Sault Ste. Marie and the District Group Health Association receive an annual lump sum payment from the Ontario Ministry of Health for each enrolled member, to finance the physician and other services provided to them. In contrast, the Quebec centers are financed by grants from the Ministry of Social Affairs and by fee-for-service payments from the Quebec Health Insurance Board.

Some of the reasons for the lack of growth of CHCs include (a) the high initial capital investment required to develop a CHC, (b) problems attracting physicians, (c) opposition by the medical profession which fears too much government control over financial arrangements and medical practice, (d) inadequate public emphasis on primary care services, and (e) lack of a fixed budget and responsibility for providing hospital services.

Summary

There is no absolute definition of health. Some people think that as long as they can work they are healthy; others think that health is the absence of disease. There are a number of factors that influence an individual's definition of health. Increasingly, however, emphasis is being placed on health as the optimum level of wellness that any particular individual can acquire. This definition suggests that, even without a disease, a person may not be healthy and that people with diseases such as diabetes can be healthy. In addition, health is a dynamic, not a static, state. An individual's degree of wellness changes constantly along the health-illness continuum. High-level wellness is at one extreme of the continuum and critical illness and death are at the opposite extremes.

There is increasing recognition of the function of the nurse in promoting health on three preventive levels: primary, secondary, and tertiary.

The term *illness* refers to a highly personalized state in which an individual feels unwell. When ill, people behave in various ways according to culturally and socially learned responses. Crying, stoicism, seeking attention, and denial are learned responses.

Five stages of illness generally occur. The first, a transition stage, occurs when the person first experiences symptoms. These may be denied and often need validation from others. During the second stage, the patient accepts and assumes the sick role. Medical care is sought if spontaneous recovery does not occur. The third stage involves confirmation of illness by the physician. In the fourth stage, once illness is verified, the sick person becomes dependent on the physician. Recommendations of the physician may or may not be accepted. The final stage is recovery or rehabilitation, which may require adjustments in life-styles. The nurse's role throughout these stages varies with the needs of the patient. Another important factor affecting a person's behavior is hospitalization. Changes in privacy, autonomy, life-style, roles, and economics all influence how a patient reacts.

The sick role has four aspects in North American society. Although sickness is considered undesirable, the patient is generally not held responsible for incurring the illness, and the sick person is excused from normal duties. The patient is obliged to get well as soon as possible, however, and is expected to seek competent help.

Two general types of health care services are provided in North America. These are restorative care for the ill or injured and preventive care that helps the healthy maintain health and avoid disease and injury. The former service predominates. A comprehensive health care delivery system should encompass four interdependent areas: health maintenance, prevention of disease and injury, diagnosis and treatment of disease and injury, and rehabilitation. Both physical and mental health and illness must be included. Health maintenance programs will probably receive greater emphasis in the future.

A wide variety of health care agencies exist in most communities. These include physicians' offices or clinics, hospitals, day-care centers, home nursing services, rehabilitation services, and nursing homes. These agencies can be classified as government or voluntary agencies. The former are financed and operated by federal, state or provincial, county, or city government; the latter by contributions from interested individuals in the community.

The health team consists of various health personnel, each offering a specialized service to patients. The composition of the health team differs with the particular needs of the patient and family. Some require the services of a social worker; others need a dietician. Almost all patients require services from nurses. The nursing team includes personnel with varied educational backgrounds and skills. Nursing teams are generally headed by registered nurses.

Associated with the sick role are certain behavior changes. Generally, sick persons are anxious and fearful of reduced functioning, changed social relationships, and death. Often regression is observed in a number of behaviors. Preoccupation and concern about oneself (egocentricity), exaggerated reactions to trivial matters, narrowed interests, and changes in the patient's perceptions need to be accepted with understanding by the nurse.

When one member of a family is ill, all other members are affected. The stress and worry incurred depend in large part on the seriousness of the illness. The roles and functions of the ill person may be reassigned. Financial problems, separation from the family, and changes in social relationships need to be handled. The more dependent the family members are on the ill person, the greater the adjustments needed. Nurses need to be aware of the effects of illness on family members as well as on the patient. These changes often create additional stress for the patient.

A number of health professions have models that convey how that profession views its discipline. Systems theory is frequently used to describe an entity, such as a person, family, or community. Nurses have used systems theory to examine interrelationships and derive principles in their practice.

Statistics reveal trends in health and the incidence of illness and death. One statistic study indicated four contributing elements to death and disease: biologic factors, life-style, environment, and the health care system. Increases in total population demand increased health care services. Successes in treating acute diseases and lower maternal death rates are two factors that have increased longevity. With increased longevity, the incidence of heart disease and other chronic diseases in the elderly has increased. The very young and the elderly require the most health care.

Mortality statistics indicate differences in causes of death among various age groups. The predominant cause of death in individuals over 40 years is heart disease, whereas accidents are the major cause in all other age groups. The incidence of homicide and suicide among adolescents and young adults is high. Morbidity statistics reveal a high incidence of alcoholism, drug addiction, sexually transmitted disease, dental disease, and psychologic illnesses. The one obvious decline is in the incidence of acute contagious diseases.

Six major problems exist in the current health-illness care system in North America. First, the care provided is fragmented. Because of increased specialization, patients can no longer see a family doctor for all of their ailments. Some patients consult as many as six specialists, become bewildered and worried, and may feel no one in the system really cares about or knows them. Second, the cost of health care is very high, necessitating programs that assist individuals to pay for health services. The cost to the public as a whole remains exorbitant. Third, rapid changes in medical science and technology quickly outdate the skills of health practitioners. Fourth, services to the poor and to minority groups are inadequate. Fifth, special needs of the elderly are increasing. Last, health services are distributed unevenly. The number of primary practice physicians is decreasing, and rural areas have lower ratios of health workers per capita than urban areas. Despite these problems, more and more people are seeking help for health problems and are using the available health services.

Health services can be regarded as the fastest growing industry in the United States. Five general types of financing for health services are voluntary health insurance plans, social insurance programs, payments by individuals, payments by industry, and charitable donations.

In response to the problems in health care delivery systems, various types of alternative health care delivery systems have developed. Examples include prepaid group practice plans, individual practice associations, and primary care networks in the United States and community health centers in Canada.

Suggested Readings

Brickner, P. W., et al. May 1976. Outreach to welfare hotels, the homebound, the frail. *American Journal of Nursing* 76:762–64.
Special programs have been established to provide professional services to "medically unreached groups"—people who cannot or will not use the current health care system.

Bullough, B. September 1976. Influences on role expansion. *American Journal of Nursing* 76:1476–81.
This article discusses some of the factors that affect the expansion of the nurse's role, including the women's movement and medicine.

Craven, R. F., and Sharp, B. H. 1972. The effects of illness on family functions. *Nursing Forum* 11(2):187–93.
This article describes the effects of illness on the contemporary American family and tells how nurses can help support the functions of the family.

Fagerhaugh, S.; Strauss, A.; Suczek, B.; and Wiener, C. November 1980. The impact of technology on patients, providers, and care patterns. *Nursing Outlook* 28:666–72.
This article discusses how technology has affected health organizations and health practices, with specific reference to the impact of technology on nursing.

Galton, L. April 1977. Questions patients ask about health and how you can answer them. *Nursing 77* 7:54–59.
The author has compiled typical patient questions and provides answers that have been supported by studies.

Luckmann, J., and Sorensen, K. C. February 1975. What patients' actions tell you about their feelings, fears and needs. *Nursing 75* 5:54–61.
Common responses of patients to illness are discussed. These responses can reveal patients' fears and needs and thus require understanding on the part of the nurse. Specific ways for the nurse to handle responses are included.

Martin, H. W., and Prange, A. J. March 1962. The stages of illness—psychosocial approach. *Nursing Outlook* 10:168–71.
This article discusses three stages of psychosocial illness: transition, acceptance, and convalescence. The nurse has a clearly defined role in each stage and needs to learn more about the psychologic aspects of illness to fulfill the nursing role satisfactorily.

Newton, L. H. June 1981. In defense of the traditional nurse. *Nursing Outlook* 29:348–54.
The author presents another point of view on the need for the autonomous nurse. Included in the article are: role components, barriers to autonomy, patient needs, needs of the hospital environment, and the feminist perspective.

Pender, N. J. June 1975. A conceptual model for preventive health behavior. *Nursing Outlook* 23:385–90.
This article analyzes the factors that promote or inhibit an individual's motivation to protect his or her health. People do not always take advantage of preventive health services, even when they are readily available.

Shaheen, P. P. June 1981. Nationalizing health care: A humanitarian approach. *Nursing Outlook* 29:358–63.
This article briefly describes health delivery systems in Canada, the Soviet Union, China, the Arab states, and the United States. National health proposals are reviewed, and future trends are discussed. The article concludes with suggestions for reform of health care in the United States.

Selected References

Health and illness

Antonovsky, A. 1972. Social class, life expectancy and overall mortality. In Jaco, E. G., editor. *Patients, physicians and illness.* 2nd ed. New York: Free Press.

Bauman, B. 1965. Diversities in conceptions of health and physical fitness. In Skipper, James K., Jr., and Leonard, Robert C., editors. *Social interaction and patient care.* Philadelphia: J. B. Lippincott Co.

Dubos, R. 1965. *Man adapting.* New Haven, Conn: Yale University Press.

———. 1978. Health and creative adaptation. *Human Nature* 74(1): entire issue.

Dunn, H. L. June 1959a. High-level wellness in man and society. *American Journal of Public Health* 49:786.

———. November 1959b. What high-level wellness means. *Canadian Journal of Public Health* 50:447.

———. 1961. *High-level wellness.* Arlington, Va.: R. W. Beatty Co.

Hover, J., and Juelsgaard, N. 1978. The sick role reconceptualized. *Nursing Forum* 17(4):406–16.

Jahoda, M. 1958. *Current concepts of positive mental health.* New York: Basic Books.

Lambert, V. A., and Lambert, C. E., Jr. 1979. *The impact of physical illness and related mental health concepts.* Englewood Cliffs, N.J.: Prentice-Hall.

Mechanic, D. 1972. Response factors in illness: The study of illness behavior. In Jaco, E. G., editor. *Patients, physicians and illness.* 2nd ed. New York: Free Press.

Parsons, T. 1951. *The social system.* New York: Free Press.

———. 1972. Definitions of health and illness in the light of American values and social structure. In Jaco, E. G., editor. *Patients, physicians and illness.* 2nd ed. New York: Free Press.

President's Commission on Health Needs of the Nation. 1953. *Building America's health.* Vol. 2. Washington, D.C.: Government Printing Office.

Rodgers, J. A. October 1981. Health is not a right. *Nursing Outlook* 29:590–91.

Rogers, C. R. 1961. *On becoming a person: A therapist's view of psychotherapy.* Boston: Houghton Mifflin Co.

Schuster, E. A. October 1976. Privacy, the patient and hospitalization. *Social Science Medicine* 10:245.

Shamansky, S. L., and Clausen, C. L. February 1980. Levels of prevention: Examination of a concept. *Nursing Outlook* 28:104–8.

Suchman, E. A. 1972. Stages of illness and medical care. In Jaco, E. G., editor. *Patients, physicians and illness.* 2nd ed. New York: Free Press.

Vincent, P. July 1975. The sick role in patient care. *American Journal of Nursing* 75:1172–73.

Health care delivery

American Academy of Nursing. 1975. *Models for health care delivery: Now and for the future.* Publication no. G–119 2M 5/75. Kansas City, Mo.: American Nurses' Association.

American Journal of Nursing. September 1976. Consumer speaks out about hospital care. *American Journal of Nursing* 76:1443–44.

Anderson, O. W. 1972. Health services systems in the United States and other countries: Critical comparisons. In Jaco, E. G., editor. *Patients, physicians and illness.* 2nd ed. New York: Free Press.

Anderson, O. W., and Andersen, R. M. 1972. Patterns of use of health services. In Freeman, H. E., et al., editors. *Handbook of medical sociology.* 2nd ed. Englewood Cliffs, N.J.: Prentice-Hall.

Archer, S. E. June 1981. National health service: Rationale and implementation. *Nursing Outlook* 29:364–68.

Benson, E. F. 1977. The consumer's right to health care: How does the nursing profession respond? *Nursing Forum* 16(2):138–43.

Colt, A. M.; Anderson, N.; Scott, H. D.; and Zimmerman, H. October 1977. Home health care is good economics. *Nursing Outlook* 25:632–36.

Dalme, F. C., and Malkemes, L. C. 1974. An analysis of the health and illness care system and some suggested renovations. In Leininger, M., editor. *Health care dimensions.* Philadelphia: F. A. Davis Co.

Enthoven, A. C. 1980. *Health plan: The only practical solution to the soaring cost of medical care.* Reading, Mass.: Addison-Wesley Publishing Co.

Glittenberg, J. December 1974. Adapting health care to a cultural setting. *American Journal of Nursing* 74:2218–21.

Isaacs, M. May 1978. Toward a national health policy: A realist's view. *American Journal of Nursing* 78:848–51.

Leavell, H. R., et al. 1965. *Preventive medicine for the doctor in his community.* 3rd ed. New York: McGraw-Hill Book Co.

Leininger, M. 1975. Health care delivery systems for tomorrow: Possibilities and guidelines. In Leininger, M., editor. *Barriers and facilitators to quality health care.* Philadelphia: F. A. Davis Co.

McIver, V. September 1980. A time to be born. A time to die. *The Canadian Nurse.* 76:38–41.

Nakagawa, H. 1974. The social organization of health care and the myth of free choice. In Leininger, M., editor. *Health care dimensions.* Philadelphia: F. A. Davis Co.

Orque, M. S. May 1976. Health care and minority clients. *Nursing Outlook* 24:313–16.

Soderstrom, L. 1978. *The Canadian health system.* London: Croom Helm.

Somers, A. R. 1971. *Health care in transition: Directions for the future.* Chicago: Hospital Research and Educational Trust.

Wald, F. S.; Foster, Z.; and Wald, H. J. March 1980. The hospice movement as a health care reform. *Nursing Outlook* 28:173–78.

Wilson, L., and Kolb, W. L. 1949. *Sociological analysis: An introductory text and case book.* New York: Harcourt, Brace and Company.

World Health Organization. 1947. *Constitution of the World Health Organization: Chronicle of the World Health Organization 1.* Geneva, Switzerland: World Health Organization.

Demographic statistics

Canadian Department of National Health and Welfare. 1974. *A new perspective on the health of Canadians: A working document.* Ottawa: Department of National Health and Welfare.

———. 1976. *Health field indicators, Canada and provinces.* Ottawa: Department of National Health and Welfare.

———. 1980. *Report of the task force to the conference of deputy ministers.* Ottawa: Minister of Supply and Services.

Statistics Canada. 1974. *Population projection for Canada and the provinces.* Ottawa: Statistics Canada.

———. 1980. Causes of death. In *Perspectives Canada III.* Ottawa: Statistics Canada.

———. 1980. *Perspectives Canada III.* Ottawa: Minister of Supply and Services.

United Nations. 1976. *Demographic year book 1975.* New York: United Nations.

U.S. Department of Health, Education, and Welfare. 1978. *Facts on life and death.* Publication no. (PHS) 79–1222. Washington, D.C.: Government Printing Office.

———. 1979. *Healthy people: The surgeon general's report on health promotion and disease prevention.* Publication no. 79–55071. Washington, D.C.: Government Printing Office.

Nursing

Bernal, H. June 1978. Levels of practice in a community health agency. *Nursing Outlook* 26:364–69.

Deloughery, G. L., and Gebbie, K. M. 1975. *Political dynamics: Impact on nurses and nursing.* St. Louis: C. V. Mosby Co.

French, J. G. March 1971. This I believe . . . about community nursing in the future. *Nursing Outlook* 19:173–75.

Orem, D. E. 1980. *Nursing: Concepts of practice.* 2nd ed. New York: McGraw-Hill Book Co.

Systems theory and models

Connally, A. C., and Van Hoozer, H. November 1980. The systems approach: A basis for course redesign. *Nursing Outlook* 28:695–98.

Daubenmire, M. J., and King, I. M. August 1973. Nursing process models: A systems approach. *Nursing Outlook* 21:512–17.

Gelein, J. L. 1979. Introduction to systems approach. In Phipps, W. J.; Long, B. C.; and Wood, N. F., editors. *Medical-surgical nursing.* St. Louis: C. V. Mosby Co.

Hazzard, M. E., and Kergin, D. J. September 1971. An overview of systems theory. *Nursing Clinics of North America* 6:385–93.

Phillips, J. R. February 1977. Nursing systems and nursing models. *Image* 9:4–7.

Putt, A. M. 1978. *General systems theory applied to nursing.* Boston: Little, Brown.

Riehl, J. P., and Roy, C. 1980. *Conceptual models for nursing practice.* 2nd ed. New York: Appleton-Century-Crofts.

Chapter 3

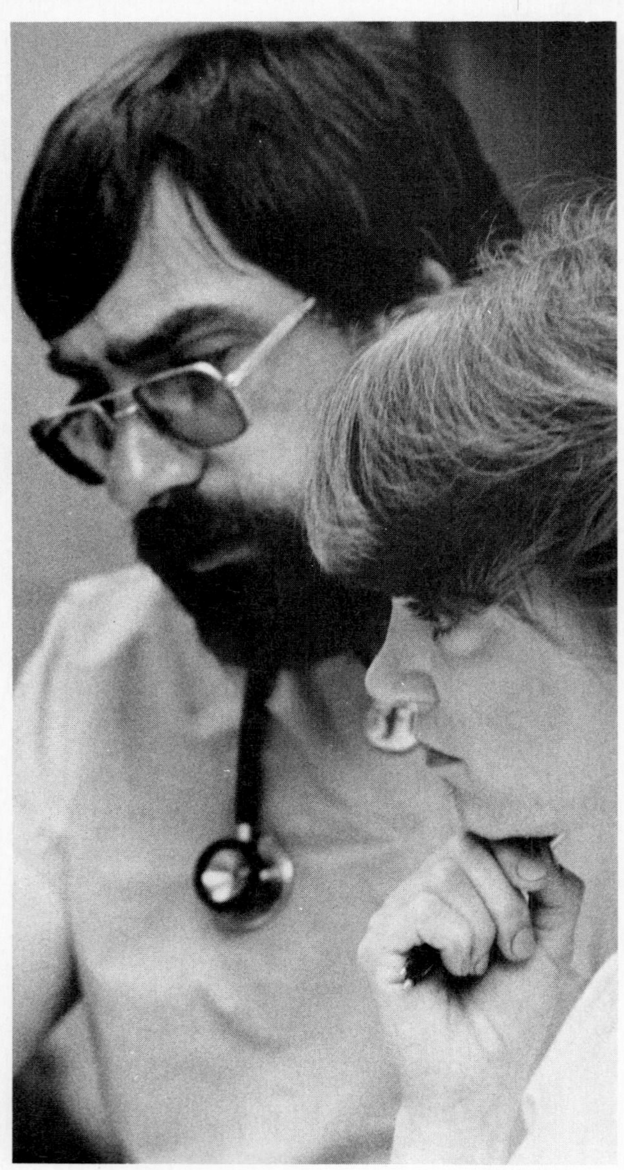

Values, Rights, and Ethics

CONTENTS

Objectives

1. Know essential facts about values, rights, and ethics
   - **1.1** Define selected terms
   - **1.2** Identify six ways in which values, beliefs, and attitudes are learned
   - **1.3** Identify Rath's process of developing values
   - **1.4** State how personal values can conflict with professional responsibilities
   - **1.5** Identify various types of rights
   - **1.6** Outline reasons for the development of statements of rights
   - **1.7** Outline essentials of the Patient's Bill of Rights established by the American Hospital Association and the Canadian National Consumer's Association
   - **1.8** Identify five essential elements of informed consent
   - **1.9** List special groups for whom statements of rights are available
   - **1.10** Identify essentials of the Canadian Nurses' Association Ethics of Nursing Research
   - **1.11** Identify Fagin's seven rights of nurses and associated obligations
   - **1.12** Identify essential student rights
   - **1.13** List the purposes of nursing ethics
   - **1.14** Describe specific aspects of the established nursing codes of ethics
2. Understand essential facts about ethical problems of nurses
   - **2.1** Categorize five broad areas of ethical problems faced by nurses
   - **2.2** Give examples of ethical problems in each area
   - **2.3** Identify essential steps in resolving ethical problems
3. Understand the nurse's role in relation to rights and ethics
   - **3.1** Identify the nurse's responsibilities in relation to patients' rights
   - **3.2** Identify the role of the nurse in patient advocacy

Terms

attitude	code of ethics	patient advocate	value
belief	ethics	right	values clarification

The values and rights of people and the ethical considerations governing behavior have received particular attention in recent years. With expansion of the nurse's role, nurses have become more aware of their own and others' values and rights. Values clarification is a process people can use to identify their own values. Nurses can also help patients to establish patterns of action based on their own values.

Patients' rights are the product of both legislation and the ethical standards of society. In the past, the patient and family were often denied fundamental rights—such as privacy, courtesy, and information—at times of illness. Patients often felt treated as the least important of all people in a health setting.

This chapter discusses the rights of patients, nurses, and students. Various ethical codes are presented together with approaches to ethical decision making. Patient advocacy is explained as a recognized role of the nurse today.

Values

A *value* can be defined as something of worth, a belief held dear by a person. A value is a personal belief about the worth, truth, or desirability of a particular idea, object, or behavior (Czmowski 1974:194). According to Simon (1973:44), "values are a set of personal beliefs and attitudes about the truth, beauty, worth of any thought, object, or behavior. They are action oriented and give direction and meaning to one's life." These definitions indicate that values are personal; codes of ethics, however, belong to a profession or to society as a whole.

Most authorities agree that values evolve from personal experiences. Values form a basis for behavior; a person's real values are shown by consistent patterns of behavior. Once one is aware of one's values, the values become an internal control for behavior.

Values have both intellectual and emotional components. The person is intellectually convinced about a value, holds it dear, and is prepared to defend it.

Children begin to learn their values at home, and values continue to develop throughout life. When a student chooses to become a nurse, that student brings preexisting values to nursing. Many of these values are probably compatible with nursing ethics, but some may not be compatible. However, values can be learned; to practice as a professional nurse, a person needs values compatible with the profession's code of ethics. Values such as respecting the dignity of people without bias, safeguarding a person's right to privacy, and accepting responsibility for one's own actions are manifested in such behaviors as conscientiously performing delegated activities and reporting errors. Nurses who value the right of privacy provide it for their patients: They curtain off areas for bathing and treatments, drape patients for certain procedures, or provide a conference area for patient consultation with a priest or for grieving family members. Other desirable values are honesty, gentleness, punctuality, and respect for others.

A personal philosophy integrates spiritual, professional, social, and esthetic values, all of which produce a code for living. Ethical values basic to nursing practice are not always a part of the nurse's personal value system. For example, a nurse who has little personal need for privacy may not be attuned to patients' needs for privacy. Yet respect for privacy is an ethical value basic to nursing, which the nursing student can learn by becoming sensitive to patients' feelings and understanding their needs.

Methods of Learning Values

According to values clarification theory, a belief or attitude can become a value only if the belief satisfies seven criteria (see page 75). A *belief* or opinion is something accepted as true by a judgment of probability rather than actuality. Beliefs are cognitive conceptual organizations. People hold beliefs that may be true or that can, with reliable evidence, be proved true. Family traditions and folklore are beliefs passed from one generation to another. Some beliefs are in fact values, because they are freely chosen and satisfy the other six aspects of values clarification. An *attitude* is a feeling tone; it is a concomitant of behavior. Attitudes are directed toward a person, object, condition, or situation. For example a child may learn attitudes such as cooperation and kindness from parents and in turn exhibit these in behavior.

Traditionally, values, beliefs, and attitudes are taught through modeling, persuading, cultural teaching, limiting choices, imposing rules, and appealing to the conscience.

Modeling

In modeling, the individual learns from examples set by others' behavior, which is imitated. Many years ago in rural America, the number of role models for children was limited because interactions were generally restricted to the family and a small local community. Today a child has many sources of role models: television, movies, peers in school, family, friends, and so on. Because there are so many role models, today's child may find learning values through modeling difficult and confusing. The child observes many kinds of behavior, often divergent and conflicting.

Persuading

Persuading or convincing has a cognitive basis. As such, it does not deal with the emotional aspects of behavior. For example, a nurse may persuade a patient to wash each morning even though he or she does not want to wash. Because the patient does not value cleanliness, old habits of washing only once a month are reestablished when the patient returns home. Thus, persuading may lead to temporary behavior change, but persuasion is not usually an effective way to develop values. Another example is a person persuaded to believe that obesity predisposes to heart disease. In spite of this knowledge, the person continues to overeat. Although the intellect has been persuaded, the emotional aspect of the behavior remains unchanged.

Cultural teaching

Religious and cultural teachings often influence behavior, particularly in the setting in which they are taught. Generally individuals are given no choice and accept these teachings on faith. In some instances these teachings become the basis for values; sometimes, however, people completely reject them when other choices become available. An example is the student who is taught at home that wearing facial makeup is sinful; she is given no choice at home or school. Later, other choices become apparent, and she decides to wear lipstick, although she does not wear lipstick when she visits home. In this instance, the religious teachings of the family and church do not become a part of her value system.

Limiting choices

Sometimes behavior is controlled by limiting a person's choices. The individual does not have free choice, but rather restricted choice. An example is the teenager who is allowed to use the family car only if it is returned by ten o'clock. The teenager has two choices that control behavior, but it is questionable whether the teenager in this situation learns any values on which to base future behavior.

Imposing rules

Persons in authority often impose rules and regulations as a way of controlling behavior. The learned behavior is usually socially acceptable in that situation and similar future situations. However, individuals may follow the rules without thinking. They behave in certain ways from fear of being caught and punished rather than from any sense of right or wrong. If such individuals are in a situation for which they have no rules, they are often confused because they have developed no values to guide behavior.

Appealing to conscience

People often learn a set of behavioral norms that they are told are right. Failure to follow these norms (inner conscience) usually results in feelings of guilt. The individual is motivated by desire to avoid guilt feelings rather than by values. For example, a mother may tell her son that she will worry if he goes out. The son has learned that to make his mother worry is wrong, so he feels guilty if he goes out. Guilt may or may not be effective in controlling behavior, but guilt is always negative and may lead to anger.

Conflict of Values and Professional Duty

With the changing scope of nursing practice and medical technology, there is an increasing chance that nursing responsibilities will conflict with the personal values of nurses. On the one hand, employers have needs and expectations for service from nurses; on the other hand, nurses have the right to be guided by their own personal values. An example of an area of conflict in the contemporary nursing scene is assisting with therapeutic abortions. Nurses have the right to refuse to participate in abortions or any procedure they consider goes against their personal values, and nurses' employment should not be jeopardized as a result. It is essential, however, that patients' welfare not suffer as a consequence.

Other areas of controversy are euthanasia, prolonging the life of nonresponsive patients by machines, and withholding blood transfusions because of an individual's religious convictions. The future promises many more situations that may conflict with personal values. To help nurses identify their own values, a system of values clarification has been established. See the next section.

Values Clarification

Values clarification is a process by which individuals find their own answers (values) to situations. It is not the transmission of "correct" values or rules, but a process of developing individual values. The principle of values clarification is that no one set of values is right for everyone.

The process of values clarification was formulated by Louis Raths in 1966, who built on the thinking of John Dewey. Raths was chiefly concerned with the *process of valuing*, not the content of the values. Valuing is composed of seven processes, which can be placed in three groups (Simon et al. 1972:19):

Prizing

1. Prizing and cherishing one's beliefs and behaviors
2. Publicly affirming them when appropriate

Choosing

3. Choosing from alternatives
4. Choosing after consideration of consequences
5. Choosing freely

Acting

6. Acting
7. Acting with a pattern, consistency, and repetition

A belief, attitude, or feeling becomes a value when all seven steps have been satisfied. The individual applies each of the seven steps to an emerging or already formed belief, behavior pattern, or attitude.

By using these seven steps in values clarification, nurses can clarify their own values and enhance their personal growth. These steps also can be applied to patient situations; the nurse can help patients identify conflict areas, examine and choose from alternatives, set goals, and act (Coletta 1978:2057).

Prizing and cherishing

Prizing or cherishing is a continuous process in which the individual asks, "Do I cherish or prize my position, belief, etc.?" Unprized beliefs may still influence behavior, but they cannot be considered values.

Publicly affirming when appropriate

Public affirmation or appropriate sharing is an indication of the quality of a value. Individuals who feel strongly about an issue may publicly stand up and share the value with others. For example, a nurse who values the autonomy of patients may refuse to obtain a signed consent form from a patient without first explaining the procedure to the patient. Thus the nurse is affirming his or her value of autonomy to others.

Choosing from alternatives

For a belief to be a value it must be chosen from among other alternatives. Individuals must consider the other options before they commit themselves to one choice.

Choosing after consideration of consequences

The individual must be able to consider the consequences of a choice—that is, the significance of the decision. The person may reject or confirm the choice because of or in spite of the consequences. For example, a nurse may refuse to give a patient a medication that the nurse believes may harm the patient. This nurse considers the consequences of her or his behavior in terms of the patient and of self. The nurse is concerned for the patient's welfare, but the refusal could result in disciplinary action. After considering all the alternatives, the nurse may confirm the choice of not giving the medication or select another course of action, such as discussing the medication with a physician before making a decision. If an individual's behavior is not the consequence of considering the results of action, it cannot be considered to reflect a value.

Choosing freely

A value must be chosen freely. Some beliefs are not freely chosen by the individual but are accepted from parents or others without much thought. These beliefs are not values. Behavior determined by fear or coercion, for example, does not reflect values.

Acting

A value involves action. Therefore a value must be incorporated into behavior. If it is not, it is not a value but a belief or an attitude.

Acting with a pattern, consistency, and repetition

Behavior must be consistent over a period of time to reflect a value. The behavior is repeated in many aspects of life. For example, a nurse who values health will eat a healthful diet and get enough sleep.

Definitions of Rights and Ethics

A *right* is a first claim to anything that is a person's due. A right may be properly demanded on the basis of justice, morality, or legality. Rights can be viewed from legal and personal points of view. In the legal view, rights provide people with a certain power to control situations; for example, a person has a right to enter a restaurant and purchase a meal. In this legal view, rights have certain attendant obligations. The individual with the right to eat in a restaurant is obliged to behave in an appropriate manner and to pay for the meal.

The personal concept of rights has much to do with ethical development, with the way one conducts one's life, with the decisions one makes, and with one's concept of right and wrong and of good and evil (Fromer 1981:2). A number of factors influence the development of a personal concept of rights: social relationships, parents, culture, and information, for example. Human rights refer to prerogatives of all humans, e.g., to express feelings, inclinations, compassions, sympathies, intelligence, and thoughts (Fagin 1975:83). Some human rights are the right to express oneself freely, to grow up, and to receive just compensation for employment.

Ethics are the rules or principles that govern right conduct. They deal with what is good and bad and with moral duty and obligation. Ethics are not unlike the law in that each deals with rules of conduct that reflect underlying principles of right and wrong and codes of morality. Ethics are designed to protect the rights of human beings.

Ethics are important in health delivery systems. In nursing, ethics provide professional standards for nursing activities; these standards protect both the nurse and the patient.

Patients' Rights

Consumers of health services are increasingly voicing their concerns about the services they want and need. Most desire more accessible services, more coordinated services, more information about their illness and care, more participation in their care, and more personalized service. In response to the public demands, bills of rights have been developed and widely distributed. Two of these are A Patient's Bill of Rights, developed by the

American Hospital Association in 1973 (see Table 3–1), and Consumer Rights in Health Care, published in Canada by the National Consumers' Association (see Table 3–2).

These statements regarding the rights of patients appear to have been influenced by several factors:

1. Increased awareness on the part of the consumer about the right to health care and to greater participation in planning that care.

2. The increasing number of malpractice suits that are receiving publicity and thus coming into the public's awareness. As a result of these, the consumer is increasingly concerned about rights, often in a protective sense.

3. Legislation that has been created in other previously protected relationships, such as the employee-employer relationship, and human rights and equal rights legislation in general.

Table 3–1 A Patient's Bill of Rights

1. The patient has the right to considerate and respectful care.

2. The patient has the right to obtain from his physician complete current information concerning his diagnosis, treatment, and prognosis, in terms the patient can be reasonably expected to understand. When it is not medically advisable to give such information to the patient, the information should be made available to an appropriate person in his behalf. He has the right to know by name the physician responsible for coordinating his care.

3. The patient has the right to receive from his physician information necessary to give informed consent prior to the start of any procedure and/or treatment. Except in emergencies, such information for informed consent should include but not necessarily be limited to the specific procedure and/or treatment, the medically significant risks involved, and the probable duration of incapacitation. Where medically significant alternatives for care or treatment exist, or when the patient requests information concerning medical alternatives, the patient has the right to such information. The patient also has the right to know the name of the person responsible for the procedures and/or treatment.

4. The patient has the right to refuse treatment to the extent permitted by law and to be informed of the medical consequences of his action.

5. The patient has the right to every consideration of his privacy concerning his own medical care program. Case discussion, consultation, examination, and treatment are confidential and should be conducted discreetly. Those not directly involved in his care must have the permission of the patient to be present.

6. The patient has the right to expect that all communications and records pertaining to his care should be treated as confidential.

7. The patient has the right to expect that within its capacity a hospital must make reasonable response to the request of a patient for services. The hospital must provide evaluation, service, and/or referral as indicated by the urgency of the case. When medically permissible, a patient may be transferred to another facility only after he has received complete information and explanation concerning the needs for and alternatives to such a transfer. The institution to which the patient is transferred must first have accepted the patient for transfer.

8. The patient has the right to obtain information as to any relationship of his hospital to other health care and educational institutions insofar as his care is concerned. The patient has the right to obtain information as to the existence of any professional relationships among individuals, by name, who are treating him.

9. The patient has the right to be advised if the hospital proposes to engage in or perform human experimentation affecting his care or treatment. The patient has the right to refuse to participate in such research projects.

10. The patient has the right to expect reasonable continuity of care. He has the right to know in advance what appointment times and physicians are available and where. The patient has the right to expect that the hospital will provide a mechanism whereby he is informed by his physician or a delegate of the physician of the patient's continuing health.

11. The patient has the right to examine and receive an explanation of his bill regardless of source of payment.

12. The patient has the right to know what hospital rules and regulations apply to his conduct as a patient.

From American Hospital Association, 1973. A patient's bill of rights, *Nursing Outlook*, February 1973, 21:82, and January 1976, 24:29. Reprinted with the permission of the American Hospital Association.

Table 3–2 Consumer Rights in Health Care

I. Right to be informed:
—about preventive health care including education on nutrition, birth control, drug use, appropriate exercise.
—about the health care system, including the extent of government insurance coverage for services, supplementary insurance plans, and referral system to auxiliary health and social facilities and services in the community.
—about the individual's own diagnosis and specific treatment program, including prescribed surgery and medication, options, effects and side effects.
—about the specific costs of procedures, services and professional fees undertaken on behalf of the individual consumer.

II. Right to be respected as the individual with the major responsibility for his own health care:
—right that confidentiality of his health records be maintained.
—right to refuse experimentation, undue painful prolongation of his life or participation in teaching programs.
—right of adult to refuse treatment, right to die with dignity.

III. Right to participate in decision making affecting his health:
—through consumer representation at each level of government in planning and evaluating the system of health services.
—the types and qualities of service and the conditions under which health services are delivered.
—with the health professionals and personnel involved in his direct health care.

IV. Right to equal access to health care (health education, prevention, treatment and rehabilitation) regardless of the individual's economic status, sex, age, creed, ethnic origin and location:
—right to access to adequately qualified health personnel.
—right to a second medical opinion.
—right to prompt response in emergencies.

From *Canadian Consumer*, April 1974, published by the Consumers' Association of Canada (CAC).

4. Consumer concern about the increasing amount of research being conducted in the health field and the increasing use of patients for educational purposes in a number of disciplines. Although patients and their families are generally willing to participate in research and educational programs, they frequently ask, "Do I have to?" In addition, some patients wonder whether the quality of their care will suffer if they do not agree to participate. See the discussion of ethics of nursing research later in this chapter.

A Patient's Bill of Rights (see Table 3–1) states that a patient has a right to an acceptable standard of care. In addition, the patient has a right to consideration while receiving that care. Therefore, the patient has a right to an explanation about what is happening, why, and when. The patient also has the right to participate in planning the care whenever possible. Every health facility should have in place a procedure for handling patient grievances. One trend in health care is patient advocacy, a function assumed by nurses in some settings. See the section on patient advocates on page 85.

Another right of patients is to understand the diagnosis, treatment, and prognosis. Therefore, patients need accurate information about their health and some understanding of medical terminology. In some instances, divulging complete information may have a negative effect on the patient, such as severe depression. The question then arises whether a patient has the right not to be informed. In this instance, the physician decides whether to inform the patient or the family.

Obtaining informed consent is the physician's responsibility in many places, although this responsibility may be delegated to nurses. The patient has a right to give or withhold informed consent before any treatment or procedure. Nurses therefore need the freedom to inform patients about the benefits and risks of a treatment.

It has also been suggested that a vital element of voluntary consent is freedom from coercion, unfair persuasions, and inducements (Besch 1979:33). Although physicians often assume the function of informing the patient, a patient advocate might be better able to inform without coercion. The patient may perceive the physician as too authoritative to question; this perception may prevent a truly voluntary decision.

How much information to disclose is a sensitive issue. A physician may have limited time or feel that full information could create anxiety for the patient. It is important to assess what information the patient needs rather than to assume needs that may not exist. Patients in addition have a right to have their questions answered and a right to information about alternative treatment. The limits on the nurse's function in this regard are unclear. In many settings, physicians are responsible for informing patients; however, increasingly nurses are assuming this responsibility. Patients also have a right to know the name of the physician in charge of their care. Patients may be confused when several physicians are treating them, as for example in an urban center where specialists practice.

Another right of patients is to change their minds and/or refuse treatments. The patient requires sufficient information to make an informed decision before signing a form of consent to surgery or other procedures. See Chapters 4 and 39 for further information on consent forms.

Informed consent has five essential elements. These were defined in the Declaration of Helsinki (see Shephard 1976:1191) adopted by the World Medical Assembly in 1964 (revised in 1975) and by the United States Department of Health and Human Services:

1. Explanation of the proposed treatment
2. Explanation of inherent risks and benefits
3. Alternatives to the proposed treatment
4. Adequate time for patient questions
5. Option to withdraw at any time

A patient may provide consent verbally or in writing. The nurse then has the responsibility to (a) be guided by the patient's expressed wishes and (b) inform the appropriate authorities in the hospital, the charge nurse and the patient's physician. The physician is responsible for informing the patient of the possible results of the patient's decision.

Patients have a right to be examined and seen by only the people directly concerned with their care. Physicians normally have responsibility for obtaining consent if, for example, a medical student needs to examine the patient. Sometimes nurses are delegated the responsibility of obtaining consent for examinations by medical students and the like. If the patient does not give consent, this fact must be reported to the appropriate hospital authority and to the physician. Patients also have a right to privacy, even after death. The degree of privacy needed by people is highly individual. See Chapter 2, page 45, for further information.

The sixth right is confidentiality. Nurses frequently receive confidential information that other members of the health team need to know. The patient should know what information is being communicated and to whom. If the patient objects, the nurse will require guidance as to how to proceed. The patient's record is the legal property of the health agency; however, in some states patients have access to their records.

Patients also have a right to consent or refuse to participate in any research or experimentation. Both the American Nurses' Association and the Canadian Nurses' Association have published guidelines for nurses who participate in research. See the section on ethics of nursing research later in this chapter.

Consumers of health care are also demanding reasonable continuity of care. Patients have a right to know what health care they will need after they are discharged from a hospital. It may be the nurse's responsibility to teach follow-up care and to make appropriate referrals to other health agencies. Patients have a right to an explanation about a bill for health care. Nurses often record billable items such as dressings, medications, and the like, and in some settings it may be the nurse's responsibility to explain a bill to a patient.

A patient also has a right to know which agency rules and regulations apply to him or her as a patient. Some agencies provide pamphlets that list visiting hours, explain cafeteria and telephone service, etc. Often nurses have responsibility for clarifying information and answering a patient's questions about hospital rules. Nurses also explain rules associated with special procedures, such as those that apply when oxygen is in use or when a patient is on protective asepsis.

Rights of Special Groups

Recently special groups have had lists of rights made public. Some of these groups are the handicapped, the dying, the retarded, and the elderly. These lists of rights reflect increased awareness of consumers' rights in general and their specific rights as members of certain groups.

In the Declaration on the Rights of Disabled Persons adopted by the General Assembly of the United Nations in December 1975, 13 points are made. See Table 3-3. This declaration defines *disability* as "deficiency, either congenital or not, in . . . physical or mental capabilities." The rights stated in this declaration do not have the force of law; however, many do have a basis in the laws of some countries. For example, statement 2 refers to the application of these rights to all people without discrimination on the basis of race, color, sex, language, religion, or other matters. This statement is similar to human rights legislation in many countries today.

The Dying Person's Bill of Rights was created at a 1975 workshop on "The Terminally Ill Patient and the Helping Person," held in Lansing, Michigan, and sponsored by the Southwestern Michigan Inservice Education Council. See Table 3-4. Amelia J. Barbus, associate professor of nursing at Wayne State University, Detroit, conducted the workshop.

The rights of the elderly were formulated as a result of a White House conference in 1961. See Table 3-5. The Declaration on the Rights of the Mentally Retarded was adopted by the United Nations in 1971. See Table 3-6. The Declaration of the Rights of the Child was adopted by the United Nations in 1979. See Table 3-7. The Pregnant Patient's Bill of Rights, published by the International Childbirth Education Association, was written by Doris B. Haire. See Table 3-8.

Table 3–3 Declaration on the Rights of Disabled Persons

1. The term "disabled person" means any person unable to ensure by himself or herself wholly or partly the necessities of a normal individual and/or social life, as a result of a deficiency, either congenital or not, in his or her physical or mental capabilities.
2. Disabled persons shall enjoy all the rights set forth in this Declaration. These rights shall be granted to all disabled persons without any exception whatsoever and without distinction or discrimination on the basis of race, colour, sex, language, religion, political or other opinions, national or social origin, state of wealth, birth or any other situation applying either to the disabled person himself or herself or to his or her family.
3. Disabled persons have the inherent right to respect for their human dignity. Disabled persons, whatever the origin, nature and seriousness of their handicaps and disabilities, have the same fundamental rights as their fellow-citizens of the same age, which implies first and foremost the right to enjoy a decent life, as normal and full as possible.
4. Disabled persons have the same civil and political rights as other human beings; article 7 of the Declaration of the Rights of Mentally Retarded Persons applies to any possible limitation or suppression of those rights for mentally disabled persons.
5. Disabled persons are entitled to the measures designed to enable them to become as self-reliant as possible.
6. Disabled persons have the right to medical, psychological and functional treatment, including prosthetic and orthetic appliances, to medical and social rehabilitation, education, vocational education, training and rehabilitation, aid, counselling, placement services and other services which will enable them to develop their capabilities and skills to the maximum and will hasten the process of their social integration or reintegration.
7. Disabled persons have the right to economic and social security and to a decent level of living. They have the right, according to their capabilities, to secure and retain employment or to engage in a useful, productive and remunerative occupation and to join trade unions.
8. Disabled persons are entitled to have their special needs taken into consideration at all stages of economic and social planning.
9. Disabled persons have the right to live with their families or with foster parents and to participate in all social, creative or recreational activities. No disabled person shall be subjected, as far as his or her residence is concerned, to differential treatment other than that required by his or her condition or by the improvement which he or she may derive therefrom. If the stay of a disabled person in a specialized establishment is indispensable, the environment and living conditions therein shall be as close as possible to those of the normal life of a person of his or her age.
10. Disabled persons shall be protected against all exploitation, all regulations and all treatment of a discriminatory, abusive and degrading nature.
11. Disabled persons shall be able to avail themselves of qualified legal aid when such aid proves indispensable for the protection of their persons or property. If judicial proceedings are instituted against them, the legal procedures applied shall take their physical and mental condition fully into account.
12. Organizations of disabled persons may be usefully consulted in all matters regarding the rights of disabled persons.
13. Disabled persons, their familes and communities shall be fully informed, by all appropriate means, of the rights contained in this Declaration.

Adopted by the General Assembly of the United Nations, December 1975.

Table 3–4 The Dying Person's Bill of Rights

I have the right to be treated as a living human being until I die.
I have the right to maintain a sense of hopefulness however changing its focus may be.
I have the right to be cared for by those who can maintain a sense of hopefulness, however changing this might be.
I have the right to express my feelings and emotions about my approaching death in my own way.
I have the right to participate in decisions concerning my care.
I have the right to expect continuing medical and nursing attention even though "cure" goals must be changed to "comfort" goals.
I have the right not to die alone.
I have the right to be free from pain.
I have the right to have my questions answered honestly.
I have the right not to be deceived.
I have the right to have help from and for my family in accepting my death.
I have the right to die in peace and dignity.
I have the right to retain my individuality and not be judged for my decisions which may be contrary to beliefs of others.
I have the right to discuss and enlarge my religious and/or spiritual experiences, whatever these may mean to others.
I have the right to expect that the sanctity of the human body will be respected after death.
I have the right to be cared for by caring, sensitive, knowledgeable people who will attempt to understand my needs and will be able to gain some satisfaction in helping me face my death.

From Amelia J. Barbus, The dying person's bill of rights, *American Journal of Nursing*, January 1975, 75:99.

Table 3–5 The Rights of Senior Citizens

1. The right to be useful.
2. The right to obtain employment, based on merit.
3. The right to freedom from want in old age.
4. The right to a fair share of the community's recreational, educational and medical resources.
5. The right to obtain decent housing suited to needs of later years.
6. The right to the moral and financial support of one's family so far as is consistent with the best interests of the family.
7. The right to live independently, as one chooses.
8. The right to live with dignity.
9. The right of access to all knowledge available on how to improve the later years of life.

From United States Department of Health, Education, and Welfare, *The Nation and Its Older People: Report of the White House Conference on Aging*, January 1961.

Table 3–6 Declaration on the Rights of Mentally Retarded Persons

1. The mentally retarded person has, to the maximum degree of feasibility, the same rights as other human beings.
2. The mentally retarded person has a right to proper medical care and physical therapy and to such education, training, rehabilitation and guidance as will enable him to develop his ability and maximum potential.
3. The mentally retarded person has a right to economic security and to a decent standard of living. He has a right to perform productive work or to engage in any meaningful occupation to the fullest possible extent of his capabilities.
4. Whenever possible, the mentally retarded person should live with his own family or with foster parents and participate in different forms of community life. The family with which he lives should receive assistance. If care in an institution becomes necessary, it should be provided in surroundings and other circumstances as close as possible to those of normal life.
5. The mentally retarded person has a right to a qualified guardian when this is required to protect his personal well-being and interests.
6. The mentally retarded person has a right to protection from exploitation, abuse and degrading treatment. If prosecuted for any offence, he shall have a right to due process of law with full recognition being given to his degree of mental responsibility.
7. Whenever mentally retarded persons are unable, because of the severity of their handicap, to exercise all their rights in a meaningful way or it should become necessary to restrict or deny some or all of these rights, the procedure used for that restriction or denial of rights must contain proper legal safeguards against every form of abuse. This procedure must be based on an evaluation of the social capability of the mentally retarded person by qualified experts and must be subject to periodic review and to the right of appeal to higher authorities.

Adopted by the General Assembly of the United Nations, December 1971.

Table 3–7 United Nations Declaration of the Rights of the Child

Preamble

Whereas the peoples of the United Nations have, in the Charter, reaffirmed their faith in fundamental human rights, and in the dignity and worth of the human person, and have determined to promote social progress and better standards of life in larger freedom,

Whereas the United Nations has, in the Universal Declaration of Human Rights, proclaimed that everyone is entitled to all the rights and freedoms set forth therein, without distinction of any kind, such as race, colour, sex, language, religion, political or other opinion, national or social origin, property, birth or other status,

Whereas the child, by reason of his physical and mental immaturity, needs special safeguards and care, including appropriate legal protection, before as well as after birth,

Whereas the need for such special safeguards has been stated in the Geneva Declaration of the Rights of the Child of 1924, and recognized in the Universal Declaration of Human Rights and in the statutes of specialized agencies and international organizations concerned with the welfare of children,

Whereas mankind owes to the child the best it has to give,

Now therefore,

The General Assembly

Proclaims this Declaration of the Rights of the Child to the end that he may have a happy childhood and enjoy for his own good and for the good of society the rights and freedoms herein set forth, and calls upon parents, upon men and women as individuals, and upon voluntary organizations, local authorities and national Governments to recognize these rights and strive for their observance by legislative and other measures progressively taken in accordance with the following principles:

Principle 1

The child shall enjoy all the rights set forth in this Declaration. Every child, without any exception whatsoever, shall be entitled to these rights, without distinction or discrimination on account of race, colour, sex, language, religion, political or other opinion, national or social origin, property, birth or other status, whether of himself or of his family.

Principle 2

The child shall enjoy special protection, and shall be given opportunities and facilities, by law and by other means, to enable him to develop physically, mentally, morally, spiritually and socially in a healthy and normal manner and in conditions of freedom and dignity. In the enactment of laws for this purpose, the best interests of the child shall be the paramount consideration.

Principle 3

The child shall be entitled from his birth to a name and a nationality.

Principle 4

The child shall enjoy the benefits of social security. He shall be entitled to grow and develop in health; to this end, special care and protection shall be provided both to him and to his mother, including adequate pre-natal and post-natal care. The child shall have the right to adequate nutrition, housing, recreation and medical services.

Principle 5

The child who is physically, mentally or socially handicapped shall be given the special treatment, education and care required by his particular condition.

Principle 6

The child, for the full and harmonious development of his personality, needs love and understanding. He shall, wherever possible, grow up in the care and under the responsibility of his parents, and, in any case, in an atmosphere of affection and of moral and material security; a child of tender years shall not, save in exceptional circumstances, be separated from his mother. Society and the public authorities shall have the duty to extend particular care to children without a family and to those without adequate means of support. Payment of State and other assistance towards the maintenance of children of large families is desirable.

Principle 7

The child is entitled to receive education, which shall be free and compulsory, at least in the elementary stages. He shall be given an education which will promote his general culture, and enable him, on a basis of equal opportunity, to develop his abilities, his individual judgement, and his sense of moral and social responsibility, and to become a useful member of society.

The best interests of the child shall be the guiding principle of those responsible for his education and guidance; that responsibility lies in the first place with his parents.

The child shall have full opportunity for play and recreation, which should be directed to the same purposes as education; society and the public authorities shall endeavour to promote the enjoyment of this right.

Principle 8

The child shall in all circumstances be among the first to receive protection and relief.

Principle 9

The child shall be protected against all forms of neglect, cruelty and exploitation. He shall not be the subject of traffic, in any form.

The child shall not be admitted to employment before an appropriate minimum age; he shall in no case be caused or permitted to engage in any occupation or employment which would prejudice his health or education, or interfere with his physical, mental or moral development.

Principle 10

The child shall be protected from practices which may foster racial, religious and any other form of discrimination. He shall be brought up in a spirit of understanding, tolerance, friendship among peoples, peace and universal brotherhood and in full consciousness that his energy and talents should be devoted to the service of his fellow men.

Adopted by the General Assembly of the United Nations, November 20, 1959.

Table 3–8 The Pregnant Patient's Bill of Rights

1. The Pregnant Patient has the right, prior to the administration of any drug or procedure, to be informed by the health professional caring for her of any potential direct or indirect effects, risks or hazards to herself or her unborn or newborn infant which may result from the use of a drug or procedure prescribed for or administered to her during pregnancy, labor, birth or lactation.
2. The Pregnant Patient has the right, prior to the proposed therapy, to be informed, not only of the benefits, risks and hazards of the proposed therapy but also of known alternative therapy, such as available childbirth education classes which could help to prepare the Pregnant Patient physically and mentally to cope with the discomfort or stress of pregnancy and the experience of childbirth, thereby reducing or eliminating her need for drugs and obstetric intervention. She should be offered such information early in her pregnancy in order that she may make a reasoned decision.
3. The Pregnant Patient has the right, prior to the administration of any drug, to be informed by the health professional who is prescribing or administering the drug to her that any drug which she receives during pregnancy, labor and birth, no matter how or when the drug is taken or administered may adversely affect her unborn baby, directly or indirectly, and that there is no drug or chemical which has been proven safe for the unborn child.
4. The Pregnant Patient has the right if cesarean section is anticipated, to be informed prior to the administration of any drug, and preferably prior to her hospitalization, that minimizing her and in turn, her baby's intake of nonessential preoperative medicine will benefit her baby.
5. The Pregnant Patient has the right, prior to the administration of a drug or procedure, to be informed of the areas of uncertainty if there is no properly controlled follow-up research which has established the safety of the drug or procedure with regard to its direct and/or indirect effects on the physiological, mental and neurological development of the child exposed, via the mother, to the drug or procedure during pregnancy, labor, birth or lactation (this would apply to virtually all drugs and the vast majority of obstetric procedures).
6. The Pregnant Patient has the right, prior to the administration of any drug, to be informed of the brand name and generic name of the drug in order that she may advise the health professional of any past adverse reaction to the drug.
7. The Pregnant Patient has the right to determine for herself, without pressure from her attendant, whether she will accept the risks inherent in the proposed therapy or refuse a drug or procedure.
8. The Pregnant Patient has the right to know the name and qualifications of the individual administering a medication or procedure to her during labor or birth.
9. The Pregnant Patient has the right to be informed, prior to the administration of any procedure, whether that procedure is being administered to her for her or her baby's benefit (medically indicated) or as an elective procedure (for convenience, teaching purposes or research).
10. The Pregnant Patient has the right to be accompanied during the stress of labor and birth by someone she cares for, and to whom she looks for emotional comfort and encouragement.
11. The Pregnant Patient has the right after appropriate medical consultation to choose a position for labor and for birth which is least stressful to her baby and to herself.
12. The Obstetric Patient has the right to have her baby cared for at her bedside if her baby is normal, and to feed her baby according to her baby's needs rather than according to the hospital regimen.
13. The Obstetric Patient has the right to be informed in writing of the name of the person who actually delivered her baby and the professional qualifications of that person. This information should also be on the birth certificate.
14. The Obstetric Patient has the right to be informed if there is any known or indicated aspect of her or her baby's care or condition which may cause her or her baby later difficulty or problems.
15. The Obstetric Patient has the right to have her and her baby's hospital medical records complete, accurate and legible and to have their records, including Nurses' Notes, retained by the hospital until the child reaches at least the age of majority, or alternatively, to have the records offered to her before they are destroyed.
16. The Obstetric Patient, both during and after her hospital stay, has the right to have access to her complete hospital medical records, including Nurses' Notes, and to receive a copy upon payment of a reasonable fee and without incurring the expense of retaining an attorney.

It is the obstetric patient and her baby, not the health professional, who must sustain any trauma or injury resulting from the use of a drug or obstetric procedure. The observation of the rights listed above will not only permit the obstetric patient to participate in the decisions involving her and her baby's health care, but will help to protect the health professional and the hospital against litigation arising from resentment or misunderstanding on the part of the mother.

Written by Doris B. Haire, published by the International Childbirth Education Association.

Nurses' Responsibilities Regarding Rights

Nurses need to recognize and protect the rights of patients and their families in these ways:

1. Respect the dignity of each patient and family.
2. Respect the right of each patient to refuse any treatment, procedure, or medication. Report any refusals to the appropriate person in the agency and to the physician.
3. Respect the right of each patient and family (support persons) to confidentiality of information.
4. Answer the patient's questions and provide information when appropriate in the setting or when delegated this function by the physician; if not permitted to answer any questions, report the questions to the appropriate person in the agency and to the physician.
5. Listen carefully to patients and their support persons and report their concerns to the appropriate person in the agency.

Nurses' Rights

Recently the idea of nurses' rights has received considerable attention. Initially this attention was focused on the right of the nurse to refuse to carry out a specific service, such as assisting with an abortion or giving a medication that the nurse considered dangerous for the patient. Now nurses' rights are being described in positive terms. Fagin (1975:82–85) lists seven rights of nurses:

1. The right to find dignity in self-expression and self-enhancement through the use of their special abilities and educational backgrounds.
2. The right to recognition for their contribution through the provision of a proper environment for practice, and through appropriate remuneration.
3. The right to a work environment that minimizes physical and emotional stress and health risks.
4. The right to control what is professional practice within the limits of the law.
5. The right to set standards of excellence in nursing.
6. The right to participate in policy making affecting nursing.
7. The right to social and political action on behalf of nursing and health care.

The rights of nurses, like other rights, are legal or ethical. Legal rights are those recognized by the legal systems, for example, fulfilling the terms of an employment contract by providing the salary stated for work provided. An ethical right is based on ethical principles or enlightened conscience. For example, a nurse has an ethical right not to assist with abortions, if they are against the nurse's beliefs. Along with legal and ethical rights come legal and ethical obligations and duties. Legal obligations are toward people or institutions defined in the law—patients and health care agencies. Ethical obligations are often felt to patients, families, and even society in general. Legal duties are related to the nurse's role and position. These are often written in regulations and legislated, for instance, in nursing practice acts. Ethical duties of nurses are written in codes of ethics of the profession.

When a nurse's rights (ethical or legal) are violated, the nurse has an obligation to discuss the matter with the appropriate person at the employing agency. If a conflict cannot be resolved, the nurse can report her or his concerns to a professional body, such as the American Nurses' Association. Most state and provincial associations have mechanisms to deal with legal and ethical issues.

Students' Rights

In 1974 in the United States, the Family Educational Rights and Privacy Act (Buckley Amendment) was passed by Congress. In it two major propositions are evident: that the records of a student should be available to that student, and that the records are private.

The specific records available to the student are educational records, not health records or the private files of teachers. Permission to see the student's file is limited to those involved in the educational process, for example, a nursing instructor who is teaching the student, or the registrar.

In addition, letters of recommendation can be kept from the student only if there is a waiver signed by the student, giving up the right to see the letter. Students do not have the right to see confidential materials obtained from parents, such as financial statements.

Students have the right to give or withhold permission for references based on information in their files. When the teacher, for example, needs access to the central file to provide reference information about graduates, the student has the right to withhold consent. References given without examining the central file do not require permission.

According to the Buckley Amendment, students have the right to challenge factual information, and a conciliation or hearing can subsequently take place.

Students also have other general rights directly involved in their nursing education. They have the right to expect that the curriculum described in the school brochure or calendar will be followed. They have a right to competent instruction in the hospital. Because students are accountable to patients for care, they must receive sufficient assistance and instruction to give safe care.

Patient Advocacy

An *advocate* pleads the cause of another or argues or pleads for a cause or proposal. Advocacy involves concern for and defined actions in behalf of another person or organizational system to bring about a change. Some nurses believe patient advocacy is an essential nursing function. Others believe that a patient advocate need not be a nurse. All, however, recognize the need of many patients to have an advocate to protect their rights and to help them speak up for themselves.

Patients' need for advocacy is generally thought to arise from the physical and psychological changes that accompany illness and hospitalization. Such changes frequently include feelings of fear or anxiety and loss of autonomy, initiative, and sense of identity. Patients who were active, independent, and responsible often become passive, dependent, and submissive. In addition many patients are worried by separation from family and friends, absence from work, unmet obligations, care of children or older parents, and accompanying financial problems.

Functions and Responsibilities

The function and responsibilities of a patient advocate are yet to be clearly defined in many agencies. Abrams (1978:260–61) outlines five plausible models or roles for the advocate:

1. *Counselor* or *lay therapist* whose function is to console patients and reduce fear, to help patients reestablish feelings of autonomy and control, to help patients recognize their feelings, and to provide companionship and attention.
2. *Adviser* whose function is to help patients make decisions about their health care. The advocate does not impose decisions or choices on patients but discusses alternative treatment plans to help patients choose options that best suit their life-styles and values.
3. *Rights advocate* whose function is to inform patients about their rights and ensure that the patients understand those rights and know how to exercise them. The advocate also makes sure that patients' rights are respected, serves as the person to whom patients report violations, and corrects or prevents them.
4. *Representative* whose function is to act as spokesperson for patients when the patient cannot do so. This function is of particular importance for patients who cannot speak for themselves, such as comatose patients, the mentally ill, and children. This function is also necessary for alert adults whose illness prevents them from representing themselves.
5. *Monitor of quality health care* whose function is to make certain patients are receiving the best care. This function includes ensuring continuity of care by making sure necessary information is transmitted to various hospital personnel, ensuring appropriate staff behavior, and ensuring appropriate therapy.

With these models and functions in mind, Abrams seriously questions whether the nurse is the best person to fulfill the role of patient advocate. She believes that patient advocacy should not be the sole responsibility of any one health professional but rather the responsibility of all health professionals. She further believes that a person who does not have loyalties and obligations within the health agency structure would be best suited for the role of patient advocate. Because of the multiple obligations and pressures on health care workers, advocacy might be necessary between patient and nurse or patient and any other health care worker.

Role of the Nurse as Advocate

The role of the nurse in patient advocacy varies from agency to agency. In some agencies a patients' representative (patient advocate) position exists. This person may or may not be a nurse. In this situation, nurses document and report inadequacies and injustices in patient care to this representative, who then initiates measures to correct them. In agencies where a patient advocate position does not exist, the nurse may assume the advocate role in various ways.

Kohnke (1980:2038) defines advocacy as "the act of informing and supporting a person so that he can make the best decisions possible for himself" and describes the role of the nurse advocate as:

1. To inform patients of their rights in a particular situation and then to make sure they have all the necessary information to make an informed decision. If the patient is unable to receive the information, the nurse must inform the patient's family or other support persons.
2. To support patients in the decisions they make.

Nurses need to present not only what the patient has a right to know but also the kinds of questions the patient should ask and of whom. The New York Hospital Patients Bill of Rights, for example, gives patients the right to feel secure about their health care program. It explains that the physician will discuss the care and course of treatment, but patients are encouraged to ask specific questions if they do not understand. Representative questions are: "What is my health problem?" "What are the results of my diagnostic tests?" "What kind of operation must I have?" "Are there alternatives?" (Cote 1981:30). See the suggested readings at the end of the chapter for further information.

Ensuring that the patient has all the necessary information to make an informed decision is a more complex matter. If the patient does not have a clear understanding of what is happening, the nurse is often the first to hear about it. Emphasis on listening and communication skills by the nurse is essential. For example, the nurse may find when conversing with a patient that the patient really has no idea about the risks involved in a procedure to be performed. As an advocate, the nurse is obligated to inform the physician or assistant about this and have the risks clarified. Even though a consent form may have been signed, the form is invalid if the patient does not understand.

Supporting the decisions that the patient makes may or may not involve action. Some patients may need active reassurance that the decision and the right to make it is theirs, regardless of pressure from others to do otherwise. It is important also for nurses to accept and support the patient's decisions even though the nurse, a family member, or another professional may consider it an unwise decision. For example, if a family member asks the nurse to convince a man that his decision to leave the hospital or not to have surgery is wrong, the nurse as an advocate needs to support the patient and must therefore refuse this request. Patients often have difficulty making decisions. With such patients, the nurse needs to emphasize giving information and support rather than offering advice.

Kosik (1972:694), a public health nurse, sees another dimension to the role of the nurse in patient advocacy—changing the system. She believes the two goals of patient advocacy are:

1. To make a person more independent by knowledge of the what, why, and how of the system
2. To change the system by revealing injustices and inadequacies

In Kosik's view, the role of the nurse is "to see that the patient knows what to expect, what [it] is his right to have, and then to display the willingness and courage to see that the system does not prevent his getting it." Kosik recognizes the fact that people become dependent on others during the early developmental periods of life and during critical and stressful periods as adults. At such times, when patients are not capable of fighting the system themselves, she believes that nurses must step in by doing and fighting for them until they are ready to take over themselves.

Efforts by the nurse to change the system may require much time, patience, and perseverance. Changing the system means attending conferences, and writing or calling nursing directors, agency administrators, and government officials. In addition it may require the nurse to "make waves," see that workers and agencies do their jobs, and even expose the indifference of some caregivers.

Codes of Ethics

A *code of ethics* provides a means by which professional standards of practice are established, maintained, and improved. It is essential to a profession. Codes of ethics are formal guidelines for professional action. They are shared by the persons within the profession and should be generally compatible with a professional member's personal values.

A code of ethics gives the members of the profession a frame of reference for judgments in complex nursing situations. No two situations are identical, and nurses are frequently in situations that require judgment about which course of action to take. A code of ethics serves as a guide in many of these situations.

When people enter the nursing profession, other members of the profession assume that they accept the established nursing codes of ethics. New nurses inherit the trust and the responsibility to carry out ethical practices and to exhibit ethical conduct.

The International Council of Nurses, American Nurses' Association, Canadian Nurses' Association, and state and provincial associations have established codes of nursing ethics. If a nurse violates the code, the association may expel the nurse from membership. Increasingly, professional nursing associations are taking an active part in improving and enforcing standards.

Purposes of nursing ethics can be outlined as follows:

1. Providing a basis for regulating the relationship between the nurse, the patient, coworkers, society, and the profession.
2. Providing a standard basis for excluding the unscrupulous nursing practitioner and for defending a practitioner who is unjustly accused.
3. Serving as a basis for professional curricula and for orienting the new graduate to professional nursing practice.
4. Assisting the public in understanding professional nursing conduct.

In 1973, the International Council of Nurses (ICN) adopted the code of ethics presented in Table 3–9, as a guide for nurses. It is meant to be understood, internalized, and used by nurses in all aspects of nursing practice. The code should be considered together with the relevant data in each situation; thus it provides assistance in setting priorities and in taking action. For the nurse practitioner, the code specifically provides assistance in making judgments and in developing attitudes appropriate to nursing.

The American Nurses' Association adopted a Code of Ethics in 1950, which was revised in 1968 and 1976. See Table 3–10. This code is designed to provide guidance for nurses by stating principles of ethical concern. Nurses have a responsibility to be familiar with the code that governs their nursing practice. In addition, nursing practice is also defined by the particular setting. In a rural, isolated setting, a nurse may be expected to assume responsibilities not normally assumed by urban nurses. For example, the nurse may assess the progress of labor and deliver the infant if the labor is normal. Only if there is a problem is the patient flown to a center for a physician's care.

Table 3–9 International Council of Nurses Code for Nurses

The fundamental responsibility of the nurse is fourfold: to promote health, to prevent illness, to restore health, and to alleviate suffering.

The need for nursing is universal. Inherent in nursing is respect for life, dignity, and rights of man. It is unrestricted by considerations of nationality, race, creed, color, age, sex, politics or social status.

Nurses render health services to the individual, the family and the community and coordinate their services with those of related groups.

Nurses and People

The nurse's primary responsibility is to those people who require nursing care.

The nurse, in providing care, promotes an environment in which the values, customs and spiritual beliefs of the individual are respected.

The nurse holds in confidence, personal information and uses judgment in sharing this information.

Nurses and Practice

The nurse carries personal responsibility for nursing practice and for maintaining competence by continual learning. The nurse maintains the highest standards of nursing care possible within the reality of a specific situation.

The nurse uses judgment in relation to individual competence when accepting and delegating responsibilities.

The nurse when acting in a professional capacity should at all times maintain standards of personal conduct which reflect credit upon the profession.

Nurses and Society

The nurse shares with other citizens the responsibility for initiating and supporting action to meet the health and social needs of the public.

Nurses and Co-workers

The nurse sustains a cooperative relationship with co-workers in nursing and other fields. The nurse takes appropriate action to safeguard the individual when his care is endangered by a co-worker or any other person.

Nurses and the Profession

The nurse plays the major role in determining and implementing desirable standards of nursing practice and nursing education.

The nurse is active in developing a core of professional knowledge.

The nurse, acting through the professional organization, participates in establishing and maintaining equitable social and economic working conditions in nursing.

From International Council of Nurses, *ICN Code for nurses: Ethical concepts applied to nursing* (Geneva, Switzerland: Imprimeries Populaires, 1973). Reprinted with permission of the ICN.

Table 3–10 American Nurses' Association Code of Ethics

1. The nurse provides services with respect for human dignity and the uniqueness of the client unrestricted by considerations of social or economic status, personal attributes, or the nature of health problems.
2. The nurse safeguards the client's right to privacy by judiciously protecting information of a confidential nature.
3. The nurse acts to safeguard the client and the public when health care and safety are affected by the incompetent, unethical, or illegal practice of any person.
4. The nurse assumes responsibility and accountability for individual nursing judgments and actions.
5. The nurse maintains competence in nursing.
6. The nurse exercises informed judgment and uses individual competence and qualifications as criteria in seeking consultation, accepting responsibilities, and delegating nursing activities to others.
7. The nurse participates in activities that contribute to the ongoing development of the profession's body of knowledge.
8. The nurse participates in the profession's efforts to implement and improve standards of nursing.
9. The nurse participates in the profession's efforts to establish and maintain conditions of employment conducive to high quality nursing care.
10. The nurse participates in the profession's effort to protect the public from misinformation and misrepresentation and to maintain the integrity of nursing.
11. The nurse collaborates with members of the health professions and other citizens in promoting community and national efforts to meet the health needs of the public.

From American Nurses' Association, *Code for nurses* (Kansas City, Mo., American Nurses' Association, 1976). Reprinted with permission.

Ethics of Nursing Research

As a profession committed to the improvement of health services to society, nursing is obligated to develop new knowledge as well as to use available knowledge and skills. Such a commitment to the development of nursing theory and to the improvement of nursing practice presupposes a commitment to research. There is, then, an obligation for nurses to undertake studies that produce broad theoretical constructs as well as studies that are directed toward more immediately tangible outcomes.

The ethics of nursing research must be consistent with the ethics of nursing practice. Nurses must not knowingly permit their services to be used for purposes inconsistent with the ethical standards of their profession.

Since nursing research necessarily involves human subjects directly or indirectly, its activities must be guided by certain ethical considerations. Codes regarding research are intended to identify some basic ethical principles that serve as guides for the nurse researcher. See Table 3–11.

Ethical Problems of Nurses

A study of the ethical problems of nurses suggests three major ethical questions in nursing (Allen 1974:22–23).

1. A question of to whom the nurse is responsible
2. A question of what course of action to take while knowing what should be done
3. A question of what can be done about an unsatisfactory level of nursing care

Ethical problems faced by nurses can also be placed in five broad areas:

1. Conflicts between professional role and personal values.
2. Problems between the nurse and peers and/or other health professionals.
3. Problems between the nurse and the patient and/or the family.
4. Problems between the nurse and the agency.
5. Problems of conflicting responsibilities.

The sections that follow give examples of specific problems in each category. In these ethical problems, the nurse has a number of options for action. The next major section, on ethical decision making, suggests a process for considering each situation and reaching a decision about how to proceed.

Table 3–11 Canadian Nurses' Association Ethics of Nursing Research

The Subject

Respect for the value of human life, for the worth and dignity of human beings, and their rights to knowledge, privacy, and self-determination must underlie research practices in nursing as in other health disciplines. The legitimacy of involving human subjects in nursing research must be assessed within the context of these values. The right of the subject to informed consent, confidentiality, positive risk value, and competence of the investigator must be assured.

Free and Informed Consent

When individuals are involved as subjects of research, the researcher must obtain free and informed consent. Informed consent implies that every effort be made to have the subject understand the purpose and nature of the research and the use or uses to which the findings will be put, in such a way that he can appreciate the implications of participation or non-participation. He must also be informed that if any significant change in purpose, nature, or use of findings is contemplated, he will also be informed and have the right to consent or refuse to participate further.

Free consent means that the relationship between the researcher and the subject, and persons or institutions involved in his care will not place him under any obligation to agree or take part in the project against his own personal inclinations. It also means that his refusal to take part, or his withdrawal after having once consented, should not lead to any repercussions or recriminations. Free consent implies informing the subject that he has the right to withdraw at any point during the research.

If the nature of the research is such that fully informing subjects before the study would invalidate results, then this fact must be stated to the subject, together with whatever explanations can be given. There must be provision for appropriate explanation to the subject on completion of the study.

If the subject for any reason is unable to appreciate the implications of participation, informed consent must be obtained from the legal guardian or an impartial committee acting on behalf of the subject. If the research should impinge on the privacy or other rights of any third party, such as the spouse of the subject, this person's consent must also be obtained.

Confidentiality

Subjects must be assured that confidentiality will be respected. Where anonymity is promised, it must be provided. Hidden coding to enable the researcher to identify individuals must not be resorted to. Every effort must be made to ensure that individuals and institutions cannot be identified.

Injury, Risk, and Priorities

Research subjects must be assured protection against physical, mental or emotional injury. Should the research involve risk of injury, such risks must be weighed against the good to be achieved. Should the risk outweigh the positive value of the research, the project must not be pursued.

Where there is conflict between the rights of the subject and the needs of the researcher for freedom of inquiry, the conflict must be resolved with priority given to the concerns and rights of the subject.

The Researcher

In order to maintain high ethical standards, the nurse researcher must possess knowledge and skills compatible with the demands of the investigation to be undertaken. The researcher has responsibility to acknowledge personal limitations and to correct misrepresentations made by others. The researcher is obligated to develop the design and procedures appropriate to the study.

The researcher is accountable in varying ways to those participating in the investigation. The purpose of the research must be honestly represented, and any uses to which the findings may be put, made known to persons or institutions involved. In order to justify the investigation, the researcher must ensure that the purposes and anticipated outcomes are compatible with the financial investment and the people and resources used.

In order to ensure the integrity of the investigation, the researcher must present the project for review to a group of professional peers. With certain studies, ongoing reviews by a peer group may be mandatory.

The Setting

The milieu in which an investigation is to be conducted must be assessed in terms of the potential for a nurse researcher to conduct a study that is consistent with these guidelines. While the board and/or administrators of an institution or agency may require approval by its research committee of a nursing study as well as of any other proposal, any such approval body should include nursing representation. There should be ongoing provisions for coping with setting-related ethical problems during the course of the investigation.

Nurse researchers ought to be the principal investigators in the study of nursing problems and must be collaborators with other researchers in the study of interprofessional problems of health care. This interprofessional involvement indicates that a common code of ethics for health research should be developed to facilitate research in nursing and its related professions.

From Canadian Nurses' Association, Ethics of nursing research, *Canadian Nurse*, September 1972, 68:23–25. Reprinted with permission.

Conflicts between Professional Role and Personal Values

In value conflict problems, the nurse knows what should be done but for various reasons either acts differently or withdraws from the situation. In all cases the nurse faces an ethical problem.

For example, a nurse whose personal value system does not support abortion has begun to develop a good personal relationship with a 13-year-old girl admitted to the hospital for a legal abortion. The girl is ambivalent about the abortion; because of her ambivalent feelings and her fear of the procedure, she wants to have the nurse's personal support. The nurse, in her professional role, needs to support the girl in going ahead with the abortion; however, as a person, the nurse is against abortion and finds it difficult to give the girl her complete support. Question: Should the nurse play a strictly professional role and support the abortion, or should she reveal her personal feelings about abortion?

A second example is a nurse who is asked to teach birth control and who opposes birth control because of personal values. Question: Does the nurse do the teaching, or does the nurse refuse?

A third example is a white nurse who is afraid to correct a black nurse's error for fear the black nurse will report the white nurse to the Human Rights Commission. Question: Does the white nurse correct the black nurse and risk labor problems and possible firing?

In each of these situations the nurse knows the correct action to take for the patient; however, the nurse's own values or fears provide ethical conflicts.

Problems between the Nurse and Peers

A nurse who faces a problem with peers or other health professionals may or may not know the course of action to take.

The first example is a nurse who sees another nurse steal medications from the nursing unit drug cupboard. The nurse who is discovered cries and explains that she needs the sleeping pills to sleep during the day while her three children are home from school. She uses them only when she is on night shift. She is the sole support of her children and needs the job. Question: Does the nurse report the theft or ignore the matter?

A second situation involves a nurse newly employed at a hospital who requests Christmas leave because his father is dying and he wants to spend Christmas with him. Under the special circumstances, the nurse is granted the time. Another nurse finds out that the first nurse's father is not dying and that he plans to spend Christmas vacation skiing with a friend. Question: Does the nurse report the skiing vacation to the nursing supervisor or forget the information?

In a third situation, a surgeon, the chief of staff of surgery, comes on a hospital nursing unit one evening to see a patient before surgery, and a nurse smells alcohol on the surgeon's breath. Question: Does the nurse report this or ignore it?

A fourth situation involves a nurse who is employed on a community mental health team. Another nurse discovers that the nurse spends most of the time at home looking after an ill mother and fabricates reports about visiting patients in their homes. Question: Does the nurse present this information to the members of the community team or discuss the situation with the nurse at fault?

Problems between the Nurse and the Patient and/or Family

In some situations, the nurse has ethical problems that involve a patient, a family, or both. In one instance, a patient requests an abortion. Her husband agrees, but he tells the nurse that he will always be tormented with the thought that he agreed to destroy a human being he helped to create. The wife tells the nurse that her husband was not the father of the unborn baby. Question: Should the nurse tell the father, the physician, or the nursing supervisor any of this information?

In a second example, an 18-year-old patient who believes he is dying tells the nurse that he wants to die with a clear conscience and confesses that at age 15 he held his brother's head under water until he drowned. He says that his parents believe his brother drowned accidentally. Question: Should the nurse tell anyone—the physician, the nursing supervisor, or the parents—this information?

A third example involving patients and their families is a nurse caring for a woman injured in an automobile accident. The husband, also in the accident, is admitted to another hospital unit and dies. The patient constantly questions the nurse about the husband. The physician directs the nurse not to tell the patient but to fabricate answers; the physician gives no reason. Question: Should the nurse fabricate answers for the patient, report the matter to the supervisor, or tell the patient the truth?

Conflicts between the Nurse and an Agency

The nurse's professional and personal ethical values may come into conflict with agency policy. In one situation, the nurse is asked by a dying patient not to call a clergyman, but the hospital policy is that the clergy are called for all dying patients. Question: Should the nurse call a clergyman or discuss this with the patient and the family?

In a second example, hospital policy is that all sedative medications are counted at the end of each shift. The nurse has already been reprimanded for staying overtime to do this. Question: Should the nurse not count the tablets but just subtract those administered to patients, or should the nurse do the count and neglect a patient who requires a change of dressing?

A third example is an upset teenager who wants information about how to obtain an abortion. The agency's policy is not to discuss abortions. Question: Should the nurse give the information to the patient or follow the agency's policy?

Problems of Conflicting Responsibilities

Nurses are repeatedly faced with conflicting responsibilities. On the one hand, the nurse is frequently an employee responsible to a hospital or health agency. On the other hand, the nurse is a professional person responsible to the professional ethics of an association and the standards of nursing practice of the profession. In addition, the nurse is responsible to and for patients and is taught to respond to their needs in a therapeutic manner.

For example, a nurse is asked by a physician not to keep a record of all the supplies used for a particular patient because the patient will have difficulty paying the bill; however, the nurse is accountable for all supplies used. Question: Should the nurse report the matter to the hospital or follow the physician's request?

In a second situation, a nurse on the evening shift is asked by a nursing supervisor to administer an intramuscular antibiotic to the supervisor, using the nursing unit stock. Question: What should the nurse do? To whom is the nurse responsible?

Resolving Ethical Problems

Several approaches to resolving ethical problems in nursing practice have appeared in nursing literature in recent years. Although codes of ethics offer general guidelines for decision making, more specific guidelines are necessary in many cases to resolve the everyday ethical dilemmas encountered by nurses in practice settings. Suggested guidelines for the nurse to resolve these problems include the following:

1. Establish a sound data base.
2. Identify the conflicts presented by the situation.
3. Outline alternative actions to the proposed course of action.
4. Outline the outcomes or consequences of the alternative actions.
5. Determine ownership of the problem and the appropriate decision maker.
6. Define the nurse's obligations.

Establishing the Data Base

To establish a sound data base the nurse needs to gather as much information as possible about the situation. Aroskar (1980:660) suggests that nurses get answers to the following questions:

1. What persons are involved and what is their involvement in the situation?
2. What is the proposed action?
3. What is the intent of the proposed action?
4. What are the possible consequences of the proposed action?

For example, Mrs. Green, a 67-year-old woman, is hospitalized with multiple fractures and lacerations caused by an automobile accident. Her husband, also in the accident, is admitted to the same hospital and dies. Mrs. Green, who was the driver of the automobile, constantly questions the primary nurse about her husband. The surgeon, however, has told the nurse not to tell the patient about the husband and to fabricate answers. The nurse is not provided with any reason for such a direction and expresses concern to the head nurse, who says the surgeon's orders must be followed.

In this example the data base includes:

Persons involved: Patient (concerned about husband's welfare), husband (deceased), surgeon, head nurse, and primary nurse.

Proposed action: Withhold information about the husband's death.

Intention of proposed action: Unknown; possibly to protect Mrs. Green from psychologic trauma, overwhelming guilt feelings, and consequent deterioration of her physical condition.

Consequences of proposed action: If information is withheld the patient may become increasingly anxious and angry and may refuse to cooperate with necessary care, delaying recovery.

Identifying Conflicts

A conflict is a clash between opposing elements or ideas. Five broad areas of ethical conflicts that confront nurses were discussed previously. The conflicts for the primary nurse in the example are:

1. Need to be honest with Mrs. Green without being disloyal to the surgeon and the charge nurse

2. Need to be loyal to the surgeon and head nurse without being dishonest to Mrs. Green
3. Conflict about the effects on Mrs. Green's health if she is informed or if she is not informed.

Outlining Courses of Action and Outcomes

Alternative courses of action to the proposed action for Mrs. Green and their outcomes might include:

1. Follow the surgeon's and charge nurse's advice and do as the surgeon suggests. The outcomes for the nurse would be (a) approval from the charge nurse and surgeon, (b) risk of being seen as nonassertive, (c) violation of own value to be truthful to Mrs. Green, (d) possible benefit to Mrs. Green's health, and (e) possible detriment to her health.
2. Discuss the situation further with the charge nurse and surgeon, pointing out Mrs. Green's rights to autonomy and information. The outcomes might be: (a) the surgeon may acknowledge the patient's right to be informed and may then inform the patient, (b) the surgeon may state that the patient's rights have no legal basis and may adhere to the original proposed action, based on a judgment about the effects of information on Mrs. Green.

Determining Ownership

In some ethical dilemmas the nurse does not make decisions about her or his own actions but assists the patient to make a decision. For example, if a patient states he does not want to have an operation, the question of ownership arises. In this example, it is obvious that the patient owns the problem and that it is his right to choose this course of action. Associated with ownership, however, is knowledge about the probability and the risk of consequences attending various courses of actions. Therefore, the nurse does not abandon the patient with this decision. The nurse has the professional knowledge and expertise to ensure that the patient makes an informed decision. Thus the patient needs information from the professional's frame of reference about the consequences of decisions.

A series of questions that evolve from decision-making theories can help nurses determine who owns a certain problem (Aroskar 1980:660):

1. Who should make the decision and why?
2. For whom is the decision being made?
3. What criteria (social, economic, psychologic, physiologic, or legal) should be used in deciding who makes the decision?
4. What degree of consent is needed by the subject (patient and other)?
5. What, if any, moral principles (rights, values) are enhanced or negated by the proposed action?

In the example of Mrs. Green, the surgeon obviously believes the decision is his or hers to make for Mrs. Green, and the charge nurse agrees. However the criteria used to decide who the decision maker should be are not clear. If the criteria were spelled out, perhaps the conflict about the effects on Mrs. Green's health from knowing or not knowing about her husband's death could be resolved. Is it psychologically advantageous for Mrs. Green to know or not to know? Is it physically advantageous? What will be the social and economic effects?

Value systems also influence the decision about problem ownership. The value of Mrs. Green's right to information about her husband will be enhanced if she is told, negated if not. Her right to autonomy will also be affected.

This example shows that there are no clearly defined right or wrong answers to ethical dilemmas. If there were, they would not be ethical dilemmas. To resolve Mrs. Green's case, it may be necessary for the involved health team members to confer and clearly establish approaches that will be in Mrs. Green's best interests. Once an approach is agreed on, the nurses and physician can devise consistent continuing methods of support for Mrs. Green. That approach may dictate actions by the nurse that conflict with her or his own value system. However, the action chosen for Mrs. Green's best interest takes precedence.

Defining the Nurse's Obligations

When determining an ethical course of action, Moser and Cox (1980:43) advise nurses to list their nursing obligations, to assess the conflicts that will arise if all obligations are met, and to determine the alternatives from which the nurse can choose. Examples of obligations are:

1. To maximize the patient's well-being
2. To balance the patient's need for autonomy and family members' responsibilities for the patient's well-being
3. To support each family member and enhance the family support system
4. To carry out hospital policies
5. To protect other patients' well-being
6. To protect the nurse's own standards of care

Summary

Personal values are learned beginning early in life from a variety of sources. A nursing student can learn values for nursing practice that have not been a part of the student's value system previously. There may be instances in which a nurse's personal values conflict with professional duty, as in attitudes toward abortion or euthanasia. Values clarification is a process that helps people identify their values.

Patients' rights are increasingly being recognized and publicized. Several factors have influenced the recognition of these rights, notably consumer demands and consumer involvement in the planning and provision of health care services. Consumers are expressing needs for personalized services, for active participation in health care planning, for greater accessibility and coordination of services, and for knowledge about health status and outcomes of health care. They expect higher standards of care, the right to refuse recommended therapies, the right to volunteer for or refuse participation in experiments, and an accounting of costs incurred for services.

In addition to the rights of all patients, the rights of special groups of consumers are increasingly recognized. These groups include the disabled, the pregnant patient, the mentally retarded, and the dying. Emphasized in lists of rights for these groups is consideration for their special needs and protection against exploitation and discrimination.

Ethics are the rules and principles that guide right conduct. Ethical codes are characteristic of professions, including nursing. With the rapid advance in medical technology, nurses are increasingly being faced with ethical issues in such areas as abortion, euthanasia, and organ transplants as well as ethical issues in daily functioning.

Nursing ethics have four broad purposes: They regulate professional relationships, provide standards of practice, serve as a basis for curricula that orient students, and educate the public about appropriate nursing practice.

Various codes of nursing have been drawn up to help nurses perform their duties. Two such codes are that of the International Council of Nurses and of the American Nurses' Association.

Special and increasing concern is being given to the ethics of nursing research. Many nurses become involved in research; this research generally involves patients. To delineate nurses' responsibilities to patients and at the same time assist with research, the Canadian Nurses' Association prepared a paper, "Ethics of Nursing Research." Points of emphasis include free and informed consent on the part of the patient and family; confidentiality of the data, including anonymity for subjects; protection of the patient from injury; and precedence of the welfare of the patient over the needs of the researcher, wherever these are in conflict. The researcher's responsibilities and accountability are described together with the setting for the research.

Nurses face a number of ethical problems in their daily nursing activities. These have been placed in five broad categories. Examples of the types of problems are given to encourage thought and discussion.

Ethical problems are not solved merely by determining right action. The right action might be evident, but the problems surrounding right action are difficult. The process of ethical decision making has been described in the literature. Guidelines for the nurse resolving ethical problems include: (a) establishing a data base, (b) identifying conflicts, (c) outlining alternative actions and their outcomes, (d) determining the appropriate decision maker, and (e) defining the nurse's obligations.

Suggested Activities

1. Select a patient in the clinical area and determine whether, in your opinion, the patient's rights, as stated by the American Hospital Association or the Consumers' Association of Canada, have been considered.
2. Talk with someone in the community and find out what this person considers to be the rights of patients.
3. Interview a registered nurse to determine what she or he views as nurses' rights. Compare your findings with other students'. Compare all the findings with the rights listed in this chapter.
4. Review the section on ethical problems of nurses, beginning on page 88. Discuss with a group of nursing students what you would do in these situations. Use the framework provided in the chapter for making a decision in each situation.
5. Select a concept that you consider a personal value. Assess this concept using the value clarification process.
6. List some of your personal values and consider whether they are compatible with the nursing ethics cited in this chapter.

Suggested Readings

Aroskar, M. A. April 1980. Anatomy of an ethical dilemma: The practice. *American Journal of Nursing* 80:661–63.

This author presents an ethical situation and analyzes it in three parts: the data base, the decision theory dimensions, and the ethical theories and positions.

Cote, A. A. January 1981. The patient's representative: Whose side is she on? *Nursing 81* 11:26–30.

This article discusses how the nurse and the patient's representative can work together to protect the patient's rights. Topics include the patient's bill of rights, informed consent, the patient's right to know and not to know, the right to decline treatment, the right to privacy, and the right to information in clinical records.

Fagin, C. M. January 1975. Nurses' rights. *American Journal of Nursing* 75:82–85.

Dr. Fagin discusses rights generally, moving from human rights and women's rights to nurses' rights.

Fay, P. April 1978. Sounding board: In support of patient advocacy as a nursing role. *Nursing Outlook* 26:252–53.

This article reveals how the concept of advocacy was introduced into a nursing curriculum. The patient's rights advocate is favored and given as an assignment for students.

Moser, D., and Cox, J. M., editors. May 1980. Perspectives: Resolving an ethical dilemma. *Nursing 80* 10:39–43.

This article presents an ethical problem encountered at St. Jude's Children's Research Center. The discussion to resolve the problem is presented with consultation by Terrence Ackerman, Department of Human Values and Ethics, University of Tennessee, and Dorothy Moser, a fellow in the Program on Human Values and Ethics at the University of Tennessee.

Nursing 74. September 1974. Nuring ethics—the admirable professional standards of nurses: A survey report. *Nursing 74* 4:35–44.

This article reports nurses' responses to a survey on ethical and interpersonal problems. It discusses what some nurses feel about distasteful patients, challenging doctors' orders, drug addiction, and sexual involvements.

Smith, S. J., and David, A. J. August 1980. Ethical dilemmas: Conflicts among rights, duties, and obligations. *American Journal of Nursing* 80:1462–66.

The authors discuss different types of conflicts confronting nurses and involving ethics. They describe the rights, duties, and obligations of nurses and offer several courses of action open to nurses faced with conflict problems.

Selected References

Ethics

Allen, M. February 1974. Ethics of nursing practice. *Canadian Nurse* 70:22–23.

American Nurses' Association. 1976. *Code for nurses with interpretive statements.* Kansas City, Mo.: American Nurses' Association.

Aroskar, M. A. April 1980. Anatomy of an ethical dilemma: The theory. *American Journal of Nursing* 80:658–60.

Canadian Nurses' Association. September 1972. Ethics of nursing research. *Canadian Nurse* 68:23–25.

Cawley, M. A. May 1977. Euthanasia: Should it be a choice? *American Journal of Nursing* 77:859–61.

Churchill, L. May 1977. Ethical issues of a profession in transition. *American Journal of Nursing* 77:873–76.

Davis, A. J., and Aroskar, M. A. 1978. *Ethical dilemmas and nursing practice.* New York: Appleton-Century-Crofts.

Fromer, M. J. 1981. *Ethical issues in health care.* St. Louis: C. V. Mosby Co.

Huttman, B. R. January 1982. No code? Slow code? Show code? *American Journal of Nursing* 82:133, 135–36.

International Council of Nurses. 1973. *ICN code for nurses: Ethical concepts applied to nursing.* Geneva: Imprimeries Popularies.

Jacobson, S. F. 1973. Ethical issues in experimentation with human subjects. *Nursing Forum* 12(1):58–71.

Johnson, P. May 1977. The gray areas—who decides? *American Journal of Nursing* 77:856–58.

Lestz, P. May 1977. A committee to decide the quality of life. *American Journal of Nursing* 77:862–64.

Levine, M. E. May 1977. Nursing ethics and the ethical nurse. *American Journal of Nursing* 77:845–49.

Nursing 74. October 1974. Nursing ethics—the admirable professional standards of nurses: A survey report. Part 2: Honesty, confidentiality, termination of life, and other decisions in nursing. *Nursing 74* 4:56–66.

Rapp, J. D. 1976. Implications of moral and ethical issues for nurses. *Nursing Forum* 15(2):168–79.

Romanell, P. May 1977. Ethics, moral conflicts, and choice. *American Journal of Nursing* 77:850–55.

Ryden, M. B. November 1978. An approach to ethical decision-making. *Nursing Outlook* 26:705–6.

Thompson, J. B., and Thompson, H. O. 1981. *Ethics in nursing.* New York: Macmillan Publishing Co.

Yeaworth, R. C. May 1977. The agonizing decisions in mental retardation. *American Journal of Nursing* 77:864–67.

Patient advocacy

Abrams, N. 1978. A contrary view of the nurse as patient advocate. *Nursing Forum* 17(3):259–67.

Donahue, P. M. 1978. The nurse a patient advocate? *Nursing Forum* 17(2):143–51.

Kohnke, M. F. November 1980. The nurse as advocate. *American Journal of Nursing* 80:2038–40.

Kosik, S. H. April 1972. Patient advocacy or fighting the system. *American Journal of Nursing* 72:694–98.

Nations, W. C. June 1973. Nurse-lawyer is patient-advocate. *American Journal of Nursing* 73:1039–41.

Rights

American Hospital Association. January 1976. A patient's bill of rights. *Nursing Outlook* 24:29 (also February 1973, *Nursing Outlook* 21:82).

American Journal of Nursing. January 1975. Dying person's bill of rights. *American Journal of Nursing* 75:99.

———. September 1976. A consumer speaks out about hospital care. *American Journal of Nursing* 76:1443–44.

American Nurses' Association. 1968. *The nurse in research: ANA guidelines on ethical values.* Kansas City, Mo.: American Nurses' Association.

———. 1975. *Human rights guidelines for nurses in clinical and other research.* ANA Publication Code no. D–46 5M 7/75. Kansas City, Mo.: American Nurses' Association.

Bandman, E., and Bandman, B. May 1977. There is nothing automatic about rights. *American Journal of Nursing* 77:867–72.

———. January 1978. Do nurses have rights? *American Journal of Nursing* 78:84–86.

Besch, L. B. January 1979. Informed consent: A patient's right. *Nursing Outlook* 27:32–35.

Canadian Consumer. April 1974. Consumer rights in health care. *Canadian Consumer* 4:1.

Dodge, J. S. October 1972. What patients should be told: Patients' and nurses' beliefs. *American Journal of Nursing* 72:1852–54.

Fagin, C. M. January 1975. Nurses' rights. *American Journal of Nursing* 75:82–85.

Kelly, L. Y. January 1976. The patient's right to know. *Nursing Outlook* 24:26–32.

Langford, T. June 1978. Establishing a nursing contract. *Nursing Outlook* 26:386–88.

May, K. A. January 1979. The nurse as researcher: Impediment to informed consent? *Nursing Outlook* 27:36–39.

Pollok, C. S., et al. April 1976. Students' rights. *American Journal of Nursing* 76:600–3.

———. April 1977. Faculties have rights, too. *American Journal of Nursing* 77:636–38.

Quinn, N., and Somers, A. R. April 1974. The patient's bill of rights: A significant aspect of the consumer revolution. *Nursing Outlook* 22:240–44.

Rozovsky, L. E. 1980. *The Canadian patients' book of rights.* Toronto: Doubleday Canada.

Shephard, D. A. December 1976. The 1975 declaration of Helsinki and consent. *Canadian Medical Journal* 115:1191–92.

Thorner, N. January 1976. Nurses violate their patients' rights. *Journal of Psychiatric Nursing and Mental Health Services* 14:7–12.

Values

Coletta, S. S. December 1978. Values clarification in nursing: Why? *American Journal of Nursing* 78:2057.

Czmowski, M. 1974. Value teaching in nursing education. *Nursing Forum* 13(2):192–206.

Raths, L. E.; Harmin, M.; and Simon, S. B. 1978. *Values and teaching.* 2nd ed. Columbus, Ohio: Charles E. Merrill Books.

Simon, S. B. 1973. *Meeting yourself halfway.* Niles, Ill.: Argus Communications.

Simon, S. B.; Howe, L. W.; and Kirschenbaum, H. 1972. *Values clarification: A handbook of practical strategies for teachers and students.* New York: Hart Publishing Co.

Uustal, D. B. February 1977. Searching for values. *Image* 9:15–17.

———. December 1978. Values clarification: Application to practice. *American Journal of Nursing* 78:2058–63.

Chapter 4

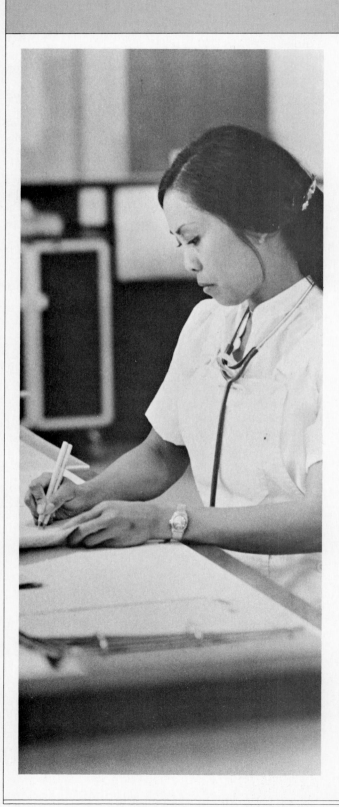

Legal Aspects of Nursing

CONTENTS

Objectives

1. Know essential facts about the law as it applies to nursing
    - **1.1** Define specific terms used in law
    - **1.2** List four basic functions of law in society
    - **1.3** Identify the origins, sources, and kinds of law
    - **1.4** Describe four basic principles of law
    - **1.5** List the functions of law in nursing
    - **1.6** Identify two kinds of legal actions
    - **1.7** Identify five steps of the judicial process
2. Understand aspects of the nurse's legal roles
    - **2.1** Identify three legal roles of the nurse
    - **2.2** Identify rights and obligations associated with the nurse's legal roles
    - **2.3** Identify essentials of the nurse's role as an expert witness
    - **2.4** Identify nine ways in which nurses can protect themselves from lawsuits
3. Understand the essentials of credentialing in nursing
    - **3.1** Identify the purpose of credentialing
    - **3.2** Explain the mechanisms of licensure
    - **3.3** Differentiate mandatory licensure, permissive licensure, and registration
    - **3.4** Differentiate certification and accreditation
4. Understand selected legal concepts as they relate to nursing
    - **4.1** Identify essential types and elements of contracts
    - **4.2** Explain the responsibilities of the nurse in witnessing a will
    - **4.3** Identify essential aspects of privileged communications
    - **4.4** Differentiate crimes and torts, and give nursing examples of each
    - **4.5** Explain the concept of fraud
    - **4.6** Differentiate malpractice and negligence
    - **4.7** Give examples of types of malpractice actions
    - **4.8** Explain the concept of invasion of privacy
    - **4.9** Compare libel and slander
    - **4.10** Differentiate assault and battery
    - **4.11** Compare false imprisonment with justifiable restraint
    - **4.12** Explain the intent of Good Samaritan acts
    - **4.13** Identify the purpose of professional liability insurance

Terms

accreditation
answer
assault
battery
burden of proof
certification
civil action
civil law
common law
complaint
contract
credentialing
crime
criminal action
criminal law
contract
decisional law
defamation
defendant
discovery (legal)
expert witness
felony
fraud
Good Samaritan act
liability
liable
libel
license
malpractice
mandatory licensure
misdemeanor
negligence
permissive licensure
plaintiff
privileged communication
public law
registration
slander
statutory law
technical assault and battery
tort
trial
will

Law is becoming so complex in today's society that its interpretation is generally a matter for experts, that is, for lawyers who specialize in a particular field of law. A nurse cannot be expected to have a complete understanding of the law. It is important, however, for nurses to understand aspects of law as it applies to nursing practice. By understanding basic concepts, the nurse has a sound basis for nursing judgments and nursing action.

The Law

Nearly every society has rules and regulations that are developed and promulgated by the society itself. These rules and regulations are the laws of the country, and they provide one aspect of social control for people. Laws can be seen as having four basic functions in a society:

1. To define relationships among the members of a society and to state which activities are permissible and which are not permissible.
2. To describe what force may be applied to maintain rules and by whom it is to be applied.
3. To provide the solution to problems.
4. To redefine relationships between persons and groups when conditions of life change.

Origins and Sources

The legal systems in both the United States and Canada have their origins in the English common law system. The *common law* has its source in the courts. Once a judge has made a decision, the decision becomes a part of the common law of the court's jurisdiction (for example, the state or district in which the court operates). The courts follow a precedent system: a lower court, for example, a local court, must follow the decisions of a higher court, for example, a state or federal court. The laws that come from this source are called *decisional laws.*

The other main source for the law is the enactments of a legislative body, such as the Congress of the United States or the Parliament in Canada. The laws passed by legislatures, whether federal, state, or provincial are called *statutory laws.*

Civil law is statutory law that deals with relations among people. It is also called *private law. Criminal law* deals with actions against the safety and welfare of the public, such as homicide and robbery. It is a part of *public law,* which deals with the relationship between an individual or individuals and the state.

Principles of Law

The system of law rests on four simple principles that are often cloaked in complex terminology (Fenner 1980: 84). These are:

1. *Law is based on a concern for justice and fairness.* The law seeks to protect the rights of one party from the transgressions of another. It sets guidelines for conduct and mechanisms to enforce those guidelines. The goal is to make known the rules of conduct that protect the rights of the parties involved and to assure a just and fair outcome.
2. *Law is characterized by change.* Social and technologic changes occur rapidly and often without predictions of problems to follow. In response to these changes, the legal system also must change. Often the legal system reacts rather than acts. For example, after technologic devices such as respirators were developed to prolong life, it became necessary for the law to change its guidelines about indications of death—from cessation of heart function to absence of electric currents from the brain for at least 24 hours.
3. *Actions are judged on the basis of a universal standard of what a similarly trained, reasonable, and prudent person would have done under similar circumstances.* It is recognized by law that not all nurses, for example, have the same capabilities, experience, or education. Therefore they are not all expected to function at the same level. However, all nurses are expected to function the same way that another nurse with similar education and experience would function. This rule of reasonable and prudent conduct forms the basis for evaluating a person's actions, e.g., for judging whether or not actions were negligent (see the discussion of negligence and malpractice on page 105).
4. *Each individual has rights and responsibilities.* Rights are privileges or fundamental powers that individuals possess unless they are revoked by law or given up voluntarily, responsibilities are the obligations associated with these rights. Failure to meet one's responsibilities can endanger one's rights. For example, a registered nurse has the right to practice nursing within the constraints of the law (nurse practice acts). If she or he fails to observe these constraints (e.g., prescribes medications or conducts a surgical procedure), the behavior is considered irresponsible and the right to practice can be revoked.

Kinds of Legal Actions

There are two kinds of legal actions: civil actions and criminal actions. *Civil actions* deal with the relationships between individuals in society; for example, a man may file a suit against a person who he believes cheated him. *Criminal actions* deal with disputes between an individual and the society as a whole; for example, if a woman shoots someone, society brings her to trial. Actions that might be of concern to nurses include those relating to wills and the estates of deceased persons. These cases are civil actions and are known specifically as *probate proceedings.*

The judicial process primarily functions to settle disputes peacefully and in accordance with the law. A lawsuit has strict procedural rules. There are generally five steps:

1. A document called a *complaint* is filed by a person referred to as the *plaintiff*, who claims that his or her legal rights have been infringed upon by one or more persons, referred to as *defendants*.
2. A written response, called an *answer*, is made by the defendants.
3. Both parties engage in pretrial activities referred to as *discovery*, in an effort to gain all the facts of the situation.
4. In the *trial* of the case, all the relevant facts are presented to a jury or a judge.
5. The judge renders a *decision* or the jury renders a *verdict*. If the outcome is not acceptable to one of the parties, an appeal can be made for another trial.

During a trial, a plaintiff must offer evidence of the defendant's wrongdoing. This is called the *burden of proof*. An additional aspect of this burden of proof is that the plaintiff must have a greater amount of convincing evidence than the defendant if the plaintiff is to prevail.

Functions of the Law in Nursing

The law serves a number of functions in nursing:

1. It provides a framework for establishing what nursing actions in the care of patients are legal.
2. It delineates the nurse's responsibilities from those of other health professionals.
3. It helps to establish the boundaries of independent nursing action.
4. It assists in maintaining a standard of nursing practice by making nurses accountable under the law.

Nurse Practice Acts

The first nurse practice acts were adopted in the United States in 1903 in New York, New Jersey, North Carolina, and Virginia. Each state in the United States and each province of Canada currently has nurse practice acts, which protect the nurse's professional capacity and legally control nursing practice through licensing. Nurse practice acts define professional nursing, and because of the number of acts there are many definitions. In 1961, the American Nurses' Association (ANA) recommended the following definition of nursing for professional nurse practice acts:

> The practice of professional nursing means the performance for compensation of any act in the observation, care and counsel of the ill, injured or infirm, or in the maintenance of health or prevention of illness of others, or in the supervision and teaching of other personnel, or in the administration of medications and treatments as prescribed by a licensed physician or dentist; requiring substantial specialized judgment and skill and based on knowledge and application of the principles of biological, physical and social science. The foregoing shall not be deemed to include acts of diagnosis or prescription of therapeutic or corrective measures.

This definition of nursing has three important points:

1. It defines nursing as performance for compensation.
2. It states what nursing is.
3. It states what nursing is not.

In recent years there has been some discussion about whether the nursing graduates from two-year programs in the general education system and diploma graduates are professional nurses. In May 1973, the Board of Directors of the ANA voted "to recognize all registered nurses as professionals" (ANA 1973:1135). This statement clarifies that, in nurse practice acts, the term *professional nurse* refers to all registered nurses unless otherwise specified.

The states and provinces also license practical nurses in much the same way as professional nurses. The major difference between the two kinds of nurses is that, through education and training, the registered professional nurse has more refined skills and knowledge and can make better judgments in relation to assessment and interpretation of data and therefore in the determination and provision of required nursing care.

Legal Roles of Nurses

Nurses have three separate, interdependent legal roles, each with rights and associated responsibilities: (a) provider of service, (b) employee or contractor for service, and (c) private citizen (Fenner 1980:86). See Table 4–1. Nurses move in and out of these roles when carrying out professional and personal responsibilities. An understanding of these roles and their rights and responsibilities promotes legally responsible conduct and practice by nurses.

Provider of Service

In the role of provider of service, the nurse is expected to provide safe and competent care so that harm (physical, psychologic, or material) to the recipient of the service is prevented. Implicit in this role are several legal concepts: (a) liability, (b) standard of care, and (c) contractual obligations.

Liability is the quality or state of being *liable*, i.e.,

Table 4–1 Nurses' Legal Roles, Rights, and Responsibilities

Role	Responsibilities	Rights
Provider of service	To provide safe and competent care commensurate with the nurse's preparation, experience, and circumstances	Right to adequate and qualified assistance as necessary
	To inform patients of the consequences of various alternatives and outcomes of care	Right to reasonable and prudent conduct from patients (e.g., provision of accurate information as required)
	To provide adequate supervision and evaluation of subordinates for whom the nurse is responsible	
	To remain competent	
Employee or contractor for service	To fulfill the obligations of contracted service with the employer	Right to adequate working conditions, e.g., safe equipment and facilities
		Right to compensation for services rendered
	To respect the rights and responsibilities of other health care participants	Right to reasonable and prudent conduct by other health care givers
Citizen	To protect the rights of the recipients of care	Right to respect by others of the nurse's own rights and responsibilities

legally responsible to account for one's obligations and actions and to make financial restitution for wrongful acts. A primary nurse or team leader, for example, has an obligation to practice and direct the practice of others under supervision so that harm or injury to the patient is prevented and standards of care are maintained. Even when a nurse is directed by a physician, the responsibility for nursing activity is the nurse's. When a nurse is requested to carry out an activity that the nurse believes will be injurious to the patient, the nurse's responsibility is to refuse to carry out the order.

The *standards of care* by which a nurse acts or fails to act are legally defined in accordance with (a) the constraints of nurse practice acts (see page 99) and (b) what would be done in similar circumstances by a reasonable and prudent professional with similar preparation and experience. A nurse, for example, would be acting illegally in diagnosing or treating a patient for a tumor, since these functions are within the scope of the physician's practice, and nurses are constrained from engaging in them. Associated with standards of care is the nurse's right to adequate and qualified assistance as required.

Contractual obligations refer to the nurse's duty of care, that is, duty to render care, established by the presence of a formal or informal contract (see the next section and the section on contracts on page 103). A nurse in some circumstances cannot be held liable for care given if a valid contractual relationship with the patient does not exist. In the contractual relationship between nurse and patient, patients have the right to expect that nurses caring for them have the competence to meet their needs. This implies that the nurse has a duty to remain competent. The nurse has the associated right to expect the patient to provide accurate information as required.

Employee or Contractor for Service

Another legal role of the nurse is that of employee or contractor for service. This role describes the nurse's rights and responsibilities as a staff nurse, private duty nurse, supervisor, consultant, independent practitioner, and member of a peer group of nurses. Implicit in this role are the legal concepts of contract law and contractual relationships.

Contract law requires that four elements be met to make a contract valid (Fenner 1980:94):

1. The act contracted for must be legal. The nurse's employment must be legal, and the duties to be performed and services provided must be within the law. For example, the nurse cannot be required to provide services that are not stated or permitted in the nurse practice act.

2. The parties to the contract must be of legal age (majority) and competent (free of mental impairment) to enter a binding agreement.

3. There must be mutual agreement about the service to be contracted for. A contract becomes invalid, for example, if the nurse does not accept an offer of hire, or if the nurse expecting to be placed in an obstetrical unit is placed in a coronary intensive care unit.

4. There must be compensation (or promise of it) for the service to be provided.

These four elements are also required for contracts made by patients (with nurses, other health professionals, or health care institutions) to be valid. For example, the activity contracted for between a patient and a hospital is health care, which is legal. Patients who are minors are not usually admitted for care without consent from their parents or legal guardians. The parties agree to the terms of the contract when the patient gives informed consent for care and the hospital offers care. The patient promises to reimburse the hospital for its services through insurance coverage or other means.

Contractual relationships vary among practice settings. For example, a private duty nurse who is not employed by a hospital functions within an independent contractor relationship with the client and is held individually liable for acts of malpractice. An independent nurse practitioner is a contractor for service, whose contractual relationship is again an independent one with the client. The nurse employed by a hospital functions within an employer-employee relationship, in which the nurse represents and acts for the hospital and therefore must function within the policies of the employing agency. This type of legal relationship creates the ancient legal doctrine known as *respondeat superior* ("let the master answer"). In other words the master (employer) assumes responsibility for the conduct of the servant (employee) and can be held responsible for malpractice by the employee. By virtue of the employee role, therefore, the nurse's conduct is the hospital's responsibility.

This doctrine does not imply that the nurse cannot be held liable as an individual. Nor does it imply that the doctrine will prevail if the employee's actions are extraordinarily inappropriate, i.e., beyond those expected or foreseen by the employer. For example, if the nurse hits a patient in the face, the employer could disclaim responsibility, since this behavior is beyond the bounds of expected behavior. Criminal acts, such as assisting with criminal abortions or taking tranquilizers from a patient's supply for personal use would also be considered extraordinarily inappropriate behavior. Nurses can be held liable for failure to act as well. For example, if a nurse sees another nurse hitting a patient and fails to do anything to protect the patient, the observer is also considered negligent.

The nurse in the role of employee or contractor for service has obligations to the employer, the patient, and other personnel. The nursing care provided must be within the limitations and terms specified. The nurse has an obligation to contract to do only those responsibilities for which she or he is competent. As an employee, the nurse is expected to uphold the good name of the employer and therefore should not spread unjustifiable criticism about the employer. The employer, in turn, is obligated to provide adequate working conditions, e.g., a safe, functional employment setting.

The nurse is expected to respect the rights and responsibilities of other health care participants. For example, although the nurse has responsibility to explain nursing activities to a patient, she or he does not have the right to comment on medical practice in a way that disturbs the patient or causes problems for the physician. At the same time, the nurse has the right to expect reasonable and prudent conduct from other health care participants.

Citizen

The rights and responsibilities of the nurse in the role of citizen are the same as any individual's fundamental rights under the legal system. Rights of citizenship protect patients from harm and ensure consideration for their personal property rights, rights to privacy, confidentiality, and other rights discussed in Chapter 3. These same rights apply to nurses. For example, nurses have the right to physical safety and need not perform functions that are considered an unreasonable risk.

Credentialing in Nursing

Credentialing is the process of determining and maintaining competence in nursing practice. The credentialing process is one way in which the nursing profession maintains standards of practice and is accountable for the educational preparation of members. Credentialing includes licensure, registration, certification, and accreditation.

Licensure

Licenses are legal documents that permit persons to offer their skills and knowledge to the public in a particular jurisdiction or area covered by the license. For a profession or occupation to obtain the right to license its members, it generally must meet three criteria:

1. There is a need to protect the public's safety or welfare.
2. The occupation is clearly delineated as a separate, distinct area of work.
3. There is an organization suitable in ability to assume the obligations of the licensing process (Sarner 1968:14).

In order to use the title *registered nurse* a nurse must be licensed by some state or province. In the United States licensure is a governmental function established under the law. Each state has a board of nursing that is empowered to grant licensure. These boards often have broad representation, usually including nurses. They have eight responsibilities, according to A. G. Stahl (1974:508):

1. To establish minimum standards for schools of nursing.
2. To survey programs in nursing to determine whether the minimum standards are being met.
3. To place programs meeting the standards on the state's approved or accredited list.
4. To select, administer, and determine the passing score on the licensing examination.
5. To grant licenses by examination and by interstate endorsement.
6. To renew licenses.
7. To prosecute licensees who are violators of the law.
8. To revoke or suspend licenses for cause.

In Canada, licensure is a legal function vested in the professional nursing association in most provinces. The one exception is Ontario, where licensure is vested in the College of Nurses under the Health Disciplines Act of the province; in that province, registration is optional. Canada has a national comprehensive licensing examination, which is offered in both French and English. Ontario, Quebec, and New Brunswick offer the examination in both languages, while the other provinces offer it only in English.

Types of licensure

There are two types of licensure: mandatory and permissive. *Mandatory licensure*, in the case of nursing, requires that anyone who practices nursing must be licensed. The only exceptions are: (a) practice in an emergency, (b) practice by nursing students as part of their education, and (c) practice by nurses employed by the federal government (nurses who practice in Veterans Administration hospitals and in public health must be currently licensed in some jurisdiction but not necessarily where the facility is). In *permissive licensure,* the titles RN and LPN are reserved for licensed practitioners, but the practice of nursing is not prohibited to others who are not licensed.

Licensure is mandatory in Prince Edward Island, Quebec, and Newfoundland in Canada, while the other provinces have permissive licensure. In the United States nursing licensure is mandatory.

License revocation

The nurses' association in each state and province has a committee, such as a board of examiners, that has the power to revoke licenses for just cause. Licenses can be revoked because of incompetent nursing practice; conviction of a crime, such as drug addiction or illegal sale of drugs; obtaining a license through deception, falsifying school records, or hiding a criminal history; and, in some areas, aiding in a criminal abortion. In each situation all the facts are generally reviewed by the committee at a hearing. In most places the nurse is entitled to be represented by legal counsel at the hearing. If the nurse's license is revoked as a result of the hearing, an appeal can be made to a court, or, in some states, an agency is designated to review the decision before any court action is initiated.

Registration

Registration is the recording or entering of certain information about individuals, i.e., formation of a list of individuals' names. In the United States, registration of nurses is a voluntary matter, accomplished by joining the professional nursing organization, the American Nurses' Association. In Canada, registration is part of provincial licensure in all provinces but Ontario. Registration does not necessarily confer the title RN.

Certification

Certification in the United States is the practice of determining minimum standards of nursing competence in specialty areas, such as maternal-child health. An individual who is certified has met predetermined standards specified by the profession. Certification programs are conducted by the American Nurses' Association and by other specialty nursing organizations.

Accreditation

Accreditation is a process in which a nongovernmental agency appraises institutions or programs to determine whether they meet established standards for service or training. In the United States, the accreditation of nursing education programs is carried out by the National League for Nursing and is voluntary. In Canada nursing education programs are approved, not accredited, by the provincial nursing associations, and approval is compulsory. The authority for approval is described in the provincial nursing acts.

Contracts

A *contract* is an agreement between two or more competent persons, upon sufficient consideration (remuneration), to do or not to do some lawful act. A contract may be written or oral; however, a written contract cannot be changed legally by an oral agreement. If two people wish to change some aspect of a written contract, this needs to be written into the contract, because one party cannot hold the other to an oral agreement that differs from the written one.

A contract is the basis of the relationship between a nurse and an employer—for example, a nurse and a hospital or a nurse and a physician. It is also the basis of the relationship that a nurse has with a patient. This latter is true whether the nurse is employed directly by the patient and family or by an agency.

A contract is considered to be *expressed* when the two parties discuss and agree orally or in writing to its terms, e.g., that a nurse will work at a hospital for a stated length of time and under stated conditions. An *implied* contract is one in which there has been no discussion between the parties, but the law considers that a contract exists. For example, when an unconscious patient receives an intravenous infusion from a nurse, the law considers that an agreement is implied between the nurse and the patient that the patient must pay for the infusion and for the nurse's services.

A nurse who is employed by a hospital works as an agent of the hospital, and the nurse's contract with patients is an implied one. However, a nurse who is employed directly by a patient, for example, a private duty nurse, may have a written contract with that patient in which the nurse agrees to provide professional services for a certain fee. If the patient is dying, the nurse can be protected by a written contract that allows collection of the fee from the patient's estate.

A nurse might be prevented from carrying out the terms of the contract because of illness or death. However, personal inconvenience and personal problems, such as the nurse's car failure, are not legitimate reasons for failing to fulfill a contract. A nurse cannot be held to a contract if the terms of the contract were misrepresented. For example, a private duty nurse might agree to look after a patient who has just had an operation; however, if the patient is also an alcoholic experiencing delirium tremens, and this information was withheld from the nurse at the time the contract was made, the nurse would not be held legally to the contract.

Informed Consent

A patient's consent to treatment is required in most instances. See the discussion of assault and battery later in this chapter. Three groups of persons cannot provide consent. In most areas, for minors to obtain treatment, consent must be given by a parent or guardian. The same is also true of an adult who has the mental capacity of a child.

The second group consists of persons who are unconscious or injured in such a way that they are unable to give consent. In these situations the consent is usually obtained from the closest adult relative. In an emergency, if consent cannot be obtained from the patient or a relative, then the law generally agrees that consent is assumed.

The third group consists of mentally ill persons. States and provinces generally provide in mental health acts or similar statutes definitions of mental illness and the rights of the mentally ill under the law as well as the rights of the staff caring for such a patient.

Wills

A *will* is a declaration by a person about how the person's property is to be disposed of after his or her death. In order for a will to be valid, the following conditions must be met:

1. The person making the will must be of sound mind, that is, able to understand and retain mentally the general nature and extent of his or her property, the relationship of the beneficiaries and of relatives to whom none of the estate will be left, and the disposition he or she is making of the property. A person therefore can be seriously ill and unable to carry out business functions, yet able to make a will.

2. The person must not be unduly influenced by anyone else.

Sometimes a patient may be persuaded by someone who is close at that particular time to make that person a beneficiary. Patients sometimes are persuaded to leave their estates to persons looking after them rather than to their relatives. Frequently, the relatives will contest the will in this situation and take the matter to court, claiming undue influence.

Nurses may be requested from time to time to witness a will. In most states and provinces, a will must be signed in the presence of two witnesses. In some situations, a mark can suffice if the person making the will cannot write a signature.

In most settings, it is required that both witnesses be present at the same time when the person is signing the will. A person who is a witness to a will should not be a beneficiary, because in most jurisdictions this affects the right to take part of the estate. If a nurse is a witness to a will, the nurse should note on the patient's chart that a will was made and the nurse's perception of the physical and mental condition of the patient. This record will provide the nurse with accurate information if the nurse is called as a witness later. The record may also be helpful if the will is contested. If a nurse does not wish to act as a witness, for example, if in the nurse's opinion undue influence has been brought on the patient, then it is the nurse's right to refuse to act in this capacity.

Privileged Communications

A *privileged communication* is information given to a professional person such as a physician. Historically, under common law, a physician who learned, for example, that a patient had a history of mental illness could be made to reveal this in a court. As a result, patients withheld some information from their physicians when it was not always in their best interests to do so. Many states solved this problem by enacting legislation that overrode the common law and provided that, under certain circumstances, a physician cannot be compelled to reveal confidential information. Some of these acts were later amended to include the clergy and spouses. Three states, New York, Arkansas, and New Mexico, have extended these statutes to include professional registered nurses (Creighton 1981:216).

Legislation regarding privileged communications is highly complicated. A nurse would be unwise to encourage disclosures or advise a patient about the subject. The privileged communication law is for the benefit of the patient; a nurse who is given confidential information should be prepared to answer questions fully and honestly if required to testify in a court of law. If the law of privileged communications is to be applied, the attorney for the patient will object to the question and the judge will resolve the problem.

The matter of privileged communications is referred to in the ANA's *Code for Nurses* (1976). It advises the nurse to seek legal counsel in regard to a privileged communication, to become familiar with the rights and privileges of the patient and the nurse.

In Canada, confidentiality of information is incorporated as an ethic in the legislation on nursing practice. Failure to maintain confidentiality can result in discipline of the nurse. The patient-physician relationship and the nurse-patient relationship are not protected under the law, except in Quebec where physicians can refuse to reveal information given by patients.

Nurses as Expert Witnesses

When called into court as a witness, the nurse has a duty to assist justice as far as possible. An *expert witness* is one who, by education or experience, possesses knowledge that the ordinary layperson does not have (Perry 1977:460). Such a witness is usually called to help a judge or jury understand evidence.

First the nurse will be sworn in, that is, will be asked to swear to tell the truth, the whole truth, and nothing but the truth, and asked to give his or her name. Then the nurse will be asked to give information about her or his education and experience. This is intended to prove the nurse's credibility.

The witness should listen carefully to each question and answer truthfully. Information should not be volunteered; facts should be presented simply. The nurse need not be afraid to say "I don't know" if this is true; an expert witness is not expected to know everything. In addition to giving facts, an expert witness can give an opinion based on knowledge and experience.

An expert witness can expect to be cross-examined by the lawyer from the opposing side. It is important that the nurse agree to testify only if he or she is in agreement with the side who asked for the testimony.

An expert witness can be paid based on a reasonable professional rate for preparation time and time spent in court.

Crimes and Torts

Crimes

A *crime* is an act committed in violation of societal law and punishable by a fine and/or imprisonment. A crime does not have to be intended in order to be a crime. For example, a nurse may accidentally give a patient an additional dose of a narcotic to relieve the patient's discomfort, but the dose may be lethal.

In most states and provinces, crimes are classified as either felonies or misdemeanors. A *felony* is a crime of a serious nature, such as murder, and punishable by a term in prison. A *misdemeanor* is of a less serious nature and is usually punishable by a fine or short-term jail sentence or both. First-degree murder and second-degree murder are felonies. The former involves the intent to murder, while the latter is murder without previous intent. In some areas second-degree murder is referred to as *manslaughter.*

If a nurse carries out an illegal practice and the patient dies, the nurse can be guilty of manslaughter. An example is the nurse who gives a medication that was not ordered by a physician, as a result of which the patient dies.

Torts

A *tort* is a wrong committed by a person against another person or against the other's property. A serious tort often becomes a lawsuit and is tried before a judge or jury, who, after hearing the evidence will order the person committing the tort to recompense the person harmed. A tort is independent of a contract. Torts, if serious, can be tried in both civil and criminal actions. A nurse who loses a patient's teeth or who gives a hot water bottle that burns a patient commits a tort. Both negligence and malpractice are torts that result either from carrying out an unreasonable act (commission) or from failing to carry out a reasonable act (omission). See the discussion of negligence and malpractice later in this chapter. Torts are classified as intentional and unintentional. The latter are also referred to as *negligence.*

Fraud

Fraud can be described as the false presentation of some fact or facts with the intention that it will be acted upon by another person. For example, if a person presents false records of education to a nursing school in order to gain admission, this is fraud; or if a nurse applying to a hospital for employment is asked to list the previous five employers and omits two employers for deceptive reasons without informing the prospective employer, this is fraud.

Negligence and Malpractice

Definitions and proof

Negligence is "the omission to do something that a reasonable person, guided by those ordinary considerations which ordinarily regulate human affairs, would do, or doing something which a reasonable and prudent person would not do" (Creighton 1981:154). *Malpractice* is that part of the law of negligence applied to the professional person: It is, in effect, any *professional* misconduct or unreasonable lack of professional skill. To clarify, a nurse in the practice of nursing could be guilty of malpractice if she or he performed a skill differently from the way other nurses would have done it and the patient was injured. Negligence would apply to any person who, for example, drove a car too quickly in snowy weather and injured a pedestrian. Malpractice and negligence are often used interchangeably; however, malpractice is reserved for professional misconduct. It is the failure of a professional person to act within the acceptable standards of his or her profession.

Proof of a nurse's negligence includes proof of all of the following: (a) the nurse's duty to the client, (b) the nurse's failure to carry out that duty, (c) an injury incurred by the client, and (d) a causal relationship between the breach of duty by the nurse and the client's injury—a relationship referred to as *proximate cause.* In cases of proven negligence, monetary damages are awarded to the plaintiff to compensate for the inconvenience and suffering experienced and, where possible, to help the person return to the state of well-being enjoyed prior to the injury.

Nurses are responsible for their own actions even though they may be employees of a health agency. The descriptions of negligence and malpractice do not mention good intentions; it is not pertinent that the nurse did not intend to be negligent. If a nurse gives an incorrect medication, even though done in good faith, the fact that the nurse failed to read the label correctly indicates malpractice.

Another significant aspect of negligence and malpractice is that both omissions and commissions are included. That is, a person can be guilty of malpractice by forgetting to give a medication as well as by giving the wrong medication.

Types of malpractice situations

Medication errors The most common nursing errors occur in the administration of medications. With the large number of medications on the market today and the variety of methods of administration, these errors may well be on the increase. Nurses are in error in not reading the label on the medication, misreading or incorrectly calculating the dosage, not identifying the correct patient, preparing the wrong concentration, or administering a medication by the wrong route (e.g., intravenously instead of orally). Some medication errors are very serious and can even cost the patient's life. If, for example, a nurse gives dicumarol to a patient recently returned from surgery, the patient could hemorrhage as a result. Nurses always need to check medications very carefully. Even after the nurse has done so, if a patient states he or she "did not have a green pill before," the nurse would be very wise to check the medication order and the medication again before giving it to the patient.

Sponge counts Sponges or other small items can be left inside a patient during an operation because the nurse either failed to count them before the surgeon closed the incision or counted them incorrectly. In either case the nurse responsible for counting the sponges can be held liable for malpractice.

Burns A relatively frequent malpractice action attributed to nurses is burning a patient. Burns may be caused by hot water bottles, heating pads, and solutions that are too hot for application. Elderly, comatose, or diabetic patients are particularly vulnerable to burns, due to decreased sensitivity. Hot objects can burn these people before they notice it. A nurse may also be held negligent for leaving a patient without taking precautions (giving warnings or providing protections), for example, when using a steam vaporizer.

Falls Accidental falls by patients, sometimes with resultant injury, occur commonly. Side rails are used on cribs, beds, and stretchers for babies and small children, and for adults when necessary, to prevent falls. If a nurse leaves the rails down or leaves a baby unattended on a bath table, that nurse is guilty of malpractice if the patient falls and is injured. Most hospitals and nursing homes have policies regarding the use of safety devices such as side rails and restraints. A nurse needs to be familiar with these policies and to use the precautions indicated to prevent this type of accident.

Failure to observe and take appropriate action In some instances nurses are guilty of malpractice when a patient's complaints are ignored. If the nurse does not report a patient's complaint of acute abdominal pain, the nurse is negligent, and an ensuing appendix rupture and death may be held the result of the nurse's malpractice. A nurse who fails to take the blood pressure and pulse and check the dressing of a postoperative patient who has just had a kidney removed has omitted important assessments and, if the patient hemorrhages and dies, may be held responsible for the death as a result of this malpractice.

Mistaken identity Identifying patients correctly is a problem, particularly in busy hospital units. It is not unknown for a nurse to prepare the wrong patient for an operation, so that a healthy gallbladder is removed, for example. These mistakes can frequently be costly to a patient and make the nurse liable for malpractice.

Loss of or damage to patients' property Items of property such as jewelry, money, and dentures are a constant concern to hospital personnel. Today agencies are taking less responsibility for property and are generally requesting patients to sign a form on admission relieving the hospital and its employees of any responsibility for property. There are, however, situations in which the patient cannot sign a waiver, and the nursing staff must follow prescribed policies about care of the patient's property. On hospital units, dentures are often a major problem; they can be lost in bedding or left on a meal tray. Nurses are expected to take reasonable precautions to preserve a patient's property, and they can be held liable for its loss or damage if reasonable care is not taken.

Invasion of Privacy

The right to privacy is the right of individuals to withhold themselves and their lives from public scrutiny. Invasion of privacy is a direct wrong of a personal nature. It injures the feelings of the person and does not take into account the effect of revealed information on the standing of the person in the community.

The right to privacy can also be described as the right to be left alone. In this context there is a delicate balance between the need of a number of people to contribute to the diagnosis and treatment of a patient and the patient's right to privacy. In most situations necessary discussion about a patient's medical condition is considered appropriate, but unnecessary discussions and gossip are considered an invasion of privacy.

A patient has a right to privacy and a right to refuse to participate in clinical demonstrations for medical and nursing personnel. In teaching hospitals it is important for health workers to obtain the patient's consent prior to any demonstration or teaching conference, to respect the right of privacy. See the discussion of patients' rights in Chapter 3 and information about privacy in Chapter 2.

Libel and Slander

Both libel and slander are wrongful actions that come under the heading of defamation. *Defamation* is communication that is false, or made with a careless disregard for the truth, and results in injury to the reputation of a person. *Libel* is defamation by means of print, writing, or pictures. *Slander* is defamation by the spoken word, stating unprivileged (not legally protected) or false words by which a reputation is damaged. A nurse has a qualified privilege to make statements that could be considered invasions of privacy of a patient, both orally and in writing, but only as a part of nursing practice and only to a physician or another health team member caring for the patient.

Truth is always a good defense to a charge of defamation. Care needs to be taken, however, to speak or write only the facts or the truth. A nurse, for example, may believe that a particular patient had been admitted to a hospital for venereal disease a year earlier; in fact, it was another patient. This information would be ground for a charge of slander if the nurse shared it with nurses from another unit.

For nurses to be protected against claims of invasion of privacy, comments about patients need to be kept to a minimum and made only to people entitled to hear them.

Assault and Battery

The terms *assault* and *battery* are often heard together, but each has its own meaning. *Assault* can be described as the attempt to touch another person unjustifiably or the threat to do so. *Battery* is the willful or negligent touching of a person (or the person's clothes or even something the person is carrying), which may or may not cause harm. In order to be actionable at law, however, the touching must be wrong in some way, e.g., done without permission, embarrassing, or causing injury.

Every person has the legal right to refuse physical contact with another. While receiving health care, a patient has the right to refuse such physical contact as an injection or an operation; personnel who proceed with contact despite such a refusal can be sued for assault and battery.

Technical assault and battery differs from criminal assault and battery in that the latter is usually carried out with intent to injure. If a person is touched and has not given implied or actual consent (for example, when the wrong limb is operated upon), a lawsuit based on technical assault and battery can result. Consent to treat a patient is therefore required.

False Imprisonment

False imprisonment is unjustifiable detention of a person that deprives him or her of personal liberty for any length of time. For example, if a nurse locks a patient in a room unjustifiably, this is false imprisonment. If it is accompanied by forceful restraint or threat of restraint it is an assault and battery (Creighton 1981:207).

Although nurses may suggest to a patient under certain circumstances that he or she remain in the room or in bed, the patient is not detained against his or her will. If the patient insists upon leaving even though it may be detrimental to health, this is the patient's right. Detention is legal only when imposed to protect the public or perhaps to protect the individual from unintended harm, for example, when a patient is high on drugs and unable to control his or her behavior. In these instances the patient cannot leave when he or she wishes.

Legal Protections for Nurses

Good Samaritan Acts

Good Samaritan acts are laws designed to protect medical practitioners, such as physicians and in some states nurses, who provide assistance at the scene of an emergency. The medical practitioners in this legislation are protected against claims of malpractice unless it can be shown that there was a gross departure from the normal standard of care or willful wrongdoing on their part. Although not all acts mention nurses, there is general agreement that when acts refer to practitioners of the healing arts, this includes nurses.

In Canada, some provinces specify in traffic acts that it is the responsibility of people to give aid at the scene of an accident. Alberta is the only province that exempts physicians and nurses from liability unless gross negligence is proved. However, lawsuits against Good Samaritans are rarely successful.

It is generally believed that a person who renders help in an emergency, at the level of helping that would be provided by any reasonably prudent person under similar circumstances, cannot be held liable. The same reasoning applies to nurses, who may be the people best prepared to help at the scene of an accident. If the level of care a nurse provides is the caliber that would have been provided by any other nurse, then the nurse will not be held liable.

Professional Liability Insurance

Because of the increase in the number of malpractice lawsuits against professional people in the health field, nurses are advised in many areas to carry their own liability insurance to protect themselves.

Coverage

Most hospitals have liability insurance that adequately covers all employees, including all nurses. However, there could be instances when the nurse is with a physician and patient, carrying out an explicit request of the physician, and she or he could be considered temporarily in the physician's employ. A physician or a hospital can be sued because of the negligent conduct of a nurse, and the nurse can also be sued and held liable for negligence or malpractice.

Liability insurance generally covers all costs of defending a nurse, including the costs of retaining an attorney. The insurance also covers all costs incurred by the nurse up to the face value of the policy, including a settlement made out of court. In return, the insurance company has the right to make the decisions about the claim and the settlement.

Instructor and student protection

Instructors of nursing and nursing students are also vulnerable to lawsuits. In hospital nursing education programs, instructors and students are often specifically covered for liability by the hospital. An instructor, however, can still be sued by a hospital in cases of negligence and malpractice. If a nursing student makes an error, the student is responsible for this action; however, the instructor is also responsible for assigning the student activities within the student's capabilities. Courts in the United States have recently found that nursing students must be competent practitioners in their activities. This finding protects patients in a health education environment.

Students and teachers of nursing employed by community colleges and universities are less likely to be covered by the insurance carried by hospitals and health agencies. It is advisable for these people to check with their employers about the coverage that applies to them. Increasingly, instructors are carrying their own malpractice insurance in both the United States and Canada. In the United States this can be obtained through the American Nurses' Association or private insurance companies; in Canada it can usually be obtained through provincial nurses' associations. Nursing students in the United States can also obtain insurance through the National Student Nurses' Association.

Self-Protection

In this era of lawsuits it is very important for nurses and nursing students to protect themselves from legal actions. The following measures are suggested:

1. Be familiar with the laws and codes of ethics that apply to nursing practice in your jurisdiction. These serve as guides to your nursing and indicate the limits ascribed to nursing.

2. Be familiar with your agency's rules and regulations that affect nursing practice.

3. Accept the concept of personal liability.

4. Maintain clinical competence in your area of practice. For students this demands study and practice before caring for patients. For graduate nurses it means continued study, including maintaining and updating clinical knowledge and skills.

5. If an incident or accident occurs, report it immediately to the responsible nurse or appropriate person, so that measures can be taken to protect the patient. Most agencies have written practices about how to proceed, including forms (e.g., an incident report) to fill out. See Chapter 22 for additional information about accidents.

6. Know your own strengths and weaknesses. If you recognize that you have difficulty calculating medication dosages, always ask someone to check your calculations before you proceed.

7. If you delegate nursing responsibilities, make sure the person to whom you are delegating understands what to do. Remember that you can be held liable if a patient is harmed by actions of the person giving the care.

8. Always record accurately and honestly. See Chapter 18 for additional information.

9. If you become involved in a legal action, obtain legal counsel to represent you.

Summary

There are different types of law in society. Common law is the accumulation of law as a result of court decisions; it is made by judges. Statutory law is enacted by legislative bodies. Civil law refers to a statutory law that affects the relations among people. Criminal law deals with the actions of individuals against the welfare of society, and as such it is a part of the public law.

Law rests on four principles: it is concerned with justice and fairness; it is characterized by change; actions are judged on the basis of a universal standard of what a similarly trained, reasonable, and prudent person would do in similar circumstances; and each individual has rights and responsibilities.

The judicial process has five distinct steps: filing of a complaint, receipt of an answer, pretrial activities, trial, and a decision. If the decision is not acceptable to a party, an appeal can subsequently be made. The trial is the formal examination of an issue in a court.

The legal roles of the nurse are: provider of service; employee or contractor for service; and private citizen. Each role has accompanying rights and responsibilities. Legal concepts associated with these roles include those delineating liability, standards of care, contractual obligations, contracts, and contractual relationships.

There are two types of nursing licensure: mandatory and permissive. With the former, a license is required for a nurse to practice the nursing profession. With permissive licensure, a license is not required by law, to practice. Nurse practice acts of each state and province legally control the practice of nursing within their jurisdictions.

A nurse enters into a contract with an employer when the nurse obtains employment and the nurse is obligated to fulfill the terms of the contract. Exceptions arise only when the nurse is ill or dies or the contract has been misrepresented. A contract is also binding on an employer.

A nurse may be asked to witness the signing of a will. A will is a declaration made by a person about how the person's property is to be disposed of after death. Nurses need to know legal conditions that govern their action as witnesses.

A privileged communication is information given to a professional person, such as information given to a physician by a patient. Nurses are advised to seek legal counsel in their own jurisdiction in regard to this aspect of the law as it applies in the nurse-patient relationship.

A crime is an act committed in violation of societal law. A tort is a wrong committed against another person or the person's property. Fraud, invasion of privacy, libel and slander, assault and battery, and false imprisonment are wrongs that nurses need to understand and avoid committing. Negligent acts and malpractice also need to be understood by nurses. Negligence applies to everyone, whereas malpractice applies to a professional person. In trials of malpractice, a nurse may be called as an expert witness. As such, the nurse is expected to testify about what is reasonable or unreasonable under the particular circumstances.

Good Samaritan acts may protect nurses. These acts are designed to override the liability of people who act in an emergency, such as at the scene of a highway accident.

Liability is the legal responsibility of a person to account for wrongful acts by making financial restitution. Because nurses can be held responsible for their own actions, many have liability insurance to protect themselves from incurring costs and other consequences of malpractice litigation. A number of steps are listed by which nurses can protect themselves from legal action.

Suggested Activities

1. Obtain information about the type of malpractice insurance available to you. Determine from your educational institution and/or hospital how or whether you are protected if a patient is harmed.
2. Select an anonymous patient's record and list all the data that would be considered privileged information. Discuss your findings with a group of other nursing students.
3. Discuss with other students how the following situation might be appropriately handled: A physician's wife is a patient on the gynecology unit of a hospital. As a nursing student on the unit, you have been instructed by her physician to make sure that information in the patient's record is not available to anyone except the patient's physician and the nursing staff. The patient's husband is a well-known physician in the hospital and asks a nursing student for his wife's record.

Suggested Readings

American Journal of Nursing. March 1976. Facing a grand jury. *American Journal of Nursing* 76:398–400.

The unnamed nurse/author describes a personal experience as a witness in an abortion case. Included in the article are eight final recommendations for nurses to follow to protect themselves.

Hemelt, M. D. October 1975. Your legal guide to nursing practice. *Nursing 79* 9:57–64.

This article discusses a number of situations that nurses encounter frequently. Issues such as informed consent, countersigning, illegible orders, resuscitation, and staffing are explored.

Mancini, M. April 1978. Laws, regulations, and policies. *American Journal of Nursing* 78:681–84.

This author discusses laws, regulations, and policies applicable to nurses. The ability to distinguish among them enables nurses to adopt rules and to influence changes when necessary.

Shannon, M. L. August 1975. Nurses in American history: Our first four licensure laws. *American Journal of Nursing* 75:1327–29.

This article cites the first four licensure laws passed in 1903, when women were not allowed to vote. They were only a beginning and provided an opening for the improved laws of today.

Williams, B. N. January 1976. Malpractice: How good is your insurance protection? *Nursing 76* 6:3, 6–7.

This author provides some legal definitions and discusses insurance protection, sources from which to acquire a policy, differences between coverage based on occurrence and on claims made, supplement "umbrella" policies, and other tips for assuring adequate protection.

Selected References

American Nurses' Association. 1961. *Legal definition of nursing*. Kansas City, Mo.: American Nurses' Association.

———. July 1973. ANA issues statement on diploma graduates. *American Journal of Nursing* 73:1135.

———. 1975. *Human rights guidelines for nurses in clinical and other research*. Publication no. D-46 5M 7/75. Kansas City, Mo.: American Nurses' Association.

———. 1976. *The code for nurses*. Kansas City, Mo.: American Nurses' Association.

Bolton, M. 1976. *Civil rights in Canada*. Vancouver, B.C.: International Self-Counsel Press.

Bullough, B. 1980. *The law and the expanding nursing role*. 2nd ed. New York: Appleton-Century-Crofts.

Creighton, H. 1981. *Law every nurse should know*. 4th ed. Philadelphia: W. B. Saunders Co.

Doll, A. January 1980. What to do after an incident. *Nursing 80* 10:73 (Canadian ed. 10:15–19).

Fenner, K. 1980. *Ethics and the law in nursing*. New York: D. Van Nostrand Co.

Good, S., and Kerr, J. C. 1973. *Contemporary issues in Canadian law for nurses*. Toronto: Holt, Rinehart and Winston of Canada.

Kelly, L. Y. January 1976. The patient's right to know. *Nursing Outlook* 24:26–32.

Murchison, I; Nichols, T. S.; and Hanson, R. 1982. *Legal accountability in the nursing process*. 2nd ed. St. Louis: C. V. Mosby Co.

Nursing Outlook. April 1979. The study of credentialing in nursing: A new approach. *Nursing Outlook* 27:263–71.

O'Sullivan, A. L. May 1980. Privileged communication. *American Journal of Nursing* 80:947–50.

Perry, S. E. March 1977. If you're called as an expert witness. *American Journal of Nursing* 77:458–60.

Sarner, H. 1968. *The nurse and the law*. Philadelphia: W. B. Saunders Co.

Shindul, J. A., and Snyder, M. E. February 1980. Legal restraints on restraint. *American Journal of Nursing* 81: 393–94.

Sklar, C. June 1980. Was the patient informed? *Canadian Nurse* 76:18, 20, 22.

Stahl, A. G. September 1974. Symposium on current legal and professional problems: State board of nursing: Legal aspects. *Nursing Clinics of North America* 9:505–12.

Wiley, L. September 1981. Liability for death: Nine nurses' legal ordeals. *Nursing 81* 11:34–43.

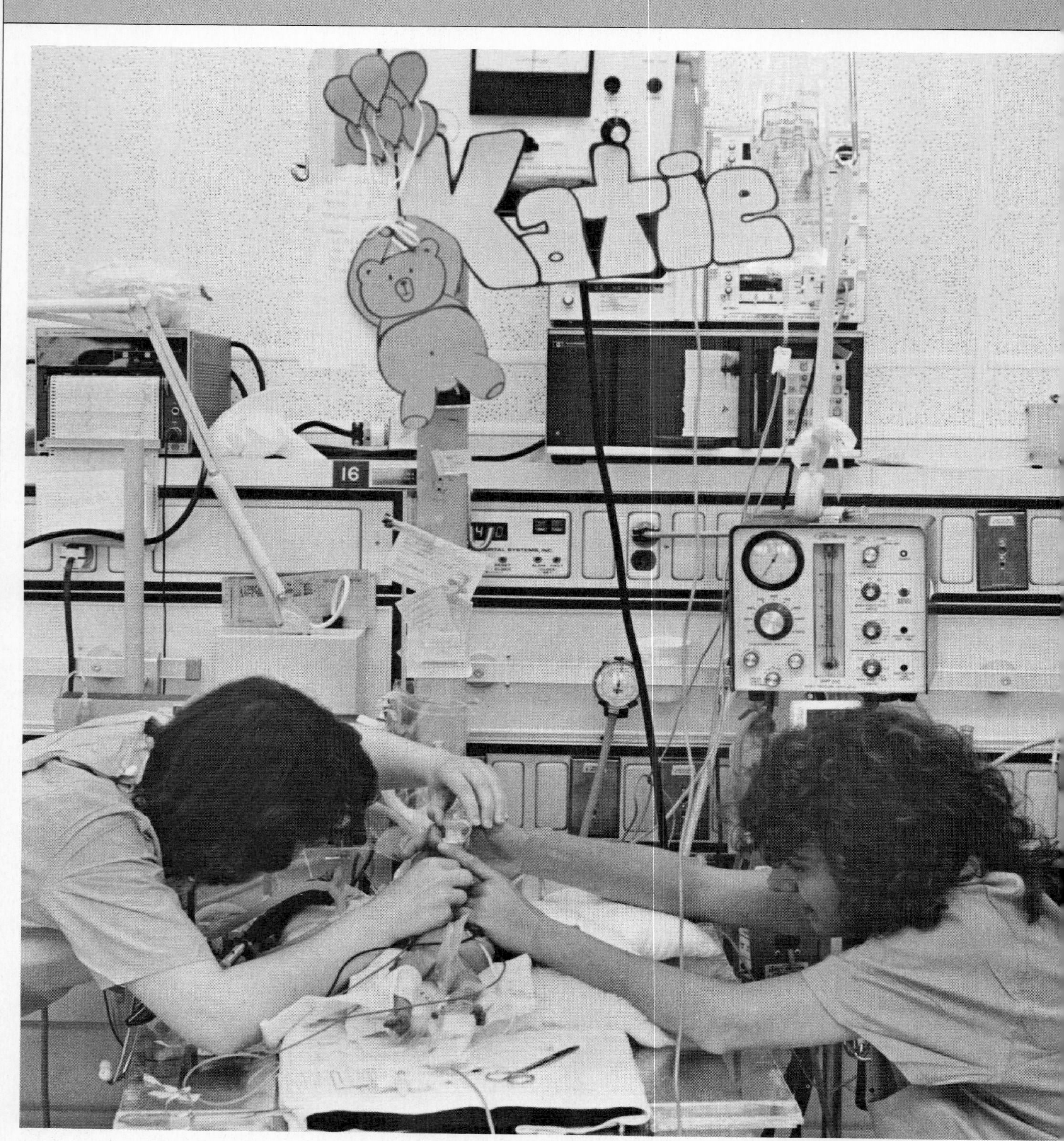
Katie
16

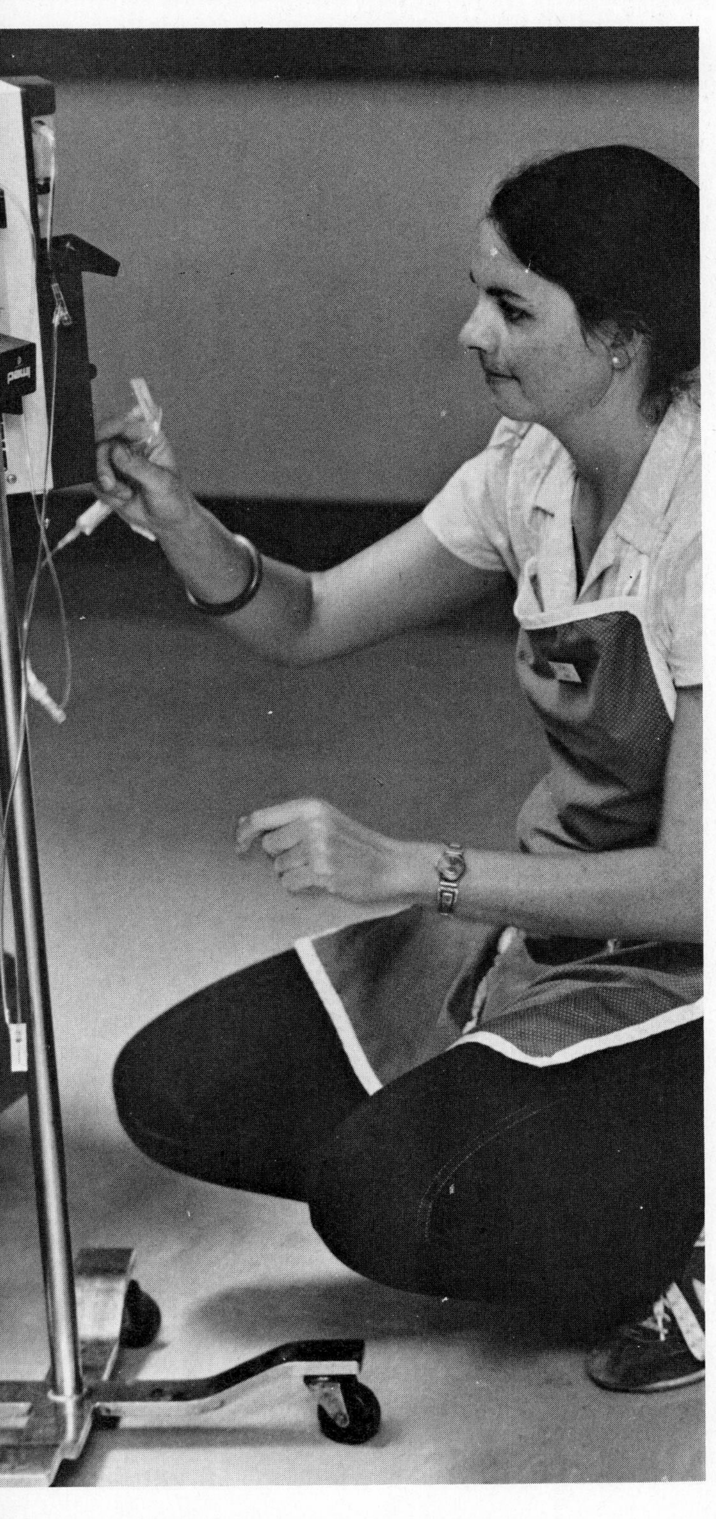

Unit II

The Nursing Process

CONTENTS

Chapter 5

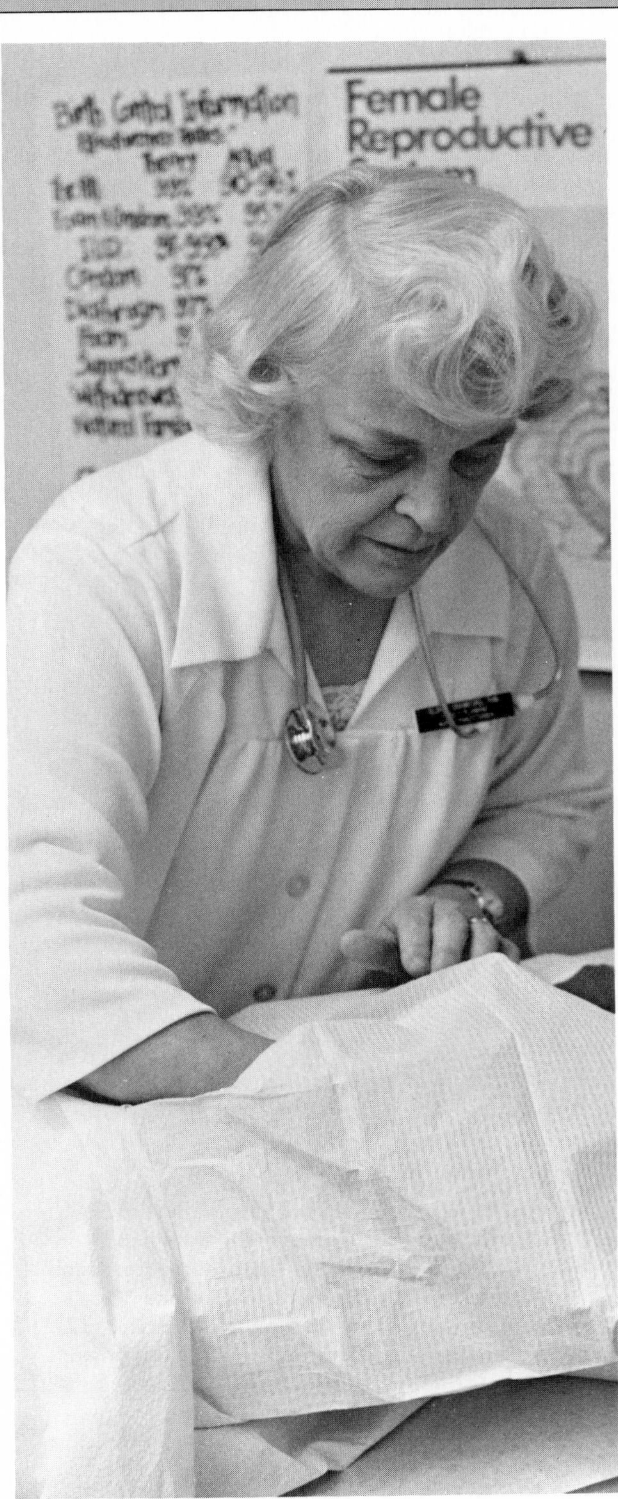

Introduction and Assessment

CONTENTS

Objectives

1. Know essential terms and facts related to the nursing process
   - **1.1** Identify the five components of the nursing process
   - **1.2** Define the five components of the nursing process
   - **1.3** Outline activities involved in each component of the nursing process
   - **1.4** Identify essential characteristics of the nursing process
   - **1.5** Describe the humanistic approach to the nursing process
2. Understand essential facts about problem solving
   - **2.1** Identify three methods of problem solving
   - **2.2** Identify four essential elements of the nursing process
   - **2.3** Identify the major elements of a cybernetic problem-solving process
   - **2.4** Identify steps involved in the Claus-Bailey systems model for problem solving
3. Understand essential terms and facts about the assessment phase of the nursing process
   - **3.1** Define data collection, data base, and baseline data
   - **3.2** Compare formal and informal methods of collecting data
   - **3.3** Give examples of objective and subjective data and variable and constant data
   - **3.4** Compare the terms *need* and *problem*
   - **3.5** Identify sources of data
   - **3.6** Identify common health areas the nurse assesses
   - **3.7** Identify essential aspects of selecting relevant data
   - **3.8** Contrast various frameworks used for assessment
   - **3.9** Identify six activities commonly employed in assessment
   - **3.10** Identify specific purposes and types of data obtained from various assessment activities

Terms

assessment
auscultation
cephalocaudal
cybernetic
data
data base
(baseline data)
data collection
diagnosis
examine
evaluation
hypothesis
inspection
intervention
need
nursing history
nursing process
objective data
observation
outcome criteria
palpation
percussion
planning
pleximeter
problem
recapitulation
subjective data

Components of the Nursing Process

The *nursing process* is a systematic, rational method of providing nursing care. It provides a framework for planning and implementing nursing care and helps the nurse use nursing knowledge, solve problems, be creative, and keep in mind the humanistic aspects of nursing when providing care. The nursing process requires specific knowledge and skills.

The term *nursing process* and the framework it implies are relatively new. In 1961, Orlando (1961:26) used the term and isolated three elements of the nursing process: (a) behavior of the patient, (b) reaction of the nurse, and (c) nursing actions designed for the patient's benefit. Later, Knowles (1967:248–72) suggested "five D's" necessary for the practice of nursing: discover, delve, decide, do, and discriminate.

In 1967, the Western Interstate Commission on Higher Education (WICHE) (1967:6) identified a nursing process with five steps: perception, communication, interpretation, intervention, and evaluation. Since that time, the concept of the nursing process and its elements have been refined further.

Today, the nursing process is usually described as having five steps or phases: assessment, nursing diagnosis, planning, nursing intervention, and evaluation. See Figure 5–1.

1. *Assessment* is collecting and organizing data about a patient or client. The data are gathered from a variety of sources and are the basis for actions and decisions taken in subsequent steps.
2. *Nursing diagnosis* is the identification and delineation of a patient's response to her or his situation. The diagnosis is stated as actual or potential problems within the scope of nursing practice.

3. *Planning* includes validating the nursing diagnosis and then planning how best to help the patient.
4. *Nursing intervention* is the implementation of the planned nursing care. Intervention may be carried out by the nurse responsible for assessment, diagnosis, and planning; intervention also may be delegated to other nursing personnel.
5. *Evaluation* is comparing the patient's response to the intervention with predetermined standards, often referred to as *outcome criteria* or *evaluative criteria.*

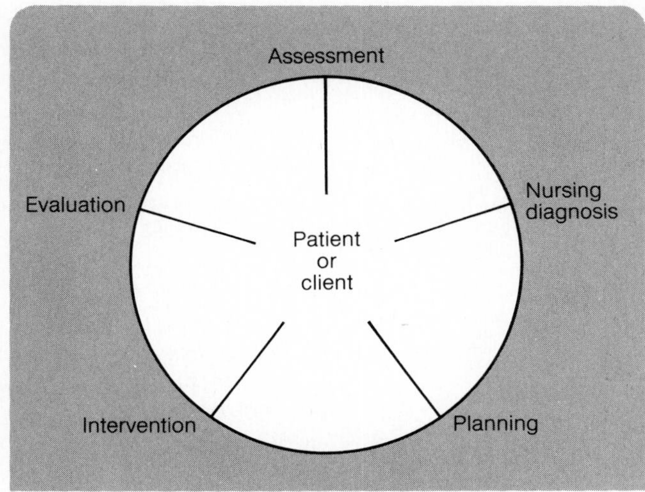

Figure 5–1 The nursing process.

Different authorities use different terms to describe these steps. In spite of these differences, the activities of the nurse within the process are similar. To avoid misunderstanding, nurses should be familiar with alternate terms that describe steps in the process. For example, *nursing diagnosis* may be called *problem identification,* and *intervention* may be called *implementation.* See Table 5–1 for terms used in this book, their definitions, and the activities involved in each phase.

The nursing process is an adaptation of problem-solving techniques and systems theory. It can be viewed as parallel to but separate from the medical process. Table 5–2 lists the two processes for comparison.

Characteristics of the Nursing Process

The nursing process has these functional characteristics:

1. It can be viewed from a systems and a humanistic perspective.
2. The system is open, flexible, and dynamic.
3. The phases of the process are interrelated.
4. Feedback is important in the process.
5. The nurse is permitted maximum flexibility and creativity.

Systems Approach

If the nursing process is viewed as the primary system, subsystems include the patient, the nurse, and the components of the process, such as data collection or nursing diagnosis. These all contribute to the end result of the system. The nursing process has input, output, and feedback as well as a purpose. Input includes assessment activities; output includes nursing diagnosis, planning, and intervention; and feedback occurs with evaluation. Feedback is an important aspect of the process. Evaluation of the intervention provides feedback, which results in either reassessment of the patient's problems or revision of the plan of intervention.

The nurse can be highly creative when using the nursing process. The nurse is not bound by standard responses but may apply problem-solving skills, creativity, critical thinking, and his or her own knowledge and skills to assist patients. The nursing process can be applied in a variety of situations. It can be used with individuals of all ages, groups, and communities.

The five steps of the nursing process are not discrete entities but overlapping, continuing subprocesses. Each one must be continually updated as the situation changes. Just as a patient's health is never static but constantly changing, the nursing process, because it is responsive to the patient's condition, is also dynamic.

Each step or phase of the nursing process affects the others; they are closely interrelated. For example, if an inadequate data base is used during assessment, the nursing diagnoses will be incomplete; this incompleteness will be reflected in the planning, implementation, and evaluation phases. Incomplete assessment necessarily means equivocal evaluation because the nurse will have incomplete criteria against which to evaluate changes in the patient and the effectiveness of interventions.

Humanistic Approach

The nurse who takes a humanistic approach to the nursing process takes into account all that is known about a patient—thoughts, feelings, values, experiences, likes, desires, behavior, and body (Lamonica 1979:xiii). This humanistic approach is the traditional "caring" aspect of nursing and as important as a systems approach and problem solving to intelligent, systematic, and logical nursing care.

Table 5–1 Definitions and Activities Associated with the Nursing Process

Term	Definition	Activities
Nursing process	A series of planned steps or phases directed toward assisting patients and their support persons.	
Assessment	Obtaining and organizing essential information about the patient.	Data collecting Nursing history Nursing examination Reviewing records Interviewing
Nursing diagnosis	A statement about the patient's response to actual or potential health problems and the etiologic and contributing factors.	Sorting data Grouping data Identifying problems Making a problem list Making inferences
Plan	A written guide for nursing intervention assisting the patient to meet health needs and coordinating the care of nursing staff.	Priority setting Goal setting Developing nursing orders Forming a nursing care plan Determining evaluation criteria
Intervention	Putting the nursing care plan into action.	Updating the data base Reviewing the plan with the patient Adjusting the plan as necessary Identifying and providing for safety precautions Determining needs for assistance Intervening as per the plan Analyzing feedback Communicating findings
Evaluation	Assessing the patient's response against predetermined standards.	Identifying the appropriate standard Collecting and organizing the data Comparing the data with the criteria Establishing conclusions

Table 5–2 Comparison of Medical and Nursing Processes

Medical process	Nursing process	Medical process	Nursing process
1. Assessment	**1.** Assessment	**2.** Intervention	**2.** Intervention
a. Medical history and physical examination	a. Nursing history	a. Physician's orders	a. Nursing orders
		b. Medical care plans	b. Nursing care plan
		c. Medical therapy	c. Nursing implementation
b. Medical diagnosis	b. Nursing diagnosis		
		3. Evaluation	**3.** Evaluation
		a. Medical prognosis	a. Nursing prognosis

Adapted from S. Carlson, A practical approach to the nursing process, *American Journal of Nursing*, September 1972, 72:1589–91.

Problem Solving

Problem solving is essential in the nursing process. How a nurse approaches a problem usually depends on the intelligence, skill, energy, and experience of the nurse and the level of difficulty of the problem. Three approaches to problem solving are trial and error, intuitive, and scientific.

Trial-and-Error Problem Solving

One way to solve problems is to try a number of possible approaches until a solution is found. However, the reason one solution works is not known when alternatives in care are not considered systematically. Trial-and-error methods in nursing care can be dangerous because the patient might suffer harm if an approach is inappropriate.

Intuitive Problem Solving

Experienced nurses develop a sense of what nursing measures might help in certain situations. This sense is in part intuitive. A nurse who bases decisions on intuition alone rather than data, however, does a disservice to the patient, even though in the past nurses sometimes solved problems successfully by intuition.

Scientific Method of Problem Solving

The scientific method in problem solving has seven steps:

1. Identifying the general problem, including defining the problem and developing hunches about it
2. Collecting all relevant data from appropriate sources
3. Formulating a *hypothesis*: an assumption made to test the logic of a proposition
4. Preparing a plan of action to test the hypothesis
5. Testing the hypothesis
6. Interpreting the test results and then evaluating the hypothesis
7. Concluding the study or revising the plan of action in the light of new data

Although the scientific method has certain applications in nursing, there are differences between the scientist's laboratory setting and the nurse's practice setting. Three of these differences are:

1. The nurse's time frame is often shorter than the scientist's. The scientist may take months or even years to carry out a study, whereas a nurse must give immediate help to a patient in pain.
2. The nurse's environment makes scientific control impossible, while the scientist strives to establish scientific controls in experiments. For example, a visiting nurse striving to control a patient's diabetes through diet and insulin injections can outline a regimen and teach the patient to administer insulin, but has no control over whether the patient will follow instructions later. The nurse often faces unpredictable events. For example, a patient may refuse certain nursing interventions. The scientist, too, may encounter unpredictable events but strives to limit them through scientific control.
3. The nurse deals with multiple, complex problems, especially since most patients have more than one problem when they are ill. The scientist isolates and studies a single aspect of a problem.

The scientific method, therefore, must be adapted for nursing practice. The nurse requires a problem-solving system that is scientific, systematic, yet flexible enough to deal with the complex situations in the health care system. Such a problem-solving system has four essential elements:

1. It is planned.
2. It is patient, family, or community centered.
3. It is problem oriented.
4. It is goal directed.

Systems Approach to Problem Solving

Bailey and Claus (1975) describe a nursing systems model for solving problems. The major elements in this cybernetic model are shown in Figure 5–2. A *cybernetic* system is one that depends on feedback to direct behavior (Bailey and Claus 1975:15).

The model proposed by Claus-Bailey has a closed feedback loop that provides feedback about the results of the actions and therefore guides subsequent actions. See Figure 5–3. The steps in this problem-solving model are:

1. *Define overall needs, purposes, and goals.* It is best to define overall goals before a problem is encountered; however, goals can be defined concurrently. The overall purposes and goals are based on the needs of the pa-

Figure 5–2 Elements of a cybernetic model.

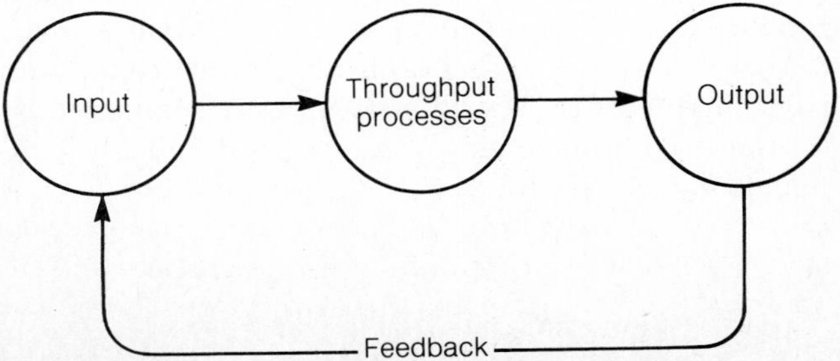

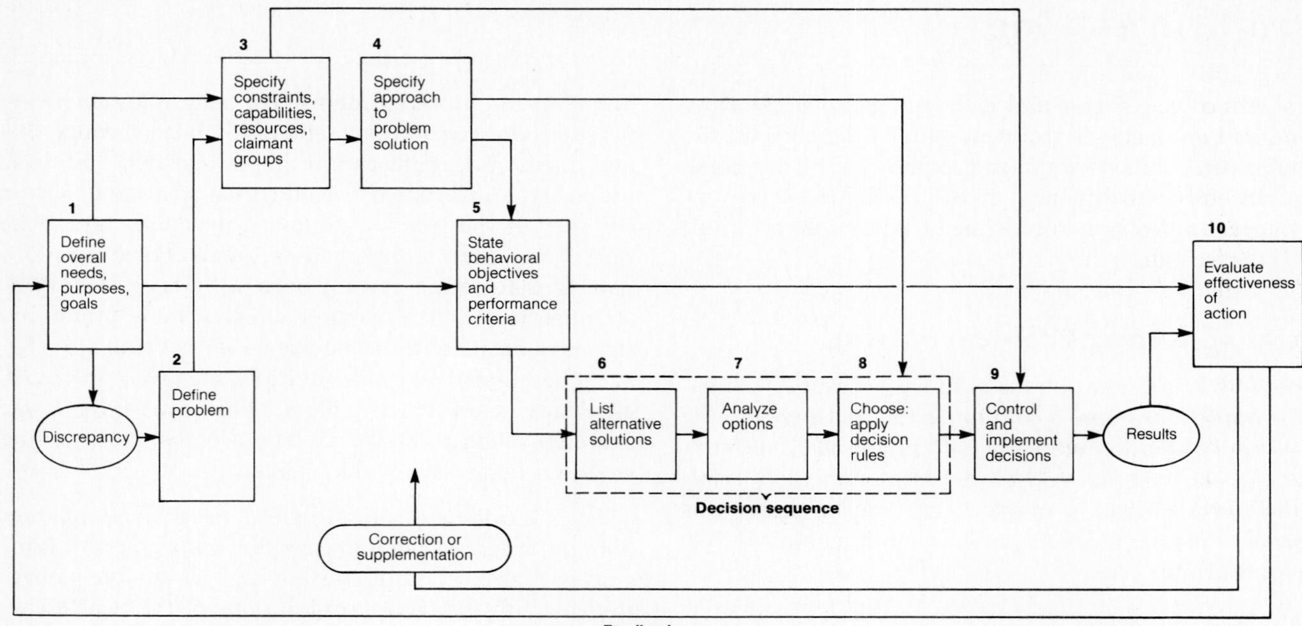

Figure 5–3 Claus-Bailey systems model for problem solution. (From J. T. Bailey and K. E. Claus, *Decision making in nursing: Tools for change* [St. Louis: C. V. Mosby Co., 1975], p. 19. Reprinted with permission.)

tient, system, institution, nurse, etc. The nature of the problem is described as a discrepancy, i.e., the difference between what is and what could be or should be.

2. *Define the problem.* Recognition of the problem implies desire for change. Accurate problem definition requires data collection. The exact nature of the discrepancy is then described, and hypotheses are developed. Hypotheses not supported by facts are eliminated, and the remaining hypotheses are plausible explanations of the nature of the discrepancy.

3. *Weigh constraints, capabilities, resources, and claimant groups.* In this step, the nurse assesses the constraints, capabilities, resources and claimant groups that affect the decision. Constraints affect the approach to the problem. For example, the constraints may be lack of time, lack of finances, or shortage of nursing personnel. By contrast, sufficient finances and availability of appropriate nursing personnel are resources. In this context, *appropriate* means that nursing personnel have the needed qualifications and expertise to achieve the stated goals and purposes.

Another consideration is how the decision will affect claimant groups such as the patient. Some decisions produce anger or anxiety, for example, because of the changes they bring. Also, people often meet change with resistance. This resistance often can be minimized by complete communication at every step and by a rationale for each decision.

4. *Specify an approach to solving the problem.* This step requires a definition of the framework for the solution. This framework needs to encompass the nurse's philosophical beliefs about nursing, e.g., a belief that it is better to help the patients develop their own solutions than to develop them for the patients.

Approaches can be one of two types: satisfying or optimizing. A *satisfying approach* is one in which the nurse chooses the first workable solution. This approach is frequently effective in emergency situations that require immediate action. The *optimizing approach* requires that the nurse find the best solution from among those available. Optimizing usually takes more time and effort than satisfying.

5. *State the specific objectives and the performance criteria.* These objectives should be stated in behavioral terms. See Chapter 17, page 419, for information about behavioral objectives. These objectives reflect the intended outcomes of the action, are listed in order of priority, and are labeled critical or noncritical. *Critical objectives* define limits that cannot be violated, such as an objective to assist a patient to void. Therefore, any action that does not meet this goal is unacceptable. *Noncritical objectives* usually involve advantages and disadvantages as the nurse perceives and values them. The nurse must determine which objectives are desirable and which are critical. By emphasizing critical objectives, nurses become more efficient and effective because the care they give reflects an awareness of the patient's most urgent needs.

6. *List alternative solutions.* The nurse uses his or her own knowledge and creativity to develop alternative solutions to the problems. To do this effectively, the nurse synthesizes experience, knowledge, and relevant information. Bailey and Claus (1975:26) suggest five methods of generating alternatives: (a) Obtain knowledge and expertise of group members, (b) gain advice from outside experts, (c) obtain advice of colleagues or other members of the organization, (d) recall past experience, and (e) form a committee to brainstorm ideas.

7. *Analyze the options.* The proposed solutions are now tested against the behavioral objectives. Each alternative action is tested against each critical objective. Alternatives that are incompatible with objectives are eliminated.

8. *Choose the best alternative.* The choice is guided by decision rules. Decision rules specify which decision is rational or optimal. The rules are based on the approach selected for a solution (step 4) and the overall purposes (step 1). For example, if an approach is to "educate patients about healthy life-style patterns" and the overall purpose is "to improve the patient's level of wellness," then alternatives that do not educate about healthy life-style patterns should be eliminated. Decision rules are frequently found in the regulations and policies of an agency.

9. *Control and implement decisions.* The nurse controls by directing and monitoring the selected solution. Important at this stage is feedback that provides information about the effectiveness of the action.

10. *Evaluate the effectiveness of the action.* At this stage, the observable results are compared with the performance criteria developed in step 5. If feedback indicates the action did not solve the problem, the decision making process needs to be repeated. It can be started again at any step in the process.

Assessment

Assessment is the first phase in the nursing process, and data collection is the primary tool used during this phase. Data collection is a continuing activity, which can be conducted both formally and informally. An example of formal data collection is the nursing history (nursing assessment); an example of informal data collection is noticing during a handshake that a patient's hand is damp. Assessment is continuous throughout the nursing process. Because the patient is always changing, data are always incomplete.

The purpose of nursing assessment is to gather information about the patient's health so that the nurse can plan individualized care. All other steps in the nursing process depend on the collection of the data, which need to be relevant and descriptive. Data are always factual, not interpretive. It is a common error to offer opinions, generalizations, and interpretations as data. For example, a nurse may describe a patient as "uncooperative" rather than record specific "uncooperative" behavior—perhaps a refusal to take a deep breath and to cough after surgery. A specific description of the behavior is more useful than an interpretation, because the causes of specific behavior can be explored. Perhaps the patient refuses to cough because he or she is afraid of rupturing a suture line, or perhaps has severe pain upon coughing.

Patients can generalize or be nonspecific. They may describe the reason for their hospitalization as a "spell" or as "chest pain." It is important that the nurse elicit specifics from the patient. For example, the chest pain needs to be described by its nature and location, how it was relieved, when it occurred, and whether it was a new experience.

Objective and Subjective Data

Objective data are detectable by an observer or can be tested by using an accepted standard. For example, discoloration of the skin, a blood pressure reading, or the act of crying are objective data. *Subjective data*, however, are apparent only to the person affected and can be described or verified only by that person. Itching, pain, and feeling worried are examples of subjective data. Objective data are sometimes called *signs* or *overt data*, and subjective data are sometimes called *symptoms* or *covert data*.

Data can also be described as *variable* or *constant*. Blood pressure, for example, varies from day to day or even by the hour and needs updating. Constant data are unchanging, for example, a date of birth.

The term *data* has a broader meaning than signs or symptoms. It also includes patient information that is not related to a disease process. In the context of the problem-oriented record, the terms *data base* and *baseline data* are often used. See page 427.

Need and Problem Defined

The terms *need* and *problem* are used in the context of the nursing process. A *need* is a requisite for living, something people require to maintain homeostasis. See Chapter 8, page 164. A *problem* is an unmet need or anything that interferes with a person's ability to meet his or her needs. For example, a patient has a need for nourishment, but the ability to meet this need may be impaired by problems such as difficulty swallowing, vomiting, or excessive intake of carbohydrates.

Areas of Assessment

The organization and approach to assessment varies considerably among experts in the field. Some nurse practice acts in the United States specify areas of assessment. Common areas of assessment are:

1. Identifying information—name, age, sex, occupation, etc.
2. Patient's perception of the illness and/or situation, including any clinical symptoms and reasons for seeking assistance
3. Stressors that affect the patient's health and the coping mechanisms employed
4. Life-style, including daily activities, schedule, etc., and how these are affected by the illness
5. Sociocultural factors that might affect health needs, e.g., spiritual beliefs and ethnic practices
6. Personal definition of health
7. Developmental level and needs
8. Basic needs (physiological and psychosocial) and the patient's ability to meet those needs
9. Resources such as strengths, abilities, support persons, assets, etc.
10. Deficits, including physical and psychosocial limitations and financial problems
11. Learning capacity, including intellectual ability, motivation, and learning skills
12. The patient's expectations of nursing or health personnel
13. Previous experience with the health care system

Sources of Data

Sources of data are *primary* or *secondary*. See Table 5–3. The patient is the primary source of data. Secondary or indirect sources are support persons, physician, written records, medical histories, etc.

Patient

The chief source of data is usually the patient unless the patient is too ill, young, or confused to communicate clearly. The patient can usually provide subjective data that no one else can offer. However, a stoical patient may understate symptoms, while another patient may exaggerate.

Table 5–3 Methods of Data Collection

Primary source	Secondary source
Informal conversation	Communication with:
Formal interview	—significant others
Nursing history	—physicians
Physical examination	—colleagues
	—other health team members
	Previous health records
	Patient records
	Reports of diagnostic tests
	Medical histories
	Admitting records

Significant Others

Significant others or support persons know the patient well and often can provide data. They may supplement information or verify information provided by the patient. They might convey information about the stresses the patient felt before the illness, family attitudes to illness and health, and the patient's home environment.

Others are an important source of data, particularly when the patient is very young, unconscious, or confused. In some cases—when the patient is an abused child, for example—the person giving information may wish to remain anonymous.

Health Team Members

Health team members are often sources of information about a patient's health. Social workers, physicians, physiotherapists, and other nurses, for example, may have information from either previous or current contact with the patient. A physician who knows the patient's home setting may provide valuable data about the family and environmental stressors.

Records and Reports

Records and reports reveal pertinent information about a patient. The patient's record, previous health records, and diagnostic reports are all sources of valuable data. Figure 5–4 shows an initial data base for a patient admitted to a hospital.

Most health institutions keep the inactive records of discharged patients, sometimes on microfilm. Health team members can refer to these records when needed.

PATIENT PROFILE

Admitted: Walking ✓ Wheelchair ___ Stretcher ___
Prostheses
Dentures Upper Hearing Aid ✓ Glasses ✓
Physical Disabilities
Temp. 37 Pulse 80 Respirations 18 BP 140/95 Height 5'4" Weight 42K.
Nutritional Preferences BRAN at Breakfast
Elimination: Urinary ✓ Bowels : pattern Once 9 a.m.
: aids
Skin Integrity Abrasion left elbow - from a fall at home.
Chronic Conditions / Past Illnesses (include current medications & treatments)

Family and/or significant other Husband + daughter Phone: 689-5454
Who will visit Husband - daily When?
Daughter - when able
Type of residence House - steps into - bedroom and bathroom on main floor.
Employment Re-tired school teacher
Difficulties caused by hospitalization States "I will be glad to get this over with".
Communication No problem if wearing hearing aids.
Cultural beliefs or practices R.C. - Communion each am. please.

Understanding of illness - by patient "In for gall-bladder surgery" - expects to stay 10 days.
- by family As above
Expectations of hospitalization To have surgery and go home.
Hobbies and/or special interests Enjoys cards + reading - has brought magazines
Discharge and Rehabilitation Plans Plans to go home - daughter will help her.

Signature M. Jones, RN. Date May 14/82

Date	Additional Information	Diagnostic Tests

Patient's statement of allergies NONE
Special considerations
Next of kin J. DOE HUSBAND
Phone 689-5454
Address 1550 E. 90th

Diagnosis	Doctors	Sur/Del/Major Tests
Cholecystitis	Admitting J. J. Smith G.P. Consulting	

Age 65 Religion RC Mar. Status M Adm. Date 5/14/82
Name (MRS) LAVINA DOE

Figure 5–4 A concise initial data base that is part of the patient care Kardex. (Courtesy of St. Paul's Hospital, Nursing Department, Vancouver, British Columbia.)

Stages of Assessment

Nursing assessment has two stages: data collection and data organization.

Data Collection

When collecting data, the nurse follows a systematic, organized framework. First, the nurse determines what and how much information is required. Next, the nurse chooses a systematic method for collecting data. A systematic approach decreases errors of omission and commission. Nurses commit errors of omission when they omit or miss something important to the diagnosis or treatment of the patient. Errors of commission occur when nurses perform nursing functions incorrectly. For example, a nurse errs by omission by failing to recognize an elderly patient's need for stimulation and not providing appropriate nursing action to meet this need. An example of an error of commission is examining the urinary bladder by palpating the upper abdomen.

There are many frameworks useful to nurses collecting data, including those by Abdellah, Henderson, McCain, and Gordon.

Abdellah's 21 problems

1. To maintain good hygiene and physical comfort
2. To promote optimal activity; exercise, rest, and sleep
3. To promote safety through the prevention of accident, injury, or other trauma and through the prevention of the spread of infection
4. To maintain good body mechanics and prevent and correct deformities
5. To facilitate the maintenance of a supply of oxygen to all body cells
6. To facilitate the maintenance of nutrition of all body cells
7. To facilitate the maintenance of elimination
8. To facilitate the maintenance of fluid and electrolyte balance
9. To recognize the physiological responses of the body to disease conditions—pathological, physiological, and compensators
10. To facilitate the maintenance of regulatory mechanisms and functions
11. To facilitate the maintenance of sensory function
12. To identify and accept positive and negative expressions, feelings, and reactions
13. To identify and accept the interrelatedness of emotions and organic illness
14. To facilitate the maintenance of effective verbal and nonverbal communication
15. To promote the development of productive interpersonal relationships
16. To facilitate progress toward achievement of personal spiritual goals
17. To create and/or maintain a therapeutic environment
18. To facilitate awareness of self as an individual with varying physical, emotional, and developmental needs
19. To accept the optimum possible goals in the light of physical and emotional limitations
20. To use community resources as an aid in resolving problems arising from illness
21. To understand the role of social problems as influencing factors in the cause of illness (Abdellah et al 1961:16–17)

Henderson's activities of daily living

1. Breathe normally
2. Eat and drink adequately
3. Eliminate by all avenues of elimination
4. Move and maintain a desirable posture (walking, sitting, lying, and changing from one position to another)
5. Sleep and rest
6. Select suitable clothing; dress and undress
7. Maintain body temperature within normal range by adjusting clothing and modifying the environment
8. Keep the body clean and well groomed and protect the integument
9. Avoid dangers in the environment and avoid injuring others
10. Communicate with others in expressing emotions, needs, fears, etc.
11. Worship according to faith
12. Work at something that provides a sense of accomplishment
13. Play or participate in various forms of recreation
14. Learn, discover, or satisfy the curiosity that leads to "normal" development and health (Henderson 1966:49)

McCain's functional abilities

Mental status

State of consciousness
Alert and quick to respond to surroundings
Drowsy and slow to respond
Semiconscious and difficult to arouse
Comatose and unable to arouse
State of automatism

Orientation
- To time
- To place
- To person

Intellectual capacity
- Level of education
- Ability to recall recent and past events

Attention span

Vocabulary level
- Use of simple, nontechnical words
- Use of complex, technical words

Ability to understand ideas
- Slow to learn meaning and make relationships
- Quick to gain meaning and make relationships
- Insight into health problems

Emotional status

Emotional reactions
- Mood
- Presence or absence of anxiety
- Defenses against anxiety, such as aggression, depression, fantasies, identification, rationalization, regression, repression, sublimation

Body image
- Effect of illness on self-concept
- Adaptation of self-concept to reality demands

Ability to relate to others
- To family
- To other patients
- To health team members

Sensory perception

Hearing
- Sensitivity to sound
  - Voice tone that distinguishes sounds: low, moderate, loud
  - Distance at which sounds are distinguished
  - Need to see speaker to distinguish sounds
- Presence of impairment
  - Partial or complete
  - Unilateral or bilateral
  - Ability to lip read
  - Use and effectiveness of supportive aid

Vision
- Acuity
- Presence of impairment
  - Partial or complete
  - Unilateral or bilateral
  - Type: hyperopia, myopia, astigmatism, colorblindness, diplopia, photophobia, nyctalopia, other
  - Use and effectiveness of supportive aid
- Enucleation
  - Unilateral or bilateral
  - Use of prosthesis

Speech
- Has auditory expression
- Aphasia
  - Verbal defect
  - Syntactical defect
  - Nominal defect
  - Semantic defect
- Anarthria
- Mute
- Laryngectomy
  - Use and effectiveness of esophageal speech
- Unusual speech patterns, such as lisping, repetition, staccato speech, stammer, stutter

Touch
- Hyperesthesia
- Anesthesia
- Paresthesia
- Paralgesia

Smell
- Anosmia
- Hyperosmia
- Kakosmia
- Parosmia

Taste
- Distinguishes: sweet, salt, sour, bitter
- Aftertaste present

Motor ability

Mobility
- Complete bed rest
- Bed rest with bathroom privileges
- Sit in chair
- Ambulatory
  - Without assistance
  - With supportive aids: person, crutches, walker
  - Use of wheel chair
  - Use of stretcher
- Posture
  - In bed
  - Upright

Range of motion
- Passive
- Active

Gait

Equilibrium

Abnormal movement
  - Clonic
  - Tonic
  - Spastic
- Flaccid
- Tic
- Ataxia

Muscle tone
- Spasm
- Contractures
- Weakness

Paralysis
  Hemiplegia
  Paraplegia
  Quadriplegia
Loss of extremity
  Location
  Extent
  Use and effectiveness of prosthesis (McCain 1965:83)

Gordon's typology of 11 functional health patterns

1. *Health-perception-health-management pattern.* Describes client's perceived pattern of health and well-being and how health is managed
2. *Nutritional-metabolic pattern.* Describes pattern of food and fluid consumption relative to metabolic need and pattern indicators of local nutrient supply
3. *Elimination pattern.* Describes patterns of excretory function (bowel, bladder, and skin)
4. *Activity-exercise pattern.* Describes pattern of exercise, activity, leisure, and recreation
5. *Cognitive-perceptual pattern.* Describes sensory-perceptual and cognitive pattern
6. *Sleep-rest pattern.* Describes patterns of sleep, rest, and relaxation
7. *Self-perception–self-concept pattern.* Describes self-concept pattern and perceptions of self (e.g., body comfort, body image, feeling state)
8. *Role-relationship pattern.* Describes pattern of role-engagements and relationships
9. *Sexuality-reproductive pattern.* Describes client's patterns of satisfaction and dissatisfaction with sexuality pattern; describes reproductive patterns
10. *Coping-stress-tolerance pattern.* Describes general coping pattern and effectiveness of the pattern in terms of stress tolerance
11. *Value-belief pattern.* Describes patterns of values, beliefs (including spiritual), or goals that guide choices or decisions (Gordon, 1982:81)

Gordon's framework, "A Typology of 11 Functional Health Patterns," organizes the data the nurse collects and is adaptable to all conceptual models. Three advantages of Gordon's framework are that it presents a short list of readily learned categories, organizes data in a way already familiar to most nurses, and steers the nurse toward nursing diagnoses, not medical diagnoses. Gordon uses the word *pattern* to signify a sequence of behavior. The nurse collects data about dysfunctional as well as functional behavior. Thus, using Gordon's framework to analyze data, nurses are able to discern emerging patterns. See the section on nursing diagnosis in Chapter 6.

Data Organization

The second phase of assessment is the organization into categories of the data collected. The nurse separates information about the patient's psychosocial life from data about her or his physical health status. By grouping data into distinct areas, the nurse can readily determine what is and what is not occurring in the patient's life. For example, a male patient's reason for resisting hospitalization becomes obvious when the nurse isolates the fact that the patient takes care of a bedridden wife at home.

Some data may need to be verified at this stage, especially contradictory data. For example, a patient may state that she vomits after each meal, while her family states she has not been vomiting. The contradiction must be resolved. It is also necessary to differentiate between pertinent data and extraneous information. Patients and their support persons often provide more information than is needed. The nurse needs to discard irrelevant information and retain only that information pertinent to the patient's health care. For example, a detailed account of a daughter's imminent wedding is not pertinent unless the patient is under stress and the nurse suspects the wedding as a stressor. Similarly, what the patient ate just before hospitalization is ordinarily not pertinent but might be very significant if the patient is admitted with an allergic reaction or a digestive problem. To be accurately selective, the nurse needs to relate all data to the patient's health needs, then eliminate data that are not relevant either directly or indirectly.

Once organized, the data are recorded in a form accessible to other members of the health team. If the data indicate the need for immediate action, information is usually conveyed verbally before it is charted. For example, a patient who is hemorrhaging from a serious cut requires immediate attention by the physician and/or nurse before detailed recording is carried out.

Assessment Activities

Six activities are common during assessment: informal conversation, observation, consultation, interview, examination, and review of records and literature. For effective assessment, the nurse needs nursing knowledge, communication skills, and psychomotor skills. See Chapter 15 for a discussion of communication; Chapter 16 for a discussion of functioning in groups; and discussions of psychomotor skills throughout the book.

Nurses use many assessment tools; for example, the nurse may use a nursing history form during an assessment interview, and a stethoscope and thermometer during a physical examination.

Informal Conversation

Nurses frequently obtain a great deal of information through informal conversation. This method of obtaining data is often underrated. In informal situations, nurses can identify attitudes and feelings which may be hidden in more formal interviews. During informal conversation, nurses usually ask few questions but guide the conversation into subject and feeling areas about which data are required.

Observation

To *observe* is to gather data by using the five senses. Although nurses observe mainly through sight, all of the senses are engaged during careful observations. Observation has two aspects: (a) noticing the stimuli and (b) selecting, organizing, and interpreting the data, i.e., perceiving it. A nurse who observes that a patient's face is flushed must relate that observation to, for example, body temperature, activity, environmental temperature, and blood pressure. Because observation involves selecting, organizing, and interpreting data, there is a possibility of error. For example, a nurse might not notice certain signs simply because they are unexpected in a certain patient or situation or because they do not conform to preconceptions about a patient's illness. Another source of error is faulty organization and misinterpretation of data. A nurse may interpret a patient's expression of sadness as fear of scheduled surgery, when in reality the patient is saddened by a television program.

Observation is a conscious, deliberate skill that is developed only through effort and with an organized approach. Nurses often need to focus on specific stimuli in a clinical situation; otherwise they are overwhelmed by a multitude of stimuli. Noticing, therefore, involves discriminating among stimuli, that is, separating stimuli in a meaningful manner. For example, nurses caring for newborns learn to ignore the usual sounds of machines in the nursery but respond quickly to an infant's cry or movement.

Nursing observations must be organized so that nothing significant is missed. Most nurses develop an individual sequence for observing events, for example:

1. Clinical signs of patient distress; e.g., pallor or flushing, labored breathing, and behavior indicating pain or emotional distress

2. The status of the patient; i.e., pulse, blood pressure, respirations, etc.

3. The functioning of associated equipment; e.g., intravenous equipment and oxygen

4. Threats to the patient's safety, real or anticipated; e.g., a lowered side rail

5. The immediate environment, including people in it

6. The larger environment; i.e., the community

Consultation

A *consultation* is a deliberation by two or more people. By consulting other members of the health team, the nurse gains additional information about a patient. Consultations are frequently oral; however, the person being consulted may prefer to contribute written information.

Consultations with health personnel who have treated the patient previously can be especially helpful. Physicians are most frequently consulted; other health team members often consulted are the social worker, laboratory technologist, dietitian, and community nurse.

Interview

An interview is a conversation with a purpose (Fenlason 1962:2). Some possible purposes are to gather data, to evaluate change, to teach, to identify problems, to provide support, and to provide counseling or therapy.

The purpose of a nursing assessment interview is to gather data. Although nurses should not lose sight of that purpose during an interview, they are sometimes obliged to postpone data collection momentarily. If, for example, a patient expresses worry about surgery, the nurse pauses to provide support. Simply to note the worry without providing support can leave the impression that the nurse does not care about the patient's concerns or dismisses them as unimportant. This impression could lessen the patient's willingness to accept assistance from the nurse at a later date.

There are two types of interviews: informal and formal.

Informal interview

An informal interview is usually shorter than a formal one. The nurse uses direct questions that address the immediate situation. For instance, nurses use the informal interview technique to assess a patient's health status after surgery: "Are you having any pain? What is it like? Show me where it is." The informal interview is also used in emergencies, when the nurse must assess the patient's health quickly and learn what events preceded the emergency. For example, when a patient is found lying on the floor of a hospital room, the nurse might interview other patients present: "When did he fall? Did he say anything? What had he been doing?

As part of the assessment process, the informal interview is also used to determine the patient's feelings and needs. For example, a nurse might ask a patient: "How are you feeling today? Is there anything I can do for you? How do you feel about this I.V.?"

Formal interview

A formal interview is structured, generally according to its purpose and the data to be obtained. There are two types of interview structures: directive and indirective or permissive.

The directive interview is highly structured and elicits specific information. The interviewer controls the interview by asking questions that call for specific responses. During an indirective interview, the interviewee establishes the direction of the interview. The interviewer clarifies and encourages communication. Open-ended statements or questions are frequently used. See Chapter 15, page 374, and the discussion of interview techniques, page 130. The indirective interview is more efficient in eliciting expressions of feeling from the interviewee than concrete responses.

A nursing assessment interview is sometimes called a *nursing history*. See Figure 5–5. The nurse uses both types of formal interview techniques when taking the nursing history. The nurse must not only obtain specific information about the patient and the illness but also determine the patient's perceptions of and feelings about the illness. To elicit perceptions and feelings, nondirective approaches are essential. The structure of the interview is determined by the framework used for data collection (e.g., Gordon's framework of 11 functional health patterns, page 126). Many agencies have their own nursing history forms.

Stages of an interview

An interview has four stages:

1. Introduction or beginning
2. Body
3. Recapitulation
4. Termination

It is important to plan an interview before beginning it. The nurse reviews what information is already available and does not ask for it again. Patients are annoyed by having to repeat information to different people. The nurse reviews the data collection form to make sure that the data to be collected are really needed and will serve some purpose related to the patient's care.

The time and place of the interview should be planned as well. The nurse chooses a time when the patient can be responsive: A person in severe pain may not want or be able to answer many questions. The nurse chooses a private place where others cannot overhear or see the patient. Most people are inhibited when answering personal questions in the hearing of others and expressing strong feelings in the sight of others. In addition, the patient should be made to feel comfortable and unhurried. Constant interruptions can distract the patient and convey the impression that the nurse is too busy to spend time with patients.

Introduction The nurse begins the interview by giving his or her name and position. This introduction gives the patient some rationale for talking with the nurse. The nurse then explains what information is needed and how it will be used. It is also important to convey where the data will be recorded and who will see it. In many situations, it is appropriate to tell the patient how long the interview will last and that she or he has the right not to provide the data. In some jurisdictions, the nurse should explain the patient's right to privileged communication with the nurse. See Chapter 4, page 104.

The following is an example of an interview introduction:

Nurse: Hello, Ms. Goodwin, I'm Ms. Fellows. I'm a student nurse, and I'll be assisting with your care here.

Patient: Hi. Are you a student from the college?

Nurse: Yes, I'm in my final year, and I'd like to sit down with you here for about 10 minutes to talk about how I can help you while you're here.

Patient: I'd be glad to talk with you. What do you want to know?

Nurse: Well, to plan your care after your operation, I'd like to get some information about your normal daily activities and what you expect here in the hospital. I'd like to make notes while we talk to get the important points and have them available to the other staff who will also look after you.

Patient: OK. I guess that's all right with me.

Nurse: If there is anything you don't want to talk about, please feel free to say so, and if there is anything you would rather I didn't write down, just tell me and it will remain confidential. Shall we start now?

Patient: Sure, now is as good a time as any.

Body The patient or client communicates what he or she thinks, feels, knows, and perceives in the body of the interview. At this stage the nurse must:

1. Listen attentively (see Chapter 15, page 372)
2. Clarify points that are not understood
3. Select the communication technique that makes both patient and nurse comfortable and elicits the data
4. Strive to build a relationship of respect, trust, concern, and interest
5. Refocus the patient if he or she wanders from the subject

VANCOUVER GENERAL HOSPITAL

NURSING ASSESSMENT

DATE ____ NURSING UNIT ____

MR., MISS, MRS. ____ UNIT NUMBER ____

SURNAME ____ GIVEN NAME ____

DOCTOR ____ (PLEASE USE BLOCK CAPITALS)

SEX ____ AGE ____

PART 1 - GENERAL INFORMATION

DATE: TIME: SOURCE OF INFORMATION:

IF NOT PATIENT, SPECIFY WHY:

MODE OF ADMISSION: AMBULATION AID(S)

VISUAL AID(S) HEARING AID(S)

DENTAL AID(S) OTHER PROSTHESIS(ES)

VALUABLES:

VITAL SIGNS: T: P:(R) (A) R: B.P.: WT: HT:

APPEARANCE & CONDITION:

PATIENT'S STATED REASON FOR HOSPITALIZATION & HISTORY OF PRESENT ILLNESS:

PAST MEDICAL HISTORY - ILLNESSES, HOSPITALIZATIONS & SURGERIES:

MEDICATIONS	DOSE	FREQ.	TIME OF LAST DOSE	INTO HOSPITAL	ALLERGIES & REACTIONS

ADDITIONAL COMMENTS:

NURSE'S SIGNATURE: ____ DATE: ____ TIME: ____

Front

PART II - BASIC NEEDS INFORMATION

	DATE	TIME	
NUTRITION			
ELIMINATION			
OXYGEN			
ACTIVITY & REST			
SECURITY			
SELF CONCEPT			
SEXUALITY			
SOCIAL SITUATION			
WORRIES & CONCERNS			

Back

Figure 5–5 A nursing assessment. (Courtesy of the Vancouver General Hospital, Vancouver, British Columbia.)

For additional information on communication techniques, see Chapter 15 and the section on techniques of interviewing later in this chapter.

Recapitulation *Recapitulation* is the repetition by the nurse of the major findings during the interview. Recapitulation serves four purposes:

1. It helps the nurse organize data.
2. It helps the nurse set priorities.
3. It lets the patient validate or correct data.
4. It clarifies the content of the communication for the patient.

Termination The interview is usually terminated by the nurse, although in some cases the patient terminates it. Nurses normally terminate interviews when they have obtained the information they need, and patients terminate interviews when they decide not to give any more information. A nurse may end an interview if for some reason—fatigue, for example—the patient cannot offer more information.

The nurse terminates the interview by indicating that no further information is required and explaining the patient's role in planning care or by saying that the interview will continue at another time. For example: "Ms. Goodwin, I will be responsible for giving you care 3 days per week while you are here. I will be in to see you each Monday, Tuesday, and Wednesday between 8 o'clock and 12 noon. At those times, we can adjust your care if we need to. When I am not here, Ms. Brown will look after you." Or: "Ms. Goodwin, it's time for you to rest. I'll come back another time to finish our talk. We need information from you and your ideas to help plan your care."

Interview techniques There are basically three types of questions with which the nurse can elicit information: (a) open-ended questions or suggestions, (b) closed questions, and (c) biased or leading questions.

An *open-ended question* or suggestion invites answers longer than one or two words. It often elicits descriptive or comparative responses and allows the patient to divulge information the patient is ready to disclose. The response may also convey attitudes and beliefs the patient holds. The chief disadvantage of the open-ended question is that the patient may spend time conveying irrelevant information.

Examples of open-ended questions and suggestions are: "How have you been feeling lately?" "Tell me how you feel about that." "How do you feel about coming to the hospital?"

Closed questions require only one- or two-word answers. Closed questions are more easily answered by the highly stressed person and the person who has difficulty communicating. The amount of information gained is generally limited. Examples of closed questions are: "What medication did you take?" "Are you having pain now?" "How long have you lived in the United States?"

Biased or *leading questions* suggest what the questioner expects in the answer. Leading questions create difficulties if the patient, from a desire to please the questioner, gives inaccurate responses. Examples of biased questions are: "You haven't had any emotional problems?" "You haven't ever had a venereal disease, have you?"

The emotional coloration of words used in questions can create bias. For example, *masturbation* has a negative connotation to some people, and hence its use in a question can create a bias.

For additional information about communication see the section on techniques for responding therapeutically in Chapter 15, page 374.

Examination

An *examination* of a patient includes physical and psychosocial aspects. A nurse examines a patient to collect objective data about that patient's health. The examination might focus on a specific problem, for example, the inability to urinate, or it may be a general examination of the patient as a whole person.

Examinations should be systematic. One frequently used approach is the *cephalocaudal* examination, from top to bottom. The examination starts at the head and ends at the toes. See Figure 5-6 for a sample head-to-toe assessment. The objective of the nursing examination is to identify the individual's coping abilities, both physiological or psychosocial. By contrast, the physician's examination is intended to detect disease. The findings of both examinations are related and at no time should be contradictory.

Visual examination of a person is called *inspection*. The nurse inspects the body in an orderly manner, focusing on one area of the body at a time. A patient's body can also be examined by touch or *palpation*. See Figure 5-7. Through palpation, the nurse is able to assess hardness, size, texture, swelling, and movability of an internal organ or part. The pads of the fingers, the most sensitive area of the fingers, are used in palpation. *Percussion* is the examination of the body by tapping it with the fingers. See Figure 5-8. The technique most commonly used today is to place one hand on the body surface with the middle finger, called the *pleximeter*, over the area to be percussed. The middle finger of the other hand is used to strike rapidly and sharply just proximal to the distal interphalangeal joint. The sound results from the vibration of the body structures adjacent to the pleximeter. Specific percussion sounds of body parts are discussed in Chapter 14.

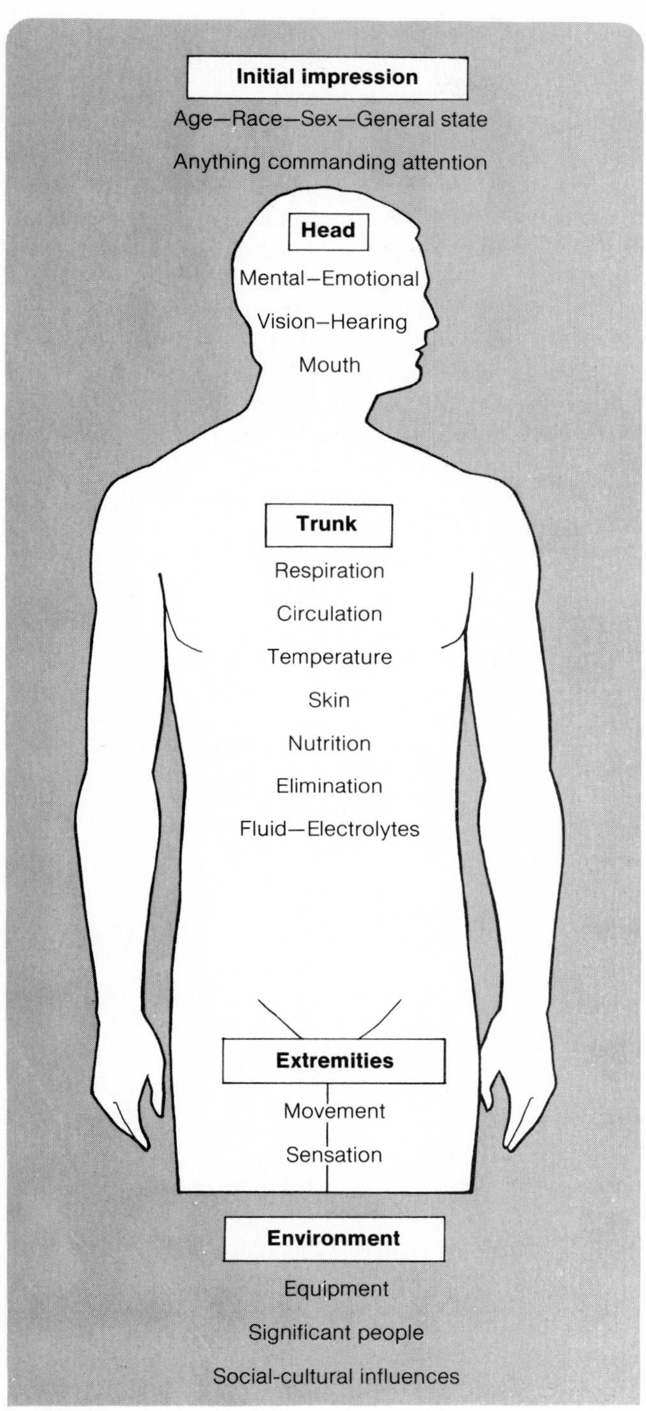

Figure 5–6 A tool for assessment. (Adapted from H. Wolff and R. Erickson. The assessment man, *Nursing Outlook,* February 1977, 25:103.)

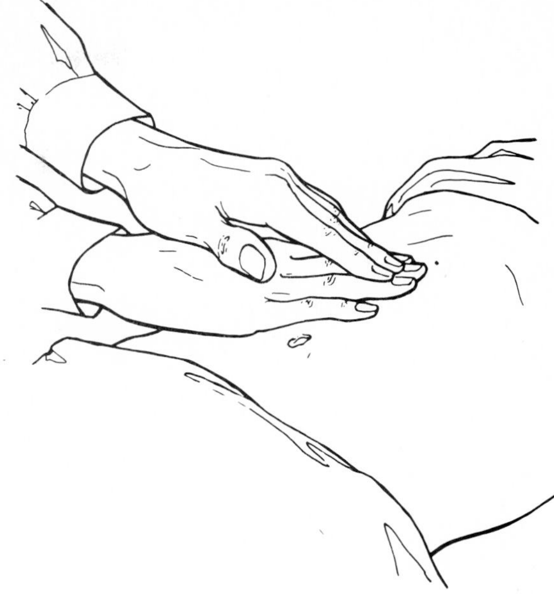

Figure 5–7 Deep palpation of the abdomen using the pads of the fingers to examine the internal organs.

Figure 5–8 Percussing the chest by striking the middle finger sharply just proximal to the distal interphalangeal joint.

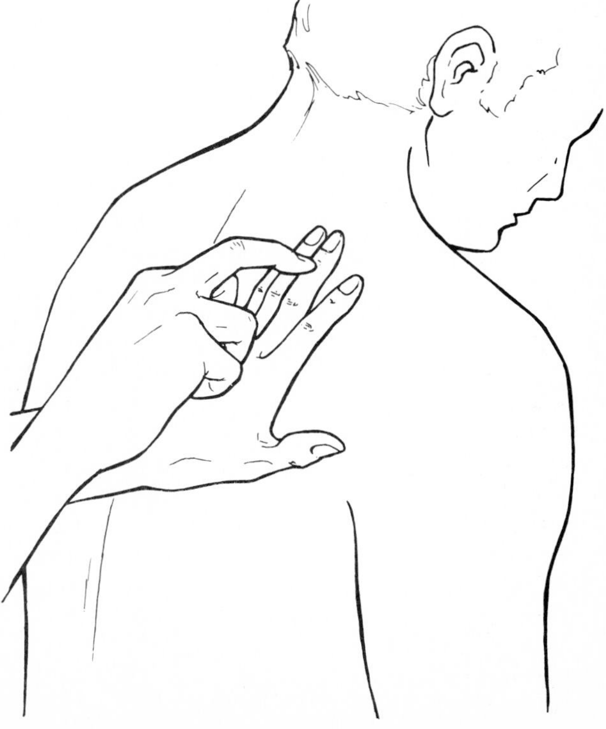

Auscultation is listening for sounds produced within the body. The sounds most frequently listened for are those of the abdominal and thoracic viscera and the movement of blood in the cardiovascular system. Direct auscultation, using the ear only, is seldom done. Indirect auscultation is generally carried out with a stethoscope.

Increasingly nurses are carrying out examinations of patients. The examination calls for interviewing and observation skills together with more specific measurements such as taking the blood pressure. For additional information about examination see Chapters 13, 14, and the appropriate subject chapter in the text.

Review of Records and Literature

Reviewing pertinent records and literature also can provide relevant data. Records can validate or contradict findings; if the latter, further action is needed to confirm the data. The following records often provide significant information:

1. Diagnostic reports
2. Reports from other members of the health team, including other nursing personnel
3. Report of the physician's examination, consultations, etc.
4. Earlier health records
5. Admission records

In addition, a search of relevant literature can help the nurse understand the patient's problems and plan nursing interventions.

Summary

The nursing process is a systematic, rational method of providing nursing care. A five-step process is frequently used: assessment, nursing diagnosis, planning, nursing intervention, and evaluation. The nursing process combines a humanistic nursing approach with a systems approach to problem solving. The process has these attributes: its steps are overlapping and continuous; each step affects the others; the system is open, flexible, and dynamic; and feedback is important in the process.

Assessment is the first phase of the nursing process, and data collection is the primary tool used. The purpose of data collection is to gather information about the patient's health. Objective data are detectable by an observer; subjective data are apparent only to the person affected. A *need* is a requisite for living, whereas a *problem* is an unmet need or anything that interferes with the individual's ability to meet needs.

The sources of assessment data can be described as primary (the patient or client) and secondary (other sources). Assessment has two stages: data collection and data organization. Six assessment activities are informal conversation, observation, consultation, interview, examination, and review of records and literature. The nursing assessment interview, commonly referred to as a nursing history, is a formal interview with direct and indirective characteristics. Interviews have four parts: introduction, body, recapitulation, and termination. A number of interview techniques are used to elicit information: open-ended questions or suggestions, closed questions, and biased or leading questions.

The nursing examination of a patient includes physical and psychosocial areas. A systematic approach commonly used is the cephalocaudal. Examination includes inspection, palpation, percussion, and auscultation. Reviewing records and literature can also provide relevant data and serve to confirm or contradict data obtained. In the latter situation, the nurse must conduct further assessment to confirm the data.

Suggested Activities

1. Compare three different nursing assessment tools and identify their similarities and differences.
2. Interview a classmate using a nursing assessment tool of your choice. Practice some interviewing techniques, and discuss with interviewers their feelings about and reactions to being interviewed.
3. Select a patient in a clinical setting and take a nursing history.
4. Obtain additional data about the patient (activity 3) from other appropriate sources. Organize all data according to a predetermined format.

Suggested Readings

Baer, E. D.; McGowan, M. N.; and McGivern, D. O. July 1977. How to take a health history. *American Journal of Nursing* 77:1190–93.

The authors discuss a health history with six sections: chief complaint or the client's reason for seeking help, the client profile, family history, past health history, history of present problems, and review of systems.

Ryden, M. B. 1977. Energy: A crucial consideration in the nursing process. *Nursing Forum* 16(1):71–82.

This article examines human energy from the standpoint of assessment, planning, implementation, and evaluation. Some questions by which to assess energy are suggested.

Wolff, H., and Erickson, R. February 1977. The assessment man. *Nursing Outlook* 25:103–7.

Nurses can use a simple, practical tool for systematic patient assessment. This head-to-toe approach has three major sections: initial impression, the patient from head to toe, and the environment.

Selected References

Abdellah, F. G., et al. 1961. *Patient-centered approaches to nursing.* New York: Macmillan Co.

Aspinall, M. J. September-October 1975. Development of a patient completed admission questionnaire and its comparison with the nursing interview. *Nursing Research* 24:377–81.

Bailey, J. T., and Claus, K. E. 1975. *Decision making in nursing: Tools for change.* St. Louis: C. V. Mosby Co.

Becknell, E. P., and Smith, D. M. 1975. *System of nursing practice.* Philadelphia: F. A. Davis Co.

Bloch, D. November 1974. Some crucial terms in nursing. What do they really mean? *Nursing Outlook* 22:689–94.

Carlson, S. September 1972. A practical approach to the nursing process. *American Journal of Nursing* 72:1589–91.

Eggland, E. T. July 1977. How to take a meaningful nursing history. *Nursing 77* 7:22–30.

Fenlason, A. 1962. *Essentials of interviewing.* Rev. ed. New York: Harper and Row.

Gordon, M. 1982. *Nursing diagnosis process and application.* New York: McGraw-Hill Book Co.

Hagar, L. October 1977. The nursing process: A tool to individualized care. *The Canadian Nurse* 73:38–41.

Hamdi, M. E., and Hutelmyer, C. M. July-August 1970. A study of the effectiveness of an assessment tool in the identification of nursing care problems. *Nursing Research* 19:354–58.

Henderson, V. 1966. *The nature of nursing.* New York: Macmillan Co.

Knowles, L. N. 1967. *Decision making in nursing—a necessity for doing: ANA Clinical Sessions 1966.* New York: Appleton-Century-Crofts.

La Monica, E. L. 1979. *The nursing process: A humanistic approach.* Menlo Park, Calif.: Addison-Wesley Publishing Co.

Little, D. E., and Carnevali, D. L. 1976. *Nursing care planning.* 2nd ed. Philadelphia: J. B. Lippincott Co.

McCain, R. April 1965. Nursing by assessment—not intuition. *American Journal of Nursing* 65:82–84. Reprinted in *Contemporary nursing series: The nursing process in practice.* 1974. New York: American Journal of Nursing Co.

McPhetridge, L. M. January 1968. Nursing history: One means to personalize care. *American Journal of Nursing* 68:68–75.

Manthey, M. E. October 1967. A guide for interviewing. *American Journal of Nursing* 67:2088–90.

Marriner, A. 1979. *The nursing process.* 2nd ed. St. Louis: C. V. Mosby Co.

Mayers, M. G. May 1972. A search for assessment criteria. *Nursing Outlook* 20:323–26.

Mitchell, P. H., and Loustau, A. 1981. *Concepts basic to nursing.* 3rd ed. New York: McGraw-Hill Book Co.

Orlando, I. J. 1961. *The dynamic nurse-patient relationship.* New York: Putnam's.

Schaefer, J. October 1974. The interrelatedness of decision making and the nursing process. *American Journal of Nursing* 74:1852–56.

Simon, J. R., and Chastain, S. September 1960. Take a systematic look at your patients. *Nursing Outlook* 8:509–12.

Smith, D. M. November 1968. A clinical nursing tool. *American Journal of Nursing* 68:2384–88.

Taylor, D. B., and Johnson, O. H. 1974. *Systematic nursing assessment: A step toward automation.* DHEW Publication no. (HRA) 74-17.

Western Interstate Commission on Higher Education. 1967. *Defining clinical content.* Graduate Nursing Programs, Medical and Surgical Nursing. Boulder, Colo.: Western Interstate Commission on Higher Education.

Yura, H., and Walsh, M. B. 1978. *The nursing process: Assessing, planning, implementing, evaluating.* 3rd ed. New York: Appleton-Century-Crofts.

Chapter 6

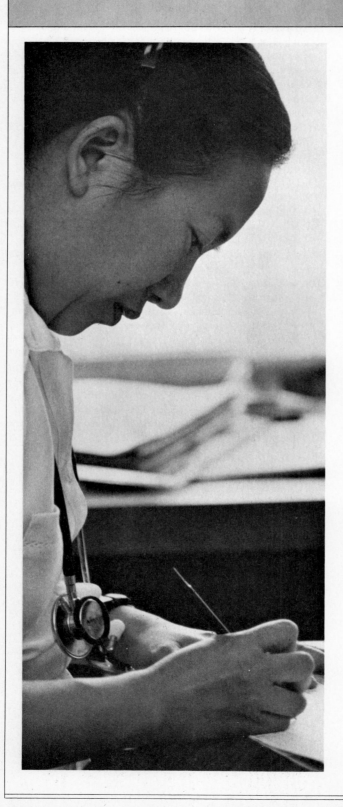

Nursing Diagnosis and Planning

CONTENTS

Objectives

1. Know essential facts about nursing diagnoses
   - **1.1** Define nursing diagnosis
   - **1.2** Identify differences between medical and nursing diagnoses
   - **1.3** Identify three essential components of nursing diagnoses
   - **1.4** Identify the two essential parts of a nursing diagnostic statement
   - **1.5** List guidelines for stating a nursing diagnosis
   - **1.6** List advantages of nursing diagnoses
   - **1.7** Identify basic steps involved in the process of diagnosing
2. Know essential facts about the planning phase of the nursing process
   - **2.1** Define terms used in planning
   - **2.2** Identify five nursing activities involved in planning
   - **2.3** Identify factors to consider when setting priorities
   - **2.4** Identify the relationship of goals to the nursing diagnosis
   - **2.5** Outline essential characteristics of patient goal statements
   - **2.6** Describe the concept of outcome criteria
   - **2.7** Identify essential characteristics of outcome criteria
   - **2.8** Identify essential components of nursing orders
   - **2.9** Describe three categories of nursing orders
   - **2.10** Describe essential aspects of a nursing care plan

Terms

actual health problem
criterion
deductive reasoning
diagnosis
goal
health problem
inductive reasoning
inference
inferential statistics
nursing diagnosis
objective
outcome criteria
potential health problem
triage

Much interest and enthusiasm is currently being generated about nursing diagnosis even though the term has appeared in the nursing literature for over a quarter of a century. Initially diagnosis as a nursing function was controversial; this task was considered to be solely in the realm of the physician. As a result, nurses tended to use the terms *problems* and *needs* rather than *nursing diagnoses.* Since 1973, however, when nursing diagnosis appeared as a function of the professional nurse in the American Nurses' Association's Standards of Nursing Practice, diagnosis as a nursing function has gained both legal and professional acceptance. Now the term is appearing in revised nurse practice acts and in health care agency statements about standards of nursing care. It is currently recognized as an essential part (the second step) of the nursing process.

Another large factor supporting the acceptance of nursing diagnosis was development of the United States National Conference Group for the Classification of Nursing Diagnoses in 1973. This group originated through the efforts of two faculty members at St. Louis University, Kristine Gebbie and Mary Ann Lavin, who perceived a need to identify their roles in an ambulatory care setting. The First National Conference held to identify nursing diagnoses was sponsored by St. Louis University School of Nursing and Allied Health Professions in 1973. Since that time national conferences have been held in 1975, 1978, and 1980. Through the efforts of these groups much progress has been made in defining, classifying, and describing nursing diagnoses. International recognition was shown by the First Canadian Conference, held in Toronto, Ontario, in 1977, and plans for a future international conference have been discussed. The results of the 1980 United States National Conference are summarized in Table 6–2 later in this chapter.

Nursing Diagnosis

Definition

The term *diagnosis,* according to the dictionary, is derived from the Greek word *diagignoskein,* which means "to distinguish." Analyzed further, *dia* means "apart" and *gignoskein* means "to know." Definitions include (a) the art of identifying a disease from its signs and symptoms, (b) a statement or conclusion concerning the nature of some phenomenon, and (c) analysis of the course or nature of a condition, situation, or problem. Although the first definition pertains to diagnoses made by physicians, the process of diagnosing is used by several professions to identify aspects of the patient's condition that are of concern to that particular profession. In fact anyone who makes a statement or conclusion about the nature of a condition, situation, or problem is diagnosing. Auto mechanics diagnose the nature or cause of automobile conditions; social workers diagnose economic and social situations; and nurses diagnose the health status of patients requiring nursing care. The term *diagnosis*, therefore, is not restricted to one particular profession and must be qualified by a professional designation, such as medical diagnosis or nursing diagnosis; that is, it is qualified by the subject matter in which the diagnostician is expert.

Several definitions of *nursing diagnosis* have been stated since the early 1950s. Each has different emphases, but all have many similarities. To Gordon (1976:1299) *nursing diagnoses*, or clinical diagnoses made by professional nurses, describe a combination of signs and symptoms that indicate actual or potential health problems that nurses by virtue of their education and experience are able, licensed, and accountable to treat. To Edel (1982:6), a *nursing diagnosis* is the statement of a potential or actual altered health status of a client, which is derived from nursing assessment and which requires intervention from the domain of nursing. Edel's definition emphasizes that the entity to be diagnosed is *health status*, which avoids the negative connotation of *problem* and allows for positive diagnoses of patients.

Implied in these definitions are the following characteristics:

1. Professional nurses (registered nurses) are the persons responsible for making nursing diagnoses. Even though other nursing personnel may contribute data to the process of diagnosing and may implement specified care, the formulation of a diagnosis lies within the realm of the professional nurse. This restriction is supported by licensing laws and national standards of practice.

2. A *health problem* is any condition or situation in which a patient requires help to maintain or regain a state of health or to achieve a peaceful death. It does not always refer to an undesirable state but does refer to a situation for which the patient needs assistance.

3. Nursing diagnoses describe (a) *actual health problems* (deviations from health), (b) *potential health problems* (risk factors that predispose persons and families to health problems) and (c) areas of enriched personal growth. Examples of actual health problems are an ineffective breathing pattern, a fluid volume deficit, or a knowledge deficit. Examples of potential health problems are risk of skin breakdown or a potential sleep pattern disturbance. Examples of areas of enriched personal growth are self-development, health management, and parenting. In general these problems encompass "actual or potential disturbances in life processes, patterns, functions, or development, including those occurring secondary to disease" (Gordon 1976:1298).

4. The domain of nursing diagnosis includes only those health states that nurses are able and licensed to treat. For example, nurses are not educated to diagnose or treat diseases such as diabeties mellitus; this task is defined legally as the practice of medicine. Yet they can diagnose a knowledge deficit, ineffective coping by the individual, alterations in nutrition, and potential for injury, all of which may accompany diabetes mellitus. These problems are within the nurse's capabilities and the scope of the nurse's licensing laws; thus, the nurse is responsible and accountable for the treatment provided for these nursing diagnoses.

Differences from Medical Diagnoses

Nursing diagnoses differ from medical diagnoses in several ways. For a summary, see Table 6–1. The medical diagnosis describes a specific disease process, which is uniform from one patient to the other. It is oriented toward pathology and lasts the duration of a patient's illness. In contrast the nursing diagnosis describes a patient's *response* to an illness or other situation, which varies among individuals. The nursing diagnosis is oriented to the individual and changes as the patient's response changes. For example, in two patients with the medical diagnosis of rheumatoid arthritis, the disease process is quite similar but the responses to it can be very different. A 70-year-old female may respond with acceptance, viewing her condition as part of the aging process. A 20-year-old female may respond with anger and hostility because of the changes this condition will make in her personal identity, body image, role performance, and self-esteem.

Another difference between the diagnoses is that medical diagnoses are described in concise phrases of two or three words and in a universally accepted format. For nursing diagnoses, however, there is no well-developed, universal taxonomy. This results in considerable variation in the terms of nursing diagnoses. Some are long and complex. It is doubtful that nursing diagnoses will ever be condensed to the size of medical diagnoses.

A nursing diagnosis may be related to a medical diagnosis, but, just as the medical diagnosis is separate and distinct, so is the nursing diagnosis. A patient who has one or more medical diagnoses and medical orders will also have one or more nursing diagnoses and nursing orders. These diagnoses and orders are complementary rather than contradictory. Nursing diagnoses relate to the nurse's *independent functions,* i.e., the areas of health care that are unique to nursing and are separate and distinct from the care included in medical management. Even though the nurse is obligated to carry out medical orders, i.e., *dependent functions,* the nurse is also obligated to diagnose and prescribe within the limits of nurse practice acts.

Components of Nursing Diagnoses

There are three essential components of a nursing diagnosis; they are referred to as the *PES format* (Gordon 1976:1299):

1. *The state of the patient or health problem* (P). This component, referred to as the *diagnostic category label* or *title,* is a description of the patient's condition (actual or potential) for which nursing therapy is given. The state of the patient is described clearly and concisely in a few words. See Table 6–2 for a list of nursing diagnoses adopted by the Fourth National Conference on Classification of Nursing Diagnoses in 1980. To be clinically useful, category labels need to be specific. Thus, quantifying or qualifying adjectives are sometimes needed to identify areas, stages, or levels of a particular problem. Where the term *specify* follows a category label in Table 6–2, the nurse is directed to state the area in which the problem occurs. For example, a knowledge deficit may be in the area of medication prescription, dietary adjustments, or disease process and therapy. Stages may be specified by using qualifying terms, such as *acute* or *chronic* (e.g., chronic ineffective breathing pattern). Numbered levels are needed to specify a problem such as impaired physical mobility. See the suggested code for functional level classification in Table 6–3.

2. *The etiology of the problem* (E). This component identifies the probable causes of the patient's state of health and gives direction to the required nursing therapy. Etiology may include behaviors of the patient, environmental factors, or interactions of the two. For example, the probable causes of impaired physical mobility include decreased strength and endurance, pain/discomfort, and musculoskeletal impairment. See Table 6–3. Differentiating among possible causes in the nursing diagnosis is essential because each may require different nursing therapies.

3. *The defining characteristics or cluster of signs and symptoms* (S). The defining characteristics provide information necessary to arrive at the diagnostic category label (component 1). Each nursing diagnostic category has a set of signs and symptoms that occur as a clinical entity. They are similar to the medical diagnostic categories. For example, the medical diagnostic category myocardial infarction (heart attack) has a standarized set of signs and symptoms that are universally understood and accepted. Likewise, the nursing diagnostic category impaired physical mobility has a standardized cluster of signs and symptoms. See Table 6–3.

Table 6–1 Characteristics of Medical and Nursing Diagnoses

Medical diagnosis	Nursing diagnosis
Describes a specific disease process	Describes an individual's response to a disease process, condition, or situation
Is oriented to pathology	Is oriented to the individual
Remains constant throughout the duration of illness	Changes as the patient's responses change
Guides medical management, some of which may be carried out by the nurse	Guides independent nursing care, i.e., nursing orders (therapies) and evaluation
Is complementary to the nursing diagnosis	Is complementary to the medical diagnosis
Has a well-developed classification system accepted by the medical profession	Has no universally accepted classification system; such systems are in the process of development

Format of a Nursing Diagnosis

The nursing diagnostic statement has two parts:

1. Statement of the patient's response
2. Contributing factors or probable causes of the response

The two parts are joined by the words *related to* or *associated with* rather than *due to.* The phrase *due to* implies a cause-and-effect relationship; one clause causes or is responsible for the other clause. In contrast, the phrases *related to* and *associated with* merely imply a relationship, and if one part of the diagnostic statement changes so may the other part; legal hazards are thus avoided. Examples of nursing diagnoses demonstrating these two parts are:

- Self-concept disturbance (response) related to role change (contributing factor)
- Potential for injury (response) related to poor vision (contributing factor)
- Ineffective breathing pattern (response) related to chest pain (contributing factor)

Table 6–2 List of Nursing Diagnoses from the Fourth National Conference, 1980

Accepted diagnoses		Diagnoses to be developed
Airway clearance, ineffective	Nutrition, alteration in: more than body requirements	Cognitive dissonance
Bowel elimination, alteration in: constipation	Nutrition, alteration in: potential for more than body requirements	Decision making, impaired/ineffective (decision made by client produces results other than or less than desired)
Bowel elimination, alteration in: diarrhea	Parenting, alteration in: actual	Family dynamics, alteration in (to be further developed as a set of family-level diagnoses, as opposed to individual-level diagnoses)
Bowel elimination, alteration in: incontinence	Parenting, alteration in: potential	A. Family role changes/shifts
Breathing pattern, ineffective	Rape-trauma syndrome: rape trauma, compound reaction, silent reaction	B. Dysfunctional coping
Cardiac output, alteration in: decreased	Self-care deficit (specify level): feeding, bathing/hygiene, dressing/grooming, toileting	C. Stress management patterns
Comfort, alteration in: pain	Self-concepts, disturbance in: body image, self-esteem, role performance, personal identity	D. Developmental transition
Communication, impaired verbal	Sensory perceptual alteration: visual, auditory, kinesthetic, gustatory, tactile, and olfactory perceptions	E. Situational transition
Coping, ineffective individual	Sexual dysfunction	Fluid volume, alteration in, excess: potential for
Coping, ineffective family: compromised	Skin integrity, impairment of: actual	Memory deficit
Coping, ineffective family: disabling	Skin integrity, impairment of: potential	Rest-activity pattern, ineffective
Coping, family: potential for growth	Sleep pattern disturbance	Role disturbance
Diversional activity, deficit in	Spiritual distress (distress of the human spirit)	Social isolation
Fear	Thought processes, alteration in	
Fluid volume deficit, actual	Tissue perfusion, alteration in: cerebral, cardiopulmonary, renal, gastrointestinal, peripheral	
Fluid volume deficit, potential	Urinary elimination, alteration in pattern of	
Gas exchange, impaired	Violence, potential for	
Grieving, anticipatory		
Grieving, dysfunctional		
Home maintenance management, impaired		
Injury, potential for; poisoning, potential for; suffocation, potential for; trauma, potential for		
Knowledge deficit (specify)		
Mobility, impaired physical		
Noncompliance (specify)		
Nutrition, alteration in: less than body requirements		

Listed by the National Conference Group for Classification of Nursing Diagnoses. From *Classification of nursing diagnoses*, Proceedings of the Third and Fourth National Conferences, pp. 281–82, by M. J. Kim and D. A. Moritz, editors. Copyright © 1982 McGraw-Hill Book Company

Table 6–3 Components of a Nursing Diagnosis

Diagnosis	Etiology	Defining characteristics
Impaired physical mobility (specify level)*	Intolerance to activity/decreased strength and endurance Pain/discomfort Perceptual/cognitive impairment Musculoskeletal impairment Depression/severe anxiety	Inability to move purposefully within physical environment, including bed mobility, transfer, and ambulation Reluctance to attempt movement Limited range of motion Decreased muscle strength, control, and/or mass Imposed restrictions of movement, including mechanical, medical protocol Impaired coordination

*Suggested code for functional level classification:
0 Completely independent
1 Requires use of equipment or assistive device
2 Requires help from another person, for assistance, supervision, or teaching
3 Requires help from another person and equipment or device
4 Dependent, does not participate in activity

From *Classification of nursing diagnoses*, Proceedings of the Third and Fourth National Conferences, p. 299, by M. J. Kim and D. A. Moritz, editors. Copyright © McGraw-Hill Book Company. Suggested code for functional level classification adapted from E. Jones et al., *Patient classification for long-term care: Users' manual*, HEW Publication no. HR–74–3107 (Washington, D.C.: Department of Health, Education, and Welfare, November 1974).

Deriving a Diagnosis from the Data Base

The key to establishing an effective diagnosis is a *thorough review* of the assessment data. If gaps are found, or the data seem illogical or contradictory, the nurse assesses the patient further, consults with other members of the health team, or uses available reference sources. The process of diagnosing is complex, involving a series of intellectual activities discussed subsequently in this chapter. Suffice it to say at this point that the nurse needs to identify which data are normal and which are abnormal, group data into meaningful categories, and then label the data with a diagnosis. In doing so, the nurse is guided by a conceptual frame of reference (nursing model), since the diagnostic focus and contributing factors vary among nursing models. See Table 6–4.

To illustrate how nursing diagnoses are developed from selected assessment data, the following example uses a 68-year-old female with a medical diagnosis of anemia and varicose ulcer. Relevant information selected from her data base includes:

History

Widow of 1 year.

Lives alone; doesn't want to burden daughter who is married; works full time as office clerk; has 2 grandchildren.

Does not smoke or drink alcohol or coffee.

Usually active in religious activities of Baptist church.

Loves gardening; has vegetable and flower garden but interest has flagged since husband died.

Doesn't like cooking for self. Tends to eat snacks (e.g., tea and toast or canned soup). Says meat is too expensive to buy.

First hospitalization

Feeling more tired than usual. Attributes this to age.

Irritable with grandchildren even though their antics are normal for their age.

Has had occasional periods of dizziness.

Unable to wear right shoe. Right foot and ankle are edematous; has "sore" that won't heal on right ankle.

Thinks the "sore" must have started from a "bump" she got while gardening, but is not sure.

Says right leg feels heavy and aches after sitting or standing for long periods.

Does not wear support stockings.

Has treated "sore" on ankle with iodine for 2 weeks.

Daughter persuaded her to contact the doctor.

Physical examination

Height: 5′ 4″

Weight: 120 lbs

Temperature: 36.2 C (97.2 F)

Pulse rate: 90 per minute

Respirations: 20 per minute at rest

Blood pressure: 120/70

Right ankle edematous, circumference 10¾″

No edema of left ankle; circumference 9½″

Ulcer (2.5 cm) on medial aspect right ankle

Veins of right leg visible and dilated

Skin from ankle to midcalf area scaly and pigmented

Laboratory data

Chest x-ray negative

Hemoglobin low

Urine negative

The following nursing diagnoses are derived from the above data base:

1. Impaired skin integrity related to decreased venous circulation
2. Potential infection related to loss of skin integrity
3. Knowledge deficit about cause of ulcer related to lack of information
4. Nutritional deficit related to social isolation and financial limitations

Table 6–6 later in this chapter matches each diagnosis with the assessment data from which it was derived.

Guidelines for Stating Diagnoses

Mundinger and Jauron (1975:97–98) offer the following guidelines for stating a nursing diagnosis, based on their experience in assisting practitioners to write diagnoses:

1. Avoid writing a diagnosis in terms of a need; instead, write in terms of a response. For example, "need for adequate fluid intake" is better stated "Deficit in fluid volume related to nausea and vomiting."
2. Avoid judgmental and legally inadvisable statements, such as "Skin breakdown related to improper positioning." This is better stated, "Impairment of sacral skin integrity related to inadequate circulation." The former statement could be a basis for legal action.
3. Ensure that both elements of the diagnostic statement do not say the same thing. For example, "Ulceration of sacral area related to skin breakdown" does not give the probable cause.
4. Avoid reversal of clauses in which the contributing factor is stated before the response. For example, in "Lack of knowledge of diabetic diet related to inability to use the food exchange system" the clauses need to be

Table 6–4 Variations of Diagnostic Focus and Contributing Factors in Selected Nursing Models

Model	Diagnostic focus	Contributing factors (etiology)
Orem's self-care agency model	Actual or potential deficit between the powers of self-care agency and the demands placed on it in relation to three self-care categories: 1. Universal 2. Developmental 3. Health deviation	Lack of knowledge, skills, interest, or motivation; disease process; or type of therapy
Roy's adaptation model	Actual maladaptation problems or potential adaptation problems in relation to four modes: 1. Physiologic 2. Self-concept 3. Role function 4. Interdependence	Coping activity that is inadequate to maintain integrity in the face of a need deficit or excess
Johnson and Grubb's behavioral system model	Behavior that does not maintain the equilibrium of eight subsystems in relation to four classifications: 1. Intrasubsystem insufficiency 2. Intrasubsystem discrepancy 3. Intersubsystem incompatibility 4. Intersubsystem dominance	Sources of stress, classified as structural (within a subsystem) or functional (from the environment)

reversed. The diagnosis should be stated, "Inability to use diabetic food exchange system (patient's response) related to lack of knowledge of diabetic diet (contributing factor)."

5. Place environmental factors, which are part of the etiology, in the second part of the diagnostic statement. For example, instead of "Noisy environment related to frequent noisy company and TV," the nurse should write, "Sleep pattern disturbance related to constant auditory stimuli (company and TV)." In the first statement the nurse has avoided diagnosing the patient's problem and has focused on the room.

6. Avoid stating diagnoses that do not provide guidance for planning nursing care actions. For example, the diagnostic statement "Inability to speak related to laryngectomy" is not helpful, since the nurse cannot undo the laryngectomy. This problem is better stated, "Communication disability related to loss of speech," which provides direction for the nurse in planning alternative communication patterns.

7. State *potential* nursing diagnoses when patient's responses to a condition or situation can be predicted or when the patient requires preventive therapies to maintain a healthy state. Predictable responses are based on known complications of a disease process or factors in the patient's history. For example, the postoperative patient requires deep breathing and coughing exercises, ambulation, and frequent position changes to prevent respiratory complications (e.g., hypostatic pneumonia and atelectasis). A potential nursing diagnosis in this situation may be stated, "risk of (prone to) atelectasis related to anesthesia and postsurgical immobility."

8. State *possible* nursing diagnoses when evidence about a response is unclear or when the related factors are unknown. A *possible diagnosis* needs to be written so that more data will be collected to support or reject the suspected response. This is similar to the "ruling out" process used in medical diagnosis.

9. Write a nursing diagnosis as soon as a pattern evolves in the patient's responses. A one-time response does not justify a nursing diagnosis; the nurse needs to accumulate sufficient data to suggest a pattern. Some diagnoses can be made on admission; others will not emerge for several days. Many patients require several diagnoses.

10. Ensure that the responses are ones that can be changed to more healthful responses through nursing interventions.

11. Word the diagnosis as concisely as possible and in terms that are specific enough to provide direction for the remainder of the nursing process, i.e., planning, intervention,and evaluation. A diagnosis of "Impaired home maintenance management related to left-sided paralysis" meets these guidelines.

Often the more critically ill the patient is, the more similar the nursing and medical diagnoses are. For example, a patient with an acute myocardial infarction may initially have a nursing diagnosis of "Chest pain and weakness related to myocardial infarction" (very like the medical diagnosis); several weeks later, the nursing diagnosis may be "Disturbed self-concept related to restricted physical activity" (quite different from the medical diagnosis).

Advantages of Nursing Diagnoses

Many advantages can be derived from the use of a nursing diagnosis (Edel 1982:8–10):

1. It strengthens the nursing process. A diagnosis identifies health status alterations from the assessment data. It provides direction for nursing interventions, because the therapies initiated are related to the diagnosis. Evaluation is then focused on the entire nursing process, including an error in diagnosis or a missed diagnosis, rather than focused on the nursing therapy only.

2. It speeds communication among nurses. Instead of relating all pertinent assessment factors to another health care worker, nurses can transmit the same amount of information through a diagnosis. Because a diagnosis consolidates a great deal of information into concise statements and includes assessment parameters, it provides a shorthand method of communication. If a nurse knows that a patient has a certain diagnosis, she or he will know what the patient's specific signs and symptoms are and what therapies are warranted.

3. It clarifies the independent functions of the nurse and increases nursing accountability. Nursing diagnoses describe and categorize the content of independent nursing practice. Ultimately, specific diagnoses will have prescribed nursing therapies associated with them, and the nurse will be accountable for those therapies. The use of diagnoses also increases the individual accountability of nurses. The nurse is required to gather more purposeful data, analyze the data with discrimination, and make scientifically based judgments (i.e., a diagnosis and plan of therapy).

4. It provides a first step for building a body of knowledge unique to nursing.

5. It provides an organizing principle and structure for nursing education, practice, and research. Once a taxonomy of nursing diagnoses is developed, educational programs can organize their curricula in relation to the nursing diagnoses and prepare students to develop diagnostic skills. The taxonomy would also provide a focus for nursing practice and research, which in turn would provide feedback for further development of nursing's unique body of knowledge.

Process of Diagnosing

Specific intellectual activities are required by nurses to arrive at a diagnosis. Several models describing this process are available from nursing literature and other professions. Three models are described in the sections that follow and summarized in Table 6–5.

Judge and Zuidema's Diagnostic Process

Richard Judge and George Zuidema (1963) describe the diagnostic process as a sequential six-step process in which decisions are made at each step. *Observation* includes the collection of data. At this step decisions are made about what data are normal and abnormal. *Description* involves tabulation of the observations, concentration and patterning of relevant findings, and the decision about what is important and what is not. *Interpretation* involves the mental activity of comparing selected data with a known body of knowledge and deciding what degree of correlation exists between the findings in this patient and the patterns described in the classification system. *Verification* involves planning a course of action to support the findings (e.g., diagnostic tests and procedures). Decisions in this step involve selecting the appropriate tests, determining their priority, and interpreting their results. *Decision* involves applying a label to the findings, i.e., the diagnosis. *Action* involves planning an appropriate course of therapy based on the diagnosis.

Gordon's Diagnostic Process

Marjory Gordon (1982:13) states that the diagnostic process is a cycle of perceptual and cognitive abilities in which observations lead to inferences which lead to further observations. This cycle continues until the nurse feels confident about naming the problem. To Gordon, the diagnostic process in its broadest sense involves four activities that occur continuously rather than sequentially:

1. Collecting information
2. Interpreting the information
3. Clustering the information
4. Naming the cluster

Underlying these activities are the intellectual activities of decision making, inferential reasoning, conceptualization, and judgment. *Data collection* is an ongoing, never ending process. Skillful data collection is essential to diagnosis. The term *skillful* implies that data collection is influenced by the nurse's clinical knowledge. This knowledge makes the nurse sensitive to cues (signals to act; information that influences decisions). The nurse must first decide whether the cues are relevant or irrelevant. If a cue is relevant, the nurse may decide that more information needs to be collected or may decide to use the cue directly in a diagnostic judgment.

Interpreting information collected involves *inference*, the derivation of a conclusion from facts or premises, and movement beyond the information to predict or explain. In fact, inferential reasoning occurs throughout the diagnostic process.

Clustering information involves a search in the nurse's memory stores for previously learned meaningful groups of clinical cues (signs and symptoms) that are associated with a diagnostic category. Gordon believes that clustering occurs in conjunction with data collec-

Table 6–5 Summary of Selected Diagnostic Processes

Judge and Zuidema's process	Gordon's process	Bircher's process
1. Observe	1. Collecting information	1. Noticing
2. Describe	2. Interpreting the information	2. Describing
3. Interpret	3. Clustering the information	3. Labeling
4. Verify	4. Naming the cluster	4. Grouping
5. Decide		5. Identifying significant relationships
6. Act		6. Noting critical attributes
		7. Selecting an organizing principle
		8. Developing criteria
		9. Developing a taxonomy
		10. Diagnosing

tion and interpretation, as evidenced in remarks or thoughts such as, "I'm getting a picture of . . ." or "This cue doesn't fit the picture."

Naming the cluster (the diagnosis) is the final act of judgment. In this process the nurse decides that the cluster is "this" and not "that." This activity occurs as a result of a cyclic process of information collection, interpretation, and clustering.

Bircher's Diagnostic Process

Andrea Bircher (1975:22–27) delineates ten steps in the process of diagnosis for nurses. Bircher believes that the first five steps are being accomplished daily in practice by professional nurses but the remaining five are in stages of development by groups of nurses, such as those involved in conferences on classifying nursing diagnoses. See Table 6–5. Until a universal taxonomy of nursing diagnoses is developed, the individual nurse making a diagnosis is faced with selecting personal organizing principles and devising a working taxonomy.

Bircher states (ibid., p. 23) that specific competencies are required for each step of the process:

1. *Noticing* requires systematic observation and the ability to detect, select, and recognize significant phenomena.

2. *Describing* requires the ability to provide a precise, objective, sequential, descriptive narrative verbally and in writing.

3. *Labeling* requires the ability to identify common elements and patterns, form concepts, and reason inferentially.

4. *Grouping* involves coding and identification of possible relationships and patterns to arrange, order, and rate phenomena according to shared characteristics.

5. *Identifying significant relationships* requires the ability to use inferential statistics and to identify values, purposes, and significance. *Inferential statistics* are statistics that are inferred by generalization from other statistics. For example, the length of 95% of a relatively large sample of American newborns was more than 48 cm (19 in). Therefore, there is a high probability that 95% of all American newborns will be longer than 48 cm.

6. *Noting critical attributes* requires the ability to identify categories that have at least one significant attribute in common.

7. *Selecting an organizing principle* requires competence in inductive and deductive reasoning and development of a first level theory to divide the information into discrete categories. *Inductive reasoning* is making generalizations from specific data. For example, a patient with a recent colostomy demonstrates behaviors such as anger, sadness, and crying. This would lead to a general conclusion of grief at actual or perceived loss and altered body image. *Deductive reasoning* is making specific observations from a generalization. For example, a patient who has had a severe cerebrovascular accident (generalization) may be expected to have a disturbance in self-concept, impaired physical mobility, and potential for injury (specific responses).

8. *Developing criteria* involves use of deductive logic to identify specific standards and patterns that must be present to assign a unit to a given category or classification system.

9. *Developing a taxonomy* requires the development of a conceptual framework that can be used to describe the system of classification, i.e., the categories and the nature of their relationship.

10. *Diagnosing* requires the ability to make a clinical inference by identifying a new phenomenon and ascertaining its nature, characteristics, and cause.

Factors Affecting Diagnostic Ability

From the three process descriptions, it is evident that nurses require specific abilities to become competent in the diagnostic process. Prior to making a diagnosis, nurses need data collection skills and a knowledge base for sorting, interpreting, and grouping the data. Diagnosis requires specific intellectual abilities, such as inferential reasoning, decision making, conceptualizing, and making judgments. In addition, competence in diagnosing is greatly enhanced by the nurse's experiential background and powers of intuition; these assist the nurse to recognize qualities and characteristics as belonging to a certain category. Because the nursing profession at present lacks a refined taxonomy or classification system for nursing diagnoses, nurses must also rely on their own philosophies and conceptual frameworks of nursing when developing nursing diagnoses. These factors are illustrated in Figure 6–1.

Planning Nursing Intervention

The plan of nursing care is the third phase of the nursing process. It is based on the first two phases: a thorough assessment of the patient and well-developed nursing diagnoses. The planning phase involves the following activities: (a) setting priorities, (b) establishing goals (objectives), (c) establishing outcome criteria, (d) writ-

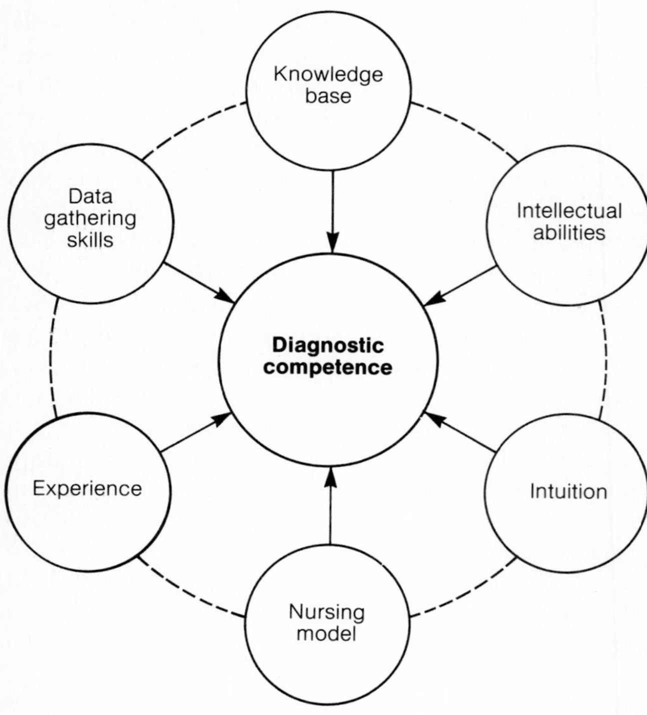

Figure 6–1 Factors that influence the nurse's ability to diagnose.

ing a plan of action (nursing orders), and (e) developing a nursing care plan.

Setting Priorities

Each of the problems that has been identified in diagnosis is assigned a rating: high, medium, or low priority. This is a nursing judgment, but it must also include the patient's views on urgency. Priorities can be analyzed according to a number of systems:

1. Triage concept
2. Maslow's hierarchy of needs
3. Patient preferences
4. Treatment plan
5. Nursing resources

Triage concept

The *triage concept* utilized in many emergency departments can be helpful in setting priorities. The term *triage*, of French origin, means picking, choosing, sorting, and selecting. In an emergency department, patients are sorted in terms of urgency rating systems or categories. Some of these systems have two categories (urgent and nonurgent), others three categories (immediate, urgent, and nonurgent), and still others five categories (life-threatening, urgent, semiurgent, nonurgent, and no need for care). For the nurse in other settings, the three-category system can be useful.

Immediate category This category has a priority 1 urgency rating and is used for patients whose problems may result in loss of a life or a body part. Examples of priority 1 problems are: cardiopulmonary arrest, severe respiratory distress, massive and uncontrolled hemorrhage, cardiac chest pain, hyperpyrexia (temperature higher than 40.5 C [105 F], and loss of consciousness. In these situations medical and nursing interventions must be provided immediately.

Urgent category This priority 2 category is used for patients whose problems require prompt care. The problems will not cause loss of a life or a body part but may produce severe impairment if left untreated for several hours. Examples of priority 2 problems are: urinary retention, lacerations without severe bleeding or neurovascular impairment, abdominal pain if vital signs are normal, noncardiac chest pain, decreased level of consciousness, fever up to 40.5 C (105 F), multiple fractures, and respiratory problems without severe respiratory impairment.

Nonurgent category This priority 3 category is assigned to patients whose problems have developed slowly and have been tolerated by the patient for a while. The problems require intervention, but time is not a critical factor. Examples of priority 3 problems include: rash, chronic headache, vaginal discharge, chronic hypertension, and constipation.

Maslow's hierarchy of needs

Abraham Maslow's hierarchy of needs as adapted by Richard Kalish (see Chapter 8) may be helpful in setting priorities. In sum, the hierarchy is:

1. Physiologic needs—food, air, water, temperature, elimination, rest, and pain avoidance
2. Need for knowledge—sex, activity, exploration, manipulation, novelty
3. Need for safety—safety, security, protection
4. Need for love and belonging—love, belonging, closeness
5. Need for esteem and self-worth
6. Need for self-actualization

From this hierarchy it can be seen that physiologic needs take precedence and that even within a category some needs are of greater importance than others. The need for air is essential for the maintenance of life; people can live longer without water than without air. Once physiologic needs are met, then other needs can assume a higher priority. The priorities of needs are continually changing, just as the patient's health status changes.

Patient preferences

The patient's preferences are also of utmost importance in determining priorities, particularly in situations that are not life threatening. What may seem relatively unimportant to the nurse may be perceived as urgent by the patient. For example, the nurse may consider that a patient's knowledge deficit takes priority over the patient's spiritual distress. To the patient, however, the priorities are reversed, and spiritual distress is more urgent. In this situation, the patient's choice takes precedence. Until spiritual distress is alleviated, the patient will probably be unwilling and unable to respond to the knowledge deficit.

Treatment plan

The patient's overall treatment plan must be considered by the nurse and the patient when setting priorities. Planned nursing interventions must be congruent with other aspects of health care. For example, a patient in shock from a severe hemorrhage must have a fluid volume deficit restored and the physical condition stabilized before social or psychologic aspects of care can be considered.

Nursing resources

Available resources also affect priorities. The nurse's caseload and the existence of emergency situations may limit the nurse to providing care that deals with only the most basic needs of each assigned patient.

Establishing Goals (Objectives)

Short- and long-term goals

A *goal* is defined by the dictionary as "the end to which a design tends or which a person aims to reach or accomplish," while an *objective* is "the aim of a maneuver or operation." The two words are often used interchangeably and will be in the context of the nursing process in this book. Simply stated, goals or objectives are hoped-for outcomes. Two types of goals are established in the nursing process: patient goals and nursing goals.

Goals for patients are stated in terms of anticipated patient outcomes, not in terms of nursing activities. Goals may be short-term or long-term. A short-term goal might be, "Patient will raise right arm to shoulder height once every 2 hours during the day." A long-term goal in the same context might be, "Patient will regain full use of right arm." Because a great deal of the nurse's time is focused on immediate needs of the patient, most goals are short-term. In addition, the nurse is better able to evaluate the patient's progress or lack of it with short-term goals.

Long-term goals are often used for patients at home with chronic health problems or in nursing homes, extended care facilities, and rehabilitation centers. Short-term goals are useful (a) for patients who require health care for only a short period of time, (b) for persons who are frustrated by long-term goals that seem difficult to attain and who need satisfaction from the success of achieving a short-term goal, and (c) by nurses who provide care for a short period of time to patients requiring care for an extended period of time (short-term goals are then set for the time the nurse is with the patient).

Relationship of goals to the nursing diagnosis

Patient goals are derived from the first clause of the nursing diagnosis, i.e., from the identified patient response (Mundinger and Jauren 1975:97), and they form the basis of evaluation criteria. For example, if "altered bowel elimination pattern" is the first clause of the nursing diagnosis, the patient goal might be stated, "Patient will achieve a normal bowel elimination pattern." More specific patient outcomes (criteria) are set from this goal, and these outcomes form the basis of evaluation. See Establishing Outcome Criteria, discussed subsequently.

The second clause of the nursing diagnosis guides the actions of the nurse (ibid.), i.e., the nursing goals. For example, if "inactivity and inadequate fiber in the diet" is the second clause related to "altered bowel elimination pattern," the nursing goals may include, "Increase patient's exercise and fiber in diet." From this nursing goal, specific nursing activities are derived, such as ambulating the patient at specified intervals, offering instruction to the patient about needed dietary adjustments, and ensuring that high fiber foods are provided in the patient's diet. For additional examples of goals, see Table 6-6 later in this chapter.

Establishing Outcome Criteria

Relationship to goals

A *criterion* is a standard or model that can be used in judging. Criteria stated in terms of outcomes, that is, alterations in the health status of patients, are standards used to determine the results of nursing interventions for the patient. They determine whether the stated goals have been achieved. These *outcome criteria* are essential to the evaluation phase of the nursing process, and their establishment is the first step in evaluation. See Chapter 7. Often, however, outcome criteria are established in the planning phase of the nursing process along with the goals. In fact, many nurses consider outcome criteria to be part of goals, and criteria are added directly to the goal statement. For example, "Patient's hydration status will be maintained (goal) as evidenced by: (a) fluid intake of at least 2500 ml daily, (b) urinary output in balance with fluid intake, (c) normal skin turgor, (d) moist oral mucous membranes (outcome criteria)." Other nurses find this method cumbersome and instead separate the statement of goals from the statement of outcome criteria.

Whichever method is used, the process of developing outcome criteria is the same; the nurse needs to ask two questions:

1. How will the patient look or behave if the desired goal is achieved?
2. What must the patient do and how well must he or she do it before successful attainment of the goal is agreed upon?

For example, a stroke patient has a nursing diagnosis of "Self-care deficit in dressing related to left-sided hemiplegia and memory impairment." Outcome criteria for this patient may include:

- Selects appropriate clothes to dress
- Puts clothes on over affected side first
- Dresses without losing balance
- Folds and places nightclothes in drawer
- Appears pleased with accomplishment

See also Table 6–6 later in this chapter.

The patient's health status and previous pattern of functioning need to be considered when establishing outcome criteria. For example, if a patient has poor vision from cataracts, it is unrealistic to specify as an outcome criterion "Measures insulin correctly." Likewise, if the previous eating pattern of an anemic patient included only vegetarian foods, it is unrealistic to specify "Eats liver 2 times per week."

Characteristics of outcome criteria

Characteristics of well-stated criteria are (Zimmer 1974:318):

1. Each outcome criterion relates to the established goal.
2. The outcome stated in the criterion is possible to achieve.
3. Each criterion is a statement of *one* specific outcome.
4. Each criterion is as specific and concrete as possible, to facilitate measurement.
5. Criteria are appraisable or measurable, i.e., the outcome can be seen, heard, felt, or measured by another person.
6. Criteria are phrased in positive rather than negative terms.

Writing a Plan of Action (Nursing Orders)

Once goals and priorities have been determined, the next step is to determine a plan for nursing action. Goal setting indicates *what* will be done; nursing intervention provides the methodology for achieving the goal, i.e., *how, where, when,* and by *whom* it will be done.

At this time the nurse may require additional information, perhaps from the patient or from resources such as current literature. The latter can add to the rationale for the nursing action. A rationale is an explanation that includes facts, principles, and knowledge.

The plan of action initially involves a decision about each problem; there are usually three alternatives open to the patient and the nurse:

1. No action is necessary or possible at this time.
2. The health problem needs to be referred to another member of the health team, a member of the family, or other personnel, such as a family priest. It is important for nurses to recognize that they cannot help the patient with all problems.
3. Nursing intervention *is* indicated to help the patient resolve the problem.

Previously the problems were placed in a hierarchic order. It is important that each problem be considered now in this sequence. For most problems a number of alternative nursing interventions are possible, and the ones that are selected need to be realistic. This judgment is generally based upon experience, knowledge, and data from other resources.

For example, if the nursing diagnosis is "Impairment of skin integrity (ulcer on medial aspect of right ankle) related to stasis of venous circulation," and the nurse's goal is "To increase venous circulation," the planned nursing interventions (also referred to as *nursing orders, nursing approaches,* or *nursing actions*) may include the following:

1. Apply elastic stockings to lower legs when patient is out of bed.
2. Elevate legs on footstool with two pillows when patient sits in chair.
3. RN to instruct re cause of impaired venous circulation.
4. Measure and record fluid intake and output.
5. Measure and record ankle circumference every 2 days.

Because of the loss of skin integrity, the patient risks acquiring an infection. Thus, another diagnosis would be "Potential infection related to loss of skin integrity" and a second nursing goal would be "To prevent infection and promote healing of the stasis ulcer." Planned nursing interventions related to this goal may include:

1. Use footboard and bed cradle in bed continously.
2. RN to apply sterile petrolatum dressing to ulcer b.i.d. (0900, 1800).
3. RN to consult physician re method of cleaning ulcer.

In choosing the most desirable nursing interventions, the nurse and the patient consider a number of criteria:

1. Will the intervention be effective?
2. Is it realistic for the patient and the nurse?
3. Is it acceptable to the patient and perhaps the family?

Nursing interventions that meet the criteria are then written in the nursing care plan or on specific nursing order sheets.

Components of nursing orders

The degree of detail included in the nursing orders depends to some degree on the health personnel who will carry out the order. It is advisable, however, to be exact in writing orders. For example, "Assess edema of left ankle daily" is not as precise as "Measure and record ankle circumference daily at 0900 hr."

Nursing orders should include five components (Little and Carnevali 1976:213):

1. Date
2. Precise action verb and possibly modifier
3. Content area
4. Time element
5. Signature

Date Nursing orders are dated when they are written and reviewed regularly at intervals that depend on the individual's needs. If a patient is acutely ill, in an intensive care unit, for example, the plan of care will be continually monitored and revised. In a community clinic, weekly or biweekly reviews may be indicated.

Action verb The verb starts the order and needs to be precise. For example, "Explain (to the patient) the actions of insulin" is a more precise statement than "Teach (the patient) about insulin." Sometimes a modifier for the verb can make the nursing order more precise. For example, "Apply spiral bandage to left lower leg *firmly*" is more precise than "Apply spiral bandage to left leg."

Content area The content is the where and the what of the order. In the above order, "spiral bandage" and "left leg" state the what and the where of the order. The nurse can also clarify in this example whether the foot or toes are to be left exposed.

Time element The time element answers when, how long, or how often the nursing action is to occur. Examples are: "Assist patient with tub bath at 0700 daily"; "Immerse patient's left arm in sterile saline soak for 1 hr"; or "Assist patient to change position every 2 hr between 0700 and 2100 hr."

Signature The signature of the nurse prescribing the order shows the nurse's accountability and has legal significance.

Categories of nursing orders

Nursing orders (plans) may be categorized (Becknell and Smith 1975:89) as:

1. Orders for nursing therapy of a problem
2. Orders for collection of additional data to define a problem better or facilitate its management
3. Orders for dissemination of information about the management of a problem

Orders for nursing therapy include those activities that maintain or restore the patient's usual patterns, alleviate symptoms, and prevent additional problems. These comprise the majority of orders. See Table 6–6 on page 148.

The collection of additional data is often necessary to define a nursing diagnosis better or to learn how to manage a problem. For example, if the nurse notices that a patient appears withdrawn, worried, and tense, the nurse needs additional data from the patient to clarify the contributing causes of this behavior. The nurse may write a tentative nursing diagnosis of "anxiety" and then write nursing orders that guide interventions toward confirming the cause. For example, a nursing order may state, "Talk with patient to determine cause of anxiety."

If the nurse needs information about how to manage a problem, data may be collected from many sources. One example is the order "RN to consult physician about method of cleaning ulcer." In other situations the nurse may consult with a pharmacist about the side effects of a medication; a dietician about the foods allowed on a certain diet; a physical therapist about appropriate exercises; etc.

Nursing orders may specify the need to distribute information about continuing management of a problem to the patient's support persons or other health team members. For example, a family member may

Table 6–6 Sample Nursing Care Plan for a Patient with a Varicose Ulcer and Anemia

Assessment data	Nursing diagnosis	Patient goal	Nursing goal	Plan/ intervention	Outcome criteria
Ulcer (2.5 cm) on medial aspect of right ankle Edema of right ankle (circumference of right ankle 10¾″, left ankle 9½″) Right leg frequently feels heavy and "aches" after sitting or standing for long periods Veins on right leg visible and dilated Skin discolored	Impairment of skin integrity related to impaired venous circulation	Skin and ankle will return to normal appearance	Improve venous circulation	• Apply elastic stocking to lower leg when out of bed • Elevate legs on footstool with 2 pillows when sitting in chair • Elevate foot of bed 6″ • Check skin color, temperature, and sensation of legs and feet b.i.d. (0900 and 1800) • Measure and record ankle circumference daily (1800 hr)	• Ulcerated area covered with granulation tissue • Circumference of right ankle reduced to 9½″ • Relief from leg discomfort
	Potential infection related to loss of skin	Ulcer will remain free of pathogens	Prevent infection and promote healing of stasis ulcer	• Use footboard and bed cradle continuously • RN to apply sterile petrolatum dressing to ulcer b.i.d. (0900, 1800) • RN to consult physician re method of cleaning ulcer • Observe ulcer at dressing changes for signs and symptoms of infection	Cultures of swabs from ulcerated area are free of pathogens

need to learn how to assist the patient in managing a long-term illness, or a visiting nurse association may need information about follow-up nursing care requirements for a patient who is being discharged.

Developing a Nursing Care Plan

The nursing care plan organizes information about the patient into a meaningful whole. Its purposes are:

1. To provide a guide to individualized care
2. To provide a means of communication to all health care workers involved in the patient's care
3. To provide a guide to what needs to be done, when, and how

Components of the nursing care plan include:

1. A concise profile of the patient, with the patient's name, medical diagnosis, religion, marital status, occupation, allergies, next of kin, etc.
2. The nursing diagnoses or problem list

Table 6–6 continued

Assessment data	Nursing diagnosis	Patient goal	Nursing goal	Plan/ intervention	Outcome criteria
Thinks she might have injured ankle while gardening Does not wear support stockings Does not relate ulcer to impaired circulation	Knowledge deficit about causes of ulcer related to lack of information	Patient will understand causes of ulcer and methods to facilitate venous circulation	Provide information re causes of ulcer and methods to facilitate venous circulation	• Instruct about causes of ulcer and impaired circulation • Instruct about methods to facilitate and maintain venous circulation, e.g.: • Elevate legs frequently • Avoid standing, sitting, crossing legs; pressure on popliteal space; garters around leg; etc. • Wear elastic stocking • Instruct about importance of skin care and preventing injury	• Describes cause of leg ulcer and edema • States measures needed to maintain venous circulation • Applies and wears support stocking • Sits with legs elevated
Low hemoglobin level Does not like cooking for self States eats "snacks" Cannot afford meat Feeling more tired than usual Irritable with grandchildren	Nutritional deficit (iron deficiency anemia) related to social isolation and financial limitations	Patient will achieve satisfactory nutritional pattern	Promote balanced diet within economical means, and if possible encourage increased socialization at meal times	• Provide information about economical, easily prepared foods rich in iron • Talk to patient about support persons with whom she could share meals	Normal hemoglobin level Increased energy shown by interest in gardening Evidence patient is eating iron-rich foods

3. The patient goals
4. Specific nursing orders and interventions
5. Outcome criteria, if not part of the goals

Often the nursing plan is part of the patient's care plan (Kardex), which also includes information about medications the patient is receiving, parenteral therapy and other treatments, current operations, and planned laboratory and diagnostic studies. See Figure 18–5 on page 433. With knowledge of the time and frequency of tests, treatments, and other activities, the nurse can organize her or his clinical assignment. This is essential when the nurse has several patients to care for.

The patient's care plan is started as soon as the patient is admitted to the health care agency by the responsible nurse (head nurse, primary nurse, or team leader). It is constantly updated and revised throughout the patient's stay, in response to changes in the patient's condition and evaluations of goal achievement.

Standardized care plans have been devised in many agencies as guides for providing essential nursing care to specified groups of patients. Because such plans are developed and accepted by the nursing staff of the agency, they serve as a basis for ensuring that minimal acceptable standards of care are provided. These plans, however, do not ensure individualized care; therefore, they should be used in conjunction with a plan developed for each patient. A sample nursing care plan for a patient with anemia and a leg ulcer associated with varicose veins is presented in Table 6–6.

Summary

The second and third phases of the nursing process are *nursing diagnosis* and *planning* respectively. Neither can be carried out effectively without the development of a comprehensive data base, i.e., effective completion of the first phase (assessment).

A nursing diagnosis differs from a medical diagnosis in several ways: (a) it describes an individual's *response* to a disease process or situation, (b) it is oriented to the individual, and (c) it changes as the patient's responses change. Three essential components of nursing diagnoses described by the PES format are:

1. State of the patient or health problem (P)
2. Etiology of the problem (E)
3. Defining characteristics or cluster of signs and symptoms (S)

To develop a nursing diagnostic statement, the nurse (after reviewing the data base) joins two related clauses together. The first clause describes the patient's response and the second clause describes the contributing factors or probable causes of the response. Guidelines for stating nursing diagnoses suggest that the nurse write in terms of a response rather than a need, make sure that the two clauses do not say the same thing, avoid diagnoses that do not provide guidance for nursing actions, differentiate potential and possible diagnoses, etc. Advantages from the use of nursing diagnoses are: the nursing process is strengthened, communication among nurses about a patient's health status is facilitated, and the independent function and accountability of the nurse are clarified.

The process of diagnosing is described in various ways by different authors. In brief, the process involves collecting information, interpreting information, clustering information, and labeling the cluster. Underlying these tasks are specific intellectual activities such as inferential reasoning (deductive and inductive) and making judgments.

The planning phase of the nursing process involves (a) setting priorities, (b) establishing goals, (c) establishing outcome criteria, if not part of the goals, (d) writing nursing orders, and (e) developing a nursing care plan.

Several systems can be analyzed when setting priorities: the triage concept (sorting problems into immediate, urgent, and nonurgent categories), Maslow's hierarchy of needs, the patient's preferences, the patient's overall treatment plan, and the availability of nursing resources.

In establishing goals, the nurse needs to relate the goals to the nursing diagnosis. Outcome criteria, essential to the evaluation phase of the nursing process, need to be established either with the goal statement or separately. These criteria must relate to the established goal, be measurable, be achievable, and be stated in positive terms.

Once priorities, goals, and outcome criteria are established, the nurse writes a plan of action (a set of nursing orders) that specifies how, when, where, and by whom the nursing interventions directed toward goal achievement will be enacted. Nursing orders have five components: date, action verb, content area, time element, and signature. They may be categorized as directing activities (a) for nursing therapy of a problem, (b) for collection of additional data, or (c) for dissemination of information. Information about the patient from all phases of the nursing process (see subsequent chapters) is organized into a meaningful whole on the patient's nursing care plan. This plan guides the nurse in providing individualized care to the patient and serves as a means of communication among all health care workers involved in the patient's care.

Suggested Activities

1. In a clinical setting, select a patient's nursing history and care plan. Then select one nursing diagnosis and list the data from the nursing history that coincide with that diagnosis.
2. Analyze the stated goal for the diagnosis in activity 1 and determine:
   - **a.** Whether it is a long-term or short-term goal
   - **b.** Whether it is a patient or nursing goal
   - **c.** Whether its subject, behavior, and conditions are realistic, clear, and concise
3. Determine whether the outcome criteria for the goal in activity 2:
   - **a.** Relate to the established goal
   - **b.** Are measurable
   - **c.** Provide guidance for the nurse
4. Select another patient's record and analyze the assessment contained in it to develop nursing diagnoses and a realistic nursing care plan. Discuss the plan with your instructor.

Suggested Readings

Dossey, B., and Guzzetta, C. E. June 1981. Nursing diagnosis. *Nursing 81* 11:34–38.

The authors describe their experiences with nursing diagnosis and how it fits into the nursing process. Included is a suggested three-step process for arriving at a nursing diagnosis, a description of how to write one, and a set of checks on whether it has been written correctly.

Gordon, M. August 1976. Nursing diagnosis and the diagnostic process. *American Journal of Nursing* 76:1298–300.

This article describes nursing diagnosis, a diagnostic category, and its components. The nomenclature of diagnostic categories is discussed, and the diagnostic process is described.

Selected References

Aspinall, M. J. July 1976. Nursing diagnosis—the weak link. *Nursing Outlook* 24:433–36.

Becknell, E. P., and Smith, D. M. 1975. *System of nursing practice.* Philadelphia: F. A. Davis Co.

Bircher, A. V. 1975. On the development and classification of diagnoses. *Nursing Forum* 14(1):10–29.

Bower, F. L. 1981. *The process of planning nursing care: A theoretical model.* 3rd ed. St. Louis: C. V. Mosby Co.

Carlson, J. H.; Craft, C. A.; and McGuire, A. D. 1982. *Nursing diagnosis.* Philadelphia: W. B. Saunders Co.

Edel, M. 1982. The nature of nursing diagnosis. In Carlson, J. H.; Craft, C. A.; and McGuire A. D., *Nursing diagnosis.* Philadelphia: W. B. Saunders Co.

Gebbie, K., and Lavin, M. A. February 1974. Classifying nursing diagnoses. *American Journal of Nursing* 74:250–53. Reprinted in American Journal of Nursing. 1976. *The nursing process in practice*, pp. 188–96. Contemporary Nursing Series. New York: American Journal of Nursing Co.

———, editors. 1975. *Classification of nursing diagnoses.* Proceedings of the First National Conference. St. Louis: C. V. Mosby Co.

Gordon, M. August 1976. Nursing diagnosis and the diagnostic process. *American Journal of Nursing* 76:1298–300.

———. 1982. *Nursing diagnosis: Process and application.* New York: McGraw-Hill Book Co.

Hilger, E. E. June 1974. Developing nursing outcome criteria. *Nursing Clinics of North America* 9:323–30.

House, M. J. July 1975. Devising a care plan you can really use. *Nursing 75* 5:12–14.

Judge, R., and Zuidema, G., editors. 1963. *Physical diagnosis: A physiologic approach to the clinical examination.* 2nd ed. Boston: Little, Brown and Co.

Kim, M. J., and Moritz, D. A., editors. 1982. *Classification of nursing diagnoses.* Proceedings of the Third and Fourth National Conferences. New York: McGraw-Hill Book Co.

La Monica, E. L. 1979. *The nursing process: A humanistic approach.* Menlo Park, Calif.: Addison-Wesley Publishing Co.

Lash, A. A. 1978. A re-examination of nursing diagnosis. *Nursing Forum* 17(4):332–43.

Little, D. E., and Carnevali, D. L. 1976. *Nursing care planning.* 2nd ed. Philadelphia: J. B. Lippincott Co.

Mundinger, M. O., and Jauron, G. D. February 1975. Developing a nursing diagnosis. *Nursing Outlook* 23:94–98.

Riel, J. P., and Roy, C. 1980. *Conceptual models for nursing practice.* 2nd ed. New York: Appleton-Century-Crofts.

Rund, D. A., and Rausch, T. S. 1981. *Triage.* St. Louis: C. V. Mosby Co.

Yura, H., and Walsh, M. B. 1978. *The nursing process: Assessing, planning, implementing and evaluating.* New York: Appleton-Century-Crofts.

Zimmer, M. J. June 1974. Guidelines for development of outcome criteria. *Nursing Clinics of North America* 9:317–21.

Zimmerman, D.S., and Gohrke, C. February 1970. The goal-directed nursing approach: It does work. *American Journal of Nursing* 70:306–10.

Chapter 7

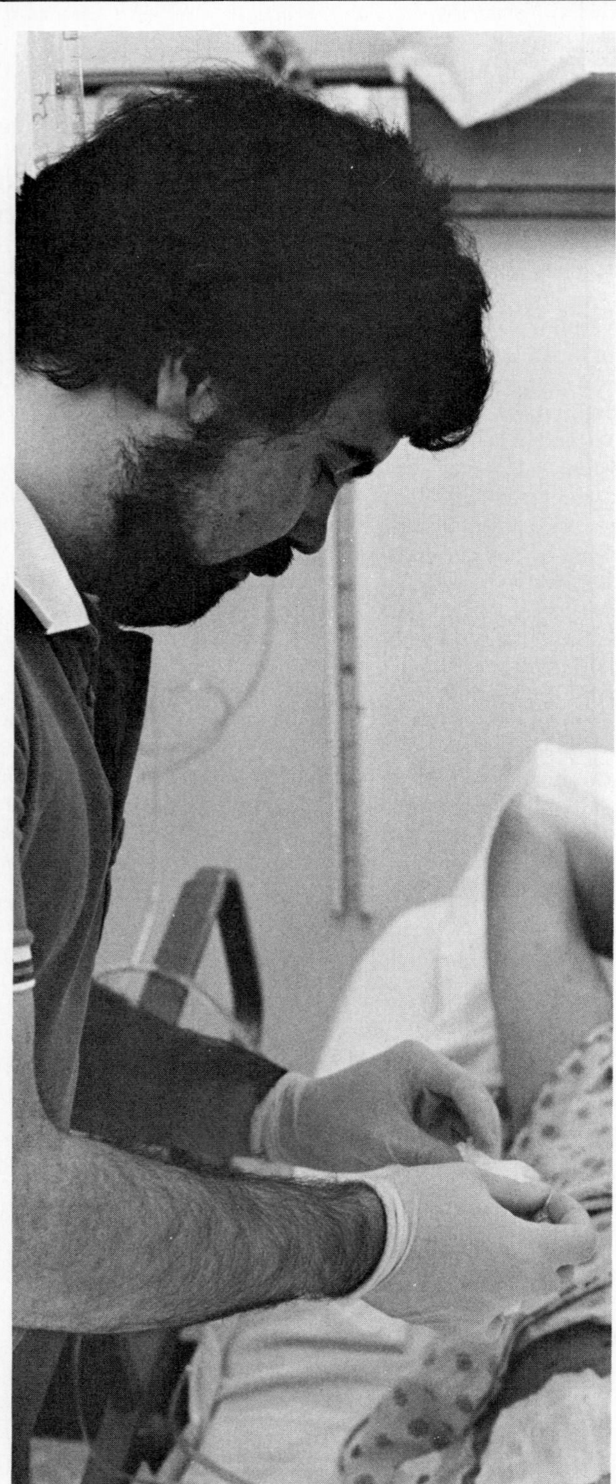

Intervention and Evaluation

CONTENTS

Objectives

1. Know essential facts about the intervention phase of the nursing process

1.1 Define nursing intervention

1.2 Identify six categories descriptive of the scope of nursing intervention

1.3 Identify nursing activities basic to nursing intervention

1.4 Identify essential steps of the intervention process

2. Know essential facts about the evaluation phase of the nursing process

2.1 Define evaluation

2.2 Identify three aspects of nursing evaluation

2.3 Identify three components of the evaluation process

2.4 Identify factors involved in modifying a nursing care plan

3. Know essential facts about nursing standards and nursing audits

3.1 Define nursing standards

3.2 Describe quality assurance

3.3 Identify the three steps in a nursing audit

Terms

concurrent audit	evaluation	nursing standards	peer review
delegate	intervention	outcome criteria	retrospective audit

Nursing intervention and evaluation are the fourth and fifth steps of the nursing process. To *intervene* means to come between. Nursing intervention, also called *nursing care,* comes between the patient and the problem. The intent of nursing intervention is to provide care that assists the patient to solve the diagnosed health problem.

Evaluation is a process of identifying the patient's progress toward achievement of established goals, using well-defined outcome criteria. It is a continuous process, giving feedback that can result in termination of the intervention, change in the intervention, or continuation of the intervention.

For evaluation on a broader scale, nursing evaluation programs have been developed in conjunction with the Professional Standards Review Organization (PSRO). These programs are intended to improve the quality of care given to patients.

Nursing Intervention

Nursing intervention consists of those activities performed by the nurse and the patient to change the effect of a problem. It is the actual action taken to affect the outcome of the problem on the patient's health. The action may be taken by the nurse; by the nurse and the patient; by other nursing personnel; or by the patient and/or support persons. If the nurse does not take the action personally, discussion and some learning usually take place before the action is taken. Nursing intervention may also be an activity by several people—the nurse and support persons, two nurses, etc. Intervention may be done directly with the patient or on the patient's behalf (for example, a nurse's referral of a patient to the community health nurse for home care).

To *delegate* is to authorize another as one's representative or to entrust authority to another. Delegating nursing activities is not a simple function; it requires the following knowledge:

1. Needs of the patient and family
2. Goals of the patient and the nurse
3. Nursing activity that can help the patient meet goals
4. Skills of various nursing personnel

During intervention, continual assessment must take place because of the changing responses of the patient. At any time, intervention may need to change in relation to the patient's response. For example, a nurse begins to teach a diabetic patient how to give his own insulin. Shortly after beginning the teaching, the nurse realizes that the patient is not concentrating on the lesson. Subsequent discussion reveals that the patient is worried about his eyesight and whether he is becoming blind. The nurse terminates the lesson, because the patient's level of stress is interfering with his learning, and makes arrangement for a physician to examine the patient's eyes. The nurse also provides supportive communication to alleviate the patient's stress, and the nursing care plan is revised appropriately.

The length of time of nursing intervention varies from a few minutes to years. For a traumatized patient entering a hospital emergency department, nursing intervention may last only a few minutes before surgery commences. For a patient in a long-term care unit, intervention can extend over years.

Scope of Intervention

Nursing activities have been classified into six categories that describe the scope of nursing practice (Brodt 1978:25):

1. Prevention of complications
2. Preservation of body defenses
3. Detection of changes in the body's regulatory systems
4. Reestablishment of the patient with the outside world
5. Implementation of the physician's prescribed diagnostic and therapeutic activity
6. Provision of comfort and safety

Nursing intervention activities comprise either dependent or independent functions. Dependent functions are a consequence of the physician's orders; independent functions result from the nurse's independent judgment. Intervention involves the creative adaptation of knowledge to the specific situation. The nurse must ensure that activities are performed safely, create minimum discomfort to the patient, and are adapted to the patient's deficits or limitations. Teaching, communicating, group process, psychomotor skills, coordination, and leadership skills are all basic to nursing intervention.

Murray and Zentner (1979:122) describe intervention as

> all those ministrations that help meet needs the individual cannot meet for himself. Intervention includes all comfort and hygiene measures; safe and efficient use of medical techniques and skills; planning and creating an environment conducive to wholeness, including protection from risk and injury; and health teaching, formal and informal. It also includes the offering of self for strength and courage in coping with problems through counseling, listening, and socializing; and utilizing information for referrals wherever indicated, either for in-agency care or as discharge planning.

Process of Intervention

The process of nursing intervention is a problem-solving process incorporating the scientific method. See Chapter 5, page 119. Because intervention is not an isolated process but overlaps with the other steps of the nursing process, data collection, diagnosis planning, and evaluating must occur along with it. In fact, in many situations intervention precedes completion of the other steps. Therefore, during intervention the following activities are normally required:

1. Review and update the data as necessary.
2. Revise the nursing care plan.
3. Establish a helping relationship with patient.
4. Determine the need for nursing assistance.
5. Implement the nursing orders.
6. Assess the patient's response.
7. Communicate the action taken and the patient's response.

Review and updating of the data

The data collected about the patient are reviewed, and any changes in the patient's health are added. Sources of updating are: (a) the patient's chart, (b) the nursing Kardex or nursing care plan, (c) the report from the previous nursing shift, (d) the physician's order book, which may have orders not yet transcribed into the patient's record, and (e) nursing unit books (the vital signs record, the discharge book, the surgery slate, etc.). These records will differ from agency to agency.

If the nurse is already familiar with data about the patient, it may be necessary only to update those data, by reviewing the records for the time since the nurse's last contact with the patient.

Revision of the nursing care plan

The nursing care plan is based on the assessment data and the established nursing diagnoses. When a patient's health status changes, i.e., physical or psychosocial responses change, the nursing care plan must be adjusted. Some of the changes that may be required are:

1. Inclusion of new nursing intervention activities based on the reviewed nursing diagnoses.
2. Time scheduling changes, for example, to arrange for longer rest periods.
3. Rearrangement of nursing activities to group similar activities, to permit longer rest and/or activity periods for the patient, for example, the nurse might assist a male patient to walk after a rest period and before a meal, so that the patient ambulates when he is rested and can sit up for his meal, if his health permits.

Establishing a helping relationship with the patient

Before commencing any nursing activity with a patient, it is important to prepare the patient. This preparation often includes planning with the patient, explaining the activity to the patient, describing the patient's responsibilities, and ensuring that the timing is appropriate for the patient.

If the nurse has not had direct contact with the patient recently, it is important to introduce herself or himself and explain her or his function. See Chapter 5, page 128, for an interview. Establishment of a helping relationship involves a series of skills discussed in Chapter 15.

Determining the nurse's need for assistance

The nurse's need for assistance may be indicated from the records used to review and update the data. Other sources for this information are the patient, the charge nurse, other nursing personnel, and the nurse's own judgment. One nurse may not be strong or skillful enough to turn an obese patient alone. Assistance is needed so that less time is required for the patient's care. Assistance may also be necessary to ensure the patient's safety, for example, while administering an intramuscular injection to a 3-year-old. If in doubt, nurses should seek aid to safeguard the patient's safety.

Once a nurse establishes that assistance is required, it is important to identify (a) the exact type of help, e.g., lifting or holding, (b) the length of time it is required, (c) when it is required, and (d) what assistance is available. The assistance must be arranged, usually by asking the appropriate person on the unit, before commencing the nursing activity.

Implementing the nursing action

Implementing the nursing orders requires skill and knowledge in the practice of nursing. The framework for implementation is the nursing care plan. During implementation, the following must be considered:

1. The patient's individuality. Individualized actions are needed, while care is taken not to violate the scientific basis of the activity. For example, a patient may prefer to have an oral medication after meals rather than before. However, this might not be justified if the medication will not act in the stomach in the presence of food.

2. The patient's need for involvement. Some patients want to be totally involved in their care, while others prefer little involvement. The amount of desired involvement is often related to the patient's energy, severity of illness, number of stressors, fear, understanding of the illness, and understanding of the intervention. A female patient with a colostomy who is very worried about her appearance may not want to be involved in care of the colostomy at that particular time.

3. Prevention of complications. When changing a sterile dressing, for example, the nurse must observe sterile technique to prevent the complication of infection.

4. Preservation of the body's defenses. For example, when turning a patient, the nurse protects the patient's skin from abrasions which could permit microorganisms to enter the body and establish an infection.

5. Provision of comfort and support to the patient.

6. Accurate performance of dependent nursing activities. The nurse takes care to administer the correct dosage of a medication by the ordered route, for example.

Assessing the patient's response

Assessing the patient's response to nursing intervention requires specific knowledge and systematic data collection. Assessment is continuous with intervention. The nurse must have sufficient clinical knowledge to differentiate between normal and abnormal, expected and unexpected, and safe and unsafe responses. This facet of intervention overlaps with evaluation, discussed later in this chapter. As a result of the assessment, the nurse can judge whether to continue the nursing action, discontinue it, or modify it.

Communicating the action taken and the patient's response

The nursing action and the patient's response are communicated both orally and in writing. Nurses usually have a specific person to whom they report—the team leader, charge nurse on the next shift, etc. For information on reporting, see Chapter 18.

Evaluation

To *evaluate* is to judge or to appraise. In the context of the nursing process, evaluation is the fifth and last step. It has been described (Bloch 1975:256–57) as covering three aspects: (a) the system, (b) the process of giving care, and (c) the outcome of that care in terms of changes in the patient. Evaluating the system reviews such factors as the physical facilities, staffing, styles of leadership, and characteristics of the caregivers. The process of giving care is evaluated in terms of what the caregiver does or by using previously developed standards. Evaluation of patient outcomes is the main focus of this chapter.

Process of Evaluation

Evaluation of patient outcomes is the process of determining to what extent the established goals have been attained. It is an exceedingly important step in the nursing process in that, as a result of the evaluation, conclusions are drawn and the nursing plan may be changed. The evaluation process has three components:

1. Identifying the *outcome criteria* (standards for measuring success) that will be used to measure achievement of the goals.
2. Gathering data related to the identified criteria.
3. Evaluating goal achievement by comparing the data collected with the identified criteria and deciding whether the goals have been attained.

Identifying outcome criteria

The identification of outcome criteria that can be used to evaluate the patient's response to nursing care was discussed in Chapter 6 on page 145. Criteria serve two purposes: they establish the kind of evaluative data that needs to be collected and they provide a standard against which the data are judged. For example, if a goal is stated, "Patient's urinary elimination pattern will be maintained," it does not indicate to the nurse what data to collect while caring for the patient. However, when criteria are added, such as, "daily fluid intake will be not less than 2500 ml, urinary output will be in balance with fluid intake, and residual urine will be less than 100 ml," any nurse caring for the patient knows what data to collect. Criteria that are clearly stated and measurable guide the next step of the evaluation process, data collection.

Collecting data

Data are collected so that conclusions can be drawn about whether goals have been reached. The nurse collects data in relation to the specified criteria, either by observing or questioning the patient or by noting observations recorded by other health care workers on the patient's record.

Collection of both objective and subjective data may be necessary. Objective data that are measured quantitatively are preferred for evaluation purposes; for example, "Respirations increased from 12 to 16 and pulse rate increased from 70 to 90 after walking around the corridor." However, the nurse often needs to collect objective data requiring interpretation and subjective data during the evaluation process. Examples of objective data requiring observation and interpretation are the degreee of tissue turgor for a dehydrated patient or the degree of restlessness of a patient with pain. Examples of subjective data include feelings of nausea or pain.

When objective data requiring interpretation are needed, the nurse may obtain the views of one or more peers to substantiate changes. When subjective data are required, the nurse must rely upon either (a) the patient's statements (e.g., "My pain is worse now than it was after breakfast") or (b) more objective indicators of the subjective data, even though these indicators may require interpretation (e.g., decreased restlessness, decreased pulse and respiratory rates, and relaxed facial muscles as indicators of pain relief). Data collected must be recorded concisely and accurately to aid the third phase of the evaluation process. Use of flow sheets and the SOAP format of problem-oriented medical records (discussed in Chapter 18) are effective.

Evaluating goal achievement

If the first two phases of the evaluation process have been carried out effectively, the phase of determining whether a goal has been achieved is relatively simple. Both the nurse and the patient play active roles in this stage. The data collected are compared with the established criteria. Did the patient drink 3000 ml of fluid in 24 hours? Did the patient walk unassisted the specified distance per day?

There are a number of possible outcomes of evaluation:

1. The patient has responded as expected.
2. Short-term goals were achieved, but intermediate and long-term goals have not yet been met.
3. No goals were achieved.
4. New problems have arisen.

The evaluation is carried out purposefully and in an organized way. It is an intellectual activity in which the patient's outcomes are assessed in terms of the identified goals.

During the evaluation the nurse can reflect on a number of questions: What factors affected attainment of the goals? Was the problem correctly identified? Why was the problem not resolved? Was the nursing intervention directed toward the stated goals? What other nursing interventions are more likely to assist the patient to attain the stated goals?

Modifying the Nursing Care Plan

If the evaluation process indicates that the outcome criteria have been met, the nursing actions may or may not be discontinued. For example, if the criterion is,

"Patient will ingest 3000 ml of fluid daily," and the goal is "Patient's state of hydration will be maintained," nursing actions need to continue even though the outcome criterion has been met. If the goal is, "Patient will safely administer his insulin daily," the nursing actions can be canceled once the specified criteria are met.

If the outcome criteria have not been met after a reasonable length of time, the nurse needs to investigate. Initially the nurse should check whether the correct nursing actions have in fact been carried out. They may not have, either because the orders were unclear to other nursing personnel or because the orders were unreasonable in terms of external constraints such as money, staff, and equipment. Next the nurse reviews whether the data base was complete and whether the nursing diagnoses were relevant to that data base. In some instances, new data may invalidate the data base, necessitating new nursing diagnoses, new goals, and new nursing actions. Another area of review is the nursing goals. It is important to check that the goals were appropriate and attainable within the circumstances. The goals need to be revised if they were inappropriate or unreachable. The nurse may also need to investigate whether the nursing actions related to the goals and whether the best nursing actions were selected for implementation.

Once any change has been made, the nursing care plan is revised, implemented, and reevaluated. Investigation of the process can start at any step, but it is important to remember that, once the problem has been identified and the change made, it must be reflected in subsequent steps of the process.

Nursing Standards

Scope and Purposes

Nursing standards, also referred to as *patient care standards*, are criteria against which care can be evaluated. Unlike an outcome criterion, a standard usually reflects a broad area of nursing practice rather than a specific patient response. Nursing standards were discussed briefly in Chapter 1. See Tables 1–3 and 1–4 for standards developed by the American Nurses' Association and the Canadian Nurses' Association respectively. These standards help nurses provide organized care that meets the patient's right to a certain quality and continuity of care. See Chapter 3, page 76. They also assist nurses to evaluate care in any health care setting.

Historical Perspective

Evaluation is not a new concept. Florence Nightingale in 1859 published an evaluation of medical and nursing care in *Notes on Hospitals*. Since that time evaluation has progressed through a number of stages. Initially it was focused on the environment, e.g., whether equipment was available at the time it was needed. Later, organizational standards in agencies were developed. For example, the ratio of nurses to patients was studied and evaluated in terms of patients' needs. From about 1952 on, the Joint Commission on Accreditation of Hospitals (JCAH) has surveyed hospitals. Its program encouraged nurses to evaluate how nursing care affected patients. Objective criteria were applied to evaluate a patient's record after discharge from the hospital. This was called a *retrospective audit*—*retrospective* meaning relating to a past event and *audit* meaning an examination or review of records.

In 1972, the United States government enacted the Bennett Amendment, which created the Professional Standards Review Organization (PSRO). This program was intended to evaluate the quality of health care partially through peer review. Nursing subsequently developed evaluation programs compatible with the PSRO. These evaluative processes may be *concurrent audits*, in that they review present practices.

Peer review is an underlying premise of the PSRO. A *peer review* is the evaluation by one's peers of the appropriateness and quality of care, in this instance a review by other nurses.

Quality Assurance Programs

Quality assurance programs in nursing are designed to improve the quality of care. Two techniques commonly employed in these programs are observation and audit. Observation was discussed in Chapter 5 on page 127. Tools are developed to provide a framework for observing the nurse over a period of time. The nursing audit is a peer review evaluation system encompassing three steps (Berg 1974:331):

1. Defining what should be (developing criteria)
2. Comparing what should be with what is
3. Identifying the gaps and taking action

A committee of nurses develops the criteria that represent what outcomes of nursing care should be present. These become the framework against which actual outcomes are measured. The criteria should be precise and stated in measurable rather than descriptive terms. They are factual statements of optimum achievement. When the patient's record is the basis of the nursing audit, the recording must include documentation about each nursing intervention and the patient's response. These records are reviewed, and complete objective data are collected.

In the second step, the data are compared to the criteria. Conformity of the two or discrepancies (gaps) may be revealed. In the third step, the causes of any gaps are analyzed and the source determined. Action is then taken to effect the changes required to eliminate the gaps. For example, analysis may reveal that there are not enough nurses to meet the established criteria or that there is insufficient equipment. Actions are then taken to improve the quality of the nursing care.

Summary

The intervention phase of the nursing process involves the activities carried out by the nurse, the patient, and support persons to assist the patient with identified problems. The scope of nursing activities can be classified into six categories: (a) prevention of complications, (b) preservation of body defenses, (c) detection of changes in the body's regulatory systems, (d) reestablishment of the patient with the outside world, (e) implementation of the physician's prescribed diagnostic and therapeutic activity, and (f) provision of comfort and safety. Nursing activities in each of these categories include teaching, communicating, group process, psychomotor skills, coordination, and leadership skills. Such activities may comprise either dependent or independent nursing functions.

The process of intervention is akin to other phases of the nursing process. Because the patient's responses change, the nurse continuously collects data, diagnoses, plans, and evaluates during this phase. Specific activities of the nurse include: (a) reviewing and updating data, (b) revising the nursing care plan as necessary, (c) establishing a helping relationship with the patient, (d) determining the need for assistance to implement nursing actions, (e) implementing the nursing orders, (f) assessing the patient's response, and (g) communicating the action taken and the patient's response.

In the evaluation phase of the nursing process, the extent to which goals have been achieved is determined. Evaluation is a three-stage process in which (a) outcome criteria are established, (b) data related to the identified criteria are gathered, and (c) conclusions are made as to whether the goals have been attained. Effective evaluation relies heavily on well-identified outcome criteria and on continuous data collection. Modification of the nursing care plan is often necessary following evaluation, since the patient's responses are continually changing (goals are achieved or not achieved). When goals are not achieved, the nurse and the patient need to reanalyze the interventions provided and even reassess the diagnosis and identified goals.

On a broader scale, evaluation of nursing care can be achieved by using written statements of patient or nursing care standards developed by professional associations. Some agencies also establish quality assurance programs to improve the quality of care provided to patients by the use of observation or auditing techniques.

Suggested Activities

1. Write outcome criteria for each of the following patient goals:

- **a.** Patient will feel relief from pain.
- **b.** Patient will achieve independence in self-care (bathing).
- **c.** Patient will achieve a normal fecal elimination pattern.
- **d.** Patient will achieve normal respiratory function.
- **e.** Patient will achieve a more positive self-concept.

While no individualized data from which to construct the criterion are supplied, the purpose of this activity is to write *specific* outcome criteria. With the assistance of other students and your instructor, determine whether the criteria stated guide the nurse in the data collection phase of the evaluation process.

2. In a health care agency explore whether a quality assurance program is operating. If one does exist, determine how it functions.

3. Determine which nursing care standards are used in your jurisdiction or agency.

Suggested Readings

Horn, B. J. March-April 1980. Establishing valid and reliable criteria: A researcher's perspective. *Nursing Research* 29:88–90.

From this researcher's point of view, criteria used to develop measures of nursing care should be (a) based on a conceptual framework, (b) reliable and valid, measuring important aspects of care, (c) relatively simple to obtain, and (d) quantifiable for reporting and comparative purposes.

Inzer, F., and Aspinall, M. J. March 1981. Evaluating patient outcomes. *Nursing Outlook* 29:178–81.
This article discusses the importance of objective methods of measuring patient progress. A study is described in which nurses developed rating scales for measuring patient progress.

Selected References

Berg, H. V. June 1974. Nursing audit and outcome criteria. *Nursing Clinics of North America* 9:331–35.

Bloch, D. July/August 1975. Evaluation of nursing care in terms of process and outcome: Issues in research and quality assurance. *Nursing Research* 24:256–63.

Brodt, D. E. 1978. The nursing process. In Chaska, N. L., editor. *The nursing profession: Views through the mist.* New York: McGraw-Hill Book Co.

Bussman, J. W., and Davidson, S. V. 1981. *PSRO: The promise, perspective, and potential.* Menlo Park, Calif.: Addison-Wesley Publishing Co.

Gold, H.; Jackson, M.; Sachs, B.; and Van Meter, M. J. October 1973. Peer review—a working experiment. *Nursing Outlook* 21:634–36.

La Monica, E. L. 1979. *The nursing process: A humanistic approach.* Menlo Park, Calif.: Addison-Wesley Publishing Co.

Little, D. E., and Carnevali, D. L. 1976. *Nursing care planning.* 2nd ed. Philadelphia: J. B. Lippincott Co.

Moore, K. R. April 1979. What nurses learn from nursing audit. *Nursing Outlook* 27:254–58.

Murray, R. B., and Zentner, J. P. 1979. *Nursing concepts for health promotion.* 2nd ed. Englewood Cliffs, N.J.: Prentice-Hall.

Taylor, J. W. June 1974. Measuring the outcomes of nursing care. *Nursing Clinics of North America* 9:337–48.

Yura, H., and Walsh, M. B. 1973. *The nursing process.* New York: Meredith Corp.

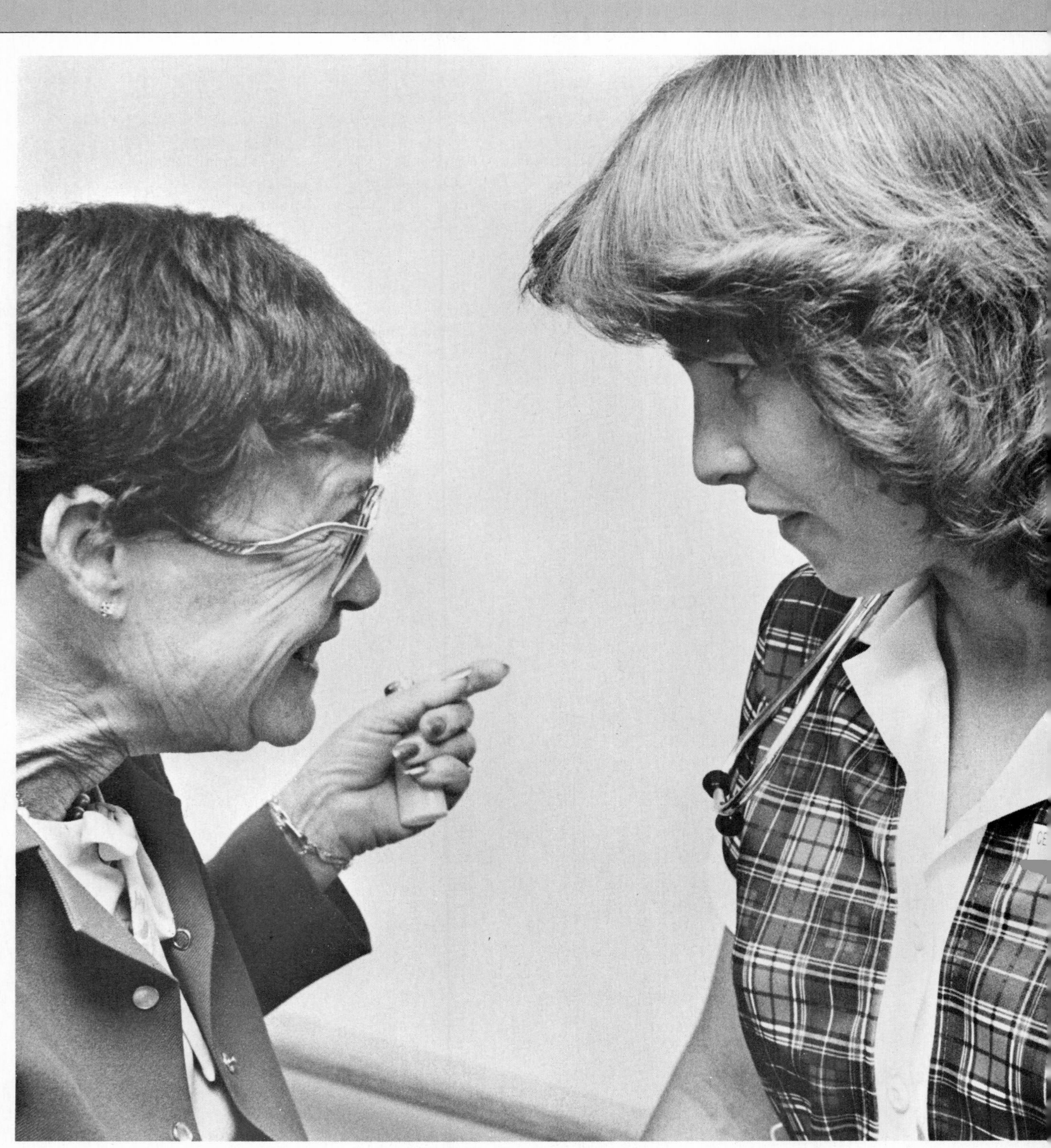

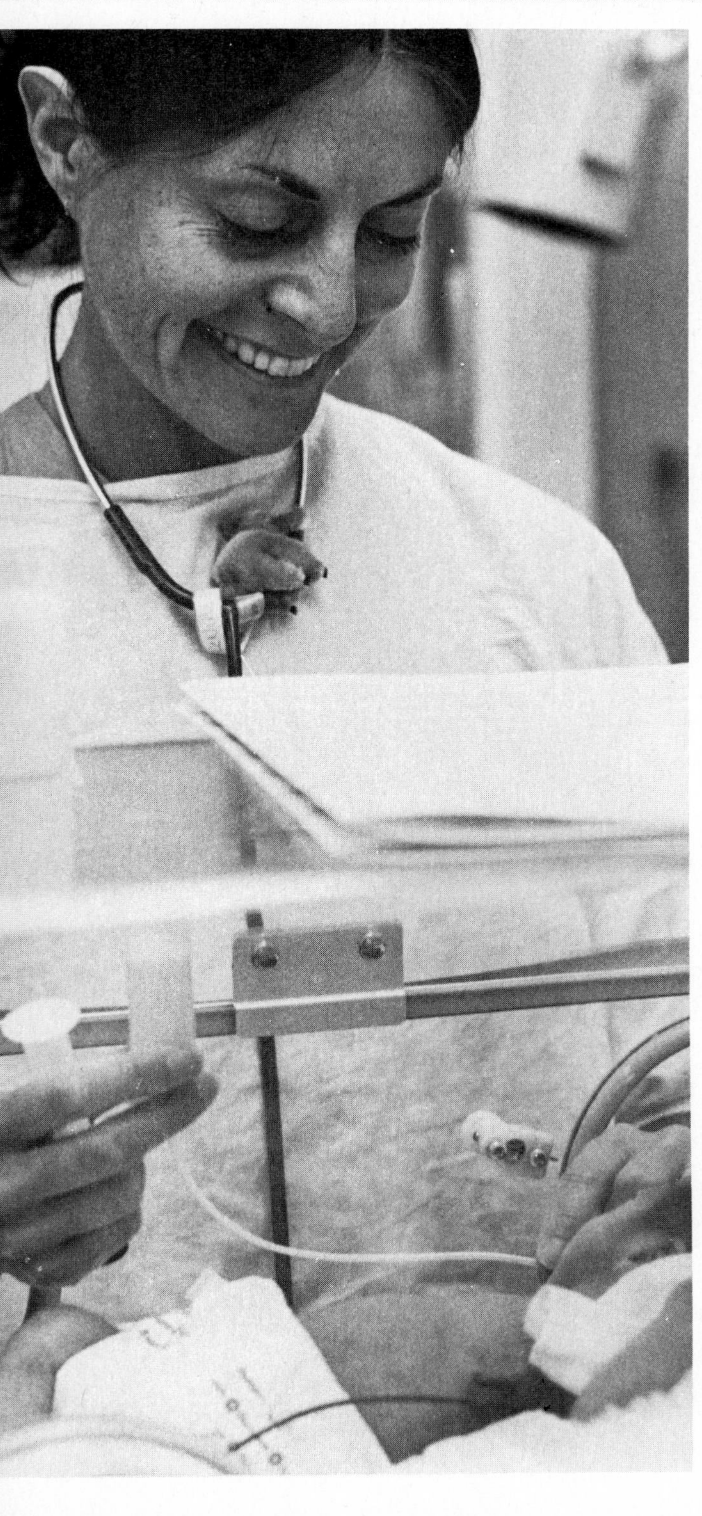

Unit III

Concepts Basic to the Nursing Process

CONTENTS

Chapter 8

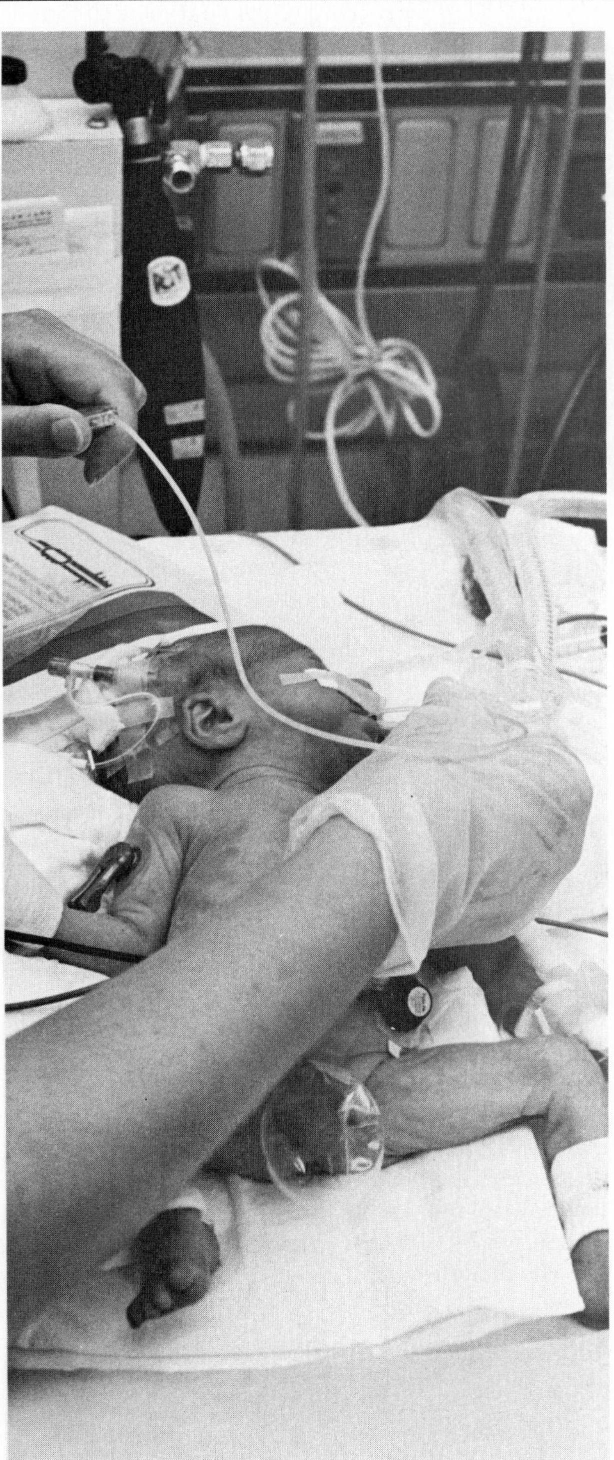

Homeostasis and Human Needs

CONTENTS

Objectives

1. Know essential facts about homeostasis, homeodynamics, and human needs

1.1 Define homeostasis, homeodynamics, and basic human needs

1.2 Outline the three essential parts of homeostatic mechanisms

1.3 List four main characteristics of homeostatic mechanisms

1.4 Outline the five major glands and two major systems of the body that maintain homeostasis

1.5 Name three homeostatic hormones secreted by the pituitary

1.6 Name two homeostatic hormones secreted by the adrenal medulla

1.7 Name two homeostatic hormones secreted by the adrenal cortex

1.8 Identify two body minerals regulated by parathyroid hormone

1.9 Describe how the respiratory and cardiovascular-renal systems regulate the body's homeostasis

1.10 List four prerequisites for the development of psychologic homeostasis

1.11 Outline seven general characteristics of basic human needs

1.12 Outline Maslow's hierarchy of needs

1.13 List Kalish's seven physiologic needs

1.14 Outline important psychosocial needs

2. Understand the concepts of homeostasis, homeodynamics, and basic human needs

2.1 Differentiate between the concepts of homeostasis and homeodynamics

2.2 Give one example of a homeostatic receptor, circuit, and effector organ

2.3 Describe the functions of ACTH, TSH, and ADH

2.4 Differentiate between a glucocorticoid and a mineralocorticoid

2.5 Compare Maslow's categories of needs with Kalish's categories of needs

2.6 Give examples that characterize the fully self-actualized person

Terms

adenohypophysis
adrenocorticotropic hormone (ACTH)
aldosterone
androgen
antidiuretic hormone (ADH)
basic human need
calcitonin
chemoreceptor
cortisol (hydrocortisone)
disequilibrium
effector organ
equilibrium
glucagon
glucocorticoid
gluconeogenesis
glycogen
hallucinate
homeodynamics
homeostasis
hypophysis
hypothalamus
insomnia
insulin
islands of Langerhans
mineralocorticoid
negative feedback
neurohypophysis
parathyroid hormone (PTH)
proprioceptor
receptor (sensor)
renin
self-actualization
thyroid hormone (TH)
thyrotropic (thyroid-stimulating) hormone (TSH)

This chapter is about homeostasis and basic human needs. Since homeostasis is a basic health concept, it will be referred to often throughout this book. An understanding of the physiologic and psychologic homeostatic mechanisms assists nursing students to understand people, especially patients, as integrated human beings.

The concept of basic human needs provides an organized approach to understanding the behavior of people. Maslow's (1968) categories and hierarchy of human needs, as adapted by Kalish (1977), provide a framework for discussion. Needs that fall within each of the categories are analyzed with emphasis on information valuable to nurses. Characteristics that describe a person whose physical and psychologic needs are met are also included.

Homeostasis

Homeostasis is derived from *homeo*, meaning "similar or like," and *stasis*, meaning "standing or stopping." The concept of homeostasis was first introduced by W. B. Cannon (1939) to describe the relative constancy of the internal processes of the body. Cannon viewed the human being as separate from his or her external environment and constantly endeavoring to maintain physiologic *equilibrium*, or balance, through adaptation to that environment. Since its introduction, the concept has broadened to include all physiologic and psychologic processes. *Homeostasis*, then, is the tendency of the body to maintain a state of balance or equilibrium while continually changing. The changes may be minor or major as the body adapts to the internal and external environments.

Changes in daily life require physiologic and psychologic adjustments in order to maintain homeostasis. A person in homeostasis is said to be in a state of health. When factors either external or internal to the body produce a *disequilibrium*, or unbalanced condition, the person is considered not healthy. The human body is extremely sensitive to changes and automatically brings into play powerful regulating mechanisms to maintain a state of balance. This state of balance operates within a narrow range. Each mechanism of the body that maintains homeostasis has the following parts:

1. A *receptor* or *sensor*, which can receive a message (input, stimulus) or sense a change in the internal or external environment. For example, three types of receptors regulate respiration: (a) The *stretch receptors* are sensory nerve terminals that are sensitive to the stretching of the tissues and are activated when the lungs are inflated; (b) the *chemoreceptors* are sensory nerve terminals that are sensitive to specific chemicals; they are located in the respiratory center and respond to changes in the oxygen, carbon dioxide, and hydrogen ion concentrations in the blood and tissue fluids; and (c) the *proprioceptors* are sensory nerve terminals that are sensitive to the movement and position of the body; they are located in the muscles and tendons, and body movement and exercise cause them to increase the respiratory rate and depth. For further information, see page 742.

2. A *circuit*, which transmits the message to an effector organ. A circuit is a number of nerve cells (neurons) that function in a reflex arc. For example, when the stretch receptors of the lungs are activated, impulses are transmitted through the vagus nerves to the brainstem and from there to the respiratory center. In this situation, the circuit that transmits the message from the stretch receptors consists of the vagus nerves and the brainstem.

3. An *effector organ*, which acts to alter the internal environment and return it to the normal homeostatic range. An effector organ is a muscle or gland that responds to nerve impulses. In the respiration example, the effector organ is the respiratory center. After the stretch receptors are activated and the impulses transmitted, the respiratory center acts to inhibit inspiration and prevent overdistention of the lungs. This homeostatic mechanism is commonly referred to as the *Hering-Breuer inflation reflex*. See Chapter 29.

Homeostatic mechanisms have four main characteristics:

1. They are self-regulating.
2. They are compensatory.
3. They tend to be regulated by negative feedback systems.
4. They may require several feedback mechanisms to correct only one physiologic imbalance.

Self-regulation means that homeostatic mechanisms come into play automatically in the healthy person. However, if a person is ill, or if a respiratory organ such as a lung is injured, the homeostatic mechanisms may not be able to respond to the stimulus as they would normally.

Homeostatic mechanisms are compensatory (counterbalancing), because they tend to counteract conditions that are abnormal for the person. An example is a sudden drop in temperature. The compensatory mechanisms are that the peripheral blood vessels constrict, thereby diverting most of the blood internally; and increased muscular activity and shivering occur to create heat. Through these mechanisms the body temperature remains stable despite the cold.

Homeostatic mechanisms tend to be regulated by negative feedback systems. This type of system is a common control mechanism for hormone levels. *Negative feedback* is a mechanism in which deviations from normal are sensed and counteracted. The deviations may be either greater or less than the normal level. By the negative feedback mechanism the biologic system is directed or adjusted back to normal. For example, an increase in the production of parathyroid hormone is stimulated by a drop in blood calcium, but, when parathyroid hormone is increased and raises the level of blood calcium, its production is then inhibited. Not all but many hormones are controlled by this negative feedback effect.

In order to correct one physiologic imbalance, several negative feedback systems may be required. For example, with hypoxia (shortage of oxygen), characteristic of people who live in very high altitudes, the concentration of red blood cells will increase and the heart rate will be faster to transport the blood and available oxygen around the body adequately.

Physiologic Homeostasis

Five major glands and two systems largely maintain the body's physiologic homeostasis. They are the pituitary gland, the adrenal glands, the thyroid gland, the

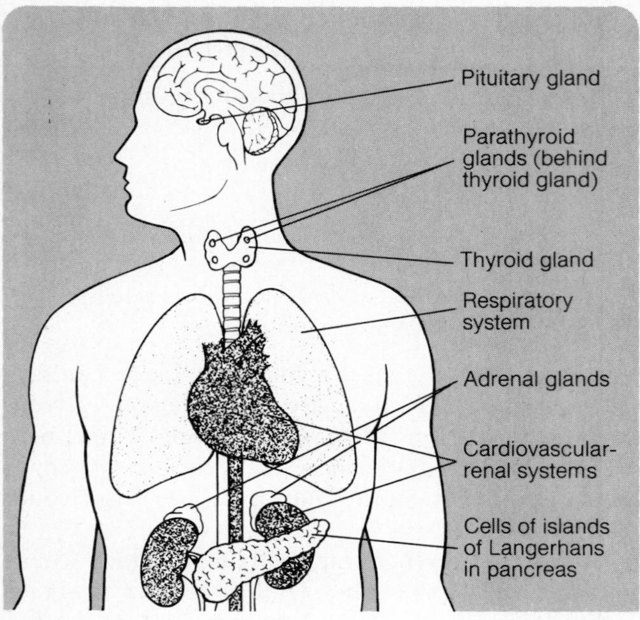

Figure 8–1 The five major glands and two major systems of the body that maintain homeostasis.

parathyroid glands, the islands of Langerhans in the pancreas, the respiratory system, and the cardiovascular-renal systems. See Figure 8–1.

Pituitary gland

The pituitary gland (*hypophysis*), although only the size of the tip of the little finger, releases several hormones in response to the body's needs. See Figure 8–2. Some of these are secreted by the anterior part of the pituitary gland (*adenohypophysis*) under the stimulus of the *hypothalamus*, a part of the nervous system. Others are stored in the posterior part of the pituitary gland (*neurohypophysis*). These latter hormones are secreted by the hypothalamus and stored in the neurohypophysis until needed.

Figure 8–2 The pituitary gland.

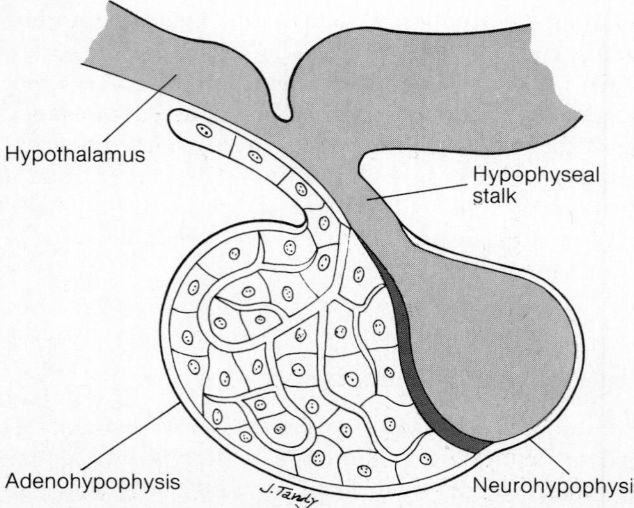

Two major hormones secreted from the anterior pituitary are *adrenocorticotropic hormone* (ACTH) and *thyrotropic* (or thyroid-stimulating) *hormone* (TSH). ACTH stimulates the adrenal cortex to produce steroids. TSH stimulates the secretion of thyroxin from the thyroid gland. The major function of thyroxin is to control the body's rate of metabolism.

From the posterior pituitary gland the homeostatic hormone stored and released is *antidiuretic hormone* (ADH). ADH controls water reabsorption in the kidney tubules and thus prevents the body fluids from becoming too concentrated. An increase in the amount of water in the bloodstream causes the blood pressure to rise; thus ADH is sometimes referred to as a *vasopressor* drug when it is given therapeutically.

Adrenal glands

The adrenal glands (see Figure 8–3) produce two very different types of hormones. The inner part of the adrenal glands, the medulla, which is part of the sympathetic nervous system, produces epinephrine (adrenaline) and norepinephrine (noradrenaline). Although the adrenal medulla is not essential for life, these hormones assist a person to meet certain emergency situations and support the sympathetic nervous system in what is known as the *fight or flight* response. This is discussed in Chapter 9.

The outer part of the adrenal glands, the cortex, secretes three kinds of adrenocortical hormones: *mineralocorticoids*, *glucocorticoids*, and *androgens*. The mineralocorticoids and glucocorticoids are the two homeostatic hormones. The most abundant mineralocorticoid is *aldosterone*, which induces sodium chloride retention, potassium excretion, and water reabsorption by the kidneys. Aldosterone is therefore an important hormone in regulating the body's fluid and electrolyte levels (see Chapter 30). Aldosterone secretion by the adrenal cortex is controlled by changes in the concentration of potassium in the blood and by a substance called *renin* that is secreted by the kidneys when the concentration of sodium in the blood falls to a low level.

Glucocorticoids, the most abundant of which is *cortisol* (*hydrocortisone*), influence the metabolism of glucose, protein, and fat and thus the production of energy for the body. The term *glucocorticoid* refers to the ability these hormones have to raise the blood sugar by mobilizing protein and fat from their storage areas and converting them into glucose. Glucocorticoids keep the blood glucose concentration high even during starvation periods and provide essential nutrients for nerve cells, which can use only glucose for energy. Another major function of the glucocorticoids is to increase a person's resistance to such physical stresses as injury, cold, pain, or fright. See Chapter 9 on the endocrine adaptive response. Glucocorticoid secretion is controlled by blood levels of pituitary ACTH. A pronounced rise in ACTH blood level is followed by an increase in the secretion of glucocorticoids.

Thyroid gland

The thyroid gland, located in the neck below the larynx, consists of two fairly large lateral lobes that are joined by a connecting portion called the isthmus. This gland stores and secretes two homeostatic hormones: *thyroid hormone* (thyroxine and triiodothyronine) and *calcitonin*. The primary physiologic actions of thyroid hormone are to regulate the body's metabolic rate and the processes of growth. Calcitonin decreases the blood's calcium concentration either by promoting the deposit of calcium into bone or by inhibiting bone breakdown, which would release calcium into the blood.

Parathyroid glands

The four parathyroid glands located behind the thyroid gland secrete *parathyroid hormone* (parathormone, PTH), which raises plasma calcium levels and lowers plasma phosphate levels. Although knowledge about this hormone and its relationship to calcium and phosphorus metabolism is still incomplete, PTH is considered invaluable for the body's homeostasis. Both calcium and phosphorus are necessary for healthy bones and teeth. Calcium is also necessary for blood coagulation when the body is injured and for proper transmission of nerve impulses.

Secretion of PTH is governed by a negative feedback system. Levels of blood calcium below normal increase the release of the hormone. PTH raises blood calcium primarily by releasing calcium from bone, where most of the body's calcium is found; it also increases the rate of calcium absorption from the intestines and calcium reabsorption by the kidneys. A dramatic example of low calcium levels is tetany, a condition in which the body's skeletal muscles are hyperirritable and in spasm. When spasm of the laryngeal muscles occurs, respiratory obstruction and death can ensue.

Islands of Langerhans

The *islands of Langerhans* are clusters of endocrine-secreting cells located in the pancreas. The islands contain two types of cells: alpha cells, which secrete glucagon, and beta cells, which secrete insulin. *Insulin* accelerates the movement of sugar (glucose), protein (amino acids), and fats (fatty acids) out of the blood and into the tissue cells. Insulin, therefore, is a key regulator, since it lowers the blood concentration of these nutrients and promotes their metabolism and use by the cells. *Glucagon*, on the other hand, tends to increase blood glucose concentration by stimulating the breakdown of liver glycogen.

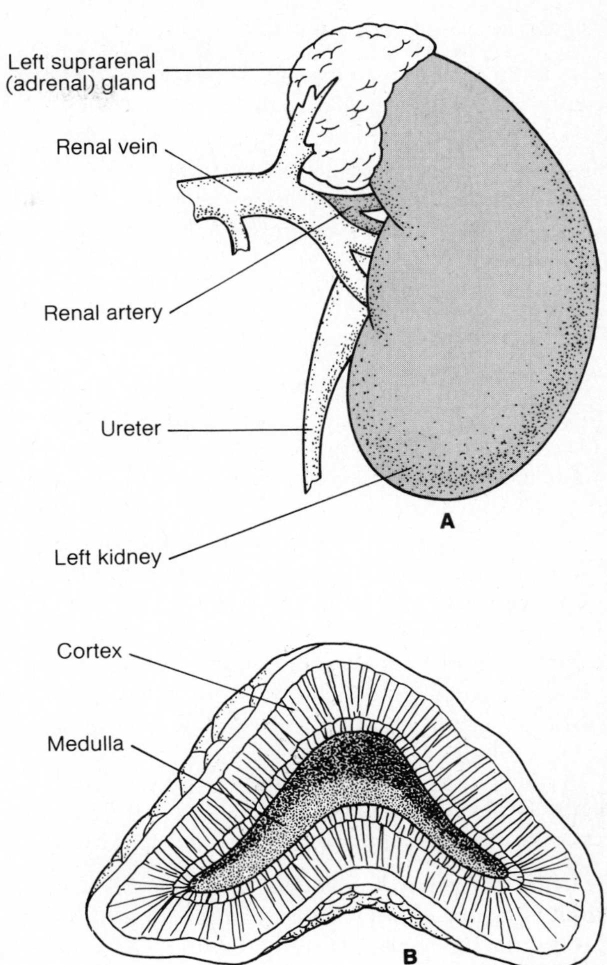

Figure 8–3 The adrenal glands: **A**, position of the gland on the kidney; **B**, cross section of the gland showing the medulla and the cortex.

Respiratory system

The respiratory system regulates intake of oxygen and exhalation of carbon dioxide. Oxygen is essential for metabolism and hence the production of energy. Elimination of carbon dioxide is also essential to maintain the body's acid-base balance, which is a very precise regulatory mechanism. For further discussion, see Chapters 30 and 31.

Cardiovascular-renal systems

The kidneys are responsible for excretion and reabsorption of many by-products of metabolism. Their role in maintaining homeostasis of the body's fluids, electrolyte levels, and acid-base balance is vital. The cardiovascular system is the transport system that provides and removes essential elements for all body cells.

Psychologic Homeostasis

The term *psychologic homeostasis* refers to emotional or psychologic balance or a state of mental well-being. It is maintained by a variety of mechanisms. Each person has certain psychologic needs, such as the need for love, security, and self-esteem, that must be met to maintain psychologic homeostasis. When one or more of these needs is not met or is threatened, certain mental mechanisms are activated to protect the person and provide psychologic homeostasis. The motivation that triggers use of these mechanisms is unconscious, not consciously determined by the person. For further information about mental mechanisms, see Chapter 9.

Psychologic homeostasis is acquired or learned through the experience of living and interacting with others. In addition, societal norms and culture influence behavior. Some prerequisites are needed for a person to develop psychologic homeostasis. These factors can be summarized as:

1. A stable physical environment in which the person feels safe and secure. For example, the basic needs for food, shelter, and clothing must be met consistently from birth onward.
2. A stable psychologic environment from infancy onward, so that feelings of trust and love develop. Growing children and adolescents also need kind but firm and consistent discipline and encouragement and support to be their own unique selves.
3. A social environment that includes adults who are healthy role models. From these individuals, the customs and values of society are learned.
4. A life experience that provides satisfactions. Throughout life people encounter many frustrations. They can deal with these better if enough satisfying experiences have occurred to counterbalance the frustrating ones.

Homeodynamics

Recently the term *homeodynamics* has been used by some to replace homeostasis. Homeodynamics implies a continual exchange of energy between human beings and the external environment. Rather than merely adapting to the environment, people interact with the environment and continually change. The concept of homeodynamics was described by Martha Rogers (1970) and is based on five assumptions:

1. Human beings are unified wholes possessing their own integrity and manifesting characteristics that are more than and different from the sum of their parts (Rogers 1970:47). That is, a person is more than and different from the total of his or her arms, legs, heart, etc.
2. People and the environment are continuously exchanging matter and energy with one another (ibid., p. 54). This continuous exchange of energy characterizes each participant as an open system. In contrast, homeostasis was considered to occur in a closed energy system. An open system is one in which there is contact with the environment and the system interacts with and is affected by the environment. All living systems are open. A closed system is not affected by the external environment; it is totally self-contained.
3. The life process evolves irreversibly and unidirectionally along the space-time continuum (ibid., p. 59). The life process is a continual series of changes incorporating the past and moving in one direction. At no time can the individual go backward.
4. This pattern and organization identify human beings and reflect their innovative wholeness (ibid., p. 65). In homeodynamics a person is viewed as a whole and each new interaction promotes change as a result of which that person becomes different. The continuous repatterning and reorganization of the person and the environment reflect a state of homeodynamics.
5. People have the capacity for abstraction, imagery, language, thought, sensation, and emotion (ibid., p. 67). This assumption is the one that differentiates humans from other living forms. Only people are sentient, thinking beings who can envisage the future.

Human Needs

Despite the fact that each individual has unique characteristics, certain basic needs are common to all people. For this book, *basic human needs* are defined as those things required by human beings in order to maintain physiologic and psychologic homeostasis.

It is important that nurses' own needs be met in order

for them to assist patients effectively. The nurse whose rest, security, love and belonging, or esteem needs are unmet will not be as effective in providing the assistance required by patients. For example, a nurse who is fatigued may lack the necessary judgment to administer medications or lack the energy to provide psychologic support to a patient who is crying.

The following characteristics apply to the basic needs of people:

1. All people have the same basic needs; however, each person's needs are modified by the culture in which the individual lives. A person's perception of a need will vary as a result of learning and the standards of the culture. For example, professional achievement may be important in a particular culture or subculture and unimportant in another.
2. People meet their own needs relative to their own priorities. For example, during a drought, a mother might give up her share of water and die in order that her child might have sufficient water to live.
3. Although basic needs generally must be met, some needs can be deferred. An example is the need for independence, which an ill person can defer until well.
4. Failure to meet needs results in one or more homeostatic imbalances, and this can eventually result in illness.
5. A need can be aroused by either external or internal stimuli. An example is the need for food. A person may experience hunger as a result of thinking about food (internal stimulation) or as a result of seeing a beautiful cake (external stimulation).
6. When a need is perceived, a person has a wide variety of responses with which to meet the need. The choice of response that a person makes is largely a result of learned experiences and the values of the culture within which the person lives. For example, the professional woman who comes home from work feeling tired may meet the need for relaxation by having a cocktail. This response reflects her experience and culture.
7. Needs are interrelated. Some needs cannot be met unless related needs are also met. The need for hydration can be seriously altered if the need for elimination of urine is not also met. Likewise, the need for security can be markedly altered if the need for oxygen is threatened by a respiratory obstruction.

There are many categories of needs. Halbert Dunn's (1958) model presents a series of needs that have to be met for the individual to achieve a state of maximum functioning or high-level wellness. Dunn's basic needs are: survival, communication, fellowship, growth, imagination, love, balance, environment, communication with the universe, philosophy of living, dignity, freedom, and space. At any specific time different needs assume a greater relative importance to the individual.

Abraham Maslow's (1970) model of human needs includes both physiologic and psychologic needs and provides a hierarchic framework for them in terms of how critical to survival they are. Maslow's five categories, in order, are (1970:37):

1. Physiologic needs
2. Safety and security needs
3. Love and belonging needs
4. Need for self-esteem
5. Need for self-actualization

Maslow's highest level, *self-actualization*, is the apex of the fully developed personality; accordingly, few people are fully self-actualized (1968:204).

Richard Kalish (1977:32) has adapted Maslow's hierarchy and suggests an additional category of needs between the physiologic needs and the safety and security needs. This category includes sex, activity, exploration, manipulation, and novelty. See Figure 8–4. Kalish emphasizes that children need to explore and manipulate their environments in order to achieve optimal growth and development. He notes that adults, too, will often seek novel adventures or stimulating experiences before considering their safety or security needs. Maslow, on the other hand, includes the pursuit of knowledge and aesthetic needs in the category of self-actualization.

In this chapter the basic human needs are subdivided into seven categories similar to Kalish's model but adapted to correspond with the material discussed in this text: (a) physiologic needs, (b) stimulation needs, (c) protection needs, (d) love and belonging needs, (e) esteem needs, (f) spiritual needs, and (g) the self-actualization need. Because spiritual beliefs are helpful in times of stress, this category is considered important for nurses. Within each category, specific needs are discussed with emphasis on the nurse's role in understanding and meeting the needs of people who are healthy or ill. Finally, the characteristics of the fully self-actualized person are considered.

Physiologic Needs

The physiologic needs encompass the basic survival requirements of humans in order to maintain biologic homeostasis and life itself. Generally, when these needs are not met, other needs, such as activity and affection, are not aroused. For most adults, being unable to meet their own needs for food and water is distressing and produces feelings of helplessness. For anyone, the inability to acquire sufficient oxygen, feeling suffocated, is a frightening experience.

Nurses are frequently called upon to assist patients of all ages to meet their physiologic needs. In terms of nursing priorities, survival needs of patients generally take precedence over other needs, such as those included in the psychologic needs category. Nurses need

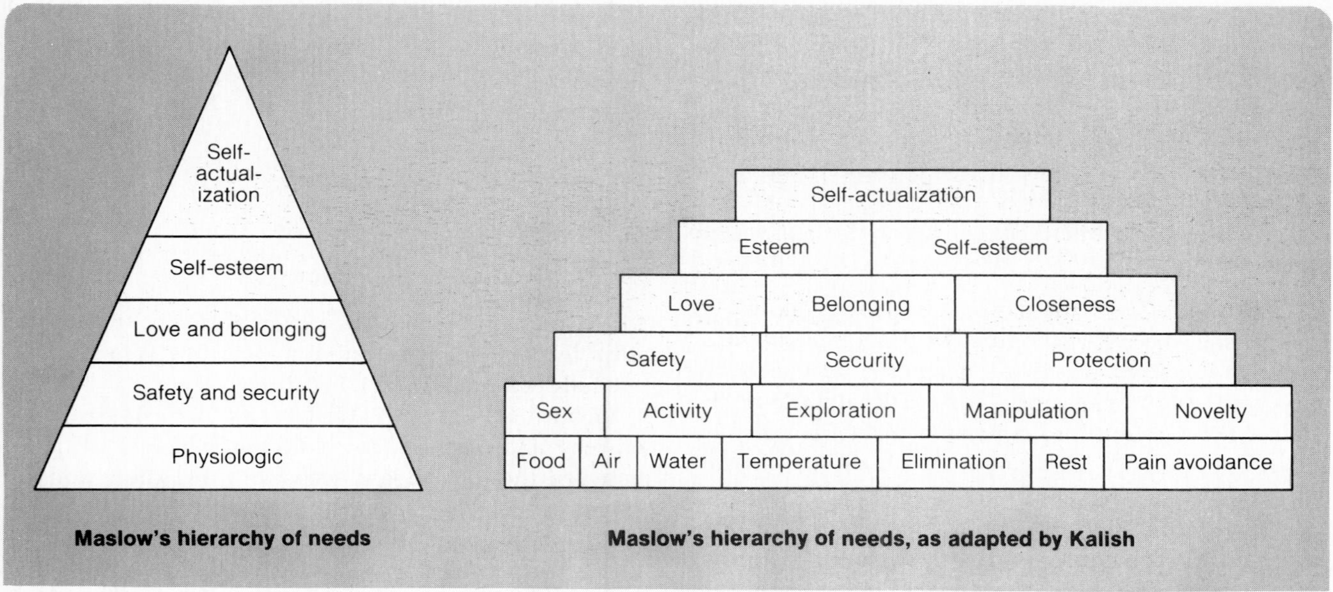

Figure 8–4 Maslow's hierarchy of needs and Maslow's needs as adapted by Kalish. (Adapted from Abraham H. Maslow, A theory of human motivation, *Psychological Review*, 1943, 50:370–96. Copyright © 1943 by the American Psychological Association, Inc. Reprinted by permission. From Richard A. Kalish, *The psychology of human behavior*, 3rd ed. [Monterey, Calif.: Brooks/Cole Publishing Co., 1973]. Reprinted by permission of the publisher. Copyright © 1973 by Wadsworth Publishing Company, Inc.)

to be sensitive to the patients' feelings, however, when assisting them with physiologic needs. For adult patients in particular, inability to meet their own needs in this area usually represents a disturbing and sometimes embarrassing degree of dependence on others. The needs included in this category are for oxygen, water, food, elimination, rest and sleep, pain relief, exercise, and temperature regulation.

Need for air (oxygen)

In normal circumstances, humans cannot survive without oxygen for more than four to five minutes without incurring irreversible brain damage. Nursing measures to ensure the free passage of oxygen into the body and subsequently to all tissues of the body are emergency measures. If a patient is unable to inhale because of an obstructed trachea or is hemorrhaging from any part of the body, essential oxygenation of the body tissues cannot be maintained.

Oxygen is vital to all the cells of the body for their metabolic activities, which provide energy. An adequate supply of oxygen to the body tissues relies upon an intact respiratory system, nervous system, and cardiovascular system. A cardiac arrest is another example of an emergency situation related to oxygenation: The heart fails to pump blood and hence deliver oxygen to body cells. There are countless other situations that are not considered emergencies but that also interfere with the oxygen supply; for example, in anemia the capacity of the blood to deliver oxygen is reduced because of the reduced supply of red blood cells to carry oxygen.

Need for water

Water is second only to oxygen as a requirement for life. Healthy people obtain water for the body by drinking fluids and ingesting food. Therefore, impairment in the availability of either or both of these sources can seriously affect a person's water supply.

Water is a universal solvent; that is, it is the basic solvent for all the chemical reactions that take place in the human body. In infants a higher proportion of the body is water than in adults. Therefore, the effects of dehydration in infants can be dramatic and serious.

Under normal conditions of activity and climate, adults have been known to survive as long as 18 days without water. However, this is an abnormally long time; as a general rule 3 to 5 days are considered the maximum time adults can function without water.

Need for food

Although people can live without food for a number of weeks, the need of the human body for food should not be underestimated. When external food sources are not available to a person, the body will use its internal resources. Carbohydrate reserves (for example, *glycogen* in the liver and muscles) are used first, followed by protein and fat reserves in the tissues. When carbohydrate reserves are depleted, the liver converts proteins and fats into glucose by a process called *gluconeogenesis.* The rate of depletion of fat continues until all fat stores are gone. The rate of protein depletion varies: It is rapid initially and then slows markedly, since fat is the prime source of energy. Shortly before death, however, when the only remaining source of energy is protein, protein depletion again becomes rapid (Guyton 1982:563).

The length of time that a person can survive without food depends to a large degree on the person's physical status. It is doubtful that any person would survive ten weeks without food. Specific nutrients are also essential needs. Lack of vitamin D is evident in a child who has the skeletal deformities of rickets.

The type of food a person is accustomed to depends largely upon cultural norms, subgroup norms within a society, and individual idiosyncrasies. For example, people of the Chinese culture are usually accustomed to rice; some people in North America enjoy snails, while others would become nauseated at the thought of eating them. Individual idiosyncrasies abound: some people like onions, others not; some like white bread, others eat only brown bread. Regardless of these cultural and individual differences, the importance of good nutrition cannot be overstated. Normal growth and development depend upon it, and both physical and mental health suffer from inadequate nutrition.

Need for elimination

In order for a person's body to function efficiently, food residues and gases need to be eliminated from the gastrointestinal tract and the waste products of metabolism must be detoxified and/or eliminated from the body. The organs involved in elimination are the kidneys, the large intestine, the lungs, and the skin. Complete malfunction of the kidneys (kidney shutdown) is a life-and-death matter.

Nurses frequently see patients who have difficulty eliminating carbon dioxide through the lungs. The accumulation of carbon dioxide in the body increases the acid content of the blood. Because body cells survive in an alkaline medium, death ensues when carbon dioxide is not eliminated adequately.

People have individual patterns for bowel evacuation. The patient who is able to maintain this pattern, for example, evacuating the bowels once a day after breakfast, is less likely to become constipated. Nurses can assist patients by helping them become aware of their normal habits and by facilitating the continuation of these habits whenever possible. Occasional irregularities brought about by a change in daily routines need not be a cause for alarm. Changes in diet and increased stress normally alter bowel evacuation.

One less obvious function of the bowel (large intestine) is to reabsorb water. This is an essential function to preserve the body's fluid and electrolyte balance. The occurrence of diarrhea in illness is an example of excessive elimination of both fluids and electrolytes.

Human skin eliminates water as perspiration with small amounts of salt (NaCl). This ability of the skin is an important mechanism in maintaining the body's temperature within a normal range.

Need for rest (sleep)

Much is still to be learned about the mechanisms and functions of sleep. What is known is that, without sufficient sleep, mental concentration and memory recall are reduced; a person becomes irritable and less able to cope with psychologic stress. Prolonged sleep deprivation can result in hallucinations while awake. To *hallucinate* is to perceive through the senses something unreal, for example, to see elephants dancing on the wall.

Insomnia (the inability to sleep) is a relatively common problem in today's society. Frequently a nurse will be called upon for supportive measures to help a patient sleep. People have individual needs for sleep and hours of sleep. Often people have ritualistic habits about sleep, such as taking a glass of warm milk or a tub bath before retiring. Being able to continue these habits whenever possible greatly assists patients to sleep.

Need for pain avoidance

The avoidance of pain is considered another basic need of humans. However, since pain is the most common symptom of illness, few patients are able to avoid it. As a result, many nursing activities are centered around providing relief measures for pain. Pain can temporarily disrupt several basic needs, such as the need for nutrition, rest, or security. The goal of nursing activities is usually to provide for comfort, rest, or sleep.

Need for temperature regulation

A relatively constant body temperature is required for body cells to function effectively. If a body temperature becomes extreme, death will occur. Since heat is always being produced in the body by metabolic processes, mechanisms are required for an equal amount of heat to be lost. The skin is one organ responsible for maintaining the body temperature at an optimum level by the processes of evaporation and perspiration. Heat is transferred from the deeper tissues to the bloodstream and then to the skin. Some heat is also lost in expired air, feces, and urine.

Nurses frequently need to assist patients when the body's homeostatic mechanisms for temperature control are not able to cope effectively with temperature changes. For specific interventions, see Chapter 13.

Stimulation Needs

Stimulation needs arise from stimuli that rouse the mind or spirit or incite a person to activity or toward a goal. As a category for basic needs of people, *stimulation* is used here in a broad sense, referring to stimulation of the emotions, the cognitive processes, and the senses. A number of activities can provide stimulation. Any change can be stimulating to a person provided the degree of change is appropriate for that person. One person might find moving to another city is a stimulating experience that affords opportunities to learn new life experiences; another person making the same move might be overwhelmed and experience acute feelings of insecurity rather than stimulation. Changes of a lesser degree, such as a new book, new clothes, or a different restaurant, can also be stimulating.

Stimulation can come from a hobby or an activity in which a person is interested. This type of stimulation can serve to balance the routine and problems of daily life. Sensory stimulants, such as a movie, the smell of newly baked bread, a beautiful sunset, or the sound of certain music, can also add interest to life.

Not all stimulation is pleasant. Adults may be bombarded by acoustic stimuli that they find unpleasant when a teenager turns on music to a high volume. Unpleasant sensory stimuli are familiar to all of us. However, even this stimulation can provoke interest, and it can help to meet some people's basic needs.

In this section three basic stimulation needs are considered: the need for activity; the need for exploration, manipulation, and novelty; and the need for sexual activity.

Need for activity

Every person has a need for some activity. Activity in this context is used to mean physical exercise and mental activity. The benefits and functions of exercise are well recognized and well publicized today. Although people can survive without it, exercise even for the immobilized improves health and prevents problems. Often the kind and the amount are determined by the person's physical and mental status.

Physical activity such as playing a game of tennis or walking along a beach in the cool of the evening can be stimulating both mentally and physically. A person often feels that vitality is restored and the mind is rested; thoughts of the experience return to give pleasure. Activities such as hobbies, knitting, and picture puzzles can also serve to stimulate mental activity and interests.

The right amount and kind of physical activity will exercise the heart by increasing its rate. As a result, deeper respirations take place, lung expansion is increased, and increased cardiopulmonary circulation occurs. Exercise also improves muscle tone and frequently increases the range and ease of movement of the joints.

For exercise to be effective, it should be regular and sustained. Generally, exercising at least three times per week is advised. People today are increasingly aware that exercise is a means to improved health and prevention of health problems. Activities such as jogging and bicycling are taking on greater importance to people of many ages.

Nurses are often challenged to assist patients to meet their needs for physical and mental activity. The means by which these needs can be met are often affected by illness. The patient who is restricted to a hospital bed from which there is no view often lacks the stimuli that most people in daily life take for granted. To such people watching television is often a therapeutic diversion and interest. The elderly person who is in the hospital and whose thoughts and words frequently come slowly, for a busy nurse, very much needs assistance in stimulation and activity.

One of the functions of a nurse is to socialize with patients; this can assist in meeting needs for stimulation. Discussions about a patient's interest in cooking or in sports often are helpful. It is important, however, that the socializing be oriented to helping the patient meet her or his needs, not the nurse's needs.

Need for exploration, manipulation, and novelty

The need for exploration and manipulation is particularly evident in the development of a child. Through exploration of the environment and manipulation of objects, a child learns how to climb trees, how to pick apples, how to dress, what a flower is, and where the rain comes from. The needs to explore and to manipulate objects that all children have is basic to much of their learning and their interests.

Novelty or newness can also offer stimulation. The face of a child who goes to her first circus or a baseball fan who attends his first World Series demonstrates the meeting of this need for novelty. Imagine how boring the days are for a long-term patient who has no new experience during a whole year. The patient sees the same people, talks about the same subjects, and frequently begins to lose interest in the surroundings—perhaps in life itself.

Need for sexual activity

Although the sexual act is essential to survival of the human species, the character of the individual's need for sex encompasses much more than this reproductive function. Already mentioned is the fact that sexual activity can be an expression of the need to give and receive love. The whole field of sexuality and sexual relationships is now being recognized and talked about. Literature abounds on the subject.

In the health field, sexuality, as it relates to a person's body image and self-concept, has many implications. In many illnesses, patients are unable to satisfy their sexual needs in the usual way. These needs may be either sublimated or expressed in flirtations or other kinds of behavior that require understanding on the part of the nurse. For both men and women, changes in body image brought about by surgical intervention or disease processes can threaten sexual relationships. For example, it is not uncommon for the woman who has had a radical mastectomy to feel anxiety about how well her love partner will accept the change. For men whose sexual organs have been removed or repaired, the psychologic trauma can often be severe. The male self-image throughout the ages has emphasized potency and virility. Even when sexual organs are not involved, as in a long-term illness, the sexual needs of patients have to be considered. In many situations the nurse can be instrumental in assessing and identifying patients' sexual problems. For patients having surgery, answering questions and explaining the effects of the surgical procedure can be helpful. For long-term patients, nurses can plan to provide privacy so that these patients can be with loved ones. In many situations the nurse may refer the patient to other health professionals who are experienced interviewers and counselors in sexual matters.

Protection Needs

Need for safety and protection

Safety needs are needs to protect oneself from physical harm. The threats to the safety of the person can be categorized as mechanical, chemical, thermal, and bacteriologic. Generally, adults meet their own safety needs in daily life, and they are seldom considered survival needs, except under unusual circumstances such as war. In illness, however, persons are frequently less able to protect themselves; their resistance to infection can be lowered, or they may be immobilized.

Patients are not always aware of the threats of injury in a hospital or health agency. Nurses therefore need to be aware of situations in which patients could be injured. Explanations to patients and appropriate safety measures generally will protect a person adequately. These measures include not only those that prevent accidents but also those that maintain cleanliness and body alignment:

1. *Measures for cleanliness.* The emphasis people place on cleanliness in North America often surpasses that necessary for safety. However, good hygienic practices facilitate the maintenance of skin integrity and the health of mucous membranes. Intact skin and mucous membranes provide a tough barrier to chemical and bacterial invasion. Much time is spent by nurses in assisting people with the hygienic practices of bathing and care of hair, teeth, and nails. Infection control measures are also frequently employed when the skin is broken, for example, by a surgical incision or a burn.

   Cleanliness can also be discussed in an environmental context. Measures for refuse and sewage disposal, measures to prevent air pollution, and measures to keep the premises free of insects and vermin all protect people from environmental hazards.
2. *Measures to maintain body alignment.* Good body alignment requires minimal muscular effort. It does not place strain on muscles, ligaments, or joints, and it favors proper functioning of all the body systems. Helping patients to maintain body alignment is of particular importance in clinical situations. Incorrect alignment can produce contractures of the ankle, knee, or hip joints, which can lead to disturbances in posture and gait.

Often people who are ill are unable to maintain suitable body alignment, because of weakness, pain, or disorientation. Nurses frequently need to assist patients to healthy positions and provide supports so that they can maintain these positions.

Need for security

The need for security can be regarded in two contexts, the physiologic and the interpersonal relationship context. Physiologic security relates to anything that poses a threat to a person's body or to life itself. The threat may be either real or imagined. For example, illness, excruciating pain, a physical attack, and acute anxiety can all bring about reactions of a protective nature.

In the interpersonal context, people also need to feel secure. Interpersonal security depends upon many factors, such as consistency in the behavior of others, awareness of the expectations or limitations of others, familiarity with people and the environment, ability to control matters concerning oneself, ability to communicate, and need to know or understand.

With consistency, people are able to predict to some degree what to expect. When expectations and limitations are clear, behavior patterns that are acceptable in a relationship are understood, forming a structure or rules that offer security. It becomes obvious that familiarity with people or places facilitates security when one experiences the opposite feelings upon meeting new people or living in strange places. Aligned with familiarity is the ability to communicate in a similar language with others.

The unknown often produces feelings of anxiety and insecurity. For example, if a patient is having surgery for a tumor that could be cancerous, until the diagnosis is known the person's security is threatened. In institutionalized health care settings, people also temporarily lose their rights to control personal matters. For example, the time and type of bath that a patient has is often prescribed by the policies of a hospital instead of the person's own preference. This lack of control may produce feelings of insecurity.

Love and Belonging Needs

Need for love and closeness

The need for love is so basic that it has been described as the bony structure of a person's emotional life (Caprio 1965:16). So much has been written on the subject of love by philosophers, poets, novelists, and behavioral scientists that the meaning of love is not always clear. Love is difficult to define. There are many kinds of love, such as mother love, romantic love, love between friends and family members, and love of God. Perhaps it is enough to understand that love is accomplished with the emotions and not the intellect, that love is a feeling—an acting response rather than an intellectual process. Love is also a strong positive feeling that is not possessive. Some characteristics of love outlined by Ashley Montagu (1975:15) are:

1. Love is not only a subjective feeling that a person has (an emotion) but also a series of acts by which one person conveys to another the feeling that he or she is deeply involved and profoundly interested in that person and the person's welfare.
2. Love is unconditional; it makes no bargains but conveys that one person is concerned for another person, that the one is there to give support and to contribute to the other's development as well as possible because the one values the other for what he or she is and as he or she is.
3. Love is supportive; it conveys that a person will always be present when the other person most needs him or her, that a person will neither condemn nor condone but will be there to offer sympathy and understanding. Whatever the other needs as a human being, that person shall have. It is tolerant but not dependent.

The need for love is met in many ways. Sexual union can be one of the most personal expressions of love between couples. For infants, the physical closeness and warmth offered by a parent during feeding times can be an expression of love. In fact, fulfillment of the need for love in small children is essential for healthy emotional development. A person's basic security comes from being loved when very young. Experiments have shown that young animals and children who lack love can exhibit unusual behavior patterns (Hurlock 1968:157).

In some situations, nurses can become the surrogate parents for young children who are in the hospital, by supplying them with the affection and physical closeness they need. With adults and elderly people the role of the nurse is less concrete. However, in all instances an interest in people's welfare and a caring and supportive attitude need to be communicated. These can be conveyed in many ways: by touching, by staying with a patient when the patient is frightened, and by listening and communicating in a friendly manner.

Need to belong

The need to belong is vividly portrayed by teenagers and their peer groups or by adults who join lodges and clubs of various kinds. This desire to affiliate with others for friendship or companionship and to share common activities, language, and dress offers a sense of identity and prestige to many people. Being a member of a group can give the individual the prestige or recognition that is given to the group as a whole. This may be more recognition than the person could ever attain alone.

The need to belong is being recognized as important in some health care settings. To avoid differentiating staff members from patients by dress, in some mental health centers, the staff uniform has been abandoned. In addition, evidence of belonging is emphasized by referring to the patients as members, thus affording them a status equal to that of staff in the mental health group. Whatever the setting, the nurse can encourage a sense of belonging in patients and their families by involving them in planning their care.

Esteem Needs

Need for self-esteem

Self-esteem is often referred to as *self-respect, self-approval*, or *self-worth*. Whatever label is used, all people need to think well of themselves. Some psychologists believe that persons need to respect themselves before they can respect others. To possess self-esteem, people must respect what they have done and what they can do. That is, they need to think they are all right, needed, and useful.

A person's self-esteem depends upon other basic needs being met. If needs such as love or security are not met satisfactorily, then the basic need of self-esteem is also threatened.

People's self-esteem is often influenced considerably by their feelings of dependence or independence. Few, if any, human beings are entirely independent or completely self-sufficient, but some have stronger needs for independence than others. Dependence and independence needs vary within the same person at different stages or times in life. For example, at birth one has little choice but to depend upon others. As growth occurs, one learns to become more independent and to balance needs to depend upon the environment and others with self-directive or self-sufficient abilities.

Illness almost always alters dependence and independence needs. Even temporary limitations on the activities a person normally carries out can decrease self-respect. It often becomes the nurse's responsibility to make decisions with the patient about balancing needs for dependence and independence in order to hasten recovery. It is important to allow patients as much control of themselves and their environment as possible to maintain their self-esteem.

Changes in the body image brought about by surgery or a disease process also seriously affect a person's self-worth. For example, a woman who is paralyzed or who has had her legs amputated is required to change her self-concept. No longer will she appear as she did before or be able to do all the things she was accustomed to doing.

Most people have feelings of inferiority and lack self-confidence from time to time. They may react in ways that attempt to bolster their self-esteem but that can alienate others. Criticism at such a time tends to exaggerate the person's behavior. A nonreactive but accepting behavior on the part of the nurse is most helpful. Acceptance differs from approval. A person's behavior can be accepted by another person, but that does not mean that the behavior is approved. Although the concept of acceptance may be easy for a nurse to understand, it is not always easy to apply. For example, it is not unusual to encounter behavior from a patient that the nurse considers offensive, such as a patient's use of sarcastic or obscene language. In these situations many nurses find it difficult to accept the patient and the behavior and not react to it. Frequently, this behavior is an attempt to gain attention in order to meet some personal needs, although the patient may not be aware of the reason behind the behavior. A nonreactive response from the nurse and an accepting attitude toward the person are required. The nurse might reply in a natural way with a statement such as, "Your words offend me, and they are not necessary; how can I help you?" Experienced nurses find that the patient's behavior frequently changes to more socially acceptable patterns when this response is given.

Need for esteem (recognition) from others

All people require social approval and recognition for what they achieve. In Western cultures much emphasis has been placed on a person's occupational role and on the acquisition of material possessions. For an individual this feeling of achievement may be oriented chiefly to a series of promotions or to the acquisition of more expensive living accommodations. The value of achievement is partly influenced by the norms of the society in which the person lives and partly by personal experiences. For example, a son whose father was very successful playing football may strive to make a million dollars in order to show his father he also can be successful even though he did not play football well. A feeling of achievement can also be gained in the performance of other roles, such as being a working mother or a responsible father and family man.

In health settings nurses have many opportunities to provide recognition for patients' achievements. Even brief statements, such as, "It's nice to see you again," or inquiries about family members can be satisfying to some patients by recognizing them as worthwhile persons. Other patients, who lack a basic sense of accomplishment, may behave in ways puzzling to a nurse in efforts to acquire some attention and recognition. For example, a person may refuse to carry out activities he is capable of doing, such as shaving or feeding himself. By anticipating a person's needs and offering praise for small achievements, a nurse may often help the person relinquish these behavioral symptoms.

Spiritual Needs

There are many other categories of needs apart from those developed by Maslow, Kalish, and Dunn. Some include spiritual needs as a separate category. These needs are often not identified by psychologists and biologists, although they have received considerable attention from philosophers and theologians. Spiritual needs have resulted in the systems of belief that are called *religions*.

Spiritual needs are closely allied to psychologic needs. They often provide strong motivations for behavior, such as the willingness of some people to fight to defend their religious practices. The spiritual needs of humans are largely met by individuals' systems of beliefs and by religious organizations in society. From these, people find answers to such questions as, "Who am I?" "Why am I here?" and "Who controls my destiny?" Spiritual needs are not completely separate entities. Close relationships exist between them and the physical and psychologic needs of people. All these needs must be considered in understanding the person as a whole. Two major spiritual needs that nurses have to consider are the need to believe and the need to hope.

Need to believe

Beliefs vary among different cultures and even among individuals in the same culture. However, the universal need exists for people to believe in someone or something, whether it is a supreme being (a supernatural entity) or something above and beyond themselves. Beliefs entrust faith, confidence, and reliance in the divine or godlike person or concept. Every system of beliefs evolves, a set of rituals for people to follow and concepts that guide a person's behavior in order to achieve its highest goal and give life some meaning.

In health and in illness, people require acceptance by others of their own particular religious values and beliefs. It is a common practice now for hospitals to include a chaplain as a member of the health team. Nurses are in a position to identify spiritual needs and should include these needs of patients in care planning. It is not uncommon for the elderly to have a particular need for religion as they come to terms with what life means to them toward the end of their life span.

Need to hope

To hope is to long for or desire something with the expectation that it will come to fulfillment. It is closely aligned with faith and trust. Hope is future oriented, suggesting that the future will be better than the present or the past. In the health care setting, hope is a common need. People hope that their surgery will be successful, or that their recovery will be speedy, or that loved ones will not suffer unnecessary discomfort. Even when the criteria of medical science suggest a poor prognosis for a patient, the person still hopes for something better. The will to live and to recover is often associated with the need to hope. People who lack hope can delay their recovery or even die prematurely. Nurses may find themselves in a paradoxical situation at times in helping patients fulfill this need. It is an easy matter when the nurse and patient hold the same degree of hope in a situation, but when the patient is hopeful and the nurse holds the opposite viewpoint (or vice versa), the nurse must still recognize and understand the patient's need.

Self-Actualization Need

Self-actualization is the final level of need according to Maslow (1968) and Kalish (1977) (see Figure 8–4). The fully self-actualized person has realized his or her full potential. Such a person has the ability to connect the past and the future to the present while living fully in the present; that is, he or she is time-competent. The self-actualized person is also inner-directed and autonomous in contrast to being other-directed. To be inner-directed means that the individual has a few basic values and principles that guide him or her, whatever the situation. To be autonomous is to be free from parental and social pressures and to apply these values or principles to behavior in a manner that appears appropriate to the individual. The other-directed individual is influenced by outside pressures, accepts guidance and direction from others, and adheres to this guidance to gain approval.

Not all people become fully self-actualized, and Maslow did not believe that intelligence is required for self-actualization. However, if all the "lower" needs have been met, an individual may aspire to become self-fulfilled or self-actualized. Maslow saw self-actualization as a product of maturity that comes about through relating to people in autonomous and time-competent ways.

The fully self-actualized person may not always be happy, successful, or well adjusted. Maslow viewed many of the subjects he believed to be self-actualized as prideful, vain, and possessing doubts and fears. However, they were able to deal positively with their fears, doubts, and failures. The following is a summary of the major characteristics of a fully self-actualized person:*

1. Is realistically oriented, a good judge of people, and one who judges them quickly.
2. Accepts self, others, and the world for what they are; is not hypocritical.
3. Has a high degree of spontaneity, is natural in behavior, and may appear unconventional.
4. Is problem-centered, not self-centered, and not very introspective.
5. Is inclined to be detached, not entirely dependent upon others; can amuse self, has a great need for privacy at times.
6. Is autonomous within self, independent, and serene.
7. Has a fresh appreciation of people and the world; is not dulled.
8. Is capable of profound inner experiences; seems detached from the world sometimes.
9. Is truly interested in the welfare of humanity.
10. Has a few special friends, is highly selective in friends, is easily moved by children.
11. Can relate to and learn from rich and poor; considers race and position not important.
12. Focuses on ends; is strongly ethical and highly moral, though standards may differ from popular ideas of right and wrong.
13. Has an inner-motivated sense of humor; does not laugh at cruelty; sees jokes in everyday things spontaneously.
14. Has a tremendous capacity to be creative, find fresh ways of doing things.
15. Is open to new experiences and resistant to conformity.

*From pp. 28–29 in *Adult Psychology*, 2nd Edition by Ledford J. Bischof. Copyright © 1976 by Ledford J. Bischof. By permission of Harper & Row, Publishers, Inc.

Characteristics of People Whose Needs Are Met

Many descriptions can be written of the characteristics of people whose basic human needs are met. Such a person may broadly be described as having a state of physical and mental well-being or health.

Physical Well-Being

A state of physical well-being encompasses fulfillment of all the previously discussed physiologic and protective needs. Lists of characteristics describing these are developed in subsequent chapters of the book. For example, how does one determine that a person is well nourished or well hydrated or physically fit? Examples of criteria that are included subsequently follow:

1. The well-hydrated person is said to have moist mucous membranes, straw-colored urine, and stable weight from day to day. See Chapter 30.
2. The well-aligned person in a standing position can be described as having toes pointed forward, head erect, and normal vertebral curves. See Chapter 23.

Mental Well-Being

There are many approaches to and definitions of mental health or mental well-being. Mentally healthy people can be considered people who are able to meet their own essential psychologic needs and cope successfully with changes related to these needs. The feeling of mental well-being is a need of all people, although some may be unaware of this. People who lament its lack desperately seek ways to acquire the feeling.

Mental health is frequently viewed as happiness, peace of mind, or satisfaction with life. Mental health is involved in every person's daily life. More specifically, it refers to how people relate to and get along with other people, such as family members, neighbors, associates, and members of the community. It also involves the manner by which a person melds ambitions, desires, abilities, ideas, and feelings in order to function effectively and meet the problems of life.

In addition to Maslow, other professionals have characterized the person enjoying mental well-being. Some of their approaches are summarized next.

Rogers's view

Carl R. Rogers (1961) writes about the "fully functioning person." The good life to which he refers is a process rather than a state of being. By this he means that it is constantly changing but moving in a direction selected freely by the person. Rogers's characteristics of the good life process can be summarized as:

1. Openness to new experiences.
2. A tendency to live fully in each moment. The experiences of that moment then help form future activities.
3. Trust in one's own judgments and reactions (Rogers 1961:183–96).

Jahoda's view

Marie Jahoda (1958) suggests the following as criteria of a mentally healthy person:

1. The person's attitudes toward self are positive; that is, the person is self-reliant, self-confident, and self-accepting.
2. The person can become aware of the meanings of his or her actions through introspection. By this process the person's behavior is accessible to the consciousness.
3. The person's self-concept is similar to the concept others have of the person.
4. The person has a sense of identity, that is, knows who she or he is and at the same time has a few doubts about it.
5. The person changes and grows throughout life.
6. The person acts in a unified manner, that is, his or her behavior is consistent throughout life (Jahoda 1958:82–95).

Glasser's view

William Glasser (1965:5–41) states that two needs are fulfilled by the mentally healthy person: the need to love and be loved and the need to feel that one is worthwhile to self and to others. A person fulfills these needs by doing what is realistic, responsible, and right.

Realistic behavior is that which the person chooses by reasoning and by considering the remote as well as the immediate consequences to self and others.

Glasser defines *responsibility* as the ability to fulfill personal needs and at the same time not deprive others of ability to fulfill their needs. In this sense a responsible person is motivated to strive and to endure privation if necessary to attain self-worth. In contrast, an irresponsible person will suffer or will cause others to suffer at some point in time. Glasser further proposes that happiness occurs most often in people who are willing to take responsibility for their own behavior.

In Glasser's terms, what is *right* is behavior that is compatible with a satisfactory standard of behavior. People need to evaluate their behavior consistently and act to improve it when it is below an acceptable standard. The person who does not do this will be unable to meet his or her own needs to feel worthwhile. There are degrees of mental health, and no one person has all the characteristics of mental health all the time.

Summary

A person in a state of homeostasis is regarded as being healthy. This means that the person's basic human needs are satisfied, including both the physiologic and the psychologic needs, and that the internal environment of the body remains relatively constant. Physiologic homeostasis operates within a narrow range by sensitive regulating mechanisms. These homeostatic mechanisms contain a receptor, a circuit, and an effector organ.

There are four main characteristics of all homeostatic mechanisms. They are self-regulating, compensatory, and generally operated by a negative feedback system; in addition, several negative feedback systems may be required to correct one physiologic imbalance.

Five major glands (pituitary, adrenals, thyroid, parathyroids, and islands of Langerhans) and two body systems (respiratory and cardiovascular–renal) are largely responsible for maintaining physiologic homeostasis. The adenohypophysis secretes ACTH and TSH, which in turn regulate the adrenal cortex to produce glucocorticoids and the thyroid gland to produce thyroxin. The body's rate of metabolism is maintained by thyroxin. The neurohypophysis is involved in maintaining the volume and concentration of body fluids through its release of ADH. The adrenal cortex secretes two major homeostatic hormones, the mineralcorticoids and the glucocorticoids. Aldosterone, the primary mineralocorticoid, causes sodium retention, thereby maintaining the body's total quantity of sodium and other electrolytes. Hydrocortisone, the primary glucocorticoid, is involved in regulating the body's fat, protein, and glucose metabolism. The thyroid gland secretes two homeostatic hormones: thyroid hormone, which regulates the body's metabolic rate, and calcitonin, which decreases the blood's calcium level. The parathyroid glands and PTH are essential in maintaining the body's calcium and phosphorus levels. The islands of Langerhans are also essential to the body's homeostasis. Insulin, secreted from the beta cells of the islands, is a key regulator in lowering the blood concentrations of glucose, proteins, and fats and promoting their utilization by the tissue cells. Glucagon, secreted from the alpha cells of the islands, acts in an opposite way to insulin by increasing the blood glucose concentration. The importance of the respiratory system and cardiovascular–renal systems in maintaining homeostasis are more obvious. The regulation of oxygen for metabolism, the transportation of all nutrients to the cells, and adequate elimination of metabolic by-products by the lungs and the kidneys are vital in maintaining homeostasis.

Psychologic homeostasis is equally important in maintaining a person's mental health. The mental mechanisms that maintain psychologic homeostasis are learned through life experiences and interactions with others. Prerequisites for the development of psychologic homeostasis include a safe and secure physical environment, a trusting and loving psychologic environment, a social environment that provides healthy adult role models, and sufficiently satisfying life experiences.

Satisfaction of specific basic human needs is essential for people to maintain homeostasis and optimal levels of well-being. The hierarchy of human needs developed by Maslow is widely recognized and with Kalish's adaptation can be useful for nurses. Seven categories of needs are outlined in this chapter. The first, physiologic needs, includes needs for oxygen, water, food, elimination, rest and sleep, pain avoidance, and temperature regulation. All these needs are basic to survival. Second, the stimulation needs of activity, exploration, manipulation, novelty, and sexual activity must be met to achieve optimal growth and development and curiosity. Third, the protection needs of safety and security emerge. These have physiologic and psychologic components. Love and belonging needs are the fourth category. Satisfaction of these provides the basis for fulfillment of higher needs, such as esteem needs, the fifth category, and the development of a self-actualized personality, the final need discussed. The spiritual needs of believing and hope are included as a separate category, since they tend to become prominent in times of stress or illness.

Although needs have been categorized into a hierarchy, people often meet their own needs relative to their own priorities. Other characteristics of needs are also recognized. One of these is that all needs are interrelated. Another is that individuals choose a variety of ways to meet their needs, modifying them in accordance with their culture or unique idiosyncrasies. Failure to meet needs, however, results in homeostatic imbalances and eventually illness. A major function of the nurse is to assist people who are healthy or ill to meet their basic needs. In times of illness the satisfaction of some needs is deferred temporarily, and a priority of needs has to be determined, with the patient when possible, in view of the illness situation.

Few people achieve self-actualization. However, optimal mental well-being can be attained. Characteristics of the self-actualized person and of mentally healthy persons are included as a guide for consideration. Generally people who are mentally healthy feel comfortable about themselves, feel right about other people, and are able to meet the demands that life presents.

Suggested Activities

1. Select one or two basic human needs from each category discussed in this chapter, and determine how well one of your patients is succeeding in fulfilling those needs or getting assistance to do so. Include whether the patient is required to alter his or her usual ways of meeting these needs.

2. Compare the various descriptions of mental well-being, and determine in a group discussion with other students which criteria you find helpful in assessing mental health.

3. Consider which patients might require particular help meeting stimulation and security needs and analyze in what ways nurses can assist them.

Suggested Readings

Byrne, M. L., and Thompson, L. F. 1978. *Key concepts for the study and practice of nursing*, pp. 10–19. 2nd ed. St. Louis: C. V. Mosby Co.

The view of a person as a set of human needs is discussed within the broader context of people and behavior. A classification of needs is suggested.

Langley, L. L. 1965. *Homeostasis.* New York: Reinhold Book Corp.

This in-depth discussion of the concept of homeostasis includes a historical perspective, general principles, and the specific homeostatic processes of body temperature, body weight, blood pressure, respiration, body fluid, hormones, and movement.

Selected References

Bischof, L. J. 1976. *Adult psychology.* 2nd ed. New York: Harper and Row.

Cannon, W. B. 1939. *The wisdom of the body.* 2nd ed. New York: Norton Publishing Co.

Caprio, F. S. 1965. *The power of sex.* New York: Citadel Press.

Chodil, J., and Williams, B. 1973. The concept of sensory deprivation. In Auld, M. E., and Birum, L. H. *The challenge of nursing: A book of readings.* St. Louis: C. V. Mosby Co.

Dunn, H. H. November 1958. What high level wellness means. *Canadian Journal of Public Health* 50:447–57.

Glasser, W. 1965. *Reality therapy.* New York: Harper and Row.

Guyton, A. C. 1982. *Human physiology and mechanisms of disease.* 3rd ed. Philadelphia: W. B. Saunders Co.

Hurlock, E. B. 1968. *Developmental psychology.* 3rd ed. New York: McGraw-Hill Book Co.

Jacob, S. W.; Francone, C. A.; and Lossow, W. J. 1978. *Structure and function in man.* 4th ed. Philadelphia: W. B. Saunders Co.

Jahoda, M. 1958. *Current concepts of positive mental health.* New York: Basic Books.

Kalish, R. A. 1977. *The psychology of human behavior.* 4th ed. Belmont, Calif.: Wadsworth Publishing Co.

Maslow, A. H. 1968. *Toward a psychology of being.* 2nd ed. New York: Van Nostrand Reinhold Co.

———. 1970. *Motivation and personality.* 2nd ed. New York: Harper and Row.

Montagu, A. 1975. A scientist looks at love. In Montagu, A., editor. *The practice of love.* Englewood Cliffs, N.J.: Prentice-Hall.

Morgan, A. J., and Moreno, J. W. 1973. *The practice of mental health nursing.* Philadelphia: J. B. Lippincott Co.

Rogers, C. R. 1961. *On becoming a person: A therapist's view of psychotherapy.* Boston: Houghton Mifflin Co.

Rogers, M. E. 1970. *An introduction to the theoretical base of nursing.* Philadelphia: F. A. Davis Co.

Selye, H. 1976. *The stress of life.* Rev. ed. New York: McGraw-Hill Book Co.

———. 1974. *Stress without distress.* Scarborough, Ont.: New American Library of Canada.

Chapter 9

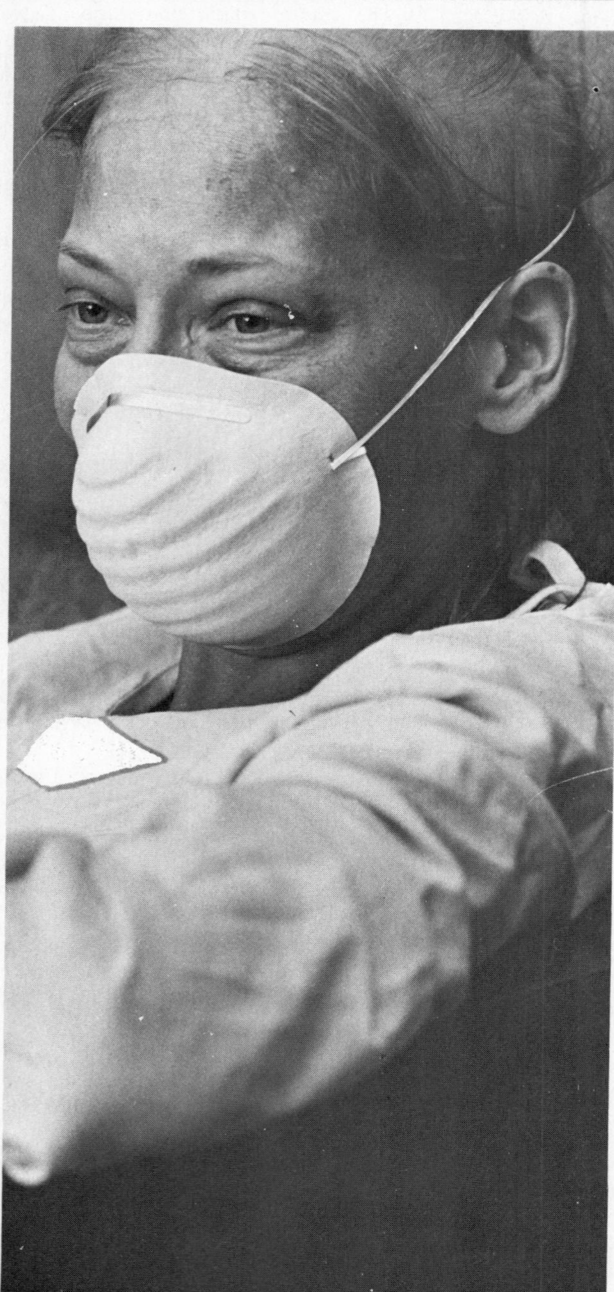

Stress and Adaptation

CONTENTS

Objectives

1. Understand essential terms and facts about stress
   - **1.1** Identify Selye's definition of stress
   - **1.2** Give examples of four variables influencing the degree to which stressors affect individuals
   - **1.3** Identify physiologic signs and symptoms of stress
   - **1.4** Identify psychologic responses to stress
   - **1.5** Identify factors influencing a person's perception of and response to stress
   - **1.6** Contrast long-term and short-term coping methods
   - **1.7** Differentiate stress from crisis
   - **1.8** Identify two types of crises
2. Understand essential facts related to adaptation
   - **2.1** Differentiate the general adaptation syndrome from the local adaptation syndrome
   - **2.2** Explain Selye's three stages of the stress adaptation syndrome
   - **2.3** Identify the body's physiologic responses associated with the general adaptation syndrome
   - **2.4** Identify tissue responses that occur in the inflammatory process
   - **2.5** Identify five types of inflammatory exudates and give examples of each
   - **2.6** Differentiate between the healing processes of regeneration and replacement with fibrous tissue
   - **2.7** Identify factors that promote tissue healing
   - **2.8** Differentiate between natural and acquired types of immunity
   - **2.9** Identify the five types of antibodies and specify their known functions
   - **2.10** Identify the four divisions of acquired immunity in terms of their antigen-antibody sources and the durations of immunity attained
   - **2.11** Identify mental defense mechanisms
3. Understand essential facts about stress and crisis assessment and intervention
   - **3.1** Identify ways the nurse can assist a person to adapt to stress
   - **3.2** Identify seven sources of support required by people
   - **3.3** Identify the four phases of crisis development
   - **3.4** Identify thoughts, feelings, and behavior indicating that a person is in a crisis state
   - **3.5** Identify essential components of an assessment interview
   - **3.6** Identify one technique used by the nurse to help people in crisis

Terms

adaptation
anaphylactic shock
antibody
antigen
antisera (immune sera)
anxiety
autoantigen
chemotaxis
cicatrix
compensation
conversion
crisis
denial
diapedesis
displacement
exudate
fantasy
fear
fibrinous exudate
general adaptation syndrome (GAS)
granulation tissue
hyperemia
identification
immunity
immunoglobulin
inflammation
introjection
leukocytosis
local adaptation syndrome (LAS)
mental defense mechanism
parenchyma
phagocytosis
projection
purulent exudate
pyogenic bacteria
rationalization
reaction formation
regeneration
regression
repression
restitution
sanguineous exudate
serous exudate
stress
stressor
stroma
sublimation
substitution
suppression
suppuration
symbolization
toxoid
vaccine

In recent years *stress* has become a household word. Parents refer to the stress of raising children, working people to the stress of their jobs. In fact, the 1970s have been described as the decade of stress. Familiarity with this word is largely due to the publications of Hans Selye (1974, 1976), whose books are widely read.

The concept of stress is important because it provides a way of understanding the person as a unified being who responds in totality (mind and body) to a variety of changes that take place in daily life. Stress is a universal phenomenon. All people experience it.

Homeostasis refers to conditions of the body that constantly vary and yet maintain stability. As a person encounters any stress, various systems of the body are brought into play in order to adjust and maintain homeostasis.

Adaptation means adjustment. In the sense that it is used in this chapter, it refers to adjustment to stress. People adapt on a number of levels, physiologically, mentally, and emotionally. The concepts of stress and adaptation are explored in this chapter.

Stress

Definitions

Stress has been defined by Hans Selye (1976:1) as "the non-specific response of the body to any kind of demand made upon it." Selye had made a number of observations about disease that resulted in his concept of stress. First he noted that, although there were characteristic or different signs and symptoms of numerous diseases, they all had many signs and symptoms in common (there appeared to be a specific syndrome), which he called *stress*. Also, there was no common cause (they were nonspecifically induced). To differentiate the cause of stress from the response to stress, Selye created the term *stressor* (1976:51). A stressor is any factor that produces stress; that is, it is a factor that disturbs the body's equilibrium.

Because stress is a state of the body, it can be observed only by the changes it produces in the body. This response of the body, the *stress syndrome*, causes certain changes in the structure and chemical composition of the body. Some of these changes are signs of change; others are signs of the body's adaptive (defense) reactions against stress. See the general adaptation syndrome and local adaptation syndrome discussed subsequently. Selye further concluded that these common signs of stress are a part of every disease process.

Some contemporary physiologists use the terms *stress* and *stressor* as Selye did. Others use the term *stress* to mean any stimulus that causes the neurons in the hypothalamus of the brain to release corticotropin-releasing hormone (CRH). This hormone stimulates the many changes in the body that are described later in this chapter.

Body Response to Stress

Selye referred to the response of the body to stress as the *stress syndrome* or *general adaptation syndrome* (GAS). This is a general response of the body, created by the release of certain adaptive hormones within the person's body. See the section on the GAS later in this chapter. The GAS, Selye found, occurred whenever an organism underwent prolonged stress. Body organs affected by stress are the gastrointestinal tract, the adrenals, and the lymphatic structures. The adrenals enlarged considerably, the lymphatic structures, such as the thymus, spleen, and lymph nodes, atrophied (shrank), and deep ulcers appeared in the lining of the stomach. In addition to a general adaptation syndrome, that is, generalized manifestations of stress, it was also proposed that the body can react by a local response. One organ or a part of the body can react alone. This is referred to as the *local adaptation syndrome*, or LAS. One example of the LAS is inflammation. See Inflammatory Adaptive Response later in this chapter.

Stress is necessary for both life and growth; that is, it is necessary for the human body constantly to adapt to its environment in order to survive. The state of stress, however, is intensified when a person is required to change activity or to increase the pace of activity in order to adapt. This process of adapting is frequently referred to as *coping*.

Stages of GAS and LAS

Selye proposed that both the GAS and the LAS had three stages (1976:38): (a) alarm reaction, (b) stage of resistance, and (c) stage of exhaustion. See Figure 9-1.

Alarm reaction (AR)

The initial reaction of the body is the alarm reaction, which alerts the body's defenses against the stressor, whether the stressor is heat, bacteria, or a verbal or physical attack from someone. The defenses of the whole body are mobilized and prepared to act to protect the body. This stage Selye divided into two parts: the shock phase and the countershock phase.

During the *shock phase*, the stressor may be perceived consciously or unconsciously by the person. In any case the autonomic nervous system reacts, and large amounts of epinephrine (adrenaline) and cortisone are released into the body. The person is then ready for fight-or-flight. This primary response is short lived, lasting from 1 minute to 24 hours.

The second part of the alarm reaction is called the *countershock phase*. During this time the body changes produced during the shock phase are reversed. It is, therefore, during the shock phase of the alarm reaction that a person is best mobilized to react.

Stage of resistance (SR)

During the second stage in the GAS and LAS syndromes, the body's adaptation takes place. In other words, the body attempts to cope with the stressor and to limit the stressor to the smallest area of the body that can deal with it. See pages 187–89.

Stage of exhaustion (SE)

During the third stage, the adaptation that the body made during the second stage cannot be maintained. This means that the ways used to cope with the stressor have been exhausted. If adaptation has not overcome the stressor, the stress effects may spread to the entire body. At the end of this stage the body may either rest and return to normal, or death may be the ultimate consequence. The choice of the end of this stage depends largely on the adaptive energy resources of the individual, the severity of the stressor, and the external adaptive resources that are provided, such as oxygen administered by mask.

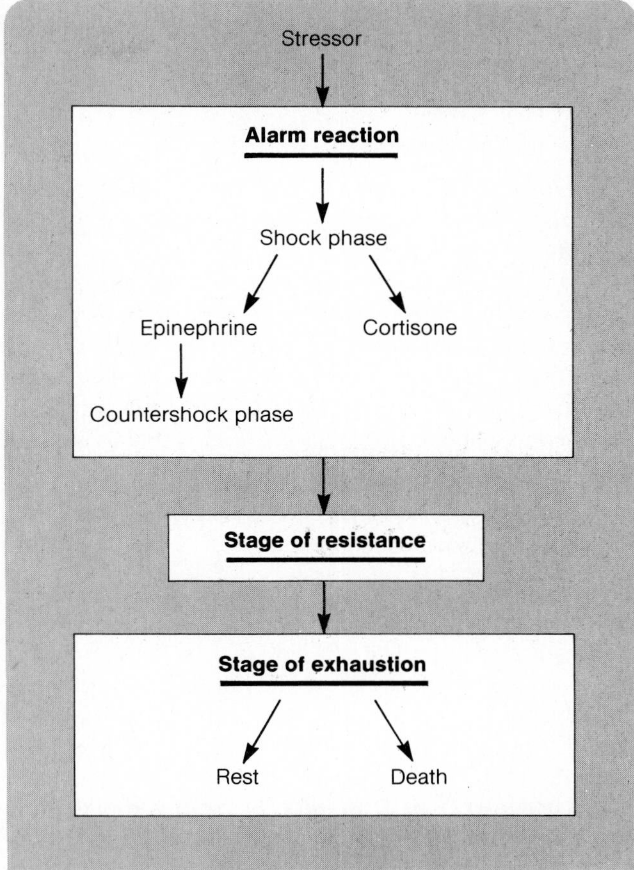

Figure 9–1 The three stages of adaptation to stress: the alarm reaction, the stage of resistance, and the stage of exhaustion.

Psychologic Response to Stress

The reaction to stressors described by Selye referred particularly to the physiologic processes of the body in reaction to acute stressors. However, adaptation can be psychologic as well as physiologic. Physiologic adaptation refers to changes in the body. Physiologic stressors either change or threaten to change the physiologic balance of the body. Psychologic adaptation refers to mental processes and behavior patterns, called *mental defense, adaptive,* or *coping mechanisms,* that are used daily to adapt to life's situations. These processes and mechanisms protect a person's self-esteem and sense of security. Just as the body's biochemical and physical processes maintain a physiologic equilibrium or homeostasis, the personality endeavors through automatic and unconscious processes to maintain psychologic stability. See the discussion of these mechanisms later in this chapter.

Stressors

Types of Stressors

Stressors are found in the internal environment (within the body) and in the external environment (outside the body). An example of a stressor within the body is a tumor of the stomach; an example of a stressor outside the body is an angry remark from a friend.

Stressors can be physiologic or psychologic. Examples of physiologic stressors are a knife wound, an overdose of heroin, and the influenza virus. Psychologic stressors include an alcoholic spouse, fear of an operation, or grief over the death of a loved one.

Factors Influencing the Effects of Stressors

The degree to which a stressor affects an individual depends on:

1. The nature of the stressor
2. The number of stressors to be coped with at one time

3. The duration of exposure to the stressor
4. Experience with a comparable stressor (Byrne 1978:73)

Nature of the stressor

The nature of the stressor has two components: (a) what the stressor means to the person, and (b) the magnitude of the stressor.

To one person an inoculation with smallpox vaccine produces a high state of stress, but for another the injection is not a stressor. The magnitude of the stressor also affects the person's response. The pain from a cut on a finger may elicit little stress, whereas the pain of an inflamed appendix produces a much greater state of stress.

Number of stressors at once

The number of stressors a person is coping with at one time can greatly affect the response. This often explains why a stressor that the nurse considers small can elicit a disproportionate response. For example, a patient in the hospital who is coping with separation from her family, the unknown outcome of her illness, and financial problems, can react angrily when the nurse brings her the wrong fruit juice. Normally, this woman would not be upset whichever juice was served; however, she is using up her coping energies on the other problems and has little left to adapt to this incident. This example also shows how a state of high stress can become a stressor itself. A patient who reacts angrily feels more stress because of this reaction. Another example is the student who is highly anxious (stressed) about an examination, and then gets a cold, an illness he rarely has and would not likely have acquired if he had not been in such a state of stress.

Duration of exposure to the stressor

Prolonged exposure to the stressor can reduce a person's ability to cope. Resistance to a stressor is low during the stage of alarm, becomes higher during the resistance stage, when the coping mechanisms are brought into action, and then drops below normal during the stage of exhaustion. Therefore, if a person's stage of resistance is extended by the duration of the stressor beyond the person's coping powers, he or she becomes exhausted and can eventually die. An example of this is a patient who is admitted to a hospital with a fractured femur. The patient survives the surgery and is healing well when he develops an acute pain in his gallbladder, necessitating another operation. By this time the patient's energy reserves have been used up, and, although the operation was successful, the patient develops an infection that delays his return home.

Experience with a comparable stressor

Experiences with a comparable stressor can be particularly significant for patients entering a hospital. For some people, contact with hospitals has been related solely to dying friends and relatives. To such patients the act of entering the hospital is particularly stressful, as they worry about whether they will die. The patients' worries in this case are completely unrelated to the reason for admission.

Ratings of Stressors

Ratings or units of stress have been applied to changes in life situations. See Table 9–1. The degree of stress a person experiences can be determined to some extent by the readjustment required for certain situations or life events.

General Adaptation Syndrome

The general adaptation syndrome encompasses a range of physiologic responses to stressors in the body as a whole. See Figure 9–2. A stressor stimulates the hypothalamus either directly or indirectly. Indirect stimulation occurs through the limbic lobe and other parts of the cerebral cortex, which in turn send impulses to the hypothalamus. For example, hypoglycemia (low blood sugar) directly stimulates the hypothalamus, while an angry dog jumping toward a person stimulates the limbic lobe or "emotional brain" and other parts of the cerebral cortex as the individual becomes fearful; these regions then send impulses to the hypothalamus. When stimulated either directly or indirectly, the hypothalamus has three main actions:

1. It releases corticotropin-releasing hormone (CRH).
2. It stimulates the sympathetic nervous system centers and the adrenal medulla.
3. It stimulates the posterior pituitary gland.

The CRH that is released then stimulates the anterior pituitary gland to release increased amounts of adrenocorticotropic hormone (ACTH). The ACTH in turn stimulates the adrenal cortex to markedly increase the release of cortisol and moderately increase the release of aldosterone. These two hormones account for some of a person's stress responses. Cortisol has the following actions, which are of particular value when there is tissue trauma:

Table 9–1 Stress Units for Life Events

Life event	Stress units (mean value)	Life event	Stress units (mean value)
Family constellation		*Individual changes*	
Death of spouse	100	Jail term	63
Divorce	73	Personal injury or illness	53
Separation	65	Death of close friend	37
Death of close family member	63	Outstanding personal achievement	28
Marriage	50	Revision of personal habits	24
Marital reconciliation	45	Minor violation of law	11
Change in family member's health	44		
Pregnancy	40	*Employment and/or school*	
Gain new member to family	39	Fired at work	47
Sexual difficulties	39	Retirement	45
Arguments with spouse	35	Business readjustment	39
Children leaving home	29	Change in job	36
Trouble with in-laws	29	Change in work responsibility	
Change in living conditions	25	(promotion or demotion)	29
Move or change in residence	20	Spouse begins or stops work	26
Change in schools, recreation, and		Begin or end school	26
church activities	20	Trouble with boss	23
Change in social activities	19		
Change in sleeping habits	16	*Financial*	
Change in number of family get-		Change in financial status	38
togethers	15	Mortgage or loan over $10,000	31
Change in eating habits	15	Foreclosure	30
Vacation	13	Mortgage or loan under $10,000	17
Holiday	12		

Suggested Score Interpretation

150–199	Mild stress: 37% of population will become ill.
200–299	Medium stress: 51% of population will become ill in two weeks.
300 and over	High stress: 79% of population will become physically ill soon.

From Ann Wolbert Burgess and Aaron Lazare, *Community mental health: Target populations* (Englewood Cliffs, N.J.: Prentice-Hall, 1976), p. 59. © 1976. Reprinted by permission of Prentice-Hall, Inc. Originally from R. H. Rahe, *Life crisis and health changes.* Report no. 67–4 (San Diego, Calif.: Navy Medical Neuropsychiatric Research Unit, 1967).

1. *Gluconeogenesis.* It forms glucose from protein and fat compounds, making energy readily available.
2. *Protein mobilization.* It causes the liver to form new proteins that can be used by damaged tissues.
3. *Fat mobilization.* It mobilizes fat to make energy available and to synthesize other compounds needed by the body.
4. *Stabilization of lysosomal membranes.* Lysosomes are the parts of a cell that contain enzymes and thus dissolve or digest most cellular compounds. When cells are damaged and the lysosome membranes are ruptured, the released enzymes cause an inflammatory response. Therefore by strengthening or stabilizing the lysosome membrane, cortisol reduces inflammation.

Aldosterone is chiefly concerned with the excretion of potassium and absorption of sodium in the kidney tubules. When excessive amounts of aldosterone are secreted, sodium is reabsorbed into the extracellular fluid of the body along with water. This adaptive mechanism conserves water for the body and maintains the blood volume.

Impulses from the hypothalamus also travel to the sympathetic nervous system centers and the adrenal medulla. The adrenal medulla secretes epinephrine and norepinephrine in response to sympathetic stimulation. These hormones act similarly to direct stimulation of the sympathetic nervous system, a reaction that has been termed the *fight-or-flight syndrome* because the body becomes ready for action as a result. Significant body's response include:

1. Increased arterial blood pressure
2. Increased blood flow to active muscles

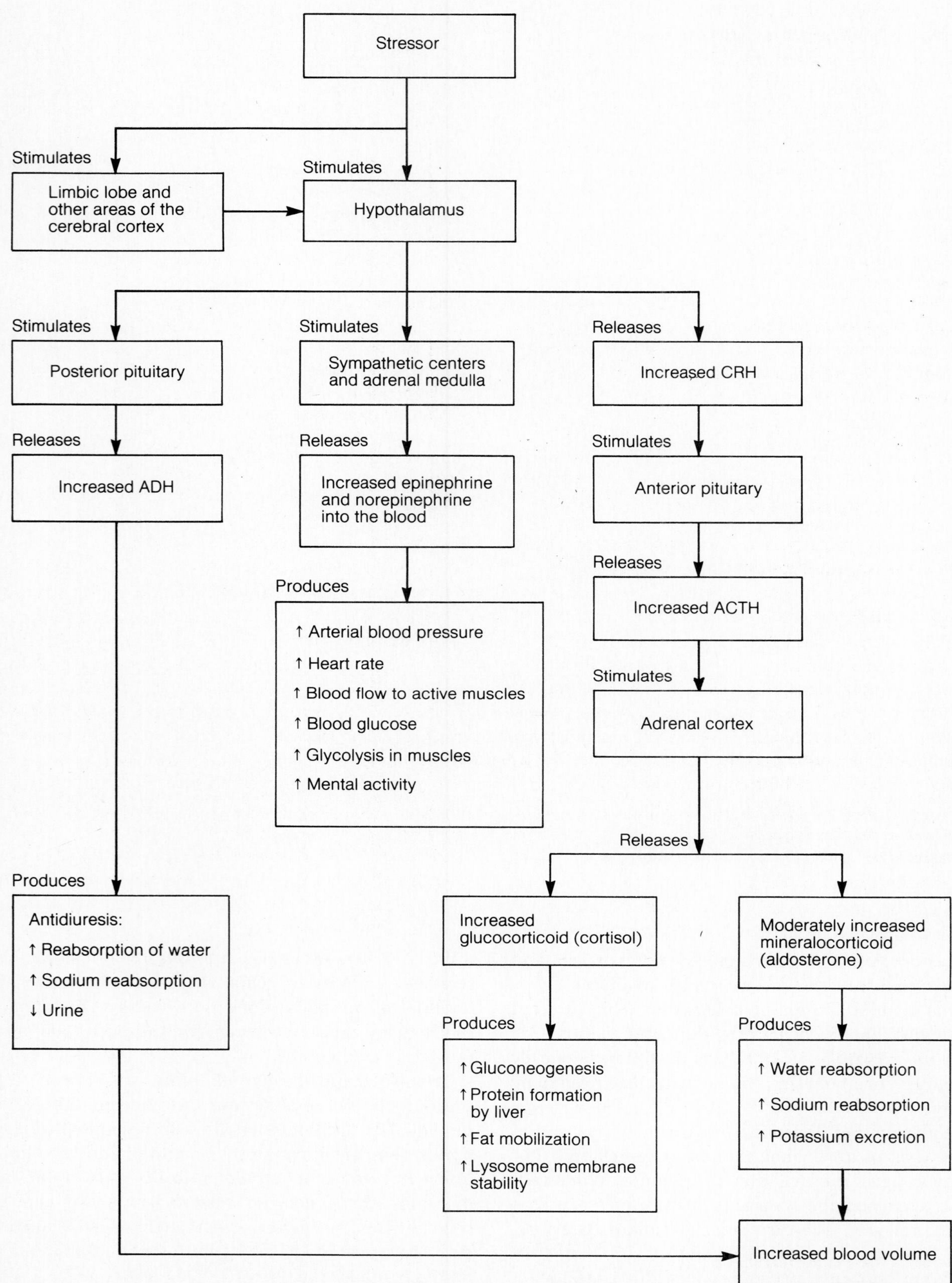

Figure 9–2 Current concepts about the body's reaction to stress.

3. Increased cellular metabolism
4. Increased blood glucose concentration
5. Increased glycolysis in muscles
6. Increased muscle strength
7. Increased mental activity (Guyton 1982:445)

Finally, impulses from the hypothalamus stimulate the posterior pituitary gland, resulting in an increased secretion of antidiuretic hormone (ADH). This in turn causes increased reabsorption of water and sodium in the kidney tubules and increased potassium excretion. The overall effects in the body from increased secretions of ADH and aldosterone are fluid retention and an increased blood volume. See Figure 9–2.

Local Adaptation Syndrome

In addition to the GAS, a large number of localized physiologic responses to stressors occur. Two of these, the inflammatory adaptive response and the immunologic adaptive response, are discussed in this chapter, while others are integrated throughout the book in discussions of specific body parts or systems or particular stressors (disease processes or trauma).

Inflammatory Adaptive Response

Inflammation is the response of the tissues of the body to injury. It is an adaptive mechanism invoked to destroy or dilute the injurious agent, to prevent further spread of the injury, and to promote repair of damaged tissue. It is characterized by five signs: pain, swelling, redness, heat, and impaired function of the part. Commonly, conditions with the suffix *-itis* refer to an inflammatory process. For example, appendicitis means inflammation of the appendix; gastritis means inflammation of the stomach. Inflammation is a local reaction and is an example of Selye's local adaptation syndrome.

Injurious stressors (inflammants) to body tissues can be categorized as physical agents, chemical agents, and microorganisms. Physical agents include mechanical objects causing trauma to tissues, excessive heat or cold (causing burn or frostbite), and radiation. Chemical agents include external irritants, such as strong acids, alkalis, poisons, and irritating gases, and internal irritants (substances manufactured within the body), such as excessive hydrochloric acid in the stomach due to altered function. Microorganisms include the broad groups of bacteria, viruses, fungi, protozoa, and rickettsiae.

The inflammatory response involves a series of dynamic events, or defenses of the tissues:

1. Cellular and vascular changes
2. Formation of inflammatory exudate
3. Repair of tissues

Cellular and vascular changes

In the first stage, constriction of the blood vessels occurs at the site of injury, lasting only a few moments. This momentary response is followed by (a) dilation of small blood vessels, (b) increased permeability of the blood vessel walls, (c) slowing of blood flow, and (d) mobilization of leukocytes.

Dilation of small local blood vessels occurs as a result of histamine released by the injured cells. Thus, more blood flows to the injured area, bringing with it large numbers of leukocytes. This marked increase in blood supply is referred to as *hyperemia* and is responsible for the characteristic signs of redness and heat.

Vascular permeability is increased simultaneously at the injured site. This is thought to occur in response to tissue necrosis, the release of chemical mediators called *kinins*, such as bradykinin, and the release of histamine. The result of this altered permeability is an outpouring of fluid, proteins, and leukocytes into the interstitial spaces. This stage is responsible for the characteristic sign of swelling (edema) and is in part responsible for the associated pain of inflammation, since pressure is created on nerve endings. Too much fluid pouring into areas such as the pleural or pericardial cavity can seriously affect organ function. In other areas, such as joints, mobility is impaired.

Slowing of blood flow occurs in the dilated vessels. This altered rate of flow facilitates the mobilization of leukocytes and their movement into the tissue spaces along with other substances.

Mobilization of leukocytes includes the two processes of margination and emigration. Normally blood cells (erythrocytes, leukocytes, and platelets) flow along the center of a blood vessel, while a cell-less stream of plasma flows around them against the walls of the blood vessel. When the blood flow slows, leukocytes aggregate or line up along this inner surface of the blood vessels. This process is known as *margination*. Leukocytes then move through the blood vessel wall into the affected tissue spaces, a process called *emigration*. The actual passage of blood corpuscles through the blood vessel wall is referred to as *diapedesis*. The reason leukocytes are attracted to injured tissue has been described by the term *positive chemotaxis*. The action of chemotaxis is not fully understood, but basically cells are drawn toward the source of chemicals released in the tissues (positive chemotaxis), or they are propelled away from the chemical (negative chemotaxis). Leukotaxine released by injured cells is thought to have positive chemotaxic properties.

In response to the exit of leukocytes from the blood vessels, the bone marrow produces large numbers of leukocytes and releases them into the bloodstream (*leukocytosis*). The exact mechanism stimulating this increase is unknown, but it is another cardinal sign of inflammation. A normal leukocyte count of 7,000 to 10,000 per cubic millimeter of blood can rise to 20,000 or more.

Having gained entrance to the tissue spaces, the leukocytes attack the injurious agent by the process of *phagocytosis*. Macrophages (reticuloendothelial cells) present in the tissue spaces assist the leukocytes in phagocytosis. Antibodies from plasma also come to the site. Their function is discussed in more detail later in this chapter. In terms of the inflammatory response, antibodies can make the inflammant more susceptible to phagocytosis.

Formation of the inflammatory exudate

In the second stage of inflammation, fluid and substances that escape from the blood vessels, as well as dead tissue cells and products that they release, produce the inflammatory *exudate*. A plasma protein called *fibrinogen* (activated by necrosin), thromboplastin, a product released from injured tissue cells, and platelets together form an interlacing network of fibrin or a clot. This fibrin mesh or clot walls off the area in an attempt to localize the inflammation. It also provides the framework for the reparative stage.

During the second stage, the injurious agent is overcome and the exudate cleared away by lymphatic drainage. When this is achieved, the reparative (third phase) begins.

Types of exudate

The nature and amount of exudate vary in accordance with the tissue involved and the intensity and duration of the inflammation. The major types of exudate are serous, catarrhal, purulent, fibrinous, and hemorrhagic (sanguineous).

A *serous exudate* is comprised chiefly of serum derived from the blood and serous membranes of the body, such as the peritoneum, pleura, pericardium, and meninges. It is watery in appearance, has few cells, and contains little or no fibrin. An example is the fluid in a blister from a burn.

Catarrhal exudate is a term formerly used to describe the inflammatory discharge of mucous membranes such as the nasopharynx or intestines. A well-known example is the fluid that runs from the nose in the common cold. This exudate is similar in appearance to serous exudate but it also contains mucus.

Purulent exudate is a thicker fluid than the serous exudate due to the presence of pus. It consists of leukocytes, liquefied dead tissue debris, and dead and living bacteria. The process of pus formation is referred to as *suppuration*, and bacteria that produce pus are called *pyogenic bacteria*. Examples are the exudates of a boil and an abscess. Purulent exudates can differ in color, some acquiring tinges of green or yellow. The colors depend to some degree on the specific causative organism. Formation of pus takes time, so this exudate is not seen in the acute stage of infections. Other inflammatory agents, such as turpentine in subcutaneous tissues, can also support pus formation. Nurses need to be specific about color and consistency when recording the presence of purulent exudates.

A *fibrinous exudate*, as the name denotes, contains large amounts of fibrin. Fibrin is produced when quantities of the large plasma protein fibrinogen combine with the thromboplastin of injured cells and with blood platelets. This type of exudate occurs in severe acute inflammations, indicating sufficient permeability and damage to capillaries to allow the escape of the large protein molecule. Excessive amounts of fibrin may form sticky membranous coatings on tissue surfaces, causing them to adhere. This is the beginning of the formation of adhesions, which most frequently develop on serous surfaces of the pleura and peritoneal membranes of the intestines.

Another term for *hemorrhagic exudate* is *sanguineous exudate*. It consists of large amounts of red blood cells, indicating damage to capillaries that is severe enough to allow the escape of red blood cells from plasma. This type of exudate is frequently seen in surgical incisions, bruises, and open wounds. Nurses often need to distinguish whether the sanguineous exudate is dark or bright. For example, a bright sanguineous exudate from a surgical incision indicates fresh bleeding and trauma, whereas dark sanguineous exudate can denote smaller and older trauma.

Nurses often observe mixed types of exudates. For example, a mucopurulent exudate can occur from the upper respiratory tract, indicating the presence of excessive mucus and pus. It is more purulent than a catarrhal exudate. A serosanguineous exudate is also commonly seen in surgical incisions and denotes serous and sanguineous exudate.

Repair of tissues (healing)

Injured tissues can be repaired by (a) regeneration or (b) replacement with fibrous tissue (scar) formation.

Regeneration is the replacement of destroyed tissue cells by cells that are identical or similar in structure and function. It involves not only replacement of damaged cells one by one but also organization of these cells so that the architectural pattern of the tissue and function are restored.

The *stroma* is the tissue that forms the framework (connective tissue) or ground substance of an organ. The *parenchyma* is a term for the essential functional elements of an organ. Functional cells must have proper relationships between stroma and parenchyma, and among their blood vessels, lymph vessels, nerves, and ducts. All must regenerate concurrently. If one component lags behind the others, a normal product will not be formed. The villain of this scenario, fibrous (scar) tissue, frequently wins, since it has the capacity to proliferate under the unusual conditions of ischemia and altered pH.

The ability to reproduce cells varies considerably from one type of tissue to another. For example, epithelial tissues of the skin and of the digestive and respiratory tracts have a good regenerative capacity, provided that their underlying support structures are intact. The same holds true for osseous, lymphoid, and bone marrow tissues. Tissues that have little regenerative capacity include nervous, muscular, and elastic tissues. These are highly specialized tissues that cannot be replaced by identically organized cells, but rather are replaced by scar tissue. Unfortunate examples are the damage to the brain from a stroke and the damage to the heart muscle from a cardiac incident. These tissues cannot be replaced.

When regeneration is not possible, repair occurs by *fibrous tissue formation*. The inflammatory exudate with its interlacing network of fibrin provides the framework for this tissue to develop. Damaged tissues are replaced with the connective tissue elements of collagen, blood capillaries, lymphatics, and other tissue ground substances. In the early stages of this process, the tissue is called *granulation tissue*. It is a fragile, gelatinous tissue, appearing pink or red because of the many newly formed capillaries. Later in the process, the tissue shrinks (the capillaries are constricted, even obliterated) and the collagen fibers contract, so that a firmer fibrous tissue remains. This is called a *cicatrix* or scar.

Although scar tissue has the positive attribute of repairing the injured area, it also can present problems. It can reduce the functional capacity of the tissue or organ. For example, scar tissue in cardiac muscle renders that area weaker. Mechanical obstructions can also arise, for example, in the healing of a duodenal ulcer. Sometimes the pyloric sphincter becomes stenosed as granulation tissue contracts into scar tissue.

Factors that favor tissue healing

1. *Minimum of injury.* The less the injury, in terms of both extent and time, the more rapid is the healing process. If few cells and blood vessels are damaged, for example, less time is required to replace the destroyed tissue.

2. *Adequate blood supply.* Because blood provides the needed products for healing, any factor restricting blood flow to the injured area hinders the healing process. Damaged or occluded arteries and restrictive bandages can inhibit blood flow. The presence of gross edema can also hinder the transport of substances in the tissue spaces.

3. *Good nutritional status.* Protein and vitamin C are the nutrients principally involved in healing of wounds. Protein is essential for the formation of new tissue. Vitamin C is thought to be necessary for the maturation of collagen fibers in the later stages of healing.

4. *Youth.* Healing is more rapid in young people than in the elderly.

5. *Absence of other stressors.* The presence of infection, foreign bodies, diabetes, or other stressors can delay healing. Radiation is said to slow the healing process after five to six days of radiation treatments.

6. *Adequate immune mechanisms.* For injuries that are induced by bacteria, the presence of appropriate immune mechanisms, facilitating phagocytosis and clearing of debris in the exudative phase, will hasten the healing process.

7. *Balance of adrenocortical hormones.* According to Selye, proinflammatory and antiinflammatory hormones exist. The latter are the glucocorticoids. An excess of these hormones inhibits inflammation, thereby slowing the healing process. Cortisone is thought to decrease the formation of collagen fibers.

Immunologic Adaptive Response

The immune response is a more specific response of the body than the inflammatory response. It is a response to foreign protein materials in the body, such as bacteria or tissues of another person, or, in some situations, even the body's own proteins. Foreign proteins in the body are called *antigens* and are considered invaders. If the proteins originate in a person's own body, the antigen is referred to as an *autoantigen*. Protective substances produced in the body to counteract antigens are called *antibodies*. They are highly specific molecules produced in response to contact with antigens. Antibodies are said to be highly specific because an antibody that is formed against a particular antigen will generally react only with that antigen.

Antibodies (immunoglobulins)

Antibodies are also referred to as *immune bodies* or *immunoglobulins*. They are part of the body's plasma proteins, specifically the gamma globulins. Laboratory methods (electrophoresis) have isolated five immunoglobulins, designated by the letters G, A, M, D, and E,

Table 9–2 Antibodies and Their Functions

Antibody	Function
IgG	Has antiviral, antitoxic, and some antibacterial actions; it is the only antibody to cross the placental barrier
IgA	Protects the mucous membranes of the gastrointestinal and respiratory tracts; found in tears, saliva, colostrum, and intestinal and bronchial secretions
IgM	Serves as A, B, and O blood groups' isoantibodies and antibodies to gram-negative microorganisms
IgD	Unknown
IgE	Combats allergic and anaphylactic responses

Table 9–3 Types of Acquired Immunity

Type	Antigen or antibody source	Duration
1. Active	Antibodies are produced by the body in response to infection	Long
a. Natural	Antibodies are formed in the presence of active infection in the body	Lifelong
b. Artificial	Antigens (vaccines or toxoids) are administered to the person to stimulate antibody production	Many years; the immunity must be reinforced by booster inoculations
2. Passive	Antibodies are produced by another source, animal or human	Short
a. Natural	Antibodies are transferred naturally from an immune mother to her baby through the placenta or in colostrum	6 months to 1 year
b. Artificial	Immune serum (antibody) from an animal or another human is injected	2 to 3 weeks

and usually written: IgG, IgA, IgM, IgD, and IgE. Each of the five has a unique structure and function. (See Table 9–2.) IgG is the most abundant immunoglobulin, constituting about 75% of the immunoglobulins in plasma. IgA and IgM constitute about 25%, and IgD and IgE comprise less than 1%.

Sources of antibodies

The major cells producing antibodies are called *plasma cells.* They are located in lymphoid tissue chiefly in the lymph nodes and the spleen. Recent research has found that the thymus gland produces most of the antibody-forming cells and thus is an important component of the immune mechanism.

Immunity

Immunity is the specific resistance of the body to infection (pathogens or their toxins). There are two major types of immunity, natural and acquired.

Natural immunity is inherited resistance to infection. It is inborn and ready made. This type of immunity may occur at the individual, species, and racial levels. Some species are more resistant than others to specific pathogens. Humans, for instance, are resistant to distemper virus, a morbid invader for cats and dogs. Racial differences also exist. For example, black people have more resistance to malaria than do white people. Even at the individual level, observations indicate that some persons are more resistant to certain infections than other persons.

Acquired immunity occurs only after a person has been exposed to a disease agent. It can be an active or passive process of the body, and in either case it may be naturally or artificially induced. See Figure 9–3. Thus there are four divisions of acquired immunity. See Table 9–3.

Active immunity

Active immunity results when a person (the host) produces his or her own antibodies in response to microorganisms or their toxins in the body. It takes time to develop and usually provides permanent or lifelong immunity.

In *naturally acquired immunity*, antibodies are actively produced within the body in response to an active infection, such as scarlet fever or chickenpox. The infectious process may be so mild (subclinical) that it goes unrecognized by the person, yet a specific active immunity results.

Artificially acquired immunity occurs when antigens are intentionally administered to the host by artificial means. The body actively produces antibodies in response to this stimulus. Antigens are administered in the form of vaccines or toxoids.

Vaccines are composed of living organisms (live vaccine), or dead organisms (killed vaccine). The use of live vaccine imitates nature's way of producing immunity. When the vaccine is administered, a very mild or subclinical infection is produced, which stimulates active antibody production. Some of these live vaccines are attenuated (weakened), that is, exposed to unnatural growth conditions in order to render them less virulent. Examples of attenuated vaccines are the Sabin polio and BCG (tuberculosis) vaccines.

Dead suspensions, or killed vaccines, are produced by subjecting virulent bacteria or viruses to an excess of heat, ultraviolet light, or certain chemicals such as phenol, formaldehyde, or alcohol. The most common types of bacterial vaccines used are those for typhoid and whooping cough. Two of the best-known viral vaccines are the Salk vaccine for poliomyelitis and the influenza vaccines.

In contrast to live and killed vaccines, *toxoids* do not use microorganisms, living or dead, but rather neutralized toxins produced by the bacteria. In some diseases the primary damage to the body is caused not by the bacteria themselves but by the exotoxins they produce. Examples are diphtheria and tetanus. Because these toxins are highly toxic, they are usually altered or inactivated by heat or chemicals before being administered to the body to induce immunity. The resulting product is called a *toxoid.*

Active immunity that is artificially acquired is not as lasting as active immunity that is naturally acquired. After a period of time, antibody levels in the plasma drop. This is why booster inoculations are required. For recommended routine immunization schedules, see Tables 22–5 and 22–6.

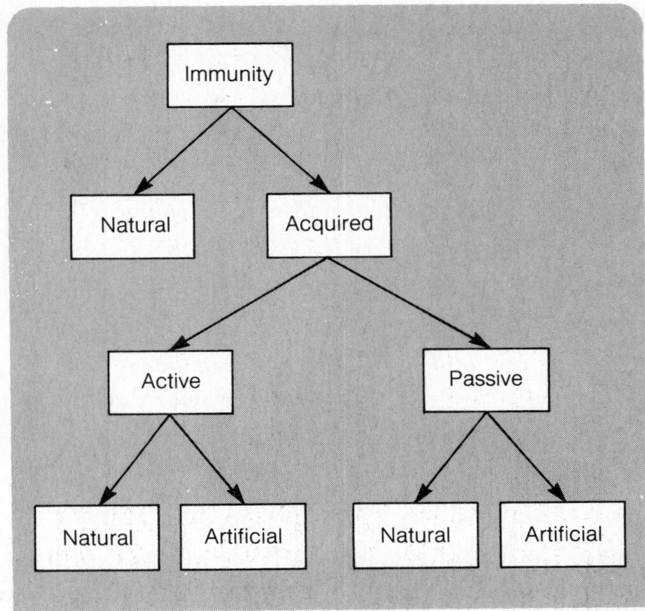

Figure 9–3 Types of immunity.

Passive immunity

Passive immunity occurs when a person receives antibodies that have been produced in the bodies of other animals or persons. Occasionally people contract diseases such as tetanus and diphtheria or are poisoned by snake bites that require immediate lifesaving responses in the form of ready-made antibodies. There is no time for the person to develop antibodies; this person must receive prepared antibodies before too much damage occurs. In other situations, a person may not be ill but has been exposed to an infectious disease and needs existing antibodies to prevent its effects before active immunity develops.

Naturally acquired passive immunity involves the diffusion of antibodies from a mother's blood across the placenta into the circulation of her unborn child. IgG molecules are small enough to pass through placental walls. Colostrum (the forerunner of breast milk) is very high in IgA and may also be significant in providing passive immunity. The infant's body is capable of producing antibodies, but less effectively than that of an older child or adult. Its chief source of antibodies is the mother, and they are transferred primarily during the third trimester of pregnancy. This type of immunity is variable; it may last 4 to 8 months against viruses and 4 to 8 weeks against some bacteria.

Artificially acquired passive immunity is achieved when antibodies produced in other humans or animals are administered to a person. Again, since the body does not participate in the antibody production, this type of immunity is short lived (2 to 3 weeks). Antibodies that are administered artificially are referred to as *immune sera* or *antisera.*

Common antisera are those against diphtheria, tetanus, gas gangrene, rabies, and botulism. Human gamma globulin is occasionally administered for the treatment of measles, hepatitis, and poliomyelitis.

Although the antisera used in passive immunity have the advantage of providing an immediate immune response, they have the potential disadvantage of producing hypersensitive reactions or allergies. Because the antisera frequently are of animal origin and are proteins, they can act as foreign material (antigens), stimulating the production of antibodies in a recipient. With subsequent injections, very severe reactions can then occur, referred to as *anaphylactic shock.*

Psychologic Adaptation

Behavioral Processes

A healthy personality requires the development of behavioral processes for adapting to life. Examples of these are communicative and problem-solving behaviors (language and thought processes). These adaptive processes are acquired through learning, as are the mental mechanisms by which the personality attempts to defend itself, enhance itself, mediate among conflicting drives, and allay tensions. Knowledge of these processes and mechanisms and their associated behavior patterns will help nurses better understand the fears and anxieties of people and how best to help patients and others.

Adaptive Mechanisms

Adaptive mechanisms are acquired during development of the personality in an attempt to defend itself, establish compromises among conflicting impulses, and allay inner tensions. A conflict can be thought of as the struggle between two parts of the personality. For example, a girl may want to skip school one day to go to a movie, yet she knows she should go to school.

Conflict produces anxiety. *Anxiety* is a state of tension about impending disaster, or a feeling of helplessness and apprehension about future events. *Fear*, in contrast, is an emotional response to an actual present danger. Once the danger is eliminated, the fear disappears.

During development of the personality, adaptive mechanisms evolve to protect a person from anxiety. These mechanisms are generally employed by the person unconsciously. Even though the mechanisms may seem maladaptive to the nurse, they have probably been employed to control anxiety and thereby maintain psychologic homeostasis. As a result, the nurse should be careful not to interfere with the mechanisms, because, if the patient is without them at that time, the patient's anxiety may be immensely increased. Emotions such as anxiety and anger are discussed in later chapters; this chapter is restricted to a description of the adaptive mechanisms.

Repression

Repression is one of the commonest mental mechanisms used to deal with conflicts. By repression, desires, impulses, thoughts, and strivings that conflict with our self-image or disturb us are put out of consciousness. They cannot be recalled or recognized, and thus we are protected from anxiety.

Experiences that involve guilt, shame, or lowering of self-esteem are most apt to be repressed. For example, a young man was engaged to be married but his fiancee terminated the engagement. The man found this embarrassing and repressed the fact that his fiancee had broken the engagement; instead he believed he had terminated the relationship himself. Another example is a patient who could not control her urine postoperatively. The patient urinated in her bed and felt ashamed and embarrassed. As a result, she completely repressed the incident so that she did not remember it upon leaving the hospital.

Identification

Identification is an important adaptive mechanism in an individual's growth. In identification, a person admires the qualities of significant people and aspires to be like them. A young boy will take over the attitudes and behavior patterns of both parents, but especially his father, whereas a young girl will frequently adopt chiefly those of her mother. Both will also adopt the behavior and attitudes of other people who are significant to them. A teenage patient may change her hairstyle so that it is like the style of a nurse whom she admires. A young boy will swear just as his uncle does. In the developmental context, successive identifications finally evolve into adult individuation, that is, a firm personal identity.

Identification can also be used as wish fulfillment for a person. An example is the person who confesses falsely to a crime; such a confession is generally based upon the person's desire to commit the crime. This mechanism is also used by people with poorly organized personalities who attach themselves to persons in whom they see desirable qualities.

In another sense, identification is projected onto another person. Again unconsciously, a person attributes traits to another person. For example, certain traits of a person might remind a nurse of a disliked relative. The other person is then quite unconsciously disliked, just as the relative is.

Empathy is a healthy form of identification. In this process, the identification is limited and temporary, but it enables one person to feel for and understand the feelings of another.

Reaction formation

Reaction formation is behavior exactly opposite to what the person is feeling. For example, a woman may show great concern for someone toward whom she is actually hostile, or an aggressive person may continually demand his rights, while really defending himself against feelings of insecurity.

Compensation

Compensation is a phenomenon of substituting behavior. Physiologically the body frequently compensates for pathologic conditions; for example, a person with a heart valve stricture will often have a hypertrophied heart muscle. In this case, the heart tries to overcome the blockage and pump blood through the valve by increasing the size of the muscle.

In behavior, people may act in a manner that compensates for some characteristic. For example, the person of short stature may show aggressive, dominating traits, to suggest strength and authority that the person's size does not convey. Extremes in this behavior are called *overcompensation*.

Compensating behavior can be highly commendable socially. For example, a boy who cannot participate in athletics may compensate by studying hard and attaining high grades.

Rationalization

Rationalization is a very common adaptive mechanism; it is designed to maintain a person's self-respect and prevent feelings of guilt. This mechanism provides rational, intellectual reasons for behavior that really has been prompted by unrecognized motives. Allied to rationalization is the sour-grapes mechanism, in which people disparage some goal that in reality they would like to attain. For example, the student who really wanted to be class president states that she wouldn't take the job if it were offered because it is a lot of work and no fun. Another example of rationalization is the patient who comes to the hospital for an operation and states that he is really pleased to be there because he will obtain a good rest.

Substitution

Substitution is a mechanism used to reduce tension when a person is frustrated (blocked from attaining a goal). In substitution, the person chooses alternative goals that are attainable and have comparable gratification. When a student is unable to attain the goal of becoming a physician, for example, she has three choices: (a) to continue to strive for and overcome obstacles to the goal, (b) to avoid the goal or flee from it, or (c) to choose a substitute goal, such as dentistry, if that is an attainable goal for her.

Displacement

Displacement is an anxiety-reducing device. In this mechanism, an emotional feeling is transferred from the actual object to a substitute. Feelings such as love and hate are apt to be displaced. For example, a child's hostility toward a parent is redirected to a teacher because it is too threatening and socially unacceptable to hate a parent. Thus, the child verbalizes hostility toward this teacher, whose negative reactions do not produce as much anxiety in the child.

Restitution

Restitution is a mechanism by which a person relieves guilt by restitutive (restorative) acts. For example, a boy breaks his sister's toy, then feels guilty, and offers to give the sister his prized frog to make up for the broken toy.

Projection

Projection is a mechanism by which a person attributes to others characteristics that the person does not want to admit are his or her own. That is, persons criticize others for traits that they themselves possess. This is frequently seen in daily life; for example, a man may criticize his neighbor for being a terrible gossip when in fact the man himself gossips but is not aware of it.

Symbolization

Symbolization is the use of objects to represent ideas or emotions that may be too painful for a person to express. To the conscious mind, the symbol is not a symbol but is real in itself. Examples might be a woman whose cat is an unconscious symbol of her child who died at birth, or a teenager who wears clothes his mother dislikes, symbolizing rebellion against his mother.

Regression

In *regression* an individual adopts behavior that was comforting earlier in life. One example is a 6-year-old child who starts bedwetting after his mother returns home with a new baby. In this example, the child unconsciously returns to an earlier behavior pattern in order to obtain his mother's attention. Another example is an elderly woman patient in the hospital who becomes more dependent upon the nurse for her needs than is physically warranted. Again, the patient is returning to an earlier level of dependence, which at one time in her life was comforting.

Denial

Denial is a mechanism by which intolerable thoughts, wishes, facts, and deeds are disowned by an unconscious refusal to recognize their existence. An example is a patient who is told he has cancer; he finds this to be an intolerable fact and denies it unconsciously, behaving as if he had never been told.

Sublimation

Sublimation is a mechanism by which the energy of unacceptable impulses is redirected into socially useful goals. The person feels anxiety from these unacceptable needs and impulses, and finds outlets for the energy behind them. The energy is frequently channeled to a vocation, art, music, or other endeavors that provide a richer life for the person and often the social group. Examples might be the physician who devotes all her energies to her practice, when at home she has a husband who is an alcoholic, or a man who devotes most of his time to charitable endeavors, rather than confronting his loneliness at work and at home.

Suppression

Suppression can be considered the opposite of repression. In suppression, a person willfully and consciously puts a thought or feeling out of mind. An example is the man who keeps ignoring a toothache, pushing it out of his mind, because he fears the pain of having a filling.

Introjection

Introjection is the opposite of projection, but it is also an unconscious mechanism. In introjection, a person takes on the character traits of another person. These traits may be desirable or undesirable. Children develop a healthy conscience in this manner by taking in the advice and warnings of parents. On the other hand, if feelings of hatred toward another person are turned inward they can create depression and even lead to suicide.

Conversion

Conversion is the mechanism of transforming (converting) a mental conflict into a physical symptom. Shameful feelings or painful emotions are first repressed and then converted into physical symptoms such as numbness or pain. The resulting physical discomfort is often accepted by the person without much distress. Thus, in reality, the person is punishing himself or herself.

Fantasy

Fantasy is likened to make-believe and daydreams. Wishes and desires are imagined as fulfilled. Imagination makes life more acceptable, and fantasy is helpful when used to determine constructive action and thought. Experiences can be relived, everyday problems solved, and plans for the future made. However, the person who uses fantasy to excess and who retreats from reality is using this mechanism in an unhealthy way.

Assessment of Increased Stress

A person who is experiencing an increased state of stress brought on by any stressor exhibits certain signs and symptoms. The stressors can be physiologic or psychosocial. Regardless of which kind of stressor is affecting the body, it responds in similar ways.

Physiologic Assessment

The following body responses result from increased sympathetic activity due to the secretion of epinephrine:

1. Pupils dilate to increase visual perception when serious threats to the body arise.
2. Sweat production (diaphoresis) is increased to control elevated body heat due to increased metabolism.
3. The heart rate increases, which leads to an increased pulse rate to transport nutrients and by-products of metabolism more efficiently.
4. Skin is pallid due to constriction of peripheral blood vessels, an effect of norepinephrine.
5. Blood pressure is elevated due to constriction of vessels in blood reservoirs such as the skin, kidneys, and most large interior organs.
6. The rate and depth of respirations increase. Epinephrine dilates the bronchioles, assisting hyperventilation.
7. Urinary output is either frequent or decreased. The former is thought to be an automatic nervous response, whereas the latter may be due to the antidiuretic hormone.
8. The mouth may be dry.
9. Peristalsis of the intestines is decreased, resulting in possible constipation and flatus.
10. Mental alertness is improved for serious threats.
11. Muscle tension is increased to prepare for rapid motor activity or defense.

Behavioral (Psychosocial) Assessment

The key to a person's behavioral response is the individual's perception. If a person perceives (a) that an event is harmful or potentially harmful and (b) that the person's skills to cope with the event are inadequate, then stress is experienced.

The psychologic responses to stressors that are manifested clinically are:

1. Reduced intellectual processes
2. Increased self-sensitivity
3. Decreased ability to cope with or master tasks
4. Decreased sense of personal effectiveness

Each of these can be observed by the nurse. It should be remembered, however, that each person has different ways of responding and may manifest only one or more behaviors in a pronounced way.

Reduced intellectual processes

Several alterations in mental processes of the stressed individual have been noted. They can be summarized as (a) decreased ability to use or remember incoming information, (b) reduced ability to think clearly, and (c) difficulty in making decisions. These responses are familiar to all of us. Most people can readily recall their responses to the stress of driving on a busy six-lane freeway. The stress of getting into the appropriate lane for an exit absorbs the driver's thoughts. Any other information offered at that time, such as a companion's joke or a comment about the surrounding scenery, will not be appreciated or used. The same holds true for a student in a sociology class studying for a microbiology exam scheduled for the next period. If the teacher asks the student to answer a question at this time, the response is likely to be "Would you please repeat the question?" or "I don't know the answer" or "I'm sorry, I wasn't listening." Recognizing this reduced ability to use incoming information, some health agencies provide simple, direct statements for patients in written form. Common examples are written information about diagnostic tests, expectations in preparation for surgery, or services provided by the hospital or health agency.

Decision making and the ability to think clearly are also difficult for stressed individuals. Nurses will frequently encounter this with patients. Some may have difficulty deciding what to eat for dinner or how to deal with an alcoholic partner. Others may question whether to keep an illegitimate newborn or delay needed surgery or an annual medical examination.

Increased self-sensitivity

Stress causes an increase in sensitivity to self, both physically and psychologically. The simple act of blushing is a common example. One manifestation the nurse may note is a person's preoccupation with body conditions such as headache or constipation. The latter is often of particular concern to elderly patients. When the sense of self is heightened, perception of the environment is reduced and may even be distorted. This can be seen when a patient expresses feelings of being talked about if he or she sees a group of doctors or nurses conferring at the nursing station, or feels he or she is the last one in a room to receive care by the nurse and expresses resentment about being neglected.

Minor events that would normally be accepted become magnified and out of proportion to the stressed person. Events such as an open window, a medication ten minutes late, or apple pie for dessert when orange sherbert was ordered can produce stress responses of tears, anger, and annoyance. It must be remembered however, that behavior is extremely complex, and the above examples cannot be generalized. Responses are highly individual and must be considered as such. Only by analyzing each situation precisely can the specific reasons for responses be understood.

Decreased ability to cope with responsibilities or to master tasks

Stress alters the ability to mobilize personal resources to cope with responsibilities or to master new tasks. Some of the first responsibilities that are frequently set aside by stressed individuals are social obligations. For example, the student who is moving from home to an apartment and who has several assignments to complete, an examination coming up, and boyfriend or girlfriend problems may not be able to contend with cooking, cleaning, shopping, and visiting friends in the usual manner. Or if social obligations take priority for this student, then the assignment may suffer or little studying may be done for the examination.

The perceived decrease in ability to master tasks is related to some degree to the reduced mental processes already discussed. People having difficulty learning new tasks confront the nurse frequently. For example, the diabetic patient may be too stressed to cope with the task of injecting her own insulin or the colostomy patient may be too upset to learn how to care for his own colostomy. It is important to realize that establishing expectations beyond what a person feels capable of doing will only increase the stress and may well result in failure to achieve the task.

Decreased sense of personal effectiveness

Closely aligned to the difficulties in achieving tasks may be feelings of worthlessness, incompetence, helplessness, bewilderment, or loss. All of these feelings suggest that the person regards himself or herself as ineffective. As a result, often relationships with others deteriorate and family ties become strained. Examples are (a) the young, active mother with anemia who feels tired and irritable and unable to take care of her three preschool children, or (b) the young executive who is barely coping with her work role but feels she is a total failure in her mother and wife roles.

Factors Influencing Stress

How a person perceives and responds to stressors is highly individual. Vulnerability to stressors is largely related to previous learning, stage of development, life events, health, and coping methods.

Previous learning

The early development of an individual, including previous experience with stressors, can influence the response and adaptation to present stressors. Many responses to stressors are learned, often from the family. For example, a child may learn to be afraid of cats because his mother is afraid. Therefore, as an adult he experiences high-level stress when encountering a cat and often responds behaviorally as he learned in childhood. Such stressors are often identifiable, but in some instances the individual may be aware of discomfort or uneasiness without being able to identify the stressor.

Stage of development

Each stage of life has particular vulnerabilities relative to stress. The various stages of childhood present particular stressors and necessitate adaptations for the individual. See Table 11-2 in Chapter 11. These developmental stressors are normally met as challenges for growth, but they may become periods of increased strain and tension without appropriate support. They may also increase a person's vulnerability to other stressors.

Life events

The events in a person's life often are related to level of stress. Table 9-1 indicated some life events and the related stress, measured in life change units. It must be remembered that the degree of stress the event presents can be highly individual. For example a divorce may be highly traumatic to one person and cause relatively little anxiety to another. What is important is that research has shown that people who have a high level of stress are often more prone to illness and have lowered ability to cope with illness and subsequent stress (Burgess and Lazare 1976:58).

A study of hospital stress, conducted by Volicer and Burns (1977:408–14), revealed that patients who entered the hospital with recent experience (within the past one to two years) of high life stress perceived and reported more changes and problems associated with hospitalization than those with low life stress in the recent past. This suggests that life stress prior to hospitalization may be an important factor in the level of stress experienced because of hospitalization itself. This study also indicated correlations between level of hospital stress and (a) age—younger patients reported higher levels of stress than older patients, (b) number of years since last hospitalization—those with recent hospitalization reported more hospital stress than others, (c) seriousness of illness—particularly for surgical patients contrasted to medical patients, and (d) sex—women indicated higher stress levels than men.

Health

Illness itself is a stressor. The individual who has been ill for a period of time may find his or her coping mechanisms exhausted and thus have little energy to cope with additional stressors. See Chapter 2 for additional information on illness and hospitalization.

Coping methods

When stressful life events are managed by effective coping methods (ways in which a person attempts to reduce stress) people learn the new coping behaviors and strengthen their emotional and problem-solving abilities. When inadequate coping methods are applied, deterioration in psychologic functioning and equilibrium occurs. Thus a person's response to stress is influenced by the person's coping methods.

Coping methods vary among individuals and are often related to the individual's perception of the stressful event. Some choose to avoid the situation, others to confront it. They may use a variety of activities, such as calling up mental defense mechanisms, seeking information, or relying on religious beliefs for support.

Bell (1977:137) defines and categorizes coping methods in two groups: long-term and short-term. *Long-term coping methods* are constructive, realistic ways of coping with stress that can effectively relieve it for long periods of time. Examples are:

- Talking with others (a friend, relative, or professional) about the problem

• Trying to find out more about the situation (seeking additional information)
• Relying on belief in a supernatural power
• Working the stress off by physical exercise
• Taking some concerted action on the basis of the person's understanding
• Making several alternative plans for handling the situation
• Drawing on past experience

Short-term coping methods are those that may reduce stress and tension to a tolerable limit temporarily but, if carried on for long periods of time, do not deal with reality and may have a destructive or detrimental effect on the person (ibid., p. 137). Examples are:

• Use of alcoholic beverages or drugs
• Daydreaming and fantasizing
• Trying to see the humorous aspects of the situation
• Not worrying, or relying on the belief that everything will work out fine
• Sleeping more
• Eating excessively
• Smoking excessively
• Getting prepared to expect the worst
• Cursing
• Crying
• Becoming involved in other activities to keep from thinking about the problem

Nursing assessment tools that include questionnaires on stressful life events and a coping methods scale can enable nurses to help patients contain present stress within limits and prevent additional stress before it becomes overwhelming.

Intervention for Stress

Stress accompanies every disease and illness. It is therefore important that nurses be able not only to recognize stress but also to assist people to cope with stress.

It has already been mentioned that stress is highly individual; a situation that to one person is a major stressor may not affect another. Some methods to help reduce stress will be effective for one person, others for another. A nurse who is sensitive to patients' needs and reactions can choose those methods of intervention that will be most effective for each individual.

The following interventions are suggested for nurses dealing with patients under stress:

1. *Be sensitive to specific situations and experiences that increase stress for patients.* Two examples might be an adult who appears highly stressed each time he receives an intramuscular injection and a child who appears frightened and highly stressed when her parents arrive at the hospital to visit her. Often a careful remark by the nurse about the stress will elicit information that the nurse or physician can use to assist the patient. In the first example, the patient's stress may be reduced by information about the injection and the technique by which it is given. Perhaps this patient was under a misconception about the content of the intramuscular syringe, the function of the drug, or the technique of administration. Specific knowledge may allay his apprehension. In the situation of the child, the nurse may learn, after establishing a relationship of trust with the child, that her parents mistreat her at home and neglect her because of their own needs. The nurse can convey this information to the physician, who may request the assistance of a community agency to investigate conditions in the home and help the parents.

2. *Orient the patient to the hospital or agency.* The nurse can help both patient and family or support persons in their adjustments. In a hospital, the patient is assisted in the role change from, for example, independent wage earner to relatively dependent patient. Family members are assisted in their adjustment by knowledge of the visiting hours and of what they can do to assist the patient.

3. *Support the patient and family at a time of illness.* By conveying caring and understanding, the nurse can help patients reduce their stress. To feel that there is someone else who helps and cares is supportive to people who are stressed. Often families require time to ventilate their worries and anxieties, before they can feel assured and less stressed.

4. *Give the patient time to ventilate feelings and thoughts.* As part of the plan of care, nurses need to allow time for patients to describe their feelings and worries if they wish. Some people find it relatively easy to talk about their feelings, while others may prove hesitant to do so. The nurse needs to be sensitive to the patient's needs and neither probe with questions nor be too busy to listen.

5. *Give the patient in a hospital some way of maintaining identity.* A person's name and clothes are important parts of his or her uniqueness as an individual. Nurses can assist patients by calling them by their correct names and by assisting them to wear their own clothes in a hospital setting, when this is possible. In the community, a nurse can help patients maintain their identity also by recognizing a new shirt or recently styled hair. All of these assist people to feel they are individuals and maintain their identities.

6. *Encourage the patient to participate in the plan of care.* Stress is frequently reduced by the feeling that the patient has some input into his or her own care and what is going to happen. Loss of the right to determine their own destiny can be very stressful to some people, particularly adults who function independently or who assume responsibility for others in their daily lives. Both adults and children can be included in formulating plans for their medical therapy and nursing care. Not only does this activity reduce stress, but also patients then have a greater tendency to comply with their care and feel they are persons of worth, which is important for their self-concept.

7. *Repeat information when the patient has difficulty remembering.* People who have a high level of stress frequently have difficulty remembering information and using the information when necessary. Nurses can assist patients by repeating information when it is requested and assisting people to apply it when they so desire. This problem is particularly true of elderly people who are stressed by the change of setting as well as by their illness.

8. *Defer as many questions to newly admitted patients as possible until later in the stay.* Hospital admission is in itself a stressor, which further heightens a patient's stress. Questions at this time can be difficult for a person to answer; recall is more difficult because of stress. Therefore, any questions that can be deferred until later will help patients reduce their stress.

9. *Encourage physical activity to dissipate stress.* If a person is able, physical activity such as folding linen can reduce stress. For patients who are restricted to bed, such activities as leather work and knitting can be helpful.

10. *Ensure that expectations are within the patient's capabilities.* Whatever the activity, whether an exercise or recreation, the nurse should make sure that it is possible for the patient to accomplish it. If an activity is beyond the patient's ability, the patient is likely to be more stressed by not achieving the goal. Frustration and depression may result. Being able to meet goals helps a patient feel personally effective, thus enhancing self-image.

11. *Bring patients and their families into contact with people in community agencies who can help them make valid plans.* People such as social workers are familiar with planning and arrangements that a patient may need to make. Their advice and assistance will enable the patient to make plans that are likely to be valid and that can be carried out. Often people are stressed needlessly because they do not know what help is available to them in the community. Plans that have a reasonable chance of success are highly desirable for a stressed person. Disappointment is likely to increase the stress of a patient and family.

12. *Reinforce positive environmental factors and recognize negative ones to help reduce stress.* A nurse can help a patient's return to homeostasis by reinforcing factors in the environment that are helpful and by recognizing but not reinforcing factors that are discouraging. A person's thoughts can dwell upon problems and difficulties, which increases stress, rather than focusing upon what can be accomplished positively, which usually decreases stress.

13. *Provide information when the patient has insufficient information.* Fear of the unknown and incorrect information can frequently cause stress. A patient may be told a fact, but the terms can be misunderstood. Additional information or clarification of information can allay misunderstanding.

14. *Assist a patient to make a correct appraisal of a situation.* Sometimes, through a lack of knowledge or misinterpretation of a sequence of events people draw incorrect conclusions. For example, if the results of a breast biopsy are not back from the hospital laboratory for two days, the patient may assume that something is seriously wrong. In fact, that length of time may be dictated by the specific test. Information from the nurse about the length of time that biopsy specimens normally take for diagnosis will often relieve a patient's stress and facilitate psychologic balance.

15. *Provide an environment in which a person can function independently to some degree without assistance.* Most adults in North America are accustomed to functioning independently and interdependently, often caring for dependents at the same time. For an adult to assume the dependent patient role even for a short time is difficult and stress producing. If patients can have some degree of independent functioning, such as using eating utensils that have been adapted so that they can feed themselves, their stress will be lowered. Patients then have an improved self-concept and feel that they are not totally helpless. The feeling of helping themselves is important for mental health and morale. Persons are often distressed to feel they are a bother.

16. *Arrange for other patients with similar experiences to visit.* Patients who have a medical condition such as a colostomy may be highly stressed and feel that they will never be able to live a normal life again. To meet another person who has a colostomy and who has successfully adjusted to this condition can lower the stress greatly. Not only are the patients reassured but they may also gain information that will assist them in rehabilitation.

17. *Communicate competence, understanding, and empathy rather than stress and anxiety.* The patient and family or support persons look upon the nurse as a source of knowledge and skill. If a nurse conveys stress or anxiety, the patient and family will be stressed about the nurse's competence and ability to function where the patient's health and life are involved. Nurses need to know themselves well and be able to function in a nondefensive manner that conveys competence and empathy, to reduce the patient's stress level.

Crisis

A *crisis* is a rapid change or an event in life that is foreign to a person's usual experience and disturbs a person's psychologic homeostasis. Crises generally do not last long and are self-limiting. People experience stressful events, predicaments, emergency situations, and crises throughout life. However there are differences and relationships among these commonly used words. *Stress* refers to tension, strain, or pressure; a *predicament* is a condition or situation that is unpleasant, dangerous, or embarrassing; and an *emergency* is an unforeseen combination of circumstances calling for immediate action (Hoff 1978:6). None of these is a crisis. Predicaments and emergencies, however, create stress, which has the potential of reaching crisis proportions. When people feel they are unable to handle the event emotionally, they are said to be in crisis.

Types of Crises

Developmental (maturational) crises

Developmental crises occur at critical points in human development. Erik Erikson (1963) identified eight developmental crises that must be resolved during the human life cycle. These are:

During infancy and childhood

1. Basic trust versus mistrust
2. Autonomy versus shame and doubt
3. Initiative versus guilt
4. Industry versus inferiority

During adolescence

5. Identity versus role confusion

During young adulthood to older adulthood

6. Intimacy versus isolation
7. Generativity versus stagnation
8. Ego integrity versus despair

These developmental crises are anticipated in a person's life and therefore the person has the opportunity to prepare for them before they occur. With appropriate support, people are normally able to meet the challenges and turmoils of these transition stages or tasks, and they mature. When support is not available, these transition phases can become crises with negative or destructive effects. Human growth is then stunted, and people may become depressed, withdrawn, or suicidal. Developmental crises are discussed in detail in Chapters 11 and 12.

Situational crises

A situational crisis may occur at any time in a person's life as a result of some unanticipated traumatic event beyond the person's control. Because it is not anticipated, the person cannot prepare for it. Common situational crises are loss of a job, loss of income, the accidental death of a loved one, the suicide of a friend, divorce, diagnosis of a terminal illness, and the need for mutilating surgery. Depending upon the person's developmental stage, personal resources, and social support system, such events may or may not result in a crisis.

People are in crisis when they suffer sudden loss or threat of loss of familiar sources of support. Seven sources of support required by people—what Norris Hansell (1976:22) calls "seven basic attachments"—are:

1. Physical need satisfaction, e.g., food, water, and shelter
2. A strong sense of self-identity
3. At least one close, mutually supportive person
4. At least one group that accepts the person as a member
5. Self-respect in one or more roles
6. Financial security
7. A meaningful set of values

Crisis Development and Sequence

The development of extreme anxiety into a crisis has four phases (Caplan 1964). Recognition of these phases can assist the nurse to prevent a potential crisis from becoming an actual crisis.

1. The person experiences feelings of stress and uneasiness in response to a traumatic event. Familiar problem-solving (coping) mechanisms are used to reduce the discomfort. For example, a 44-year-old man receives a diagnosis of terminal cancer but adjusts to this with the support of his wife and by continuing to work.
2. The person experiences greater stress due to continuation of the stimulus causing the initial rise in tension or addition of another stressor. In this phase the

person's usual problem-solving mechanisms fail, and the potential for a crisis state increases. In the example above, the man's financial resources may be threatened with increasing medical expenses and loss of time at work. He may also have learned that his son has been expelled from college and convicted on a marijuana charge.

3. The person experiences even more tension, which necessitates mobilization of both internal and external resources and unfamiliar ways to cope with the increased stress. If the person's inner strength and social support resources are sufficient at this stage, a crisis state can be prevented. It may, however, be necessary for the person to change unattainable goals to attainable ones. For example, the man's role as financial provider may have to be altered. Perhaps his son and his wife will need to take jobs to ease the financial burden. To facilitate this adjustment, other social support systems may become necessary, e.g., homemaker services.

4. The person experiences major disorganization and emotional homeostatic imbalance—a state of actual crisis. In this phase internal resources and outside support systems are lacking and tension rises to an unbearable level. The person's problem is unresolved.

According to Parad and Resnick (1975:4), the sequence of a crisis involves three time periods: precrisis, crisis, and postcrisis. In the precrisis period, the person is handling the stress in a way that meets most basic needs. This period may be likened to Caplan's first three phases of crisis development. The crisis period is characterized by trial-and-error disequilibrium responses and altered patterns of thinking, feeling, and acting. This period is likened to Caplan's fourth phase of crisis development. See the discussion of assessment of crisis on this page. The crisis period generally lasts from a few days to a few weeks. Unable to endure the emotional turmoil, the person moves toward actions that will resolve the crisis.

In the postcrisis period, there can be three outcomes. First, if previously developed coping mechanisms were sufficient, the person returns to the level of emotional homeostasis experienced before the crisis. Second, if the person's coping mechanisms were insufficient, the person experiences less emotional stability than previously. Third, if the person's coping mechanisms were more than adequate, as a result of the crisis the person gains emotional strength and stability.

Crisis Intervention

Crisis intervention is a short-term helping process that focuses on resolution of the immediate problem. A basis of crisis intervention is the problem-solving method or the nursing process. This involves four steps: assessing the problem, planning the intervention, intervening, and evaluating the results.

Assessment

The signs (thoughts, feelings, and actions) of people in crisis are obviously individual and vary considerably. Examples are:

- Heightened feeling of anxiety
- Fear of losing control and losing one's mind
- Anger at a loss or injustice
- Guilt
- Embarrassment at not being able to cope
- Sense of dread, hopelessness, and helplessness
- Sense of detachment or distance from others
- Distorted perception of what is happening
- Inability to make decisions
- Inability to solve problems
- Inability to recall facts
- Inability to put facts into logical order
- Inability to perform normal functions
- Inability to concentrate
- Withdrawal from social contacts
- Making demands to avoid being alone
- Impulsive, reckless, or lawless behavior
- Behavior inconsistent with thoughts and feelings
- Rejection of available help
- Alcohol or drug abuse
- Suicidal or homicidal tendencies

The assessment interview provides the nurse with the opportunity to (a) identify the crisis, (b) determine the person's perception of the crisis event, (c) determine how much stress the person is experiencing, (d) establish methods of coping or identify support resources, and (e) determine whether there is an obvious or potential threat to the life of the individual experiencing crisis or to the lives of others.

Because the person is often under considerable tension and strain, he or she will be particularly sensitive to the nurse's attitudes and reactions. It is important, therefore, that the nurse initially establish a trusting, helping relationship. See Chapter 15, page 380.

To identify the crisis, the nurse needs to pay close attention to the person's first phrases, since the crisis may be stated in the presenting complaint. If it is not stated at that time, the nurse listens attentively for the critical issue throughout the interview. It is important to determine the circumstances under which the event occurred, the people involved, their thoughts and reactions, and significant events since the traumatic event.

The person's perception of the crisis event is also essential information. The nurse needs to ascertain what meaning the crisis has to the person in terms of his or her developmental stage, life-style, and personal feelings and goals.

To determine how much stress the person is experiencing, the nurse needs answers to the following questions (Hoff 1978:53):

1. To what extent has the crisis disrupted the person's normal life pattern?
2. Is she or he able to go to school or hold a job?
3. Can the person handle the responsibilities involved in the activities of daily living—for example, eating and personal hygiene?
4. Has the crisis situation disrupted the lives of others?
5. Does the person seem to be on the brink of despair?
6. Has the high level of tension distorted the person's perception of reality?

The person's previous methods of coping and external support systems are also assessed. The nurse needs to determine whether the person's usual support system is present, absent, or exhausted, and what resources are appropriate from the nurse or agencies to meet the person's assessed needs.

The risks of suicide or assault and homicide are also assessed. If the crisis has life and death dimensions, emergency services may have to be mobilized on behalf of the person or family members. Assessment of homicidal danger should always be carried out in consultation with an experienced professional crisis counselor and should include the following:

1. History of homicidal threats
2. History of assault
3. Current homicidal threats and plan
4. Possession of lethal weapons
5. Use or abuse of alcohol or drugs
6. Disruption of meaningful social relationships, e.g., infidelity or threat of divorce
7. Threats of suicide following homicide

If assessment reveals the presence of one or several of the above, the person is a probable risk for assault or homicide (Hoff 1978:32).

Assessment of suicidal danger should include (Hoff 1978:120–26):

1. Plan for suicide
2. History of suicide attempts
3. Alcohol and drug abuse
4. Isolation physically and emotionally
5. Unexplained change in behavior
6. Recent loss (e.g., of spouse, job, or status)
7. Depression

Planning, intervention, and evaluation

Plans to assist the person in crisis are based on the assessment information and need to be developed in collaboration with the person and other significant people in his or her life. The goal of intervention is to help the person restore psychologic equilibrium. Interventions need to be as brief as possible and focus on the immediate problem contributing to the crisis.

Crisis intervention and evaluation require knowledge, skill, and experience beyond the scope of this chapter. Summarized here are several techniques the nurse can use to facilitate the person's psychologic equilibrium (Hoff 1978:61–65):

1. Listen actively and with concern.
2. Encourage the open expression of feelings.
3. Help the person gain an understanding of the crisis.
4. Help the person gradually accept reality.
5. Help the person explore new ways of coping with the problems.
6. Link the person to a social network.
7. Help the person make decisions about what problem needs to be solved, how it is to be solved, when and where it should be solved, and who should be solving it.
8. Reinforce newly learned coping devices, and encourage a follow-up contact after resolution of the crisis.

Summary

Selye defines stress as a state manifested by a nonspecific response of the body to any kind of demand made upon it. The body's responses to stress are categorized as the general adaptation syndrome (GAS) and the local adaptation syndrome (LAS). Both have three stages: (a) the alarm reaction, (b) the stage of resistance, and (c) the stage of exhaustion. These adaptive reactions described by Selye are physiologic ones. However, individuals also respond with psychologic adaptive reactions.

Stressors are factors that disturb the body's equilibrium. They may be external or internal, physiologic or psychologic. The effect of stressors depends on four factors: (a) the nature of the stressor—its magnitude and its specific meaning to a person; (b) the number of stressors the person has to cope with at the same time (the more stressors, the greater the response); (c) duration of exposure to the stressor (the longer it endures, the more exhausted become the person's powers of resistance); and (d) the person's experience with comparable stressors.

Adaptation to stress can be general or specific. The general adaptation syndrome involves the endocrine and sympathetic nervous systems. Stressors initially stimulate the hypothalamus directly or indirectly. The hypothalamus in turn stimulates the posterior pituitary gland, the sympathetic nervous centers, and the adrenal medulla, and through the release of CRH it also stimulates the anterior pituitary gland. Through a series of steps, processes such as increased reabsorption of water in the kidney tubules and the fight-or-flight syndrome are initiated.

Two local adaptation syndromes are the inflammatory and immunologic adaptive responses. The inflammatory response is a major example of the LAS. Its purpose is to destroy and localize injurious agents and to repair resulting damage to the tissues. Three stages of this process are (a) cellular and vascular change, (b) formation of inflammatory exudate, and (c) repair of tissues. The first stage is characterized by hyperemia and the observable signs of swelling, redness, heat, pain, and impaired mobility. Blood vessels dilate and become more permeable, plasma proteins move into the tissues, blood flow slows, and leukocytes marginate, emigrate, and attack the stressor by phagocytosis. The second stage produces the exudate, consisting of fluid and other substances from the blood vessels, dead tissue cells, and their by-products. The inflammation is localized by the formation of a fibrin mesh or clot. Exudates vary with the tissue involved and the intensity and duration of the inflammation. Major types of exudate are serous, catarrhal, purulent, fibrinous, and hemorrhagic. The third and final stage of inflammation is repair of the tissues by either regeneration or fibrous tissue substitution. The latter process involves the formation of granulation tissue and a cicatrix (scar tissue).

Several factors influence the character and speed of tissue healing. Included are the degree of injury, adequacy of the blood supply, nutrients available, age of the person, presence of other stressors, adequacy of immune mechanisms, and balance of adrenocortical hormones.

The immunologic response is a highly specific adaptive response, involving the formation of antibodies (immunoglobulins) to counteract foreign proteins in the body called *antigens*. Five immunoglobulins, designated by the letters G, A, M, D, and E, have been isolated, each having specific functions.

Immunity may be either natural or acquired. The former is an inborn species, racial, or individual resistance, while the latter occurs through exposure to disease agents. Acquired immunity is referred to as active when the host produces his or her own antibodies either naturally or artifically in response to vaccines or toxoids. Passive immunity occurs when antibodies produced by other animals or persons are administered to a person. Passive immunity can be acquired naturally by a fetus or newborn from antibodies synthesized by the mother. Artificial means to produce passive immunity are immune sera or antisera. Active immunity has the advantage of a longer duration, but passive immunity has the advantage of immediate or rapid immunity.

Psychologic adaptive responses are referred to as *mental defense mechanisms* or *coping mechanisms.* They protect the person by relieving inner tensions or conflicts and anxiety. The behavioral responses are primarily employed by unconscious means. They may be effective or ineffective means of adapting to life situations. In other words, each mechanism can be considered in terms of healthy use or unhealthy use.

Excessive levels of stress can be assessed. Some physiologic responses are diaphoresis, increased heart and respiratory rates, skin pallor, and urinary frequency. Usual psychologic responses are reduced intellectual processes, increased self-sensitivity, decreased ability to cope with or master tasks, and decreased sense of personal effectiveness.

Nurses must be able not only to recognize stress but also to intervene to assist people to cope with stress. Several methods can be selected according to the needs of the person at a given time. The nurse has to be sensitive to specific situations that increase the person's stress. Some general measures to reduce stress include orienting patients to the hospital or agency, providing time for patients to ventilate their feelings and thoughts, preserving the patient's identity, encouraging participation in the plan of care, repeating information as necessary, encouraging physical activity, and arranging for other patients with similar experiences to visit.

A crisis is a sudden event that disrupts a person's equilibrium to the point where assistance is required to help the coping mechanisms. Two types of crises are classified: developmental and situational. Crisis development has four phases that nurses need to recognize. A crisis can also be viewed as having three time periods: precrisis, crisis, and postcrisis. The nurse can be instrumental in assessing patients in crisis, helping them to identify and plan ways to deal with the crisis, and facilitating their psychologic equilibrium.

Suggested Activities

1. Try to assess your own level of stress within the past few months according to Table 9–1, and determine your individual stress score.

2. Select a friend or patient who you think is undergoing physical and psychologic stress, and compare the signs and symptoms he or she is experiencing or manifesting with those described in this chapter.

3. In a clinical or home situation, select a person and apply some of the methods suggested in this chapter to help a person adapt to stress. Evaluate their effectiveness.

4. In a clinical setting, select a patient with an inflammation. Assess the patient's signs and symptoms, and determine what factors are facilitating or hindering the healing process.

5. With a group of students, describe and share examples of situations in which patients, family members, friends, and yourself have used specific mental defense mechanisms.

Suggested Readings

Peterson, M. H. September 1972. Understanding defense mechanisms: Programmed instruction. *American Journal of Nursing* 72:1651–74.
This programmed instruction provides the nursing student with means to learn human defense mechanisms. Situations are described in which mechanisms are employed, and the student is asked to identify the mechanism.

Richter, J. M., and Sloan, R. November 1979. Stress: A relaxation technique. *American Journal of Nursing* 79:1960–64.
These authors discuss the whats and hows of progressive relaxation exercises. The sequence of steps to be followed is outlined.

Scully, R. May 1980. Stress in the nurse. *American Journal of Nursing* 80:912–15.
The author discusses individual and group responses to stress. She groups nurses' sources of stress into four areas: patient care, tensions within the staff group, outside forces, and unrealistic self-expectations. Ways to control stress are discussed.

Shields, L. September-October 1975. Crisis intervention: Implications for the nurse. *Journal of Psychiatric Nursing and Mental Health Services* 13:37–42.
The author describes the four phases of crises with examples of the four levels of intervention.

Storlie, F. J. December 1979. Burnout: The elaboration of a concept. *American Journal of Nursing* 79:2108–11.
Burnout is identified as a disparity between the real and the ideal. Why nurses may become automated shells instead of feeling persons is examined.

Tierney, M. J. G., and Strom, L. M. May 1980. Stress: Type A behavior in the nurse. *American Journal of Nursing* 80:915–18.
This article describes the personality profile of the stress-susceptible person identified in the work on Type A behavior and heart disease by Friedman and Rosenman (1974). Suggestions for the nurse about how to relieve job stress are provided.

Selected References

Anthony, C. P., and Thibodeau, G. A. 1979. *Textbook of anatomy and physiology.* 10th ed. St. Louis: C. V. Mosby Co.

Bell, J. M. March-April 1977. Stressful life events and coping methods in mental-illness and -wellness behaviors. *Nursing Research* 26:136–40.

Burgess, A. W., and Lazare, A. 1976. *Community mental health: Target populations.* Englewood Cliffs, N.J.: Prentice-Hall.

Byrne, M. L., and Thompson, L. F. 1978. *Key concepts for study and practice of nursing.* 2nd ed. St. Louis: C. V. Mosby Co.

Caplan, G. 1964. *Principles of preventive psychiatry.* New York: Basic Books.

Dharan, M. October 1976. The immune system: Immunoglobulin abnormalities. *American Journal of Nursing* 76:1626–28.

Erikson, E. H. 1963. *Childhood and society.* 2nd ed. New York: W. W. Norton and Co.

Friedman, M., and Rosenman, E. H. 1974. *Type A behavior and your heart.* Greenwich, Conn.: Fawcett Publications.

Guyton, A. C. 1982. *Human physiology and mechanisms of disease.* 3rd ed. Philadelphia: W. B. Saunders Co.

Hansell, N. 1976. *The person in distress.* New York: Human Services Press. Cited in Hoff, L. A. 1978. *People in crisis: Understanding and helping.* Reading, Mass.: Addison-Wesley Publishing Co.

Hoff, L. A. 1978. *People in crisis: Understanding and helping.* Reading, Mass.: Addison-Wesley Publishing Co.

Kjervik, D. K., and Martinson, I. M. 1979. *Women in stress, a nursing perspective.* New York: Appleton-Century-Crofts.

Kolb, L. C. 1977. *Modern clinical psychiatry.* 9th ed. Philadelphia: W. B. Saunders Co.

Levine, S. 1971. Stress and behavior. In *Readings from Scientific American: Physiological psychology.* San Francisco: W. H. Freeman and Co.

McLean, A. A. 1979. *Work stress.* Reading, Mass.: Addison-Wesley Publishing Co.

Morgan, A., and Moreno, J. W. 1973. *The practice of mental health nursing: A community approach.* Philadelphia: J. B. Lippincott Co.

Nysather, J. O.; Katz, A. E.; and Lenth, J. L. October 1976. The immune system: Its development and functions. *American Journal of Nursing* 76:1614–17.

Parad, H. J., and Resnick, H. L. P. 1975. A crisis intervention framework. In Resnick, H. L. P., and Ruben, H. L., editors. *Emergency psychiatric care.* Bowie, Md.: Charles Press.

Sedgwick, R. September-October 1975. Psychological responses to stress. *Journal of Psychiatric Nursing and Mental Health Services* 13:20–23.

Selye, H. 1974. *Stress without distress.* Scarborough, Ont.: New American Library of Canada.

———. 1976. *The stress of life.* Rev. ed. New York: McGraw-Hill Book Co.

Volicer, B. J., and Burns, M. W. November-December 1977. Preexisting correlates of hospital stress. *Nursing Research* 26:408–15.

Weissman, I. L.; Hood, L. E.; and Wood, W. B. 1978. *Essential concepts in immunology.* Menlo Park, Calif.: Benjamin/Cummings Publishing Co.

Chapter 10

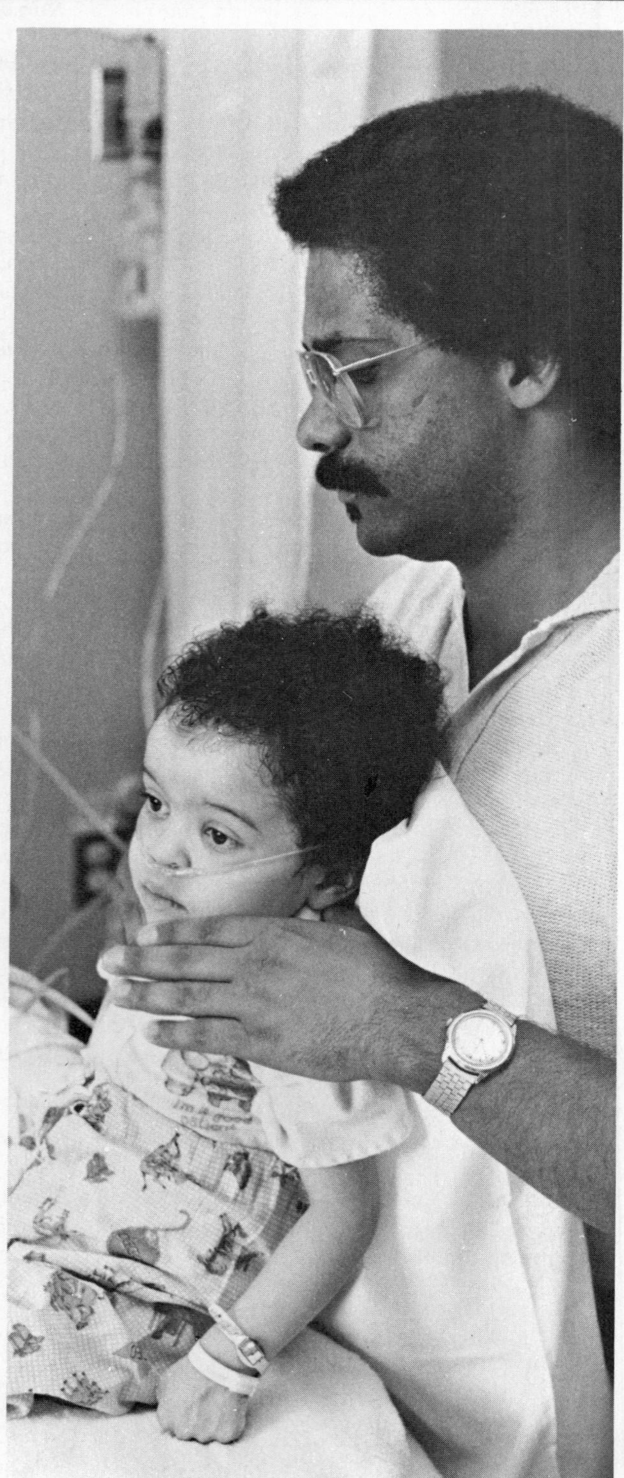

Human Values and Culture

CONTENTS

Objectives

1. Know essential facts about humanism, culture, and ethnicity

  1.1 Define selected terms

  1.2 Describe the concept of humanism

  1.3 Identify universal attributes of humanism

  1.4 Identify seven characteristics of culture

2. Understand aspects of the health needs of multicultural groups

  2.1 Relate the incidence of specific diseases to certain ethnic groups

  2.2 Identify problems unique to ethnic minorities in the provision and use of physical and mental health care services

  2.3 Identify social characteristics common to all ethnic groups that require consideration by health care providers

3. Understand essential health-related beliefs and practices of four North American cultural groups (Afro-Americans, Native American Indians, Asian Americans, and Hispanic Americans)

  3.1 Identify unique health and illness beliefs of each cultural group

  3.2 Identify unique illness practices of each cultural group

  3.3 Identify specific characteristics and values of each cultural group that may influence nursing assessment and intervention

4. Understand essential facts about low- and high-income groups and the health care system as subcultures

  4.1 Identify health-related beliefs and values of high-income groups

  4.2 Relate health-related beliefs and practices of low-income groups to effects of poverty

  4.3 Compare the differences in values between the health care culture and minority ethnic cultures

  4.4 Identify aspects of culture shock

Terms

culture
culture shock
ethnic group
ethnicity
ethnoscience
geographic poverty
holism
humanism
ideational
invisible poverty
material culture
nonmaterial culture
race
visible poverty

Humanism and culture are of particular importance in the United States and Canada, where there are many cultural groups. Nurses need to understand that human values and beliefs are often culturally determined, and thus a patient may not see things the way the nurse does. In this chapter, four of the many North American cultural groups are considered with specific reference to their health care needs and perspectives: American Indians, Afro-Americans, Asian Americans (particularly Chinese Americans), and Hispanic Americans (particularly Mexican Americans).

Issues about humanistic values and health have not been fully explored or resolved. For example, recent laws on abortions in the United States and in Canada are being challenged by some cultural and religious groups who contend that an unborn child has rights that are violated by abortion. With advances in technology and other social changes, nurses will be challenged to preserve human values of diverse ethnic groups while providing needed nursing care.

Humanism

Humanism is concern for human attributes, for those characteristics that are considered human. Some of these attributes are universal, that is, they occur in all cultures. Examples of humanistic behaviors are empathy, compassion, and sympathy toward other people and respect for life. Other characteristics are related to a person's culture, varying from one culture or subgroup to another. They involve beliefs and values that are learned and transmitted from generation to generation.

Humanism has received increased attention in nursing in response to the technologic advances that have affected nursing practice. Humanism in nursing refers to an attitude and an approach to the patient and support persons recognizing them as human beings with human needs, rather than as "the appendectomy in Room 192" or "the catheterization in bed 6A."

Holistic is another term used in nursing to refer to the entire person—recognizing that people respond as entire beings. *Holism* is the view that a person is more than a sum of many parts; the biologic, psychosocial, and spiritual aspects of the individual must be considered. For example, nurses see that an individual responds as a whole to an infected foot. The person's interpersonal relationships may change as pain makes the person more inner-directed. Limited functioning may cause loss of time from work and restricted recreation. Medications may necessitate changes in food intake and elimination of alcohol. The person may need to stop smoking to increase circulation to the foot. In addition, the person may be worried about the medical costs. Just as the physiologic and psychologic aspects of the individual must be considered, so must the sociologic factors, including cultural influences.

North American societies are multiethnic (i.e., they have diverse ethnic groups within them). They are person-centered in their humanism and include a human rights concept. This means that individuals are seen as autonomous and have certain rights and freedoms; in fact, each person has the right to be treated as an individual. This can be contrasted with societies in which the tribe or the family is the primary unit endowed with values and rights, not the person. Other characteristics of American humanism—though not necessarily unique to it—are belief in helping the poor and the suffering and respect for the ways and values of others, even if these differ from one's own.

Ethnicity and Culture

Definitions

Ethnicity is the condition of belonging to a specific ethnic group. An *ethnic group* is a set of individuals who share a unique cultural and social heritage passed on from one generation to another (Henderson and Primeaux 1981:xx). Ethnicity thus differs from race. *Race* refers to a system of classifying humans into subgroups according to specific physical and structural characteristics. The characteristics include skin pigmentation, stature, facial features, texture of body hair, and head form (ibid., p. xix). The three racial types that are commonly recognized are Caucasoid, Negroid, and Mongoloid. However, because of the mixture of races in North America, the three groups meld together, and there are many commonalities among groups. See Figure 10–1. Culture should not be confused with race or ethnic group. *Culture* is the beliefs and practices that are shared by people and passed down from generation to generation. Anthropologists have traditionally divided it into material culture and nonmaterial culture. *Material culture* consists of objects (such as dress, art, religious artifacts or eating utensils) and the ways these are used. *Nonmaterial culture* consists of beliefs, customs, languages, and social institutions. Races have different ethnic groups, and the ethnic groups have different cultures. It is therefore important to understand that all white or black people do not have the same culture. North America has people of different ethnic groups and different cultures. Their cultural beliefs and practices can affect health and illness and thus become an important consideration for nurses.

Characteristics of Culture

1. *Culture is learned.* It is not instinctive or innate. It is learned through life experiences after birth.

2. *Culture is inculcated.* It is transmitted from parents to children over successive generations. All animals can learn, but only humans can pass culture along. Language is the chief vehicle of culture. Through language children can learn knowledge in a relatively short time compared to the time it may have taken their forebears to develop it.

3. *Culture is social.* It originates and develops through the interactions of people.

4. *Culture is adaptive.* Cultures tend to adapt to the environment over a period of time. Customs, beliefs, and practices change slowly, but they do adapt to the social environment and to the biologic and psychologic needs of people. As life conditions change, some traditional forms in a culture may cease to provide satisfaction and are eliminated. For example, if it has been customary for family members of different generations to live together (extended family), yet education and employment often require children to leave their parents and move to other parts of the country, the extended family norm may change.

5. *Culture is integrative.* The elements in a culture tend to form a consistent and integrated system. For example, religious beliefs and practices influence and are influenced by family organization, economic values, and health practices.

6. *Culture is ideational. Ideational* means forming images or objects in the mind. The group habits that are

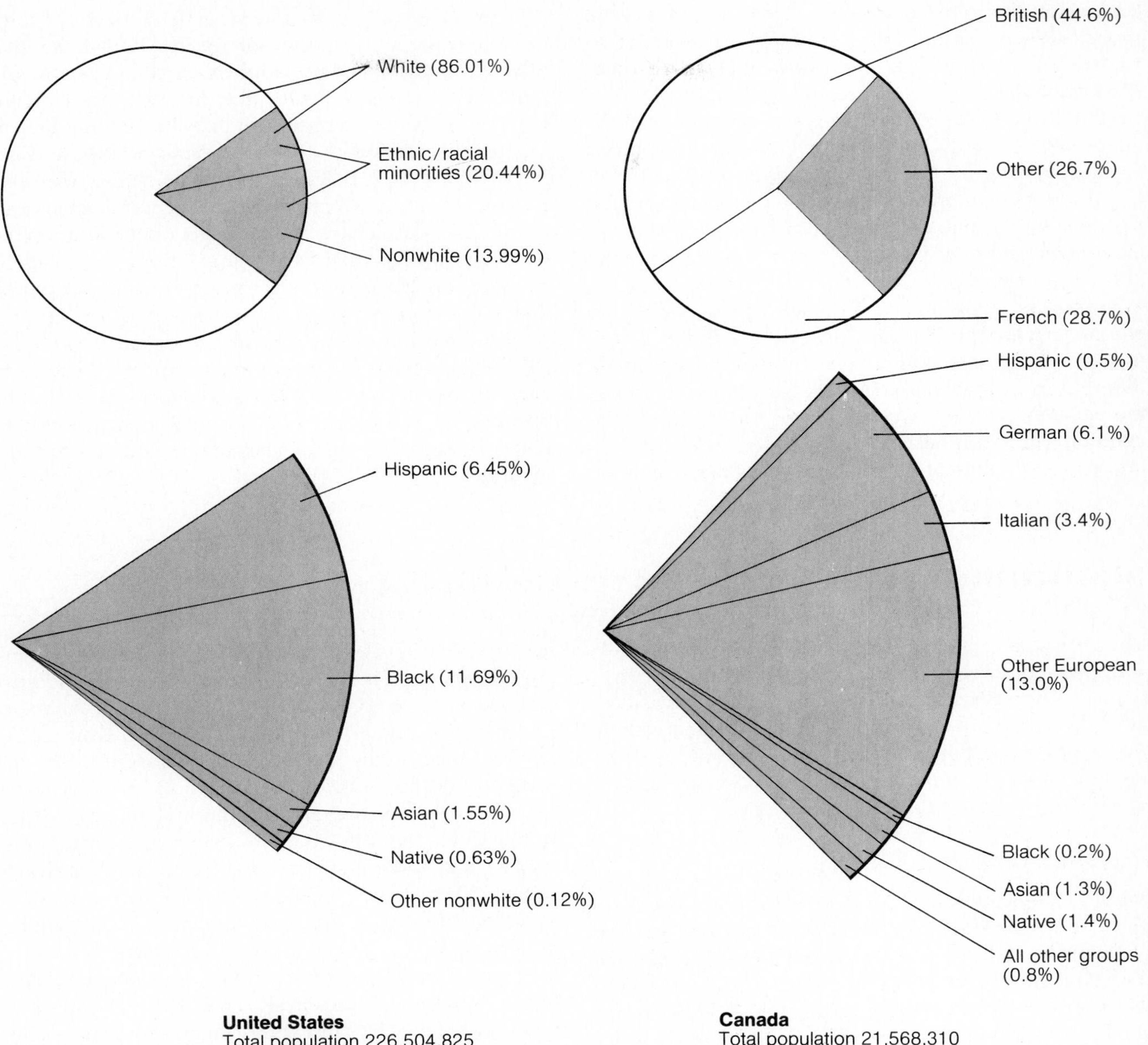

Figure 10–1 Estimates of the distribution of population by ethnic/racial origin based on the United States 1970 census and the Canadian 1971 census. (Information from U.S. Department of Commerce, Bureau of the Census, *Population profile of the United States, 1980,* Series P-20, no. 363 [Washington, D.C.: Government Printing Office, June 1981], p. 9; Statistics Canada, *Census of Canada* [Ottawa: Minister of Supplies and Services, 1981], p. 137.

part of culture are to a considerable extent ideal norms or patterns of behavior. People do not always follow those norms. The norms of their culture may in fact be different from the norms of society as a whole.

7. *Culture is satisfying.* Cultural habits persist only as long as they bring some satisfaction of people's needs. Gratification strengthens habits and beliefs. Once they no longer bring gratification, they may disappear.

Ethnoscience

Ethnoscience is "the systematic study of the way of life of a designated cultural group with the purpose of obtaining an accurate account of the people's behavior and how they perceive and interpret their universe" (Leininger 1970:168). Anthropologists have for years studied cultural groups' own perceptions of and knowledge about their world. However, ethnoscientists use a more rigorous method of systematic data collection to provide an accurate collection and analysis of data. Ethnoscientists attempt to provide an inside view of a culture from the way the people of the culture talk about it. They study and classify data about a cultural or subcultural group so that their report is meaningful to both people within the culture and people outside the culture who try to understand it. Emphasis is placed on the person's point of view, the person's vision, and the person's world.

Nurses can apply much of the knowledge gained by ethnoscientists, specifically about the health-illness behavior systems of people from cultural backgrounds different from their own. In the past decade or more, the patient's personal view of illness has received recognition and emphasis. Nurses have, as a result, implemented methods to discover how well patients understand their illnesses, how patients perceive they can be helped by health personnel, and how illness has affected them and their families. In recent years cultural views affecting health practices and beliefs have been receiving greater recognition. The fact that beliefs and practices about health vary among cultures and the implications of this for nursing have also received greater attention. To provide effective nursing services to patients, data about the patient's personal and cultural views regarding health and illness are needed. Nursing care plans need to consider the patient's world and daily experiences; nurses need to try to see and hear the world as their patients do to make valid assessments. Specific cultural data can provide scientific generalizations about health and illness behavior in different cultures. Patients' needs and behaviors can be better understood when particular health norms are identified.

Multicultural Considerations for Health Care

The provision of quality health care to all North Americans is a desired goal. Because of the multicultural nature of American society, it is essential that consideration be given to the unique health needs of ethnic minority groups. Following are some general considerations that can help nurses develop an awareness and sensitivity to some of these specific needs.

Physical Health

Studies have shown that some ethnic groups are more prone to certain diseases than others. The diseases may be inherited or acquired (environmentally induced). Acquired conditions that are common to most ethnic minority groups are malnutrition, tuberculosis, parasitosis, neoplasms, and diseases of the digestive tract (Parreno 1976:14). Other diseases have a higher incidence in specific ethnic groups. Some of these are:

1. *Sickle cell anemia* occurs in about 1 out of every 400 Afro-Americans. This type of anemia, caused by a genetic hemoglobin abnormality, is characterized by elongated, sickle-shaped red blood cells that break down more rapidly than the normal cells (which are round, biconcave disks).

2. Puerto Ricans and Filipinos have a high incidence of *gout*. This is a disease in which uric acid levels increase in the bloodstream, resulting in the deposit of uric acid crystals in the joints or other tissues. Swelling, inflammation, and pain occur.

3. The tendency toward *hypertension* is higher in Filipino males, Afro-Americans, and American Indians.

4. *Lactase deficiency* occurs more often in Afro-Americans, Asian Americans, and American Indians. Lactase is an enzyme necessary for the breakdown of lactose, a sugar (disaccharide) derived from milk. Without lactase, the lactose remains unsplit in the intestines, and the individual experiences an intolerance to milk. Unsplit disaccharides remaining in the intestine retain fluid and can cause diarrhea, gas formation, nausea, and abdominal cramps. Many individuals learn early in life to avoid ingesting dairy products or learn to ingest only fermented milk products such as buttermilk, yogurt, ripened cheese, and cottage cheese.

5. *Acatalasia* occurs mostly in Asians, such as the Japanese, Koreans, and Chinese. This is a rare inherited deficiency of the enzyme catalase in body tissues, particularly in erythrocytes, bone marrow, the liver, and the skin. It results in an increased susceptibility to tissue damage by normal microbial flora and is most often first detected in the mouth.

6. *Coccidioidomycosis* (valley fever), a fungal infection acquired by the respiratory route, is more common in Afro-Americans and Filipinos than in other ethnic groups.

7. *Sarcoidosis* occurs ten times more frequently among blacks than among whites. The term *sarcoid* means fleshy. Sarcoidosis is a granulomatous disorder of unknown cause. It is characterized by epithelioid cell granulomas (tumorlike masses or nodules) on various parts of the body. Most frequently the lymph nodes, spleen, lungs, skin, eyes, and small bones of the hands and feet are involved.

Mental Health

Current psychiatric therapy emphasizes responsibility to oneself to be comfortable, to grow, and to be competent and successful (Osborne 1976:20). Individualism is stressed. However, for most people of minority groups, basic concerns and usual interactions are with family and friendship groups. These people do not place individualism above family and friends. They often want others whom they can depend upon for support, and they stress the social component of the human race. Therapies are therefore needed that include significant other people in the environment, especially the family. The term *family* is not restricted to the American nuclear family of a couple and their children but often includes the extended family, such as aunts, uncles, grandparents, and godparents especially in Hispanic cultures. These people provide the primary support system for minority group patients. Of the many systems of therapy, those that are done in groups may be effective modes for such patients.

In mental health therapy for members of minority cultures, the racial identity and unique cultural experiences of the patients cannot be ignored. Sometimes the predisposing and precipitating causes of the illness may be rooted in problems associated with being a minority in a complex, rapidly changing, large social system. At other times, problems may be related to the person's human needs, such as socialization, and to relationships with others, even within the cultural group. Some problems may be related to a composite of racial or cultural and individual or humanistic factors. Therefore, nurses require an understanding of the unique differences of cultural groups.

Patients belonging to certain ethnic groups may not possess qualities compatible with some theories of psychiatry, and this needs to be considered. For example, many therapies rely upon such personality and intellectual characteristics as good verbal skills, adequate ego strength for introspection, and the ability to delay gratification (Leininger 1970:168). Not all ethnic groups value or develop these qualities. It is said, as a result, that minority group patients receive physiologic or custodial therapies more frequently than majority white American patients. Even the definitions and conceptions of mental health and mental illness can vary among cultural groups. For example, minority group people who have high incomes may think in terms of self-actualization, whereas those with low income may think in terms of survival in meeting demands of daily life.

The use and the availability of mental health services to minority groups are variable. Some ethnic groups consider it almost taboo to discuss emotional problems with outsiders, including therapists and nurses. Others view therapeutic resources as irrelevant to their specific needs and inaccessible. Some view mental illness as caused by evil spirits and curses, for which burning candles, herbal remedies, etc., are more credible therapies. Many psychiatrists operating on a fee-for-service basis charge fees that are out of reach to many members of minority groups. Even if a resource is accessible and is utilized, minority group patients may question the usefulness of the resource, particularly if the therapist or nurse is representative of the majority group society.

Certain common feelings and behaviors, although not unique to minority groups and not experienced by all minority group patients, are appropriate to consider when planning and implementing mental health therapy with patients of any group that finds itself in the minority (Osborne 1976:22–24):

1. Feelings of inferiority and inadequacy
2. Incompetent behaviors
3. Anger and hostility
4. Withholding and withdrawal
5. Selective inattention
6. Overcompensation

Feelings of inferiority and inadequacy can result from prejudice and racism in a society. The effects of racism are often denials of adequate resources such as housing, education, jobs, and health services, which limit the group's ability to achieve its aspirations. Feelings of inferiority then arise in members of the disadvantaged group in specific situations such as competing for a job with members of the majority group.

Incompetence is the behavioral outcome of feelings of inferiority and inadequacy. The person may be unable to perform certain activities or may manifest behaviors that do not achieve the goals mutually set by the person and the health care team. Judgments of incompetence are often made when a minority person is competing against majority group people in situations ruled by the majority group. For example, a minority group person may be judged by an IQ test that has racial and cultural biases.

Anger is generated from reflections about judgments of incompetence and feelings of inferiority, but, because the minority group person fears retribution by the majority, this anger is frequently suppressed rather than expressed. Suppressed anger results in *hostility* and depression, which have a corrosive effect, diffusing into and marring many of the person's relationships. A great deal of energy is expended to keep this anger suppressed. It may not be expressed toward threatening authoritative figures; rather, it may be expressed in acting out behavior, such as speeding in cars or verbally or physically abusing persons less able to retaliate. Hostility may be expressed as paranoid ideas reinforcing the view that members of the majority group have feelings of ill will toward the minority group person.

Feelings of hatred are usually focused more on specific persons or objects.

Withholding and withdrawal are behaviors that eventually occur when feelings of anger accumulate. Withholding is not sharing feelings and experiences with others. Withdrawal behavior often denies the existence of a situation or denies that available help is relevant to the person. Anger may therefore lead to missed clinic appointments or avoidance of health care workers.

Selective inattention, also referred to as *cognitive screening*, is a behavior that minority people may manifest to remove frustrating or insulting situations and events from their awareness. The advantage of this is that they can then pursue their goals without expending energy in responding to situations that provoke feelings of inferiority or inadequacy. Overuse of this mechanism, however, can lead to muted emotional responses in many situations.

Overcompensation is an attempt to perform in a way superior to that of the majority of the population. In other words, the person concludes that in order to succeed in this society he or she must perform better than is expected of a majority group person. This can lead to family problems if, for instance, the job requires much time and effort. It may even create more conflict with majority colleagues who do not have the motivation to perform as well.

Social Considerations

Each cultural group establishes norms, values, and beliefs that assist the functioning of that particular group. In North America, people have a tendency to assume that anything different from their own culture is inferior. Yet there is richness and value in each culture. For example the Appalachians who live in an 80,000 square mile area in Alabama, Georgia, Kentucky, North Carolina, Tennessee, and West Virginia have their own culture. Their churches are of the Pentecostal and Holiness type and include faith healing practices and visions. While their folklore reveres fighting, drinking, and wife stealing, Appalachians also value individualism and self-reliance, in contrast to the urban American value of the "organization man." Appalachians are highly traditional and resist change, whereas the values of progress and development prevail in most of the United States.

Although the history and reasons underlying certain practices may not always be clear, nurses need to appreciate and to accept cultural differences, to view these differences as positive elements, and to modify nursing interventions accordingly. The values, beliefs, and practices of each culture are deeply rooted and have worked effectively through time for the particular group. Nurses need to be more open to the experiences of people from different cultures to learn their unique characteristics.

Because each culture has unique differences (see subsequent sections), the nurse needs to assess the following variables:

1. Language barriers
2. Food habits
3. Perceptions of illness
4. Illness practices
5. Time orientations
6. Concepts of the family
7. Male/female norms

Language barriers

Some patients may not speak English fluently enough to express their needs or wishes or to understand all that is said to them. This can be particularly frustrating and anxiety producing when a person is ill and can neither state problems nor understand instructions. It is most difficult for people to convey their emotions about threatening situations in a second language, a crucial factor in cases of emotional and psychiatric illness. Language barriers also arise between people using the same language. The idiomatic English of a regional or cultural group may not be readily understood outside the group. For example, *belly* can mean the abdomen or the entire cavity from nipple line to pubes.

Food habits

Eating habits and food choices vary considerably from one culture to another. Hospitalized patients often have very little choice about the food they are served. Family members could be encouraged to bring in special meals within the limitations of the patient's diet. Instructions about meal planning for special diets at home may have to be given to younger family members who are more fluent in English or given by a health worker of the same culture, who can act as an interpreter.

Perceptions of illness

Some cultures view illness as part of life's inevitable suffering, to be borne without complaint. Others are convinced that illness is an imbalance in a person's energy field. Cultural perceptions may influence how persons respond to prescribed care or medical treatment.

Illness practices

Ways of curing illness are often closely allied to the culture's perception of the cause of illness. Those who believe their illness is God's punishment may refuse pain killers and even some nursing care, since they believe they must atone for their sins. Other practices may include supplication or atonement rituals with God or specific saints, such as repeating rosary prayers specified times and chanting. Penitence may be done by fasting for a number of days or walking on the knees to a certain cathedral. Some patients may prefer a person skilled in the use of herbs to a physician, or a combination of the two. Efforts on the part of health personnel to convince some patients that their mental illness may be due to a biochemical imbalance or that a physical illness may be due to an infectious process can be futile.

Time orientations

In contrast to the majority North American culture, which places great value on the future, some minority groups place high value on the present, the here and now. It is important that nurses recognize this concept and plan nursing interventions with a here-and-now orientation. Instruction about long-term goals or health needs cannot be overlooked, however. It presents a challenge to health professionals to educate people to anticipate the future as a realistic dimension of life.

Concepts of the family

The minority patient's concept of family can differ from that of white middle-class culture. The minority group family may include the nuclear family plus uncles, aunts, grandparents, cousins, and godparents—the extended family. Associated with this may be the concept that family members are most important and must be helped at all costs. When health care is offered to persons with this concept, it is important to consider the total family needs. Occasionally some family members' needs may take a priority detrimental to the patient. For example, a mother may not think that purchasing elastic stockings for her own ankle edema is as important as purchasing food for a relative who is unemployed. The public health nurse in this instance may have to see that the relative's needs are met before dealing with the mother's needs.

Cultures that emphasize that the needs of the extended family are as important as personal needs may also hold the belief that personal and family information must stay within the family. Some cultural groups are very reluctant to disclose family information to outsiders, including physicians and nurses. This can present difficulties for psychiatrists and mental health workers who view family interaction patterns as the locus of emotional problems

Male/female norms

In some cultures men must be strong and brave. They cannot cry or complain of discomfort and must always control emotions such as fear. For women, modesty is valued, and females cannot have their bodies inspected or touched by a strange man, not even a physician. If a female holding such a belief must be examined by a male physician, a female nurse needs to be present. This modesty is often manifested even in the presence of other women. Care must be taken to cover female patients as much as possible during examination procedures.

Native American Indians

The total American Indian, Eskimo, and Innuit population in the United States in 1980 was 1,418,195 (U.S. Department of Commerce, Bureau of the Census 1980:9), and in Canada in 1977 was 295,898 (Statistics Canada 1981:138). In both countries responsibility for health services for Indians rests with the federal government. There are, however, differences in health care among geographic locations in the United States. For example, Indians living in the eastern states and in most urban areas are not covered by the services of the Indian Health Service, whereas Indians living on reservations in the western states are eligible for such services (Spector 1979:286).

Because over 300 different tribes of Native American Indians exist in the United States, each with its own language, folkways, religion, mores, and patterns of interpersonal relationships, caution needs to be taken in generalizing about the Indian culture. Moreover, generations of contact with non-Indians have diluted each purely Indian ethnic group. In terms of health care, this variability needs to be considered. For example, the Native American Indian who lives in isolation on a reservation may hold to traditional beliefs of cure provided by the medicine man, while the urban Native American Indian who lives away from the reservation may respond more to the values of modern medicine provided by the majority culture. It is not uncommon for Indians to accept both kinds of health practices concurrently.

A Native American Indian's cultural identity can

no longer be determined from physical appearance. Some persons who are only one-eighth Indian by blood view themselves as more traditionally Indian than persons who have less dilution of ancestry. For this reason Indians are sometimes classified as "functional" or "nonfunctional" (Spruce 1972:6). Functional Indians have an intimate understanding of their people gained through socialization from childhood. Their behavior is dictated by the accepted patterns of Indian neighbors. They think of themselves as being Indian and are considered by the group to be Indian. In contrast, nonfunctional Indians, even if full-blooded, know little or nothing about the traditions of culture of the Indian people, hold the beliefs of the majority white culture, and consider themselves non-Indian.

Despite the many variations among tribes and individuals, some similarities of all Indian cultures can be considered and are discussed in the following sections. See also Table 10–1 on page 220.

Health and Illness Beliefs

Native American Indians tend to value harmonious relations with the world around them. Each rock, tree, animal, flower, and person is equally respected, and all are seen to coexist in harmony. A state of health exists when a person is in total harmony with nature. The earth is considered a living organism that has a will and desire to be well, but, just as human beings may be healthy or less healthy, so the earth's health may vary. It is believed that when people harm the earth they harm themselves, and vice versa. Thus, Native American Indians believe they should treat the body with respect and should treat the earth with respect.

Many Native American Indians view illness as an imbalance between the person who is ill and the natural or supernatural forces around the person, rather than as an altered physiologic state. Causes of illness relate to this concept. Native American Indians believe that if one interferes with this harmony by abusing or offending another person or thing, one may become ill. Even bad thoughts or wishes, such as jealousy or anger, by another person may cause illness. In addition, supernatural or spiritual forces may be involved. In the Papago tribe of southern Arizona, for example, many persons believe that ghosts of the dead, returning as owls or other animals of night, bring sickness. All animals are believed to have supernatural powers, which they can use to send sickness (Winn 1976:281).

American Indians do not relate disease causation to germ theory. A survey of American Indian registered nurses from 23 tribes revealed that none of these tribes had a word for *germ* (Henderson and Primeaux 1981:243). This makes it difficult for American Indians to understand the cause of tuberculosis, for example. Some Navajo Indians believed that the signs and symptoms caused by tuberculosis were the result of lightning. If lightning struck a tree and a person used the wood from that tree for firewood or other purposes, it would cause abscesses to develop in the lungs (Wauneka 1976:236).

Illness Practices

Various curative and preventive rituals may be conducted to restore balance when illness occurs. Some of these may be carried out by medicine men, others by family members. Sacred foods such as cornmeal may be sprinkled on people's shoulders before they enter a home to prevent flu or cold germs from entering the home. This sacred food or other substance, such as tobacco or feathers, may be sprinkled around an ill person's bed for a period of time. It is important for nurses to provide privacy for such ceremonies and to inquire about the length of time the substance is to be left in place, how to dispose of it, and, if it must be disturbed, exactly how and where the nurse may do so. Items such as herbs or mixtures are frequently placed near the patient on the bedside stand or on the bed; some may be worn by the patient. Nurses need to acquire permission from the patient, family, or medicine man, if these have to be removed.

Healing ceremonies, sometimes referred to as *sings* or *prayers*, may be requested. These vary in length from ½ hour to 9 days. Space and privacy need to be provided for such ceremonies. Usually in the hospital the sing lasts less than 1 hour. A medicine man may also be requested to perform curative rituals, which vary with the signs and symptoms of the patient.

Death and Loss

Native American Indians are less concerned with the future than are whites of the majority culture. The quality of life in the here and now is more important than longevity. Native American Indians accept that they will die as part of the life cycle and do not worry about how or when or why. They know they will join another world of long-ago ancestors when the Spirit intends. Funerals generally take place in the home and are associated with a large feast and gifts for relatives of the deceased. Proper burial rituals according to tribal tradition are important to American Indians.

Associated with burial is the belief of wholeness. Thus, when limbs are amputated, Indians may want to reclaim them and retain them for appropriate burial when the person dies. Indians also fear the spirits of the dead. It is important to the dying Indian patient and his or her family that people, e.g., relatives, be present.

Verbal and Nonverbal Communication

Native American Indians sometimes are labeled non-motivated, uninterested, or shifty-eyed because they may not look directly into the eyes of another person. This practice is based on their respect for the other person's privacy and the other person's soul. It is believed that direct eye contact is disrespectful, intrudes on individual privacy, and may even take the other's soul away.

Associated with this belief is the Native American Indian's commitment to autonomy. Each person has the right to speak only for himself or herself and each person's actions should be self-initiated. Thus, the nurse who tries to obtain a patient's history from close family members may have difficulty. Family members may believe they have no right to give personal information about another; they do not mean to be uncooperative but are following an unwritten ethical code.

Kinship

The family, relatives, and friends are important to Indians. During illness the patient is comforted when many relatives and friends visit. This conveys caring and enduring bonds of support. Being present is generally more important than talking, and it is not uncommon for large numbers of people to congregate. Most often one person likes to remain near the patient for long periods. The Native American Indian's kinship system can be confusing to nurses of other cultures. A child, for example, may have several mothers or several sets of brothers or sisters who are not direct-line relatives but are considered such according to the tribe. These people are all important to the patient who is ill. The aged, particularly, are looked upon for counsel and wisdom. Friendship ties are strong and can be as meaningful as those of the family or extended family in sustaining the patient's recuperative powers.

Time Orientation

American Indians tend to be casual about time, compared to people of other cultures. Their lives are less rigidly controlled by the clock. An Indian will sleep when tired, eat when hungry, and disregard a health appointment during the fishing season. This has many implications when nurses give health care instructions, such as to take medications every 6 hours.

Health Problems and Care

The leading causes of death in the Indian population are accidents, suicide, diabetes, alcoholism, and homicide (Primeaux 1977:58–59). At least one-third of the Native American Indian population is poverty stricken. Associated with this income level are poor living conditions, malnutrition, tuberculosis, and high maternal and infant death rates. Native Indians have the highest infant mortality rate in the United States, even though their birth rate is almost twice that of the general population. This is attributed to the high incidence of diarrhea in young babies and the harsh environment in which they live (Spector 1979:285).

Recent data also suggest that the clinical picture for diseases such as diabetes, hypertension, and alcoholism is different for American Indians. For example, the diabetic Indian patient who has a blood sugar of 500 mg/ml may remain asymptomatic. The normal blood sugar is 80 to 100 mg/ml (West and Kalbsleisch 1970). Indian youths also acquire hypertension, gastric ulceration, and liver cirrhosis at earlier ages than do non-Indians.

When caring for Native American Indian patients, nurses need to consider the following:

1. Although most American Indians recognize the value of Anglo-Western health care, many continue to use traditional medicine and cures either independently or in conjunction with such care.

2. Indian medicine and religion cannot be separated. Native American Indians make no distinction between physical and mental illness or the mind and the body. They live the concept of wholeness.

3. Tribal healing ceremonies and practices are highly ritualistic, religious ways to deal with sickness and death.

4. Tribal rituals that include extended "family" members are the way that Indians share all aspects of life.

5. Each tribe has foods or other substances that have symbolic meanings.

6. Characteristics such as not looking someone in the eye should not be labeled as disrespect, inattention, lack of interest, or avoidance.

7. Communication with Native American Indians needs to include an awareness of the following factors:

   a. The person's custom of speaking only for himself or herself.

   b. Use of extensive questions during history taking may be construed as an intrusion of individual privacy. The history taker may need to rely on observation techniques and make declarative statements to the patient such as, "You have an obvious cough that keeps you awake at night."

   c. Note taking may pose a barrier to communication, since Indians tend to value conversation, story telling, and listening.

   d. Native Americans often use a very low tone of voice, and the listener is expected to pay attention.

Afro-Americans

With the arrival of the first African slaves in Jamestown, Virginia, in 1619, a history of deprivation on this continent began for blacks. Even after slavery was abolished, black people endured severe economic and social deprivation. The struggles to overcome these deprivations continue today. However, Afro-American culture now is more similar to the white culture than it was 300 years ago. There is a large middle class and a large lower class. United States Census Bureau statistics for 1977 show that the majority of black families/households have incomes of $10,000 or less. There are strong kinship bonds in both low-income and more prosperous black families. These families provide financial support, assist with child care, and serve as buffers against racism and discrimination during children's growing years. A black family may show much cohesion and sharing, particularly in times of trouble.

Often a significant member of a black family must be consulted before important decisions are made. This person may be a father, mother, aunt, son, or grandparent. Nurses need to be sensitive to the fact that a decision may not be made until this person is consulted.

When Afro-Americans who are not familiar with the health care system enter it, they may show defensive behaviors such as hostility and suspicion. These attitudes are often adopted in expectation of being demeaned in some manner. It is important for nurses to recognize the reasons for these responses and learn to relate to all patients as worthy human beings.

The 1980 United States census found that blacks comprised 11.6% of the total population (U.S. Department of Commerce, Bureau of the Census 1980:9). Their numbers are greater than the total population of Canada. In Canada in 1971, blacks made up 0.2% of the population (Statistics Canada 1981:137).

Food Habits and Health Beliefs

Food habits are partly influenced by heritage and by economic factors. Hogs, chickens, corn, and beans were native products in the early history of the southern United States. The land did not lend itself to pastures for grazing cattle. Parts of the hog that were not considered desirable to the white masters were given to the black slaves to eat. These included the head, feet, brains, chitterlings (intestine), maw (stomach), and fatback (layers of fat). Today many blacks still prefer these meats as well as chicken because they are less expensive than beef and because they are part of the Afro-American cultural heritage.

Some blacks believe that certain combinations of foods and drugs can cause severe illness or even death. A few examples are:

1. Eating fish and milk or ice cream at the same meal.
2. Drinking milk when a person (particularly a child) has a high fever.
3. Having a penicillin injection after drinking whiskey (Martin 1976:54).

Afro-Americans may believe traditionally that health is maintained by proper diet, which includes a hot breakfast. Some believe that laxatives are important to keep the system running and open (Spector 1979:235). A person who is a practicing Black Muslim does not eat pork or pork products.

Many black families continue to use folk health practices (Henderson and Primeaux 1981:210) and home remedies. Voodoo and witchcraft practices occur to a minor extent. Thus the cause of illness may be thought of by a few as the result of a hex. Spiritualists or sorcerers may sometimes be consulted, or patients may vacillate for treatment between Western physicians and witch doctors or spiritualists who can remove spells. Historically churches have been a bulwark of support for blacks. Hence religious practices and Bible reading often continue during hospitalization.

It is important for nurses to understand the values held by a black patient and that person's definition of health. Traditional definitions in black culture stem from the African view of life as a process rather than a state. All things, whether living or dead, were believed to influence each other (Spector 1979:231). Health meant being in harmony with nature; illness was a state of disharmony. Therefore illness could be treated in a number of ways, including reliance on the power of a "healer." These beliefs and practices may or may not apply to a particular Afro-American patient. However, nurses should be aware of any cultural differences and take these into consideration when planning care. See also Table 10–1 on page 221.

Health Problems

The life expectancy of the black population is lower than that of the white population. For persons born in 1976, the average life expectancy for black males was 61.3 years, contrasted with 69.8 years for white males; for black females it was 72.7 years, contrasted with 77.5 years for white females. Other statistics reveal:

1. The death rate of black mothers at childbirth is 8.5 per 10,000 live births, compared to 2 per 10,000 for white mothers.
2. The infant mortality rate for blacks is double that of the white population.
3. The death rate from childhood diseases is six times greater for blacks than for whites (McVeigh 1970).

Specific diseases are more common among blacks due to environmental and hereditary factors:

1. The incidence of tuberculosis is three times greater for blacks than for whites.
2. Hypertension is a major killer.
3. Sickle cell anemia occurs in 1 per 400 blacks; 1 in 12 carries the trait.
4. Uterine cancer is twice as common in black females as in whites.
5. Malnutrition is a serious problem among blacks.
6. Diabetes mellitus is relatively common in the black population.

Asian Americans

The term Asian American refers to persons of American citizenship whose parents or ancestors originate from one or more Asian countries, e.g., China, Japan, Korea, and Vietnam. Recently the term *Pacific Asian* has been used to include descendants of the Pacific islands, such as the Philippines, Samoa, and Guam, as well as the other Asian countries. See Figure 10–2 for the population breakdown of Asian Americans.

It is difficult to classify many Asians because they are of mixed national parentage. For example, the person's parents may be Chinese and Korean or Japanese and Filipino. In addition most Asians view themselves as belonging to particular subgroups and ethnic groups and generally dislike being viewed as a member of another group. For example, the Chinese Americans and Japanese Americans in Hawaii consider themselves different from the "mainlanders," i.e., those in the United States. Japanese Americans also subgroup themselves by numbers of generations in the United States: Issei (first), Nisei (second), Sansei (third), and Yonsei (fourth); Kibei is the name for a subgroup of Nisei educated in Japan.

Because of the wide diversity of groups of Asians, full coverage of their views is beyond the scope of this book. This section will focus on Chinese health beliefs and practices, since the traditions of many other Asians derive in part from them. First, however, some general traditional Asian values and behaviors are outlined, recognizing that a wide range of behaviors exists among and within groups.

General Traditional Asian Values and Beliefs

Chang (1981:260–75) outlines the following general Asian values and behaviors:

1. Traditionally, the Asian household consisted of the extended kinship family in which grandparents, parents, siblings, uncles, aunts, and cousins lived together. Although this is rare in North America today, members of traditional families often maintain strong emotional bonds. It is not unusual, therefore, for hospitalized Asians to have many family members visit them.

2. The traditional Asian family is male dominated. Where elderly persons are housed in the family, they are usually the husband's parents. Asian women historically occupied an inferior position to men, and sons were more welcome in a family than daughters. Even in modern families, sons may receive preferential treatment to daughters. It is wise, therefore, for nurses to ascertain the opinion of the father, or in his absence the eldest son, on health care issues requiring decision making.

3. Traditionally, there is unquestioning respect for and deference to authority. It is expected that each in-

Figure 10–2 Population breakdown of Asian Americans in the United States. (From U.S. Department of Commerce, Bureau of the Census, Race of the population by state, *Supplementary reports, census of population*, p. 7, table 1 [provisional statistics], Series PC80 S1-3 [Washington, D.C.: Government Printing Office, April 1, 1980].)

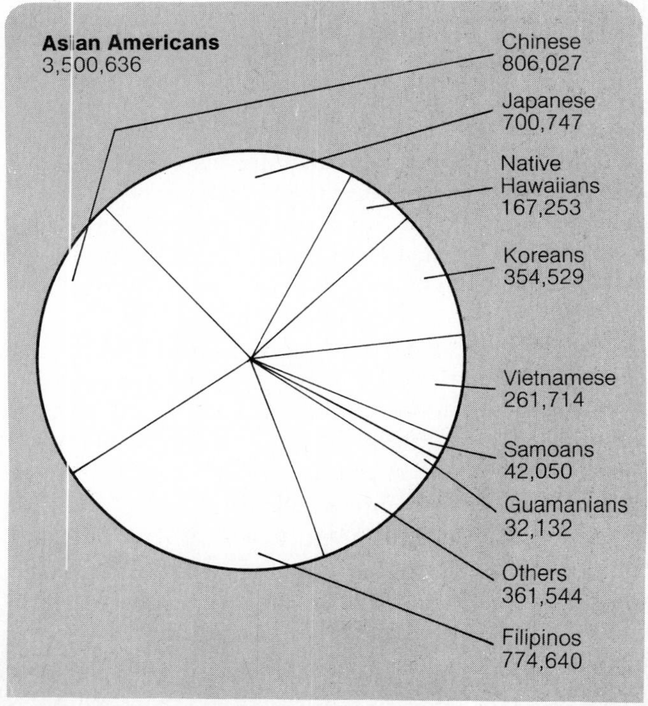

dividual will maintain filial piety (devotion and loyalty to family authority). Asian families are considered a continuum from past to future. Membership includes not only the present generation but also the ancestors and the unborn. Failure to comply with familial authority, duty, and obligations, to pay obedience to the family, and to engage in behavior that gives the family and the ethnic group a good name results in feelings of shame and guilt.

4. Interactions in the Asian family tend to be less verbal than in the white middle-class family, and praise of self or of members of one's own family is considered poor manners. This behavior of Asians is often misconstrued as lack of self-esteem or as belittling of family members. This does not imply that the nurse should not offer appropriate praise; but she or he should accept a self-deprecating response as a cultural variant.

5. Asians strongly emphasize harmony and avoidance of conflict in groups. In contrast to the behavior of whites, who may consider the individual most important, the behavior of Asians may not benefit the individual but instead be best for the situation and for others in the group. Often behavior is described as quiet, obedient, unassertive, reticent, agreeable, and reserved. For example, an individual may remain quiet or simply nod the head, often to avoid conflicts in ambiguous, embarrassing, or anxiety-producing situations. This behavior may be more apparent in Asian women due to their socialization. Asians avoid direct confrontations in which one of the parties must lose face; to do so, they may blame themselves for a mistake even when facts indicate that it was the other person's error.

6. Asian respect for those in authority positions such as doctors, teachers, and nurses often evokes a "yes" response that is different from the American connotation of the word. Asians tend to answer "yes" to be polite and to mean "I don't want to cause embarrassment." For example, in response to a nurse's question, "Is that clear?" an Asian patient may say "yes" because it is considered impolite to say "No, it is not clear," since this may imply that the nurse is either confused or unable to communicate. It is wise, therefore, for nurses to ask questions that require more than a "yes" or "no" answer.

7. Outward signs of feelings are discouraged. Asians are taught patterns of self-control and bravery even in situations of emotional conflict, hardship, and pain. This has implications for nurses when assessing pain in such patients and when assisting Asians with emotional crises. Often Asians express feelings of caring by their physical presence and attendance in times of illness rather than by an outward verbal expression of feelings.

8. Asians characteristically avoid attracting special attention to themselves. This inconspicuousness is related to their culture, which emphasizes harmony, consideration of others' rights and feelings, avoidance of behavior that would dishonor the family, and respect for and obedience to those in authority.

Chinese Health Beliefs and Practices

The Chinese in the United States and Canada are largely concentrated on the west coasts of the countries, on the east coast of the United States, and in large cities such as New York and Chicago. The Chinese population can be considered in three groups: (a) people who were born in rural villages in China and immigrated to North America 40 to 50 years ago; (b) new immigrants who have come within the past 20 years, from several Asian countries and Hong Kong; (c) Chinese born in North America who are descendants of 19th-century immigrants. Chinese in the first group are still largely oriented to Chinese folk medicine, while those in the third group are oriented to Western medical practices but still may be influenced by their elders in regard to health care. Those in the second group often practice a mixture of Chinese folk and Western medicine.

Prior to the revolution in China, the Chinese family was patriarchal and patrilineal. Respect for ancestors and parents was important, and obedience to the family was practiced. The Chinese family was frequently an extended one with several generations living in one household. Family clans were strong social organizations and were formed of people of the same bloodline with the same surnames. People who came to North America 40 to 50 years ago set up the same traditional families, based on associations to which they were accustomed in China.

Following the revolution, traditional family practices and superstitions became less evident in China and among immigrants. Family ties continue to be strong; however, the nuclear family now is seen more commonly in Chinese American society.

Campbell and Chang (1973:245–49) outline the following health beliefs and practices of the Chinese. Chinese folk medicine originated with Taoist philosophy. It proposes that the universe and health are regulated by two forces, the *yin* and the *yang*. The yin is a negative, female force; some of its characteristics are darkness, cold, and emptiness. The yang represents the positive, the male, light, warmth, and fullness. When these two energy forces are in balance, health exists. When a person has too much yin, he or she is nervous and is predisposed to digestive disorders. Too much yang, on the other hand, causes dehydration, fever, and irritability.

The Chinese do not consider their bodies to be personal property. The body is viewed as a gift provided by parents and ancestors and thus must be cared for. Various parts of the body are controlled by yin and yang. The inside, front part of the body, and five solid organs (*ts'ang*) that collect and store secretions—i.e., the liver, heart, spleen, lungs, and kidneys—are controlled by yin. The outside, back part of the body, and five hollow organs (*fu*) that excrete—i.e., the gallbladder, stomach, large and small intestines, and bladder—are controlled by yang. Yin stores the vital strength of life; yang protects the body from outside forces. A person who does not balance yin and yang properly will have a short life. Illness occurs when an imbalance of yin and yang exists. The sole cause of disease is considered to be disrupted harmony.

The Chinese also believe that there are six different pulses (three in each hand); each has its own characteristics and is related to various body organs. Specific pulses are associated with certain disease conditions, such as pregnancy, epilepsy, and oncoming death.

Chinese folk medicine uses herbs and acupuncture. A folk medicine diagnosis is made chiefly by observation, questioning, listening to the body, and taking the pulse. The prescription is a combination of herbs, which are obtained from a Chinese pharmacy. Acupuncture, or a cold treatment, is used chiefly to treat muscular and skeletal disorders and diseases in which there is excessive yang. Needles are inserted into the body at specific points along certain internal channels, which are called *meridians.* The internal organs are believed to be connected to the skin points and to the meridians; the acupuncture helps to balance the energy that flows within them.

The concept of yin and yang is also involved in a balanced meal. Yin is cold and includes fruits, vegetables, cold drinks, and hot (in temperature) melon soup. Yang is hot, for example, soups containing ginger and scrambled eggs. In Chinese culture the concepts of hot and cold have nothing to do with the temperature of the food. A Chinese patient who is ill with a hot disease, such as an eye infection, will want treatment with cold foods rather than hot foods in order to get well.

Chinese people of the older generations may also believe that their blood is not replaceable. Therefore, they are often very reluctant to give blood even for a blood test. Like many other people, the elderly Chinese often believe that a hospital is a place to go to die rather than to get well.

Specific health problems are more commonly found among the Chinese population: eye problems, tuberculosis, dental caries, malnutrition, and mental illness. Some of these are directly related to the poor environmental conditions of North American Chinatowns rather than to an inherited predisposition.

Some patients follow both Western and Chinese medical advice at the same time. This can produce problems if the therapies are not correlated. For example, a patient may be receiving the same drug from an herbal pharmacy that is prescribed by the Western physician, thus taking a double dose. Chinese patients should be encouraged to tell a doctor whether they are taking or receiving other therapy.

Folk medicine practices are often carried out during pregnancy. For example, use of soy sauce may be restricted so that the baby's skin will not be very dark, or a mother may refuse to take iron because it will harden the bones and make delivery of the baby difficult.

Following are some differences between Western practice and Chinese folk medicine (see also Table 10-1 on page 221):

1. One dose of an herbal medicine is thought to cure a person or make the person feel better. Thus, the vast number and dosages of medicines prescribed by some Western physicians are puzzling to Chinese patients.

2. Herbs are generally boiled in water for a prescribed time before being ingested, rather than prepared as capsules or pills.

3. Chinese patients may change physicians during an illness in order to find the best cure. When they do so, they may not tell the former doctor because they do not want the doctor to lose face.

4. The Chinese do not understand or react well to numerous diagnostic procedures that are painful. They believe that a physician should be able to make a diagnosis solely on the basis of a physical examination. Many may leave the Western system to avoid distasteful procedures.

5. Most Chinese believe that it is best to die with the body intact. This belief originates with Confucius, who taught that only those shall be truly revered who at the end of their lives return their physical bodies whole and sound. As a result Chinese patients may refuse surgery and donation of organs after death.

Hispanic Americans

Hispanic Americans have their origins in a number of Spanish-speaking countries: Mexico, Spain, Cuba, Puerto Rico, and the nations of Central and South America. Hispanic Americans comprised about 6.4% (14,605,883) of the population in the United States in 1980 (U.S. Department of Commerce, Bureau of the

Census 1981:9). In Canada it is estimated that only 27,515 people have Spanish as their mother tongue (Statistics Canada 1981:137). The family is the basic social unit of Hispanic Americans and provides the main support system at time of illness.

One of the largest groups for whom Spanish is the dominant tongue is the Chicano (Mexican American) population. Chicanos may refer to themselves as Spanish American, Mexican American, Latin American, Latino, or Mexican; some resent being called Latins. Chicano identifies all Americans of Mexican descent.

Puerto Ricans, another group of Hispanic Americans, numbered about 1,823,000 in the United States in 1980 (U.S. Department of Commerce, Bureau of the Census 1980:5). They live chiefly on the east coast. Like the Chicanos, the Puerto Ricans have their own culture, although there are similarities between the two.

Because a full discussion of each Hispanic American culture and its health care implications is beyond the scope of this book, the following pages focus on Chicano beliefs and practices.

Health and Illness Beliefs

Many Mexican Americans entered the United States during the early 1900s and brought with them the values, beliefs, and practices of rural Mexico; others are more recent immigrants. Folk concepts of health and illness that they had when they came to the United States continue to affect the thinking of some second- and third-generation Chicanos today. See also Table 10–1 on page 220.

Chicanos may hold the following health-related beliefs to varying degrees:

1. Certain foods help good health and others can produce poor health. An example of the former is tea made from fresh orange leaves; examples of the latter are rice and coffee, which should not be taken during an evening meal.
2. A person must be in tune with God to maintain good health. Thus, a person who is chronically ill is believed to have offended God and is being punished.
3. Health means being free of pain and being robust, even obese, rather than thin.

Chicanos are generally proud people. Those who are socially and economically deprived may well have low self-esteem and be reluctant to accept care for which they cannot pay. Therefore, Chicano patients in the hospital may not ask for help when they have pain; a young Mexican American male may react with hostility rather than passivity in response to nursing intervention to uphold his self-image.

Chicanos look upon the hospital as a place to die. Thus, they may avoid hospitals when they can and enter only with great fear, feeling that death is imminent. Illness is generally regarded not as a personal affair but as a family affair. Therefore, when a person is ill, many relatives generally gather around and visit. Restricting visitors can cause mistrust; nurses need to deal with such a requirement in the context of illness as a matter for the entire family. See Figure 10–3.

As a cultural group, Chicanos are very modest. Usually they consider bathing, defecating, and urinating to be very personal matters, yet they may be shy about asking a nurse to leave at such times. The sensitive nurse will provide complete privacy when possible.

Illness is seen as an imbalance in the individual's body or as a punishment for wrongdoing. The causes of illness can be grouped into four categories (Spector 1979:251):

1. *Imbalance between "hot" and "cold" or "wet" and "dry."* The four humors or body fluids that must be in balance are: blood (hot and wet), phlegm (cold and wet), yellow bile (hot and dry), and black bile (cold and dry). When these fluids are not in balance, illness results. Treatment in hospitals can be based on hot and cold principles. For example, illnesses that are classified as hot are treated with food, drugs, and drinks, which are classified as cold.
2. *Magic or supernatural forces.* Mal de ojo (evil eye) is disease caused by forces outside the body, such as a person's admiration for a part of another person's body, e.g., the hair. The victim can lose the admired part or fall ill. In some places mal de ojo is thought to be prevented by having the admirer touch the admired person while complimenting him or her, and it is believed to be cured with eggs in a ritual. The symptoms of mal de ojo include headaches, fever, fatigue, and prostration.
3. *"Dislocation" of body parts.* One example of a disease of "dislocation" is empacho. This is a disease, primarily seen in children, that produces swelling of the abdomen as a result of intestinal blockage. It is thought to be caused by overeating foods such as soft bread and bananas.
4. *Strong emotional states.* Susto is a disease of emotional origin—fright caused by natural phenomena such as lightning or loud noises. The symptoms have been described as insomnia, restlessness, and nervousness. It is a common folk disease that is difficult to cure, but it can be treated with herbal tea. Espanto is a disease with symptoms similar to susto. Its origin is fright caused by seeing supernatural spirits or events and can be likened to being "spooked" in American slang. Coraje is rage, a response to a particular situation. The victim may continually scream, cry, or yell and display hyperactivity.

Many Chicanos, when they are ill, may believe a folk medicine diagnosis rather than a Western diagnosis, even though they may also seek help from a Western

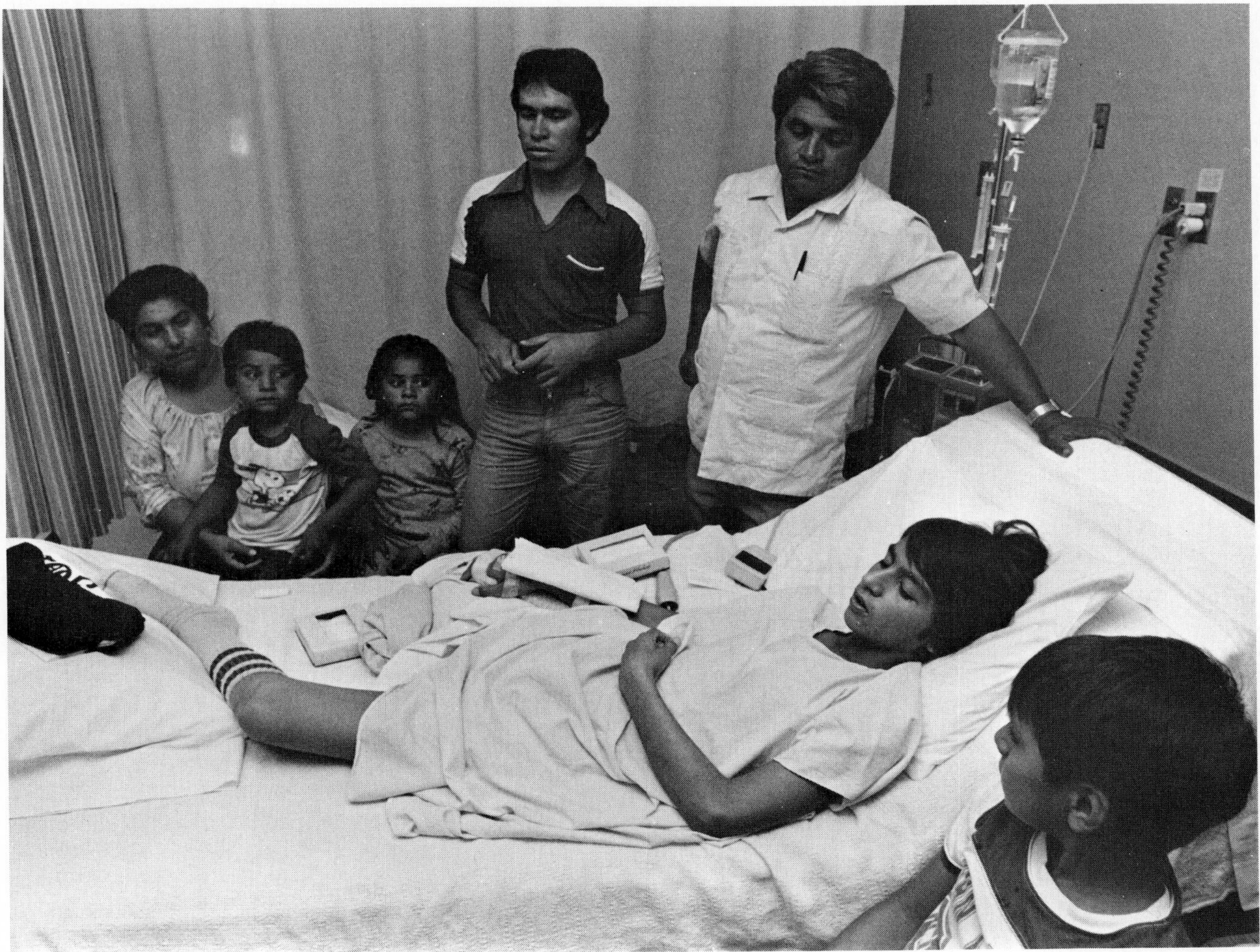

Figure 10–3 Illness is a matter of concern for an entire Chicano family.

physician. Healers within the Chicano community can be either male (a curandero) or female (a curandera). They offer a number of treatments; one of the most frequently used involves herbs in tea. Chicanos have a personal relationship with the curandero, in contrast to the relations in a hospital.

Puerto Rican beliefs about health and illness are not unlike those of Chicanos. Their diseases are also classified as hot and cold; however, food and medications are classified as hot (caliente), cold (frio), and cool (fresco) (Spector 1979:259).

Diet

Traditionally Chicanos eat foods such as beans and tortillas. For patients requiring a special diet this can present problems and requires special planning in consultation with dietitians. For example, Hispanics generally prefer rice to potatoes. The manner of preparing the rice is important; it differs from the Asian method. The diet of many low-income Mexican Americans often contains a high proportion of starches: tortillas, beans, corn, etc. It is usually possible to plan diets to meet patients' preferences and thus increase the chances that the food will be eaten.

Health Barriers

Hispanic Americans encounter a number of barriers to health care: language, poverty, and time orientation. To Hispanic Americans time is relative; the exact time is not a primary consideration. This hinders effective use of a health care system that values promptness for appointments and specific intervals between doses of medications. Language is another major barrier for many Hispanic Americans seeking help from the

Table 10–1 Comparison of Health-related Factors and Subcultures

	Definition of health	Cause of illness—is prevention possible; if so, how?	Name of healer, healing practices	Problems of entry to health care system	Communication patterns	Sexuality and family life	Beliefs about death
Navajo Indian	Harmony between individual, earth, and supernatural, as well as the ability to survive difficult circumstances[1,2]	Disease is disharmony and can be caused by violating taboo or attack by witch; illness prevented through elaborate religious rituals; do not believe in germ theory[1,2]	Medicine man, who is more than average human being, is therefore influential figure; medicine man diagnoses and treats problem; treatments include yucca root, massage, herbs, and chanting; his chant states person will get well, and person believes him[1,2]	Language; will first visit medicine man; general beliefs are not compatible with health care system and structure; problems also include money and past experiences of disrespect; fear of spirits of dead may influence decision to leave hospital early[1,2]	Time of silence after each speaker to show respect and reflection on what they said; little eye contact; time orientation not very strict; recording of conversation invasion of privacy[1,2]	Family, extended family, and tribal ties strong; cooperation emphasized; consider children as individuals as soon as they can talk, therefore can make own decisions[1,2]	Fear of spirits of dead; children and family should be with dying person[1]
Hispanic-American	Gift from God, also good luck; can tell healthy person by robust appearance and report of feeling well[1,3,4]	Illness is punishment from God for wrongdoing, to be suffered; it can be prevented by eating well, praying, being good, and working; wearing medals may help; physically, illness is an imbalance between "hot" and "cold" properties of body[1,3,4]	Healer called curandero; cures hot illness with cold medicine and reverse; classification of hot and cold diseases varies; penicillin is hot medicine; massages and cleanings are common[4]	Language; will first go to woman for advice, then if needed, to "señora," then to curandero, then to physician; many migrant workers are Hispanic, and frequent moves may make access to medical care difficult; belief that hospital is place to go to die causes underuse of system; modesty may result in woman bringing friend to physician with her[1,3,4]	Confidentiality and modesty important; too many questions are insulting; it is more acceptable to make tentative statement to which they can respond; time orientation not strict; politeness essential[1,3–5]	High degree of modesty, may prefer home births for this reason; men are breadwinners, women homemakers; women are healers, men make all decisions[1,3–5]	Afterlife of heaven and hell exists

Traditional black	Harmony with nature, no separation of mind and body[4]	Disease is disharmony caused by spirits and demons; it can be prevented through good diet, rest, cleanliness, and laxatives to clean out system; some use of copper and silver bracelets for prevention	Some belief in voodoo still prevalent; religious healing practiced; geophagia (eating of clay) and pica (eating of starch) practiced[4,6]	May seek folk or religious healer first; money and type of service affect decision; emergency room frequent entry point; black women have high "non-compliance" rate[4,6]	Racism toward blacks still prevalent; common names for symptoms should be known by health worker; time orientation not strict	Matriarchy prevalent; almost 30% of black families have woman head of household; therefore women make decisions[4,6]	Death is passage from evils of this world to another state; blacks have shorter life expectancy than national average[6]
Chinese-American	Balance of yin and yang (negative and positive energy forces); healthy body is gift from parents and ancestors[4,7,8]	Illness caused by imbalance of yin and yang, which may be due to overexertion or prolonged sitting; disease is prevented through better adaptation to nature[4,7]	Acupuncture and moxibustion (which is a therapeutic application of heat to skin) restore balance of yin and yang; herbal remedies such as ginseng used for many illnesses; healer is called physician[4,7]	Language; traditional Chinese physicians were paid to keep their patients well and cared for sick without fees because illness indicated they had failed in their job; Chinese physicians are available in community and may encourage patients to use Western physician; family spokesman may accompany patient to Western physician[4,7]	Open expression of emotions not acceptable; therefore might not complain about pain or symptoms; may smile when does not understand[4,7]	Women subservient to men; patriarchal family; ancestor worship and respect for obedience for parents observed; divorce considered disgrace[1,4,5]	Reincarnation[7]

(For notes, see page 223.)

Table 10–1 continued

	Definition of health	Cause of illness—is prevention possible; if so, how?	Name of healer healing practices	Problems of entry to health care system	Communication patterns	Sexuality and family life	Beliefs about death
Low income	Functional definition; if you can work, you are healthy[5,9]	Belief that illness is not preventable; fatalism common; future orientation minimal because present problems are too great[1,5,9]	Will often rely on folk healers and remedies because of belief and problems gaining access to health care system[5]	Use of public funding may limit access and type of care; present time orientation and beliefs about prevention may cause delay in obtaining care; inability to afford health insurance; may lose day's pay to go to physician[5,9]	May use slang and language of subculture; may view providers as authoritarian; time orientation not strict[5]	Many single-parent families with woman head of household[9]	Depends on culture and religion
High income	No data available	General belief in prevention of illness through diet, exercise, and good health habits; motivators such as previous experience or family tradition are influential in actual practice of prevention[5]	Combination of traditional practices of religion and culture, frequent use of health care system and self-help information[5]	Access not too difficult, usually through private physician; most have health insurance through employer[5]	Most like health care culture; cannot be expected to understand jargon	Women more likely to have career by choice than financial necessity	Depends on culture and religion

Health care culture	Optimal level of functioning; more than absence of disease; physical, emotional, social, and mental health included[5]	Scientific approach to cause of illness; prevention involves periodic physical examinations, laboratory studies, inoculations, as well as avoiding smoking and overeating, etc.[4]	Healing done by physician, usually takes place in office or hospital; treatments based on scientific knowledge and are frequently embarrassing or uncomfortable; often emotional component of disease is ignored[4]	Physician is main access to system; focus is basically curing illness rather than prevention; encouragement given to population to seek care as soon as symptoms appear; consider health care system as only provider	Widespread use of jargon and specialized language; large percentage of workers from middle class; often expect gratitude for care given; time orientation strict; written records kept[4]	Hierarchy, with physicians making decisions	Death usually means workers have failed to do their job; elaborate means are used to keep people alive; ethical and legal questions are being discussed and tested

[1]Data from Brownlee, A. T.: 1978. Community, culture, and care: a cross-cultural guide for health workers, The C.V. Mosby Co., St. Louis.

[2]Data from Wood, R.: 1976. The American Indian and health. In Ethnicity and health care, NLN publ. no. 14-1625, pp. 29–35.

[3]Data from Gonzales, H.: 1976. Health care needs of the Mexican American family. In Ethnicity and health care. NLN publ. no. 14–1625, pp. 21–28.

[4]Data from Spector, R.: 1979. Cultural diversity in health and illness, Appleton-Century-Crofts, New York.

[5]Data from Murray, R., and Zentner, J.: 1975. Nursing assessment and health promotion through the life span, Englewood Cliffs, N.J.

[6]Data from Martin, B.: 1976. Ethnicity and health care: Afro-Americans. In Ethnicity and health care, NLN publ. no. 14–1625, pp. 47–55.

[7]Data from Wang, R.: 1976. Chinese Americans and health care. In Ethnicity and health care, NLN publ. no. 14–1625, pp. 9–18.

[8]Data from Channing, G.: 1955. What is a Christian Scientist? In Rosten, L., editor: A guide to religions of America. Simon & Schuster, New York.

[9]Data from Fromer, M.: 1979. Community health care and the nursing process. The C. V. Mosby Co., St. Louis.

health care delivery system. Some do not speak English, and communication is difficult and embarrassing in a system where the English language predominates. In addition some Hispanic Americans belong to the poverty group in American society. They may not have knowledge of available health resources in the community or the money to use them. See the discussion of low-income groups as a subculture below.

Income Groups as Subcultures

The "poor" and the "rich" are viewed by some as subcultures of the dominant society. To describe the lower classes or the upper classes of society as subcultures, it is necessary to study both the strengths and the weaknesses of their life situations and behaviors. Unfortunately many studies dealing with poverty-stricken people tend to focus on only the negative aspects, and little has been written about the health care beliefs, practices, and problems of the rich.

High-Income Groups

Beliefs and behaviors of the rich tend to vary according to whether the persons come from second- or third-generation wealth. Second-generation wealthy persons (new rich), who are close to their parents' value systems, tend to value the "work ethic" (Henry and DiGiacomo-Geffers 1980:1426). These persons in their early years had fewer economic advantages and participated in the struggle to get ahead. In contrast the third-generation rich (older rich) tend not to value work (ibid.). They have been accustomed to wealth from birth, were raised largely by hired help, and grow up expecting great freedom with little discipline. Common characteristics of persons within this group who seek psychotherapy have been cited by Grinker (1978: 913) as:

- Feelings of emptiness and boredom
- Superficiality; absence of values, goals, ideals
- Low self-awareness; lack of introspection
- Lack of empathy
- Disinterest in work
- Chronic mild depression
- Intense pursuit of pleasure and excitement
- Belief that they can be happy only with persons like themselves
- Belief that use of their wealth (buying, spending, travel) will solve their emotional problems

Beliefs about health, illness, and death among the rich depend on their specific religion and culture. Generally the rich tend to (a) believe in the prevention of illness through diet, exercise, and good health habits; (b) make frequent use of the health care system and self-help information, and (c) have ready access to the health care system through private physicians. See Table 10–1 on page 222.

Specific problems nurses may encounter with the hospitalized rich are outlined by Henry and DiGiacomo-Geffers (1980:1428):

1. Demands by the patient or family members that are not related to health care. Being accustomed to highly responsive hired help, the rich person tends to have the same expectations of nurses, who then feel they are being treated like servants. This type of behavior is often an attempt to gain attention and to control the unfamiliar, uncertain environment.
2. Restrictions on the times when the nurse can provide care, because of luxuries that are considered necessities by the patient but often considered unnecessary by nurses. For example, some patients routinely have hour-long manicure appointments.
3. A concern with appearance that produces expectations for exceptional treatment. Outward appearance is often of critical importance to nationally known people, who are accustomed to being in the limelight. Prior to surgery, some may refuse to remove makeup or dentures; this necessitates their removal after general anesthesia.
4. A need to structure the environment and make it more appealing. In some cases, hospital rooms are literally redecorated. Drapes and bedcoverings may be changed, paintings hung on the walls, and the room stocked with expensive personal supplies such as liqueurs and floral arrangements.
5. Requests for care by only persons of their own ethnic background. Such expectations are often relinquished when the patient understands the need for assigning nurses with appropriate skills for the patient's care.

Low-Income Groups

The status of being poor is often referred to as the "culture of poverty," a phrase coined by anthropologist Oscar Lewis in the 1960s. Lewis (1966:19) defined the culture of poverty as a subculture of Western society with its own values and behaviors that differ from those of the nonpoor and that are passed on from generation to generation. This subculture transcends ethnic and regional boundaries. Characteristics of the poor include:

- Lack of participation in the larger society
- Hostility toward and mistrust of bureaucratic institutions
- Inadequate use of health services
- Long periods of unemployment
- Use of public assistance
- Authoritarian, mother-centered families that do not value childhood
- Abandonment of mothers and children by fathers
- Lack of privacy
- Disciplining of children by physical violence
- Orientation to the present
- Fatalistic attitudes
- Strong feelings of helplessness, dependence, and inferiority (ibid., pp. 19–25)

Lewis's portrayal of the poor as a subculture is challenged by other researchers, who believe this cultural viewpoint is negative, makes no attempt to question why these features exist, and fails to recognize the role of the larger society in perpetuating poverty. Some research has shown, for example, that the poor have the same values as the rest of society and that the traits Lewis identified may not be cultural but rather responses to situational circumstances. For example, the negative work behaviors associated with the lower class are not culturally derived but situationally induced. It has been shown that the poor have a strong work ethic, want to work, and do work when given equal opportunity (Mason 1981:83). Lack of societal incentives interferes with the poor obtaining and holding a job. Situational theorists believe, therefore, that if society were rid of poverty, the former poor would demonstrate middle-class attitudes and behaviors.

Still other researchers suggest that all members of a society share general, abstract values but that specific, concrete values differ among subgroups and social classes. This viewpoint combines the cultural and situational perspectives of poverty into an adaptational perspective. In other words, the poor are considered a special subgroup of society in response to social structures that make it impossible for them to actualize the values and behavior forms of the dominant society.

Poverty defined and described

Poverty has been defined and described by various people in several ways (Spector 1979:142–46):

1. It is a condition of being in want of something that is needed, desired, or generally recognized as having some value.

2. It is a condition whose essence is inequality.

3. It is both visible and invisible. *Visible poverty* refers to a lack of money or material resources such as housing and clothing. *Invisible poverty* refers to social and cultural deprivation, such as limited employment opportunities and lack of or inferior educational opportunities, medical services, and health care facilities.

4. It is a relative term that reflects a judgment made on the basis of standards prevailing in the community. What is considered poverty in one community may be regarded as wealth in another. For example, a person with a television set may be considered poor in one community and wealthy in another community.

Factors influencing poverty

Geographic and social factors influence poverty. *Geographic poverty* refers to the existence of "pockets of poverty." In the United States these pockets occur in dense urban areas (e.g., the ghettos) and in rural regions such as Appalachia, the Deep South, the lower Southwest and northern New England. Unless people move out of such regions of poverty, they are likely to remain destitute, since social mobility, education, and employment opportunities are scarce. In spite of reform efforts, local governments have been ineffective in improving the conditions in such areas. Massive outside assistance is required to upgrade services in education, sanitation, health, employment, job training, transportation, welfare, etc.

Social factors of poverty include demographic characteristics that determine the social position a person occupies. Such characteristics are race, age, family structure and size, education, income, and type of work. In terms of race, Afro-Americans, American Indians, and Hispanic Americans are overrepresented in poor populations. For example, in 1971 blacks accounted for 11% of the national population but 29% of the poverty population; whites accounted for only 9% of the poor. Statistics for Hispanics were similar to those for Afro-Americans (Spector 1979:145). People over 65 years of age also account for a substantial number of the impoverished, and the number is increasing in direct relationship to inflation. About one-third of the total poverty population is comprised of youths and children due to the poverty of their parents. Families in which the mother provides the major support are generally more poverty stricken than families in which the father provides the major support, since employment opportunities and incomes for females are substantially less than for males. Large families with set incomes also are more impoverished. Lower educational attainment and lack of educational opportunities contribute to lower employment opportunities and income. The typical low-income person has less than an eighth grade education and, if employed, works at an unskilled occupation.

Health considerations

Low-income families often define health in terms of work; if people can work they are healthy. They tend to be fatalistic and believe that illness is not preventable. Because their present problems are so great and all efforts are exerted toward survival, an orientation to the future may be lacking. Most low-income people do not have regular preventive medical checkups, because they cannot afford them. It is more important to them to work than to lose a day's pay visiting a physician. Reliance on public assistance and inability to afford health care insurance limit both the low-income person's access to health care and the type of care available. See also Table 10–1 on page 222.

The environmental conditions of poverty-stricken areas also have a bearing on overall health. Slum neighborhoods are overcrowded with people and with buildings in a state of deterioration. Neglect and disorder are common. Sanitation services tend to be low. Many streets are strewn with garbage, and alleys are overrun by rats. Fires and crime are constant threats. Recreational facilities are almost nonexistent, forcing children to play in streets and alleys. Parents who can work usually work long hours and earn barely enough for subsistence. They are often too tired to spend much time with their children, even though they love them. As a result, preschool children often come and go as they please, and elder siblings assume the role of parent for younger children. With all of these problems confronting the poverty stricken, it is little wonder that frustration tolerance levels are low, physical abuse is used as the form of discipline, and value is placed on encouraging children to seek employment rather than complete their education.

Contrary to the beliefs of some, poverty-stricken patients have the same needs and feelings as other people. They are sensitive, concerned, and easily embarrassed. When admitted to health care agencies, they are often treated with humiliating, patronizing, and prejudicial behavior by professional caregivers. Because prejudice is usually based on fear of the unknown, and fear is based on insecurity, it is important for nurses to examine their own values and attitudes. Nurses need to become culturally sensitive and to accept and respect the differences in the life-styles of others.

Health Care System as a Subculture

It is important for nurses to remember that the health care system can be considered a subculture in society. This system has rules, customs, and a language of its own. When individuals obtain an education in health care, they become enculturated into the system. But patients who enter the system may experience culture shock if it is very different from their own. For example, the health care culture values cleanliness; thus, nurses wash their hands often and expect their patients to wash daily. This value may not be shared by all patients, and the practice of washing daily may be a new one for some patients.

The health care culture has its own definition of health; often it is defined as "an optimal level of functioning." See Chapter 2 for additional information. Diagnosis and prescription are usually carried out by physicians, often in offices, clinics, or hospitals. Healing practices are based on scientific knowledge. Treatment procedures are frequently embarrassing or uncomfortable. The emotional component of disease is often ignored (Wold 1981:140).

Jargon is widely used in the system and tends to make patients feel more like outsiders. Many health care workers are from the middle class; they often expect gratitude for the care they give. Strict time orientation is adhered to and highly valued, which may conflict with the patient's culture. Written records kept in the system may also conflict with patients' cultural beliefs.

Traditionally, death has often meant to health care workers that they have failed. This belief is currently being reconsidered. Measures were often taken to preserve the lives of patients but seldom to facilitate death. Currently, clinical nurse specialists called *thanatology nurses* work with families and patients coping with a terminal illness. See also Table 10–1 on page 222.

If nurses recognize that they have been enculturated into the health care system, they can often identify the values of the system that they have adopted. It is then easier to recognize how a patient's values differ from those of the system. These differing values may be a source of anxiety or frustration to patients and their families. See the next section.

Culture Shock

Culture shock is the reaction that occurs in many people when they enter an unfamiliar situation where former patterns of behavior are ineffective. Culture shock can occur when members of one culture are abruptly moved to another culture or setting, for example, when people of Asian background and upbringing suddenly move to the United States, or when patients are abruptly thrust into the health care subculture. When this occurs, a number of stressors impinge on the individual.

Types of Stressors

1. *Communication.* Often there is a change in the system of verbal and nonverbal communication.
2. *Mechanical differences.* These include habits and activities of daily living, which often change with a change in environment. Even tasks such as shopping for food or using the telephone can be unfamiliar.
3. *Isolation.* There appears to be a sense of isolation inherent in any situation totally populated by strangers (Brink 1976:128). When moving from one culture to another, people immediately experience friendlessness and nonrelatedness.
4. *Customs.* Often new customs need to be learned, including systems of etiquette and role behaviors.
5. *Attitudes and beliefs.* Attitudes and values about life and behavior frequently differ between cultures. People may find that beliefs they have always taken for granted are radically different in another culture.

Phases of Culture Shock

Brink and Saunders (1976:129–30) describe four phases of culture shock:

1. *Phase one.* The initial phase is identified as one of excitement and is called the *honeymoon phase.* People are stimulated by being in a new environment. Behavior that indicates this varies with the ethnic origin of the person and the individual personality. Some patients, for example, may express their excitement outwardly, while others are quiet. People try to learn the norms of behavior appropriate for the new environment and often ask questions.
2. *Phase two.* Once the individual feels somewhat comfortable in the new environment, phase two begins. The person then realizes that he or she is actually in the environment. This awareness is often accompanied by feelings of frustration and embarrassment because of errors the individual makes. Accompanying this may be feelings of inadequacy, which can diminish the individual's self-concept and self-esteem. To these feelings is added loneliness. Although there may be many people around, there may be no one who enhances the individual's feelings of self-worth. Feelings of anxiety and inadequacy may be expressed through periods of withdrawal or anger.
3. *Phase three.* During the third stage the individual seeks new patterns of behavior appropriate to the environment. He or she makes friends and can often give newcomers advice. Current friendships take on importance and occupy much of the individual's conversation. At this time, ties to the old culture become weaker.
4. *Phase four.* In the fourth phase, the individual functions comfortably and effectively. If the person returns to the former culture during this phase he or she may experience reverse culture shock.

Summary

Although humanism is universal, its specific characteristics are learned and vary from one culture to another. Since North American society is composed of many cultural groups, it is important that nurses recognize the specific beliefs and values of different ethnic groups that relate to health and illness.

Several physical health problems are common to most ethnic minority groups. These include malnutrition, tuberculosis, neoplasms, and some digestive diseases. Other diseases occur with greater frequency among specific groups, although not unique to an ethnic group. Examples are the higher incidence of sickle cell anemia in Afro-Americans, gout in Puerto Ricans, and lactose deficiency in Asian Americans.

Variables among groups need to be considered in providing mental health care to individuals of differing cultures. Different definitions of mental health may be held by various minority groups. Therapies often need to include not only the immediate family but also extended family members. Because behavior has individual and cultural components, both facets must be considered when assessing predisposing and precipitating causes of illness. Some feeling and behavior patterns are common to racial minority groups but are not necessarily unique to them. These include feelings of inferiority, which result in inappropriate behavior according to standards of the dominant culture, and feelings of anger, which are generally withheld and suppressed. Persons from minority groups often resort to selective inattention and overcompensation.

Social factors must also be considered in providing health care. General considerations for cultural groups include language barriers, different food habits, and unique views of health, illness, and treatment. Time orientations and male/female norms also vary. All of these factors directly influence the effectiveness of nursing intervention. Awareness of the specific differences in health-related beliefs and practices of various ethnic and subcultural groups is essential for meaningful nursing care. Four large ethnic groups of North America are Native American Indians, Afro-Americans, Asian Americans, and Hispanic Americans. Two subcultures are the high-income group and the low-income group. Each group is unique in its family orientation, concepts of time, life, and death, beliefs about causes of illness, curative practices for illness, dietary habits, and specific health problems. The importance of understanding and accepting differences from a nurse's own beliefs is emphasized. An understanding of the health care system as a subculture is also important to nurses. The differences of this subculture from minority ethnic or subcultural groups can induce culture shock in those suddenly thrust into the system as patients and create misunderstandings between those seeking help and those wishing to help.

Suggested Activities

1. With a group of nursing students of various ethnic and socioeconomic backgrounds, discuss and list some of the health practices or folk beliefs that you learned from your family or friends.

2. In a clinical area, select a patient of a different ethnic background from your own.

- **a.** Attempt to learn more about his or her unique customs and beliefs.
- **b.** Determine how the nursing care could be adjusted or accommodated to his or her differences.

3. With a group of people discuss your attitudes about spiritualism and witchcraft practices as means of treatment for health problems.

Suggested Readings

Campbell, T. and Chang, B. April 1973. Health care of the Chinese in America. *Nursing Outlook* 21:245–49.
This article includes some insights into Chinese beliefs and customs such as the concept of yin and yang, food habits, the relationship of food to disease, practices during pregnancy, and attitudes about medications and hospitalization.

Ellis, D. and Ho, S. L. March 1982. Attitudes of Chinese women towards sexuality and birth control. *Canadian Nurse* 78:28–31.
Focusing on issues of sex and birth control, these authors interviewed a group of Chinese women about menstruation, masturbation, contraception, and coitus during pregnancy.

Gonzales, H. H. 1976. Health care needs of the Mexican-American. In *Ethnicity and health care*, pp. 21–28. Publication no. 14–1625. New York: National League for Nursing.
Health care needs unique to Mexican-Americans are discussed, including health superstitions; concepts of modesty, hospitals, and charity; and dietary needs. The health care needs of Mexican-Americans as distinct from the needs of the dominant culture are also described.

Hodgson, C. June 1980. Transcultural nursing: The Canadian experience. *Canadian Nurse* 76:23–25.
This author discusses the concepts of transcultural nursing as applied in the Canadian North with traditional Indian and Innuit cultures. She believes that separating culture from illness is like separating mind from body.

Kniep-Hardy, M., and Burkhardt, M. A. January 1977. Nursing the Navajo. *American Journal of Nursing* 77:95–96.
Suggestions are offered for adapting and individualizing nursing care for a Navajo patient. Several beliefs and customs are included.

Kwok, A. W. H. March 1982. Culture conflict: A study of the problems of Chinese immigrant adolescents in Canada. *Canadian Nurse* 78:32–34.
This author interviewed two Vietnamese and one Chinese adolescents about the conflicts they encounter not only as adolescents but also as individuals having to deal with two cultures. The values in one culture often violate those in the other.

Primeaux, M. January 1977. Caring for the American Indian patient. *American Journal of Nursing* 77:91–94.
This article describes some common cultural beliefs that pertain to health care for Native Americans. Health rituals, child-rearing practices, and many other specific values and beliefs are discussed.

Rosenblum, E. H. August 1980. Conversation with a Navajo nurse. *American Journal of Nursing* 80:1459–61.
This author converses with a graduate nurse who is a Navajo and a member of the largest Indian tribe in the United States. The matrilineal clanship system of the Navajo and other aspects of the culture are discussed.

Thomas, D. N. 1981. Black American patient care. In Henderson, G., and Primeaux, M., editors. *Transcultural health care*, pp. 209–23. Menlo Park, Calif.: Addison-Wesley Publishing Co.
The author discusses the socioeconomic, sociocultural, language, religious, hygiene, and dietary implications of the Black American patient for nursing intervention.

Selected References

Anderson, A. B., and Frideres, J. S. 1981. *Ethnicity in Canada: Theoretical perspectives.* Toronto: Butterworths.

Brink, P. J., editor. 1976. *Transcultural nursing: A book of readings.* Englewood Cliffs, N.J.: Prentice-Hall.

Bush, M. T.; Ullom, J. A.; and Osborne, O. H. March–April 1975. The meaning of mental health: A report of two ethnoscientific studies. *Nursing Research* 24:130–38.

Chang, B. 1981. Asian-American patient care. In Henderson, G., and Primeaux, M., editors. *Transcultural health care.* Menlo Park, Calif.: Addison-Wesley Publishing Co.

Chen-Louie, T. T. 1980. Bicultural experiences, social interactions, and health care implications. In Reinhardt, A. M., and Quinn, M. D., editors. *Family-centered community nursing: A sociocultural framework*, vol. 2. St. Louis: C. V. Mosby Co.

Clark, M. 1970. *A community study: Health in the Mexican-American culture.* 2nd ed. Berkeley: University of California Press.

Comer, J. P., and Poussaint, A. F. 1975. *Black child care: How to bring up a healthy black child in America, a guide to emotional and psychological development.* New York: Simon and Schuster.

DeGracia, R. T. August 1979. Cultural influences on Filipino patients. *American Journal of Nursing* 79:1412–14.

Dudley, L. P., and Smith, J. J., editors. 1970. *The American annual.* New York: Americana Corp.

Fawcett, M. J., editor. 1977. *The Corpus almanac of Canada.* Toronto: Corpus Publishers Services.

Flaskerud, J. H. May-June 1980. Perceptions of problematic behavior by Appalachians, mental health professionals, and lay non-Appalachians. *Nursing Research* 29:140–49.

Glillenberg, J. June 1981. Variation in stress and coping in three migrant settlements—Guatemala City. *Image* 13:43–46.

Gordon, V. C.; Matousek, I. M.; and Lang, T. A. November 1980. Southeast Asian refugees: Life in America. *American Journal of Nursing* 80:2031–36.

Grinker, R. R. August 1978. The poor, rich: The children of the super-rich. *American Journal of Psychiatry* 135:913.

Henderson, G., and Primeaux, M., editors. 1981. *Transcultural health care.* Menlo Park, Calif.: Addison-Wesley Publishing Co.

Henry, B. M., and DiGiacomo-Geffers, E. August 1980. The hospitalized rich and famous. *American Journal of Nursing* 80:1426–29.

James, S. M. November 1978. When your patient is black West Indian. *American Journal of Nursing* 78:1908–9.

Leininger, M. M. 1970. *Nursing and anthropology: Two worlds to blend.* New York: John Wiley and Sons.

———. 1974. Humanism, health and cultural values. In Leininger, M., editor. *Health care dimensions.* Philadelphia: F. A. Davis Co.

Lewis, O. October 1966. The culture of poverty. *Scientific American* 215:19–25.

Macdonald, A. C. June 1981. Folk health practices among north coastal Peruvians: Implications for nursing. *Image* 13:51–55.

McVeigh, F. J. May 1970. The life conditions of Afro-Americans. *Afro-American Studies* 1:45–49.

Martin, B. J. W. Ethnicity and health care: Afro-Americans. In *Ethnicity and health care.* 1976. New York: National League for Nursing.

Mason, D. J. October 1981. Perspectives on poverty. *Image* 13:82–85.

Meleis, A. I. June 1981. The Arab American in the health care system. *American Journal of Nursing* 81:1180–83.

Murillo-Rhode, I. 1976. Unique needs of ethnic minority clients in a multiracial society: A socio-cultural perspective. In *Affirmative action: Toward quality nursing care for a multiracial society.* Publication no. M-24 2500 5/76. Kansas City, Mo.: American Nurses' Association.

Nakane, C. 1973. *Japanese society.* Harmondsworth, England: Penguin Books.

Noble, G. P. October 1978. Social considerations in northern health care. *Canadian Nurse* 74:16, 18.

O'Brien, M. E. June 1981. Transcultural nursing research—alien in an alien land. *Image* 13:37–39.

Osborne, O. H. 1976. Unique needs of ethnic minority clients in a multiracial society: A psycho-social perspective. In *Affirmative action: Toward quality nursing care for a multiracial society.* Kansas City, Mo.: American Nurses' Association.

Parreno, H. 1976. Unique needs of ethnic minority clients in a multiracial society: A biological perspective. In *Affirmative action: Toward quality nursing care for a multiracial society.* Kansas City, Mo.: American Nurses' Association.

Primeaux, M. H. March 1977. American Indian health care practices: A cross-cultural perspective. *Nursing Clinics of North America* 12:55–65.

Rotkovitch, R. 1976. Ethnicity and health care—the Jewish heritage. In *Ethnicity and health care.* New York: National League for Nursing.

Schaefer, O. October 1978. Health in our time? *Canadian Nurse* 74:32–36.

Shubin, S. June 1980. Nursing patients from different cultures. *Nursing 80* 10:78–81 (Canadian ed. 10:26–29).

Spector, R. E. 1979. *Cultural diversity in health and illness.* New York: Appleton-Century-Crofts.

Spruce, B. B. 1972. The cultural patterns and values of the American Indian and their relation to health and illness. In *Becoming aware of cultural differences in nursing.* Speeches presented during the 48th annual convention of the ANA. Kansas City, Mo.: American Nurses' Association.

Statistics Canada. 1981. *Census of Canada.* Ottawa: Minister of Supplies and Services.

Stern, P. N. June 1981. Solving problems of cross-cultural health teaching: The Filipino childbearing family. *Image* 13:47–50.

U.S. Department of Commerce, Bureau of the Census. March 1980. Persons of Spanish origin in the United States. *Current Population Reports.* Series P–20, no. 361. Washington, D.C.: Government Printing Office.

———. June 1981. *Population profile of the United States, 1980.* Series P–20, no. 363. Washington, D.C.: Government Printing Office.

Valentine, V. F., and Vallee, F. G. 1968. *Eskimo of the Canadian artic.* Toronto: McClelland and Stewart.

Wang, R. M. 1976. Chinese Americans and health care. In *Ethnicity and health care.* New York: National League for Nursing.

Wauneka, A. D. 1976. Helping a people to understand. In Brink, P. R., editor. *Transcultural nursing: A book of readings.* Englewood Cliffs, N.J.: Prentice-Hall.

Wenzel, G. October 1978. A changing relationship. *Canadian Nurse* 74:12–15.

West, K., and Kalbsleisch, J. September 1970. Diabetes in Central America. *Diabetes* 19:656–63.

White, E. H. March 1977. Call of the minority patients. *Nursing Clinics of North America* 12:27–40.

Winn, M. C. 1976. A proposed tuberculosis program for Papago Indians. In Brink, P. J., editor. *Transcultural nursing: A book of readings.* Englewood Cliffs, N.J.: Prentice-Hall.

Wold, S. J. 1981. *School nursing: A framework for practice.* St. Louis: C. V. Mosby Co.

Wood, R. 1976. The American Indian and health. In *Ethnicity and health care.* New York: National League for Nursing.

Chapter 11

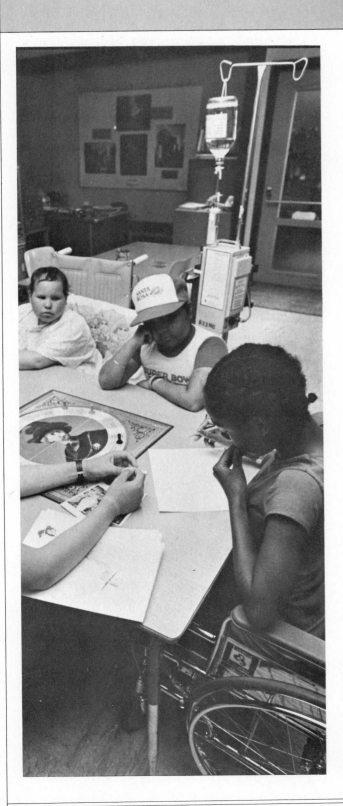

Early Growth and Development

CONTENTS

Objectives

1. Know essential facts about stages of development and growth cycles
    - **1.1** Identify Piaget's four stages of cognitive development
    - **1.2** Describe the processes of assimilation, accommodation, and adaptation
    - **1.3** Describe Freud's five stages of development
    - **1.4** Identify Erikson's eight stages of development
    - **1.5** List Havighurst's six periods of development
    - **1.6** Identify fundamental principles of growth and development
    - **1.7** Identify four distinct growth cycles
2. Understand selected facts related to physical growth from birth to 12 years
    - **2.1** Give reasons for measuring the chest and head circumference of newborns and infants
    - **2.2** Give reasons for measuring length or height and weight of infants and children
    - **2.3** Identify factors that cause asymmetry of the scalp in newborns
    - **2.4** Identify normal times for closure of two prominent skull fontanelles
    - **2.5** Identify times of eruption of temporary and permanent teeth
    - **2.6** Explain visual abilities present at birth and subsequent changes throughout infancy and childhood
3. Understand selected facts related to behavioral development from birth to 12 years
    - **3.1** Describe nine reflexes normally present at birth
    - **3.2** Identify changes in motor abilities throughout infancy and childhood
    - **3.3** Identify language and speech abilities present at birth and subsequent changes in childhood
    - **3.4** Identify changes in sleep patterns from birth to 12 years of age
    - **3.5** Identify changes in emotional responses from birth to 12 years of age
    - **3.6** Identify variations in sleep patterns from birth to 12 years of age
    - **3.7** Identify changes in the social development of infants and children
    - **3.8** Identify changes in the cognitive and intellectual development of infants and children
    - **3.9** Identify changes in moral and religious development throughout infancy and childhood
4. Know the role of the nurse in regard to the growth and development of persons from infancy through adolescence
    - **4.1** Identify data required to assess developmental changes
    - **4.2** Identify essential needs to maintain health of individuals in various stages of early growth and development

Terms

accommodation (Piaget)
adaptation (Piaget)
adaptive or defense mechanism
anal stage (Freud)
assimilation (Piaget)
Babinski reflex
caput succedaneum
cephalhematoma
cognitive development
displacement
ectoderm
ego (Freud)
Electra complex (Freud)
embryonic phase
endoderm
fetal phase
fontanelle
genital stage (Freud)
growth
hydrocephalus
id (Freud)
identification
imagination
incorporation
intelligence
introjection
lanugo
latency stage
libido (Freud)
macrocephaly
malingering
maturation
meconium
mesoderm
microcephaly
milia
Moro reflex
normocephaly
Oedipus complex (Freud)
oral stage (Freud)
palmar grasp reflex
phallic stage
placing reflex
plantar reflex
rationalization
regressing
repression
ritualistic behavior
rooting reflex
stepping reflex
sucking reflex
superego (Freud)
suture
swallowing reflex
symbolization
tonic neck reflex
trimester
unconscious mind (Freud)
vernix caseosa

A knowledge of growth and development is essential for nurses to identify developmental and health needs. The terms *growth* and *development* are often used interchangeably, but they are different. *Growth* refers to an increase in weight and height, an increase in physical size. *Development* is the increasing capacity and skill of a person to function. *Maturation* refers specifically to the development of traits, which are passed on from one generation to another by the genes.

Each person demonstrates an individual *rate* of growth. The *pattern* of growth, by contrast, is more predictable; for example, infants stand before they walk. Growth and development include physical, social, mental, emotional, sexual, and spiritual aspects, all of which are interrelated.

Growth and development are discussed in this chapter and subsequent chapters. Chapters 11 and 12 treat the following stages of growth and development:

Intrauterine
Neonate (birth to 28 days)
Infant (1 month to 1 year)
Toddler (1 to 3 years)
Preschooler (4 to 5 years)
School-age child (6 to 12 years)
Adolescent
Adulthood
  Young adult
  Pregnant woman
  Middle-aged adult
Elderly adult

Stages of Development

A great deal has been written about human development. Chapters 11 and 12 provide a brief overview of some of the theories of development and the essential knowledge associated with growth and development that is considered important for nursing students. Growth and development as they relate to specific nursing topics are discussed in the appropriate subsequent chapters. The reader is referred to the suggested readings and references at the end of both chapters for additional information.

Theories of Development

Piaget

Jean Piaget's theories are concerned chiefly with cognitive or intellectual development. Piaget proposes that cognitive development is an orderly process with four successive stages. In each of the four developmental stages, the person uses three primary methods: assimilation, accommodation, and adaptation.

Assimilation is the process through which humans encounter and react to new situations by using the mechanisms they already possess. In this way people acquire new knowledge and skills as well as insights into the world around them.

Accommodation is a process of change whereby cognitive processes mature sufficiently to allow the person to solve problems that were unsolvable before. This adjustment is possible chiefly because new knowledge has been assimilated.

Adaptation, or coping behavior, is the ability to handle the demands made by the environment.

Piaget's cognitive developmental process is divided into four major stages: the sensorimotor stage, the preoperational stage, the concrete operations stage, and the formal operations period. A person develops through each of these stages, and each stage has its own unique characteristics. See Table 11-1.

Freud

Sigmund Freud, whose writings and research were very popular in the 1930s, introduced a number of concepts and stages of development that are still used today. The concepts of the unconscious mind, defense mechanisms, and the id, ego, and superego are Freud's. The *unconscious mind* is the mental life of a person of which the person is unaware. This concept of the unconscious was one of Freud's major contributions to the field of psychiatry. *Defense mechanisms*, or *adaptive mechanisms* as they are more commonly called today, are the result of conflicts between inner impulses and of the anxiety that attends these conflicts. The *id* is the source of instinctive and unconscious urges, which Freud considered chiefly sexual in nature. The id is also the source of all pleasure and gratification. The *ego* is formed by the person to make effective contact with these social and physical needs. Through the ego, the id impulses are satisfied. The third aspect of the personality, according to Freud, is the *superego*. This is the conscience of the personality, a control on the id. The superego is the source of feelings of guilt, shame, and inhibition. See Chapter 9 for additional information on adaptive processes and mental mechanisms (pages 192–94.)

Table 11–1 Piaget's Developmental Stages (Cognitive)

Stage	Ages	Significant behavior
Sensorimotor	0 to 2 years	Preverbal behavior; coordinates simple motor actions; perceives through different senses
Preoperational	3 to 7 years	Egocentrism; associates objects representative of concepts; elaborates concepts; asks questions
Concrete operations	7 to 11 or 12 years	Solves concrete problems; begins to understand relationships such as size; understands right and left; cognizant of viewpoints
Formal operations	11 to 15 or 16 years	Lives in the present and the nonpresent; concerned about the possible; capable of scientific reasoning; can use formal logic

Summarized from J. Piaget, *Origins of intelligence in children* (New York: W. W. Norton and Co., 1963).

Freud's stages of development are:

1. Oral—the 1st year
2. Anal—the 2nd and 3rd years
3. Phallic—the 4th and 5th years
4. Latency—the school-age years (6 to 12 years)
5. Pregenital and genital—adolescence and adult years (12 years and after)

Freud proposed that the underlying motivation to human development is an energy form or life instinct, which he called *libido*.

Each of the stages of development during the first 5 years is associated with a part of the body. During the first or *oral stage*, the mouth is the principal area of activity. It is the main source of pleasure, primarily as a result of eating. Feelings of dependence arise in the oral stage, and they tend, according to Freud, to persist throughout life. The *anal stage* occurs when the child is learning toilet training. Many character traits such as creativity, stinginess, and cruelty are said to have their sources during this stage. During the *phallic stage* sexual and aggressive feelings associated with the genital organs come into focus. Masturbation offers pleasure at this time, and the Oedipus or Electra complex occurs. The *Oedipus complex* refers to the male child's attraction for his mother and hostile attitudes toward his father. The *Electra complex* is the female child's attraction for her father and hostility toward her mother. *Latency stage* describes the quiet years during which impulses tend to be repressed. Following latency comes adolescence and the reactivation of the pregenital impulses. The person usually displaces these impulses and subsequently passes into the final stage of maturity of an adult, the *genital stage*.

Erikson

Erik H. Erikson describes eight stages of development. See Table 11–2. These stages relate to psychosocial development. Life is pictured as a sequence of levels of achievement. Successful achievement of these developmental levels can be supportive to the person's ego; failure to achieve can be damaging. The ego is the conscious core of the personality.

Erikson further states that although one stage may be attained, the person may fall back and need to approach it again. Erikson's eight stages reflect both positive and negative aspects of the critical life periods. The resolution of the conflicts at each stage enables the person to function effectively in society. These stages are discussed further in Chapter 32.

Havighurst

Robert J. Havighurst suggests six periods or stages of development. There are also nine or ten tasks, both psychosocial and motor, delineated for each age period. Havighurst, unlike Erikson, believes that once a person masters a task, it is retained for life. He also states that the developmental tasks must be achieved before a person can be successful with later tasks (Havighurst 1972:2).

Havighurst's six periods of development are:

1. Infancy and early childhood
2. Middle childhood
3. Adolescence
4. Early adulthood
5. Middle age
6. Later maturity

See Table 11–3 showing the periods and the related developmental tasks.

Table 11–2 Erikson's Eight Stages of Development

	Age	Conflict	Some positive behavior
1.	Early infancy (birth to 1 year)	Basic trust versus mistrust	Shows affection, gratification, recognition
2.	Later infancy (1 to 3 years)	Autonomy versus shame and doubt	Dependent upon parents but views self as a person apart from parents
3.	Early childhood (4 to 5 years)	Initiative versus guilt	Shows imagination, imitates adults, tests reality, anticipates roles
4.	Middle childhood (6 to 11 years)	Industry versus inferiority	Has sense of duty, develops social and scholastic competencies, undertakes real tasks
5.	Puberty and adolescence (12 to 20 years)	Identity versus role confusion	Is self-certain, experiences sexual polarization, is role experimenter, has ideologic commitment
6.	Early adulthood (20 to 40 years)	Intimacy versus isolation	Shows capacity to commit oneself to others and capacity to love and work
7.	Middle adulthood (41 to 64 years)	Generativity versus stagnation	Productive and creative for self and others
8.	Late adulthood (65 years on)	Integrity versus despair	Appreciates continuing of past, present and future, accepts life cycle and style, accepts death

Summarized from E. H. Erikson, *Childhood and society*, 2nd ed. (New York: W. W. Norton and Co., 1963).

Table 11–3 Havighurst's Six Periods of Developmental Tasks

	Period	Tasks
1.	Infancy and childhood	Learning to walk; learning to talk; learning to take solid foods; learning to control the elimination of body wastes; learning sex differences and sexual modesty; achieving physiologic stability; forming simple concepts of social and physical reality; learning to relate oneself emotionally to parents, siblings, and other people; learning to distinguish right and wrong and developing a conscience
2.	Middle childhood	Learning physical skills necessary for ordinary games; building wholesome attitudes toward oneself as a growing organism; learning to get along with age mates; learning an appropriate masculine or feminine social role; developing fundamental skills in reading, writing, and calculating; developing concepts necessary for everyday living; developing conscience, morality, and a scale of values; achieving personal independence; developing attitudes toward social groups and institutions
3.	Adolescence	Accepting one's physique and accepting a masculine or feminine role; developing new relations with age mates of both sexes; achieving emotional independence of parents and other adults; achieving assurance of economic independence; selecting and preparing for an occupation; developing intellectual skills and concepts necessary for civic competence; preparing for marriage and family life; acquiring values and ethical systems in harmony with an adequate scientific world picture; desiring and achieving socially responsible behavior
4.	Early adulthood	Selecting a mate; learning to live with a marriage partner; starting a family; rearing children; managing a home; getting started in an occupation; taking on civic responsibility; finding a congenial social group
5.	Middle age	Achieving adult civic and social responsibility; establishing and maintaining an economic standard of living; assisting teenage children to become responsible and happy adults; developing adult leisure-time activities; relating oneself to one's spouse as a person; accepting and adjusting to physiologic changes of middle age; adjusting to aging parents
6.	Later maturity	Adjusting to decreasing physical strength and health; adjusting to retirement and reduced income; adjusting to death of spouse; establishing an explicit affiliation with one's age group; meeting social and civic obligations; establishing satisfactory physical living arrangements

Summarized from R. J. Havighurst, *Developmental tasks and education*, 2nd ed. (New York: David McKay Co., 1952).

Duvall

Duvall conceives of developmental tasks in eight categories through the family life cycle. The eight categories are: married couple, childbearing years, preschool years, school-age years, teenage years, families as launching centers, middle-aged parents, and aging family members. The developmental tasks in these categories are largely family oriented.

Principles of Development

There are a number of principles of development that are fundamental to understanding growth and development.

1. Growth is a continuous process determined by maturation, which is predetermined for the individual. Each person normally passes through each successive stage of development. On occasion there are individual exceptions, usually minimal, commonly due to environmental influences.

2. All humans follow the same pattern of growth and development, but each person does so in his or her own way. These individual differences are due chiefly to three broad factors: the rate or way in which maturation takes place, inherited factors, and environmental influences, which include learning.

3. Human development is the result of both learning and maturation. Learning can either help or hinder the maturational process, depending on what is learned. Maturation is the growth of the functional aspects of the body. The maturation of a person depends chiefly on heredity. Although the maturational rate is inherited, it can be affected by such factors as nutrition and parental attitudes.

4. Each developmental stage has its own characteristics. For example, Piaget suggests that in the sensorimotor stage (birth to 2 years) children learn to coordinate simple motor tasks. See Table 11–1.

5. During infancy and early childhood basic attitudes, life-styles, traits, and patterns of growth are formed. The role the child plays in the family largely determines whether the child becomes a leader, a follower, or a nonresponder in life. The person's physical and psychologic traits have their bases in the early stages of living.

6. As children develop, they master certain skills and learn certain behavior patterns; these are called *developmental tasks*. Some of the tasks they need to learn are necessary for survival, such as learning to take solid food. See Table 11–3. Others are secondary to survival, but pertinent to living in a society, such as learning to get along with peers. Society's expectations of the individual person change with each stage of development. For example, a 2-year-old child is not expected to be able to write with a pencil, but a 6-year-old child is expected to learn this skill.

7. A child's readiness to learn depends on his or her degree of maturation. The body must mature sufficiently before a person can perform certain skills. For example, a child must develop fine motor coordination before he or she can learn to write. Eyesight must also be sufficiently developed for the child to read.

8. Development proceeds generally from the head downward, and from the trunk of the body to the extremities. Thus before a child walks, the child can first hold the head up and then sit up without assistance.

9. Reactions of a person are initially gross and undifferentiated and then become more specific. For example, a baby's initial response is one of crying; responses become more specific as the child learns to laugh and to cry and then to speak words.

10. Development is unevenly paced. For example, a child's physical growth is accelerated during the 1st year and again in the preadolescent period.

11. Culture, ethnicity, and race can affect growth and development. For example, Oriental and Black children tend to be smaller than Caucasian children of the same age. In addition, cognitive development differs greatly in various subcultures. For example, American Indian children are often brought up without schedules, and thus the concept of time is often slower to develop in them than in Caucasian children. The latter's day usually is marked by scheduled activities, which they learn to associate with time.

There is a tendency for children to be preoccupied with the skills they are learning. For example, when children are learning to talk, they will talk a great deal, thus practicing word pronunciation.

Growth Cycles

Growth is a predictable rhythmic progression; it does not occur regularly, but it does occur in cycles. There are four distinct growth periods, two in which there is rapid growth and two in which there is slow growth. The first occurs from birth and lasts until about 2 years; this is a period of rapid growth. The second period, terminating at about puberty, is a period of slow growth. The third period is one of rapid growth again, beginning between 8 and 11 years and terminating at about 16 or 17 years. The fourth is a slow growth period from 17 years until maturity (about 21 years).

Intrauterine Development

Intrauterine development lasts approximately 9 calendar months (10 lunar months) or 38 to 40 weeks, depending on the method of calculation. (A lunar month is 28 days.) If the time is calculated from the day of conception, this stage of life is 38 weeks or 9½ lunar months. If the time is calculated from the 1st day of the last menstrual period, its average length is 10 lunar months or 40 weeks. This time span is not precise, however. Many pregnancies terminate within 1 to 2 weeks before or after the estimated date. To determine an expected day of confinement (EDC) according to Nägele's rule, one counts back 3 calendar months from the 1st day of the last menstrual period and adds 7 days. For example, if the last menstrual period began on April 5, one counts back 3 months to January 5 and adds 7 days. The EDC is then January 12 of the next year.

For conception to take place, the ovum leaves its graafian follicle (ovulation). It is surrounded by a mucopolysaccharide fluid (zona pellucida) and is propelled along the fallopian tube by cilia of the tube. An ovum can be fertilized within 24 to 48 hours after ovulation. During ovulation, the viscosity of the cervical mucus is reduced. Reduced viscosity facilitates the movement of the spermatozoa.

The normal ejaculation of semen contains several million spermatozoa. These spermatozoa are ejaculated at the cervix or move by flagella to the cervix of the uterus within 90 seconds. The spermatozoa cluster around the ovum, and hyaluronidase is released, which dissolves the corona radiata, a sphere of follicle cells surrounding the zona pellucida. One sperm penetrates the cell membrane of the ovum, resulting in conception.

Important in intrauterine development is the formation of the placenta, which normally starts at about the third week. Amniotic fluid surrounds the fetus in utero. A pregnant woman usually has about 30 ml of fluid at 10 weeks and perhaps 1000 ml at 38 weeks, although this amount is variable.

The placenta functions as an endocrine gland and to transport materials between the fetus and the mother. Nutrients as well as oxygen, carbon dioxide, water, and electrolytes move through the placenta. Many drugs, including narcotics and antibiotics, pass through the placenta. Amniotic fluid has a number of functions:

1. It protects the fetus from trauma by equalizing pressures that can occur as a result of a blow to the mother.
2. It permits the fetus to move and thus allows musculoskeletal development.
3. It separates the fetus from the fetal membranes that surround the fetus.
4. It helps even growth of the fetus.
5. It helps maintain a relatively constant fetal temperature.
6. It is a source of oral fluid for the fetus.
7. It functions as a system to collect excretions.

The intrauterine stage of life can be divided into two phases, the embryonic and the fetal (Vaughan et al. 1979:17). The embryonic phase is the period during which the fertilized ovum develops into an organism with most of the features of the human. This period is considered to extend for either the first 8 weeks, or the first 12 weeks or first trimester of pregnancy. Those authorities who consider the embryonic phase to be 12 weeks believe that some organs develop after 8 weeks.

This embryonic phase derives its name from the Greek word *embryo*, meaning "swell." The fetal phase extends from the first 8 or 12 weeks until birth. The Latin term *fetus* means "young one." From about 20 weeks on, the fetus is considered viable, that is, able or likely to live if born. Before 20 weeks, the fetus is considered previable or unlikely to live if born.

Traditionally, pregnancy has been divided into three periods called *trimesters*, each of which lasts about 3 months. Each trimester marks certain landmarks for developmental changes in the mother and the fetus. The phases of intrauterine life, therefore, can also be considered in trimestral terms. The embryonic phase is the first trimester, and the fetal phase includes the second and third trimesters.

Embryonic Phase

The rapidity of cell division and differentiation of the fertilized ovum (zygote) is remarkable. By 12 weeks the fetus weighs 15 to 20 gm and is about 7.5 to 9.0 cm (3 to 3.5 in) long. It has a sex that can be distinguished, a heartbeat, and a definite human form. The head is very large; the limbs are small with identifiable fingers and toes. Facial features such as nose, mouth, and ears are distinct, and some ossification of the bones has started.

Within the first 3 weeks of life, tissues differentiate into three layers—the *ectoderm* (outer layer), *mesoderm* (inner layer), and *endoderm* or *entoderm* (inner layer). The ectoderm and endoderm are formed in the 2nd week; the mesoderm forms in the 3rd week. From these layers are formed all of the body's complex organs and systems as a series of outpouchings, inpouchings, foldings, and tubular formations. Examples follow:

1. Ectoderm: central and peripheral nervous systems; epithelium of the internal and external ear, nasal cavity, sinuses, mouth, and anal canal; hair follicles; nails and tooth enamel; oral glands; sweat and sebaceous glands

Table 11–4 Fetal Development During the First Trimester

Lunar month	Lunar week	Developmental occurences
1	4	Cells divide actively from zygote The three primary layers form (10th to 14th day) Fetal heart beats can be heard (7 weeks) Digestive tract begins to form
2	8	Heart development is complete (8 weeks) Length of fetus 2.5 to 3 cm crown to rump
3	12	Bones are clearly outlined (12 weeks) Some swimming motions occur Fingers and toes differentiated Fetal circulation Bile secretion begins Liver produces red blood cells Lungs acquire shape Skin is pink and delicate Fetus weighs 45 gm (12 weeks) Length of fetus 8 cm crown to rump

Adapted from S. B. Olds, M. L. London, P. A. Ladewig, and S. V. Davidson, *Obstetric nursing* (Menlo Park, Calif.: Addison-Wesley Publishing Co., 1980), pp. 150–51.

Table 11–5 Fetal Development During the Second Trimester

Lunar month	Lunar week	Developmental occurrences
4	16	Hard tissues of teeth, central incisors form Mother can detect fetal movement Intestines begin to collect meconium Eyes, ears, and nose are formed
5	20	Fetal antibody levels (IgG type normally) are detectable Fetus actively sucks
6	24	Brain structure resembles mature brain Respiratory movement may occur Eye structure complete Fetus weighs 650 gm Length of fetus 23 cm crown to rump

Adapted from S. B. Olds, M. L. London, P. A. Ladewig, and S. V. Davidson, *Obstetric nursing* (Menlo Park, Calif.: Addison-Wesley Publishing Co., 1980), pp. 150–53.

2. Mesoderm: dermis; skeleton; connective tissue (cartilage, bone, and joint cavities); cardiovascular system (blood and bone marrow); genitourinary system (kidneys, ureters, gonads, and genital ducts); muscles; linings of cavities (pericardial, pleural, and peritoneal); teeth except enamel; adrenal cortex; lymphatic tissue
3. Endoderm: epithelial lining of the digestive tract (except portions arising from the ectoderm); epithelial lining of the respiratory tract (larynx, pharynx, trachea, and passages including the alveoli); epithelium of the tongue, tonsils, and auditory tubes; epithelium of the thyroid, parathyroid, and thymus; urethra and the urinary bladder except the trigone; primary tissue of the pancreas and liver; vagina (parts)

Concurrently during the first 3 weeks three other events occur:

1. The embryo is implanted.
2. Placental function starts. The placenta is a flat, disc-shaped organ, which is highly vascular. It normally forms in the upper segment of the endometrium of the uterus. Its functions are to exchange nutrients and gases between the fetus and the mother.
3. The fetal membranes differentiate.

Table 11–4 is a summary of this embryonic phase.

Fetal Phase

This phase of development is characterized by a period of rapid growth in the size of the fetus. Haase's rule offers a guide for estimating the approximate size of the fetus in centimeters each month of the intrauterine life. The length of the fetus during its first 5 months is determined by squaring the number of lunar months. For example, a 3-month fetus is approximately 9 (3 × 3) cm long, and a 5-month fetus is 25 (5 × 5) cm long. After the 5th month, the size of the fetus is estimated by multiplying the month by five. Thus a 7-month fetus is 35 (5 × 7) cm long, and a 9-month fetus is 45 (5 × 9) cm long.

At the end of the second trimester or 6 lunar months, the fetus resembles a small baby. Because very little fat is present beneath the skin, the skin appears wrinkled, red, and transparent. Underlying vessels are visible. A protective covering called *vernix caseosa* begins to develop over the skin. This is a white cheeselike substance that adheres to the skin and can become ⅛ inch thick by birth. *Lanugo*, a fine downy hair, also covers the body. At about 5 months, the mother first perceives movement by the fetus, and the first fetal heartbeat may be heard. The amount of activity varies among fetuses. There is some evidence that activity may be related to the mother's emotions by the transfer of epinephrine and other hormones through the placenta. Very few fetuses born before or at the end of 6 months survive. See Table 11–5.

At the end of the third trimester (9½ lunar months) the fetus has developed to approximately 50 cm (20 in) and 3.2 to 3.4 kg (7.0 to 7.5 lb). Black, American Indian, or Oriental newborns often have lower birth weights than Caucasians. The lanugo has disappeared, and the skin is a more normal color and appears less wrinkled. More subcutaneous fat makes the baby look more rotund; the last 2 months in utero are largely devoted to accumulating weight. The fetus born in the last trimester prior to full term has varying chances for survival. Those born at 7 months weigh about 1.1 kg (2.5 lb) and have approximately a 10% chance of survival; at 8 months the fetus weighs about 1.8 kg (4 lb) and has a 75% chance. See Table 11–6.

Table 11–6 Fetal Development During the Third Trimester

Lunar month	Lunar week	Developmental occurrences
7	28	Nervous system begins to regulate some body processes Eyebrows and eyelashes are present Testes descend into scrotal sac Fetus can suck
8	32	More reflexes present Skin is red and wrinkled
9	36	Hair fuzzy or woolly Sebaceous glands are active
10	40	Moderate to profuse silky hair Lanugo present on shoulders, upper back Creases cover soles Fetus weighs 3200 gm or more Length of fetus 40 cm crown to rump

Adapted from S. B. Olds, M. L. London, P. A. Ladewig, and S. V. Davidson, *Obstetric nursing* (Menlo Park, Calif.: Addison-Wesley Publishing Co., 1980), pp. 152–53.

Neonates (Birth to 28 Days)

The chief task of neonates is to adapt to their new environment. The first step in this process is breathing, an accomplishment that must occur within 30 seconds of birth if asphyxia is to be avoided. Neonates are completely dependent on others; they have no voluntary control over their movements, and their only emotion is a state of excitement. Their lives are dominated chiefly by reflexes.

Physical Development

Appearance

Newborn babies (Figure 11–1) usually have puffy eyelids and a flat broad nose. The lower jaw appears small and the neck very short. The shoulders slope, and the abdomen appears large and rounded with a protruding umbilical stump. The legs are bowed and appear short and out of proportion to the head, which makes up 21% of the total body surface. The arms appear long in proportion to the rest of the body. Lanugo may be apparent, particularly on the shoulders, back, and extremities. The vernix caseosa is obvious in the skin folds but will rub off naturally after a few days.

The skin of newborns is thin and appears delicate and often pink or reddish in Caucasians. They may have *milia*, which are small white spots on the nose and forehead. These are collections of sebaceous secretions, which usually disappear about 3 weeks after birth. Black, Oriental, and dark-skinned babies usually have bluish brown areas on their lower back called Mongolian spots. These will fade without treatment.

Figure 11–1 A newborn infant showing the short bowed legs, protruding abdomen, and the drying umbilical stump. (Courtesy of the City of Vancouver Health Department.)

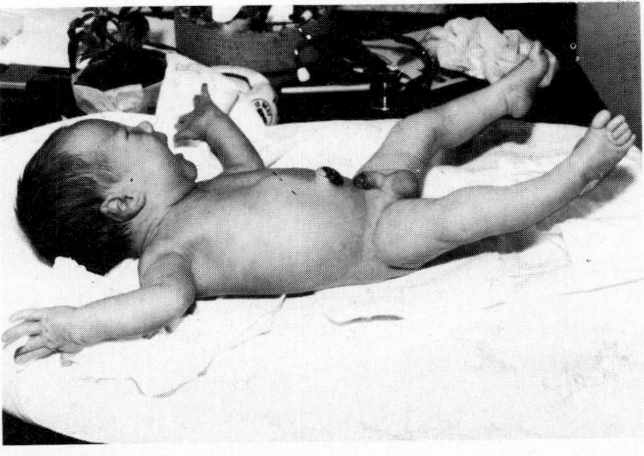

Table 11–7 Apgar Scoring System to Assess the Newborn

Sign	Score 0	Score 1	Score 2
1. Heart rate	Absent	Slow (below 100 per minute)	Above 100 per minute
2. Respirations	Absent	Slow, irregular	Regular rate, crying
3. Muscle tone	Flaccid	Some flexion of extremities	Active movements
4. Reflex irritability	None	Grimace	Cries
5. Color	Body pale or cyanotic	Body pink (for black babies, pink mucous membranes), extremities blue	Body completely pink in whites, pink mucous membranes in blacks

Physiologic jaundice of the newborn generally occurs between 3 and 4 days after birth because of excess red blood cells in the baby's blood, which are left over from fetal life. This jaundice normally disappears by 2 weeks. Jaundice that occurs within 24 hours of birth, however, must be monitored carefully because it may be caused by an incompatibility between the baby's blood and the mother's blood.

Newborn babies can be assessed by the Apgar scoring system. It provides a numerical indicator of physical status, that is, of the baby's capacities to adapt to extrauterine life. Each of five signs has a maximum score of 2, so that the total score achievable is 10. A score under 7 suggests that the baby is having difficulty, and a score under 4 indicates that the baby's condition is critical. Apgar scoring is usually carried out 60 seconds after birth and is repeated in 5 minutes. Those with very low scores require special resuscitative measures and care. See Table 11–7.

Table 11–8 Average Normal Vital Signs and Measurements of Newborns

Weight	3.4 kg or 3400 gm (7.5 lb)
Length	50 cm (20 in) head to heel
Head circumference	34 to 36 cm (13.5 to 14.5 in)
Pulse	70 to 170 beats per minute at rest
Blood pressure	65 to 90 mm Hg systolic 30 to 60 mm Hg diastolic
Temperature	36.1 to 37.7 C (97 to 100 F) by axilla
Respiratory rate	40 to 60 breaths per minute (average 35)

Weight

At birth most babies weigh between 2.7 to 3.8 kg (6.0 to 8.5 lb). Black infants tend to weigh less than Caucasians. Some of this birth weight (about 10%) is lost the first few days due to fluid loss. Children can be expected to double their weights by 6 months of age and to weigh about 10 kg (22 lb) at 1 year and 13.6 kg (29 lb) at 2 years. A number of factors, such as mother's nutrition, mother's age, and heredity, can affect birth weights.

Just after birth, a baby loses weight due to fluid loss and the excretion of meconium from the intestines. This weight loss is normal, and infants usually regain weight in about 1 week. After the 1st week, babies usually gain weight. Table 11–8 gives average measurements and average vital signs. Chapter 14 describes how infants are weighed.

Length

The average Caucasian newborn in the United States is about 50 cm (20 in) long. Black infants tend to be shorter than Caucasians at birth (Clark 1981:81). This range is from 47.5 to 52.5 cm (19 to 21 in). Female babies are on the average smaller than male babies.

Two recumbent lengths are the crown to rump length (the sitting length) and the head to heel length (from the top of the head to the base of the heels). See Figure 11–2. Normally the crown to rump length is approximately the same as the head circumference.

Head growth

The skull is measured at its greatest diameter from above the eyes to the occipital protuberance. Steel, cloth, or disposable paper tapes can be used. If a cloth tape is used, it should be checked periodically against a metal standard, since cloth tends to stretch with use.

Assessment of skull circumference is of particular importance in infants and children to determine the growth rate of the skull and the brain. An infant's head should be measured at every visit to the physician or nurse until the child is 2 years. Head measurement of infants 3 years or older usually does not need to be done routinely; however, this measurement should be taken during initial examinations of young children. See Figure 11–3.

Normal head circumferences (*normocephaly*) are often related to chest circumferences. At birth the average head circumference is 35 cm (14 in) and generally varies only 1 or 2 cm (0.5 in). The chest circumference of the newborn is usually less than the head circumference by about 2.5 cm (1 in). As the infant grows, the chest circumference becomes larger than the head circumference. At about 9 or 10 months the head and chest circumferences are about the same, and after 1 year of age the chest circumference is larger.

Abnormalities in head circumferences are referred to as *macrocephaly* (a large head) or *microcephaly* (a small head). The former is often the result of excessive cerebrospinal fluid within the skull (*hydrocephalus*).

Skull shape and fontanelles

Most newborn babies have misshapen heads due to the molding of the head that occurs during vaginal deliveries. Molding of the head is made possible by *fontanelles* (unossified membranous gaps) in the bone structure of the skull and by overriding of the *sutures* (junction lines of the skull bones). Within a week the newborn's head usually will regain its symmetry, a fact that reassures parents.

The eight bones of the cranium are separated by sutures, which gradually ossify during childhood. These bones are the frontal bone, the occipital bone, two parietal and two temporal bones, and the sphenoid and ethmoid bones. See Figure 11–4. Six fontanelles are present at birth, but the two most prominent ones are the frontal (anterior) and the occipital (posterior) ones. The latter is the smaller of the two (1 to 2 cm in diameter) and is generally closed by 2 months. The posterior fontanelle may not be palpated for a few hours after birth because of the overriding of the sutures during delivery. The larger anterior fontanelle (4 to 6 cm in diameter and diamond-shaped) can increase in size for several months after birth. After 6 months, the size gradually decreases until closure occurs between 10 and 18 months.

Examination of the head of infants for symmetry of shape and for palpation of the fontanelles is best achieved while the infant is sitting comfortably in the mother's lap. Normally, in a crying, coughing, or vomiting infant, the anterior fontanelle has a certain tenseness, fullness, and bulging, indicating increased intracranial pressure. Continual bulging is abnormal and associated with tumors or infections of the brain or hydrocephalus due to obstruction of the cerebrospinal fluid circulation in the ventricles. Depression of the anterior fontanelle generally indicates dehydration.

Asymmetry of the scalp can be caused by a number of factors. Frequently a newborn will have disfiguring localized swellings over a portion of the scalp at birth or shortly after birth. *Caput succedaneum* is an edematous swelling of the soft tissues of a part of the scalp that was encircled by the cervix before the latter became fully

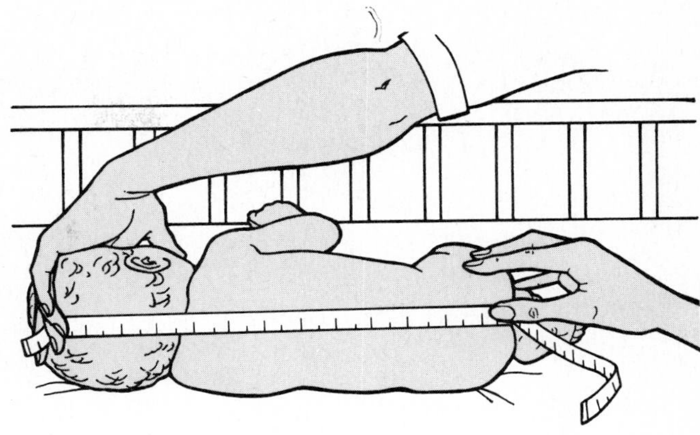

Figure 11–2 Measuring an infant crown to rump.

Figure 11–3 An infant's head circumference is measured around the skull above the eyebrows.

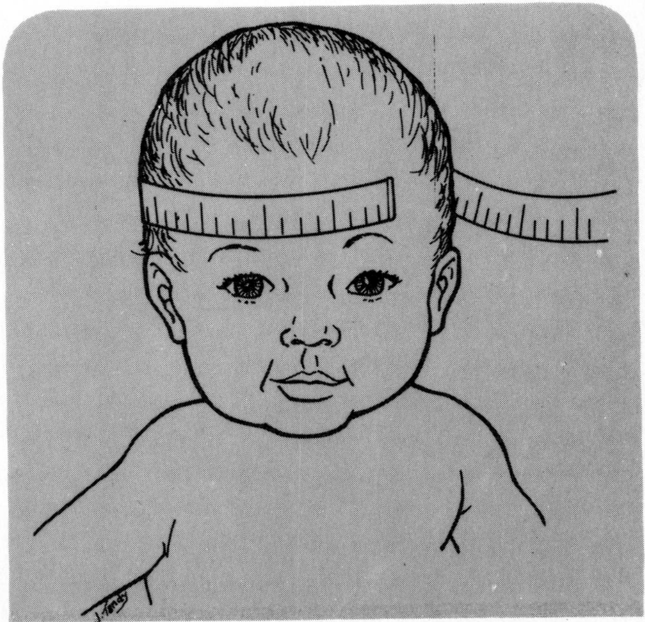

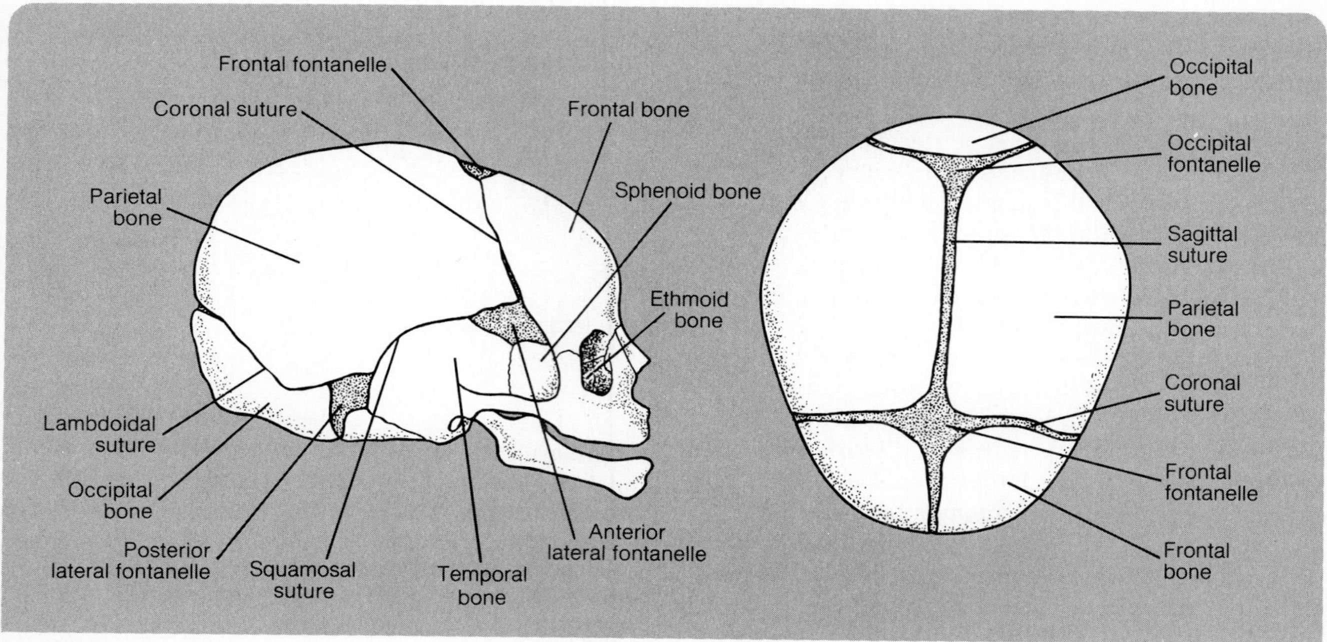

Figure 11–4 The bones of the skull showing the fontanelles and suture lines.

dilated. This condition commonly occurs over the occipitoparietal region (the presenting part of the fetus) and disappears spontaneously within a few days of birth. Bilateral symmetrical swellings of the scalp can also occur in difficult deliveries that require the use of forceps.

Another type of swelling of the scalp in the newborn is called *cephalhematoma*. This differs from caput succedaneum in that the swelling occurs directly over a bone or portion of it and is not visible until several hours after delivery. The cause is an effusion of blood between the periosteum and the bone (subperiosteal); it most commonly occurs over the parietal bones. This hematoma increases gradually in size for about a week and then slowly disappears. Misshaping of the head can also be caused by premature closure of the cranial sutures. Flattening of a part of the scalp frequently occurs in infants who almost always sleep in the same position.

Chest circumference

The chest circumference is measured by placing the tape around the chest at the level of the lower aspect of the scapula posteriorly and over the nipple line anteriorly. Often three measurements are taken and the average is recorded. The newborn's chest circumference is normally 30.5 to 33 cm (12 to 13 in).

Teeth

Newborn babies are normally born without visible teeth.

Vital signs

Newborns have unstable vital signs. Their temperature fluctuates from 36.1 to 37.7 C (97 to 100 F) because their heat regulating system is not fully developed. The pulse of the baby at birth ranges from 70 to 170 beats per minute at rest. Respirations are irregular, shallow, and quiet, ranging from 40 to 60 breaths per minute. Blood pressure of the newborn normally ranges from 60 to 90 mm Hg (millimeters of mercury) systolic and 30 to 60 mm Hg diastolic (see Table 11–8).

Feces

Meconium is the first fecal material passed by the newborn. It normally appears up to 24 hours after birth and is black, tarry, odorless, and sticky. Transitional stools, which follow for about a week, are generally greenish yellow; they contain mucus and are loose.

Eyes

The eyes of the newborn are usually tightly closed. To view the infant's eyes, the nurse holds the infant in a supine position and then gently lowers the baby's head. the eyes will then usually open. The eyes should be assessed for subconjunctival hemorrhages that may appear on the sclera. The cornea is examined for clarity. It is not uncommon for newborns to have a searching nystagmus or strabismus, which may persist intermittently for up to 4 to 6 months.

Senses

The newborn infant is sensitive to touch. Through touch the newborn perceives warmth, love, and security as well as the opposite of these. The newborn is also sensitive to temperature extremes and pain; however, babies react diffusely and cannot isolate the discomfort. The pain of an open safety pin in the buttock, for example, will not be isolated in the buttock.

Visual abilities are present at birth; the newborn can follow large moving objects and can react to changes in the intensity of light. The baby blinks in response to bright light and to sound.

The pupils of the newborn respond slowly, and the eyes cannot focus on close objects. Hearing is indistinct at birth because of the retention of fluid in the middle ear. The newborn does not differentiate sounds for some time but will have a startle reaction (Moro reflex) to a loud noise (see the following section on infant reflexes). The senses of smell and taste are not developed, although the newborn reacts to acid, bitter, salt, and sweet tastes by grimacing.

Reflex ability

The reflexes of the newborn are unconscious, involuntary responses. They are neither learned nor consciously carried out. They are nervous system reflexes to a number of stimuli. The degree of stimulation that is required to produce a reflex, for example the sucking reflex, varies considerably among newborns. Some newborns respond with vigor to the slightest stimulus, while others respond more slowly.

Ten main reflexes are normally present at birth. They are rooting, sucking, swallowing, Moro, palmar grasp, plantar, tonic neck, placing, stepping, and Babinski. In addition, yawning, stretching, sneezing, burping, and hiccuping are all present at birth.

The *rooting* and *sucking reflexes* are both used in feeding. The former is elicited by touching the baby's cheek; this causes the baby's head to turn to the side that was touched. The sucking reflex occurs when the baby's lips are touched. The *swallowing reflex* can be observed when the infant swallows any liquid obtained from sucking.

The *Moro reflex* (startle reflex) is often assessed in order to estimate the maturity of the central nervous system. A loud noise, a sudden change in position, or an abrupt jarring of the crib elicits this reflex. The infant reacts by extending both arms and legs outward with the fingers spread, then suddenly retracting the limbs. Often the infant cries at the same time.

The *palmar grasp reflex* occurs when a small object is placed against the palm of the hand, which causes the fingers to curl around it. The *plantar reflex* is similar in that an object placed just beneath the toes causes them to curl around it.

The *tonic neck reflex* (TNR) or fencing reflex is a postural reflex. When a baby who is lying on his or her back turns his head to the right side, for example, the left side of the body shows a flexing of the left arm and the left leg. This reflex is observed during the 1st week after birth.

The *placing reflex* is seen when a baby is held vertically with legs separated. When one foot is moved to touch the edge of a table, the baby automatically flexes the knee and hip of the same leg and tries to place the foot on the surface of the table.

The *stepping reflex* (walking or dancing reflex) can be elicited by holding the baby upright so that the feet touch a flat surface. The legs then move up and down as if the baby were walking. This reflex usually disappears at about 2 months.

A newborn baby also has a positive *Babinski reflex.* When the sole of the foot is stroked, the big toe rises and the other toes fan out.

Infant reflexes disappear during the 1st year of life. After age 1, the infant exhibits a negative Babinski, that is, the toes curl downward; positive Babinski after age 1 indicates brain damage.

Behavioral Development

Motor development

Motor development is the development of the baby's ability to move and to control the body. Movement begins before birth at about the 3rd month, when the fetus is able to move arms and legs spontaneously. After birth, activity increases gradually to include sucking, breathing, swallowing, and uncoordinated body movement. Newborn babies defecate and urinate with no controls.

Language and speech development

Neonates cry when they are uncomfortable, usually because they are hungry. By 1 month they begin to make cooing sounds.

Sleep

Newborns can be expected to sleep from 18 to 22 hours a day. It is normal during sleep for them to suck and move their arms. They usually awaken about every 4 hours, eat, and then go back to sleep.

Emotional development

In newborn babies the capacity to react emotionally is already present. The first sign of emotion is usually that of excitement in response to a strong external stimulus, for example, a loud noise. This response becomes differentiated into a response of pleasure and one of displeasure. Pleasure can be elicited by rocking or patting, while displeasure can be elicited by an abrupt change of position.

Learning adaptive mechanisms

Adaptive mechanisms are learned behavioral responses. They assist a person to adjust to the environment, and they assist in emotional development. Neonates have no adaptive mechanisms. When babies are born, they are neither moral nor immoral. They are amoral in that their behavior is neither guided nor influenced by moral considerations.

Assessing Developmental Changes

Stage: Neonate
Developmental task: Adjusting to birth

1. Has the temperature regulating system adjusted to the environment?
2. Has the infant established a sucking and swallowing mechanism so that he or she can obtain nourishment?
3. Have the bowels and bladder started to eliminate waste products?
4. Is the infant's physical development normal? (See previous section.)
5. How does the infant notify others when he or she is uncomfortable?
6. Does he or she sleep 18 to 22 hours per day?
7. Does the infant react with excitement to external stimuli?

Needs

Neonates have five special needs after respiration is established. These are stabilization of body temperature, eye care, cord care, protection against infection and trauma, and nourishment.

Providing warmth

Immediately after birth, the baby's body temperature drops, usually because the temperature of the delivery room is lower than the temperature inside the uterus. Failure to provide warmth at this time can lead to increased metabolic rate, which, if prolonged, can result in an increased consumption of glucose, subsequent hypoglycemia, and consequent brain damage. Wrapping the newborn in a warm blanket or using radiant infant warmers or incubators helps newborns establish a normal temperature. They continue to require protection from abrupt temperature changes because their temperature regulation is poorly developed. A draft-free room at a temperature of between 20.0 to 24.4 C (60 to 76 F) is considered appropriate.

Eye care

It is legally required in most places to treat newborns' eyes with a germicide that destroys the gonorrhea organism that can be present if the mother is infected. The usual germicide is a 1% solution of silver nitrate, two drops in each eye. A few minutes after the drops are inserted, the eyes are irrigated with warm distilled water. Today, penicillin is also used. It is administered as an ophthalmic ointment or intramuscularly. It is important to record the administration of the medication on the appropriate record.

Cord care

During a baby's first 24 hours of life, the cord needs to be observed for bleeding. The cord usually heals in about 1 week by dry healing. It is customary to clean the cord daily, usually after bathing the baby, with a 60% alcohol solution to facilitate healing and prevent infection. The stump must be observed closely for any signs of infection. Washing it with mild soap and water and thorough drying help prevent infection.

Protection against infection and trauma

Although newborns receive some antibodies from their mothers, they have very little resistance to infection. For this reason nurses wash their hands before handling a baby and, in some areas, wear masks and sterile gloves. Persons with respiratory or skin infections normally avoid contact with a newborn baby.

To protect the infant against trauma, vitamin K is often administered into the vastus lateralis muscle. See Chapter 37 on intramuscular injections.

The eyes are also checked for infection and trauma. The vulva is cleaned from anterior to posterior to prevent pathogens from entering the urethra and vagina.

Nourishment

Newborns are frequently put to the mother's breast within 1 hour of the delivery. Bottle feeding of sterile water is postponed until sucking and swallowing are coordinated. Water and supplementary feedings are normally not offered to a breast-feeding infant because they may interfere with breast feeding and lactation.

Newborn babies may become hungry shortly after they are born, or they may not develop an appetite for 1 or 2 days. Behavior such as restlessness, crying, and moving the head can indicate hunger. Infants in the nursery often are taken to the mother on demand (every 2 to 3 hours). Bottle-fed babies are offered 60 to 88 ml (2 to 3 oz) of formula after they establish sucking, gagging, and swallowing reflexes. For added information on infant feeding see Chapter 26.

Infants (1 Month to 1 Year)

The period of infancy is one of tremendous growth. (See Table 11–9 for common terms used to describe developmental stages.) One-year-old babies should weigh about three times their birth weight and may be able to walk with help.

Physical Development

Weight

Infants are twice their birth weight by 6 months and three times their birth weight by 12 months.

Height

By 6 months, they gain another 13.75 cm (5.5 in). By 12 months, they add another 7.5 cm (3 in). Rate of increase is largely influenced by the baby's size at birth and by nutrition.

Head growth

By 12 months, head circumference has increased about 33% over the birth size.

The posterior fontanelle between the parietal bones and the occipital bone closes from 4 to 8 weeks after birth. The anterior fontanelle (between the frontal and parietal bones) closes between 10 and 18 months.

Teeth

At about 5 to 6 months, the infant's first teeth appear.

Vital signs

Pulse averages 120 beats per minute between 1 month and 11 months. Respirations are 30 breaths per minute at 1 month. Temperature at 1 month is between 36.1 and 37.8 C (97 to 100 F). The average blood pressure at 1 month is 80 mm Hg systolic. The normal blood pressure at 1 year is 65 to 125 mm Hg systolic, 40 to 90 mm Hg diastolic.

Vision

By 3 months, vision develops so that both eyes are coordinated both horizontally and vertically. At 4 months the infant recognizes familiar objects and follows moving objects.

Behavioral Development

Motor development

By 3 months, infants can raise the head from a prone position, and by 6 months they can sit without support. See Figure 11–5. At 12 months, they can turn the pages of a book, stand alone for a moment, walk with help, and help with dressing.

Language development

By 1 month, an infant coos with pleasure and starts to babble a little by the second or third month. By 6 months, they chatter in nonsense syllables and continue to do so into the 2nd year. By 12 months some children can say a few words they have heard, such as *Mummy* and *Daddy*.

Sleep

By 4 months, normal infants sleep 8 hours or more at a time and require 16 to 18 hours each day. The average amount of sleep required by 6-month-olds is about 12 hours at night and 3 to 4 hours during the day. At 12 months, they sleep about 14 out of 24 hours, including one or two naps.

Social development

By the 2nd month, infants enjoy playing with objects and with people. They vocalize in response to the parents' voices. By 6 months, infants begin to perceive

Table 11–9 Developmental Stages

Stage	Ages
Neonatal	Birth to 28 days
Infancy	1 month to 1 year
Toddler	1 to 3 years
Preschool	3 to 5 years
Juvenile (schoolchild)	6 to 9 years
Preadolescence (prepubescence)	Girls 10 to 12 years; boys 12 to 14 years
Puberty	Girls 12 to 14 years; boys between 14 and 18 years
Adolescence	Girls 12 to 18 years; boys 14 to 20 years
Young adult	20 to 40 years
Middle-aged adult	40 to 65 years
Elderly adult	65 years and over

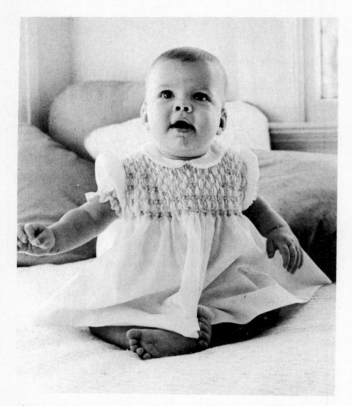

Figure 11–5 An infant sits without support at 6 months of age.

strangers, and by 9 months they interact by playing peek-a-boo and similar games. By 12 months, they recognize the meaning of *yes* and *no*. Infants are still egocentric, concerned only with themselves.

Cognitive and intellectual development

Cognitive refers to such processes as remembering, thinking, perceiving, abstracting, and generalizing. It is the development of a logical method of looking at the world and utilizing perceptual and conceptual abilities. *Intelligence*, by contrast, is the ability to learn. *To learn* is to acquire knowledge, to retain knowledge, and to respond to new situations and to solve problems.

From 4 to 8 months, infants begin to have perceptual recognition. By 6 months, they respond to new stimuli, and they remember certain objects and look for them for a short time. By 12 months, infants have a concept of both space and time. They experiment to reach a goal such as a toy on a chair.

Emotional development

At 1 month, the emotional response of infants is generally restricted to tension and occasional panics. The latter are exhibited by crying, arching the back, and flexing and extending the extremities. Infants also experience satisfaction chiefly from nourishment and when they are cuddled, held, and rocked. At 3 months, they need to suck to meet emotional needs, and by 6 months other members of the family are important in meeting their emotional needs. At 6 months, infants smile at the mother and family members, and they are able to wait a short time when they are hungry. By 6 months, infants have a beginning sense of self and often may be seen pulling at their toes as they learn to associate parts of the body with the concept of self.

Moral and religious development

At this early stage of development, children associate right and wrong with pleasure and pain. What gives them pleasure is right, since they are too young to reason otherwise.

Learning adaptive mechanisms

In infancy and toddlerhood several adaptive mechanisms are used to mediate anxieties. Three of these are symbolization, incorporation, and displacement.

Symbolization occurs when a mental image is created to stand for something. For example, being fed symbolizes security and pleasure. *Incorporation* occurs when people or objects are internalized and become a part of understanding. For example, *mother* is internalized; this internalization becomes the basis for the separation anxiety that infants normally experience at about age 9 months. *Displacement* is the transfer of emotions from the original person or object to another; for example, infants admitted to the hospital transfer the emotions they had for parents to the nurse.

Assessing Developmental Changes

Stage: Infancy
Developmental task: Basic trust versus mistrust
Does the infant:

1. Take nourishment satisfactorily?
2. Sleep normally?
3. Eliminate feces normally?
4. Permit his or her parents to go out of sight without undue anxiety or rage?
5. Indicate a separateness even though he or she is dependent on others? How does the infant let the parents know about his/her needs?
6. Differentiate between familiar and strange people, objects and environments?
7. Show affection? How does he or she respond to affection?

8. Reflect physical changes? (See previous sections.)
9. Exhibit an awareness of the environment? Do the infant's eyes follow moving objects? Does he or she reach for objects?

Needs

The needs of infants for food, sleep, play, immunizations, accident prevention, and mothering often have implications for nursing practice.

Nutrition

The early nourishment of infants is entirely liquid. Human milk is considered the ideal food for babies, and it is gradually supplemented with vitamins and more solid foods. See Chapter 26 for further information on nutrition.

Sleep

Sleep is an important need of infants because the bones, muscles, senses, nervous system, and internal organs develop during sleep. The sleep requirements of infants were discussed earlier in this chapter. The nurse is also referred to the section on developmental variables of rest and sleep, Chapter 25.

Play

Infants play with their toes and hands and assume many positions. Colorful hanging toys, particularly toys that move, are important from birth to about 3 months. After that infants require toys they can grasp and put into the mouth but cannot swallow, for instance, a large wooden spoon, stuffed toys, and small plastic animals. By age 1, they like building blocks and other toys they can pull apart and move around. They also enjoy playing in the sand or dirt; they fill pails and dump small loads of sand. When infants begin to walk, they like push-and-pull toys, such as wagons, and pounding toys, such as drums.

Immunizations

Immunizations are needed to protect infants from specific communicable diseases: diphtheria, pertussis, and tetanus. Immunization is provided in a combined form (DTP)—diphtheria, tetanus toxoids, and pertussis vaccine. Infants also require the orally administered poliomyelitis vaccine. In the United States and Canada infants usually receive DTP and poliomyelitis vaccine at approximately 2, 4, and 6 months. Measles-rubella vaccine or a combined measles-mumps-rubella vaccine is recommended at age 1 year, as well as a tuberculin test for contact with the tuberculosis bacillus. In some areas, smallpox vaccine is also given between the 3rd and 12th months. See Chapter 22 for further information.

Accident prevention

Accidents are the leading cause of morbidity and mortality of infants. Drowning, poisoning, suffocation, and falls are the most common accidents among infants. For example, an unwatched baby may roll off a table; thus infants need vigilant surveillance even during ordinary activities. Parents often require assistance to become aware of potential dangers in their homes, and nurses in hospitals need to be actively involved in accident prevention. See Chapter 22 for additional information.

Mothering

Mothering is the care usually provided by a mother, but mothering can be provided by another person. It involves loving care, handling, stroking, and cuddling the child. From the 3rd to the 15th month mothering is essential for both physical and intellectual growth. Infants deprived of mothering in this stage of development will not learn to form significant relationships or to trust others. Erikson sees this stage as characterized by the conflict of basic trust versus mistrust. See Table 11–2. Sometimes infants who are institutionalized for a long period suffer maternal deprivation and fail to grow even though there is no physiologic reason for the lack of growth. It is important that nurses provide mothering to hospitalized infants and to infants separated from the people who normally perform this function. The effect of the deprivation depends on the age of the child when deprived, the length of the deprivation, and similar factors. Maternal deprivation does not always cause a child to grow into a delinquent or an adult with many problems. People can learn and adapt to their environments in spite of this trauma.

Toddlers (1 to 3 Years)

Toddlers develop from having no voluntary control to being able both to walk and speak. They also learn to control their bladder and bowels, and they acquire all kinds of information about their environment.

Physical Development

Appearance

Two-year-old children lose the baby look. See Figure 11–6. Toddlers are usually chubby. The face appears small in comparison to the skull; but as the toddler grows, the face seems to grow from under the skull and appears better proportioned.

Growth

During the 2nd year, the rate of growth usually slows, and toddlers may gain only another 7.5 cm (3 in). The brain is 70% of its adult size by the time the infant is 2 years old.

Teeth

Toddlers are likely to have between 16 and 20 (all) of their deciduous teeth at 2 years of age. It is also during this period that the permanent teeth, with the exception of the second and third molars, begin to calcify.

Figure 11–6 A busy toddler appears slimmer than an infant.

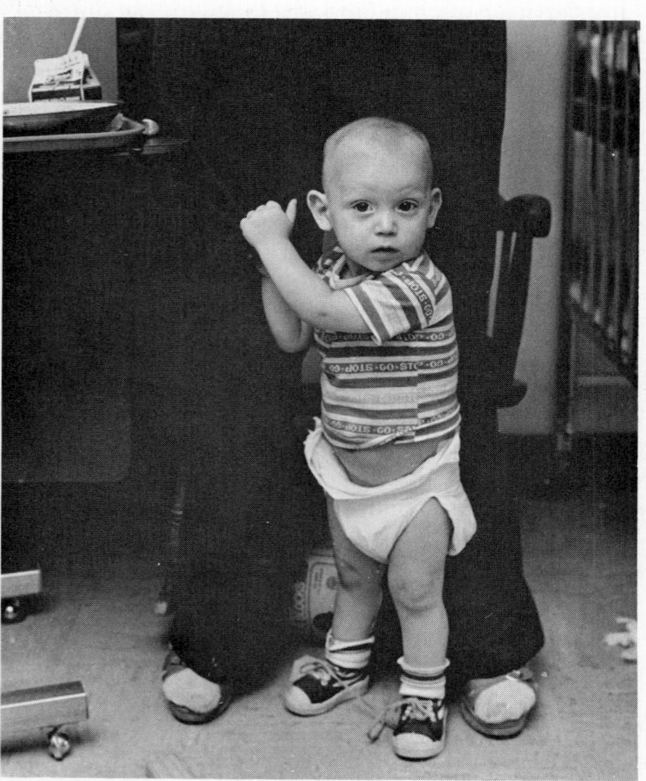

Vital signs

At 2 years, the toddler's temperature stabilizes at 37.2 C (98.9 F), which is considered normal. Respiration slows to about 25 breaths per minute, and the pulse averages 110 beats per minute. The blood pressure of the 2-year-old averages 75 to 100 mm Hg systolic and 40 to 90 mm Hg diastolic. By 3 years the temperature is 37.1 C (98.7 F), the pulse is 100 beats per minute, and the respiration rate is about 25 breaths per minute. The 3-year-old's blood pressure is normally 95 mm Hg systolic and about 60 mm Hg diastolic.

Weight

Two-year-olds can be expected to weigh approximately four times their birth weight. At 3 years, toddlers weigh about 15 kg (33 lb).

Senses

Visual acuity is fairly well established by 1 year; however, it is continually refined until the age of 6 years, when it becomes 20/20. Full binocular vision is usually established by 1 year. The senses of hearing, taste, smell, and touch become increasingly developed and associated with each other.

Touch is a very important sense to the toddler. He or she is often soothed by tactile sensations. When toddlers are hospitalized or ill, it is often the nurse's function to cuddle, hold, or rock them.

Posture

Toddlers have a pronounced lumbar lordosis and a protruding abdomen. The abdominal muscles develop gradually as the toddler grows, and the abdomen flattens.

Behavioral Development

Motor development

At the age of 18 months, babies can pick up small beads and place them in a receptacle. They can also hold a spoon and a cup and walk upstairs with assistance. They will probably crawl down the stairs.

At 2 years, toddlers can hold a spoon and put it into the mouth correctly. They are able to run; their gait is steady; and they can balance on one foot and ride a tricycle.

By 3 years, most children are toilet trained, although there still may be the occasional accident when playing or during the night.

Language and speech

Most children learn to imitate words in the 2nd year, when sufficient cortical maturity has taken place. By 2 years, they usually can arrange several words into a sentence. Three-year-olds speak almost constantly. They practice speaking in bed and during play. They imitate adults and can express feelings, thoughts, desires, and problems in words. Logic is elusive, so not all their words at any one time relate to the same activity.

Sleep

Rest and sleep continue to be important to toddlers. They still require 12 hours of sleep at night during the 2nd year as well as a nap of several hours during the day, or a total sleep requirement of about 15 or 16 hours per day. Three-year-olds also require a similar amount of sleep, anywhere from 9 to 13 hours each night, perhaps a reduction of 1 to 2 hours from their need at 2 years. Three- and 4-year-olds may have dreams and nightmares that awaken them.

Social development

At 2 years, children are very possessive of their toys. They are dependent on their parents and react strongly to separation from them. By age 3, toddlers are learning to play with their peers.

Cognitive development

By 2 years, children have developed considerable cognitive and intellectual skills. They have learned about the sequence of time. They have some symbolic thought; for example, a chair may represent a place of safety, while a blanket symbolizes comfort. Concepts start to form in late toddlerhood. A concept develops when the child learns words to represent classes of objects or thoughts. An example of a concrete concept is *table*, representing a number of articles of furniture, which are all different but all tables. Between the ages of 3 and 5 years, toddlers become concerned with the concept of death. They often think of death as a simple departure from home.

Emotional development

At 18 months, toddlers imitate their parents and play games. They indicate displeasure over a wet diaper. By 2 years, routine is very important; toddlers find change disturbing and often cry when routine is changed. Toddlers' emotions of love and hate are often extreme.

Toddlers begin to develop their sense of autonomy by asserting themselves with the frequent use of the word *no*. They are often frustrated by restraints to their behavior; between ages 1 and 3 children may have temper tantrums. However, they slowly gain control over their emotions, usually with the guidance of their parents.

The period of the development of a sense of autonomy (1 to 3 years) is a time of expanding social contacts. Toddlers are curious and ask many questions. Children at this age are often creative, although the products of this activity may not be perfect.

Moral and religious development

During the 2nd year of life, children begin to know that some activities elicit affection and approval. They also recognize that certain rituals, such as repeating phrases from prayers, also elicit approval. This provides children with feelings of security. By 2 years of age, toddlers are learning what attitudes their parents hold about religious and moral matters. Three-year-old children may repeat short prayers at bedtime.

Assessing Developmental Changes

Stage: Toddler
Developmental task: Autonomy versus shame and doubt
Does the toddler:

1. Indicate adjustment to daily routines such as play periods and sleep times?
2. Demonstrate appropriate practices for nutrition?
3. Start to develop bowel and bladder control?
4. Exhibit physical skills appropriate for his or her age?
5. Begin to play and communicate with children and others outside the immediate family?
6. Express likes and dislikes or exhibit any other autonomous behavior?
7. Demonstrate learning of some of the religious practices of the family?

Needs

The needs of toddlers for sleep, accident prevention, and nutrition must be met when they are ill.

Sleep

Sleep is an important need of children 2 to 3 years old. Three-year-olds usually sleep through the night but need one nap during the day. Nursing plans should include this time for rest.

Accident prevention

Accidents are a leading cause of morbidity and mortality of toddlers. Drowning, poisoning, suffocation, and falls are the most common accidents experienced by toddlers. For example, a toddler may swallow liquid household cleaners if they are left in reach.

Precautions need to be taken to keep medicines, cleaners, and the like out of the reach of toddlers. Parents may need to learn to lock cupboards or to place dangerous substances out of reach. See Chapter 22 for additional information.

Nutrition

Toddlers' nourishment is basic to their health and growth. During the 2nd year of life, the average toddler will gain 0.2 kg (0.5 lb) per month (Endres and Rockwell 1980:74). The hospitalized toddler also needs to have nutritional needs met. Because of their growth and activity, toddlers' food needs are proportionately greater, by body size, than an adult's. For additional information, see Chapter 26.

Preschoolers (4 and 5 Years)

Physical Development

By the time children are 4 or 5 years old, they appear taller and thinner than toddlers because children tend to grow more in height than in weight. See Figure 11–7.

Figure 11–7 The preschool child appears taller and slimmer than the toddler.

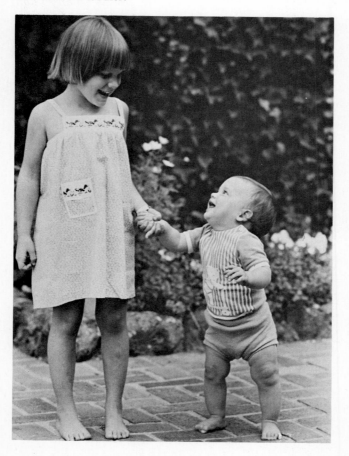

Weight

Weight gain in preschool children is generally slow. By 5 years, they have added only another 3 to 5 kg (7 to 12 lb) to their 3-year-old weight, increasing it to somewhere between 18.1 and 20.4 kg (40 and 45 lb).

Height

Preschool children grow about 5 to 6.25 cm (2.0 to 2.5 in) each year. Thus by 5 years of age, they double the birth length and measure 100 cm (40 in).

Body proportions

The preschooler's brain reaches almost its adult size by 5 years. The extremities of the body grow more quickly than the body trunk, making the child's body appear somewhat out of proportion.

Vital signs

The vital signs of preschoolers are normally a pulse rate of about 100 beats per minute, respiratory rate of about 23 breaths per minute, and blood pressure 80 to 120 mm Hg systolic and 45 to 85 mm Hg diastolic. Body temperature is between 37.2 and 37.0 C (100 and 98.6 F).

Vision

Preschool children are generally hyperopic (farsighted). As the eye grows in length, it becomes emmetropic (it refracts light normally). If the eyes become too long, the child becomes myopic (nearsighted).

Posture

The posture of preschoolers gradually changes. The posture becomes transformed as the pelvis is straightened and the abdominal muscles become stronger. Thus the preschooler appears slender with erect posture.

Behavioral Development

Motor development

By 5 years of age, children are able to wash their hands and face and brush their teeth. They are self-conscious about exposing their body and go to the bathroom without telling others.

Typically, preschool children run with increasing skill each year. By 5 years of age, they run skillfully and can jump three steps. Preschoolers can balance on their toes and dress themselves without assistance.

Language and speech

By 4 years of age, children tend to believe that what they know is right. They tend to be dogmatic in their speech. Four-year-olds love nonsense words such as *jump-jump* and can string them together much to an adult's exasperation. At 4, children are aggressive in their speech and capable of long conversations, often mixing fact and fiction.

By 5 years of age, speaking skills are well developed. Children use words purposefully and ask questions to acquire information. They do not merely practice speaking as 3- and 4-year-olds do, but speak as a means of social interaction. Exaggeration is common among four- and five-year-olds.

Sleep

Preschoolers are still a bundle of energy. During nap time in the afternoon, they are more likely to rest than to sleep. At night, they are likely to sleep more peacefully than toddlers.

Social development

Preschool children gradually emerge as social beings. At the age of 3 or 4 they learn to play with a small number of their peers. They gradually learn to play with more people as they grow older.

Cognitive and intellectual development

Concepts start to form in late toddlerhood or the early preschool years. Preschoolers become concerned about death as something inevitable, but they do not explain it. They also associate death with others rather than in relation to themselves.

Most children at the age of 5 years can count pennies; however, the opportunity to spend money usually does not occur until they attend school. Reading skills also start to develop at this age. Young children like fairy tales and books about animals and other children.

At this age the preschooler may experience conflict with the introduction of a new baby into the family. Parents' time and affection are now shared, and the preschooler may react jealously.

Relationships

Preschoolers participate more in the family than they did previously; however, they also start to play with their peers. In associations with neighbors, family guests, and baby sitters, too, they learn about relationships.

The phase of close emotional relationship with both parents changes to the phase Freud referred to as the Electra or Oedipus complex (Engel 1962:90–104). At this time, the child focuses feelings of love chiefly on the parent of the opposite sex, and the parent of the same sex may receive some hostile feelings. At this time, the child begins to develop sexual interests. The child becomes interested in clothes and hair styles.

Emotional development

According to Erikson, the major problem of preschoolers is attaining a sense of initiative: They must learn what they can do. As a result, preschoolers imitate behavior, and their imagination and creativity become lively.

Preschoolers also become increasingly aware of themselves. They play with their bodies largely out of curiosity. They know where the body begins and ends as well as the correct names for the different parts. By 5 years of age, they are able to draw a person including all the features. Preschoolers also learn about their feelings; they know the words *cry, sad, laugh* and the feelings related to them. They also begin to learn how to control their feelings and behavior.

Learning adaptive mechanisms

During the preschool years, four adaptive mechanisms are learned: identification, introjection, imagination, and repression. *Identification* occurs when the child perceives the self as similar to another person and behaves like that person. For example, a boy may internalize the attitudes, behavior, and gender of his father. *Introjection* is similar to identification. It is the assimilation of the attributes of others. When preschoolers observe their parents, they assimilate many of their values and attitudes.

Imagination is an important part of preschoolers' life. The preschooler has an active imagination and fantasizes in play; for example, a chair becomes a beautiful throne to a girl and she is the ruler. *Repression* is removing experiences, thoughts, and impulses from awareness. Thoughts related to the Oedipus or Electra complex are generally repressed by the preschooler.

Moral and religious development

Preschool children hear others discuss moral and religious topics, but they learn better from the example set by their parents than from what they hear. Preschoolers accept the religion of parents without question. Many parents send their preschool children to Sunday school. Children are aware of religious occasions more as holidays than as times of worship and observance.

Preschoolers generally have a developing conscience and behave well with very little prompting.

Assessing Developmental Changes

Stage: Preschooler
Developmental task: Initiative versus guilt
Does the preschooler:

1. Appear active and relaxed during activities?
2. Possess physical skills appropriate for the age?
3. Demonstrate that he or she is toilet trained?
4. Participate as a family member?
5. Handle unusual or potentially dangerous situations, such as an angry dog?
6. Demonstrate autonomy by doing certain things without help?
7. Exhibit appropriate emotional expressions in different situations?
8. Respond to others' expectations about behavior?

Needs

The needs of the preschooler are primarily accident prevention, nutrition, dental care, play, and guidance. These needs have nursing implications.

Accident prevention

Accidents continue to be the major cause of mortality among preschool children. These children are active, often clumsy, and therefore susceptible to injury. Accidents can be prevented in two ways: control of the environment and education of the child. Parents may need to learn to control the environment, for instance, by keeping matches out of the child's reach, putting toys away when they are not being used, and safeguarding swimming pools and other potentially dangerous areas. The education of the preschooler involves many aspects of daily living. Three of these are learning how to cross streets, learning traffic signals, and learning bicycle safety practices.

Nutrition

Preschool children still need milk in addition to a balanced diet of fruit, vegetables, bread, cereals, and meat or fish daily. Children eat much like adults except that they need smaller quantities. Generally a preschooler's age is a good guide to the size of a serving: 4-year-olds eat 4 Tbsp servings of foods from each group at each meal; 5-year-olds eat 5 Tbsp servings.

Preschoolers also require sufficient protein for the growth of new tissues. A child who weighs 13.6 kg (30 lb) requires 37 gm of protein daily as well as 30 mg of vitamin C. The latter is found in fruits, fruit juices, and some vegetables. One medium orange contains 55 mg of vitamin C.

Preschool children also require snacks, usually in the morning, afternoon, and evening. A snack might be a glass of milk and a sandwich. They usually eat one food at a time and often dislike coarse-textured foods and strong-tasting foods.

Nurses caring for hospitalized or ill children need to be aware of children's special nutritional requirements.

Dental care

Regular dental examinations are essential at this age; caries develop quickly in young children. Examinations usually are initiated at about 2½ years. It has been estimated that 80% of children have some tooth decay. Deciduous teeth guide the entrance of permanent teeth; therefore, abnormally placed or lost deciduous teeth can cause the misalignment of permanent teeth. Dental care also involves teaching children to brush after each meal and before retiring. For additional information on dental care, see Chapter 21.

Play

Preschoolers spend most of the day playing. Play serves a number of purposes:

1. Children learn to cooperate with others.
2. Focus changes from family to peers.
3. Children develop strength and coordination.
4. Abundant energy is dispersed.
5. Children have an avenue to express initiative and imagination.

Play is also fun to preschoolers. They take it seriously but express joy and pleasure during play. Play at this age is loosely organized. Preschoolers who are hospitalized can frequently have play time included in their nursing plans.

Guidance

Guidance is an essential need of preschoolers. They require both guidance and discipline that is consistent and fair. Through guidance, they gain a sense of security and the feeling that their parents care about them. It is important that parents follow through with a punishment once it is imposed; a child confined to his or her room for 1 hour should stay the full hour. In a hospital setting, nurses often must provide the guidance normally given by parents.

School-Age Children (6 to 12 Years)

The school-age period starts when children are about 6 years of age, when the deciduous teeth are shed, and includes the preadolescent (prepuberty) period. It ends at about 12 years with the onset of puberty. Puberty is the age when the reproductive organs become functional and secondary sex characteristics develop. Because the average age of onset of puberty is 10 for girls and 12 for boys, some people define the school-age years as 6 to 10 for girls and 6 to 12 for boys. Skills learned during this stage are particularly important in relation to work later in life and willingness to try new tasks.

Starting school is significant for a number of reasons; for one, children are able to compare their skills to those of their peers. They also receive impressions of how their skills are perceived by others—the teacher, the school nurse, and their peers. These perceptions can bolster a child's self-image or can weaken feelings of self-worth. In general, the period from 6 to 12 years is one of rapid and dramatic change.

Physical Development

Appearance

School-age children at 7 years gain weight rapidly and thus appear less thin than previously. Individual differences due to genetic influences and environment are generally obvious at this time.

Weight

At 6 years, boys tend to weigh about 21 kg (46 lb), about 1 kg (2 lb) more than girls. The weight gain of school children from 6 to 12 years of age averages about 3.2 kg (7 lb) per year, but the major weight gains occur from age 10 to 12 for boys and from age 9 to 12 for girls. By 12 years of age, boys and girls weigh on the average 40 to 42 kg (88 to 95 lb); girls are usually heavier. See Table 11–10. These are average weights, and wide variations exist.

Height

At 6 years, both boys and girls are about the same height, 115 cm (46 in). They are about 150 cm (60 in) by 12 years. Refer to Table 11–10. Before puberty, children of both sexes have a growth spurt, girls between 10 and 12 years and boys between 12 and 14 years. Thus girls may well be taller than boys at 12 years, although the boys are usually stronger. The extremities tend to grow more quickly than the trunk, thus school-age children's bodies appear somewhat ill-proportioned.

Table 11–10 Approximate Average Heights and Weights, School-Age Children (6 to 12 years)

	Weight				Height			
	Boys		Girls		Boys		Girls	
Age	kg	lb	kg	lb	cm	in	cm	in
6	21	46	20	44	116	46	115	46
7	23	50	22	48	121	48	121	48
8	26	57	25	55	127	50	126	49
9	29	63	28	61	132	52	132	52
10	32	70	33	72	137	54	137	54
11	36	79	38	83	142	56	145	57
12	40	88	42	95	150	59	152	60

Adapted from U.S. Department of Health, Education, and Welfare. Public Health Service, *NCHS growth curves for children, birth–18 years: United States*, DHEW Publication no. (PHS)78-1650 (Hyattsville, Md.: National Center for Health Statistics, 1977), pp. 58–63.

Teeth

Permanent teeth start to appear between 6 and 7 years of age, and dental caries also can appear. Thus regular dental checkups are needed. By the age 13 or 14, children have most of their permanent teeth with the exception of their third molars (wisdom teeth), which erupt between 17 and 24 years of age.

Vital signs

At age 6, both boys and girls have these average vital signs: body temperature, 37.0 C (98.6 F), pulse rate, 75 to 115 beats per minute; respiratory rate, 21 breaths per minute; and blood pressure, 85 to 115 systolic, 50 to 60 diastolic. By 12 years, children have a body temperature, pulse, and respiration rate similar to those of adults. Body temperature still averages 37 C (98.6 F). A 12-year-old boy's pulse is between 65 and 105 beats per minute when resting; a girl's, between 70 and 110 beats per minute. The respirations are about 19 breaths per minute, and blood pressure measures from 95 to 135 mm Hg systolic and 50 to 70 mm Hg diastolic.

Vision

The depth and distance perception of children 6 to 8 years of age is accurate. By age six, children have full binocular vision: The eye muscles are well developed and coordinated, and both eyes can focus on one object at the same time. Because the shape of the eye changes during growth, the farsightedness of the preschool years gradually changes to 20/20 vision during the school-age years; 20/20 vision is usually well established between 9 and 11 years of age. In later childhood, myopia is not uncommon; that is, the child is able to see clearly only objects that are close. This problem is generally corrected by eyeglasses.

Posture

By 6 years, the thoracic curvature starts to develop, and the lordosis disappears. Full adult posture is not assumed, however, until after the complete development of the skeletal musculature during the adolescent period.

Reproductive and endocrine changes

Very little change takes place in the reproductive and endocrine systems until the prepuberty period. During prepuberty, at about ages 9 to 13, endocrine functions slowly increase. This change in endocrine function can result in increased perspiration and more active sebaceous glands. As a result, acne may develop, particularly on the face, neck, and back.

Certain physical changes occur in both boys and girls during prepuberty. Some of the changes in approximate sequence are as follows:

For the boy:

1. The testes and scrotum increase in size.
2. The skin over the scrotum changes color; it becomes reddened and stippled.
3. The breasts may enlarge slightly, but this growth disappears in a few months.
4. Sparse, downy pubic hair grows at the base of the penis. This hair darkens, thickens, and spreads upward from the penis and to the thighs by about age 16 to 18.
5. The penis gradually enlarges in both width and length. Development of the genitals to adult size takes about 5 to 6 years.
6. Spontaneous erections may occur under various kinds of stimulation.

For the girl:

1. The pelvis and hips broaden.
2. The breast tissues develop and may be tender. At first the nipple is slightly elevated, at 7½ to 8 years of age. The areolae become somewhat protuberant and enlarged between the ages of 9 and 11 years.
3. Fat is deposited on the hips, thighs, and breasts.
4. The initial growth of pubic hair occurs at about 10½ years.
5. Vaginal secretions become milky and change from an alkaline to an acid pH, and menstruation may occur toward the end of the 12th year (Murray and Zentner 1979:164, Whaley and Wong 1979:637).

Behavioral Development

Motor development

During the middle years (6 to 10), children perfect their muscular skills and coordination. By 9 years, most children are becoming skilled in games of interest, such as football or baseball. These skills are often associated with school, and many of them are learned there. By 9 years, also, most children have sufficient fine motor control for activities such as building models or sewing.

Language and speech

Sentence length increases for most children until the age of 9½, at which time sentence length stabilizes or decreases slightly. Boys tend to lag behind girls in speech development. They usually speak with shorter sentences, and their grammar is less correct. See a discussion of factors influencing language development in Chapter 15 for further information.

Children between 8 and 12 years often boast to win peer approval. Children between 8 and 12 also engage in name calling; frequently, it is done to gain attention and to impress others with the child's superiority. Another common development is tattling, a form of criticism in which children project and blame their own shortcomings on someone else. Children consider tattling one of the worst crimes, and peer censure is generally severe.

Social development

As they grow older, schoolchildren learn to play with more children at one time. Usually the 6- or 7-year-old is a member of a peer group. This group can replace children's families in teaching attitudes and can be a great influence. During late childhood, children join a gang, a small group of peers, which is formed by the children themselves. It is usually informal and transitory, and the leadership changes from time to time. During this period of socialization with others, children gradually become less self-centered and selfish and more cooperative and conscious of the group.

Cognitive and intellectual development

Money is a concept that gains meaning for children when they start school. By the time they are 7 or 8 years old, children usually know the value of most coins.

The concept of time is also learned at this age. By 6 years of age, children enter school; the schedule in school helps them to learn time periods, but it is not until 9 or 10 years of age that children are able to understand the long periods of time in the past. Knowing the time of day and the day of the week are relatively easy for children because they relate time to routine activities. For example, a girl may go to school Monday through Friday, play on Saturday, go to Sunday school on Sunday morning, and go out with her father Sunday afternoon. Children are beginning to read a clock by the time they are 6 years old.

Later in childhood reading skills are usually well developed, and what a child reads is largely influenced by the family. By 9 years of age most children are self-motivated. They compete with themselves, and they like to plan in advance. By 12 years, they are motivated by inner drive rather than by competition with peers. They like to talk and to discuss different subjects, and they like to debate.

During school-age years, the child learns to identify with the parent of the same sex and learns the behaviors associated with the role of that parent. At this time, the child probably has some conflict with siblings, although this conflict is less severe than it is for the preschooler. Again, the school-age child may resent a new baby, and may also resent the freedom given older brothers and sisters. Parents who compare siblings' accomplishments and talents can cause resentment and rivalry.

Emotional development

According to Erikson's stages of emotional development, from 6 to 11 years the conflict is industry versus inferiority.

In school, children have the restraints of the school system imposed on their behavior and learn to develop controls. Children compare their skills with those of their peers in a number of areas, including motor development, social development, and language. This comparison assists in the development of self-concept. Schoolchildren can sometimes be cruel in their honesty, and teachers often need to intercede to assist children who have limitations.

Learning adaptive mechanisms

The schoolchild develops a number of adaptive mechanisms that help the child adapt. Four of these are regression, malingering, rationalization, and ritualistic behavior.

Regression is returning to a form of behavior that was suitable at an earlier age. For example, the child who is anxious about starting school may start bedwetting at night or perhaps revert to baby talk. *Malingering* is a familiar mechanism to schoolchildren. It is pretending to be ill rather than facing something unpleasant; the child who feels sick the morning before a test may be malingering.

Rationalization is an attempt to justify behavior by logical reason and explanation. A girl who does not make the swimming team may rationalize to her parents by saying she really did not try hard because she doesn't want swimming to interfere with her piano lessons.

Ritualistic behavior is demonstrated by schoolchildren in many settings. For example, a child may walk down the sidewalk without stepping on a crack. Clubs and gangs often have rituals for their members. These rituals become very important to schoolchildren even though they usually do not persist for a long time. For example, the boy who must have a shower every morning may forget this ritual after a few weeks.

Moral and religious development

During the school years children may see God as a human being. They expect their prayers to be answered. They may ask many questions about God and religion in these years and will generally believe that God is good and always present to help. In the period just before puberty, children become aware that their prayers are not always answered and become disappointed. At this age, some children reject religion, while others continue to accept it. This decision is largely influenced by the parents. If a child continues religious training, the child is ready to apply reason rather than blind belief in most situations.

Assessing Developmental Changes

Stage: School-age child
Developmental task: Industry versus inferiority
Does the school-age child:

1. Apply himself or herself to given tasks in the school and with peers?
2. Begin to solve problems?
3. Become a cooperative family member?
4. Become less dependent on the family?
5. Control strong and impulsive feelings?
6. Begin to understand the importance of sharing with family and peers?
7. Begin to learn how to save and spend money?
8. Think of self as likable and healthy?

Needs

Immunizations

During the school-age years, children need boosters for those immunizations given in infancy. Generally, they are given against tetanus, diphtheria, and poliomyelitis. Local health departments have their own recommended schedules, which are revised regularly in light of medical advances. See the schedules in Chapter 22.

Some physicians recommend that girls receive the rubella vaccine before puberty to prevent the possibility of rubella during pregnancy and subsequent congenital defects. Boys need to be protected against mumps, thus preventing subsequent sterility, which can occur as a result of contracting mumps later in life.

Nutrition

School-age children eat four or five times a day, including a snack after school. Children need a protein-rich food at breakfast to sustain the prolonged physical and mental effort required at school. Studies reveal that children who eat well-balanced breakfasts have better attitudes and school records than those who omit breakfast (Pipes 1981:173). Undernourished children become fatigued easily and face a greater risk of infection, resulting in frequent absences from school.

The average school-age child generally requires:

1. 4 servings per day of milk or milk products (1 serving equals 1 cup).
2. 2 or more servings per day of meat (1 serving equals 6 to 8 Tbsp).
3. 4 or more servings per day of cereals and breads (1 serving equals ½ to 1 cup or 1 or 2 slices).
4. 4 or more servings per day of green or yellow vegetables and fruits (1 serving equals ⅓ to ½ cup).

Exercise and rest

By the time children enter school, they probably do not need a nap in the afternoon. Sleep needs also are less. A 6-year-old may require 11 hours of sleep, while an 11-year-old may need only 9 hours. See Chapter 25, page 626, for further information.

School-age children need exercise to build muscles and develop fine motor coordination. Parents often introduce children of this age to healthful and enjoyable physical activities. For example, the 10-year-old boy who plays golf with his parents not only obtains good exercise but also shares an activity with persons who are important in his life.

Play

School-age children have more friends than preschoolers. In early school years they like to playact familiar roles, such as police officer or teacher. By the age of 9 or 10 years, they become more interested in skill games, such as football or baseball. Boys and girls of this age separate for play activities and form preadolescent gangs. Membership in the gang is strictly regulated. Often membership in a gang or club is predicated on a skill, such as tying knots, or a ritual, such as making a finger bleed without acknowledging pain. At this age most children have a best friend. This is usually someone of the same sex; the child shares feelings, thoughts, and activities with the friend.

Accident prevention

See accident prevention for the school-aged child in Chapter 22.

Guidance

Schoolchildren can discuss matters of discipline with their parents. They may need several alternative courses of action and probably more guidance than discipline. It is important not to embarrass children by disciplining them in front of others. Children also may be confused if a parent provides two messages at once. For example, when a father tells his son that he should not lie, but then tells a lie in front of the child, the child receives two messages.

Summary

With a knowledge of growth and development the nurse is able to:

1. Assess the developmental needs of people
2. Anticipate developmental stressors of people
3. Determine the growth and developmental capacities of people

There are a number of approaches to growth and development. A brief overview of some of these is given early in the chapter. Each stage poses developmental tasks or problems. Failure to master these tasks can result in impaired development and often impaired functioning in life; for example, the infant who fails to develop basic trust may have difficulty establishing close relationships later in life.

The first stage of growth and development is intrauterine development, which begins with conception and ends with the birth of a baby, usually 10 lunar months (9 calendar months) later. The intrauterine stage can be divided into phases, the embryonic and fetal. During these stages three tissue layers differentiate to develop a human being.

The neonatal stage lasts from birth to 28 days. During this period the baby adapts to the environment and establishes basic physiologic processes such as respiration and digestion. Assessment of the newborn is done with the Apgar scoring system. This system assesses heart rate, respirations, muscle tone, reflex irritability, and color; each characteristic is given a numerical value of 0, 1, or 2.

Infancy lasts from age 1 month to 1 year. During this time, the infant needs to develop basic trust. The infant's birth weight will triple, and at 1 year of age the infant may be walking with help. The infant has many needs for which nurses must plan, such as nutrition, sleep, play, immunization, protection from accidents, and mothering.

Toddlerhood lasts from age 1 to age 3. The toddler learns to control bladder and bowels. The basic need is to develop a sense of autonomy. Toddlers are normally curious about their environment, but they need assistance so that this curiosity does not result in injury. Because of growth and activity at this age, nourishment is important. Another important need of the toddler is sleep; during sleep tissues form.

Preschoolers (ages 4 and 5) run and jump; they are a bundle of energy. Their developmental need, according to Erikson, is to show initiative. The preschooler's posture changes from that of the toddler, and language and speech continue to develop. Preschoolers often believe that what they know is right. Preschoolers develop healthy routines and master other skills such as eating, climbing, and learning healthy emotional expressions.

The school-age stage starts at 6 years and terminates with puberty. The important task during this period is industry. Permanent teeth start to appear between 6 and 7 years, and most permanent teeth with the exception of the third molars are present by the age of 12. Between the ages of 8 and 12 years, endocrine functions slowly increase and prepuberal physical changes occur. Nursing intervention during this period includes consideration of immunizations, nutrition, play, and the prevention of accidents.

Social and emotional development are particularly significant during the school years. Children gradually learn to be less self-centered and more cooperative through social relationships with peers. Emotional development is demonstrated with increasing control. Through feedback from peers, among others, children develop self-concepts.

Suggested Activities

1. Visit a playground, schoolyard, or beach where there are children of various ages. Select several children to observe, and describe their activities in terms of their developmental stages.
2. Visit a newborn baby at home. Assess developmental changes as outlined in this textbook.
3. Visit a preschooler or a school-age child who is a patient in a hospital. Assess the child's particular needs, including health needs and developmental status.
4. Visit a classroom of children about the same age. Observe the children for developmental differences.

Suggested Readings

Comer, J. P., and Poussaint, A. F. 1975. *Black child care: How to bring up a healthy black child in America.* New York: Simon and Schuster.

This book describes developmental needs with particular reference to black children. The sections include the infant, the preschool child, the black child in school, the elementary-school-age child, and the adolescent.

Ilg, F. L., and Ames, L. B. 1955. *The Gesell Institute's child behavior from birth to ten.* New York: Harper and Row.

This classic pocket book provides information about how a child grows; ages and stages and individuality are stressed. Part Two deals with specific subjects such as eating behavior, sleeping, and dreams and fears.

Selected References

Block, G. J.; Nolan, J. W.; and Dempsey, M. K. 1981. *Health assessment for professional nursing: A developmental approach.* New York: Appleton-Century-Crofts.

Clark, A. L. 1981. *Culture and childrearing.* Philadelphia: F. A. Davis Co.

Endres, J. B., and Rockwell, R. E. 1980. *Food, nutrition, and the young child.* St. Louis: C. V. Mosby Co.

Engel, G. L. 1962. *Psychological development in health and disease.* Philadelphia: W. B. Saunders Co.

Erikson, E. H. 1963. *Childhood and society.* 2nd ed. New York: W. W. Norton and Co.

Fong, B. C., and Resnick, M. R. 1980. *The child: Development through adolescence.* Menlo Park, Calif.: Benjamin/Cummings Publishing Co.

Havighurst, R. J. 1972. *Developmental tasks and education.* 3rd ed. New York: David McKay Co.

Kozier, B., and Erb, G. L. 1982. *Techniques in clinical nursing: A comprehensive approach.* Menlo Park, Calif.: Addison-Wesley Publishing Co.

Murray, R. B., and Zentner, J. P. 1979. *Nursing assessment and health promotion through the life span.* 2nd ed. Englewood Cliffs, N.J.: Prentice-Hall.

Piaget, J. 1963. *Origins of intelligence in children.* New York: W. W. Norton and Co.

Pipes, P. L. 1981. *Nutrition in infancy and childhood.* St. Louis: C. V. Mosby Co.

Sahler, O. J. Z., and McAnarney, E. R. 1981. *The child from three to eighteen.* St. Louis: C. V. Mosby Co.

U.S. Department of Health, Education, and Welfare, Public Health Service. November 1977. *NCHS growth curves for children, birth–18 years: United States.* DHEW Publication no. (PHS)78-1650. Hyattsville, Md.: National Center for Health Statistics.

Vaughan, V. C.; McKay, R. J.; Behrman, R. E.; and Nelson, W. E. 1979. *Nelson textbook of pediatrics.* 11th ed. Philadelphia: W. B. Saunders Co.

Whaley, L. F., and Wong, D. L. 1979. *Nursing care of infants and children.* St. Louis: C. V. Mosby Co.

Chapter 12

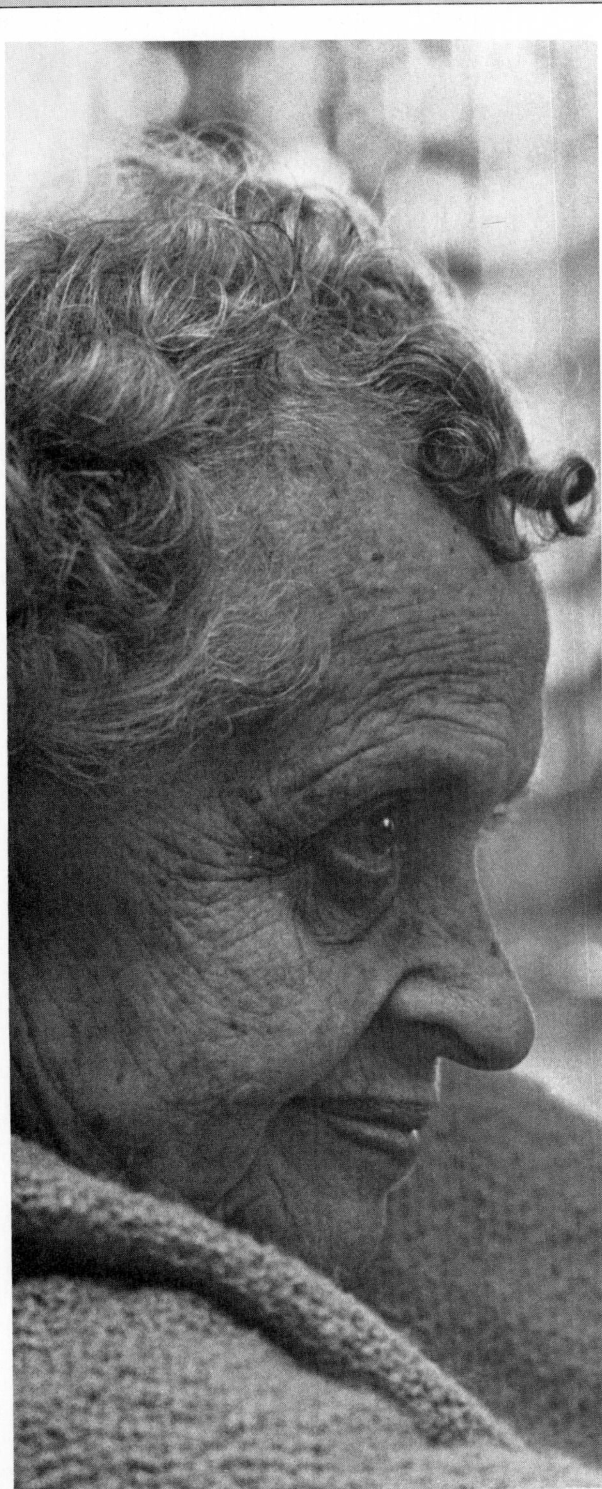

Development from Adolescence to Late Adulthood

CONTENTS

Objectives

1. Know selected information related to the growth and development of adolescents and adults
    - **1.1** Identify the major psychosocial tasks of adolescents
    - **1.2** Identify normal times for the development of secondary sex characteristics in adolescents
    - **1.3** Identify factors influencing mate selection by young adults
    - **1.4** Outline purposes of becoming engaged
    - **1.5** Identify factors that predict whether a relationship will be successful
    - **1.6** Describe the major psychosocial tasks required of young couples
    - **1.7** Identify characteristics of the mid-life crisis
    - **1.8** Outline physiologic changes that occur with aging
    - **1.9** Identify essential psychosocial tasks of middle-aged adults
    - **1.10** Identify the developmental tasks of the elderly
2. Know essential facts about pregnancy and the puerperium
    - **2.1** Identify physiologic changes of pregnancy
    - **2.2** Identify some emotional changes that occur during pregnancy
    - **2.3** Outline common physical problems related to pregnancy
    - **2.4** Identify changes that occur in the reproductive system and the breasts during the puerperium
    - **2.5** Describe two stages of emotional changes that occur during the puerperium
    - **2.6** Identify the major physical needs of women during the puerperium
    - **2.7** Identify three major problems that occur during the puerperium
3. Know the role of the nurse in regard to the growth and development of persons from adolescence through old age
    - **3.1** Identify data required to assess developmental changes
    - **3.2** Identify needs essential to maintain health in persons from adolescence to old age
    - **3.3** Identify ways to prevent common health problems in persons from adolescence to old age

Terms

adolescence
anorexia nervosa
Braxton Hicks contractions
bulimia
cataracts
climacteric
colostrum
cystocele
engorgement
generativity
gerontology
homogamy
human chorionic gonadotropin (HCG)
human placental lactogen
involution
kyphosis
lightening
lochia
menarche
menopause
Montgomery's glands
morning sickness
osteoporosis
oxytocin
papule
pica
postpartum depression
preeclampsia
presbycusis
presbyopia
primigravida
ptyalism
puberty
puerperium
pustule
rectocele
senescence
show
striae gravidarum

Adolescents

Adolescence is a critical period in development. Its length varies from one culture to another. In America adolescence is longer than in some cultures, extending to 18 years of age for girls and to 20 years for boys. *Adolescence* is the period during which the person becomes physically and psychologically mature. At the end of adolescence the person is ready to enter adulthood and assume its responsibilities.

Puberty is the stage of adolescence in which many physiologic changes take place and the sex organs mature. In boys the maturing process takes about 2 years or more, while in girls it takes about 6 months. For girls puberty normally starts between 12 and 14 years and for boys between 14 and 18 years.

Physical Development

Appearance

The adolescent period is preceded by the prepuberal period, during which the second growth spurt starts. The first growth spurt is from birth to 1 year. This physical growth continues into the adolescent period. During the second growth spurt, the bony structure grows faster than the muscles and internal organs. As a result, the young adolescent is clumsy and poorly coordinated. The feet and hands grow early, giving them an ungainly appearance. Often the adolescent feels tired because the heart and lungs have not developed sufficiently to supply the body's needs for oxygen.

In boys, secondary sexual characteristics develop, and other physical changes take place. Some of these, in order of appearance, are:

1. Sweating from the axillae
2. Enlargement of the testes and the penis
3. Appearance of facial hair at about 14 or 15 years
4. Voice change at about 14 or 15, shortly after the appearance of the facial hair

Growth is fastest for boys at about 14 years, and the maximum height is often reached at about 18 or 19 years. Some men add another 1 or 2 cm to their height during their 20s, as the vertebral column gradually continues to grow. During the period of 10 to 18 years of age the average American male doubles his weight, gaining about 30 kg (67 lb) and grows about 34 cm (13½ in) (Suitor and Hunter 1980:95).

Physical growth during adolescence is greatly influenced by a number of factors. Some of these are heredity, nutrition, medical care, illness, physical and emotional environment, family size, and culture. Generally, people in the United States have grown taller in recent years. This increase in average height is thought to be due largely to many of the above factors.

In girls a number of physical changes take place during adolescence:

1. The *menarche* (the initiation of menstruation) occurs 9 months to 1 year after the peak growth rate has passed, between 12 and 13 years. It is usually another year to 18 months before the ovulatory cycle has matured sufficiently to allow conception.
2. The breasts continue to develop until about 13 years.
3. Pubic hair appears at about 11 years, and axillary hair appears later.

The fastest rate of growth in girls occurs at about age 12; they reach their maximum heights at about 15 to 16 years. During ages 10 to 18, the average American female gains about 22 kg (49 lb) and grows about 24 cm (9 in) (Suitor and Hunter 1980:95).

During adolescence both sexes experience increased secretions from the apocrine glands in the skin, sometimes resulting in acne. (Increased secretions begin in prepuberty.)

Vital signs

During adolescence the pulse rate drops about 10 beats per minute in both boys and girls. The usual pulse rate for boys of 14 years is between 60 and 100 beats per minute; by age 18 the pulse drops to between 50 and 90 beats per minute. The usual pulse rate for girls of 14 is between 65 and 105 beats per minute; it drops to between 55 to 95 beats per minute by age 18.

Adolescents' blood pressure increases until age 14 or 15, when it levels off. At that age, systolic values range between 100 to 140 mm Hg, and diastolic values range between 50 and 70 mm Hg (Whaley and Wong 1979:1601).

Psychosocial Development

The adolescent is faced with seven major psychologic tasks during this period:

1. Relating with the family
2. Establishing a self-concept that remains stable
3. Adjusting to his or her sexual role
4. Establishing a value system that is appropriate for life
5. Making a career or vocation choice
6. Developing cognitive abilities
7. Relating with a peer group

Family relationships

About the age of 15 years many adolescents gradually draw away from the family and gain independence. This need for independence and the need for family support sometime result in conflict within the adolescent and between the adolescent and the family. The young person may appear hostile or depressed at times during this painful process.

At this age adolescents prefer to be with their peers rather than their parents and may seek advice from adults other than their parents. Parents sometimes are bewildered at this stage of development; instead of reducing controls, they increase them, which results in rebellion by the adolescent.

Adolescents also have to resolve their ambivalent feelings toward the parent of the opposite sex. As part of resolution, adolescents may develop brief crushes on adults outside the family—teachers or neighbors, for example. Adolescents sometimes adopt some of the attributes of the adults with whom they are infatuated. This modeling can be helpful in the maturing process.

Some of the discord in the family at this time is due to the generation gap. The values of the adolescent may differ from those of the parents. This difference may be difficult for the parents to understand and to accept.

Adolescents still need guidance from their parents, although they appear neither to want it nor to need it. However, adolescents need to know that their parents care about them and that their parents still want to help them. Restrictions and guidance need to be presented in a manner that makes adolescents feel loved. They need consistency in guidance and fewer restrictions than previously. They should have the independence they can handle yet know that their parents will assist them when they need help.

Stable self-concept

During this period, the body changes rapidly. Rapid change makes developing a stable identity difficult. Adolescents are usually concerned about their bodies, their appearances, and their physical abilities. Hair styling, skin care, and clothes become very important.

The adolescent needs to learn an accurate self-concept; one that accepts both personal strengths and weaknesses. Adolescents need to learn to build on their strengths and not be preoccupied by defects such as acne. They gain self-concepts largely from the impressions that others have of them. If others accept defects—for example, a lost finger—adolescents accept those defects more readily.

Sexual role adjustments

Sexual identification begins at about 3 or 4 years of age and is established during adolescence. Adolescents are active sexually. Masturbation is the most common form of activity, but heterosexual and even homosexual activity are not uncommon. Boys have a higher sex drive than girls in late adolescence and therefore often become more experienced.

Premarital intercourse and pregnancies are on the rise among adolescents. In one report from Hawaii, 25% of the 400 women who had abortions were adolescents (Gedan 1974:1856). Adolescence is also a time for forming ideas about what qualities are desired in a mate. During this time young people choose the criteria they use later in the selection process.

Establishing a value system

During adolescence persons examine the values, standards, and morals they hold. Adolescents may discard the values they have adopted from parents in favor of values they consider more suitable.

By the age of 16 years the adolescent is likely to have made a decision about religion. Some teenagers meet others of the same age at church or church-sponsored activities; youth groups serve social and recreational as well as religious purposes.

Career choice

In North America most adolescents are free to choose a vocation. They take their first steps toward a future career in high school by selecting one program of studies over another.

The career choice is important not only in terms of employment but also in terms of life-style, status, and economic compensation. Many young people continue their education in college and may postpone the career choice until then.

Cognitive development

The adolescent becomes more informed about the world and environment. Adolescents use new information to solve everyday problems and can communicate with adults on most subjects.

Cognitive abilities mature during adolescence. The adolescents' capacity to absorb and use knowledge is great. They can be highly imaginative. Study habits and learning skills developed in adolescence are used throughout life. Adolescents also develop their own areas for learning; they explore interests from which they may evolve a career plan. Career plans and hobbies may be influenced by sexual roles. In the past, for instance, automobile mechanics was the province of males; sewing, of females. In recent years, however, male-female interests are melding.

Peer group relationships

During adolescence peer groups assume great importance. The peer group has a number of functions. It provides a sense of belonging, pride, social learning, and sexual roles. Most peer groups have well-defined, sex-specific modes of acceptable behavior. In adolescence the peer groups change with age. They start as single-sex groups, evolve to mixed groups, and finally narrow to couples who share activities.

Dating helps prepare adolescents for marriage by teaching them how to act with members of the opposite sex. In the United States dating starts early, often by 11 years for girls and later, perhaps 15, for boys, although dating ages vary with culture and social class and the subsequent pressures from society. Some adolescents initially date in groups of couples and eventually progress to going on dates alone.

Needs

Nutrition

The growth spurt during adolescence means increased nutritional needs. Adolescents have tremendous appetites; a boy between the ages of 11 and 14 may need as many as 2800 kcal daily; a girl, 2400 kcal (Suitor and Hunter 1980:95). There is an increased need for protein, calcium, and vitamin D. An adequate diet for an adolescent is 1 quart of milk per day as well as appropriate amounts of meat, vegetables, fruits, breads, and cereals. See Chapter 26. Even when adolescents eat nutritionally sound meals and meet their needs for specific nutrients, they may still require extra calories. This need prompts frequent snacking of high-calorie foods such as cookies, doughnuts, and soft drinks. Parents can promote better lifelong eating habits by encouraging children to eat healthful snacks.

Rest and sleep

Most adolescents require 10 hours of sleep each night to prevent undue fatigue and susceptibility to infections. Sometimes teenagers also need to rest during the day. Often quiet activities such as reading are good respite from the physically active life.

Sexual education

Teenagers want to know about sex. One study of 417 high school students assessed what teenagers believed their needs were and what knowledge they already possessed. Most of the students had obtained their first information about sex from friends or from reading while in grade school. The family and school were the other major sources of information (Inman 1975: 217–19).

Some teenagers wanted sex information from both parents, and some wanted the church to be involved. White students had more formal knowledge than nonwhite students, and Protestants and boys had more informal knowledge than Catholic students and girls.

The subjects teenagers wanted included in sex education classes were:

1. Sexually transmitted disease
2. Biology of sexes and reproduction
3. Pregnancy
4. Birth control (requested by boys)
5. What boys think of girls and development of a sexual code of conduct (requested by girls)

Assessment

The assessment of growth and development of the adolescent deals primarily with the development of secondary sexual characteristics and with self concept and sexuality. See Table 12–1. According to Erikson the developmental task of the adolescent is identity formation versus identity confusion.

Common Health Problems

Obesity

Obesity is a common problem of the preadolescent period and continues to be a problem in the adolescent period. It is estimated that 10% to 16% of people between the ages of 10 and 19 years are obese.

Obese adolescents are frequently discriminated against in many ways. They are usually rejected by their peers, badgered by their parents, and ridiculed on television and in the movies. Many feel ugly and socially unacceptable. Depression is not unusual among obese adolescents.

Treatment of obesity in this age group includes education on nutrition as well as assessment of psychosocial problems that may produce overeating.

Acne

Acne is a common problem of the preadolescent and adolescent periods due to increased activity of the sebaceous glands. Noninflammatory acne appears as open and closed whiteheads and blackheads. Inflammatory acne appears as inflamed skin together with *pustules* and *papules*. A pustule is a visible collection of pus within the epidermis. A papule is a superficial circumscribed elevation of the skin. Inflammatory acne may cause scarring.

Thorough cleansing of the skin is important in the treatment of acne. A well-balanced diet and avoidance of fatigue, stress, and excessive perspiration are also desirable. Teenagers who find acne a problem are advised to consult a physician.

Accidents

The major cause of death during the adolescent period is accidents, in particular motor vehicle accidents. Obtaining a driver's license is an important event in the life of an adolescent in the United States and Canada, but the privilege is not always wisely handled. Head injuries and fractures are frequent outcomes of automobile and motorcycle accidents.

Adolescent pregnancy

Unplanned pregnancies during adolescence are not uncommon. Education about contraceptive measures is recommended for adolescents. Pills, diaphragms, intrauterine devices (IUDs), the rhythm method, and

Table 12–1 Assessment of Growth and Development: The Adolescent

Assessment data	Normal findings*	Assessment data	Normal findings*
Physical		*Psychosocial*	
Height	Varies with ethnic group and individual differences, maximum height attained in boys by age 18 and in girls by age 16	Developmental task: identify formation versus identity confusion	
Weight	Varies with frame and age, average weight gain from age 10 to 18 in girls is 22 kg (49 lb) and in boys 30 kg (67 lb)	Self-concept and sexuality	Accepts changes in body image Identifies and accepts personal strengths and weaknesses Develops concept of male and female roles Develops sexual code of conduct Begins to establish criteria about suitable mate Understands essentials about reproduction, intercourse, and birth control
Musculature	Muscles develop more slowly than skeleton resulting in poor coordination		
Secondary sexual characteristics	*Females*: Pubic hair appears at about age 11 Menarche occurs at about age 12 to 13 Breasts develop until age 13 Axillary hair appears at about age 13 *Males:* Testes and penis enlarge from about age 11 to 14 Pubic hair appears at about age 12 Nocturnal emissions begin at about age 14 Facial and axillary hair appear at about age 14 Voice changes at about age 15	Family and peer relationships	Seeks some parental guidance and views parents as friends Has peer relationships with both sexes Participates in activities with both sexes Begins dating
		Independence	Makes decisions regarding future and career Develops own set of values and moral standards Makes decision about value of religion
		Wellness	Carries out preventive health care practices that promote exercise, rest, and nutrition
Vital signs	Temperature: 37 C (98.6 F) Pulse: For boys decreases from 60 to 100 beats per minute at age 14, to 50 to 90 per minute at age 18. For girls decreases from 65 to 105 beats per minute at age 14, to 55 to 95 beats per minute at age 18 Respirations: 12 to 20 breaths per minute Blood pressure: stabilizes at age 15 to 100 to 140 mm Hg systolic and 50 to 70 mm Hg diastolic		

*Findings represent trends in some instances and not exact values. Individual differences must be considered in assessment.

condoms are preventive measures. See Chapter 33. The incidence of abortion is notable among this group, and those who choose to carry through with their pregnancies have unique needs and problems. Adolescents are high-risk mothers, physiologically and emotionally. Rearing a child as an unwed single parent or placing a child for adoption can precipitate an emotional crisis.

Sexually transmitted disease

Syphilis and gonorrhea are the most common sexually transmitted diseases (venereal diseases). Gonorrhea has been continually on the increase since 1957. More than half of the people reported to have gonorrhea are between 15 and 24 years old. The increase appears due to two major factors: changing sexual mores of the young and increased male homosexuality.

Because the term *venereal disease* elicits feelings of guilt, shame, and fear in many people, medical help is frequently not sought as early as it should be. Table 12-2 describes the early symptoms of gonorrhea and syphilis. Syphilis and gonorrhea are generally curable if the person receives the prescribed treatment, usually penicillin injections. Other sexually transmitted diseases being recognized as major public health problems are genital herpes and nonspecific urethritis.

Table 12-2 Symptoms of Gonorrhea and Syphilis

	Male	Female
Gonorrhea*	Painful urination; urethritis with watery white discharge, which may become purulent	May be asymptomatic; or vaginal discharge, pain, urinary frequency
Syphilis†	Chancre, usually on glans penis, which is painless and heals in 4–6 weeks; secondary symptoms in 6 weeks to 6 months after chancre heals—skin eruptions, low-grade fever, inflammation of lymph glands	Chancre on cervix, etc., heals in 4–6 weeks; symptoms same as male

*Symptoms usually appear in 3–9 days after contact. Gonorrhea is usually treated with aqueous procaine penicillin.

†Symptoms usually appear in 10–60 days after contact. Syphilis is usually treated with benzathine penicillin or procaine penicillin G in oil.

Gastric problems

It is not unusual for adolescents to complain of indigestion and gastric problems. These complaints may be due to the increase in gastric acidity that takes place during adolescence. Occasionally a gastric ulcer develops as a result of increased acidity as well as increased stress during adolescence.

Drug abuse

Mood swings and emotional problems are common in adolescence. Drug abuse is on the rise among teenagers, some of whom have emotional problems. Many adolescents take drugs for the experience, to belong to a group and thus relieve loneliness, or to prove they are courageous. Some of the drugs used are alcohol, glue and similar substances, barbiturates and amphetamines, hallucinogens, and marijuana. Marijuana is used widely by both adolescents and adults. Its use is a controversial issue, and marijuana advocates believe it should not be grouped with the more dangerous drugs.

Teenagers who habitually use drugs create problems not only for themselves but also for the people with whom they associate. These teenagers may need help from physicians and other professionals, such as psychiatrists who specialize in adolescent problems.

Anorexia nervosa

Under social pressure to be slim, some adolescents severely limit their food intake to a level significantly below that required to meet the demands of normal growth. *Anorexia nervosa* is a severe psychophysiologic condition usually seen in adolescent girls and young women. It is characterized by a prolonged inability or refusal to eat and rapid weight loss in persons who believe they are fat even though they are emaciated. Anorexics may also induce vomiting and use laxatives and diuretics to remain thin. This illness is most effectively treated in the early stages by psychotherapy that also involves the parents. Hospitalization may be necessary when the effects of starvation become life-threatening.

Bulimia

Bulimia is an increasing problem among teenagers. It is an uncontrollable compulsion to consume enormous amounts of food and then expel it by self-induced vomiting or by taking laxatives. For example, the afflicted person may consume a whole cake, a dozen doughnuts, and a half dozen apple turnovers before inducing vomiting. After prolonged periods of alternatively gorging on food and vomiting, the person no longer needs to induce vomiting; it becomes an uncontrollable reflex. Voluntary organizations are established in some regions to assist individuals with bulimia.

Suicide and homicide

Suicide and homicide are two of the leading causes of death among teenagers. Adolescent males are more likely to commit suicide than adolescent females, and blacks are more likely to commit homicide than whites. Suicides by firearms, drugs, and automobile exhaust gases are the most common.

Most suicidal persons give verbal or behavioral warnings prior to suicide, and certain tendencies or behaviors are suspect. For example, most people who commit suicide have made previous attempts, are severely depressed, and are at odds with themselves and those close to them. Such individuals need to be referred to professional help.

Homicide is more common among the poor than other economic classes, and both killers and their victims are more likely to be men than women. Often homicide is associated with alcohol abuse and occurs most frequently at night and on weekends. Factors influencing the high homicide rate include economic deprivation, family breakup, and the availability of firearms, which are the most frequently used weapons. Cutting or stabbing tools are the next most frequently used weapons.

Young Adults

The adult phase of development encompasses the years from the end of adolescence to death. Because the developmental tasks of young adults differ from those of older adults, adulthood is often divided in three phases—the young adult phase, the middle-aged adult phase, and the elderly adult phase. In this book young adults are defined as people 20 to 40 years old; middle-aged adults, as 40 to 65; and elderly adults, over 65. In addition, a section is included about the pregnant woman, although pregnancy is not unique to this period of development.

Physical Development

Persons in their early 20s are in their prime years physically. The musculoskeletal system is well developed and coordinated. This is the period when athletic endeavors reach their peak. Indeed, after 40 years, most athletes are considered old.

All other systems of the body are also functioning at peak efficiency. The circulatory system is well developed so that pregnant women, for example, are able to provide additional blood supplies to the placenta. The reproductive system is fully developed. The woman's menstrual cycle is regular, and sexual organs are sufficiently mature to cope with childbearing. The man's sexual maturity, reached in adolescence, remains at a peak so that the sexual urge remains high throughout this phase. In summary, physical change, with the exception of pregnancy, is minimal during this phase; psychosocial development, by contrast, is great. Changes that occur during pregnancy will be discussed subsequently.

Psychosocial Development

Young adults face a number of new experiences and changes in life-style. They must now make decisions for themselves, and many of the decisions made now influence the person's life-style in years to come. The expectations of the young adult are often taken for granted, since they are well defined in most cultures. Choices must be made about education and employment, about whether to marry or remain single, about starting a home, and about rearing children. Social responsibilities include forming new friendships and assuming some community activities.

Selecting education and employment

Today, education is more important than ever. It enhances employment opportunities, enriches leisure time, and ensures economic survival. Occupational choice and education are largely inseparable. Education influences occupational opportunities; conversely, an occupation, once chosen, can determine the education needed and sought.

In the past, young men were encouraged more than young women to pursue advanced education, particularly college education. Traditionally, education was deemed unnecessary for women in the roles of wife and mother. This notion is being challenged today. Also, the role of the woman is changing, and many now choose to assume more active, civic roles in society.

Staying single

Remaining single is becoming the life-style of more and more North Americans. Many people choose to remain single, perhaps to pursue an education and then to have the freedom to pursue their chosen vocations.

The single status does, however, present some problems. People in their 20s and 30s often feel social pressures to get married. Often young single persons as well as older single adults need support for their single status and verification that they are contributing members of society.

Because single adults often live alone or with other adults who are employed, problems can present themselves when single persons are ill. Finding someone to drive them to a hospital or to help with shopping and meals during recuperation can be major challenges. A support system for a single adult may take more organization than the support system of a married person.

Choosing a mate

Deciding on a mate is a difficult task. It is in many ways more complex and confusing than other tasks required of the young adult. In North America there is emphasis on falling in love as a basis for mate selection. However, the multiple aspects of love make it difficult for some people to recognize and to know the meaning of love. Numerous definitions of love are available in literature, but the one important aspect of love is that it is lasting. Love survives times of frustration, strained relationships, and sadness, as well as times of happiness and achievement. It evolves out of interaction and requires adjustments and readjustments of the personalities of the people involved. There is a desire to do all one can to make the other person's life meaningful. In contrast, infatuation is sexually stimulating and exciting, but it is too shallow to nurture total personal growth of either partner and lasts only a short time.

Multiple factors other than love influence mate selections, such as age, religion, race, social class, and common interests. Several theories (Kaluger and Kaluger 1979:380) explain why people choose certain partners:

1. Nearness or proximity
2. Concept of the ideal mate
3. Complementary needs
4. Homogamy
5. Compatibility

Proximity is said to be a major influencing factor. People usually meet other people through work, school, church, or recreational activities. Because of familiar associations, people are drawn toward each other.

The *concept of the ideal mate* also guides choice of mates. Consciously or unconsciously, people seek the ideal mate, who possesses qualities desired in a husband, wife, or partner in parenthood. Some people are able to list these desired qualities.

The theory of *complementary needs* suggests that persons are attracted to those with different characteristics. Each partner wishes to have the characteristics of the other and believes the other can help the partner become the person he or she wants to be—or at least that one partner can complement the other.

Homogamy—the mating of like with like—is an opposite theory. People with similar social, racial, religious, and economic backgrounds seek each other and marry.

Couples who are *compatible* enjoy a wide variety of activities together and have similar value systems. They communicate and respond deeply to each other. The partners understand and accept each other and are thus said to be supplementary rather than complementary.

Marriage

Many questions arise when the young adult contemplates marriage: What does marriage really mean? Why get married? When should a couple get married? What behavior is expected of married people? There are no universal answers to these questions. The answers rest largely with each couple and with the society in which they live.

The purposes of engagement (Duvall 1977:190) perhaps also apply with some adaptation to a couple who decide to live together without marrying:

1. Placing themselves as a couple in their own eyes and the eyes of both families and friends
2. Working through systems of communication that encourage exchange of confidences and increase the degree of empathy and the ability to predict each other's responses
3. Planning for marriage, if they are mutually agreeable, and deciding where and how their life together will be lived

Before marriage the couple meets and gets to know in-laws and shares as a couple social activities with them.

Most people are married at least once in their lives. Although the traditional marriage is between a man and a woman, other forms of marriage are emerging, such as the communal or group marriage in which all members are married to each other and all of them become parents to all the children. Another type of marriage is the homosexual marriage, which may not be childless; for example, the couple may adopt a child. Although change can and does occur, the traditional family is the one largely accepted by society and law. The discussion in this book, therefore, will be restricted to this relationship.

The marriage contract is a legal one, with certain legal prerequisites. These are different in various states and provinces. There are minimum age requirements for men and women. Generally the age for women is lower than for men. Prior marriages must be dissolved, and marriage to certain blood relatives is banned. The marriage relationship is allowed by the issuance of a marriage permit and formalized by a ceremony, but by law it can also exist without formal entry into a marriage contract. The latter is the common-law marriage.

What ingredients predict a successful relationship? Many studies suggest predictors of good relationships, but many variables exist among individuals. One significant predictor of success for new couples is the happiness of the parents in their own relationships.

Other predictors of success include personal happiness and consistent discipline during childhood, a year-long or longer acquaintanceship of the partners, parental approval, common interests and cultural background, desire for children, and a sense of equality in relationships or at least clearly differentiated roles. Sexual education and sexual experiences prior to the relationship are not significant factors.

A couple's developmental tasks (Duvall 1977:195) are as follows:

1. Learn to live together as a couple
2. Find, furnish, and maintain a home of their own
3. Establish mutually satisfactory ways of supporting themselves
4. Allocate responsibilities each partner is willing and able to assume
5. Develop a satisfactory sexual relationship
6. Plan for possible children
7. Interact with in-laws, relatives, and the community

Learning to live together

New couples are generally reasonable with and considerate of each other. Adjusting to each other may necessitate giving up some old habits and developing different ways or different times to do things. For example, one partner may be an early riser and like to shower in the morning, but the other is accustomed to staying up late and likes a bath in the evening. Accommodating to food preferences, meal hours, sleeping with the window open or closed, taking time to relax or read the paper, sharing the television, entertaining others, and going out or staying in are other examples.

A relationship cannot be described as an equal give-and-take situation. In most instances one partner gives more in certain aspects than in others. A major factor in determining the success of a relationship is the quality of adjustments that are made by each for the other. Couples need to accept a state of continual adjustment and a partnership in which all things will *not* be agreed upon. Conflicts inevitably arise. Learning to accept and understand each other as persons and learning to communicate and solve problems together is essential.

Communicating in mature and healthy ways is easier for some couples than others. Most couples tend to develop a private, intimate communication system of words, gestures, and symbols. Words of endearment, gestures of affection, and symbols such as a favorite song become the couple's own private language. However, it is more difficult to develop effective ways of handling negative feelings such as anger and disappointment. Being silent or sullen, withdrawing in anger, weeping, or pretending that a problem does not exist are common patterns of behavior when conflicts arise. However, such behavior does little to solve problems. The problem tends to be perpetuated unless a system of caring and communicating is developed together. Although it is difficult to be objective when feelings are intense, young couples can learn constructive ways of coping—for example, using cooling-down periods and finding effective ways to talk about their problems. When there is communication, couples usually can arrive at mutually agreeable solutions.

In developing a philosophy for living, the young couple need not agree on every issue that arises. For example, they may have opposing views on a political issue and may vote according to their own convictions. Countless issues arise during which the couple weaves a philosophy of life, including racial issues, religious issues, childrearing practices, civic responsibilities, ways of dealing with the neighbors, and the way the house is maintained.

Deciding about household tasks and finances

Today the division of household responsibilities is clearly a decision of the couple themselves. Traditionally the roles of the man and woman were outlined for them. The man was the sole breadwinner, and the woman was the housekeeper. The trend today involves the sharing of many tasks; the woman is often a wage earner along with the man, particularly before children are born. The man is now often involved in many of the household tasks, such as cooking, grocery shopping, cleaning house, and washing the dishes. The division or sharing of tasks, however, involves mutual decision making and examination of past and present influences. Who looks after the garbage? Who washes the car? Who mows the lawn? Who does the laundry? Who pays the bills? Who feeds the dog? Flexibility in division of tasks is often necessary for working couples. Even though a general pattern of tasks is decided on, temporary adjustments may often become necessary. For example, a couple whose employment involves shift work may switch tasks periodically.

Financing the household also requires discussion and planning. Traditional roles—the man holds the purse strings and the woman knows little about money—are rare today. Often joint bank accounts are established, and decisions about what to spend for food, furniture, rent, or home mortgages, for example, are made cooperatively. Long-term and short-term budgets can present a challenge to the young couple who strive to stretch the dollar and realize some of their dreams.

Developing satisfying sexual relations

Sexual drives and attitudes differ among individuals. The frequency of sexual intercourse is variable, as is the nature of love-making. For example, sensitivity to touch, levels of arousal, and length of orgasm are all variable among individuals. Attitudes influence and preferences dictate the activities a couple performs. Some desire tactile or oral stimulation prior to sex; others prefer less or no foreplay. The environment may be important to some; they may find dim lighting, quiet surroundings, or soothing music necessary during sex. Certain aromas arouse some people, hence the use of certain perfumes. The sexual act can be a most intimate, fulfilling form of communication; the effort to learn to give and receive love is rewarded. Couples who learn about their partners' desires and preferences and accept differences can usually achieve mutual fulfillment in sexual relations. It is important for couples to realize that lovemaking need not always include intercourse and orgasm.

Planning for children

Planned parenthood and birth control measures are common today. For additional information on birth control see Chapter 33. Most couples, however, have their first child within the first few years. Some couples are not interested in having children.

The advantages of planned parenthood are underscored by the experience of couples who have an unplanned or unwanted baby. The unplanned baby can create a crisis. Educational goals, plans for a home, financial independence from parents, and time to enjoy each other at leisure can all be disrupted. Little time is allowed for the psychologic preparations required to assume the role of parent.

Promoting relationships with relatives and friends

Frequently social ties established prior to living together are interrupted for one or both partners. The woman may move to a new location with her mate or vice versa. Even if the couple does not move, former activities and associations are often not maintained with the same frequency. The couple often must find new social activities. These are often chosen on the basis of common interests with other couples, the social prestige the activities offer, the amount the couple can spend on entertainment, and the occupational contacts of the couple. Having the boss to dinner or going to the company dance may take precedence over going to dinner and a dance alone. A couple often undergoes a change in family orientation. They are each no longer a member of one family but are now a member of three—his, hers, and their own. Some couples retain close family ties, whereas others see parents only occasionally. However, most couples assume some responsibility for keeping in touch with their families, and many receive financial help, help with child care, or other assistance from parents. The couple's new roles as partners can create some frustrations and conflicts in the early years. The man and woman are now each other's first concern, and both must learn to place the mate above parents and other family members. Most couples develop effective relationships with parents-in-law. The concept of family is expanded for both partners, although the roles are different—increasingly independent.

Assessment

The assessment of growth and development of the young adult chiefly encompasses psychosocial aspects. According to Erikson the developmental task of the young adult is intimacy versus self-isolation. For a summary of selected developmental assessments, see Table 12–3.

Common Health Problems

There are a number of health problems that appear in this age group: accidents, upper respiratory tract infection, stress reactions such as suicide and homicide, alcoholism, and drug abuse and addiction are just a few.

Accidents

Accidents are a leading cause of death. In 1977 motor vehicle accidents were the leading cause of mortality in the 15 to 24 year age group (U.S. DHEW 1979:46). Alcohol consumption was associated with many of these fatalities.

Nursing has a preventive function in this regard, in particular relative to those attitudes that allow people to drive recklessly and while intoxicated.

Upper respiratory tract infections

Upper respiratory tract infections occur more frequently in young adults than any other acute illness. Nursing function is largely preventive—reducing the individual's susceptibility by supporting body defenses through adequate nutrition, rest, liquids, and exercise. It also includes reducing susceptibility by teaching the dangers of alcohol, cigarettes, and contaminants. When

Table 12–3 Assessment of Growth and Development: Young Adult

Assessment data	Normal findings*	Assessment data	Normal findings*
Physical		*Psychosocial*	
		Developmental task: intimacy versus self-isolation	
Weight	Varies with frame and age. Refer to Tables 14–1, 14–2, for normal weights	Self-image	Stabilized self-image; likes self and the direction in which life is going Career selection supports self-image and provides satisfaction
Height	Varies with ethnic group and individual differences, slight increase in height may occur in early 20s in males	Independence	Establishes self separate from parents
Musculature	Muscle mass increases gradually to maximum amount in early 20s, then declines slightly	Wellness	Establishes practices, such as diet and exercise, that promote optimum level of wellness
Vision	Trend toward myopia until about 30 years	Intimacy	Has been or is involved in an enriching intimate relationship
Adipose tissue distribution	Some women slim after full maturation	Social activity	Has friends and a meaningful social life
Vital signs	Temperature: 98.6 F (37.0 C) Pulse: 60 to 100 beats per minute Respirations: 16 to 20 breaths per minute Blood pressure: 110 to 140 mm Hg systolic, 60 to 80 mm Hg diastolic	Philosophy	Is developing a philosophy for living and values and ethical standards to support this philosophy

*Findings represent trends in some instances and not exact values. Individual differences must be considered in an assessment.

ill, the young adult should be encouraged to obtain medical treatment rather than risk chronic respiratory problems later in life.

Stress reactions (suicide and homicide)

Suicide is the third leading cause of death among teenagers and young adults. Homicide accounts for 10% of all deaths among teenagers and young adults—7% of all deaths among whites and nearly 30% among blacks in this age group (U.S. DHEW 1979:50–51). Preventive measures for suicide involve three areas (Murray and Zentner 1979:301):

1. Educating the public about the early signs of suicide
2. Establishing significant relationships for high-risk people
3. Encouraging young adults to participate in social activities thus preventing isolation

Nursing counseling services and crisis facilities (see Chapter 9) can often assist young adults at times of high stress to make important decisions and constructive adaptations to their environments, thereby decreasing the incidence of suicide and homicide.

Alcoholism and drug abuse

The misuse of drugs and alcohol has implications in many areas including suicide, homicide, accidents, family disruption, and poor job and school performance.

The preventive role of nursing is to increase public awareness of the problems resulting from the abuse of alcohol and drugs. Referrals to counseling agencies can assist many people.

Pregnant Women

The announcement of the first baby can be a joyful experience. The couple feel the pride of knowing they can conceive and anticipate the experience with pleasure. Pregnancy is not welcomed by all couples, however. The child may be unwanted or untimely, and pregnancy can induce many fears in one or both partners. Even those who feel positively about pregnancy need to adjust to the idea of parenthood. The demands of being a parent differ significantly from the demands of being a mate. The young couple must now prepare for the expected baby, adjust present living arrangements, and learn how to care for an infant. See Figure 12–1.

Pregnancy is a responsibility shared by both partners. The expectant mother can do much to include the father in this event. The father can be encouraged to help select a physician, to participate in clothing purchases for the mother and baby, and in general to share plans. The father can take part in the decision of whether to breastfeed. Many educational programs are offered for prospective parents. Both partners have the opportunity to share knowledge about medical services during pregnancy and childbirth, care of the pregnant woman and newborn, physical and mental changes associated with pregnancy, and what each prospective parent can do to have a child successfully. Fathers can help support the mother during pregnancy. Fathers can encourage good health practices and be tolerant of the physical and emotional changes that occur during pregnancy.

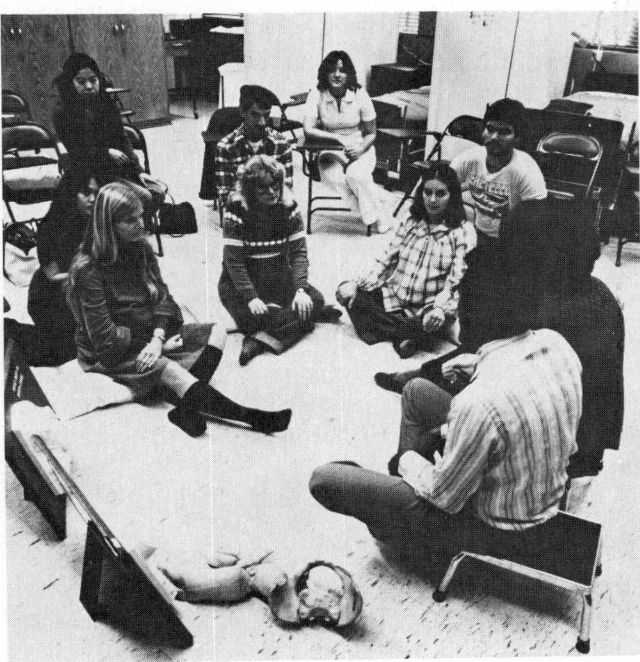

Figure 12–1 Expectant couples learn prenatal exercises.

Physiologic Changes of Pregnancy

Cessation of menses

Normally the high levels of estrogen and progesterone produced during the menstrual cycle drop rapidly, causing the lining of the uterus to slough off in menstrual flow. After fertilization, however, these hormones are maintained at high levels to retain the rich lining of the uterus, and the woman does not menstruate. Menstrual periods can be missed for many reasons other than pregnancy, such as the stress of a final exam or severe physical illness. When two successive menstrual periods are missed, however, pregnancy is a probability.

Uterine changes

During pregnancy, the uterus becomes enlarged, anteflexed, and soft. Softening of the cervix (Goodell's sign) occurs due to increased vascularity about the time the second menstrual period is missed. Normally the cervix is about as rigid as the tip of a nose, but during pregnancy it feels as soft as ear lobes or lips. The isthmus (the lower part of the body of the uterus between the cervix and the fundus) softens more than the cervix (Hegar's sign) by about the 6th week and is another important sign of pregnancy. By bimanual examination (two fingers of one hand inserted into the vagina and the other hand palpating the abdomen) the lower uterine segment can be compressed relatively easily against the abdominal wall so that the examiner's internal and external fingers almost touch each other.

Braxton Hicks contractions of the uterus occur throughout pregnancy. These are painless intermittent contractions that may or may not be consciously recognized by the pregnant woman until 35 to 36 weeks. They occur at intervals of 5 to 10 minutes throughout pregnancy and often account for the experience of false labor. The purpose of the contractions is to enlarge the uterus. The contracting and relaxing muscles enlarge, and estrogen stimulates this enlargement.

Vaginal changes

The mucous membrane of the vagina becomes bluish or violet in color because of an increased blood supply (Chadwick's sign). Normally the vagina has a pink tint. This color change occurs at about 4 weeks, but the discoloration remains after delivery; therefore it is helpful in diagnosing pregnancy only in a *primigravida* (a woman who is pregnant for the first time). In addition, the acidity of the vagina increases to protect against invading pathogens, and the vaginal secretions become thick and more profuse. In the cervical canal a thick, tenacious mucous plug forms, another protective device against pathogens throughout pregnancy. This mucous plug is expelled during labor, and the expulsion is referred to as *show*.

Breast changes

Pregnant women experience sensations of tingling, fullness, stretching, throbbing, and even soreness in their breasts as they enlarge. Increased pigmentation of the nipple and of the area surrounding the nipple (areola) occurs and is particularly extensive in brunette women. The areola also becomes puffy and widens about an inch in diameter. Sebaceous glands in the areola enlarge during pregnancy and become protruded and prominent. These are referred to as *Montgomery's glands.* The breasts begin to secrete small amounts of *colostrum*, the watery precursor of milk. Blood vessels not noticed before pregnancy tend to become prominent as pregnancy advances, an indication that the blood supply is richer.

Skin changes

Striae gravidarum, often referred to as *stretch marks*, frequently appear on the abdominal wall, the breasts, the buttocks, and the thighs. These appear as pink or reddish streaks and are caused by hormonal changes. The extent of striae formation varies considerably in women, and a very few women do not develop any. After labor the pink coloration of striae changes to the glistening white appearance of a scar. Striae are seen in conditions other than pregnancy that distend the abdominal wall.

Weight gain

A total weight gain of from 9.9 to 13 kg (22 to 30 lb) occurs steadily throughout pregnancy, although wide individual variations exist. This additional weight is attributed to the causes shown in Table 12–4. As pregnancy progresses there is an increased tendency toward salt retention and concomitant water retention. Normally this fluid and salt are eliminated after delivery. For some women, sudden or rapid increase in this fluid retention in the last trimester is an indication of the onset of toxemia of pregnancy.

Table 12–4 Weight Gain in Pregnancy

	Kilograms	Pounds
Fetus	3.4	7½
Placenta	0.4	1
Amniotic fluid	0.9	2
Uterus	1.1	2½
Breasts	1.4	3
Increased blood volume	0.9–1.8	2–4
Extravascular fluid and fat	1.8–4	4–9

From S. B. Olds, M. L. London, P. A. Ladewig, and S. V. Davidson, *Obstetric nursing* (Menlo Park, Calif.: Addison-Wesley Publishing Co., 1980), p. 225.

Other changes

Many other changes occur in the pregnant woman adapting to the needs of the fetus. The total blood volume increases by approximately one-third, and the production of red blood cells by the bone marrow is increased. The latter places extra demands on the body's iron reserves for hemoglobin formation. The increase in blood volume also has its effect on the cardiac output, since more blood per minute must be pumped.

Gastrointestinal functions are altered to some degree during pregnancy by progesterone, which slows the action of smooth muscle. Increased fluid absorption thus occurs, and constipation is more likely than before. Pressure on the gastrointestinal tract also leads to the common symptoms of constipation, heartburn, and flatulence. Urinary output is increased and has a lower specific gravity than usual. Because of endocrine influences and pressure from the expanding uterus, the ureters soften and dilate. As a result the ureters do not propel urine as satisfactorily, and urinary stasis is common. The bladder itself functions effectively throughout pregnancy.

Metabolic changes also occur during pregnancy, particularly in carbohydrate metabolism. Usually the fasting blood sugar levels are lower and the pancreas secretes increased amounts of insulin. The renal threshold for sugar is often lowered during pregnancy and may result in elevated levels of sugar in the urine. This occurrence, however, should always be reported to the physician.

Several endocrine changes occur during pregnancy. The placenta, in addition to diffusing substances from mother to fetus, is the major endocrine gland during pregnancy. *Human chorionic gonadotropin* (HCG) is produced in the first trimester from chorionic villi, which are part of the basic formation of the placenta. This output normally persists up to the 12th week of pregnancy. HCG stimulates the ovaries to continue the production of estrogen and progesterone by the corpus luteum, both of which are needed to maintain the endometrium. Because HCG is excreted in the urine in the first trimester, its presence in the urine is used as a basis for the immunologic pregnancy test.

By the 16th week of pregnancy the placenta is formed, and it becomes the major source of estrogen and progesterone. When estrogen and progesterone are metabolized, they are excreted as estriol and pregnanediol. The presence of these substances in the urine indicates that the fetal and maternal well-being and placental diffusion are satisfactory. Both estrogen and progesterone are known to influence the growth of the uterus and the changes of the body and the breasts. The placenta also secretes *human placental lactogen* (chorionic somatomammotropin), which influences growth of fetal cells and prepares the breasts for lactation.

Oxytocin is released by the posterior pituitary gland. This hormone is a strong uterine muscle stimulant that helps the uterus to contract before, during, and after delivery and thus reduces the possibilities of hemorrhage. Oxytocin also produces the letdown reflex in ejection of milk from the breasts. Stressors can inhibit the production of oxytocin, resulting in less milk production. Therefore minimizing stress is an important consideration for nursing mothers.

The adrenal cortex enlarges during pregnancy. A significant increase is noticed throughout pregnancy in the production of aldosterone, which regulates the retention of sodium by the kidneys. This sodium retention along with water can result in hidden or obvious edema.

Emotional Changes of Pregnancy

Ambivalence

Emotional changes of pregnancy parallel the physiologic changes. In the early months of pregnancy it is not unusual for the expectant mother to have some mixed feelings of pleasure and displeasure. Initially it takes time to accept the surprise of being pregnant. Even when a child is wanted and planned for, there is no best time to become prepared. For some, the timing may be awkward. The woman may need to postpone or interrupt school or a job. Nurses can often encourage expectant mothers to express their feelings of ambivalence and reassure them that the feelings are perfectly normal and usually resolve themselves with time.

Mood swings

Rapid emotional swings from sadness to happiness occur largely as a result of hormonal changes. Increased irritability and sensitivity need to be understood and accepted by both partners. Very trivial remarks from the father may cause the mother to burst into tears for no reason other than that she is pregnant.

Change in body image

In the second trimester the pregnant woman notices that her abdomen is bulging and that her clothes feel snug. These changes make some women feel increasingly uncomfortable and unattractive. It is important for the family to help the woman with these feelings. These can be compounded by her need for increased love and affection. Again her partner can be instrumental by demonstrating his love and by helping her as much as possible.

Passivity and introversion

Passivity and introversion characteristically occur about the second trimester and reach a peak by approximately the 7th month. The mother fantasizes about her baby and begins to spend more time thinking about herself and less about others (introversion), and she is less active in making decisions and doing things (passiveness). She would rather others did things for her, preferring to receive rather than give.

Changes in sexual desire

It is important for both parents to be aware of changes in sexual desire. In the first trimester there may be little difference in sexual activity, or there may be less activity if one or both partners fears spontaneous abortion. In the second trimester sexual desire may increase. The woman may desire intercourse more frequently and may experience more orgasms than when she was not pregnant. Sexual interest may decrease in both partners during the third trimester. Sexual activity is not contraindicated at this time, but unfounded fears of harming the baby may exist. Because this vacillation occurs, it is important for the couple to have some understanding of what is happening.

Physiologic Needs of the Pregnant Woman

Nutrition

During pregnancy, a woman's caloric needs increase slightly from the prepregnancy stage. For moderately active women these caloric needs become about 2200 to 2400 kcal daily. The pregnant adolescent needs additional calories, particularly during periods of her own rapid growth. Adequate calories preserve protein for tissue growth.

Nutritional quality is as important as sufficient caloric intake during pregnancy. Throughout the antenatal period, protein requirements are doubled, and other specific nutrients—such as iron, calcium, and vitamins A, B, and C—need to be increased. See Chapter 26 for additional information about nutrition during pregnancy.

Rest

Rest is of particular importance during pregnancy, in particular during the last 6 weeks. Getting rest may be difficult for the woman who has young children, but planned rest periods are important. During the last 6 weeks, the unborn baby will probably feel heavy to the woman, since she is carrying additional weight. This added weight and the other discomforts of pregnancy, such as swollen ankles, varicosities, and backache, increase the need for planned rest periods and exercise. During the last few weeks of pregnancy urinary frequency may interrupt sleep.

Pregnant women can learn positions that assist relaxation and promote rest. One of these, the semiprone position, is discussed in Chapter 23. Other positions and exercises to promote rest and relaxation are discussed in Chapter 24.

Exercise

Exercise is important during pregnancy, and the usual daily activities generally suffice. Walking is encouraged, however, because it stimulates circulation. Normally, activity is not restricted except upon the physician's advice.

Common Problems During Pregnancy

Most of the problems encountered in pregnancy are related to the physiologic changes that occur and are therefore often referred to as discomforts without pathology. Not all women experience all problems or have them to the same degree.

Nausea and vomiting

About 50% of women experience nausea and vomiting, particularly in the first trimester of pregnancy. This problem is often referred to as *morning sickness*, since the symptoms frequently occur when the woman gets up in the morning. The symptoms are not restricted to this time of day, however. The cause of nausea and vomiting is unknown. Some think it is because of the high levels of progesterone, estrogen, and chorionic gonadotropin, particularly the former two hormones, since some women on birth control pills experience the same problem. A few others believe nausea and vomiting have a base in emotions such as ambivalence about pregnancy. Morning sickness has been known to occur in the man along with the woman. Still others think it may be due to the lowered blood sugar or to an increase in saliva called *ptyalism*. Mouth secretions become more acidic during pregnancy, and the salivary glands are stimulated to produce large quantities of saliva. The nurse can recommend that the woman do the following:

1. Eat smaller, more frequent, high-protein meals to prevent the stomach from becoming empty.
2. Keep crackers or an apple at the bedside, and eat them before rising. This is an attempt to elevate the blood sugar.
3. Eat some foods high in carbohydrates after arising.
4. Seek the advice of the physician. Some medications may be prescribed.

Ginger ale or cola drinks may settle the stomach but have limited nutritional value.

Breast soreness

Breast soreness is due to the changes induced by progesterone and estrogen. The nurse can have the patient do the following:

1. Wear a good brassiere with wide shoulder straps that supports the breasts upward and inward.
2. Anticipate buying a larger brassiere. Both brassiere and cup size usually enlarge two sizes.
3. Pad the inside of the brassiere with soft cotton or the like to alleviate nipple soreness.

Fatigue

Most women feel some fatigue, particularly in the early months of pregnancy, because of metabolic changes. In later pregnancy, the extra weight and postural changes are largely responsible. The woman can get the extra rest required by planning an earlier bedtime hour and by resting throughout the day as needed. Learning to conserve energy when carrying out household tasks is also helpful. For example, it is less tiring to sit rather than to stand for ironing.

Urinary frequency

The need to urinate more frequently is common in the first trimester because the enlarging uterus is posterior to and presses on the bladder. There is little that can be done about this problem. It resolves itself when the uterus rises into the abdominal cavity. Urinary frequency again occurs after *lightening* in the third trimester. Lightening is the descent of the uterus into the pelvic cavity. It usually occurs 2 to 3 weeks before labor.

Constipation

Constipation is a common problem of pregnant women commencing in the second trimester. Contributing factors are the pressure of the expanding uterus on the bowel and the increased reabsorption of water. Both contribute to alterations in bowel motility and stool consistency (drier stools).

The nurse can intervene by having the patient do the following:

1. Increase the fluid intake.
2. Obtain adequate exercise.

3. Ingest foods containing roughage.
4. Avoid taking mineral oil, since it interferes with the absorption of fat-soluble nutrients, and avoid enemas and laxatives because they can induce premature labor.

Flatulence is often associated with constipation. Avoiding such gas-forming foods as fried foods, parsnips, corn, and sweet desserts; ingesting small amounts of food at frequent intervals; and chewing food thoroughly are helpful suggestions. Small amounts of yogurt are helpful.

Heartburn

Slight regurgitation of the acid contents from the stomach into the esophagus occurs during the second and third trimesters. The acid irritates the esophageal mucosa, resulting in a burning sensation. The nurse can have the patient do the following:

1. Drink milk between meals.
2. Take small, frequent meals.
3. Avoid highly spiced or fried foods.

Food craving

Craving for certain foods is referred to as *pica* and may be caused by physiologic, psychologic, or social factors. Pica is a well-known phenomenon often humorized in literature and movies. The stories about the expectant father getting up in the middle of the night to purchase strawberries or pickles are exaggerations of this craving. Some women in the southern United States are influenced by culture to ingest clay or large amounts of laundry starch. Nurses can provide counseling in regard to food cravings. Intervention may be necessary if a woman is not receiving a nutritionally balanced diet.

Backache

Backache during pregnancy is due in large part to changes in body mechanics, change in posture, and overexertion. In the first trimester backache is associated with stretching of the uterosacral ligaments. The nurse can have the patient do the following:

1. Pay continual attention to posture.
2. Wear supportive shoes with low heels.
3. Take rest periods after standing for long periods.
4. Do the pelvic rock exercise frequently (see Chapter 24).

Muscle cramps

Spasmodic, painful muscle cramps in the legs sometimes occur as a result of fatigue, tension, chilling, or the drinking of too much milk. Relief can be obtained by straightening the leg (pushing down on the knee) and by stretching the toes upward. Frequent elevation of the legs and adequate warmth may prevent cramps to some extent. Excessive quantities of milk contribute to increased phosphorus absorption, which results in cramping. One solution is to reduce milk consumption, although the patient may then need to take additional calcium in pill form. Another solution is to take aluminum hydroxide with the milk to remove some of the phosphorus.

Edema

Some swelling of the lower extremities is common during the third trimester. It is aggravated by hot weather, by standing for long periods, and by the presence of varicose veins. Relief is usually obtained by elevating the limbs frequently.

Edema that is pronounced in the early morning and that involves the face or other parts of the body should be brought to the physician's attention. This latter situation could be the beginning of *preeclampsia*, a condition characterized by increasing hypertension, albumin in the urine, and generalized edema. It can occur during pregnancy or early in the puerperium.

Puerperium

The *puerperium* is that period from delivery to about 6 weeks after delivery. A number of changes take place during this time. These changes involve the reproductive system, the breasts, and the woman's emotions.

Reproductive system changes

During this period the uterus, which after delivery can be felt at the level of the umbilicus, becomes smaller and descends in the pelvic cavity. By the tenth day postpartum, it is usually below the level of the symphysis pubis. This decrease in the size of the uterus is called *involution*.

Also during this time, the lining of the uterus forms anew. The top layer sloughs off, and the endometrium regenerates. Regeneration is generally almost complete by 6 to 10 days except at the placental site, which takes about 6 weeks to heal. The old layer of the uterus that is sloughed off is discharged from the body as *lochia*.

Lochia has three stages:

1. *Lochia rubra* is the reddish to pinkish red discharge from the day of delivery to the 3rd or 4th day postpartum.
2. *Lochia serosa* is a pink to brown discharge that occurs from about the 4th to the 10th day postpartum.
3. *Lochia alba* is a discharge of white or yellow ap-

pearance. It appears at about the 10th day and may last 3 to 6 weeks.

Breast changes

The woman's breasts are normally soft the first 2 days after delivery. About the 3rd day they become fuller and firmer, or *engorged. Engorgement* is caused by the hormone prolactin, which is formed in the anterior pituitary gland. This hormone causes the production of milk, which together with increased lymph and blood circulation to the breasts causes engorgement.

Emotional changes

Emotional changes during the puerperium can be divided into two stages: the taking-in phase and the taking-hold phase (Rubin 1961:753–55).

During the *taking-in phase*, which lasts 2 or 3 days after delivery, the woman appears passive and dependent. She will make few or no decisions, and most of her needs are expressed in terms of herself. Not only does she often show preoccupation with food, but she also needs at this time to repeat the details of the delivery frequently. In this way she integrates the experience of the delivery with the reality of her living.

During the *taking-hold phase* the woman appears more decisive and autonomous. She is more interested in her baby and in people around her. At this time also she is concerned that her own body function properly. For example, bowel control can be a problem. The mother requires reassurance at this time that she is performing well as a mother and that her body problems are normal, if in fact they are. This period lasts about 10 days.

The *postpartum depression* is another emotional reaction, which can occur about the 3rd day or just after the woman comes home. She may say she feels let down, and she may cry readily for no reason that is apparent to her. There are a number of theories as to the cause of this depression, but as yet there is no known cause. At this time, the woman needs understanding and attention from nurses as well as increased affection from her family. Usually this emotional reaction passes without serious consequences.

Learning mothering is a gradual process, and mothers need time to adjust to their new babies. Being at home alone with a new baby is a reality of recent generations. Previously mothers had parents and grandparents to share the care of newborns and household responsibilities. Postpartum groups are now established to assist new mothers in adjusting to the demands of their roles as wife and mother. In these groups, mothers learn to accept limits on what they can realistically expect to accomplish; for instance, some household tasks have to be postponed.

Physiologic Needs During the Puerperium

The major physical needs of the woman during the puerperium are nutrition and protection from infection, which involves breast and perineal care.

Nutrition

If a woman breastfeeds her baby, her nutritional needs change. The diet recommended is similar to the one recommended for pregnant women. The woman will require, along with a well-balanced diet, an additional 500 kcal per day for 3 months for the production of milk. She will also need additional protein (20 gm), bringing the total protein requirement to about 80 to 85 gm daily. Another additional requirement is for increased fluids, to 3000 ml daily. For additional information see the section on pregnancy and lactation in Chapter 26.

Protection from infection

Breast care Breast care for the nursing mother involves two primary aspects: support of the breasts between feedings and nipple care.

A mother requires a supportive brassiere after delivery. Generally, it is worn 24 hours a day. A breast binder can be used in place of a brassiere. If the breasts are engorged, the infant should be put to the breast every 3 hours. Excess milk can be manually expressed to relieve the pressure.

If the woman does not plan to breastfeed, ice bags are generally applied to the breasts. In some instances, medications, such as chlorotrianisene (Tace), are ordered, and analgesics may be indicated.

For the breastfeeding mother, care of the nipples is of utmost importance. Nipples need to be kept clean and exposed to the air for 10 minutes after feedings to keep them dry. A heat lamp may be applied a few times a day to ensure drying. Creams can be applied after drying to help keep the nipple soft. At the first indication of cracking of the nipple, nipple shields are advised to prevent undue irritation from feeding. They are recommended for the first few minutes of suckling, but they then need to be removed because they prevent complete emptying of the breast (Worthington-Roberts, Vermeersch, and Williams 1981:216).

Perineal care Care of the perineum includes observation of the lochia (page 275) and the perineum itself. The amount of lochia discharged is generally about 200 g. If the initial flow is heavy, two perineal pads may be needed; they are changed every hour. The flow of lochia can be described as heavy, moderate, or light. A moderate flow saturates one perineal pad in about an hour.

The perineum needs to be observed for contusions. The suture line, if there is one, is observed for approximation of the skin edges, bulging, edema, or undue redness. For information on perineal care, see Chapter 21.

Common Problems During the Puerperium

Perineal sutures

Painful perineal sutures can be a source of discomfort to a patient, who may be reluctant to exercise because she anticipates pain. Heat lamps or peri-lights relieve discomfort and hasten healing. For information on infrared lamps and heat lamps, see Chapter 40.

Sitz baths are also used to hasten healing. They are used frequently by postpartum patients both in the hospital and at home. See Chapter 40.

Constipation

It is not uncommon for women to have difficulty defecating after delivering a baby. During pregnancy, the intestines are crowded by the enlarged uterus; after delivery the intestines once again occupy their normal position in the body. In this larger space, the muscle tone of the intestines is greatly reduced, and constipation can result. Fecal softeners are frequently ordered by the physician together with an enema or a suppository about the 3rd day.

Hemorrhoids

Hemorrhoids are frequently aggravated and can become painful during the puerperium because of pressure by the baby on the rectal blood vessels and the expulsive pushing efforts of the mother during delivery. Warm compresses, sitz baths, anesthetic ointments, and witch hazel relieve the discomfort of hemorrhoids.

Middle-Aged Adults

The middle years, from 40 to 65, have been called the years of stability and consolidation. It is a time in most people's lives when children have grown and moved away or are moving away from home. Thus partners generally have more time for and with each other and time to pursue interests they may have deferred for years.

Mid-Life Crisis

Gail Sheehy (1977) suggests that the transition into middle life is as critical as adolescence. She outlines characteristics of the mid-life crisis and calls the decade between the ages of 35 to 45 the "deadline decade."

According to Sheehy, most women pass through the mid-life crisis between 35 and 40, and most men between 40 and 45. This crisis occurs when a person recognizes he or she has reached the halfway mark of life. Although people of these ages are reaching their prime, there is a beginning recognition that time is at a premium and that life is finite. Youthfulness and physical strength can no longer be taken for granted.

Sheehy (ibid., p. 44) describes this mid-life crisis as an "inner crossroads" or "footbridge" leading to the second half of life. It is an "authenticity" crisis in which people face the discrepancy between their youthful ambitions and their actual attainment. To overcome this crisis, people need to reexamine their purposes and reevaluate ways to use their abilities and energies from now on. In Sheehy's words, it is a time when people ask, "Why am I doing all this? What do I really believe in? Is this all there is?" The parts of self that have been previously suppressed now need to be expressed. Both men and women in mid-life crises sense a feeling of urgency and perhaps despair when they look at those options they have set aside and realize that aging and ill health may soon hinder such opportunities.

Lillian Rubin (1979:6), in her study of 160 women between the ages of 35 and 54 and from all walks of life, describes mid-life for women as a time of endings and also a time of beginnings. The words of one woman (a 44-year-old student and homemaker married 22 years to a businessman) clearly express this beginning and ending and her strong desire to change her primary tasks of marriage and motherhood to something more, something new: "Twenty years of kids and doctors and chauffeuring and PTA and bridge and all that talk, talk, talk about nothing is enough. I got so I knew I couldn't stand another afternoon of that kind of talk. Enough! There's got to be more to life than hot flashes and headaches" (ibid., p. 155). Rubin does not define mid-life for women as a stage tied to a chronological age. Rather, it is that point in the life cycle of the family when the children are grown and gone, or nearly so, and when perhaps for the first time in her adult life a woman can attend to her own needs, desires, and development as a separate and autonomous being (ibid., p. 7).

Women often respond to a mid-life crisis by entering the job market or attending college. Men may respond by seeking second careers, by seeking promotions into management, by departing from well-established base lines (such as marriage), or by becoming more interested in developing themselves personally. Some people become self-destructive. When people confront the mid-life crises constructively, they can feel revitalized; the middle years of life can be the happiest years of one's life. When people do not make changes through this transition stage, they experience a sense of staleness and feelings of resignation.

Some characteristics of the mid-life crisis include:

1. Feeling bored, burdened, restless, and unappreciated
2. Dissatisfaction with the way one's life has developed
3. Ambivalence and uncertainty about the future
4. Dismay about signs of aging
5. Fear that time will be insufficient to accomplish goals
6. Feelings of self-doubt
7. Need to search for self, i.e., establish a true identity
8. Worry about health
9. Feelings of sadness, loneliness, or depression

Physiologic Changes

A number of changes take place during the middle years. At 40, most adults can function as effectively as they did in their 20s. However, during ages 40 to 65, physical changes do take place. Some of these are as follows:

1. Gray hair appears.
2. Crease lines appear at the lateral aspects of the eyes (laugh lines).
3. Fatty tissue is redistributed in men and women; men tend to develop fat on their abdomens, and women also deposit fat around the middle of the body.
4. Energy is more slowly recovered and more quickly expended. Vigor and endurance start to deplete at about 40 years.
5. Hearing acuity decreases and sight diminishes; reading glasses or bifocals may be needed.
6. Skeletal muscle bulk decreases at about 60 years.
7. General slowing of metabolism results in weight gain.
8. Hormonal changes take place in both men and women (see following section).

Hormonal changes

Both men and women experience decreasing hormonal production during the middle years. The *menopause* refers to the so-called change of life in women, when menstruation ceases. The *climacteric* (andropause) refers to the change of life in men, when sexual activity decreases. Sometimes *climacteric* is also used to refer to that time in the life of women when conception is no longer possible.

The menopause usually occurs anywhere between ages 40 and 55. The average is about 47 years. At this time, the ovaries decrease in activity until ovulation ceases. There are a number of menstrual patterns that can signal the menopause. Four of these are:

1. Periods remain regular, but menstrual flow decreases.
2. Periods will occur irregularly, and some periods are missed.
3. Menstrual flow ceases abruptly.
4. Menstrual flow occurs irregularly, with irregular amount of menses.

During this time the ovaries decrease in size, and the uterus becomes smaller and firmer. Progesterone is not produced, and the estrogen levels fall. Although the pituitary gland continues to produce the luteinizing hormone (LH) and the follicle-stimulating hormone (FSH), the ovaries do not respond. As a result of the lack of feedback, the pituitary gland increases the production of the gonadotropins, in particular FSH. This disturbed endocrine balance accounts for some of the symptoms of the menopause. Common symptoms are hot flashes, chilliness, a tendency of the breasts to become smaller and flabby, and a tendency to become obese. Insomnia and headaches also occur with relative frequency. Psychologically, the menopause can be an anxiety-producing time, especially if the ability to bear children is an integral part of the woman's self-concept.

In men there is not a change comparable to the menopause in women. Androgen levels decrease very slowly; however, men can father children even in late life. The psychologic problems that men experience are generally related to the fear of getting old and to retirement, boredom, and finances.

Psychosocial Development

At this time, adults usually face a number of adjustments in relation to their relationships and their activities. Husbands and wives generally have more time for leisure activities. Relationships with families change. Children move away and marry and have children of their own. Parents are elderly and often have additional needs. Thus people in their 40s and 50s often find themselves grandparents, enjoying their grandchildren but having few responsibilities for them, and at the same time assisting with the care of their own elderly parents. At this time people often face the death of a parent and as a result come to terms with their own aging and inevitable death.

For adults who are career oriented, these years often represent the peak professional and occupational performance. Adults have many experiences behind them, which, together with intellectual skills, permit them to be effective in many areas, such as financial and career endeavors.

Retirement plans are also essential for middle-aged people. It is important that feelings about retirement be considered and that thought be given to ways in which increased leisure time is used. Middle-aged people who plan ahead for the financial needs of retirement and establish new ways to keep active often adapt to the retirement situation more effectively than those who do not.

Generativity versus stagnation

Until recently the developmental tasks of middle-aged adults have received little attention. Erik Erikson (1963:266) viewed the developmental choice of the middle-aged adult as generativity versus stagnation. *Generativity* is defined as the concern for establishing and guiding the next generation. In other words, there is concern about providing for the welfare of humankind that is equal to the concern of providing for self. People in their twenties and thirties tend to be self- and family-centered. In middle age, the self seems more altruistic, and concepts of service to others and love and compassion gain prominence. These concepts motivate charitable and altruistic actions, such as church work, social work, political work, community fund-raising drives, cultural endeavors, etc. Marriage partners have more time for companionship and recreation; thus marriage can be more satisfying in the middle years of life. There is time to work together in volunteer activities or for one partner to go out for lunch, and for the other to go fishing. Generative middle-aged persons are able to feel a sense of comfort in their life-style and receive gratification from charitable endeavors. Erikson believes that persons who are unable to expand their interests at this time and who do not assume the responsibility of middle age suffer a sense of boredom and impoverishment, i.e., stagnation. These persons have difficulty accepting their aging bodies and become withdrawn and isolated. They are preoccupied with self and unable to give to others. Some may regress to younger patterns of behavior, e.g., adolescent behavior.

Changing self-image and self-concept

The middle-aged person looks older and feels older. People usually accept the fact that they are aging; however, a few try to defy the years by their dress and even their actions. It is at this time that some men and women have extramarital affairs and even marry younger partners.

A new freedom to be independent and follow one's individual interests arises. Sheehy (1977) describes this change as a movement from "us-ness" to "me-ness." Prior to this period, the marriage partner or lover and other persons were crucial to a definition of self. Now the middle-aged person does not make comparisons with others, no longer fears aging or death, relaxes his or her sense of competitiveness, and enjoys the independence and freedom of middle age. Other people's opinions become less important, and the earlier habit of trying to please everyone is overcome. The person establishes ethical and moral standards that are independent of the standards of others. The focus shifts from inner self and being to outer self and doing. Religious and philosophical concerns become important.

Developing alternative abilities

The stereotyped image of women at mid-life as lonely, depressed, and clinging pathetically to the past—"the empty nest syndrome"—is a fallacy, according to a study by Rubin. Almost all of the women she spoke with responded to the pending or actual departure of their children with a decided sense of relief (Rubin 1979:15). Even women who were divorced were relieved to be freed of the responsibilities of mothering and happy to be able to call their lives their own.

In middle age, the interests set aside in favor of family and career can be renewed and developed. Hobbies such as photography, collecting antiques, or painting may develop into serious work. Some people who deferred education now pursue it or take refresher and other courses to keep abreast of changes. Some women enter the work force. Many middle-aged people feel a mixture of excitement and fear about these new undertakings.

Needs

Nutrition

The major object in nutrition during the middle years is to maintain a balanced diet and at the same time decrease the caloric intake. Decreased metabolism together with decreased activity mean a decreased need for calories. For each decade after 25 years, there should be a 7.5% reduction in total calories consumed (Wil-

Table 12–5 Assessment of Growth and Development: Middle-Aged Adult

Assessment data	Normal findings*
Physical	
Weight and height	Refer to Tables 14–1 and 14–2 for normal weights, slight gains are common
Appearance	Graying hair and facial creases
Adipose tissue distribution	Redistribution of fat around abdomen
Menopause	Change in menstrual pattern; hot flashes or other symptoms such as headaches or insomnia
Vision	Need for reading glasses or bifocals
Vital signs	Temperature: 98.6 F (37 C) Pulse: 60 to 100 beats per minute Respirations: 16 to 20 breaths per minute Blood pressure: 100 to 140 mm Hg systolic, 60 to 80 mm Hg diastolic
Psychosocial	
Developmental task: generativity versus stagnation	
Self-image and concept	Accepts physical changes in appearance Increased charitable and community contributions Increased independence and renewed sense of self-identity Renewed interest in previously set aside hobbies or career goals Career provides satisfaction
Philosophy	Has meaningful philosophy of life
Marriage and family relationships	Increased time spent with spouse Views spouse as companion and lover Encourages independence of children Assists aging parents as required
Social activity	Enjoys leisure time Develops new friendships with people over wide age range
Retirement plans	Has considered feelings about retirement and how to deal with it
Wellness	Follows preventive health care practices such as rest, exercise, and healthful diet

*Findings represent trends in some instances and not exact values. Individual differences must be considered in an assessment.

liams 1981:474). Emphasis needs to be placed on balanced meals of foods from the four basic food groups (see Chapter 26) and on low-calorie and low-cholesterol foods. People over 50 often need to avoid excessive salt intake because of the high incidence of heart failure and hypertension in this age group.

Rest and exercise

Rest and sleep are important in middle years. Middle-aged adults have less vitality than previously and tire at a point when in their twenties they would have continued to be physically active. Regular exercise must be balanced with rest and sleep. Exercise slows the aging process, assists in maintaining joint mobility, and promotes blood circulation to body tissues. Exercise needs to be taken regularly and should be appropriate to the person's physical condition.

Assessment

Assessment of the growth and development of the middle-aged adult focuses largely on the self-image and self-concept, marriage and family relationships, and social activities. See Table 12–5.

Common Health Problems

Obesity

Obesity is a common but preventable problem and one that is intimately associated with other problems, such as atherosclerosis and digestive disorders. Middle-aged people need fewer calories than before and should eat accordingly. Regular exercise is also advisable, not only as a means of weight control but also to improve cardiorespiratory functions.

Osteoarthritis

Complaints of arthritis increase in the middle years and continue to increase with age. Stiffness of joints, swelling, and pain are common complaints. Obesity frequently accompanies this type of arthritis.

Excessive use of alcohol

The excessive use of alcohol presents a multifaceted problem to the individual and to society. Use of the drug is part of the life-style of many Americans and Canadians. Excessive use can result in unemployment, disrupted homes, accidents, and diseases. It is estimated that in the United States there are four million people who are dependent on alcohol and can be considered alcoholics.

Depressive disorders

At this period in life, men and women face a number of psychologic stresses. Women experience the menopause and thus termination of the childbearing ability. Their children are grown and usually leave home, leaving some women with more time than they had previously. The married woman now focuses on her husband and her own desires and ambitions. The change in the role of the woman can make her question her usefulness, and sometimes new challenges cause anxiety or depression.

Men also face stressors that can cause problems. Worries about economic security, retirement, and the quality of the husband-wife relationship are common sources of stress. As the man strives to adjust to change, he often experiences anxiety.

Cardiovascular diseases

Cardiovascular diseases are the leading cause of death of middle-aged people in the United States. Included in this group are coronary heart disease, atherosclerosis, and other vascular diseases. Preventive measures include regular exercise, keeping an appropriate weight, low-cholesterol diets, and abstinence from smoking.

Neoplasms

Cancer accounts for considerable mortality and morbidity in both men and women. It is the second leading cause of death among people between the ages of 25 and 64 in the United States. The patterns of cancer types and incidences for men and women have changed over the past several decades. Over one-third of the deaths due to cancer occur between the ages of 35 to 64. Men have a higher incidence of cancer of the lung, intestines, bladder, and stomach than women. In women breast cancer is highest in incidence followed by uterine, intestinal, lung, cervical, and rectal cancer. See Figure 12–2.

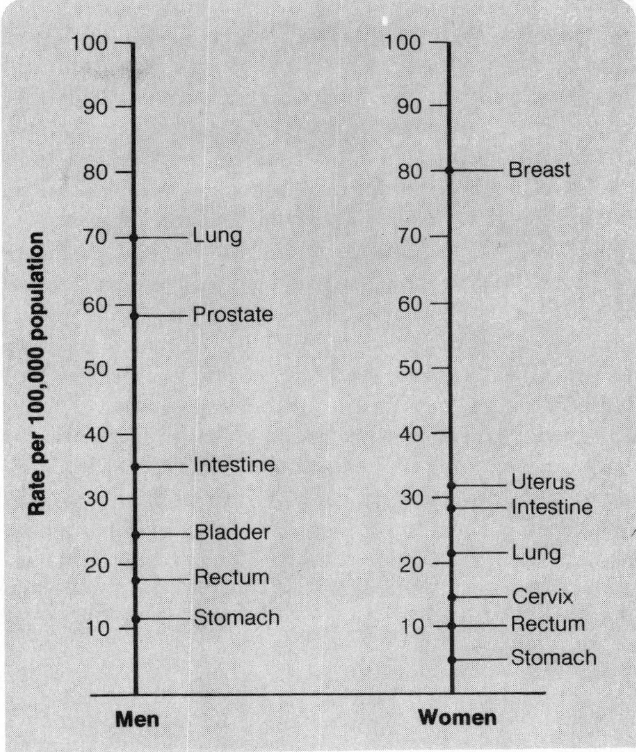

Figure 12–2 Cancer incidence rate by site: United States, 1977. (From U.S. Department of Health, Education, and Welfare, Public Health Service, *Healthy people: The surgeon general's report on health promotion and disease prevention*, DHEW Publication no. (PHS)79–55071, [Washington, D.C.: Government Printing Office, 1979], p. 61.)

Elderly Adults

Scientific interest in aging became keen during the 1930s. It was then that the term *gerontology* was adopted. Gerontology is the scientific study of the problems of aging in all its aspects—biologic, psychologic, sociologic, and clinical. Since then literature and conferences on gerontology in all its aspects have abounded. As a result much has been learned about the process of human aging, including the physical and psychosocial changes, illness in later years, and dying.

Physiologic Development

Different parts of the human body begin to decline at different ages and deteriorate at different rates. The basic mechanisms underlying the decline and deterioration are not known.

Integument

Obvious changes occur in the integument (skin, hair, nails) with age. These changes often present concerns in relation to self-image more than acute physical problems. These changes include wrinkles, dryness, loss of fullness, and increased itchiness of the skin and baldness or thinning and graying hair. The skin also becomes paler and blotchy and loses its elasticity. Fingernails and toenails become thickened and brittle, and in women over 60 years, facial hair increases.

These skin changes accompany progressive losses of underlying adipose and muscle tissue and loss of elastic fiber. Initially adipose tissue is redistributed from the extremities to the hips and abdomen in middle age. Generalized loss of adipose tissue progresses along with muscle atrophy, creating a wrinkled and wasted appearance. Bony prominences become visible, a double chin develops, and lower eyelids appear puffy. In elderly women the breasts become smaller and may sag, if large and pendulous, causing chafing where the skin surfaces touch. Loss of subcutaneous fat also decreases the elderly person's tolerance of cold.

Itching increases due to dryness of the skin and to deterioration of the nerve fibers and sensory endings. Decreased blood flow to the skin causes pallor and blotchiness. Baldness is thought to be due to decreased blood flow to the skin. The loss of hair color is due to a decrease in the number of functioning pigment-producing cells.

The ways people respond to these changes varies among individuals and cultures. For example, one person may feel distinguished with gray hair, while another may feel embarrassed by it. Most women dislike their facial hair because hirsute women do not conform to the feminine cultural ideal of North America.

Body temperature

Body temperature is lower in the elderly adult due to a decrease in the metabolic rate. It is not uncommon for an elderly adult to have a temperature of 35 C (95 F), particularly in the early morning when the body's metabolism is low. This fact has implications for nurses assessing the elderly adult for fever. For example, a temperature of 37.5 C (99.5 F) can represent a marked fever in some elderly people, although it represents only a mild fever in young adults. It is important that the normal temperature of each individual person be known as a baseline for assessing changes.

One of the body's normal compensating reactions to a fall in heat production is the contraction of the surface blood vessels and shivering. Because elderly adults have a diminished shivering reflex and do not produce as much body heat from metabolic processes, they tolerate prolonged exposure to cold poorly. At the other extreme, the body compensates for higher temperatures by slowing down muscular activity to produce less heat and by dilating surface blood vessels and sweating to increase losses of body heat. Older people, however, have sluggish sweating and circulatory mechanisms and therefore cannot cope with heat as well as younger people. For example, they do not tolerate working in moderately high temperatures for prolonged periods. It is therefore important for the elderly adult to have a constant, comfortable environmental temperature.

Skeleton

Slight loss in overall stature occurs with age due to atrophy of the discs between the spinal vertebrae. This can be exaggerated by muscular weakness resulting in a stooping posture and *kyphosis* (humpback of the upper spine). *Osteoporosis*, a decrease in bone density, along with increased brittleness of bone, makes the elderly adult prone to serious fractures, some of which are spontaneous. Since the incidence of osteoporosis is higher in elderly women, the effects of the menopause on the skeleton are being investigated. Frequently female hormones are given to women to treat this problem. Other causes of osteoporosis are thought to be lack of activity and inadequate calcium intake or inability to metabolize calcium.

In the joints some degenerative changes occur, which make movement stiffer and more restricted. Stiffness is aggravated by inactivity; for example, if persons sit too long, their joints become stiff and they have difficulty standing and walking. Although these skeletal changes do restrict the activity of the elderly adult, prevention of severe disability is possible.

Muscles

With aging there is a gradual reduction in the speed and power of skeletal or voluntary muscle contractions. The capacity for sustained muscular effort is also decreased. Great individual differences in muscular efficiency are apparent throughout life. Exercise can strengthen weakened muscles, and up to about age 50 the skeletal muscles can increase in bulk and density. After that time there is a steady decrease in muscle fibers, ultimately leading to the typical wasted appearance of the very old person. Thus elderly adults often complain about their lack of strength and how quickly they tire. Activities can still be carried out, but at a slower pace. Prolonged muscular efforts may be sustained by older people provided they take judicious rest pauses and avoid capacity or peak performance.

The effects of age on the smooth or involuntary muscles such as the stomach, the colon, the respiratory tubes, and the bladder are small in contrast to the effects on the skeletal muscles, with the exception of the blood vessels. These muscles function relatively normally until late *senescence.*

Senses

Vision Obvious changes around the eye are the shrunken appearance of the eyes due to loss of orbital fat, the slowed blink reflex, and the looseness of the eyelids, particularly the lower lid because of poorer muscle tone. Other changes result in loss of visual acuity, less power of accommodation to darkness and dim light, loss of peripheral vision, and difficulty in discriminating similar colors. The degenerative change in the eyes leading to the relative inflexibility of the lens is called *presbyopia.*

As the lens of the eye ages it becomes more opaque and less elastic. By the age of 80 all elderly people have some lens opacity (*cataracts*) that reduces visual acuity. Surgical removal of cataracts is common at this age. Accompanying this are changes in the ciliary muscles, which control the shape of the lens. These changes reduce the power of the lens to adjust to near and far vision. It is thought that changes in the nervous system play a part in reducing the diameter of the pupil, thereby restricting the amount of light entering the eye. This slows the reaction time to decreases in light or illumination, a problem compounded at night with driving. Reduced blood supply due to arteriosclerosis can diminish retinal function. Reduced peripheral vision also is thought to be a result of arteriosclerosis.

Many elderly adults require eyeglasses for close work. It is not uncommon for elderly people to buy inexpensive magnifying eyeglasses from department stores. Nurses should encourage elderly adults to have routine eye examinations by a physician and use appropriate eyeglasses. Many places now offer free eye examinations and eyeglasses to elderly people.

Hearing The loss of hearing due to senescent change is called *presbycusis*. Presbycusis comes about through changes in the structure of the inner ear: changes in nerve tissues in the inner ear and a thickening of the eardrum. Gradual loss of hearing is usual among the aging and more common among men than women, perhaps because men are more frequently in noisy work environments. Hearing loss is usually greater in the left ear than the right and greater in the higher frequencies than the lower. Thus, elderly adults with hearing loss usually hear speakers with low, distinct voices best. Elderly adults have more difficulty compensating for hearing loss than the young, who pay closer attention to the lip movements of the speaker.

Nurses can assist elderly people who are hard of hearing by the following measures:

1. Speaking more loudly and in a lower tone
2. Speaking slowly and sometimes using alternative words
3. Using facial expressions that convey moods and feelings, thus helping comprehension
4. Encouraging patients to use hearing aids when appropriate

Other senses Older persons have a poorer sense of taste and smell and are less stimulated by food than the young. Taste buds in the tongue are reduced in number, and the olfactory bulb at the base of the brain atrophies. (The olfactory bulb is responsible for smell perception.)

The sense of balance decreases with age, resulting in the greater incidence of falls and accidents in elderly persons. Changes occur also in the sensations of pain and temperature, as evidenced by the increased tolerance of the older person to these sensations.

Voice

Changes in the voice occur throughout life as a result of hardening and decreased elasticity of the laryngeal cartilages. These processes are completed by middle age. With age, the laryngeal muscles atrophy and vocal cords slacken. The voice becomes higher pitched, less powerful, and restricted in range. These changes are generally unnoticed unless greater demands on capacity, such as singing or public speaking, are made. Noticeable changes, such as slower speech and eventual slurring, are the result of central nervous system changes rather than the local mechanisms.

Respiration

Respiratory efficiency is reduced with age. The lungs contain a smaller volume of air due to the musculoskeletal changes in the chest wall that reduce the size of the chest. There is a greater volume of residual air left in the lungs after expiration and a decreased capacity to cough efficiently because of weaker expiratory muscles. Mucous secretions tend to collect more readily in the respiratory tree due to decreased ciliary activity. Thus susceptibility to respiratory infections is notable in elderly adults.

Dyspnea occurs frequently with increased activity, such as running for a bus or carrying heavy parcels up stairs. This dyspnea occurs in response to an oxygen debt in the muscles. Intense exercise is followed by short, heavy, rapid breathing, which is an attempt to repay this oxygen debt in the muscles. Although this is a normal response, it occurs more quickly in the aged because delivery and diffusion of oxygen to tissues is often diminished by changes in both respiratory and vascular tissues.

Circulation

The working capacity of the heart is diminished with age. This is particularly evident when increased demands are made on the heart muscles such as during periods of exercise or emotional stress. The valves of the heart tend to become harder and less pliable, resulting in reduced filling and emptying abilities. In addition, the pumping action of the heart is reduced due to changes in the coronary (cardiac) arteries, which supply progressively smaller amounts of blood to the heart muscle. These changes are evidenced by shortness of breath on exertion and pooling of blood in the systemic veins.

Changes in the arteries occur concurrently. The elasticity of smaller arteries is reduced by the thickening of their walls and increased calcium deposits in the muscular layer. Reduced arterial elasticity often results in diminished blood supply to, for instance, the legs and the brain, resulting in pain on exertion in the calf muscles and dizziness, respectively.

Blood pressure measurements often indicate increases in both systolic and diastolic pressures, partly as a result of the inelasticity of the systemic arteries. Variations in the pulse rate of the aged also occur. A rate of 70 to 80 beats per minute is quite usual.

Digestion and elimination

The digestive system is significantly less impaired by aging than other body systems. Previously mentioned was the diminished ability to taste and smell, which contributes in part to a lack of appetite. Gradual decreases in digestive enzymes occur; examples are ptyalin in salivary secretions, which converts starch; pepsin and trypsin, which digest protein; and lipase, a fat-splitting enzyme. Yet digestive functioning and absorption of food are relatively unimpaired. The common complaints of heartburn, gas, and indigestion are largely due to other disease processes or to dietary excesses, such as highly spiced or fried foods.

The majority of elderly adults have poor teeth or wear dentures and therefore may have difficulties masticating food. Foods that require extensive chewing, such as meat and fresh vegetables or fruit, may as a result be avoided, leading to nutritional deficiencies.

Constipation is a common complaint of older people. However, the aging process has little if any effect on the bowels, which retain their ability to function normally. Thus constipation is usually a result of poor fluid intake, inadequate roughage in the diet, and insufficient exercise.

The excretory functions of the kidney are diminished with age, but usually not significantly below normal levels unless a disease process intervenes. Blood flow can be reduced by arteriosclerotic changes so that renal function is decreased. With age the number of functioning nephrons (the basic functional units of the kidney) is reduced to some degree, thus affecting the kidney's filtering abilities.

More noticeable changes are those related to the bladder. Complaints of urgency and frequency are common. In men these changes are often due to an enlarged prostate gland and in women to weakened muscles supporting the bladder or weakness of the urethral sphincter. The capacity of the bladder and its ability to empty completely are diminished with age. This explains the need for elderly adults to arise during the night to void (nocturnal frequency) and the retention of residual urine, predisposing to bladder infections.

Sexual organs

In men degenerative changes in the gonads are very gradual. The ability of the testes to produce sperm remains into old age, although there is a gradual decrease in the number of sperm produced. The ability to have sexual intercourse also remains until late in life, and therefore satisfying sexual activities need not be altered. However, a gradual reduction in the frequency of sexual intercourse occurs. In women, by contrast, the degenerative changes in the ovaries are noticed by the abrupt cessation of menses in middle age during the menopause.

Changes in the gonads of elderly women result from the reduction of the ovarian hormones. Some changes, such as the shrinking of the uterus and ovaries, go unnoticed. Other changes are obvious. The breasts atrophy, and lubricating secretions of the vagina are reduced. Reduced natural lubrication is the cause of painful intercourse, which often necessitates the use of lubricating jellies.

Nervous system

The idea that a person's intellectual capacities decrease with age is a fallacy. Elderly people are able to follow desired intellectual pursuits. Many colleges and universities now provide special lecture series for elderly people in a variety of subjects. Grandparents have been known to graduate from universities at the same time as their grandchildren.

The person's reaction time is slowed with age because of the diminished conduction speed of nerve fibers. Reaction time can be delayed further by decreased muscle tone as a result of diminished physical activity. Elderly people compensate for this reaction difference by being exceptionally cautious, for instance, in their driving habits, which exasperate some impatient young drivers. Because sensory nerve endings in the skin also change with age, old people are less sensitive to touch, and safety precautions are necessary, for example, when a hot-water bottle is applied.

Psychosocial Development

Duvall (1977:390) summarizes the developmental tasks of elderly people as follows:

1. Making satisfactory living arrangements
2. Adjusting to retirement income
3. Establishing comfortable routines
4. Maintaining love, sex, and marital relationships
5. Keeping active and involved
6. Remaining in touch with other family members

7. Safeguarding physical and mental health
8. Finding meaning in life

Kart and associates, by contrast, discuss three tasks described by Peck (1955) as paramount in old age: First, elderly people must establish new activities so that the loss of accustomed roles is less keenly felt. Second, they must select activities that transcend the physical limitations of old age. Third, individuals may make contributions that extend beyond their own lifetimes, thereby providing a meaning for life (Kart et al. 1978:180).

Housing for elderly people

According to a Chinese saying, the house with an old grandparent harbors a jewel. However, in North American society most aging people live apart. Most think it unwise to live with married sons and daughters, since overcrowded and tense situations can arise. It is also difficult for some elderly people to assume a new role while still living with their children—relinquishing the authority they had and allowing them to become independent.

Deciding where to live in the retirement years is a very individual matter, influenced by many factors, but to a large degree it is based on these five:

1. Income
2. Proximity to family and friends
3. Convenience to transportation services, medical services, shopping areas, and recreational pursuits
4. Loss of a spouse
5. Degree of health and independence

Many aging couples prefer to retain their own homes so that children and grandchildren can return for holidays. Others move from larger to smaller homes or apartments after their children are financially independent. Sometimes large homes are a financial burden and require too much upkeep for aging couples. It is not uncommon for people to move to warmer climates. Florida, Arizona, and southern California are becoming retirement meccas. Moving to a new area may isolate elderly people from family and friends. It is interesting to note, though, that some retired couples meet several of their old friends when they move to a popular retirement region. Moving also requires adjustment to new and unfamiliar settings, which is beneficial for some people but not to all. Coping with change is more difficult as age advances. For example, some persons prefer to retain their familiar butcher and hairdresser than to look for a new one.

The following are some considerations about housing for elderly adults:

1. One-story houses are best for people with physical impairments such as cardiac disease or arthritis.
2. Stairways need solid handrails, and bathtubs should be equipped with handbars to prevent falls.
3. Good lighting is essential, since the older person's eyes adjust less quickly to changes in light. Particular attention should be paid to lighting in hallways, stairways, closets, and at the bedside.
4. A well-heated and draft-free home is best, since elderly adults do not tolerate temperature changes well. Thermostat and humidity controls are recommended.
5. Doors need to be wide enough for wheelchairs and walkers.
6. Throw rugs should not be used or should be tacked down, and nonskid material should be put into bathtubs and shower stalls.
7. Cupboards should be low enough to reach without standing on a stool or chair.
8. An outside sitting area that is partly sheltered from sun and wind is useful.
9. Access to shopping areas, church, and transportation services is essential to many.
10. Homes need to offer privacy and a certain degree of quiet, although some older people, particularly those with visual loss, need increased auditory input. The visually impaired get much of their sensory input from noise.
11. Homes should be near others and near to medical services.

About 5% of elderly adults become increasingly dependent and need to live in institutions (U.S. DHEW 1979:74). These lodgings vary in many ways and offer varying degrees of independence to the residents. All provide meals, but vary in giving other services, such as assistance with hygiene and dressing, physical therapy or exercise, recreational activities, transportation services, and medical and nursing supervision. Many of these lodgings are costly and require that younger family members help pay the cost. Governments now are increasingly recognizing the need to provide additional low-cost lodging services for elderly people.

Retirement

Today, a majority of the people over 65 are unemployed, a sharp contrast from the early 1900s, when the majority continued to work. At present, most industries and professions make retirement mandatory, although this policy is currently being questioned by some. Some who are self-employed continue to work until ill health intervenes. Work offers these people a better income, a sense of self-worth, and the chance to continue long-established routines. Some need to work for economic reasons.

Retirement requires many adjustments. These adjustments include:

1. Adapting to a lower income
2. Finding new ways to remain active
3. Adjusting to being home together all day
4. Maintaining social relationships

Lowered income Some of the financial needs of elderly people diminish considerably. Less money is needed for clothing, entertainment, and work, and many have planned ahead so that homes are owned outright. However, costs continue to rise, and for some it is difficult to make ends meet. For some people, food and medical costs alone are a financial burden. It is said that when older people speak about their greatest need, it is not happiness or health, but money. Money allows them to be independent and look after themselves.

Sources of income vary from state to state or province to province. In general, the elderly person derives money from independent income if working, from social security plans, from investment incomes, from retirement pensions, and from private pensions. There are additional income supplements for those in need in many states and provinces. Other incomes are allocated for widows, for example. It is estimated that many pensioners are existing at near poverty levels. As a result, young people are being encouraged to start saving for retirement as early in life as possible.

Special benefits are increasingly being offered to elderly people in many areas. Some of these include bus passes and theater passes at reduced costs. Some areas even provide free health services.

Figure 12–3 Retirement allows elderly people to pursue interests that were previously put aside for child rearing and work.

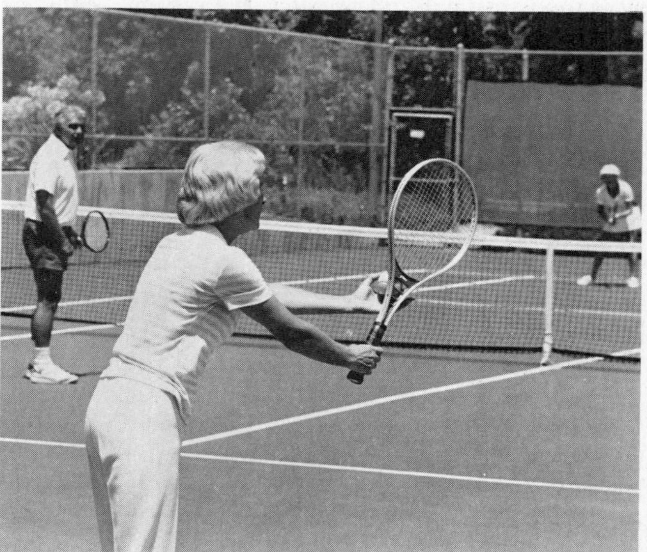

Keeping active Retirement can be a time when projects or recreational activities deferred for a long time can be pursued. See Figure 12–3. Pensioners are no longer governed by an alarm clock and can get up when they please. The enjoyment of staying up later is another luxury. Few elderly people, however, spend much time resting or sleeping. Being accustomed to activity most of their lives, most elderly find many outlets: jobs, community projects, volunteer services, intellectual or recreational pursuits, or hobbies such as stamp collecting or fishing. Travel opportunities are expanding.

The life-style of later years is to a large degree formulated in youth. This fact was recognized by Robert Browning: "Grow old along with me! / The best is yet to be, / The last of life, for which the first was made." People who attempt to refocus and enrich their lives all of a sudden at retirement usually find themselves in difficulty. Those who learned early in life to live well-balanced and fulfilling lives are generally more successful in retirement. The woman who has been concerned only with the accomplishments of her children or the man who has been concerned only with the paycheck and his job status can be left with a feeling of emptiness when children leave and the job no longer exists. The later years can foster a sense of integrity and continuity, or they can be years of despair.

Being home all day Many couples worry about one change retirement brings: Both the man and woman are home all day. If the woman has been a homemaker all her life, her job does not change. The retired man, however, does not have this established routine. Adjustments, therefore, are often required in household activities during retirement. Tasks may be shifted or shared. Many men assume some of the dishwashing and cooking responsibilities, and women may share some of the gardening activities. With the constant concerns regarding failing health, this shifting of tasks and sharing of responsibilities can be advantageous if one spouse becomes ill. The other can then function relatively independently.

Maintaining social relationships The social life of older people varies considerably. Married couples and members of higher socioeconomic groups tend to be socially more active than the widowed or those of lower socioeconomic status. Aging also influences social life. The span of social relationships narrows with age, and the individual relies more heavily on the family for companionship. This narrowing is due largely to loss of work associates, poor health, and eventual death of friends, relatives, and mates.

Many communities offer social activities to meet the needs of elderly people. Golden Age Clubs, lodges, and churches provide many opportunities for the elderly to maintain old friendships and to establish new ones.

Younger family members can do much to enhance the social life of elderly people. The joy of being a grandparent is matched by the joy of having one. Without the pressures of parenthood, many elderly people find their new roles as grandparents more satisfying than their old roles as parents. Close and meaningful family relationships are rewarding and fulfilling experiences for aging people.

Facing bereavement and dying

Well-adjusted aging couples thrive on companionship. Many couples rely increasingly on their mates for this company and may have few outside friends. Great bonds of affection and closeness can develop during this period of aging together and nurturing each other.

When a mate dies, the remaining partner inevitably experiences feelings of loss, emptiness, and loneliness. Many are capable and manage to live alone; however, reliance on younger family members increases as age advances and ill health occurs. Some widows and widowers remarry, particularly the latter, perhaps because widowers are less inclined to maintain a household than widows.

Women face bereavement and solitude more often than men, since their life spans are usually longer. The brevity of life is constantly reinforced by the death of friends. It is a time when one's life is reviewed with happiness or regret. Feelings of serenity or guilt and inadequacy can arise. Independence established prior to loss of a mate makes this adjustment period easier. A person who has some meaningful friendships, economic security, ongoing interests in the community, or private hobbies and a peaceful philosophy of life copes more easily with bereavement. Successful relationships with children and grandchildren are also of inestimable value. Facing death and dying is discussed in Chapter 36.

Needs

The needs of elderly people are influenced by the physical changes that occur with age and the developmental tasks that arise in the last years of life. Following is a brief summary of these needs. Each need is discussed in more detail in later chapters, for example, Chapter 25 on rest and sleep, Chapter 26 on nutrition, and Chapter 36 on dying.

Physical needs

Protection Accident prevention is a major consideration for elderly people. Because vision is limited, reflexes are slowed, and bones are brittle, climbing stairs, driving a car, or even walking requires caution. Safety precautions in homes of the elderly are discussed on page 285.

Driving, particularly night driving, requires caution because accommodation of the eye to light is impaired and peripheral vision is diminished. Older persons need to learn to turn the head before changing lanes and should not rely on side vision, for example, when crossing a street. Driving in fog or other hazardous conditions should be avoided.

Fires are a hazard for the elderly person with a failing memory. The older person may forget that the iron or stove is left on or may not extinguish a cigarette completely.

Because of reduced sensitivity to pain and heat, care must be taken to prevent burns when the person bathes or uses heating devices. Elderly people are also intolerant to cold and need warm clothing and often a blanket over their extremities. At night, woolen socks are safer for cold feet than hot-water bottles.

Nutrition Elderly adults need well-balanced diets. However, smaller servings with fewer calories are appropriate because of the reduction in metabolic rate and exercise. A diet high in protein, moderate in carbohydrates, and low in fat is recommended. Malnutrition is not uncommon in elderly people because many have bad teeth, many cannot afford the cost of food (particularly protein), and many eat alone. Also, appetite can be reduced by a dulled sense of taste and smell.

Elimination Constipation is not infrequent among the elderly. A cup of hot water or tea taken at a regular hour in the morning is helpful for some. For most, an assessment of fluid intake, exercise, and diet will help in deciding on a remedy. Adequate roughage in the diet, adequate exercise, and six to eight glasses of fluid daily are essential preventive measures for constipation.

Nocturnal frequency is also a common problem. Many older people learn to deal with this by restricting their fluid intake in the latter part of the evening, particularly those fluids that stimulate voiding, such as coffee or alcohol. Eventually most men require prostatic surgery to relieve increasing urinary frequency throughout the day, and some women require vaginal surgery for *cystoceles* or *rectoceles*. A cystocele is a protrusion of the urinary bladder through the vaginal wall. A rectocele is the protrusion of part of the rectum through the vaginal wall. Both of these conditions produce pressure and reduce bladder capacity, thereby creating urinary urgency and frequency.

Exercise and rest A regular program of moderate exercise is recommended for elderly adults. Walking, golfing, gardening, bowling, and bicycling are common activities. These can be performed at a leisurely pace. It is important that exercise not be too strenuous and that rest periods be taken as needed. Rapid breathing and accelerated heart beat should disappear within a few minutes after exercise; exercise should refresh rather than fatigue. People who are too disabled to engage in active exercise can implement a program of isometric exercises to maintain joint mobility and muscle tone. Exercise is also essential to maintain bone calcification. See Chapter 24.

Older people require more rest than before because they tire more easily. Often sleep habits change. Naps taken frequently throughout the day can cause difficulty sleeping at night. Measures to promote rest are discussed in Chapter 25. Encouraging plenty of fresh air and exercise helps facilitate sleep at night.

Hygiene Elderly persons should avoid daily bathing because their skin is dry and thin. Attention needs to be given to bony prominences exposed to pressure and to skin folds, which increase with loss of adipose tissue and cause abrasion from friction of skin surfaces. Soothing creams and oils can be applied for dryness. Excessive hair on the face of elderly women needs removal. Nails that become brittle, particularly the toenails, may need attention from a podiatrist, an individual who specializes in the care of the feet.

Sex Sexual drives persist into the 70s, 80s, and 90s provided good health is retained and there is an available and interested partner. Men have greater sexual drives than women. However, the frequency of sexual activity declines with age. Sometimes a chronic cardiac or respiratory illness interferes with sexual energy, and counseling may be required from a physician or nurse about sexual restrictions.

Health promotion Health care for elderly people includes medical supervision and dental supervision. Cardiovascular and respiratory diseases are common. Routine eye tests are needed to check for glaucoma, cataracts, and arteriosclerotic changes of the retina. Audiometric (hearing) studies are usually also included. Those who have eyeglasses and hearing aids need to have them checked at regular intervals. Regular visits to the dentist can help the older person to keep his or her teeth in good shape or to be fit with dentures.

Health services available to the elderly vary from place to place. Some elderly people's organizations routinely offer free eye examinations. Some nursing homes do not have dental services. Some communities offer comprehensive services through neighborhood geriatric clinics, visiting nurse services, and social services. The nurse who is aware of the available community resources can be instrumental in informing and referring people for appropriate care.

Psychologic needs

Independence Most elderly people thrive on independence. It is important to them to be able to look after themselves even if they have to struggle to do so. Although it may be difficult for younger family members to watch the oldster completing tasks in a slow, determined way, the aging need this sense of accomplishment. Children will often notice that the aging father and mother with diminishing vision cannot keep the kitchen as clean as formerly. The aging father and mother likewise may be slower and less meticulous in carpentry tasks or gardening. To maintain the elderly adult's sense of self-respect, nurses and family members need to encourage them to do as much as possible for themselves. Many young people err in thinking that they are helpful to older people when they take over for them and do the job much faster and more efficiently.

Some older people who are ill appear to enjoy the dependent role of being waited on and attended to. Nurses need to show an interest in such people as persons and set realistic, achievable goals. Praise and recognition for each accomplishment, no matter how small, are important. Success at getting out of bed independently or feeding oneself, if recognized by the nurse, can encourage people to achieve more and more. Some people may be afraid that they are not going to get better; others may feel that dependence brings them more recognition and importance. The nurse needs to understand each person's feelings and concerns before helping the older person toward independence. If patients know, for example, that an increasing level of wellness is possible and that as much attention by the nurse will be offered when they attempt tasks independently as when they are dependent, they probably will feel better about progressing on the road to independence.

Respect Aging people need to be recognized for their unique individual characteristics. It can be more difficult to recognize these differences, since elderly people have less energy than the young to show how they are different. Perhaps this is one reason elderly people tend to talk about past accomplishments, jobs, deeds, and experiences.

The ability to think, to reason, and to make decisions is important to recognize. Most elderly people are willing to listen to suggestions and advice, but they do not need to be ordered around. The nurse can support a decision by an elderly patient even if eventually the decision is reversed because of failing health.

Thoughtfulness, consideration, and acceptance of one's waning abilities are appreciated by old people. For example, having dinner out in a well-lighted restaurant or not expecting grandmother to baby sit for too many hours, if at all, are actions that recognize the diminishing vision and energy of older people.

The values and standards held by older people need to be accepted, whether they are related to ethical, religious, or household matters. For example, it is wise to respect an older person's decision to use a washboard rather than an automatic washing machine, to hang up the laundry outside rather than use a dryer, or to cook on a wood stove.

Assessment

The assessment of the development of the elderly person encompasses both physical and psychosocial aspects. According to Erikson the developmental task of the elderly person during later maturity is ego integrity versus despair. For a summary of selected developmental assessments see Table 12–6.

Common Health Problems

The common health problems of elderly adults include chronic illnesses such as arthritis (44% of those over 65 years), reduced vision (22%), hearing impairments (29%), heart conditions (20%), and hypertension (35%) (U.S. DHEW 1979:75).

Programs in the community are directed toward (a) early detection of illness; (b) services such as dietary counseling, eye care, foot care and routine medical care; and (c) activities that encourage exercise and social interaction to help prevent social isolation.

Nurses can assist elderly people maintain as much independent function as possible. Elderly patients can also learn certain skills that assist them to function as fully as possible within their limitations. In some instances, episodes of acute illness or injury—e.g., influenza, burns, and falls—can be prevented.

Table 12–6 Assessment of Growth and Development: Elderly Person

Assessment data	Normal findings*
Physical	
Weight	Decreased from that at age 50
Height	Decreased from height as young adult
Musculature	Some atrophy and loss of muscle tone
Vision	Presbyopia, cataracts
Adipose tissue distribution	Usually fat stores are decreased after 80 years
Vital signs	Temperature: 36 C (96.8 F) or higher Pulse: 70 to 80 beats per minute Respirations: above adult normal (16+ to 20+ breaths per minute) Blood pressure: as for middle aged-adult (100 to 140 mm Hg systolic, 60 to 80 mm Hg diastolic) or slightly higher
Psychosocial	
Developmental task: ego integrity versus despair	
Ego integrity	Makes decisions about where and how to live Adjusts life-style to retirement income
Intimacy	Continues close relationship with partner Maintains relationships with family and friends
Socialization	Develops new friendships and maintains old ones
Self-worth	Identifies how life is meaningful to self and others
Philosophy	Copes with loss of friends, partner, etc. through death Develops a philosophy that incorporates thoughts about death

*Findings represent trends in some instances and not exact values. Individual differences must be considered in an assessment.

Summary

Adolescence is a critical period of development in which people become physically and psychologically mature. In America, adolescence extends to 18 years for girls and to 20 years for boys. Because the skeleton grows more rapidly than muscles at this stage of development, many young adolescents appear poorly coordinated. Often they feel tired until the heart and lungs develop sufficiently to meet the body's increased growth needs. Major physical changes noted in boys are the appearance of facial hair (14 to 15 years), voice changes shortly thereafter, and gradual enlargement of the penis and testes. In girls the menarche occurs at about 12 to 13 years of age, the breasts mature gradually, and maximum height is reached by 16. Physical growth during adolescence is influenced by heredity, nutrition, and physical health. Thus the major needs of this group include nutrition (increased calories, protein, calcium, and vitamin D), rest, and sleep up to 10 hours a day. Sexual education is also needed and should include information about sexually transmitted diseases, the reproductive process and pregnancy, birth control measures, and sexual codes of conduct.

Seven major psychologic tasks face adolescents. These include relating with their parents at a time when they are gaining independence and yet need guidance; developing a stable self-concept that recognizes both strengths and weaknesses; adjusting to sexual roles; establishing appropriate life value systems; selecting a vocation or career; developing cognitively; and relating effectively with the peer group. Common health problems affecting adolescents include obesity, acne, accidents, pregnancy, sexually transmitted disease, gastric indigestion and acidity, drug abuse, and suicide and homicide.

Adulthood encompasses the years from the end of adolescence to the end of life. Young adults are people between 20 and 40 years of age; middle-aged adults are people between 40 and 65 years of age. Young adults are at peak efficiency physically, and physical changes are minimal throughout this period with the exception of pregnant women. Psychologic development offers several new experiences. Selecting educational pursuits or employment, choosing a mate, and getting engaged or married are some major experiences. After marriage, if this is chosen, newlyweds also face many adjustments. Learning to live together as a couple, delineating household tasks and financial matters, developing gratifying sexual relations, planning for children, and promoting relationships with family and friends are essential tasks.

The experience of pregnancy means additional adjustments for couples. They prepare to assume the parental role, and both partners need to share the responsibilities of preparing for a baby, adjusting living conditions, and learning to care for a baby.

Physical changes induced by pregnancy involve not only the reproductive organs but many other bodily systems. Menstruation stops due to the high levels of progesterone and estrogen after fertilization occurs. The uterus becomes enlarged and anteflexed and softens at the cervix (Goodell's sign) and at the isthmus (Hegar's sign). Braxton Hicks contractions occur throughout pregnancy. Vaginal changes include changed coloration (Chadwick's sign), increased acidity, and profuse, thick vaginal secretions. Tingling and throbbing sensations occur in the breasts as they enlarge. Pigmentation of the nipples and areola increases, Montgomery's glands appear, and blood vessels increase in prominence. Striae gravidarum frequently appear on the abdomen, breasts, buttocks, and thighs.

Other changes include blood volume and red blood cell increases, alterations in gastrointestinal functioning, increased urinary elimination, decreased fasting blood sugar levels, the secretion of HCG and human placental lactogen by the placenta, and adrenal enlargement with increased production of aldosterone. A total weight gain of up to 13 kg (30 lb) occurs during pregnancy.

Emotional changes parallel the physiologic changes. Included are feelings of ambivalence in the early stages of pregnancy, rapid mood swings due to hormonal changes, discomfort about body image changes, passive and introverted behavior, and changes in sexual desire.

The major needs of pregnant women are nutrition, rest, and exercise. Common discomforts include nausea and vomiting, breast soreness, fatigue, urinary frequency, constipation, heartburn, food cravings, backache, muscle cramps, and edema. Specific suggestions for the relief of each discomfort are listed.

During the puerperium, the uterus undergoes involution, the endometrium regenerates, and lochia is discharged, progressing through three stages of color (rubra, serosa, and alba). The breasts become engorged about the 3rd day under the influence of prolactin. Emotional changes include a taking-in phase and a taking-hold phase. Postpartum depression is not uncommon. The major physical needs of women during this period are nutrition and protection from infection, which includes breast care and perineal care. The common problems are painful perineal sutures, constipation, and hemorrhoids.

The transition into middle life begins with an awareness that one's life is finite and that time is at a premium. The middle-aged adult undergoes a number of physical changes. Gray hair, facial crease lines, and fat deposits on the abdomen appear. Energy is quickly expended, and metabolic activity decreases. Hearing acuity may diminish, and visual changes often require the use of bifocals. The menopause and the climacteric are the major endocrine changes. Psychologic changes accompany these physical changes, such as anxiety about aging and fears of sexual changes. Nutrition, rest and sleep, exercise, and acceptance of a changing self-image are the major needs of middle-aged people. Common health problems include obesity, osteoarthritis, excessive use of alcohol, cardiovascular disease, neoplasms, and depressive disorders.

The elderly person is faced with progressive physical deterioration but can also enjoy an enriched life-style. Obvious physical changes include skin inelasticity and thinness; muscle weakness; joint stiffness; flexed posture; shortened stature; impaired sight, hearing, taste, and smell; poor coordination and balance; slowed speech; and delayed reaction times. Other measurable changes include increased blood pressure, reduced respiratory efficiency, and lowered body temperature.

Several psychologic adjustments are required of elderly people. Changes in housing are usually necessitated by reduced income, widowhood, or limited independence and are influenced by proximity of family and friends, transportation, health, and other services. Housing needs of elderly adults include adequate heating, lighting, and safety handrails. Retirement years offer many pleasures but also require many adjustments. Establishing ways to keep active, adjusting to being home all day, and maintaining social relationships are some of these. Many communities offer social activities and lodging facilities for elderly people. Facing bereavement, solitude, and dying are major adjustments of this period.

The major needs of elderly people correlate with the physical changes that occur with aging and with the psychologic adjustments required for the last years of life. Included are protection from accidents, adequate nutrition, balanced rest and exercise, attention to elimination, independence, and self-respect.

Suggested Activities

1. Select an elderly patient. Assess his or her health and living problems. Compare these with the needs common to that stage of development.
2. With reference to Erikson's or Duvall's stages of development, briefly analyze your own development.
3. Interview an adolescent. Assess his or her developmental needs and problems.

Suggested Readings

Adolescents

Abrams, B. March 1981. Helping pregnant teenagers eat right. *Nursing 81* 11:46–47.
The nutritional needs of the pregnant teenager are discussed together with some possible problems and suggestions regarding nourishment.

Admire, G., and Byers, L. April 1981. Counselling the pregnant teenager. *Nursing 81* 11:62–63.
The phases of counseling are outlined together with some of the particular needs of the pregnant teenager.

Bartel, C. H. March 1981. Old enough to get pregnant . . . Too young to have babies. *Nursing 81* 11:44–45.
The physiologic changes that occur during pregnancy are reviewed, and the implications for adolescents are discussed.

Boyle, M. P.; Koff, E.; and Gudas, L. J. November/December 1981. Assessment and management of anorexia nervosa. *American Journal of Maternal Child Nursing* 6:412–18.
The disease process and the cause of anorexia nervosa are discussed as well as a profile of an anorexic adolescent. Common fantasies and family dynamics are included as well as the nursing interventions often required.

Campbell, C. E., and Herten, R. J. September 1981. VD to STD: Redefining venereal disease. *American Journal of Nursing* 81:1629–35.
This article redefines venereal disease (VD) as sexually transmitted disease (STD). It describes a variety of diseases that fall into this category, including herpes progenitalis, trichomoniasis, and nonspecific urethritis. Included with the article is a table about diseases and colored photographs of the etiologic organisms and the clinical pictures they present.

Nelms, B. C. November/December 1981. What is a normal adolescent? *American Journal of Maternal Child Nursing* 6:402–5.
The author describes the phases of adolescence, areas of influence, and developmental tasks. Included is a table of guidelines for assessing the adolescent.

Young Adults

David, M. L., and Doyle, E. W. December 1976. First trimester pregnancy. *American Journal of Nursing* 76:1945–48.
This article discusses the reasons for the changes in the pregnant woman's body and what can be done to make her pregnancy easier. Included is a table of commonly used antiemetics for pregnant women.

Diekelmann, N. L. August 1976. The young adult: The choice is health or illness. *American Journal of Nursing* 76:1272–77.
Nurses can help young adults to recognize the importance of health maintenance and promotion by encouraging them to develop proper sleeping, eating, and exercising habits and fulfilling emotional tasks. Many problems can occur in later life if attention to health is lacking between the ages of 20 and 35.

Dresen, S. E. August 1976. The young adult adjusting to single parenting. *American Journal of Nursing* 76:1286–89.
The nature of the crisis of single parenting is discussed; some available resources that can provide counseling services and help are included. Several people who have been through this crisis offer advice.

Hammons, C. February 1976. The adoptive family. *American Journal of Nursing* 76:251–57.
This article discusses some of the stresses inherent in adoption and stresses to the adoptive family. Successful adoption depends on how well the parents perform their special tasks of telling the child that he or she is adopted and how well they assist the child in identity formation.

Hott, J. R. September 1976. The crisis of expectant fatherhood. *American Journal of Nursing* 76:1436–40.
This article emphasizes that pregnancy is a crisis for the man as well as the woman.

Obrzut, L. A. J. September 1976. Expectant fathers' perception of fathering. *American Journal of Nursing* 76:1440–42.
Increasingly, fathers are becoming more involved in childbearing and childrearing. However, fathers do not always describe the role of fathering as nurses do.

Wuerger, M. K. August 1976. The young adult: Stepping into parenthood. *American Journal of Nursing* 76:1283–85.
Five goals of parental growth by which the nurse can assess

the status of the family are given. The skills of parenting are not always easily learned.

Middle-Aged Adults

Diekelmann, N. L. June 1975. Emotional tasks of the middle adult. *American Journal of Nursing* 75:997–1001.

This article outlines four areas in which middle-aged adults become more self-oriented. Specific examples of how several couples and singles view these years enhance the content.

Diekelmann, N. L., and Galloway, K. June 1975. A time of change. *American Journal of Nursing* 75:994–96.

Psychologic, physical, environmental, value, and social changes occur in the middle-aged adult. The nurse's role in teaching and preparing families for these changes is outlined.

Dresen, S. E. June 1975. The full life. *American Journal of Nursing* 75:1008–11.

This article focuses on the experiences of one woman during the menopause and the middle adult years.

———. June 1975. The sexually active middle adult. *American Journal of Nursing* 75:1001–5.

This article includes sexual patterns in middle age and some associated problems. It discusses the relationship between a good marriage and satisfactory sexual activity. An emphasis is that the nurse gain self-awareness about his or her own attitudes and feelings before attempting to counsel or help people with sexual problems.

Galloway, K. June 1975. The change of life. *American Journal of Nursing* 75:1006–11.

The problems and concerns of both men and women at the change of life are outlined as well as the nurse's role in helping people cope with these changes.

Graber, E. A., and Barber, H. R. October 1975. The case for and against estrogen therapy. *American Journal of Nursing* 75:1766–71.

These obstetric and gynecologic specialists caution that more scientific facts are needed to support the estrogen therapy that is frequently prescribed for postmenopausal women.

Hargreaves, A. G. October 1975. Making the most of the middle years. *American Journal of Nursing* 75:1772–76.

This article discusses some of the reactions to middle age. The outcomes of crises in midlife are influenced by the kind of help offered by family, friends, and caregivers.

Johnson, L. June 1975. Living sensibly. *American Journal of Nursing* 75:1012–16.

Changes in patterns of diet and exercise are required of the middle-aged adult. Routine preventive care, in addition, can promote healthier and happier people.

Owen, B. D. June 1975. Coping with chronic illness. *American Journal of Nursing* 75:1016–18.

Increased adjustments are required of the middle-aged adult when he or she is ill.

Peplau, H. E. October 1975. Mid-life crises. *American Journal of Nursing* 75:1761–65.

Role changes, physical changes, and new social needs are potential stressors in the middle years. Nurses can help people recognize some of these stressors and help them to resolve these and enjoy what can be a productive period of life.

Prock, V. N. June 1975. The mid-stage woman. *American Journal of Nursing* 75:1019–22.

The middle years may be more stressful for women, resulting in lowered self-esteem.

Elderly Adults

Burnside, I. M. October 1975. Listen to the aged. *American Journal of Nursing* 75:1801–3.

Much can be learned from the aged about living and dying; about problem solving, grief, sensory deprivation, and survival; and about how to be courageous, loving, and generous.

———. March 1977. Recognizing and reducing emotional problems in the aged. *Nursing 77* 7:56–59.

General, verbal, and physical signs of emotional problems in the aged are offered. Specific nursing measures to reduce the effects of anxiety, grief, loneliness, and paranoia are given.

Cohen, S. October 1981. Programmed instruction: Sensory changes in the elderly. *American Journal of Nursing* 81:1851–80.

This programmed instruction includes descriptions of the changes that occur in the senses with age. It includes ways in which nurses can provide sensory stimulation and assess sensory changes.

Conti, M. L. August 1970. The loneliness of old age. *Nursing Outlook* 18:28–30.

This article reveals some interesting insights about loneliness. Inclusion in a group is not the answer to everyone's loneliness.

Cooper, S. July/August 1981. Common concern: Accidents and older adults. *Geriatric Nursing* 2:287–90.

This article describes falls, motor vehicle injuries, fires, and burns as they relate to elderly people.

Greenberg, B. December 1973. Reaction time in the elderly. *American Journal of Nursing* 73:2056–58.

Practical suggestions are offered by this author, a nurse, about the nursing care of elderly people and how it relates to studies concerning reaction times.

Harmon, V. C. February 1975. Rx for RN retirement: Speaking out. *Nursing 75* 5:22–23.

Like everyone else, nurses are subject to birthdays, and recurring birthdays eventually lead to retirement. Six basic prescriptions are offered that can help nurses maintain a healthy perspective on retirement.

Macdonald, M. I. April 1977. Practical concerns for nursing the elderly in an institutional setting. *The Canadian Nurse* 73:25–30.

Physical and psychosocial needs of elderly adults are closely intertwined. The author itemizes the physical and psychosocial care goals by first listing the changes that occur with aging; then she discusses related nursing care measures.

Martin, D. May/June 1981. Enjoyable activity for everyone. *Geriatric Nursing* 2:210–13.

The author describes a stimulation program for people living in a nursing home.

Morlok, M. A. April 1977. Community resources for the elderly—Day therapy centre: The role of the primary care nurse. *Canadian Nurse* 73:50–51.

This article describes some services in Hamilton, Ontario, that help elderly adults delay the need for institutionalized care and the role of a primary nurse as a nursing team leader and patient advocate.

Ross, M. May 1981. Nursing the well elderly. *Canadian Nurse* 77:50, 53–55.

The author describes a program developed to assist a group of elderly people identify health issues of concern to them and obtain nursing assistance to cope with these issues.

Schattschneider, H. April 1977. Community resources for the elderly: Day hospital. *Canadian Nurse* 73:47–49.

This article describes some services in Edmonton, Alberta, that help maintain people in their own homes and communities.

Selected References

Beaton, S. R. 1980. Reminiscence in old age. *Nursing Forum* 19:270–83.

Block, G. J.; Nolan, J. W.; and Dempsey, M. K. 1981. *Health assessment for professional nursing: A developmental approach.* New York: Appleton-Century-Crofts.

Butler, R. N., and Lewis, M. I. 1981. *Aging and mental health.* 3rd ed. St. Louis: C. V. Mosby Co.

Crandall, R. C. 1980. *Gerontology: A behavioral science approach.* Menlo Park, Calif.: Addison-Wesley Publishing Co.

Duvall, E. M. 1977. *Marriage and family development.* 5th ed. Philadelphia: J. B. Lippincott Co.

Ebaugh, F. G., editor. 1981. *Management of common problems in geriatric medicine.* Menlo Park, Calif.: Addison-Wesley Publishing Co.

Erikson, E. H. 1963. *Childhood and society.* 2nd ed. New York: W. W. Norton and Co.

Fong, B. C., and Resnick, M. R. 1980. *The child: Development through adolescence.* Menlo Park, Calif.: Addison-Wesley Publishing Co.

Gedan, S. October 1974. Abortion counseling with adolescents. *American Journal of Nursing* 74:1856–58.

Harvey, K. January/February 1977. The empty cradle: Caring perceptively for the relinquishing mother, part 1. *American Journal of Maternal Child Nursing* 2:24–28.

Inman, M. 1975. What teen-agers want in sex education. Reprinted in A. B. O'Connor, editor. *Contemporary nursing series: Nursing of children and adolescents.* New York: American Journal of Nursing Co.

Kaluger, G., and Kaluger, M. F. 1979. *Human development: The span of life.* 2nd ed. St. Louis: C. V. Mosby Co.

Kandell, N. December 1979. The unwed adolescent pregnancy: An accident? *American Journal of Nursing* 79:2112–14.

Kart, C. S.; Metress, E. S.; and Metress, J. F. 1978. *Aging and health: Biologic and social perspectives.* Menlo Park, Calif.: Addison-Wesley Publishing Co.

Kellett, A. 1975. Update on aging: Its problems, its promises. *Image* 7(3):10–21.

Marshall, D. March/April 1981. Common concern: Toward a stimulating retirement. *Geriatric Nursing* 2:143–45.

Murray, R. B., and Zentner, J. P. 1979. *Nursing assessment and health promotion through the life span.* 2nd ed. Englewood Cliffs, N. J.: Prentice-Hall.

Olds, S. B.; London, M. L.; Ladewig, P. A.; and Davidson, S. V. 1980. *Obstetric nursing.* Menlo Park, Calif.: Addison-Wesley Publishing Co.

Peck, R. 1955. Psychological developments in the second half of life. In Anderson, J., editor. *Psychological aspects of aging.* Washington, D.C.: American Psychological Association.

Rubin, L. B. 1981. *Women of a certain age: The midlife search for self.* New York: Harper and Row.

Rubin, R. December 1961. Puerperal change. *Nursing Outlook* 9(12):753–55.

Sheehy, G. 1977. *Passages: Predictable crises of adult life.* New York: E. P. Dutton and Co.

Smith, D. W., and Bierman, E. L., editors. 1973. *The biologic ages of man: From conception through old age.* Philadelphia: W. B. Saunders Co.

Stone, V. October 1969. Give the older person time. *American Journal of Nursing* 69:2124–27.

Suitor, C. W., and Hunter, M. F. 1980. *Nutrition: Principles and application in health promotion.* Philadelphia: J. B. Lippincott Co.

Sutterley, D. C., and Donnelly, G. F. 1973. *Perspectives in human development: Nursing throughout the life cycle.* Philadelphia: J. B. Lippincott Co.

U.S. Department of Health, Education, and Welfare. Public Health Service. 1979. *Healthy people: The surgeon general's report on health promotion and disease prevention.* U.S. DHEW (PHS) Publication no. 79-55071. Washington, D.C.: Government Printing Office.

Vaughan, V. C.; McKay, R. J.; and Behrman, R. E., editors. 1979. *Nelson textbook of pediatrics.* 11th ed. Philadelphia: W. B. Saunders Co.

Whaley, L. F., and Wong, D. L. 1979. *Nursing care of infants and children.* St. Louis: C. V. Mosby Co.

Wiley, L. April 1980. Nursing care of a suicidal adolescent. *Nursing 80* 10:56–59.

Williams, S. R. 1981. *Nutrition and diet therapy.* 4th ed. St. Louis: C. V. Mosby Co.

Worthington-Roberts, B. S.; Vermeersch, J.; and Williams, S. R. 1981. *Nutrition in pregnancy and lactation.* 2nd ed. St. Louis: C. V. Mosby Co.

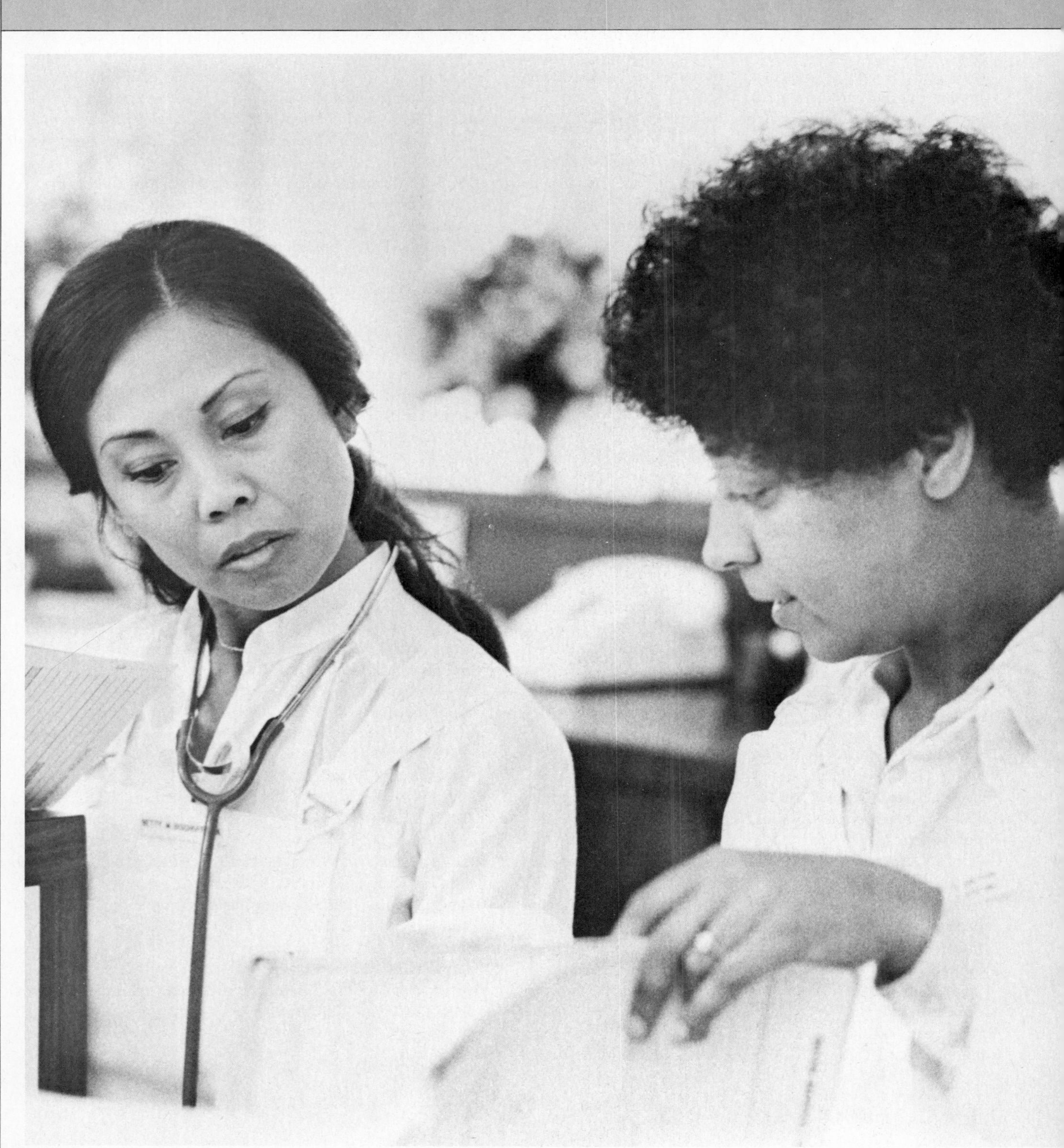

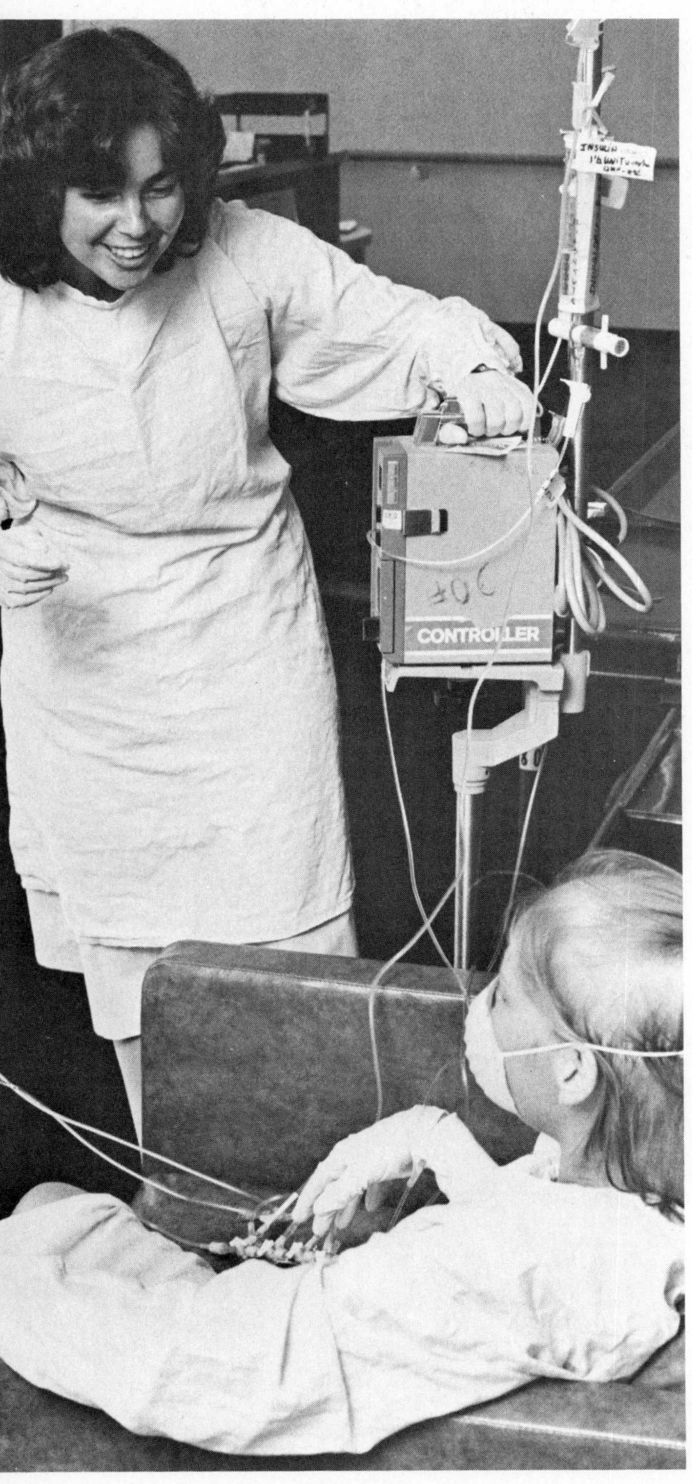

Unit IV

Skills Basic to the Nursing Process

CONTENTS

Chapter 13

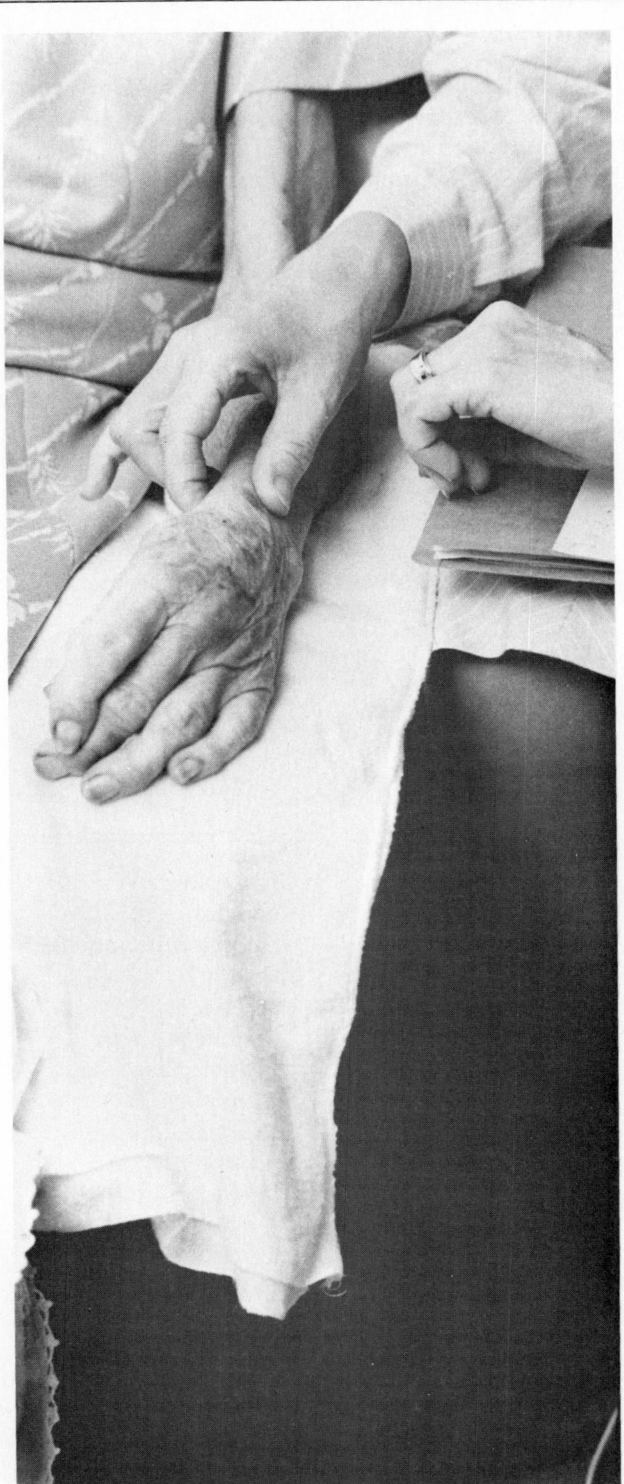

Assessing Vital Signs

CONTENTS

Objectives

1. Know essential facts about the body's vital signs and thermoregulation
    - **1.1** Define selected terms associated with the vital signs
    - **1.2** Identify the changes that occur in the vital signs as age increases
    - **1.3** Identify three ways the body produces heat
    - **1.4** Identify four ways the body loses heat
    - **1.5** Name the body's main thermoregulatory organ and the mechanism by which it operates
    - **1.6** Identify some major factors that affect body temperature, pulse, respirations, and blood pressure
    - **1.7** Identify four factors that control blood pressure
2. Understand essential facts related to assessment methods used to measure vital signs
    - **2.1** Compare the relationship between oral, rectal, and axillary measurements of body temperature
    - **2.2** Identify situations in which measurements of body temperature by mouth, rectum, and axilla are indicated and contraindicated
    - **2.3** Identify recommended times for accurate measurement of body temperature
    - **2.4** Identify alternative methods of measuring body temperature
    - **2.5** Identify eight sites commonly used to assess the pulse and reasons for their use
    - **2.6** Identify qualitative data needed to assess pulse and respirations
    - **2.7** Explain how to locate the apex of the heart
    - **2.8** Identify factors influencing the areas of maximum intensity of fetal heart tones
    - **2.9** Give reasons for selected steps of vital signs procedures
3. Demonstrate skill in performing procedures for assessing the vital signs for patients of all ages
    - **3.1** Assemble all necessary equipment before the procedure
    - **3.2** Carry out essential medical aseptic practices such as hand washing, appropriate cleaning and disinfection of equipment, etc.
    - **3.3** Prepare the patient, physically and psychologically
    - **3.4** Implement steps to acquire the vital signs measurements accurately and safely
    - **3.5** Record the vital signs measurements accurately

Terms

apnea
arrhythmia
basal metabolic rate
blood pressure
bradycardia
bradypnea
chemical thermogenesis
circadian rhythm
conduction
convection
diaphoresis
diastole
diastolic pressure
dyspnea
eupnea
exhalation (expiration)
fever (pyrexia)
hyperpyrexia
hypertension
hyperventilation
hypotension
hypothermia
hypoventilation
inhalation (inspiration)
Korotkoff's sounds
lumen
obligatory heat
orthostatic hypotension
pulse
pulse deficit
pulse pressure
pulsus regularis
radiation
rales
respiration
souffle
sphygmomanometer
stridor
systole
systolic pressure
tachycardia
tachypnea
vaporization
ventilation
vital (cardinal) signs

Chapter 5 discusses assessment as part of the nursing process. This chapter deals specifically with skills used to assess vital physiologic functions.

Nurses have always assessed their patients' conditions generally, but they are employing increasingly specific techniques to ascertain health status. In some agencies nurses carry out the complete physical examination and report their findings to the physician on the patient's record. See Chapter 14. Nursing students need to become familiar with the policies and practices in a specific agency before initiating particular assessment techniques.

This chapter discusses the assessment of the vital signs of a patient of any age.

Vital Signs

The *vital* or *cardinal signs* are body temperature, pulse, respirations, and blood pressure. These signs, which should be looked at in total, monitor the functions of the body; the signs reflect changes in function that otherwise might not be observed.

Some variation in an individual's vital signs is normal. The time of day, the amount of exercise the patient has taken before assessment, the patient's age and emotional status, and even the eating of a meal can affect some of the vital signs. As a basis for assessing changes in a patient's condition, the vital signs are usually taken on initial contact with a nurse or physician. The record of these initial signs constitutes baseline data for subsequent comparison.

Body Temperature

The *body temperature* is the balance of the heat that is produced and the heat that is lost from the body. Heat is produced by the metabolism of food, in particular by the cellular activity of the muscles and the secreting glands. Exercise, shivering, or the unconscious tensing of muscles produce heat. In addition, heat production can be increased or decreased by the presence of disease, an important fact to remember when assessing body temperature.

Heat Production

Food metabolism and activity

The metabolism of food produces heat referred to as *obligatory heat.* This rate of metabolism is referred to as the *basal metabolic rate* (BMR). Additional activity such as exercise adds to the BMR, that is, to the heat produced. *Shivering,* which is the contraction of the skeletal muscles, can increase heat production of the body as much as five times (Guyton 1982:554).

Increased thyroxine production

The hypothalamus, in response to cooling, is stimulated to release the thyrotrophin-releasing factor. This factor stimulates the release of thyrotrophin from the adenohypophysis, which in turn stimulates the output of thyroxine by the thyroid gland. This thyroxine increases the rate of cellular metabolism throughout the body and thus increases heat production.

Chemical thermogenesis

Chemical thermogenesis is the stimulation of heat production through the circulation of norepinephrine and epinephrine or through sympathetic stimulation.

Heat Loss

Heat is lost from the body through four major methods: radiation, conduction, convection, and vaporization. Sweating, panting, lowering the environmental temperature, and wearing less clothing all promote heat loss through one or more of these methods.

Radiation

Radiation is a method of transfer of heat from the surface of one object to the surface of another without contact between the two objects. One object contains more heat than the other; the former loses heat through radiation. A person standing in front of an open freezer experiences heat loss through radiation.

Conduction

Conduction is the transfer of heat from one molecule to another. Again, a temperature gradient is implied: The heat transfers to a molecule of lower temperature. Conductive transfer cannot take place without contact between the molecules and normally accounts for minimal heat loss except, for example, when a body is immersed in ice water for a period of time.

Convection

Convection occurs with the movement of air. As the air near a body becomes warmed, it moves away to be replaced by cooler air, which is subsequently warmed by heat from the body. When a room is cooled by currents from fans and open windows, convection is the mechanism for heat transfer. Convection and conduction are less important than radiation and vaporization in heat loss from the body.

Vaporization

Vaporization or evaporation is the fourth method of heat loss. Vaporization occurs continuously through the respiratory tract and through insensible perspiration from the skin. Body sweating increases heat loss by this method, providing that the surrounding air is not saturated (unable to hold more water vapor). For further information regarding sweat, see Chapter 30.

Balanced Body Heat Production and Loss

A healthy body is able to maintain an almost constant temperature despite changing environmental conditions. Temperature control is such that a healthy person's body temperature rarely varies more than 0.77 C (1.4 F).

The main thermoregulatory organ is the hypothalamus. Body heat regulation involves the relative concentrations of sodium and calcium ions within and around the posterior hypothalamus. Body temperature is maintained through a negative feedback system. See the discussion of homeostasis in Chapter 8. The temperature of the body is sensed, and specific motor reactions respond to that temperature.

Factors Affecting Body Temperature

Age

Age affects body temperature to some degree. See Table 13–1. A newborn's body temperature mechanism is imperfect. As a result, the baby is greatly influenced by the temperature of the environment and must be protected from extreme changes. In the newborn, the normal body temperature fluctuates between 36.1 and 37.7 C (97 and 100 F). In fact, a child's temperature

Table 13–1 Variations of Vital Signs by Age

Age	Average temperature	Pulse rate at rest		Respiratory rate	Blood pressure
		Average	*Range*		
Newborn	36.1–37.7 C 97.0–100.0 F (axilla)	120	70–170	35	65–90 systolic, 30–60 diastolic by flush technique: 30–60
1 year	37.7 C 99.7 F	120	80–160	30	65–125 systolic, 40–90 diastolic
2 years	37.2 C 98.9 F	110	80–130	25	75–100 systolic 40–90 diastolic
4 years		100	80–120	23	80–120 systolic 45–85 diastolic
6 years	37.0 C 98.6 F (oral)	100	75–115	21	85–115 systolic 50–60 diastolic
8 years		90	70–110	20	90–120 systolic 50–65 diastolic
10 years		90	70–110	19	95–125 systolic 50–70 diastolic
12 years		Male 85 Female 90	65–105 70–110	19	95–135 systolic 50–70 diastolic
14 years		Male 80 Female 85	60–100 65–105	18	100–140 systolic 50–70 diastolic
16 years		Male 75 Female 80	55–95 60–100	17	
18 years		Male 70 Female 75	50–90 55–95	17	
Adult		Same as 18 years		16	110–140 systolic 60–80 diastolic
Elderly	36.0 C 96.8 F	Same as 18 years		16+	Same as adult

Pulse rates: From V. C. Vaughan and J. R. McKay, editors, *Nelson textbook of pediatrics*, 10th ed. (Philadelphia: W. B. Saunders Co., 1975), p. 1003.

Respiratory rates: From L. F. Whaley and D. L. Wong, *Nursing care of infants and children* (St. Louis: C. V. Mosby Co., 1979), p. 1601.

Blood pressure: From M. S. Brown and M. A. Murphy, *Ambulatory pediatrics for nurses* (New York: McGraw-Hill Book Co., 1975), p. 186.

continues to be more labile than an adult's until puberty. A 2-year-old's body temperature is about 37.2 C (98.9 F); a 12-year old's, an average of 37 C (98.6 F), the same as an adult's.

In elderly adults, body temperature drops to an average of 36 C (96.8 F). Thus, elderly people have less heat to lose than younger adults before reaching *hypothermia* (very low temperature) levels. *Accidental hypothermia* (a rectal body temperature below 35 C, or 95 F) is associated most frequently with exposure to cold outdoors. However, recent studies (Kolanowski and Gunter 1981:362) indicate that many elderly people, particularly those over 75 years, are at risk of hypothermia (in this case temperatures below 36 C, or 96.8 F) for a variety of reasons:

1. Lack of central heating in their homes or inadequate heating due to high fuel costs. The mean room temperature at which most elderly people feel comfortable is 24.3 C (75.8 F). When environmental heat is low, they may wear heavy clothing indoors, take warm baths, and use heating pads to keep warm.
2. Inadequate diets resulting in inadequate body heat production.
3. Loss of subcutaneous fat resulting in inadequate thermal body insulation.
4. Lack of activity, which is necessary for heat production.
5. Tendency towards *orthostatic hypotension*, which is predictive of the loss of thermoregulatory efficiency, since it correlates with abnormal patterns of peripheral blood flow.

These factors have several implications for nursing practice (Kolanowski and Gunter 1981:365):

1. Shake the thermometer down to its lowest point before taking the elderly person's body temperature. Although most thermometers are calibrated to 34 C (94 F), the "shake-down" level is between 35 to 35.5 C (95 to 96 F).
2. Use a low-reading thermometer, if available. An oral mercury thermometer calibrated from 90 to 106 F is available.
3. If a very low oral temperature is measured, check the patient's rectal temperature to rule out hypothermia.
4. Teach the patient measures to increase body temperature, such as wearing additional clothing, eating an adequate diet, and taking moderate activity.

Time of day

The human, like many animals, has variations in vital signs, such as temperature and blood pressure. These variations occur cyclically over 24 hours. This cycle is called *circadian rhythm*. It is observable in the body temperature, which can vary as much as 1.1 to 1.6 C (2 to 3 F) between the early morning and the late afternoon. The point of highest body temperature is usually reached between 1600 and 2000 hours (4 and 8 P.M.), and the lowest point is reached during sleep between 0400 and 0600 hours (4 and 6 A.M.).

The variation in rhythm is chiefly accounted for by variations in muscular activity and digestive processes, which are at a minimum in the early morning, while people are sleeping. Nurses and others who work at night often note an alteration in their temperature rhythms. Some people adapt readily to nocturnal employment, and their cycles change accordingly. Others take longer to adapt and change their cycles only with difficulty.

Sex

A person's sex affects his or her body temperature. The increased level of progesterone during ovulation raises the body temperature of a woman about 0.3 to 0.5 C (0.5 to 1 F). In addition, estrogen and testosterone also increase the basal metabolic rate. Because estrogen causes an increase in the deposition of adipose tissue, women are usually better insulated than men, and thus women maintain internal body temperature more efficiently than men.

Emotions

Extremes in emotional states and behavior can affect the body temperature. Just as heightened emotions can increase body temperature, lack of affect, such as apathetic depression, can lower heat production.

Exercise

Body temperature can become considerably elevated as a result of muscular activity. For example, trained athletes after strenuous activity show a temperature increase of as much as 2.7 C (5.0 F). Vigorous chewing of gum for a few minutes can also raise an oral temperature as much as 0.5 C (1.0 F).

Food, fluids, and smoking

Drinking hot or cold fluids and smoking can alter oral temperature reading temporarily. For example, taking ice water can lower the oral temperature about 0.9 C (1.6 F). It is recommended, therefore, that at least 30 minutes elapse between intake of food or fluids or smoking and measurement. For the same reason, the measurement of a rectal temperature should be delayed for at least 15 minutes following an enema.

Environment

The environment can also affect a person's temperature, even an adult's. Although it is not a major factor, on a hot day a patient in the hospital may register an elevated oral temperature for no reason other than environment.

Assessing Body Temperature

A person's body temperature can be measured in three places: the mouth, the rectum, and the axilla. Each of these measures vary somewhat. A rectal temperature is about 0.4 C (0.7 F) higher than an oral temperature. An axillary temperature is on average 0.6 C (1 F) lower than an oral one.

Oral (per ora)

Hospital and health agency personnel most frequently take patients' body temperatures orally. Placing the thermometer in the mouth is the most convenient and generally the least disruptive to the patient. This method is generally contraindicated for the following patients:

1. Babies and children under age 6, who can be unpredictable; there is a danger of the thermometer breaking in their mouths.
2. Patients who have oral pathology or surgery or who have difficulty breathing through their noses.
3. Patients who are confused, irrational, or have convulsive disorders, who may also break an oral thermometer.
4. Patients who are receiving oxygen through a mask or nasal cannula. (Recent evidence, however, suggests that taking oral temperatures of patients receiving oxygen by nasal cannula may not be inappropriate.)

Figure 13–1 Fahrenheit and centigrade thermometers showing normal adult temperature (98.6 F and 37 C).

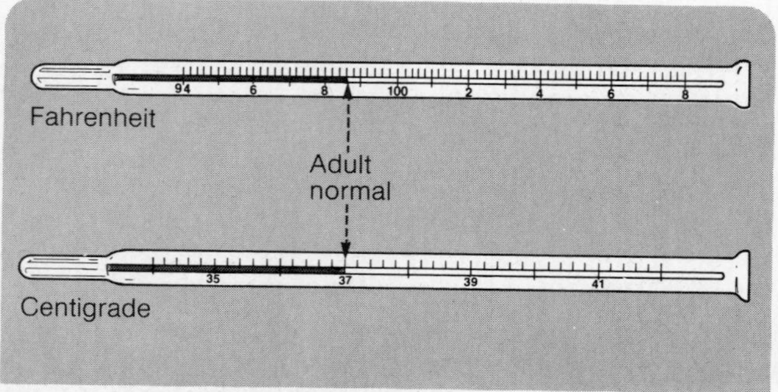

To take an oral temperature reading, the nurse places the thermometer under the patient's tongue, where it registers heat largely from the small blood vessels at the surface under the tongue. Critical to the accurate measure of the temperature is the time that the thermometer is left in place before it is read. Literature provides differing instructions in regard to oral readings. It has been recommended that a sheathed or unsheathed mercury thermometer remain in place 3 minutes (Graves and Markarian 1980:323). It is also recommended that the nurse wait 30 minutes if the patient has ingested hot or cold substances or has been smoking (Erickson 1980:104).

There are a number of thermometers available for measuring body temperature orally. The most common type is the glass tube that contains a column of mercury. The principle underlying the thermometer is that with heat the mercury expands, thus extending the column inside the glass tube, where the mercury level can be measured against marked calibrations.

Thermometers are calibrated in either one of two scales: centigrade or Fahrenheit degrees. The scale of a centigrade thermometer usually extends from 34 to 42 C. A Fahrenheit scale usually extends from 94 to 108 F. See Figure 13–1. It is unusual for body temperatures to occur above or below these ranges.

It is sometimes necessary for the nurse to convert a Fahrenheit reading to centigrade and vice versa. To convert from Fahrenheit to centigrade, one deducts 32 from the Fahrenheit reading and then multiplies by (5/9). That is:

$$C = (\text{Fahrenheit temperature} - 32) \times 5/9$$

To convert from centigrade to Fahrenheit, one multiplies the centigrade reading by the fraction 9/5 and then adds 32. That is:

$$F = (\text{centigrade temperature} \times 9/5) + 32$$

There is other equipment available for taking a patient's temperature. An electric thermometer has been developed that registers a body temperature in a few seconds. Electric thermometers are often used in acute care settings, such as intensive care units. Another device used to measure body temperature is a disposable tape. When applied to the skin, usually of the forehead or abdomen, the temperature-sensitive tape responds by changing color. The tape is removed and discarded after the color has been noted. This method is particularly useful at home and for infants whose temperatures are to be monitored for any reason. There are also chemical disposable thermometers in which a temperature-sensitive chemical is impregnated into a series of calibrated dots that change color in accordance with the temperature.

Procedure 13–1 Assessing Body Temperature by Mouth

Equipment

1. An oral thermometer. Oral thermometers may have a blunt or a narrowed bulb. In some agencies oral thermometers are distinguished from others by white or silver bulbs.
2. Soft tissues to wipe the thermometer if clean plastic sheaths are not used.
3. A pencil or pen to record the temperature.
4. A book, record, or worksheet on which to record the temperature.

Intervention

1. Wash hands.

   Rationale The nurse washes the hands to remove microorganisms, which should not be transmitted to the patient.

2. Explain to the patient what you plan to do. Adjust the explanation to the patient's need.

   Rationale By explaining, the nurse (a) reassures the patient by giving knowledge of what will happen, (b) identifies the patient, and (c) ascertains that this method of taking the temperature is appropriate.

3. **a.** If using a mercury thermometer: Remove the thermometer from its container. If the thermometer is stored in disinfectant, wipe off the solution from the thermometer with a soft tissue or rinse it under cold water. Wipe from the bulb end to fingers in a rotating fashion. Discard the tissue.

   Rationale Disinfectant can irritate mucous membrane and taste unpleasant. Cold water is used because hot water causes the mercury to expand and can break the thermometer. The thermometer is wiped from the cleanest to the least clean area. Rotating ensures that all sides are wiped.

   b. If using an electric thermometer: Assemble the kit and disposable probe covers. Place a cover on the probe. Warm up the machine by switching the on button, if not kept on.

4. Check the temperature reading on the thermometer. If necessary, shake down a mercury thermometer by holding it between the thumb and forefinger at the end farthest from the bulb. Sharply snap the wrist downward. Repeat until the mercury is down. The mercury level should be below 35 C (95 F).

5. Ask the patient to open his or her mouth, and place the thermometer at the base of the tongue to the right or left of the frenulum (posterior sublingual pocket).

   Rationale The thermometer needs to reflect the core temperature of the blood in the larger blood vessels of the posterior pocket.

6. Ask the patient to close the lips, not the teeth, around the thermometer.

   Rationale A patient who bites the thermometer can break it.

7. Leave the thermometer in place according to agency policy.

   Rationale The nurse must allow sufficient time for the temperature to register. The recommended time is 3 minutes. If an electric oral thermometer is used, the patient holds thermometer under the tongue about 10 to 20 seconds.

8. Remove the thermometer.

9. Remove the plastic sheath or wipe with a tissue starting at the end held by the nurse, and wipe in a rotating manner toward the bulb. Discard the tissue. If using an electric thermometer, remove and discard the probe cover.

   Rationale The thermometer is wiped from the area of least contamination to that of greatest contamination.

10. Read the temperature. If using a mercury thermometer, hold it at eye level and rotate it until the mercury column is clearly visible. See Figure 13–2. The upper end of the mercury column registers the patient's body temperature. Each long line on the thermometer reflects 1 degree. Each short line indicates 0.2 degree.

11. Wash the mercury thermometer in tepid soapy water, rinse it in cold water, dry it, and then disinfect it.

    Rationale Organic material such as mucus must be removed before the thermometer is placed in disinfectant. Organic materials on the thermometer can inhibit the action of the disinfectant solution. Effective disinfectants are

Procedure 13–1, continued

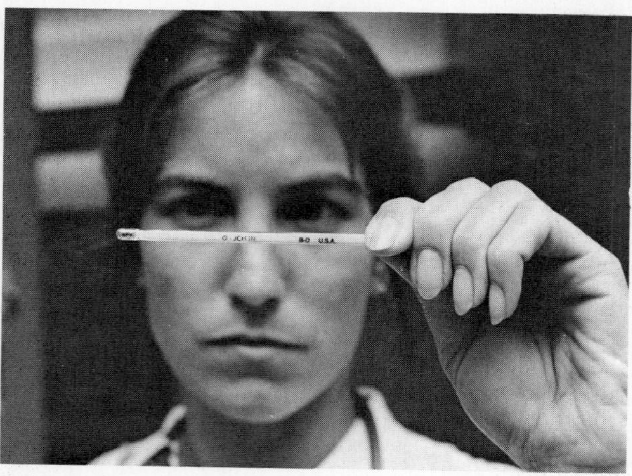

Figure 13–2

ethyl alcohol 70%, benzalkonium chloride (Zephiran chloride) 1:1000, and synthetic phenols.

12. Shake down the thermometer and return it to its container. Many agencies store the thermometer in a small container of disinfectant at the bedside; others place it in a large container in the utility area. Some agencies also have special equipment for spinning down the mercury levels.

13. Wash hands.

14. Record temperature in the book or on the record or worksheet.

Rationale Recording the temperature immediately ensures it is not forgotten.

Rectal (per rectum)

Temperatures taken in the rectum are considered highly accurate reflections of the body's temperature. Rectal temperatures are not affected by the ingestion of hot or cold fluids or by mouth breathing as are oral temperatures but may be affected by enemas or rectal suppository insertion.

Rectal temperatures are indicated for (a) children under age 6, although some agencies discourage its use for infants under 2 years of age, because of possible rectal perforation, and (b) the unconscious or irrational and confused patient. They are generally contraindicated for patients who have rectal pathologic conditions or who have had rectal surgery and in some agencies for patients with myocardial infarctions and convulsive disorders.

The rectal thermometer is usually left in place 2 or 3 minutes before it is read. In this way the most accurate reading is obtained.

Procedure 13–2 Assessing Body Temperature by Rectum

Equipment

1. A rectal thermometer. In some agencies the rectal thermometers have round, blue-colored bulbs.
2. Soft tissues to wipe the thermometer.
3. Lubricant to lubricate the thermometer in order to ease insertion into the rectum.
4. A pencil or pen to record temperature.
5. A book, record, or worksheet on which to record the temperature.

Intervention

1. Follow steps 1 to 4 in Procedure 13–1, page 303.

2. Assist the patient to assume a lateral position, but allow infants to remain in a supine position. Provide privacy before folding the bedclothes back to expose the buttocks.

Rationale Privacy is essential since exposure of the buttocks embarrasses most patients.

3. Place some lubricant on a piece of tissue. Then apply lubricant to the thermometer. For an adult, lubricate 2.5 to 4 cm (1 to 1.5 in) of the bulb end of the thermometer. For an infant, lubricate 1.5 to 2.5 cm (0.5 to 1 in).

Rationale The lubricant facilitates the insertion of the thermometer without irritating the mucous membrane.

Procedure 13–2, continued

4. With one hand raise the patient's upper buttock to expose the anus. If the patient is an infant, hold both of his or her ankles by one hand and raise the legs to expose the anus.

5. Ask the patient to take a deep breath and insert the thermometer into the anus anywhere from 1.5 to 4 cm (0.5 to 1.5 in), depending on the age and size of the patient (for example, 1.5 cm for an infant, 4 cm for a large adult). Do not force insertion of the thermometer.

   Rationale Inability to insert the thermometer into a newborn could indicate the rectum is not patent. Having the patient take a deep breath relaxes the external sphincter muscle, thus easing insertion. The end of the thermometer should not be embedded in feces.

6. Hold the thermometer in place for 2 minutes (Nichols 1972) or for the length of time recommended by agency policy. Hold an electric thermometer in place 10 to 20 seconds.

7. Remove the thermometer.

8. Follow steps 9 to 14 in Procedure 13–1, page 303.

Axillary (per axilla)

The axillary temperature is measured in the armpit, or axilla. It is the least accurate of the three methods, although it is safer than the oral method and more convenient and safer than the rectal method. If the axilla has recently been washed, the nurse should delay about 10 minutes before taking the temperature, because the friction of rubbing the axilla dry may influence the reading.

The thermometer is left in place 10 minutes before it is read. It sometimes may be necessary for the nurse to hold the thermometer in place for that time. Taking temperatures by axilla is standard practice in some newborn nurseries; the first body temperature following birth, however, is usually taken per rectum.

Procedure 13–3 Assessing Body Temperature by Axilla

Equipment

1. An axillary thermometer. Oral thermometers are usually used in most agencies.
2. Soft tissues to wipe the thermometer.
3. A towel to wipe the axilla.
4. A pencil or pen to record the temperature.
5. A book, record, or worksheet on which to record the temperature.

Intervention

1. Follow steps 1 to 4 in Procedure 13–1, page 303.

2. Expose the patient's axilla. If the axilla is moist, dry it with a patting motion.

   Rationale Friction created by rubbing can raise the temperature of the axilla.

3. Place the thermometer in the patient's axilla.

4. Assist the patient to place the arm tightly across the chest.

   Rationale This position keeps the thermometer in place.

5. Leave the thermometer in place for 10 minutes. Remain with the patient and hold the thermometer in place if the patient is irrational or very young.

6. Remove the thermometer.

7. Follow steps 9 to 14 in Procedure 13–1, page 303.

Fever

An elevated body temperature is called a *fever* or *pyrexia*. A very high fever—40.5 C (105 F) or more—is *hyperpyrexia*, or *hyperthermia*. There are three types of fevers: (a) intermittent, (b) remittent, and (c) relapsing.

An *intermittent* or *quotidian fever* is one in which the body temperature is elevated but returns to normal sometime in a 24-hour period. It is not unusual for an intermittent fever to be highest in the late afternoon or evening and lowest in the early morning.

A *remittent fever* is one in which there is a wide range of temperatures over the 24-hour period, all of which are above normal.

In a *relapsing fever*, short febrile periods of a few days are interspersed with periods of 1 or 2 days of normal temperature.

A fever can also be described according to the type of onset and the type of termination. A fever can start gradually or suddenly, and the temperature can return to normal either suddenly (*crisis*) or gradually (*lysis*).

Fevers are caused by an increase in heat production, a decrease in heat loss, or a combination of both. For every 1 C rise in body temperature, heat production increases 13%. The highest temperature at which a person can survive is thought to be about 46 C (114.8 F). However, when the body temperature rises above 41 or 42 C (106 or 108 F), body cells are damaged (Guyton 1981:89).

Assessing clinical signs of fever

The clinical signs of a fever vary, depending on the stage of the fever, that is, the onset, the course, or the termination.

Signs during the *onset* of a fever are:

1. Chills; the patient complains of feeling cold.
2. Shivering due to strong skeletal muscle contractions.
3. Pallid skin due to peripheral vasoconstriction.
4. "Gooseflesh" appearance of the skin due to contraction of the arrector pili muscles.
5. Increased pulse rate due to increased cardiac rate.
6. Rising rectal temperature even though skin reading is cool.

Signs during the *course* of a fever are:

1. Patient does not complain of feeling hot or of feeling cold.
2. Complaints of headache.
3. Flushing of the skin due to peripheral vasodilation, which permits heat loss.
4. Patient's skin feels warm to the touch.
5. Sweating, in some instances.
6. Irritability or restlessness due to irritation of the central nervous system.
7. Disorientation and confusion with extremely high temperatures; in children, convulsions.
8. Generalized weakness and aching of body parts.
9. Weight loss, with a prolonged fever.
10. Anorexia, nausea, and vomiting.
11. Dehydration of the skin and mucous membranes, particularly in babies, young children, and elderly patients. See the section on dehydration, Chapter 31.

Signs during the *termination* of a fever are:

1. *Diaphoresis* (profuse perspiration), which permits rapid heat loss by vaporization
2. Reddening of the skin due to vasodilation
3. Possible dehydration

Nursing interventions for patients with fever

The following nursing interventions may be implemented, unless specifically not recommended, for patients who have a fever. During the period of chills, provide additional bedclothes and note the onset and duration of the chill. During the stage of diaphoresis, increase the circulation of air in the room to promote heat loss by vaporization. Because bedclothes become wet with diaphoresis, it is important that they be changed as necessary. It is also important to make sure that sufficient bedcovers are applied to prevent chilling.

Encouraging the patient to increase fluid intake is essential to prevent potential dehydration due to excessive fluid loss from diaphoresis (see Chapter 31 for further information about fluid loss). The patient's fluid intake and output should also be measured and recorded (see Chapter 30).

In addition to monitoring the patient's temperature, the nurse needs to assess the patient's pulse and respirations. The pulse rate and respiratory rates increase in direct association with the increase in the basal metabolic rate and demands for oxygen that accompany a temperature rise. The pulse rate can increase 10 to 15 beats per minute with each 1 C rise in temperature. The physician should be notified of the patient's vital and clinical signs so that appropriate diagnostic procedures, e.g., a blood culture, may be implemented.

Pulse

The *pulse* is the pulse wave of blood created by the contraction of the left ventricle of the heart. A pulse can be palpated on certain superficial areas of the body, for example, where an artery passes over or alongside a bone. By slight pressure on the artery the pulse wave can be felt as the blood is pumped around the body.

Pulse Sites

A pulse is commonly taken at a number of sites: temporal, carotid, apical, brachial, radial, femoral, popliteal, and pedal (dorsalis pedis). See Figure 13-3. The most commonly used is the radial site.

Temporal pulse

The temporal pulse is taken at a site superior and lateral to the eye. At this site the temporal artery passes over the temporal bone of the head. This site is often used when the radial pulse is inaccessible.

Carotid pulse

The carotid pulse is felt at the side of the neck. If an imaginary line is drawn from the lobe of the ear down along the anterior border of the sternocleidomastoid muscle, the carotid pulse can be felt along this line. It is likely to be felt most clearly near the angle of the jaw. This site is commonly used in cases of cardiac arrest.

Apical pulse

The apical pulse is auscultated at the apex of the heart. Its location, which varies slightly according to the age of the patient, is discussed on page 310. The apical pulse site is commonly used for infants and children up to 3 years and to determine discrepancies with the radial pulse in patients of all ages.

Brachial pulse

The brachial pulse can be felt on the inner aspect of the biceps muscle. It is found a few centimeters below the axilla on the inner aspect of the arm or medially in the antecubital space. This site is commonly used when assessing blood pressure.

Radial pulse

The radial pulse is found on the inner aspect of the wrist on the radial or thumb side. It is the most commonly used site because it is readily accessible, usually with little disturbance to the patient.

Femoral pulse

The femoral pulse is found in the groin about at the midpoint of the inguinal ligament. This site is often used for infants and children or to assess the adequacy of circulation to the leg.

Popliteal pulse

The popliteal artery can be palpated behind the knee. It is a difficult pulse to find, but the assessment is facilitated if the patient flexes the knee and the nurse's fingers are pressed into the center of the popliteal space. This site may be used when assessing blood pressure.

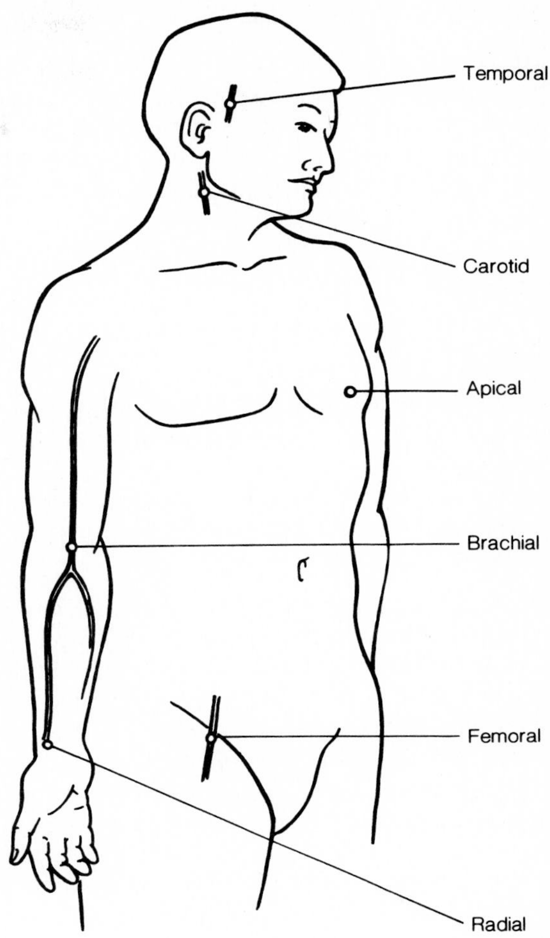

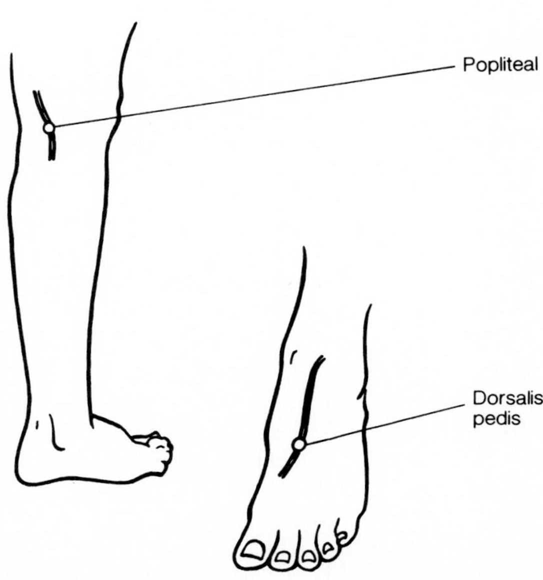

Figure 13–3 Eight sites commonly used for assessing a pulse.

Pedal (dorsalis pedis) pulse

This pulse in the foot, the dorsalis pedis pulse, can be felt by palpating the instep of the foot on an imaginary line drawn from the middle of the ankle to the interdigital space between the big toe and the second toe. It is often assessed to determine the circulation to the foot.

Reasons for Taking a Pulse

There are two basic reasons for taking a patient's pulse:

1. To assess the adequacy of the blood flow to a certain area, for example, to assess blood flow to a foot by taking the pedal pulse.
2. To assess the rate, rhythm, volume, and tension of a pulse, which may reflect a general problem, such as a slow heart rate.

Peripheral pulses are all pulses other than the centrally located apical pulse. Generally, the peripheral pulses are used to assess the adequacy of blood flow to a particular area. Nurses are expected to check these pulses for a variety of reasons; for example, they take a dorsalis pedis pulse after the application of a leg cast to assess circulation of the blood flow to the patient's foot or assess the radial pulse after surgical procedures to an elbow.

When nurses assess the rate, rhythm, volume, and tension of a pulse, it is customary to use the radial site because of its convenience for most people. If the radial pulse is not readily available—for example, if a patient has both arms bandaged—a temporal or carotid pulse is customarily taken.

Factors Affecting Pulse Rate

The rate of the pulse is expressed in beats per minute. A pulse rate varies according to a number of factors: age, sex, exercise, emotions, heat, and body position, for example.

Age

The pulse of a newborn baby averages 120 beats per minute with a wide range of variability from 70 to 170. As age increases, the pulse rate gradually decreases to its adult rate of about 70 to 75 beats per minute. Unless a disease process exists, the pulse rate is stabilized at the adult level for the rest of a person's life. Refer to Table 13–1 for specific variations in pulse rates from birth to adulthood.

Sex

The pulse rate tends to vary somewhat between men and women of similar ages. After puberty, the average male's pulse rate is slightly lower than the female's.

Exercise

The pulse rate normally increases with activity. Increased need for oxygen by the muscles during exercise results in an increased heart rate to deliver that oxygen through the bloodstream. The rate of increase in the professional athlete is often less than in the average person because of greater cardiac size, strength, and efficiency.

Emotions

The heart rate alters in response to changes in both the sympathetic and parasympathetic divisions of the autonomic nervous system. Emotions such as fear, anger, and worry, as well as the perception of pain, stimulate the sympathetic system. As a result, the heart rate as well as the contractility of the heart are increased. The parasympathetic stimulation slows the heart and the contractility of the atria. Digitalis is a drug frequently used to stimulate the parasympathetic system, specifically the vagus nerve.

An excessively fast heart rate is referred to as *tachycardia*. A rate of over 100 beats per minute in an adult is considered tachycardia. *Bradycardia* refers to a slow rate of heart contraction, usually any rate below 60 beats per minute.

Heat

The prolonged application of external heat as well as fever also can accelerate the heart (pulse) rate. The pulse rate increases in response to the lowered blood pressure, which in turn is a result of a peripheral vasodilation response to the heat.

Body position

Prolonged assumption of a horizontal position can also result in increased pulse rates. The normal blood volume in the extremities is diminished, and a greater blood volume circulates centrally. Thus, the heart has to beat more rapidly to pump this added blood volume.

Assessing Pulse Rhythm

The *rhythm* of the pulse is the pattern of the beats and the intervals between the beats. Equal time elapses between beats of a normal pulse; this is called *pulsus regularis*. A pulse with an irregular rhythm is referred to as an *arrhythmia*.

Arrhythmia may be characterized by random, irregular beats or by a predictable pattern of irregular beats.

Assessing Pulse Volume

A pulse *volume* refers to the force of blood with each beat. Usually, pulse volume is the same with each beat.

A normal pulse can be felt with moderate pressure of the fingers, and it can be obliterated with greater pressure. A forceful or full blood volume that is obliterated only with difficulty is called a *full* or *bounding* pulse. A pulse that is readily obliterated with pressure from the fingers is referred to as *weak, feeble,* or *thready.*

Assessing the Arterial Wall

The arterial walls can also be palpated with the fingers. Elderly people often have inelastic arteries, which may feel twisted and irregular. Normally, arteries are straight and smooth.

By palpating an artery, the nurse is able to feel beading or roughness in the artery more clearly. To palpate an artery, the nurse places two fingers over the artery and compresses it firmly. The finger distal to the heart is then moved along the artery; that section of the artery is temporarily emptied of blood. An artery that is very hard may feel gritty to the touch.

Assessing the Peripheral Pulse

To assess the pulse, the nurse should first make sure that the patient is in a comfortable position. If the patient has been active, the pulse observation should be deferred for 10 to 15 minutes until the patient has had time to rest.

Procedure 13–4 Assessing the Peripheral Pulse

Equipment

1. A watch with a second hand to count the pulse rate.
2. A pencil or pen to record pulse data.
3. A book, record, or worksheet on which to record pulse data.

Intervention

1. Wash hands.

   Rationale Washing removes any microorganisms, which should not be transmitted to the patient.

2. Explain to the patient what you plan to do. Adjust the explanation to the patient's need.

   Rationale Explaining reassures the patient by giving knowledge of what will happen and allows the nurse to identify the patient.

3. Select the pulse point. Normally, the radial pulse is taken unless it cannot be exposed or circulation to another body area is to be assessed.

4. Place three middle fingertips lightly and squarely over the pulse point.

   Rationale Using the thumb is contraindicated because the thumb has a pulse that the nurse could mistake for the patient's pulse.

5. Count the pulse for 30 seconds and multiply by 2 if the pulse is regular. If it is irregular, count for 1 full minute. Count 1 full minute for an infant's apical pulse (see page 310).

   Rationale To be assessed correctly, an irregular pulse requires a full minute's count.

6. Assess the pulse rhythm by noting the pattern of intervals between the beats.

   Rationale A normal pulse has an equal time period between each beat.

7. Assess the pulse volume. A normal pulse can be felt with moderate pressure.

   Rationale Normally, the pressure of the blood with each beat is equal. A forceful pulse volume is full; an easily obliterated pulse is weak.

8. Palpate the arterial wall by compressing the artery firmly and running a finger distal to the heart along the artery.

   Rationale Palpating the wall allows the nurse to assess the artery. A normal arterial wall is smooth and straight.

9. Assist the patient to a comfortable position.
10. Wash hands.
11. Record the pulse rate, rhythm, and volume, and the condition of the arterial wall.

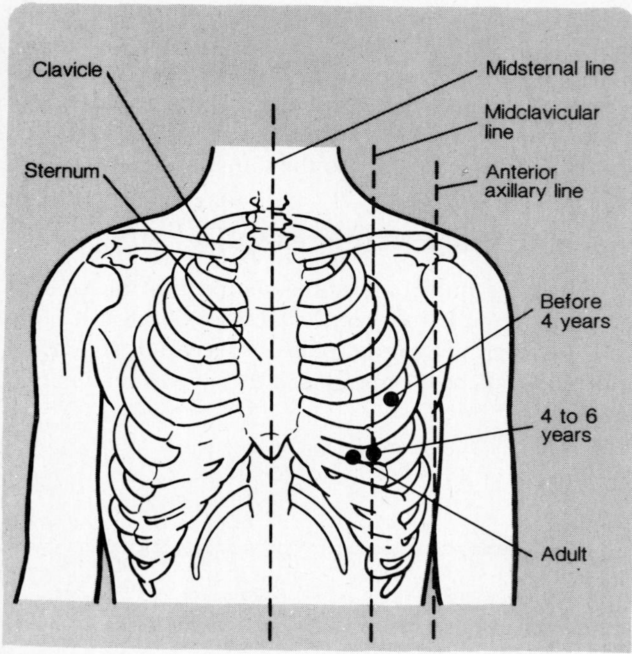

Figure 13–4 The location of the apical pulse for a child under 4 years, a child 4 to 6 years, and an adult.

Assessing the Apical Pulse

Nurses use the apical pulse site (apex of the heart) to assess the pulse rate of infants and children up to 2 or 3 years of age. Nurses also use this site to monitor the heart's action in adults with cardiac arrhythmia or those receiving cardiac medications. For example, the apical pulse, not the radial pulse, should be measured in patients receiving digitalis preparations. The apical pulse should also be assessed if an adult's radial pulse rate is 60 beats per minute or less.

Locating the apical pulse

Location of the apical pulse varies slightly with age. In an adult, it is located on the left side of the chest, no more than 8 cm (3 in) to the left of the sternum (breastbone) and under the fourth, fifth, or sixth intercostal space (area between the ribs). Another way to locate the apex is to find the midclavicular line (MCL), an imaginary line dropping straight down from the center of the clavicle (collarbone). See Figure 13–4. Normally, the apex lies inside or on the MCL at the fourth, fifth, or sixth intercostal space. In men, the MCL usually passes through the nipple.

To locate the center of the clavicle, the nurse first feels for the medial end of this bone where it joins the sternum. This joint can be felt more readily if the patient moves the shoulder forward. Next, the nurse locates the lateral end of the clavicle, where it joins the shoulder, by feeling along the front edge of the clavicle until a bony prominence or notch is felt at the shoulder. Midway between these identified points on the sternum and shoulder is the center of the clavicle.

In a child 7 to 9 years of age, the apical pulse is located between the fourth and fifth intercostal spaces. In children younger than 4, it is left of the MCL; in children between 4 and 6 years, it is at the MCL. See Figure 13–4.

Measuring the apical pulse

To assess a patient's apical pulse rate, the nurse needs a watch with a second hand and a stethoscope with a bell-shaped or flat disc diaphragm to listen to the heartbeats. See Figure 13–5. If the nurse is uncertain about

Figure 13–5 A stethoscope with two types of diaphragms.

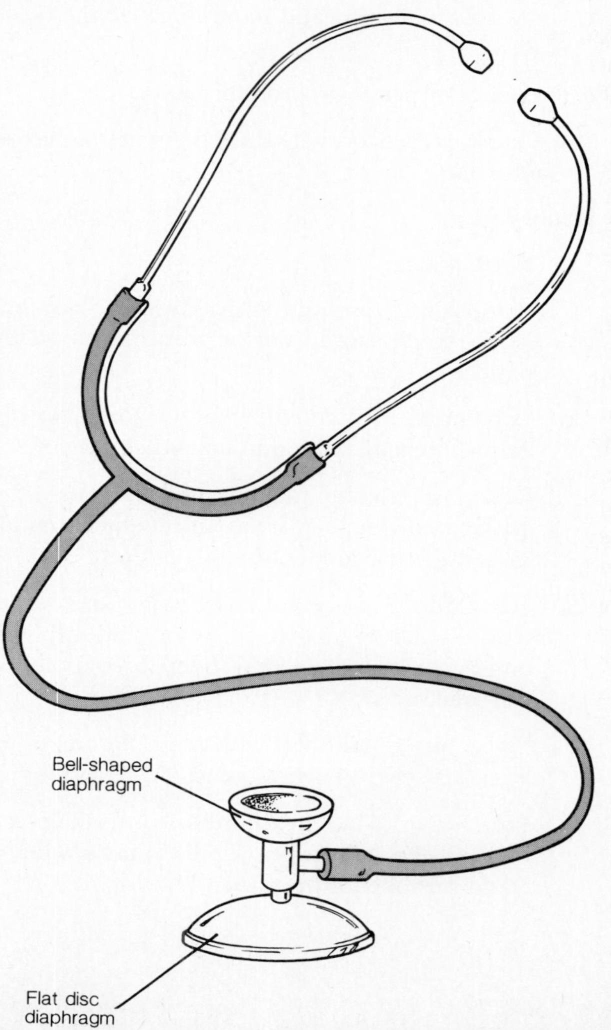

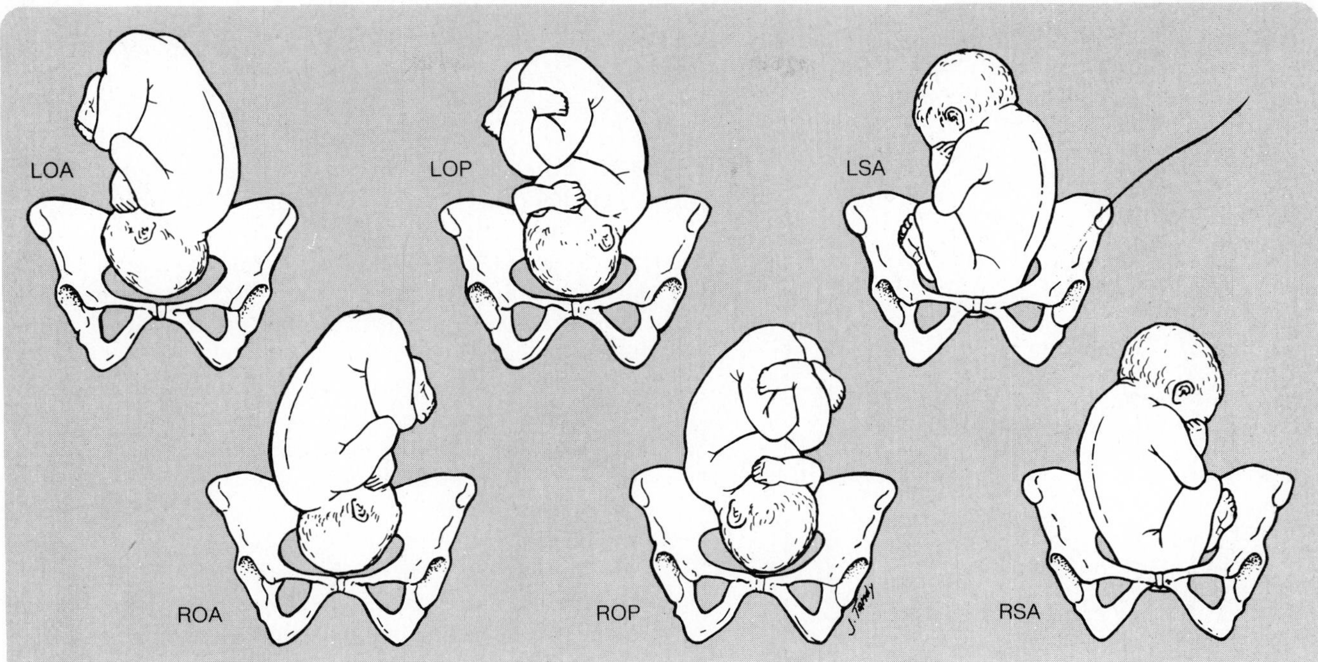

Figure 13–6 Six presentations and positions of the fetus during childbirth are: left occiput anterior (LOA), right occiput anterior (ROA), left occiput posterior (LOP), right occiput posterior (ROP), right sacrum anterior (RSA), and left sacrum anterior (LSA).

the cleanliness of the earpieces and diaphragm, they should be cleaned with an antiseptic gauze prior to use. Only the diaphragm needs to be cleaned if the nurse's own stethoscope is used.

The nurse warms the diaphragm of the stethoscope by holding it in the palm of the hand for a moment before placing it over the apex of the patient's heart. The heartbeat is counted for 30 seconds. If irregular, the apical pulse should be counted for 60 seconds to check the count. Each heartbeat will be heard as a *lubb-dupp*. The *lubb* is the closure of the atrioventricular valves (the tricuspid and mitral valves), and the *dupp* is the closure of the semilunar valves (pulmonary and aortic valves). Any beats in addition to these should also be counted. For further information see also the sections on heart size and location and heart sounds in Chapter 14. In addition to assessing the heart rate, the nurse also needs to note the strength of the heartbeat and its rhythm.

Assessing the Apical-Radial Pulse

Physicians or nurses may order an apical-radial pulse to assess cardiovascular function in adult patients. Normally, the apical and radial rates are identical. An apical pulse rate greater than the radial pulse rate can indicate that the thrust of the blood from the heart is too feeble for the wave to be felt at the peripheral pulse site, or it can indicate that vascular disease is preventing impulses from being transmitted. Any discrepancy between the two pulse rates needs to be reported promptly. In no instance will the radial pulse be greater than the apical pulse.

Two nurses working together or one nurse alone can assess a patient's apical-radial pulse. When two nurses are available, one counts the apical pulse at exactly the same time as the other nurse counts the radial pulse. Usually one nurse signals when to begin counting with a hand motion, and each person counts for 1 full minute. Discrepancies between the two pulses are noted. The difference between the apical and radial pulse is referred to as the *pulse deficit*.

Assessing Fetal Heart Tones

Fetal heart tones (FHT) are generally first heard by auscultation sometime between the 18th and 20th week of the pregnancy. The fetal rate is usually between 120 and 160 beats per minute. Fetal pulse can be detected during the early months of pregnancy over the mother's symphysis pubis; however, later in the pregnancy, the fetal pulse location varies with the position of the fetus.

The fetus can assume several positions in utero. Therefore, to obtain the fetal heart rate, the nurse must first determine the position of the fetus by palpating the mother's abdomen. See Figure 13–6 for six common presentations and positions of the fetus during birth.

In vertex presentations (when the head is nearest the

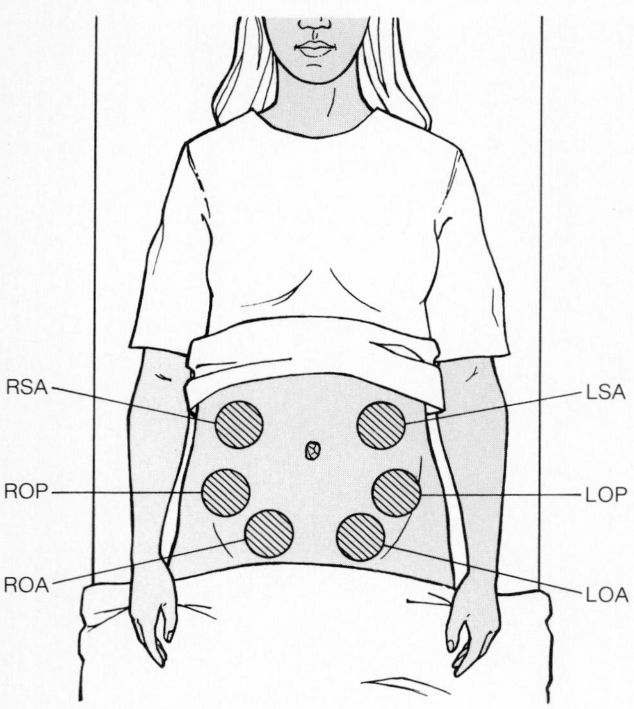

Figure 13–7 Circles indicate areas of maximum intensity of fetal heart tones for various fetal positions: right occiput anterior (ROA), right occiput posterior (ROP), right sacrum anterior (RSA), left sacrum anterior (LSA), left occiput posterior (LOP), and left occiput anterior (LOA).

Figure 13–8 The nurse can listen to the fetal heart using a bell stethoscope held by rubber bands.

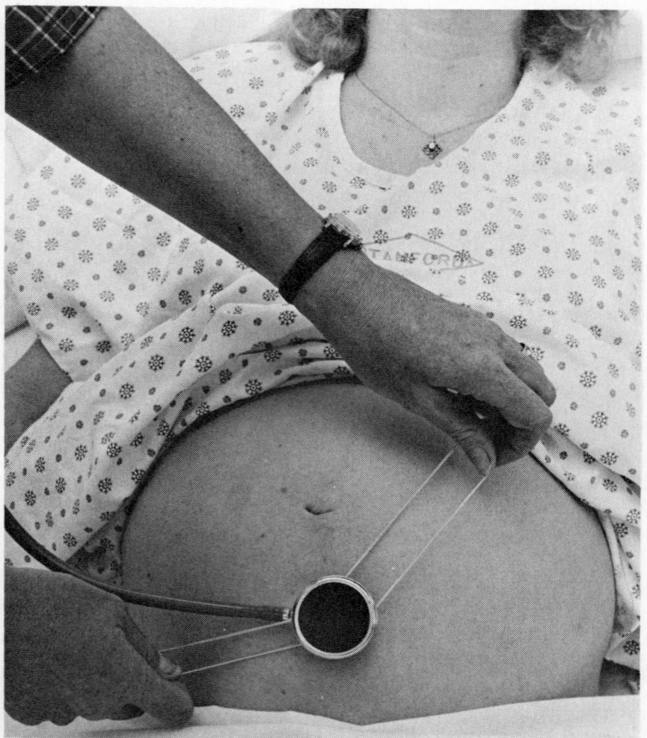

cervical opening and presents first), the fetal heart sounds are most audible in a lower quadrant of the abdomen. If the fetus is in this position, the heart sounds are heard through the back of the fetus unless it is a face position, in which case the tones are transmitted through the fetus's chest. For left occipital anterior (LOA) and left occipital posterior (LOP) positions, auscultation of the left lower quadrant usually produces the most audible tones. By contrast, in sacral-anterior presentations the fetal heart sounds are generally loudest to the right and left above the mother's umbilicus. See Figure 13–7.

To listen to the fetal heart, the nurse can use an ordinary bell stethoscope held by rubber bands. See Figure 13–8. A head stethoscope can augment the sounds, however, since sounds are transmitted not only to the nurse's eardrums but also by bone conduction through the headpiece the nurse wears. See Figure 13–9. Special fetal heart stethoscopes are also available. These have large weighted bells for fetal heart auscultation, and some are interchangeable in that a smaller bell can be attached to monitor the mother's blood pressure.

When counting the fetal heart rate, the nurse listens and counts for 1 minute. Two other blowing or whizzing sounds referred to as *souffles* may be heard during fetal heart auscultation. One is the funic (umbilical cord) souffle; the other is the uterine souffle. The funic souffle, a sharp hissing sound, is caused by blood rushing through the umbilical cord and is equivalent to the fetal heart rate; that is, about 140 beats per minute. It is not heard in every person (about 15%) and occurs when the umbilical arteries are subjected to pressure, torsion, or tension. The uterine souffle, a softer blowing sound, is due to blood propelled by the maternal heart through

Figure 13–9 The fetal heart tones can be assessed by using a head stethoscope.

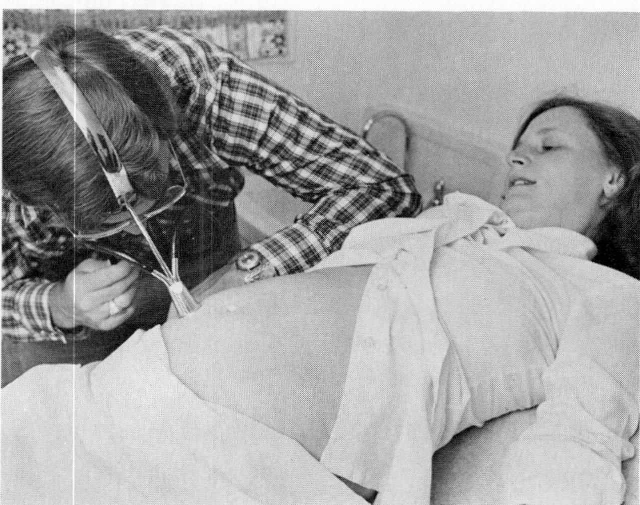

large dilated blood vessels of the uterus. Thus, it synchronizes with the maternal heart rate; for example, 75 beats per minute. It can be heard distinctly when the lower portion of the uterus is auscultated. The nurse can distinguish between the fetal heart tones and the maternal heart rate by palpating the maternal radial pulse while listening to the fetal heart tones. Later in pregnancy, other sounds also become audible, such as the gurgling of gas in the mother or sounds produced by fetal movement.

Assessment of fetal heart sounds is of particular importance in the first and second stages of labor. The fetal heart is monitored generally every 30 to 60 minutes in the first stage and every 5 minutes in the second stage. Fetal distress is indicated when the rate slows to below 100 beats per minute for as long as 30 seconds. During labor, the fetal heart rate normally slows (physiologic bradycardia) after the onset of a contraction, but this slowing normally ends 10 or 15 seconds before the contraction is completed. Because the uterine muscle is tense during a contraction and because lying still during a contraction is difficult for the mother, assessment of the fetal heart rate may be difficult. Electronic and ultrasound techniques are being used increasingly for high-risk mothers, such as those with diabetes or a previous history of stillbirths.

Respirations

Respiration is the act of breathing; it includes the intake of oxygen and the output of carbon dioxide. Reference is often made to *external respiration* and *internal respiration.* The former refers to the interchange of oxygen and carbon dioxide between the alveoli of the lungs and the pulmonary blood. Internal respiration, by contrast, takes place throughout the body; it is the interchange of these same gases between the systemically circulating blood and the cells of the body tissues.

The term *inhalation* or *inspiration* refers to the intake of air into the lungs. *Exhalation* or *expiration* refers to breathing out or the movement of gases from the lungs to the atmosphere. *Ventilation* is another word that is used to refer to the movement of air in and out of the lungs. *Hyperventilation* refers to very deep, rapid respirations; *hypoventilation* refers to very shallow respirations.

There are basically two types of breathing that nurses observe, *costal* or thoracic breathing and *diaphragmatic* or abdominal breathing. Costal breathing involves chiefly the external intercostal muscles and other accesory muscles such as the sternocleidomastoid muscles. It can be observed by the movement of the chest upward and outward. By contrast, diaphragmatic breathing chiefly involves the contraction and relaxation of the diaphragm, and it is observed by the movement of the abdomen, which occurs as a result of the diaphragm's contraction and downward movement.

Respirations are observed to determine (a) rate, (b) depth, (c) rhythm, and (d) character.

Assessing Respiratory Rate

The respiratory rate varies according to a number of factors, such as exercise and the presence of disease. It also varies normally with the age of the person. Refer to Table 13-1. To assess the rate, follow Procedure 13-5. The normal rate of respirations for an adult is between 16 to 20 breaths per minute. In the older adult, however, the respiratory rate increases, and respirations are generally shallow. These changes are due primarily to two physiologic changes of aging:

1. Decreasing elasticity of the lungs
2. Impaired gaseous exchange between the alveoli and the pulmonary capillaries

A number of terms are used to describe respiratory rate. Normal effortless breathing is referred to as *eupnea.* A respiratory rate greater than 24 breaths per minute is called *tachypnea.* A count of fewer than 10 respirations per minute is described as *bradypnea.* The complete absence of respirations is *apnea,* which is often described in time periods, for example, 30 seconds of apnea. Prolonged apnea results in death.

Assessing Respiratory Depth

The depth of a person's respirations can be established by watching the movement of the chest. Respiration is generally described as either deep or shallow. Deep respirations are those in which a large volume of air is inhaled and exhaled, inflating most of the lungs. Shallow respirations involve the exchange of a small volume of air and often the use of minimal lung tissue.

The depth of respirations can also be measured accurately by the use of pulmonary equipment. See the discussion of pulmonary capacities in Chapter 29. It is also sometimes necessary to assess the symmetry of chest expansion by palpation. This technique is described in Chapter 14 on page 336.

The capacity of the lungs varies with sex, age, stature, physical development, and body position. Men generally have a greater lung capacity than women of the same age. Variance by age is obvious: Babies have less vital capacity than children, children less than adolescents, and adolescents less than adults. However, elderly people usually have less vital capacity than young adults.

Stature affects lung volume: Tall, thin people usually have a greater vital capacity than obese people. The athlete in top condition usually has a vital capacity that is above normal.

Body position also affects the amount of air that can be inhaled. People in a supine position experience two physiologic processes that suppress respiration: an increase in the volume of the intrathoracic blood and compression of the chest. Consequently, patients in a supine position have poorer lung aeration, which can predispose to the stasis of fluids and subsequent infection.

Assessing Respiratory Rhythm

Respiratory rhythm refers to the regularity of the expirations and the inspirations. Normally, respirations are evenly spaced. Respiratory rhythm can be described as regular or irregular.

Assessing the Character of Respirations

The character of respiration refers to those aspects of breathing that are different from normal, effortless breathing. Two of these are the amount of effort a patient requires to breathe and the sound of breathing.

Usually, breathing does not require noticeable effort; some patients, however, breathe only with decided effort. Difficult breathing is referred to as *dyspnea*. Dyspnea is usually evidenced by the obvious effort of the accessory muscles, such as the sternocleidomastoid, to maintain respirations.

The sound of breathing is also significant. Normal breathing is silent, but there are a number of abnormal sounds that are obvious to the nurse's ear. Wheezing occurs when the airway is constricted; wheezing is usually more apparent on expiration than inspiration. Acute constriction of the trachea produces a harsh crowing sound on inspiration called *stridor*. This usually reflects respiratory distress. *Rales* or *rhonchi* are bubbling or crackling sounds that are evident with respiration. These sounds occur as a result of the presence of fluid in the lungs and are most clearly heard with a stethoscope. See Chapter 14, pages 336–39, for auscultation and percussion methods used to assess lung sounds and Chapter 29, page 745, for further information about abnormal breath sounds.

Procedure 13–5 Assessing Respirations

Equipment

1. A watch with a second hand to count the respiratory rate
2. A pencil or pen
3. A book, record, or worksheet

Intervention

1. Wash hands.

   Rationale The nurse washes the hands to remove microorganisms, which should not be transmitted to the patient.

2. Inform the patient about measuring his or her temperature, pulse, and blood pressure.

   Rationale An explanation about assessing respirations could cause the patient to alter his or her respiratory pattern.

3. Place a hand against patient's chest and observe the chest movements. This is conveniently done directly after taking the pulse.
4. Count the respiratory rate for 30 seconds if the respirations are regular. Count for 1 full minute if they are irregular.
5. Observe for depth. During deep respirations a large volume of air is exchanged; during shallow respirations a small volume is exchanged.
6. Observe the respiratory rhythm, which may be regular or irregular.
7. Observe the character of respirations—the sound they produce and the effort they require.
8. Wash hands.
9. Record the respiratory rate, depth, rhythm, and character.

Blood Pressure

Arterial blood pressure is a measure of the pressure exerted by the blood as it pulsates through the arteries. Because the blood moves in waves, there are two blood pressure measures: the *systolic* pressure, which is the pressure of the blood as a result of contraction of the ventricles, that is, the pressure at the height of the blood wave; and the *diastolic* pressure, which is the pressure when the ventricles are at rest. Diastolic pressure, then, is the lower pressure, present at all times within the arteries. The difference between the diastolic and the systolic pressures is called the *pulse pressure.*

Blood pressure is measured in millimeters of mercury (mm Hg). This measurement registers on a *sphygmomanometer*, which reflects the pressure of air in a rubber cuff wrapped around a patient's extremity, for example, the upper arm.

Factors Controlling Blood Pressure

Cardiac output

Cardiac output is the amount of blood ejected from the heart per minute during ventricular contraction. At rest, the left ventricle normally puts out about 70 ml; this is the stroke volume. Cardiac output is normally about 5 liters; that is, 70 ml multiplied by the number of contractions per minute (70) equals 4900 ml, or 5 liters per minute.

Cardiac output increases with fever and exercise, and the systolic pressure may increase as a result. However, cardiac output can be decreased as a result of heart disease, and the systolic pressure may then be low.

Blood volume

An increased or decreased blood volume also affects blood pressure. Normally, an adult has about 6 liters of blood in the circulatory system. Loss of blood volume due to hemorrhage or dehydration results in a lowered systolic and diastolic pressure. Excessive blood volume, perhaps the result of a quickly administered blood transfusion, can result in an increased blood pressure.

Elasticity of the arterial walls

Arterial walls normally have some elasticity, which permits them to yield somewhat during systole and then retract during diastole. (*Systole* is the period of contraction of the ventricles of the heart. *Diastole* is the period of relaxation of the heart's ventricles.) With arteriosclerosis, the arteries lose much of their elasticity and become rigid. This condition is frequently seen in elderly people. As a result, the systolic pressure is generally elevated because the arteries do not yield to the pressure, and the diastolic pressure is generally lower because the arteries have limited retractability upon ventricular relaxation.

Size of the arterioles and capillaries

The size of the arterioles and the capillaries determines in great part the peripheral resistance to the blood in the body. A *lumen* (plural: lumina) is a channel within a tube. The smaller the lumina the greater the resistance. Normally, the arterioles are in a state of partial constriction. Increased vasoconstriction raises the blood pressure, whereas decreased vasoconstriction lowers the blood pressure.

Factors Affecting Blood Pressure

Age

Blood pressure increases with age. See Table 13–1 for variations in blood pressure by age.

Exercise

Exercise increases the cardiac output and hence the blood pressure. Therefore, a patient needs to be resting when blood pressure is taken if the reading is to be reliable.

Emotional and physical stress

Emotions, such as anxiety and fear, and physical stress, such as moderate pain, can also increase the blood pressure. Stimulation of the sympathetic nervous system results in increased cardiac output and vasoconstriction of the arterioles. However, severe pain can cause a fall in the blood pressure and subsequent shock. In this case the vasomotor center is inhibited, and vasodilation takes place.

Assessing Blood Pressure

There are two methods of assessing blood pressure, the direct and the indirect methods. Direct measurement involves the insertion of a catheter into the brachial, radial, or femoral artery. Arterial pressure is displayed in wavelike forms on an oscilloscope. Generally, physicians insert the catheters, and nurses are responsible for monitoring the pressure readings. This pressure reading is relatively accurate.

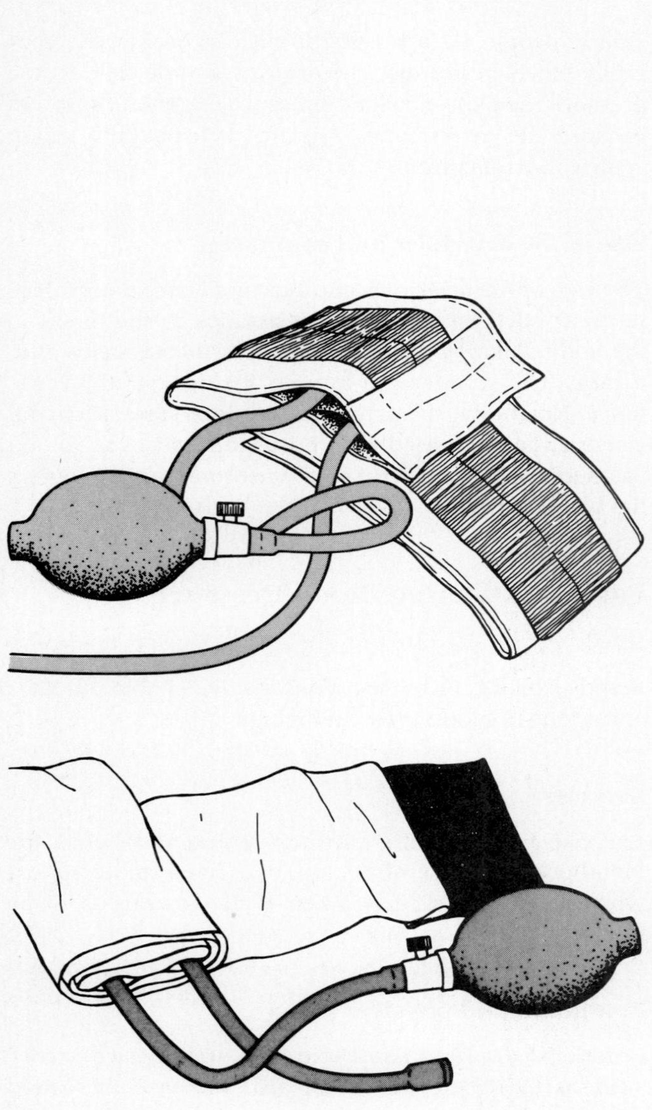

Figure 13–10 Two kinds of blood pressure cuffs.

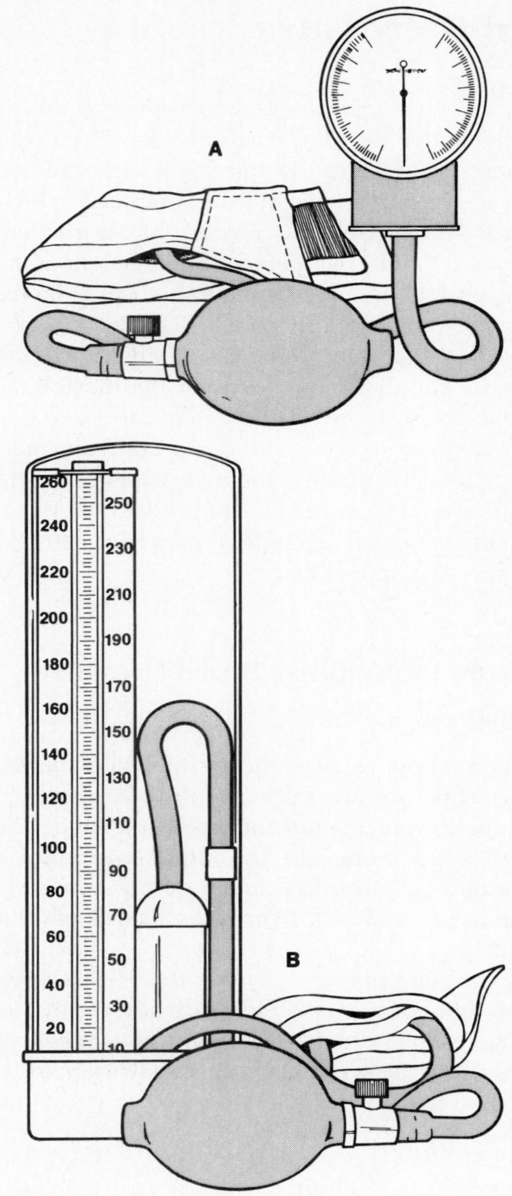

Figure 13–11 Blood pressure equipment: **A,** aneroid manometer and cuff; **B,** mercury manometer and cuff.

The indirect method of taking the blood pressure, in this case arterial blood pressure, is commonly carried out by nurses. The equipment required is a stethoscope and a sphygmomanometer with a cuff. The cuff is a rubber bag that can be filled with air. It generally is covered with a cloth and has two rubber tubes attached to it. One tube is attached to the rubber bulb that blows up the cuff. The other tube is attached to a manometer indicating the pressure of air within the cuff. See Figure 13–10.

There are two types of manometers commonly used. One is the aneroid manometer. It has a calibrated dial with a needle that points to the calibrations. The second type of manometer is a tube or cylinder filled with mercury. The nurse reads this manometer by looking directly (at eye level) at the meniscus of the mercury column. If the nurse views the column of mercury from above or below, distortions in the reading can result. See Figure 13–11.

Blood pressure cuffs come in six standard sizes. Some cuffs hook together; others wrap or snap in place. To get an accurate reading, it is particularly important to use a cuff of the appropriate size and length. The cuff should be wide enough to cover about two-thirds of the upper arm or thigh or be 40% of the circumference of the midpoint of the limb. The cuff needs to be long enough to completely encircle the limb. Too narrow a cuff can result in erroneously high readings, while too wide a cuff can produce low readings.

In some settings electronic equipment is used, which eliminates the need to use a stethoscope. As the pressure in the cuff decreases, a light flashes on to indicate the systolic and diastolic readings.

For a blood pressure measurement the patient normally assumes a sitting position with the arm slightly flexed and the forearm supported at heart level. For most people there is very little difference in the blood pressures between sitting, standing, and supine positions. However, in specific people where there is a difference and a variety of positions are used it is recommended that the exact position be specified, that is L (lying), St. (standing), Sit (sitting). In instances where there is a difference in the blood pressure between the two arms, the arm used should also be specified, for example, RA (right arm 160/120).

When taking a blood pressure using a stethoscope the nurse should identify five phases in the series of sounds. These sounds are called Korotkoff's sounds. First the cuff is pumped up to about 30 mm Hg above the point where the last sound is heard; that is until the blood flow in the artery is stopped. The pressure is then released slowly (2 to 3 mm Hg/second). While the pressure in the cuff is slowly released the nurse observes the pressure readings on the manometer and relates these to the sounds heard through the stethoscope. The following phases are identified:

Phase I. The period initiated by the first faint clear tapping sounds. These sounds gradually become more intense. To ensure that one is not hearing an extraneous sound at least two consecutive tapping sounds should be identified.

Phase II. The period during which the sounds have a swishing quality.

Phase III. The period during which the sounds are crisper and more intense.

Phase IV. The period during which the sounds become muffled and a soft blowing quality is heard.

Phase V. The point where the sounds disappear (American Heart Association, 1980, *Recommendations for Human Blood Pressure Determination by Sphygmomanometers,* p. 11).

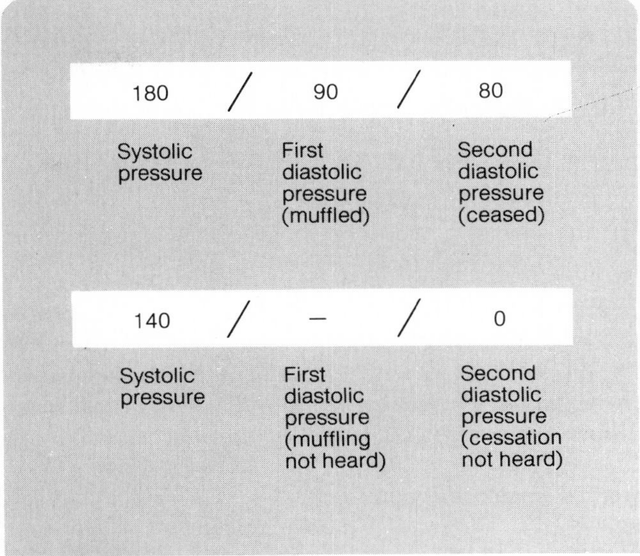

Figure 13–12 Recording a blood pressure reading, including systolic pressure, first diastolic pressure, and second diastolic pressure.

The American Heart Association recommends that the systolic pressure be considered the point where the first tapping sound is heard. In adults the diastolic pressure is the point where the sounds become inaudible (phase V). In children however the diastolic pressure is recommended to be the onset of phase IV, where the sounds become muffled. In agencies where the fourth phase is considered to be the diastolic pressure of adults, three measures are recommended (systolic pressure, diastolic pressure, and fifth phase). These may be referred to as systolic, first diastolic, and second diastolic pressures.

If the practice of the agency is to use the fourth phase (muffled sounds) as the diastolic blood pressure it is recommended that the fifth phase also be recorded. The fifth phase (second diastolic pressure) may be zero; that is the muffled sounds are heard even when there is no air pressure in the blood pressure cuff. In some instances muffled sounds may not be heard at all, in which case a dash is inserted where the reading would normally be recorded. See Figure 13–12.

Procedure 13–6 Assessing Blood Pressure

Equipment

1. A stethoscope. The ear attachments are to be cleaned with disinfectant, if others have worn it.
2. A blood pressure cuff of the appropriate size (newborn, infant, child, small adult, adult, large adult, thigh).
3. A sphygmomanometer.

Procedure 13–6, continued

Preparation

1. Wash hands.

   Rationale The nurse washes the hands to remove any microorganisms which should not be transmitted to the patient.

2. Help the patient assume the appropriate position. A sitting position is normally used unless otherwise specified. The arm should be slightly flexed with the forearm supported at heart level.

   Rationale The blood pressure is normally similar in sitting, standing, and lying positions although it can vary in certain persons.

3. Expose the upper arm. Usually an arm is used however the thigh or leg can be used in certain instances.

Intervention

1. Wrap the cuff evenly around the upper arm so that the center of the bladder (expandable bag) is applied directly over the medial aspect of the arm. For an adult the lower border of the cuff should be about 2.5 cm (1 in) above the antecubital space. For an infant the lower edge can be nearer the antecubital space.

   Rationale The bladder inside the cuff must be directly over the artery to be compressed if the reading is to be accurate.

2. Palpate the brachial artery with the finger tips. The brachial artery is normally found medially in the antecubital space.

3. Close the valve on the pump by turning the knob clockwise.

4. Pump up the cuff until the brachial pulse can no longer be felt.

   Rationale At that pressure the blood cannot flow through the artery.

5. Note the pressure on the sphygmomanometer at which point the pulse can no longer be felt. This will give an estimate of the maximum pressure required to measure the systolic pressure.

6. Release the pressure completely in the cuff and wait one to two minutes.

   Rationale To give the trapped blood in the veins time to be released.

7. Put the ear attachments of the stethoscope in the ears. Insert the ear attachments so that they tilt slightly forward.

   Rationale Sounds are sharper when the ear attachments lie along the direction of the ear canal.

8. Ensure that the stethoscope hangs freely from the ears to the diaphragm.

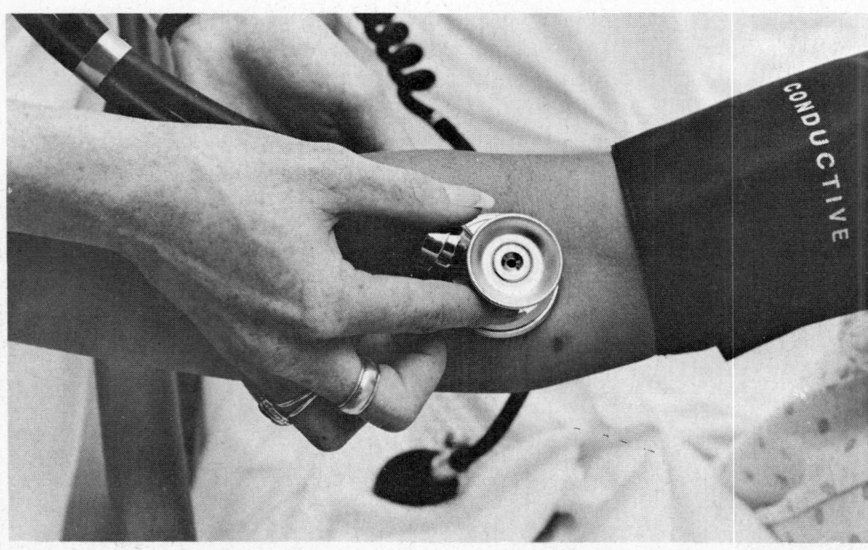

Figure 13–13

Procedure 13–6, continued

Rationale Rubbing the stethoscope against an object can obliterate the sounds of the blood with an artery.

9. Place the diaphragm of the stethoscope over the brachial pulse. The diaphragm can be held with the thumb or first few fingers (see Figure 13–13).

10. Pump up the cuff until the sphygmomanometer registers about 30 mm Hg above the point where the brachial pulse disappears.

11. Release the valve on the cuff carefully so that the pressure decreases at the rate of 2 to 3 mm Hg/second.

Rationale If the rate is faster or slower an error in measurement may occur (American Heart Association, p. 11).

12. As the pressure falls identify the five phases and relate each to the manometer reading.

13. Deflate the cuff rapidly and completely and wait one to two minutes before repeating.

Rationale To permit the trapped blood to be released from the veins.

14. Repeat steps 10 to 12 once or twice as necessary to confirm the accuracy of the reading.

15. Remove the cuff from the patient's arm.

16. Assist the patient to a comfortable position.

17. Wash hands.

18. Record the blood pressure according to agency policy. Record two pressures in this form 130/80 when 130 is systolic and the 80 is the fifth phase or diastolic pressure. Record three pressures in this form: 130/110/90 when 130 is systolic, 110 is fourth phase, and 90 is fifth phase.

Summary

Although nurses have always assessed their patients' conditions, increasingly specific techniques are being employed to determine health status. These techniques include those that assess physical health status. An outline of the physical assessment techniques to determine vital signs as well as influencing factors and points of emphasis follows:

I. Body temperature
  A. Influencing factors
    1. Age
      a. Newborns: fluctuations between 36.1 and 37.7 C
      b. 2 years: 37.2 C
      c. 6 years: 37.0 C
      d. 12 years: 37.0 C
      e. Adults: 37.0 C
      f. Elderly: 36 C
    2. Time of day
      a. Lowest in the morning
      b. Highest in the evening
    3. Sex: body temperature increased by ovulation
    4. Emotions: temperature increased by heightened emotions
    5. Exercise: elevates body temperature
    6. Temperature of environment: direct relationship to body temperature
  B. Sites of measurement
    1. Oral
      a. Taken for 2 to 8 minutes
      b. Contraindicated for infants, young children, nose breather, the confused, those with oral surgery, and in some agencies, for patients receiving oxygen by cannula or mask
    2. Rectal
      a. Indicated for the very young, unconscious, or confused patient
      b. Contraindicated for patients with rectal pathologic conditions or trauma
      c. Taken for 2 or 3 minutes
      d. Must be held in place
    3. Axilla
      a. Least accurate of the three methods
      b. Taken for 10 minutes
  C. Types of fever
    1. Intermittent (quotidian)
    2. Remittent
    3. Relapsing
  D. Symptoms of fever
    1. During fever onset
      a. Shivering and chills
      b. Increased pulse rate
      c. Pallor and skin coldness
      d. Gooseflesh
      e. Convulsions with high temperature

2. During fever course
   a. Skin feels warm
   b. Flushing
   c. Headache, irritability, restlessness
   d. Disorientation with high temperature
   e. Weakness
   f. Dehydration
3. During fever termination
   a. Increased diaphoresis
   b. Skin redness

II. Pulse measurement
   A. Pulse sites
      1. Temporal
      2. Carotid
      3. Brachial
      4. Radial
      5. Femoral
      6. Popliteal
      7. Dorsalis pedis
      8. Apical
   B. Factors influencing pulse rates per minute
      1. Age
         a. Newborns: fluctuates between 70 and 170 beats per minute
         b. 2 years: 80 to 130
         c. 12 years: boys, 65 to 105; girls, 70 to 110
         d. 18 years: boys, 50 to 90; girls, 55 to 95
         e. Adults: same as 18 years
         f. Elderly: 70 to 80 or same as 18 years
      2. Sex: lower pulse rates in men than women
      3. Exercise: increases pulse rates
      4. Emotions: tachycardia with sympathetic nervous system stimulation
      5. Heat: pulse rate elevated by prolonged external heat
      6. Body position: pulse rate increased by prolonged horizontal position
   C. The apical and apical-radial pulses
      1. Apical pulse used for newborns, infants, children up to 2 or 3 years of age, and adults with cardiac problems
      2. Apical-radial pulse ordered for adults who have heart problems
      3. Locations of the apical pulse vary with age
   D. Fetal heart sounds
      1. Heard by 18 to 20 weeks of pregnancy
      2. Normal fetal heart rate: 120 to 160 beats per minute
      3. Sounds heard predominantly through the back of the fetus
      4. Locations of sounds: depend on the fetal position
      5. Sounds differentiated from souffles (the funic and the uterine)
      6. Assessment of utmost importance during labor

III. Respirations
   A. Variations in respiratory rate by age
      1. Newborns: 30 to 40 breaths per minute, irregular and shallow
      2. Adult: 16 to 20
      3. Elderly: same as adult or increased rate and shallow
   B. Measurements in addition to rate
      1. Depth: observed by movement of the chest or by the use of pulmonary equipment
      2. Capacity: see Chapter 29, pulmonary volumes
      3. Rhythm: normally regular
      4. Character: normally silent and effortless
         a. Note abnormal sounds of breathing (rales or rhonchi)
         b. Notable effort by accessory muscles of respiration and dyspnea

IV. Blood pressure
   A. Measured in mm Hg
      1. Systolic pressure
      2. Diastolic pressure
   B. Factors controlling blood pressure
      1. Cardiac output
      2. Blood volume
      3. Elasticity of arterial walls
      4. Size of arterioles and capillaries
   C. Factors influencing blood pressure
      1. Age
         a. Newborn has systolic pressure of 65 to 90 mm Hg and a diastolic pressure of 30 to 60 mm Hg
         b. Adult has systolic pressure of 110 to 140 and a diastolic pressure of 60 to 80
      2. Exercise increases blood pressure
      3. Stress: moderate stress increases blood pressure but severe stress may lower the pressure
   D. Methods of measurement
      1. Direct
      2. Indirect by use of stethoscope, cuff, and sphygmomanometers: the aneroid manometer or the mercury manometer
      3. Electronic equipment without a stethoscope
   E. Abnormalities
      1. Hypertension: above 140 systolic (adults)
      2. Hypotension: below 100 systolic (adults)

Suggested Activities

1. Select three patients of differing ages. Take their vital signs (temperature, pulse, respirations, and blood pressure) and compare them.

2. Determine the policies governing taking vital signs at a local health agency. Compare these with the data obtained by other students at other agencies.

3. At a physician's office, listen to fetal heart sounds. Determine the location at which the sounds are most distinct. Relate your findings to the position of the fetus.

Suggested Readings

Abbey, J. C., et al. August 1978. How long is that thermometer accurate? *American Journal of Nursing* 78:1375–76.
This study shows the need to test the accuracy of new, used, and stored thermometers.

Adelman, E. M. February 1980. When the patient's blood pressure falls . . . . What does it mean? What should you do? *Nursing 80* 10:26–33.
This article discusses causes of hypotension and provides guidelines for the nurse to follow when hypotension is suspected. In addition six mistakes that produce abnormally low blood pressure readings are listed.

American Journal of Nursing. October 1965. Correcting common errors in blood pressure measurement, programmed instruction. *American Journal of Nursing* 65: 133–64.
A programmed unit of instruction for learning about blood pressure.

———. January 1979. Patient assessment. Pulses, programmed instruction. *American Journal of Nursing* 79: 115–32.
This programmed unit of instruction deals with the assessment of major pulses (radial, brachial, pedal (dorsalis pedis), posterior tibial, carotid, femoral, popliteal) and the significance of relevant findings.

Blainey, C. G. October 1974. Site selection in taking body temperature. *American Journal of Nursing* 74:1859–61.
This article discusses rectal temperatures and their advantages and disadvantages. Blainey also discusses oral (sublingual) and other temperatures. The author concludes that the sublingual site provides the most accurate reflection of body temperature under normal conditions.

Castle, M., and Watkins, J. February 1979. Fever: Understanding a sinister sign. *Nursing 79* 9:26–33.
This article includes case examples of remittent and constant fever, intermittent fever, and relapsing fever. The nurse's role in caring for the fever patient is outlined.

Jarvis, C. M. April 1976. Vital signs: How to take them more accurately and understand them more fully. *Nursing 76* 6:31–37.
This article gives in-depth meanings of the vital signs.

Rosenberg, H. August 1981. Malignant hyperpyrexia. *American Journal of Nursing* 81:1484–86.
This life-threatening condition occurs in certain individuals on exposure to certain anesthetic agents. Diagnosis and treatment are discussed.

Tate, G. V., et al. September 1970. Correct use of electric thermometers. *American Journal of Nursing* 70:1898–99.
This article points out that distrust of the electric thermometer may be related to the nurse's insecurity in using it or to the sensitivity of the instrument itself. Correct ways to operate the thermometer are discussed.

Warren, F. M. April 1975. Blood pressure readings: Getting them quickly on an infant. *Nursing 75* 5:13.
The author describes the flush method of obtaining a blood pressure reading.

Whitner, W., et al. January/February 1970. The influence of bathing on the newborn's body temperature. *Nursing Research* 19:30–36.
The study by this author set out to test 2 hypotheses: (a) Infants bathed on admission to the nursery would tend to show a greater initial decrease in body temperature, and (b) bathing would tend to produce a more rapid return toward the desired level of body temperature.

Selected References

Bell, S. April 1969. Early morning temperatures? *American Journal of Nursing* 69:764–66.

Brown, M. S., and Murphy, M. A. 1975. *Ambulatory pediatrics for nurses.* New York: McGraw-Hill Book Co.

Erickson, R. May-June 1980. Oral temperature differences in relation to thermometer and technique. *Nursing Research* 29:157–64.

Felton, G. January-February 1970. Effect of time cycle change on blood pressure and temperature in young women. *Nursing Research* 19:48–58.

Graas, S. October 1974. Thermometer sites and oxygen. *American Journal of Nursing* 74:1862–63.

Graves, R. D., and Markarian, M. F. September-October 1980. Three-minute time intervals when using an oral mercury-in-glass thermometer without J-temperature sheaths. *Nursing Research* 29:323–24.

Guyton, A. E. 1981. *Textbook of medical physiology.* 6th ed. Philadelphia: W. B. Saunders Co.

———. 1982. *Human physiology and mechanisms of disease.* 3rd ed. Philadelphia: W. B. Saunders Co.

Hill, M. N. May 1980. Hypertension: What can go wrong when you measure blood pressure. *American Journal of Nursing* 80:942–45.

Jarvis, C. M. April 1976. Vital signs: How to take them more accurately and understand them more fully. *Nursing 76* 6:31–37.

Kolanowski, A., and Gunter, L. September/October 1981. Hypothermia in the elderly. *Geriatric Nursing* 2:362–65.

Murray, R. B., and Zentner, J. P. 1979. *Nursing assessment and health promotion throughout the life span.* 2nd ed. Englewood Cliffs, N.J.: Prentice-Hall.

Nichols, G. A. June 1972. Taking adult temperatures: Rectal measurement. *American Journal of Nursing* 72:1092–93.

Nichols, G. A., and Kucha, D. H. June 1972. Taking adult temperatures: Oral measurement. *American Journal of Nursing* 72:1090–93.

Nichols, G. A., and Verhonick, P. J. November 1967. Time and temperature. *American Journal of Nursing* 67:2304–6.

Vaughan, V. C., and McKay, J. R., editors. 1975. *Nelson textbook of pediatrics.* 10th ed. Philadelphia: W. B. Saunders Co.

Whaley, L. F. and Wong, D. L. 1979. *Nursing care of infants and children.* St. Louis: C. V. Mosby Co.

Chapter 14

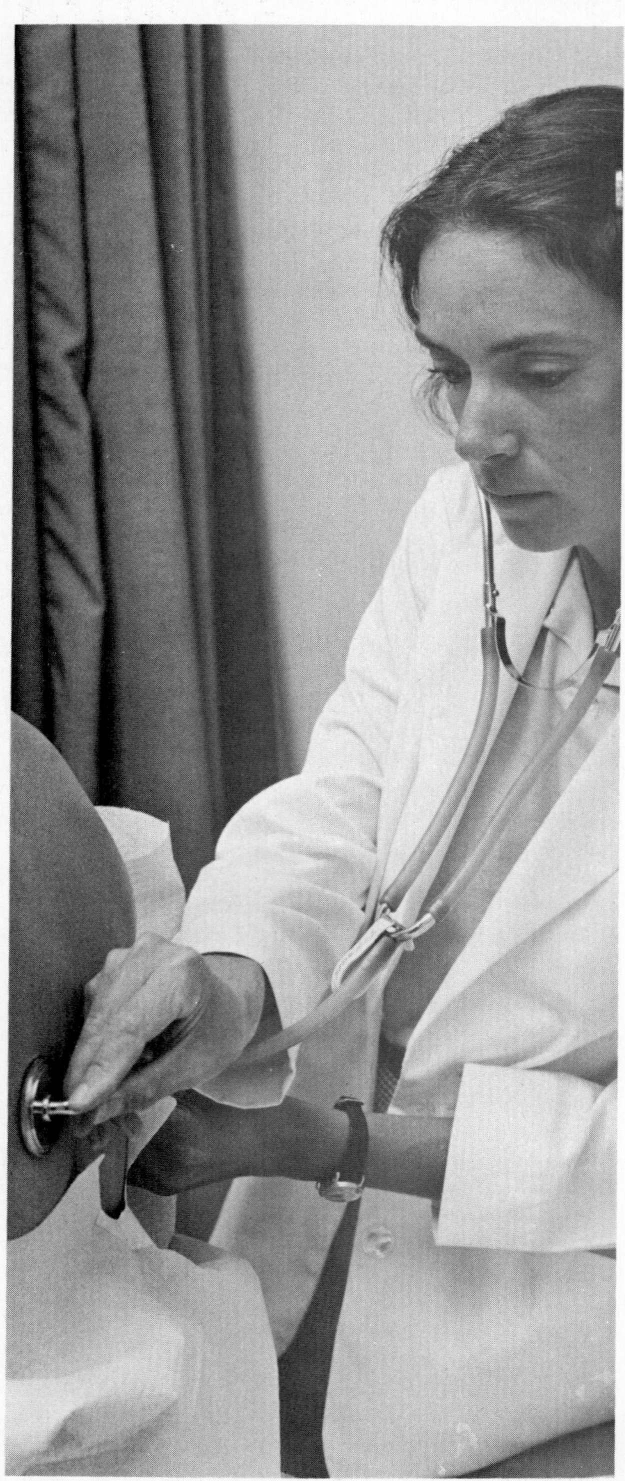

General Assessment Skills

CONTENTS

(Continued on next page)

Objectives

1. Know essential terms and facts about assessment of a patient's neck, eyes, ears, nose, and throat

- **1.1** Define selected terms
- **1.2** Identify ways to assess the range of motion of the neck
- **1.3** Identify significant chains of lymph nodes in the neck
- **1.4** Describe the method used to palpate the thyroid gland
- **1.5** Identify essential data to obtain when observing and palpating the jugular veins and carotid arteries
- **1.6** Identify essential data to obtain when inspecting the external structures of the eye
- **1.7** Identify the appearance of essential structures viewed during a funduscopic examination of the eye
- **1.8** Describe normal visual acuity of children and adults
- **1.9** Describe the cover test used to test eye movement in children
- **1.10** Describe the appearance of a normal tympanic membrane
- **1.11** Describe Rinne's and Weber's tests to assess hearing acuity
- **1.12** Describe Romberg's test to assess balance
- **1.13** Identify essential data to obtain when inspecting the nose and palpating facial sinuses
- **1.14** Identify essential data to obtain when inspecting the mouth and pharynx

2. Know essential terms and facts about assessment of a patient's chest (thorax, lungs, heart, breasts, and axillae)

- **2.1** Define selected terms
- **2.2** Identify normal and abnormal contours of the chest
- **2.3** Describe the method used to assess symmetry of expansion of the thorax
- **2.4** List assessment data that can be obtained by chest percussion
- **2.5** Identify three normal chest percussion sounds and their locations
- **2.6** Describe normal breath and voice sounds heard by auscultation
- **2.7** Identify essential data to obtain when inspecting the precordium
- **2.8** Describe the first and second heart sounds
- **2.9** Identify four valvular areas used to auscultate the heart
- **2.10** Identify essential data to obtain when inspecting the breasts and the axillae

3. Know essential terms and facts about assessment of a patient's abdomen, genitals, and rectum

- **3.1** Define selected terms
- **3.2** Identify quadrants and nine regions of the abdomen used for descriptive purposes
- **3.3** Identify data that can be obtained by abdominal auscultation, palpation, and percussion
- **3.4** Identify essential data to obtain when inspecting and palpating the genitals, rectum, and anus

4. Know essential terms and facts about assessment of a patient's extremities and neurologic and mental-emotional status

- **4.1** Identify essential data to obtain when inspecting the extremities
- **4.2** Identify normal reflex responses of the extremities
- **4.3** Identify methods of testing selected cranial nerves
- **4.4** Identify ways to assess mental and emotional status
- **4.5** Identify selected coordination and balance tests
- **4.6** Identify ways the sensory system is assessed
- **4.7** Identify data to obtain when assessing the motor system

5. Demonstrate beginning skill in the following assessment techniques:

5.1 Palpation of an adult's neck for lymph nodes
5.2 Palpation of an adult's thyroid gland
5.3 Inspection of external eye structures
5.4 Tests of pupillary reaction
5.5 Funduscopic examination of the eye
5.6 Snellen chart test of visual acuity
5.7 Otoscopic examination of the ear
5.8 Rinne's and Weber's tests for hearing acuity
5.9 Romberg's test for balance
5.10 Inspection of the nose
5.11 Palpation of facial sinuses
5.12 Inspection of the mouth and pharynx
5.13 Percussion of the chest
5.14 Inspection of the precordium
5.15 Cardiac auscultation for the first and second heart sounds
5.16 Inspection and palpation of the breasts
5.17 Palpation of the axillae
5.18 Auscultation of the abdomen
5.19 Palpation of the liver and spleen
5.20 Percussion of the liver and spleen
5.21 Inspection of the genitals and rectum
5.22 Palpation of the rectum
5.23 Inspection of extremity reflexes
5.24 Assessment of mental-emotional status
5.25 Assessment of the sensory system
5.26 Assessment of the motor system

Terms

adventitious breath sounds
aneurysm
atelectasis
athetosis
barrel chest
bronchial sounds
bronchophony
bronchovesicular sounds
bruit
cataract
consensual reaction (eyes)
cover test
dullness
ectropion
egophony
emphysema
entropion
exophthalmos
fasciculation
fibrillations
flaccid paralysis
flatness
funnel chest
hyperopia
hyperresonance
intensity
kyphosis
murmur (cardiac)
mydriatic
ophthalmoscope
osteoporosis
pectoriloquy
pigeon chest
pitch
pitting edema
pleural rub
precordium
presbyopia
rales
reflex
resonance
rhonchi
scoliosis
stereognosis
strabismus
stye
tactile (vocal) fremitus
tics
tonometer
tremors
tympany
vesicular sounds
vocal resonance

General assessment skills are skills nurses use in the physical examination of patients. This examination, which encompasses both physical and psychosocial aspects of the individual, is adjusted to a patient's needs. It may be: (a) a complete physical examination, as on admission to a health agency; (b) an examination of a body system such as the urinary system, integument, etc.; or (c) an examination of a body part, e.g., the urinary bladder when urinary retention is suspected. Assessment skills are also adjusted to the individual's age; for example, the height of infants is measured when they are supine, and children's vision is tested with a special Snellen chart until they learn the alphabet.

Certain assessment is performed during common nursing interventions. For example, nurses assess patients' skin as a matter of course when they bathe patients. This kind of assessment is discussed throughout this book, under specific subject headings.

Chapter 5 also discusses assessment, including general methods used during the physical examination and laboratory tests. The intent of Chapter 14, however, is to delineate areas of assessment and emphasize normal findings, although some abnormal findings are included for comparison. Although the word *nurse* has been used throughout this chapter to denote the examiner, it is recognized that some aspects of the physical examination are not carried out by nurses in some jurisdictions.

General Impression

The general impression that an individual presents includes appearance and health state. The patient's height, weight, and vital signs are also determined at this time.

The nurse observes weight relative to height, posture, facial expression, movements, behavior, and any obvious abnormalities. Posture can indicate mood. For example, a slumped position may reflect depression; too rigid and upright a position, anxiety. Facial expressions may reveal patients' attitudes to their illnesses. Expressions can reflect anxiety, pain, anger, or disinterest. The facial skin may indicate certain health problems (see Chapter 21). The behavior of the patient may reflect nervousness, e.g., wringing the hands, continual shifting of the feet, etc. Any obvious, unusual behavior is observed as part of the general impression; perhaps the patient paces the room or verbalizes anger or fear about illness.

Height and Weight

Height and weight are standard measures frequently taken in physicians' offices, schools, and hospitals. Height is a measure of a child's growth, and weight is in many ways a measure of general health for all people.

Chapter 11 gives height and weight ranges up to age 12 years. Because of the growth spurt before puberty, prepubescent girls are often taller than boys of the same age. Boys reach their maximum height at age 18 or 19 years; girls, at about 15 or 16 years. Elderly adults usually decrease in overall stature due to the atrophy of the intervertebral discs.

Length and Height

For information about newborn lengths, see Chapter 11. To measure the length of a baby who cannot stand, the nurse places the baby supine on a hard surface with the soles of the feet supported in an upright position. The baby's knees are extended, and the nurse measures the length from the soles of the feet to the vertex (the top of the head). The head should be in such a position that the eyes face the ceiling.

After infancy, patients stand against a wall or on a scale to be measured. One method is to have the patients place the heels, back, and head against a wall. The nurse places a small flat board on top of the patient's head, with the edge of the board against the wall. The distance from the floor to the board is the patient's height. When the patient stands on a height scale, the nurse raises an L-shaped, sliding arm until it rests on the top of the patient's head. The height is read on the vertical part of the arm.

Weight

Patients' weight is more likely to vary from the norm than height. Genetic influences, diet, and activity are some factors that affect weight. For information about normal weights, see Tables 14–1 and 14–2, and Chapters 11 and 12.

Table 14–1 Weight According to Frame (Indoor Clothing), Women 25* and Over

Height†			Small frame		Medium frame		Large frame	
Feet	*Inches*	*cm*	*Pounds*	*Kilograms*	*Pounds*	*Kilograms*	*Pounds*	*Kilograms*
4	10	147.3	92–98	41.7–44.5	96–107	43.5–48.5	104–119	47.2–54.0
4	11	149.9	94–101	42.6–45.8	98–110	44.5–49.9	106–122	48.1–55.3
5	0	152.4	96–104	43.5–47.2	101–113	45.8–51.3	109–125	49.4–56.7
5	1	154.9	99–107	44.9–48.5	104–116	47.2–52.6	112–128	50.8–58.1
5	2	157.5	102–110	46.3–50.0	107–119	48.5–54.0	115–131	52.2–59.4
5	3	160.0	105–113	47.6–51.3	110–122	49.9–55.3	118–134	53.5–60.8
5	4	162.6	108–116	49.0–52.6	113–126	51.3–57.2	121–138	54.9–62.6
5	5	165.1	111–119	50.3–54.0	116–130	52.6–59.0	125–142	56.7–64.4
5	6	167.6	114–123	51.7–55.8	120–135	54.4–61.2	129–146	58.5–66.2
5	7	170.2	118–127	53.5–57.6	124–139	56.2–63.0	133–150	60.3–68.0
5	8	172.7	122–131	55.3–59.4	128–143	58.1–64.9	137–154	62.1–69.9
5	9	175.3	126–135	57.2–61.2	132–147	59.9–66.7	141–158	64.0–71.7
5	10	177.8	130–140	59.0–63.5	136–151	61.7–68.5	145–163	65.8–73.9
5	11	180.3	134–144	60.8–65.3	140–155	63.5–70.3	149–168	67.6–76.2
6	0	182.9	138–148	62.6–67.1	144–159	65.3–72.1	153–173	69.4–78.5

Courtesy of the Metropolitan Life Insurance Company.

*For women between 18 and 25, subtract 0.5 kg (1 lb) for each year under 25.

†With shoes on—5.1 cm (2-in) heels

Table 14–2 Weight According to Frame (Indoor Clothing), Men 25 and Over

Height*			Small frame		Medium frame		Large frame	
Feet	*Inches*	*cm*	*Pounds*	*Kilograms*	*Pounds*	*Kilograms*	*Pounds*	*Kilograms*
5	2	157.5	112–120	50.8–54.4	118–129	53.5–58.5	126–141	57.2–64.0
5	3	160.0	115–123	52.2–55.8	121–133	54.9–60.3	129–144	58.5–65.3
5	4	162.6	118–126	53.5–57.2	124–136	56.2–61.7	132–148	59.9–67.1
5	5	165.1	121–129	54.9–58.5	127–139	57.6–63.0	135–152	61.2–68.9
5	6	167.6	124–133	56.2–60.3	130–143	59.0–64.9	138–156	62.6–70.8
5	7	170.2	128–137	58.1–62.1	134–147	60.8–66.7	142–161	64.4–73.0
5	8	172.7	132–141	59.9–64.0	138–152	62.6–68.9	147–166	66.7–75.3
5	9	175.3	136–145	61.7–65.8	142–156	64.4–70.8	151–170	68.5–77.1
5	10	177.8	140–150	63.5–68.0	146–160	66.2–72.6	155–174	70.3–78.9
5	11	180.3	144–154	65.3–69.9	150–165	68.0–74.8	159–179	72.1–81.2
6	0	182.9	148–158	67.1–71.7	154–170	69.9–77.1	164–184	74.4–83.4
6	1	185.4	152–162	68.9–73.5	158–175	71.7–79.4	168–189	76.2–85.7
6	2	188.0	156–167	70.8–75.8	162–180	73.5–81.6	173–194	78.5–88.0
6	3	190.5	160–171	72.6–77.6	167–185	75.8–83.9	178–199	80.7–90.3
6	4	193.0	164–175	74.4–79.4	172–190	78.0–86.2	182–204	82.6–92.5

Courtesy of the Metropolitan Life Insurance Company.

*With shoes on—2.5 cm (1-in) heels

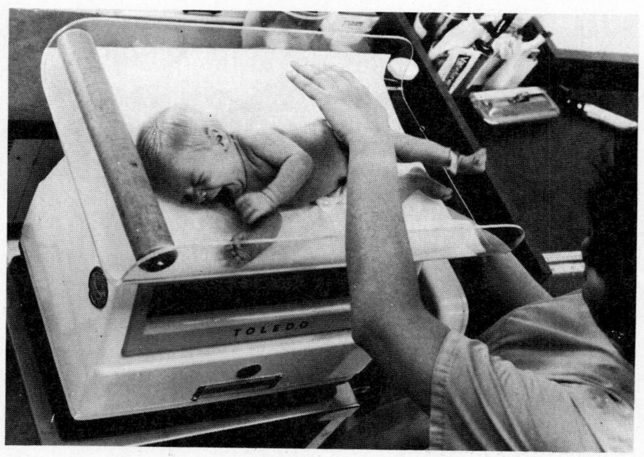

Figure 14–1 Weighing an infant.

Several types of scales are used to weigh babies. Hospitals usually have scales with a container in which the baby is placed to be weighed. Some scales are portable. It is important to weigh a baby unclothed or to weigh the clothes separately and subtract their weight.

Before placing an infant on a scale, the nurse drapes the scale to prevent cross-infection. The nurse balances the draped scale, if necessary, and places the unclothed infant on the tray. Holding one hand about 2.5 cm (1 in) over the baby, the nurse uses the other hand to adjust the scale. See Figure 14–1. The weighed infant is returned to the crib and covered. The nurse then records the weight. For additional information about weighing infants, see Kozier and Erb (1982:512–15).

Patients who can stand are generally weighed on a standing scale. The person stands on a platform, and the weight is read from a dial on the scale. Patients are usually weighed without shoes. A clean paper towel on the platform helps keep the feet clean. Patients who cannot stand can be weighed on a scale with canvas straps used to lift the patient mechanically. See Chapter 23, page 578.

Skin, Hair, and Nails

Part of assessment is observation of all skin surfaces, hair, and nails. Usually the nurse assesses these gradually while observing parts of the body for other data. The skin is observed for color, texture, temperature, and lesions. Lesions warrant particular attention during assessment. See Table 14–3 for descriptions of different types of lesions. See Chapter 21 for assessment of skin, hair, and nails.

Table 14–3 Primary Skin Lesions

Type	Description	Size	Example
Macula	Flat circumscribed area of color with no elevation of its surface	1 mm to several cm	Freckles
Papule	Circumscribed solid elevation of skin	Less than 1 cm	Acne
Nodule	Solid mass extending deeper into dermis than papule	1–2 cm	Pigmented nevi
Tumor	Solid mass larger than nodule	Over 2 cm	Epithelioma
Cyst	Encapsulated fluid-filled mass in dermis or subcutaneous layer	Over 1 cm	Epidermoid cyst
Wheal	A relatively reddened, flat, localized collection of edema fluid	1 mm to several cm	Mosquito bite; hives
Vesicle	Circumscribed elevation containing serous fluid or blood	Less than 1 cm	Herpes; chickenpox
Bulla	Larger fluid-filled vesicle	Over 1 cm	Second-degree burn
Pustule	Vesicle or bulla filled with pus	1 mm to 1 cm	Acne vulgaris

Head and Neck

When examining the head and neck, the nurse assesses skull shape, skull circumference, fontanelles of infants, hair, scalp, face, skin, eyes, ears, mouth, and throat. The neck is examined for mobility, pulsation, symmetry, and enlarged underlying structures. The nurse uses only observation and palpation, except when examining the eyes and the ears. See Chapter 11 for assessment of infants' skull shape, circumference, and fontanelles. See Chapter 21 for assessment of the hair, scalp, face, and skin.

Neck

First, the nurse assesses the skin of the neck. The nurse then assesses its range of motion by asking the patient to flex, extend, hyperextend, and rotate the head. If necessary—for example, if the patient is too young to understand directions—the nurse can move the patient's head and neck through these motions. Older children can be asked to follow with head motions the path of a light moved up, down, and sideways. Control of the head is assessed in infants. Normally, infants 3 months or younger show some head lag when pulled from a sitting to a lying position. Head lag in children older than 3 months suggests a neuromuscular defect such as cerebral palsy.

Lymph Nodes

To allow the nurse to examine the lymph nodes, the patient flexes the neck forward slightly. The nodes are palpated with the pads of the middle and index fingers.

Lymph nodes occur in a number of places in the body; however, the most palpable are in the neck region. Lymph nodes tend to occur in chains or groups. Figure 14–2 shows the significant chains in the neck area. They are:

1. Preauricular: in front of the tragus of the ear
2. Postauricular (posterior auricular): in front of the mastoid process but behind the auricle of the ear

Figure 14–2 The major lymph nodes in the neck.

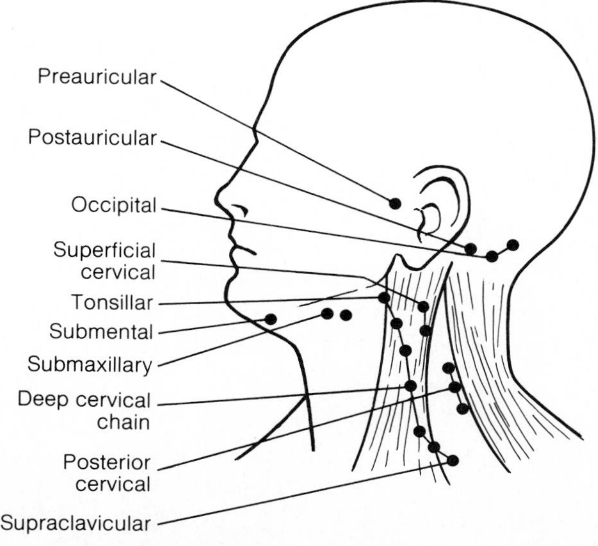

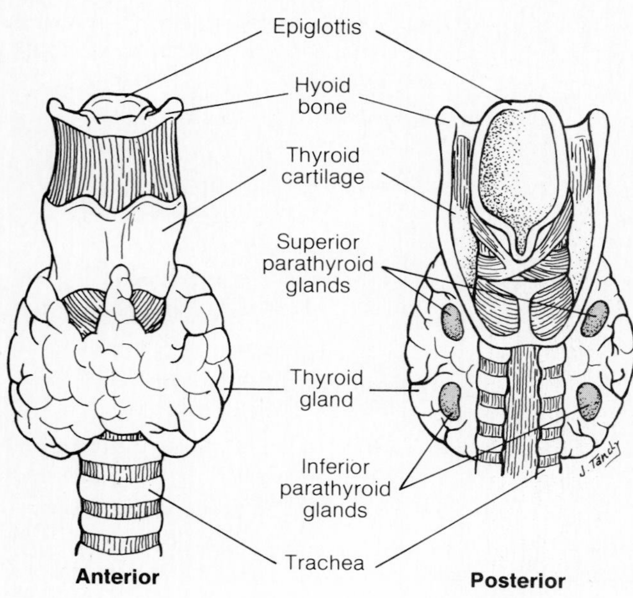

Figure 14–3 Anterior and posterior views of the thyroid gland.

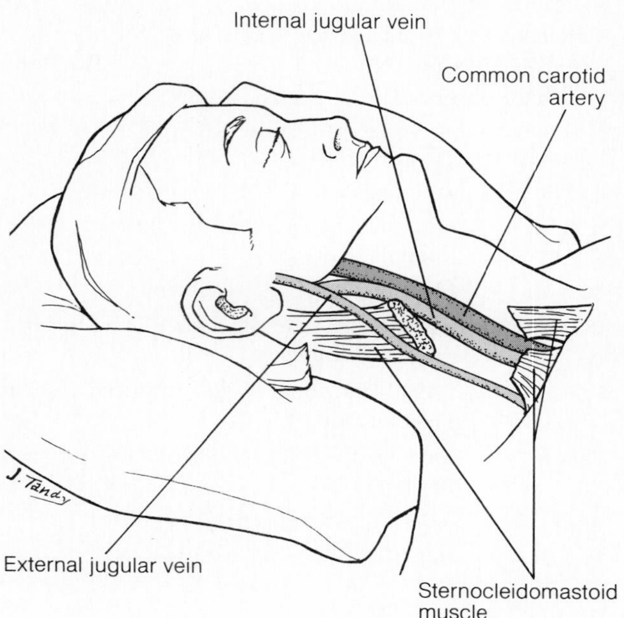

Figure 14–5 The jugular veins and the common carotid artery.

3. Occipital: at the base of the skull posteriorly
4. Submaxillary: along the mandible halfway between the angle of the jaw and the chin
5. Tonsillar: at the angle of the mandible
6. Submental: behind the tip of the mandible in the midline, under the chin
7. Superficial cervical: along the sternocleidomastoid muscle
8. Posterior cervical: along the anterior aspect of the trapezius muscle
9. Deep cervical: under the sternocleidomastoid muscle (may not be palpable)
10. Supraclavicular: above the clavicle, in the angle between the clavicle and the sternocleidomastoid muscle

Figure 14–4 Palpating the thyroid gland.

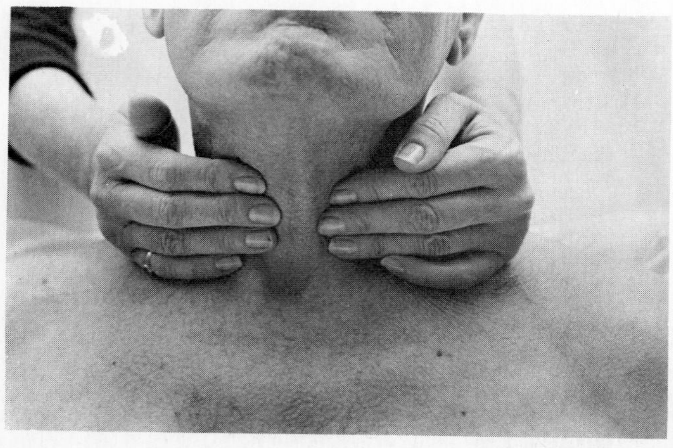

Larynx and Trachea

Further examination (inspection and palpation) of the neck should reveal that the larynx and trachea lie in the midline. In very thin people and in males, the thyroid cartilage of the larynx is seen halfway between the chin and the sternal notch.

Thyroid Gland

The thyroid gland is attached to the trachea just below the larynx. See Figure 14–3. It is not normally visible except in very thin people or when enlarged. To palpate the thyroid gland, the nurse stands behind the patient, places the fingers on the thyroid, and asks the patient to swallow. See Figure 14–4. The nurse can feel the size of the gland and the presence of nodules as the gland moves upward when the patient swallows.

Jugular Veins and Carotid Arteries

The external jugular veins run from the angle of the jaw across the sternocleidomastoid muscles to the suprasternal notch (see Figure 14–5). Normally these veins are not distended when the patient sits but fill when the patient is in the back-lying position. Their palpation provides an indication of the patient's central venous pressure. Jugular veins that appear distended upon palpation while the patient is in a sitting position may indicate a disease process, such as congestive heart failure.

The common carotid arteries ascend the neck alongside the internal jugular veins on the anterior aspect of the sternocleidomastoid muscles. Carotid pulsations can often be observed in very thin people and palpated by pressing the carotid artery on the lower aspect of the neck. It should not be pressed in the upper part of the neck because of its proximity to the carotid sinus; a sudden increase in the blood pressure within the sinus causes a slowing of the heart rate. Both arteries should not be pressed at the same time because of the danger of interfering with the blood flow to the brain.

Eyes

An examination of the eyes needs to include an assessment of the external structures: eyebrows and eyelashes, eyelids, eyeballs, conjunctivae, sclera, cornea and iris, and pupils. Assessment is not complete until the fundus is examined with an ophthalmoscope and visual acuity is tested, either by having the patient read an eye chart or less accurately by having the patient read a newspaper. Eye movement is also assessed.

External Structures

Eyebrows

The eyebrows are normally present over both eyes. Tweezing eyebrows is a normal practice today for men and women; the complete absence of eyebrows, however, is abnormal and needs to be noted.

Eyelashes

Eyelash follicles need to be observed for infection, which produces a red stye. A *stye* (hordeolum) is inflammation of one or more sebaceous glands of the eyelid. Patients usually describe styes as painful.

Eyelids

Eyelids need to be observed primarily for discoloration, edema, lesions, and positional faults. Edema is readily seen on the eyelids because this skin is thin and loosely attached to the underlying tissues. Positional faults include *ectropion* (a rolling out of the lid) and *entropion* (an inturned lid). The former usually requires surgical intervention; the latter is normally present in Oriental children and is generally harmless unless the cornea becomes abraded by the eyelashes.

Eyeballs

The eyeballs are observed to see whether they are situated deeply in the eye socket or whether they protrude abnormally from the socket. Patients who are dehydrated or emaciated often appear to have sunken eyeballs, while patients with hyperthyroidism may have protruding eyeballs. The latter is called *exophthalmos*.

The nurse palpates the eyeball with the finger when the eye is closed to assess the relative hardness or softness of the eyeball. Patients with glaucoma have abnormally hard eyeballs due to the increased pressure of the aqueous humor. The exact pressure is assessed by a physician using a *tonometer*. Particularly soft eyeballs can often be detected in a patient who is dehydrated.

Conjunctivae

The conjunctivae of the eye are observed for inflammation and for paleness and cyanosis in dark-skinned people. The lower portion of the conjunctiva can be observed by pulling down gently on the skin just below the eye. The upper conjunctiva is observed by everting the upper eyelid. The patient looks downward while the nurse holds the lid by the eyelashes and pulls it down and outward. Then the nurse places an applicator against the upper border of the eyelid and everts the lid over the applicator by moving the eyelashes toward the eyebrow.

The conjunctivae of the newborn may have small hemorrhages, which normally disappear relatively soon after birth. See Figure 14–6 for parts of the eye.

Sclera

The sclera of the eyes are observed chiefly for their color. They should be white and clear. Jaundice will be reflected in a yellow tinge to the sclera. The sclera of newborns usually have a slightly bluish tinge, and the sclera of black patients is frequently slightly brownish. A bluish sclera can indicate glaucoma.

Cornea and iris

These structures are chiefly observed for irregularities and abrasions. The cornea is normally clear and smooth. Shining a flashlight from the side can sometimes reveal these defects. Clouding or opaqueness of the cornea is considered abnormal.

Pupils

Normal pupils are round and of equal size. Pupils normally dilate in a darkened environment and constrict in

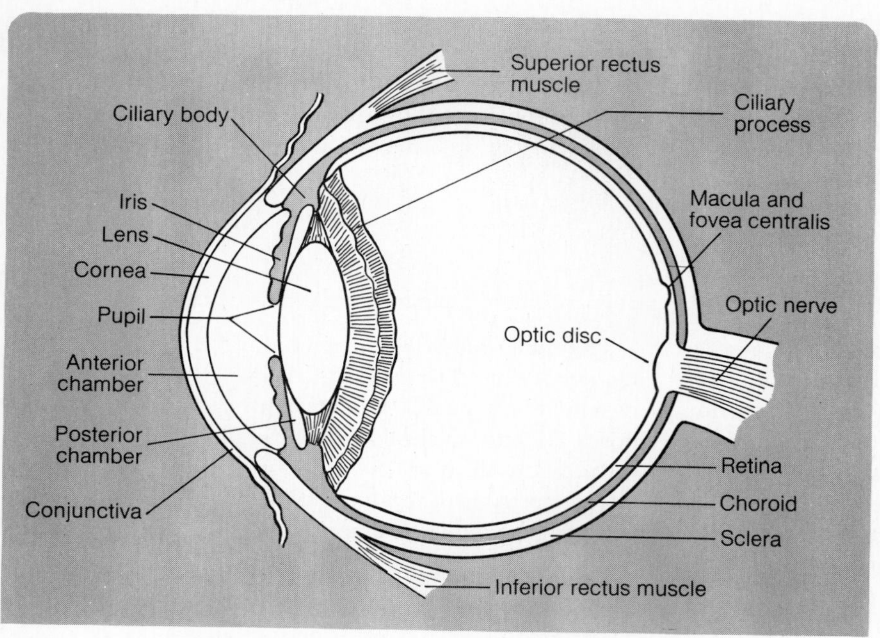

Figure 14–6 The anatomic structures of the right eye.

Figure 14–7 The ophthalmoscope is a lighted instrument used to examine the interior of the eye.

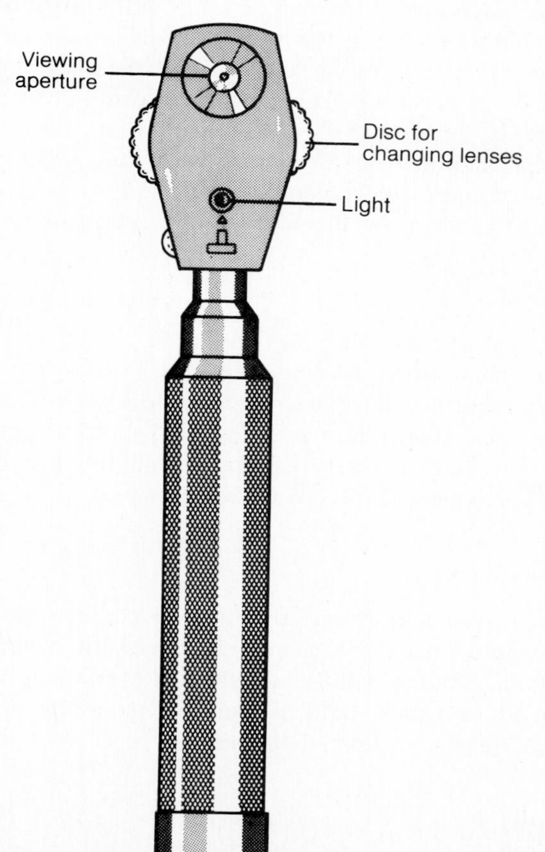

a bright light. Pressure on the brain from, for example, a cerebral hemorrhage can result in uneven pupils, and certain drugs make the pupils constrict regardless of light.

To test the reaction of the pupils, the room is darkened and a flashlight beam is directed from the side into the pupil. Usually the pupil dilates in the darkened room and contracts quickly with the sudden light. When the light shines directly into the pupil, it should constrict quickly; the other pupil should also constrict, but more slowly. This response is called *consensual reaction*. To make sure that the second pupil is not also reacting to direct light, the examiner places a hand on the bridge of the patient's nose.

Fundus

To examine the interior of the eye, the nurse uses an *ophthalmoscope* (Figure 14–7). This instrument focuses a beam of light into the eye. It also has a series of lenses with which the nurse can focus on various parts of the eye.

The room is darkened, and the patient assumes either a supine or sitting position and looks straight ahead without moving the eye. The nurse holds the ophthalmoscope with the right hand and looks with the right eye into the right eye of the patient. The left eye is then used to look into the patient's left eye. Normally, when the light enters the eye the nurse sees a reddish orange reflected light. By changing the focus of the ophthalmoscope, the nurse should be able to see each structure of the eye clearly. If there is a pathologic condition that interferes with the passage of the light, for example, a cataract, the nurse will see dark lines.

Funduscopic examinations may be deterred on infants until age 2 to 6 months unless other assessments, such as the neurologic examination, suggest pathologic conditions. For proper visualization a *mydriatic* is required. Generally the drops are instilled three times before the test at 15-minute intervals. The baby can lie supine on the examining table or be held on an adult's lap or upright over one shoulder. The optic disc of infants is paler than that of adults, and edema of the optic disc is rare even with increased intracranial pressure, since the sutures and fontanelles are not ossified and will permit fluid collection.

Retina

The retina of the eye has certain features that the nurse needs to identify during assessment. The optic disc is the central point on the retina. The sensor organs come together at this point, forming the optic nerve, which goes to the brain. The optic disc is normally a flat, round, white or grayish area. When there is increased intracranial pressure, the disc may appear to bulge or push forward into the eye.

Blood vessels can also be seen on the retina. The arterioles appear red, while the venules are reddish purple. They are normally distributed over the retina forming wide curves. In some pathologic conditions, they may appear narrowed in places and tortuous. See Figure 14–8 for a normal ocular fundus.

The macula of the eye will also be seen lateral to the disc. It is yellow and most readily seen in brunettes, whose retinas are normally darker red than those of fair persons. The cones are most greatly concentrated at the macula; thus it is the point of maximum visual acuity and the point of central vision.

Usually the structures of the eye and abnormalities are described by their position on an imaginary clock. For example, a hemorrhage of the right eye might be described as at "7 o'clock," that is, below the disc, and "out one disc diameter."

Lens and chambers

If the lens is opaque, it appears as a grayish white opacity, often impairing visualization of the retina. Bleeding into the posterior eye chamber may also give a reddish haze to the structures in the eye.

In middle-aged and elderly adults, eyesight often deteriorates. This is frequently due to an opacity of the lens, called a *cataract*. *Presbyopia* (ineffective powers of accommodation) occurs as a result of hardening of the lens. *Hyperopia* (farsightedness) commonly occurs in middle age.

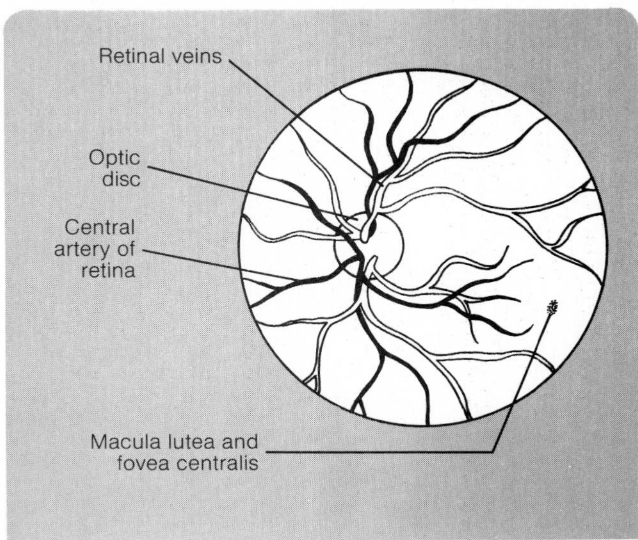

Figure 14–8 The fundus of a left eye.

Intraocular pressure

Intraocular pressure is the pressure of the fluid inside the eyeball. Pressure is commonly tested by a tonometer after the eye is anesthetized. The examiner places the tonometer against the cornea and takes the pressure. A normal intraocular pressure is 10 to 30 mm Hg.

Visual Acuity

The ability of the person to see can be tested with the Snellen chart. With children 3 years or older, a Snellen E chart can be used. After children know the alphabet, the regular Snellen chart can be used. Each eye is tested separately.

Visual acuity is stated in terms of the test distance of 20 feet. Normal vision is stated as 20/20. Vision of 20/40 means that the person can read at 20 feet what a person with perfect vision can read at 40 feet. A child's visual acuity changes with age; at 3 years vision is 20/40, at 4 and 5 years it changes to 30/40, and by 6 years it is usually 20/20. During adolescence, myopia tends to increase, often requiring correction by eyeglasses.

Eye Movement

The eyes normally move synchronously to the right and left, upward and downward, and diagonally. All children over 6 months of age require screening tests to detect *strabismus*, commonly referred to as squint or crossed eyes. In strabismus, the eye movements are not coordinated and deviate from the normal visual axis. Some deviations are readily apparent; others are very subtle and detectable only when the child's eyes are fatigued.

The *cover test* assesses subtle strabismus. The child is asked to focus the eyes on an object about 1 foot away and to keep the eyes very still for the duration of the test. The nurse then holds a card in front of one eye for several seconds, removes it quickly, and observes the eye that was covered. This test is repeated for the other eye and can be repeated for both eyes focused on a more distant object. If the eye jerks after the cover is removed, some strabismus exists.

Ears

There are three major aspects of assessment of the ears: first, observation of the external ear structures, ear canal, and tympanic membrane; second, a test of hearing acuity; and third, a test of balance.

External Ear

The external structures of the ear can be observed for skin lesions, pus, and blood. The nurse uses an otoscope to view the external canal. This lighted instrument has a funnel-shaped part that is inserted into the external auditory canal. To insert the otoscope, one must straighten the ear canal. The auricle of an adult is pulled upward and backward. The auricle of an infant is pulled downward. See Figure 14–9.

The otoscope lets the nurse observe cerumen in the canal as well as the tympanic membrane. The latter appears as a light gray, translucent membrane. Any abnormalities of the tympanic membrane such as perforations, scars, bulging, and discharges need to be reported. Figure 14–10 shows a normal tympanic membrane.

A child must be carefully restrained during otoscopic assessment. Infants under 1 year of age can lie on their backs on the examining table with their heads turned to one side and their arms placed over their heads. An adult holds the child's arms securely at the elbows. The nurse then leans over the infant's chest and examines the ear with both hands. Young children sit on an adult's lap, with their legs restrained between the adult's knees and their arms restrained against their chest. The adult uses the free hand to hold the child's head against the adult's chest. Older children generally cooperate when standing or sitting.

Hearing

Hearing acuity can be tested roughly with a wristwatch. The nurse's hearing is compared to the patient's, if the nurse's hearing is normal. A watch is held to the patient's ear and slowly withdrawn until the patient can no longer hear the ticking. This distance is then compared to the distance at which the nurse can no longer hear the watch.

Figure 14–9 Straightening the external auditory canal: **A,** infant; **B,** adult.

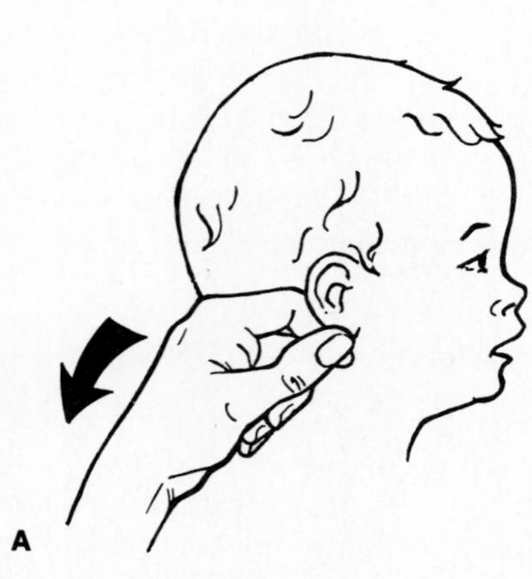

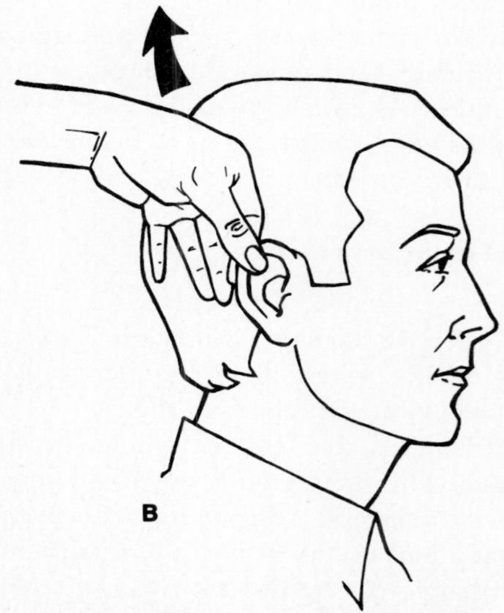

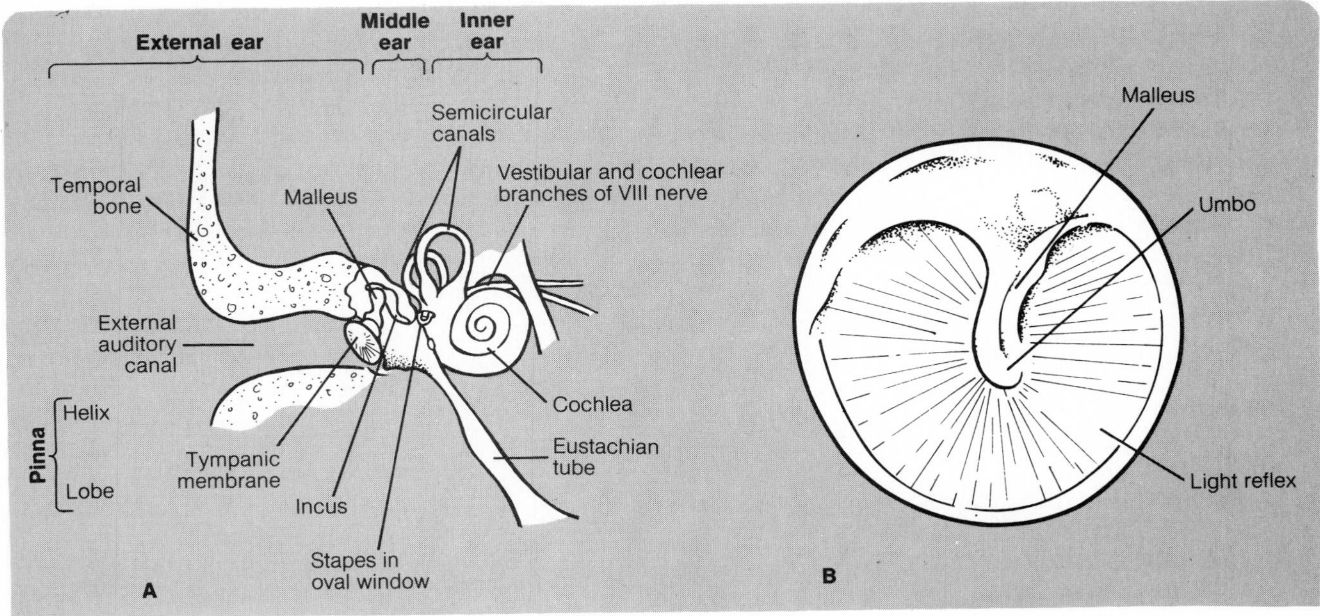

Figure 14–10 The ear: **A,** anatomic structures; **B,** right tympanic membrane.

Rinne's test compares air conduction to bone conduction, one ear at a time. The nurse places the narrow end of a vibrating fork against the mastoid bone behind the ear. When the patient can no longer hear the fork, the pronged end is immediately placed in front of the auditory meatus, where the tone should be heard approximately twice as long. When air-conducted sound is heard twice as long as bone-conducted sound, the test is interpreted as *Rinne positive* (AC>BC). Otherwise the test is *Rinne negative* (AC≤BC), a sign of conductive loss due to impaired sound transmission through the auditory canal, tympanic membrane, and ossicular bones to the cochlea and auditory nerve.

Weber's test assesses bone conduction by testing lateralization of sounds. A softly tuned vibrating fork is placed on the midline of the patient's forehead, and the patient indicates in which ear the sound is heard loudest. If the sound is heard in the affected ear, the patient has conductive loss; if in the unaffected ear, a sensorineural (perceptive) hearing loss.

Balance

A common test for balance is the Romberg test. For further discussion see the section on the cerebellum later in this chapter.

Nose

The nurse can examine the nasal passages very simply with a flashlight, but observes the external nares for crusts or discharges beforehand. Also, the nurse assesses the size, shape, and symmetry of the nose. Observation of the nasal passages can then be carried out. The patient tips the head back, and the examiner shines the flashlight in each nostril. Sometimes the otoscope is inserted carefully into each nostril. The otoscope should never be forced if an obstruction is encountered. The nurse notes obstructions as well as discharges in the nostrils. The mucous membrane is normally pink. Color variations, such as the redness of inflammation or the grayness of an allergy, are also noted.

Normally the nasal septum lies in the midline dividing the two nasal passages. The inferior and middle concha and the middle meatus are observed for color, exudate, swelling, and polyps. See Figure 14–11. Any deviation or protuberance of the septum is noted. After this, the nurse assesses the openness of the passage by pressing one side of the nose so that one nostril is closed and then asking the patient to close the mouth and breathe out through the other nostril. The nurse assesses the other nostril in the same way and notes obstructions in either passage.

The examiner palpates the sinuses for tenderness by pressing up on the frontal and maxillary sinuses. See Figure 14–12. Frontal and maxillary sinuses are illu-

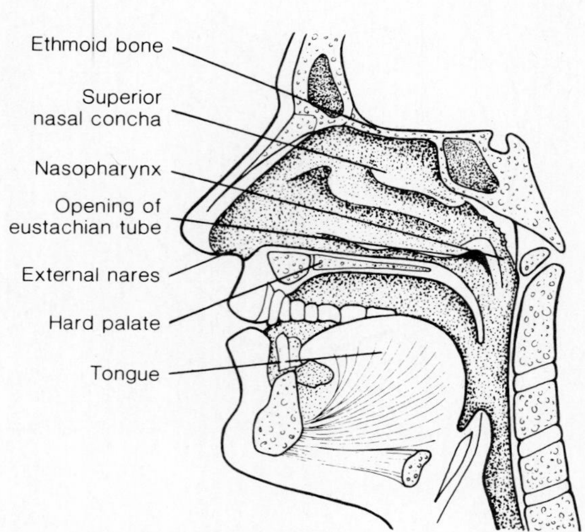

Figure 14–11 Anatomic structures of the nasal cavity.

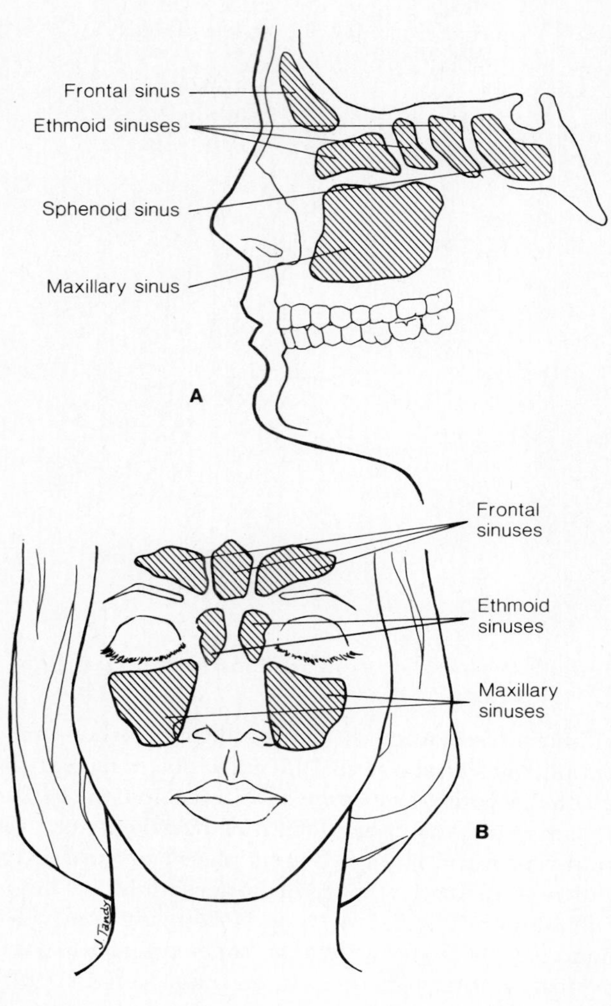

Figure 14–12 The facial sinuses: **A,** lateral view; **B,** frontal view.

minated in this way: In a darkened room, the nurse places a flashlight against the inner aspect of the supraorbital ridge of the frontal bone to illuminate the frontal sinus. Normally, the light shines through the bone and outlines the sinus. To illuminate the maxillary sinus, the nurse places the flashlight in the patient's mouth and directs the beam first to one side of the hard palate and then to the other. The patient closes the mouth around the flashlight during this examination.

Mouth and Pharynx

First, the nurse observes the lips for color and moisture and notes abnormalities, such as undue redness, swelling, and crusts. A tongue depressor and a flashlight or otoscope are used for detailed observation after the patient removes dentures, if necessary. The examiner uses a tongue depressor or gloved finger to retract the lips and cheeks. The mucous membranes are observed for ulceration, bleeding, swelling, redness, and, in some instances, pus. The teeth are observed for discoloration and caries. A foul odor in the patient's mouth can indicate an infective process.

The tongue should lie in the midline of the mouth. When the patient sticks out the tongue, it should remain on the midline and not have a tremor. The tongue is assessed for color, moisture, and lesions. Normally, the top of the tongue has a velvety appearance given by the tastebuds and small furrows. The tongue of a dehydrated person may have deep furrows that run anterior to posterior.

The examiner should assess the parotid and submaxillary (submandibular) salivary glands. The openings of the parotid glands are opposite the second upper molar, and the submaxillary glands open on the floor of the mouth at the base of the tongue. See Figure 14–13.

The nurse palpates the glands with a gloved finger and notes enlargements. Slight compression should produce a flow of clear saliva. The absence of saliva flow sometimes indicates an obstruction in the salivary duct.

The throat or pharynx is also observed. Often the throat is best viewed one side at a time to avoid initiating the gag reflex. The nurse places the tongue depressor at the back and side of the tongue while the patient sticks out the tongue. The mucous membranes should be pink and smooth, and the uvula should be in the midline. Behind the fauces on each side is a tonsil. See Figure 14–13. The presence of pus or large amounts of mucus is noted; they might be evidence of an infection in the nasopharynx or sinuses.

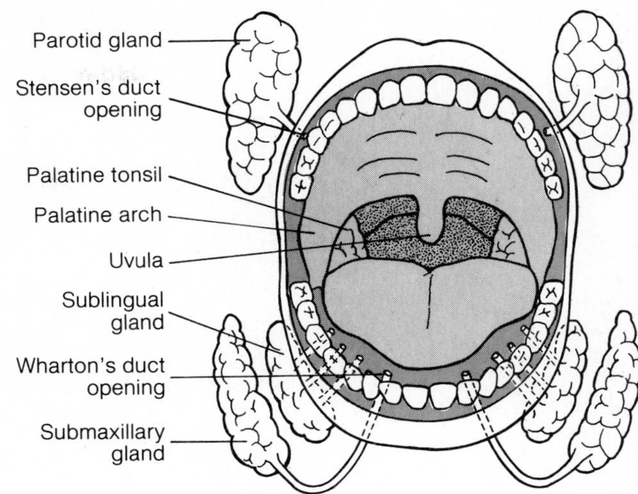

Figure 14–13 Structures of the mouth.

Thorax and Lungs

To assess the chest, the nurse examines the thorax, lungs, heart, breasts, and axilla. The nurse uses observation (inspection), auscultation, palpation, and percussion during the chest examination. The patient removes all clothing to the waist and assumes a sitting position.

Inspection

The chest is inspected for posture, shape, and symmetry of expansion.

Posture

The patient's posture is important to note. Some people with chronic respiratory problems tend to bend forward or even prop their arms on a support to elevate their clavicles. This posture is an attempt to expand the chest fully and thus breathe with less effort.

Shape

In the infant, the thorax is rounded; that is, the diameter from the front to the back (anteroposterior, A-P) is equal to the transverse diameter. It is also cylindrical, having a nearly equal diameter at the top and the base. When a child reaches 6 years, the anteroposterior diameter has decreased in proportion to the transverse one. In adults, the thorax is oval. Its anteroposterior diameter is two times smaller than its transverse diameter. The overall shape of the thorax is elliptical; that is, it has a smaller diameter at the top than at the base. In the elderly, kyphosis and osteoporosis alter the size of the chest cavity as the ribs move downward and forward.

The shape of the chest is assessed from the front, sides, and back. There are several deformities of the chest. See Figure 14–14. *Pigeon chest* (pectus carinatum), a permanent deformity, is caused by rickets. Pigeon chest is characterized by a narrow transverse diameter, an increased anteroposterior diameter, and a protruding sternum. A *funnel chest* (pectus excavatum), a congenital defect, is the opposite of pigeon chest in that the sternum is depressed, narrowing the anteroposterior diameter. Because the sternum points posteriorly in patients with a funnel chest, abnormal pressure on the heart may result in altered function. A *barrel chest*, in which the ratio of the anteroposterior to lateral diameter is 1 to 1, occurs normally in some short, stocky persons. Barrel chests, however, are also seen in patients with thoracic *kyphosis* (excessive convex curvature of the thoracic spine) and *emphysema* (chronic pulmonary condition in which the air sacs, or alveoli, are dilated and distended).

The examiner notes spinal deformities, such as kyphosis or *scoliosis* (lateral deviation of the spine), during examination of the thorax. In addition, the nurse looks for changes in the exterior chest wall, such as bulges caused by cardiac enlargement or neoplasms. Depressions in the chest may be the result of the surgical removal of some ribs.

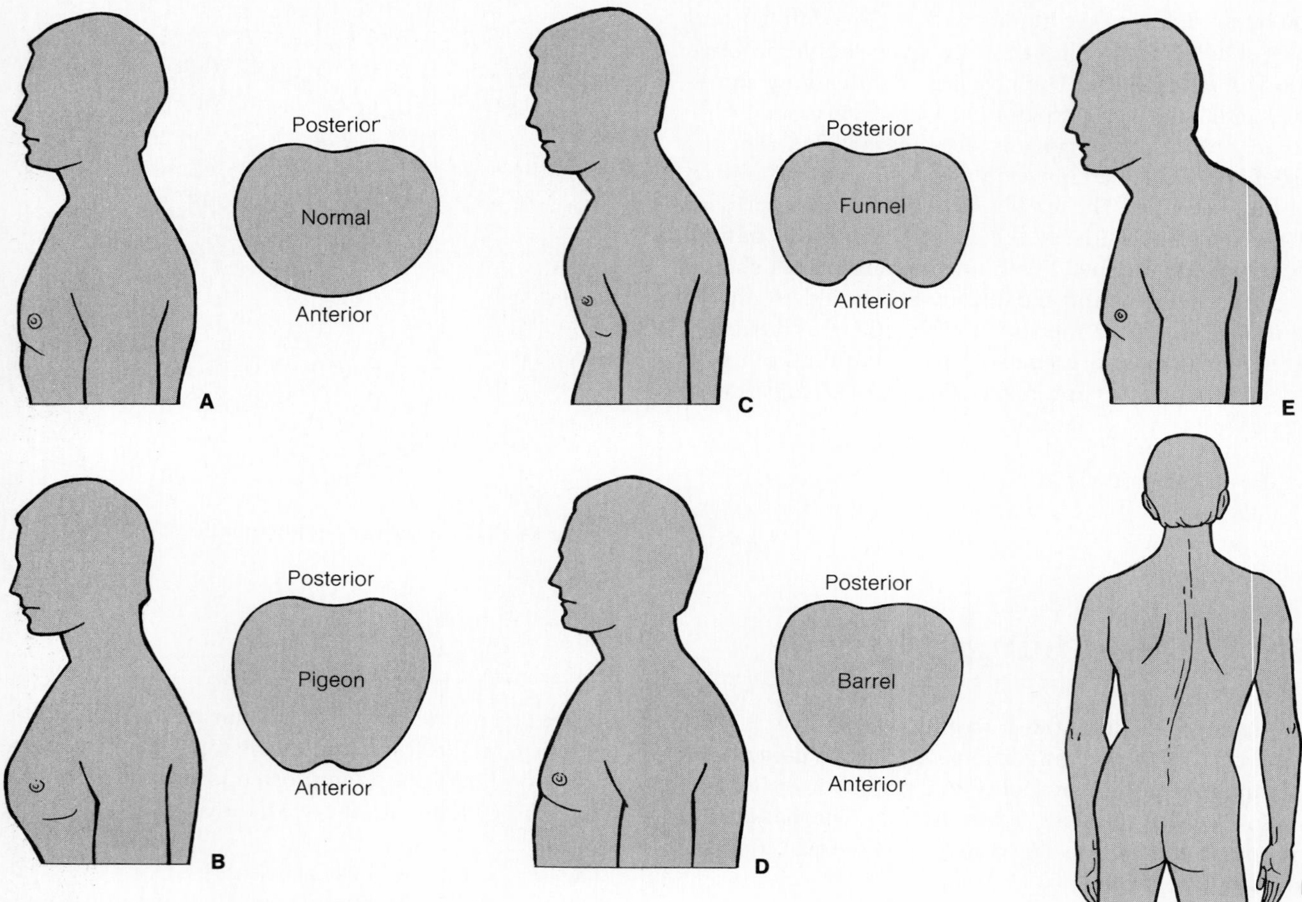

Figure 14–14 Chest shapes: **A,** normal chest; **B,** pigeon chest; **C,** funnel chest; **D,** barrel chest; **E,** kyphosis; **F,** scoliosis.

Symmetry of expansion

The nurse palpates the thorax to assess the symmetry of chest expansion. First, the examiner places both hands on the lower part of the posterior chest with the thumbs adjacent to the spine and the fingers stretched laterally. See Figure 14–15. During a deep inspiration the thumbs normally move an equal distance apart from the spine at the same time. The nurse assesses expansion of the upper thorax in a similar way, and assesses the anterior thorax by placing the fingers laterally along the lower rib cage with the thumbs extending along each costal margin and pointing to the sternum. Wide variations between the upper and lower chest expansions are noted. Asymmetry of expansion can be due to such factors as *atelectasis* (collapse of a lung), fractured ribs, or acute pleurisy. During assessment of chest expansion, the nurse notes bulging or retraction of intercostal spaces.

Percussion

When the chest is percussed, the underlying tissues vibrate and produce audible sounds. The denser the underlying tissue, the more it vibrates with percussion. Therefore, a lung filled with air vibrates less than a lung without air. Percussion of the chest enables the nurse to determine (a) the relative amount of air, liquid, or solid material in underlying lung tissue, (b) the positions and boundaries of organs such as the heart and liver, and (c) the excursion of the diaphragm.

Three normal percussion sounds over the thorax are resonance, dullness, and tympany. *Resonance*, the lower-pitched, hollow sound, is produced over normal lung tissue. *Dullness*, a higher-pitched thud, is produced over the heart or liver. *Tympany* is a musical drumming produced over the stomach or intestinal organs that enclose air or gas. See Figure 14–16.

Two abnormal sounds produced by percussion are

hyperresonance and flatness. *Hyperresonance* is a lower-pitched sound than resonance and occurs over a lung portion abnormally filled with air. Hyperresonance may signal severe emphysema or a pneumothorax. *Flatness* is an extreme dullness and therefore is higher pitched. This sound can be simulated by percussing the thigh, which is a totally nonaerated tissue. Some authorities use the term *flatness* to describe the normal sound over the heart or liver. Many, however, consider flatness an abnormality and prefer the term *dullness* to describe the normal percussion sound over the heart or liver.

Any dullness heard over areas that are normally resonant is also considered abnormal. When large amounts of fluid, pus, or blood collect in the lung (alveolar spaces or pleural spaces), percussion produces dullness rather than resonance. Dullness may signal many conditions, among them, pneumonia, pulmonary edema, or tumors.

The percussion technique is discussed in Chapter 5 on page 130. For anterior chest percussion, the patient sits erect; for posterior percussion, the patient sits and leans forward, crossing the forearms and resting them on the thighs so that the scapulae are separated.

The nurse percusses the thorax systematically, starting superiorly and progressing inferiorly. See Figure 14-17. Parallel areas of each side of the chest are percussed at each level, anteriorly and posteriorly, so that one side can be compared with the other. Percussion sounds vary considerably from one patient to another because of variations in the amount of fat, muscle, and bone. The top of each shoulder is percussed as well to assess the resonance over each lung apex. The scapular areas and sternum are avoided, since the skeleton obscures the normal sounds.

The nurse determines the intensity, pitch, and duration of each percussion sound. See Table 14-4 for descriptions of percussion sounds. *Intensity* (amplitude) refers to the loudness or softness of the sound. Areas of normal resonance over aerated lung tissue produce sounds of moderate to loud intensity, while areas over relatively nonaerated tissue produce dull or flat sounds of soft intensity. Areas of hyperresonance and tympany are loud. *Pitch* refers to the number of vibrations per second or the frequency of vibrations. Vibrations are rapid in dense areas, such as over the liver and heart, resulting in high-pitched sounds. Slow vibrations occur over normal lung tissue and produce low-pitched sounds. *Duration* refers to the length of time a sound is heard. Resonance produces longer sounds than dullness and tympany. Any asymmetry of percussion sounds warrants further assessment, since percussion provides a gross assessment only.

The location of the heart and the liver is determined

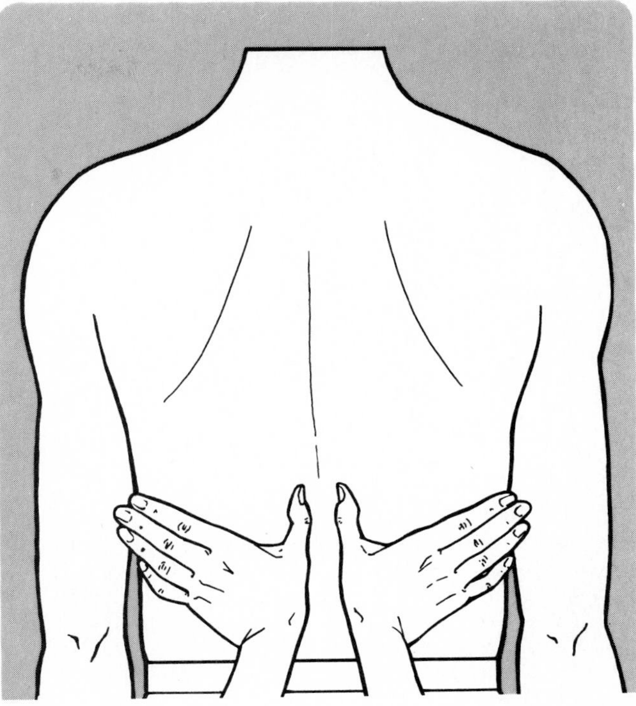

Figure 14–15 The position of the hands on the posterior chest to test for symmetry of chest expansion.

Figure 14–16 Normal percussion sounds of the thorax.

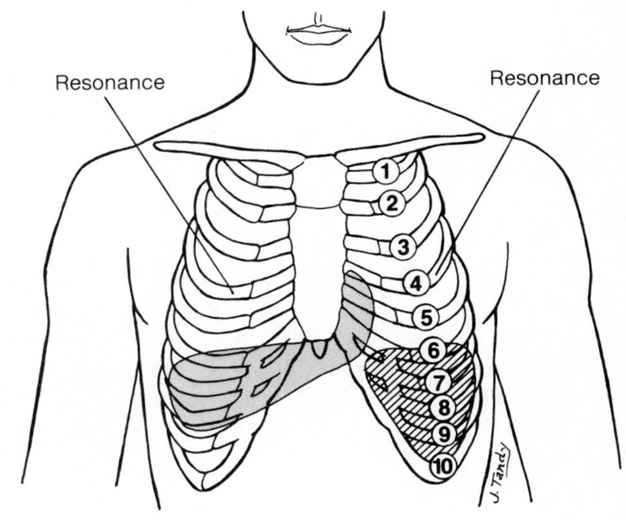

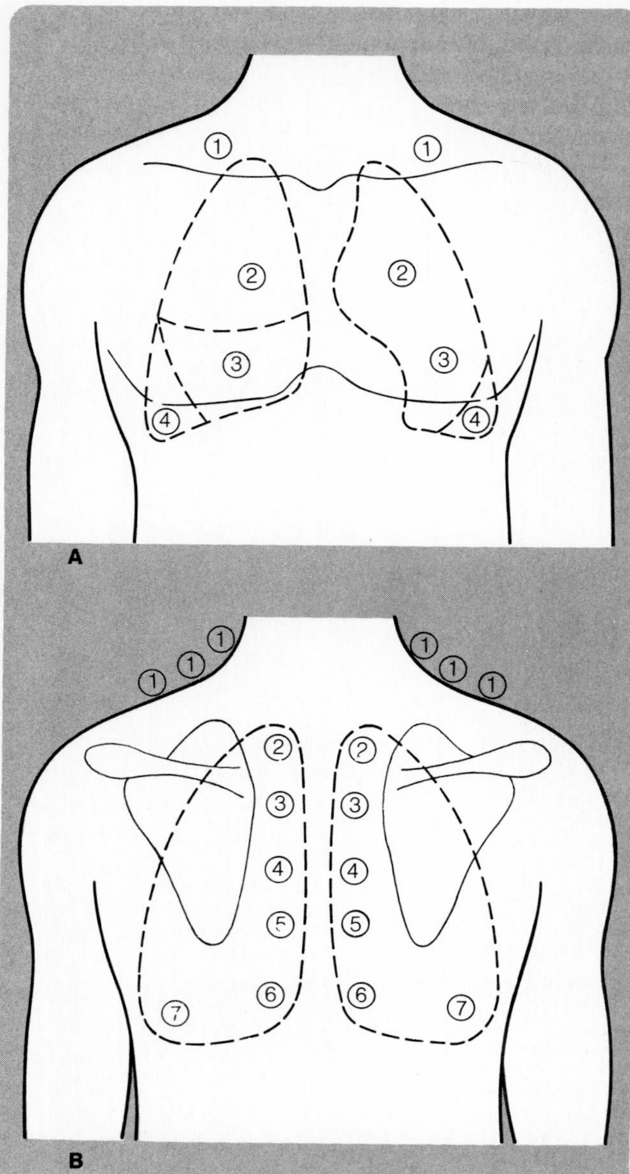

Figure 14–17 Chest percussion sequence on the: **A,** anterior chest; **B,** posterior chest.

by percussing the anterior chest. The upper border of the liver is normally at the right fourth or fifth intercostal space and is found readily by percussing down from the right midclavicular line. See page 310. The heart location is discussed later in this chapter.

Excursion of the diaphragm is determined by percussing the posterior chest. Normal excursion is 3 to 5 cm in females and 5 to 6 cm in males. The nurse notes the difference between the levels of dullness during a deep inspiration and a deep expiration. The patient is asked to hold in a deep breath while the nurse percusses downward until the quality of the percussion tone changes from resonant to dull. This area is then marked on the chest. The patient is then asked to exhale completely and not draw breath again until the nurse repeats the percussion procedure and marks the place where the tone changes.

Auscultation

Lung sounds include breath sounds, voice sounds, and adventitious sounds (abnormal sounds). Lung sounds can be heard with or without a stethoscope. Normal breathing is quiet; but using a stethoscope, the examiner can hear breath sounds as soft air vibrations. Some sounds can be heard only with a stethoscope.

When auscultating the chest, the examiner, particularly if a beginning student, should be in a quiet room. The nurse listens for the character and quality of the breath sounds and of the whispered voice as well as for adventitious sounds.

Breath sounds

Normal breath sounds are of three major types: vesicular, bronchial, and a combination of the two, bronchovesicular.

The *vesicular sounds* can be likened to a sigh and/or a soft, quiet rustle or swish. These sounds are produced in the alveoli and the terminal bronchioles and are therefore heard over most lung areas during respiration. Vesicular sounds are loudest during inspirations

Table 14–4 Percussion Sounds

Sound	Intensity	Pitch	Duration	Example of location
Resonance	Loud	Low	Long	Normal lung
Dullness	Medium	Medium	Moderate	Liver, heart
Tympany	Loud	High (distinguished mainly by musical timbre)	Moderate	Stomach filled with gas (air)
Hyperresonance	Very loud	Very low	Very long	Infant's lung or emphysematous lung

because the flow of air is more rapid and because the air is transported into smaller and smaller channels. Expiration is more passive and one and one-half times longer than inspiration and creates less air turbulence and less sound.

The *bronchial sounds* are loud, harsh, hollow blowing sounds heard normally over the trachea and major bronchi; that is, along the vertical line below the neck over the sternum. They are louder during expiration.

The *bronchovesicular sounds*, which are a combination of the two, are heard over parts of the chest where a bronchus is near lung tissue, in the upper anterior chest on each side of the sternum or posteriorly between the scapulae.

When assessing breath sounds, the nurse first warms the diaphragm of the stethoscope in the palms of the hands and then places it firmly against the patient's chest wall. The patient is asked to breathe quietly with the mouth open. (Deep breathing converts vesicular sounds into bronchovesicular sounds.) The patient breathes with open mouth to prevent the interference of sounds produced in the nares and nasopharynx. The chest is auscultated systematically, much as the chest is percussed. See Figure 14–18 for the auscultation sequence.

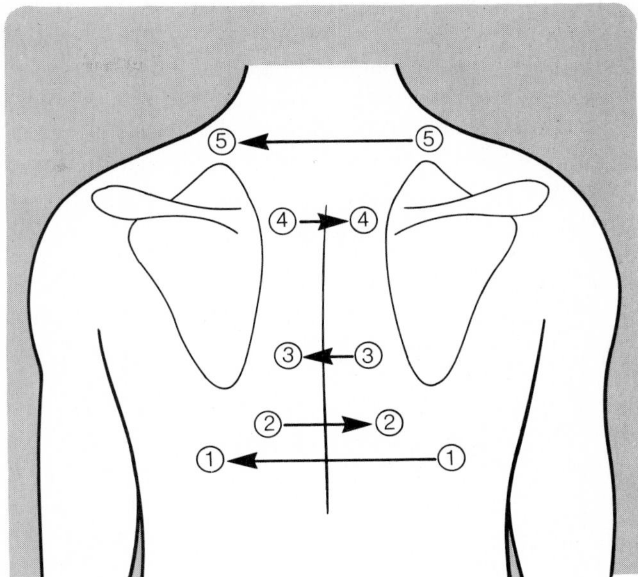

Figure 14–18 Auscultation of the posterior chest.

Voice sounds

Voice sounds are assessed only when lung pathology is suspected. Talking produces vibrations in the larynx, which are transmitted through the respiratory system to the chest wall. These vibrations are referred to as *vocal resonance* when heard with a stethoscope or *tactile* or *vocal fremitus* when felt by the palms of the hands during palpation. Voice sounds are best heard or felt in the superior portion of the chest wall rather than at the base. Audibility varies among individuals and is more pronounced in males and people with thin chest walls. Normally, when a person repeats a phrase (e.g., "ninety-nine, ninety-nine"), the examiner hears muffled sounds and cannot distinguish the words spoken. Sounds normally decrease in intensity and clarity as they pass through the bronchi and alveolar tissue. If the sounds are loud and the words distinguishable, the finding suggests consolidation of the lung tissue, that is, that the lung tissue has become more solid. Consolidation facilitates transmission of sound and can be due to an infectious process such as pneumonia.

To determine tactile fremitus, the nurse places the palms of the hands and fingers symmetrically against the chest wall. Four major areas are assessed: posterior chest, anterior chest, right and left lateral thoracic areas, and the apices. The nurse asks the patient to count or to say (not whisper) a few words. Normally, the nurse feels a mild vibration. Fremitus should be felt equally on each side. Any increase, decrease, or absence needs to be noted. Fremitus increases when lung tissue is consolidated. Decreased or absent fremitus means that air is not conducted and may signal that a bronchus is obstructed or that the pleural space is thickened or enlarged with fluid or air, such as in a pneumothorax.

To determine vocal resonance, the nurse uses a stethoscope and assesses the same four areas assessed for tactile fremitus. Three abnormal voice sounds are *bronchophony* (an increase in vocal resonance), *whispered pectoriloquy*, and *egophony*. Pectoriloquy is exaggerated bronchophony. The patient is asked to *whisper* a series of words, and if heard distinctly, pulmonary consolidation is confirmed. *Egophony* is a type of bronchophony in which the voice has a nasal, bleating quality. The patient is asked to say words with final long *e* sounds, such as *Tennessee*. Egophony causes the long *e* to be heard as long *a*, and the patient says *Tennessay* for *Tennessee*.

Adventitious breath sounds

Descriptions of the adventitious breath sounds, not normally heard over the chest, vary to some degree in the literature. Some of the common sounds, however, are discussed.

Rhonchi *Rhonchi* is a Greek term meaning "wheezing sounds." These sounds are generally heard more prominently during expiration, when the air passages are normally contracted. Rhonchi are continuous, coarse, wheezy, whistling sounds produced in the large bronchi by air passing through mucus and/or narrowed air passages. The pitch varies in accordance with the size of the bronchus. Larger bronchi produce a lower pitch than smaller ones. Any disease process that narrows the lumen of a bronchus—e.g., asthma, tumors, accumulation of mucus, and edema—causes rhonchi.

Rales *Rale* is a French term meaning "a rattle" and is a sound heard chiefly during inspiration. Rales are sounds produced by the bubbling of air through fluid in the alveoli or air passages. They can be described as a shower of bubbling sounds, short and interrupted. The pitch of rales also varies with the location. Those produced in the alveoli are high pitched and sound close to the ear. Those produced in the bronchioles are crackling and lower pitched and are not unlike the fizzing of a carbonated beverage. When rales are heard, the patient should be asked to cough. If the rales are accentuated or do not disappear, fluid accumulation due to congestive heart failure or inflammatory disease such as pneumonia is suspected.

Sometimes rales are also referred to as *creps* or *crepitations.* Some people use the term solely to describe the rales produced in the terminal airways and liken it to the sound of cellophane being crumpled.

Pleural rub The pleural rub is a coarse, leathery, or grating sound produced by the rubbing together of the surfaces of the pleura, and thus it is often referred to as a *friction rub.* It occurs when these surfaces are inflamed and is generally heard over the lower lateral areas of the thorax, particularly the anterior portion, where there is greater chest expansion. It is important that the nurse hold the diaphragm of the stethoscope firmly when auscultating. Sliding the bell can produce artificial sounds similar to a rub. A pleural rub can be simulated by placing the palm of the hand tightly over the ear and then rubbing the back of that hand with one finger of the other hand.

Heart

Heart function can be assessed to a large degree by findings in the history, by symptoms such as shortness of breath, by the patient's general appearance (cyanosis and edema of the legs suggest impaired function), and by pulse rate, rhythm, and quality. Direct examination of the heart, however, offers more specific information, including the heart sounds, the heart size, and findings such as lifts, heaves, or murmurs. Nurses assess heart function through observation (inspection), palpation, and auscultation, in that sequence. Auscultation is more meaningful when other data are obtained first. Procedures are the same for infants, children, and adults.

Inspection and Palpation

The area of the chest overlying the heart is the *precordium.* The nurse inspects and palpates the precordium to determine the presence and extent of normal or abnormal pulsations, which may be seen as the apex beat (impulse), or as lifts or heaves. Heart activity and size are reflected by such manifestations. Both inspection and palpation are carried out while the patient is supine. The nurse stands at the patient's right side.

In the average adult the base of the heart (both atria) lies slightly to the right of the sternum and toward the back, while the apex of the left ventricle lies to the left of the sternum and points forward. The apex touches the anterior chest wall at or medial to the left midclavicular line (MCL) and at or near the fifth left intercostal space (LICS). See Figure 13–4, page 310.

An apical impulse can be seen in about 50% of the adult population. The apical impulse is a good index of cardiac size. If the heart is enlarged, this impulse is lateral to the MCL. The nurse records the distance between the apex and the MCL in centimeters. If the apical beat cannot be observed, the apex may be located by palpation, but not always. The apex of a newborn lies in a more horizontal position than the adult's and can be palpated in the third or fourth intercostal space. It is normal for the apex of infants to be lateral to the MCL. See Figure 13–4, page 310, for apical pulse locations.

An abnormal lift or heave may be noticed in some people. These terms, often used interchangeably, refer to a lift along the sternal border with each heartbeat. A lift occurs when cardiac action is very forceful and should be confirmed by palpation with the palm of the hand. Enlargement or overactivity of the left ventricle produces a heave lateral to the apex, while enlargement of the right ventricle produces a heave at or near the sternum. All pulsations are described by their location in an intercostal space and their distance from the midsternal, midclavicular, or axillary lines.

Auscultation

Several heart sounds can be heard by auscultation. Only the first and second heart sounds will be emphasized in this text. The normal first two heart sounds are produced by closure of the valves of the heart.

S_1 and S_2

The first heart sound (S_1) occurs when the atrioventricular (A-V) valves close. These valves close when the ventricles have been sufficiently filled. Although the right and left A-V valves do not close simultaneously, the closures occur closely enough to be heard as one sound (S_1), a dull, low-pitched sound.

After the ventricles empty their blood into the aorta and pulmonary arteries, the semilunar valves close, producing the second heart sound (S_2). S_2 has a higher pitch than S_1 and is also shorter. These two sounds, S_1 and S_2, occur within 1 second or less, depending on the heart rate.

Associated with these sounds are systole and diastole. Diastole is the period in which the ventricles are relaxed. It starts with the second sound and ends at the subsequent first sound. Systole is the period in which the ventricles are contracted. It begins with the first heart sound and ends at the second heart sound. Systole is usually shorter than diastole. Normally no sounds are audible during these periods.

When auscultating the heart, the nurse stands at the patient's right side. The patient assumes two positions, the upright and the recumbent positions, for the examination. Certain sounds are more audible in certain positions. The nurse then places the stethoscope on the patient's chest and auscultates the entire precordium.

Although the two heart sounds are audible anywhere on the precordial area, they are heard best over specific valve areas. See Figure 14–19. These areas are the tricuspid valve area, which is near the lower sternum; the mitral valve area, which is located at the cardiac apex; the aortic valve area; and the pulmonic valve areas. The aortic area is located in the second right intercostal space (RICS) near the sternal border, and the pulmonic area is in the second LICS at the sternal border.

Auscultation should not be limited to these areas. The nurse needs to locate these areas and then move the stethoscope to find the most audible sounds for each particular patient. Both sounds need to be distinguished in every area of auscultation. It is also necessary when auscultating to concentrate on one particular sound at a time in each area: the first heart sound, then the second heart sound, followed by systole, and then diastole.

Normally both cardiac sounds are heard loudest in the aortic area. S_2 is distinctly louder. The intensity or loudness of the sounds is described as normal, absent, diminished, or accentuated. The quality of sounds can be described as sharp, full, booming, or snapping.

Best results are achieved if the nurse auscultates systematically, starting at the aortic area, then the pulmonic, the tricuspid, and the mitral. A stethoscope with a bell and a diaphragm attachment are needed for adequate auscultation. The bell attachment transmits lower-pitched sounds best, while the diaphragm transmits the higher-pitched sounds best. The bell attachment should be used for the tricuspid and mitral valve areas. The heart sounds heard over these valve areas are described and compared in Table 14–5.

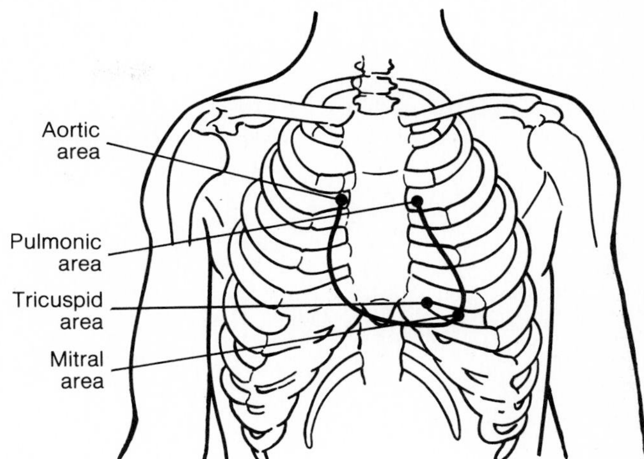

Figure 14–19 Placements of the stethoscope to auscultate for heart sounds.

In infants the first heart sound is usually louder than the second heart sound at the apex. Murmurs are frequently heard at the left sternal border because of the newborn's changing circulatory system. Repeated follow-up is required to assess abnormalities. Other cardiovascular signs such as respirations, color, and pulses will usually confirm any abnormality. Note in Table 14–5 that S_2 is usually louder in the pulmonic area in children and young adults and that by about age 30 most adults have a louder S_2 in the aortic and pulmonic areas. As part of the auscultation procedure, therefore, the loudness of S_2 should be compared between the aortic and pulmonic areas. When the pulmonic S_2 is louder than the aortic S_2 in adults over age 40, the finding is abnormal. The loudness of S_2 in the pulmonary area relates to the blood pressure in the pulmonary artery, while the loudness of S_2 in the aortic area relates to the arterial blood pressure in the systemic circulation. Thus when the pulmonary artery pressure increases, as in patients with some chronic obstructive lung diseases, the loudness of S_2 pulmonic also increases. In contrast, the S_2 aortic sound is louder than normal in patients with hypertensive disease.

Cardiac murmurs

Murmurs result when blood flow becomes turbulent within the heart due to valvular defects or abnormal openings between the compartments of the heart. Not all murmurs indicate cardiac disease. Murmurs are

Table 14–5 Heart Sounds

Sound	Description	Area: *Aortic*	*Pulmonary*	*Tricuspid*	*Mitral*
S_1	Dull, low-pitched and longer than S_2	Less intensity than S_2	Less intensity than S_2	Louder than S_2 or equal	Louder than S_2 or equal
S_2	High-pitched, snappy, and shorter than S_1	Louder than S_1	Louder than S_1 in children and young adults; abnormal if louder in adults over 40	Less intensity than S_1 or equal	Less intensity than S_1 or equal
Systole	Normal silent interval between S_1 and S_2				
Diastole	Normally no sounds; interval between S_2 and next S_1				

described in relation to their location of maximum intensity, quality (e.g., loud, harsh, rumbling), and timing according to the phase of the cardiac cycle. Diastolic murmurs are usually considered abnormal. Murmurs relating to the valves are usually heard over the valvular areas.

Breasts

The breasts of men, women, and children need to be examined. Men and children have some glandular tissue beneath each nipple, while mature women have glandular tissue throughout the breast. The breasts of newborns may be slightly enlarged due to maternal hormones. This usually disappears in a few days. During adolescence, asymmetrical development is not unusual, and boys may have some breast development in early adolescence.

During pregnancy, both breasts become enlarged. In the 2nd month the areolae normally become raised, pigmented, and edematous. It is not unusual for some colostrum to be expressed from the breasts during the 3rd month. During a breast examination, the nipples are observed for discharge, crusting, edema, retraction, and disease. Although retraction is not necessarily indicative of any disease process, it needs to be noted.

The breasts are observed for size, shape, and position, and then the two breasts are compared according to these criteria. Size varies according to age, heredity, endocrine functions, and amount of adipose tissue.

Breasts must also be palpated for masses. Women today are encouraged to palpate their own breasts regularly. Women are advised to examine their own breasts at least once a month, preferably after menstruation or on the first day of the calendar month if they are not menstruating. For information on breast self-examination, see Chapter 33, page 874. Nurses can use the technique described in Chapter 33 to examine a patient's breasts.

Axillae

The axillae are usually examined for enlarged lymph nodes, infections, and bulges.

To palpate the axillae, the nurse helps the patient relax the arm, perhaps by resting it on a table. The nurse presses the fingers as far up toward the apex of the axilla as possible and brings them downward, pressing against the chest wall. Nodes in the central area of the axilla and toward the thorax may be palpated in this manner. The central nodes are the most readily palpable. If the thoracic nodes are palpable and/or either group of nodes feels enlarged, this finding is reported. The procedure is then repeated on the other axilla.

Abdomen

There are a number of organs in the abdominal cavity, some of which extend beyond the normal boundaries of the abdomen. There are two ways to describe relative locations in the abdomen: by quadrants or by nine areas. To divide the abdomen into quadrants, a vertical line is made from the xiphoid process to the pubic symphysis, and a horizontal line is drawn across the umbilicus. These quadrants are labeled upper left quadrant, upper right quadrant, lower right quadrant, and lower left quadrant. See Figure 14–20. The second method, division into nine areas, uses two vertical lines that extend superiorly from the midpoints of the inguinal ligaments and two horizontal lines, one at the level of the edge of the lower ribs and the other at the level of the iliac crests. See Figure 14–21.

Generally the following structures lie in the quadrants:

Right upper quadrant: liver, gall bladder, kidney at the back, part of the colon and small intestine

Left upper quadrant: stomach, pancreas, spleen, kidney at the back, part of the colon and small intestine

Left lower quadrant: colon, rectum, and urinary bladder

Right lower quadrant: colon, appendix, rectum, and urinary bladder

Nurses use four methods to examine the abdomen: observation, auscultation, palpation, and percussion. The patient is supine, with a pillow under the head and the knees slightly flexed and supported by another pillow.

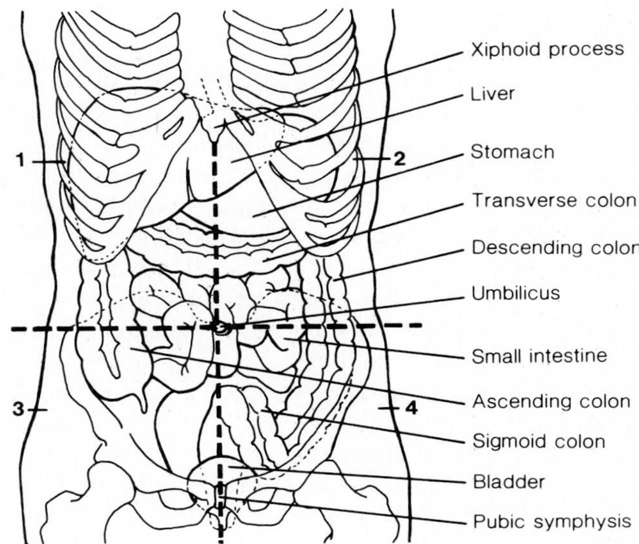

Figure 14–20 The four abdominal regions and the underlying organs: **1,** right upper quadrant; **2,** left upper quadrant; **3,** right lower quadrant; **4,** left lower quadrant.

Figure 14–21 The nine abdominal regions: **1,** epigastric; **2, 3,** left and right hypochondriac; **4,** umbilical; **5, 6,** left and right lumbar; **7,** suprapubic or hypogastric; **8, 9,** left and right inguinal or iliac.

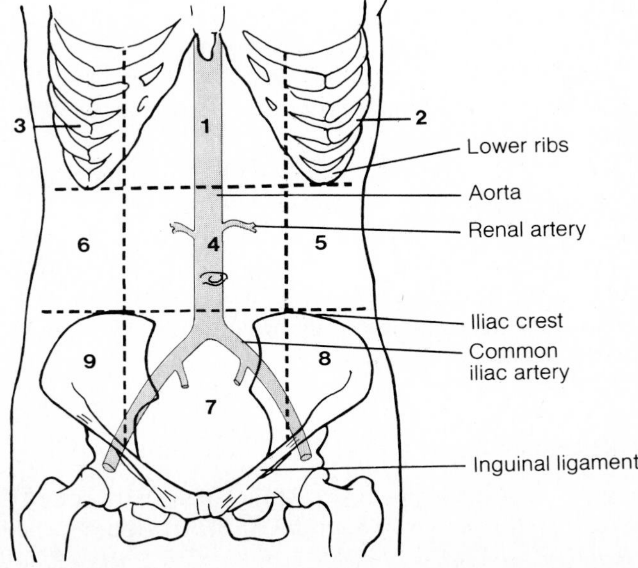

Observation

The abdomen is observed for skin rashes, lesions, scars, and generalized or localized swelling. Examiners should not touch the abdomen during observation.

In the newborn it is normal for the abdomen to protrude slightly due to the undeveloped abdominal muscles. The abdomen of a standing child normally protrudes, but the protuberance disappears when the child lies down.

Normally the abdomen is flat; in the obese adult, however, the abdomen assumes a rounded appearance. Localized swellings may indicate a hernia. These are most common above and below the inguinal ligaments, along the midline, and near any scars from previous operations.

Normally, peristalsis of the intestines cannot be observed through the abdominal wall; however, in acute intestinal obstruction, waves may be seen. This finding is abnormal and needs to be reported.

It may be possible to see the fetus move during the later stages of pregnancy.

Auscultation

There are two abdominal sounds for which the nurse must listen: bowel sounds and vascular bruits. In the pregnant woman fetal sounds are also assessed. A *bruit* is a murmur or sound, which is frequently abnormal.

Using a stethoscope, the nurse can hear bowel sounds in all four quadrants. (It is important to warm the stethoscope before placing it on the abdomen.) These sounds are caused by gas and food moving along the intestines. When the intestine is not functioning correctly, the bowel sounds may be heard at a slow rate, for example, one per minute. This slow rate may signal paralytic ileus, an occasional after-effect of surgery. When the patient has diarrhea, the bowel sounds occur at a very fast rate, perhaps as frequently as every 3 seconds. This is referred to as hypermotility. For further information on assessing bowel sounds, see Chapter 27, page 688.

Bruits

The examiner listens for bruits in each quadrant and along the midline, where a problem of the abdominal aorta may be heard. Bruits may resemble blowing or swishing sounds. Bruits originate in the arteries and veins and are heard by auscultation. They can reflect a partial obstruction of the blood or a particularly turbulent flow of blood, as in an aneurysm. (An *aneurysm* is a dilation of the wall of an artery, vein, or the heart.)

Bruits heard over the epigastric area can mean an aortic aneurysm. Bruits over the lower side quadrants can mean narrowing of the renal arteries. For the locations of the major abdominal arteries, see Figure 14–21.

Fetal heart sounds

About the 5th month of pregnancy, fetal heart sounds can usually be heard. They are assessed with a fetoscope, an instrument like a stethoscope. See Chapter 13 for additional information.

Palpation

Palpation can be either superficial or deep. Before palpation, the nurse must warm the hands. The nurse who performs deep palpation must have short fingernails that will not injure the patient. In superficial palpation the abdominal wall is pressed, but no effort is made to feel more deeply. The nurse palpates the muscle layer with the palmar surface of the four fingers. This layer is normally firm but also yields to pressure. Observed protuberances can also be palpated in this manner for size, hardness, mobility, and tenderness.

Deep palpation is carried out on the entire abdomen to detect tenderness and masses. The nurse presses the fingers more deeply, often using both hands. Each quadrant is deeply palpated, and certain structures are identified.

The liver edge can frequently be detected about 5 cm (2 inches) below the costal margin in the right upper quadrant at the midclavicular lines. While the patient inhales deeply, the nurse presses down firmly with the fingers. If the liver edge is not detected, the nurse and patient repeat the procedure. This procedure should not be painful, although it is normal for the liver edge to be tender to pressure. Pain may signal an inflammation or infection of the liver or the gall bladder or both. The nurse also examines the liver edge to assess its texture—smooth or nodular—and its position in the abdominal cavity.

The nurse should also check in the left upper quadrant for the spleen. It is found in the same manner as the liver; however, a normal spleen is rarely palpable. A diseased spleen may be sufficiently enlarged to feel. In newborns, the tip of the spleen can be felt beneath the left costal margin, and the liver edge is felt about 2 cm below the right costal margin. Children are examined much as adults, but special attention is paid to tenderness in the right lower quadrant (appendicitis) and to protuberances indicative of inguinal hernias.

The kidneys are also not always palpable except in very thin people. See Chapter 28 for a discussion of kidney and urinary bladder palpation.

Tenderness of an abdominal area needs to be carefully assessed and accurately described. It is important to find the point where the tenderness is greatest (point of maximum tenderness).

Percussion

Percussion is used to detect gas, fluid, and/or masses. Abdominal percussion is similar to chest percussion. If the urinary bladder is distended, percussion produces dull sounds rather than the normally resonant sounds. However, percussion of the colon when gas is present produces a tympanic sound in contrast to the usually dull sound around the umbilicus. Tympany over the gastric area is also normal.

Percussion can help the nurse assess the size of the

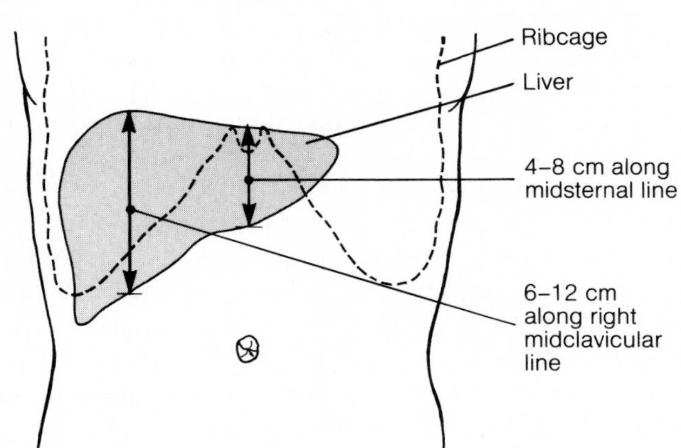

Figure 14–22 The position of the liver in relation to the right midclavicular line and the midsternal line.

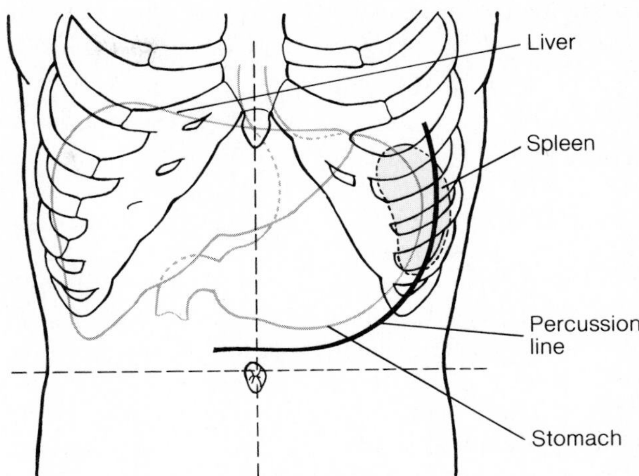

Figure 14–23 The position of the spleen and its percussion line.

liver and the spleen. The nurse begins percussion in the right upper quadrant and moves downward along the midclavicular line (see Figure 14–22) to locate the upper border of the liver. The liver produces a dullness upon percussion, usually at about the fifth to seventh intercostal space. Percussion continues downward until it produces tympany, indicating the lower liver border. The liver is normally about 6 to 12 cm (2.3 to 5 in), averaging 10 cm (4 in), along the midclavicular line. If the liver extends further than 10 cm it is often enlarged. The liver normally descends about 2 cm (0.75 in) in the abdominal cavity when the patient inhales deeply.

To percuss the spleen, the nurse has the patient assume a right lateral position. The spleen then falls in front of the stomach and the colon. The nurse starts percussion in the left lower thorax and moves through the left upper abdominal quadrant to the right upper quadrant in a slightly diagonal direction. See Figure 14–23. Percussion above the spleen produces a dull sound. Normally, the spleen is about 7 cm (2.8 in) long and under the left lower ribs.

For a discussion of abdominal percussion to assess fluid levels, see Chapter 27, page 689.

Genitals and Rectum

Infants, Children, and Adolescents

Nurses assess the genitals of newborns for normalcy. Nurses examine newborn boys to check that a urinary meatus is on the glans penis and that the meatus is patent. The testes are also palpated within the scrotum. Undescended testes are noted. Normally, both testes have descended at birth. The vaginal orifice of newborn girls is also inspected. Any discharge is noted and recorded, although a reddish discharge may be normal. The first rectal temperature is taken with particular care in case the anus is closed (imperforate anus).

Nurses need to play close attention to problems involving the genitals of children. Bed wetting may be the result of a urinary infection or anxiety. Young boys' scrotums are palpated to check for descended testicles. The external genitals of the female child are usually inspected, but a pelvic examination is usually not performed.

During assessment of male adolescents it is most important to establish the descent of the testicles into the scrotum; undescended testes are noted. Assessment of adolescent girls is limited to an inspection of the external genitalia unless the girl is sexually active. If so, a Papanicolaou test (Pap test) is advised once a year to detect cancer of the cervix and uterus. See the following section for information about taking a specimen for a Papanicolaou test. If the adolescent is sexually active and has an increased or abnormal vaginal discharge, specimens should be taken to check for sexually transmitted disease.

Adult Female Genitals

To examine the genitals of the adult female, the nurse helps the woman assume a lithotomy position either in bed or on an examining table, where she can place her feet in stirrups. For a lithotomy position, the patient lies on her back with the knees flexed and the hips externally rotated. The patient's hips are usually brought down to the bottom end of the examining table to expose the perineal area. Appropriate draping and a pillow for her head help make the patient comfortable. Some women prefer to have the head of the bed elevated to 35°.

The external genitalia are first examined for lesions, rashes, inflammation, and swelling. Any discharge such as pus or blood is noted.

A vaginal speculum is required for a thorough assessment of the vagina and cervix. The size of the speculum used depends on the size of the vagina. Women who have had children probably need a large speculum; elderly women and very young women require a small speculum; and women who have not had children need an average speculum.

The nurse dons gloves, warms the speculum for the patient's comfort, and lubricates it to ease insertion. The speculum can be lubricated with water or a lubricant unless the latter is contraindicated because it would harm the quality of a specimen to be taken. The nurse inserts the speculum with the blades closed and pointing upward. When the blades are in the vagina, the nurse turns the speculum handle down and opens the blades. See Figure 14–24 for the parts of the vaginal speculum.

Figure 14–24 A vaginal speculum used to examine the vagina and cervix.

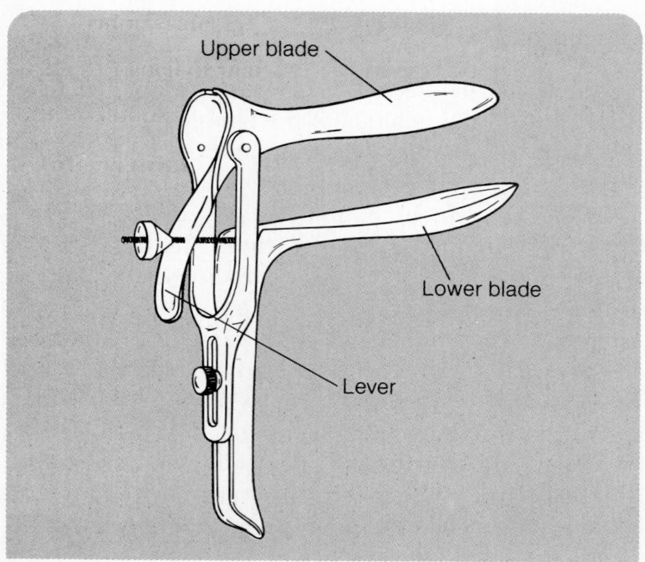

A flashlight helps the nurse observe the color, shape, and firmness of the cervix. Normally, it is pale pink, round, smooth, and firm in the nonpregnant woman. At this time a specimen is usually taken for a Papanicolaou smear.

The Papanicolaou test, often referred to as a Pap smear or a cytologic examination, was developed by Dr. George Papanicolaou to detect cancer of the cervix. Now the test is also used to detect early cancer of the gastrointestinal, respiratory, and renal tracts and occasionally cancer of the breast. The Papanicolaou test is also used currently to assess a patient's response to chemotherapy and radiation therapy. The specimen required may be cervical scrapings, bronchial secretions obtained during a bronchoscopy, urine sediment, sputúm, aspirated gastric secretions, or fluid discharged from the mammary glands.

Once obtained, the specimen is placed on a slide, which is then fixed by immersion in equal parts of a water and ethyl alcohol (95%) solution. The slide is dried, stained, and examined under a microscope for sloughed-off cells. The results of the smear are reported on a five-point scale: class I, normal; class II, probably normal; class III, doubtful; class IV, probably malignant; and class V, malignant.

The nurse removes the speculum after the smear and examines the internal organs manually. (In some settings, the manual examination is carried out before the speculum is inserted.) Usually the nurse puts gloves on one or both hands and lubricates the tips of the first and middle fingers. With the fourth and fifth fingers curled into the palm and the thumb stretched out, the nurse inserts the two lubricated fingers into the vagina. The nurse raises the arm so that the fingers follow the vagina, which angles backward.

The cervix can be palpated readily. Usually a finger cannot enter the cervical canal; if it does enter, this fact is noted and recorded.

With the other hand on the patient's abdomen (bimanual examination) and pressing by starting below the umbilicus and working downward, the nurse can feel the fundus of the uterus with the fingers in the vagina. The fundus is generally anterior to the cervix. It is normally mobile and has a smooth, regular surface. Its size should also be noted.

The fallopian tubes and ovaries can also be palpated. The hand on the abdomen presses about midway on the inguinal ligament, and the hand in the vagina presses to the right or left and toward the abdominal wall to detect each ovary. The size of the ovary, its firmness, and the regularity of the surface of the ovary are assessed. If the ovary feels tender to the patient, the nurse records the fact.

Usually a fallopian tube cannot be palpated; however, any enlargement is reported. The nurse then removes the hand from the vagina, takes off the glove, and helps the patient to a comfortable position.

Pelvic examination of the woman may provide evidence of pregnancy. Three signs are (a) Goodell's sign, (b) Chadwick's sign, and (c) Hegar's sign. See Chapter 12 for information about these signs.

Adult Female Rectum and Anus

During examination of the rectum and anus, the female patient can remain in a draped, dorsal recumbent position with her knees flexed. See Figure 14–25.

First the nurse inspects the anus for protruding hemorrhoids (distended veins, which appear as red bodies), fissures, and cracks. When the patient bears down as if to defecate, other hemorrhoids may become visible.

To palpate the anus and rectum, the nurse puts on a glove and lubricates the index finger. The nurse asks the patient to bear down and slips the lubricated finger through the anus into the anal canal. The muscle around the anus will tighten, but this should not be painful to the patient. The nurse moves the finger up the rectum to palpate both the anterior and the posterior walls and checks for masses. See Figure 14–26. The nurse describes masses by their location, size, firmness, mobility, smoothness, tenderness, and regularity.

The nurse can palpate the cervix from the anterior wall of the rectum. It should feel smooth, round, firm, and movable and should not be tender to palpation. During pregnancy, the cervix becomes larger and softer. After the rectal examination, the nurse removes the glove, washes hands, and records the observations.

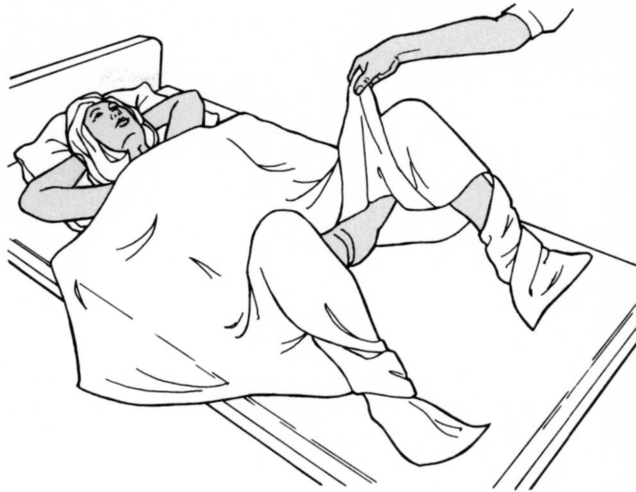

Figure 14–25 A dorsal recumbent position with knees flexed and hips externally rotated.

Adult Male Genitals

Nurses wear gloves when examining the male genitalia to prevent infection of nurse or patient. The reason for gloves needs to be explained tactfully to the patient.

The male pubic area is examined for the absence or thinness of the pubic hair. Missing hair can be indicative of cirrhosis of the liver or other problems. Normally, pubic hair does not grow on the penis, but at the base of the penis.

The nurse examines the penis for lesions, swellings, and discharges. The foreskin (prepuce) of uncircumcised males is drawn back to expose the glans, which is normally reddish. Ulcers, particularly on the glans or just inside the urinary meatus, are noted. The nurse can usually open the meatus by applying slight pressure near the tip of the glans.

The scrotum usually has loose, wrinkled skin. Palpated testes are normally oval, firm, smooth, and freely movable within the scrotum. The testes are usually 4 cm (1.5 in) long and 2.0 to 2.5 cm (0.8 to 1 in) wide, varying from one end to the other, like a chicken egg. The epididymis can be felt at the lower aspect of the testis and extends along the posterior surface. The spermatic cord can also be palpated. It extends from the superior pole of the testis upward and enters the inguinal canal and subsequently the abdominal wall.

The nurse observes the scrotum for lesions and palpates the testes for swelling, masses, and inflammation, noting the size, mobility, position, firmness, and surface

Figure 14–26 Anatomic structures of the female reproductive tract with index finger inserted for examination of the rectum.

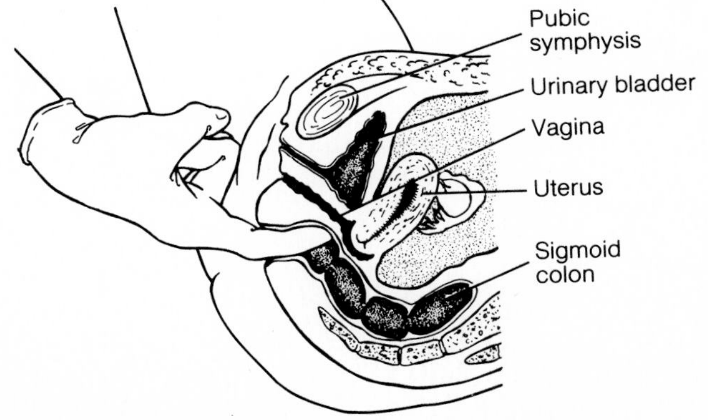

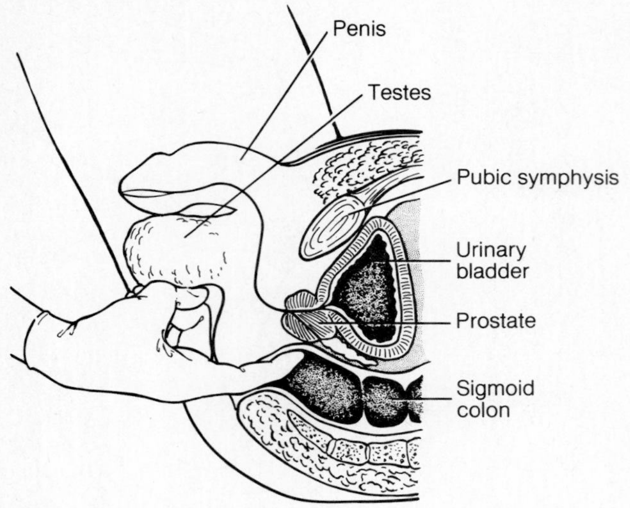

Figure 14–27 Anatomic structures of the male reproductive tract with the index finger inserted to examine the rectum.

regularity of masses. The nurse palpates the inguinal region for enlarged lymph nodes by pressing the fingers along a line from the base of the penis up toward the crest of the ilium. Any weakness should also be noted at this time as a sign of a possible inguinal hernia.

Adult Male Rectum and Anus

For this examination the patient can assume one of several positions. The most comfortable one is probably a lateral position with the upper leg acutely flexed. The anus of males is inspected much as the anus of females: the nurse inserts a gloved finger into the rectum for the rectal palpation. The prostate gland can be palpated on the anterior wall of the rectum. See Figure 14–27. Each lobe of this gland is felt for masses, consistency of size of the two lobes, firmness, and tenderness. It is important to examine the rectal wall for nodules or masses.

Extremities

General Assessment

The extremities (the arms and legs) are inspected, palpated, and moved. First the skin is observed. The limb is assessed for any unusual joint angle, which could indicate a current or old bone fracture. The joints are next moved to assess range of motion. See the discussion of movement of the joints in Chapter 24. The joints are also assessed for size and redness. The nurse notes complaints of pain by the patient.

Muscles are observed for tremors or unsteadiness. A fine tremor can sometimes be observed by asking the patient to extend the arms toward the front for a few minutes. Each extremity is observed.

The feet and legs are also observed for shape, color, and edema (excess fluid). The swelling may be tense and hard, stretching the skin, or it may be possible to press the skin and produce an indentation that disappears in a few minutes. The latter is called *pitting edema*. The nurse inspects the legs for varicose veins—distended, bluish veins, which may be tortuous and lumpy and tender to the touch.

Until about 2 years of age a child will appear somewhat bowlegged. For additional information about the feet, see Table 23-2, page 562.

Reflexes

A *reflex* is an automatic response of the body to a stimulus. See Chapter 11 for a discussion of reflexes normally present at various ages.

Figure 14–28 Testing the biceps reflex.

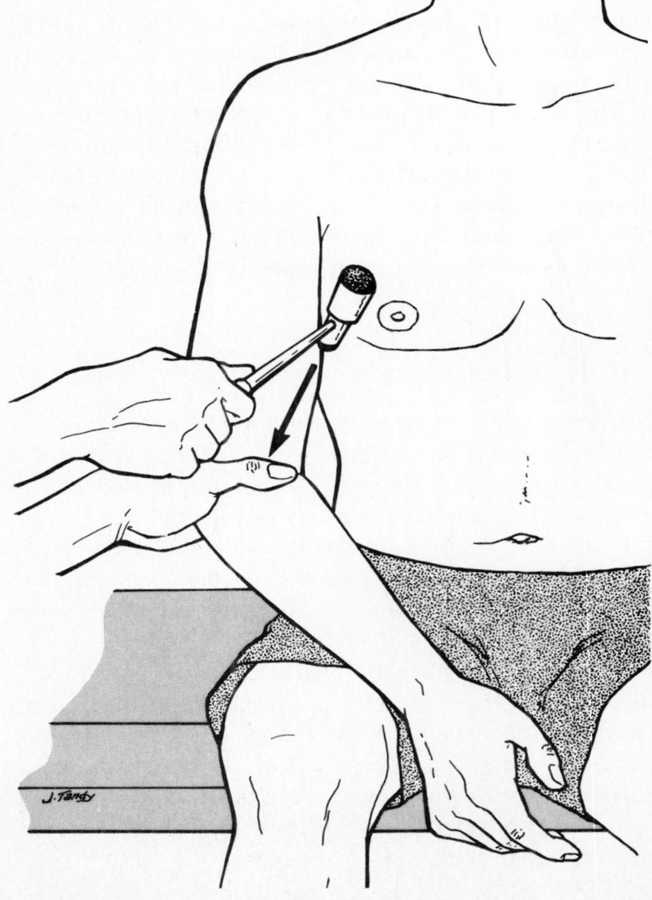

Reflexes are tested using a percussion hammer. They are described on a scale of 0 to + + + +. 0 means no reflex, + is minimal activity (hypoactive), + + is a normal reflex, + + + is more active, and + + + + means maximum activity (hyperactive). It is important to compare one side of the body with the other when assessing reflexes.

Several reflexes are normally tested during a physical examination. These are (a) the biceps and triceps reflex, (b) the patellar reflex, (c) the Achilles reflex, and (d) the plantar reflex.

Biceps and triceps reflexes

The biceps reflex is tested with the nurse's thumb on the biceps tendon while the patient's arm is supported. When the nurse's thumb is tapped with the hammer, the biceps muscle normally contracts noticeably. See Figure 14–28.

In the triceps reflex test, the patient relaxes the arm, which is supported by the nurse. The nurse taps the patient's arm with the hammer just above the olecranon process. Normally, the forearm will straighten. See Figure 14–29.

Figure 14–29 Testing the triceps reflex.

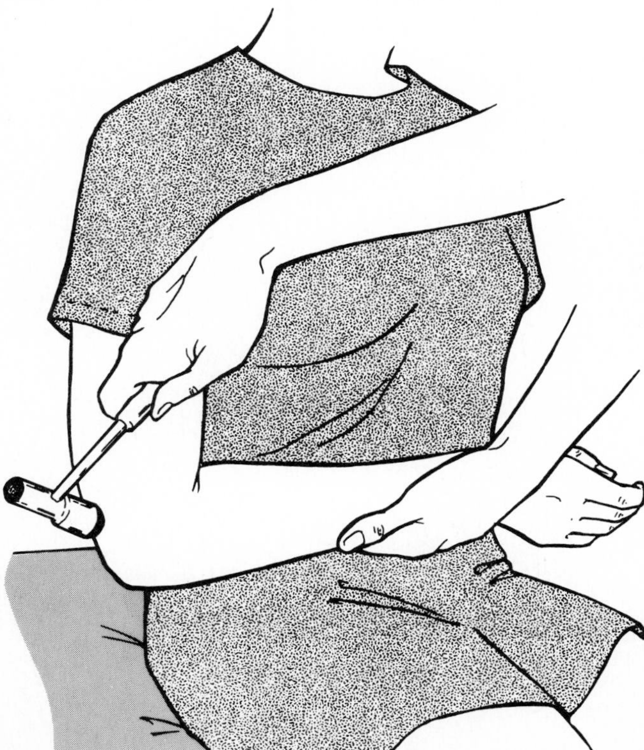

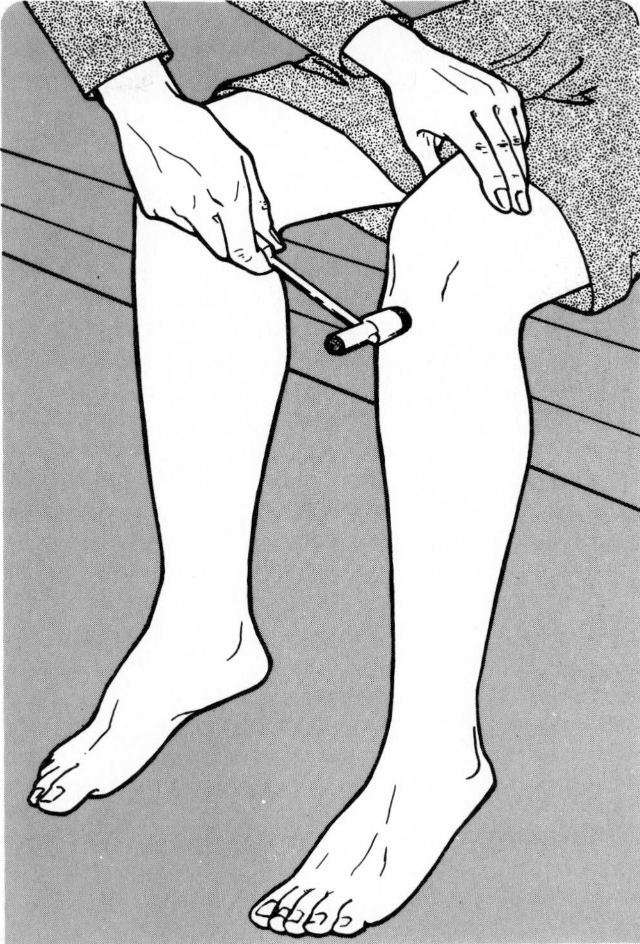

Figure 14–30 Testing the patellar reflex.

Patellar reflex

To test this reflex, the nurse has the patient sit on the edge of a table so that the legs hang freely. The hammer strikes the area just below the patella, and normally the lower leg kicks forward. See Figure 14–30.

Achilles reflex

The patient assumes the position for the patellar reflex test. The nurse supports the toes slightly and taps the Achilles tendon. The normal response is a downward jerk of the foot. See Figure 14-31.

Plantar reflex

To test the plantar or Babinski reflex, the nurse strokes the sole of the foot with a thumb nail or the sharp end of a percussion hammer. See Figure 14-32. Normally, all five toes bend downward; this reaction is negative Babinski. In an abnormal response, positive Babinski, the toes spread outward and the big toe moves upward. Positive Babinski is abnormal after age 1.

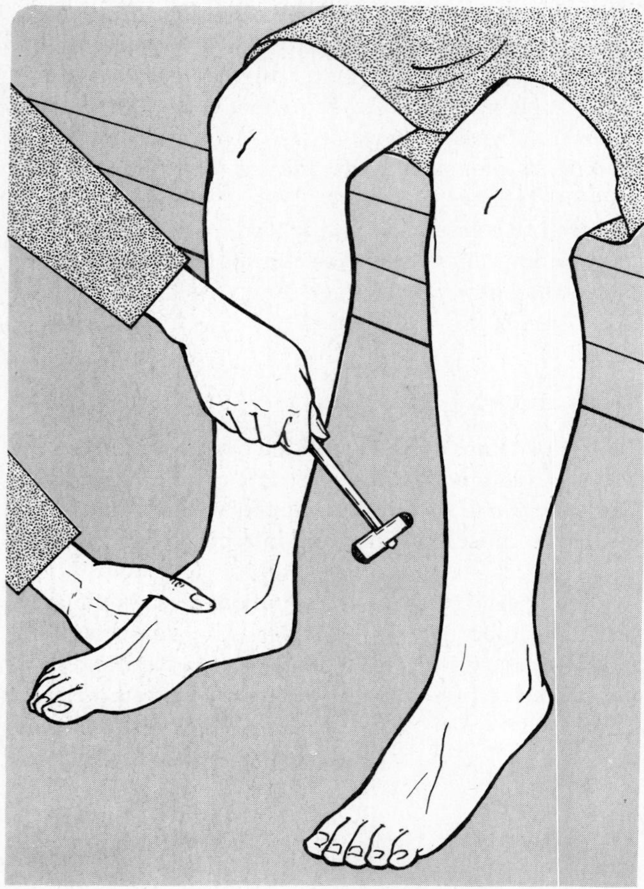

Figure 14-31 Testing the Achilles reflex.

Figure 14-32 Plantar reflex: **A,** the line of stroking; **B,** negative Babinski (normal); **C,** positive Babinski (abnormal).

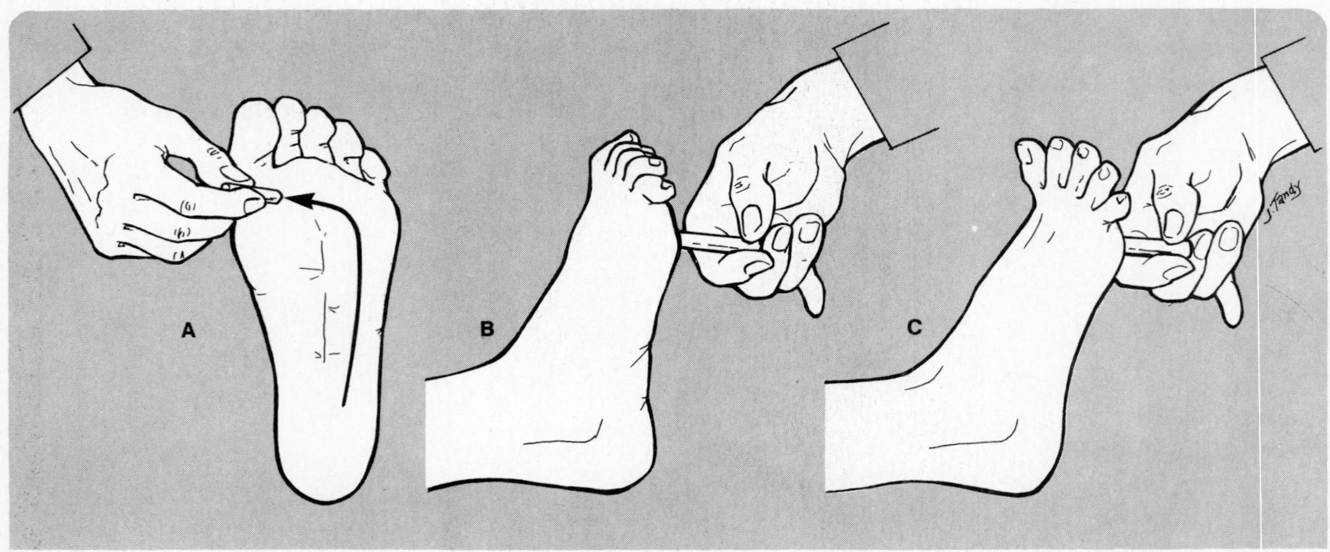

Neurologic and Mental-Emotional Assessment

Neurologic assessment includes examination of the reflexes and the cranial nerves and the functions of the cerebrum, the cerebellum, and the sensory and motor systems. The reflexes have been previously described in the assessment of the extremities.

Cranial Nerves

Assessment of the functions of the twelve pairs of cranial nerves is included to a large degree in an examination of the head and neck. A neurologist usually conducts specific examination of these nerves if needed. However, the routine neurologic assessment of a basic physical examination includes assessment of some of these cranial nerves. For the specific functions of each cranial nerve see Table 14–6. The nurse needs to be aware of these functions to detect abnormalities.

The sense of smell (cranial nerve I) and the sense of taste (cranial nerves VII and IX) are not routinely tested. Vision and eye movements have been previously discussed. These activities involve cranial nerves II, III, IV, and VI. The cranial nerves V (trigeminal) and VII (facial) are not routinely tested other than by observing facial expression and symmetry of facial movements and of the face at rest. Any weakness of the face is made more obvious by having the patient close the eyes tightly, wrinkle the forehead, and show the teeth. Only the cochlear branch of nerve VIII (vestibulocochlear) is routinely tested, that is, hearing ability. The vestibular branch concerned with balance is not routinely tested but will be subsequently discussed as it relates to assessment of cerebellar functions. Swallowing, the gag reflex, tongue movement, and phonation, involving cranial nerves IX, X, and XII, are routinely included in examination of the mouth. Nerves IX and X are tested at the same time. Each side of the pharynx is touched with a tongue blade, and normally, when the pharyngeal muscles contract, the patient gags. Another test is to have the patient say "ah." The soft palate normally moves. Imperfect movement suggests difficulty with nerves IX and X. Nerve XII (hypoglossal) can be readily examined by having the patient protrude the tongue as

Table 14–6 Functions of the Cranial Nerves

Nerve	Name	Type of nerve	Function
I	Olfactory	Sensory	Smell
II	Optic	Sensory	Vision and visual fields
III	Oculomotor	Motor	Extraocular eye movement (EOM) and movement of sphincter of pupil and ciliary muscles of lens
IV	Trochlear	Motor	EOM, specifically moves eyeball downward and laterally
V	Trigeminal	Motor and sensory	
	Ophthalmic branch	Sensory	Sensation of cornea, skin of face, and nasal mucosa
	Maxillary branch	Sensory	Sensation of skin of face and anterior oral cavity (tongue and teeth)
	Mandibular branch	Motor and sensory	Muscles of mastication; sensation of skin of face
VI	Abducens	Motor	EOM, moves eyeball laterally
VII	Facial	Motor and sensory	Facial expression; taste (anterior tongue)
VIII	Vestibulocochlear (acoustic)		
	Vestibular branch	Sensory	Equilibrium
	Cochlear branch	Sensory	Hearing
IX	Glossopharyngeal	Motor and sensory	Gag reflex, tongue movement, taste (posterior tongue)
X	Vagus	Motor and sensory	Sensation of pharynx and larynx; swallowing and phonation
XI	Accessory	Motor	Head movement; shrugging of shoulders
XII	Hypoglossal	Motor	Protrusion of tongue

far as possible. Deviation of the tongue toward either side suggests paralysis. Cranial nerve XI (accessory), which is the motor nerve of the sternocleidomastoid muscle, can be tested by asking the patient to shrug the shoulders while the nurse presses down on them with the hands. Any weakness is noted.

Cerebral Functioning (Mental Status)

The highest functions of the nervous system are carried out in the brain. These functions include intellectual (cognitive) as well as emotional (affective) functions. A large part of the mental status assessment is included in the history taking. If disorders of speech, behavior, memory, or thought are detected, a more extensive examination is required. Some of the major areas of mental assessment follow.

Behavior and appearance

The patient's dress and hygiene, appropriateness of gestures and facial expression, ability to relax and relate to persons and things in the environment, and attentiveness to the nurse all provide clues about mental status. The posture a person assumes and the quality and quantity of speech also provide significant clues. For example, is the patient's posture tense, slumped, or relaxed? Does the patient speak quickly, loudly, clearly, coherently? Speech is a complex act involving the tongue, mouth, palate, larynx, respiratory system, cerebrum, and cerebellum. Thus, disturbances of speech may or may not relate to the nervous system.

Nurses assess newborns and infants by observing the overall appearance, activity, alertness, and the cry. Some postural deviations, such as marked hyperextension of the head, continual turning of the head to one side, stiffness of the neck, or extension of the extremities can indicate severe intracranial problems.

Consciousness

The state of consciousness or level of alertness is often determined at the beginning of the physical examination. It varies from a state of alertness to coma. These levels are assessed by describing the patient's response to various verbal and physical stimuli. See Table 35–1, page 901.

Emotional state

Assessment of the emotional state, mood, or affect is made by observation and by questioning. Appropriate or inappropriate responses throughout the interview are observed. For example, being overly cheerful in response to bad news, laughing while discussing a serious topic, or crying when talking about a pleasant topic are inappropriate affect. The patient's approachability and openness should be noted. Is the patient overly active (euphoric, agitated, or hostile) or underactive (flat or unresponsive)?

The nurse may need to question the patient about mood. For instance, the nurse may ask if the patient sleeps well at night, gets discouraged, feels down, or cries frequently. The patient's answers help the nurse determine whether the patient is depressed. Other questions then may determine the depth of a depression. For example, a nurse may ask whether the patient ever feels life is not worth living or whether things are getting too bad for the patient to cope. Affirmative answers to these questions warrant other questions such as, "Have you ever thought of killing yourself or tried to kill yourself?" and "How did you do it or how do you plan to do it?" By gradually leading up to questions of suicide, the nurse can gauge the depth of depression.

Intellect

Intellectual or cognitive functions include orientation, memory, concentration, calculation, knowledge, judgment, and thought processes.

Orientation The patient's orientation to time, place, and person is determined by tactful questioning. Orientation is easily assessed by asking the patient the city and state of residence, time of day, date, day of the week, duration of illness, and names of family members. More direct questioning may be necessary for some people, such as "Where are you now?" or "What day is it today?" or "What is your name?" These questions are readily accepted by most people if initially the nurse asks, "Do you get confused at times?"

Memory Three categories of memory are tested: immediate recall, recent memory, and remote memory. Immediate recall can be tested by having the person repeat a series of digits spoken slowly, such as 7-4-3-5-6-7-2. Most people recall seven digits easily. Recent memory can be tested by having the patient relate events that occurred that same day, such as how the patient got to the clinic. This information should be validated, however. Also, the nurse can ask the patient to recall information given early in the interview, such as the name of a doctor. Remote memory can be tested by having the patient relate events from the past, such as surgery performed on the patient several years before.

Concentration and calculation The ability to concentrate or attention span can be tested by asking the patient to repeat a series of digits forward and backward. Most adults are able to recall correctly five to eight digits forward and four to six digits backward. Consecutive digits or digits of easily recognized dates (such as 1980) should be avoided in this test. Concentration can also be tested by other tests of varying difficulty, such as having the patient recite the alphabet or count backward from 100.

The ability to calculate can be tested by having the patient subtract 7 or 3 progressively from 100; that is, 100, 93, 86, 79, or 100, 97, 94, 91. This standard test is often referred to as the *serial sevens* or *serial threes* test. Normally one adult can complete the serial sevens test in about 1½ minutes with three or fewer errors. Because calculating ability is affected by educational level and by language or cultural differences, this test may be inappropriate for some. These patients can be asked to add or to subtract small numbers.

Knowledge A patient's knowledge is also influenced by cultural background and education. In addition, it is closely related to memory. A series of questions may be asked, such as "What are the five largest cities in America?" "When are potatoes planted?" or "What are the four seasons of the year?" Vocabulary can also be assessed by asking the patient the meaning of various words such as *extract, imitate, microscope*, and *multiple*.

Judgment To test judgment, nurses ask relatively simple questions and take into consideration the person's cultural background. Direct questions can be asked about what a person would do in certain situations, such as being stopped for failing to observe a stop sign or after breaking a piece of borrowed equipment. Another test is to have the person pick from a series a word that does not relate to the others. For example: large, small, and red; or up, left, and down.

Thought processes When taking the nursing history, the nurse notes the relevance and organization of the patient's thought processes. For example, the patient may appear to be listening to or looking at stimuli undetected by the nurse or display other bizarre behavior. If so, the nurse asks questions to learn whether the patient is hallucinating or having delusions.

Patients with insight recognize that they see or hear things or are aware that their delusions are not justified. Others do not reveal insight, and the examiner can ask whether the patient actually believes the delusions or ever questions the reality of the hallucinations. These questions can elicit anger and the response, "Do you think I'm crazy?" In such cases, it is important that the nurse acknowledge the responses as unusual but avoid telling the patient that he or she is normal or abnormal.

Cerebellum

The center for balance and muscle coordination is in the cerebellum. Many tests can be used to assess normal functioning of this center. A few are outlined below.

Coordination tests

These tests familiar to nurses are referred to as the finger-to-nose test, the alternating motion test, and the heel-to-shin test. For the finger-to-nose test, the patient is asked to abduct and extend the arms at shoulder height and to rapidly touch the nose alternately with one index finger and then the other. The patient repeats the test with the eyes closed if the test is performed easily. In abnormal responses, the patient misses the nose and may bring the finger beyond the nose (past-pointing).

Alternating motions are coordinated by the normal person, but are slow and incorrect in persons with cerebellar dysfunction. For this test, the patient can be asked to use one hand to rub the abdomen with circular movements and the other to pat the top of the head. Another way of examining alternating motion is to have the patient sitting in a chair tap the floor with the toes and at the same time rapidly pronate and supinate the hands.

The heel-to-shin test is carried out while the patient is supine on the examining table. The patient is asked to rapidly move the right heel down the shin bone of the left leg to the left ankle. The patient repeats the test, using the left heel and right leg.

Balance tests

Balance or equilibrium tests are conducted while the patient walks or stands. The nurse notes abnormalities of gait, such as a staggering or unsteady gait not unlike that of intoxicated people. Disequilibirum is best assessed when the patient is standing with the eyes open and the feet together. If the patient does not lose balance or does not begin to fall with eyes open, the patient closes the eyes and repeats the test. It is important to be prepared to help patients who begin to fall. The test conducted with the eyes closed is referred to as *Romberg's sign*. If disequilibrium is noted, the nurse records a Romberg positive.

Sensory System

The sensory functions include touch, pain, vibration, position, temperature, and discrimination. The first three are routinely tested in a few locations. Generally the face, arms, legs, hands, and feet are tested for touch and pain, although all parts of the body can be tested. If the patient complains of numbness, peculiar sensations, or paralysis, sensation should be checked more carefully over flexor and extensor surfaces of limbs. Abnormality of touch or pain should then be mapped out clearly by examining responses in the area about every 2 cm (1 in). This is a lengthy procedure. A more detailed neurologic examination includes position sense, temperature sense, and discrimination.

Superficial touch

The sensation of touch is tested with a wisp of cotton. Because sensitivity to touch varies normally with specific skin areas, it is important to compare the sensation in symmetrical areas of the body, such as the cheeks. The patient is asked to close the eyes and to respond whenever the cotton touches the skin.

Pain

The sharpness or dullness of pain can be tested by using the point and the blunt end of a safety pin. The patient is asked to close the eyes and to say which end of the safety pin is touching. Areas of reduced or heightened sensations should be noted, although responses can be somewhat subjective and difficult to assess. When sensations of pain are dulled, temperature sense is usually also impaired, since distribution of these nerves over the body is similar. Thus, testing sensitivity to temperature may prove more reliable. Distal and proximal areas should be compared.

Vibration

The vibratory sense is tested with a tuning fork held firmly against a bone. Bones commonly used are at the thumb side of the wrist, the outside of the elbow, the ankle on either side, and the knee. Routinely the distal bones of an extremity are tested first. If some impairment is noted, the more proximal bones are also tested. The nurse may test other bones, such as the sternum or the iliac crests.

To perform the vibratory test, a tuning fork is struck fairly hard and held against the patient's chin. The patient should feel the vibration or buzz. Then the wrists and ankles are similarly tested, and the patient states whether he or she feels the vibration and when it stops. The nurse's own responses to the test serve as a comparison. If the nurse believes the patient is confusing the pressure of the fork against the skin with its vibrations, the tuning fork can be struck but placed on the patient only after the vibrations stop; the patient then should not report vibrations.

Position

The patient closes the eyes while the nurse tests the sense of position. Commonly the middle fingers and the large toes are tested. To test the fingers, the nurse supports the patient's arm with one hand and holds the patient's palm in the other. To test the toes, the nurse places the patient's heels on the examining table.

It is important for the examiner to grasp the finger or toe firmly between the thumb and index finger and to exert the same pressure on both sides of the toe or finger while moving it. The nurse moves the finger or toe until it is up, down, or straight out and asks the patient to identify the position. The nurse can use a series of brisk up-and-down movements before coming to rest suddenly in one of the three positions. Normal persons can easily determine the position of their fingers and toes.

Temperature

Temperature sensation is determined by touching the skin with test tubes filled with hot or cold water. The patient identifies which tube feels hot and which cold. If the pain sensation test is normal, it is not necessary to conduct this test.

Discrimination

The ability to discriminate can be tested in several ways. One way is to have the patient discriminate between one- and two-point stimuli. The skin is stimulated alternately with two pins simultaneously and then one pin. Since the fingertips are particularly sensitive, the normal person can differentiate between a one- and two-point stimulus within 2 to 3 mm, while on the chest differentiation occurs at about 75 mm apart.

Another test for discrimination assesses the ability to recognize objects by touching them. This ability is referred to as *stereognosis*. The nurse places familiar objects, such as a key, paper clip, or coin, in a person's hand, and asks the patient to identify them. If the patient has a motor impairment of the hand and is unable to voluntarily manipulate an object, the examiner can write a number or letter on the patient's palm and ask the patient to identify it.

Two other tests of discrimination are referred to as point localization and the extinction phenomenon. Point localization involves having the patient close the eyes and stimulating a point on the skin with a pin. The patient is then asked to open the eyes and point to the place touched. The extinction phenomenon involves the simultaneous stimulation of two symmetrical areas of the body such as the thighs, the cheeks, or the hands. Normally, both points of stimulus are felt.

Motor System

The motor system is assessed by determining the function of the voluntary skeletal muscles, including tonus, size, strength, and involuntary movements.

Tonus

Normally the muscles feel firm and are maintained in a state of slight contraction, that is, they have a normal tone. This tone is maintained by the central nervous system acting through the peripheral nerves. When muscle tone is lacking, the muscles become relaxed, flabby, and weak, and eventually they atrophy, resulting in *flaccid paralysis*. Involuntary movements, such as a localized twitching, are often associated with atrophy and flaccidity. These involuntary movements are referred to as *fibrillations* or *fasciculations*. Normal persons also experience fibrillations periodically, such as the quivering of an arm or the twitching of an eyelid.

Rigidity and *spastic paralysis* refer to muscles that have increased tone; the latter is more severe. The muscles feel firmer and harder than normal. A spastic muscle is difficult to move, springing back sometimes when the examiner lets go of the muscle. A rigid muscle usually offers increased resistance but can be moved with relative ease by the nurse. Sometimes a cogwheel rigidity occurs: The muscle vacillates between increased tone and normal tone.

When assessing muscle tone, the nurse can palpate muscles for firmness and in addition note restrictions in active movement. Various joints of the body can also be passively moved through their ranges of motion. For example, to test the arm muscles, the nurse grasps the patient's wrist firmly with one hand and uses the other to alternately straighten and bend the patient's arm at the elbow. Slight resistance to movement is normal. This procedure is repeated for other joints, such as the fingers, wrist, shoulder, knee, or ankle.

Muscle size

Slight asymmetry in muscle size can be normal. The nurse notes significant asymmetry in corresponding left and right muscle groups, which are observed during assessment of the neck and extremities.

Muscle strength

Muscle power can be tested against gravity or the examiner's resistance. The latter is commonly used. The patient moves each joint in every direction, and the nurse restrains the motions with his or her hands. For example, the patient extends the wrist while the nurse opposes this movement. Muscle strength varies among individuals; therefore, the examiner must use judgment to determine relative weakness. Both extensor and flexor muscle groups should be checked. See Chapter 24 for normal range of joint movements.

Involuntary movements

Abnormal muscle movements can be readily observed in adults. Some terms used to describe abnormal movements are fasciculation, tics, tremors, and athetosis. Fasciculations have been previously described. *Tics* are also twitching of muscles but are repetitive and often occur in the face or upper trunk. *Tremors* are involuntary rhythmic movements. Some tremors are more pronounced on movement or activity; others, at rest. The former are intention tremors; the latter, resting tremors. *Athetosis* refers to involuntary twisting and writhing movements, such as those of patients with cerebral palsy.

Summary

I. General impression
   A. Appearance
      1. Posture
      2. Facial expression
      3. Behavior
   B. Height and weight
II. Skin, hair, and nails
   A. Color
   B. Texture
   C. Temperature
   D. Lesions
III. Head and neck
   A. Skull shape and circumference
   B. Range of neck motion
   C. Lymph nodes
   D. Larynx and trachea
   E. Thyroid gland
   F. Jugular veins and carotid arteries
IV. Eyes
   A. External structures
      1. Eyelash follicles for styes
      2. Eyelids for discoloration, edema, lesions, ectropion, and entropion
      3. Eyeballs for sunkenness or exophthalmos or excessive pressure by tonometry
      4. Conjunctivae for inflammation
      5. Sclera for discolorations
      6. Cornea and iris for irregularities and abrasions
      7. Pupils for reaction

B. Fundus of the eye by ophthalmoscope:
1. Retina
a. The optic disc (normally flat, round, and white or grayish)
b. Blood vessels (arterioles red, venules reddish-purple)
c. Macula (normally yellow)
2. Lens and chamber
a. Opacity
b. Bleeding
c. Intraocular pressure
C. Visual acuity assessed by Snellen charts
D. Eye movements normally synchronous in all directions

V. Ears
A. Visual inspection for skin lesions, pus, or blood
B. Otoscopic inspection
1. Excessive cerumen in ear canal
2. Tympanic membrane (normally light gray and translucent)
C. Hearing acuity
1. Wristwatch test
2. Rinne's test
3. Weber's test
D. Balance

VI. Nose
A. External structures
1. Encrustations or discharges
2. Symmetry
B. Internal structures by a flashlight or otoscope
1. Color of the mucous membrane
2. Position of the nasal septum
3. Patency of the nasal passages
4. Sinuses

VII. Mouth and pharynx
A. Mouth
1. Color, moisture, and character of the lips
2. Status of the oral mucous membranes
3. Condition of the teeth and gums
4. Presence of malodor
5. Tongue movement and appearance
6. Salivary glands
B. Pharynx
1. Condition of the mucous membranes
2. Position of the uvula
3. Appearance of the tonsils

VIII. Chest
A. Thorax and lungs
1. Posture as a clue to respiratory problems
2. Chest shape and symmetry in accordance with age variations
3. Symmetry of expansion by palpation
4. Lung percussion sounds
5. Location of the heart and liver by percussion
6. Lung sounds by auscultation
7. Excursion of the diaphragm by percussion
B. Heart
1. Heart size and location by percussion
2. Heart sounds by auscultation over specific valve areas
3. Presence of cardiac murmurs
C. Breasts
1. Symmetry of size, shape, and positions (asymmetry is not unusual in adolescence)
2. Abnormal discharges
3. Palpation for tumors
D. Axillae
1. Palpation of nodes
2. Palpation for bulges
3. Infections

IX. Abdomen
A. Observation for skin rashes, lesions, scars, and edema
B. Observation for localized swellings or generalized protuberances
C. Observations for contractions during labor or peristalsis during acute bowel obstructions
D. Auscultation for bowel sounds, vascular bruits, and fetal heart sounds
E. Palpations to detect tenderness, masses, and the position of the liver and spleen
F. Percussion to determine the presence of gas, fluid, or masses and the size of the liver and spleen

X. Genitals and rectum
A. Genitals
1. Observation for patency of the urinary meatus in newborns
2. Palpation of the scrotum to check for descent of testes in newborns and boys
3. Observation for abnormal vaginal discharge
4. Papanicolaou smear in mature females
5. Inspections for venereal disease for all adults
6. Pelvic examination for females
7. Palpation of scrotum for masses and swelling
8. Palpation of inguinal canal for lymph node enlargement or hernia in males
B. Rectum
1. Observation for imperforate anus prior to rectal temperature assessment in newborns
2. Inspection of the anus for protruding hemorrhoids or fissures
3. Palpation of anterior wall to assess the prostate gland or the cervix
4. Palpation of rectal walls for nodules or masses

XI. Extremities
A. Inspection of the skin for color and edema
B. Range of joint motions
C. Observation for muscle tremors
D. Observation for varicosities
E. Status of reflexes using a percussion hammer

1. Biceps and triceps reflex
2. Patellar reflex
3. Achilles reflex
4. Plantar reflex

XII. Neurologic and mental-emotional assessment
A. Examination of the reflexes
B. Tests for cranial nerve function
C. Observations of mental status during history taking
1. Behavior and appearance
2. Level of alertness
3. Emotional state
4. Intellect, including orientation, memory, concentration, calculation, knowledge, judgment, and thought processes
D. Coordination tests
1. Finger-to-nose
2. Alternating motion test
3. Heel-to-shin test
E. Balance tests
F. Sensory function tests
1. Superficial touch
2. Pain
3. Vibration
4. Position
5. Temperature
6. Discrimination
G. Motor function tests
1. Tonus
2. Muscle size
3. Muscle strength
4. Observation of involuntary movements

Suggested Activities

1. In a laboratory setting, practice auscultation and percussion of a classmate's chest.
2. Percuss a classmate's liver and spleen and estimate their size.
3. Choose a patient, and, using a stethoscope, assess lung and heart sounds.
4. Using an ophthalmoscope, examine the interior of a classmate's eyes. Make a diagram of your findings.
5. Visit a community health nurse in a school. Observe or note the assessment tests used in this setting.
6. Visit a nursing home. Select an elderly patient and assess his or her emotional and intellectual status.

Suggested Readings

Derbes, V. J. March 1978. Rashes: Recognition and management. *Nursing 78* 8:54–59.
The author has updated his March 1973 article. He discusses rashes nurses may encounter, how to recognize them, and the nurse's role in treatment.

McVan, B., editor. April 1977. What the nose knows: Odors. *Nursing 77* 7:46–49.
This article includes the physiology of the sense of smell, different odors, and their sources. Deodorants are also discussed as well as measures to reduce body odors.

Sloboda, S. September 1977. Understanding patient behavior. *Nursing 77* 7:74–77.
A psychological assessment is described including self-concept, perception, stress, and loss. Listening attentively, being objective, and using open-ended statements are advised.

Yoos, L. May/June 1981. A developmental approach to physical assessment. *Maternal Child Nursing* 6:168–70.
The author describes some guidelines for assessing infants, 9-month to 12-month babies, toddlers, preschoolers, school-aged children, and adolescents. The suggestions are related to the developmental stages of Erikson and Piaget.

Selected References

Alexander, M. M., and Brown, M. S. Physical examination series. Parts 1–18. *Nursing 73, 74, 75,* and *76.*

Bates, B. 1979. *A guide to physical examination.* 2nd ed. Philadelphia: J. B. Lippincott.

Block, G. J.; Nolan, J. W.; and Dempsey, M. K. 1981. *Health assessment for professional nursing: A developmental approach.* New York: Appleton-Century-Crofts.

Derbes, V. J. March 1973. Rashes: Recognition and management. *Nursing 73* 3:44–49.

Gillies, D. A., and Alyn, I. B. 1976. *Patient assessment and management by the nurse practitioner.* Philadelphia: W. B. Saunders Co.

Jarvis, C. M. May 1977. Perfecting physical assessment: Part 1. *Nursing 77* 7:28–37. June 1977. Part 2. 7:38–45. July 1977. Part 3. 7:44–53.

Kahn, H. October 1974. Visual dysfunctions. Some easy tests for detecting them in children. *Nursing 74* 4:26–27.

King, P. A. October 1980. Foot problems and assessment. *Geriatric Nursing* 1:182–86.

McFarlane, J. December 1974. Pediatric assessment and intervention. Some simple how-to's for ambulatory settings. *Nursing 74* 4:66–68.

Malasanos, L.; Barkauskas, V.; Moss, M.; and Stoltenberg-Allen, K. 1981. *Health assessment.* 2nd ed. St. Louis: C.V. Mosby Co.

Murray, R. B., and Zentner, J. P. 1979. *Nursing assessment and health promotion through the life span.* 2nd ed. Englewood Cliffs, N.J.: Prentice-Hall.

Roach, L. B. November 1972. Color changes in dark skins. *Nursing 72* 2:19–22.

Slessor, G. April 1973. Auscultation of the chest—a clinical nursing skill. *The Canadian Nurse* 69:40–43.

Chapter 15

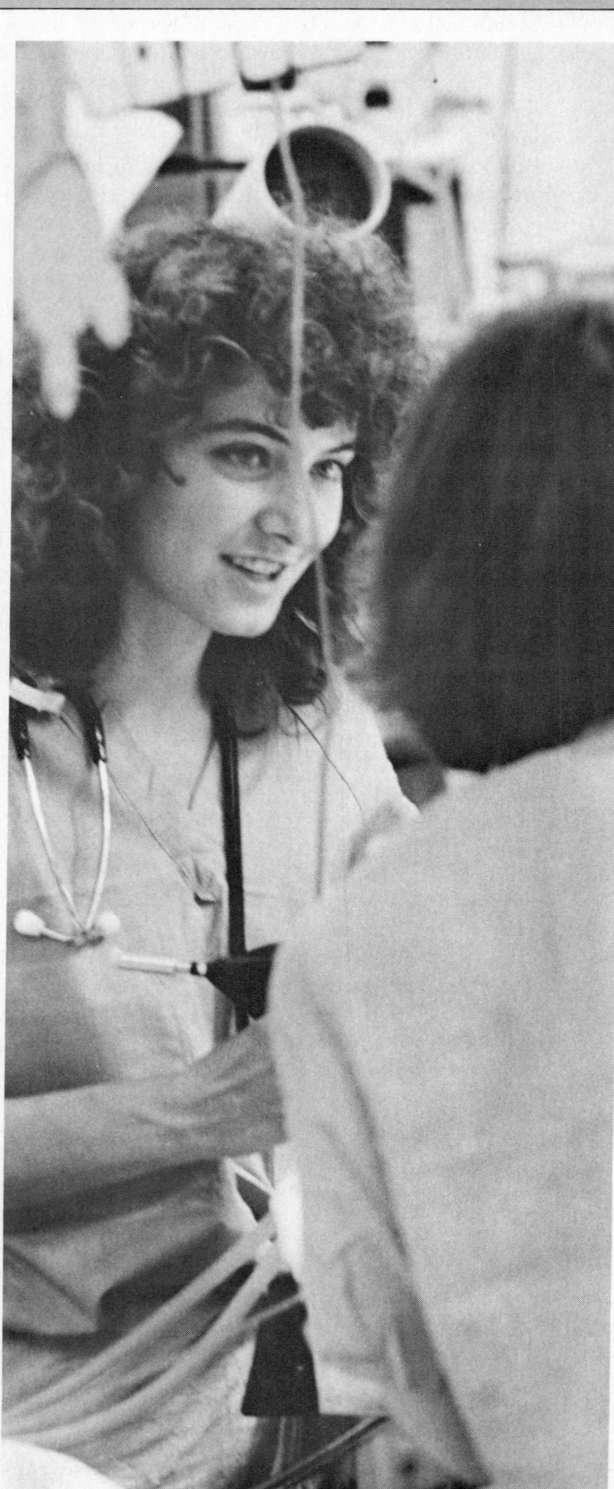

Communicating Effectively

CONTENTS

(Continued on next page)

Objectives

1. Understand essential facts about communication, the communication process, and language development

- **1.1** Differentiate between verbal and nonverbal communication
- **1.2** Identify five characteristics of effective verbal messages
- **1.3** Identify various attributes and limitations of nonverbal communication
- **1.4** Identify aspects of nonverbal behavior that need to be assessed
- **1.5** Explain the four elements of the communication process outlined in this chapter
- **1.6** Identify ways in which selected factors influence the communication process
- **1.7** Outline aspects of communication (language) development
- **1.8** Identify factors that influence language development
- **1.9** Identify ways in which language development can be stimulated

2. Know essential facts about effective and ineffective methods used by nurses when communicating with patients

- **2.1** Describe attentive (active) listening
- **2.2** Outline five ways in which the nurse conveys physical attending
- **2.3** Describe techniques the nurse can use to respond therapeutically to the patient
- **2.4** Describe responses the nurse may give that inhibit the patient's communication

3. Know essential facts about an effective nurse-patient relationship

- **3.1** Outline general guidelines for helping relationships
- **3.2** Describe empathy
- **3.3** List behaviors associated with genuineness
- **3.4** Identify four phases of the nurse-patient relationship
- **3.5** Identify essential elements of each phase of the nurse-patient relationship

4. Evaluate the nurse-patient communication interaction

- **4.1** Write a process recording of an interaction with a selected patient
- **4.2** Analyze the interaction

Terms

babbling
communication
congruence
decode
echolalia
egocentric speech
empathy
encoding
feedback (in communication)
holophrastic speech
lalling
monologue
nonverbal communication
paraphrasing
perception checking
personal space
probing
process recording
proxemics
reflexive vocalization
semantics
socialized speech
territoriality
verbal communication

The term *communication* has various meanings, depending on the context in which it is used. To some, communication is the interchange of information between two or more people; in other words, the exchange of ideas or thoughts. This kind of communication uses methods such as talking and listening or writing and reading. However, it can also use painting, dancing, and story telling. Thoughts are conveyed to others not only by spoken or written words but also by gestures or body actions.

Communication may have a more personal connotation than the interchange of ideas or thoughts. It can be a transmission of feelings, or a more personal and social interaction between people. In this context, communication often is synonymous with relating. Frequently one member of a couple comments that the other is not communicating. Some teenagers complain about a generation gap—being unable to communicate with understanding or feeling to a parent or authority figure. Sometimes a nurse is said to be efficient but lacking in something called *bedside manner*. For the purpose of this text, *communication* is any means of exchanging information or feelings between two or more people. It is a basic component of human relationships.

The intent of any communication is to elicit a response. Thus, communication is a process. It includes all the techniques by which an individual affects another. It has two main purposes: to influence others and to obtain information. Whether verbal or nonverbal, communication can be described as helpful (therapeutic) or unhelpful (nontherapeutic). The former encourages a sharing of information, thoughts, or feelings between two or more people. The latter hinders or blocks the transfer of information and feelings.

To communicate effectively with patients and their support persons, nurses need to become skilled in therapeutic communication techniques and in developing helping relationships.

Kinds of Communication

Communication is generally categorized into two basic kinds, verbal and nonverbal. *Verbal communication* uses the spoken or written word; *nonverbal communication* uses other forms such as gestures or facial expressions. Although both kinds of communication occur concurrently, the majority of communication is nonverbal. This may be surprising to those who associate communication with only verbal expression. Learning about nonverbal communication is thus an important consideration for nurses in developing effective communication patterns and relationships with patients.

Verbal Communication

Verbal communication is largely a conscious effort in that people choose the words they use. The words used vary among individuals according to culture, socioeconomic background, age, and education. As a result, countless possibilities exist in the way ideas are exchanged. An abundance of words can be used to form messages. In addition, a wide variety of feelings can be conveyed when talking. The intonation of the voice can express animation, enthusiasm, sadness, annoyance, or amusement, to name some examples. The number of different intonations heard when people say "hello" or "good morning" illustrates the variety that is possible. The pacing or rhythm of a person's communication is another variable. Monotonous rhythms or very rapid rhythms can be products of lack of energy or interest or of anxiety or fear.

Characteristics of effective verbal messages

When choosing words to say or to write, nurses need to consider several criteria of effective communication. These include (a) simplicity, (b) clarity, (c) timing and relevance, (d) adaptability, and (e) credibility.

Simplicity The best teachers can state complex ideas in simple words. The same holds true for persons communicating everyday concerns. Simplicity includes the use of commonly understood words, brevity, and completeness.

Many people have a tendency to overcommunicate. Their messages are wordy, contain too many extraneous explanations, or use words that are highly academic, technical, or slangy. In the world of nursing, many complex technical terms become natural to nurses. However, these terms can often be misunderstood even by informed laypeople. Words such as *discombobulate* or *cholecystectomy* may be meaningful to the speaker and easy to use but are ill-advised when communicating with most patients. Nurses need to learn to select simple words intentionally even though effort is required to do so. For example, instead of saying to a patient, "The nurse will be catheterizing you tomorrow for a urine specimen," it is better to say, "Tomorrow a sample of your urine is needed, and it will be necessary to collect it by putting a tube into your bladder." The latter statement is likely to produce a response from the patient about why it is needed and whether it will hurt or be uncomfortable. The former statement may simply make the patient wonder what the nurse means.

Another consideration related to simplicity is brevity. Most people have heard others give lengthy explanations of events, to which they respond, "Get to the point." By using short sentences and avoiding unnecessary material, brevity can be achieved. This is of particular importance in writing. Busy people do not have the time to read several pages before discovering the main issue or recommendations. Reports or memos need to be concise and condensed into a single paragraph or page, if possible.

The opposite of overcommunicating is undercommunicating. Shortcuts for the sake of simplicity can lead to incomplete or unclear communication. For example, initials or abbreviations such as b.i.d. (twice a day) or ICU (intensive care unit) should be avoided unless the nurse is certain that the initials will be readily understood. Because clarification is required, abbreviations can waste the listener's or reader's time. At the first use, names should be expressed in full; later they can be shortened when the nurse is sure that the patient or reader knows the meanings.

Clarity *Clarity* means saying exactly what is meant. It also is aligned with meaning what is said. The latter involves a blending of the speaker's behavior (nonverbal communication) with the words that are spoken. When the words and the behavior blend together or are unified, the communication is regarded as consistent or congruent.

The goal of clarity is to communicate so that people know the what, how, why (if necessary), when, who, and where of any specific event. Without these, people are left to make assumptions. To ensure clarity in communication, the nurse also needs to speak slowly and enunciate words well. It may be helpful to repeat the message and to reduce distractions such as surrounding noises.

Some common pitfalls that can produce unclear communications are ambiguous statements, generalizations, and opinions. For example, "Men are stronger than women" is both a generalization and an opinion, and the term *stronger* is open to several interpretations. Another example is a nurse's statement to a patient, "Mrs. Smith, you need to keep busy today." The specific actions Mrs. Smith is expected to carry out and the reasons for them are open to many interpretations.

Timing and relevance No matter how clearly or simply words are stated or written, the timing needs to be appropriate to ensure that words are heard. Moreover, the messages need to relate to the person or to the person's interests and concerns. Consider the woman whose children are crying and whose doorbell is ringing while she is on the telephone. This is not the best time for the person on the other end of the telephone to try to make a sale, even if the woman is interested.

Nurses need to be aware of both relevance and timing when communicating with patients. This involves being sensitive to the patient's needs and concerns. For example, if a female patient is enmeshed in fear of cancer, she may not hear the nurse's explanations about the expected procedures before and after her gallbladder surgery. In this situation it is better for the nurse first to encourage the patient to express her concerns and deal with those; at another time the necessary explanations are provided.

Another pitfall is to ask several questions at once. For example, a nurse enters a patient's room and says in one breath, "Good morning, Mrs. Brody. How are you this morning? Did you sleep well last night? Your husband is coming to see you before your surgery, isn't he?" The patient no doubt feels bombarded and confused and wonders which question to answer first, if any. A related pattern of poor timing is to ask a question and then not wait for an answer before making another comment. To Mr. Ramirez the nurse says, "How is that swollen leg this morning? I'm getting your bath water now before the doctor comes."

Adaptability Spoken messages need to be altered in accordance with behavioral cues from the receiver. This adjustment is referred to as *adaptability*. Moods and behavior may change minute by minute, hour by hour, or from day to day. In this sense the nurse needs to avoid routine or automatic speech. What the nurse says and how it is said must be individual and carefully considered. This requires astute assessment and sensitivity on the part of the nurse.

Credibility *Credible* means worthy of belief, trustworthy, and reliable. It may be the most important criterion of effective communication. A nurse's credibility to patients depends in part upon the opinion of others. If other health workers and patients regard the nurse as trustworthy, then the patient will. Developing trust is discussed later in this chapter in the section on phases of the helping relationship.

To become credible, the nurse needs to be knowledgeable about the subject matter being discussed and to have accurate information. The nurse also needs to convey confidence and certainty in what she or he is saying. This is often referred to as *positivism*. People tend to perceive confidence, which is more dynamic and emphatic, as more credible than hesitance or uncertainty, which is less forceful and less active. However, caution needs to be taken not to sound overconfident or authoritarian. This can be prevented by stating messages in a constructive way focused on being helpful to patients.

Reliability, the third aspect of credibility, is developed by being consistent, dependable, and honest. People value the nurse who acknowledges limitations and can say, "I don't know the answer to that, but I'll find someone who does, and you can talk to that person."

Nonverbal Communication

Nonverbal communication is sometimes called *body language*. It includes gestures, body movements, and physical appearance, including adornment. The majority of communication is nonverbal. Nonverbal communication often tells others more about what a person is feeling than what is actually said, because nonverbal behavior is controlled less consciously than verbal behavior. As a result, listeners tend to rely on body language more than on words. Nonverbal communication either reinforces or contradicts what is said verbally. For example, a nurse may say to a patient, "I'd be happy to sit here and talk to you for a while," yet she glances nervously at her watch every few seconds. The actions are contradicting the verbal message. The nonverbal behavior, suggesting "I am very busy," is more likely to be believed.

Certain limitations exist in nonverbal communication. Observers cannot always be sure of the feelings being expressed by nonverbal behavior. On the one hand, the same feeling can be expressed nonverbally in more than one way. For example, anger may be communicated by aggressive or excessive body motion, or it may be communicated by a frozen stillness. On the other hand, a variety of feelings, such as embarrassment, pleasure, or anger, can be expressed by a single nonverbal cue, such as blushing (Johnson 1972:104).

Observing and interpreting the patient's nonverbal behavior are essential skills for nurses. Observation skills use the senses of seeing, hearing, touching, and smelling. Interpreting the observations requires validation with the patient, using specific communication techniques discussed subsequently in this chapter.

The nurse's own nonverbal behavior is under constant scrutiny by patients. It is therefore necessary for nurses to gain awareness of their actions and to learn to convey understanding, respect, and acceptance to patients.

Assessing nonverbal behavior

To observe nonverbal behavior efficiently, a systematic approach needs to be used. Generally the nurse assesses the person's overall physical appearance, including adornments, posture, and gait, and then assesses specific parts of the body such as the face and the hands.

Physical appearance The person's appearance includes physical characteristics and manner of dress. Physical characteristics can denote the person's state of health. Skin color and texture, length of fingernails, weight, and deformities causing physical limitations are a few examples. The skin may appear dry, mottled, or pale. Weight may indicate malnourishment. Nails may be well manicured or extremely short. Whatever is observed, the nurse needs to exercise caution in interpretation. For example, pale skin may be normal for that person. Nails may be short because they were bitten nervously or because they were broken by hard manual labor.

Clothing and adornments are sometimes rich sources of information about a person. The choice of apparel is highly personal. Clothing may convey social and financial status, culture, religion, group association, and self-concept. Adornments such as jewelry, perfume, and cosmetics reveal additional information.

How a person dresses is often an indicator of how the person feels. People who are tired or ill may not have the energy or the desire to maintain their normal grooming. The nurse also needs to be alert to sudden changes in a person's dress. When a person who is known for immaculate grooming becomes lax about appearance and stays in nightclothes all day, this may suggest a loss of self-esteem or a physical illness. Hair care or nail care may be lacking, and dress may be inappropriate. Appropriateness of dress also depends upon context. A swimsuit worn to a beach party is appropriate, whereas a swimsuit worn to a formal dinner party is not.

In acute general hospital settings, indications that a patient is feeling better often relate to dress, particularly personal adornment. A male patient may request a shave or a female patient may request a mirror and her lipstick.

Posture and gait The way people walk and carry themselves are often reliable indicators of self-concept, current mood, and health. Erect posture and an active, purposeful stride suggest a feeling of well-being. Slouched posture and a slow, shuffling gait suggest dejection or physical discomfort. Tense posture and a rapid, determined gait suggest anxiety or anger. Likewise, the sitting or lying postures of patients can communicate feelings.

Facial expression No part of the body is as expressive as the face. See Figure 15–1. Feelings of joy, sadness, fear, surprise, anger, and disgust can be conveyed by facial expressions. The muscles around the eyes and the mouth are particularly expressive. Although actors learn to control these muscles to convey emotions to audiences, facial expressions generally are not consciously controlled.

Patients are quick to notice the nurse's facial expression, particularly when the patients feel unsure or uncomfortable. The patient who questions the nurse about a feared diagnostic result will watch the nurse's face to see if the nurse looks at him or her to answer or looks away. The patient who has disfigurement will examine the nurse's face for signs of disgust. Nurses, like actors, need to be aware of their facial expressions, and what they are communicating to patients. Although it is impossible to control all facial expressions, the nurse must learn to control feelings such as fear and disgust in certain situations.

Many facial expressions convey a universal meaning. The smile conveys happiness. Contempt is conveyed by the mouth turned down, the head tilted back, and the eyes directed down the nose. No single expression can be interpreted accurately, however, without considering (a) other reinforcing physical cues, (b) the setting in which it occurs, and (c) the expression of others in the same setting. For instance, when a person is smiling at others who are intently watching an accident victim on the street, the smile could convey contempt.

Eye contact is another essential element of facial communication. Mutual eye contact acknowledges recognition of the other person and a willingness to maintain communication. Often the eye initiates contact with another person with a glance, capturing the person's attention prior to communicating. Eye contact is generally averted or avoided when a person feels weak or defenseless. The communication received may be too embarrassing or too dominating. Animals are known to succumb to dominance by averting first their eyes and then their presence. See also the discussion of eye contact in Native American Indian cultures, on page 213.

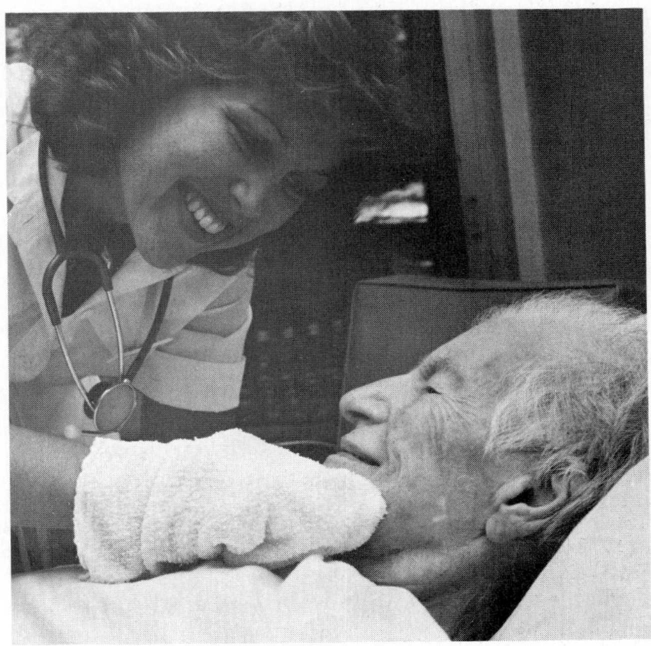

Figure 15–1 The nurse's facial expression communicates warmth and caring.

Hand movements and gestures Like faces, hands are expressive. They can communicate feelings at any given moment. Envision a relative waiting for word about a patient in surgery. Anxious people may wring their hands or pick their nails; relaxed persons may interlock their fingers over their laps or allow their hands to fall over the ends of armrests. Hands also communicate by touch. Hitting someone in the face or caressing another person communicates obvious feelings.

Hands are frequently involved in gestures. The handshake, the victory sign, the wave good-bye, the hand motion to ask a visitor to sit down are gestures that have relatively universal meanings. Some gestures, however, are socially accepted in one culture but not in another. European women walk together holding hands as a sign of friendship; in North American society, for two women to hold hands is usually regarded as unacceptable. Even the same gesture can have different meanings in different cultures. The "shoo away" or "go away" gesture of the hands in North America means "come here " or "come back" in some Japanese cultures.

Hands are also very expressive in illustrating or stylizing verbal communication. The French and Italian cultures are noted for using their hands in this manner. Instead of describing in words alone the shape and size of an object, the hands are manipulated to reinforce the verbal message.

For people who have special communication problems, such as the deaf, the hands are invaluable in communication. Many deaf people learn sign language. Ill persons who are unable to reply verbally can similarly devise a unique communication system using the hands. The patient may be able to raise an index finger once for "yes" and twice for "no." Other signals can often be devised by the patient and the nurse to denote other meanings.

Gestures often involve body parts other than the hands. In some cultures a gentleman may bow before a lady; two European men greet each other by embracing and touching opposite cheeks alternately; men and women kiss to say hello or goodbye.

The Communication Process

A number of models have been used to explain the communication process. The purpose of a model is to break down the process of communication into its essential components so that it can be better understood. A communication model has two main parts: people and messages. In face-to-face communication there is a

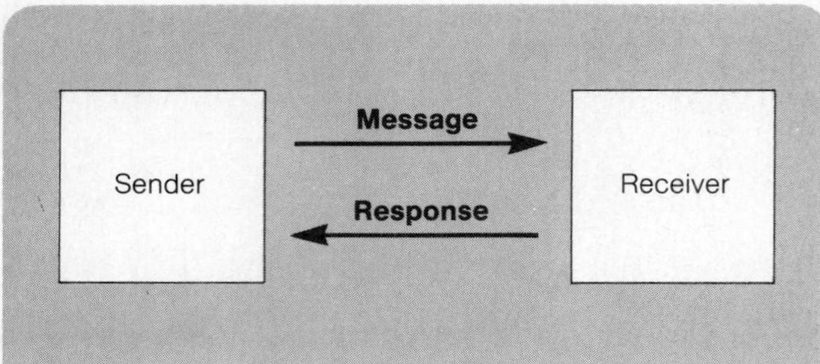

Figure 15–2 The communication process.

sender, a message, a receiver, and a response (feedback). See Figure 15–2. In its simplest form, communication is a two-way process involving the sending and the receiving of a message. Since the intent of communication is to elicit a response, the process is ongoing; the receiver of the message then becomes the sender of a response message while the original sender then becomes the receiver. Several sequential models have been proposed for the communication process, incorporating from four to six elements but sender, message receiver, and response are essential to all models.

Sender

The sender or person who wishes to convey a message to another is sometimes called the *source-encoder*. This term includes the concept that the person sending the message first must have an idea or reason for communicating (source) and second must put the idea or feeling into a form that can be transmitted. *Encoding* involves the selection of specific signs or symbols (codes) to transmit the message, such as the use of English or French words, the specific arrangement of the words, and the tone of voice and gestures to use. For example, if the receiver speaks English, English words will usually be selected. If the message is "No, Johnny, you may not have any more cookies before dinner!" the tone of voice selected will be one of firmness, and a shake of the head or a pointing index finger can reinforce it.

Message

The second component is the message itself—what is actually said or written, the body language that accompanies the words, and how it is transmitted. Various channels can be used to convey messages, and frequently combinations are used. It is important that the channel be appropriate for the message and one that will make the intent of the message clear.

Talking face-to-face with a person may be more effective in some instances than telephoning or writing a message. Recording messages on tape or communicating by radio or television may be more appropriate for larger audiences. Written communication is often appropriate for long explanations or for a communication that needs to be preserved. The nonverbal channel of touch is often highly effective.

Receiver

The receiver, the third component, is the listener, sometimes called the *decoder*. This person must perceive what the sender intended (sensation) and then analyze the information received (interpretation). Perception involves use of all the senses to receive all verbal and nonverbal messages. To *decode* means to relate the message perceived to the receiver's storehouse of knowledge and experience and sort out the meaning of the message. Whether the message is decoded accurately by the receiver, according to the sender's intent, depends largely on their similarities in knowledge and experience. For example, Johnny may perceive the message accurately—"No more cookies for me right now." However, if experience has taught him that he can help himself to the cookie jar without punishment, he will interpret the message differently from the way his mother intended it.

Response

The fourth component, the response, is the message that the receiver returns to the sender. It is also called *feedback*. Feedback can be either positive or negative. Nonverbal examples are a nod of the head or a yawn. Either way, feedback allows the sender to correct or reword a message. In the case of Johnny, the receiver may cry, or move away from the cookie jar, or say, "Well, Judy had three cookies and I only had two." The sender then knows the message was interpreted accurately. However, now the original sender becomes the receiver, who is required to decode and respond.

The receiver is not the sole source of feedback. Communicators constantly receive *internal feedback* from themselves. Internal feedback is often used for written messages. For example, after composing a letter, a person will read it silently or out loud to see how it sounds; or a person who makes a social blunder (faux pas) may instantly realize the mistake and say, "That isn't what I really meant" or "I didn't mean it that way."

Factors Influencing the Communication Process

In addition to the factors mentioned previously, such as variations in a person's sociocultural background, language, age, and education, and the limitations and attributes of nonverbal communication, the following factors affect the communication process: ability of the communicator; perceptions; personal space; territoriality; roles, relationships, and purposes; time and place; attitudes; and emotions and self-esteem.

Ability of the communicator

The person's ability to speak, hear, see, and comprehend stimuli influences the communication process. People who are hard of hearing may require messages that are short, loud, and clear. Those who are unable to read or write will be unable to comprehend written information. Some, because of disease processes, are unable to see or to speak, and individual methods for communication need to be devised with them.

The receiver of a message also needs to be able to interpret the message. Mental faculties can be impaired for such reasons as brain damage or use of sedative drugs or alcohol.

Even if a patient is free of physical impairments, the nurse needs to determine how many stimuli the patient is capable of receiving in a given time frame. Frequently the receiver is expected to assimilate too much information. The nurse may be talking too quickly or presenting too many ideas at once. This is of particular importance when offering health instruction.

Perceptions

Because each person has unique personality traits, values, and life experiences, each will perceive and interpret messages differently. For example, the nurse may draw the curtains around a crying woman and leave her alone. The woman may interpret this as "The nurse thinks I shouldn't cry and will upset the other patients" or "The nurse doesn't like crying" or "The nurse respects my need to be alone." It is important in many situations to validate or correct the perceptions of the receiver.

Personal space

Personal space is the distance people prefer in interactions with others. *Proxemics* is the study of distance between people in their interactions. Middle-class North Americans use definite distances in various interpersonal relationships, along with specific voice tones and body language. Communication thus alters in accordance with four distances, each with a close and a far phase, that have been described by Hall (1969:45):

1. Intimate: 7.5–45.0 cm (3–18 in)
2. Personal: 0.4–1.2 m (1.5–4.0 ft)
3. Social: 1.2–3.7 m (4–12 ft)
4. Public: beyond 3.7 m (12 ft)

Intimate distance communication is characterized by body contact, heightened sensations of body heat and smell, and vocalizations that are low. Vision is intense, restricted to a small body part, and may be distorted. Intimate distance is frequently used by nurses. Examples occur in cuddling a baby, touching the sightless patient, positioning patients, observing an incision, and restraining a toddler for an injection. It is a natural protective instinct for people to maintain a certain amount of space immediately around them, and the amount varies with individuals. When someone who wants to communicate steps too close, the receiver automatically steps back a pace or two. In their therapeutic roles, nurses often are required to violate this personal distance. However, it is important for them to be aware when it will occur and to forewarn the patient, if possible. In many instances the nurse can respect (not come as close as) a person's intimate distance. In other instances, the nurse may choose this distance to communicate warmth and caring.

Personal distance is less overwhelming than intimate distance. Voice tones are moderate, and body heat and smell are noticed less. Physical contact, such as a handshake or touching a shoulder, is possible. More of the person is perceived at a personal distance, so that nonverbal behaviors, such as body stance or full facial expressions, are seen with less distortion. Much communication between nurses and patients occurs at this distance. Examples occur when nurses are sitting with a patient, giving medications, or establishing an intravenous infusion. Communication at a close personal distance can convey involvement by facilitating the sharing of thoughts and feelings. At the outer extreme of 1.2 m (4 ft), however, less involvement is conveyed. Bantering and some social conversation are usual at this distance.

Social distance is characterized by a clear visual perception of the whole person. Body heat and odor are imperceptible, eye contact is increased, and vocalizations are loud enough to be overheard by others. Communication is therefore more formal and is limited to seeing and hearing. The person is protected and out of reach for touch or personal sharing of thoughts or feelings. Social distance allows more activity and movement back and forth. It is expedient in communicating with several people at the same time or within a short time. Examples occur when nurses make rounds or wave a greeting to someone. Social distance is important in accomplishing the business of the day. However, it is frequently misused. For example, the nurse who stands in the doorway and asks a patient "How are you today?" will receive a more noncommittal reply than the nurse who moves to personal distance to inquire.

Public distance requires loud, clear vocalizations with careful enunciation. Although the faces and forms of people are seen at public distance, individuality is lost. Instead, a general notion is perceived about a group of people or a community.

Territoriality

Territoriality is a concept of the space and things that an individual considers belong to him or her. Territories marked off by people may be visible to others. For example, a patient in a hospital often considers that his or her territory is bounded by the curtains around the bed unit or the walls of a private room. This human tendency to claim territory must be recognized by all health care workers. Patients often feel the need to defend their territory when it is invaded by others; for example, when a visitor removes a chair to use at another bed, the visitor has inadvertently violated the territoriality of the patient whose chair was moved.

The way in which territoriality affects the communication process is seen in the following example. Mrs. Brown, an elderly woman, had been hospitalized in an extended care unit for 3 months. A nurse removed the overbed cradle from her bed, because, in the nurse's opinion, Mrs. Brown no longer had a need for it, and it was needed for a newly admitted patient's bed. Mrs. Brown got angry with the nurse and voiced loudly, "That's mine and belongs on my bed. If you take it away I'll report you to the administrator." The nurse continued to transfer the cradle and responded, "You can't report me, and you don't need this." The outcome was that Mrs. Brown's anger toward the nurse increased; she became distrustful and withdrew from further interactions with that nurse.

Roles, relationships, and purposes

The roles and the relationship between the sender and receiver affect the communication process. Roles such as nursing student and instructor, patient and physician, or parent and child will affect the content and responses in the communication process. Choice of words, sentence structure, and tone of voice vary considerably from role to role. In addition, the specific relationship between the communicators is significant. The nurse who meets with the patient for the first time will communicate differently from the nurse who has previously developed a relationship with that patient.

The intended purpose of a communication also alters interactions with others. For example, if the purpose is to acknowledge another's presence, the nurse may say, "Hello, how goes it today?" but if the purpose is to assess the person's pain and the effect of an analgesic, several more specific questions and responses are necessary.

Time and setting

The time factor in communication includes what precedes and follows the interaction. The setting of the interaction is a related factor. The patient in a hospital who is anticipating surgery or who has just received news that a spouse has lost a job will not be very receptive to information. A patient who has had to wait for some time to express needs may respond quite differently from one who has endured no waiting period. The setting also influences communication. If the room lacks privacy or is hot, noisy, or crowded, the communication process can break down.

Nurses' use of time can facilitate or inhibit a patient's communication. The nurse who tells a patient "I'll be back in a moment" while delivering medications is likely to convey "I haven't time now" or "I've got work to do." This inhibits patient communications. Some patients learn that requests need to be made as soon as the nurse appears. Often their request is accompanied by an apology for taking the nurse's time. If this nurse says to the patient, however, "Would you tell me now what your concern is about, and then when I've finished delivering medications I'll come back and help you with it," the communication process is facilitated.

The concept of time also has cultural connotations. Caucasians, for example, tend to emphasize punctuality and think in terms of the hour, the day, the week, or the month. American Indians, on the other hand, are governed more by events of nature, such as the season. Appointments for child care or health screening programs will usually be kept by the former group. The latter group, however, may well defer appointments when nature beckons regardless of how well the communication was offered in advance. Priority for them may be that "the salmon are running" or "the geese are flying."

Attitudes

Attitudes convey beliefs, thoughts, and feelings about people and events. They are communicated convincingly and rapidly to others. Attitudes such as caring, warmth, respect, and acceptance facilitate communication, whereas condescension, lack of interest, and coldness inhibit communication.

Caring and *warmth* are terms frequently used to describe the attitudes of people. They convey a feeling of emotional closeness, in contrast to impersonal distance. Caring is more enduring and intense than warmth. It conveys deep and genuine concern for the person. Warmth, on the other hand, conveys friendliness and consideration shown by acts of smiling and attention to physical comforts (Brammer 1973:31). Caring involves giving feelings, thoughts, skill, and knowledge. It requires psychologic energy and the risk of little in return, yet it usually reaps the benefits of greater communication and understanding.

Respect is an attitude that emphasizes the other person's worth and individuality. It conveys that the person's hopes and feelings are special and unique even though similar to others in many ways. People have a need to be different from others and at the same time to be similar to others. Being too different can be isolating and threatening.

Acceptance emphasizes neither approval nor disapproval. The nurse willingly receives patient's honest feelings and actions without judgment. An accepting attitude allows patients to express personal feelings freely and to be themselves. The nurse may find that acceptance has to be restricted in certain situations when the patient's actions are personally harmful or harmful to others.

In contrast, *condescension* is an attitude that conveys superiority over the other person. It magnifies the patient's differences and inequality. Patients who feel helpless often perceive nurses to be in an elevated position with their knowledge and skill as helpers. In these instances, the nurse may convey condescension by an air of superiority and intellectualism. One common condescending act by nurses is to call patients "honey" or "dear" whether they are male or female, young or old. This makes the nurse a superior mother and the patient an inferior child.

Lack of interest also inhibits communication by saying "I'm not concerned" or "What you say is not important." This attitude is conveyed when the nurse forgets part of the patient's conversation or does not concentrate on it sufficiently to respond. The nurse may be tired after a long day's work or in a hurry to complete tasks.

Coldness is the opposite of caring and warmth. This attitude can be conveyed to patients by nurses who appear more interested in the technical and procedural aspects of nursing than in the concerns of the person receiving the therapy. For example, the nurse who is more concerned about the neatness of the patient's bed than about the patient's restlessness, or one who focuses more on the efficient functioning of a cardiac monitor than on the patient's anxiety conveys an attitude of coldness. A rigid body posture, the nurse's tone of voice, and the *way* things are said (in contrast to *what* is said) can also convey a nurse's lack of genuine concern for the patient.

Emotions and self-esteem

All kinds of emotions can influence a person's ability to communicate. Most people have experienced overwhelming joy or sorrow that is difficult to express in words. Anger may produce loud, profane vocalizations or controlled speechlessness. Fright may produce screams of terror or paralyzed silence.

Emotions also affect a person's ability to interpret messages. Large parts of a message may not be heard, or the message may be misinterpreted when the receiver is experiencing strong emotion. This situation occurs frequently in nursing. For example, the patient feeling great fear may not remember all the preoperative instructions offered by a nurse.

Self-esteem also influences communication patterns. People whose self-esteem is high communicate honestly, with confidence, and with *congruence* (agreement or coinciding) between verbal and nonverbal messages. For example, a nurse explaining the importance of preoperative exercises would present a sincere and serious facial expression. Those with low self-esteem or under high stress tend to give double messages, that is, their verbal and nonverbal messages are incongruent (lack consistency). For example, while explaining about a patient's colostomy to the patient's family, a nurse laughs. Many patterns of communication are used to alleviate feelings of low self-esteem.

Development of Communication

The development of communication, from the cry of the infant to the verbal fluency of the adult, is a complex process. The art of language is learned by sharing ideas and feelings with others. The precise ways by which children learn socialized speech are not fully understood. Various theories of language development have been proposed, which are beyond the scope of this book. This section describes the various sounds and phases of children's language.

Phases of Development

Prelinguistic phase

The first sound of a newborn is the birth cry as air moves across the vocal cords. This is a reflexive response associated with the air pressure and the temperature changes of extrauterine life. Although infants are speechless for almost one year, they do communicate their needs. Within two to three weeks after birth parents can describe notable differences in the cries of their infant. Babies cry in one way when they are hungry and in a different way when they are wet, tired, in pain, or wanting attention. The hunger cry may start out in a plaintive way and become increasingly demanding. The cry of pain is usually a sudden yell, because the baby is startled about what is happening. The cry of discomfort or the need for attention may sound like complaining, because it goes on and on. Some babies will cry jerkily when they are put down to sleep. Some become loudly demanding, but when a parent does not appear they settle down with progressively fading crying spurts. Each mother and father soon learn to communicate in response to the child's unique sounds. Infants also make comfort sounds. Smiling is noted in a number of infants as early as the second week of life. Soon after, some begin small throaty cooing sounds while feeding or bathing. Babies usually make these comfort sounds when they are contented, for example, when they are cuddled or when others talk to them.

Until the age of 10 months to 1 year the infant's sounds are not related to language and therefore are considered *prelinguistic*. These early sounds are actually exercise for the vocal cords. The first sounds are vowels or gurglings from the throat. When the mouth is opened, air is exhaled, resulting in various happy noises such as "uuuuuuu" or "eeeeeeeee." To produce consonant sounds such as "b" or "k," infants need sufficient motor development to manipulate their lips, tongue, throat, and voice at the same time. These sounds therefore appear less frequently and later than vowel sounds. The consonants are then combined into syllables with the vowel sounds. Such sounds as "da" and "ge" are then heard.

The prelinguistic phase includes reflexive vocalization, babbling, and echolalia. *Reflexive vocalization* is a term for the nondescriptive sounds infants make in response to various stimuli and environmental conditions. These are the discomfort cries and the comfort coos.

Babbling begins when infants become aware that they are making noises. They delight in producing and repeating sounds, particularly when they are enjoying themselves. They spend more time making noises and will talk to themselves when alone. Babbling often occurs just after waking up or before going to sleep. It is as if they are practicing self-produced sounds. By about 7 months babbling includes some sounds infants have picked up from their environment. Hearing and the sounds they produce are now associated. This is referred to as *lalling:* infants are repeating sounds they have heard.

Echolalia is the repetition or echoing of sounds just spoken by another. This involves definite acoustic awareness. Whole sequences of the sound may be strung together, such as "dadadadada." At this point there is no meaning associated with the infants' sounds, but they have learned to manipulate their tongue, lips, and throat and to imitate sounds spoken by others. Language and speech development proceed at a faster pace if the parent at this time repeats the baby's sounds. The baby in turn echoes the parent's sounds.

First words

The first word of the infant is a notable event for proud parents. By about 10 to 12 months of age children develop a *passive* understanding of the language. They will respond to a few familiar words such as "no" and familiar names—their own and those of family members and household pets. Even when family members are not present, children will turn to look for them when their names are mentioned.

Active use of language follows. The first words that children use may be unrecognized by parents, since children often invent their own first words. A word such as "nenene" may mean many things to a child. It may mean comfort when spoken softly, or it may mean a scolding or wrongdoing when spoken sharply. The word "mama" may mean food, comfort, warmth, and love. To understand this early language, it is necessary to listen to what children say in relation to what they are doing and their situation. Whole messages can be involved in one word based on the tone or manner of voice. This is not surprising, since babies respond to their mother's tone of voice as early as 4 or 5 weeks after birth, when they are comforted by soothing, soft tones. Although the words are not understood, it is known that babies respond differently to the same word said with different intonations at the age of 4 to 5 months.

True speech begins at 12 to 18 months of age, when the child correctly uses a conventional word or facsimile of the word. It is used with intent, and a response is anticipated; a child may bang a cup on the high chair and say "wawa" (water). This type of speech is referred to as *holophrastic speech* (one word expresses a whole sentence). "Wawa" means "I want some water." "Bath" means "I want to take a bath now." Generally children can say about four words at 15 months, about ten words at 18 months, and about fifty words by 2 years. The vocabulary that children understand is much larger. They can respond to commands such as "Give that to me" and "Touch your nose."

First sentences

By 2 years of age children learn to put words together. This period is considered the beginning of complete speech, the use of different word combinations in grammatical form.

In the beginning, only two words are combined; later three-word and four-word sentences appear, until full adultlike sentences are constructed. The child's sentences, like the first words, have personal meanings and do not follow the rules of grammar. Examples are: "See plane," "Kitty sleep," "Dat mine." Some peculiar combinations can be made up, such as "Bye-bye shoe." Regardless of the combinations, a certain order exists in the child's language. Some words will always appear at the beginning of a phrase and others at the end. "See" is usually at the beginning and "it" is usually at the end.

Learning to use the past tense and to create questions is more complex. Most of the early phrases spoken use the present tense. When learning the past tense children provide much amusement for adults. They initially put an "ed" on every verb, saying things like "Dolly eated" or "Mommy boughted it." As the child grows older, questions are formulated. Three stages are involved in transferring a statement into a question (Bee 1975: 147–49). These can be exemplified using the statement "Daddy is driving a blue car." Although dozens of words can be used to phrase a question, the word "why" will be used to illustrate the three changes:

1. The word "why" must be added: "Daddy is driving a blue car why?"
2. The word "why" then needs to be moved to the beginning of the statement: "Why daddy is driving a blue car?"
3. Then the verb "is" needs to be moved to follow the word "why": "Why is daddy driving a blue car?"

The earliest questions of a child do not change the sentence structure. Instead inflections are used at the end of a phrase, such as "See tree?" raising the voice as the child says "tree." Then questions will occur without verbs, such as "Where my coat?" followed by ones with verbs but not subjects, such as "Why can't do it?"

Children also have various ways of dealing with some consonants. One child who could not pronounce "f" to say her uncle Fred's name constructed the name "Pete" to avoid her difficulty. Another child pronounced Valerie as "Bralerie."

Egocentric and socialized speech

The French psychologist Jean Piaget (1952) categorized the conversation of children from ages 4 to 11 into egocentric and socialized speech. *Egocentric speech* is self-centered, noncommunicative speech. Children talk merely to please themselves or to please anyone who happens to be there to hear. Although the conversation is not directed to anyone in particular, the talking is about the child's thoughts and activity of the moment. The child is thinking out loud. Three categories of egocentric speech are repetition, monologue, and collective monologue. An example of *repetitive speech* is provided by 4-year-olds in a nursery school.

Judy: I've got a red block.
Tracey: I've got a red block.
Judy: I've got a red block.
Tracey: I've got a red block.

The *monologue* refers to a long speech that occurs when there is no listener. For example, the preschooler who is building a castle with blocks will mutter, "This big red block goes here . . . that's good . . . and now this green block goes there . . . uh . . . let's see, I'll put it this way . . . now, where's the bridge? That will keep the bad guys out." In contrast, the *collective monologue* involves the presence of others. Children speak with awareness of another child's presence, but they are indifferent to what others are saying.

In contrast to Piaget, the Russian psychologist Lev Vygotsky (1962:16–17) proposes that egocentric speech is a form of self-guidance and assists the child in problem-solving situations. He believes that egocentric speech is both goal oriented and communicative. It is the state between external speech and what he refers to as "silent inner speech" (ibid., p. 149). Egocentric or external speech goes underground and becomes internalized as thought processes.

Socialized speech refers to the exchange of thoughts with others. It includes questions, answers, commands, and criticism of others. In school-age children the use of egocentric speech gradually diminishes, and communicating thoughts to other people becomes predominant.

Semantic development

Semantics is the study of the meanings of words in a given language. Increasing attention has been given to semantic development in recent years. The words children use do not always indicate their meaning to adults. A preschooler said before his birthday that he did not want his birthday in January. After his parents explored what bothered him about having his birthday in January, his response was, "I want my birthday here at home on the farm." Although the child had the vocabulary, his personalized meaning referred to a place.

Children learn the meanings of concrete words and their categories first; later abstract words and their categories are understood. A child learns "chair" and "table" before learning the meaning of the category "furniture," or learns "apple" and "orange" before learning the category "fruit." Abstract words such as "quality" or "relation" are learned primarily after the preschool years.

Other words in the English language that have double meanings are also difficult for preschoolers. Such words as "sweet" or "crooked" can have either a physical or psychologic meaning. They are not fully comprehended until about age 10. See Table 15-1 for a summary of language development.

Factors Influencing Language Development

Growth in language development is affected by a number of factors: intelligence, sex, bilingualism, status as a single child or twin, parental stimulation, and socioeconomic components.

Table 15-1 Language Development

Stage	Normal behavior
Newborn	At birth—cries as air passes over vocal cords. Within 2 to 3 weeks—cries become differentiated.
Infant	At 2 to 3 months—babbling begins. At 7 months—repeats sounds heard from environment. At 10 to 12 months—responds to few familiar words; single words are pronounced. At 15 months—can say about four words.
Toddler	At 2 years—initially has over 50-word vocabulary; this increases progressively to about 800-1000 words by 3 years. Associates symbols with form, e.g., words, pictures. Grammatical errors are common.
Preschooler	At 4 years—vocabulary has grown to about 1600 words. Sentences are complete. By 5 to 6 years—most infantile pronunciations have disappeared.
School-age child	At 6 years—has command of most sentence structures. Speech is less egocentric. Vocabulary continues to increase; comprehension exceeds use. Slang and swear words become part of vocabulary. At 8 to 12 years—boasting commonly occurs.
Adolescent	Uses language of subgroup. Speech reflects consideration of hypotheses.
Adulthood	Has full speech skills. Language often reflects specialized education.

Intelligence

Brighter children begin to talk earlier than those with lower intelligence. Vocabulary development of intelligent children occurs more rapidly, and they articulate better and use sentences that are longer and grammatically more correct. Mentally defective children show notable lags in vocabulary growth.

Sex

During the first year there is not much difference in the sounds produced by boys and girls. After this time girls tend to be superior in both the rate of vocabulary development and articulation. In later school years boys tend to equal girls in reading abilities and be superior in use of certain words. Females on the whole exceed males in grammatical word usage and spelling tests.

Bilingualism

Research has contradicted the belief that a child of a bilingual home is hindered in language development. Lambert and Tucker (1972) found that language development was not retarded in bilingual children over a 7-year period. The bilingual children also scored high on tests of creativity.

Status as a single child or twin

Evidence suggests that twins and triplets exhibit certain aspects of retarded language development, particularly during the preschool years. It is thought that (a) twins may receive less verbal stimulation from parents, (b) they grow up so close together that they understand each other's speech patterns early, and (c) they lack the motivation to verbalize with others. The school years are apparently instrumental in resolving these problems (Helms and Turner 1976:164).

Parental stimulation

Vocabulary growth occurs at a more rapid pace in children who are spoken to more frequently by their parents. Less rapid growth has been noted in children who spend most of their time with other children and who watch a great deal of television. The kind of stimulation offered by parents is significant. (Bee 1975:166). An only child may show rapid growth of communication skills largely due to interaction with the parents, whereas the youngest of six children may have less communication with parents and hence develop communication skills more slowly. Children who have mothers described as "object oriented and noncritical" acquire language more rapidly. These mothers tend to talk and ask questions about the child's toys rather than criticizing what the child is doing with the toys. In contrast, children who have mothers described as "critical and intrusive" display inhibited language development. These mothers focus on giving their children directions (commands and demands) about what to do with their toys. Vocabulary is enhanced in children who travel away from their homes and who have contact with several different adults.

Socioeconomic components

The social and economic family setting in which the child is reared affects language development. Children from upper-class families, such as those whose parents are lawyers and doctors, use many more words even by age 3 than children from lower social classes, where the parents are unskilled workers. The caliber of conversation overheard by youngsters is an influencing factor in their choice of vocabulary and sentence structure. Middle-class and upper-class families tend to discourage the use of profane language or slang; instead, proper word usage and grammar are encouraged and often rewarded by praise. Homes that expose their children to a variety of educational aids also increase the child's language development. The effects of lack of development are noted in homes without magazines, books, newspapers, encyclopedias, radios, or a television set.

Although differences exist in language development among social classes, lower-class children should not be regarded as inferior. These children possess a fully developed language that is similar to a dialect. They are able to articulate well in their own cultural setting but not as well with middle-class or upper-class children. The converse also applies. Upper- and middle-class children have difficulty articulating in dialects outside their own cultural settings.

Stimulating Children's Language Development

Nurses can be instrumental in assisting parents to become active stimulants in language development and helping children when they are hospitalized. The following interventions are suggested:

1. *Improve the parental model.* Parents can be encouraged to provide the best possible instruction and to become good models. Some parents may need to attend English classes; others may need encouragement to acquire educational aids such as storybooks.

2. *Encourage verbal and nonverbal means of communication.* Children need different verbal experiences, such as rhyming games, reading aloud, and songs, with accompanying nonverbal gestures, such as smiling and laughing. See Figure 15–3. Expanding upon the child's remarks, drawing, painting, and musical endeavors also are vital parts of learning the communication process.

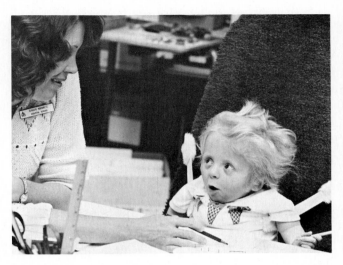

Figure 15–3 Development of a child's language is stimulated by reading together.

3. *Provide experiences to talk about.* Children talk when they have something to talk about. Whenever possible, parents and/or nurses need to provide pets, toys, picture books, numbers, and colors that the child can experiment with and talk about.

4. *Encourage listening.* Articulation skills of children can be enhanced by teaching them to pay attention and to listen to sounds. Parents can encourage these by having children listen to and repeat nursery rhymes or jingles or asking questions such as "What was that sound?"

5. *Encourage speech as a substitute for action.* Children's ability to express themselves verbally can be enhanced when parents direct them to say what they want rather than respond to physical action. The child who tugs at a playmate's tricycle can be instructed by the parent to express a want verbally by the remark, "Tell him what you want; perhaps he will let you have it."

6. *Use exact terms.* Children learn to distinguish color, size, shape, position, and ownership of objects when exact terms are used. Parents can be encouraged to say, "Bring the big red ball from the playroom table," rather than "Bring that thing from over there—you know what I mean." Asking a child to "Put away your toys" instead of "the toys" can clarify property problems.

Assessing Communication

When nurses assess the communication of patients, they need to include language development, nonverbal behavior, and communication style.

Language Development

The nurse assesses the following aspects of language development:

1. The language skills presented by the patient, compared to the language skills normally expected.
2. Adequacy of the language skills in relation to the individual's need.
3. The chief method of communicating, e.g., words or gestures.
4. Obstacles to language development, such as deafness or absence of environmental stimuli.
5. Specific forms of language impairment, e.g., a school-age child's inability to write or lack of abstractions in the language of an adult.
6. Cultural influences on language development, e.g., the language used in the home or customs about when and how to speak.

Nonverbal Behavior

In assessing nonverbal communication, the nurse considers:

1. Gestures used by the individual.
2. Posture and facial expressions employed.
3. Use of touch as a means of communication. See the discussion of touch later in this chapter.
4. The interpersonal distance with which the person feels comfortable, e.g., whether the person assumes an intimate distance for most discussions.
5. The grooming and appearance of the individual. These may affect the communication process, e.g., when dress is inconsistent with a setting or presents a stereotype that may evoke biases.

Style of Communication

A person's style of communication is often affected by such factors as his or her health, culture, education, stress level, fatigue, and cognitive ability. In assessing communication style, the nurse considers the following:

1. The vocabulary of the individual, particularly any changes from the vocabulary normally used. For example, if a person who normally never swears starts using swear words, this may indicate an increased stress level, illness, etc.
2. The use of symbols and gestures to communicate. Some uses of symbols and gestures are culturally determined; for example, a Puerto Rican girl may be taught not to look an adult in the eyes, as a sign of respect and obedience not as a sign of guilt.
3. The presence of characteristics such as hostility, aggression, assertiveness, reticence, hesitance, anxiety, or loquaciousness in the communication.
4. Difficulties with verbal communication, such as stuttering, inability to pronounce a particular sound, or lack of clarity in enunciation.

Nursing Intervention: Listening and Responding

Attentive Listening

It is essential, in therapeutic communication, that nurses listen and respond to patients purposefully and deliberately. Attentive listening is listening actively, using all the senses, as opposed to listening passively with just the ear. It is probably the most important technique of all. Attentive listening is an active process that requires energy and concentration. It involves paying attention to the total message, both verbal messages and nonverbal messages that can modify what is spoken, and noting whether these communications are congruent. Attentive listening absorbs both the content and the feeling the person is conveying, without selectivity. This means that the listener does not select or listen to solely what he or she wants to hear; the nurse does not focus on her or his needs but rather on the patient's needs. Attentive listening conveys an attitude of caring and interest, thereby encouraging the patient to talk. In summary, attentive listening is a highly developed skill, but fortunately it is one that can be learned by nurses with practice.

How attentive a nurse is in listening to patients can be conveyed in various ways. Common responses are a nod of the head, uttering "uh huh" or "mmm," repeating the words that the patient has said, or saying "I see what you mean." Each nurse will have characteristic ways of responding. Caution needs to be taken not to sound insincere or phony.

Gerard Egan (1975:65–67) has outlined five specific ways that convey physical attending. Egan defines physical attending as the manner of being present to another or being with another. Listening, in his frame of reference, is what a person does while attending. The five actions of physical attending, which convey a "posture of involvement," are:

1. *Face the other person squarely.* This position says, "I am available to you." Moving to the side lessens the degree of involvement.

2. *Maintain good eye contact.* This was discussed in the section on facial expression earlier. Mutual eye contact, preferably at the same level, recognizes the other person and denotes a willingness to maintain communication. Eye contact neither glares at nor stares down another but is natural.

3. *Lean toward the other.* People move naturally toward one another when they want to say or hear something—by moving to the front of a class, by moving a chair nearer a friend, or by leaning across a table with arms propped in front. Whispering a secret into someone's ear is an extreme example. Likewise, the nurse conveys involvement when he or she leans forward, closer to the patient.

4. *Maintain an open posture.* The nondefensive position is one in which neither arms nor legs are crossed. It conveys that the person wishes to encourage the passage of communication, as the open door of a home or an office does.

5. *Remain relatively relaxed.* Total relaxation is not feasible when the nurse is listening with intensity. The term *relative* acknowledges that the nurse can show relaxation by taking time in responding, allowing pauses as needed, balancing periods of tension with relaxation, and using gestures that are natural. See Figure 15–4. The nurse who feels tight and tense will generally offer responses too quickly to the patient and prevent a free flow of thoughts and feelings.

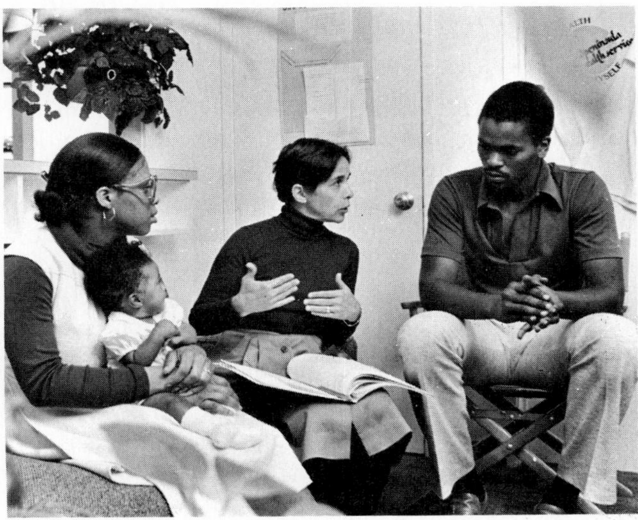

Figure 15–4 The nurse conveys attentive listening through a posture of involvement.

These five attending postures need to be adapted to the specific needs of patients in a given situation. For example, leaning forward may not be appropriate at the beginning of an interview. It may be reserved until a closer relationship grows between the nurse and the patient. The same applies to eye contact. This is generally uninterrupted when the communicators are very involved in the interaction. At times, however, eye contact may need to be interrupted.

Responding

Nurses can learn much by examining and becoming aware of their own reactions (feelings) and responses. Although it is difficult for nurses to see their own nonverbal communication other than by videotape feedback, much can be learned by reflecting on what was heard, what the nurse said, and when and how it was said. Methods such as role playing, process recordings, and audio tapes can be useful.

Nurses need to respond not only to the content of a patient's verbal message but also to the feelings expressed. It is important to understand how the patient views the situation and feels about it, before responding. This understanding is called *empathy* and is discussed in the section on effective nurse-patient relationships later.

The content of the patient's communication is the words or thoughts, as distinct from the feelings. Sometimes people can convey a thought in words while their emotions contradict the words, i.e., they are incongruent. For example, a patient says, "I am glad he has left me; he was very cruel." However, the nurse observes that the patient has tears in her eyes as she says this. To respond to the patient's *words* the nurse might simply rephrase them, saying, "You are pleased that he has left you." To respond to the patient's *feelings*, the nurse would need to acknowledge the tears in the patient's eyes, saying, for example, "You seem saddened by all this." Such a response helps the patient to focus on her feelings. In some instances, the nurse may need to know more about the patient and her resources for coping with these feelings.

Sometimes patients need time to deal with their feelings. Strong emotions are often draining to a person. Yet feelings usually need to be dealt with before a person can cope with other matters, such as learning new skills or planning for the future. This is most evident in hospitals when patients learn that they have a terminal illness. Some require hours, days, or even weeks before they are ready to start other tasks. The degree of assistance that patients require varies considerably. Some need only time to themselves, others need someone to listen, others need assistance identifying and verbalizing feelings, and others need assistance making decisions about future courses of action. A number of techniques are used to help patients. These are discussed in the next section.

Techniques for Responding Therapeutically

Several techniques can be used to facilitate therapeutic communication that promotes understanding by both the sender and the receiver. These techniques also assist in the formation of a constructive relationship between the nurse and the patient, although use of the techniques is no guarantee of effective communication. So many factors are involved in communication that the nurse would be ill-advised to rely solely on any one or even several techniques. Not all people feel comfortable with all techniques, and skill in using them appropriately is essential. It is important that the nurse be comfortable with the technique used and convey sincerity to the patient. A phony or false response is usually quickly identified by patients and hinders the development of an effective relationship.

Paraphrasing

Paraphrasing, also called *restating,* involves listening for the patient's basic message and then repeating those thoughts and/or feelings in similar words. Usually fewer words are used. Paraphrasing conveys that the nurse has listened and understood the patient's basic message. It may also offer the patient a clearer idea of what he or she said. The patient's response to the paraphrase may tell the nurse whether the paraphrase was accurate or helpful. (It may be necessary for the nurse to ask for a response.)

Patient: I couldn't manage to eat any of my dinner last night—not even the dessert.

Nurse: You had difficulty eating yesterday.

Patient: Yes, I was very upset after my family left.

Clarifying

Clarifying is a method of making the patient's message more understandable. It is used when paraphrasing is difficult, when the communication has been rambling or garbled. To clarify the message the nurse can (a) make a guess and restate the basic message, or (b) confess confusion and ask the patient to repeat or restate the message (Brammer 1973:85). In the latter instance the nurse might say, "I'm puzzled" or "I'm not sure I understand that" and "Would you please say that again?" or "Would you tell me more?"

If the reason for not understanding the message was the nurse's inattention, it is best to admit it and apologize. "I'm sorry, I was distracted by . . ." or "I was thinking about . . ." When possible, the nurse should discuss the distraction with the patient.

Nurses sometimes need to clarify their own messages to patients. The need to do so is generally discovered from the patient's nonverbal feedback. Then the nurse might ask a question or say, "It seems to me I didn't make that clear" and repeat or rephrase the message. Sometimes only one word or phrase in a message needs clarifying.

Clarifying also includes *verifying what is implied.* In this instance, the patient implies or hints at something without actually saying it. The nurse then tries to clarify the patient's statement without interpreting it.

Patient: There is no point in asking for a pain pill.

Nurse: Are you saying that no one gives you an analgesic when you have pain?

or

Nurse: Are you saying that your pills are not helping your pain?

Another clarifying technique is *perception checking* or *consensual validation.* This verifies the accuracy of the nurse's listening skills by giving and receiving feedback about what was communicated. It involves paraphrasing what the nurse thinks she or he heard and asking the patient for confirmation. It is important to allow the patient to correct inaccurate perceptions. The advantage of frequent perception checking is that inaccurate perceptions are corrected before communications become confused and misunderstandings arise. Examples of perception checking are: "You sound annoyed with me—is that correct?" or "You seem to have some doubts about the decision you made, and I'd like to see if what I'm hearing is accurate."

Using Open-ended Questions and Statements

An *open-ended question* is one that leads or invites patients to explore (elaborate, clarify, or illustrate) their thoughts or feelings. It allows patients the freedom to talk about what they wish. It also places responsibility on patients to explore and to understand themselves in contrast to receiving advice from another (Brammer 1973:87–89). Examples of open-ended questions are: "How did you feel in that situation?" "What do you think she meant by that remark?" "Would you describe more about how you relate to your child?" "What would you like to talk about today?" Examples of open-ended statements are "I'd like to hear more about that" and "Tell me about . . . ."

These questions or statements requires more than a "yes" or "no" or other short response, such as "yesterday" or "I don't know." They encourage patients to discover what their thoughts and feelings truly are. Such questions usually begin with "what" or "how." Questions that begin with "when," "where," "who," "do (did, does)" or "is (are, was)" tend to produce short answers that impede self-exploration. However, nurses need to use this latter type of question in situations that require information gathering, such as taking a nursing history.

Focusing

Focusing is used when the patient's communication is vague, when the patient is rambling, or when the patient seems to be talking about numerous things. Focusing can be compared to using a telephoto lens, which focuses sharply upon a certain aspect of the view; similarly the nurse assists or leads the patient to focus on one specific aspect of a communication. It is important for the nurse to wait until the patient thinks he or she has talked about the main concerns before attempting to focus. The focus may be an idea or a feeling; however, a feeling is often emphasized to help the patient recognize an emotion disguised behind words.

> Patient: My wife says she will look after me but I don't think she can, what with the children to take care of, and they're always after her about something—clothes, homework, what's for dinner that night.
>
> Nurse: You are worried about how well she can manage.

Being Specific, Tentative, and Informative

When responding to another person's comments, it is helpful to make statements that are (a) specific rather than general, (b) tentative rather than absolute, and (c) informative rather than authoritarian. Examples are: "You scratched my arm" (specific statement); "You're as clumsy as an ox" (general statement); "You seemed unconcerned about Mary" (tentative statement); "You don't give a damn about Mary and you never will" (absolute statement); "I haven't finished yet" (informative statement); "Stop interrupting!" (authoritarian statement).

In being informative, the nurse needs to present facts or specific information simply and directly. If the nurse does not know some fact, this is also stated simply, together with a suggestion about where or how the information can be obtained.

> Patient: I don't know the visiting hours.
>
> Nurse: The visiting hours are 9 A.M. to 9 P.M. each day.
>
> Patient: When will my doctor be in?
>
> Nurse: I don't know, but Ms. Lu, the charge nurse will be here in a few minutes, and she may know.

Another way to be informative is to make an observation. This indicates that the nurse has noticed a change of behavior but is not placing a value judgment upon it. For example: "You have washed your hair" (neutral observation); "Your hair looks better now that you have washed it" (value judgment); "You are holding your arm carefully; is it painful?" (observation; verifying implication).

Using Touch

Certain forms of touching indicate affection. For example, cheek patting, hand patting, and putting an arm over the person's shoulder are valued forms of affection in North America. The "laying on of hands" is a common expression indicating curative and comforting actions. This expression is often attributed to individuals in the healing professions such as religion, medicine, and nursing. Tactile contacts vary considerably among individuals, families, and cultures. Some families have a great deal of tactile contact among members. Other families, even within the same culture, have minimal contact. Appropriate forms of touch can be helpful in reinforcing caring feelings by the nurse. See Figure 15–5. The use of touch alone often says much more

Figure 15–5 Appropriate forms of touch can communicate caring.

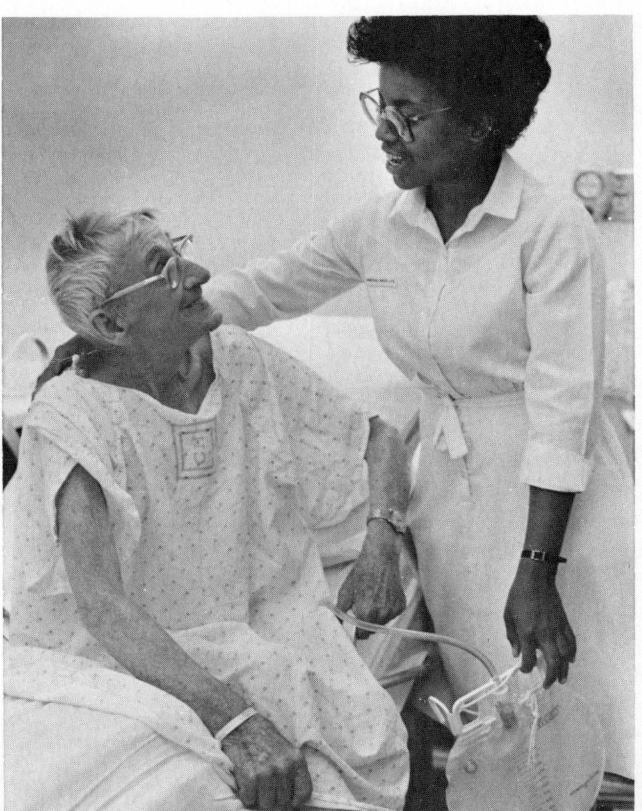

than words for patients such as those who are terminally ill or who are unable to speak, for whatever reason. It is important, however, for the nurse to be sensitive to the differences in attitudes and practices related to touch among individuals, including the nurse's own attitudes.

Using Silence

In everyday conversations natural pauses or silences are often accepted without thought. The listener attentively waits until the talker resumes conversation. These natural pauses are generally taken to recall a name or event or to put thoughts or feelings into the most accurate words possible. Pauses or silences that extend for several seconds or minutes, however, make some listeners extremely uncomfortable. The listener often interjects with thoughts, questions, or explanations to reduce the discomfort. This puts words into the other person's mouth, so to speak. The unfortunate result is that self-expression is blocked for the initial communicator.

When people are ill, communication about how they feel is often difficult for them. Many prefer to remain stoically silent until they are sure that the nurse is interested or to be trusted. Once communication is initiated, it may be expressed awkwardly with many pauses. The nurse needs to learn to be silent in these situations and to wait patiently until the person is able to put thoughts and feelings into words.

Clarifying Reality, Time, or Sequence

Sometimes it is important for nurses to clarify reality when a patient has misrepresented it. This assists the patient to differentiate the real from the unreal.

Patient: Someone took my magazine last night.
Nurse: Your magazine is here in your drawer.

Patient: There is a dead mouse in that corner.
Nurse: It is a discarded washcloth, not a mouse.

It may also be necessary to clarify a sequence of events or a time period:

Patient: I vomited this morning.

Nurse: Was that after breakfast?

Patient: I feel that I have been asleep for weeks.

Nurse: You had your operation Monday, and today is Tuesday.

Providing General Leads

By providing a general lead, the nurse encourages the patient to verbalize and at the same time choose the topic of conversation.

Patient: I am sure glad yesterday is over.

Nurse: Perhaps you would like to talk about it.

or

Nurse: Would it help you to discuss your feelings?

Summarizing

Summarizing the main points of a discussion is a useful technique near the end of an interview, after a significant discussion, or to review a health teaching session. It clarifies for both the nurse and the patient the relevant points discussed and often acts as an introduction to future care planning. For example, the nurse might say, "During the past half hour we have talked about . . . . Tomorrow afternoon we may explore this further" or "In a few days, I'll review what you have learned about the actions and effects of your insulin." A word of caution about summarizing: No new material should be added.

Nontherapeutic Responses

Nurses need to recognize nontherapeutic techniques that interfere with effective communication. These include failing to listen; unwarranted reassurance; using judgmental responses; being defensive; agreeing or disagreeing; and probing, testing or challenging.

Failing to Listen

Because listening is the most effective technique to facilitate communication, the opposite, failure to listen, is the primary inhibitor to communication. It says to the patient, "I'm not interested" or "I'm bored" or "You are not important." It suggests that the nurse needs to be entertained, that the nurse's needs require attention, or that the nurse prefers to discuss topics that concern herself or himself.

Unwarranted Reassurance

Statements such as "You'll feel better soon," "I'm sure everything will turn out all right," "Don't worry," and "You're looking better each day" are futuristic and intended to provide hope for the patient. However, they disregard the patient's feelings of the moment and in many instances are said when there is no hope of improvement. The patient who fears death, for example, needs to express these concerns rather than have them dismissed with false reassurance. The nurse who offers reassurance in this manner needs to examine her or his own feelings and recognize that this type of response is of more help to the nurse than to the patient.

Judgmental Responses

Passing judgment on the patient implies that the patient *must* think as the nurse thinks—the patient's values must be the same as the nurse's—if the patient is to be accepted. Several responses that fall into this category are discussed in the next sections.

Approval and disapproval

Approving or disapproving responses, such as "That's good (bad)," "You shouldn't do that," and "That's not good enough," tell patients they must measure up to the nurse's standards rather than to their own goals. Perhaps what the nurse considers "bad" the patient considers "good."

Approving or disapproving responses can also be nonverbal. For example, a patient may have managed to bathe herself completely without the nurse's assistance for the first time. Although this activity took time and effort, she is feeling pleased. The nurse, who thinks she took too long, says nothing but hurriedly makes her bed.

Common advice

Giving common advice removes decision-making control from the patient to the nurse. It suggests that the patient is inferior and less wise than the nurse. Moreover, it fosters dependence and often the advice is not followed. Note that the adjective *common* is used, not *expert*. This differentiation is significant, since giving expert advice can be therapeutic. Brammer (1973:108) writes:

> Advice can be helpful if it is given by trusted persons with expert opinions based on solid knowledge of a supporting field such as law, medicine, or child rearing. Sometimes . . . patients need a recommended course of action supported by wide experience and . . . facts.

Common advice, on the other hand, refers to matters dealing with individual choice. For example, when patients ask, "should I move from my home to a nursing home?" "I'm separated from my wife; do you think I should have sexual relations with another woman?" "Do you think I should have an abortion?" or "Should I give up my baby to an adoption agency?" offering advice such as "If I were you . . ." is unwise for the nurse. The patient needs support to make his or her own decisions.

Stereotypes

Stereotyping responses place the patient into categories that negate his or her uniqueness as an individual. "Stereotypes are generalized and oversimplified beliefs we hold about various groups of people, which are based upon experiences too limited to be valid" (Hein 1973:81). The less one knows about a person, the more the tendency to stereotype. Examples of stereotyping statements are: "Two-year-olds are brats," "Women are complainers," or "Men don't cry." Communication between nurse and patient can be inhibited depending on how emotionally charged the stereotype is for the nurse. For example, if the nurse is not deeply committed to the "brat" theory, the communication pattern with a 2-year-old who is cooperative may be only temporarily affected. On the other hand the nurse who has marked feelings about men who cry will probably ignore the individualism of a male patient who expresses his grief.

Another common error is to offer meaningless stereotyped responses to patients:

Patient: I'm sure having a lot of pain.

Nurse: Really? Most people don't have pain after this type of surgery.

Patient: I don't have the energy I'd like to have.

Nurse: Rome wasn't built in a day.

Defensive Responses

Many patients offer opinions or comments about their care, directed toward the nurse, the nurse's colleagues, or the institution. Feeling threatened or attacked, the nurse may become defensive and prevent the patient from expressing feelings. Following are two examples:

Patient: The food here is lousy.

Nurse: It's a lot better here than in the county hospital. You should consider yourself lucky.

Patient: Those night nurses must just sit around and talk all night. They didn't answer my light for over an hour.

Nurse: I'll have you know we literally run around on nights. You're not the only patient, you know.

These responses prevent the patient from expressing true concerns. The nurse is saying, "You have no right to complain." Defensive responses protect the nurse from admitting weaknesses in the health care services, including personal weaknesses.

Agreement and Disagreement

Agreeing and disagreeing imply that the patient is either right or wrong and that the nurse is in a position to judge this. They can deter the patient from thinking through his or her position. Disagreement sometimes causes the patient to defend a position.

Patient: I don't think Dr. Broad is a very good doctor. He doesn't seem interested in his patients.

Nurse: Dr. Broad is head of the Department of Surgery and is an excellent surgeon.

Probing, Testing, and Challenging Responses

Probing, testing, and challenging are often considered hostile responses. *Probing* is asking for information chiefly out of curiosity rather than with the intent to assist the patient. Usually probing is considered prying, and the patient feels that his or her privacy is not being respected. Often asking "why" is probing and can place the patient in a defensive posture:

Patient: I was speeding along the street and didn't see the stop sign.

Nurse: Why were you speeding?

Patient: I didn't ask the doctor when he was here.
Nurse: Why didn't you?

Testing is questioning by nurses to make patients admit to something. With testing, the nurse usually asks a question that permits the patient only limited answers. Testing often meets the nurse's need rather than the patient's. Examples of testing questions are: "Who do you think you are?" which forces the patient to admit that his or her status in the health care agency is that of "only a patient," and "Do you think I am not busy?" which forces the patient to admit that the nurse really *is* busy.

Challenging is giving a response that makes a patient prove his or her statement or point of view. Usually the patient's feelings are not considered, and he or she feels the necessity to defend a position. Challenging a patient's perceptions rarely changes them; often it strengthens them, because the patient feels forced to find proof to support the position.

Patient: I felt nauseated after that red pill.

Nurse: Surely you don't think I gave you the wrong pill?

Patient: I feel as if I am dying.

Nurse: How can you feel that way when your pulse is 60?

Patient: I believe my husband doesn't love me.

Nurse: You can't say that; why, he visits you every day.

Effective Nurse-Patient Relationships

An effective nurse-patient relationship is referred to by some as a *therapeutic relationship* and by others as a *helping relationship*. Helping is a growth-facilitating process in which one person assists another to grow in the direction the assisted person chooses (Brammer 1973:3). Several terms are used to describe the persons involved in a helping relationship: *helper* and *helpee; giver* and *receiver;* and *counselor* and *client.* For purposes of consistency, in this text the term *nurse* or *helper* will refer to the person who gives the help, and the term *patient* will denote the person receiving the help. However, we recognize that various people in all walks of life act as helpers and receivers of help.

Developing Helping Relationships

Although special training in counseling techniques and psychiatry is advantageous for nurses to become effective helpers, there are many ways of helping patients that do not require special training. Shanken and Shanken (1976:24–27) have outlined 11 of these:

1. Listen actively.
2. Help to identify what the person is feeling.
3. Put yourself in the other person's shoes.
4. Be honest.
5. Do not tell a person not to feel.
6. Do not tell a person what he or she should feel.
7. Do not make excuses for the other person.
8. Be personal.
9. Use your ingenuity.
10. Try to summarize to the person at the end of the interview.
11. Know your role and your limitations.

Active listening was discussed previously. It involves being attentive, clarifying, paraphrasing, and asking questions to understand the other person accurately.

Helping patients to identify their feelings requires feedback from the nurse about how the patient appears. Often patients who are troubled are unable to identify or to label their feelings and consequently have difficulty working them out or talking about them. Responses by the nurse such as "You seem angry about taking orders from your boss" or "You sound as if you've been lonely since your wife died" can assist patients to recognize what they are feeling and to talk about it.

Putting oneself into another person's shoes is referred to as *empathy*. According to Egan (1975:76) empathy involves the ability to:

> (1) *discriminate:* get inside the other person, look at the world through the frame of reference of the other person and get a feeling for what the other's world is like; and (2) *communicate* to the other this understanding in a way that shows the other that the helper has picked up both his *feelings*, and the *behavior and experience* underlying these feelings.

Empathy therefore requires more than sharing past similar feelings and events that people have all experienced, such as fright or depression. The nurse needs to understand the patient's world as if the nurse were inside it, to see it through the patient's eyes, and to feel as the patient feels. Empathy is valuable in supporting patients to explore their situation and to move toward resolution of their problems. Feelings of closeness and understanding gradually evolve between patient and nurse. Neither person, however, loses a sense of self.

Four steps have been identified in the process of empathy (Ehmann 1971:77–78). All the steps occur rapidly and tend to overlap.

1. *Identification.* To understand the feelings and situation of another, the helper must first lose consciousness of self and become engrossed in the personality and situation of the other person (identification). The nurse needs to relinquish a certain amount of self-control to achieve this.

2. *Incorporation.* At a step beyond identification, the experiences of the other person are taken into the helper's self (incorporation). The experience, however, is still recognized as belonging to the patient.

3. *Reverberation.* The next step involves understanding the feelings of the other. There is interaction between the nurse's feelings from past experience and the experience incorporated from the patient. Because humans have the same potential for feelings, the experiences people share need not be identical for them to understand associated feelings.

4. *Detachment.* In the last step the nurse returns to her or his own identity. The results of the three preceding steps are then combined with other knowledge about the patient, and all information is used collectively as a basis for responding to the patient.

The value of *honesty* was previously mentioned as an aspect of credibility. In effective relationships nurses honestly recognize any lack of knowledge by saying, "I don't know the answer to that right now"; openly discuss their own discomfort by saying, for example, "I feel uncomfortable about this discussion"; and admit tactfully that problems do exist, when a patient says such things as "I'm a mess, aren't I?"

Nurses *should not tell a patient not to feel.* Feelings expressed by patients often create discomfort for nurses. Common examples occur when the patient expresses anger or worry or cries. When the nurse is uncomfortable, common responses are, "Don't worry about it, everything will be fine" or "Please don't cry." These responses inhibit the patient's expression of feelings. Unless feelings are extremely inappropriate, it is best to encourage ventilation (voicing) of them. This allows them to be expressed in words and examined objectively. Indirectly it tells patients "Your feelings are not that awful, since I am not bothered by them."

Nurses *need to avoid telling patients what they should feel.* Statements that indicate to patients how they should feel, rather than how they actually do feel, in essence deny patients' true feelings and suggest that they are inappropriate. Examples are: "You shouldn't complain about pain; many others have gone through this same experience stoically," and "You should be glad that you are alive and not worry about the loss of your arm."

It is *not helpful to make excuses for the other person.* When a person reacts with an intense feeling such as anger or grief and seems to have lost control of behavior to the astonishment or discomfort of others, a common error is to explain the behavior by offering excuses. Examples are : "Well, Mr. Brown, you're upset about not finishing your lunch, but the dietitian and I gave you too much," or "I guess you've had a tough session in physical therapy." These responses discourage and divert the person from discussing feelings of anger or inadequacy. The helper has made assumptions about the reasons for the patient's behavior and therefore inhibits exploration of what is really being experienced and felt by the patient.

Not all people feel comfortable about *offering personal statements* about themselves to strangers or to those they do not know well. Used with discretion, however, personal statements can be helpful in solidifying the rapport between the nurse and the patient. The nurse might offer such comments as "I recall when I was in (a similar situation) and I felt angry about being put down." Egan (1975:35) states that the helper "must be spontaneous, open. He can't hide behind the role of counselor. He must be a human being to the human being before him." Egan refers to this as *genuineness* and outlines five behaviors that are components of it (ibid., pp. 90–94):

1. The genuine helper does not take refuge in the role of counselor.

2. The genuine person is spontaneous.

3. The genuine person is nondefensive.
4. The genuine person displays few discrepancies—that is, the person does not think or feel one thing but say another.
5. The genuine person is capable of deep self-disclosure (self-sharing) when it is appropriate.

Caution needs to be exercised by nurses when making references about themselves. These statements must be used with discretion. The extreme of matching each of the patient's problems with a better story of the nurse's own is of little value to the patient.

Nurses can *use their ingenuity to help identify options* for patients. There are always many courses of action to consider in handling problems. Whatever course is chosen needs to achieve the patient's goals, be compatible with the patient's value system, and offer the probability of success. These actions are not explored until the relationship is well established (see Phases of the Helping Relationship, next) and the exploration is done jointly by patient and nurse. The patient needs to choose the ways to achieve goals; however, the nurse can assist in identifying options. For example, a widower may ask for help because he is depressed and anxious about retirement. The nurse could suggest that he:

- Read books and articles on retirement
- Consider working part-time at his former employment
- Talk to other senior citizens about retirement
- Move in to live with a child and grandchildren
- Join a senior citizens' club
- Renew old hobbies, such as gardening or golf
- Join a counseling group
- Move from his house to an apartment
- Remarry
- Move into a senior citizens' lodge
- Join a volunteer service group
- Increase church activities
- Get involved in politics
- Write articles for the local newspaper
- Make plans to travel more extensively

The ingenious nurse will help the patient to select acceptable alternatives. For example, if this man loves animals, young children, and story telling, the nurse might direct his thoughts toward activities such as acquiring a puppy, writing children's stories, or volunteering at the public library.

Summarizing at the end of a discussion or interview is the process of tying together several thoughts and feelings into one or two statements. It is broader than paraphrasing and includes both what was said and how it was said. Several purposes are achieved by summarizing: (a) it helps to terminate the interview, (b) it reassures the patient that the nurse has listened, (c) it checks the accuracy of the nurse's perceptions, (d) it clears the way for new ideas, and (e) it assists the patient to note progress and forward direction (Brammer 1973:94). Sometimes patients may spontaneously offer a summary; at other times the nurse must initiate it or ask the patient to do so. The nurse may say, "Let's look at what has happened in this interview; what do you think has been accomplished?"

Every person has unique strengths and problems. It is important for nurses to *recognize their role and their limitations* and to be as open about them as necessary. When the nurse feels unable to handle some problems, the patient should be informed and referred to the appropriate health professional.

Phases of the Helping Relationship

The relationship process can be described in terms of four sequential phases, each of which is characterized by identifiable tasks and skills. Progression through the stages must occur in succession, as each builds on the one before. Nurses can identify the progress of a relationship by understanding these phases: preinteraction phase, introductory phase, working (maintaining) phase, and termination phase.

Preinteraction phase

In most situations the nurse has information about the patient before the first face-to-face meeting. Such information may include the patient's name, address, age, medical history, and/or social history. Tasks of this phase for the nurse include reviewing pertinent knowledge, considering potential areas of concern, and developing plans for the initial interaction. For example, prior to meeting a young pregnant woman in her home, a nursing student may need to review the normal physical changes that occur with pregnancy and related needs and discomforts. If the woman is in the first trimester of pregnancy, the nurse may anticipate areas of concern about urinary frequency, nausea, fatigue, or feelings of ambivalence, which are common discomforts during this period. Planning for the initial visit may generate some anxious feelings in the nurse. By recognizing these feelings and identifying specific information to be discussed, positive outcomes will evolve. It is wise for the nurse to recognize limitations at this stage and to seek assistance as required.

Introductory phase

The introductory phase is also referred to as the *orientation phase* or the *prehelping phase*. The tone is set during this phase for the rest of the relationship phases. Some of the tasks of this phase were discussed in Chapter 5 for the nursing assessment interview. Three stages of this introductory phase are: (a) entry—

preparing the patient and opening the relationship; (b) clarification—stating the problem or concern and reasons for seeking help; and (c) structure—formulating the contract and the structure (Brammer 1973:55).

Other important tasks of the introductory phase include getting to know each other and developing a degree of trust.

Opening the relationship Initially the nurse and the patient need to identify each other by name as a friendly gesture and to open the relationship. When the nurse initiates the relationship, it is important to explain her or his role to give the patient an idea of what to expect. When the patient initiates the relationship, the nurse needs to help the patient express concerns and reasons for seeking help. Vague, open-ended questions, such as "What's on your mind today?" are helpful at this stage. The nurse needs to be aware that it is not easy for all patients to receive help. Thus, a relaxed, attending attitude on the part of the nurse is important. Providing a setting with minimal distractions and disturbances is also helpful.

Clarifying the problem Initially the patient may not see the problem clearly. To clarify the problem, the nurse needs to use such techniques as attentive listening, paraphrasing, and clarifying, discussed previously in this chapter. A common error at this stage is to ask too many questions of the patient.

Structuring and formulating the contract A contract includes the obligations to be met by both the nurse and the patient. These commitments are agreed upon verbally and need to evolve naturally. Contracts need to cover:

1. Location, frequency, and length of meetings.
2. Overall purpose of the relationship.
3. How confidential material will be handled.
4. Duration and indications for termination of the relationship.

The first three points were described in Chapter 5. Determining the duration of the relationship and indications for termination depends in part upon conditions outside the relationship. For example, many relationships are terminated when the patient is discharged from the hospital or when the nursing student ends clinical rotation. In these situations the nurse and the patient need to discuss these limits. When outside controls do not exist, both participants need to agree upon indications for termination. These are largely determined by the purpose of the relationship. An example is the nurse who terminates the relationship after the patient has learned how to care for his colostomy and is able to resume a life-style acceptable to himself.

Developing trust During the initial parts of the introductory phase the patient may display some resistive behaviors and some testing behaviors. *Resistive behaviors* are those that inhibit involvement, cooperation, or change. Three major reasons for their occurrence are (a) difficulty in acknowledging the need for help and thus a dependent role, (b) fear of exposing and facing feelings, and (c) anxiety about the discomfort involved in changing problem-causing behavior patterns. *Testing behaviors* are those that examine the nurse's interest and sincerity. For example, a patient may refuse to talk, to test whether the nurse will stay with her for the prescribed period of time.

By the end of the introductory phase, the patient begins to develop trust in the nurse. Both participants also begin to view each other as unique individuals. Characteristics of trusting individuals include (a) a feeling of comfort with growth in self-awareness, (b) an ability to share this awareness with others, (c) acceptance of others as they are without needing to change them, (d) openness to new experiences, (e) consistency between words and actions, and (f) ability to delay gratification (Thomas 1970:118).

Working phase

When the nurse and the patient begin to view each other as unique individuals, they begin to appreciate this uniqueness and care about each other. *Caring* is sharing deep and genuine concern about the welfare of another person. Once caring develops, the potential for empathy increases. The purpose of the working phase is to accomplish the tasks that have been outlined in the introductory phase.

The working phase has three successive stages: (a) responding and exploring, (b) integrative understanding and dynamic self-understanding, and (c) facilitating and taking action (Egan 1975:34–40). A summary of these stages and the specific skills required by both participants follows. Each stage builds on the previous one; therefore, they must occur in succession.

Responding and exploring During the introductory phase, emphasis was placed on the listening or attending skills of the nurse. These skills must be continued in the working phase of the relationship, but in addition the nurse now must respond to the patient in ways that assist the patient to explore thoughts, feelings, and actions.

The nurse requires four skills for this first stage:

1. *First-level empathy.* The nurse must communicate (respond) in ways that indicate she or he has listened to what was said and understands how the patient feels. The nurse responds to content or feelings or both, as appropriate.

2. *Respect.* The nurse must show respect for the patient, willingness to be available, and desire to work with the patient.
3. *Genuineness.* This was discussed earlier in this chapter.
4. *Concreteness.* The nurse must assist the patient to be concrete and specific rather than speaking in generalities. When the patient says, "I'm stupid and clumsy," the nurse narrows the topic to the specific by pointing out, "You tripped on that scatter rug."

In self-exploration, the patient explores feelings and actions associated with problems. This is also referred to as *self-disclosure.*

During this first stage of the working phase, trust and rapport are enhanced. The intensity of interaction increases, and feelings such as anger, shame, or self-consciousness may be expressed. If the nurse is skilled in this stage and if the patient is willing to pursue self-exploration, the outcome is a beginning understanding on the part of the patient about behavior and feelings.

Integrative understanding and dynamic self-understanding In this second working stage, patients achieve an objective understanding of themselves and their world (dynamic self-understanding). This ultimately enables patients to change and to take action. More self-exploration occurs, and more information is produced. As a result of this, isolated pieces of information can now be integrated into larger contexts that reveal behavior patterns or themes.

To acquire integrative understanding about the patient, the nurse needs the following skills in addition to those of the first stage:

1. *Advanced-level empathy.* The nurse responds in ways that indicate an understanding not only of what is said but also of what is hinted at or implied nonverbally. Isolated statements become connected.
2. *Self-disclosure.* The nurse willingly but discreetly shares personal experiences.
3. *Confrontation.* The nurse points out discrepancies between thoughts, feelings, and actions that inhibit the patient's self-understanding or exploration of specific areas. This is done with empathy, not judgmentally.

The skills required by the patient include:

1. *Nondefensive listening.* The patient, with support from the nurse, develops the skill of listening.
2. *Dynamic self-understanding.* The patient gains insight into personal behavior, and this understanding forms the basis for changing behavior.

Facilitating and taking action Ultimately the patient must make decisions and take action to become more effective. The responsibility for action belongs to the patient. The nurse, however, collaborates in these decisions and may offer options or information.

When planning action programs, the patient needs to learn to take risks, that is, to accept that either failure or success may be the outcome. Whatever action is taken needs to fall within the patient's capabilities.

Short-term and long-term goals are considered, and it is essential that the nurse offer support at this time. Successes need to be reinforced, and failures need to be recognized realistically. The fact that new problems may arise during this period also needs consideration. Often solving one problem raises new ones. Each new problem then needs to be dealt with by beginning at the first stage of the working phase (responding and exploring).

Termination phase

Terminating the relationship is often expected to be difficult and filled with ambivalence. However, if the previous phases have evolved effectively, the patient can accept this phase of the relationship without feelings of anxiety or dependence. The patient generally has a positive outlook and feels able to handle problems independently. However, because caring attitudes have developed, it is natural to expect some feelings of loss, and each person needs to develop a way of saying good-bye.

Many methods can be used to terminate relationships. Summarizing or reviewing the process can produce a sense of accomplishment. This may include sharing reminiscences of how things were at the beginning of the relationship, compared to now. It is also helpful for both the nurse and the patient to express their feelings about termination openly and honestly. Thus termination discussions need to start in advance of the termination interview. This allows time for the patient to adjust to independence. In some situations referrals are necessary, or it is appropriate to offer an occasional standby meeting to give support as needed.

Evaluating Communication

Techniques that enhance or interfere with therapeutic communication were discussed earlier in this chapter. For nurses to evaluate the effectiveness of their own communications with patients, process recordings are frequently used. A *process recording* is a verbatim (word for word) account of a conversation. It can be taped or written, and it includes all verbal and nonverbal interactions.

One method of writing a process recording is to make three columns on a page. The first column lists what the patient said and did, the second what the nurse said and did, and the third contains comments, such as how the nurse felt and the patient's interpretation of the nurse's responses. See Table 15–2.

Table 15–2 Sample Process Recording

Mary Jane Adams, a nursing aide, reports to Irene Olsen, the staff nurse, that Sandra Barrett, the patient in room 815, had finished only her orange juice when Ms. Adams collected the breakfast trays. Mrs. Barrett had been admitted two days earlier for diagnostic studies. Concerned about her patient, Miss Olsen walks down the corridor to room 815, knocks, and enters. Mrs. Barrett turns away from the window, tears in her eyes, as Miss Olsen enters.

Patient	Nurse	Comments
	Good morning, Mrs. Barrett.	Acknowledging.
Hello.		
	I understand you didn't eat your breakfast.	Making a specific statement, but ignoring the nonverbal.
I wasn't hungry.		
	Is something wrong?	Asking a closed-ended question that fails to facilitate exploration.
No. (Eyes fill with tears.)		
	You look sad; as if you're about to cry.	Giving feedback.
(Cries.)		
	I'll sit here a while with you. (Sits down.)	Offering self.
(Continues to cry.)	(After a 30-second pause): Sometimes it's hard to share the things you're concerned about with someone you don't know well. I'd like to be able to help.	Empathizing. Supporting. Offering self.
(Angrily): You can help me by telling me the truth.		
	(Leans forward and maintains eye contact.)	Actively listening and demonstrating interest.
Everyone beats around the bush when I ask them what's wrong with me. The head nurse said, "What do *you* think is wrong?" That kind of put-off drives me up the wall!		
	You're angry because you're not getting any answers. It seems as if the staff knows something about your condition and they're keeping it from you.	Paraphrasing.
They all seem to be in cahoots. Nobody tells me anything. (Pause.) (Softly): If the news was good, they wouldn't beat around the bush.		
	I'm wondering if you're worried that because people haven't answered your questions it means that you have a serious illness?	Paraphrasing.
Good news is always easy to give.		

(Continued on next page)

Table 15–2 continued

Patient	Nurse	Comments
	Yes, people do seem to be able to deliver good news easier and faster. I also know that we don't have any news—good or bad—to give you because none of the laboratory or X-ray results are back yet. I know that doesn't help answer your questions, but I hope it relieves you a bit from worrying that there is some bad news that's being withheld.	Giving information. Supporting.
Well, when my father-in-law had surgery for a bleeding ulcer, the X-ray and laboratory results were available immediately.		
	When there's a question of emergency surgery being needed, then tests results are asked for immediately. Usually, though, it's preferable to wait for an accurate reading and a thorough written report.	Giving information.
Are you absolutely sure?		
	You don't sound convinced.	Acknowledging the implied.
Listen, I don't mean to give you a hard time. It's just that . . . it may not seem like an emergency to my doctor or the lab people, but it sure is to me. I can't stand not knowing. I don't know the results of the tests I had yesterday. I don't know how many more tests I have to have. Will I have to have surgery? When can I go home?		
	The problem you need help with now is finding out the answers to four questions: What are the results of yesterday's tests? Is your doctor considering any other tests for you, and if so what are they? Is surgery being planned? And when can you go home? Let's try to figure out how you can get the answers to these questions.	Summarizing. Encouraging problem-solving.
Well, I can't call my doctor on the phone. All his receptionist will do is take the message. And, anyway, I'm afraid that he'll be offended if he thinks I'm complaining about him. You won't tell him, will you?		
	No, not unless you and I decide together that it would be the best solution.	Encouraging collaboration.

Table 15–2 continued

Patient	Nurse	Comments
I suppose I could just try to forget about it and be patient, just like everyone tells me to.		
	You've tried that, but you're still worried, fearful, and angry. Let's think of some other possibilities.	Encouraging further exploration.
Maybe you could call his office for me! Since you're a nurse, they'll probably put your call right through.		
	So far there are three possible solutions—calling his office yourself, waiting until he comes to visit you later this afternoon, or having me call his office. Are there any other possible solutions that we haven't considered?	Focusing on solutions.
I can't think of any others.		
	Okay, then, which do you think would be best?	Demonstrating respect for the patient.
I guess I'd feel better if you called his office. I just don't want him to think that I'm criticizing him.		
	You're concerned about what he might think of you because of this phone call. Let's discuss how I should handle the call and what I should say.	Paraphrasing. Encouraging collaboration and problem-solving.

After a few minutes they develop a plan for calling Mrs. Barrett's physician, and Miss Olsen makes the call. The physician has decided to call both the laboratory and the X-ray department for the results of Mrs. Barrett's tests and promises to phone her as soon as he learns the results. They will discuss further possible tests and treatment plans that afternoon when he makes his hospital rounds. Mrs. Barrett asks Miss Olsen to stay with her while she receives the physician's telephone call about the test results.

Courtesy of Carol Ren Kneisl, Associate Professor, Graduate Program, Mental Health/Psychiatric Nursing, State University of New York at Buffalo.

Once a process recording has been completed, it should be analyzed in terms of (a) the direction and development of the interaction (process), and (b) the content. The nurse's interaction can be analyzed for process according to a number of questions:

1. Was the patient's verbal and nonverbal behavior really heard and seen?
2. Were any cues missed?
3. Were the nurse's verbal responses and behavior congruent?
4. Did the patient respond to the nurse or independently of the nurse?
5. Did the communication process flow smoothly?
6. Were the nurse's responses consistent with what the nurse observed and heard? Or were they unrelated, exaggerated, or underresponsive?
7. Were the nurse's responses therapeutic or nontherapeutic? See the previous sections on responding therapeutically or nontherapeutically.

Each response can also be analyzed for content in terms of facilitating or inhibiting communication. See Table 15–2 for a sample analysis.

Summary

Communication incorporates all means of exchanging information between two or more people and is a basic component of human relationships. It is usually categorized as verbal and nonverbal. Verbal communication is effective when the criteria of simplicity, clarity, timing, relevance, adaptability, and credibility are met. Nonverbal communication, however, often reveals more about a person's thoughts and feelings than verbal communication. It includes physical appearance, posture and gait, facial expressions, hand movements, and other gestures. When assessing nonverbal behaviors, the nurse needs to consider cultural influences and be aware that a variety of feelings can be expressed by only one nonverbal expression. In effective communication, verbal and nonverbal expressions are congruent.

Communication is a two-way process involving the sender of the message and the receiver of the message. Because the sender must encode the message and determine the appropriate channels for conveying it, and because the receiver must perceive the message, decode it, and then respond, the communication process includes four elements: (a) sender, (b) message, (c) receiver, and (d) feedback.

Many factors influence the communication process: the ability of the communicator, perceptions, personal space (intimate, personal, social, and public distance), territoriality, roles and relationships, purposes, time and setting, attitudes, emotions, and self-esteem.

The development of communication is a complex process. Normal descriptions of the sounds and phases of children's language are outlined for the nurse to use when assessing individuals. Sounds of the newborn, the prelinguistic phase, passive and active use of language, true speech, and sentence construction are outlined. Egocentric speech, which includes the monologue and the collective monologue, and socialized speech are defined. Semantic development starts with concrete words such as "table," followed by abstract words such as "quality." Factors that influence language development are intelligence, sex, bilingualism, single child versus twin status, parental stimulation, and socioeconomic components. Nurses can assist parents in stimulating the language development of children by encouraging verbal and nonverbal communication, listening, use of speech as a substitute for action, use of exact terms, and other techniques.

There are three broad areas for assessing communication: language development, nonverbal behavior, and style of communication. Many techniques facilitate therapeutic communication. These include attentive listening, paraphrasing, clarifying, using open-ended questions and statements, focusing, being specific, using touch and silence, clarifying reality, time, or sequence, providing general leads, and summarizing. In contrast, techniques that inhibit communication include offering unvalidated reassurance, stating approval or disapproval, giving common (not expert) advice, stereotyping, and being defensive.

The effective nurse-patient relationship is described as a growth-facilitating process. Eleven guidelines for developing helping relationships have been identified. Four phases of the helping relationship include the preinteraction phase, the introductory phase, the working phase, and the termination phase. Each has a specific purpose or goal and requires specific skills of the nurse.

Process recordings are frequently made by nurses to evaluate their own communication. Using them, nurses can analyze both the process and the content of the communication.

Suggested Activities

1. In a clinical situation, analyze your ability to provide information to a patient using the criteria outlined in this chapter for giving effective verbal messages.
2. Visit an ethnic family or restaurant and observe cultural differences in the use of nonverbal expressions.
3. Using a process recording, analyze an interaction with a patient, and identify techniques that facilitated or inhibited communication. Indicate your own feelings regarding the use of specific techniques, emphasizing those with which you feel comfortable and those you tend to avoid.
4. In a clinical situation, observe the frequency, purpose, and effectiveness of touch used by several staff members. Discuss and compare your findings with a group of classmates.
5. Assess the language development of an infant and a preschool child.
6. In a laboratory setting, select a classmate and over a period of weeks alternate roles of being the patient and the nurse. Select some real-life problems for discussion, such as difficulty relating to older patients or anxiety about starting a new clinical experience. Throughout these interactions, analyze the course of your relationship. Emphasize listening skills and empathizing.

Suggested Readings

Communication

Bentz, J. M. January/February 1980. Missed meanings in nurse/patient communication. *American Journal of Maternal-Child Nursing* 5:55–57.
This article presents some terms commonly used about pregnancy and birth and the false images they can imply. The author also presents seven suggestions for clear communication.

Dreher, B. September/October 1981. Overcoming speech and language disorders. *Geriatric Nursing* 2:345–49.
The author describes the effects of stroke, degenerative diseases, and laryngeal cancer upon patients' speech. Methods of improving communication with the person who has a speech impairment are suggested, and descriptions of surgical prostheses for laryngectomies and esophageal speech are given.

Forrest, J. W. July 1972. Student termination: Saying goodbye. *Nursing Papers* 4:23–28.
This article (in a journal by the School for Graduate Nurses, McGill University, Montreal) outlines the process of termination and the feelings that student nurses experience when saying good-bye to patients. The role of the faculty adviser as an integral part of this experience is included.

Kelly, H. S. November 1979. The sense of an ending. *American Journal of Nursing* 69:2378–81.
The author likens the ending of a relationship to grief after bereavement. Devices such as substitution, rationalization, and fantasy are used to avoid the pain of separation.

Kron, T. November 1972. How we communicate nonverbally with patients. *Canadian Nurse* 68:21–23.
This article emphasizes the importance of the nurse's nonverbal communication in conveying self-confidence, interest, respect, and approval to patients. Pertinent examples are given.

MacDonald, M. R. June 1977. How do men and women students rate empathy? *American Journal of Nursing* 77:998.
This article reveals the empathy ratings of men and women in nursing contrasted to those of men and women not in nursing. The results are contrary to what many would think.

Travelbee, J. February 1963. What do we mean by rapport? *American Journal of Nursing* 63:70–72.
The basic ingredients of rapport are outlined in this article. Nurses are constantly reminded that they need to develop rapport with patients but often are unable to explain its meaning.

Territoriality and personal space

Stillman, M. J. October 1978. Territoriality and personal space. *American Journal of Nursing* 78:1670–72.
Territoriality and personal space are explained, with some applications to patients in hospitals.

Touch

Goodykoontz, L. 1979. Touch: Attitudes and practice. *Nursing Forum* 18(1):4–17.
Communicating through touch, procedural touch, and nonprocedural touch are described. Factors that influence touch and the approaches to using touch are presented.

Krieger, D. May 1975. Therapeutic touch: The imprimatur of nursing. *American Journal of Nursing* 75:784–87.
The author describes therapeutic touch and gives a summary of its history. A study involving therapeutic touch is also described.

Lynch, J. J. June 1978. The simple act of touching. *Nursing 78* 8:32–36.
This article describes a study in which the therapeutic effects of touch were identified.

Selected References

Communication

Almore, M. G. June 1979. Dyadic communication. *American Journal of Nursing* 79:1076–78.

Bee, H. 1975. *The developing child.* New York: Harper and Row.

Brammer, L. M. 1973. *The helping relationship: Process and skills.* Englewood Cliffs, N.J.: Prentice-Hall.

Clark, C. C. 1977. Psychotherapy with the resistant child. *Perspectives in Psychiatric Care* 15(3):123–25.

Collins, M. 1981. *Communication in health care: Understanding and implementing effective human relationships.* 2nd ed. St. Louis: C. V. Mosby Co.

Cooper, J. April 1979. Actions really do speak louder than words. *Nursing 79* 9:29–32 (United States ed. 9:113–16).

Cosper, B. December 1977. How well do your patients understand hospital jargon? *American Journal of Nursing* 77:1932–34.

Davis, A. J. 1981. *Please see my need.* Charles City, Iowa: Satellite Books.

Devillers, L. March 1982. What to do when you just can't communicate. *Nursing Life* 2:34–39.

Egan, G. 1975. *The skilled helper: A model for systematic helping and interpersonal relating.* Monterey, Calif.: Brooks/Cole Publishing Co.

Ehmann, V. 1971. Empathy: Its origin, characteristics and process. *Perspectives in Psychiatric Care* 9(2):72–80.

Evans, E. D., and McCandless, B. D. 1978. *Children and youth psychosocial development.* New York: Holt, Rinehart and Winston.

Hein, E. C. 1973. *Communication in nursing practice.* Boston: Little, Brown and Co.

Helms, D. B., and Turner, J. S. 1976. *Exploring child behavior.* Philadelphia: W. B. Saunders Co.

Herth, K. June 1974. Beyond the curtain of silence. *American Journal of Nursing* 74:1060–61.

Johnson, D. W. 1972. *Reaching out: Interpersonal effectiveness and self-actualization.* Englewood Cliffs, N.J.: Prentice-Hall.

Jungman, L. B. June 1979. When your feelings get in the way. *American Journal of Nursing* 79:1074–75.

Kramer, M., and Schmalenberg, C. November 1977. Constructive feedback: Are you and your coworkers getting the message? *Nursing 77* 7:20–21 (United States ed. 7:102).

Kratzer, J. B. December 1977. What does your patient need to know? *Nursing 77* 7:70–71 (United States ed. 7:82).

Lambert, W. E., and Tucker, G. R. 1972. *Bilingual education of children: The St. Lambert experiment.* Boston: Newbury House.

Landreth, C. 1967. *Early childhood.* New York: Alfred A. Knopf.

Long, L., and Prophit, P. 1981. *Understanding/responding: A communication manual for nurses.* Belmont, Calif.: Wadsworth Publishing Co.

Mitchell, A. C. February 1978. Barriers to therapeutic communication with black clients. *Nursing Outlook* 26:109–12.

Piaget, J. 1952. *The language and thought of the child.* London: Routledge and Kegan Paul.

Ramaekers, M. J. June 1979. Communication blocks revisited. *American Journal of Nursing* 79:1079–81.

Shanken, J., and Shanken, P. February 1976. How to be a helping person. *Journal of Psychiatric Nursing and Mental Health Services* 14:24–28.

Shubin, S. November 1976. Familiarity: Therapeutic? Harmful? When? *Nursing 76* 6:18–24.

Sundeen, S. J., et al. 1981. *Nurse-client interaction: Implementing the nursing process.* 2nd ed. St. Louis: C. V. Mosby Co.

Thomas, M. 1970. Trust in the nurse-patient relationship. In Carlson, Carolyn E., editor. *Behavioral concepts and nursing intervention.* Philadelphia: J. B. Lippincott Co.

Toth, S. B., and Toth, A. September 1980. Empathetic intervention with the widow. *American Journal of Nursing* 80:1652–54.

Van Dersal, W. R. December 1974. How to be a good communicator—and a better nurse. *Nursing 74* 4:57–64.

Veninga, R. November 1978. Are you a successful communicator? *Canadian Nurse* 74:34–37.

Vygotsky, L. S. 1962. *Thought and language.* Cambridge, Mass.: MIT Press.

Wright, J. May 1976. Deaf but not mute. *American Journal of Nursing* 76:795–99.

Interviewing and counseling

Edinburg, G. M., et al. 1975. *Clinical interviewing and counseling: Principles and techniques.* New York: Appleton-Century-Crofts.

Kesler, A. R. September 1977. Pitfalls to avoid in interviewing patients. *Nursing 77* 7:70–73.

Meadow, L. and Gass, G. Z. February 1963. Problems of the novice interviewer. *American Journal of Nursing* 63:97–99.

Territoriality and personal space

Allekian, C. I. May/June 1973. Intrusions of territory and personal space: An anxiety-inducing factor for hospitalized persons—an exploratory study. *Nursing Research* 22: 236–41.

Brown, B. G. July 1972. The language of space: A silent component of the therapeutic process. *Nursing Papers* (School for Graduate Nurses, McGill University, Montreal) 4:29–34.

Hall, E. T. 1969. *The hidden dimension.* Garden City, N.Y.: Doubleday and Co.

Touch

Blondis, M. N., and Jackson, B. E. 1977. *Nonverbal communication with patients: Back to the human touch.* New York: John Wiley and Sons.

Ernst, P., and Shaw, J. September/October 1980. Touching is not taboo. *Geriatric Nursing* 1:193–95.

Krieger, D.; Peper, E.; and Ancoli, S. April 1979. Therapeutic touch: Searching for evidence of physiological change. *American Journal of Nursing* 79:660–62.

Lynch, J. J. June 1978. The simple act of touching. *Nursing 78* 8:32–36.

Macrae, J. April 1979. Therapeutic touch in practice. *American Journal of Nursing* 79:664–65.

Montagu, A. 1971. *Touching: The human significance of the skin.* New York: Harper and Row.

Quinn, J. F. April 1979. One nurse's evolution as a healer. *American Journal of Nursing* 79:662–64.

Ujhely, G. B. 1979. Touch: Reflections and perceptions. *Nursing Forum* 18(1):18–32.

Chapter 16

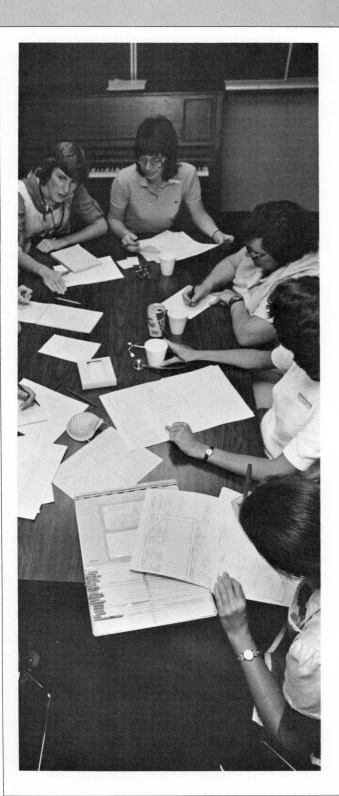

Functioning in Groups

CONTENTS

Objectives

1. Know essential facts about groups
   - **1.1** Define selected terms
   - **1.2** Identify differences between primary and secondary groups
   - **1.3** Identify features of formal, semiformal, and informal groups
   - **1.4** Identify structural and functional characteristics of groups
   - **1.5** Describe three stages of group development
   - **1.6** Identify features of effective groups
2. Understand essential facts about forces influencing group dynamics (process)
   - **2.1** Identify forces that influence group dynamics
   - **2.2** Outline attitudes and behaviors indicating group commitment
   - **2.3** Identify advantages and disadvantages of three leadership styles
   - **2.4** Explain the concept of diffused leadership
   - **2.5** Identify behaviors of an effective leader
   - **2.6** Identify five methods of decision making
   - **2.7** Identify ways in which effective decisions are made
   - **2.8** Identify three categories of functional roles of group members
   - **2.9** Identify behaviors associated with member roles
   - **2.10** Explain how the sociogram can be used to ascertain group interaction patterns
   - **2.11** Outline attitudes and behaviors indicating group cohesiveness
   - **2.12** Explain the concept of power
   - **2.13** Identify some kinds of power
3. Understand essential factors about common group problems and interventions to handle them
   - **3.1** Differentiate between productive and nonproductive conflict
   - **3.2** State reasons for nonproductive conflict
   - **3.3** Identify ways the group leader can resolve productive conflict
   - **3.4** Identify ways the group leader can handle nonproductive conflict
   - **3.5** Identify indications of inadequate group decision making
   - **3.6** Identify common causes of group apathy
   - **3.7** Identify ways the group leader may deal with group apathy
   - **3.8** Identify ways the group leader may intervene when a member monopolizes the group
4. Understand essential facts about assertiveness
   - **4.1** Identify five effects of assertiveness as stated by Alberti and Emmons
   - **4.2** Differentiate among aggressive, nonassertive, and assertive responses
   - **4.3** Identify selected assertiveness techniques
5. Know essential facts about group self-evaluation
   - **5.1** Identify the purpose of feedback
   - **5.2** Identify essential feedback information
   - **5.3** Describe the role of a group productivity observer

Terms

apathy
assertiveness
assimilation
authority
cohesiveness
commitment
conformity
dyad
group
group dynamics (process)
homogeneity
influence
mores
norms
polarization
power
primary group
role
sanctions
secondary group
sociogram
tone

An understanding of groups and group dynamics is essential to nurses, who conduct their professional activities largely within groups of various types and sizes. The nurse's behavior in such groups is affected by many factors: group structure, the nurse's role, the leadership style, power structures, and the behavior of other group members. To function effectively in groups, whether they are patient and family groups or interdisciplinary groups, nurses need to be able to analyze the effects of certain factors on group dynamics and observe specific characteristics of groups. This chapter is designed to assist the nurse to become a more effective group member or group leader.

Groups

People are born into a group (i.e., the family) and interact with others at all stages of their lives in various groups: peer groups, work groups, recreational groups, religious groups, etc. A *group* is defined as two or more persons who have shared needs and goals, who take each other into account in their actions, and who thus are held together and set apart from others by virtue of their interactions.

Much of a nurse's professional life is spent in a wide variety of groups, ranging from *dyads* (two-person groups) to large professional organizations. As a participant in a group, the nurse may be required to fulfill different roles: member or leader, teacher or learner, adviser or advisee, etc.

Groups exist to help people achieve goals that would be unattainable by individual effort alone. For example, groups can often solve problems more effectively than one person, by pooling the ideas and expertise of several individuals; and information can be disseminated to groups more quickly than to individuals. In addition, groups often take greater risks than do individuals. Just as responsibilities for actions are shared by group members, so are the consequences of actions. The overall effectiveness of groups in attaining goals depends on many factors, discussed in this chapter.

Types of Groups

Groups are classified as either primary or secondary, according to their structure and type of interaction. *Primary groups* are small, intimate groups in which the relationships among members are personal, spontaneous, sentimental, cooperative, and inclusive. Examples are the family, a play group of children, informal work groups, and friendship groups. Members of a primary group communicate with each other largely in face-to-face interactions and develop a strong sense of unity or "oneness." What belongs to one person is often seen as belonging to the group. For example, a success achieved by one member is shared by all and is seen as a success of the group.

Primary groups set standards of behavior for the members but also support and sustain each member in stresses he or she would otherwise not be able to withstand. Expectations are informally administered and involve primarily internal constraints imposed by the group itself. To its members, the primary group has a value in itself, not merely as a means to some other goal. The group has a sense of "we" and "our" to it, in contrast to "I" and "mine." Affective relationships are stressed.

The role of the primary group, particularly the family, in health care is increasingly recognized. It is to the primary group that people turn for help and support when they have health problems. Treatment and health care of individuals therefore are developing an expanded focus that includes the family.

Secondary groups are generally larger, more impersonal, and less sentimental than primary groups. Examples are professional associations, task groups, ad hoc committees, political parties, and business groups. Members view these groups simply as means of getting things done. Interactions do not necessarily occur in face-to-face contact and do not require that the members know each other in any inclusive sense. Thus, there is little sentiment attached to such relationships. Expectations of members are formally administered through impersonal controls and external restraints imposed by designated enforcement officials. Once the goals of the group are achieved or change, the interaction is discontinued.

Levels of Group Formality

Formal groups

Groups may be classified as formal, semiformal, or informal. The most common example of the formal group is the work organization. People become familiar with many different formal work groups during their lifetimes and spend a major part of their working hours in such groups. Formal groups usually exist to carry out a task or goal rather than to meet the needs of group members. Traditional features of formal groups include:

1. Authority is imposed from above.
2. Leadership selection is assigned from above and made by an authoritative and often arbitrary order or decree (fiat).
3. Managers are symbols of power and authority.
4. The goals of the formal group are normally imposed at a much higher level than the direct leadership of the group.
5. Fiscal goals have little meaning to the members of the group.
6. Management is endangered by its aloofness from the members of the work group.
7. Behavioral *norms* (expected standards of behavior), regulations, and rules are usually superimposed. The larger the turnover rate of members, the greater the structuring of rules.
8. Membership in the group is only partly voluntary.

9. Rigidity of purpose is often a necessity for protection of the formal group in the pursuit of its objectives.
10. Interactions within the group as a whole are limited, but informal subgroups are generally formed.

Semiformal groups

Some examples of semiformal groups are churches, lodges, social clubs, PTAs, and some labor unions. Many of a person's social needs and ego needs are satisfied by membership in these groups. The groups are similar in form to formal groups, but exhibit slight differences. Features of semiformal groups include:

1. The structure is formal.
2. The hierarchy is carefully delineated.
3. Membership is voluntary but selective and difficult to achieve.
4. Prestige and status are often accrued from membership.
5. Structured, deliberate activities absorb a large part of the group's meeting time.
6. Objectives and goals are rigid; change is not recognized as desirable.
7. In many cases, the leader has direct control over the choice of a successor.
8. The day-to-day operating standards and methods (group norms) are negotiable. Because most people become bored at quibbling about norms, leaders can often "railroad" acceptance of a list of norms they desire.

Informal groups

All people, from childhood on, have membership in numerous informal groups. These groups provide much of a person's education and develop most cultural values. Fives types of groups are representative of the numerous informal groups in existence:

1. *Friendship groups.* The first groups formed in life are friendship groups. They are often formed on the basis of common interests. Many arise out of semiformal group interactions or are formed spontaneously from work organizations.
2. *Hobby groups.* Hobby groups bring together a wide variety of people from all walks of life. The differences in members' personalities and backgrounds are largely ignored in the interests of the hobby itself.
3. *Convenience groups.* Many examples of convenience groups are found both in and out of the work setting. Two examples are the car pool and the child-care group organized by mothers.
4. *Work groups.* Informal work groups can make or break an organization. Managers need to be sensitive to such groups and cultivate their cooperation and good will. Friendships often arise out of such groups between a new member and the first person who makes him or her feel a welcome addition to the group.
5. *Self-protective groups.* Self-protective groups can be found anywhere but are particularly common in work organizations. They arise spontaneously out of a real or perceived threat. For example, a supervisor may approach a worker too strongly and find a group of workers organizing a united front against the threat. Such groups dissipate as soon as the threat has subsided.

Features of informal groups include:

1. The group is not bound by any set of written rules or regulations.
2. Usually there is a set of unwritten laws and a strong code of ethics.
3. The group is purely functional and has easily recognized basic objectives.
4. Rotational leadership is common. The group recognizes that only rarely are all leadership characteristics found in one person.
5. The group assigns duties to the members best qualified for certain functions. For example, the member who is recognized as being effective during times of stress will be called upon for guidance when threats or problems arise; the person who is recognized as outgoing and socializing will be assigned responsibilities for planning parties etc.
6. Judgments about the group's leader are made quickly and surely. The leader is replaced when he or she makes one or more mistakes or does not get the job done efficiently.
7. The group is an ideal testing ground for new leadership techniques, but there is no guarantee that such techniques can be transferred effectively to a large, formal organization. For example, management by committee originated in small, informal group structures.
8. Behavioral norms are developed either by group effort or by the leader and adopted by the group.
9. Deviance by one member from the group's behavioral norms is more threatening to the perpetuation of small, informal groups than to large, formal, heterogeneous groups. Conformity and group solidarity are important for the protection and preservation of small groups.
10. Group norms are enforced by *sanctions* (punishments) imposed by the group on those who violate a norm. Examples are the withholding of privileges or isolation of the offender from the group. Different values are placed on norms, however, in accordance with the values of the leader. One leader may regard an action as a gross violation, while another leader may find it quite acceptable.
11. Interpersonal interactions are spontaneous.

Characteristics of Groups

Many characteristics of groups are associated with the type and level of formality of the specific group, as discussed earlier in this chapter. Groups of all kinds, however, have certain structural and functional characteristics that need to be understood before the nurse can gain a perspective on the interactions that occur between individual members and the group. These characteristics are outlined and described in Table 16–1.

Structural properties refer to the ways in which persons in a group are involved in (a) ordered arrangements, (b) that define and regulate their behavior, and (c) that provide a patterned constancy and stability to their behavior together. Structural properties of a group are defined independently of the particular persons who are members. Thus a change in group membership does not create a change in group structure. For example, a hospital has ordered arrangements of personnel whose behavior is defined and regulated in prescribed role and power structures. Even when personnel change, the structure remains the same or similar.

Functional properties relate to operational and procedural methods of functioning and to group process or dynamics as determined by group norms, climate, tone, etc.

Table 16–1 Characteristics of Groups

Characteristic	Description	Characteristic	Description
Structural		*Functional*	
Size	Number of members. Ranges from two members to infinity. The smaller the group, the less formal the relationship.	Norms	Expected standards of behavior based on the group mores (values). May be established by: (a) tradition, (b) imposition by the highest authority or immediate supervisor of the group, (c) cooperation between the leader and the group, or (d) group action.
Membership methods	How people become members of the group. May be ascribed or assigned. Ascribed membership means voluntary choice, e.g., membership in a hobby club. Assigned membership means involuntary draft, e.g., membership in the armed forces. Permeability (access to membership in the group by outsiders) varies from highly selective to highly permissive.	Homogeneity	Degree of likeness of attitudes and beliefs among members.
		Sanctions	Measures used to enforce normative behavior. Range from light censure to expulsion from the group.
Relationship to other groups	Whether the group functions autonomously from or in concert with other groups; whether it is a separate organization or a subgroup of a larger structure.	Tone	Pleasant or unpleasant atmosphere sensed in a group.
Stability	The degree of permanence of a group and the sense of continuity felt by the group.	Cohesiveness	Degree of group unity (oneness); sense of members being "we." Forces that tend to hold the group together include: (a) perceived threats from outside, (b) leadership that communicates and reinforces group objectives, (c) homogeneity, and (d) identification by members with the group's objectives.
		Climate	Unwritten traditions, habits, relationships, practices, rules, beliefs, and attitudes that become characteristic of a group.
		Conformity	Actions in accordance with specified standards of authority or of the group.

Stages of Group Development

There are three stages of group development: the initiation, functional, and dissolution stages. The *initiation stage*, when a group first forms, involves interactions in which members become familiar with one another, determine a method of operation, and establish their roles within the group. Tasks predominate, and behavior is tested. The group is viewed more as a series of individuals than as a unified whole, and differences among individuals are more evident than similarities. People seek a place in the group in relation to others in various ways: some hang back as observers; others are highly extroverted, relating with excessive good humor and amicability. As the group forms, a testing process begins, in which people gradually increase their personal exchanges and contacts and try to find out about one another's attitudes, values, and readiness to be contacted. At this stage the group may appear to be acting effectively. It is progressing with its tasks, and there appears to be a friendly comradeship among members. However, this condition is only superficial, arising from experiences established before the group was formed.

The *functional stage* occurs when the members feel comfortable with one another. It is during this phase that group properties such as *tone, homogeneity, cohesiveness,* and *conformity* develop and increase. See Table 16–1 for definitions. Group goals are established, and *polarization* (movement by members toward a common goal) occurs. Individual behavior is less obvious due to the process of *assimilation* (the blending of attitudes and beliefs among members); a group unified in approach becomes evident. The tasks to be achieved are also evident.

The *dissolution stage* occurs when group members no longer see a need for the group. Group goals may or may not have been attained, and group properties such as cohesion and assimilation may not have been achieved. Members may feel a sense of relief or frustration about dissolution. Relief may be felt if (a) the degree of members' dependence on the group for meeting their needs is low, (b) the potency (importance) of the group for its members is minimal, (c) the climate of the group was tense, and (d) group cohesion did not occur. Frustration or anxiety will be felt if dependence on and potency of the group were high and if the climate and group cohesion were pleasant and agreeable.

Features of Effective Groups

Two characteristics are recognized as descriptive of an effective group (Francis and Young 1979:6):

1. It produces outstanding results and succeeds in spite of difficulties.
2. The members feel responsible for the output of their group and act to clear obstacles.

To be effective, a group must achieve three main functions:

1. Accomplish its goals
2. Maintain its cohesion
3. Develop and modify its structure to improve its effectiveness

The many factors that influence these functions can be analyzed and used to evaluate the effectiveness or ineffectiveness of groups. See Table 16–2.

Assessing Group Dynamics (Process)

During the past decade the terms *group dynamics* and *group process* have frequently appeared in literature and discussions among group workers, educators, and professional organizations. *Group dynamics* (or *process*) are forces in the group situation that determine the behavior of the group and its members (Jenkins 1974:5). They are a way of looking at groups. Every group has its own unique dynamics and constantly changing pattern of forces, just as each individual has unique forces from within that shape the person's character. To study the dynamics of a group, several factors, in addition to group structure and organization, may be analyzed: (a) commitment, (b) leadership style, (c) diffused leadership function, (d) decision-making methods, (e) member behaviors, (f) interaction patterns, (g) group cohesiveness, and (h) power.

Commitment

The members of effective groups have a *commitment* (agreement, pledge, or obligation to do something) to the goals and output of the group. Because groups demand time and attention, members must give up some autonomy and self-interest. Inevitably conflicts arise between the interests of individual members and those of the group. However, members who are committed to the group feel close to each other and willingly put themselves out for the group. Some indications of group commitment are:

1. Members feel a strong sense of belonging.
2. Members enjoy each other.
3. Members seek each other for counsel and support.
4. Members support each other in difficulty.

Table 16–2 Comparative Features of Effective and Ineffective Groups

Factor	Effective groups	Ineffective groups
Atmosphere	Informal, comfortable, and relaxed. It is a working atmosphere in which people demonstrate their interest and involvement.	Obviously tense. Signs of boredom may appear.
Goal setting	Goals, tasks, and objectives are clarified, understood, and modified so that members of the group can commit themselves to cooperatively structured goals.	Unclear, misunderstood, or imposed goals may be accepted by members. The goals are competitively structured.
Leadership and member participation	Shift from time to time, depending on the circumstances. Different members assume leadership at various times, because of their knowledge or experience.	Delegated and based on authority. The chairperson may dominate the group or the members may defer unduly. Member participation is unequal, with high-authority members dominating.
Goal emphasis	All three functions of groups—goal accomplishment, internal maintenance, and developmental change—are emphasized.	One or more functions may not be emphasized.
Communication	Open and two-way. Ideas and feelings are encouraged, both about the problem and about the group's operation.	Closed or one-way. Only the production of ideas is encouraged. Feelings are ignored or taboo. Members may be tentative or reluctant to be open and have "hidden agendas" (personal goals at cross-purposes with group goals).
Decision making	By consensus, although various decision-making procedures appropriate to the situation may be instituted.	By the highest authority in the group with minimal involvement by members, or an inflexible style is imposed.
Cohesion	Facilitated through high levels of inclusion, trust, liking, and support.	Either ignored or used as a means of controlling members, thus promoting rigid conformity.
Conflict tolerance	High. The reasons for disagreements or conflicts are carefully examined, and the group seeks to resolve them. The group accepts basic disagreements that cannot be resolved and lives with them.	Low. Attempts may be made to ignore, deny, avoid, suppress, or override controversy by premature group action.
Power	Determined by the members' abilities and the information they possess. Power is shared. The issue is how to get the job done.	Determined by position in the group. Obedience to authority is strong. The issue is who controls.
Problem solving	High. Constructive criticism is frequent, frank, relatively comfortable, and oriented toward removing an obstacle to problem solving.	Low. Criticism may be destructive, taking the form of either overt or covert personal attacks. It prevents the group from getting the job done.
Self-evaluation as a group	Frequent. All members participate in evaluation and decisions about how to improve the group's functioning.	Minimal. What little evaluation there is may be done by the highest authority in the group, rather than by the membership as a whole.
Creativity	Encouraged. There is room within the group for members to become self-actualized and interpersonally effective.	Discouraged. People are afraid of appearing foolish if they put forth a creative thought.

From H. S. Wilson and C. R. Kneisl, *Psychiatric nursing*, 2nd ed. (Menlo Park, Calif.: Addison-Wesley Publishing Co., 1982), p. 221.

5. Members value the contributions of other members.
6. Members are motivated by working in the group and want to do their tasks well.
7. Members express good feelings openly and identify positive contributions.
8. Members feel that the goals of the group are achievable and important.

Leadership Style

Three leadership styles have been described: autocratic, democratic, and laissez-faire. The three are often blended in a selective combination to fit the situation, the needs of the leader, and the needs of the group, rather than being implemented continuously in pure form.

Autocratic leadership

In autocratic leadership the leader makes the decisions for the group. This style is likened to dictatorship and presupposes that the group is incapable of making its own decisions. The leader determines policies and gives orders and directions to the members. Autocratic leadership generally has negative connotations and often makes group members dissatisfied. It may, however, be a necessary style of leadership when urgent decision making is required, or when group members do not wish to participate in making a decision.

Democratic leadership

In democratic leadership the leader participates as a facilitator, encouraging group discussion and decision making. This supportive style increases group productivity and satisfaction. It presupposes that group members are capable of making decisions, are motivated to do so, and value independence. Democratic leadership generally has positive connotations, but it requires time for consultation and collaboration. It may not always be the most effective method.

Laissez-faire leadership

In laissez-faire leadership the leader participates minimally and often only on request of the members. This style is described as a "hands-off" approach. It recognizes the group's need for autonomy and self-regulation. It is most effective after a group has made a decision, is committed to it, and has the expertise to implement it. The leader acts as a resource person and consultant.

Diffused leadership

Diffused leadership can be described as an approach to group leadership in which functions are distributed. This concept recognizes that the leadership function is not held irrevocably by one person but rather is distributed among the group members. To clarify this concept, Francis and Young (1979:63) distinguish the roles of group manager (the formal head of the group) from those of group leader. Managers have special responsibilities and functions recognized by the organization and vital to the group's performance as an energizing and creative force. However, group leadership is a broad function. Different members come to the fore in their areas of strength to suit the tasks at hand. To determine which group members carry out leadership functions, the following questions may be asked:

1. Who starts the meeting or the work?
2. Who contributes additional information to help the group carry out its functions?
3. Who represents the group with other groups?
4. Who encourages contributions from group members?
5. Who provides support to members with difficult situations?
6. Who clarifies thoughts expressed in discussions?
7. Who keeps the discussions relevant?

Effective leadership

Much has been written about effective leadership and style. Listed below are some statements descriptive of effective leaders—they:

- Use a leadership style that is natural to them
- Use a leadership style appropriate to the task and the members
- Assess the effects of their behavior on others and the effects of others' behavior on themselves
- Are sensitive to forces acting for and against change
- Express an optimistic view about human nature
- Are energetic
- Are open and encourage openness, so that real issues are confronted
- Facilitate personal relationships
- Plan and organize activities of the group
- Are consistent in behavior toward group members
- Delegate tasks and responsibilities to develop members' abilities, not merely to get tasks performed
- Involve members in all decisions
- Value and use group members' contributions
- Encourage creativity
- Encourage feedback about their leadership style

Decision-making Methods

Five methods of decision making have been identified:

1. *Individual or authority rule decisions.* The designated leader of the group makes the decision and group members or others involved in the decision are expected to abide by it. Authority rule decisions may be made without discussion or consultation with the group or may be made after discussing the issue and eliciting the group's ideas and views. Decisions made without discussion are often advantageous for simple, routine matters. Those made after discussion are advantageous in that they use the resources of the group and gain the benefits of discussion. However, this type of decision making does not develop a commitment in members to implement the decision, and it fails to resolve controversies among members.
2. *Minority decisions.* A few group members meet to discuss an issue and make a decision that is binding for all. This method of decision making is advantageous when the total group is unable to meet together due to time pressures. It is useful for routine decisions. Its limitations are similar to those of decision making by authority rule. Often executive committees of large groups exercise minority control in decision making.
3. *Majority decisions.* More than half of those involved make the decision. This method is commonly used in large groups when complete member commitment is unnecessary. It is an effective method to close a discussion on issues that are not highly important for the group and when sufficient time is lacking for a decision by consensus.
4. *Consensus decisions.* Each group member expresses an opinion, and a decision is made by which members can abide, if not in whole, at least in part. This type of decision making takes a great deal of time and energy and therefore is not effective when time pressures are great or when an emergency is in progress. It is useful, however, when important and complex decisions requiring commitment from all members need to be made. This method has several advantages: (a) it produces creative, high-quality decisions, (b) it elicits commitment by all members and responsibility for implementing action, (c) it uses the resources of all members, and (d) it enhances the future decision-making ability of the group.
5. *Unanimous decisions.* Each group member agrees on the decision and can support the action to be taken. This method is commonly used for issues that are highly important to the group and require complete member commitment. Unanimous decisions are not practical for simple, routine matters or controversial issues, however.

Effective decisions

Making sound decisions is essential to effective group functioning. Effective decisions are made when:

1. The group determines which decision method to adopt.
2. The group listens to all the ideas of members.
3. Members feel satisfied with their participation.
4. The expertise of group members is well used.
5. The problem-solving ability of the group is facilitated.
6. The group atmosphere is positive.
7. Time is used well, i.e., the discussion focuses on the decision to be made.
8. Members feel committed to the decision and responsible for its implementation.

Member Behaviors

The degree of input by members into goal setting, decision making, problem solving, group evaluation, etc., is due in part to the group structure and leadership style, but members, too, have responsibilities for group behavior and participation. Each member participates in a wide range of *roles* (assigned or assumed functions) during group interactions. These roles have been categorized as (a) task roles, (b) maintenance or building roles, and (c) self-serving roles.

Task roles

A task role is related to the task of the group. Its purpose is to enhance and coordinate the group's movement toward achievement of its goals. Task roles and the behaviors associated with them include:

1. *Information and opinion giver:* offers facts, opinions, ideas, suggestions, and relevant information to help group discussion
2. *Information and opinion seeker:* asks for facts, information, opinions, ideas, and feelings from other members, to help group discussion
3. *Starter:* proposes goals and tasks to initiate action within the group
4. *Direction giver:* develops plans on how to proceed, and focuses attention on the task to be done
5. *Summarizer:* pulls together related ideas or suggestions; restates and summarizes the major points discussed
6. *Coordinator:* shows relationships among various ideas; harmonizes activities of various subgroups and members

7. *Diagnoser:* identifies sources of difficulties the group has in working effectively and blocks to progress in accomplishing the group's goals
8. *Energizer:* stimulates a higher quality of work from the group
9. *Reality tester:* examines the practicality and workability of ideas; evaluates alternative solutions, and applies them to real situations to see how they will work
10. *Evaluator:* compares group decisions and accomplishments with group standards and goals (Wilson and Kneisl 1982)

Maintenance or building roles

The maintenance role is related to maintaining or building the group's continuity, cohesion, and stability. Roles and behaviors associated with this include:

1. *Encourager of participation:* warmly encourages everyone to participate, giving recognition for contributions, demonstrating acceptance and openness to the ideas of others; is friendly and responsive to group members
2. *Harmonizer and compromiser:* persuades members to analyze their differences of opinion constructively, searches for common elements in conflicts, and tries to reconcile disagreements
3. *Tension reliever:* eases tensions and increases the enjoyment of group members by joking, suggesting breaks, and proposing approaches to group work that will be fun
4. *Communication helper:* shows good communication skills and makes sure that each group member understands what other members are saying
5. *Evaluator of emotional climate:* asks members how they feel about the way in which the group is working and about each other, and shares own feelings about both
6. *Process observer:* watches the process by which the group is working and uses those observations to help examine the group's effectiveness
7. *Standard setter:* expresses group standards and goals, to make members aware of the direction of work and of progress toward the goal, and to get open acceptance of group norms and procedures
8. *Active listener:* listens and serves as an interested audience for other members; is receptive to others' ideas; goes along with the group when not in disagreement
9. *Trust builder:* accepts and supports the openness of other group members, reinforces risk taking, and encourages individuality
10. *Interpersonal problem solver:* promotes open discussion of conflicts between group members, to resolve them and increase group togetherness (Wilson and Kneisl 1982)

Self-serving roles

Self-serving roles often present obstacles to effective group functioning. The self-serving role is aimed at satisfying the individual's needs and does not enhance group effectiveness. Examples of self-serving roles and behaviors are:

1. *Aggressor:* deflates the status of others by expressing disapproval of their values, acts, or feelings, by attacking the group or the problem it is working on, or by joking aggressively
2. *Blocker:* tends to be negative and stubbornly resistant; attempts to maintain or bring back issues after group has rejected or bypassed them
3. *Recognition seeker:* calls attention to self through boasting, reporting on personal achievements, acting in unusual ways, or struggling not to be placed in an "inferior" position
4. *Self-confessor:* uses the group as an audience for expression of personal, non-group-oriented feelings, insights, or ideologies
5. *Playboy:* displays lack of involvement in the group's processes through cynicism, nonchalance, horseplay, and other more-or-less studied forms of irrelevant behavior
6. *Dominator:* tries to assert authority or superiority by engaging in flattery, claiming a superior status or the right to attention, giving directions authoritatively, and interrupting the contributions of others
7. *Help seeker:* attempts to evoke a sympathy response from other group members or from the whole group, through expressions of insecurity, personal confusion, or self-depreciation beyond "reason"
8. *Special interest pleader:* speaks for some underdog—the small businessperson, the grass roots community, the housewife, labor, etc.—usually cloaking personal prejudices or biases in a stereotype that best fits the individual's need (Wilson and Kneisl 1982)

Bales's system of verbal behavior analysis

Another system for observing and analyzing group members' verbal behaviors was proposed by R. F. Bales in 1950. It is a 12-category system organized into two major areas, *task* issues and *socioemotional* or *maintenance* issues:

I. Communication involving task issues
  A. Giving or sending material to others
    1. *Gives suggestion:* takes some lead and direction in task matters, focuses the group's attention on a problem, develops an agenda, etc. This implies a problem of control.
    2. *Gives opinion:* expresses a feeling or wish; gives serious evaluation and analysis or com-

mentary on the task. This relates to problems of evaluation.

3. *Gives orientation:* provides information and clarification of points and issues; helps to orient the group to its task; repeats, clarifies, and confirms information. This relates to problems of communication.

B. Asking for or receiving material from others

4. *Asks for suggestion*: emphasizes need for some direction, e.g., requests an agenda. This involves a concern about control as in category 1.

5. *Asks for opinion:* seeks to elicit or to encourage reactions on the part of others; tries to elicit opinions from others on various items and issues that come before the group. This involves a concern about evaluation as in category 2.

6. *Asks for orientation:* seeks factual information; seeks repetition or clarification of still confusing matters. This involves a concern about communication as in category 3.

II. Communications involving maintenance issues

A. Socioemotionally positive expressions

7. *Shows solidarity:* acts in a generally supportive and friendly way; helps others; expresses harmony and unity. This relates to problems of reintegration.

8. *Shows tension release:* jokes, laughs, and shows satisfaction. This relates to problems of tension reduction.

9. *Agrees:* shows passive acceptance; concurs; complies with others; understands others; is receptive and interested. This relates to problems with decision making.

B. Socioemotionally negative expressions

10. *Shows antagonism:* defends or asserts self; is unfriendly; deflates others' status; indicates alienation from others, boredom, noncaring, or lack of concern. This relates to problems of reintegration as in category 7.

11. *Shows tension:* withdraws and hangs back from issues; shows fear or apprehension, e.g., inappropriate laughter, excessive hesitation, tremor, or blocking of speech. This relates to problems of tension reduction as in category 8.

12. *Disagrees:* withholds help, passively rejects others; shows disbelief in others' comments or ideas; is nonresponsive. This relates to problems with decision making as in category 9.

Interaction Patterns

Interaction patterns can be observed and ascertained by a *sociogram*, a diagram of the flow of verbal communication within a group during a specified period, e.g., 5 or 15 minutes. This diagram indicates who speaks to whom and who initiates the remarks. Ideally the interaction patterns of a small group would indicate verbal interaction from all members of the group to all members of the group. See Figure 16–1. In reality, however, such an interaction pattern does not occur. See Figure 16–2. This second diagram illustrates that not all communication is a two-way process. The lines with arrows at each end indicate that the statement made by one person was responded to by the recipient; the short lines drawn near one of the arrows indicate who initiated the remark. One-way communication is indicated by lines with an arrow at only one end. Remarks made to the group as a whole are indicated by arrows drawn to only the middle of the circle. By using a sociogram, nurses can analyze strengths and weaknesses in a group's interaction patterns. Used in conjunction with member behavior tools, this can offer considerable data about the group's dynamics.

Cohesiveness

Cohesive groups possess a certain group spirit, a sense of being "we," and a common purpose. Groups lacking in cohesiveness are unstable and prone to disintegra-

Figure 16–1 An ideal small group interaction pattern, in which members interact with all other members.

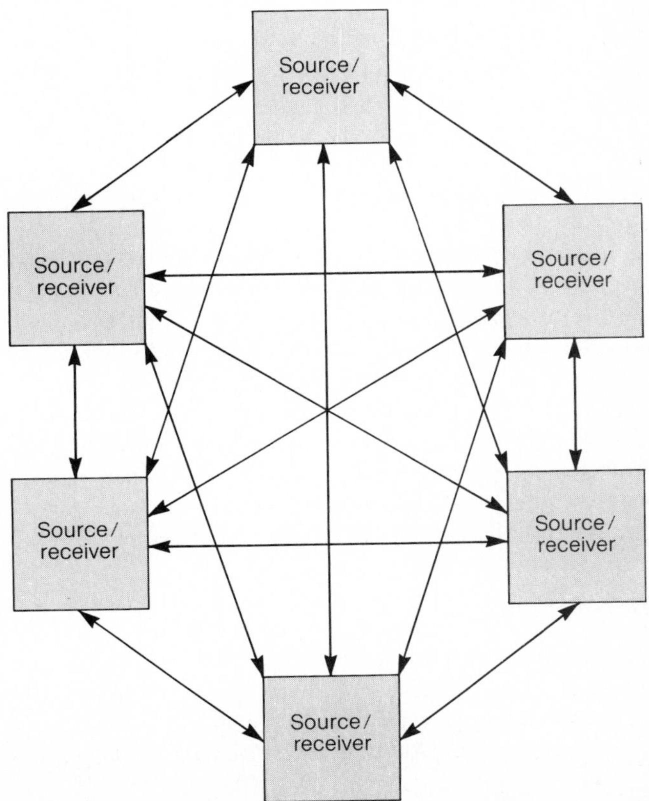

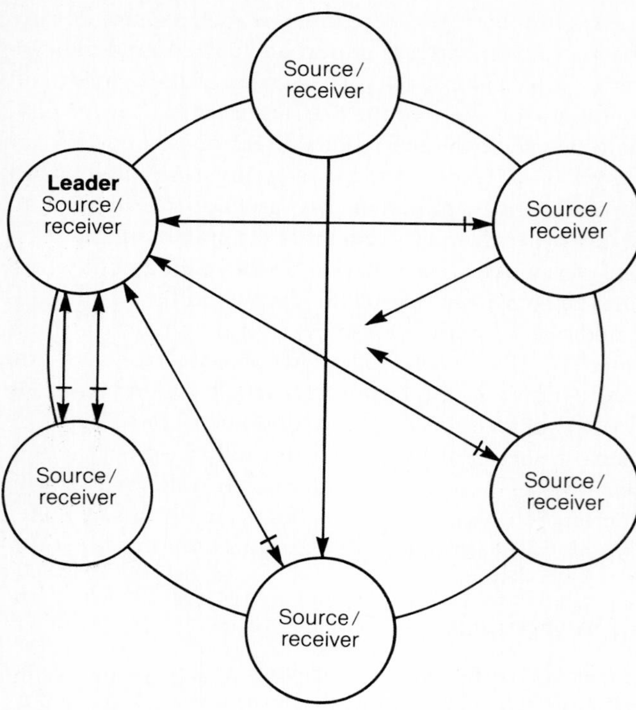

Figure 16–2 A sociogram indicating the flow of verbal communication within a group during a specific period. Note that five questions or comments calling for a response were directed at the leader.

tion. The following membership attitudes and behaviors and group properties characterize high-cohesion groups (Wilson and Kneisl 1982):

Membership attitudes and behaviors

1. Members like each other, trust one another, and are friendly and willing to interact.
2. Members receive support from the group and praise one another for accomplishments.
3. Members have similar attitudes and beliefs.
4. Members are loyal to the group and defend it against outside criticism.
5. Members readily accept assigned roles and tasks.
6. Members influence each other and value being influenced by others.
7. Members feel satisfied and secure.
8. Members attend meetings, arrive on time, and stay in the group.

Group properties

1. Group goals are valued and are consistent with the goals of individuals.
2. Group activities are handled by group action.
3. Group actions are interdependent and cooperative.
4. Group goals that are difficult to achieve are met by persistent efforts.
5. Participation is high.
6. Commitment is high.
7. Communication is high.
8. "We" is frequently heard in discussions.
9. Group productivity is high.
10. Group norms are adhered to and protected.
11. Leadership style is appropriate.

Power

Patterns of behavior in groups are greatly influenced by the force of power. *Power* can be defined as the ability to influence another person in some way or the ability to do something, whether it is to decide the fate of a nation or to decide that a certain change in policy or practice is necessary. Claus and Bailey (1977:17) define power in terms of three interrelated elements: *ability* (based on strength of the person), *willingness* (based on positive energy), and *results*, such as affecting the behavior of others (produced by action). The relationship of the three is pyramidal: *strength* (the basis of ability) supports *energy* (the basis of willingness to use the ability), which in turn supports *action* (the basis of results). See Figure 16–3.

Many people have a negative concept of power, likening it to control, domination, and even coercion of others by muscle and clout. However, power can be viewed as a vital, positive force that moves people toward the attainment of individual or group goals. The overall purpose of power is to encourage cooperation and collaboration in accomplishing a task.

Figure 16–3 The tripartite and pyramidal nature of power according to Claus and Bailey (1977).

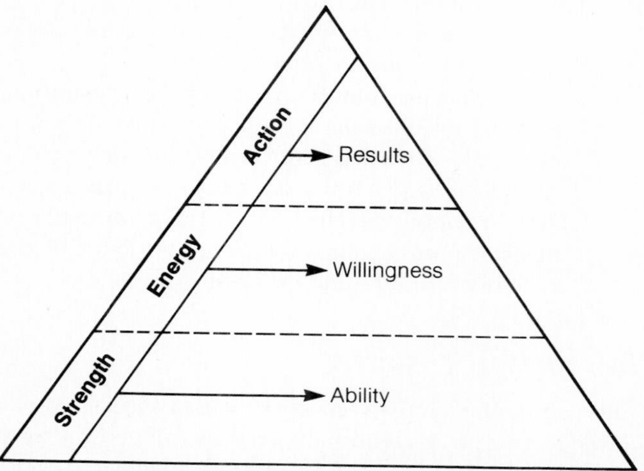

Power versus influence and authority

Often the terms *power, influence,* and *authority* are used interchangeably, but they need to be differentiated. *Power* is the source of influence, whereas *influence* is the result of proper use of power. *Authority* is the official or legitimized right to use a given amount or type of power, i.e., the right to act and the right to command (Claus and Bailey 1977:21). Authority may be either delegated or acquired.

Stages of power orientation and development

Four stages of power orientation and development are categorized by McClelland (1975:14). See Table 16–3.

Kinds of power

Four kinds of power have been identified:

1. *Legitimate power.* A person has legitimate power when group members believe this person ought to have influence over them (endorsed power) because of the person's position in the group or organization (authorized power). Authorized power may be either formal or informal. *Formal authorized power* usually resides in positions in organizations and arises historically through custom or delegation. *Informal authorized power* originates from an individual's personal power base.
2. *Referent power.* A person has referent power when group members identify with and want to be like that person. Members do what that person wants because they like and respect the person and want to be liked in return.
3. *Informational power.* A person has informational power when group members believe that the person has access to useful information not available to other members in the group.
4. *Expert power.* A person has expert power when group members see the person as having some special knowledge or skill.

Dimensions and levels of power

Rollo May (1972:99) defines power as the ability to cause or prevent change and asserts that it has two dimensions: *potentiality* (latent power) and *actuality.* Latent power is power that has not yet developed fully but has the ability to cause a change at some future time.

Five levels of power are categorized by May (ibid.):

1. The power to be
2. Self-affirmation
3. Self-assertion
4. Aggression
5. Violence

When lower levels of power are ineffective for attaining goals or needs, a person feels powerless and moves to a higher, more destructive level of power, such as aggression and violence.

Table 16–3 Stages of Power Orientation and Development

Stage	Object of power	Source of power	Characteristics
1	Self: to feel stronger	External phenomena (God, mother, leader) strengthen self	Desire to talk, to share, and to nurture
2	Self: to strengthen, control, direct self	Self; internal phenomena (autonomy, will power) strengthen self	Desire for knowledge of how to control things better; emphasis on outward control of expressions of anger; attempts to be independent
3	Others: to influence others	Self; internal phenomena (assertiveness, desire to experience power) strengthen self	Concern with prestige and possessions; having a goal of power rather than achievement
4	Others: to serve or influence others	External phenomena (religion, law, group values) strengthen self	View of power-related actions in terms of duty or responsibility to a higher authority; development of loyalty

From D. C. McClelland, *Power: The inner experience* (New York: Irvington Publishers, 1975).

Common Group Problems

Conflict

Conflict, a normal stage in the life of most groups, refers to disagreement, impatience, and argument among members. It can be either productive or nonproductive, and group leaders need to distinguish destructive conflict from constructive conflict by making observations and interpretations (diagnoses).

Productive conflict

Conflict is productive and beneficial when members feel involved, when the issue being discussed is important to them, and when they are working intensively on a problem. Productive conflict contributes to problem solving as long as the goal is clearly understood. Observations that indicate a conflict is productive, according to Sampson and Marthas (1977:269) include:

1. Members have an agreed upon goal in mind and are working toward it.
2. Members make comments that are relevant to the task.
3. Members encourage all to participate, even those with different points of view.
4. Members listen to and hear others even though they may be impatient with one another and disagree with the suggestions made.
5. The bases for disagreements are examined and evaluated openly and critically.
6. Problems are solved by rational discussion and compromise and do not tend to recur.

Nonproductive conflict

Conflict that is nonproductive leads the group astray and hinders the achievement of group goals. Three common reasons (or diagnoses) for this type of conflict, identified by Bradford, Stock, and Horwitz (1974:38), are:

1. The group has been given an impossible task or the task is not clear, and members are frustrated because they feel unable to meet the demands on them.
2. The main concern of members is to find status in the group and to deal with their personal and individual tasks rather than the group problem.
3. Members are operating from unique, unshared points of view and may have competing loyalties to and conflicting interests in outside groups.

Each of these diagnoses for nonproductive conflict has typical signs. See Table 16–4.

Interventions

Conflict-handling interventions depend on both the who and the what of the conflict, the group climate, and whether the conflict is perceived as productive or nonproductive. Interventions that occur within a climate of group cohesion and trust are most effective. Where such a climate does not exist, the leader first needs to facilitate its development. Early diagnosis of conflict and early intervention are also essential. Early intervention can thwart an escalating cycle of nonproductive conflict and form a basis for using constructive conflict effectively in the future.

1. *Productive conflict resolution.* According to Sampson and Marthas (1977:272), the group leader has three tasks in resolving productive conflict:

a. *Supporting and legitimizing disagreement and conflict.* Supporting disagreement helps members realize that they can disagree without losing their integrity and that the disagreement can be useful for problem solving. The leader may say, for example, "I think there are disagreements being expressed on this problem, and I consider it a sign of a healthy group."

b. *Clarifying the basis and the meaning of the conflict.* In this step the leader assists members to focus on the basis of their disagreement. For example, the leader may say, "I realize the two of you are disagreeing, but I'm not exactly sure what the disagreement is about. Could each of you take a minute to say what your position is?" Once the basis of the conflict is identified, all members are encouraged to discuss it further.

c. *Negotiating a compromise.* After the basis of the conflict is identified, the group leader and members are ready to examine acceptable solutions. It is helpful to focus first on the commonalities members share rather than emphasizing ways in which they differ. A compromise is then developed for the opposing perspectives. For example, if two members feel that they are both overloaded and unable to give anyone more time, a compromise may be reached in which one person is given some assistance for the overload, thus freeing that person to provide assistance to the other.

2. *Nonproductive conflict resolution.* Resolving nonproductive conflicts is more complex. In some instances, the conflict needs to be avoided or played down rather than confronted. This is a matter of careful judgment on the part of the group leader. Strategies that can be employed if the leader decides it is more beneficial for the group to face the issue directly (ibid., p. 271) include:

a. *Interpreting.* The leader explains her or his view of the problem. For example, the leader might say, "I think the group is having trouble making a decision because there are some distinct conflicts among several members. Before we try to accomplish any other task I think we had better take some time and look at those conflicts."

b. *Reflecting.* With this strategy, the leader points out certain behaviors of the members or points out his or her own feelings. To *reflect behavior* the leader may say, "I've noticed that several persons have been very quiet for some time, that others are talking a great deal but usually at cross-purposes, and that as a group we seem unable to focus our efforts on any thing except disagreeing." To *reflect feeling* the leader may say, "I'm not sure how anyone else feels, but I'm feeling frustrated and annoyed over the constant bickering. I know we have a job to do, and I'd like to get on with it."

c. *Confronting.* With this strategy, the leader calls the group's attention to what she or he perceives is taking place with one or more members. For example, the leader may say, "Mrs. Purple, I think you are angry because . . . , and you seem to feel . . . . Is that why you are so distressed?" or "I think that Mr. Black and Ms. White are each trying to gain some points in this discussion, but this is not helping us deal with the task at hand. I wonder if you two could either cool it for a while or let us all explore your behavior with you?"

Inadequate Decision Making

Inefficient decision making generally arises if (a) the decision is threatening to the group because of unclear consequences, fear of reactions of other groups, and fear of failure by the members, or (b) the decision is too difficult or has been requested prematurely and the group lacks faith in itself. According to Bradford, Stock, and Horwitz (1974:44), indications that group decision making is inadequate include:

1. There is continued effort to leave the decision making to others, i.e., the leader, a subgroup, or an outside source.
2. Group members refuse responsibility.
3. A decision is challenged after it is made.
4. The group is divided and unclear about what the decision is.
5. The group almost makes decisions but retreats at the last minute.
6. Members frequently ask for definition and redefinition of minute points.
7. Members vacillate between making decisions too rapidly and not deciding anything.
8. Group discussion wanders, often into abstraction.

Table 16–4 Diagnoses and Indications of Nonproductive Group Conflict

Diagnosis	Indications
The group has been given an impossible task	Every suggestion made seems impossible Some members feel the group is too small Members think the group does not have the knowledge or experience to get anywhere Members feel pushed for time Members are impatient with one another Members have different ideas about what the group is supposed to do
The main concern of members is in finding status in the group	Members take sides and refuse to compromise Ideas are attacked before they are completely expressed There are subtle attacks on leadership and personal attacks on members There is much clique formation There is no concern about finding a goal or sticking to a point
Members operate from unshared points of view and may have competing loyalties to outside groups	Members take sides and refuse to compromise on general terms Members do not listen to one another The group goal is stated in very general terms Each member pushes his or her own plan Members disagree on suggestions and do not build on previous suggestions

From L. P. Bradford, *Group development* (La Jolla, Calif.: University Associates, 1974), pp. 38–40.

Apathy

Apathy (nonparticipation or silence) varies from complete indifference to the group task and signs of boredom to lack of genuine enthusiasm, inability to mobilize much energy, lack of persistence, and being satisfied with poor work. Apathy can affect either an individual or the group as a whole. An apathetic group may be the result of an autocratic leadership style or several other factors, discussed in the next section.

Indications of apathy, familiar to most people, include:

1. Members arrive late and are frequently absent.
2. The participation level is low; conversation drags.
3. Members yawn, doze, slouch, and are restless.
4. The concentration level is low, and often the point of the discussion is lost.
5. Decisions are made too quickly, and there is failure to follow through on decisions.
6. Members are reluctant to assume additional responsibility.
7. Suggestions for adjournment are abundant, and arrangements for the next meeting are neglected.

Causes

Some common causes of apathy identified by Bradford, Stock, and Horwitz (1974:44) are:

1. *The task facing the group does not seem important to members,* even though it is important to someone, e.g., the group leader or the larger organization of which the group is a part. In this situation, members may raise questions about what their job really is, what "they" (others) want the group to do, and what the reason for doing the task is. Suggestions may be made that the group work on something else.
2. *The group has inadequate problem-solving procedures or capabilities.* This situation is revealed when:
- **a.** No one can suggest the first step in getting started on the task.
- **b.** Members are unable to stay on a given point.
- **c.** The same points are made over and over.
- **d.** Little attention is given to fact-finding or use of special resources.
- **e.** Minimal consideration is given to evaluating the possible consequences of decisions reached.
- **f.** Private discussions are held in subgroups.
- **g.** Members feel their abilities are inadequate to carry out the task.

3. *Members feel powerless about influencing final decisions.* This situation is indicated when:
- **a.** Members express the view that someone with more authority and power should be at the meeting.
- **b.** Members feel that decisions arrived at will be "meaningless," group efforts will just be wasted, and someone outside the group will not really listen to the ideas of the group.
- **c.** Members try to get the group leader to understand and listen rather than try to reach a consensus decision by the group.
- **d.** Members feel that the management of the organization is pretending to be democratic by asking for their participation.
- **e.** Discussions arise about power structures either inside the group (i.e., the leader or a subgroup) or outside the group.

4. *A conflict among a few members dominates the group.* In this situation a few members control the conversation but never agree, and they appeal to others for support, while the less dominant members withdraw from participation and become apathetic.

Interventions

Nonparticipation or apathy of one or a few members is sometimes best handled by nonintervention. Sometimes such silences are not a reflection of something in the immediate group setting but rather of some past traumatic experience in the person's life. For example, after expressing an idea previously, this person may have been told, "That was a stupid thing to say," or "You should know better than that." Having been hurt once in a group, such persons feel insecure about their views and are reluctant to express themselves again in groups.

Continued nonparticipation or apathy, however, needs to be dealt with by the leader, after a careful assessment of whether the apathy is a reflection of leadership style, task issues, or interpersonal conflicts. Sampson and Marthas (1977:259) offer the following suggestions for dealing with apathy:

1. For apathy reflecting the members' opinion that the task is unimportant, the leader may suggest, "I think there is general boredom with today's task. Do people feel that what we are doing is not really relevant or important?" After members have responded, the leader needs to ask, "What things would you prefer the group to do?"
2. For apathy due to members' feelings of inadequacy about handling the task or lack of the structure and organization needed for problem solving, the leader may ask, "Are people feeling generally that the group is not up to handling the task we are facing?" or "I think, because we're not really sure of what to do or how to go about dealing with the task facing us, that it may be helpful if we break up the task into smaller parts, decide what the important issues are, and develop a method for dealing with each part."

3. For apathy based on an interpersonal issue such as anger or fear and expressed by silence, the leader needs to decide whether to let the silence simply pass or to intervene. If generally responsive group members suddenly become silent, it is important to note which issue or topic immediately preceded the silence. Sometimes a conflict among a few members has been uncovered or the group has been pushed into discussing a topic considered irrelevant or threatening. In this situation the leader may say, "I am wondering whether people are angry at what I've done," or "Are some of you anxious about bringing up that topic, since it may bring out bad feelings?"
4. For apathy due to an autocratic leadership style, the leader must implement measures to change the style and assist the group to work through and change their relationship with him or her.

Monopolizing Member

Because most group meetings have time restraints, domination of the discussion by one member seriously deprives others of their chances to participate. A sense of injustice develops, and ultimately the frustration and anger of members may be directed toward the group leader, who in the members' opinion should be doing something to stop that person's behavior.

Indications

Signs of monopolization include:

1. Compulsive, incessant talking
2. Interruption of others who start to talk
3. Tendency to complete others' sentences
4. Inability to listen
5. Inability to keep still
6. Apparent belief that the act of talking is more important than what is said
7. Responses of restlessness, inattentiveness, and anger deflected to the leader by other members

There may be several reasons for monopolizing behavior (e.g., anxiety or a need for attention, recognition, and approval). Whatever the reason, the goal of the leader is to assist the person to moderate his or her participation in the group. Often compulsive talkers are unaware of their behavior and its effect on others and need help to look at what they are doing and the consequences.

Interventions

The following intervention strategies for groups in general are suggested by Sampson and Marthas (1977:254):

1. *Interrupt simply, directly, and supportively.* This strategy is an initial attempt to get the person to hear others. The leader may say, "Thank you very much, David; I don't like to cut you off right now, since that is an interesting and valuable idea, but I feel it is important for us to hear from everyone about this issue. Perhaps after the others have had a chance to convey their thoughts, we can return to you."
2. *Reflect the person's behavior.* This strategy is an attempt to help the person become aware of the monopolizing behavior. The leader may say, "Lisa, we are really having difficulty hearing from everyone today because you are using up considerable time talking. I wonder if you are aware of this?"
3. *Reflect the group's feelings.* This strategy is an attempt to help the person become aware of the effects of his or her behavior on others. The leader may say "Todd, I've noticed that you have been talking so much today that few others have been able to participate. I've also realized that I am getting frustrated and bored, I haven't kept up with what you are saying, and I finally stopped listening. I really do want to hear what you have to say, as well as what others have to say, and I wonder if other people are having the same trouble?"
4. *Confront the person and/or the group.* This strategy can be directed toward the individual or toward the group to help members realize their own responsibility for the problem. To confront the individual, the leader may say, "Mary, could you please be quiet for a few minutes and let other people have the floor?" To confront the group, the leader may say, "I've noticed that Mary is talking so much that none of you others have had a chance to participate. I am wondering why all of you have allowed Mary to dominate this discussion and whether you want to take more responsibility for working in this group?"

Group Self-Evaluation

Groups need to set up mechanisms for feedback of information to the members about their method of operation. Only when a group acquires information about itself can it make adjustments to improve its efficiency. Several mechanisms can be set up for group feedback and self-evaluation: use of a group productivity observer, use of a group self-evaluation guide, general open discussion initiated by the group leader prior to the end of the meeting, or combinations of the above.

Some groups establish a rotating position for a group

productivity observer, just as positions are established for a recorder; others acquire the assistance of an outsider specially trained in this area. The responsibility of this person is to observe the group during its discussions, rather than participate, and to provide feedback to the group about perceptions of the group's behavior. The observer notes the general atmosphere of the group, leadership techniques, orientation of the group, participation by members, and any factor considered to affect the productivity of the group. See Table 16–5 for a sample group self-evaluation guide that can be used by the observer.

The provision of feedback requires skill by the observer in presenting comments. It is helpful to present

Table 16–5 Example of Group Self-Evaluation Guide

Criteria	Comments
A. Group direction and orientation	
1. How much was achieved?	Only ⅓ of agenda covered. Too much time spent on irrelevant material.
2. How clear are goals and purposes?	A few members not clear about purposes.
3. How clear is procedure to achieve goals?	No discussion about how to try to achieve task.
4. Was sufficient relevant information available?	Yes.
B. Group motivation and unity	
5. What degree of interest is there in task?	A few do not think problem is important.
6. Was interest maintained throughout?	Interest lagged when one member made lengthy lecture.
7. Is group united in purpose?	Feelings of unity not evident in two members.
C. Group atmosphere	
8. Formal?	
9. Informal?	Yes
10. Permissive?	Yes
11. Inhibited?	
12. Cooperative?	Yes
13. Competitive?	
14. Friendly?	Yes
15. Hostile?	
D. Member contributions	
16. What is degree of participation by members?	All participated. Some monopolization by one member.
17. Were contributions relevant, factual, and problem-centered?	Most were.
18. Were members listening to what others said?	A few were not, at point of high interest in discussion.
19. How did special members serve group?	
a. Leader	Facilitated discussion. Could have handled dominating member better. Let group wander too much.
b. Recorder	Asked for clarification of some points. Assisted group to focus on issue.
c. Resource person	Provided essential clarifying information.
d. Others	Two members criticized four out of five ideas while they were being suggested. After that, fewer suggestions were offered.
20. How did majority of members feel about meeting?	
a. Poor	
b. Mediocre	Yes
c. Okay	
d. Good	
e. Excellent	

Adapted from David H. Jenkins, Feedback and group self-evaluation, in Leland P. Bradford, editor, *Group development* (La Jolla, Calif.: University Associates, 1974), pp. 84–86.

objective data first and then phrase comments in the form of tentative hypotheses, alternative solutions, or expressions of the observer's feelings. This allows group members the chance to reject a comment if they are not ready to handle it. The observer can be viewed as "in error." For example, the observer of the group meeting evaluated in Table 16–5 might comment (Jenkins 1974:82):

Objective data: During the time we were trying to suggest solutions to problems, two of us seemed impatient to tear a new idea apart. Out of five suggestions made, four were immediately criticized. Right after that, suggestions for solutions lagged.

Alternative solution: I was wondering at the time whether more and better ideas might have emerged if we had withheld our critical comments until after most of the ideas about solutions were on the blackboard.

Open discussion needs to follow such comments.

Assertiveness in Nursing Interactions

Because nurses work with both formal and informal groups in much of their nursing practice, it is particularly important that they communicate clearly and effectively. Types and techniques of communication were discussed in Chapter 15. Communication that reflects the power of the nurse as a professional person is assertive behavior. *Assertiveness* is expression of oneself openly and directly without hurting others. It provides feelings of control and self-confidence for the communicator. Assertive nurses are able to present their feelings and values, stand up for themselves, and claim their rights.

Some nurses may have difficulty being assertive because they believe that they must provide tenderness and compassion to all people at all times, i.e., always meet others' needs. However, this is an unrealistic expectation.

Effects of Assertiveness

According to Alberti and Emmons (1974:3), assertiveness with individuals and groups facilitates:

1. Prompt coping with problems
2. Achievement of group goals
3. Communication of power within oneself
4. Communication of competence and self-confidence
5. Reduction of anxiety or tenseness in key situations

Assertive, Nonassertive, and Aggressive Responses

Assertive behavior has been described as falling between nonassertiveness and aggressive behavior on a continuum (ibid., p. 11). Nonassertive or passive nurses appear hesitant and unsure of themselves. Their feelings are hidden, for fear of hurting others or being hurt. Because nonassertive nurses do not ask or know how to ask, they often do not obtain what they want and thus become frustrated. This frustration after a period of time often results in explosive aggressive behavior, which helps the nurse feel better for only a short time. Aggressive nurses, at the other extreme, make their feelings known, often at others' expense. Although this behavior can result in change, it can be harmful to the individual eventually, as others respond negatively to the nurse's behavior.

The example that follows illustrates the different types of responses in a typical nursing situation.

Situation

Charge nurse: Miss Eammons, why can't you ever take your blood pressures on time? This is the fourth day this week that they have not been taken.

Aggressive response

Nurse: It's not my fault they are late. You're always interrupting my work with extra duties.

Nonassertive response

Nurse: Yes, I'm sorry. We've been short staffed, and I have a very heavy load.

Assertive response

Nurse: I didn't know that all the blood pressures were late. I'd like to check that further. Could we discuss this in your office before you leave today?

Assertive Techniques

These assertive techniques can help nurses:

1. Include positive and negative information in a statement: "I like your plan but . . . ."
2. Start the statement with "I," and avoid generalizations such as "we all believe" or "it seems like a good idea."
3. Express your own beliefs and rights: "I believe that . . . ."
4. Express your thoughts and feelings directly, to reinforce your identity: "I feel you are . . . " or "I want you to . . . ."

5. When replying negatively, state "I won't . . ." not "I can't . . . ." The latter implies lack of power, whereas the former communicates assumption of responsibility.
6. Give assertive statements (Bakdash 1978: 1712):
  a. Simple assertive: "I think . . . ."
  b. Empathic assertive: "I realize you are very tired, but . . . ."
  c. Confrontive assertive: "You said you could bathe Mr. Greene, but you didn't . . . ."
  d. Soft assertive: "I am very grateful you did that for me, and I think . . . ."
  e. Persuasive assertive: "I agree with most of what you said, but I also think . . . ."

When an individual says something that the nurse perceives as negative or a "put-down," the following assertive responses can be given to provide time:

1. "I need to think about this for a few minutes."
2. "It seems to me that . . . " and a clear statement of personal feelings.
3. Silence as an answer, giving no verbal response.

Three assertive methods of coping with criticism are fogging, negative assertion, and negative inquiry (Smith 1975: 104–32). *Fogging* is agreeing in principle to a statement made by another. In this technique, the nurse listens carefully to the criticism and accepts it without becoming defensive or anxious.

Patient: You can't do anything right.
Nurse: You're not satisfied with my work, Mr. Milos.

Negative assertion is the assertive expression of those attributes that are negative about oneself.

Patient: You didn't give that injection well.
Nurse: I didn't give it very smoothly.

Negative inquiry asks for additional information about the critical statements.

Charge nurse: You look messy today.
Nurse: What do you mean?
Charge nurse: You look untidy.
Nurse: Do you mean my uniform is wrinkled?

To learn assertiveness, nurses can take workshops or study articles on the subject (see the Selected References at the end of this chapter). This section is intended only to introduce the subject to nursing students.

Summary

Nurses work within groups of various types and sizes and need to learn to become effective group members and leaders. Groups are classified as either primary or secondary, according to their structure and type of interaction. In small, intimate, primary groups, relationships are spontaneous, personal, and sentimental. In larger secondary groups, relationships are impersonal and less sentimental. Groups are also described as formal, semiformal, or informal; each has unique features.

Although group properties are related to the type and level of formality of the group, all kinds of groups have certain structural and functional characteristics. Structural properties relate to the ordered arrangements that define and regulate the behavior of persons in the group, whereas functional properties relate to operational and procedural methods of functioning or group process.

Groups develop in three stages: the initiation stage, in which tasks predominate and member behaviors are tested; the functional stage, in which members feel comfortable with one another and functional group properties develop and increase; and the dissolution stage, in which group members no longer see a need for the group. Several features of effective groups have been identified; in general, such groups may be said to produce outstanding results, succeed in spite of difficulties, and have members who feel responsible for the output of the group.

Each group has its own unique dynamics (processes), which can be analyzed and assessed for effectiveness or ineffectiveness: commitment of members, leadership style, decision-making methods, member behaviors, interaction patterns, cohesiveness, and power forces. Nurses need to learn causes of and interventions for common group problems—conflict, inadequate decision making, apathy, and monopolizing members.

Group self-evaluation is essential to improve the efficiency of the group. Several feedback mechanisms can be set up: use of a group productivity observer, use of a group self-evaluation guide, general open discussion initiated by the group leader, or combinations of the above.

To be effective in group interactions nurses need to develop assertive behavior. Assertive, nonassertive, and aggressive behaviors can be distinguished. Specific assertive techniques can help nurses in their practice.

Suggested Activities

1. Select a small work group of which you are a member.
  a. Using the criteria in Table 16–2 on page 395 or the evaluation guide in Table 16–5 on page 406, analyze its effective and ineffective features.
  b. Determine which group members carry out leadership functions.
  c. Determine how effectively decisions are made.
  d. Determine the interaction patterns, using a sociogram.
  e. Determine the power sources.

2. For the group in activity 1, ascertain the roles a few members assume, e.g., task, maintenance, or self-serving roles.
3. With a group of students, share situations in which you felt you reacted in a nonassertive manner. Discuss assertive techniques that you could have used.

Suggested Readings

Donnelly, G. January 1978. The assertive nurse or how to say what you mean without shaking or shouting. *Nursing 78* 8:65–69 (Canadian ed. 8:65–68).
This mental health specialist provides hints on how nurses can make their communication open, clear, and direct.

Kron, T. October 1976. How to become a better leader. *Nursing 76* 6:67–68 (Canadian ed. 6:6–7).
Tips on how to improve leadership ability are provided. Techniques, qualities, and rules for leadership are included.

Larson, M. L., and Williams, R. A. August 1978. How to become a better group leader? Learn to recognize the strange things that happen to some people in groups. *Nursing 78* 8:65–72 (Canadian ed. 8:12–15).
These authors outline several nonfunctional or problem behaviors of group members: deserter, nontalker, interrogator, smoke-screener, rescuer, scapegoat, seducer, and angry aggressor. Effective ways for the group leader to deal with them are outlined.

McConnell, E. A. October 1978. What kind of delegator are you? *Nursing 78* 8:105–6 (Canadian ed. 8:12–14).
Five ineffective delegators and four nondelegators are described.

Small, L. L. July 1980. Finding your leadership style in groups. *American Journal of Nursing* 80:1301–3.
This author analyzes and critiques her experiences as a group leader.

Selected References

Alberti, R. E., and Emmons, M. L. 1974. *Your perfect right.* 2nd ed. San Luis Obispo, Calif.: Impact Publishing Co.

Bakdash, D. P. October 1978. Becoming an assertive nurse. *American Journal of Nursing* 78:1710–12.

Benne, K. D., and Sheats, P. 1974. Functional roles of group members. In Bradford, L. P., editor. *Group development.* La Jolla, Calif.: University Associates.

Bloom, L. Z.; Coburn, K.; and Pearlman, J. 1975. *The new assertive woman.* New York: Dell Publishing Co.

Bradford, L. P., editor. 1974. *Group development.* La Jolla, Calif.: University Associates.

Bradford, L. P.; Stock, D.; and Horwitz, M. 1974. How to diagnose group problems. In Bradford, L. P., editor. *Group development.* La Jolla, Calif.: University Associates.

Browne, S. E. March 1980. Group leadership experiences for students. *Nursing Outlook* 28:166–69.

Claus, K. E., and Bailey, J. T. 1977. *Power and influence in health care: A new approach to leadership.* St. Louis: C. V. Mosby Co.

Donnelly, G. F.; Mengel, A.; and Sutterley, D. C. 1980. *The nursing system: Issues, ethics, and politics.* New York: John Wiley and Sons.

Francis, D., and Young, D. 1979. *Improving work groups: A practical manual for team building.* San Diego, Calif.: University Associates.

Hamm, S. R. December 1980. The influence of formal and informal organization within a modern hospital. *Supervisor Nurse* 11:38–40.

Jenkins, David H. 1974. Feedback and group self-evaluation. In Bradford, L. P., editor. *Group development.* La Jolla, Calif.: University Associates.

McClelland, D. C. 1975. *Power: The inner experience.* New York: Irvington Publishers.

Marley, M. S. May 1980. The making of a group. *Journal of Gerontological Nursing* 6:275–79.

May, Rollo. 1972. *Power and innocence: A search for the sources of violence.* New York: W. W. Norton and Co.

Moniz, D. October 1978. Putting assertiveness techniques into practice. *American Journal of Nursing* 78:1713.

Reeves, Elton T. 1970. *The dynamics of group behavior.* New York: American Management Association.

Sampson, E. E., and Marthas, M. S. 1977. *Group process for the health professions.* New York: John Wiley and Sons.

Smith, M. J. 1975. *When I say no, I feel guilty.* New York: Bantam Books.

Wilson, H. S. and Kneisl, C. R. 1982. *Psychiatric nursing.* 2nd ed. Menlo Park, Calif.: Addison-Wesley Publishing Co.

Chapter 17

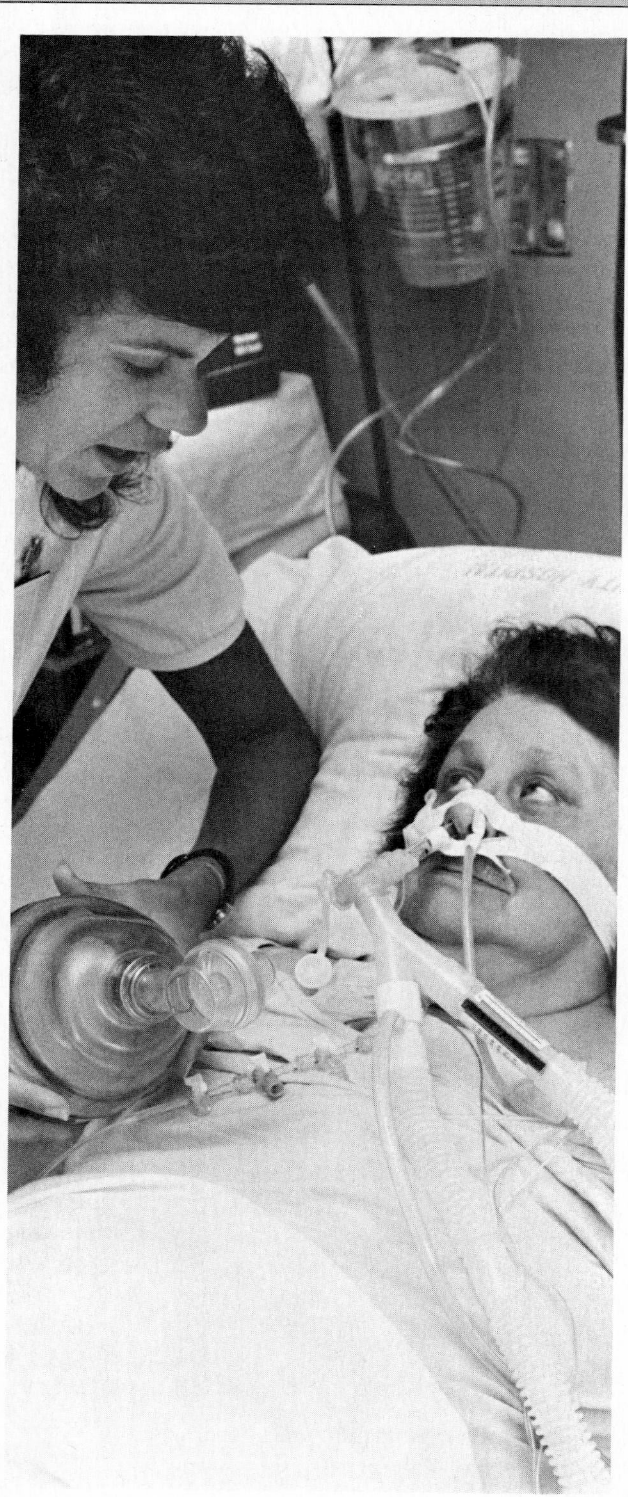

Teaching and Learning

CONTENTS

Objectives

1. Know essential facts about teaching and learning
   1.1 Define terms commonly used in the teaching and learning context
   1.2 Identify six principles that facilitate learning
   1.3 Outline internal factors that affect learning
   1.4 Outline external factors that affect learning
   1.5 Identify developmental learning needs at various ages
   1.6 Identify five essential principles of teaching
   1.7 Describe three levels at which health teaching is directed
2. Understand essential facts about the nursing process as it is applied to meeting the learning needs of patients
   2.1 Identify essential sources of data to assess the learning needs of patients
   2.2 Identify criteria used to assess a patient's readiness to learn
   2.3 Identify essential steps in planning teaching activities for patients
   2.4 Identify essential aspects of well-written learning objectives
   2.5 Relate appropriate methods of teaching to types of learning required by patients
   2.6 Identify ways in which learning can be evaluated

Terms

compliance
feedback
learning
learning need
motivation
teaching

A major nursing function is to assist patients and their families to meet their learning needs. This teaching function applies to needs related to both health and illness. A *learning need* is a need to change behavior. The behavior is often observable activity, such as taking a medication, administering insulin by hypodermic syringe, or following a diet. The areas of learning with which nurses are concerned are:

1. Developmental learning needs
2. Learning needs related to promoting health
3. Learning needs related to restoring health
4. Learning needs related to gaining new skills and knowledge as a result of impaired functioning
5. Learning ways of coping with a terminal illness

People continually acquire knowledge and learn new skills. This is most apparent during childhood, when so much is learned in a relatively short time. Nurses are frequently involved in developmental learning, such as assisting the parent of a 2-year-old with toilet training. For an adult the learning may be related to new experiences, such as illness, or to a change of environment, such as entering the hospital.

Promoting health is a nursing function that frequently involves teaching patients and/or their support persons. This type of teaching transmits knowledge and, in some instances, skills. An example of the former is knowledge about calories and the caloric values of specific foods taught to an obese person. Related skills would be cooking attractive meals for a low-calorie diet or a program of exercises to assist weight loss.

Learning related to restoring health is frequently needed by hospitalized patients. The man who has had surgery may need to learn to care for his incision; the woman who has a paralyzed arm will need to learn exercises to regain muscular functioning in the arm. Generally this type of learning need is readily identified by nurses, since it relates directly to the patient's illness.

Patients who have impaired functioning may need to learn new skills in daily living. Patients who have diabetes need to learn to give themselves insulin by hypodermic injection, to test their urine for glucose, and to cut their nails without cutting the skin and consequently incurring an infection. The patient who has had one leg amputated needs to learn to strap on an artificial leg and to walk with it. Learning of this type assists people to resume their daily activities with as few limitations as possible.

Teaching by nurses may assist patients and their families to cope with their health problems. If the teaching is well done, the patient often becomes able to function without the nurse. This independence can be one measure of the patient's learning.

Learning

Learning is defined as a permanent change in behavior. This change is the result of planned activities, not a maturational process. The behavior may be observable or unobservable. Following a diet is observable behavior, whereas thinking about an infant's stimulation is unobservable.

An important aspect of learning is the individual's agreement to learn, commonly referred to as *compliance*. For learning to take place, compliance must be present. Compliance is best illustrated when the person accepts and recognizes the need to learn and willingly expends the energy required to learn. On the other hand, when an individual has not complied, learning will not take place.

There are three basic types of learning: psychomotor, cognitive, and affective. Psychomotor learning includes physical skills. Skills such as walking, talking, and eating are learning tasks for some patients. Often exercises and training programs are designed to assist the patient in reeducating muscles. Learning and relearning these skills usually takes both practice and time; 2-year-old children who are learning to walk fall many times before they walk steadily.

Cognitive learning includes knowledge and understanding. Cognitive skills include the capacity to learn, to retain knowledge, to organize information, and to solve problems. These skills vary considerably from person to person. *Knowledge* is the remembering of previously learned materials (Gronlund 1978:28). *Understanding* or *comprehension* is the ability to grasp the meaning of a word. Understanding is a higher level cognitive skill than knowledge. A patient's family may need to understand what a diabetic coma is, how to identify it, and what to do about it; a new parent may need to understand when and how to feed an infant.

Affective learning includes attitudes, appreciations, and values. A patient may need to learn new attitudes about an illness or about people. For example, a father may need to learn an accepting attitude about his teenage daughter's life-style, to replace his anger. Attitudes are often reflected in behavior and may need to be changed before the behavior can change. Patients who have a colostomy may need to develop an accepting attitude toward it before they can learn to care for it effectively. Attitudes and values can often be learned from others. Thus, colostomy patients may learn attitudes from others who have colostomies.

Learning Principles

When nurses assist individuals to meet their learning needs, it is important for them to apply principles that facilitate and maximize learning:

1. A person's interest and motivation to learn are increased when the person understands the relevance of the learning. When someone understands why learning is necessary and accepts that the method of teaching is appropriate for the task, learning is facilitated. On the other hand, if patients do not accept the necessity of learning a particular technique, for example, or find the teaching method "stupid" or "boring," learning will be impeded.

2. Understanding of the learning is increased by proceeding from the simple to the complex. Progressing from the simple to the complex enables the learner to comprehend the new information, assimilate it with previous learning, and form new understandings. *Simple* and *complex* are relative terms, varying with the level at which the person is learning. What might be simple for one person may be complex for another.

3. Anxiety affects learning, attention span, and retention of facts. A high level of anxiety impairs retention of facts, reduces the capacity to attend, and impairs learning. An extremely low level of anxiety, on the other hand, decreases interest or motivation to learn. For optimum learning, an individual needs to experience sufficient anxiety to be motivated without perceiving pressure.

4. Active involvement in the learning process makes learning more meaningful. If the learner actively participates, for example, through discussion, learning is faster and retention is better. Passive learning, such as listening to a lecture or watching a film does not foster optimal learning.

5. Success in learning helps the individual accept failure. Once learners have succeeded in accomplishing a task or understanding a concept, they gain a sense of self-confidence in their ability to learn. This reduces their anxiety about failure and can motivate greater learning. The learners then have increased confidence with which to accept failure.

6. Feedback that accompanies practice helps performance improve. Practice is necessary to learn psychomotor skills, but unless the practice is accompanied by feedback learners can repeat their mistakes, and their performance will stay at the same level. *Feedback* is information relating a person's performance to the desired goal. It has to be meaningful to the learner. Support of desired behavior through praise, positively worded corrections, and suggestions of alternative methods are ways of providing positive feedback. Negative feedback using ridicule, anger, or sarcasm can cause people to withdraw from learning. These responses can be viewed as types of punishment; they may cause reactions such as avoidance of the teacher to avoid punishment.

Factors That Affect Learning

Internal factors

Anxiety A greatly elevated anxiety level can impede learning. Patients or families who are very worried may not hear spoken words or may retain only part of the communication. Mild anxiety, however, can often increase learning by focusing attention.

Extreme anxiety might be reduced by medications or by information that relieves uncertainty. Patients who appear to be disinterested and to have no concern may need to hear about possible problems to increase their anxiety slightly and thus facilitate their learning.

Physical status Impaired physical status, such as fatigue, weakness, and hunger, can affect a person's ability to learn. Patients who have just had an operation may need to devote all their energy just to breathing or moving themselves and thus have no inclination to learn about next week's diet. Learning has to be timed according to patients' readiness and energy level. By providing rest periods and comfort, nurses can help such patients conserve their physical stamina to meet other needs. It is important to recognize that secondary needs such as learning can be met only after primary needs such as breathing, eating, and resting have been met.

Age Age is a primary consideration in learning. The very young have obvious limitations to what and how they learn. A child's nervous system and musculoskeletal system must be sufficiently developed for certain learning to take place. Therefore, parents need to learn skills and knowledge for a child's care. The parents of a newborn may need to learn how to bathe the baby safely; parents of a 3-year-old may need to learn to change a dressing on an incision.

Older children can often learn skills and acquire knowledge about their health. Teenagers, for example, may need and want help dealing with facial acne; they can learn to follow a diet, wash with a special soap, and avoid squeezing blackheads and pimples. Adults can learn to look after their health if they perceive the need. Elderly people sometimes have difficulty learning new skills or new ways of doing things. It may be hard for older persons to remember to take a medicine every 4 hours, and they may need to have the times written down as a reminder. It is helpful for the nurse to write down the date and time in especially large letters for patients with impaired vision. Then, after taking the medicine the patient can cross out the time, to serve as a reminder that the medicine was taken.

Motivation *Motivation* is desire; in the case of learning, it is the desire to learn. Motivation is generally greatest when a person recognizes a need and believes that through learning this need will be met. It is not adequate for the nurse to see and express the need; it must be experienced by the patient. Often the nurse's task is to assist the patient to work through a problem and identify the need personally. Sometimes patients or families need help identifying elements in the situation before they can see a need. Patients who have heart disease may need to know the effects of smoking and being overweight before they recognize a need to stop smoking or adopt a weight reducing diet. Adolescents may need to know the consequences of an untreated venereal disease before they see the need to obtain treatment. The readiness of the person is critical to learning. Motivation must be present when the individual is ready to learn.

Communication skills Communication skills involve the person's ability to perceive, understand, and convey thoughts and feelings to others. People's abilities to do this vary. One patient may have a large sophisticated vocabulary; another may know only simple words. The ability to understand health needs is also affected to a large degree by the person's value system about health. People who do not care about keeping their teeth intact probably will not learn to brush them regularly.

Senses The acuity of the senses affects a person's ability to learn. The person who has difficulty seeing may be unable to learn by reading a brochure; the person who is hard of hearing may be unable to learn through participation in a group discussion.

Education and experience The ability to learn is affected by education and experience. Learners' vocabularies may relate to their backgrounds. Words such as *feces* or *emesis* may be familiar to some people and strange to others. Parents who have four children will have different needs in learning to care for a handicapped baby than parents learning to care for their first child. Familiarity with the language can also be an important factor. A patient who was born in Korea may have difficulty with the English language. Even those born in the United States or Canada may be more familiar with the language of their parents, such as Spanish, Chinese, or French, than with English. Nurses need to watch for language barriers and not assume that people born in the United States or Canada are comfortable with the nurse's language.

External factors

Physical environment Environmental factors include heat, light, temperature, ventilation, noise, and supports such as chairs and tables. An environment for optimum learning needs to have adequate lighting free from glare, a comfortable room temperature, and good ventilation. Most students know what it is like to try to learn in a hot, stuffy room; the subsequent drowsiness interferes with concentration. Noise can also distract. Loud voices, interruptions by others, and outside traffic can interfere with listening and thinking. For the best learning in a hospital, nurses may try to choose a time when visitors are not present and interruptions are unlikely. Privacy is essential for some learning, for example, when a patient is learning to irrigate a colostomy. The presence of other people can embarrass the patient and thus interfere with learning.

It is equally important for the patient to be comfortable while learning. Pain and fatigue can hinder concentration on the subject. If a group of patients is attending a class such as a baby bath demonstration, each person needs to have a chair that provides good support and comfort as well as a clear view of the demonstration.

Timing The time for learning, the length of the learning period, and the intervals between learning periods are of great importance. The best time for the patient needs to be chosen. If a patient is rested in the morning, this may be the best time for that patient to learn. For another person it may be the evening or half an hour after taking an analgesic. Nurses need to identify the best time for the patient or family and use that time. If repeated learning sessions are needed, it is often helpful to schedule them at the same time each day. The patient can then anticipate the lesson and prepare for it.

The length of learning periods greatly affects learning. If periods are too long, patients lose their ability to concentrate; periods that are too short may not offer enough time to master a skill or to understand the information.

The interval between learning periods should depend on the patient's needs. For a patient who wants to learn quickly, learning sessions in the morning, afternoon, and evening may be appropriate; for another, once a day or every other day may suffice. The intervals should not be so long that patients forget from one session to another; neither should they be so close together that patients do not have time to assimilate what they are learning.

Timing also has to be considered relative to the learning need. For example, a patient who is being discharged from the hospital and has to irrigate his own colostomy at home will need to learn these skills sufficiently ahead of discharge to practice the irrigation in the nurse's presence and ask questions regarding his care. However, the learning will be less effective if it is done before the patient is aware of his needs upon discharge and before he can even think of going home.

Teaching methods and aids The method used to convey knowledge and skills will depend largely on how the patient best learns. Usually a combination of hearing, seeing, and doing is best. Handling equipment and practicing with the nurse present assist patients in gaining skill and confidence. For specific teaching methods, see page 420.

Content The content to be learned should relate to the learner's needs, not the nurse's. A patient may want and need to know only simple anatomy regarding a colostomy, not detailed knowledge. The vocabulary the nurse uses should be appropriate for the learner. Words such as *feces* and *void* may not be understood, whereas *bowel movement* and *pass urine* may be understood by adults, and *pooh pooh* and *pee pee* by children. It is very important that nurses assess what words patients do use in this regard.

The learning content needs to follow a logical sequence, starting at the place where the patient has some information and logically progressing toward the objectives for the learning. When learning is planned over a number of sessions, it is best each time to review what has already been covered and answer any questions that the patient may have. This way the patient is always starting learning from a base, and the nurse is in no doubt about what the patient already knows.

The content of the learning needs to be specific. It is not sufficient to say "a few times," since this can have different meanings to people; the nurse needs to say "three times" or whatever is appropriate. In teaching patients to take medications, the specific hours need to be planned. For example, an antibiotic may be required four times a day, every 6 hours around the clock, not four times between 8:00 A.M. and 10:00 P.M..

Developmental Learning Needs

People learn from the day of birth to the day of death. Some learning is done with conscious effort; other learning is done with minimal effort and awareness. For example, a patient in a hospital may be unaware that she is learning the times for her medications, and only when they do not come does she consciously realize that they are normally delivered at a certain hour. The learning needs of people change to some degree when they are ill or injured. They often become secondary needs, as physiologic needs take priority. The adolescent who is studying hard for a scholarship may well forget that fact when he is in acute pain. Suddenly relief from pain takes precedence over studying.

Nurses need to be aware of the normal learning needs of patients and their families during the life cycle and to support these needs when appropriate. See Figure 17-1.

Infants (Birth to 2 Years)

From birth to 2 years, infants learn voluntary control over movements. They learn to hold a spoon and put it in their mouths. They also learn to control bladder and bowels, to chatter nonsensically, and to say a few words. They learn to sleep during the entire night and to respond to certain objects. By 18 months, they imitate their parents. At this age routines are very important.

For children who are in the hospital at this age, nurses need certain information so that they can help the children with their adjustments and learning needs. To know the child's stage in developmental tasks is important. See Table 11-3, page 235. Maintaining routines, when possible, and using words the child knows assist the child to adjust. With a change in environment, an infant may seem to forget some learning as a result of anxiety, but this is usually temporary. It is best handled by the nurse with supportive, understanding, and noncritical responses.

It is also helpful to know what foods the child is accustomed to eating, likes, and dislikes.

Preschool Children (2 to 5 Years)

During the preschool period, children become social beings. They usually are toilet trained by the age of 3, although they may still have accidents occasionally. They learn to manage their own clothes, and by 5 years of age many have learned to be modest about exposing their bodies to others. This requires tactful handling by the nurse caring for the preschool child.

Preschool children learn to brush their teeth and wash themselves alone. In the hospital, the nurse should allow them the time to carry out the tasks they have learned, if they are well enough. During these years children learn to talk with others, and by 5 years of age they ask the nurse questions to obtain information. It is important to answer their questions in words that they understand.

By the age of 3 or 4, children want to play with their peers, whereas at 2 years they prefer solitary play. Children from 2 to 5 like to look at picture books and to have stories read to them. For the nurse to know a child's favorite bedtime story can be helpful to the adjustment in the hospital.

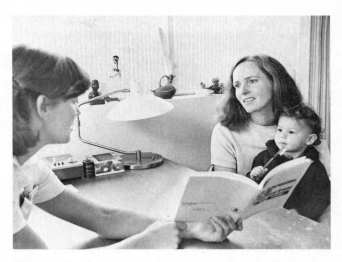

Figure 17-1 A new mother discusses her child's nutrition with the nurse at a community child health clinic.

Preschool children focus their feelings chiefly on the parent of the opposite sex. Thus, in a hospital, a boy will probably look to a female nurse for support, while a girl will look to a male nurse. Children also play with their bodies and want to know the names of the different parts. This interest may be heightened when they are ill, because of others' interest in their bodies. They will ask the nurse the names of equipment and what the nurse is doing, expecting answers.

Children at this age have learned to like certain foods and may dislike strong-tasting or coarse-textured foods. This information will help the nurse provide the child with proper nourishment. Some preschool children may have learned that they do not have to do what they are asked. This can usually be corrected by adequate explanations to accompany requests and by following through with a stated alternative. For example, if a child refuses to practice her arm exercises after the nurse has said that she cannot watch a program on television unless she does so, then it is important to follow through as announced. See Table 11-3, page 235.

School-Age Children (6 to 10 years)

Children from 6 to 10 have learning needs concerning the skills of daily activities, games such as football and baseball, and communication with peers and others in their social sphere.

Physical activity is usually important to children at this time, and any impairment in their ability to participate with their peers will usually require special support and understanding from parents as well as nurses. School-age children require activity of one sort or another. Physical activity at this age serves to develop fine coordination.

The peer group is very important at this age. It is then

that children learn to play and work with others. Through this activity they become less self-centered and more conscious of others in a group. School-age children are aware of death as a concept, may experience anxiety about death, and may require support at such times.

At this age children ask questions, and they like to be busy. It is often challenging for nurses to provide activities that are within the energy tolerance of hospitalized children and yet meet their needs to learn and to accomplish some task.

Adolescents (11 to 19 Years)

The learning needs of adolescents that are of concern to nurses largely center around four areas: sexual roles, learning to care for and use the body effectively, grooming, and achieving emotional independence. Adolescents need to learn role behavior, and often a role model provides much of this information. An adolescent girl may learn a great deal from a female nurse; a boy may learn from a male nurse. Often learning to care for the body is a major concern. Hair styling, skin problems, and dress become very important. It is during this period that adolescents learn what they want in a future mate.

It is equally important for adolescents to learn some emotional independence from their parents. They still need guidance, and they may seek this from another adult. Adolescents want to know about sex, including information about venereal disease and birth control. They also have learning needs about the use of drugs and alcohol. See Table 11–3, page 235, on developmental tasks during adolescence.

Young Adults

Adults in their 20s and 30s who become ill have learning needs largely related to the changes in their health and environment. For the young couple expecting a baby, learning needs concern what is happening, what they can expect, and how they can best prepare for the baby. The physical and emotional changes associated with pregnancy need to be understood as well as changes related to body image and sexual desire. The couple needs to learn about the woman's diet, need for rest, and exercises. After the birth of the baby, the parents have many learning needs about care of the mother and the child. See Chapter 12.

Young adults who become hospitalized may be experiencing for the first time not only being in a hospital but also being seriously ill. They have learning needs about expectations of the sick role, the routines of the hospital, and adjustments they may need to make in life-style after discharge.

Middle-Aged Adults

During middle age, adult learning needs primarily relate to adjustments necessitated by health problems, physiologic changes, and anticipated retirement.

A number of common health problems in this age group may involve learning a new life-style: obesity, excessive use of alcohol, depressive disorders, and cardiovascular disease. The patient who is hospitalized at this time because of a heart condition may need to know about a diet, obtaining adequate rest and exercise, and making adjustments in settings that produce stress, for example, employment. Further learning is related to the developmental tasks of middle age. See Table 12–5, page 280.

Elderly Adults

The special learning needs of the elderly are largely associated with their diminishing physical capacities. Aging affects most of the body's tissues, requiring the person to accommodate to the changes. See Chapter 12. In addition, a few elderly people have reduced mental capacities as a result of reduced blood flow to some areas of the brain and increased atherosclerosis. They may think more slowly, have trouble remembering, and, in some instances, have some difficulty thinking and reasoning.

Elderly people need to learn to take precautions to prevent accidents, for example, having adequate lighting, handrails, and a floor area free from clutter. These and other precautions are discussed in Chapter 12.

When elderly persons are admitted to the hospital, they need to learn what is expected of them just as other patients do. Nurses sometimes take for granted that patients know or will find out for themselves where the bathroom is and how to use the call light. This assumption may not be warranted. A change in environment for elderly persons may create some degree of confusion, particularly for those with impaired vision or hearing. Thus they require repeated orientations as to time, place, and person for a while. It is often difficult for an elderly person to change—to learn new ways of doing things or a new diet. However, most can change with the help of the nurse. Often teaching material needs to be repeated a number of times. Special aids to learning, such as a detailed list of foods to eat, also can help the elderly person learn and remember.

Teaching

Teaching is a system of activities intended to produce learning. The teaching process is intentionally designed to produce specific learning. Teaching is considered one of the functions of nurses. In some states in the United States teaching is included in the legal definition of nursing, making it a required function under the law.

The teaching-learning process involves dynamic interaction between teacher and learner. Each participant in the process communicates information, emotions, perceptions, and attitudes to the other.

Teaching involves three phases: planning, implementing, and evaluating. See the sections on these phases later in this chapter. It also involves a type of communication for which there are specific goals. For example, patients who need to administer their own eye drops or to change an incision dressing share these goals with the nurse. Another aspect of teaching is the relationship between the teacher and the learner. It is essentially one of trust and respect. The learner trusts that the teacher has the knowledge and skill to teach, and the teacher respects the learner's ability to attain the recognized goals. Once a nurse starts to instruct a patient or family, it is important that the teaching process continue until the participants reach the goals, change the goals, or decide that the goals will not help the patient or family meet the learning objectives.

Principles of Teaching

The following principles may be helpful to nursing students:

1. Teaching activities should help the learner meet individual learning objectives. If certain activities do not assist the learner, these need to be reassessed; perhaps other activities can replace them. For example, a patient may not be able to learn to handle a syringe by explanation only. The patient may learn more effectively by handling the syringe.

2. Rapport between teacher and learner is essential. A relationship that is both accepting and constructive will best assist the patient to learn.

3. The teacher who can use the patient's previous learnings in the present situation encourages the patient and facilitates the learning of new skills. For example, a person who already knows how to cook can use this knowledge when learning about a special diet.

4. A teacher must be able to communicate clearly and concisely. The words the teacher uses need to have the same meaning to the learner as to the teacher. For example, a patient who is taught not to put water on an area of the skin may think a wet washcloth is permissible for washing the area. In effect, the nurse needs to explain that no water or moisture should touch the area.

5. The teaching activities need to be oriented around the learning objectives. Thus information and skills not related to the learner's objectives need to be eliminated from the teaching process. If they remain, they may confuse the learner or be a distraction from effective learning.

Teaching Patients and Support Persons

Teaching patients and their support persons is conducted on three levels: promoting health, preventing illness, and coping with illness or disability.

Promoting health

Teaching that promotes health is carried out both in the community and in health institutions. Its goal is to encourage high-level wellness in individuals, including physical and psychologic development. Examples of teaching strategies for promoting health include dietary classes for pregnant women, mental health counseling for family members, and exercise classes for middle-aged adults.

Preventing illness

Teaching to prevent illness is designed to avoid complications from an illness or to prevent people from incurring some illnesses. Dietary classes in the community for obese persons can help prevent future complications of obesity. Teaching a family member to wash hands after contact with a child who has an infected hand can prevent transmission of the infection. Teaching adolescents the problems associated with drug abuse and sexually transmitted diseases are other examples of preventive teaching.

Coping with illness and disability

Patients and their support persons may need to learn how to live with an illness or disability that cannot be cured. This teaching may include nursing techniques as well as activities of daily living. Teaching a family how to communicate with an aphasic father, how to dress a wife who has hemiplegia, or how to administer a child's insulin are examples.

Assessing Learning Needs

Assessment of learning needs can be divided into three steps: (a) obtaining data, (b) identifying learning needs, and (c) identifying readiness and ability to learn.

Obtaining Data

Data for assessing learning needs come from two main sources:

1. *The patient and/or family.* Their perceptions of the needs are highly significant and must be considered initially in any learning plan. Sometimes conveying information can suffice to relieve patients of worry. Hospitalized patients can also tell the nurse about problems in the home that concern them. For example, a patient who is to remain in bed except to use the bathroom may explain that his bedroom is on a different floor of the house from the bathroom. Often adjustments in living such as moving the bed to another room can resolve this problem relatively easily.
2. *The patient's record.* When a patient has been cared for by members of a health team, the health record will provide recent data. It will also probably include information about possible eventual outcomes and how the patient is adjusting to illness. The record provides useful information on financial resources, employment, daily living habits, and other pertinent matters. See Chapter 18.

Included in the data will be information on how the patient's progress will be evaluated after discharge from a hospital. Often this involves a plan for visits by a member of the health team and perhaps follow-up teaching.

Identifying Learning Needs

After all the data have been collected, the nurse identifies the specific learning needs of the patient and/or family. It is important to identify those needs that the patient recognizes and those of which the patient is unaware. Part of the teaching plan can be to make the patient aware at a time when he or she is ready. These needs should be noted so that the patient and the nurse can deal with them at an appropriate time. Sometimes, in the course of gaining knowledge or skills, patients become ready to recognize needs that they initially would deny or find impossible to comprehend. Often by asking questions the patient will indicate the need to learn.

Sometimes a need to learn is reflected in patient behavior that nurses find difficult. The patient appears angry or orders the nurses around. These behaviors may well reflect a need for the patient to control the environment; but the patient can be taught more acceptable ways of coping with the environment.

Identifying Readiness and Ability to Learn

The third phase in assessment of learning needs is identifying the patient's or family's readiness and ability to learn. The factors discussed in the following sections can be examined to assess these facts.

Age

Age provides information on the person's developmental status. Simple questions to school-age children and adolescents will elicit information on what they know. Observing children in play provides information about their motor and intellectual development as well as relationships with other children. For the elderly person, conversation and questioning may reveal memory deficiencies and learning difficulties. These are often associated with sensory limitations such as deafness, which can be ascertained.

Education and socioeconomic status

The patient's level of education and socioeconomic status give the nurse some idea about the health beliefs and behavior of that person. Is oral care part of the person's system of health behavior, or does she never brush her teeth? This information also assists the nurse to evaluate the person's intellectual capacity. For example, a person who has had a university education can be expected to have a larger working vocabulary than a person who does not read. If an adult patient has had no schooling and can neither read nor write, this needs to be considered in relation to learning needs.

Physical status

Is the patient physically ready to learn? Does the patient have sufficient strength to learn to walk? Often patients who have been acutely ill may feel stronger than they really are and quickly tire after slight exertion. Patients may need to try to walk to realize how weak they are and what their limits are at the time.

Emotional status

Does the patient want to learn and have the psychologic energy to do so? When people are ill, they often go through a number of stages, from denial and disbelief to acceptance. These stages are described by Kübler-Ross in relation to death and dying (1970:38–137):

1. *Denial and isolation*—involving disbelief and withdrawal from others
2. *Anger*—which is projected into the environment, often at random
3. *Bargaining*—including wishing, in hope of postponing a future event such as disability
4. *Depression*—including a sense of loss
5. *Acceptance*—including adaptation to the situation

A patient's ability and desire to learn are largely related to the stage of the illness. People learn most effectively when they have reached the stage of acceptance and have some sense of their own identity and control.

Planning Teaching

When the nurse plans teaching, it is important to identify the following:

1. The learner(s)
2. Where the teaching will be done
3. The time during which the teaching is best carried out
4. The length of time available for the teaching
5. The exact nature of the cognitive, psychomotor, and/or affective learning required, i.e., the goals and objectives
6. The most desirable teaching method
7. The degree of expertise required by the learner
8. Whether an environment for learning first has to be established
9. The method of evaluating the learning

It is important to identify not only the learners but also their individual learning needs. Teaching normally starts at the level of the learner, and this varies considerably among people. The teaching may be best carried out in privacy or in a group. Timing can be very important, especially for patients who have limited energy and tire easily. Patients who are anxious may have difficulty concentrating for long periods and thus need short learning periods.

The exact nature of the learning can affect the type of teaching method used. Reading, watching a film, demonstrating, and discussing are possible methods. For some patients, a climate for learning must be created before actual learning can take place. A climate for learning is an environment or atmosphere conducive to an individual's learning. For example, some patients learn better sitting up than lying down; most learn better if the radio is turned off. It is important to understand what the patient perceives as important and to deal with that before proceeding to other learning needs. Evaluating the learning is also important, and methods of evaluation need to be planned before the teaching activity is implemented.

Planning involves a number of stages: setting goals, setting priorities, planning the learning content, and selecting methods of teaching.

Setting Goals and Objectives

The words *goals* and *objectives* are used interchangeably by some educators and distinguished by others. Used interchangeably, they can be considered both immediate and long-term aims intended to be accomplished in a learning situation. However, a *goal* is often meant to be the more general term, describing a long-range and general intended learning outcome, while an *objective* is used to mean a specific, immediate, or short-range intended outcome of a learning situation.

Setting goals and objectives is done by the patient or support persons and the nurse. Often the patient can identify the goals that are most meaningful personally and about which the nurse has little information. Objectives relate to immediate needs of a patient, such as perineal care after birth of a baby. Goals relate to long-term needs, such as the need of an obese new mother to lose weight. In this case, the goal may be a specific weight loss through diet and exercise.

The patient or family and the nurse should set the learning objectives together. The learner who is actively involved in planning at this stage is more likely to follow through in meeting the objectives. In some instances, the patient might be grateful to the nurse for doing most of the planning, for example, when the patient is very weak but needs to learn quickly. If a patient wants and needs to learn responsibility for medications, yet has difficulty concentrating upon the subject, a written plan for the patient that is discussed for short periods will often be most helpful.

The objectives for learning should be both specific and observable in terms of behavior. A specific goal might be "to take 60 mg furosemide (Lasix) upon identifying ankle edema." An objective needs to be stated in terms of patient behavior not nurse behavior. For example, "The patient will write his own diets as instructed" (patient behavior), not "To teach the patient about his diet" (nurse behavior). Objectives should contain three types of information (Mager 1975:21): performance, conditions, and criteria.

Performance

Performance or behavior describes what the learner will be able to do after mastering the objective. The objective must reflect an observable activity. The performance may be visible, e.g., walking, or invisible, e.g., adding a column of figures. However, it is necessary to be able to deduce whether an unobservable activity has been mastered from some performance that represents the activity. Therefore, the performance of an objective might be written: "Writes the total for a column of figures in the indicated space" (observable), not "Adds a column of figures" (unobservable).

Conditions

In some instances it is necessary to state the conditions under which a performance is to be carried out so that the objective is clear. For example, "Walks to the end of the hall and back without crutches" describes a performance clearly; "without crutches" is a condition of the objective.

Nurses always need to determine the conditions in which an activity will be carried out. Then the objectives for the learning plan can reflect those conditions. For example, if a patient lives alone and must irrigate his own colostomy, then "Irrigate his colostomy *independently* as taught" would be correct.

Criteria

Criteria state the standards of performance that are considered acceptable. Each objective should specify a standard against which the performance can be measured. Examples include speed, quality, and accuracy.

For patients, quality is often used in the objective. For example, "as instructed," "as listed," "as described" all refer to quality as determined by someone. Learners need to understand the criteria so that they can evaluate their performance validly. Sometimes it is necessary to clarify criteria for them. For additional information on objectives and criteria, see Chapter 6.

Setting Priorities

The priorities for learning are set by the patient or support persons and the nurse. The final priority list results from a combination of the patient's perceived needs and the nurse's professional judgment. For example, exercising an arm may take priority over bathing; taking a medication regularly for hypertension may take priority over sleeping.

Planning Learning Content

Learning content needs to be written as a plan. It may consist of a detailed statement, an outline, or a few words. However the plan is written, it should be meaningful to all people involved. The content is what needs to be learned, such as how to irrigate a colostomy or how to transfer independently from a wheelchair to a tub. It can often be divided into elements or steps.

Selecting Methods of Teaching

The methods of teaching should be suited to the individual patient's needs. There are many methods of conveying knowledge, feelings, and skills. See Table 17–1. To a baby, the sense of touch and warmth is highly significant. To a child, manipulating objects can be meaningful. For adults, a combination of hearing, seeing, and doing is highly effective. Some people can conceptualize from verbal instruction, while others need to see and do for themselves.

Some teaching methods involve group learning, where people can learn from each other as well as from the teacher. Other methods use individual instruction. This permits the nurse to teach at the patient's pace, and it is particularly appropriate for learning that the patient might find embarrassing, such as learning to perform a urinary catheterization on oneself. Often there are aids to assist patients with special learning needs. For example, a variety of special syringes can assist a visually impaired person draw up insulin for injection (Boyles 1977).

Demonstration is widely used as a method of teaching for both individuals and groups. It can be planned or informal; the latter is most often used in one-to-one instruction. During the demonstration it is important for the nurse to follow a step-by-step method. If the patient appears confused, the nurse should stop and clarify the step before proceeding.

Audiovisual aids are also helpful for teaching. Charts, posters, films, and tapes are generally available. The nurse must remember to choose materials appropriate to the learner's level. A film with many medical terms might confuse rather than assist the viewer.

The method of teaching is usually related to the type of learning to take place—i.e., psychomotor, affective, or cognitive learning.

Psychomotor learning

To learn psychomotor skills, such as administering insulin using a syringe, usually involves four phases:

1. Teaching in relation to fear, anxiety, etc., if this is present. Often this phase requires considerable interaction by the patient with the nurse and/or discussions in a small supportive group.

2. Teaching the cognitive basis for the skill. The nurse may do this through discussions with the patient, furnishing reading materials, showing films, etc.

Table 17–1 Selected Teaching Methods

Method	Major type of learning	Characteristics
Explanation or description (e.g., lecture)	Cognitive	Teacher controls content and pace. Feedback is determined by teacher. May be given to individual or group. Encourages retention of facts.
One-to-one discussion	Affective, cognitive	Encourages participation by learner. Permits reinforcement and repetition at learner's level. Permits introduction of sensitive subjects.
Answering questions	Cognitive	Teacher controls most of content and pace. Teacher must understand question and what it means to learner. Can be used with individuals and groups. Sometimes teacher needs to confirm whether question has been answered by asking learner, e.g., "Does that answer your question?"
Demonstration	Psychomotor	Often used with explanation. Can be used with individuals, small or large groups. Does not permit use of equipment by learners.
Group discussion	Affective, cognitive	Learner can obtain assistance from supportive group. Group members learn from one another.
Practice	Psychomotor	Allows repetition and immediate feedback. Permits "hands-on" experience.
Printed and audiovisual materials	Cognitive	Forms include books, pamphlets, films, programmed instruction, and computer learning. Learners can proceed at their own speed. Nurse can act as resource person, need not be present during learning.
Role playing	Affective, cognitive	Permits expression of attitudes, values, and emotions. Can assist in development of communication skills. Involves active participation by learner.

3. Demonstration of the psychomotor skill by the nurse. This may be done for a group or an individual.
4. Repeated practice of the skill by the patient with feedback from the nurse.

Some people learn best through seeing—they are visually oriented; others learn best through hearing—having the skill explained. This attribute of the patient should be considered during the planning phase. If it is not identified until the teaching plan has been implemented, it may be a reason to revise the plan.

Affective learning

Learning of affective content is accomplished through interaction with the nurse, often one-to-one or in a small supportive group. To learn new attitudes, interests, and values usually requires considerable time and does not occur as a result of an explanation or a class lecture.

Cognitive learning

Teaching for cognitive learning involves the transmission of knowledge to a person or group. The source of the information may be the nurse, reading materials, films, etc. Common methods of teaching this type of learning are verbal explanations to one person or a small group and lectures to larger groups.

Implementing Teaching

The teaching plan is implemented using the planned strategy. See the section on teaching methods earlier. During implementation it may be necessary to revise the plan, for example, if the patient tires sooner than anticipated or is faced with too much information too quickly.

Sometimes the teaching plan must be adjusted because the patient's needs change or external factors intervene. The nurse and the patient may have planned for the patient to learn to administer his own insulin at a particular time, but when the time comes the nurse finds that the patient wants additional information before actually giving the insulin. The nurse alters the teaching plan and discusses the desired information, provides written information, and defers teaching the psychomotor skill until the next day. It is important for the nurse to be flexible in implementing any teaching plan.

During implementation there are three major concerns: timing, environment, and teaching method. The time for learning must be appropriate for the patient, particularly in terms of fatigue and anxiety. The environment needs to be suitable for the learning with particular reference to the appropriateness of privacy. Teaching methods were discussed previously in this chapter.

When implementing a teaching plan, the nurse may find the following activities helpful:

1. Determine that the time is suitable for the patient. Distractions, such as visitors or the presence of other health personnel, can inhibit learning.
2. Arrange for the appropriate environment, e.g., a private room or a classroom.
3. Gather all the instructional resources that will be needed. If the nurse has to leave to obtain forgotten equipment, this is distracting to the learner.
4. Adjust the teaching when unforeseen factors intervene. For example, a patient who protests "I don't know why I need to learn this" may not be ready to learn to give an injection.
5. Be sensitive to signs that the learner has had enough. People can become overwhelmed by information before the nurse anticipates that they will.
6. Decide how and when to follow up the learning, i.e., to reinforce a new skill and to provide feedback.
7. Determine when and how to evaluate the learning. Although evaluation is planned beforehand, it may be necessary to adjust the plan if, for example, the patient has become fatigued.

Evaluating Learning and Teaching

Evaluating is an ongoing process in which the patient, the nurse, and perhaps the family members assess what has been learned. The evaluation phase in the teaching-learning process must include:

1. The most effective feedback mechanism
2. Reinforcement or correction of the patient's learning
3. Evaluation of the nurse's teaching

Feedback in the teaching-learning context is information given to the learner about the effectiveness of the learning; that is, how the learning compares with its purpose and goals. Feedback is most successful when behavior is compared with predetermined criteria. On a paper-and-pencil test, feedback can show that the learner answered seven questions correctly out of ten. In learning a psychomotor skill, comparing the learner's performance of the skill against a list of criteria tells how well the learner has learned the skill

Feedback can be positive or negative. Positive feedback is similar to reward. In the example of the paper-and-pencil test, positive feedback places emphasis on the seven questions answered correctly. Negative feedback is, in a sense, a reprimand; it stresses what was *not* learned rather than what was learned. Motivation to learn can be affected by feedback in highly individual ways. Some people are more motivated with positive feedback while others are more motivated by negative feedback.

The nurse's reinforcement or correction of learning must also be timed appropriately for the patient. Generally it is best provided directly after the learning but only if the patient can assimilate the message. If the patient feels overwhelmed with information, it may be better left for another time.

Evaluation of the nurse's teaching should also take place. This includes a consideration of all the factors in the process, including the timing, the teaching method, the amount of information, and whether it was helpful. The nurse may find, for example, that the patient was overwhelmed with too much information, was bored, or was motivated to learn more.

There are many ways in which learning can be identified:

1. The patient's questions and comments indicate a certain knowledge.
2. The patient gives answers to direct questions.
3. The patient demonstrates a skill such as giving a baby bath.
4. Members of the family and other health team members observe the patient's newly learned behavior.
5. The patient says he or she understands.

Evaluation is one means by which the patient can be encouraged in learning. Even the smallest advances are worthy of positive feedback from the nurse, which will encourage the patient. Feedback at frequent intervals is important so that the patient does not practice incorrectly or retain incorrect information. When evaluating, nurses need to be objective, that is, to be without personal bias, and to focus on the task, not the person. For example, it is better to say, "You handled the syringe well" rather than, "You are good at injections," or "You small-boned people have an easy time with syringes."

The evaluation needs to be measured against the objectives of the learning. If the objectives are not being reached, this may necessitate changing the teaching plan. It may well be that the patient's needs must be reassessed or that factors not considered before are interfering with the learning or that the teaching methods need to be changed for that particular patient. Often the patient can tell the nurse where the difficulty is and what needs to be changed. The nurse and the patient can then revise the teaching plan accordingly and continue.

Summary

Nurses are concerned with three types of learning in relation to patient care: cognitive, affective, and psychomotor. Patients and their support persons have learning needs related to their development as well as needs directly related to health. Thus the teaching function of the nurse is important in assisting normal development and in assisting patients to meet needs related to health.

Learning is a permanent change in behavior. Relative to health needs, nurses are concerned with three types of learning: psychomotor, cognitive, and affective learning. Learning is affected by many factors, some of which hinder it and some of which assist it. It is important for nurses to identify these factors in a particular situation and implement learning when it is most likely to be successful.

Developmental learning needs were discussed in Chapters 11 and 12. They vary with each age group and among persons within a particular group. Teaching is a process that assists people to learn. There are a number of principles that may be helpful to the nurse who is teaching.

Assessing learning needs and readiness to learn are the first steps in teaching. They are followed by drawing up a teaching plan and then implementing that plan. The learning and teaching are evaluated, and, if indicated, the plan is changed. Positive feedback is often important to encourage the patient about progress, particularly when learning is slow.

Suggested Activities

1. Interview a person in the community. Establish the developmental learning tasks of that person. Compare these with the developmental tasks of that age group as described by Havighurst on page 235.
2. In a hospital interview a patient convalescing after surgery. Assess the patient's learning needs, and develop a plan to assist him or her to meet these needs.
3. Assess the readiness to learn of the patient in activity 2.
4. Implement the plan in activity 2, and evaluate the learning.

Suggested Readings

Aiken, L. H. September 1970. Patient problems are problems in learning. *American Journal of Nursing* 70:1916–18.
The nurse's teaching function begins with the assessment of patient problems. Teaching is a continuous process in which the nurse helps patients learn to cope with problems in their environment.

Kratzer, J. B. December 1977. What does your patient need to know? *Nursing 77* 7:82 (Canadian ed. 7:70–71).
This article describes setting up a teaching plan, collecting data, and implementing the plan. A complete patient education form is included.

Murray, R., and Zentner, J. February 1976. Guidelines for more effective health teaching. *Nursing 76* 6:44–53.
The role of health teacher is a constant challenge for the nurse. A wide variety of factors affect learning, and many teaching techniques can be used.

Selected References

Bille, D. A. December 1980. Educational strategies for teaching the elderly patient. *Nursing in Health Care* 1:256–59.

Bloom, R. S. 1975. Stating educational objectives in behavioral terms. *Nursing Forum* 14(1):30–42.

Boyles, V. A. September 1977. Injection aids for blind diabetic patients. *American Journal of Nursing* 77:1456–58.

deTorney, R. 1971. *Strategies for teaching nursing.* New York: John Wiley and Sons.

Eaton, S.; Davis, G. L.; and Benner, P. E. September 1977. Discussion stoppers in teaching. *Nursing Outlook* 25:578–83.

Fuhrer, L. M., and Bernstein, R. November 1976. Making patient education a part of patient care. *American Journal of Nursing* 76:1798–99.

Gronlund, N. E. 1978. *Stating objectives for classroom instruction.* 2nd ed. New York: Macmillan Publishing Co.

Kübler-Ross, E. 1970. *On death and dying.* New York: Macmillan Publishing Co.

McKeehan, K. M., editor. 1981. *Continuing care: A multidisciplinary approach to discharge planning.* St. Louis: C. V. Mosby Co.

Mager, R. F. 1975. *Preparing instructional objectives.* Belmont, Calif.: Fearon Publishers.

Mager, R., and Pipe, R. August 1976. You really oughta wanna . . . or how not to motivate people. *Nursing 76* 6:65 (Canadian ed. 6: 7, 10).

Pugh, E. J. 1976. Dynamics of teaching-learning interaction. *Nursing Forum* 15(1):47–58.

Redman, B. K. 1980. *The process of patient teaching in nursing.* 4th ed. St. Louis: C. V. Mosby Co.

———. September 1981. Patient education in hospitals: Developmental issues. *Journal of Nursing Administration* 11:28–30.

Smith, D. M. February 1971. Writing objectives as a nursing practice skill. *American Journal of Nursing* 71:319–20.

Chapter 18

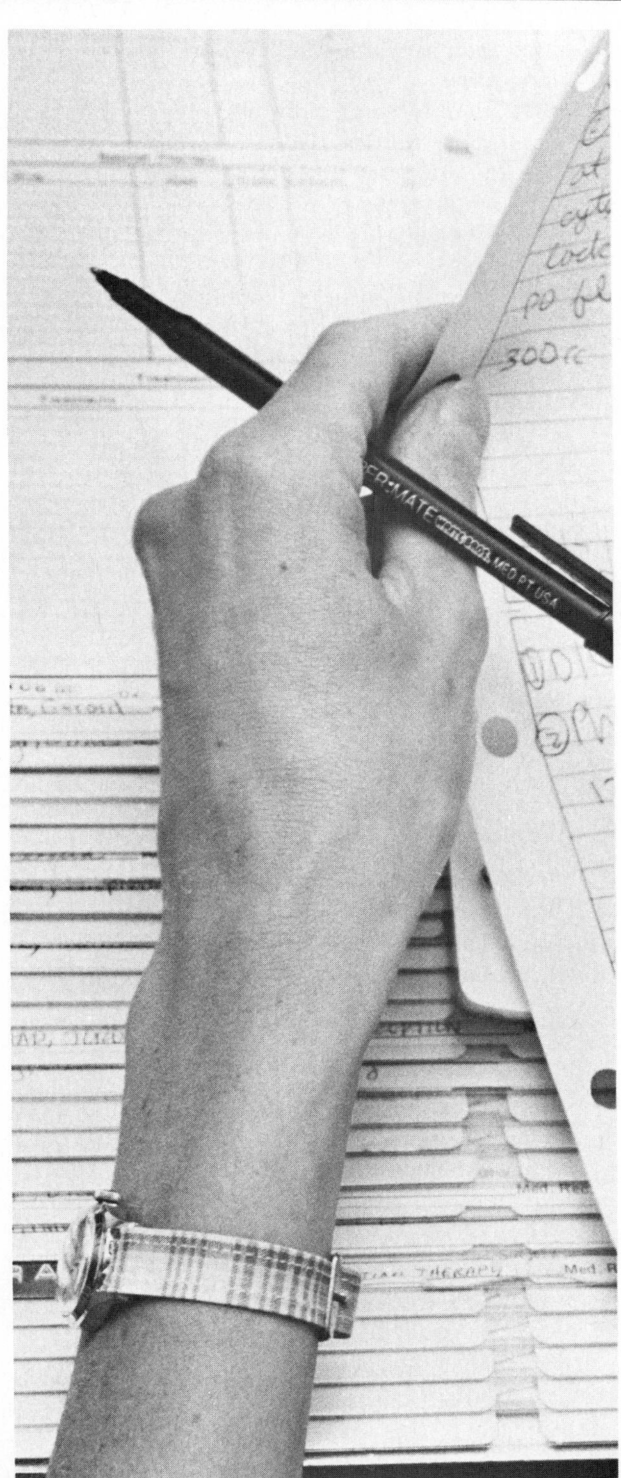

Recording and Reporting

CONTENTS

Objectives

1. Know essential facts about patient records
   1.1 Define selected terms
   1.2 Identify four reasons health team members communicate about patients
   1.3 Describe six purposes of patient records
   1.4 Name four basic components of the problem-oriented record (POR)
   1.5 Identify essential aspects of the four basic components of POR for the patient and for involved health personnel
   1.6 Identify the systematic format for writing SOAP progress notes
   1.7 Describe three kinds of progress notes related to POR
   1.8 Identify six parts of the traditional patient record
   1.9 List the kinds of information included on the traditional patient record
   1.10 List the advantages of the Kardex record
2. Know essential facts about recording and reporting
   2.1 Identify essential guidelines for nurses recording patient data
   2.2 Identify some legal factors to consider when recording
   2.3 Identify commonly accepted terms, symbols, and abbreviations used in recording
   2.4 Identify essential guidelines for nurses reporting patient data
3. Know essential facts about computerized information systems
   3.1 Describe some advantages of computerized information systems to the nurse and to the patient
   3.2 Identify essential components of an integrated information system
   3.3 Identify some implications of computerized information systems to health care agencies

Terms

audit
data base
peer review
problem-oriented record (POR)

Communication among health team members is vital to good patient care. Generally, health team members communicate through discussions, reports, and records. A discussion is an informal oral consideration of a subject by two or more members of the health team, often leading to a decision. A report is an oral or written account by one member to others in the health team; for instance, nurses always report on patients at the end of a hospital work shift. A record is always written; it is a formal, legal documentation of a patient's progress and treatment.

Accurate, complete communication serves several purposes:

1. It helps coordinate care given by several people.
2. It prevents the patient from having to repeat information to each health team member.
3. It promotes accuracy in the provision of care and lessens the possibility of error.
4. It helps health personnel make the best use of their time by avoiding overlapping of activities.

Reasons for Records

Traditionally, written records have been an important aspect of care. All health agencies keep written records, although the form of the record may vary considerably from place to place.

A patient's record or chart is a written record of health status and health care. It describes the patient's health, specifies diagnostic and therapeutic measures employed, and records the patient's response to these measures. The record is usually kept current as long as the patient attends the health agency.

The patient's record has a number of purposes: communication, legal documentation, research, education, statistics, and audit.

1. *Communication.* The record is the vehicle by which members of the health team communicate. Although

health team members also communicate orally, the record is efficient and permanent. An accurate record helps nurses prevent such errors as inadvertently administering a medication twice. The record also allows health team members on different shifts to convey meaningful information about the patient to one another.

2. *Legal documentation.* The patient's record is a legal document that is admissible in court as evidence. In some jurisdictions, the record is not admitted as evidence if the patient objects on the grounds that such evidence violates the confidentiality of the physician-patient relationship.

A record is usually considered the property of the agency, although increasingly the patient, upon request, has a right to the information in the record. The Patient's Bill of Rights supports this right. See Chapter 3. Legal decisions in California uphold this right (Creighton 1981:116). Some agencies, however, do not permit the patient access to the record; thus, the nurse follows the policy of his or her agency.

3. *Research.* The information in records can be a valuable research tool. For example, researchers may study treatment plans for a number of patients with the same illness to ascertain which plan might be of greatest benefit to a particular patient.

A record made years previously may shed light on a current problem. Patients usually have incomplete recollection of a past illness and its treatment, but the record generally reveals accurate data perhaps forgotten by the patient. Records are also very important where experimental drugs and treatments are being used.

4. *Statistics.* Statistic information from patient records can help an agency anticipate and plan for future needs. For example, agency management might analyze past admission statistics when deciding which services to expand or curtail. Some statistics are required by law, such as the records of births and deaths; these are filed with a government agency and become a part of local, national, and international statistics.

5. *Education.* Students in various health disciplines use patient records as tools in education. A record frequently provides a comprehensive view of the patient, the illness, and the assistance provided. Medical records are used to educate nurses, physicians, dietitians, and people in most of the health disciplines.

6. *Audit.* The patient's record is used also to monitor the quality of care the patient receives and the related competencies of the people giving that care. Specifically, a *nursing audit* monitors nursing care; it is often a retrospective audit in that the care has already been given. This care is then measured against established standards.

The nursing audit, when carried out by other nurses, is sometimes called a *peer review.* Many agencies have audit committees that monitor individual nurse practice. Audits are also carried out by outside groups that accredit institutions.

Various aspects of care are assessed in nursing audits: data base, identification of the health problems, goals of the nursing intervention, nursing interventions chosen, and evaluation of goal attainment. Included in this audit are the skills of the nurse as well as the judgment and knowledge the nurse used in providing care.

Problem-Oriented Records

The *problem-oriented record* (POR) or problem-oriented medical record (POMR) is an increasingly used recording system. It is also referred to as the *Weed system* after its originator, L. L. Weed. This system provides a patient-centered problem-solving approach to care, one that all health disciplines contributing care to the patient can use. The record first lists all of the patient's identified problems at a point in time and specifies the therapy planned for each identified problem. This record, because it integrates the care given by all health team members, differs from the traditional patient record, which segregates medical, nursing, and other problems in different sections.

The POR has the following basic components: (a) defined data base, (b) complete problem list, (c) initial plan for each identified problem, and (d) progress notes.

Defined Data Base

The *data base* is all the information known about the patient when he or she first enters the health care agency. It includes nursing history and assessment, medical history, and data from the physical examination. To these are added social and family data from other sources, such as the social worker, and baseline laboratory and radiographic data. Important in the data is the chief complaint of the patient. Most agencies use a standardized form that helps personnel obtain a complete data base.

Problem List

The problem list is a careful listing of the problems presented by the patient. Some problems are obvious on initial contact with the patient; others are discovered as additional data are gathered.

The initial problem list is usually made by the physician or the person who assumes primary responsibility for the patient's care. Other members of the health team add to the list if they discover further problems in the course of giving care.

The problem list, if complete, includes socioeconomic, psychologic, and physiologic problems. The list is attached to the front of the patient's record. Each problem is labeled and numbered so it can be identified throughout the record. This list has been likened to an index or table of contents. See Figure 18–1. Problems are also usually listed according to their status, such as active or inactive.

If a problem is potential rather than actual, it is usually entered on the progress notes rather than on the problem list. Only when the problem becomes active is it added to the list.

Plans

The initial list of plans is made with reference to the active problems. Each plan is numbered to correspond to its related problem and has three parts: diagnostic workup, therapy, and patient education.

In the *diagnostic workup,* the physician indicates what needs to be done first. This indication of priority helps with planning, prevents duplication, eliminates some distress for the patient, and often saves time and money. Included in the diagnostic workup may be plans to collect further data to establish a medical

Figure 18–1 A sample patient's problem list. (Courtesy of the Medical Records Committee of the Medical Board of the University of Maryland Hospital, Baltimore, Maryland.)

UNIVERSITY OF MARYLAND HOSPITAL

PATIENT'S PROBLEM SHEET

PROBLEM NUMBER	DATE OF ONSET	DATE PROBLEM RECORDED	ACTIVE PROBLEMS	INACTIVE/RESOLVED PROBLEMS	DATE RESOLVED
1	Aug. 31 1982	Sept. 1 1982	Suddenly Passed Out Scalp Laceration		9/1/82 9/8/82
2	2 yrs. +	Sept. 2 1982	Diabetes Mellitus – Uncontrolled Long Standing Out of Control		Controlled 10/5/82
3	10 yrs.	Sept. 1 1982	Obesity	March, 1983	
4	Sept. or Oct. 1982	Sept. 1 1982	Pre Tibial Varicose Ulcers Walked into furniture Sept. & Oct, 1981	Feb, 1983	Feb, 1983
5	1 yr. + or	Sept. 4 1982	Family Problems – Because "he is always sick"	Feb, 1983	Feb, 1983
6	Gradual Onset ?time	Sept. 4 1982	Impotence (complete)		April 83
7	Nov. 24 1982	Nov. 25 1982	I "don't care." I am "down in the dumps" I cannot eat the way I want		April, 83
8	2 wks.	Jan. 3 1983	Toe Nails Get Sore Especially Rt. Big Toe	Feb 15, 1983	
9	June 10 1983	June 10 1983	Congestive Heart Failure { Dyspnea Leg Edema Tender Abdomen	June 24, 1983	
10	3 days	June 10 1983	Cloudy Smokey Urine		
		Current	Summation of Patient's Problems as of July 15, 1983 (over)		

3020

Date	Time	Problem
12-25-83	1800	#1 Anginal Pain
		S c/o severe substernal pain radiating
		to (L) shoulder and down arm—
		States a compressing sensation
		and tightness is felt in the chest
		O BP 90/40, P 140. Appears ashen-colored,
		skin cold and clammy to touch
		A Anxious and in pain
		P Place on bedrest. Start O_2 per nasal
		cannula at 5 L/min. Notify physician.
		— Pat A. Sung, R.N.

Figure 18–2 Progress notes that show the SOAP format.

or nursing diagnosis or to assist in the therapeutic management of the patient.

The *therapy* aspect of the planning includes the physician's orders, which often specify drug therapy and treatments. The orders are also numbered according to the problem they address. This organization gives the reader (the nurse) considerable information about the plan, including the reason for a physician's specific order.

The *patient education* aspect of the plan lists skills that will help the patient manage the illness and outlines an education plan.

Progress Records

Progress records are the fourth part of the POR. These notes are made by all members of the health team involved in a patient's care: for example, the nurse, occupational therapist, dietitian, physician, and social worker. In many settings, all health team members annotate the same progress record.

SOAP is a systematic format for writing progress records. SOAP is an acronym for **s**ubjective data, **o**bjective data, **a**ssessment, and **p**lanning. Compiling *subjective data* includes reporting what the patient perceives and the way the patient expresses it. Subjective data help team members see the patient as a person and identify emotional responses, such as anger or frustration, that might be used therapeutically (Woody and Mallison 1973:1173).

Objective data include vital signs, observations made using the senses, laboratory and radiographic findings, as well as responses to other diagnostic and therapeutic measures, such as medications.

During the *assessment stage,* the observer interprets the subjective and objective data and draws conclusions. Team members make assessments based on their specialized knowledge.

In the traditional method of recording, nurses are not usually expected to draw conclusions and make interpretations. Thus, many nurses find assessment difficult to learn. It involves the use of a knowledge base as well as logical thinking.

The fourth stage of SOAP, *planning,* involves a revision of the initial plan. Plans have three major aspects: educational, diagnostic, and therapeutic. The revised plan may indicate a need for immediate change or for future changes in any of these aspects. The plans incorporate what the patient has been taught and what the patient has learned. Each plan is signed, dated, and timed by the person writing it. See Figure 18–2.

Recording Progress on PORs

Three kinds of progress records are generally recognized: (a) narrative notes, (b) flow sheets, and (c) discharge notes.

1. *Narrative notes.* Narrative notes record the patient's progress day-to-day. They are keyed to the related patient problems and filled out by all members of the health team who give care. The caregiver who has nothing new to report writes "as above" in the notes.

2. *Flow sheets.* Flow sheets are used when a patient's progress, as reflected by such specific or operative variables as pulse, blood pressure, medications, or progress in learning a new skill, must be reported accurately and concisely. In these cases, narrative notes would be too long, but the flow sheet, a graphic record, reflects the patient's condition quickly. Figure 18–3 is an example of a nurse's flow sheet. The time parameters for flow sheets can vary from minutes to months. In an intensive care unit, a patient's heart rate may be monitored by the minute; in an ambulatory clinic, a patient's blood glucose may be recorded once a month. Once a problem on a flow sheet is resolved, a narrative note is written.

3. *Discharge notes.* The discharge note is written by the physician or by another member of the health team, depending on the policy of the health care agency. In a home visiting service or community clinic, a nurse may write the discharge note. The discharge note refers to the problems identified earlier and describes the degree to which each problem has been resolved. If the patient is referred to another agency, the referral is documented on the discharge note. In some agencies, nurses fill out a nursing discharge profile, which contains patient information relevant at the time of discharge.

Figure 18–3 A nurse's activity flow sheet.

Date/Time → Param/Rx ↓	0100	0130	0200	0230	0300	
B/P	80/50/40	80/55/40	75/50/30	60/40/20	60/40/20	
Apical pulse	122	115	130	140	142	
Dressing	Dry	Small serous	Mod. Sero-Sanguineous	Mod. Sero-Sanguineous	Mod. Sero-Sanguineous	
Resp.	22	22	26	28	28	
Foley Drainage	60ml. cl. amber	—	40ml. cl. amber	—	25ml. cl. amber	

Traditional Patient Records

The traditional patient record is a source-oriented record, that is, each category of caregiver or source fills out his or her own individual record. Information about a particular problem is therefore distributed throughout the cumulative record, and a problem identified by one caregiver is not always followed up by other health team members. For example, a physician who does not read the nurses' notes may not learn that a patient has a great fear of injections. That knowledge could affect the physician's orders.

Patient Charts

Traditional patient charts generally have six parts: admission sheet, face sheet, physician's order sheet, history sheet, nurses' notes, and other special reports and records.

The *admission sheet* is a part of the record in most agencies. It generally contains specific data about the patient, including an identification number. Most hospital admission sheets contain the following information: the patient's full name, address, date of birth, name of attending physician, sex and marital status, nearest relative, occupation and employer, hospital payment arrangements, religious preference, date and hour of admission to the hospital, hospital unit or agency of admission, previous hospital admission or call, admitting diagnosis or problem, and identification number.

The *face sheet* is the front sheet of the chart. It has a number of uses; for instance, it is frequently used to list the patient's allergies.

The *doctor's order sheet* is a written record of the physician's orders. The physician is expected to date and sign each order or to sign once for several orders written at the same time. Often agencies flag a patient's chart to indicate to the nurse that there is a new order.

When a physician gives orders about a patient by

telephone, the person who receives the order writes it on the sheet, writes the date and time, signs the order, and indicates that it was given by telephone. Often the physician is expected to countersign the telephone order within 24 or 48 hours of giving the order.

The *history sheet* is a record of the patient's health history written by the physician. Often the physician also uses this sheet to record progress notes and any future plans for the patient.

The *nurses' notes* are a record of nursing interventions. Nurses also record on these notes their assessments of patients and evaluations of the effectiveness of interventions. Nurses' notes contain the following kinds of information:

1. Assessment of the patient by various nursing personnel, for example, assessment of skin color or odor of urine
2. Nursing interventions ordered by the physician, such as medications or treatment
3. Nursing interventions initiated by the nurses themselves, for example, special skin care or health teaching
4. Evaluation of the effectiveness of nursing interventions
5. Specific measures carried out by the physician, for example, shortening a drain in an incision
6. Visits by members of the health team, such as a consulting physician

Special reports and records also become a part of a patient's chart. These often include radiographic reports, laboratory findings, reports of surgery, and anesthesia records. Often nurses use data from these reports to formulate a plan of nursing care.

Clinical flow sheets similar to those used in POR records include graphic records for vital signs, medications, fluid intake and output, and other data (e.g., appetite and fecal elimination) monitored regularly. See Figure 18–4 for a sample graphic observation record.

Kardex Records

The Kardex is a widely used, concise method of recording significant data about a patient. An advantage of the Kardex is that it makes patient data quickly accessible to members of the health team. The system is a series of cards, which are usually kept in a portable index file. A card can be quickly turned up to reveal significant data about a patient. Often Kardex data are written in pencil and changed frequently to be up to date. See Figure 18–5. The Kardex is not a legal document.

Guidelines for Recording

The following guidelines assist the nurse to annotate the patient's chart in either the traditional or the problem-oriented recording system.

1. *Brevity.* Entries should be brief, yet all pertinent data must be included. Extra words, such as the patient's name and the word *patient,* should be omitted, since the patient's identity is obvious. Correct terms and acceptable abbreviations and symbols are used. See Appendix A.
2. *Accuracy.* All data recorded must be accurate and specific. Notation of time is an important part of accuracy. In some settings, time is recorded according to the 24-hour clock (military clock). This method avoids confusion between A.M. and P.M. See Figure 18–6. The nurse charts the exact time a patient takes a medication, not the approximate time, that is, "1425 hours," not "about 1400 hours." It is also important that all pertinent information be included on the record; the omission of significant data is regarded as an inaccuracy.
3. *Legibility.* All recording must be legible. Records are normally kept in ink because pencil does not provide a permanent record. Black ink may be required for photocopying purposes. Print or script writing is acceptable. Correcting an error in charting is discussed later in this chapter.
4. *Correct spelling.* Spelling is important to accuracy. Two decidedly different medications may have similar spellings, for example, Digoxin and Digitoxin.
5. *Differentiating between observation and interpretation.* The nurse must record observations accurately and differentiate them from interpretations. For example, "the patient is crying" is an observation, but "the patient is depressed because of his illness" is an interpretation. If, however, the patient expresses anxiety, he or she should be quoted directly on the chart: "I am worried about my gut."
6. *Consecutive lines.* Records are chronological and made on consecutive lines. When an entry does not fill the entire line, a straight line is drawn through to the end of the line to prevent inserts. Capital letters begin each thought, and periods complete each thought, for example, "Is dyspneic on exertion. Appetite is poor."
7. *Signature.* The nurse's legal signature must be used in many jurisdictions. This usually includes the nurse's first name, middle initial, legal last name, and abbre-

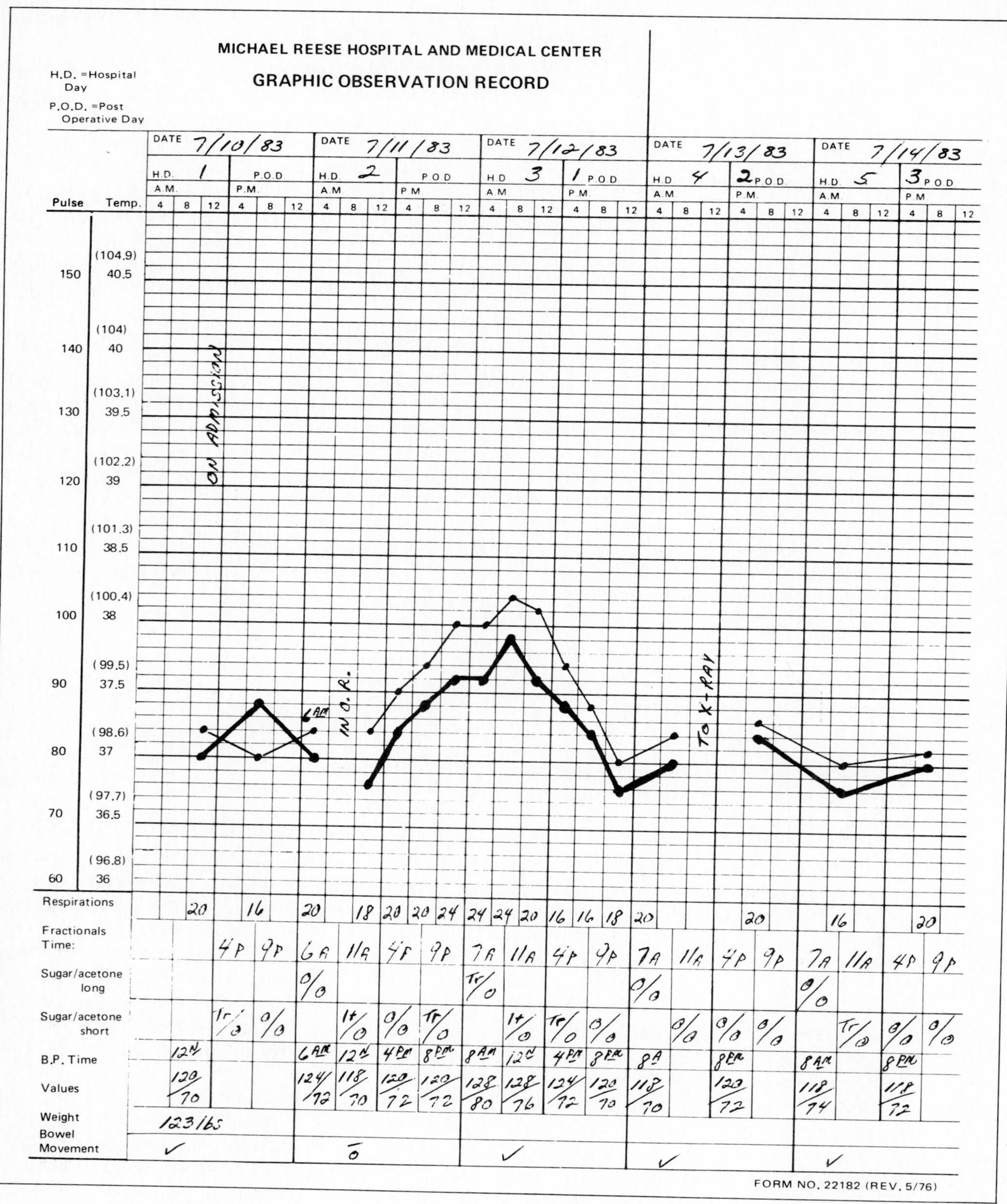

Figure 18–4 A sample graphic observation record. Normally the pulse is shown in red. The pulse line here has been widened to distinguish between the two lines. (Courtesy of Michael Reese Hospital and Medical Center, Chicago, Illinois.)

X-MATCH

DATE	MEDICATIONS	TIME	DATE	I.V.'s
JULY 4	MYLANTA 15cc q.2.h.	06-08-10 12-14-16		
"	HALDOL 1mgm. T.I.D.	08-14-20		
"	FROSST 292 - CRUSHED FOR PAIN	P.R.N.		
"	BIONETS TO SUCK	P.R.N.		
"	SLIDING SCALE TORONTO INSULIN			
	5% GIVE 12 UNITS.			
	3% " 10 "			
	2% " 8 "			TREATMENTS/PROCEDURES
	2%-0 " 0 "		JULY 4	CLINITEST T.I.D. & H.S. – 07-11 17-H.S
JULY 11	AZOGANTRISIN $\dot{\overline{\text{T}}}$ Q.I.D.	06-11 16-22	JULY 8	IRRIGATE FOLEY CATH. DAILY ½ N.S
JULY 4	H.S. MED. DALMANE 30 mgm.	H.S.		
JULY 14	AMITRIPTYLYNE (ELAVIL) 25 mgm	H.S		

NAME	ROOM	DOCTOR	015
FOO MUI SENG	306-A	T.Y. TUNG.	

DATE	No.	PROBLEM LIST	RESOLVED	DATE	OTHER RELEVANT DATA (Include x-rays and tests)
JULY 17	#1	PT. STILL VERY DEPRESSED			DATE OF BIRTH
	#2	L-SIDED WEAKNESS		JULY 17	CHEST PHYSIO.
	#3.	COMMUNICATION PROBLEMS		JULY 14	BARIUM MEAL ✓
					HEALTH CARE CONSULTANTS
DATE REVIEWED					

(Continued on next page)

Figure 18–5 A nursing Kardex. This is the top card. It is folded where the broken line appears. The bottom card is shown on page 434. (Courtesy of Mount Saint Joseph Hospital, Vancouver, British Columbia.)

DIET
- [x] Regular CHINESE
- [ ] Soft
- [ ] Fluid
- [ ] Clear Fluid
- [ ] N.P.O.
- [ ] Other

FEEDING
- [x] Self ̄c SOME ASSISTANCE
- [ ] Assist

FLUIDS
- [ ] I. & O.
  .... Am't Daily
- [ ] I.V.
- [ ] Preferred Fluids

ELIMINATION
- [ ] B.R.
- [x] Commode
- [ ] Ostomy
- [ ] Incontinent
- [ ] Condom
- [ ] Catheter
  Size #16 Date JULY 6
  30cc BALOON
- [ ] Other Specify:

ACTIVITY
- [ ] Up ad lib
- [ ] B.R.P.
- [ ] Amb c asst
- [ ] Walker
- [x] Chair T.I.D 08-12-16
- [ ] Dangle
- [ ] Bed rest

HYGIENE
- [x] Self ̄c SOME ASSISTANCE
- [ ] Partial
- [ ] Bed
- [ ] Tub
- [ ] Shower
- [ ] Mouth Care

SAFETY
Side Rails
- [x] Constant
- [ ] Night Only

Other

PROSTHESIS
- [ ] Glasses
- [ ] Hearing Aid
- [ ] Dentures
- [ ] Other - Specify

V.S. FREQUENCY
- [x] B.P. } O.D @ 0800
- [x] T.P.R. }
- [ ] Other - Specify

SPECIAL CONSIDERATIONS:
(L)-SIDED WEAKNESS

ALLERGIES

DISCHARGE AND REHAB. PLANS: DATE REVIEWED

DATE	PROBLEM AND SHORT TERM GOAL	APPROACH
JULY 17	#1 PT. WILL BE LESS DEPRESSED, PARTICIPATE MORE IN A.D.L. – ↑ HER SELF-ESTEEM	(1) SHOW CARING BY BEING PATIENT AND UNDERSTANDING. (2) BE CONSISTENT IN INVOLVING HER AS MUCH AS POSSIBLE IN A.D.L – AND PRAISE HER WHEN SHE ACCOMPLISHES THEM. (3) MAINTAIN A ROUTINE OF CARE + EXPECT HER TO DO HER SHARE.
JULY 17	#2 PT. WILL BE ABLE TO PARTICIPATE AS MUCH AS POSS. IN A.D.L AND BE AWARE OF POSITIONING OF (L) LIMBS	(1) ASSIST PT. WHENEVER NECESSARY (2) EXPECT PARTICIPATION IN A.D.L. (3) KEEP PT. AWARE OF LEFT LIMB POSITIONS.
JULY 17	#3 PT. WILL UNDERSTAND PROCEDURES ETC.	(1) GET INTERPRETER WHEN NEC. (2) SPEAK SLOWLY

Next of Kin: HUSBAND - FOO YUNG TOY | S.I. | Isolation

Occupation: HOUSEWIFE | Surgery: JULY 4 - ESOPHAGOSCOPY

Age	Religion	Mar. Status	Adm. Date	Diagnosis
61	NIL	M.	JUNE 21/78	(1) ACID INGESTION (2) DIABETES (3) OLD (LT) C.V.A.

Name:	Hosp. No.	Accom.	Doctor	016
FOO MUI SENG		(W) P SP	T.Y. TUNG	

Figure 18–5 continued

viated title or position; for example, Angela I. Marcos, RN. The following title abbreviations are often used, but nurses are advised to check the practice in their agencies.

RN registered nurse
LVN licensed vocational nurse
LPN licensed practical nurse
NA nursing assistant
NS (SN) nursing student (student nurse)

8. *Where and when to chart.* Nurses record information in accordance with agency policies. Some specific data, such as vital signs, medications, or appetite, are recorded on clinical flow sheets. Any abnormal data on these records are often repeated on the nurses' notes with additional relevant details. Nurses record all medications and treatments after they are administered to the patient, not before. The nurse records the time of treatment, not the time of annotation. In many agencies, the nurse's first entry is the duration of his or her tour of duty, for example, 0900 to 1600 hours. Specific times accompany subsequent entries.

Frequency of recording depends primarily on the patient's degree of illness and therapies administered. General guidelines include:

1. Record immediately after initial or other assessments, for instance, when the patient is admitted to the agency or transferred from the operating room, recovery room, or other area, or on the initial shift assessment.

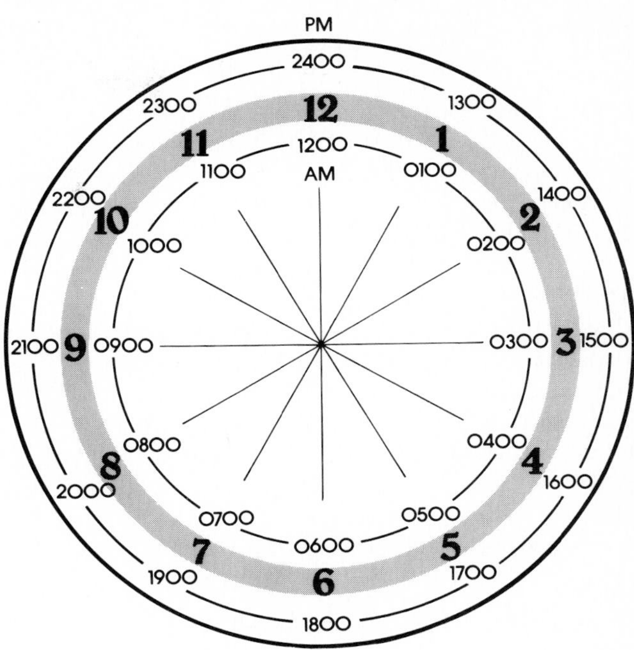

Figure 18–6 The 24-hour clock.

2. Record analgesics immediately after administration, and record their effectiveness subsequently.
3. Record immediately prior to leaving the patient for extended periods of time, such as lunch or coffee breaks, particularly when the patient's condition is critical.

Legal Considerations

The patient's record can be admitted as evidence in a court of law. Nurses insure the legal status of the document by following certain practices. If a nurse makes an error in recording, he or she draws a line through the error and adds the correct material. In some settings, the nurse also writes "error" and his or her initials or name nearby. Erasures on a legal document are generally avoided.

Nurses chart nursing intervention as a record of what they have done for the patient. However, in settings where problem-oriented recording is used, nursing intervention is added to the progress notes (Creighton 1981:327).

It is also important for all health-team members to use abbreviations recognized and accepted by their agencies; standardized abbreviations eliminate the possibility of misinterpretation.

Terms, abbreviations, and symbols may differ somewhat from one agency to another, and often a hospital has an official list of abbreviations to be used in recording. Professionals in some specialty areas use terms, abbreviations, and symbols specific to that specialty. The nurse is advised to become familiar with the terms used in a particular agency before charting, writing, or interpreting reports. See Appendix A.

Problem-oriented charting necessarily raises issues of the legal limits of nursing practice. The issues are complex: The POR makes nurses in part responsible for diagnosis and therapy. Where does that responsibility begin and end? Nurses are advised to consult the legal definitions of nursing in their respective states and provinces. Nurses need to practice within the guidelines set by those definitions if their activities are to be legal.

Reporting

Reports can be either oral or written. The purpose of reporting, in general, is to communicate specific information to a person or group of people. A report should be concise. A good report includes pertinent information, but not extraneous detail.

These guidelines can help nurses prepare and present reports about patients:

1. Start with the patient's name so that the listeners or readers can immediately relate the subsequent information to the subject patient, for example, "Ms. Jessie Jones has a reddened area on her left hip," not "There is a reddened area on the left hip of Ms. Jessie Jones."

2. Report only pertinent information; do not include data irrelevant to patient care.

3. Provide exact information, such as "Ms. Jessie Jones received Demerol 100 mg intramuscularly at 2000 hours (8 P.M.)," not "Ms. Jessie Jones received some Demerol during the evening."

4. When reporting about a series of patients, follow a particular order; for example, by room number in a hospital or by time of appointment in a community clinic.

5. When reporting about one patient, present the pertinent information in this order: assessment, nursing diagnoses, planning, intervention, and evaluation. For example, "Mr. Ronald Oakes states he has an aching pain in his left calf. Inspection revealed no other signs. Calf pain is related to altered blood circulation. Rest and elevation of his legs on a footstool for 30 minutes provided relief."

Computerized Information Systems

In the past decade computers have become part of our daily lives. They have changed nurses' lives, too. Many North American hospitals now use computer systems. Computers speed the processing of orders for tests and treatments, return results to the nursing unit quickly, and free the nurse from transcriptions and paper work. It has been estimated that before hospitals had computerized systems head nurses spent 58% of their time, staff nurses 36% of their time, and nursing assistants 7% of their time processing patient data (Cook and McDowell 1975:49).

There are many types of computer systems and many variations in equipment. Some computers operate independently in one department alone. Others are integrated hospital information systems that channel information within and between departments. The integrated system coordinates the efforts of all departments so that an optimum level of patient care is achieved. See Figure 18–7 for a computerized laboratory data report.

Components of an Integrated System

The components of an integrated information system include:

1. A large main computer, which may be located outside of the hospital and used by several other agencies.

2. Terminal(s), an instrument with a video display screen and a keyboard similar to a typewriter's. Each nursing unit and other departments has one or more terminals. See Figure 18–8.

3. A printer, associated with the terminal, that can print on paper a copy of information appearing on the screen. See Figure 18–9.

Communicating with the Terminal

To use the terminal, the nurse first types a personal identification code on the keyboard or inserts an identification card into a slot. The computer checks that the nurse's code is legitimate, thereby safeguarding the system from unauthorized users. Once the nurse's code is verified, a list of transactions available is displayed on the screen. The screen displays three kinds of data.

1. Words or phrases to select in composing a message to put into the computer

2. Completed messages

3. Computer responses to the user's request for patient data or other information

To communicate with the terminal, the nurse makes a series of transactions known as *menus,* i.e., selects words needed to input a message or command. The nurse selects the words by touching the screen with a light pen or by pressing a button. The nurse types in words or phrases not offered as a choice on the screen. The completed message (command) then appears on the screen. If the message is correct, the nurse releases the message to the computer by pressing an "enter" key. In this way, medical and nursing orders (requisitions for service) are transmitted to the laboratory, pharmacy, radiology, central supply, and any other department connected to the system. In less than 1 minute, the computer processes the message by printing requisitions in the appropriate departments and duplicates in other departments concerned. For example, if the patient needs a special radiologic test before which certain medications and dietary adjustments are required, the computer prints a requisition for the test

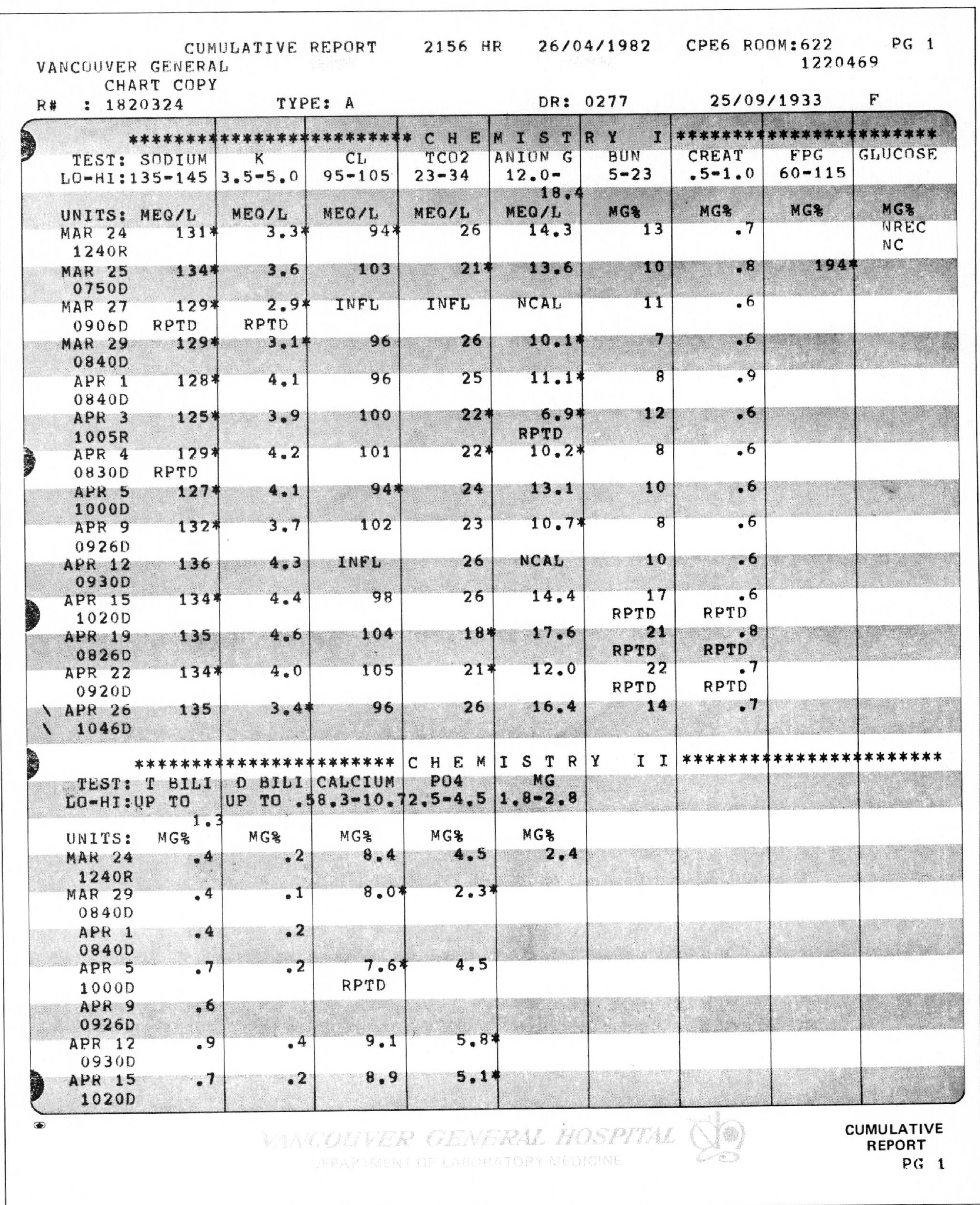

CUMULATIVE REPORT 2156 HR 26/04/1982 CPE6 ROOM:622 PG 1
VANCOUVER GENERAL 1220469
CHART COPY
R# : 1820324 TYPE: A DR: 0277 25/09/1933 F

****************************** C H E M I S T R Y I ******************************

TEST:	SODIUM	K	CL	TCO2	ANION G	BUN	CREAT	FPG	GLUCOSE
LO-HI:	135-145	3.5-5.0	95-105	23-34	12.0-18.4	5-23	.5-1.0	60-115	
UNITS:	MEQ/L	MEQ/L	MEQ/L	MEQ/L	MEQ/L	MG%	MG%	MG%	MG%
MAR 24 1240R	131*	3.3*	94*	26	14.3	13	.7		NREC NC
MAR 25 0750D	134*	3.6	103	21*	13.6	10	.8	194*	
MAR 27 0906D	129* RPTD	2.9* RPTD	INFL	INFL	NCAL	11	.6		
MAR 29 0840D	129*	3.1*	96	26	10.1*	7	.6		
APR 1 0840D	128*	4.1	96	25	11.1*	8	.9		
APR 3 1005R	125*	3.9	100	22*	6.9* RPTD	12	.6		
APR 4 0830D	129* RPTD	4.2	101	22*	10.2*	8	.6		
APR 5 1000D	127*	4.1	94*	24	13.1	10	.6		
APR 9 0926D	132*	3.7	102	23	10.7*	8	.6		
APR 12 0930D	136	4.3	INFL	26	NCAL	10	.6		
APR 15 1020D	134*	4.4	98	26	14.4	17 RPTD	.6 RPTD		
APR 19 0826D	135	4.6	104	18*	17.6	21 RPTD	.8 RPTD		
APR 22 0920D	134*	4.0	105	21*	12.0	22 RPTD	.7 RPTD		
\ APR 26 \ 1046D	135	3.4*	96	26	16.4	14	.7		

****************************** C H E M I S T R Y I I ******************************

TEST:	T BILI	D BILI	CALCIUM	PO4	MG
LO-HI:	UP TO 1.3	UP TO .5	8.3-10.7	2.5-4.5	1.8-2.8
UNITS:	MG%	MG%	MG%	MG%	MG%
MAR 24 1240R	.4	.2	8.4	4.5	2.4
MAR 29 0840D	.4	.1	8.0*	2.3*	
APR 1 0840D	.4	.2			
APR 5 1000D	.7	.2	7.6* RPTD	4.5	
APR 9 0926D	.6				
APR 12 0930D	.9	.4	9.1	5.8*	
APR 15 1020D	.7	.2	8.9	5.1*	

VANCOUVER GENERAL HOSPITAL
DEPARTMENT OF LABORATORY MEDICINE
CUMULATIVE REPORT
PG 1

Figure 18–7 A computerized cumulative laboratory data report. (Courtesy of Vancouver General Hospital, Vancouver, British Columbia.)

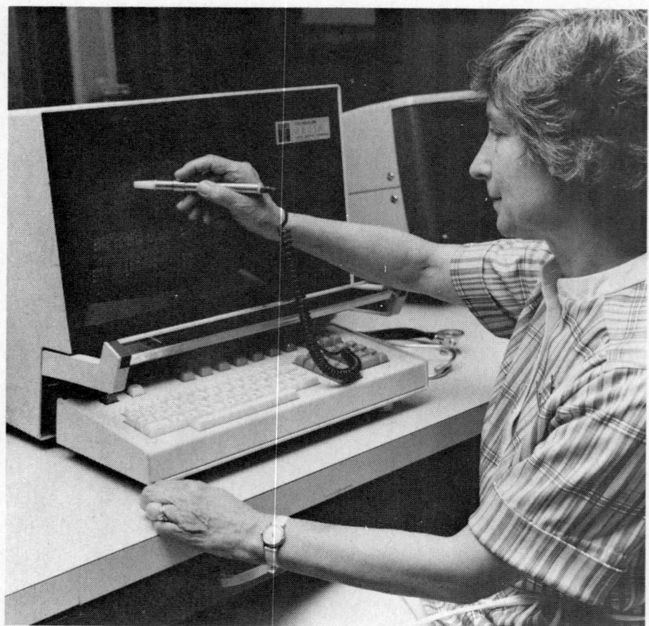

Figure 18–8 A computer terminal in a hospital nursing unit.

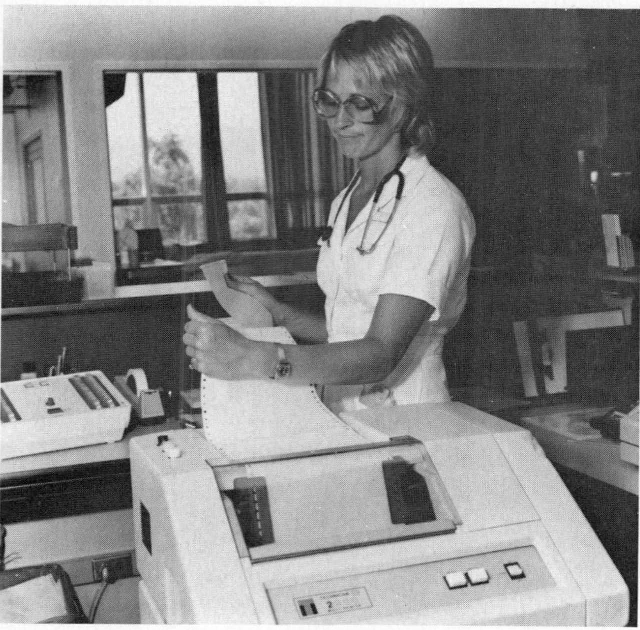

Figure 18–9 A computer printer in a nursing unit.

in the radiology department, a requisition for the medications in the pharmacy, a requisition in the dietary department, and a billing copy in the business office. In addition, this data is automatically added to various worksheets discussed subsequently.

Besides requisitioning services, the nurse can use the terminal and printer to generate worksheets necessary for planning and organizing patient care and to record data on the patient's permanent records. Examples of these worksheets are the nursing care plan, the laboratory specimen pick-up list, and the medication administration schedule. The medication schedule eliminates the need for medication cards. The computer also records data on the patient's permanent record. For example, after administering a medication the nurse calls up the medication list on the video display terminal and enters the name of the medication and the time and dosage given into the permanent record.

Implications of Information Systems

The computer age is here, and nurses will no doubt use automated information systems increasingly. Nurses often contribute to the programming and planning of such systems. Nurses have expressed these concerns about computerized systems (Johnson and Stegen, 1982:9):

1. How will the confidentiality of the data collected be maintained?
2. Will all personnel using the computer receive adequate training?
3. To what degree will health professionals and patients accept such a system?
4. Will computer code name or numbers be acceptable as a signature in a court of law?
5. Will computer information systems compromise the quality of patient care?
6. Will nurses continue to make independent judgments about nursing or will they take direction from the computer?

Summary

Health team members must communicate effectively to provide coordinated, high-quality care. When there is accurate communication, all health-team members are informed about patient needs, and overlapping of activities is avoided.

Written records serve several purposes. They ensure transmission of information to all health workers caring for a patient. Records are a source of research, educational, and statistical data. In addition, records allow the audit of patient care standards. Patient records are admissible as evidence in a court of law.

The POR (Weed system) is increasingly recognized as a method that provides a patient-centered problem-solving approach to care. All health disciplines cooperate in recording the patient's problems, therapy, and progress on integrated records. The POR has four basic components: a defined data base, a complete problem list, an initial plan for each identified problem, and progress notes. The defined data base incorporates initial assessments by the physician, nurse, and other health workers. The problem list includes both active and inactive physiologic, psychologic, and socioeconomic problems. Initial plans include a diagnostic workup, therapy, and patient education. Progress notes follow the systematic SOAP format and include narrative notes, flow sheets, and discharge notes.

Traditional patient records are source-oriented records in that each category of health worker keeps separate records. Traditional records generally have six parts: admission sheet, face sheet, doctor's order sheet, medical history sheet, nurses' notes, and other special records such as the laboratory record. The Kardex record is widely used for a quick access to current data about patients.

Record entries should be brief, accurate, legible, chronological, made on consecutive lines, and appropriately signed. Record entries are made after nursing interventions and usually when the patient is admitted or transferred. Because the record is a legal document, nurses sign their full legal names and use standard terms and abbreviations.

Reports about patients need to be concise and pertinent. Guidelines are included.

Computerized information systems are being used increasingly in health care agencies. They free nurses from transcriptions and paper work, but they give rise to concerns about confidentiality, quality of patient care, autonomy of nursing judgments, need for training, acceptance by the public and the profession, and legality. Nurses can make a significant contribution when these systems are planned and programmed.

Suggested Activities

1. Review a traditional patient record. Note the information it includes.
2. Review a problem-oriented record, and compare it with a traditional patient record. Compare specifics of content and recording method.
3. Establish a problem-oriented record for a member of your class who relates a specific health problem to you.
4. Select a patient. Use the SOAP format to fill out a progress record for a 5-day period.

Suggested Readings

Eggland, E. T. February 1980. Charting: How and why to document your care daily—and fully. *Nursing 80* 10:38–43.
Eggland explains the purposes of daily charting and the mechanics and ways to chart in specific instances, for example, when the patient refuses a treatment. Eggland also gives information about nurses' notes and errors and a list of do's and don'ts of daily charting.

Kerr, A. H. February 1975. Nurses' notes: "That's where the goodies are!" *Nursing 75* 5:34–41.
This article explains the importance of nurse's notes and provides charting guides for the nurse. The chart as a means to improve nursing care is explored in the article.

Lambert, K. 1974. Basic principles of the problem-oriented system. In *The problem-oriented system—a multidisciplinary approach.* 1974. Pub. no. 20–1546. New York: National League for Nursing.
The POR can be adapted to a variety of settings. Information is provided about the data base, problem list, initial plan, and progress notes (plan of action). Examples of the various records are provided.

Selected References

Abruzzese, R. S. 1974. The nursing process and the problem-oriented system. In *The problem-oriented system—a multidisciplinary approach.* 1974. Pub. no. 20–1546. New York: National League for Nursing.

Ansley, B. August 1975. Patient-oriented recording: A better system for ambulatory settings. *Nursing 75* 5:52–53.

Berni, R. and Readey, H. 1978. *Problem-oriented medical record implementation allied health peer review.* 2nd ed. St. Louis: C. V. Mosby Co.

Bloom, J. T., et al. November 1971. Problem-oriented charting. *American Journal of Nursing* 71:2144–48.

Cook, M., and McDowell, W. January 1975. Changing to an automated information system. *American Journal of Nursing* 75:46–51.

Creighton, H. 1981. *Law every nurse should know.* 4th ed. Philadelphia: W. B. Saunders Co.

Johnson, I., and Stegen, A. January-February 1982. Will the computer be the new "nurses" aid? *Registered Nurses Association of British Columbia News* 14:8–9.

Larkin, P. D., and Backer, B. A. 1977. *Problem-oriented nursing assessment.* New York: McGraw-Hill Book Co.

Schell, P. L., and Campbell, A. T. August 1972. POMR—not just another way to chart. *Nursing Outlook* 20:510–14.

Schmidt, A. March–April 1981. Predicting nurses' charting behavior, based on Fishbein's model. *Nursing Research* 30:118–23.

Sklar, C. February 1981. You and the law: When nurses fail to communicate. *The Canadian Nurse* 77:47–48.

Ulisse, G. C. 1978. *POMR application to nursing records.* Menlo Park, Calif.: Addison-Wesley Publishing Co.

Vaughan-Wrobel, B. C., and Henderson, B. 1976. *The problem-oriented system in nursing: A workbook.* St. Louis: C. V. Mosby Company.

Weed, L. L. 1971. *Medical records, medical education and patient care: The problem-oriented record as a basic tool.* Cleveland: Case Western Reserve University Press.

Woody, M., and Mallison, M. July 1973. The problem-oriented system for patient-centered care. *American Journal of Nursing* 73:1168–75.

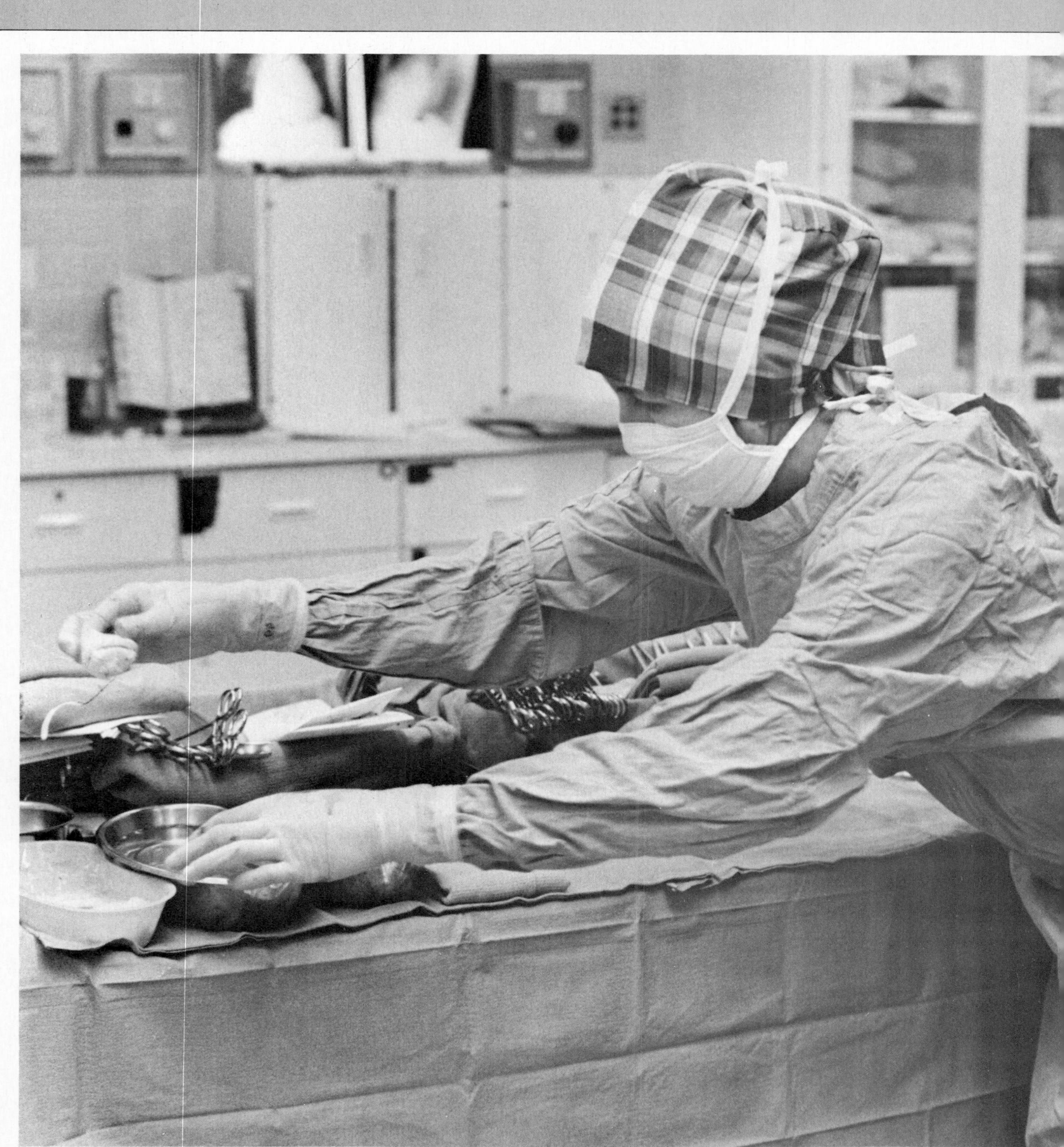

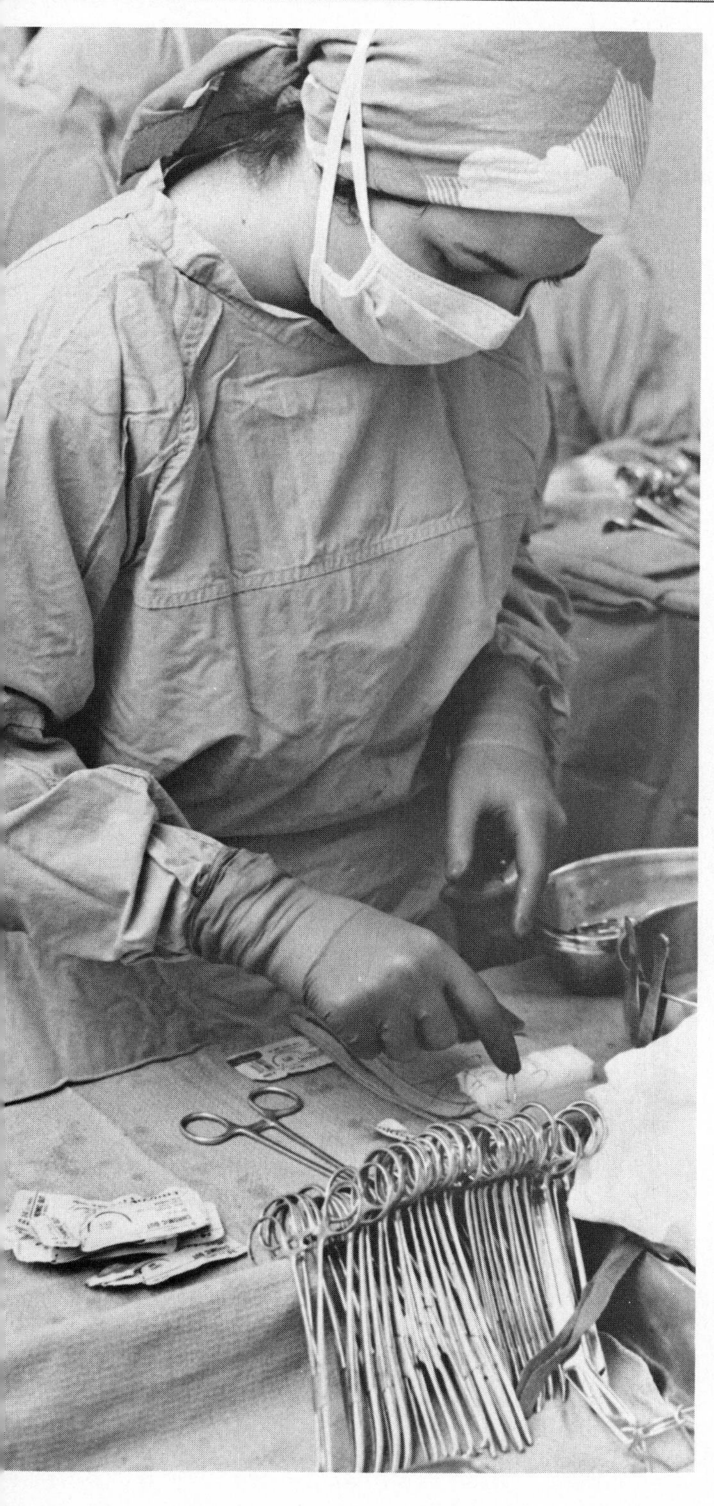

Unit V

Protective Measures Related to Nursing Practice

CONTENTS

Chapter 19

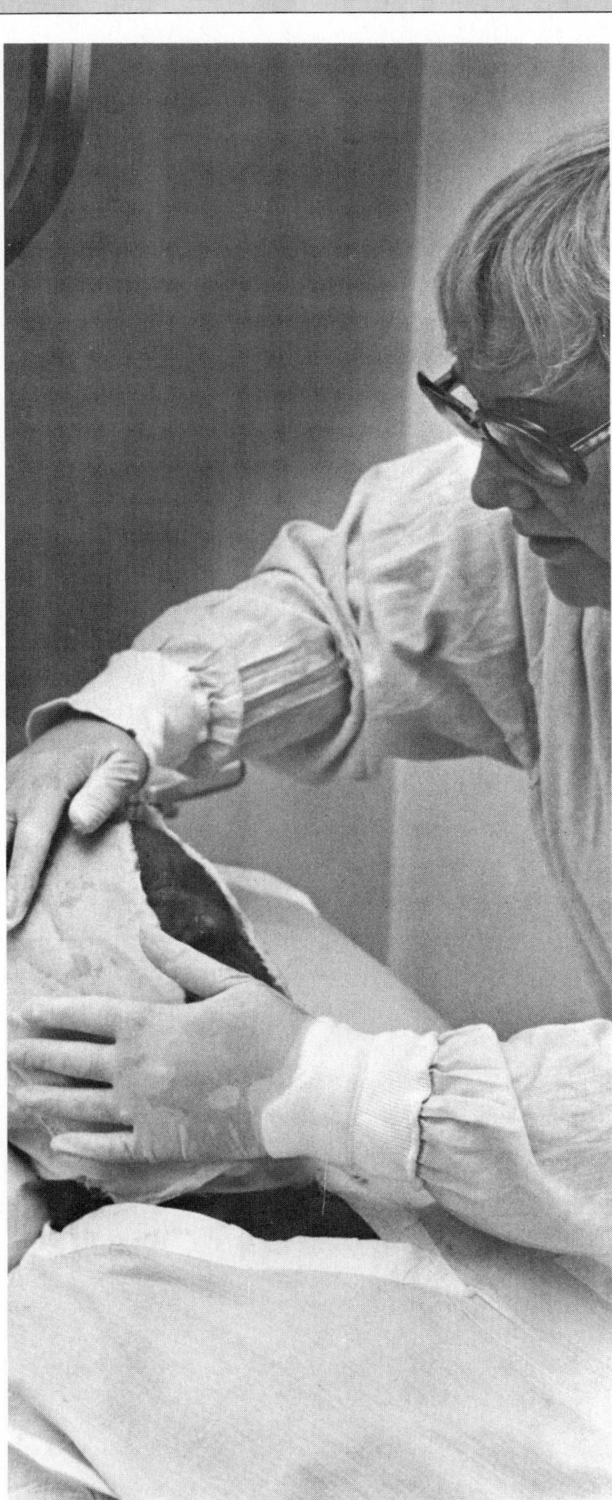

Medical Asepsis: Infection Control

CONTENTS

Objectives

1. Know essential terms and facts about infections
   - **1.1** Define selected terms
   - **1.2** Identify six groups of microorganisms that can cause an infection
   - **1.3** Identify causes of nosocomial infections
   - **1.4** Identify six components of the chain of infection
   - **1.5** List factors influencing a microorganism's capability of producing disease
   - **1.6** Describe environmental conditions favorable to the growth of microorganisms
   - **1.7** Identify exit methods of microorganisms from six parts of the body
   - **1.8** Identify vehicles that transmit microorganisms to people
   - **1.9** Identify body barriers to the entrance of microorganisms
   - **1.10** Identify three stages of infection
2. Know essential data required by the nurse to assess a patient's susceptibility to an infection or to assess a patient with an infection
   - **2.1** Identify factors affecting a person's susceptibility to an infection
   - **2.2** Identify signs of localized infection
   - **2.3** Identify signs of systemic infection
3. Know nursing interventions that prevent infections
   - **3.1** Identify measures to strengthen the body's barriers against infection
   - **3.2** Identify measures to minimize the number of microorganisms present (i.e., personal hygiene)
   - **3.3** Identify essentials of hand washing
   - **3.4** Identify essential steps in cleaning articles soiled with organic material
   - **3.5** Identify appropriate methods to disinfect and sterilize selected objects
4. Understand essential facts about protective aseptic techniques
   - **4.1** Identify five types of protective asepsis
   - **4.2** Identify precautions taken in each type of protective asepsis
   - **4.3** Identify psychological problems associated with protective asepsis
   - **4.4** Identify essential steps of protective aseptic techniques
   - **4.5** Give reasons for selected steps of protective aseptic techniques
5. Perform protective aseptic techniques safely so that patients, self, and others are protected
   - **5.1** Wash hands appropriately
   - **5.2** Initiate protective aseptic precautions
   - **5.3** Don and remove face masks appropriately
   - **5.4** Don and remove gowns appropriately
   - **5.5** Don and remove gloves appropriately
   - **5.6** Carry out double-bagging effectively
   - **5.7** Handle used equipment effectively
   - **5.8** Dispose of refuse appropriately
   - **5.9** Assess patients' vital signs safely
   - **5.10** Administer medications to the patient safely
   - **5.11** Collect specimens effectively
   - **5.12** Transport patients safely
   - **5.13** Handle patients' money, letters, and documents appropriately

Terms

aerobe
anaerobe
antibiotic
antiseptic
asepsis
autogenous
carrier
clean
communicable disease
contaminate
culture
disinfection
etiology
fomite
iatrogenic
incubation period
infection
medical asepsis
microorganism
nosocomial
parasite
pasteurization
pathogen
phagocyte
portal
prodromal stage
protective asepsis
reservoir
sensitivity
spore
sterilization
surgical asepsis
trauma
vector
vehicle
virulence

Microorganisms (organisms of microscopic size) are everywhere in the environment: on the skin, in the intestinal tract, in the air, in the soil, and on clothes. Most of these microorganisms do not produce disease; those that do are called *pathogens.*

An *infection* is the invasion and physiological response of the body to pathogenic organisms that multiply and overcome the flora normally present. If the infection can be passed on readily to others—for example, anthrax or typhoid fever—it is referred to as a *communicable disease* or *infectious disease.*

Trauma is injury to the body. Trauma can be physical, such as a cut by a piece of glass; trauma also describes injury caused by invading microorganisms. Thus, an infectious process can be described as trauma. Often physical trauma is accompanied by the trauma of infection, as when a cut becomes infected.

Etiology is the study of causes; the etiology of infectious disease is the identification of the invading microorganisms. Control of the spread of pathogens and protection of people from infectious diseases and infections are practiced on four levels: international, national, community, and individual.

An example of infectious disease control at the international level is the protection people must have against certain diseases before they can visit certain countries. Similarly, there are health regulations about the reentry into the country of American and Canadian citizens traveling abroad.

National regulations govern, for example, the interstate and interprovincial transportation of food. These regulations protect people from receiving contaminated food. There are also regulations regarding pollution of water, air, and the environment as a whole, subjects currently receiving a great deal of publicity.

On a community level, there are regulations regarding the disposal of sewage and the purity of drinking water, for example. These regulations are designed to protect people from infectious disease.

Protection from infection is also very much an individual responsibility. Individuals protect themselves not only by hygienic practices, such as oral hygiene as a preventive measure against periodontal disease (see Chapter 21, which discusses personal hygiene), but also by assuming individual responsibility for sound diet and proper exercise.

This chapter is concerned mainly with the nursing implications of caring for patients with infections. See Chapter 22 for information about communicable diseases and their prevention.

Asepsis

Asepsis refers to the absence of all disease-producing microorganisms. Asepsis is largely a relative term in that the complete absence of all pathogenic microorganisms is difficult to sustain for prolonged periods. When hands are washed with a disinfectant, they can be considered aseptic; that is, pathogenic organisms have been removed or destroyed. However, some nonpathogenic microorganisms in all probability are still present on washed hands. *Sterilization* is the absence of *all* forms of microorganisms, including bacteria, viruses, spores, and fungi. Unlike human skin, such objects as forceps can be sterilized—freed of all microorganisms.

There are two types of asepsis: medical and surgical. *Medical asepsis*, or *clean technique*, is those practices that limit the number of microorganisms and their growth and spread. Medical asepsis includes all practices intended to confine a specific microorganism to a specific area. Aseptic measures are protective measures in that they are meant to prevent infections or the spread of infections.

Surgical asepsis, or *sterile technique*, is intended to keep all microorganisms from a specific area; surgical asepsis includes practices that destroy all microorganisms and their spores. (A *spore* is a round or oval structure, with a tough resistant capsule, assumed by some microorganisms; this structure is formed in response to adverse conditions and is highly resistant to destruction.) An example of surgical aseptic practice is the technique used to clean and dress a surgical wound to prevent microorganisms from entering the patient's body through the incision.

Infections

Infections occur when pathogenic organisms of sufficient numbers and virulence invade a susceptible host. A susceptible person is one with certain characteristics that make him or her more likely than most to contract an infection. See the section on assessing susceptibility later in this chapter.

Microorganisms vary in their abilities to produce disease; that is, in their *virulence*. In the environment there are normally five groups of microorganisms that can cause disease: bacteria, viruses, fungi, protozoa, and rickettsiae. Microorganisms also vary in the severity of the diseases they produce and their degree of communicability. For example, the common cold virus is more readily transmitted than the bacillus (*Mycobacterium leprae*) that causes leprosy.

Nosocomial infections are those infections contracted in hospitals. These infections have received increasing attention in recent years. They are considered more difficult to prevent and treat, more unpredictable, and more resistant to cure than infections contracted in the community (Norton 1981:813). Nosocomial infections occur in about 5% of all persons admitted to hospitals and in about 8% of persons in long-term care facilities (Norton 1981:815). Table 19–1 outlines common types and sources of infections in hospitals. There are several causes of nosocomial infections:

1. Diagnostic or therapeutic procedures. The infection is *iatrogenic*—caused by the physician.
2. The presence in hospitals of resistant strains of such microorganisms as *Serratia marcescens*, which causes urinary tract, respiratory, and wound infections (Bond 1981:2184). These organisms have become highly resistant to antibiotics ordinarily used.
3. The use of antibiotics. Antibiotics destroy many of the microorganisms normally present in the intestine, thus enabling resistant strains to take hold. Normal intestinal flora play a significant role in competitively excluding pathogens, thus preventing disease.
4. Changes in the diet and activity of patients because they are hospitalized. These changes alter the normal flora of the body and facilitate the establishment of more resistant hospital strains.

Table 19–1 Common Sources of Infection in Hospitals

Microorganism	Source	Mode of transmission*	Infection or disease
Bacteria			
Staphylococcus aureus	Nares, skin, hair	Contact, vehicles, airborne, autogenous	Infected wounds, pneumonia, abscesses, cellulitis, food poisoning
Streptococcus, beta-hemolytic Group D	Colon, vagina of adult females	Contact, vehicles, autogenous	Urinary tract and wound infections
Streptococcus viridans	Naso-oro-pharynx	Autogenous	Bacterial endocarditis
Toxigenic *Escherichia coli*	Colon	Contact, vehicles	Enteritis
Bacteroides species	Colon	Contact, autogenous	Peritonitis, abscesses
Serratia species	Colon, perineum	Direct, airborne	Pneumonia, bacteremia, urinary tract and wound infections
Fungi and Yeasts			
Candida albicans	Mouth, colon, genital tract, skin	Contact, vehicles, autogenous	Moniliasis, dermatitis
Viruses			
Herpes viruses	Lesions of the mucous membrane, skin, blood	Contact, vehicles	Sexually transmitted disease, cold sores
Hepatitis A	Feces, blood, urine	Contact, vehicles	Infectious hepatitis
Hepatitis B	Feces, blood, body excretions and fluids	Contact, vehicles, airborne, possibly vectors	Serum hepatitis

*Modes of Transmission

Contact — direct contact involves close proximity of people, i.e., direct touch, by hands or body or through droplet spray from the mouth and nose.
— indirect contact involves contact with personal articles of an infected individual such as tissues or dentures. It also includes contact with pathogens on articles such as bed linen.

Vehicles — this route of transmission is through food, water, medications, or blood from infected persons.

Airborne — includes droplets from the respiratory tracts of infected persons or carriers, contaminated dust and microorganisms shed into the environment from hair, skin, wounds or perineal area.

Vectors — includes contaminated or infected mosquitos, fleas, ticks, flies, etc.

Autogenous — infection from the patient's usual microbial flora.

Adapted from C. O. Hargiss and E. Larson, How to collect specimens and evaluate results and Guidelines for prevention of hospital acquired infections, *American Journal of Nursing*, December 1981, 81:2166–83 and from G. B. Bond, *Serratia*: An endemic hospital resident, *American Journal of Nursing*, December 1981, 81:2183–86.

Chain of Infection

Six factors or elements are involved in the infectious process:

1. Etiologic agent, or pathogen
2. Source of the pathogen, or *reservoir*
3. Method of escape of the pathogen from the source, or exit
4. Method of transmission
5. Method of entry, or *portal*
6. Susceptibility of the person (host) to the pathogen

Etiologic Agent

Microorganisms and parasites are the sources of infection. A *parasite* is an animal or plant that lives in or on another and obtains its nourishment from it. Some microorganisms, such as the gonococcus bacillus, are parasites. The extent to which any microorganism or parasite is capable of producing a disease depends on these factors:

1. Number of organisms
2. Virulence and potency of the organisms
3. Source of the organisms
4. Their ability to enter the body
5. Their ability to establish themselves within the body

Body discharges may contain pathogens. To test a discharge for pathogens, the nurse obtains a specimen and sends it to the laboratory, where the pathogen is cultured and tested for sensitivity to certain medications. The laboratory technologist places some of the specimen in a test tube or Petri dish containing a medium conducive to the growth of the pathogen. After a certain time, which varies with the incubation period of the pathogen, the technologist observes the pathogen under the microscope and identifies it. The technologist may then test the pathogen's sensitivity to certain medications, for instance, by placing discs impregnated with antibiotics on culture plates with microorganisms. The technologist gauges the effectiveness of each antibiotic by the size of the ring—a circle of killed microorganisms—around each disc.

Laboratory technologists usually culture microorganisms and test their sensitivity to medications, but nurses generally obtain specimens. For further information on obtaining specimens, see Kozier and Erb (1982:543–97).

Some microorganisms, such as the smallpox virus, have the ability to infect almost anyone on first contact. By contrast, microorganisms such as the tuberculosis bacillus attack a relatively small number of the population, often people who are poorly nourished and living in unsanitary conditions. Some animals and humans are *carriers*, that is, they carry pathogenic organisms in their bodies although they are not ill themselves. They can pass the pathogen along to other people. For example, some persons harbor the typhoid bacillus in the gallbladder, excrete it in feces, but do not manifest any symptoms of the disease themselves.

Sources and Source Characteristics

There are many sources or reservoirs of pathogens. They may be other humans, the patient's own normal microbial (*autogenous*) flora, plants, animals, or the general environment. Quite commonly people serve as the source of infection for others. The person with, for example, an influenza virus frequently spreads this infection to others. Sometimes people carry a pathogen, yet are not ill. Only when resistance is lowered by fatigue and other factors does an infection emerge.

Insects, birds, and other animals are common sources of infection. The *Anopheles* mosquito is the source of the malaria parasite. Food, water, milk, and feces also can be reservoirs of pathogens, for example, contaminated chicken at a club luncheon.

The reservoir of the pathogen must have certain characteristics for the organisms to live and grow. Some of these follow:

Food

All living microorganisms require nourishment. Some require organic matter, whereas others use carbon dioxide and simple inorganic compounds as foods.

Water

Most living organisms require water, although their needs vary widely. For example, certain bacteria in the spore form can live without water for years.

Oxygen

Some microorganisms (*obligate aerobes*) require oxygen, for example, *Staphylococcus aureus*. Others, such as the tetanus bacillus (*Clostridium tetani*), cannot live in the presence of oxygen. These are referred to as *obligate anaerobes*. *Obligate* means "obliged."

Temperature

Organisms thrive in environments within certain temperature ranges and are killed if the temperature rises above or falls below the boundaries of that range. Temperature is an important factor during asepsis.

pH

Microorganisms are sensitive to changes in pH. Most grow best in an environment between pH 5 and 8.

Light

Microorganisms are either inhibited or killed by ultraviolet rays. Sunlight is the best source for ultraviolet light.

Antibiosis

An *antibiotic* is a chemical agent produced by one microbe and able to inhibit or kill other microbes. Antibiotics are used frequently to combat infections; for example, penicillin is used to treat syphilis.

Exit from the Source

Before an infection can establish itself, the pathogen must leave the reservoir (the source) and enter the host. If the reservoir is within a human, the pathogen has a number of exits, depending on the pathogen and the exact site of the reservoir.

Respiratory tract

The respiratory tract is one of the most common exit routes for pathogens. While a person sneezes, coughs, breathes, and talks, pathogens can leave the tract through the nose and the mouth.

Gastrointestinal tract

The gastrointestinal tract is another site of exit. Pathogens can be expelled in feces; through drainage, such as gallbladder drainage; and even in vomitus. One example is the typhoid bacillus, which in some patients is carried in the gallbladder and/or the large intestine and expelled in the feces.

Urinary tract

The urinary tract (the kidneys, the bladder, and the urethra) can be a reservoir of pathogens that exit in the urine.

Reproductive tract

Pathogens in the reproductive tract of women exit by the vagina. In men, they exit through the urinary meatus. Thus, pathogens of the reproductive tract may exit in the urine of males, while in females they exit in vaginal discharges.

Blood

Circulating blood may be a reservoir of pathogens, such as the virus of B or non-H, non-B hepatitis. Any escape of blood from the circulatory system provides an exit for such pathogens.

Tissues

The tissues of the body also can be a reservoir for pathogens, and thus any opening into the tissues can serve as the exit. For example, wounds can become infected and produce drainage that contains a high concentration of pathogens.

Method of Transmission

Once a pathogen has escaped its reservoir, it must have a means of transmission to another person or host. Various methods of transmission carry organisms to a host. Some of these are (a) direct contact, (b) air, (c) fomites, (d) food and water, and (e) insects and other animals.

Direct contact

Direct contact with an infected person permits the transfer of a pathogen to a second person. For example, kissing, sexual intercourse, or touching provide the opportunity for pathogens to transfer.

Air

The air can readily serve as a vehicle for some pathogens. Sneezing, for example, sprays pathogens into the air, where they can be inhaled by others. Pathogens can attach themselves to dust particles in the air and be carried quickly to other people even over some distance.

Fomites

A *fomite* is an object other than food that can harbor microorganisms. For example, organisms can be transferred on dishes, silverware, forceps, and dressings. Disposable equipment in hospitals and modern methods of disinfection have reduced this mode of transmission considerably in recent years.

Food and water

Food and water are also vehicles for pathogens. Cities in the United States and Canada have laws that protect the public from contaminated food and water. However, in remote areas of the country contaminated water can still serve as a vehicle. An example is the virus of infectious hepatitis, which may be transmitted through water.

Insects and other animals

Insects and other animals can spread such pathogens as the *Salmonella* bacillus, which is naturally present in domestic animals but causes gastroenteritis in humans. Flies carry microorganisms also; thus they contaminate food and fluids with which they come in contact. A fly, for example, may pick up pathogens from the feces of soiled diapers, and then transmit them to various exposed foods. A *vector* is an animal that transfers pathogens from a reservoir to a host.

Portal of Entry

Before a person can become infected, a pathogen must enter the body. The skin serves as a barrier to infections; however, any break in the skin can readily serve as a portal of entry. Microorganisms can enter the body through the same routes they use to leave the body. See the section on exits from the source.

Course of an Infection

The course of an infection can be divided into three stages: the incubation period, the period of illness, and the convalescent period.

Incubation Period

The *incubation period* is the time between the entry of the pathogen into the body and the onset of the symptoms of the infection. During this time the organism adapts to the person and multiplies sufficiently to produce disease. The length of incubation varies greatly, depending on the pathogen. For example, rubella (measles) develops in 10 to 14 days, whereas tetanus (lockjaw) takes from 4 to 21 days to develop.

Period of Illness

The period of illness can be divided into two stages: the prodromal stage and the full illness stage. During the *prodromal stage* the patients manifest some early signs of illness. The signs are usually nonspecific: Patients may have fever, feel tired and irritable, and may complain of malaise. It is during this stage that persons are most infectious and most likely to spread the disease. A prodromal stage usually lasts a short time, hours or days at the most. Following this is the full illness stage, in which more specific signs and symptoms develop. The severity of the symptoms and the length of the illness vary with the pathogen and the host.

Convalescent Period

During the convalescent period, the symptoms disappear and there is a return to health. Depending on the severity of the illness and the patient's general condition, the length of convalescence can vary from a few days to months.

Nursing Assessment

Nursing assessment related to the prevention of infections and care of patients who have infections includes assessment of the individual's susceptibility and of the clinical signs of an infectious process.

Susceptibility

Whether an organism causes an infection depends on a number of factors already mentioned. One of the most important factors is susceptibility, which is affected by (a) stress, (b) nutritional status, (c) fatigue, (d) sex, (e) heredity, (f) age, (g) medical treatment and health habits.

Stress

Stress can influence susceptibility to infection. The person exposed to stressors for a long period of time may have little energy left for coping with infection. For example, a person recovering from a major operation is more likely to develop an infection than a healthy person who has not had surgery.

Nutritional status

The nutritional status directly affects the health of body tissues and hence susceptibility to infection. Unhealthy tissues are more likely to become infected and are slower to heal. Protein is an essential element in the growth of tissues. Some infections, such as tuberculosis, are found frequently among poorly nourished people.

Fatigue

Fatigue also affects susceptibility to disease. A tired person's coping mechanisms are less effective; such a person has lower than normal resistance to stressors. A common example is the overworked, overtired person who becomes vulnerable to the cold virus.

Sex

Sex affects susceptibility to some infections. For example, pneumonia occurs more frequently in men, whereas scarlet fever is more often seen in women.

Heredity

Some people have a genetic susceptibility to certain infections. For example, some people may be deficient in immunoglobulins, which play a significant role in the internal defense mechanism of the body.

Age

Age is also a major factor in susceptibility to infections. A neonate receives from the mother antibodies that provide protection for the first 2 or 3 months. These gradually provide decreasing protection. Infections are one of the major causes of death of newborn children. Growing children normally develop their own immunoglobulins. A young child readily acquires colds, common infectious diseases, and intestinal infections. An only child may experience these chiefly upon entering nursery school, while a child with older brothers and sisters acquires these infections earlier. In adults, viral diseases are a common reason for intermittent illness. The immune responses become weaker with age, so that the elderly person, like the young child, acquires infections more readily.

Medical treatment

Some forms of medical treatment, because of their effects, can predispose a person to infection. For example, radiation treatments destroy tissue, thereby rendering it more vulnerable to infections. Treatment for leukemia lowers the white blood cell count and thus lowers resistance.

Health habits

Good health habits—bathing, oral hygiene, hand washing, hair and nail care, and washing after urination and defecation—lower an individual's susceptibility to infection. Poor health habits mean increased numbers of microorganisms on the body. If injury or illness occurs, these microorganisms are present to infect the body. In addition, people with poor health habits can transmit microorganisms to others, for example, when giving nursing care or when handling food.

Clinical Signs

An infection can be localized or systemic. A *localized infection* is limited to a particular body part or area, e.g., a finger, whereas a *systemic infection* affects the entire body.

Clinical signs of a localized infection are:

1. Swelling
2. Redness
3. Pain or tenderness
4. Heat at the infected area
5. Loss of function of the body part affected

For additional information regarding localized responses and description of exudate see the section on inflammatory adaptive responses in Chapter 9, page 187, and the description of a clean healing wound in Chapter 40, page 1031.

Clinical signs of a systemic infection are:

1. Fever (a symptom associated with most infections)
2. Lassitude, malaise
3. Anorexia, nausea
4. Headache
5. Lymph node enlargement and tenderness
6. Vomiting and diarrhea

For additional information about inflammation see the section on the general adaptation syndrome in Chapter 9, page 184.

Nursing Intervention: Preventing Infections

The nurse's responsibilities for preventing infections include:

1. Teaching individuals measures to prevent infection, including
   a. Measures that strengthen the body's barriers against infection
   b. Measures that encourage personal hygiene
2. Hand washing
3. Ensuring appropriate cleaning, disinfection, and sterilization of contaminated objects

Teaching Individuals Preventive Measures

Strengthening the body's barriers against infection

A number of measures can be taken to strengthen the body's infection barriers:

1. *Immunization.* The immunologic system is the body's major defense against infections. The body gradually builds up natural defenses against pathogens with which it comes in contact; immunizations give additional protection. See the section on immunizations in Chapter 22, page 547.
2. *Nutrition.* A balanced diet enhances the health of all body tissues. Proper diet helps keep the skin intact and able to repel microorganisms. Adequate nutrition also enables tissues to maintain and rebuild themselves. Proper nourishment helps keep the reticuloendothelial system functioning well. This is the system of connective tissue cells (phagocytes) that combat and prevent infections by ingesting microorganisms, other cells, or foreign matter. There are three types of phagocytes: reticuloendothelial cells, which line the liver, spleen, and bone marrow; macrophages, which wander in the tissues; and microglia, which are located in the central nervous system.
3. *Adequate rest and sleep.* Rest and sleep are essential to health and to one's ability to perform usual activities. See Chapter 25 for additional information.
4. *Normal stress level.* Elevated stress predisposes a person to infection. A balance, for example, between work and recreation is important. See the section on psychologic homeostasis in Chapter 8, page 168.

Encouraging hygiene

Personal hygiene, if practiced in daily living, minimizes the number of microorganisms present and decreases the likelihood of acquiring an infection.

1. *Hand washing.* Washing one's hands after urination and defecation prevents the transfer of microorganisms to other objects and food. Hand washing before handling food also prevents contamination of the food and subsequent ingestion of the organisms by others. See the section on hand washing immediately following.
2. *Perineal care.* Females should clean the rectum and perineum after elimination by wiping from the area of least contamination (the urinary meatus) to the area of greatest contamination (the anus). This method of wiping helps to prevent genitourinary infections. See the section on perineal and genital care in Chapter 21, page 503.
3. *Regular bathing.* Bathing removes microorganisms from the skin surface and helps prevent infections. See Chapter 21, page 491.
4. *Brushing teeth regularly.* See the section on oral hygiene in Chapter 21, page 509.
5. *Blowing the nose.* Blowing the nose and sneezing clear microorganisms from the upper respiratory tract. They also help remove organisms and dust caught in the cilia (tiny hairlike processes inside the nose). Children need to be taught not to pick their noses. This practice contaminates the hands and may damage the mucous membrane that lines the nose.
6. *Coughing.* Coughing helps remove organisms and dust from the lower portions of the respiratory tract. When coughing, one should cover the mouth with a tissue, to avoid spraying organisms into the air, where they can infect others.
7. *Nail care.* Carefully cutting the nails and not the side tissue maintains the integrity of the nail-skin barrier and so prevents the entry of organisms. The tissue around nails may also need regular lubrication with oil to prevent drying and cracking.

Hand Washing

Hand washing is important wherever people are ill, including hospitals. It is considered one of the most effective infection control measures. The goal of hand washing is to remove microorganisms that might be transmitted to patients, visitors, or other health personnel.

Nurses wash their hands:

1. Before and after contact with a patient
2. After contact with any contaminated equipment, such as a bedpan
3. At the start and end of delivering nursing care

4. Before leaving for coffee or a meal
5. Before charting or preparing medications
6. Before handling any sterile equipment, such as a syringe (see Chapter 20)

Patients wash their hands:

1. Before eating
2. After using the bedpan or toilet
3. After the hands have come in contact with any known infected material, such as sputum or drainage from a wound

Health personnel wash their hands:

1. Before and after contact with a patient
2. After contact with equipment or supplies used by a patient
3. Before charting
4. Before handling sterile supplies, such as intravenous equipment (see Chapter 20)

Visitors wash their hands:

1. After contact with a patient who has an infection
2. After contact with any contaminated equipment or supplies
3. Before handling food

The recommended duration of hand washing for nurses is as follows:

1. Two minutes at the start and end of nursing duty
2. One minute after contact with contaminated equipment, before leaving for coffee or a meal, and before charting or preparing medications
3. Thirty seconds between patients
4. Three minutes before handling sterile equipment

Procedure 19–1 Hand Washing

Equipment

1. Soap. Most hospitals supply soaps that contain a germicide. Liquid soaps are frequently supplied in dispensers at the sink.
2. Running water. It is best to use warm water. Very hot water opens the pores in the skin and allows the soap to irritate the skin more readily.
3. Towels. Nurses usually dry their hands with paper towels; they discard the towels in the appropriate container immediately after use.

Intervention

1. File the nails short.

   Rationale Short nails are less likely to harbor microorganisms and scratch a patient.

2. Remove jewelry, except a plain wedding band, from the hands and arms. Some nurses slide their watches up above their elbows. Others pin the watch to the uniform so that it can still be used.

   Rationale Microorganisms can lodge in the settings of jewelry. Proper cleaning of the hands and arms is facilitated.

3. Check hands for breaks in the skin, such as hangnails or cuts. Report cuts to the instructor or responsible nurse before beginning work, or check agency policy about such cuts. Use lotions to prevent hangnails and cracked, dry skin. A nurse who has open sores may have to change work assignments or wear gloves to avoid contact with highly infectious materials.

4. Stand in front of the sink. Do not lean on the sink or splash water on your uniform. Flex your knees slightly if the sink is low.

   Rationale Microorganisms thrive in moisture. Dampness can contribute to contamination of the uniform.

5. Turn on the water. There are four types of faucet controls:

   a. Hand-operated handles. Use paper towels when turning these. See Figure 19–1.

   Rationale Towels protect the hands from possible contamination.

   b. Knee levers. Move these with the knee to regulate flow and temperature. See Figure 19–2.

   c. Foot pedals. Press these with the foot to regulate flow and temperature. See Figure 19–3.

   d. Elbow controls. Move these with the elbows, instead of the hands. This type of handle is most frequently used for surgical asepsis. See Chapter 20.

Procedure 19–1, continued

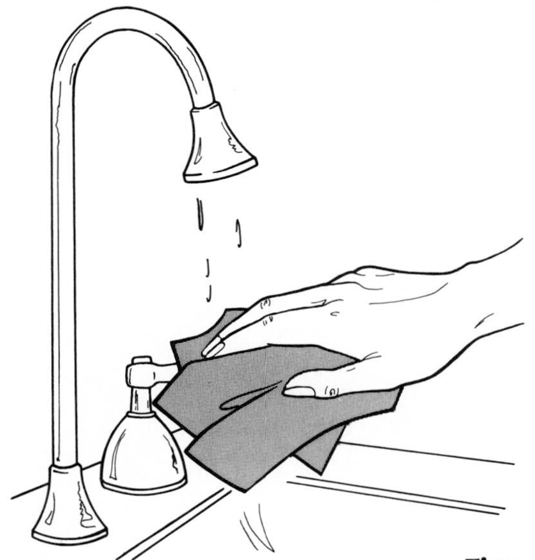

Figure 19–1

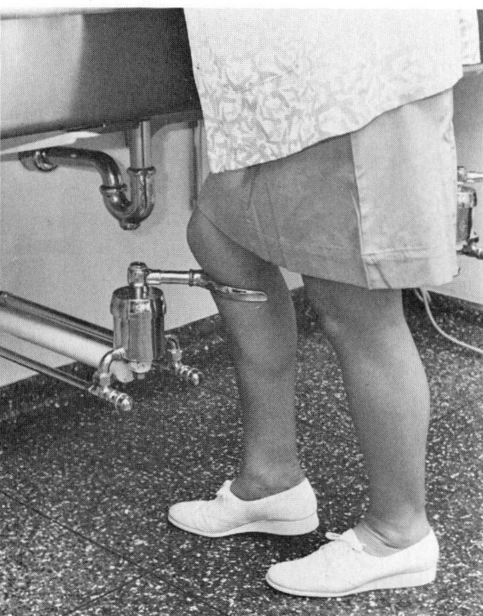

Figure 19–2

6. Adjust the flow so that the water is warm.

   Rationale Warm water is not as irritating as hot water, which opens the pores. Open pores are more easily irritated by soap. Warm water removes less of the protective oil of the skin.

7. Wet the hands and lower arms thoroughly by holding them under the running water. Hold the hands lower than the elbows so that the water flows from the arms to the fingertips.

   Rationale The water should flow from the least contaminated to the most contaminated area, and the hands are more contaminated than the lower arm.

8. Apply soap to the hands. If the soap is liquid, apply 2 to 4 ml (1 tsp). If it is bar soap, rub it firmly between the hands and rinse the bar before returning it to the dish.

   Rationale Rinsing the bar removes microorganisms.

9. Use firm, rubbing, circular movements to wash the palm, back, and wrist of each hand. Interlace the fingers and thumbs and move the hands back and forth. See Figure 19–4. Continue this motion for 10 to 15 seconds.

   Rationale The circular action helps aids remove microorganisms. Interlacing the fingers and thumbs cleans the interdigital spaces.

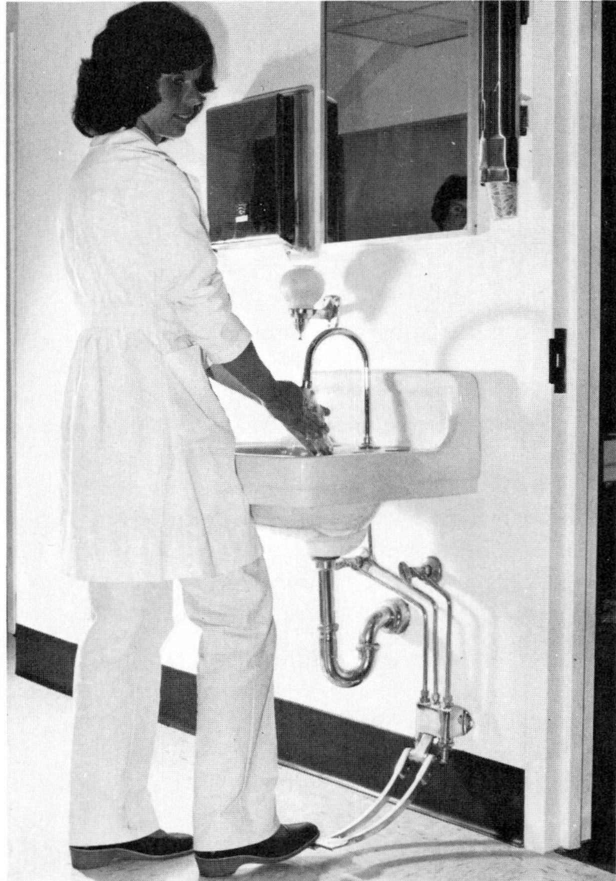

Figure 19–3

Procedure 19–1, continued

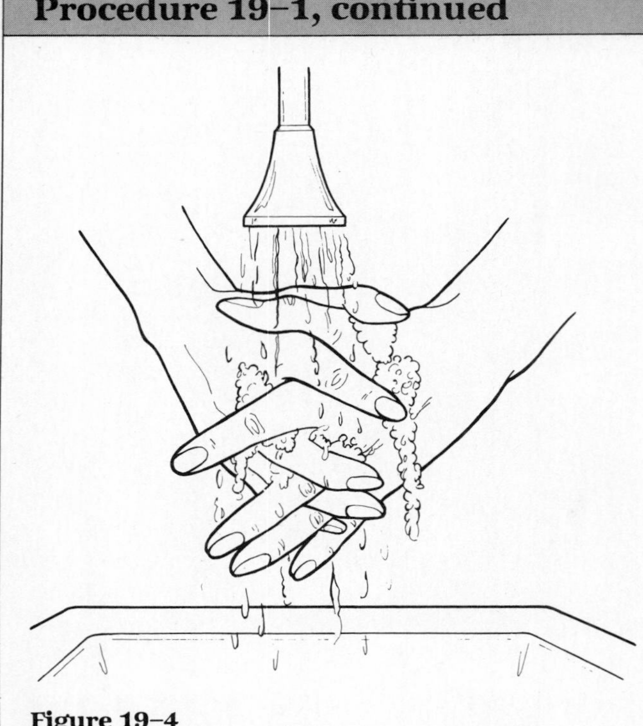

Figure 19–4

10. For a 1-minute hand wash, repeat steps 7 through 9. For 2- and 3-minute hand washes, repeat steps 7 through 9 but extend the washing time. See the durations recommended on page 452.
11. Dry the hands thoroughly with the towel. Discard the paper towel in the appropriate container.

    Rationale Moist skin becomes chapped readily; chapping produces lesions.
12. Turn off the water. Use paper towels to grasp hand-operated controls when turning the water off.
13. Apply lotion to the hands if the skin appears dry.

    Rationale Lotion can keep the skin of the hands and fingers from becoming dry and cracked.

Cleaning, Disinfecting, and Sterilizing

Cleaning

Cleanliness inhibits the growth of microorganisms. An object is considered *clean* when it is free of pathogenic organisms. An object that is not free of pathogens is considered dirty or *contaminated.* Most objects used by nurses, whether artery forceps or drawsheets, can be cleaned by rinsing them in cold water to remove any organic material, washing them with hot soapy water, then rinsing them again to remove the soap. The following steps should be followed when cleaning in a hospital or home setting where pathogens exist.

1. Rinse the article with cold water to remove organic material. Hot water coagulates the protein of organic material and tends to make it stick to the article. Examples of organic material are blood and pus.
2. Wash the article in hot water and soap. Soap has an emulsifying action and reduces surface tension, which facilitates the removal of dirt. Washing dislodges the emulsified dirt.
3. Use an abrasive, such as a stiff-bristled brush, to clean equipment with grooves and corners.
4. Rinse the article well with hot water.
5. Dry.
6. Disinfect or sterilize if indicated.

Disinfecting and sterilizing

Disinfection is a process by which most microorganisms are destroyed, with the exception of spores. Spore-forming organisms such as *Bacillus anthracis* (which causes anthrax) and *Clostridium tetani* (which causes tetanus) are killed by *sterilization.* It is therefore important to know what type of pathogen is present and how it is destroyed. Various methods exist for disinfecting and sterilizing hospital objects:

1. *Hot-air oven.* Hot-air ovens are used to sterilize glassware and some metal objects in hospitals. Objects are subjected to dry air at a temperature of 180 C (356 F) for 2 hours; all microorganisms and spores are thus destroyed.
2. *Steam.* Steam under pressure and free steam (moist heat) are used to sterilize objects. The autoclave uses steam at 17 pounds pressure, 121 C (250 F) for 30 minutes. Microorganisms (including spores) exposed to

this pressure and temperature for 30 minutes are destroyed. Autoclaving is used to sterilize surgical dressings, surgical linens, parenteral solutions, and metal and glass objects.

Free steam, 100 C (212 F), is used for objects that would be destroyed at the higher temperature and pressure of the autoclave. Usually it is necessary to steam the article for 30 minutes on 3 consecutive days. The intervals are required so that the spores not killed at that temperature will return to their vegetative state and again become vulnerable to the heat.

3. *Radiation.* Ultraviolet light rays are also used for disinfection and sterilization. They are used in some hospitals and in industry. They provide a relatively safe and quick method for killing microorganisms.

4. *Ultrasonic waves.* In this method inaudible sound waves, above 20,000 cycles per second, are used. They break up microorganisms and sterilize objects.

5. *Chemical methods.* Several chemicals work either by interfering with the metabolism of microorganisms or by destroying the molecules of the organisms. There are basically two types of anti-infectives: (a) those applied for local action, such as disinfectants and *antiseptics*, and (b) those with a systemic action, such as antibiotics and specialized agents. An example of the latter is para-aminosalicylic acid, which is effective against the tuberculosis bacillus.

6. *Pasteurization.* Pasteurization is used in the disinfection of milk and similar substances. They are heated to a moderate temperature for a specific time. One method heats the product at 71 C (160 F) for 15 seconds. The product is then cooled and placed in the containers.

7. *Ethylene oxide gas.* Ethylene oxide gas sterilization is also used in some institutions. Microorganisms are destroyed when subjected to a temperature of 43.3 C (110 F) in a concentration of ethylene oxide of 440 mg/liter. This type of sterilization is generally used for delicate plastic or rubber objects that can be harmed by higher temperatures. Examples of articles sterilized by gas are oxygen or suction gauges, blood pressure apparatus, stethoscopes, sheepskins, motors, plastic drinking glasses, and catheters.

Nursing Intervention: Protective Aseptic Techniques

When a person is ill with an infection, the usual measures that are taken in health to prevent infections continue to apply. In addition, both in the home and in the hospital, it is necessary to restrict the spread of the pathogens from the infected person to others. The problem of confining the organisms and subsequently killing them or inactivating them involves a number of practices referred to earlier in the chapter.

Protective aseptic techniques include those practices carried out to prevent the transfer of organisms to any person or object that comes in contact with the infected person. A nurse caring for an infected patient needs to take precautions against acquiring the patient's pathogens. Care should be taken that dishes, equipment, and body discharges do not serve to transmit the pathogens to others. Protective asepsis is accomplished by destroying pathogens after they leave the body.

Protective aseptic techniques are called barrier techniques in some agencies. In the past, they were called isolation techniques; however, this name has fallen into disuse because of its negative connotation of isolating the patient physically and psychologically and the negative effect isolation can have on patients and support persons.

The need for protective asepsis arises when a patient has or is suspected of having a communicable disease or infection or when he or she is very susceptible to infections. The purpose is to keep pathogens within a defined area by establishing mechanical barriers (such as a closed room or a bed unit) to prevent their escape. Of course, pathogens are more effectively isolated in a separate room than in part of a room because airborne spread is more readily restricted in a closed space. Ideally, a protective asepsis room is serviced by clean entry rooms with washing sinks and storage space for supplies and has hand washing facilities and a private bathroom for the patient.

Types of Protective Asepsis

Because communicable diseases are transmitted in various ways, different types of precautions are necessary. The Center for Disease Control (U.S. DHEW 1975) has outlined five procedures that prevent the spread of microorganisms by various means. The type of protective asepsis (isolation) is identified by a color-coded placard placed on the door of the patient's room. The five categories are: respiratory, enteric, wound and skin, strict, and reverse.

Respiratory protective asepsis

Respiratory protective asepsis is indicated when the pathogens can be spread on droplets from the respiratory tract. In this type of asepsis, nurses generally wear masks and, if the patient is an infant, gowns, in the event the infant patient drools. To prevent the spread of infection, nurses teach patients proper tissue techniques; for example, patients should always cover their noses and mouths with several layers of tissue when they sneeze and cough, and they should dispose of these immediately in the appropriate receptacle.

Visitors also need to learn why masks are used and how to wear and discard them properly.

In some agencies patients also wear masks when they are transported or wherever they come in contact with people. When the patient is masked, the nurse need not mask. Table 19–2 presents a summary of types of protective asepsis and precautions.

Respiratory protective asepsis is indicated for patients who have respiratory illnesses, such as active pulmonary tuberculosis, pertussis (whooping cough), and pneumonia due to *Staphylococcus aureus.* Precautions must be taken when acquiring sputum specimens. Specimen containers should have close-fitting lids and be double-bagged before they are sent to the laboratory.

Enteric protective asepsis

Enteric protective asepsis is indicated when pathogens can be transmitted in the feces. The pathogen is transmitted when another ingests it. In some instances throat secretions or vomitus may be a source of pathogens; these also require special precautions in handling. In most settings, it is appropriate for the patient to use the usual toilet and bedpan; feces and urine are then treated to kill the microorganisms. However, the bathroom is not used by other patients. Usually, leftover food and fluids of patients on enteric protective asepsis are also disposed of in the toilet.

For this type of aseptic practice, nurses need not wear masks, but it is recommended they wear gloves and gowns when handling feces and urine containers and soiled linen. To destroy pathogens before disposing of excreta, the nurse adds 0.5 to 1.0% chloride of lime solution to the excreta, which then stands for 1 hour. This type of protective asepsis is indicated for patients who have diseases such as typhoid fever, salmonellosis, hepatitis, and dysentery (amebiasis).

Some patients who are carriers of the typhoid bacillus can live safely and comfortably at home. The only precaution they need take is to put chloride of lime solution in their feces before emptying the toilet. Special precautions are required when needles and syringes are used in the treatment of patients with viral hepatitis. Disposable needles and syringes should be placed in labeled, puncture-resistant containers. These containers are then incinerated or safely discarded.

Wound and skin protective asepsis

This type of protective asepsis is appropriate when pathogens are found in wounds and can be transmitted directly by contact with the wound or with articles contaminated by the wound, such as dressings or linen. The techniques are intended to retain the pathogens in a wound area and prevent transmission to other parts of the patient or to another patient.

Usually gowns are worn for this type of asepsis; in some cases gloves are also worn. Masks (respiratory precautions) are recommended for some specific pathogens, such as *Staphylococcus coagulase* positive and *Streptococcus*, beta-hemolytic group A. Important in this type of protective asepsis is the safe disposal of dressings, clothes, and equipment used to treat the wound. This type of asepsis is indicated for patients with abscesses, boils, or infected burns. Gas gangrene requires strict isolation measures.

Strict protective asepsis

Strict protective asepsis is indicated where the pathogen can be spread by contact and by air. It is used for all highly communicable diseases that can produce serious disease in other susceptible persons. Those in contact with the patient usually wear gowns, masks, and gloves, and the patient usually has a single room. Strict protective asepsis is indicated for patients with diphtheria, smallpox, and rabies.

Reverse protective asepsis

This is also referred to as *reverse barrier technique.* Its objective is to protect an uninfected patient with lowered resistance from potential pathogens in the environment. In this instance, the pathogens are kept *out* of a designated area. One way of accomplishing this asepsis is to enclose the patient in a large plastic bubble into which purified air is circulated.

This technique is indicated for patients who are particularly susceptible to infections, for example, patients with defective immunologic reactions, patients taking immunosuppressive drugs for cancer therapy, or patients with leukemia.

Psychologic Problems of Protective Asepsis

Patients on protective asepsis can develop several problems as a result of their isolation from others. Two of the most common are sensory deprivation and feelings of inferiority. Sensory deprivation occurs when the en-

Table 19–2 The Five Recommended Types of Isolation and Precautions*

Type of isolation	Purpose	Private room	Gowns	Masks	Gloves	Articles
Strict	To prevent the transmission of pathogens spread both by contact and by airborne sources	Necessary; door must be kept closed	Must be worn by all persons entering room; for smallpox, coverings for cap and shoes are also recommended	Must be worn by all persons entering room	Must be worn by all persons entering room	Discard or wrap before sending to central supply for disinfection or sterilization
Respiratory	To prevent airborne infection and contaminated articles (e.g., tissues) from respiratory droplets that are coughed, sneezed, or exhaled	Necessary; door must be kept closed	Not necessary	Must be worn by all persons entering room	Not necessary	Discard or disinfect articles contaminated with secretions
Protective (Reverse Isolation or Barrier Technique)	To protect an uninfected patient with lowered resistance from any pathogens in the environment	Necessary; door must be kept closed	Must be worn by all persons entering room	Must be worn by all persons entering room	Must be worn by all persons having direct contact with the patient; use sterile gloves for burn patients	Sterilize some articles that come in direct contact with the patient prior to use, e.g., linen for a burn patient
Enteric	To prevent the transmission of pathogens in the feces	Necessary for children only	Must be worn by all persons having direct contact with the patient	Not necessary	Must be worn by all persons having direct contact with infected area or articles contaminated by fecal material	Disinfect or discard articles contaminated with urine and feces using special precautions
Wound and Skin	To prevent the transmission of pathogens transmitted by direct contact with wounds or articles contaminated by wounds (e.g., dressings or linen)	Desirable	Must be worn by all persons having direct contact with the patient	Not necessary except during dressing changes	Must be worn by all persons having direct contact with the infected area	Special precautions are necessary for instruments, dressings, and linen

*For *all* types of isolation, the hands must be washed on entering and leaving the room.

From B. Kozier and G. Erb, *Techniques in clinical nursing: A comprehensive approach* (Menlo Park, Calif.: Addison-Wesley Publishing Co., 1982), p. 851.

vironment lacks normal stimuli for the patient, e.g., frequent communication with others. Such patients are usually in private rooms; also, because donning a gown may be necessary before entering the room, support persons may not visit as often as usual. In addition, visits by other patients are usually discouraged. The clinical signs of sensory deprivation are described on page 906.

Patients can have feelings of inferiority because of the infection itself, the reason for the precautions. In North America, many people place a high value on cleanliness, and sometimes patients with infectious diseases feel "contaminated," "dirty," and somehow at fault. While this is obviously not true, in our social context the infected person can feel inferior to others and blame himself or herself for the disease.

Nurses need to provide care that prevents these two problems and/or deals with them positively. Nursing intervention needs to include:

1. Assessment of the individual's need for stimulation.
2. Provision of measures to help meet these needs, including regular communication with the patient; diversions, such as toys for a child and books, television, or radio for an adult; stimulation of the sense of taste with a variety of food; and stimulation of the visual sense by providing a view or an activity to watch.
3. Explanations about the infection and the associated procedures to help patients and their support persons understand and accept the situation.
4. No conveyance to the patient of annoyance about the protective aseptic precautions or of revulsion or disgust because of the infection. Warm, accepting behavior is particularly important for patients on protective asepsis.

Initiating Protective Asepsis

The equipment required for protective asepsis depends primarily on the type of protection required, the ability of the patient to participate responsibly in the procedures, and the physical facilities of the agency. Practices vary, and thus the necessary equipment and supplies also vary. For example, nurses usually wear masks when caring for patients who are on respiratory protective asepsis, but they need not wear them when caring for patients on enteric protective asepsis. Some patients are able to cooperate with the precautions; others—e.g., a confused adult—cannot. Nurses may not need to gown to measure the body temperature of a rational patient; gowning for the same procedure is essential if the patient is confused.

The physical facilities of the agency can affect the equipment and supplies required. Some hospitals have specially designed rooms on the nursing unit. These rooms have in place most of the equipment needed for protective asepsis; so very little setting up is required. The technique described below includes the equipment normally required when setting up a unit.

Assessing the patient

Not all the assessment practices described below are normally carried out while a unit is being set up; some practices are appropriate at that time, and others while protective asepsis is being implemented.

1. Determine the capacity of the patient to understand and to cooperate with the practices.
2. Assess the patient's understanding of the procedures and his or her need for information.
3. Continually assess the patient's need for stimulation while on protective asepsis. Be aware of the clinical signs of sensory deprivation: boredom, inactivity, slowness of thought, daydreaming, increased sleeping, disorganized thought, anxiety, panic, and hallucinations. See Chapter 35 for additional information on stimulation.

Preparing the patient and support persons

Explain the practices and the reasons for them to the patient. If appropriate, provide explanations and demonstrations after the patient is moved to the unit or after the equipment has been set up.

Be reassuring and supportive to the patient. If the patient is to be moved to a protective asepsis unit assist him or her to gather clothing and personal effects.

Explain the practices that support persons need to carry out, e.g., gowning. Demonstrating procedures is often helpful. Arrange diversionary activities for the patient as appropriate and a teaching plan as needed for the patient and his or her support persons.

Assembling the equipment

Wash hands before assembling the equipment so as not to transmit any microorganisms to the patient. The following equipment is usually needed:

1. A sink with a liquid germicidal soap dispenser for washing hands and cleaning used articles.
2. Paper towels near the sink.
3. At least one waste container lined with plastic. See the section on double-bagging on page 462.
4. A laundry hamper to collect used linen.
5. A table on which to place supplies, e.g., a stethoscope and thermometer.
6. A toilet for the disposal of excreta. In some agencies garbage is also put in the toilet. In other agencies, there is a hopper in addition to a toilet for the disposal of waste products.

7. A tub or shower for the patient.
8. A rack for hanging the gowns if they are reused (reuse is not recommended by the U.S. Center for Disease Control).
9. Bedside supplies for the patient, e.g., tissues, drinking water, cup, etc.
10. A cart outside the unit with clean supplies such as gowns, plastic bags, isolation tags, disinfectant solutions, masks, plastic disposal bags, etc.
11. A sign on the door indicating what precautions should be taken or saying "Visitors inquire at the desk."

Donning and Removing Face Masks

Masks are generally used to prevent the spread of microorganisms to and from the respiratory tract. Nurses wear masks for two reasons: to prevent the passage of organisms from their own respiratory tracts to the patient or to prevent inhaling pathogenic microorganisms from the patient. Sometimes patients, too, wear masks so they will not inhale pathogenic microorganisms in the air or in droplets coughed, sneezed, or exhaled by others. Similarly, patients sometimes wear masks so they will not exhale pathogens.

Masks are made of a variety of materials such as cotton or glass fiber; disposable masks are being used increasingly. Masks should be worn only once and then discarded to ensure effective filtering of microorganisms. Masks that become wet are less effective and should also be discarded. Masks should be worn no more than 1 hour at a time.

Masks need to cover both the mouth and the nose and fit tightly around the face to prevent escape of microorganisms around the sides. If a person wears glasses, the upper edge of the mask should fit under the glasses to help prevent the glasses from clouding over. A mask is put on with clean hands prior to donning a gown.

As a precaution the nurse dons a mask before entering the unit. The mask is removed after the hands have been washed if gloves were not worn. See Chapter 20, Procedure 20–2 on page 476. After use, a disposable mask is discarded in a plastic-lined waste container. Reusable masks are usually placed in a moisture-resistant bag designated for that purpose, where they await washing and sterilization. Some agencies require that a bag be hung on the door of the room to remind personnel to don and remove masks. For additional information, see Kozier and Erb (1982:98–100).

Gowning

Gowning technique is used for two main reasons: (a) to cover clothes so that they will not become contaminated by pathogens from a patient and (b) to cover clothes so that microorganisms on the clothing will not be transferred to a patient; for example, a mother wears a gown when she visits her sick newborn baby in the nursery.

Gowns are worn for all categories of protective asepsis except respiratory. Gowns used in hospitals open down the back and usually have a tie at the neck and one or two other ties at the back. Some agencies provide disposable paper gowns that are fastened by tapes. Protective asepsis gowns need to be long and wide enough to cover all the clothing worn under them and preferably have sleeves with tight-fitting cuffs and a belt or tie for the waist. It is best to put on a clean gown each time care is given to the patient and discard it before leaving the patient's room.

When taking a gown off, the nurse needs to ensure that the hands, which are contaminated, do not touch anything but the gown until they are washed. The outside of the gown (the contaminated side) should not touch the nurse's clothing or any clean, uncontaminated objects. The hands are then washed. See Procedure 19–1.

In certain settings and situations, e.g., the nursery, gowns are occasionally reused rather than discarded. When putting on a used gown, the nurse keeps in mind that the inside of the gown is clean and the outside is contaminated. The neck band and the fasteners at the neck are also considered clean. The gown is usually hanging on a stand designated for that purpose; the nurse picks it up from the inside and then slides hands and arms down the sleeves. If the hands will not move easily through the cuffs, the nurse can pull the sleeve over the hand with the opposite hand, which is still in the sleeve. The second hand may then be pushed through, or the sleeve can be pulled on by taking a clean paper towel and grasping that second sleeve on the outside. However, it is important that both hands remain clean and not touch the outside of the gown. If the hands become contaminated, they need to be washed before the neck of the gown is secured. The gown is then fastened at the neck; the gown is overlapped, left over right side, as much as possible at the back, and then the waist tie or belt is secured. See Figure 19–5.

To remove a gown that is to be kept for reuse, the nurse first unties the waist ties, then washes the hands before untying the neck and taking off the gown, being careful to touch only the inside of the gown. Still holding it on the inside, the nurse hangs it on the rack. The neck ties are clean and are permitted to fall down on the inside of the gown. When the nurse holds the gown with both hands inside the shoulders at the shoulder seams, the hands can be brought together and then one shoulder of the gown inverted over the other. This ensures that the clean part of the gown is on the outside. The gown is then hung outside the protective aseptic unit on a rack ready for reuse. See Figure 19–6.

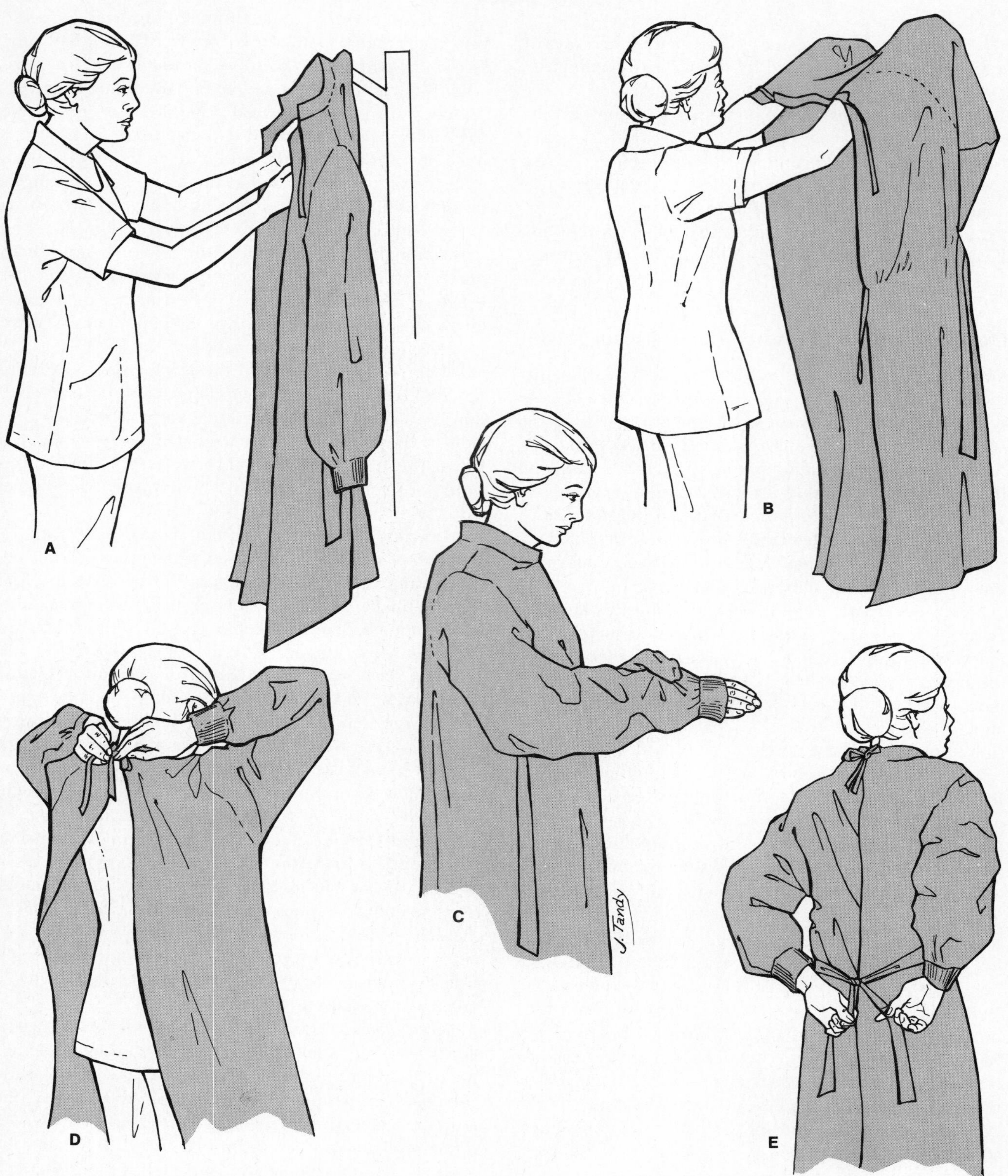

Figure 19–5 Donning a used gown for protective asepsis: **A,** reach to the inside at the shoulders; **B,** slide the arms down inside the sleeves; **C,** pull the hands through the cuffs; **D,** tie the gown at the neck; **E,** fasten the gown at the back, the left side (clean) over the right side (contaminated). Note the hands remain clean until **E.**

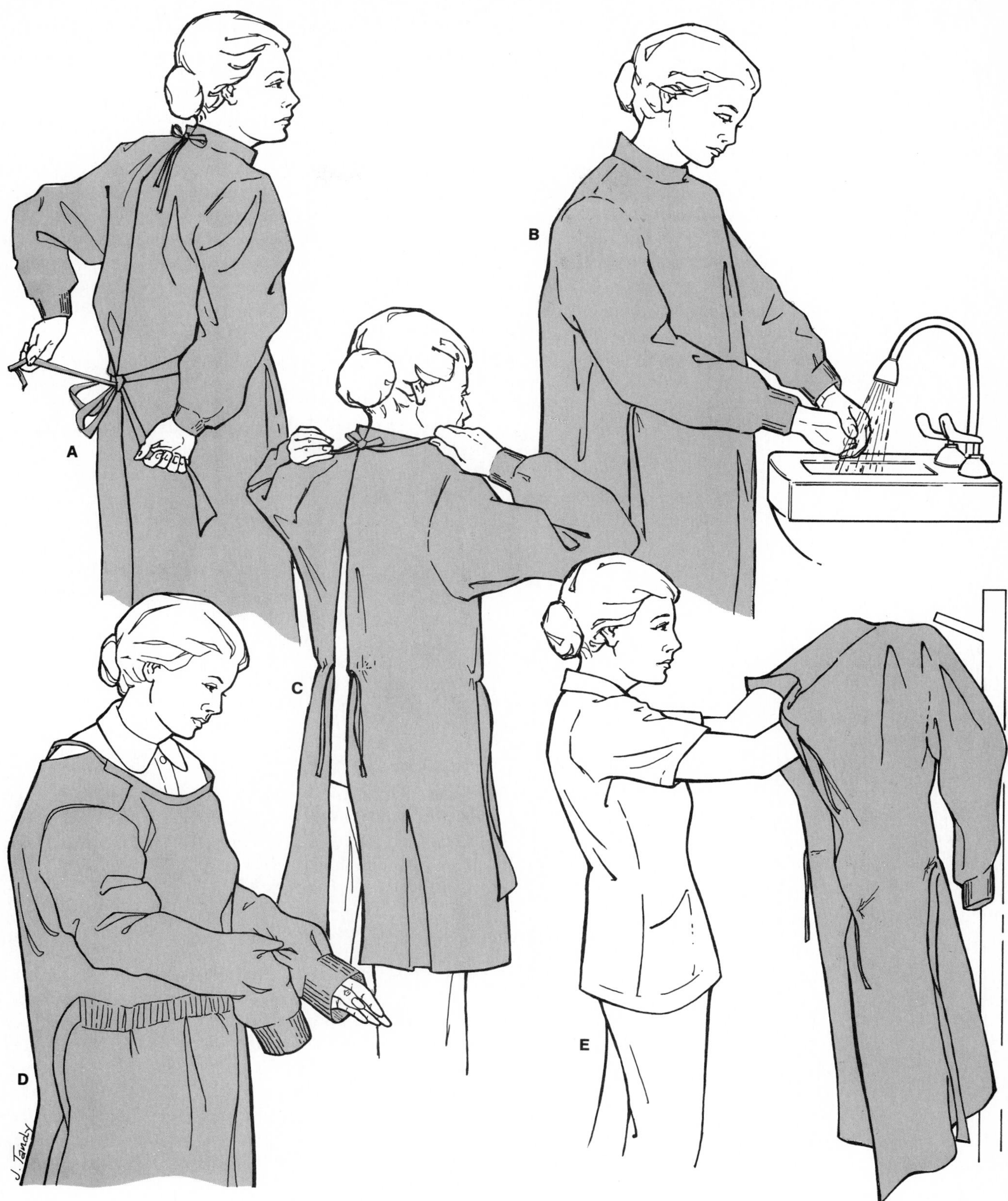

Figure 19–6 Removing and retaining a gown for protective asepsis: **A,** untie the waist ties; **B,** wash hands; **C,** untie the neck ties; **D,** remove the arms from the sleeves by touching the inside of the sleeve only; **E,** hang the gown on a rack.

Some agencies are now using disposable gowns, which are used once and then destroyed. These are usually disposed of in a covered garbage can. For detailed techniques for donning and removing a gown, see Kozier and Erb (1982:855–61).

Donning and Removing Gloves

Gloves are used in medical asepsis to protect the nurse from pathogens. They serve as a barrier to infection when a nurse is handling feces or wound drainage, which may contain highly virulent microorganisms.

The gloves used for this purpose are usually clean but not sterile and are often disposable. Generally, the nurse removes the gloves in the patient's unit, when the nurse is finished handling the contaminated articles; the nurse does not wear gloves while giving further care. For additional information about donning and removing gloves, see Kozier and Erb (1982:118–21, 862).

Double-Bagging

Clothes, linens, and contaminated articles are normally sealed in a single bag that is impervious to microorganisms. The outside of the bag remains clean. Double-bagging is indicated when the outside of the bag does not remain clean. This means that the first bag is placed inside another bag, the outside surface of which is kept free of the pathogenic organisms. The bag is labeled to indicate that it contains contaminated linens and taken to a laundry isolation storage area or chute.

Figure 19–7 In double-bagging, the outside of the outer bag remains clean, and the inner bag is contaminated.

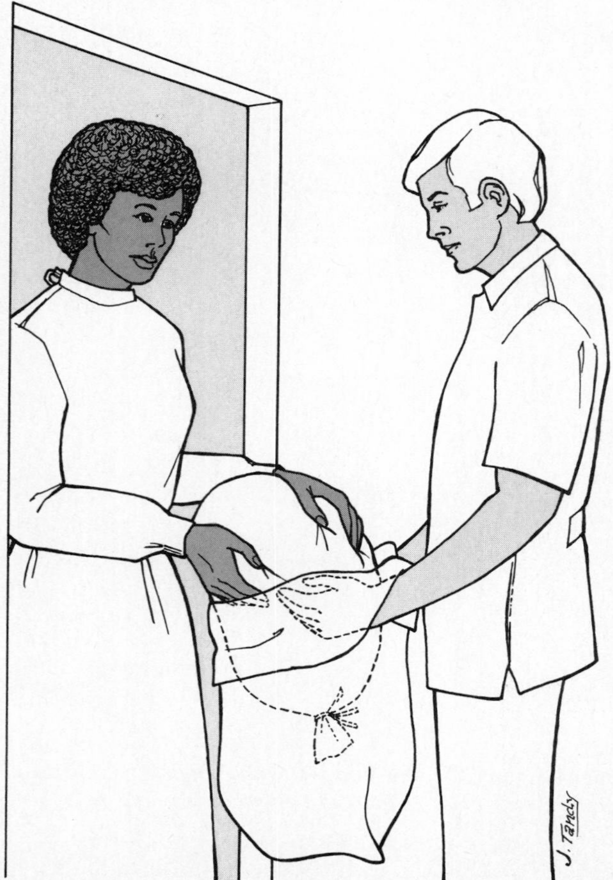

To double-bag linen, the nurse needs an assistant who holds the outside bag. The nurse inside the room, who may gown and mask if indicated, closes the top of the first bag securely and drops it into the outer bag. As an added precaution, the nurse may put the first bag into the outer bag tied end first (see Figure 19–7). The assistant cuffs the upper part of the second bag so that the hands are well covered and receives the soiled bag from the nurse in the room. Care is taken not to contaminate the outside of the outer bag. This is done by holding the outer bag so that the contaminated part of the cuff is innermost (see Figure 19–7). The assistant then closes the bag securely and tags it appropriately, according to agency policy. In some agencies, the outer bags are colored. For additional information see Kozier and Erb (1982; 862–64).

Most hospital laundries have standard laundering techniques that safely disinfect the linens by killing most microorganisms. Linens contaminated by spore-forming organisms require special treatment, usually with steam at a high temperature, to ensure disinfection.

Refuse Disposal

Refuse such as used dressings is handled much as used linen; that is, two people double-bag it in moisture resistant bags. Once double-bagged, the refuse is taken directly to the incinerator.

Disposal of Food and Contaminated Dishes

Food left on a tray is normally discarded in the patient's toilet or in the patient's plastic-lined garbage receptacle. Dishes and trays may then be placed in a plastic bag that is sealed and marked "contaminated" before returning it to the kitchen to be handled by dishwashing personnel with gloved hands. Some hospitals use disposable plastic or paper dishes that are discarded in the refuse container lined with a plastic bag. Silver cutlery may be washed, dried, folded in a paper towel, and left in the patient's room.

A patient on protective asepsis usually keeps his or her own tray; the dishes are transferred to the patient's tray from the tray on which the food is delivered. In this way, the tray does not have to be disinfected after each meal.

Handling Contaminated Equipment

When a patient is on protective asepsis, it is usual to leave the equipment that is used regularly, such as a thermometer, blood pressure cuff, stethoscope, and tourniquet, in the patient's room until the patient is discharged or until protective asepsis is no longer necessary.

Much equipment used in most hospitals today is disposable, thereby lessening the need for concurrent disinfection (disinfection of equipment used while the patient is ill). In most cases, it is necessary merely to bag disposable equipment safely and have it destroyed. Most hospitals have incinerators for this purpose.

Equipment that cannot be discarded, such as special instruments, is washed, double-bagged, and sealed. Paper bags are used for steam sterilization; plastic bags are used for gas sterilization.

Assessing Vital Signs

The sphygmomanometer, thermometer, and stethoscope are kept in the patient's room for the duration of protective asepsis. A thermometer can be stored in a test tube taped to the mirror over the sink. The test tube is filled with a cotton fluff, to protect the tip of the thermometer, and disinfectant solution, which is changed daily. Some agencies advocate the use of a clean thermometer or one with a clean protective sheath each time a temperature is taken. Agency practices need to be ascertained and followed.

To assess the pulse and respiration of a patient whose environment is suspected of being contaminated, the nurse must place the watch on a paper towel on the patient's overbed table. The nurse gowns and takes the vital signs, then removes the gown and washes both hands. When picking up the watch, the nurse touches only the top or clean surface of the paper towel. The nurse discards the towel before leaving the room but can first use it to grasp the handle to open the door of the room.

If a blood pressure cuff for the sole use of the patient is not supplied, it is necessary to have the patient whose hygiene practices are unsafe put on a clean, long-sleeved gown before the pressure is taken. In this way, the cuff touches only the clean gown. After determining the blood pressure, the nurse places the apparatus on clean paper towels. Any surfaces that have been in contact with infected secretions, for example, the bell of the stethoscope, are sprayed with disinfectant after the nurse has degowned and washed both hands. The apparatus is not used again until the appropriate time has elapsed for disinfection, usually 20 minutes. Vital signs are charted on a piece of paper left on the cart outside the room. Kept outside, the paper is not infected. For additional information see Kozier and Erb (1982: 864–68).

Administering Medications

All medications are prepared according to agency practices and taken to the unit. The medication tray and card may be left outside the room, and the medication taken into the room. The nurse need not gown to administer oral medications if the patient's hygienic practices are safe. The medicine cup is discarded in the wastebasket or patient's bedside paper bag. The nurse washes hands prior to leaving the room and then charts the medications.

To administer injectable drugs, the nurse must don a gown when the patient's hygienic practices are unsafe. Only the prepared syringe and needle are taken into the room. Most agencies now use disposable needles and syringes. Used syringes and needles are not put into wastebaskets in the patient's room but are usually placed in specially provided covered containers at the nursing station. If necessary, they are wrapped in clean paper towels before they are taken from the patient's room. In some agencies, an appropriately labeled can is placed in the patient's room and used to receive the contaminated needles. Only the needles are placed in the can; the disposable syringes are placed in the garbage receptable.

Collecting Specimens

The outside of the specimen container is kept clean. When a patient's hygienic practices are unsafe the lid of the container is left on the isolation cart outside the room, and the open container is taken into the patient's bathroom and placed on clean paper towels. The nurse then puts on a gown and acquires the specimen, e.g., urine or feces. The nurse pours the urine from the bedpan into a graduate pitcher and then pours some into the specimen container, taking care not to contaminate the outside of the container. Tongue blades are used to transfer stool specimens into the appropriate container; the blades then are wrapped in paper towels and discarded in the waste basket. The bedpan is cleaned and returned to the bedside unit. Throat swabs are placed in the designated container. The nurse then washes hands, removes the gown, and washes hands again. The nurse takes the specimen out of the room, covers it, and labels it twice to denote the type of specimen and the fact that it is a specimen, for instance, from a patient on respiratory protective asepsis. In some agencies, the policy is to swab the outside of the specimen container with a disinfectant; in others, to place it in a paper bag before it is sent to the laboratory.

Transporting Patients

Sometimes it is necessary to transport patients on protective asepsis, for instance, to the radiography department. Before the patient is moved, the nurse gives the patient a clean gown and robe and, if respiratory precautions are in effect, a mask or tissues and bag so that the patient can follow proper tissue technique. The nurse places a clean sheet over the stretcher or wheelchair, making sure that all areas the patient might touch are covered. Stretcher straps can be fastened over the clean sheets. When the patient is transported back to his or her room, the linen is placed in the patient's hamper, and the transport vehicle is sprayed with disinfectant if necessary.

Handling Patients' Personal Effects

Collecting money from a protective asepsis area does not usually require special precautions, but the money may be sprayed with disinfectant to alleviate any apprehension on the part of personnel. Coins may be placed on clean paper towels on the cart outside the room, sprayed, and allowed to stand. Outgoing mail likewise does not require disinfection, except in cases of smallpox. The nurse may need to remind the patient to keep the letters free of expectorations or secretions. Thus, the patient may need to wear a mask while writing the note. Some agencies advocate that envelopes be sealed and stamped at the nurse's station.

Sometimes patients need to sign documents. In instances where the patient's hygienic practices are unsafe, the nurse can place the document on the patient's overbed table on clean paper towels, where the patient can read it without touching it; or the patient may touch it if he or she has washed hands. Before the patient signs the document, the nurse may place a paper towel over it, leaving exposed just the space required for signature. The patient can use his or her own pen or the nurse's pen, which can then be sprayed or wiped with disinfectant. The nurse takes the document outside with one hand, discards the paper towels, and washes hands.

Nursing Evaluation

The effectiveness of medical protective asepsis can be evaluated by determining if microorganisms are being transmitted to others or contained within a designated area. For example, the pathogen infecting one patient's abdominal incision ordinarily would be cultured and tested for sensitivity to several antibiotics. If that same pathogen appears in another patient's incision or on the hands of health personnel, the effectiveness of the medical aseptic practices could be questioned.

Evaluating the effectiveness includes:

1. Determining if the source of infection is being controlled or destroyed, e.g., through adequate treatment, protective aseptic precautions for wound discharge, etc.
2. Determining if the susceptibility of the host is decreasing, e.g., through proper nourishment, health habits, etc.
3. Determining if the transmission of the pathogenic organisms is being blocked, e.g., through hand washing, double-bagging, etc.

Summary

Medical aseptic practices are involved in all nursing activities, since microorganisms are always present in the environment. A knowledge of medical asepsis and an awareness of how microorganisms are transmitted are essential for safe nursing practice. The chain of infection involves the etiologic agent, the source, the exit, the method of transmission, the portal of entry, and the susceptibility of the person.

Many factors affect a person's susceptibility to infection. Among them are stress, nutritional status, fatigue, sex, heredity, age, medical treatment, and health habits.

There are three stages during the course of an infection: the incubation period, the period of illness, and the convalescent period. During the period of illness, signs and symptoms are evident. Localized infections are noted by the signs of inflammation: swelling, redness, heat, pain, and loss of function. Systemic symptoms include fever, malaise, anorexia, headache, and lymph node enlargement.

Many measures are employed to prevent infections and to maintain health. Some environmental measures include preventive programs for immunization, regulations about food transportation and pollution of air and water, and sanitation of sewage. Individual preventive measures are employed to strengthen the body's barrier against infections and to minimize the number of microorganisms present. Examples of measures that strengthen the body's barriers are adequate nutrition, immunization, and adequate rest. Personal hygiene minimizes the numbers of microorganisms.

Preventing infections in ill persons requires medical

aseptic practices such as hand washing, cleaning, disinfection, and sterilization. Methods of disinfection include hot-air ovens, steam, radiation, ultrasonic waves, chemical methods, and pasteurization.

Protective aseptic techniques vary according to the way specific pathogens are transmitted. Five types of protective asepsis are respiratory, enteric, wound and skin, strict, and reverse protective. Except for reverse protective asepsis, the purpose of each of these techniques is to limit pathogens to a defined area. The nurse needs to be aware of the special needs of patients on protective asepsis. In addition, nurses need to know how to prepare a protective asepsis unit.

Specific protective aseptic techniques include gowning, applying and removing face masks, and gloving. Nurses caring for patients on protective asepsis need to use special techniques when handling linen, disposing of food and refuse, disinfecting equipment, assessing vital signs, administering medications, collecting specimens, transporting the patient, and handling the patients personal effects.

Suggested Activities

1. Set up a protective asepsis unit in the nursing laboratory. Have a classmate take the role of a patient in the unit and take his or her pulse and blood pressure and serve a tray as for a meal.
2. Review the practices used for protective asepsis in one hospital. Compare the practices with those followed in other agencies and with those presented in this book.
3. Interview a patient who is or has been on protective asepsis in a hospital. Find out how that person viewed the experience.

Suggested Readings

Castle, M. May 1975. Isolation: Precise procedures for better protection. *Nursing 75* 5:50–57.

Photographs and step-by-step techniques are used to outline procedures in protective asepsis.

Garner, J. S., and Kaiser, A. B. April 1972. How often is isolation needed? *American Journal of Nursing* 72: 733–37.

Results of a survey of infections in hospitals are given, and the types of isolation practices indicated for communicable disease are discussed.

Hargiss, C. O., and Larson, E. December 1981. Guidelines for prevention of hospital acquired infections. *American Journal of Nursing* 81:2175–83.

This article describes many nosocomial infections and methods for reducing the incidence of these infections. Particular attention is paid to urinary tract infections, surgical wounds, respiratory tract infections, and bacteremia. A table of common skin cleaning agents is included.

Selected References

Aspinall, M. J. October 1978. Scoring against nosocomial infections. *American Journal of Nursing* 78:1704–7.

Bond, G. B. December 1981. Infection control: Serratia—An endemic hospital resident. *American Journal of Nursing* 81:2183–86.

Brandt, S. L., and Benner, P. March 1980. Infection control in hospitals: What are the challenges? *American Journal of Nursing* 80:432–34.

Dubay, E. C., and Grubb, R. D. 1978. *Infection: Prevention and control.* 2nd ed. St. Louis: C. V. Mosby Co.

Fox, M. K.; Langner, S. B.; and Wells, R. W. September 1974. How good are hand washing practices? *American Journal of Nursing* 74:1676–78.

Garner, J. S., and Simmons, B. T. July/August 1983. CDC Guidelines for isolation precautions in hospitals. *Infection Control* 4:245–325. Special Supplements.

Greene, V. W. November 1969. Microbial contamination: Control in hospitals. *Hospitals* 43:78.

Hardy, C. S. August 1973. Infection control: What can one nurse do? *Nursing 73* 3:18–21.

Hargiss, C. O., and Larson, E. December 1981. Infection control: How to collect specimens and evaluate results. *American Journal of Nursing* 81:2166–74.

Jenny, J. November 1976. What you should be doing about infection control. *Nursing 76* 6:78–79.

Litsky, B. Y. 1973. *Hospital sanitation: An administrative program.* Chicago: Modern Hospital Press, McGraw-Hill Publications Co.

McInnes, M. 1975. *Essentials of communicable disease.* 2nd ed. St. Louis: C. V. Mosby Co.

Nadolny, M. D. March 1980. Infection control in hospitals: What does the infection control nurse do? *American Journal of Nursing* 80:430–31.

National League for Nursing. 1975. *Infection control.* Publication no. 20-1582. New York: National League for Nursing.

Norton, C. F. 1981. *Microbiology.* Reading, Mass.: Addison-Wesley Publishing Co.

Streeter, S.; Dunn, H.; and Lepper, M. March 1967. Hospital infection: A necessary risk? *American Journal of Nursing* 67:526–33.

U.S. Department of Health, Education, and Welfare. 1975. *Isolation techniques for use in hospitals.* 2nd ed. DHEW Publication No. (CDC) 76-8314.

Chapter 20

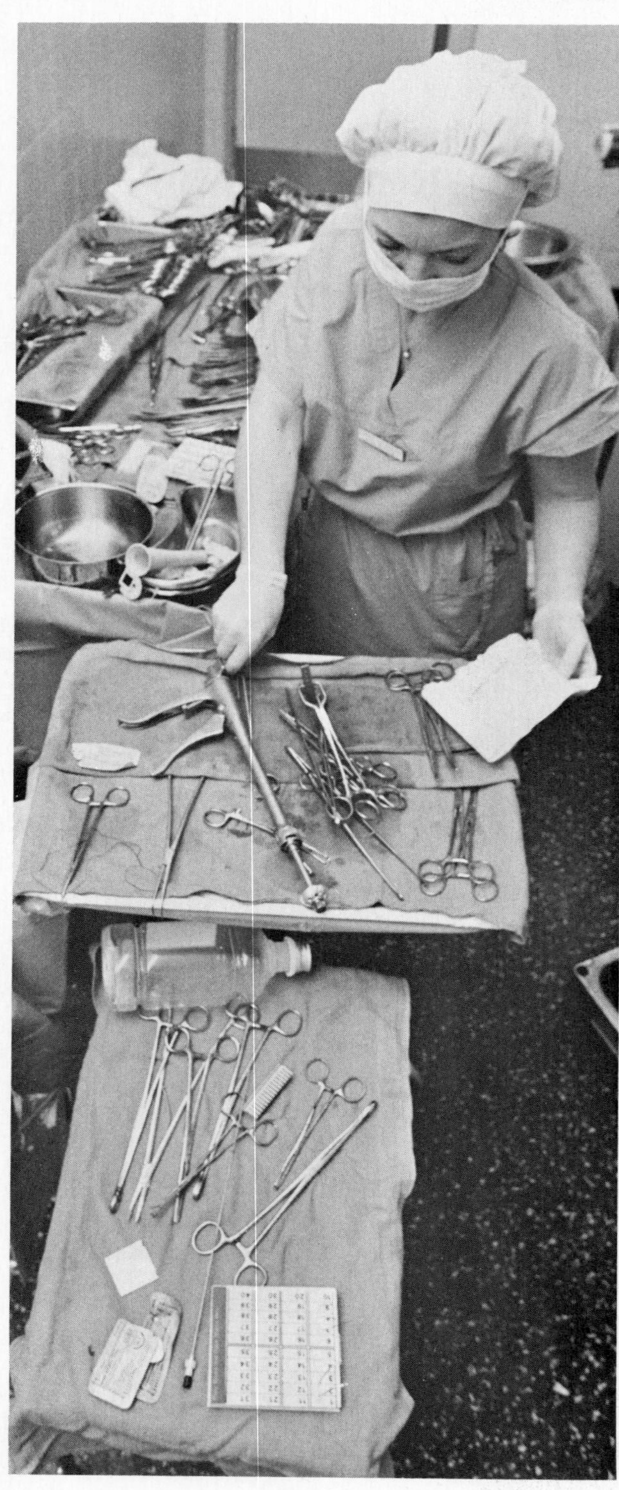

Surgical Asepsis

CONTENTS

Objectives

1. Know essential terms and facts about surgical asepsis
   1.1 Define selected terms
   1.2 List basic principles of surgical asepsis and examples of related practices
2. Assess essential data prior to surgical asepsis
   2.1 Identify the educational needs of patients
   2.2 Identify the precautions necessary to maintain surgical asepsis
3. Perform surgical aseptic techniques correctly
   3.1 Wash hands correctly
   3.2 Open sterile wrapped packages
   3.3 Handle sterile forceps correctly
   3.4 Pour sterile solutions safely
   3.5 Apply sterile drapes correctly
   3.6 Don and remove face masks correctly
   3.7 Don sterile gloves correctly
   3.8 Don a sterile gown correctly

Terms

clean
contamination
hemostat
sterile
sterile field
surgical asepsis (sterile technique)

Surgical asepsis, also called *sterile technique*, consists of measures designed to render and maintain objects free from microorganisms, including all pathogens, spores, and nonpathogens. It also includes practices designed to keep all microorganisms away from an area, such as a patient's wound. Surgical asepsis is employed in many situations, such as in operating and delivery rooms, and for such procedures as changing surgical dressings, inserting urinary catheters, and administering injections and intravenous solutions. *Contamination* refers to the presence of pathogenic microorganisms. *Clean* is defined as the condition in which microorganisms but not pathogens are present. Therefore, an unsterile condition may be clean or contaminated. An object is *sterile* only when it is free of all microorganisms. A *sterile field* is a sterile area, such as the area of a sterile towel or container. In surgical asepsis it is not uncommon to refer to an item that becomes unsterile as contaminated, i.e., it has microorganisms that may or may not be pathogenic.

Some practices—for example, sterilization, masking, and gowning—used in medical asepsis (see Chapter 19) are also used in surgical asepsis. However, in surgical asepsis the purpose is to keep microorganisms away from a particular area—e.g., the urinary bladder—rather than within a given area as, for example, in respiratory protective asepsis. Therefore the methods of washing hands and putting on gloves and gowns are different in surgical asepsis than in medical asepsis.

Sterile supplies are handled with sterile forceps or with the hands if they are in sterile gloves or enveloped in a sterile drape, but never with the naked hand. Prior to handling sterile equipment, the nurse in all instances needs to scrub hands and forearms thoroughly, and, in some situations, needs to wear a mask, a sterile gown, sterile gloves, and a cap.

Basic Principles of Surgical Asepsis

Whenever the skin barrier is broken or whenever a body cavity considered free from organisms is entered, sterile technique is employed. In all situations, these basic principles apply:

1. *Sterile objects become contaminated unless touched only by other sterile objects.* In other words:

Sterile to sterile = Sterile

Sterile to clean = Contaminated

Sterile to contaminated = Contaminated

Sterile to questionable = Contaminated

2. *Sterile items out of the range of vision or below the waist level of the nurse are considered contaminated.* Sterile objects not in view can be accidentally touched by unsterile objects. Thus, nurses never leave a sterile field unattended. They hold objects in view above waist level, and do not turn their backs on a sterile field.

3. *Sterile objects are contaminated by airborne sources.* The environment in which sterile technique is carried out must be as clean as possible. Such areas are usually damp cleaned with detergent germicides to reduce the number of contaminants in the area and to reduce their transfer by air currents. Most institutions provide a room used only for clean and sterile techniques. Clothing worn by personnel must also be clean.

Headgear, when worn, needs to cover the hair completely to prevent particles and organisms dropping from the hair.

People disperse airborne contaminants in droplets from the mouth and nose, especially when they talk, laugh, sneeze, or cough. Therefore, nurses minimize talking over sterile fields or wear masks so as to not contaminate the field. A nurse who has a mild upper respiratory infection should not perform sterile measures or should double-mask while doing such tasks.

Air currents are produced by moving objects. Therefore, traffic must be kept to a minimum, and items should not be moved over a sterile field. When nurses open sterile bundles or packages, they do not reach over the sterile field, since particles can drop from the nurse's arm. Once a sterile item is exposed, the nurse refrains from reaching over it and moves economically to reduce air currents. Moving sterile objects as little as possible also minimizes chances of contamination.

4. *Moist or damp sterile fields are considered contaminated if the surface below them is not sterile or if the surface has been exposed to the air for a length of time.* Once moisture penetrates a sterile object such as a drape, capillary action draws microorganisms from the unsterile surface to the sterile surface. To prevent this, sterile trays are often used beneath sterile objects so that when disinfectants and other liquids are added to the sterile field, they are confined to the sterile area. In this way, capillary action from an unsterile surface is made impossible. However, sterile covers that become moistened are considered contaminated by airborne contaminants. Therefore, nurses should avoid spills when they pour solutions in or near a sterile field.

5. *Objects are rendered sterile by the processes of dry and moist heat, chemicals, and radiation.* Sterility is maintained by storing sterile articles in double wrappers but only for prescribed periods of time. Storage areas need to be clean and dry.

6. *Fluids flow in the direction of gravity.* Wet forceps are always held with the tips down. If the tips are held up, the fluid will flow toward the handle, become contaminated by the hands, and then flow back down and contaminate the tips when the forceps are pointed downward. The surgical hand scrub also applies this principle. When scrubbing, the nurse holds the hands higher than the elbows to prevent contaminants from the forearms reaching the hands. Hands are dried from the fingertips toward the elbows (from the cleanest to the least clean area).

7. *The edges of a sterile field are considered contaminated.* Because opened drape edges are in contact with an unsterile surface, a 2.5 cm (1 in) margin around a drape is considered contaminated. When nurses open disposable packages or remove lifting forceps from a container of disinfectant they avoid touching the edges of the container with the forceps because the edges are in contact with the air and thus are considered contaminated.

8. *Wound exudates are considered contaminated, and dry wounds are considered clean.* Sterile swabs used to clean a wound become contaminated and are therefore discarded away from the sterile field in a separate receptacle, such as a moisture resistant bag. When cleaning wounds, the nurse uses each swab only once. The wound is cleaned from the center outward toward the skin and from incisions toward drain sites (from the cleanest to the least clean area).

9. *Conscientiousness, alertness, and honesty are necessary in maintaining surgical asepsis.* When an object is contaminated, its appearance is unchanged. Only the person who saw it become contaminated knows and only that person knows to correct the situation.

Assessment Prior to Surgical Asepsis

Nurses frequently carry out procedures requiring surgical asepsis, e.g., urinary catheterizations and surgical dressing changes. Before any such procedures, the nurse needs to assess the following:

1. What the patient needs to know about surgical asepsis

2. What precautions the patient must take

Educational Needs

Patients often need to be taught how to maintain sterile technique during specific procedures. For example, they may need to learn the following:

1. To refrain from coughing, sneezing, and talking near a sterile field. Coughing, sneezing, and talking can emit pathogens from the respiratory tract and thus contaminate the sterile field.

2. To refrain from touching sterile supplies or a sterile field and so contaminating it.

Patient Precautions

The nurse needs to assess the particular needs of the patient before the procedure requiring surgical asepsis, so that equipment and supplies will remain sterile. Incontinent patients may need to urinate or defecate and then wash before the procedure. Patients with respiratory infections need to mask before any surgical aseptic procedures begin.

Surgical Aseptic Techniques

Nurses use several techniques to ensure surgical asepsis. The following eight techniques are frequently part of procedures—for example, urinary catheterization—that call for surgical asepsis. One of those techniques, the surgical hand wash, is especially important because it is a first step in many nursing procedures.

Hand Washing in Surgical Asepsis

Surgical aseptic hand washing differs from medical aseptic hand washing in that the hands are held higher than the elbows. The elbows are considered more contaminated than the hands, and the washing and rinsing water runs from the cleanest to the least clean area (from the hands to the elbows).

The fingernails are trimmed short so they can be cleaned easily. Sleeves are kept above the elbows, and the wristwatch is removed. All rings are removed because they harbor microorganisms and can be damaged by the soap and water.

Surgical aseptic hand washes in hospital clinical areas, by contrast to those in operating rooms, usually last 1 minute—a wash and rinse of 25 to 30 seconds repeated once. The length of the scrub in an operating room depends on agency practice; it may be as long as 10 minutes for the first scrub of the day.

Following a surgical hand wash or scrub, the nurse holds the hands above the elbows and away from the body.

Procedure 20–1 Technique for Surgical Hand Washing

Equipment

1. A germicidal soap or detergent. Most agencies supply liquid detergent beside the sink. The detergent is often dispensed by a foot pedal.
2. A deep sink with foot, knee, or elbow controls for the water and a faucet high enough so that the hands and forearms can be positioned under it. See Figure 20–1. For a description of the types of faucet controls, see Procedure 19–1, page 452.
3. Towels for drying the hands. Many agencies supply paper towels, which are discarded after use.
4. A file, orange stick, or other tool for cleaning the nails.

Intervention

1. Turn on the water and adjust the temperature to lukewarm.

   Rationale Warm water removes less protective oil from the skin than hot water. Soap irritates the skin more when hot water is used.

2. Wet the hands and forearms under running water, holding the hands above the level of the elbows so that the water runs from the fingertips to the elbows. See Figure 20–2.

   Rationale The hands will become cleaner than the elbows. The water should run from the least contaminated to the most contaminated area.

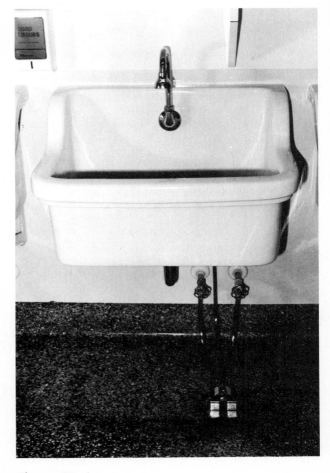

Figure 20–1

Procedure 20–1, continued

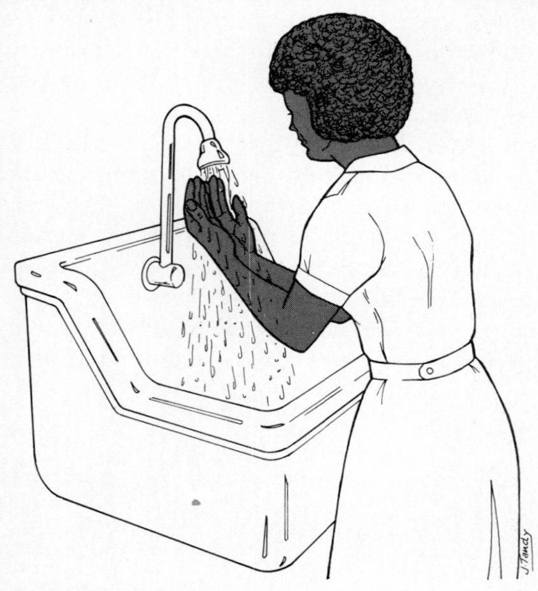

Figure 20–2

3. Apply 2 to 4 ml (1 tsp) soap to the hands.

4. Use firm, rubbing, circular movements to wash the palms and backs of the hands, the wrists, and the forearms. Interlace the fingers and thumbs and move the hands back and forth. Continue washing for 20 to 25 seconds.

   Rationale Circular strokes clean most effectively and rubbing ensures a thorough mechanical cleaning action. The areas between the fingers need to be cleaned.

5. Hold the hands and arms under the running water to rinse thoroughly, keeping the hands higher than the elbows.

   Rationale Soap remaining on the skin is irritating. The nurse rinses from the cleanest to the least clean area.

6. Check the nails and clean them with a file or orange stick if necessary. Rinse the nail tool after each nail is cleaned.

   Rationale Sediment under the nails is removed more readily when the hands are moist. Rinsing the nail tool prevents the transmission of sediment from one nail to another.

7. Repeat steps 3 through 5.

8. Use a towel to dry one hand thoroughly from the fingers to the elbow. Use a rotating motion. Use a new, clean towel to dry the second hand in the same manner.

   Rationale Moist skin readily becomes chapped and subject to open sores. Thorough drying also makes it easier to don sterile gloves. The nurse dries the hands from the cleanest to the least clean area.

9. Discard each towel in the waste container.

10. Turn off the water. If the faucet has hand controls, use the elbows, if possible; otherwise use a dry paper towel when touching the handle.

    Rationale Touching the handle directly contaminates the hands.

11. Keep the hands in front of you and above your waist.

    Rationale This position maintains their cleanliness and prevents accidental contamination.

Opening Sterile Wrapped Packages

Sterile packages of such items as dressing gauzes, catheterization trays, or dressing sets are commercially prepared in paper or plastic containers. In hospitals, a double-thickness linen or special paper may be used to wrap nondisposable items. Sterile equipment is stored in clean, dry areas to preserve its sterility. If the equipment is moist or damp, it is considered contaminated and should not be used. The sterilization dates should also be checked to ensure that the wrapped item has not been kept beyond the sterilization period. Frequently, chemical indicator tape is used to fasten sterile packages. These indicator strips change color during the sterilization process, indicating that the contents are sterilized. If the color change is not evident, the package is considered unsterile.

Sterile packages may be opened by (a) placing them on a clean, dry surface and unwrapping them in such a way that the sterility of the contents, including the inside of the wrapper, is maintained or (b) by holding the outside of the package with one hand and unwrapping it with the other hand. Prior to opening any sterile item, the nurse's hands must be thoroughly washed.

Sterile items are packaged so that the package can be opened without contaminating the contents. A large, clean working area above waist level must be used. The indicator tape on the package is removed rather than torn and is discarded. Tape that is not removed from a cloth wrapper creates problems in the laundry.

The package is placed so that it can be opened away from the body. The flap farthest from the nurse is opened first, but the nurse takes care not to reach over the sterile field. See Figure 20–3. The nurse needs to hold the arm out at the side or lateral to the package. Then the side flaps are opened (Figure 20–4), and the flap nearest the nurse is opened last (Figure 20–5). When opening the flaps, the nurse takes care not to touch the inside of the wrapper. Usually the corners are turned outward; so the nurse can grasp these easily and avoid touching the inside. When opening the last flap, the nurse stands well back from the package—15 to 30 cm (6 to 12 in)—to avoid contamination from the nurse's uniform. If space on the table is limited, it may be necessary to fan fold this flap so that it remains above the waist level of the nurse. Some sterile sets have an additional inner wrapping. This is opened in similar fashion, but sterile forceps must be used.

In some situations, it may be necessary to close or loosely wrap a sterile package. For example, after solutions have been added to a dressing set, the set may need to be rewrapped for transport to the bedside. A sterile package is wrapped in the *reverse* order to that of unwrapping. The proximal flap is closed first to prevent reaching across the sterile field, the side flaps next, and the distal flap last.

Opening smaller or light items

Smaller items can be opened by holding them in one hand and opening them with the other hand in the same manner described above. The sterile item can then be transferred to a sterile field or handed to another person.

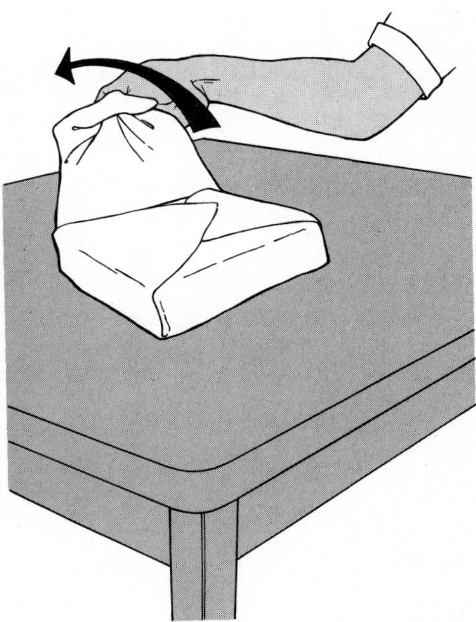

Figure 20–3 Opening the first flap of a sterile wrapped package.

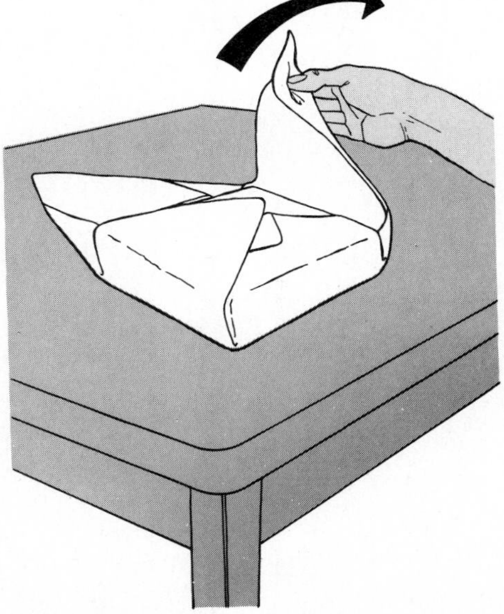

Figure 20–4 Opening the second flap to the side.

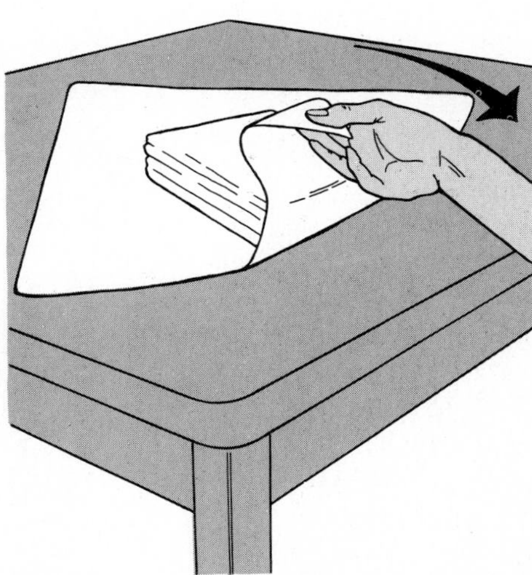

Figure 20–5 Pulling the last flap toward the nurse by grasping the corner.

Before the transfer, it is important to enclose the hand holding the package in the sterile wrapper. The hand is enclosed by grasping all corners of the wrapper with the other hand and securing them above the wrist level of the first hand. See Figure 20–6. The item can then be dropped safely onto a sterile field or, with arm extended, handed to another person who is wearing sterile gloves.

Opening commercially prepared packages

Many disposable items, such as syringes and some dressings, are dispensed in sterile paper packages. Usually one end of this package has some unsealed edges, which the nurse grasps (one in each thumb and index finger) and peels apart, taking care not to touch the inside of the wrapper. This wrapper can often be laid on a table surface sterile side up and used as a sterile area, or it may be discarded, depending on the needs of the moment. See Figure 20–7. For additional information, see Kozier and Erb (1982: 104–110).

Handling Sterile Forceps

There are many styles of forceps used for handling sterile supplies. Some of the forceps used most commonly by nurses are:

1. *Hemostat* or artery forceps with straight or curved tips. See Figure 20–8.
2. Thumb or tissue forceps with or without teeth. See Figure 20–9.
3. Handling or sponge forceps, also referred to as a transfer or pickup forceps. See Figure 20–10.

Regardless of the type of forceps used, the following principles apply in their use. Forceps are useful in many situations that require the transfer of sterile items from one place to another, for example, moving sterile cotton balls or gauzes from a large sterile stock container onto a dressing or catheterization tray.

The practice of storing lifting forceps in germicidal solution and storing sponges and gauzes in large metal containers is decreasing, since the sterility of these is questionable. If forceps, sponges, and gauzes are stored in these ways, the nurse needs to ascertain that the containers are sterilized and the solutions changed at least daily.

1. *Sterile forceps are always held above and in front of the waist* to prevent inadvertent contamination out of the nurse's range of vision.
2. *The tips of the forceps are considered sterile and need to be held down*, particularly when they become wet. If the forceps tips tilt upward, liquids flow from the sterile tips to unsterile hands, become contaminated, and then flow back when the tips are tilted downward, contaminating them. The nurse needs to learn to abduct the elbows when handling forceps. This abduction keeps forceps tips in the downward position.
3. *The handles of forceps are considered contaminated except when handled with sterile gloves*. When they are held by the naked hand, forceps are placed onto sterile trays with the tips inside the sterile field and the handles outside or at the edge of the sterile field. Every part of the forceps is placed inside the sterile field when the nurse is wearing sterile gloves.
4. When removing sterile items from a container, *the forceps tips and/or the item should be kept away from*

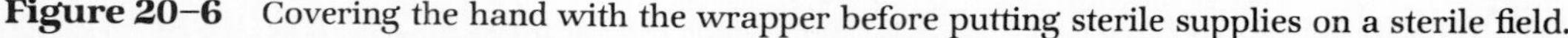

Figure 20–6 Covering the hand with the wrapper before putting sterile supplies on a sterile field.

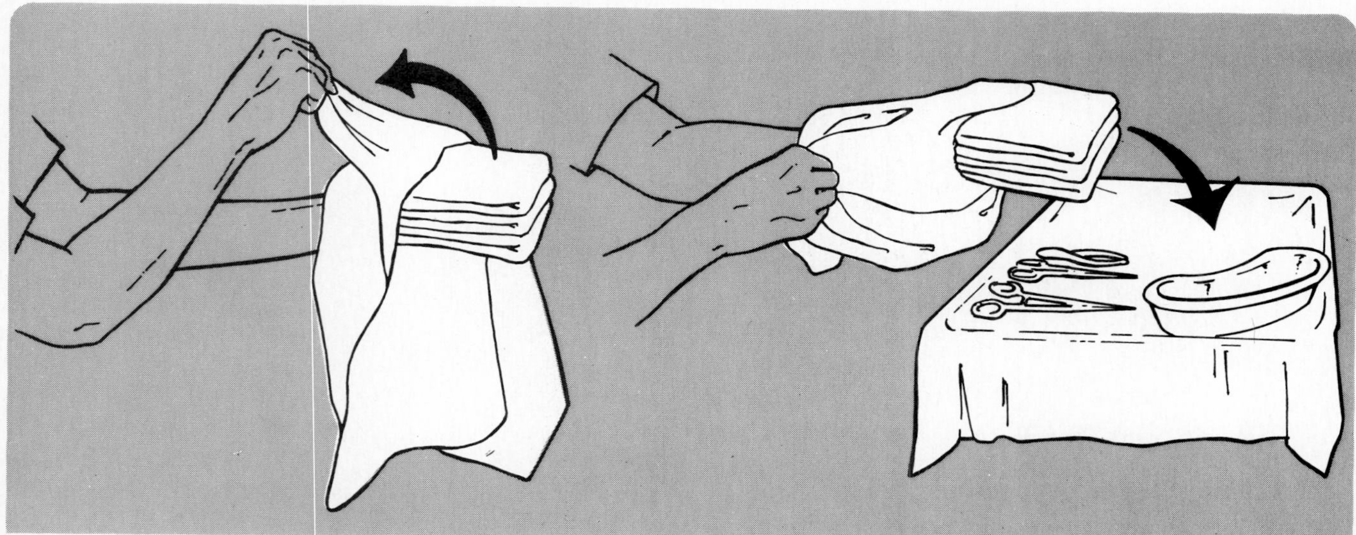

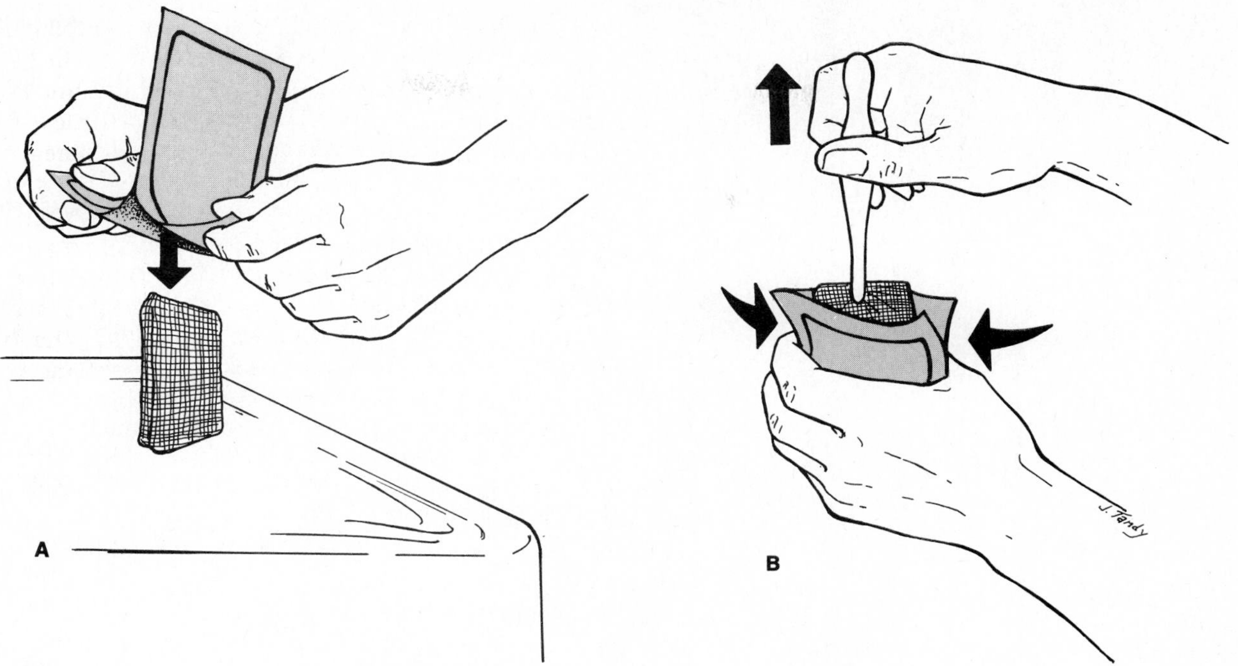

Figure 20–7 Opening a commercially prepared sterile package: **A,** onto a sterile field; **B,** by cupping the package and using forceps.

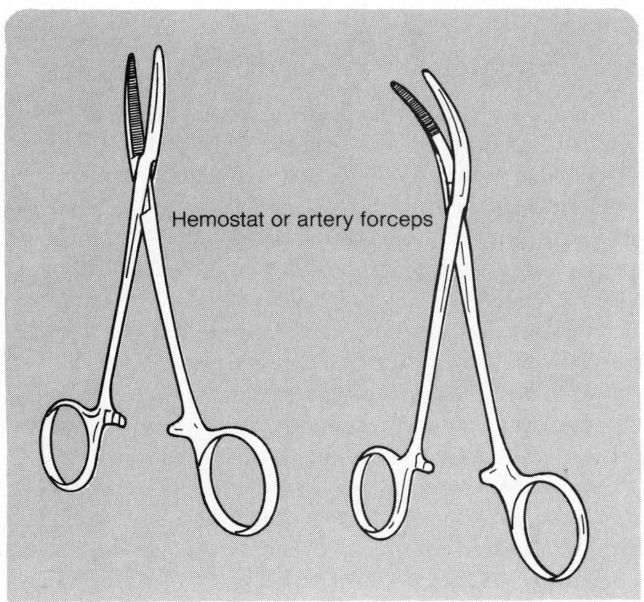

Figure 20–8 Hemostat forceps (straight and curved).

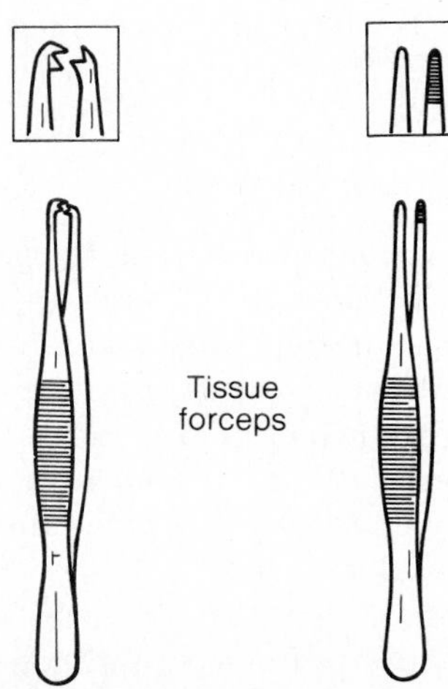

Figure 20–9 Tissue forceps (toothed and plain).

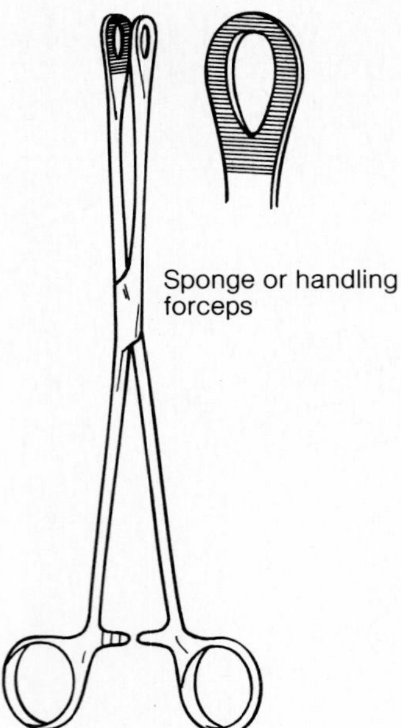

Figure 20–10 Pickup forceps.

the edges of the container or disposable package. The edges are exposed to air and are considered contaminated. Thus, when a nurse lifts forceps from a container of germicidal solution, he or she avoids touching the forceps against the sides and top edges. When removing gauzes from commercially prepared paper packages, the nurse pulls the flaps well apart or cups the package.

5. *Forceps tips moistened with germicidal solution should not touch a sterile field.* Sterile articles are dropped gently onto a sterile field. Excess moisture on the forceps tips can be removed by gently tapping the tips while holding them in the downward position over the solution container. Caution is needed to avoid touching the top edges of the container, which are contaminated. For additional information see Kozier and Erb (1982: 111–13).

Pouring Sterile Solutions

Nurses often handle sterile solutions. Many solutions are contained in sterilized solution bottles, such as those for intravenous fluids, and in vials or ampules, which are used for parenteral medications. The methods of handling these are discussed in Chapters 31 and 37, respectively. Frequently, nurses need to pour a sterile solution from a large or small bottle into another container, such as a solution basin.

Flasks or bottles containing sterile solutions are considered sterile on the inside and contaminated on the outside. Thus, when the cap of a bottle is removed, only the outer unsterile surface is touched. Because the inner part of the cap, including the inner rim, is sterile, the cap, once removed, is placed top down, i.e., inner aspect uppermost, on the table or held with the inner side pointed downward. This principle also applies to lids of large containers that hold other sterile materials, such as gauzes or cotton fluffs. Microorganisms in the air are less likely to contaminate the inside of a lid that is held downward than one held upward.

Before pouring the sterile solutions, nurses pour a small amount of solution into a sink or waste container to clean the lip of the bottle. The bottle should be held with the label on the upward side to avoid wetting it. When the solution is poured, care must be taken not to contaminate the receiving basin by contact with the outside of the bottle. Undue splashing of solution may contaminate underlying sterile drapes. It is important also to avoid reaching over the sterile field. Therefore, the nurse holds the bottle outside the sterile field as much as possible and keeps the top of the bottle at a reasonable distance from the receiving container. This distance varies with the size of the bottle. A distance of 10 to 15 cm (4 to 6 in) is recommended for large bottles, but the distance can be decreased for smaller bottles. The nurse recaps the solution flask touching only the outside of the cap.

Applying Sterile Drapes

Sterile drapes are often used to expand a sterile field. Extensive draping procedures are used in the operating rooms, and the student is referred to agency policies for these techniques.

Many sterile sets such as dressing, catheterization, or special diagnostic sets (lumbar puncture) are equipped with sterile drapes. Sizes of drapes vary, but commonly they are approximately 30 cm by 45 to 60 cm (1 ft by 1½ to 2 ft). Some drapes are plain pieces of cloth or paper. Others have holes in the center; these are called fenestrated drapes. Placement of drapes varies with the number of drapes and the procedure used.

Many drapes are placed in sterile packages in such a way that the nurse can pick up the drape by one corner with the bare hand without contaminating the rest of the drape. See Figure 20–11. Care must be taken not to contaminate it with the nurse's uniform. See Figure 20–12. By lifting the drape with one hand, the nurse can grasp the opposite corner of the drape with the other hand. See Figure 20–13. The drape is then placed so that the side farthest from the nurse is positioned first and the side nearest the nurse, last. See Figure 20–14. This prevents the nurse from reaching across the sterile field. If gloves are used to handle drapes, care must be taken to avoid contamination of fingertips on the bedclothes. This is done by enclosing the fingertips in the corners of the drape prior to placing the drape.

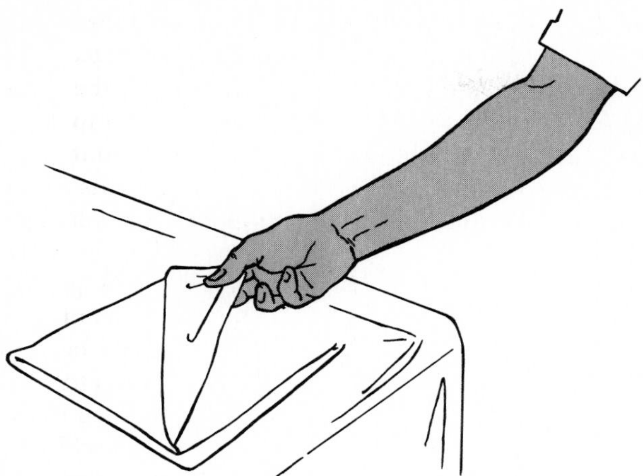

Figure 20–11 Picking up a sterile drape at one corner.

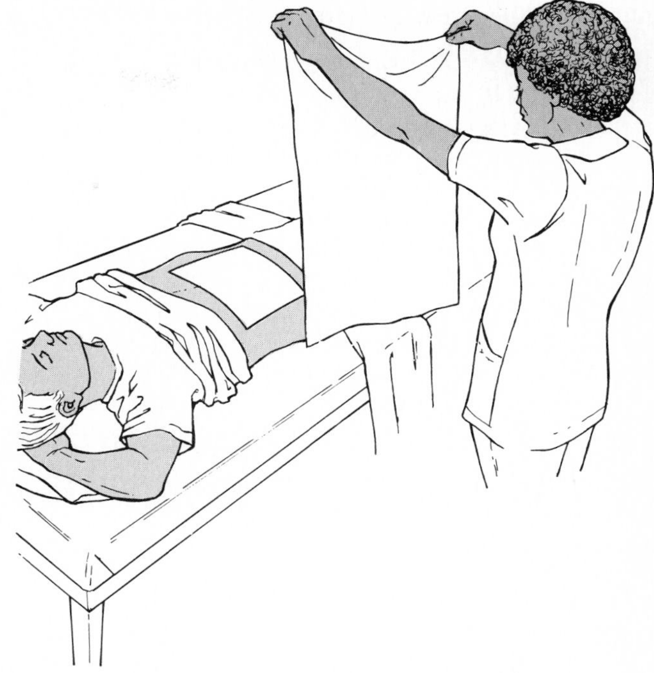

Figure 20–13 Holding the drape at two corners.

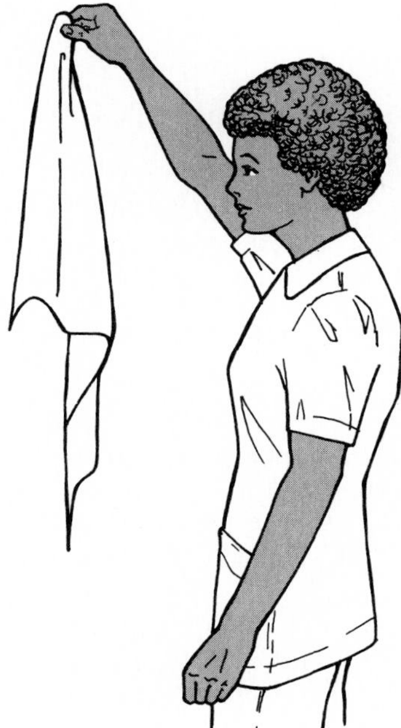

Figure 20–12 Holding the drape away from the nurse.

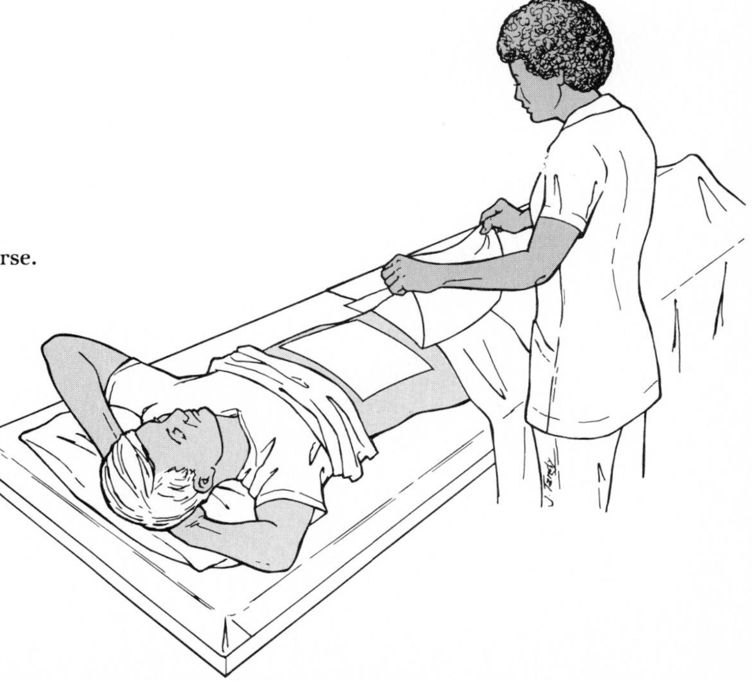

Figure 20–14 Laying drape down on the far side first.

Donning and Removing Face Masks

Because the face and hair are contaminated, a cap is donned first, if required; next a face mask is donned; and then hands are washed. Masks must cover both the nose and mouth in sterile technique. They are removed after completion of the sterile procedure.

Masks made of cotton and similar materials may be washed and reused; those made of less durable materials are discarded after use. Disposable masks are being used increasingly. Some masks have a metal strip that molds the mask over the bridge of the nose. When this strip is fitted snugly over the nose, very little air escapes around the edges of the mask. This kind of mask is particularly advantageous for people who wear eyeglasses, since it prevents the glasses from fogging. Many disposable masks have elasticized side loops that fit over the ears and facilitate rapid donning and removal.

Nurses wear face masks for two reasons:

1. To prevent the spread of microorganisms from their own respiratory tracts to patients
2. To prevent inhaling pathogenic microorganisms from an infectious patient (see Chapter 19)

Procedure 20–2 Donning and Removing a Face Mask

Equipment

Face mask

Intervention

To don the face mask

1. Pick up the mask by its upper ties (or side loops) near where they are attached to the mask. Position the mask over the bridge of the nose. See Figure 20–15.

   Rationale Holding the mask by its ties maintains the cleanliness of the facial portion of the mask.

2. Tie the upper strings at the top of the back of the head or slip the loops over the ears.

   Rationale By tying the upper strings first, the nurse prevents accidental contamination of the inner side of the mask. Fastening the mask over the top of the head prevents it from slipping.

3. Tie the lower strings snugly around the nape of the neck. Be sure that the lower part of the mask is well under the chin. See Figure 20–16.

4. If the mask has a metal strip, adjust this firmly over the bridge of the nose.

   Rationale A secure fit prevents both the escape of microorganisms around the edges of the mask and the fogging of eyeglasses.

5. Avoid talking, sneezing, or coughing, if possible.

   Rationale These activities increase the number of microorganisms in the mask and the possibility of their escape through the mask.

To remove the mask

6. Remove gloves or wash hands if they are contaminated.

   Rationale This step is taken to avoid contaminating the hair and neck.

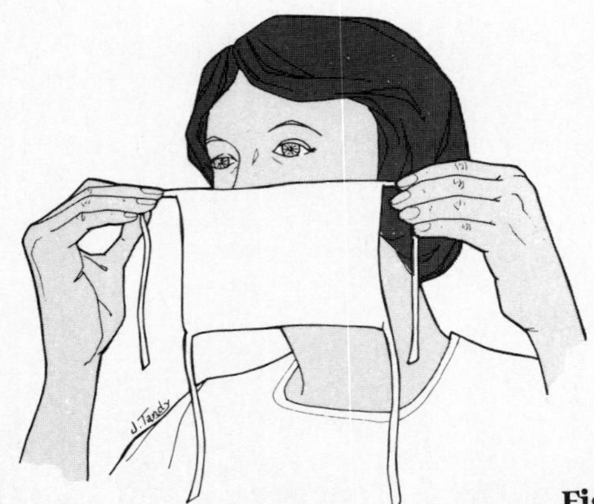

Figure 20–15

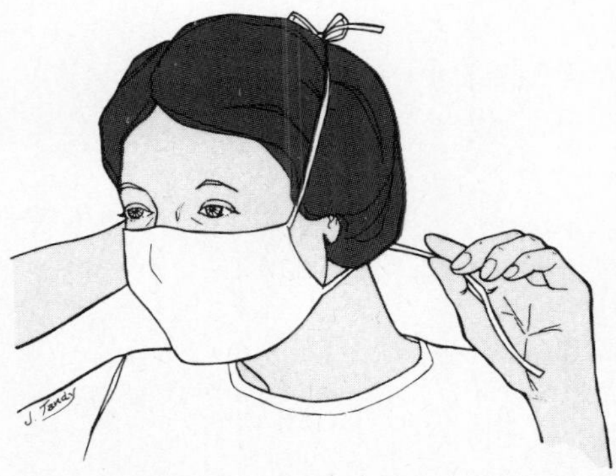

Figure 20–16

Procedure 20–2, continued

7. Unhook the side loops from the ears, or untie the lower strings.
8. Untie the top strings.
9. Holding the top strings or side loops, remove the mask and bring the strings or loops together so that the inner part of the mask folds upon itself.

   Rationale The nurse avoids touching the most contaminated part of the mask, the area in contact with the face.
10. Discard a disposable mask in the waste container. Put a reusable mask in the laundry hamper.
11. Wash hands if they became contaminated accidentally by touching the main part of the mask.

   Rationale Washing prevents the spread of microorganisms to others.

Donning Sterile Gloves

Sterile gloves are packaged with a cuff of about 5 cm (2 in). A surgical scrub must precede gloving. There are two methods for donning sterile gloves: the open method and the closed method. The open method is most frequently employed in clinical areas, not the operating room; the closed method requires that the nurse wear a sterile gown and is frequently used in operating rooms.

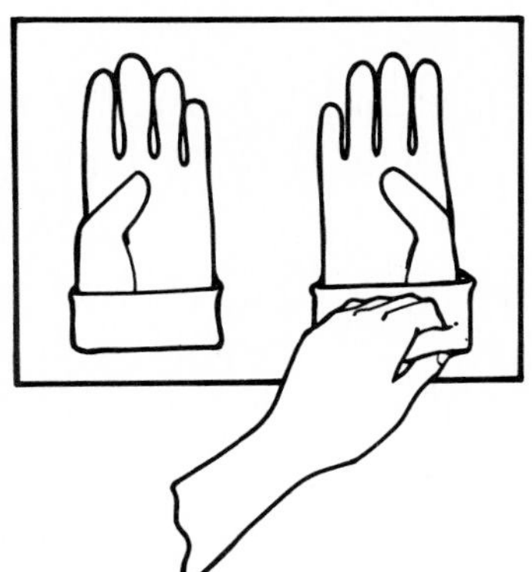

Figure 20–17 Picking up the first glove by its cuff.

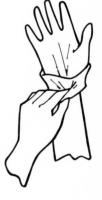

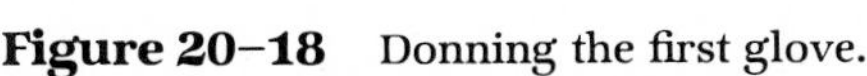

Figure 20–18 Donning the first glove.

Open method

To put on the first glove, the nurse grasps the glove by its cuff (on the palmar side) with the thumb and first finger of one hand, being careful to touch only the inside of the glove. See Figure 20–17. This technique is used because the outside of the glove must remain sterile, and the nurse's hand is considered contaminated. The other hand is then inserted into the glove, and the glove is pulled in place by the hand grasping the cuff. See Figure 20–18. The cuff is left turned down, and care is taken not to touch the outer part of the glove.

To put on the second glove, the nurse uses the sterile gloved hand. The nurse picks up the second glove by inserting the gloved fingers under its cuff. See Figure 20–19. This technique preserves the sterility of the outside of both gloves. The nurse then pulls on the second glove, paying particular attention that the gloved thumb does not touch the palmar skin or wrist of the second hand. The thumb of the first hand is held up and back. See Figure 20-20. The cuffs of both gloves may then be unfolded by touching only the sterile sides.

If a sterile gown is also being worn, this same technique can be used, but the cuffs are pulled well up over the cuffs of the sleeves. See the section on gowning technique in this chapter.

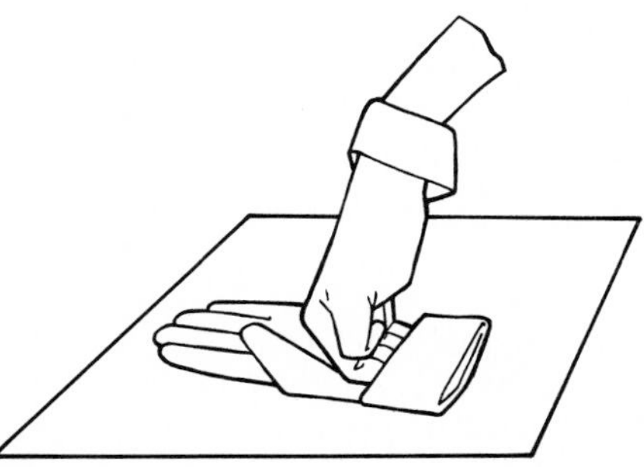

Figure 20–19 Picking up the second glove under the cuff.

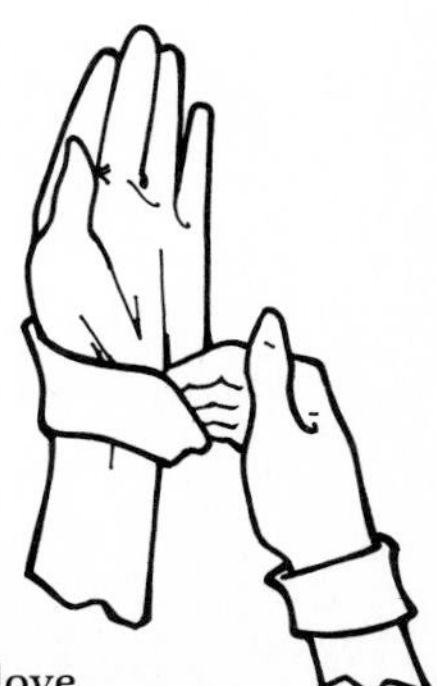

Figure 20–20 Donning the second glove.

Closed method

This method can be used only when a sterile gown is worn, as in the operating room, because the gloves are handled through the sleeves of the gown. The gown is first put on so that the hands are in only as far as the cuff seam of the sleeve, and the gown is tied by another person. To put on the gloves, the nurse first grasps the inside of one sleeve cuff with the thumb and index finger. One glove is then picked up and placed palm side down on the palm of the other (still sleeved) hand, with the fingers of the glove pointing toward the elbow. The cuff of the glove and the gown cuff lie together. The glove is then put on. For a right glove, the left hand (still covered by the sterile gown) grasps the top edge of the glove cuff, and the right hand (also covered by the sterile gown) grasps the bottom edge of the glove cuff. The left hand then pulls the glove onto the right. Care must be taken not to expose the fingers. The left glove is put on in the same manner, except that the gloved right hand can now handle the glove.

Donning a Sterile Gown

Sterile gowns are worn in the operating room and the delivery room and when open wound technique is used, as for the burned patient. The gown may be picked up from a sterile pack, or it may be handed to the nurse by someone who is already gowned and gloved. Gowns are folded inside out and touched only on the inside so that the outside remains sterile. When a gown is donned, the parts considered sterile are the area above the anterior waist and the anterior aspects of the sleeves. Parts of the gown considered unsterile are the backs of the sleeves, all areas below the waist, the collar area, and the areas under the arms. The gown is put on after the head turban and mask, and after the surgical scrub.

Procedure 20–3 Donning a Sterile Gown

Equipment

Sterile gown.

Intervention

1. Remove watch and rings.

   Rationale Jewelry can harbor microorganisms.

2. Wash hands (surgical hand wash).

   Rationale Washing removes microorganisms.

3. Pick up the gown by grasping the folded gown at the neck band. Stand well back (30 cm or 12 in) from the sterile bundle. The neck area and the inside of the gown are then considered contaminated.

4. Hold the gown out at arm's length and allow it to unfold naturally. See Figure 20–21. The inside of the gown (the armholes) must face the wearer.

   Rationale Shaking the gown can bring it in contact with unsterile objects or create air currents that could contaminate it.

5. Hold the gown by the open inside shoulder seams and put each hand alternately into the armholes.

6. Extend the arms. Keep the hands at shoulder height when you put them through the armholes. See Figure 20–22.

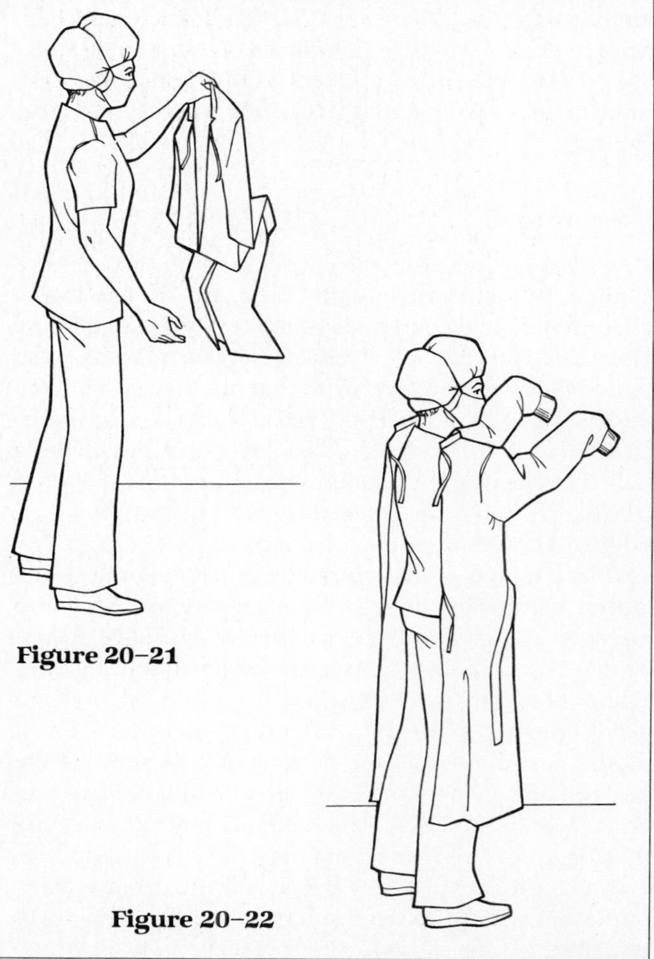

Figure 20–21

Figure 20–22

Procedure 20–3, continued

Rationale This position holds the gown in place and lessens the chance of contaminating the gown.

7. An unsterile person (circulating nurse) then pulls the sleeves onto your arms by working from behind and inside the gown. The sleeves may be pulled over the hands, or they may be pulled so that the seams of the cuff are at the fingertips.

   Rationale If the cuff seam is at the fingertips, the closed method of gloving can be used. See the explanation of the closed method of gloving.

8. The unsterile nurse fastens the neck and folds or holds closed the edges of the gown.

9. The unsterile nurse fastens the waist ties from behind. These ties are grasped at the tip after the gown wearer bends at the waist. See Figure 20–23.

   Rationale Bending allows the ties to fall free and away from the sterile gown.

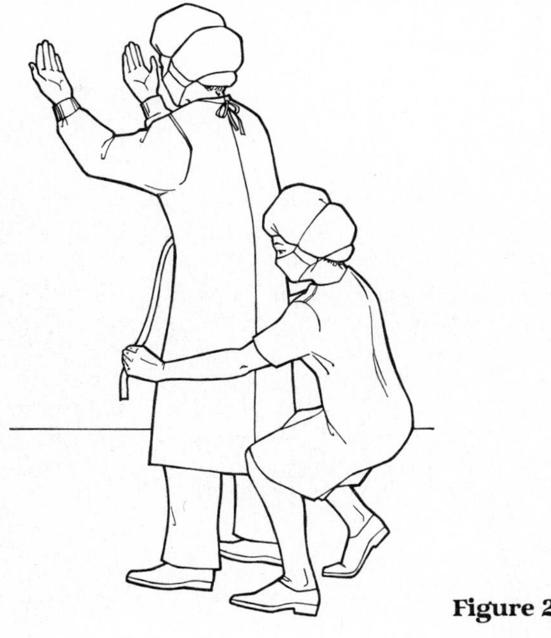

Figure 20–23

Summary

Surgical aseptic practices are intended to eliminate all microorganisms, including spores, from a designated area. Surgical hand washing should precede all techniques that involve surgical asepsis. Although the hands cannot be sterilized, most microorganisms can be removed by washing the hands correctly. Sterile gowns, sterile gloves, and masks are frequently donned to maintain surgical asepsis. Caps that cover the hair are sometimes donned also.

An important aspect of maintaining surgical asepsis in the presence of patients is their education about these practices. For example, patients must learn not to touch sterile equipment. Nurses assess patients before asepsis to determine individual needs; for example, a patient with a respiratory infection may need to mask near a sterile field. The techniques for hand washing, opening sterile packages, handling forceps, pouring solutions, using drapes, masking, gloving, and gowning are frequently used by nurses in the ordinary course of duty.

Suggested Activities

1. In a laboratory setting, practice sterile techniques with a partner. The partner can assist you to evaluate your performance in the following: (a) surgical hand wash, (b) donning and removing a mask, (c) donning and removing sterile gloves, and (d) donning a sterile gown.
2. In the laboratory set up a sterile field using a sterile towel. In this field, (a) open a sterile wrapped package, (b) pour sterile solutions, and (c) open commercially prepared sterile packages.
3. Practice handling different types of forceps with each hand. Practice closing and opening them and using them to lift and set down sterile equipment.

Suggested Readings

Kozier, B., and Erb, G. 1982. *Techniques in clinical nursing: A comprehensive approach.* Menlo Park, Calif.; Addison-Wesley Publishing Co.

Chapter 5 treats practices and principles of surgical asepsis.

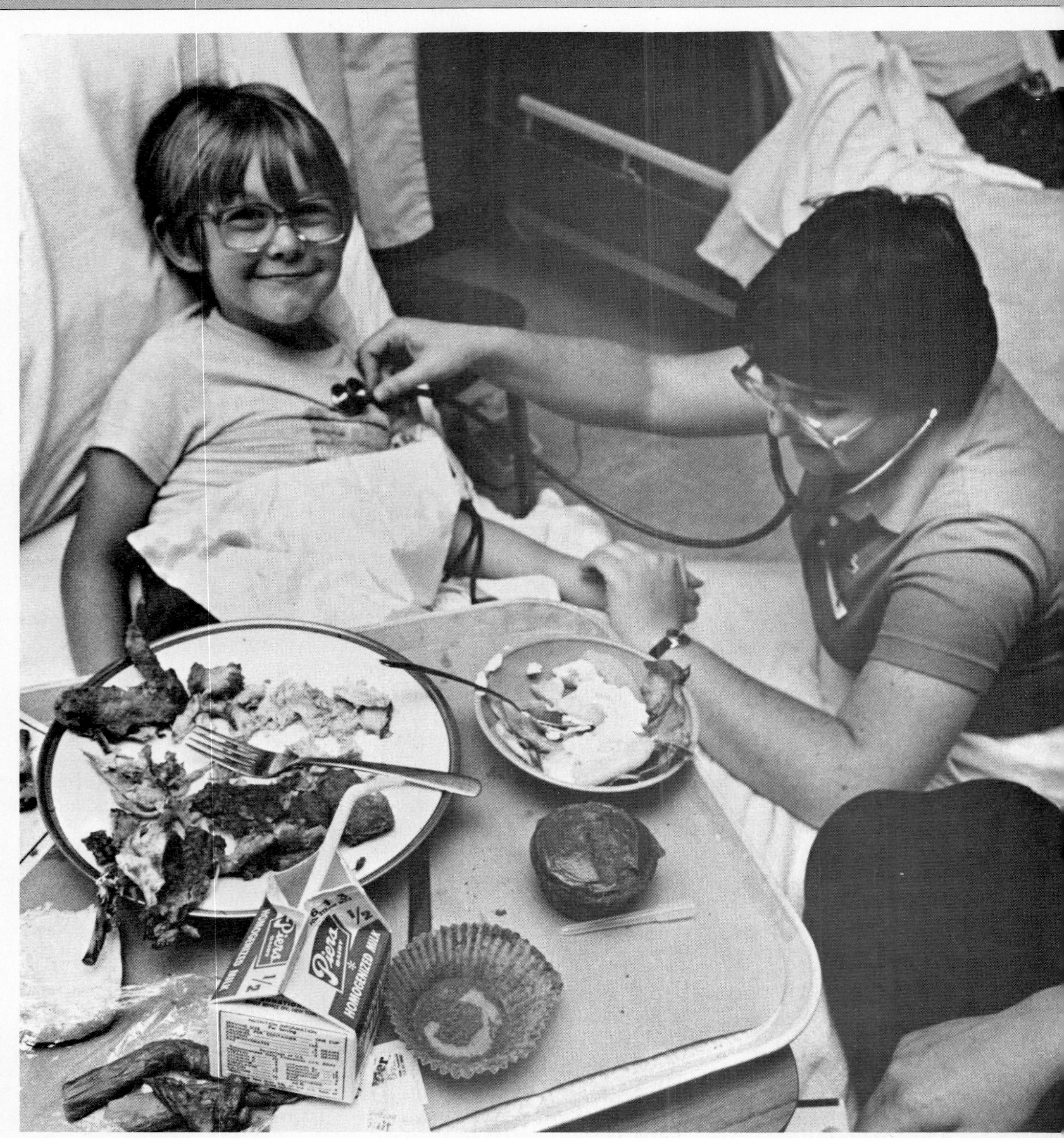
Piera
1/2
HOMOGENIZED MILK

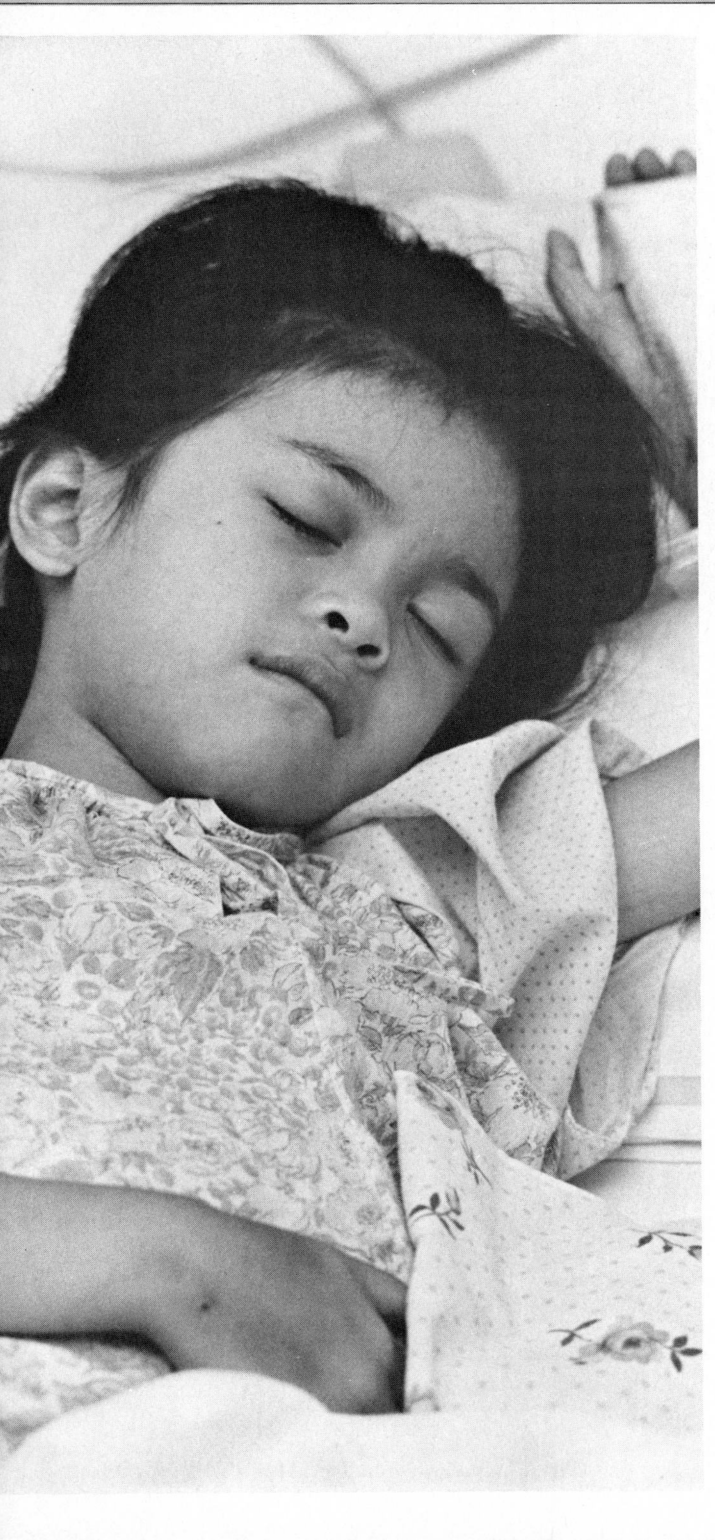

Unit VI

Physiologic Needs of Patients

CONTENTS

Chapter 21

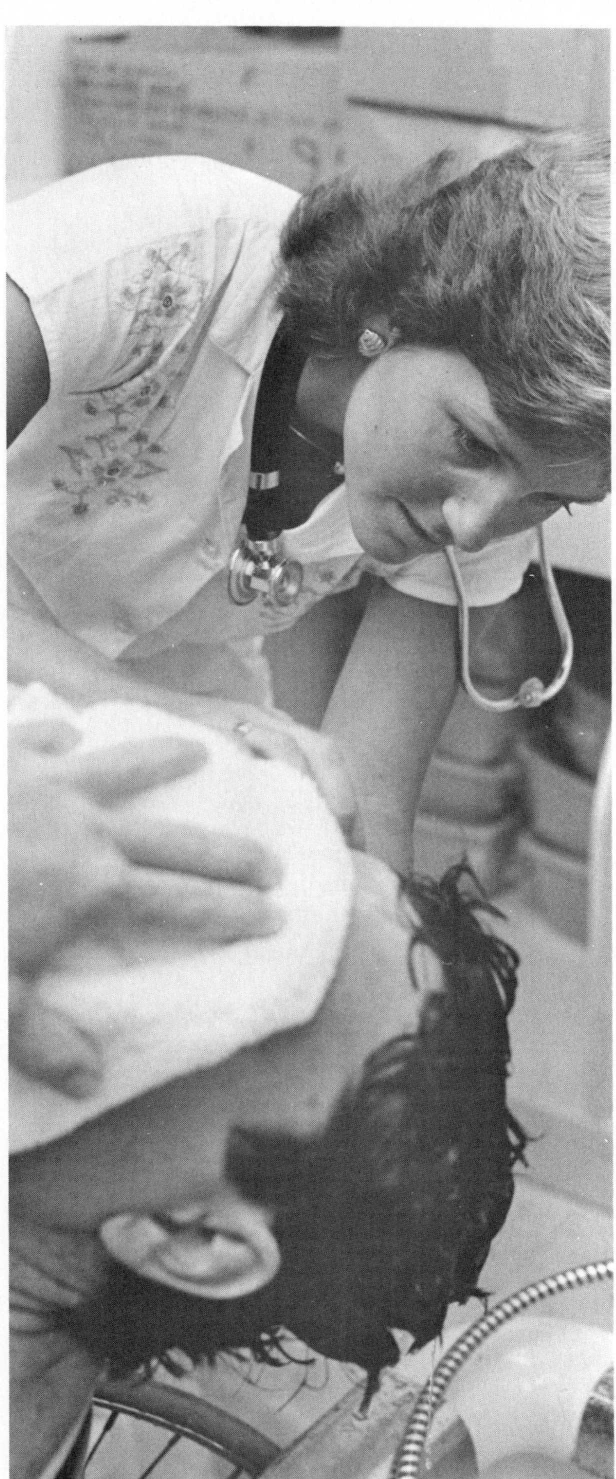

Personal Hygiene

CONTENTS

(Continued on next page)

Beds
Bed Positions
Bed Unit Equipment
Changing Beds
Special Bed Equipment
Specialized Beds

Objectives

1. Understand essential physiologic facts about the skin, feet, nails, mouth, hair, and eyes

- **1.1** Define selected terms
- **1.2** Identify three layers of the skin
- **1.3** Identify three ways in which the skin rids itself of pathogens
- **1.4** Identify five major functions of the skin
- **1.5** Identify four major functions of mucous membrane
- **1.6** Identify specific structures of a tooth
- **1.7** Identify specific structures of the mouth
- **1.8** Identify specific structures of hair

2. Know essential facts about assessment of the skin, mouth, hair, nails, and eyes

- **2.1** Identify normal and abnormal data obtained during physical examination of the skin, feet, nails, mouth, hair, and eyes
- **2.2** Describe variations in the appearance of the skin, nails, and mucous membranes of whites and blacks
- **2.3** Identify developmental changes in the skin, teeth, hair, and nails
- **2.4** Identify factors influencing personal hygiene practices

3. Know facts about common problems and nursing diagnoses associated with the skin, feet, nails, mouth, hair, and eyes

- **3.1** Identify common problems and nursing diagnoses related to the skin
- **3.2** Describe decubitus ulcers
- **3.3** Identify factors that render a person susceptible to skin breakdown
- **3.4** Identify common problems and nursing diagnoses associated with the feet and nails
- **3.5** Identify common problems and selected nursing diagnoses of the mouth
- **3.6** Identify common problems and selected nursing diagnoses related to the hair and scalp
- **3.7** Identify common refraction problems of the eye (see Chapter 14)

4. Understand essential facts about planning and implementing nursing interventions for the skin, feet, nails, mouth, hair, and eyes

- **4.1** Identify nursing goals related to nursing interventions
- **4.2** Identify outcome criteria for evaluating nursing interventions
- **4.3** Identify guidelines for interventions related to the skin
- **4.4** Identify the purposes of bathing
- **4.5** Identify various types of cleaning baths
- **4.6** State the rationale for essential steps in the procedure for bathing an adult in bed
- **4.7** Identify essential aspects of skin care for newborns and infants
- **4.8** Identify essential preventive measures for decubitus ulcers
- **4.9** Identify essential aspects of treating decubiti
- **4.10** Explain four techniques used in back rubs
- **4.11** Identify essential steps in perineal and genital care
- **4.12** Identify essential steps in catheter care
- **4.13** Identify measures to prevent foot problems
- **4.14** Identify essential steps in nail care
- **4.15** Identify essential steps in brushing and flossing teeth
- **4.16** Explain specific ways in which hospitalized patients are assisted with oral hygiene
- **4.17** Identify safety measures involved in denture care
- **4.18** Identify essential steps in brushing, combing, and shampooing hair
- **4.19** Identify essential aspects of eye care
- **4.20** Identify essential steps in applying and removing contact lenses
- **4.21** Identify safety and comfort measures underlying bedmaking procedures

5. Demonstrate beginning skill in assisting patients with hygienic measures

- **5.1** Assist patients with bathing
- **5.2** Provide back rubs
- **5.3** Assist patients with perineal and genital care
- **5.4** Assist patients with foot care
- **5.5** Provide nail care
- **5.6** Assist patients with oral hygiene
- **5.7** Clean dentures
- **5.8** Give special mouth care
- **5.9** Apply and remove patients' contact lenses
- **5.10** Assist patients with hair care
- **5.11** Give patients shampoos
- **5.12** Make occupied and unoccupied beds

Terms

abrasion
acne vulgaris
alopecia
ammonia dermatitis
apocrine sweat gland
arrector pili muscles
athlete's foot
Beau's line
body image
callus
cementum
cerumen
clubbing (of nails)
comedo (plural: comedone)
corn
crown (of tooth)
cyanosis
debride
decubitus ulcer
dental caries
dentin
dentures
dermis
ecchymosis (plural: ecchymoses)
eccrine sweat gland
emaciation
enamel (of tooth)
epidermis
erythema
eschar
excoriation
flushing
frenulum
gingiva
gingivitis
glossitis
hair follicle
hair shaft
halitosis
hemangioma
hirsutism
hygiene
hyperextension bed position
hypodermis
incurvated (ingrown) nail
integumentary system
ischemia
jaundice
keratized cells
lanugo
louse (plural: lice)
mastication
melanin
milia
miliaria rubra
mongolian spots
mucous membrane
necrotic
palate
pallor
paronychia
parotitis
periodontal disease
petechiae
pilosebaceous follicle
plantar wart
reverse Trendelenburg's bed position
sebaceous gland
sebum
smegma
sordes
stomatitis
sudoriferous gland
sulcular technique
terminal hair
tick
tinea pedis
Trendelenburg's bed position
turgor
uvula
vellus
vernix caseosa

Hygiene can be defined as a science of health and its maintenance. Personal hygiene is the care that people themselves take in regard to health. In the literature many types of hygiene are described: mental, oral, sexual, and social are just a few of the subdivisions.

Hygiene is a highly personal matter attached to individual values and practices. It is influenced by cultural, social, familial, and individual factors, as well as by the person's knowledge of health and hygiene and perceptions of personal comfort and needs. People may or may not be aware of their individual needs. A person with particularly odorous feet is likely to be aware of this problem; however, people with underarm perspiration odors may need assistance, for example, from a nurse, to cope with the problem.

When people are ill, hygienic practices frequently become secondary to other functions, such as breathing, which are usually taken for granted. One sign that a formerly ill or depressed patient is feeling better is an interest in shaving, hair care, or makeup.

Hygiene practices involve care of the skin, hair, nails, teeth, oral and nasal cavities, and perineal and genital areas. The skin, hair, and nails are referred to commonly as the *integumentary system*.

Skin

The skin covers the entire surface of the body and thus is the largest organ of the body. At body orifices such as the ears, eyes, nose, rectum, and vagina, the skin is continuous with the mucous membrane that lines these orifices. Skin varies in thickness from about 0.5 mm over the ear lobes to 1.5 mm on the palms of the hands and soles of the feet.

Composition

The skin is made up of three major layers: the epidermis (outer layer), the dermis or corium, and the subcutaneous tissue or hypodermis. The *epidermis* is made up of five layers in most areas of the body, none of which has blood vessels in it. The outermost layer of the epidermis is the stratum corneum or horny layer, which is continually being shed. It consists of dead cells referred to as *keratized cells*, because they are converted to protein before being shed. The other layers of the epidermis are the stratum lucidum, stratum granulosum, stratum spinosum, and the deepest layer, the stratum germinativum. It is in this last layer that new cells are formed and start to move toward the surface; it is also here that *melanin* is formed, which gives skin its dark pigment. Exposure to the sunlight stimulates melanocytes to produce melanin, which gives some people a tan. Certain races have more active melanocytes and hence darker pigmentation to the skin than others. The distribution of pigmentation in dark-skinned people varies considerably. People from the Mediterranean area tend to have very blue lips. Blacks usually have a bluish pigmentation to their gums either evenly distributed or in patches. The observable portion of the sclera of the eyes may also have melanin deposits.

The *dermis* is situated under the epidermis. It is a tough, elastic, flexible tissue, which is highly vascular and contains nerves and nerve endings. The pink tint of skin is due to blood vessels in the dermis. Hair follicles, sweat glands, and oil-supplying glands (*sebaceous glands*) are situated in this layer of the skin. The sebaceous glands secrete *sebum*, an oily substance that lubricates the skin.

Below the dermis is the *hypodermis*. It is a loosely knit connective tissue containing blood and lymph vessels, nerves, and fat globules. It serves to anchor the other skin layers and provides the springy base for the skin.

The normal skin of a healthy person has microorganisms on it that are not harmful. Adults usually have some resident micrococci, bacteria of the genera *Corynebacterium* and *Propionibacterium*, and a genus of fungi, *Pityrosporon*. Children also have gram-positive, spore-forming rods and *Neisseria* bacteria.

Transient microorganisms vary considerably from one person to another. They do not maintain themselves on the skin. Normally the skin can rid itself of pathogenic microorganisms in three general ways: (a) the drying and (b) the chemical effects of the fatty acids in the sebum, and (c) the normal skin pH of 5 to 6, which is too acidic for many microorganisms (Cahn 1960:944).

Functions

The skin serves five major functions:

1. It regulates the body temperature.
2. It protects underlying tissues from drying and injury by preventing the passage of harmful microorganisms. The skin and mucous membrane are considered the body's first line of defense.
3. It secretes *sebum*, which has antibacterial and antifungal qualities.
4. It contains nerve receptors, which are sensitive to pain, temperature, touch, and pressure, thus transmitting these sensations.
5. It aids in vitamin D production.

Sweat Glands

Sudoriferous (sweat) glands are on all body surfaces except the lips and part of the genitals. The body has from two to five million, which are all present at birth. They are most numerous on the palms of the hands and the soles of the feet. Sweat glands are classified as apocrine and eccrine. The *apocrine glands*, located in the axillae and pubic areas, are of little use. Bacteria act upon the sweat produced by these glands, causing odor. The *eccrine* glands are important physiologically. The sweat they produce cools the body through evaporation. Sweat is made up of water, sodium, potassium, chloride, glucose, urea, and lactate.

Assessment of the Skin

Assessment of an individual's skin includes examination of the physical attributes of the skin, consideration of developmental changes, and determination of the individual's hygiene practices and the factors influencing them.

Physical examination

Normal skin has a number of characteristics:

1. It exhibits variations in pigment or color.
2. It has good tissue turgor and is smooth, soft, and flexible.
3. It has a variety of pigmented spots.
4. It shows no evidence of cyanosis, jaundice, or pallor.
5. It feels warm to touch.

Color Skin color varies from person to person and from one area of the body to another. Normal skin tones can range from ivory to deep brown (sometimes called *black*). Some people have hues of pink, yellow, or orange. A description of skin color needs to include deviations from the normal, including increased pigmentation. The skin may reflect pallor, flushing, jaundice, or cyanosis. *Pallor* is a whitish-grayish tinge. In a black-skinned person, pallor can appear as ashen gray and in a brown-skinned person as yellowish-brown. In both instances, the skin appears to have lost its underlying red tones. *Flushing* is redness, which may be generalized or restricted to a particular area. In a dark-skinned person, flushing due to a fever may appear at the tips of the ears. *Jaundice* is a yellow tinge to the skin and is often most readily seen in the sclera of the eyes, in both dark- and light-skinned people. However, in darkly pigmented people jaundice of the sclera needs to be distinguished from deposits of subconjunctival fat; the latter generally appear more concentrated further from the cornea. The color of the mucous membrane of the hard palate can be checked for jaundice to confirm it. *Cyanosis* is a bluish color on the lips, around the mouth, in the nails when they are pressed downward, over the cheekbones, and on the earlobes. In black- and brown-skinned people, cyanosis is difficult to detect. Repeated experience observing the patient's palms, soles, nail beds, and lips often enables the nurse to detect it. The palpebral (eyelid) conjunctiva will also show cyanosis.

Increased or decreased pigmentation is another observation nurses need to note. Some increased pigmentation is perfectly normal and temporary—for example, brown patches on the forehead and cheeks of some pregnant women (chloasma gravidarum, commonly called the *mask of pregnancy*). This particular pigmentation usually disappears spontaneously after childbirth. However, changes in pigmentation may also indicate disease processes.

Texture and turgor Although there is some variation in normal skin, it is usually smooth, soft, and flexible. Skin that is dry, flaking, wrinkled, or holding excessive moisture may reflect serious problems.

Turgor refers to fullness. Skin turgor can be assessed by picking up and pinching the skin. Healthy skin springs back into position, whereas a dehydrated person's skin remains pinched for a short time.

Pigmented spots People have a variety of pigmented areas on their bodies. Infants with black and brown skins often have *mongolian spots*—dark bluish areas on the back or buttocks due to the presence of pigmented cells in the deeper skin layers. They disappear in early childhood. Light-skinned people may have freckles on the face and other parts of the body.

Temperature Palpation of the skin reveals to the nurse whether it is a normal warm temperature or unusually hot or cold. Skin temperature may be similar throughout the body or particular to one area, such as a foot that feels cold due to decreased blood flow.

Lesions Many types of lesions occur on the skin. The nurse's main responsibility is to describe them accurately, including (a) distribution and location, (b) size, (c) contour, and (d) consistency. See Table 14–13 on page 327, which describes the different types of primary skin lesions.

Excoriations and abrasions An *excoriation* is the loss of superficial layers of the skin. For example, if a nurse scratches a patient while palpating with long fingernails, the scratch is an excoriation. An *abrasion* is the wearing away of a structure such as the skin or teeth, often by friction (for example, when a patient is dragged instead of rolled across a bed).

Developmental changes

In early embryonic life the skin is a single layer of cells. Other layers develop quickly. The fetus's skin is covered by a substance called *vernix caseosa*, a whitish, cheesy material seen on newborns. It usually disappears in the first day. The skin of an infant is thinner than an adult's, it is usually mottled, and in whites it varies from pink to red and becomes ruddy when the baby cries. Babies who are genetically dark-skinned are lightly pigmented at birth. Skin pigmentation gradually increases until about 6 or 8 weeks. Sweat glands of babies begin to function at about 1 month of age.

In adolescence the sebaceous glands increase in activity as a result of increased levels of hormones (androgens). This is thought to be one factor responsible for the development of acne, a common skin problem of adolescents. For further information, see page 489 in this chapter.

The older adult also experiences skin changes. The skin tends to be thinner and drier, with fine wrinkling and some inelasticity. This process appears anytime from 40 years on. The elderly person's skin typically shows wrinkles, sagging, pigmentations, and keratotic spots usually on areas exposed to the sun. The skin is less resilient, that is, when pinched it returns to place more slowly than the skin of a younger person.

Factors influencing skin care

Each individual has unique hygiene practices concerning bathing, tooth and mouth care, hair care, the control of body odors, and the use of cosmetics. These practices are influenced by the individual's body image, sociocultural factors, the expectations of the person's social group, and the person's knowledge level, developmental status, personal preferences, and health.

Body image *Body image* is the continually changing concept that an individual has of his or her own body. One man may view his body as trim, clean, and neatly groomed, whereas another sees himself as untidy and ungroomed. The view affects to some degree the hygienic practices of the individual. People who see themselves as clean and neatly groomed are likely to have established practices to support this view.

Sociocultural factors Many sociocultural factors affect hygienic practices. The individual's economic resources affect such practices as the use of cosmetics. Cultural patterns influence the frequency of bathing. For example, in some European cultures a full tub bath is normally not taken more than once a week, whereas in North America people may bathe once a day if water and facilities are available.

Expectations of the person's social group A number of social groups, e.g., family, work groups, and friends, may affect a person's hygienic practices. Early in life children learn practices from their parents, and these are often continued in adult life. Some practices relate to physical conditions, such as the availability of hot water and the number of people in the family, as well as to family customs. Perhaps a father believes the use of deodorant is unmanly. His sons may adopt this attitude or, on the contrary, use deodorants because of other influences. Teenagers who want to be accepted by their peers will wash frequently and use advertised deodorants and hair creams. If the school football hero uses a particular toothpaste, boys who admire him may use it. A person's colleagues at work often have expectations that affect hygiene practices. Nurses usually expect other nurses to be clean and without body odor, whereas members of a male logging crew may consider body odor masculine and the use of deodorants effeminate.

Knowledge level The information an individual possesses about hygiene affects his or her practices. Knowledge about the effect of personal appearance on others, the various methods to maintain hygiene, and the implications of hygienic practices for health can alter a person's practices.

Developmental status Hygiene practices vary with an individual's stage of development. Many adolescents spend considerable time on their appearance, reflecting the values of their peer group. A 4-year-old, in contrast, may enjoy being dirty and resist parents' efforts to encourage washing.

Personal preferences Preferences often reflect a person's values and are highly individual. They can dictate the brand of soap used, the frequency of bathing, and the choice of a bath rather than a shower. For some people, to be in a tub of water is a luxury to be enjoyed after a day of work; to others, it is a waste of time that could be used to better advantage. Nurses' own personal preferences should not affect their assessment of appropriate behavior for patients in light of their health status. For example, a nurse may believe that daily bathing is appropriate, while a patient is accustomed to bathing once a week. If bathing once a week does not affect the patient's health, the nurse should not try to change the pattern. The nurse needs to intervene if a patient's hygiene practices warrant change for health reasons. A female patient, for example, who repeatedly has infections in the skin creases of the groin and under the breasts needs to learn to wash and thoroughly dry those areas each day, rather than once a week.

Health state People who are very ill often are unable or lack the energy to bathe or brush their teeth, for example. They require assistance to carry out many hygienic activities. It is important for nurses to know exactly how much a patient can safely do and how much assistance is required.

Nursing Diagnoses: Common Skin Problems

Nurses frequently observe problems of the skin. Some need to be brought to a physician's attention; others require minimal care; and still others eventually disappear without intervention. Nursing diagnoses of skin problems requiring intervention can be categorized as (a) actual impairment of skin integrity, and (b) potential impairment of skin integrity (Kim and Moritz 1982:312).

Actual impairment of skin integrity

Skin integrity may be either disrupted or destroyed. Disruptions involve surface layers of the skin, while destruction may involve all layers.

Disruptions of skin integrity The following are common examples of skin disruptions:

1. *Miliaria rubra* (prickly heat rash) in infants appears as small, red, irritated lesions most often on the face, neck, trunk, and diaper areas. It is due to excess heat. Usually if the baby is kept cooler, often with fewer clothes, the rash disappears.

2. *Milia* (milk spots) in newborns are white spots due to plugged sebaceous glands. They are commonly present on the newborn's face, particularly across the nose and cheeks. They normally disappear in a few weeks with no treatment.

3. *Mongolian spots* are bluish discolorations usually seen in the sacral area of dark-skinned babies. They generally disappear without treatment as the baby gets older.

4. *Hemangiomas* are vascular lesions present at birth. There are a number of types, most of which disappear eventually. However, nurses should refer the child to a physician for accurate diagnoses of the type and treatment if it is indicated. In observing a hemangioma, the nurse notes and records the size, shape, exact color (such as pink or port wine color), and elevation (whether flat or raised from the skin).

5. *Diaper rash*, also referred to as *ammonia dermatitis*, is caused by skin bacteria reacting with urea, a product related to ammonia and excreted in the urine. This reaction is irritating to the baby's perineum and buttocks, causing them to appear red and sore. Diaper rash can usually be prevented by keeping the buttocks clean and dry. Protective ointments such as baby oil or petroleum jelly (Vaseline) may be preventive but are not usually needed. Pastes that are difficult to remove should be avoided. A good treatment for diaper rash is to expose the baby's buttocks to the air and to a 40-watt gooseneck lamp placed 30 cm (12 in) away. This can be done several times a day for about 30 minutes. The lamp provides drying as well as warmth for the baby. Boiling the diapers removes the bacteria; however, most detergents now have antibacterial agents in them. Thorough rinsing is critical to remove the detergent.

6. *Erythema* (redness) is associated with a variety of rashes, infections, and drug reactions. It is also an early sign of impaired circulation resulting from prolonged pressure. See the discussion of decubitus ulcers on page 497.

7. *Petechiae* are tiny, pinpoint, nonraised, round, red or purple areas in the skin, due to intradermal or submucous hemorrhages or tiny thrombi. They are often associated with chronic diseases of the heart and lungs. Petechiae do not blanch with pressure and often fade within a few days.

8. *Ecchymoses* are collections of blood beneath the skin, commonly known as *bruises*. Initially an ecchymosis is bluish-purple, firm, and tender; as the blood is absorbed it becomes yellowish and softens.

9. *Acne vulgaris*, the etiology of which is still unclear, is a common problem of adolescents. It involves the *pilosebaceous follicles* (the hair follicle and sebaceous gland complex) of the "flush areas" of the skin (face, neck, shoulders, upper chest, and back). Two types of acne are categorized: noninflamed and inflamed. In *noninflamed acne*, the pilosebaceous follicle becomes obstructed and dilated, causing a comedo to form. A *comedo* (plural: *comedones*) is a mass consisting of keratin, lipids, fatty acids, and bacteria. Comedones may be either closed or open. Closed comedones are whiteheads with no visible opening. Open comedones have a visible opening and appear as blackheads, due to discoloration of the fatty acids by oxidation from the air. Noninflamed acne may disappear or may become inflamed as a result of infection. *Inflamed acne* results when the pilosebaceous follicles rupture and papules, pustules, nodules, and cysts appear. Acne can result in severe skin destruction and scarring if left untreated.

A number of factors are involved in the development of acne: heredity, increased levels of hormones (androgens), emotional stress, and cold winter weather are some. There is no positive evidence that certain foods are a factor, although some adolescents may report that symptoms are aggravated after they eat certain foods.

Treatment of acne varies according to the types of lesions. Medical and nursing goals are prevention of comedo formation, removal of existing comedones, control of infection, and prevention of scar formation. General intervention for all types of acne includes meticulous cleanliness of the skin (to prevent infection), adequate rest, moderate exercise, reduction of stress, consumption of a balanced diet, removal of any foci for infection, avoidance of cosmetic creams or oils that add to the plugging of follicles, and avoidance of exposure to excessive humidity or heat, which can cause exacerbations of symptoms in severe acne. Medical therapies for acne vary considerably and are beyond the scope of this book.

Destruction of skin integrity Examples of destruction of skin integrity are burns and decubitus ulcers. The subject of burns is beyond the scope of this book; decubitus ulcers are discussed in detail on page 497.

Potential impairment of skin integrity

Many factors make persons susceptible to skin breakdown and ulcerations, particularly over the bony prominences of the body:

1. *Alterations in nutritional status*, such as emaciation and insufficient protein intake. *Emaciation* is a wasted appearance due to extreme weight loss. In emaciated individuals, subcutaneous fat is insufficient to provide padding or support over bony prominences to withstand normal stress or pressure. Individuals with inadequate protein intake are also prone to skin breakdown since protein is essential for the building, maintenance, and repair of all body tissues.

2. *Physical immobility.* Normally people change position frequently, even during sleep. When position cannot be altered, e.g., if the person is paralyzed or unconscious, or when it is not altered for prolonged periods (1 or 2 hours), blood circulation, which carries essential nutrients to the skin, is reduced. Without essential nutrients, tissues of the skin are ultimately destroyed.

3. *Altered hydration.* In dehydrated individuals, the skin becomes excessively dry, and skin turgor (firmness and elasticity) is diminished. Both conditions make the skin less resistant to injury.

4. *Altered sensation.* Loss of sensation in a body area may be the result of paralysis or other neurologic disease. With loss of sensation, a person's ability to discern injurious heat and cold and to feel the tingling (pins and needles) that signals loss of circulation is impaired. This makes the person prone to skin damage.

5. *Presence of secretions or excretions on the skin.* An accumulation of secretions such as perspiration and sebum or excretions such as urine or feces is irritating to the skin, harbors microorganisms, and makes an individual prone to skin breakdown and infection.

6. *Mechanical devices.* The presence of restraints, casts, or braces that create pressure or a shearing force can alter skin integrity considerably.

7. *Altered venous circulation.* Stasis of venous blood in the lower extremities, which is associated with varicose veins, can cause stasis dermatitis (inflammation of the skin) on the feet and around the ankles. This dermatitis is characterized by redness, dryness, itching, and swelling. Ultimately skin tissues become *ischemic*

(deficient of blood) and *necrotic* (dying), and ulcerations form. See Figure 21–4 later in this chapter.

Examples of nursing diagnoses

1. Impaired skin integrity related to:
   a. Prolonged immobility
   b. Acne vulgaris
   c. Drug reaction
   d. Urinary incontinence
   e. Burns
   f. Malnutrition
   g. Altered venous circulation
   h. Altered sensation
   i. Shearing force of cast
2. Risk of (potential) impaired skin integrity related to:
   a. Prolonged immobility
   b. Urinary incontinence
   c. Malnutrition
   d. Altered venous circulation
   e. Altered sensation

Planning and Intervention for the Skin

Nursing goals

The overall nursing goal is to maintain the integrity of the skin. Subgoals are:

1. To prevent the accumulation of secretions and excretions
2. To prevent infections
3. To stimulate circulation of the blood
4. To enhance the patient's self-esteem

Planning

Planning for assisting a patient with personal hygiene includes consideration of: the patient's personal preferences, health, and limitations; the time; and the equipment, facilities, and personnel available. Patients' personal preferences—about when and how they bathe, for example—should be followed as long as they are compatible with the patient's health needs, the equipment available, etc. Nurses need to provide whatever assistance the patient requires because of individual limitations. The nurse may provide help directly or delegate this task to other nursing personnel. In some instances patients say they can perform activities, e.g., shaving, that they should not or cannot do. Nurses need to be guided by the health needs of the patient, which are often specified on the nursing care plan.

Planning involves establishing outcome criteria. For suggestions, see page 497.

Guidelines for interventions

1. *An intact, healthy skin is the body's first line of defense.* It protects the body from invasion by microorganisms and from harmful agents such as chemicals. Nurses need to ensure that all skin care measures prevent injury and irritation. Scratching the skin with jewelry or long, sharp fingernails is avoided. Harsh rubbing or use of rough towels and washcloths can cause tissue damage, particularly when the skin is irritated or when circulation or sensation is diminished. Bottom bedsheets are kept taut and free from wrinkles to reduce friction and abrasion to the skin. Top bed linens are arranged to prevent undue pressure on the toes. When necessary bed cradles or footboards are used to keep bedclothes off the feet.
2. *The degree to which the skin protects the underlying tissues from injury depends on the general health of the cells, the amount of subcutaneous tissue, and the dryness of the skin.* Skin that is poorly nourished and dry has less ability to protect and is more vulnerable to injury. When the skin is dry, lotions or creams with lanolin are applied, and bathing is limited to once or twice a week. For backrubs, lotion is used, rather than alcohol. The greater the amount of subcutaneous tissue, the more padding there is, particularly over bony prominences. Nurses also assess the patient's nutritional and fluid intake. When either one is deficient, measures are taken to improve it.
3. *Moisture in contact with the skin for a period of time can result in increased bacterial growth and irritation.* After a bath, the patient's skin is dried carefully, paying particular attention to potential irritation areas, such as the axillae, the groin, beneath the breasts, and between the toes. A nonirritating dusting powder, such as cornstarch, tends to reduce moisture and can be applied to these areas after they are dried. If patients are incontinent of urine or feces or if they perspire excessively, immediate cleaning is provided to prevent skin irritation.
4. *Body odors are caused by resident bacteria of the skin acting on body secretions.* Cleanliness is the best deodorant. Commercial deodorants and antiperspirants can be applied only after the skin is cleaned. Deodorants diminish odors, whereas antiperspirants reduce the amount of perspiration. Neither is applied immediately after shaving, because of the possibility of skin irritation. They are also withheld from skin that is already irritated.
5. *Skin sensitivity to irritation and injury varies among individuals and in accordance with their health.* Generally speaking, skin sensitivity is greater in infants, very young children, and the elderly. A person's nutritional status also affects sensitivity. Excessively emaciated or obese persons tend to experience more skin irritation and injury. The same tendency occurs

among individuals with poor dietary habits and insufficient fluid intake. Even in healthy persons, skin sensitivity is highly variable. Some people's skin is sensitive to chemicals in skin care agents and cosmetics. Hypoallergenic cosmetics and soaps or soap substitutes are now available for these people. The nurse needs to ascertain whether the patient has any sensitivities and what agents are appropriate to use.

6. *Agents used for skin care have selective actions and purposes.* Commonly used agents are described in Kozier and Erb (1982:351, Table 12–1).

Bathing and Skin Care

Purposes of bathing

Bathing has a number of functions. The skin is physiologically bathed continuously with sebum and perspiration from the sebaceous and sudoriferous glands, respectively. Sebum and perspiration have protective functions: Sebum prevents dryness, and perspiration provides a slightly acid medium, which discourages bacterial growth. These two processes, however, can be injurious or disadvantageous if bathing is not carried out regularly, so that perspiration, sebum, and dead skin cells accumulate. Excessive perspiration interacts with bacteria on the skin, causing body odor, considered offensive in some cultures. An accumulation of sebum on the skin can be irritating in itself, since it assists the growth of bacteria. Large numbers of bacteria on the skin can cause problems, particularly when the skin integrity is interrupted, for example, by a cut. Dead skin cells also harbor bacteria. Bathing, then, removes accumulated oil, perspiration, dead skin cells, and some bacteria. The quantity of oil and dead skin cells produced can be appreciated when nurses observe the skin of a person after the removal of a cast that has been on for 6 weeks. The skin will be crusty, flaky, and dry underneath the cast. Applications of oil over several days are usually necessary to remove the debris.

Excessive bathing, on the other hand, can interfere with the intended lubricating effect of the sebum, causing dryness of the skin. This is an important consideration for people who produce limited sebum.

In addition to its cleaning value, bathing also stimulates circulation. A warm or hot bath dilates superficial arterioles, bringing more blood and nourishment to the skin. Vigorous rubbing has the same effect. Rubbing with long smooth strokes from the distal to proximal parts of extremities is particularly effective in facilitating venous blood flow.

Bathing also produces a sense of well-being for people. It is refreshing and relaxing and frequently boosts a person's morale, appearance, and self-respect. Some people take a morning shower for its refreshing, stimulating effect. Others prefer an evening bath because it is relaxing. These effects are more prominent when a person is ill. For example, it is not uncommon for patients who have had a restless or sleepless night to feel relaxed, comfortable, and sleepy after a morning bath.

The effectiveness of bathing in eliminating some body odors can also be important. The apocrine glands, which produce sweat, are situated in the axillae and pubic areas and appear at puberty. Their secretions are decomposed by bacterial action, resulting in a prominent odor that is often distasteful to others. Apocrine glands are thought to secrete less after menopause and to enlarge and become more active before and after monthly menses. The use of antiperspirants to control perspiration and odor from the axillae is prevalent in North America. On occasion the nurse may recommend its use to persons with problem perspiration.

The bathing procedure can offer opportunities for the nurse to assess ill patients. The nurse can observe the condition of the patient's skin and physical conditions such as sacral edema or rashes. The skin is said to mirror health, but it is not always an accurate index. While assisting a patient with a bath, the nurse can also assess the patient's mental and emotional state, for example, orientation to time and ability to cope with the illness. Learning needs, such as a diabetic patient's need to learn foot care, can also be assessed.

Kinds of baths

There are generally two categories of baths given to patients: cleaning and therapeutic. Cleaning baths are given chiefly for hygienic purposes whereas therapeutic baths are given for a physical effect, such as to soothe irritated skin or to treat an area (e.g., the perineum).

Cleaning baths

1. *Complete bed bath.* The nurse washes the entire body of a dependent patient in bed.

2. *Self-help bed bath.* A patient confined to bed is able to bathe himself or herself with help from the nurse for washing the back and perhaps the feet.

3. *Partial bath (abbreviated bath).* Only the parts of the patient's body that might cause discomfort or odor, if neglected, are washed: the face, hands, axillae, perineal area, and back. Omitted are the arms, chest, abdomen, legs, and feet. The nurse provides this care for dependent patients and assists self-sufficient bedridden patients by washing their backs. Some ambulatory patients prefer to take a partial bath at the sink. The nurse can assist them by washing their backs.

4. *Tub bath.* Tub baths are preferred to bed baths, since washing and rinsing are easier in a tub. Tubs are also used for therapeutic baths. The amount of assistance offered by the nurse depends on the abilities of the patient. Many agencies have specially designed tubs for dependent patients. These tubs greatly facilitate the work of the nurse in lifting patients in and out of the tub and offer patients greater benefits than a sponge bath in bed.

5. *Shower.* Many ambulatory patients are able to use shower facilities and require only minimal assistance from the nurse.

Therapeutic baths A therapeutic bath is usually ordered by a physician. Medications may be placed in the water to come in contact with parts of the body, often large skin areas. A therapeutic bath is generally taken in a tub one-third or one-half full, about 114 liters (30 gal). The patient remains in the bath for a designated time, often 20 to 30 minutes. If the patient's back, chest, and arms are to be treated, these areas need to be immersed in the solution. The bath temperature is generally ordered by the physician; 37.7 to 40.5 C (100 to 105 F) is frequently used for adults and 40.5 C (105 F) is usually ordered for infants. See Kozier and Erb (1982:353) for types of therapeutic baths.

Time and frequency of bathing

The time of day and frequency of bathing are highly variable. Some people prefer morning baths, whereas others prefer the evening. The environment and activity of the person dictate the frequency of bathing. If the weather is hot or if a person engages in athletic endeavors, more than one bath may be taken daily. The age of the person also dictates frequency. Elderly people rarely require bathing more than once or twice a week because of the reduction in the amount of their skin oil and perspiration.

When people are ill, the frequency of bathing may need to be increased. Very ill patients may require at least one bath daily. People confined to bed are not subjected to the air currents that normally help to evaporate perspiration. This is accentuated for patients who have high fevers and are diaphoretic. In contrast, some illnesses decrease body perspiration.

Usually hospital policies prescribe the frequency of baths. Full baths and complete bed linen changes may be offered twice a week for patients, and partial baths, that is, of the face, hands, axillae, back, and pubic areas are offered the rest of the time. *This does not preclude additional baths if necessitated by illness or in the nurse's judgment.* Institutions commonly schedule baths in the morning. For patients who are accustomed to bathing in the evening before retiring, this routine may be a source of frustration.

Procedure 21–1 Bathing an Adult in Bed

Equipment

1. Two bath towels, one for the face and one for the remainder of the body.
2. A washcloth.
3. Soap in a soap dish.
4. A basin for the wash water.
5. Hygienic supplies such as lotion, powder, and deodorant.
6. A bath blanket to cover the patient during the bath.
7. Water between 43 and 46 C (110 and 115 F) for adults. The water should feel comfortably warm to the patient. People vary in their sensitivity to heat. Most patients will verify a suitable temperature.
8. A clean gown or pajamas as needed.
9. Additional bed linen and towels, if required.
10. A bedpan or urinal.

Intervention

1. Explain what you plan to do. Adjust the explanation to the patient's needs.

   Rationale This reassures the patient by providing knowledge of what will happen, identifies the patient, and allows the nurse to assess whether any special equipment is needed, such as a razor.

2. Make sure the room is free from drafts by closing windows and doors.

   Rationale Air currents increase loss of heat from the body by convection.

3. Provide privacy by drawing the curtains or closing the door.

   Rationale Hygiene is a personal matter.

4. Offer the patient a bedpan or urinal.

   Rationale The patient will be more comfortable after voiding, and voiding is advisable before cleaning the perineum.

Procedure 21–1, continued

5. Wash hands.

Rationale This prevents transmission of microorganisms to the patient.

6. Place the bed in the high position.

Rationale This avoids undue strain on the nurse's back.

7. Remove the top bed linen, and replace it with the bath blanket. If the bed linen is to be reused, place it over the bedside chair. If it is to be changed, place it in the linen hamper.

8. Assist the patient to move near you.

Rationale This facilitates access without undue reaching and straining.

9. Remove the patient's gown.

10. Make a bath mitt with the washcloth (see Figure 21–1):

a. Triangular method: (1) Lay your hand on the washcloth; (2) fold the top corner over your hand; (3, 4) fold the side corners over the hand; (5) tuck the second corner under the cloth on the palmar side to secure the mitt.

b. Rectangular method: (1) Lay your hand on the washcloth, and fold one side over your hand; (2) fold the second side over your hand; (3) fold the top of the cloth down, and tuck it under the folded side against your palm to secure the mitt.

Rationale A bath mitt retains water and heat better than a cloth loosely held.

11. Place one towel across the patient's chest.

12. Wash the patient's eyes with water only, and dry them well. Use a separate corner of the washcloth for each eye, and wipe from the inner to the outer canthus.

Rationale Use of separate corners prevents transmitting microorganisms from one eye to the other. Cleaning from the inner to the outer canthus prevents secretions from entering the nasolacrimal ducts.

13. Ask whether the patient wants soap used on the face. Wash and dry the patient's face, neck, and ears.

Rationale Soap has a drying effect, and the face, which is exposed to the air more than other body parts, tends to be drier.

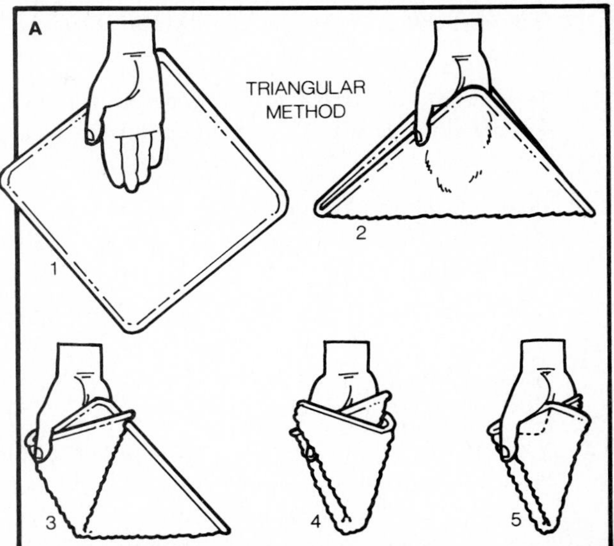

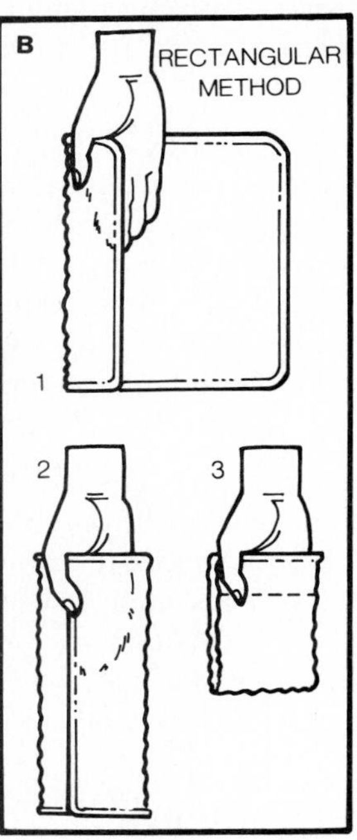

Figure 21–1

14. Place the bath towel lengthwise under the patient's arm. Wash and dry the arm, using long, firm strokes from distal to proximal areas (from the point furthest from the body to the point closest). Wash the axilla well. Repeat for the other arm. Exercise caution if an IV is pres-

Procedure 21–1, continued

ent, and check its flow following movement of the arm.

Rationale The bath towel protects the bed from becoming wet. Firm strokes from distal to proximal areas increase venous blood return.

15. Place the patient's hands in the basin. Wash and dry them, paying particular attention to the spaces between the fingers.

Rationale Many patients enjoy immersing their hands in the basin and washing themselves. The nurse can place the basin directly on the bed with a towel under it.

16. Fold the bath blanket down to the patient's pubic area and place the towel alongside the chest and abdomen. Wash and dry the patient's chest and abdomen, giving special attention to the skin fold under the breasts. Keep the patient's chest and abdomen covered with the towel between the wash and the rinse. Replace the bath blanket when the areas have been dried.

Rationale It is important to avoid undue exposure when washing the patient's chest and abdomen. For some patients, it may be preferable to wash the chest and the abdomen separately. In that case, the bath towel is placed horizontally across the abdomen first and then across the chest.

17. Wrap one leg and foot with the bath blanket, ensuring that the pubic area is well covered. Place the bath towel lengthwise under the other leg, and wash that leg. Use long, smooth, firm strokes, washing from the ankle to the knee and from the knee to the thigh. Dry that leg, reverse the coverings, and repeat for the other leg.

Rationale Washing from distal to proximal areas stimulates venous blood flow.

18. Wash the feet by placing them in the basin of water. Dry each foot. Pay particular attention to the spaces between the toes. If you prefer, wash one foot after that leg, before the other leg is washed.

19. Obtain fresh, warm bath water.

Rationale The temperature of the water in the basin cools relatively rapidly, and the water becomes soapy. It needs to be changed often.

20. Assist the patient to turn to a prone or side-lying position. Place the bath towel lengthwise alongside the patient's back and buttocks. Wash and dry the back, buttocks, and upper thighs, paying particular attention to the gluteal folds. Give a back rub. See page 501.

Rationale The towels are handled in the same manner as for the abdomen and chest, to avoid undue exposure of the patient.

21. Assist the patient to the supine position, and clean the perineum. See page 503.

Rationale Many patients prefer to clean their own perineums, if they are able, because it is embarrassing to have this done by another person.

22. Assist the patient to use any hygienic aids desired, such as powder, lotion, or deodorant.

23. Help the patient to put on a clean gown or pajamas. If intravenous apparatus is attached, place the sleeve of the gown over the infusion bottle first.

24. Assist the patient with hair, mouth, and nail care. See the discussions later in this chapter. Some patients prefer or need mouth care prior to the bath.

25. Make the patient's bed. See page 524.

26. Assist the patient to a comfortable position.

27. Place the call light and other needed items within easy reach of the patient.

Rationale This avoids the risk that the patient will fall while reaching for them.

28. Clean and dry the bath basin and soap dish. Replace all equipment in the bedside unit. If the bath blanket is not soiled, store it for future use.

29. Record on the patient's chart significant observations made during the bath (such as excoriation in the folds beneath the breasts or reddened areas over bony prominences) and progress in relief of previous problems.

30. Report to the responsible nurse any abnormal or unusual data, such as difficult breathing on exertion, abnormal color, or excoriated or reddened skin areas.

Skin care for the newborn

Practices in skin care of the newborn vary from agency to agency. When the baby is first admitted to the nursery, some agencies offer an admission bath; others remove any blood or vernix caseosa from the infant's face for aesthetic reasons only, then diaper and wrap the baby loosely in a blanket. The newborn's temperature-regulating mechanisms are undeveloped, so measures to avoid chilling are important. Hexachlorophene soap was previously used for admission baths to prevent staphylococcus infections in nurseries. However, its use has been largely discontinued, since it was suggested that central nervous system damage follows repeated use. After the newborn's status is stabilized, daily hygienic care includes a sponge bath (optional) until the cord falls off, cleaning the genitals and buttocks with diaper changes, cord care, and, for some male infants, circumcision care. If sponging is done, small soft washcloths or cotton balls should be used. The vernix caseosa usually disappears in about 24 hours. If it persists in creases and folds, it can become an irritant and needs to be removed with gentle wiping with a cotton ball moistened with warm water.

The cord falls off spontaneously, usually in 5 to 8 days, but it may last up to 2 weeks. Attempts should *not* be made to remove it. To encourage drying of the cord and to discourage infection, the base of the cord is wiped once a day with alcohol. In most nurseries the cord is left exposed to the air; however, in some agencies a small gauze dressing is applied. This needs to be changed when soiled.

For babies who are circumcised, the penis must be inspected for bleeding, although most incisions heal rapidly. If the baby is diapered lightly over the penis, bleeding will be noticeable on the diaper if it occurs. Immediately after a circumcision the area is covered with sterile gauze saturated with petroleum jelly. This gauze may be left on until it falls off spontaneously or it may be removed when the infant voids; the area is then cleaned gently with moistened cotton balls, and a new dressing is applied each time the diaper is changed.

Smegma, a curdlike secretion, may collect under the prepuce of the glans in male babies and between the labia in female babies. This can be removed with a moistened cotton ball. For females one swab should be used for each stroke, moving from the front of the body toward the back.

Babies are usually clothed in a shirt and a diaper, although the shirt may or may not be necessary depending on the temperature of the environment. Babies do not perspire for the first month nor do they respond with gooseflesh; therefore the nurse must use judgment about clothing babies appropriately. If they are too hot, they develop miliaria rubra (prickly heat, a rash) on the face, neck, and/or places where skin surfaces touch.

Infant bathing

Sponge baths are given to infants until the cord stump disappears and the umbilicus is well healed. Then tub baths may be given. The general bathing measures previously discussed should be employed for the infant's bath, paying particular attention to preventing undue exposure.

Sponge bath The equipment required for sponging the baby depends on agency facilities and policies. Generally included are a shirt, a diaper, safety pins, a soft washcloth, cotton balls, a towel, a paper bag for soiled cotton balls, facial tissue or toilet tissue to remove feces, and a basin of water at 38 to 40.5 C (100 to 105 F). The water should feel slightly warm to the inside of the wrist or the elbow. Optional materials include alcohol to apply at the base of the cord stump, mineral oil or petroleum jelly for protection against diaper rash, and mild soap. If soap is used, it should be used sparingly, since it can be drying to a baby's skin. Cotton-tipped applicators are contraindicated, because they can break when the baby moves, causing injury to the mucous membranes of the nose or to an eardrum. Powders are also avoided, since the baby may inhale them while they are being shaken from the container. Powders also tend to cake with moisture and cause skin irritation.

The infant's face, neck, ears, and scalp are cleaned before the baby is undressed. The baby's eyes, behind the ears, and neck creases can be wiped with a cotton ball. The eyes are wiped from the inner canthus to the outer canthus using one cotton ball for each stroke. The inside of the ears can be cleaned with a rolled wisp of cotton, dampened and rotated gently in the ear. To clean the baby's scalp, the nurse slides one hand under the baby until the baby's head is well supported in the palm, and picks up the baby securely. The baby's head is held over the basin, soaped, rinsed, and dried thoroughly.

The infant's shirt is then removed and the trunk, arms, and legs are washed. The infant is turned to wash the back. Alcohol may be applied at the base of the cord stump before putting the shirt back on. To put on an open-fronted shirt, the nurse lays the baby in the shirt and then reaches through a sleeve and grasps the baby's arm to pull it through the sleeve. For a pullover shirt, the nurse pulls the neck opening rapidly over the baby's head and then pulls the arms through the sleeves.

The baby's buttocks and perineum are cleaned last. First excess feces are removed with facial tissue or toilet tissue. The genital area is cleaned from front to back. The circumcised area should not require special care, and the trend is *not* to retract the foreskin of uncircumcised male infants. The folds between the labia and around the scrotum should receive particular attention

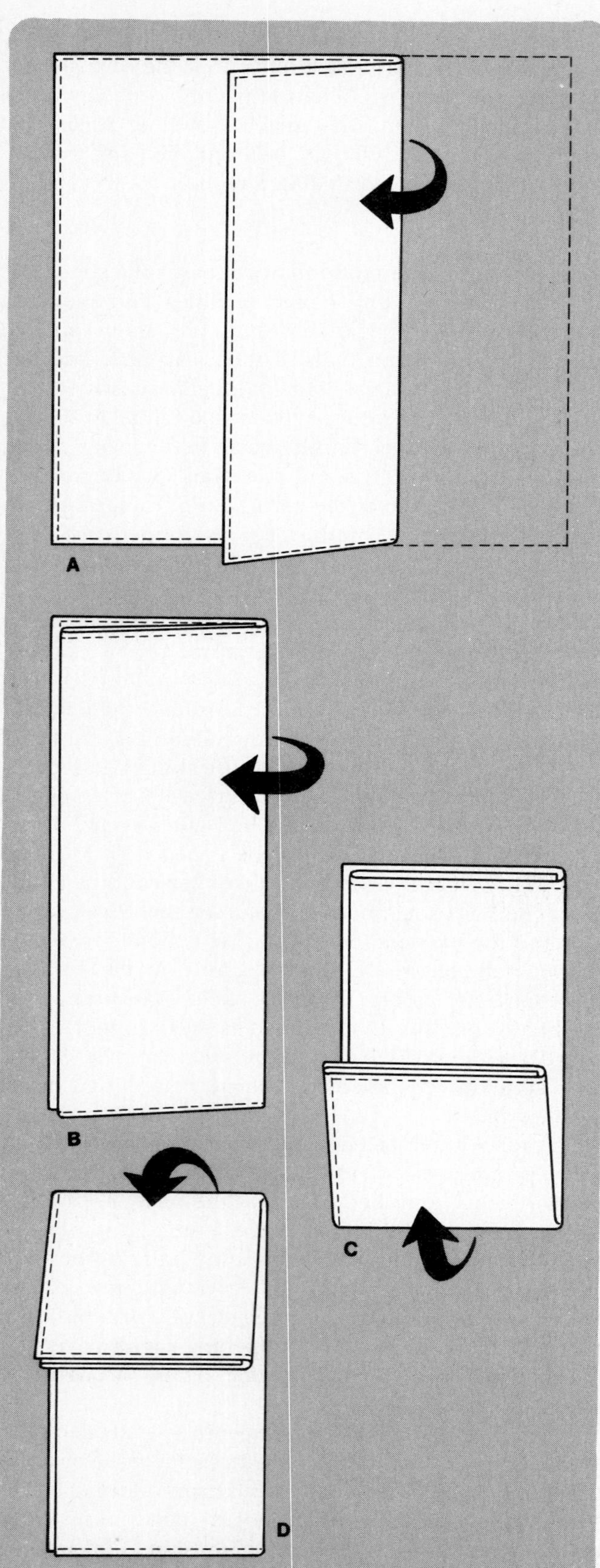

Figure 21–2 The rectangular method of folding a diaper: **A, B,** fold the diaper into a rectangle by bringing the sides over; **C,** fold the bottom edge up to provide thickness in front; **or D,** fold the top edge down to provide thickness at the back.

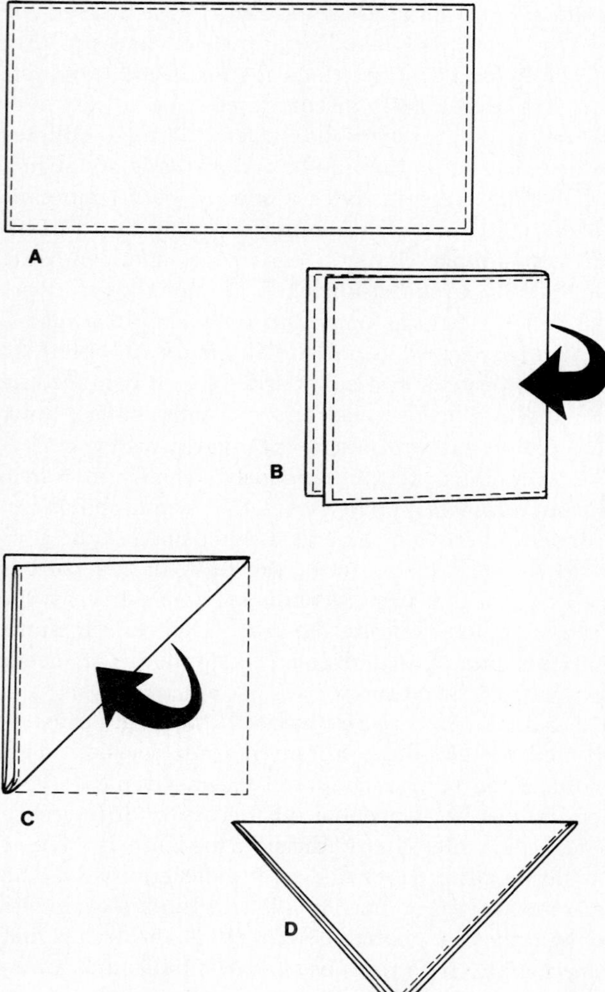

Figure 21–3 The triangular method of folding a diaper: **A,** fold a square cloth to a rectangular shape; **B,** fold the cloth again to the correct size square; **C,** bring opposite corners together to form a triangle; **D,** turn the triangle so that the fold is at the baby's waist.

and be dried thoroughly. A baby's skin usually does not need oil on the perineum. However, if the skin is excessively dry or excoriated, petroleum jelly or mineral oil can offer protection. To fold a diaper, see Figures 21–2 (rectangular method) and 21–3 (triangular method).

Tub bath Infants can be given tub baths when the umbilicus is well healed, usually within the first 2 weeks of life. This can be a pleasurable experience for the baby. Preparation of the environment and of supplies is the same as for the sponge bath. It is important to keep safety pins out of the infant's reach and to have all supplies available. Infants must never be left alone in a bassinette even for a few seconds, because they do move and can fall.

Before putting the baby into the bath, the face, neck, eyes, and scalp are washed in the manner described for the infant sponge bath. The baby is then undressed and excess feces wiped away.

The baby is submerged gradually in the tub and held firmly with one hand. The baby is then soaped and rinsed with the nurse's free hand. If the baby appears to be enjoying the experience, the bath can be offered in a leisurely manner. When removed from the tub, the baby is wrapped completely in a towel and gently patted dry. Special attention is given to drying body creases. The baby is then dressed.

Evaluation: Outcome Criteria

Outcome criteria for skin care interventions may include:

1. No evidence of reddened skin areas.
2. Skin has good tissue turgor and is smooth, soft, and flexible.
3. Skin temperature is warm.
4. Patient has no complaints of localized discomfort.
5. No evidence of abrasions, excoriations, etc.; or, evidence of healing (e.g., reduced size of impairment) is present.
6. Patient is able to bathe self in bed without becoming dyspneic.

Decubitus Ulcers

Decubitus ulcers (also called *pressure sores, bed sores,* or *decubiti*) are ulcerations of the skin. They are chiefly due to deprivation of oxygen and essential nutrients to an area because of prolonged pressure that occludes the blood supply to the tissues. Although they are not a common problem, the potential for them to develop is great, and preventive measures need to be carried out continuously. Decubitus ulcers are frequently seen in the elderly, who have difficulty moving in bed or in a chair, and in very emaciated or paralyzed patients.

Decubiti can be categorized as superficial and deep (Ahmed 1980:113). *Superficial* ulcers start with an excoriation caused by a shearing force (such as sliding up and down in a bed or chair), friction from movement on rough surfaces (such as a wrinkled sheet), and maceration produced by urine, feces, or excessive perspiration. (ibid., p. 114). Untreated superficial ulcers become infected and painful, but if treated they heal within a few days.

Deep ulcers start as ischemic areas in the muscle or subcutaneous layers and then surface to the skin as black blisters, which change to thick, hard *eschar* (slough). See Figure 21–4. What is apparent to the eye is misleading in terms of the degree of damage, since destruction of the underlying tissues is extensive. The visible eschar is composed of dried plasma, proteins, and dead cells. If this eschar is not removed, the *necrotic* process (dying of the tissues) spreads and becomes a focus of infection.

A number of conditions predispose patients to develop decubitus ulcers. Prolonged pressure is considered the primary cause. Other predisposing factors are moisture, a break in the skin surface, poor nutrition, impaired circulation to the area, lack of subcutaneous and adipose tissue to pad bony prominences, lack of sensation in the area so that the patient cannot feel the tingling (pins and needles) of loss of circulation, and the presence of pathogens.

Figure 21–4 A stasis ulcer of the legs appears similar to a pressure ulcer. (Courtesy of the City of Vancouver Health Department.)

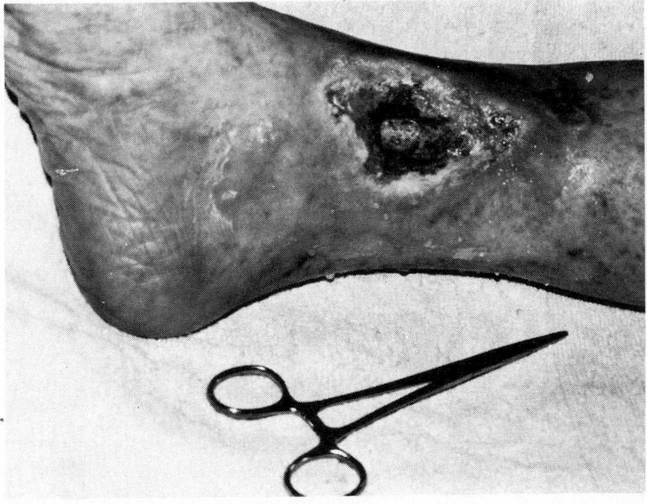

Assessment of risk patients

Assessment of patients at risk for the development of decubiti is essential for prevention. Kerr et al. (1981:27) have devised a pressure assessment scale with five categories: physical condition, mental condition, activity, mobility, and continence. This scale needs to be used weekly or whenever there is a change in the patient's condition or situation. Patients at risk (ibid., p. 24) include:

1. Those with paralysis from either brain or spinal cord injury. Incidence rates for these people are as high as 80%, due to their extensive loss of sensory and motor function.
2. Those with a reduced level of awareness, such as unconscious or heavily sedated patients (those taking analgesics, barbiturates, or tranquilizers). In these patients, the usual perceptions stimulating changes of position are reduced or absent.
3. Those who are malnourished and whose diet is insufficient in protein and ascorbic acid (vitamin C). Good nutrition is thought essential to promote normal tissue maintenance and healing.
4. Those who are over age 85. These patients have problems with mobility and incontinence and are generally lean. Changes in the circulatory system due to aging also reduce the system's capacity and ability to carry essential nutrients to the skin.
5. Those who are confined to bed or to a wheelchair, particularly if they are dependent on others for movement.

Intervention

Nursing goals Nursing goals for patients at risk for *potential skin breakdown* are:

1. Prevention of prolonged skin pressure
2. Elimination of shearing forces and friction
3. Provision of adequate nutrition (protein and vitamin C)
4. Removal of skin secretions and excretions

Nursing goals for patients with *actual skin breakdown* include all of the above plus:

5. Prevention of infection
6. Removal of necrotic tissue (for deep ulcers)
7. Promotion of healing

Preventive measures

1. Change the patient's position at least every 2 hours even when a special support mattress is used, so that another body surface bears the weight. Four body positions can usually be used: prone, supine, and right and left lateral (side-lying) positions. See Chapter 23. Prolonged pressure on bony prominences is considered the primary cause of decubiti. See Figure 21–5 for pressure areas in various positions assumed by bed patients. Prolonged low pressure is potentially more dangerous than high pressure for a short duration, since it is prolonged pressure that alters the tissue's blood supply (Ahmed 1980:113).
2. Provide good nutrition for the patient, particularly a diet high in protein and vitamin C. Elderly people have increased protein requirements (up to 0.6 gm per kg of body weight) to maintain proper nitrogen balance (Kerr et al. 1981:26).
3. Keep the patient's skin clean and dry, and protect damaged skin from irritation and maceration by urine, feces, sweat, incomplete drying after a bath, soap, and alcohol.
4. Apply powders (rather than astringents, such as alcohol or witch hazel) on tissues with limited blood flow. Astringents constrict the blood vessels and thus inhibit the supply of blood and essential nutrients to the skin.
5. Lubricate dry skin areas to prevent cracking. Superfatted soaps and oils may be used.
6. Avoid massaging bony prominences with soap. Research has indicated that the alkalis in soap produce swelling, drying, and loss of natural oils of the skin, thus facilitating skin damage. In addition, prolonged exposure to soap alters the pH of the skin, one of its natural defense barriers (Kerr et al. 1981:25). Vigorous massage over bony prominences is avoided, since it increases tissue damage in deep ulcers that are not apparent to the eye (ibid., p. 24).
7. Provide a smooth, firm, wrinkle-free foundation on which the patient can lie.
8. Use foam rubber pads and sheepskins under pressure areas such as the sacrum and heels, and elevate the heels above the bed surface.
9. Avoid the use of rubber rings. Donut-shaped, inflated rubber rings were traditionally placed around actual or potential pressure areas to prevent pressure over bony prominences or actual decubiti. These rings put a great pressure on areas of contact, however, and blood flow is restricted in both direct contact areas and the enclosed area.
10. Use a special mattress, such as an alternating pressure, eggshell, or flotation mattress, to decrease pressure on body parts.
11. Teach patients to be aware of discolored areas and of sensations such as tingling, which can indicate pressure.
12. Be alert to early symptoms of pressure sores, particularly over bony prominences: redness or whiteness of an area, tenderness, an unpleasant sensation frequently described as burning, coldness of the area, and localized edema.

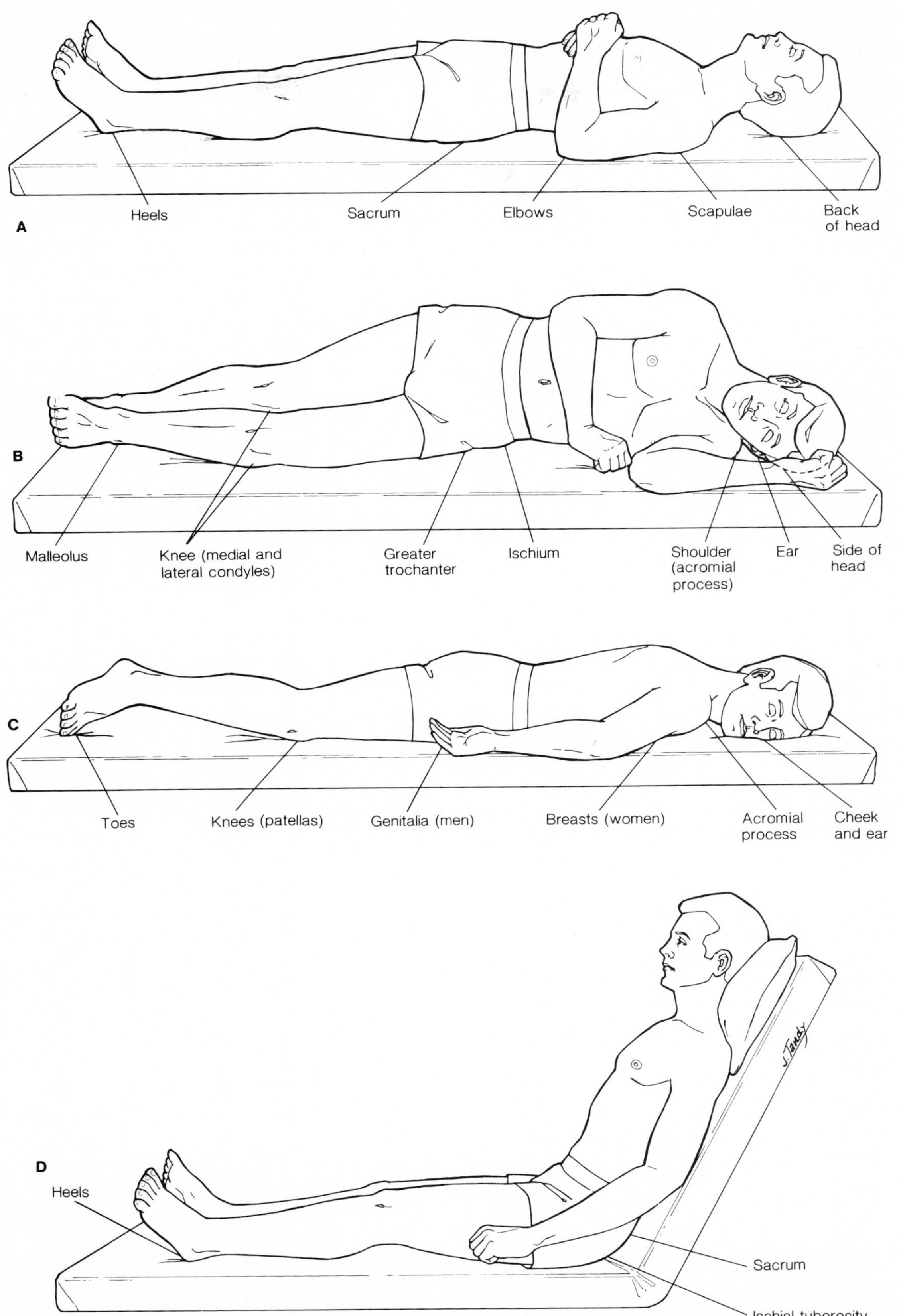

Figure 21–5 Body pressure areas in: **A,** supine position; **B,** lateral position; **C,** prone position; **D,** Fowler's position.

Treatment

Pressure sores are a challenge for nurses to cure because of the number of variables involved (e.g., risk factors, types of ulcers, and degrees of impairment) and because numerous treatment measures are advocated. Interventions need to be selected from the following:

1. Take a wound culture as soon as the ulcer is noticed, to ascertain the specific invading organisms, and then weekly or whenever increases in drainage appear or healing is delayed. If infection is present, antiseptics are preferred to local or systemic antibiotics. Locally applied antibiotics have not proved effective (Morley 1981:29; Ahmed 1980:115), and systemic antibiotics do not reach the desired site of action because the blood supply to the ulcer is disrupted (Ahmed 1980:115). Antiseptics are discussed subsequently.

2. *Debride* (remove foreign and contaminated or devitalized material from) deep ulcers to remove necrotic tissue, which impedes the healing process and provides an excellent culture medium for bacteria. Debridement may be achieved by chemical or surgical means:

a. Chemical debridement uses enzyme ointments such as collagenase (Santyl), fibrinolysin and desoxyribonuclease (Elase), and sutilains (Travase). Use of enzymes requires a physician's order. Collagenase, an enzyme that digests collagen, may be more effective than Elase or Travase, since 79% of the necrotic and living tissue is collagen, and in the normal healing process a small amount of collagenase is produced. Thus, collagenase ointment seems to simulate and enhance the body's normal self-debridement process for healing wounds (Barrett and Klibanski 1973:849; Ahmed 1980:114). Because enzymes do not penetrate thick hard eschar, either the eschar is softened for several days or weeks with continuous saline soaks or the eschar is surgically scored or crosshatched to permit the enzyme to penetrate. Once the eschar is softened, it is removed with forceps or scissors. Generally collagenase dressings are changed daily or whenever soiled; Elase twice daily; and Travase up to 4 times daily (Judd 1981:33). Before applying enzymes, the nurse cleans the ulcer with normal saline or hydrogen peroxide to remove old ointment and digested material. The enzyme ointment is applied to only the ulcerated area, since it can irritate normal skin and damage new granulation tissue. Surrounding skin may be protected with zinc oxide, karaya paste, or petroleum jelly. Generally a moist gauze dressing is applied over the area and covered with a waterproof (e.g., plastic) pad. Ahmed (1980:114) cautions that antiseptics or detergents containing metal ions or acidic substances should not be used in conjunction with enzymes. Tincture of iodide, Merthiolate, Furacin, and hexachlorophene inactivate collagenase, and Burow's solution inhibits enzyme action by altering the pH. When debridement is complete (i.e., the wound appears clean), the enzyme ointment is discontinued and other measures to promote healing (discussed subsequently) are initiated.

b. Surgical debridement is performed by a physician. It may be done with or without anesthetic. The wound is surgically excised with a scalpel blade. This procedure may have to be repeated several times until the wound remains clean. Surgical debridement has the disadvantage of increasing ulcer size and increasing the patient's risk of infection and hemorrhage. Following debridement, the ulcer should appear clean and pink and reveal evidence of healing by secondary union (see Chapter 40, page 1030). Because the ulcer is susceptible to infection, every effort is then exerted to maintain a clean wound and promote healing. In some instances surgical closure using skin grafts may be necessary.

3. Promote healing by keeping the ulcer moist and preventing infection. Wounds need moisture to heal; thus, dehydrating solutions, such as liquid antacids, are avoided (Ahmed 1980:114). Heat lamps and hair driers were erroneously recommended in previous years to dry the surface of the ulcer; they are contraindicated. Various measures are advocated:

a. Saline or Betadine soaks may be applied to a superficial ulcer to keep the wound moist (Ahmed 1980:114).

b. Op-site, a commercially prepared, transparent, self-adhesive film, may be applied to superficial ulcers and some deep, draining or necrotic ulcers (Chrisp 1977:1202; Ahmed 1980:117). This preparation acts like skin in that it isolates the ulcer from contaminants and keeps it moist. It is also permeable to air, is waterproof (it can be washed if soiled), and allows freedom of movement. Before Op-site is applied, the wound and surrounding skin are cleaned with saline solution or water and thoroughly dried to ensure proper adhesion. The Op-site is applied without tension over the ulcer and at least 2.5 cm (1 in) over the surrounding skin. It is left in place 5 to 7 days or until seepage or an odor appears. The application is repeated until the ulcer has healed. When removing the Op-site, the nurse takes care to remove only the nonadherent portion, since an attempt to remove adherent portions may tear the skin. In some instances, the nurse may need to cut a hole in the center and apply the new piece over it.

c. Gelfoam powder and sponges, applied with a dressing, are effective for small or medium-sized clean ulcers but not for draining or hard, necrotic ulcers. Draining or necrotic wounds must be cleaned or debrided before applying Gelfoam. Gelfoam powder seems more advantageous for healing than Gelfoam sponge, since it adheres well to the ulcer. Some authorities recommend changing the Gelfoam dressing daily; others, every 3 to 7 days (Ahmed 1981:116; Lang and McGrath 1974:461). If the dressing is changed every 3 to 7 days, the ulcer must be inspected daily to ensure that it is free of drainage.

d. Silver nitrate 1:400 dressings, covered with a plastic wrap and secured with nonallergenic tape, can be used for superficial ulcers involving only the epidermis. Higher strengths of silver nitrate may cause bleeding (Morley 1981:30).

e. *Karaya powder* (a vegetable gum) is advocated for clean or draining superficial and deep ulcers but not for hard, leathery eschar. The procedure outlined by Wallace and Hayter (1974:1094) is: (1) irrigate the ulcer with saline or 3% hydrogen peroxide solution (any karaya adhering is left in place), (2) encircle the wound with a karaya gum ring, and (3) cover the ulcer and karaya ring with Saran wrap. The Saran wrap is opened every 8 hours to add more karaya powder, and the entire procedure is repeated daily.

f. Stomahesive, another vegetable gum, may be used for clean and draining superficial and deep ulcers and is effective in debriding hard, necrotic eschar (Ryan 1976:299). This preparation is similar to Op-site but thicker, and it is applied in the same way.

g. Debrisan (molecular chains of dextran beads) is a product used for infected, draining ulcers only. The dry, porous beads absorb bacteria, proteins, fibrin, and toxins. When drainage stops, the ulcer may be grafted or other therapies that promote healing initiated (Ahmed 1980:116).

h. Antiseptics such as povidone-iodine (Betadine) in ointment or solution form, merbromin (Mercurochrome) in 5% or 10% solutions, Helafoam, an aerosol foam of povidone-iodine, and sodium hypochlorite solution (Hygeol) are effective for draining infected or clean ulcers. They do not, however, penetrate hard eschar. Betadine can be applied at any stage of the healing process (even prior to debridement), since its antiseptic properties are effective in the presence of pus, necrotic tissue, serum, or blood. Often the ulcer is cleaned with Betadine solution and then packed with gauze impregnated with Betadine ointment. If only solution is used, dressings are changed twice daily; if ointment is used, dressings are changed daily (Judd 1981:33). Patients need to be watched for allergy to iodine prior to the use of Betadine. Mercurochrome solution can also be applied at any stage of the healing process, but is not as strong as Betadine. It is said to stimulate the formation of granulation tissue, however (ibid.). Helafoam requires less frequent application than other forms of Betadine. It is advocated in conjunction with Betadine Viscous Formula Antiseptic Gauze Pads, which prolong the foam's action (Ahmed 1980:116). Hygeol solution (1:12 to 1:20 dilution) is effective for dermal ulcers only. It may be caustic to some persons and must be used with caution on soft tissue where bleeding is suspected (Judd 1981:33).

Many other measures have been used to treat decubitus ulcers, but their therapeutic value is questionable or not established, and they therefore should be avoided. These include applications of granulated sugar, sugar and egg white mixture, and insulin. The therapeutic value of granulated sugar is unknown. A sugar and egg white mixture has been found to have no therapeutic value and may even retard normal healing (Ahmed 1980:18). However, a paste of powdered cane sugar, lanolin, and compound benzoin tincture in specified amounts may have some therapeutic value when used to treat clean ulcers (ibid.). The effectiveness of insulin (10 I.U. of regular insulin) applied topically is highly questionable. Moreover, insulin can be absorbed through the ulcer, causing hypoglycemic (low blood sugar) reactions (Gerber and Van Ort 1981:1159).

Clearly, treatment of decubiti is a complex matter. It requires strict sterile technique (see Chapter 20). Very superficial ulcers may heal within a few days; deep, necrotic ulcers may take several months. The nurse must set specific outcome criteria to evaluate the effects of therapy. If after a specified period of time (e.g., 14 or 21 days) the criteria have not been met, the therapy must be reevaluated.

Back Rubs

The back rub is a massage of the back, with two chief objectives: to relax and relieve tension (sedative effect) and to stimulate blood circulation to the tissues and the muscles. Friction from the rubbing produces heat at the skin surface. This causes the peripheral blood vessels in the area to dilate, thus increasing the blood supply to the area. Because tissues are under pressure when a patient is in bed and muscles are usually relaxed, stimulation of the circulation is essential so that the tissues obtain the necessary nutrients and oxygen.

There are four techniques that can be used in a back rub:

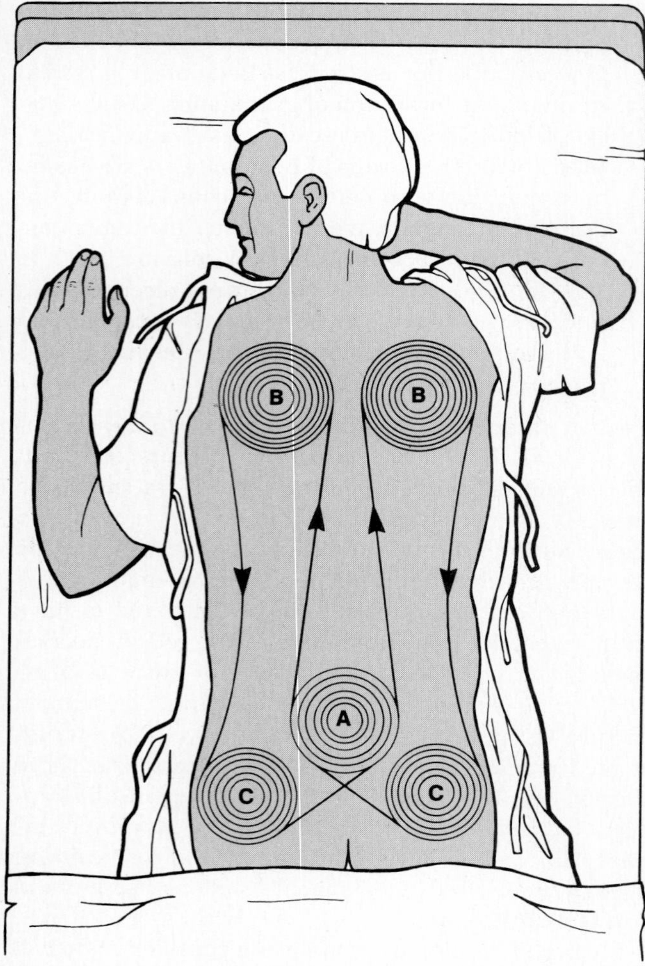

Figure 21–6 A back rub technique massaging bony prominences: **A,** start with a circular motion over the sacrum; **B,** move both hands up the medial aspect of the back, and massage the two scapulae with a circular motion; **C,** move both hands down the lateral aspects of the back, and massage the two iliac crest areas.

1. *Effleurage* is a smooth, long stroke, moving the hands up and down the back. The hands are moved lightly down the sides of the back, maintaining contact with the skin, and then moved firmly up the back. This rub has a relaxing, sedative effect if slow, light pressure is used.
2. In *tapotement*, the little-finger side of each hand is used in a sharp hacking movement on the back. Care must be taken not to hurt the patient with this type of rub. It is not advised for debilitated patients or patients who have pathologic conditions of the back.
3. *Petrissage* is a large pinch of the skin, subcutaneous tissue, and muscle, quickly done. The pinches are taken first up the vertebral column and then over the entire back. Tapotement and petrissage are primarily stimulating, especially if they are done quickly with firm pressure.
4. *Three-handed effleurage* is a smooth, stroking motion that gives the patient an impression of three hands. The nurse starts at the base of the patient's neck and moves to the lateral aspect of the shoulder. The other hand then makes the same movement to the other shoulder before the first hand is removed from the shoulder to return to the base of the neck. This rub is particularly effective in relieving tension of the neck muscles.

A number of preparations can be used for back rubs. Emollient creams and lotions are frequently used. These lubricate the skin. Alcohol preparations are cooling, but they are used infrequently today. They are refreshing, and they toughen skin by hardening the skin protein, but they tend to dry the skin, and very dry skin is likely to crack. Alcohol preparations are particularly undesirable for use on elderly patients, whose skin is usually dry. Patients who are dehydrated and poorly nourished may also find an alcohol back rub disadvantageous.

The position of choice for a back rub is the prone position (lying on the stomach). The second preferred position is the side-lying position; its disadvantage is the difficulty of massaging the lateral aspect of the hip on which the patient is lying. This necessitates turning the patient to the other side.

In addition to the four types of rubs described, a back rub using long smooth strokes up and down the back combined with circular motions over the bony prominences (see Figure 21–6) is relaxing and stimulates blood circulation to the tissues and muscles in the area. The hands and lotion are warmed first. Then, with lotion on both hands, rubbing commences with circular motion over the sacrum. The hands move up the center of the back and massage the skin over the scapulae with circular movements. The hands move down the back on the lateral aspects and massage the right and left iliac crest areas in a circular motion. This pattern is repeated for 3 to 5 minutes, depending on the patient's needs.

Other pressure points on the body that generally benefit from massage and the application of lotions are the elbows, knees, and heels. Sometimes massage of the anterior aspects of both iliac crests of very thin patients is also indicated.

During the back rub the nurse observes any reddened areas that do not disappear after a few minutes of massage, any breaks in the skin, and any bruises. They should be reported and recorded. Often these conditions predispose to decubitus ulcers. See the discussion earlier in this chapter.

Nurses are advised not to rub tender, reddened areas on the lower legs of patients, particularly the calves.

Redness, tenderness, and heat, particularly along the course of a vein, may indicate a thrombus (blood clot) in the area. Any massage might dislodge the clot, which could travel to the heart or the lung, causing a myocardial or pulmonary embolus. This can present a very serious problem.

Perineal and Genital Care

Perineal care is an embarrassing procedure for most patients. Nurses also may find it an embarrassment initially, particularly if the patient is of the opposite sex. Today male nurses frequently give total care to male patients requiring genital care. Most patients who require a bed bath from the nurse are able to clean their genital areas with minimal assistance. The nurse may need to hand the moistened washcloth and soap to the patient, rinse the washcloth, and provide a towel. Because many people do not use anatomic terminology for the genitals and perineal area, it may be difficult for nurses to explain to patients what is expected. Most patients understand what is meant if the nurse simply says, "I'll give you a washcloth to finish your bath." Elderly patients may be familiar with the term *private parts*. Whatever expression the nurse chooses, it should be one that the patient understands and that is comfortable for the nurse to use.

For female patients

When providing perineal care for female patients, the nurse places a towel under the patient's hips parallel to the legs and positions the patient with knees flexed and spread well apart. One end of the towel is used to dry the anterior perineum and the other the posterior perineum. The legs are draped with a bath blanket to avoid undue exposure. When cleaning the perineum, the nurse first washes the area between the thighs and the labia. This can be done with a washcloth. The area is well rinsed and dried. Then the labia are spread, and the folds between the labia majora and labia minora are well cleaned, using disposable cotton balls or separate corners of the washcloth, wiping from the pubic to rectal areas. For menstruating women it is advisable to use cotton balls or gauze. Some nurses at this point place the patient on a bedpan and rinse the perineum well with a pitcher of warm water. This action ensures removal of the soap. The perineum is then dried thoroughly, because microorganisms can grow and accumulate in moist, dark areas. To clean between the buttocks, the nurse helps the patient to turn on her side. The area is cleaned well, paying particular attention to the anal region. If the patient is incontinent, it is important to clean the area with toilet tissue as much as possible before washing it. It is poor technique to use a soiled washcloth to clean the patient. After drying the area, powder can be applied sparingly. If the skin appears excoriated, petroleum jelly or a protective ointment can be applied.

For male patients

The nurse assists a male patient to the same position as a female for genital care. The upper thighs are washed and dried first. The penis is washed with firm strokes. In uncircumcised males the foreskin is retracted, and the glans and prepuce are washed and dried to prevent accumulation of smegma. Smegma that accumulates not only causes an offensive odor but also facilitates bacterial growth. The outside of the foreskin, the scrotum, and the medial aspects of the thighs are washed and dried well. The buttocks are cleaned in the same manner as a female's, with the patient lying on his side.

Because of the sensitivity of the penis to manipulation there is always the possibility that the patient may have an erection during this procedure. It is recommended that this possibility and ways of dealing with it be discussed beforehand by nursing students. Some suggestions are: leave the room for a short period and return later to complete the bath; ignore the erection and complete the bath; or clean the scrotum before the penis although the scrotum may be more soiled (Gibbs 1969:125).

Should the nurse wear gloves when giving perineal care? Those opposed to gloves feel that their use suggests to the patient that he is dirty and distasteful. Those who favor gloves suggest that the area becomes more soiled bacteriologically without gloves. Each nurse needs to judge which method to employ for the individual patient. The important point is that perineal care has to be provided effectively.

Catheter care

When nurses give perineal care to patients with indwelling catheters, it is particularly important to observe the area around the urinary meatus for inflammation, swelling, odor, or discharge. Catheter care is normally given after perineal and genital care. Catheter care kits, containing gloves, cotton balls or swabs, antiseptic solution, and antibiotic ointment (such as neomycin or hydrocortisone), may be available. The perineal-genital area is cleaned with the antiseptic solution as described previously; then, using another swab, the catheter is cleaned, using a circular motion, starting at the meatus and extending about 10 cm (4 in) along the catheter. The antibiotic ointment is applied around the base and along 2.5 cm (1 in) of the catheter to protect the urethra from infection.

Feet and Nails

The feet are essential for ambulation and merit attention even when patients are confined to bed. Each foot contains 26 bones, 107 ligaments, and 19 muscles. These structures function together for both standing and walking.

During childhood, the bony structure of the feet and the small muscles are easily damaged by tight, binding stockings and ill-fitting shoes. In fact, in China, it was customary for a girl baby's feet to be bound, to limit their growth. This practice was outlawed by Chou En-lai in the 1930s. For normal development, it is important that the arches be supported and that the bony structure and the feet grow with no external restrictions.

The fingernails and toenails are epidermal appendages. Like the hair and the apocrine, eccrine, and sebaceous glands, they are directly related to the epidermis; they are made of epidermal cells that have been changed to keratin. Today the nails have little functional value except for cosmetic purposes. Nails usually grow regularly, about 1 mm per week, but this growth may stop at times of severe stress or illness. When the patient's nails begin to grow again, a deep line will become visible across the nail. This is called *Beau's line.* A lost fingernail takes 3½ to 5½ months to regenerate, and a toenail takes 6 to 8 months.

Assessment of Feet and Nails

Assessment of the feet and nails entails physical examination, including examination of the functional ability of the feet to walk and stand, assessment of developmental changes, and assessment of personal practices related to foot and nail care.

Physical examination

Feet Each foot is examined for swelling, redness, deformity, and abnormal growth or abrasions. The patient's ability to perform range-of-motion exercises with each ankle, foot, and set of toes (see Chapter 24) is also assessed.

A number of foot problems that produce considerable discomfort are commonly observed. Among these are calluses, corns, unpleasant odors, plantar warts, fissures between the toes, and fungus infections such as athlete's foot.

A *callus* is a thickened portion of epidermis, a mass of keratotic material. It is flat and usually found on the bottom or side of the foot over a bony prominence. Calluses are usually caused by pressure from shoes. Calluses can be softened by soaking in warm water with Epsom salts, and they can be removed by an abrasive substance such as a pumice stone. Creams with lanolin can also be used to keep the skin soft and prevent the formation of calluses.

A *corn* is a keratosis caused by friction and pressure from a shoe. It commonly occurs on a toe, usually the fourth or fifth toe, and usually on a bony prominence such as a joint. Corns are usually conical (circular and raised). The base is the surface of the corn and the apex is in deeper tissues, sometimes even attached to bone. Corns are generally removed surgically. They are prevented from reforming by relieving the pressure on the area and massaging the tissue to promote circulation.

Unpleasant odors occur as a result of perspiration and its interaction with microorganisms. Regular and frequent washing of the feet and wearing clean hosiery help to minimize odor. Foot powders and deodorants also help prevent this problem.

Plantar warts appear on the sole of the foot. These warts are caused by the virus *papovavirus hominis.* They are moderately contagious. They are frequently painful and often make walking difficult. The treatment ordered by a physician may be curettage, freezing with solid carbon dioxide several times, or repeated applications of salicylic acid.

Fissures between the toes occur frequently as a result of dryness and cracking of the skin. The treatment of choice is good foot hygiene and administration of an antiseptic to prevent infection. Often a small piece of gauze is inserted between the toes in applying the antiseptic and left in place to assist healing by allowing air to reach the area.

Athlete's foot or *tinea pedis* (ringworm of the foot) is caused by a fungus. The symptoms are scaling and cracking of the skin, particularly between the toes. Sometimes small blisters form containing a thin fluid. In severe cases the lesions may also appear on other parts of the body, particularly the hands. Treatments vary from potassium permanganate soaks using a 1:8000 solution, to commercial antifungal ointments or powders. Prevention is important. Common preventive measures are: permitting feet to be well ventilated, wearing clean socks or stockings, and not going barefoot in public showers.

Nails Nails should be examined for shape, thickness, smoothness, color, and length. The tissue around the nails is inspected for dryness, breaks in the skin, inflammation, and paronychia (discussed later).

Caucasians normally have pink nails and nail beds. Normal nails blanch when pressed but quickly turn pink when pressure is released. In dark-skinned people, the nail may be pigmented along the edges or in lines along the nail, and the rate of return of nail bed color may be more significant than the color. Nails are normally convex in shape and smooth.

It is important to note any *clubbing*, an elevation of the proximal aspect of the nail and softening of the nail bed, which spreads from the nail to the terminal phalanx. With more advanced clubbing, the terminal aspect of the finger becomes wider and rounder and the nail becomes more curved. Clubbing frequently results from a long-term lack of oxygen.

Incurvated nails (ingrown toenails) are a relatively common condition. The toenail grows so that it impinges into the soft tissue. The symptoms are pain with walking and when pressure is put on the nail, tenderness, and sometimes redness if inflammation has started in the soft tissues. The usual treatment is to remove the part of the nail that has curved into the tissue and to clear any debris and callus tissue in the area. The nail groove is then packed in such a way that the nail will grow forward rather than into the soft tissue. Any secondary infection is generally treated with an antibiotic ointment or powder.

Paronychia is an inflammation of the tissue surrounding the nail. Acute paronychia is called *thecal whitlow*; it is a painful red swelling that develops quickly. It usually follows a hangnail or injury. This condition occurs most frequently in people who have their hands in water a great deal, and it is three times more common in patients who have diabetes. Prevention by careful manicuring that does not injure the adjacent soft tissue is stressed. If a hangnail develops and is not infected, it can be carefully flattened and held in place with collodion. Often oil rubbed into the tissue around the nail will lubricate the tissue and prevent hangnails.

Developmental changes

Feet At birth a baby's foot is relatively unformed. The arches are supported by fatty pads and do not take their full shape until 5 or 6 years of age. Feet are not fully grown until about age 20. Healthy feet remain relatively unchanged during life. However, the elderly often require special attention for their feet. Reduced blood supply, accompanying arteriosclerosis, for example, can make the foot prone to infection following trauma.

Nails Nails are normally present at birth. They continue to grow throughout life, and they change very little until people are old. At that time the nails tend to be tougher, more brittle, and in some cases thicker. The nails of an elderly person will normally grow less quickly than those of a younger person, and they may be ridged and have grooves.

Personal practices

Personal hygienic practices for the feet are of particular importance when the patient has an infection or abrasion, diabetes mellitus, or impaired circulation to the extremities. The latter two conditions predispose patients to infections. These patients need to learn nail and foot care to prevent problems. Other patients normally care for their own feet and nails. After learning about a patient's personal foot and nail care practices, the nurse can identify learning needs of the patient.

Nursing Diagnoses: Foot and Nail Problems

Foot and nail disorders often interfere with the patient's mobility (ambulation) or create a risk of infection. Patients who have diabetes or vascular disturbances are particularly prone to infection if the integrity of the skin or nails is impaired. Such patients require specific instruction about care of the feet and nails. Examples of nursing diagnoses for actual or potential foot and nail problems are:

1. Impaired mobility related to:
   a. Painful corn on left small toe
   b. Painful plantar wart
   c. Painful ingrown toenail
2. Risk of infection related to:
   a. Impairment of skin integrity (fissure between toes)
   b. Diabetes or vascular disturbance

Planning and Intervention for Feet and Nails

Nursing goals

The overall nursing goal is to maintain the skin integrity of the feet and a well-groomed appearance of the nails. Subgoals are:

1. To maintain the cleanliness of the skin
2. To prevent foot odors
3. To prevent infections of the skin

Planning

Planning to assist a patient with foot care involves consideration of the best time for that care and development of a teaching plan to meet the patient's learning needs.

Intervention

Foot care Many foot problems can be prevented by having patients follow simple guidelines:

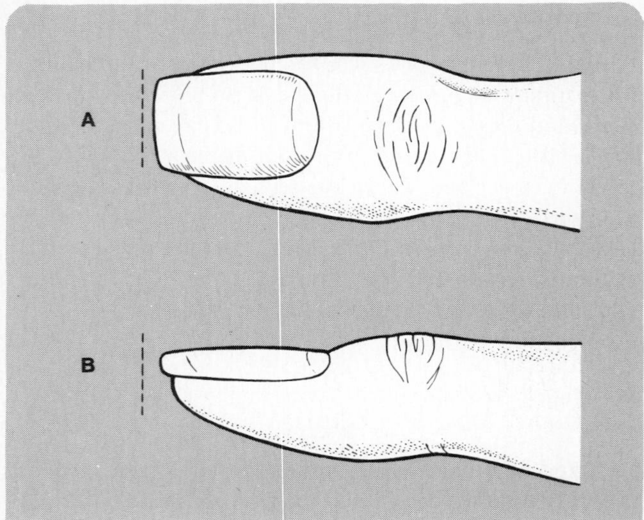

Figure 21–7 Trimming or filing straight across the nail beyond the end of the finger or toe.

1. Wear correctly fitting shoes that neither restrict the foot nor rub on any area; rubbing can cause corns and calluses. For the elderly, an oxford or slip-on style is advised with 2.5 to 5 cm (1 to 2 in) heels (King 1980:186).
2. Wash the feet daily, and dry them well.
3. To prevent or control an unpleasant odor due to excessive perspiration on the feet, wash frequently and change socks and shoes. Special deodorant sprays are also helpful.
4. Wear clean stockings or socks daily.
5. Avoid walking barefoot in public showers and change areas, to prevent contracting common infections such as athlete's foot.
6. Avoid excessive drying of the skin of the feet. Use creams or lotions to moisten the skin or soak the feet in warm water with Epsom salts. This will soften calluses, which can then be removed with an abrasive such as pumice stone. An effective lotion for reducing dryness is a mixture of lanolin and mineral oil (ibid.).

Nail care When a patient requires help with nail care, the nurse needs a nail cutter or sharp scissors, a nail file, an orange stick to push back the cuticle, hand lotion or mineral oil to lubricate any dry tissue around the nails, and a wash basin with water to soak the nails if they are particularly thick or hard.

One hand or foot is soaked, if needed, and dried; then the nail is cut or filed straight across beyond the end of the finger or toe. See Figure 21–7. Patients who have diabetes or circulatory problems should have their nails filed, rather than cut. After the initial cut or filing, the nail is filed to round the corners, and the nurse cleans under the nail. Then the cuticle is gently pushed back, taking care not to injure it. The next finger or toe is cared for in the same manner. Any abnormalities, such as an infected cuticle or inflammation of the tissue around the nail, are recorded and reported. See Kozier and Erb (1982:295–300) for additional information.

Evaluation: Outcome Criteria

Outcome criteria for foot and nail care may include:

1. No evidence of calluses or corns.
2. Skin around nails is intact.
3. No evidence of inflammation on feet or around nails.
4. Patient has cut nails as instructed.

Mouth

Mucous membrane, which is continuous with the skin, lines the digestive, urinary, reproductive, and respiratory tracts and the conjunctiva of the eye. It is an epithelial tissue, and it forms mucus, concentrates bile, and secretes or excretes enzymes, for example, in the digestive tract. It serves four general functions:

1. Protection
2. Support for associated structures
3. Absorption of nutrients into the body (in the digestive tract)
4. Secretion of mucus, enzymes, and salts

The mouth (oral cavity) is bordered by the lips anteriorly, the cheeks laterally, and the pharynx posteriorly. The cheeks contain several accessory muscles of *mastication* (chewing), which keep food from escaping the masticating motions of the teeth. The tongue, containing numerous taste buds, extends from the floor of the mouth and is attached to it by a fold of mucous membrane called the *frenulum*. The tongue helps to mix saliva, keeps food pressed between the teeth for chewing, and pushes food into the pharynx for swallowing. The *palate* (roof of the mouth) has two parts: the anterior portion (hard palate) and the posterior portion (soft palate), which ends in a free projection called the *uvula* that marks the opening of the mouth into the pharynx.

The mouth contains two sets of *dentures* (teeth), which are discussed under Developmental Variables on page 507. Teeth are necessary to masticate food, so that it can be swallowed and digested in the stomach. Each tooth has a number of parts: the crown, the root, and the pulp cavity. The *crown* is the exposed part of the tooth, which is outside the gum. It is covered with a hard substance called *enamel*. The internal part of the crown below the enamel is ivory colored and is referred to as *dentin*. See Figure 21–8. The *root* of a tooth is embedded in the jaw, and it is covered by a bony tissue called *cementum*. The *pulp cavity* in the center of the tooth contains the blood vessels and nerves.

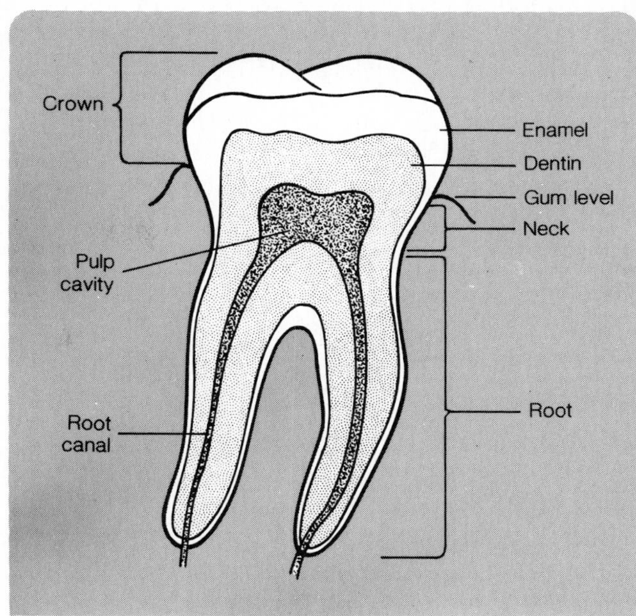

Figure 21–8 The parts of a tooth.

Assessment of the Mouth

Assessment of an individual's mouth includes examination of its physical characteristics, consideration of developmental changes, and determination of the person's hygienic practices, including factors that influence them.

Physical examination

Physical examination of the mouth includes inspection and palpation techniques. The status of the lips, mucous membrane, tongue, teeth, and *gingiva* (gums) is assessed.

Lips Lips are inspected for color, texture, contour, and ability to move. Lip color varies with race and heredity. The lips of Caucasians are normally pink in color and soft, moist, and smooth in texture. People from the Mediterranean area tend to have darker lips. The nurse asks the patient to open the mouth and then notes any discoloration (such as pallor), blisters, swelling, cracks, or scales. The symmetry of contour is also observed. To determine lip movement, the patient is asked to purse the lips as if to whistle.

Mucous membranes Mucous membranes in light-skinned patients are normally pink, moist, and smooth. The hard palate is a lighter shade than the soft palate. In both light- and dark-skinned patients, hyperpigmentation of the mucous membranes of the mouth can occur. Black patients often have a normal bluish pigmentation of the gums and a brown freckled pigmentation of the gums, buccal cavity, and borders of the tongue (Roach 1977). To inspect the mucous membrane, the nurse retracts the cheeks with a tongue blade or an index finger covered with a piece of gauze. Any ulcerations, discoloration, white patches, nodules, excessive redness, and irritations are noted.

Tongue The tongue normally is moist, slightly coated, and a reddish color. The nurse notes dryness, excessive roughness or smoothness, fissures, ulcerations, and white or red patches.

Teeth Healthy teeth appear aligned, smooth, and white. The nurse notes missing teeth, dental caries, discolorations, the presence of partial or complete artificial dentures and how they fit, and the state of fillings.

Gums The gums are normally pink in color. Black people may have a bluish pigmentation to their gums, either evenly distributed or in patches. The nurse notes excessive redness, swelling, bleeding, tenderness, or receding gum lines.

Developmental changes

Teeth start to develop in the fetus at the 7th week and appear at about 5 months of fetal age. Temporary or deciduous teeth generally begin to show above the gum 5 to 8 months after birth.

By the time children are 2 years old, they usually have all 20 of their temporary teeth. See Figure 21–9. At about age 6 or 7, children start losing their deciduous teeth, and these are gradually replaced by the 32 permanent teeth. See Figure 21–10. By age 25, most people have all their permanent teeth.

By the time adults have reached advanced years, they may have very few of their permanent teeth left, and many have dentures. About 75% of elderly people have lost all their own teeth by age 70 (Anderson 1971:110). This is attributed mostly to periodontal disease rather than to dental caries; however, caries are also common in the middle-aged adult. Preventive dental care is important.

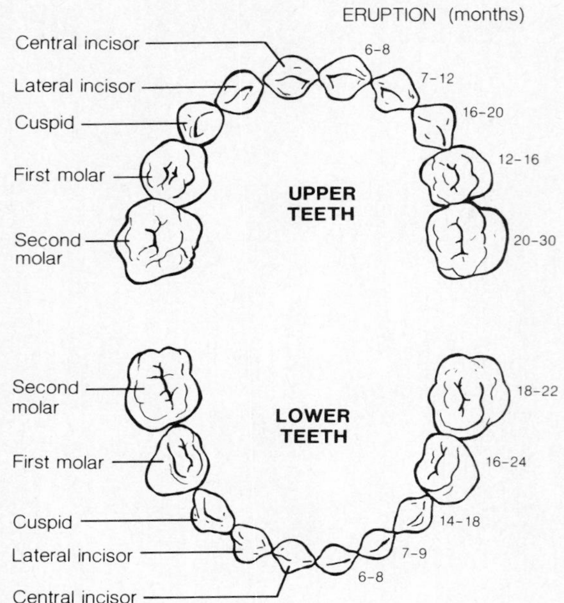

Figure 21–9 Temporary teeth and their times of eruption (stated in months).

Figure 21–10 Permanent teeth and their times of eruption (stated in years).

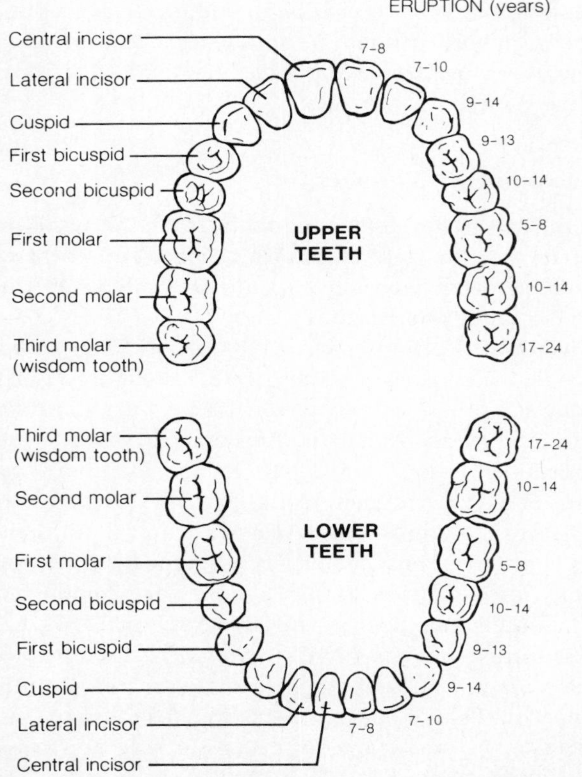

The age when people lose teeth or have them removed is highly individual. It depends on many factors, including dental care, diet, and dental hygiene practices (such as the frequency of brushing).

Oral hygienic practices

Oral hygienic practices include brushing teeth or cleaning dentures, flossing teeth, and the use of fluoride. When assessing a person's specific practices, the nurse determines the patient's frequency of cleaning and methods used.

Specific practices are influenced largely by:

1. *Personal preferences.* Great variation exists in the types of toothpaste, mouthwashes, denture cleaners, and types of dental floss available and selected.
2. *Sociocultural factors.* Early practices learned from parents often become well-established habits. For example, children who are encouraged to clean and/or rinse their teeth after every meal and at bedtime will often retain this practice as adults. Peers in work or social settings may also be a substantial influence, as evidenced by the numerous television commercials asserting the social benefits of cleaner, whiter teeth and fresh breath.
3. *Knowledge level.* A person's knowledge about the most effective ways to brush and floss teeth, the use of fluoride to prevent dental caries, the implications of infrequent oral hygiene, and the need for regular dental examinations often needs updating or reinforcement.
4. *Developmental status.* Children can start to brush their teeth by 2 years of age, when all deciduous teeth have appeared. They require much supervision and assistance, however.
5. *Health state.* Impaired health may alter a person's ability to manage oral hygiene self-care. The degree of assistance required needs to be determined.

Nursing Diagnoses: Common Oral Problems

Symptoms of oral problems

The following symptoms described by patients or observed in the mouth can reflect a problem that requires the assistance of a physician, dentist, or nurse:

1. *Halitosis* (bad breath)
2. Inflamed, swollen, receding, and/or bleeding gums
3. Discomfort or pain in a tooth when eating or drinking hot or cold fluids
4. Pain in a part of a jaw
5. Crusts on the mucous membranes

Common problems

Dental disease is common in North America. A study in 1960–62 found that the average American had 20 to 32 teeth either missing, filled, or decayed. It is estimated that three out of four adults who have their natural teeth show evidence of *periodontal disease* (a disease process around the teeth). It is further estimated that 800 million cavities as a result of tooth decay are unfilled (Milgrom 1975:29–30).

The most common oral problem in younger people is the occurrence of *dental caries* (tooth cavities). Dental caries is a pathologic process in which the enamel and the dentin gradually dissolve, eventually involving the pulp of the tooth. The underlying cause of dental caries is thought to be the presence of enzyme-producing bacteria of the lactic acid bacilli group. These bacteria, which are present in saliva, convert carbohydrates to lactic acid, which in turn dissolves tooth enamel, allowing for bacterial invasion and caries formation. The number of lactic acid bacilli can be reduced by the intake of fluoridated water or by topical application of fluoride, thus reducing dental caries.

Periodontal disease (pyorrhea) is a disease of the tissues that support the tooth. These tissues include the cementum, the periodontal ligament, the alveolar bone, and the gingiva. Often periodontitis, inflammation of the periodontal tissue, occurs as an extension of gingivitis (discussed below). Initially in the process of periodontal disease, plaque forms on the teeth, particularly at the gum line. Plaque is made up of mucin, carbohydrates, and the microorganisms normally found in the mouth. Mucin is the chief constituent of mucus and is a glycoprotein substance.

Stomatitis is an inflammatory condition of the mouth. Glossitis and gingivitis are localized forms. *Glossitis* is inflammation of the tongue (glossa), and *gingivitis* is inflammation of the gums (gingiva).

Parotitis is inflammation of the parotid salivary gland. It can occur in patients who have maintained poor oral hygiene, such as those unable to provide their own care because of paralysis and who have not received assistance.

Many pathogenic organisms can cause these inflammations: streptococci, herpes simplex viruses, and measles viruses. The inflammatory process can extend to the salivary glands, which empty into the oral cavity. Good oral hygiene, which includes brushing and flossing the teeth, helps prevent these inflammations. When a patient is taking very few or no fluids and little or no food, it is of utmost importance that oral hygiene be maintained as a preventive measure.

Halitosis may be the result of poor oral hygiene, or it may be caused by a disease process. If it is the result of bacterial action on food particles, cleaning the teeth, cleaning between the teeth, and the use of a mouthwash are helpful. If the cause is systemic, hygiene is of limited help.

Establishing nursing diagnoses

Mouth problems are often indications of other nursing diagnoses. For example, dry mucous membranes are often associated with fluid volume deficits. Dental caries, periodontal disease, inflammatory conditions, and halitosis may be regarded as health maintenance (or promotion) deficits or nutritional deficits that can be related to not following a recommended hygienic regime or lack of knowledge. If the patient is incapacitated by a disease process, the nursing diagnosis is often stated as a self-care deficit related to the specific impairment produced by the illness—e.g., "Self-care deficit (oral hygiene) related to severe arthritis."

Planning and Intervention for Mouth Care

Nursing goals

The overall nursing goal is to maintain the integrity of the teeth and oral mucous membrane. Subgoals are:

1. To remove food particles from around and between the teeth
2. To remove dental plaque
3. To enhance the patient's sense of well-being
4. To prevent infections of oral tissues

Planning

Planning interventions to assist a patient with oral hygiene includes consideration of the patient's personal preferences, the patient's health status and limitations, and the supplies available. Establishment of outcome criteria is a necessary part of planning. For suggested criteria, see the section on evaluation on page 513.

Oral Hygiene

Good oral hygiene includes daily stimulation of the gums, mechanical scrubbing of the teeth, and flushing of the mouth. Checkups by a dentist every 6 months are also recommended. The nurse is often in a position to help people, young or old, ill or well, to maintain oral hygiene by helping or teaching them to carry out oral practices, by inspecting whether hygiene has been carried out, particularly with children, or by actually providing hygienic measures for patients who are ill or

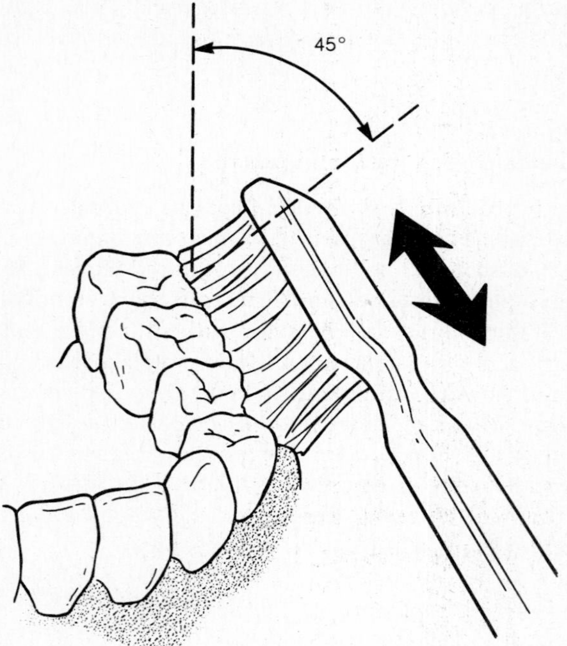

Figure 21–11 The bristles of the toothbrush are held against the teeth at a 45° angle.

Figure 21–12 The tips of the bristles penetrate under the sulcus of the gum.

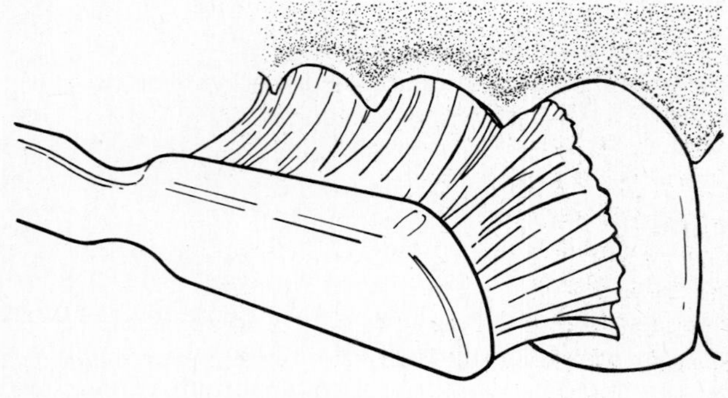

incapacitated. The nurse can also be instrumental in identifying and referring problems that require the services of a dentist. The following measures combat tooth decay:

1. Brush the teeth thoroughly after meals and at bedtime. Assist children or inspect their mouths to be sure the teeth are clean.
2. Floss the teeth daily.
3. Ensure an adequate intake of nutrients, particularly calcium, phosphorus, vitamins A, C, and D, and fluoride.
4. Avoid sweet foods and drinks between meals. Take them in moderation after meals.
5. Eat coarse, fibrous foods (cleansing foods), such as fresh fruits and raw vegetables.
6. Take a fluoride supplement daily until age 14 or 16 as an alternative to fluoridated water.
7. Have topical fluoride applications as prescribed by the dentist.
8. Have a checkup by a dentist every 6 months.

Brushing teeth

Thorough brushing of the teeth is important in preventing tooth decay. Teeth should be brushed at least four times a day—after meals and at bedtime. Use of a medium or soft multibristled brush is advised, since it minimizes the chance of trauma to the gums. The mechanical action of brushing removes food particles that can harbor and incubate bacteria. It also stimulates circulation in the gums, thus maintaining their healthy firmness.

The technique most recently recommended for brushing teeth is called the *sulcular technique*. It removes plaque and cleans under the gingival margins. Use of a soft-bristled, small toothbrush is required. The brush is held against the teeth so that the bristles are at a 45° angle. See Figure 21–11. The tips of the outer bristles should rest against and penetrate under the gingival sulcus of the gums. See Figure 21–12. The brush will clean under the sulci of only two or three teeth at one time. The bristles are moved back and forth using a vibrating or jiggling motion, from the sulcus to the crown of the tooth. This process is repeated until all outer and inner surfaces of the teeth and sulci of the gums are cleaned. Biting surfaces of the teeth are cleaned by moving the brush back and forth over them in short strokes.

An abundant variety of toothpastes are marketed, any of which can be used in the cleaning process. They are flavored and scented to make them pleasant tasting. However, an effective dentifrice can be made by combining two parts of table salt to one part of baking soda.

After the teeth are brushed, the mouth is rinsed with water to remove dislodged food particles and excess dentifrice. Many antiseptic mouthwashes are marketed, and some people prefer these for rinsing. If brushing cannot be done after the intake of food, vigorous rinsing of the mouth with water is recommended.

Children should be taught the habit of brushing their teeth by age 2, when the teeth appear. Because children cannot manage this independently for several years, parents are advised to do the brushing for them. A small stool can be provided in the bathroom for the child to reach the sink, and a special place for the child's toothbrush can enhance positive attitudes about this habit.

Dental flossing

Daily flossing of the teeth is advised. It is especially beneficial in preventing the formation of plaque and

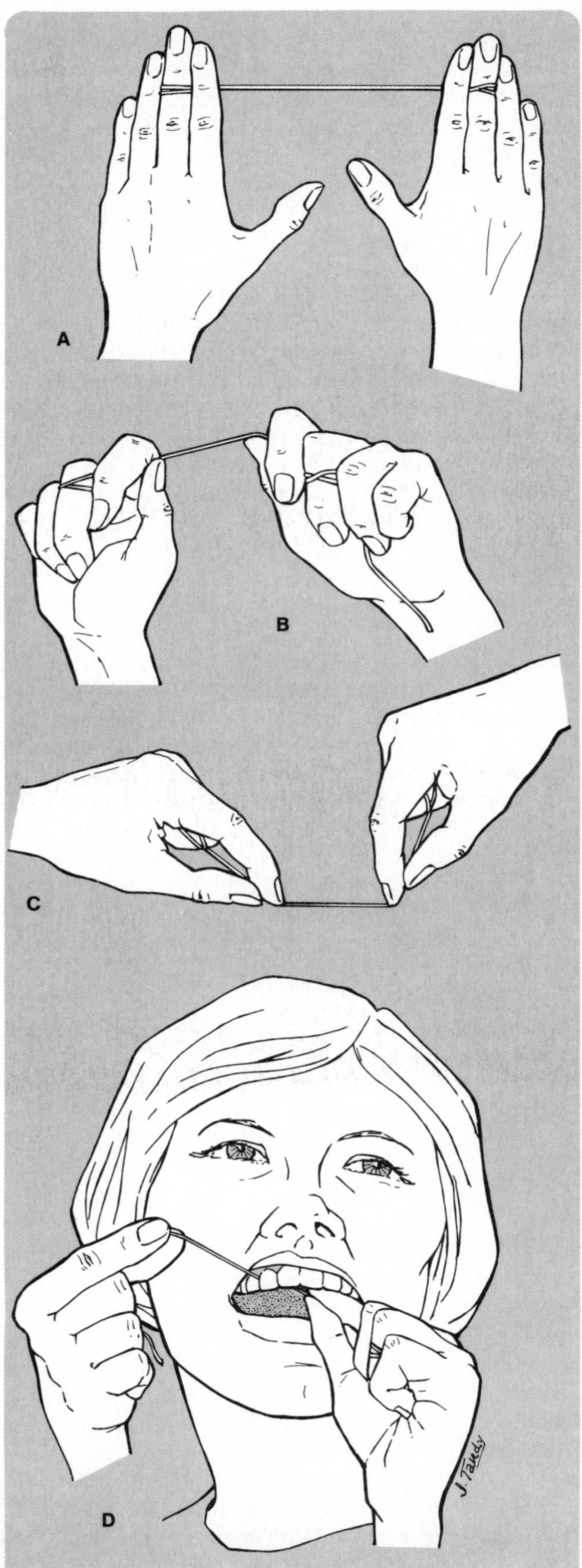

Figure 21–13 Flossing teeth: **A,** hold the floss between the third fingers of the hands; **B,** floss the upper teeth using the thumbs to stretch the floss; **C,** floss the lower teeth using the second fingers to stretch the floss; **D,** move the floss back and forth between the teeth. Do not force the floss. Floss gently to the gum surface.

removing it from the teeth, particularly at the gum line. A method for flossing is described in Figure 21–13.

Use of fluoride

The use of fluoride is known to prevent dental caries, although by itself it does not eliminate tooth decay. Many regions have water supplies that contain fluoride. Children who drink fluoridated water when their teeth are forming can develop a resistance to cavities that carries over to adult life. Some benefit is also received if a child starts drinking fluoridated water even after the teeth are formed. For people who do not have access to fluoridated water, a fluoride solution can be applied to the teeth at regular intervals by a dentist or dental hygienist. Using toothpaste and mouthwash that contain fluoride can help in preventing tooth decay.

Fluoride supplements are also recommended as an alternative to fluoridated water, starting at 1 month and continuing until age 14 or 16 years. Some preparations are combined with vitamins, but these are not necessary. Prevention of tooth decay depends on regular ingestion of fluoride. Recommended dosages of liquid fluoride supplement (8 drops = 1 mg fluoride ion) where there is little or no fluoride in the water are:

2 weeks to 2 years	2 drops (0.25 mg) daily
2 to 3 years	4 drops (0.5 mg) daily
3 to 16 years	8 drops (1 mg) daily

Patients need to be cautioned about the effects of overfluoridation, one of which is a mottled discoloration of the tooth enamel. The supplement can be acquired without a prescription and can be taken with water, milk, or juice. It needs to be kept out of the reach of children.

Dental examinations

It is recommended that children be taken to the family dentist by age 2½ or 3, to become accustomed to going to a dentist and to begin topical fluoride applications. By this age 50% of children have tooth decay, and prompt treatment is necessary. Small cavities in primary teeth can progress to large ones within a few months. Unlike bones that can heal themselves, teeth must be filled. Nothing but a filling will arrest tooth decay. The dentist can also offer advice at this time about care of the child's teeth and can identify any problems.

Some people hold the illusion that it is not necessary to fill primary teeth, since they will inevitably be replaced. The nurse can be instrumental in teaching the facts in this situation. It is important that primary teeth be looked after, since some must last up to 12 years. Primary teeth are needed as guides for permanent tooth eruption, for stimulating natural growth of the jaws, for an attractive appearance, and for normal speech development. Primary teeth that are lost earlier than prescribed by nature can cause permanent teeth to erupt out of line. Once a tooth is lost, adjacent teeth drift over to close the space, and they may interfere with eruption of the underlying permanent tooth. When the space for the new permanent tooth is narrowed, that tooth is forced to grow either in toward the tongue or out toward the cheek. A temporary space maintainer can be inserted by the dentist until the permanent tooth erupts, to prevent malalignment.

Assisting hospitalized patients

When patients are hospitalized, it is the nurse's responsibility to assist them in carrying out oral hygiene. Most ambulatory patients can do this independently. Most bedridden patients require little assistance other than provision of a glass of water, dentifrice, a mouthwash if desired, a kidney basin for rinsing the mouth, and a towel to wipe the mouth. Afterward, the nurse needs to clean the patient's toothbrush and kidney basin. Patients who are fasting for surgery or diagnostic tests greatly appreciate oral hygiene. Their mouths are dry, and they feel thirsty. Oral hygiene can do much to alleviate their thirst.

Dependent patients Patients who are unconscious need oral hygiene provided for them. Unconscious patients are positioned laterally with the head of the bed lowered to prevent aspiration of the oral care fluids. A kidney basin or a towel is placed under the patient's chin.

For edentulous patients, the gums, cheeks, roof of the mouth, and tongue are thoroughly cleaned, while the cheeks are retracted with one hand. Commercially prepared applicators soaked with oil and lemon juice can be used for cleaning. If these are not available, a gauze square rolled around the index finger and dipped in an oil and lemon juice preparation or an antiseptic mouthwash is also effective. Only small amounts of solution are needed to moisten the mucous membranes. Large amounts of fluid are avoided because they can be aspirated by patients who have swallowing difficulties. Excess fluid is drawn out by gravity if the patient is in an appropriate position. The patient's mouth is then dried, and a lubricant such as petroleum jelly can be applied to the lips.

For dentulous patients, in addition to the above measures, the nurse needs to brush the patient's teeth. Brushing someone else's teeth requires some practice in order to apply sufficient pressure for cleaning the teeth but not so much pressure that the gum tissue could be injured. Rinsing the mouth, if warranted, can be accomplished using a rubber-tipped bulb syringe and water.

Hemiplegic patients Patients who have hemiplegia frequently require assistance from the nurse because food particles tend to collect in the affected side of the mouth. Due to loss of sensation and muscle power on one side of the mouth, these patients often have difficulty doing a thorough cleaning.

Care of dentures

Most patients in a hospital can clean their own dentures. However, for the incapacitated or the bedridden elderly or confused patient, it becomes the nurse's responsibility.

To remove upper dentures, the nurse grasps them at the front with the thumb and index finger, using a piece of tissue or gauze. They may need to be moved slightly up and down to overcome the suction effect on the roof of the mouth. Lower dentures are readily removed by retracting the cheek, turning them slightly, and pulling them out between the lips on one side and then the other. Partial plates and removable bridges may also need to be taken out by the nurse. Dentures must be handled carefully, since they can break if dropped or knocked against metal water taps. Most agencies supply special containers for patients' dentures, which are labeled with the patient's name and stored at the bedside. Dentures are cleaned with a toothbrush and dentifrice and then well rinsed with water. Replacing dentures in the patient's mouth is facilitated if the dentures are moist. Water, saline, or commercial preparations can be used to soak dentures during the night.

Special oral care

Disease processes and inadequate nutrition can alter the normal moist mucous membranes of the mouth and the tissues of the lips. For example, dehydration can cause halitosis (bad breath), furry tongue, and sordes. *Sordes* is the accumulation of foul matter (food, microorganisms, and epithelial elements) on the teeth and lips. In order to remove sordes it is necessary to use special cleaning solutions such as hydrogen peroxide. If hydrogen peroxide is used, it must be diluted with an equal amount of water. Prolonged action of full-strength hydrogen peroxide makes the gums and mucosa spongy. After the cleaning, the peroxide solution is rinsed from the mouth. Special mouth care usually means increased frequency of mouth care and increased mechanical cleaning and lubrication.

Evaluation: Outcome Criteria

Outcome criteria for oral hygiene interventions may include:

1. Lips are smooth, moist, and intact.
2. Mucous membranes are moist and smooth.
3. Tongue is moist, slightly coated, and reddish in color.
4. Patient brushes teeth four times a day.
5. Patient flosses teeth daily.

Hair

Hair grows on the whole body surface except on the palms of the hands, the soles of the feet, the dorsal surfaces of terminal phalanges, and parts of the genitals (the inner surface of the labia and inner surface of the prepuce of the glans penis).

Surface hair is of two types: the *vellus*, which is the fine, nonpigmented hair covering large areas of the body, and *terminal hair*, which is longer, coarser, and pigmented. Hair grows at varying rates and is shed at varying times. The scalp of the average person loses between 20 and 100 hairs per day. Body hair is shed in 3 to 4 months, whereas hair in beards lasts 3 or 4 years (Brown et al. 1973:39).

The visible part of a hair is called the *hair shaft*. The root is in a tube known as a *hair follicle*. There are muscles known as *arrector pili muscles* attached to the hair follicles. When these contract, the skin assumes a gooseflesh appearance. Sebaceous glands, which secrete sebum, grow from the walls of hair follicles. Sebum is produced in greater quantities on the scalp and the face than elsewhere on the body.

Assessment of the Hair

Assessment of an individual's hair includes physical examination of the hair, consideration of developmental changes, and determination of the individual's hair care practices and the factors influencing them.

Physical examination

Normal, natural hair is black, brown, red, yellow, or shades of these colors. Hair fibers vary in shape—they may be straight, spiral, wavy, or helical. This variation makes the texture of the hair straight, wavy, kinky, or woolly. Hair also varies from fine to coarse. Black-skinned people often have thicker, drier, curlier hair than white-skinned people.

Normal hair has resilience and is evenly distributed. People with severe protein deficiency (kwashiorkor) have faded hair colors that appear reddish or bleached and coarse, dry hair texture. Some therapies for cancer cause *alopecia* (baldness), and some disease conditions affect the coarseness of hair.

Hair is assessed for:

1. The evenness of hair growth over the scalp and, in particular, any patchy loss of hair.
2. Texture, i.e., whether it is coarse or silky.
3. Oiliness, i.e., whether it is dry or greasy.
4. Thickness or thinness.
5. Presence of infections or infestations on the scalp, including flaking, sores, lice, nits (louse eggs), and ringworm.
6. Sutures in the infant's skull. Sutures in the newborn can be felt as ridges, since overriding of the bones occurs during delivery. Flattening occurs by about 6 months, and some infants normally have wide spaces. After 6 months, ridges or breaks in the cranial bones usually indicate fractures.
7. The presence of hair on the body. *Hirsutism* is the presence of unusually dark, thick hair on the body. It has little significance in men but should be noted in children and women.

Developmental changes

Newborns may have *lanugo* (the fine hair on the body of the fetus, also referred to as *down* or *woolly hair*) over their shoulders, back, and sacrum. This generally disappears, and the hair distribution becomes noticeable on the eyebrows, head, and eyelashes of young children. Some newborns have hair on their scalps; others are free of hair at birth but grow hair over the scalp during the first year of life.

Pubic hair usually appears in early puberty followed in about 6 months by the growth of axillary hair. Boys develop facial hair in later puberty.

In adolescence the sebaceous glands increase in activity as a result of increased hormone levels. As a result, hair follicle openings enlarge to accommodate the increased amount of sebum, and the adolescent's hair may become more oily.

In elderly people the hair is generally thinner, grows more slowly, and loses its color as a result of aging tissues and diminishing circulation. Men often lose their scalp hair and may become completely bald. This phenomenon may occur even when a man is relatively young. The older person's hair also tends to be drier than normal. With age, axillary and pubic hair becomes finer and scanter, in contrast to the eyebrows, which become bristly and coarse. Most women develop hair on their faces, which may be a problem to them.

Factors affecting hair care

Each person has particular ways of caring for hair, influenced by a number of factors. Some shampoo it daily, e.g., under the shower; others shampoo once a week or even less often. Black-skinned people often need to oil their hair daily because it tends to be dry. Oil prevents the hair from breaking and the scalp from drying. A wide-toothed comb is usually used, because finer combs pull and break the hair. Some people brush their hair vigorously before retiring, others comb their hair frequently. For additional information about factors influencing hair care, see Factors Influencing Skin Care on page 487.

Common problems

Ticks *Ticks* are small parasites that bite into tissue and suck blood. They take many forms and can adapt themselves to various conditions. The genera *Ornithodoros* and *Dermacentor* are found in North America. They can attach to human beings and are found frequently in the hair. They can be as large as 1.3 cm (0.5 in) and appear gray-brown. They attach to a person with the apparatus by which they suck blood and should not be torn off, because the sucking apparatus will be left in the skin and become infected. If oil is poured on the tick, it loses its hold, because it is deprived of oxygen, and it withdraws its sucker.

Ticks transmit several diseases to people, in particular, Rocky Mountain spotted fever and tularemia.

Lice *Lice* are parasitic insects that infest mammals. Hundreds of varieties of lice infest humans. Three that are particularly common are *Pediculosis capitis* or the head louse, *Pediculosis corporis* or the body louse, and *Pediculosis pubis* or the crab louse.

Pediculosis capitis is found on the scalp and tends to stay hidden by the hairs; similarly, *Pediculosis pubis* stays in pubic hair. *Pediculosis corporis* tends to cling to clothing, so that, when a patient undresses, the lice may not be in evidence on the body; these lice suck blood from the person and lay their eggs on the clothing. The nurse can suspect their presence in the clothing from three chief symptoms: (a) the person habitually scratches, (b) there are scratches on the skin, and (c) there are hemorrhagic spots on the skin where the lice have sucked blood.

Head and pubic lice lay their eggs on the hairs; the eggs look like oval particles, similar to dandruff, clinging to the hair. Bites and pustular eruptions may also be noticed at the hair lines and behind the ears.

Lice are very small, grayish white, and difficult to see. The crab louse in the pubic area has red legs. Lice may be contracted from infested clothes and direct contact with an infested person.

The treatment now used in most areas is gamma benzene hexachloride (Kwell). It comes as a cream, a lotion, and a shampoo. For head lice the hair is washed with the shampoo and the bed linens are changed. This treatment is repeated 12 to 24 hours later if needed. For pubic and body lice, the patient takes a bath or shower, dries, and applies the lotion or cream—to the entire body surface for body lice, and to the pubic area and adjacent areas for pubic lice. After 12 to 24 hours, the lotion is washed off, and clean clothing and linens are supplied.

Dandruff Dandruff appears as a diffuse scaling of the scalp often accompanied by itching. In severe cases it involves the auditory canals and the eyebrows. Mild cases of dandruff can usually be treated effectively with a commercial shampoo specifically recommended for dandruff. In severe or persistent cases, the patient may need the advice of a physician.

Hirsutism Hirsutism is the growth of excessive body hair. The acceptance of body hair in the axillae and on the legs is largely dictated by culture. In North America the well-groomed woman, as depicted in magazines, has no hair on her legs or under her axillae (although this idea is changing). In many European cultures it is not customary to remove this hair to be considered well groomed.

Excessive facial hair on a woman is thought unattractive in most Western and Oriental cultures. For example, some Japanese brides follow the custom of shaving their faces the day before the wedding.

The cause of excessive body hair is not always known. Elderly women may have some on their faces, and women during menopause may also experience the growth of facial hair. The causes of these conditions may involve the endocrine system. It is also thought that heredity influences both the pattern of hair distribution and the production of androgens by the adrenal glands.

There are a number of ways of removing hair: waxing, pulling with tweezers, shaving with a razor, applying depilatory lotions, and electrolysis. In the waxing process, warm wax is poured on the area and allowed to harden. The hairs become embedded in the wax and come away from the skin when the wax is removed. Tweezers are commonly used to remove excess hair from the eyebrows and the face. This can be a time-consuming project if there is a great deal of hair, and it needs to be repeated when the hair grows back, often in 2 to 3 weeks. Shaving with a razor is done frequently for leg and axilla hair. It is an inexpensive and effective method, but it must be repeated frequently. Depilatory creams and lotions destroy the hair shaft through a chemical action, so that the hair wipes away easily. This method of hair removal is expensive compared to shaving. In the initial use of a product, it is important to assess the amount of skin irritation it causes. It is advisable to put lotion on a small area initially and observe for signs of irritation. Electrolysis is the only permanent way of removing hair. The hair follicle is destroyed by means of an electric current. Usually, repeated treatments on a follicle are needed before it is completely destroyed. This method of treatment is relatively expensive.

Planning and Intervention for Hair Care

Nursing goals

The overall nursing goal is to maintain the well-groomed appearance of the hair. Subgoals are:

1. To prevent tangles
2. To enhance the individual's feelings of self-esteem by maintaining the hair attractively and neatly
3. To stimulate blood circulation to the scalp
4. To maintain cleanliness of the hair and scalp

Planning

Planning for assisting a patient with hair care includes consideration of the patient's personal preferences, health, and energy resources, and the time, equipment, and personnel available. Often patients like to have hair care following a bath, before visitors, and/or before retiring. At some agencies shampoos can be given to patients only after a physician's order.

Planning involves establishing outcome criteria. For suggestions, see Evaluation later in this chapter.

Hair Care

Brushing and combing

Hair needs to be brushed daily in order to be healthy. Brushing has three major functions: It stimulates the circulation of blood in the scalp, it distributes the oil along the hair shaft, and it helps to arrange the hair for the patient, although most people use a comb for this.

Long hair may present a problem to patients when they are unable to go to a hairdresser for a long period. To prevent it from matting, it needs to be combed at least daily. Some patients are pleased to have it tied neatly in the back or braided until other assistance is available or until they feel better and can look after it.

Shampooing

The cleanliness and grooming of both men's and women's hair is frequently related closely to their sense of well-being. Often after patients begin to feel better, having their hair done is a boost to morale and positive feelings about their appearance.

The frequency with which a person needs to shampoo is highly individual, depending to a large degree on the person's activities and the amount of sebum secreted by the scalp. Oily hair tends to look stringy and dirty, and it feels unclean to the person.

There are a wide variety of shampoos on the commercial market, and most patients have their own favorite brands. If a person's hair tends to tangle after it is washed, a cream rinse after the shampoo can prevent this. A black-skinned person's hair needs to be combed with a wide-toothed comb before it dries, to avoid tangling. Following a shampoo many women and some men like to have their hair rolled on curlers and styled. Some hospitals also provide hair driers.

A patient who is unable to sit up at a sink for a shampoo may be able to lie on a stretcher with the head at the edge of a water basin. A nurse assisting a patient with a shampoo needs to rinse all the shampoo solution from the hair, particularly a dandruff shampoo, which may damage the hair and irritate the scalp if it remains.

Evaluation: Outcome Criteria

Outcome criteria for hair care may include:

1. No evidence of extreme dryness or oiliness.
2. Hair appears neat, clean, and well groomed.
3. No matting or tangles in hair.
4. No evidence of dandruff, lice, scalp redness, or excoriations.
5. Patient can comb and brush hair with left arm.

Eyes

The eyes are extremely important organs, but they require no special care in daily living. The lacrimal glands, situated in a depression in the frontal bone at the upper outer angle of the eye orbit, produce lacrimal fluid, which continually washes the eyes. This fluid empties into the lacrimal sac, which is situated in the inner canthus. From the lacrimal sac the fluid drains through the lacrimal duct to the inferior meatus of the nose. The fluid keeps the eyeball moist and helps wash away foreign particles. Excessive lacrimal fluid forms tears. For additional information about the eyes, see Chapter 14.

Assessment of the Eyes

Relative to patient hygiene, the eyes are assessed for redness of the conjunctiva and the presence of secretions that can dry on the lashes as crusts. The dependent patient needs assistance wiping these crusts away. Other aspects of eye assessment are discussed in Chapter 14.

Normally patients do not have hygiene practices for the eyes unless they have a special appliance such as an artificial eye (discussed later in this chapter).

Planning and Intervention for Eye Care

In newborns the eyes are treated soon after birth to prevent ophthalmia neonatorum (gonorrheal conjunctivitis). Penicillin and silver nitrate are the drugs of treatment. Treatment is mandatory by law in all states in the United States. The method of instilling the drops and wiping the eyes is the same for babies as for children and adults. See Chapter 37.

Dried secretions on the lashes may need to be softened and wiped away. In hospitals this is usually done with a sterile cotton ball moistened with sterile water or normal saline. The nurse wipes from the inner canthus of the eye to the outer canthus, to prevent the particles and fluid from draining into the nasolacrimal duct. In the home, it is usually not necessary for the fluid to be sterile, and the excess fluid is usually wiped away with a soft tissue.

Evaluation: Outcome Criteria

Outcome criteria for eye care may include:

1. No evidence of conjunctival redness.
2. No evidence of secretions.

Other Care Related to the Eyes

Care of artificial eyes

Patients who have artificial eyes usually have their own ways to remove and clean them and to clean the socket and surrounding tissues. Nurses should ask patients how they wish to do this and what equipment they require.

If a patient is unconscious or for some reason is unable to do this, the nurse needs to assist. To remove the artificial eye from the socket, the nurse pulls the lower lid down and exerts slight pressure just below the eye. This will usually break the suction, and the eye will come out. The nurse must make sure to catch the eye and not scratch it in any way.

Another method to remove the eye uses a small rubber bulb (syringe bulb or medicine dropper bulb). The bulb is first squeezed to create a suction effect, and then the tip is placed directly on the eye. This suction counteracts the pressure holding the eye in place, causing the eye to come away with the bulb.

Artificial eyes are usually washed with warm normal saline. The eye socket and the surrounding tissues are also washed with the solution, cleaning from the inner canthus to the outer canthus.

The eye can be reinserted by pulling the lower lid down and slipping the eye gently into its socket. It should fit neatly under the upper lid.

Care of eyeglasses

Most eyeglasses manufactured today are impact resistant. That is, with a forceful blow they will not fragment as glasses did in years past. Plastic is also being used in eyeglasses today. It is safe but also is easily scratched.

Most patients have their own way of washing and drying their glasses. If nurses are required to clean glasses, they can do so with warm water, and then wipe the glasses dry with a soft tissue. If the patient has plastic lenses, the use of tissue may be contraindicated, and a special cloth or paper is used for wiping.

Care of contact lenses

A contact lens is a small oval disk that fits directly on the eye. It may be a hard or soft lens. Most people have special small containers for their contact lenses when they are not wearing them. Contact lenses have several advantages over eyeglasses for some people. First, they cannot be seen, and thus have a cosmetic value. Second, they can be highly effective in correcting some types of

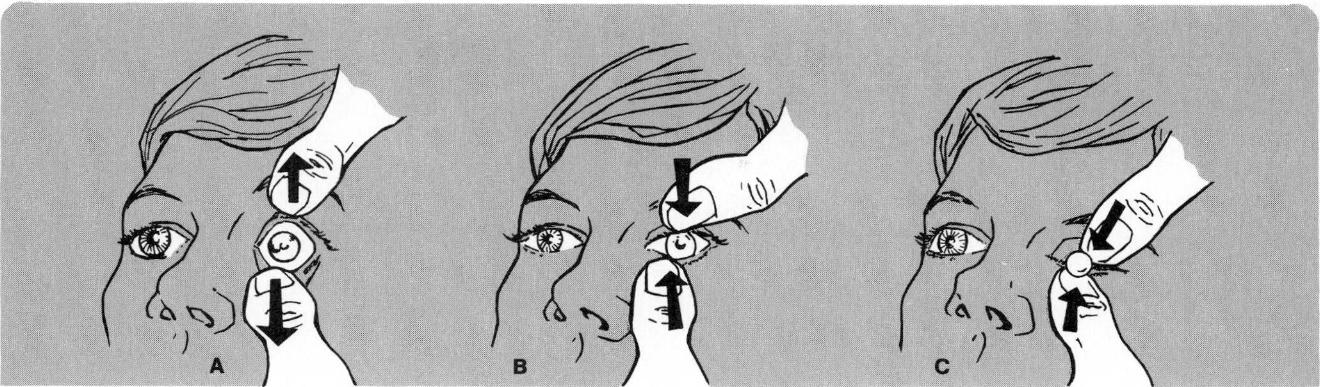

Figure 21–14 Removing a hard contact lens for a patient: **A,** spread the eyelids apart; **B,** bring the eyelids to the edge of the lens; **C,** move both lids closer together, pressing the lower lid more firmly under the lens to tip the lens out.

astigmatisms when there is a problem in the curvature of the cornea. Third, they can be safer than eyeglasses in activities such as sports and physically active jobs.

Contact lenses should not be worn continually because of irritation to the eyes. They are normally worn for a maximum of 12 to 15 hours daily and removed when sleeping, swimming, and in very smoky environments. If a patient cannot remove his or her own contacts, the nurse assumes this responsibility to prevent damage to the eyes.

Removal of contact lenses Contacts are normally worn directly over the cornea of the eye. To remove a hard lens for a patient, the nurse separates the upper and lower eyelids, one with each thumb, until they are beyond the edges of the lens. Pressure is exerted toward the bony orbit above and below the eye, not directly on the eye. Next, the lower eyelid margin is gently moved up toward the lens, and the upper eyelid margin is moved down to the lens edge. The lower lid margin is then pressed more firmly under the contact lens while the top is held stationary. The lens will tip with this pressure and lift out on the bottom edge. If both eyelids are moved toward each other, the lens will slide off the eye and out. See Figure 21-14. If a lens is not directly over the cornea, it should be moved back to the proper place prior to removal. This can be done with gentle pressure on the eyelid, moving in the direction indicated.

To remove a soft contact lens, the nurse asks the patient to look upward. The lower lid is retracted with the nurse's middle finger and the tip of the index finger is placed on the lower edge of the lens. The nurse slides the lens down to the inferior aspect of the eye and compresses the lens slightly between the thumb and index finger. Rolling the thumb and index finger together causes the lens to double up and air to enter underneath the lens. The lens can then be removed from the eye.

Insertion of contact lenses Lenses are stored in special containers that either are dry or contain a solution. Each lens slot is labeled, for the right or left eye. It is essential that the correct lens be applied to the eye, since lenses are ground to fit the individual eye. Prior to insertion, a contact lens should be cleaned with a sterile, nonirritating solution. Wetting agents are then applied to the lens. Use of saliva as a wetting agent should be discouraged, since it harbors many pathogens. To insert the contact lens, the nurse places it on the tip of the index finger, separates the eyelids sufficiently to expose the area, and places the lens directly over the cornea. See Figure 21–15. This is best done by having the patient either lie on the back or bend the head backward. Soft lenses can be inserted by flexing the lens between the thumb and the index finger. The edge should be erect and pointing slightly inward if the lens is in the correct position for application. The nurse then places the lens directly on the cornea.

Figure 21–15 Separating the upper and lower eyelids with the thumb and index finger to insert a contact lens.

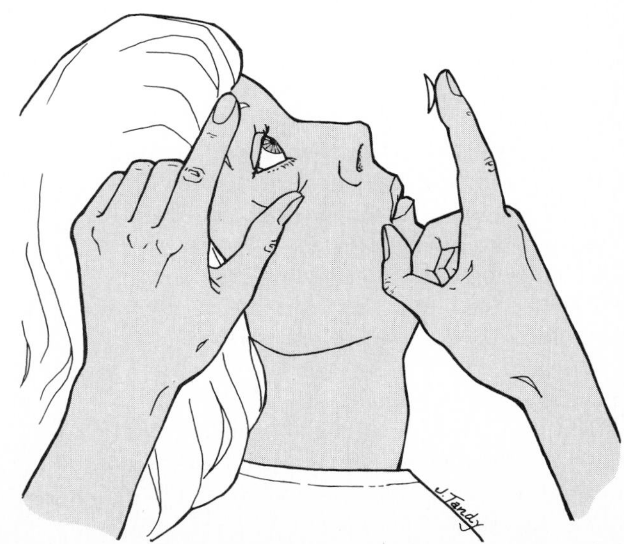

Nose and Ears

The nose and the ears require minimal care in normal hygiene. For babies and small children, a small piece of absorbent cotton moistened with warm water and twisted between the fingers can be used to clean the nostrils and the external ear canals. It is inserted and then rotated inside the orifice to catch any foreign materials. Neither sticks nor bobby pins should be used because of the danger of abrading the mucous membrane or puncturing the eardrum.

A common problem of the ears is accumulation of *cerumen* (earwax) in the external auditory canal. This may cause difficulty hearing and discomfort when it hardens. The treatment is to syringe the ears, and this is generally carried out by a physician. For additional information, see Chapter 14.

Beds

Ill persons are frequently confined to a bed, sometimes for weeks or months. The bed then becomes an important piece of furniture, and the patient's ability to rest and sleep is often directly related to it.

There are different types of beds. Patients who are ill at home may find their own beds quite satisfactory as long as the periods of illness are brief. A hospital bed has characteristics particularly suited to people who are in bed continuously or for a long time. Some of the chief characteristics are:

1. It is equipped to save a patient energy. Many hospital beds are motorized, so that by pushing a button the patient can raise or lower the head or the foot.
2. It is made so that a nurse can easily reach a patient in bed. Most hospital beds are 66 cm (26 in) from the floor and can be raised above that by a motor or lever. A nurse then does not need to bend over as far as for most home beds. The hospital bed is 0.9 m (3 ft) wide and 1.8 m (6.5 ft) long. Thus it is narrower than a normal bed.
3. The mattress is generally firm, to provide good body support. Special mattresses are also available, including sponge rubber, alternating pressure, eggshell, and water mattresses. Hospital mattresses are generally covered with a water repellent material so that they do not soil readily.
4. A rubber or plastic drawsheet can be used over the middle area of the bed, to protect the mattress and bottom sheet from drainages. These drawsheets are seldom used routinely today.
5. Linen is generally long and wide enough so that it tucks under well, and the bed stays in a comfortable, neat condition for a relatively long time.
6. Linens and blankets are of durable quality, to withstand many washings.
7. The bed is easily moved. Each leg has a caster, usually made of hard rubber, that turns easily, making it possible to move the bed without jarring the patient.

Nurses need to be able to make hospital beds in different ways in order to suit specific purposes. For example, it is often necessary to make a bed while the patient remains in it (occupied bed), or to make a bed for a patient who is having surgery (anesthetic bed). Although in most instances nurses delegate bed making to other personnel, a nurse should know how to make beds quickly and expediently, disturbing a patient as little as possible.

Hospital beds are either open or closed. An open bed is one currently being used by a patient; generally the top covers are folded back to make it easier to get in. A closed bed is not being used and has the top covers under the pillows.

Bed Positions

Hospital beds can be adjusted to a number of positions. The most common are:

1. *Fowler's and semi-Fowler's positions.* See Chapter 23.
2. *Trendelenburg's position.* The head of the bed is lowered, the foot of the bed is elevated, and the mattress remains unbent. See Figure 21–16. Pins are usually placed in the extendable legs at the foot of the bed. Sometimes blocks, often referred to as *shock blocks*, are placed under the legs at the foot of the bed. This position is contraindicated in shock, head injury, chest injury, and respiratory cases.
3. *Reverse Trendelenburg's position.* This is the opposite of Trendelenburg's position. The head section is elevated, and the foot is lowered, while the mattress remains unbent. See Figure 21–17. The legs at the head of the bed may be placed on blocks.
4. *Hyperextension position.* Both the head and the foot sections are lowered 15° to create an angle in the bed foundation. See Figure 21–18. This position is some-

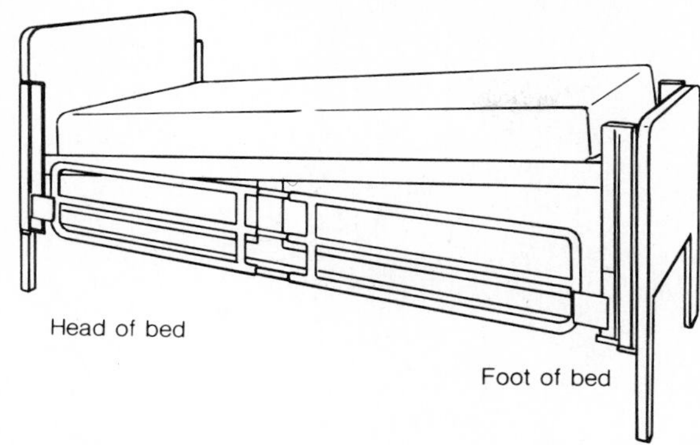

Figure 21–16 A bed in Trendelenburg's position.

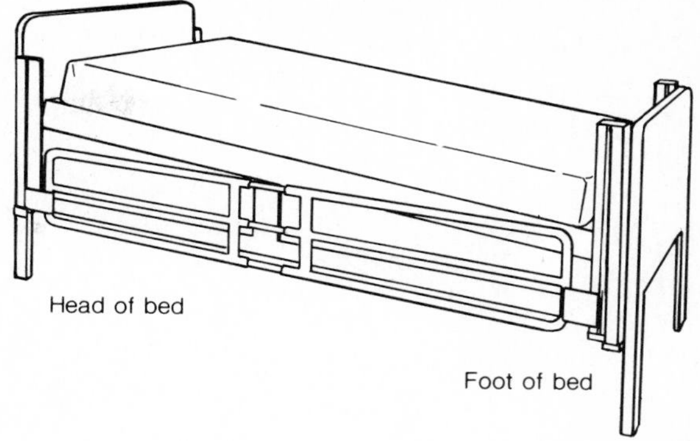

Figure 21–17 A bed in reverse Trendelenburg's position.

times used for patients who have spinal fractures but only on the specific order of the physician.

Bed Unit Equipment

Hospital beds usually are accompanied by a bedside table and an overbed table for the patient's use. The bedside table has a drawer and a cupboard. The drawer is used for the patient's personal possessions. The cupboard usually contains a washbasin and a kidney basin. A rod on the back of the table holds the patient's towels and washcloths. The overbed table fits over the bed. A patient can sit in bed and eat from the table in relative comfort. Most overbed tables can be raised or lowered, to meet the patient's needs.

One or two chairs are generally part of the hospital bed unit, together with a closet or locker, lights, and a signal at the bed. When the switch is pulled or the button is pressed, the signal turns on a light outside the patient's room and in other places on the hospital unit, e.g., the nursing office, to indicate to the nursing staff that a patient requires assistance.

Changing Beds

An unoccupied bed can be either closed or open. Generally the top covers of an open bed are folded back to make it easier for a patient to get in. Open and closed beds are made the same way, except that, for a closed bed, the top sheet, blanket, and bedspread are drawn up to the top of the bed under the pillows.

Mitering bed corners

Mitering is used at most corners of the bed for the sheets, blankets, and bedspread. The purpose of mitering is to secure the bedclothes while the bed is occupied. The following steps are required:

1. Tuck the bedcover (sheet, blanket, and/or spread) in firmly under the mattress at the bottom or top of the bed. See Figure 21–19.
2. Lift the bedcover at point 1 and bring it up so that it forms a triangle with the side edge of the bed, and the edge of the bedcover is parallel with the end of the bed. See Figure 21–20.
3. Tuck the part of the cover that hangs below the mattress under the mattress (see Figure 21–21), while holding the cover at point 1 against the mattress.
4. Bring point 1 down toward the floor while the other hand holds the fold of the cover against the side of the mattress. See Figure 21–22.
5. Remove the hand, and tuck the remainder of the cover under the mattress, if appropriate. See Figure 21–23. The sides of the top sheet, blanket, and bedspread may be left hanging freely rather than tucked in. The bedspread is mitered separately and left hanging freely if the top sheet and blanket are tucked in.

Figure 21–18 A bed in hyperextension position.

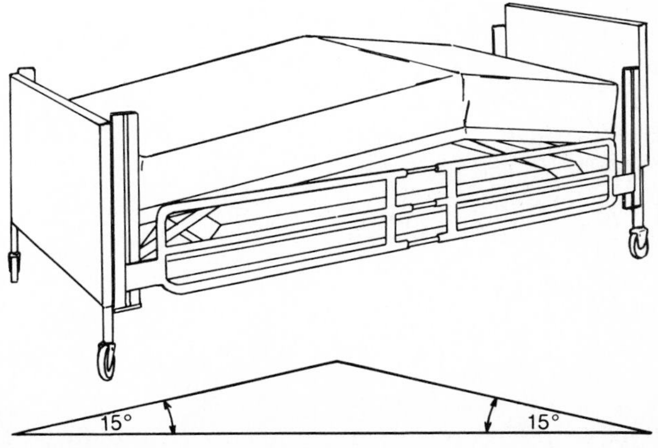

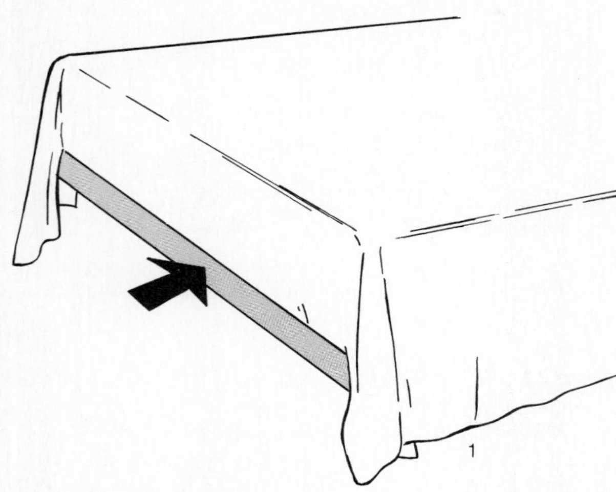

Figure 21–19 The bedcovers tucked in to prepare for mitering the corner.

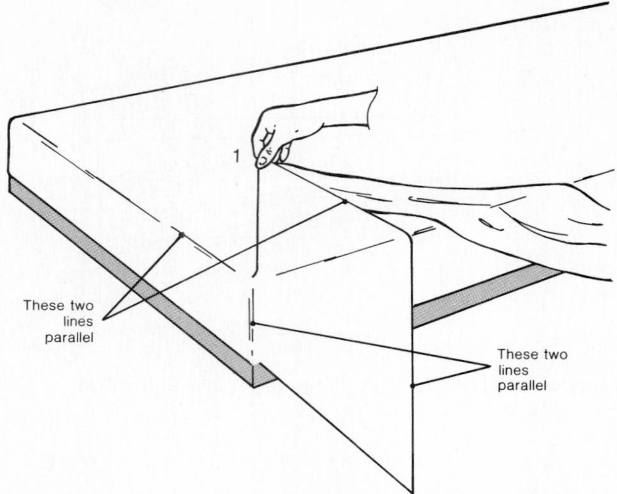

Figure 21–20 Lifting the cover to form a triangle.

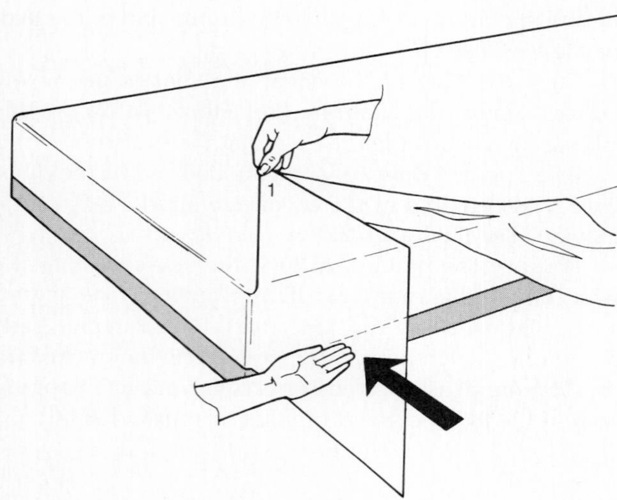

Figure 21–21 Tucking the hanging edge under the mattress.

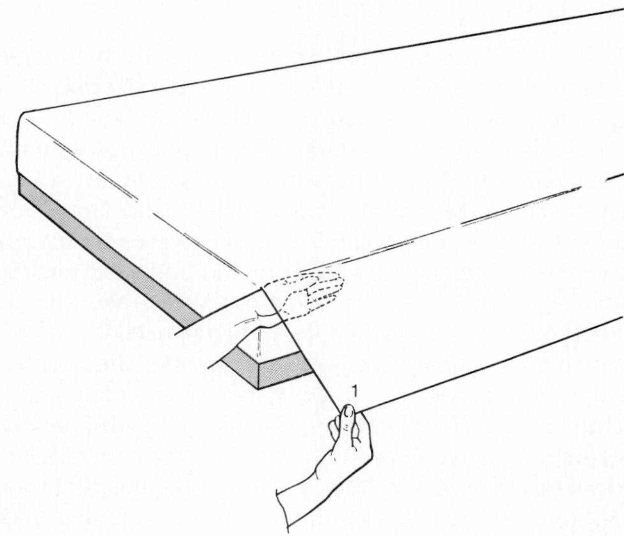

Figure 21–22 Bringing the top of the triangle down.

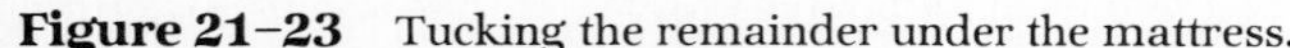

Figure 21–23 Tucking the remainder under the mattress.

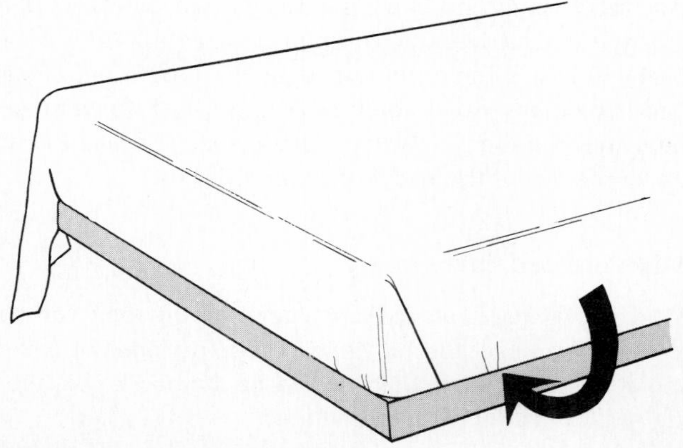

Procedure 21–2 Changing an Unoccupied Bed

Equipment

1. A mattress pad, if used. Some agencies do not use pads, so the nurse needs to check agency practice. Some mattress pads are attached to the bed by elastic or ties at the corners. Some lie freely on the mattress.
2. Two large sheets. Fitted sheets which do not require mitering are being used increasingly in hospitals.
3. A plastic or rubber drawsheet, if required, to place across the center of the bed to protect the bottom sheet from drainage, urine, or feces. Some agencies use drawsheets only when they are required in a nurse's judgment.
4. A cloth drawsheet to be placed over the plastic or rubber drawsheet, if required.
5. One blanket.
6. One bedspread.
7. Two pillowcases for the two head pillows. Additional pillowcases may be needed if additional pillows are used.

Preparation

Wash hands before obtaining the linen. Place the fresh linen on the patient's chair or overbed table. Do not use another patient's bed; it is important to prevent cross-contamination (the movement of microorganisms from one patient to another via the linen). Explain the procedure to the patient, and make sure that this is an appropriate and convenient time for the patient to be out of bed. Assist the patient to a comfortable chair. Close the windows if there is any air movement, to reduce the spread of microorganisms. Screen the bed if it is in a room with other beds. Screening decreases the spread of microorganisms from the bed linens when they are moved. Raise the bed to a working height at which you need not bend to reach the bed. This height reduces or prevents back strain.

Intervention

Stripping the bed

1. Starting at the side on which you have the clean linen, loosen the bedding, including the foundation, starting at the head, moving down the bed, working around the foot, and moving up to the other side of the head. Remove the signal, if it is attached to the linen.
2. Return to the first side.
3. Remove the pillowcases, if soiled, and place the pillows on the bedside chair near the foot of the bed.

   Rationale The bedside chair can be used to hold bedding that can be reused.
4. Using both hands, grasp the top edge of the spread, one hand at the center, the other at the mattress edge. Fold it in half by bringing the top edge even with the bottom edge.

   Rationale Linens folded this way are readily reapplied to the bed later.

   If it is soiled, place it in the linen hamper, if the agency has portable linen hampers that can be taken to the bed unit. If the agency has a central disposal chute for linen, tuck the soiled spread in at the foot of the bed, and collect all the soiled linen at the bed to take to the chute.
5. Pick up the spread carefully by grasping it at the center of the middle fold and the bottom edges.

   Rationale Shaking the bedclothes will spread microorganisms.
6. Lay the spread over the back of the bedside chair if it is to be reused. Take care to prevent the bed linen from touching your uniform.

   Rationale The uniform can transmit microorganisms to other patients.
7. Repeat steps 4–6, first for the blanket and then for the top sheet.
8. Pick up the cotton drawsheet at the center of the top and bottom edges, and lay it over the back of the bedside chair or discard it in the hamper if it is soiled.
9. Repeat step 8 for the plastic or rubber drawsheet.
10. Repeat steps 4–6 for the bottom sheet.
11. Move the mattress up to the head of the bed by grasping the mattress lugs and using good body mechanics. If there are no lugs, grasp the lower edge of the mattress.

Procedure 21–2, continued

Making the bed

12. Standing at the same side of the bed as the linen supply, place the mattress pad on the bed.

13. Smooth the mattress pad so that it is free of wrinkles.

Rationale Wrinkles can irritate the patient's skin and feel uncomfortable.

14. Working from the foot of the bed, place the bottom sheet, folded into four layers, on the bed so that the vertical center fold of the sheet is at the center line of the mattress and the bottom edge of the sheet extends about 2.5 cm (1 in) over the end of the mattress. Open the sheet across the bottom of the bed, and then pull the top layer up to the top of the bed, so that the sheet is fully spread. (Agency practice may vary on methods of folding and spreading sheets on beds. This is one common method. In some agencies the sheet is spread over only one side of the bed at a time.)

Rationale Unless a contour sheet is used, the sheet is not tucked in at the bottom so that it can readily be changed without removing the top bedcovers.

15. Move to the head of the bed on the same side. Tuck the excess sheet under the mattress at the near side of the head of the bed. If a contour sheet is used, fit it under the corner of the mattress.

16. Miter the bottom sheet at the top corner on that side, and tuck the sheet under the mattress side, working from the head of the bed to the foot. See Mitering Bed Corners earlier in this chapter.

17. Lay the plastic or rubber drawsheet on the bed, folded in half, with the center fold at the center line of the bed. Fanfold the uppermost half of the drawsheet at the center of the bed. Place the top edge of the drawsheet 30 to 37 cm (12 to 15 in) from the head of the bed.

18. Tuck the drawsheet in on the near side.

19. Repeat steps 17–18 for the cloth drawsheet, making sure that it completely covers the rubber or plastic sheet at both top and bottom edges.

Rationale Any exposed plastic or rubber can be irritating to the patient's skin.

20. Move to the opposite side of the bed.

21. Starting at the head of the bed, tuck the excess bottom sheet under the head of the mattress.

22. Pulling the sheet firmly, miter the side corner at the head of the bed or fit a contour sheet under the mattress corner.

23. Tuck the bottom sheet in, working toward the foot of the bed. Pull the sheet firmly so that there are no wrinkles in it.

24. Pull the plastic or rubber drawsheet over firmly, and tuck it in at the side.

25. Repeat step 24 for the cotton drawsheet.

26. Return to the first side of the bed. The foundation of the bed is now complete.

27. Place the top sheet on the bed so that the vertical center fold is at the center line of the bed, the top edge is even with the top edge of the mattress and the hems of the sheet are uppermost.

Rationale With the hems facing up, the edges of the sheet will not rub against the patient's skin.

28. Spread the sheet over the bed as described in step 14 or according to agency practice.

29. Tuck in the sheet at the bottom of the bed on the near half (optional).

30. Make either a vertical or a horizontal toe pleat in the sheet:

a. Vertical toe pleat: Standing at the foot of the bed, make a fold in the sheet 5 to 10 cm (2 to 4 in), perpendicular to the foot of the bed. See Figure 21–24. Tuck the remainder of the end of the sheet in at the foot of the bed.

b. Horizontal toe pleat: Make a fold in the sheet 5 to 10 cm (2 to 4 in), across the bed, 15 to 20 cm (6 to 8 in) from the foot. Tuck the sheet in at the foot.

Rationale A toe pleat provides additional room for a patient's feet. It is an optional comfort measure. Additional toe space can also be provided by loosening the top covers around the feet after the patient is in bed.

31. Place the blanket on the bed so that the top edge is about 15 cm (6 in) from the head of the bed and the center fold is at the center of the bed.

Procedure 21–2, continued

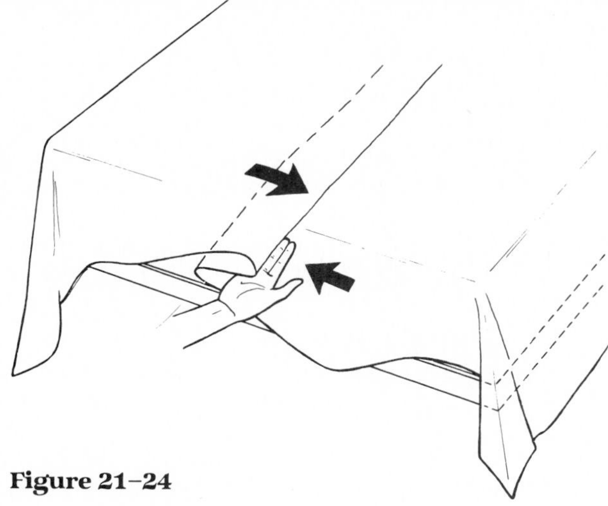

Figure 21–24

Rationale This allows a cuff of sheet to be folded over the blanket and spread.

32. Tuck the blanket in at the foot of the bed on the near side. Make a toe pleat if needed. See step 30.

33. Put the bedspread on the bed so that the center fold is at the center of the bed and the top edge extends about 2.5 cm (1 in) beyond the blanket. Tuck the top edge of the spread under the top edge of the blanket. See Figure 21–25.

34. Fold the top of the top sheet down over the spread, providing a cuff of about 15 cm (6 in). Smooth the spread, working from the top to the foot of the bed.

Rationale The cuff of sheet protects the patient's face from rubbing against the blanket or bedspread, thus preventing skin irritation.

35. Tuck in the spread at the foot of the bed on the near side.

36. Miter the corner of the bed using all three layers of linen (top sheet, blanket, and spread). Leave the side of the spread hanging freely.

Rationale Mitering makes the corner of the bedclothes secure even though they are left hanging freely to permit easy access by the patient.

37. Walk around the foot of the bed to the far side, pulling the blanket and spread over the bed. Work toward the head of the bed on the second side.

38. Fold the remainder of the spread under the top of the blanket. Fold the remainder of the top sheet over the spread to make a cuff.

39. Going to the foot of the bed tuck in the top sheet, blanket, and spread at the bottom of the bed on the second side. Maintain the toe pleat if one was made.

40. Miter this corner as in step 36.

41. Moving to the first side of the bed put clean pillowcases on the pillows:

a. Grasp the closed end of the pillowcase at the center with one hand.
b. Gather up the sides of the pillowcase, and place them over the hand grasping the case. Then grasp the center of one short side of the pillow through the pillowcase.
c. With the free hand, pull the pillowcase over the pillow.
d. Adjust the pillowcase so that the pillow fits into the corners of the case and the seams are straight.

Rationale A smoothly fitting pillowcase is more comfortable than a wrinkled one.

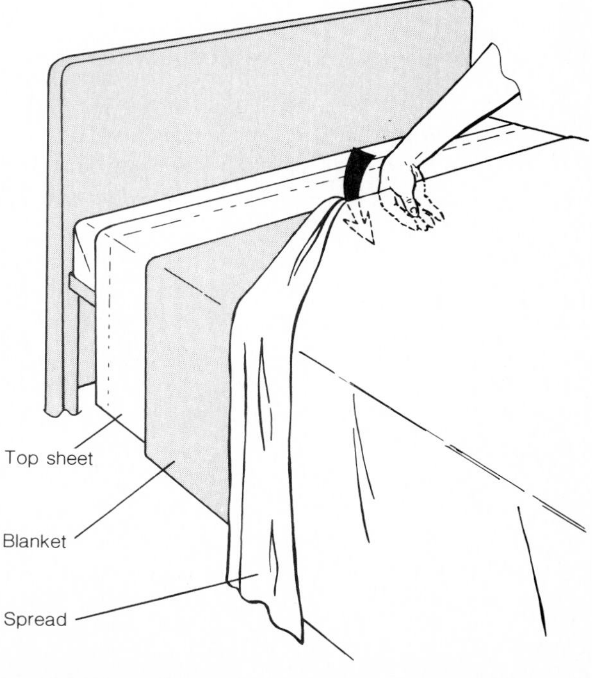

Figure 21–25

Procedure 21–2, continued

42. Place the pillows at the head of the bed in the center, with the open ends of the pillowcases facing away from the door of the room.

Rationale This provides a neat appearance.

43. Attach the signal cord so that the patient can conveniently use it. Some cords have clamps that attach to the sheet or pillowcase. Others are attached by a safety pin.

44. If the bed is currently being used by a patient, either fold back the top covers at one side or fanfold them down to the center of the bed.

Rationale This makes it easier for the patient to get into the bed.

45. Put the bedside table and the overbed table in order so that they are available to the patient.

46. Put the bed in the low position. (Place the bed in the high position if the patient is returning by stretcher.) Draw back the screens and/or open the room door. Open the windows, if appropriate.

47. Remove the soiled linen according to agency policy.

48. Wash hands to prevent the transfer of microorganisms to others.

Changing an occupied bed

When changing an occupied bed, the nurse needs to work quickly, disturb the patient as little as possible, and assist the patient to keep proper body alignment and comfort. It is easier to make a bed when it is flat; however, this may not be possible if the patient needs to maintain another position. For example, a patient who is having difficulty breathing may not tolerate a supine position, and the bed must be made with the head elevated for the patient's safety and comfort.

One method that is widely used to make an occupied bed is:

1. Loosen the top covers at the foot of the bed.
2. Remove the top bedding with the exception of the sheet. Fold the top edge to the bottom edge and then fold across the bed in quarters.
3. Put a bath blanket over the top sheet. Have the patient hold it, or tuck it under the patient's shoulders. Then remove the sheet by pulling it out from under the bath blanket. Bath blankets provide warmth needed by most patients.
4. Place the soiled linen on the seat of the chair or in the linen hamper.
5. Move the mattress up to the top of the bed. Some patients can assist by grasping the head of the bed and pulling themselves up. If the patient is unable to help, a second person is usually needed to grasp the lugs of the mattress on the other side of the bed; both people then slide the mattress upward. A nurse might be able to do this alone by going from one side to another, sliding the mattress a little each time. It is usually not possible for one person to move a mattress under a heavy, helpless patient.
6. Assist the patient to the far side of the bed. A side-lying position is considered best in that it frees a considerable portion of the bed.
7. Loosen the foundation of the bed on the near side and near half at the head of the bed. Fold the linen at the center of the bed against the patient's back.
8. Place the clean linen on the bed with the excess for the other half of the bed fanfolded in the center. Place the bottom sheet with the bottom edge extending 2.5 cm (1 in) beyond the end of the mattress and the top tucked under the mattress. There should be 30 to 45 cm (12 to 18 in) of sheet under the top of the mattress, to keep the sheet secure when the head of the bed is elevated.
9. Miter the top corner and tuck in the side of the bottom sheet.
10. Tuck the plastic drawsheet and the linen drawsheet under the mattress.
11. Have the patient turn to the clean side of the bed. Complete the far side in the manner used for the first side. Pull the sheets tightly to make them wrinkle-free.
12. Place the top sheet on the bed and remove the bath blanket.
13. Place the blanket and spread on the top of the bed and miter the bottom corners. A toe pleat is usually made in the top bedclothes. See Procedure 21–2, step 30. Tuck the spread under the blanket at the top edge, and fold the top sheet at least 5 cm (6 in) over the blanket and spread at the head of the bed.
14. Put clean pillowcases on the pillows. If there is a

soft and a firm pillow, place the soft pillow on top of the firm pillow.

15. Assist the patient to a comfortable position.

Changing a crib

Cribs are changed in a similar fashion to a bed. The major difference is that no drawsheets are used, because most crib mattresses have plastic covers. The crib sides are kept in the raised position when the nurse is not actually working at that side.

Preparing a surgical bed (recovery, anesthetic, or operative bed)

A surgical bed is made for a patient who has had an operation, or in some hospitals, for any patient who has received an anesthetic (e.g., during a bronchoscopy). The objectives of this type of bed are:

1. To provide as clean an environment as possible.
2. To provide a bed into which a patient can easily move or be transferred.
3. To provide a bed that can be readily changed with minimal disturbance to the patient if it becomes soiled, for example, with vomitus.

Surgical beds are made in various ways in different settings. The following practices are used in most places:

1. All clean linen is used for the bed.
2. The foundation of the bed is made as for other beds.
3. A plastic sheet and an additional linen drawsheet may be put on the top of the bed where pillows are usually placed. In some agencies a disposable pad is used.
4. The top covers are not tucked under the mattress. They are generally folded up on the sides and the end, making a 14 cm (6 in) cuff, and fanfolded lengthwise either to the side of the bed or to the center. They may also be fanfolded widthwise to the bottom of the bed.
5. Pillows are usually placed on the bedside chair.
6. The bed is left in a high position to meet the level of the stretcher and facilitate transfer of the patient.

Special Bed Equipment

A number of devices are commonly used with a hospital bed: bed boards, side rails, footboards, bed cradles, and intravenous rods.

Bed boards

A bed board, or *fracture board* as it is sometimes called, is a board placed directly under a mattress to give added support to a patient's body. Physicians often order bed boards for patients with back injuries. Other patients who are accustomed to sleeping with bed boards will be uncomfortable without one on the bed.

The bed board is usually the size of the mattress. Some are one-piece flat boards, while others are hinged so that the head of the bed, and sometimes the knees, can be elevated.

Side rails

Side rails, or safety sides, are used on both hospital beds and stretchers. They are of various shapes and sizes and are usually made of metal. Devices to raise and lower them differ. Often one or two knobs are pulled to release the side and permit it to be moved. When side rails are being used, it is important that the nurse *never* leave the bedside while the side rail is lowered.

Side rails have a number of functions:

1. To prevent patients from rolling or falling out of bed (this is a danger particularly for the elderly, young children, restless patients, and unconscious patients)
2. To give some patients, especially the elderly, the blind, and the sedated, a sense of security
3. To provide a hand hold with which a patient can move up in bed or turn over
4. If they are half rails, to provide a sense of security for the patient while in bed and to provide support for getting out of bed

Footboards

A footboard is a flat panel, often made of wood or plastic, that is placed at the foot end of a bed. Footboards are often made in an L shape, so that the base of the L fits under the foot of the mattress. Some footboards are adjustable—the board can be moved up the mattress to adjust to the patient's height. If a board cannot be adjusted, sandbags and rolled pillows or blankets can be used to fill the space between the patient's feet and the board.

The functions of footboards are:

1. To provide support for the patient's feet, maintaining a natural foot position while the patient is in bed
2. To keep the top bedcovers off the patient's feet, relieving pressure from the weight of the covers
3. To facilitate foot comfort, for example, when a patient has a painful foot

Without the support of a footboard, a patient's feet will "drop" from the normal right angle with the legs to a plantar flexion position with the toes pointing toward the foot of the bed. Prolonged assumption of this position results in permanent shortening of the muscles and tendons at the back of the ankles. When that happens, the patient is unable to stand flat-footed on the floor, and walking is seriously impaired.

Bed cradles

A bed cradle, sometimes called an *Anderson frame*, is a device designed to keep the top bedclothes off the feet, legs, and even abdomen of a patient. The bedclothes are arranged over the device and may be pinned in place. There are several types of bed cradles. One of the most common is a metal rod in an arch shape that extends from one side of the bed to the other. Part of the cradle fits under the mattress, and a small metal bracket presses down on the mattress to keep the cradle in place. The rods on some cradles run above one leg and extend over only half of the bed.

Intravenous rods

Intravenous rods (poles, stands, or standards), usually made of metal, are used to support intravenous infusion containers while fluid is being administered to a patient. These rods were traditionally freestanding on the floor beside the patient's bed. Now hospital beds often have intravenous rods attached to the bed. Some models even feature a metal container for storing the rod, as part of the bed. A bed may have four or six places where a rod can fit.

Specialized Beds

A number of specialized beds are designed to meet specific patient needs. The water bed or flotation bed has a mattress that consists of a plastic bag filled with water. The principle behind the use of this bed is displacement: The body loses an amount of weight equal to the liquid displaced; therefore the body weight is lightened, and there is less pressure on weight-bearing areas (Pfaudler 1968:2352). A similar bed is the alternating pressure bed or air bed. This mattress is filled with air, and the pressure automatically changes on the different body areas.

A Stryker frame or Foster frame is another specialized bed. It is used for patients who are unable to move, for example, as a result of fractured vertebrae. The patient lies on a canvas piece attached to a metal frame. When the patient needs to turn, a similar frame is placed on top of him or her and attached to the lower frame. The frame is unlocked and turned so that the patient's position is reversed. The upper frame over the patient is then removed.

Another type of bed, the CircOlectric bed, is fastened to a circular frame. It functions electrically and can be operated by the patient. One of its major advantages is that it permits a patient to assume a standing position without exertion.

Specialized beds use specially fitted sheets over the mattress. If a fitted sheet is not available, a drawsheet or plain sheet can be used and folded to cover the mattress.

Specialized beds are frequently frightening to patients and their support persons. It is important for nurses to explain how the bed works and give a demonstration before the patient uses the bed, if possible.

Summary

The total picture of hygiene includes mental, sexual, social, oral, and personal aspects. Hygiene practices are influenced to a large degree by family influences. When people become ill, hygienic practices often assume a secondary role to other vital body needs such as rest or breathing. The nurse then assumes responsibility for hygienic care of patients.

Major functions of the skin are to regulate temperature, protect underlying tissues, secrete sebum, contain nerve receptors, and aid in vitamin D production. Normal integument is assessed to provide baseline data, but developmental differences and personal practices must also be considered.

Some skin problems observed by nurses need to be brought to the attention of a physician; others require nursing intervention; and still others spontaneously disappear. Miliaria rubra, milia, mongolian spots, hemangiomas, and diaper rash are common among infants. Acne is prevalent among adolescents, and erythema, petechiae, ecchymoses, and skin ulcers are common in adults. Six guidelines related to the care of the skin assist the nurse in planning and intervention.

The major purposes of regular bathing and skin care are (a) removal of dead skin cells, excessive perspiration, and sebum, which, if left to accumulate, harbor bacteria; (b) stimulation of circulation; (c) providing a sense of well-being; and (d) eliminating body odors. Assisting patients with bathing can allow the nurse to assess the patient's state of health. The frequency of bathing is largely determined by the patient's preferences, age, degree of illness, and agency policies. Nurses frequently bathe patients in bed. They also give sponge and tub baths to newborns and infants.

Prevention of decubitus ulcers is a major nursing function for bedridden patients. Treatments are numerous, ranging from antiseptic applications to debridement and soaking.

The back rub is an essential part of hygiene care for patients confined to bed. Four techniques can be used when massaging backs: effleurage, tapotement, petrissage, and three-handed effleurage.

For patients who are incapacitated, the nurse needs to provide perineal and genital care. This procedure can create embarrassment for both the patient and the nurse, and nurses need to master techniques for providing the care for female and male patients. The perineal area is cleaned and dried thoroughly, because microorganisms grow in damp dark places.

Common problems of the feet are calluses, corns, unpleasant odors, plantar warts, fissures between the toes, and fungus infections. Six interventions are designed to prevent these problems. The nails also require regular attention to prevent incurvation and paronychia.

Good oral hygiene includes daily dental flossing and mechanical scrubbing of the teeth and flushing of the mouth four times a day. Dental checkups are recommended every 6 months starting at 2½ to 3 years of age. Fluoride supplements are recommended as an alternative to fluoridated water from 1 month of age to 14 years. Common oral problems are dental caries, periodontal disease, glossitis, gingivitis, stomatitis, parotitis, and halitosis. Hospitalized patients often require assistance from the nurse to maintain oral hygiene. Nurses need to know how to position the unconscious patient, care for dentures, brush a patient's teeth, and use commercially prepared cleaners. Halitosis and sordes require special mouth care measures.

Hair care includes daily combing and brushing and regular shampooing. The black person's hair may also require lubrication. Dandruff, ticks, and lice are problems frequently seen by the nurse.

Eye care is normally minimal. Dried secretions on the lashes or inner canthus need softening and removal. Newborns initially require eye medications to prevent ophthalmia neonatorum. The nurse also needs to be cognizant of hygiene measures related to artificial eyes, eyeglasses, and contact lenses.

The nose and ears also require minimal care. For infants these orifices are cleaned with moistened absorbent wisps of cotton.

Changing beds is part of hygiene for hospitalized patients. It is important that beds be clean and comfortable for ill patients. Special beds include surgical beds, the Stryker frame, and the CircOlectric bed.

Suggested Activities

1. In a health agency, explore the recommended oral hygiene practices.
2. When caring for a patient in a hospital, assess what hygiene practices the patient carries out. Explain how these differ from your own practices, and consider why.
3. Identify a situation in which you can offer health guidance about a hygiene matter to a patient of any age.
4. In a long-term care setting, identify the special arrangements made to assist patients to meet their hygiene and grooming needs. Compare your findings with the practices in an acute hospital setting.
5. Visit a local school nurse, and determine the specific hygiene practices the children are taught.
6. In a hospital setting, make an occupied bed and provide needed skin care. Discuss in a group what problems you encountered.

Suggested Readings

Davis, M. April 1977. Getting to the root of the problem. *Nursing 77* 7:60–65.
This article describes hair care for a black patient, including selecting the right comb and some basic grooming techniques. Removing tangles and preventing matting are discussed.

Gannon, E. P., and Kadezabek, E. March 1980. Giving your patients meticulous mouth care. *Nursing 80* 10:14–19.
The authors describe examining the mouth and throat, helping with mouth care, providing mouth care to unconscious patients, removing and cleaning dentures, and using special patient aids. Photographs are provided throughout the article.

Kerr, J. C.; Stinson, S. M.; and Shannon, M. L. July/August 1981. Pressure sores: Distinguishing fact from fiction. *Canadian Nurse* 77:23–28.
The authors discuss some of the myths about pressure sores, patients at risk, and prevention and treatment. A chart categorizing pressure sore treatments and an assessment scale are provided.

MacMillan, K. March 1981. New goals for oral hygiene. *Canadian Nurse* 77:40–43.
Problems of the mouth commonly associated with hospitalized patients are described. Good oral hygiene and nursing measures for mouth care are discussed.

Michelsen, D. July 1978. Giving a great back rub. *American Journal of Nursing* 78:1197–99.
The author describes a 15-step technique, referred to as a *back massage*, which stimulates circulation and relieves muscle tension. Photographs accompany the steps of the technique.

Morley, M. July/August 1981. 16 steps to better decubitus ulcer care. *Canadian Nurse* 77:29–31.
The author, a skin care nurse coordinator, outlines the do's and don't's of decubitus ulcer care.

Wallace, G., and Hayter, J. June 1974. Karaya for chronic skin ulcers. *American Journal of Nursing* 74:1094–98.
The karaya procedure is outlined in detail, accompanied by detailed photographs of deep decubitus ulcers that learners are advised to see.

Zucnick, M. M. May 1975. Care of an artificial eye. *American Journal of Nursing* 75:835.
This article presents the steps involved in removing, cleaning, and inserting an artificial eye. Five photographs illustrate the technique.

Selected References

Skin

Barnhill, S. E., and Chenoweth, E. E. March 1966. Cleansing the perineum. *American Journal of Nursing* 66:566.

Brown, M. S., et al. September 1973. Physical examination. Part 3: Examining the skin. *Nursing 73* 3:39–43.

Cahn, M. M. July 1960. The skin from infancy to old age. *American Journal of Nursing* 60:993–96.

Carney, R. G. June 1963. The aging skin. *American Journal of Nursing* 63:110–12.

Davis, E. D. November 1970. Give a bath? *American Journal of Nursing* 70:2366–67.

Gibbs, G. E. January 1969. Perineal care of the incapacitated patient. *American Journal of Nursing* 69:124–25.

King, P. A. September/October 1980. Foot problems and assessment. *Geriatric Nursing* 1:182–86.

Kozier, B., and Erb, G. 1982. *Techniques in clinical nursing.* Menlo Park, Calif.: Addison-Wesley Publishing Co.

Roach, L. B. November 1972. Assessment of color changes in dark skins. *Nursing 72* 2:19–22.

———. March 1974. Assessing skin changes: The subtle and the obvious. *Nursing 74* 4:64–67.

———. January 1977. Color changes in dark skin. *Nursing 77* 7:48–51.

Roberts, S. L. April 1975. Skin assessment for color and temperature. *American Journal of Nursing* 75:610–13.

Temple, K. D. October 1967. The back rub. *American Journal of Nursing* 67:2102–3.

Decubitus ulcers

Ahmed, M. C. December 1980, Special Report. Choosing the best method to manage pressure ulcers. *Nurses' Drug Alert* 4(15):113–20.

Barrett, D., and Klibanski, A. May 1973. Collagenase debridement. *American Journal of Nursing* 73:849–51.

Berecek, K. March 1975. Treatment of decubitus ulcers. *Nursing Clinics of North America* 10:171–210.

Chrisp, M. August 4, 1977. New treatment for pressure sores. *Nursing Times* 73:1202–5.

Clark, M. O., et al. March 2, 1978. Pressure sores. *Nursing Times* 74:363–66.

Dyson, R. June 15, 1978. Bed sores—the injuries hospital staff inflict on patients. *Nursing Mirror* 146:30–32.

Gerber, R. M. and Van Ort, S. R. June 1981. Topical application of insulin to pressure sores: A questionable therapy. *American Journal of Nursing* 81:1859.

Gruis, M. L., and Innes, B. November 1976. Assessment: Essential to prevent pressure sores. *American Journal of Nursing* 76:1762–64.

Gusnell, D. J. January–February 1973. An assessment tool to identify pressure sores. *Nursing Research* 22:55–59.

Harrin, J., and Hargest, T. March 1970. The air-fluidized bed: A new concept in the treatment of decubitus ulcers. *Nursing Clinics of North America* 5:181–87.

Judd, C. O. July/August 1981. The prevention and treatment of pressure sores. *Canadian Nurse* 77:32–33.

Kerr, J. C.; Stinson, S. M.; and Shannon, M. L. July/August 1981. Pressure sores: Distinguishing fact from fiction. *Canadian Nurse* 77:23–28.

Lang, C., and McGrath, A. March 1974. Gelfoam for decubitus ulcers. *American Journal of Nursing* 74:460–61.

Miller, M. E., and Sachs, M. L. 1974. *About bedsores: What you need to know to help prevent and treat them.* Philadelphia: J. B. Lippincott Co.

Morley, M. H. October 1973. Decubitus ulcer management—a team approach. *Canadian Nurse* 69:41–43.

———. July/August 1981. 16 steps to better decubitus ulcer care. *Canadian Nurse* 77:29–31.

Nursing 77 (Kauchak-Keyes, M. A., consultant). September 1977. Four proven steps for preventing decubitus ulcers. *Nursing 77* 7:58–61.

Pfaudler, M. November 1968. Flotation, displacement and decubitus ulcers. *American Journal of Nursing* 68:2351–55.

Rubin, C. F.; Dietz, R. R.; and Abruzzese, R. S. October 1974. Auditing the decubitus ulcer problem. *American Journal of Nursing* 74:1820–21.

Ryan, D. M. February 26, 1976. Pressure sores: Treatment using stomahesive. Part 5. *Nursing Times* 72:299–300.

Stilwell, E. J. November 1961. Pressure sores—one method of care. *American Journal of Nursing* 61:109–10.

Van Ort, S. R., and Gerber, R. M. January-February 1976. Topical application of insulin in the treatment of decubitus ulcers: A pilot study. *Nursing Research* 25:9–12.

Verhonick, P. J. August 1961. A preliminary report of a study of decubitus ulcer care. *American Journal of Nursing* 61:68–69.

Wallace, G., and Hayter, J. June 1974. Karaya for chronic skin ulcers. *American Journal of Nursing* 74:1094–98.

Mouth

Anderson, H. C. 1971. *Newton's geriatric nursing.* 5th ed. St. Louis: C. V. Mosby Co.

Block, P. L. July 1976. Dental health in hospitalized patients. *American Journal of Nursing* 76:1162–64.

Dyer, E. D., et al. July 1976. Dental health in adults. *American Journal of Nursing* 76:1156–59.

Milgrom, P. The quality of general medical services by dentists. In Leininger, M., editor. 1975. *Barriers and facilitators to quality health care.* Philadelphia: F. A. Davis Co.

Roach, L. B. January 1977. Color changes in dark skin. *Nursing 77* 7:48–51.

Schweiger, J. L.; Lang, J. W.; and Schweiger, J. W. April 1980. Oral assessment: How to do it. *American Journal of Nursing* 80:654–57.

Slattery, J. July 1976. Dental health in children. *American Journal of Nursing* 76:1159–61.

Hair

Brown, M. S., et al. September 1973. Physical examination. Part 3: Examining the skin. *Nursing 73* 3:39–43.

Giles, S. F. 1972. Hair, the nursing process and the black patient. *Nursing Forum* 11(1):78–88.

Beds

Geriatric Nursing. January/February 1981. A water bed that works . . . and costs only pennies. *Geriatric Nursing* 2:42–43.

Piper, D. A. November 1968. Weightless ward. *American Journal of Nursing* 68:2360–61.

General

Ebersole, P., and Hess, P. 1981. *Toward healthy aging: Human needs and nursing response.* St. Louis: C. V. Mosby Co.

Forbes, E., and Fitzsimons, V. 1981. *The older adult: A process for wellness.* St. Louis: C. V. Mosby Co.

Gordon, M. 1982. *Manual of nursing diagnosis.* New York: McGraw-Hill Book Co.

Kim, M. J., and Moritz, D. A. 1982. *Classification of nursing diagnoses.* New York: McGraw-Hill Book Co.

Chapter 22

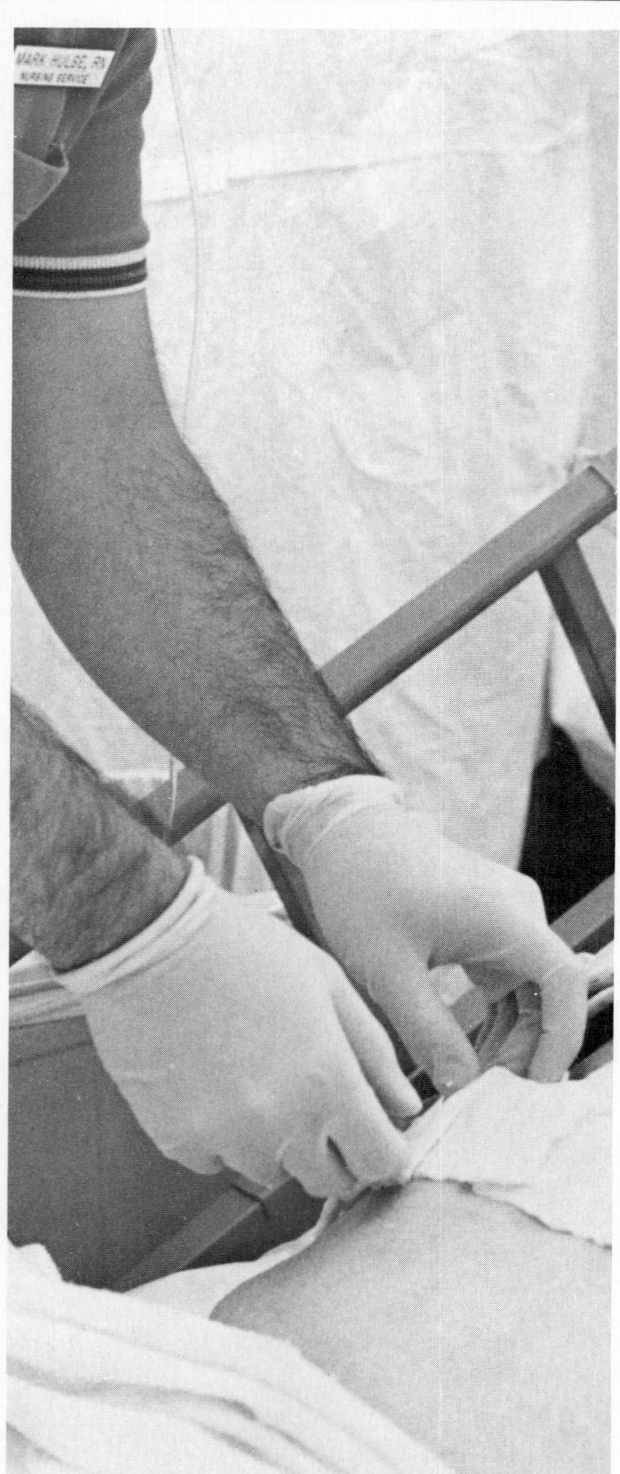

Protection

CONTENTS

Objectives

1. Understand essential measures to prevent accidents and communicable disease

- **1.1** Identify characteristics of a safe environment
- **1.2** List six essential environmental sanitation measures
- **1.3** Identify essential safety precautions for each developmental stage
- **1.4** Identify essential precautions to prevent falls
- **1.5** Identify situations in which restraints are warranted
- **1.6** Outline guidelines for selecting and applying restraints
- **1.7** Identify legal implications of restraints
- **1.8** Identify various types of restraints
- **1.9** Identify essential steps in the event of a fire
- **1.10** Identify types of fire extinguishers appropriate for class A, B, and C fires
- **1.11** Identify measures to reduce electric hazards
- **1.12** Identify precautions to prevent poisoning in children
- **1.13** Outline essential steps in the event of poisoning
- **1.14** Identify precautions to prevent asphyxiation
- **1.15** Identify precautions to prevent exposure to radiation
- **1.16** Identify immunization requirements for various ages

2. Know essential information to assess persons at risk of injury

- **2.1** Identify patients at risk for physical injury
- **2.2** Identify associated environmental hazards

Terms

antibody	dynamic electricity	humidity	static electricity
antigen	electron	immunity	Td
asphyxiation	epidemic	immunization	TOPV
communicable disease	epidemiology	induration	toxoid
DT	grounding	MMR	vaccine
DTP	hapten	pandemic	vector

People's need for protection is lifelong. The environment contains many hazards, both seen and unseen. The automobile, which may run down a pedestrian, is an obvious hazard. Microorganisms and radiation are unseen hazards.

The need for a safe environment is a national, community, and individual concern. Nurses are voicing their thoughts individually and collectively about such issues as air and water pollution and the safety of foods, cosmetrics, and medications. The need for safety on the highways is underscored by newspaper reports of morbidity and mortality from automobile accidents. Increasingly, governments are being pressed to take action and legislate in these areas to make the environment safer. In addition, people are also becoming aware of safety hazards in their communities. Regulations to control the speed of boats on lakes used for swimming, local ordinances curbing the burning of refuse, and stricter local regulation of industrial pollution are all indications of increasing awareness of the need for safety in the environment.

Traditionally, nurses have thought of safety in relation to a patient's immediate environment, and this awareness is no less important today in spite of the broader focus on human protection. A primary concern of nurses is awareness of what constitutes a safe environment for a particular person and how this environment can be achieved. The blind person may need railings; the crawling baby, a protective gate at the head of the stairs; and the elderly person, secure footing and an uncluttered floor. Nurses thus focus attention on preventing accidents and injury as well as on assisting the injured.

The word *environment* usually refers both to physical and abstract qualities of one's surroundings. The focus of this chapter is achieving safety in the physical environment.

Safe Environments

An environment is safe when the likelihood of illness or injury due to environmental factors is reduced as much as possible. People function safely and feel secure in a safe environment. Maslow (1968) states that the safety and security needs of people are second only to physiologic needs such as food, air, and water. See Chapter 8. Characteristics of a safe environment include (a) appropriate temperature and humidity, (b) adequate lighting, (c) orderly arrangement of furniture or other objects, (d) freedom from excessive noise, (e) freedom from pathogenic microorganisms, and (f) absence of special hazards such as fire, radiation, electricity, and chemicals. Special hazards are discussed on pages 542–47.

Temperature

The temperature of the environment affects the comfort and safety of its inhabitants. In extreme heat or cold, people become less alert, have slowed thought processes, and are in danger of physical injury, such as burn or frostbite. How people define comfort in temperature varies among individuals and cultures. Most North Americans are comfortable in indoor temperatures between 20 and 22 C (68 and 72 F). Extremes in environmental temperatures can affect people's behavior; people are more likely to be impatient and lose their temper, to work less efficiently, and to become ill more quickly when subjected to extreme temperatures (Hillman 1973:692). An individual's age, level of activity, and health largely determine what temperature feels comfortable. Inactive, ill, very young, and elderly persons frequently prefer warmer environments.

Humidity

Humidity is the amount of moisture, expressed as a percentage, in the air. Most people are comfortable when the humidity is between 30% and 60%. When the humidity is high, the evaporation rate of perspiration decreases; conversely, when the humidity is low, perspiration evaporates faster. In some situations, a high-humidity environment is provided as a therapeutic measure. For example, steam inhalations increase the humidity of the air inhaled and thus facilitate breathing.

Air-conditioned settings are characterized by low humidity. As a result, people who live and work in such settings often have dry mucous membranes of the nose and throat, and an increased incidence of irritation and infection.

Light

Adequate lighting is important for accomplishing daily tasks with minimum eye strain. An adequately lit environment is neither dim nor glaring and has no deep shadows. Some people are more sensitive to bright light than others. A patient may prefer a soft light, whereas the nurse may need a brighter light to perform nursing tasks safely.

Night lights help prevent falls in darkened homes. They help people walk to the bathroom safely, especially in unfamiliar surroundings. Night lights should not shine in sleepers' eyes, and yet they should light walkways.

Orderly Arrangement

Two common hazards are clutter and objects placed out of easy reach. Many falls are caused by clutter and wet spots on floors, equipment crowded around beds or chairs, and furniture or equipment that obstructs access to beds, chairs, bathrooms, or railings in corridors. Weakened patients frequently rely on hospital corridor railings when walking with or without ambulation aids. Overbed tables, bedside stands, or call lights placed out of reach frequently cause falls. Thus, order, neatness, an uncluttered environment, and placement of objects within reach are essential to safety.

Noise Control

Noise can be an environmental hazard. Sound levels above 120 decibels (units of loudness) are painful and may damage people's ears. Tolerance of noise is largely individual. The rural dweller may find the city noisy, whereas the city dweller may be oblivious to urban sounds. Adults often find teenager's music uncomfortably loud.

Noise pollution is a concern in modern industrial societies. Some suggest that hearing loss among elderly people may be due in part to the noise of the urban environment.

The ill and injured are frequently sensitive to noises that normally would not disturb them. Loud voices, the clatter of dishes, and even a nearby television can disturb patients, some of whom react angrily.

Noise can be minimized in several ways. Acoustic tile on ceilings, walls, and floors as well as drapes and carpeting absorb sound. Background music can mask noise and have a calming effect on some people.

Control of Pathogens

Pathogens, microorganisms capable of producing disease, are a continual threat to safety. People who are not immunized or weakened by illness are particularly vulnerable. See the section on immunizations later in this chapter.

Environmental Sanitation

Sanitation has a direct effect on health. Contaminated food or water can cause widespread illness. Some environmental sanitation concerns follow.

Water Purification

Nearly all water is polluted while falling as rain or running over the surface of the ground or through the soil. Pollution by wastes further contaminates many water supplies. The most significant diseases spread by contaminated water are typhoid fever, dysentery, paratyphoids, infectious hepatitis, and cholera. The incidence of these diseases has declined in recent years, primarily due to (a) water treatment including filtration and chlorination, (b) protection of water supplies, (c) improved waste disposal methods, and (d) immunizations during epidemics.

The presence of fluoride in the water in minute quantities (0.6–1.7 mg/liter) has been found to reduce the incidence of dental caries significantly.

The U.S. Public Health Service has established purity standards for drinking water; these are enforced by state departments of health.

Pollution Control

Air pollution is the presence in the outdoor atmosphere of contaminants such as dust, fumes, gas, mist, odor, smoke, or vapor in sufficient quantities and of sufficient duration to be harmful to humans, plants, or animals. Air pollution is an increasing problem in all countries where urban growth has meant industrial development and greater numbers of automobiles.

Health problems associated with air pollution include respiratory disease and eye, nose, and throat irritations.

Smoking is also generally recognized as a health hazard. The incidence of lung cancer and heart disease is higher in smokers than nonsmokers. Some people believe that cigarette smoke is also a health hazard even when not directly inhaled but merely in the environment. Increasingly, nonsmokers are asking to be segregated from smokers in theaters, restaurants, trains, and airplanes.

Pollution of the environment is an increasingly acknowledged problem. The inappropriate disposal of industrial wastes and nuclear wastes endangers the lives and health of people, animals, and plants. In all industrialized societies, waste disposal is a major problem that requires careful planning.

Disposal of Human Wastes

A very important aspect of environmental sanitation is disposal of human wastes. Sewage contains microorganisms, such as *Escherichia coli* (E coli), which normally inhabits the intestines of humans, and *Aerobacter aerogenes* and *A. cloacae*, also found in feces and in soils. Diseases transmitted through sewage include typhoid fever, paratyphoid, poliomyelitis, and hepatitis.

In rural areas, sewage is usually disposed of in cesspools and septic tanks. Filtration, dilution, or activated sludge are three commonly used methods. The purposes of sewage treatment are (a) to make the sewage inoffensive, (b) to eliminate the danger of contaminating water and bathing areas, and (c) to prevent the destruction of fish and wildlife.

Milk Pasteurization

Pasteurization is the application of heat to milk to destroy disease-producing microorganisms. Unpasteurized milk can spread tuberculosis, diphtheria, dysentery, streptococcal infections, and Q fever. Milk must not only be free of disease, it must also be clean, with relatively few bacteria. To be safe and clean, milk must be given by healthy cows in clean barns, handled by clean, healthy workers working in clean surroundings with clean utensils, processed in separate milk rooms, and pasteurized.

Food Sanitation

Contaminated food can cause serious illness and death. The five types of contaminants are as follows:

1. Animal parasites, such as tapeworms that may infest meat or fish

2. Microorganisms, such as the bacteria that cause typhoid fever and dysentery
3. Toxins, which are produced by certain bacteria in food, for example, *Clostridium botulinum*
4. Poisonous plants, such as toadstools
5. Poisonous sprays

Laws govern the preparation, storage, transportation, and sale of food, including the sanitation of eating and drinking establishments.

Insect and Rodent Control

Insects are significant transmitters of disease. A *vector* is animate (often an animal) and transmits disease. Some significant vectors are mosquitoes, which pass on malaria, encephalitis, and yellow fever; flies, which convey bacteria from excreta to food; and cockroaches, which can contaminate food with bacteria from sewage. Fleas and lice that harbor microorganisms also can transmit disease, such as typhus.

There has been a worldwide effort to control the mosquito that transmits malaria. The incidence of malaria in the United States is low because of protection of rural homes from mosquitoes, drainage of swamp waters where mosquitoes breed, mass medication, and spraying. Other insects are also controlled by sprays.

Rats and other rodents are also a potential source of disease, such as hemorrhagic jaundice and amebic dysentery. It is estimated that the rat population in the United States equals the human population. Rats can be controlled in two ways: adequate garbage disposal to limit their food supply and poisons, such as the coumarin anticoagulant, Warfarin sodium.

Incidence and Causes of Accidents

In Canada, accidents, not disease, are the leading cause of death in people 1 to 44. More than 2500 children 20 or younger died from accidents in 1977 (Statistics Canada 1981:146). Countless other children had accidents of a less serious nature. See Table 22–1.

Table 22–1 Accidental Deaths in Canada, 1977

Age	Number	Rate*
1 to 4 years	387	28.0
5 to 19 years	2,253	35.0
20 to 44 years	3,881	45.2
45 to 64 years	2,091	46.9
65 years and over	2,434	117.6

*Per 100,000 population

From Statistics Canada, *Canada year book 1980–81* (Ottawa: Minister of Supplies and Services, 1981), pp. 146–47.

Table 22–2 Accidental Deaths in the United States, 1976

Age	Number	Rate*
1 to 4 years	3,439**	27.9
5 to 14 years	6,308**	17.0
15 to 24 years	24,316**	59.9
25 to 44 years	22,399**	40.8
45 to 64 years	19,000	43.5
65 years and over	23,961	104.5

*Per 100,000 population in specified age group
**Leading cause of death in specified age group

From U.S. Department of Health, Education, and Welfare, *Facts of life and death* (Hyattsville, Md.: Department of Health, Education, and Welfare, 1978), pp. 33–38.

In the United States, motor vehicle accidents are the major cause of death in white adolescents, 15 to 24 years. Homicide is the major cause in all other adolescents in the same age group (U.S. DHEW 1978:45). Accidents are among the ten leading causes of death in people of all ages. Among adults 25 to 64, all accidents, including motor vehicle accidents, rank fourth after heart disease, cancer, and strokes (ibid., p. 55). Among people of 65 and older, accidents rank seventh after heart disease, malignant neoplasms, cerebrovascular disease, influenza and pneumonia, arteriosclerosis, and diabetes mellitus (ibid., p. 38). See Table 22–2 for accidental death rates in the United States.

The eight major causes of accidental death among children and adults are listed in order of prevalence in Table 22–3.

Table 22–3 Major Causes of Accidental Death, United States, 1976

Type	Number	Rate*
Motor vehicle	47,038	21.9
Falls	14,136	6.6
Fires and flames	6,338	3.0
Drowning	5,645	2.6
Poisoning	4,161	1.9
Suffocation	3,033	1.4
Surgical and medical complications	3,009	1.4
Firearms	2,059	1.0

*Per 100,000 population

From U.S. Department of Health, Education, and Welfare, *Facts of life and death* (Hyattsville, Md.: Department of Health, Education, and Welfare, 1978), p. 45.

Assessing Risk of Physical Injury

The ability of people to protect themselves from injury is affected by a number of factors. Each of these factors needs to be assessed by nurses when they are planning care or teaching patients to protect themselves.

Age

Age is an important factor affecting people's ability to protect themselves. Through knowledge and accurate assessment of the environment, people learn to protect themselves from many injuries. Children walking to school learn to stop before crossing the street and wait for oncoming traffic. They also learn not to touch a hot stove. For the very young, learning about the environment is essential. Only through knowledge and experience do children learn what is potentially harmful.

Parents normally attach a great deal of importance to teaching children what is potentially dangerous and at the same time childproofing the home environment. Safety precautions adequate for an older child or an adult are not adequate for a young child. For example, the young child who cannot read is likely to mistake lye or medications for candy. Accordingly, it is most important to place these hazards out of reach of the young child.

Elderly people also can have special problems protecting themselves from injury. Often the balance of elderly people is impaired by their flexed posture, which places their center of gravity forward. See Chapter 23. Once balance is lost, it is not readily regained. An elderly person may need to learn to stand up slowly, thus avoiding the fall that can result from a quick, sudden movement. Slowness of movement and diminished sensual acuity also contribute to the likelihood of injury. Elderly persons may neither see nor hear an oncoming car. The may not see a footstool. They may also be unable to pull themselves out of a bathtub safely.

Life-Style

Life-style is a significant factor affecting safety. Fifty percent of deaths are due to unhealthy behavior or life-style. See Chapter 2. Factors that place people at risk are: unsafe work environments, where workers are in danger from machinery, industrial belts and pulleys, and chemicals; residence in neighborhoods with high crime rates; access to guns and ammunition; insufficient income to buy safety equipment or make necessary repairs; and access to illicit drugs, which may also be contaminated by harmful additives. Risk-taking behavior is a factor in accidents. For example, some people disregard safety recommendations by driving automobiles at high speeds and refusing to wear seatbelts in automobiles, headgear on motorcycles, or flotation jackets in boats.

Sensory Perception

Accurate perception of environmental stimuli is vital to safety. These stimuli, which are received by sensory receptors of the body, travel through the nerves to the central nervous system. In a reflex action, such as jerking the hand away from a hot object, some of the impulses travel directly to motor neurons, which then convey the impulses to the muscles that effect the sudden, quick withdrawing of the hand. At the same time, other sensory impulses travel to the cerebral cortex; and the person, now aware of the stimulus, initiates further impulses that result in voluntary muscle movement. Impairment of any of these areas—the sensory receptors, sensory pathways, the internuncial neurons that transmit the impulse from the sensory pathways to the motor pathways, the motor pathways, or the cerebral cortex—can diminish ability to respond normally to environmental stimuli.

People with impaired touch perception, hearing, taste, smell, and vision are highly susceptible to injury. A person who does not see well may trip over a toy or not see a signal cord at a hospital bed unit. Deaf persons do not hear a siren in traffic, and persons with impaired olfactory sense may not smell burning food or escaping gas. Paralysis and other neurologic impairments diminish touch perceptions. A paralyzed person may not feel a burn from a burning hot-water bottle, and a person whose sense of taste is impaired may not detect contaminated food.

Lack of sleep can diminish sensual acuity. A fatigued driver may fail to see a sign on the side of the highway, or a tired parent may forget to place cleaning solution out of the reach of a toddler.

Awareness

Patients with impaired awareness include:

1. Unconscious or semiconscious persons. There are varying levels of consciousness, that is, levels of lack of response to environmental stimuli. One unconscious patient, for example, may respond to painful stimuli, whereas another may not. See Table 35–1, page 901.
2. Disoriented persons, who may not understand where they are or what to do to help themselves.
3. Persons who perceive stimuli that do not exist. For example, during alcohol withdrawal, a person may believe worms are crawling on the bed.

4. Persons whose judgment is altered by medications, such as narcotics, tranquilizers, hypnotics, and sedatives.

Mobility

Persons who have paralysis, muscle weakness, and poor balance or coordination are obviously prone to injury. Patients with spinal cord injury and paralysis of both legs may be unable to move even when they perceive discomfort. Hemiplegic patients or patients with leg casts often have poor balance and fall easily. Patients weakened by illness or surgery are not always fully aware of their condition. It is not uncommon for patients to believe themselves able to walk and fall while trying. Nurses need to consider mobility when assessing a patient's potential for injury. Mobility increases the possibility of injury. For example, a slippery floor does not threaten the bedridden patient's safety as it does the ambulatory patient's.

Emotional State

Extreme emotional states can alter ability to perceive environmental hazards. The acutely anxious or angry person has reduced perceptual awareness. Depressed persons may think and react to environmental stimuli more slowly than usual. People worried about their own or loved ones' illnesses are less aware than usual of potential dangers in the environment, such as a street curb or an oncoming automobile.

Ability to Communicate

Obviously, people with diminished ability to receive and convey information are at risk. Aphasic patients and people with language barriers are among them. For example, the person unable to interpret the sign "No smoking—oxygen in use" may cause a fire.

Previous Accidents

It has been recognized for some time that some people are accident prone. These people have accidents more frequently than the average person. Some children cut themselves and fracture bones more often than their peers. Some adults drive a car for 15 years without an accident, while others have at least one accident each year.

Predisposition to accidents is thought to have an emotional basis. One theory is that emotional tension impairs a person's perceptions and judgments, thus making that person more likely to have an accident. Some propose that accidents may fulfill masochistic and hostile needs or fulfill desires to be cared for by others.

Safety Knowledge

Information is crucial to safety. Patients in hospitals and other unfamiliar environments frequently need specific safety information. Unfamiliar equipment, such as oxygen tanks, intravenous tubing, and hot packs, is a potential hazard. Nurses need to teach patients what safety precautions to take when oxygen is in use, how to maintain intravenous infusions, etc. See Chapters 29 and 31. Knowledge and use of safety precautions is essential in daily living. Specific precautions for various age levels are listed later in this chapter.

Nursing Diagnoses

Kim and Moritz (1982:294–97) categorize nursing diagnoses for patients at risk for accidental injury as follows:

1. Potential for trauma (physical injury)
2. Potential for poisoning
3. Potential for suffocation

Many factors—some individual, some environmental—increase these potentials:

- Age or developmental stage
- Impaired sensory acuity
- Impaired mobility
- Alterations in level of awareness
- Insufficient education (safety or drug)
- Disregard for safety precautions
- Impaired balance or coordination
- Muscle weakness
- Language barriers
- Improper storage of toxic agents
- Air pollutants
- Noxious substances
- Unsafe equipment
- Cluttered environment
- Inadequate lighting
- Access to illicit drugs or weapons
- Exposure to dangerous machines
- Risk-taking behavior

Planning and Intervention for Safety

Nursing Goals

The overall nursing goal is to prevent injury to a patient. Subgoals are:

1. To teach appropriate safety practices
2. To make the environment safe
3. To support the patient and support persons psychologically
4. To maintain skin integrity
5. To maintain joint mobility

Planning

The nurse planning safety measures must consider the age, knowledge level, and sensory deficits of the patient. The nursing care plan should include two aspects: educating patients and modifying the environment. The latter can involve not only arranging the environment but also limiting the environment in some ways.

Education

Most accidents are due to negligence and preventable. This section deals with accidental hazards to the lives and health of people in different age groups. The nurse needs to be aware of these hazards and play a preventive role. Making patients aware of safety precautions is an ongoing nursing function.

Infants

Although infants are completely dependent on others for care, they soon learn to roll from side to side, put objects in their mouths, and crawl. They are oblivious to such dangers as falling or ingesting harmful substances. Infants need constant surveillance by adults, who must provide protective measures.

Nurses need to educate others about the special safety needs of infants. The following list outlines safety precautions that adults caring for infants should take.

1. Provide only soft, large toys that do not have parts the infant can remove and swallow.
2. Always have the sides of the crib up when not handling the baby. The rungs of the crib sides need to be closely spaced, so that the baby cannot get her or his head between them.
3. Hold the baby at feeding time. The infant could choke if left alone with a bottle.
4. Put pins, needles, buttons, and nails out of reach of the baby. It is natural for infants to put such objects in their mouths.
5. Use guard rails at the top and bottom of the stairs when the baby starts to crawl.
6. Cover electric outlets, and install safety outlets if possible. Babies like to explore these places.
7. Do not leave a baby alone in the bath, bed, table, or anywhere there is a danger the child may roll off.
8. Do not hang a pacifier or anything that might cause strangulation around an infant's neck.
9. Do not put pillows, plastic, or anything that might suffocate a baby in the crib.
10. Restrain babies who ride in automobiles.

Toddlers

Toddlers are curious and like to feel and taste everything. They walk unsteadily at age 2. Toddlers like to climb and explore and are fascinated by such potential dangers as garden pools and busy streets. As a result, toddlers need constant supervision and protection. Training in safety can begin when the child is a toddler.

Nurses need to educate others about precautions they should take when caring for toddlers:

1. Place knives, other sharp tools, and matches safely out of the toddler's reach.
2. Place hot pots on the back burners, away from the toddler's reach.
3. Keep cleaning solutions, insecticides, and medicines in locked cupboards.
4. Do not let toddlers play near deep ditches, wells, and pools.
5. Teach the toddler the words *no* and *don't.* Make the child understand these words often signify danger and must be obeyed.
6. Ensure that the toddler is protected from electrical outlets.
7. Make sure that windows and balconies are made safe, for instance, sturdily screened.
8. Make children who ride in cars wear seat belts and sit in the back seat.
9. Do not leave toddlers unattended in bathtubs or pools.

Preschoolers

It is important to teach preschoolers accident prevention and safety rules, particularly since at this age they become increasingly independent. Preschoolers are very active; they run, climb, and often act before they think. They like to imitate their parents, and adults can teach safety through example.

The following checklist helps nurses teach adults

caring for preschoolers the special safety education needs of that age group:

1. Teach preschoolers to cross streets safely and to obey traffic lights.
2. Teach them to play on sidewalks or grass rather than in driveways, streets, or railroad tracks.
3. Teach them to swim and to understand that water can be dangerous.
4. Teach them not to run with sharp utensils or with hard objects in their mouths.
5. Encourage them to put their toys away so that they and others will not trip over them.
6. Teach them the dangers of ingesting vegetation, peeling paint or plaster, and other possibly poisonous substances.
7. Teach them not to put small objects in the mouth, nose, and ears.

School-age children

By the time children attend school, they are learning to think before they act. They often prefer adult equipment to toys. They want to be active with other children in such activities as bicycling, hiking, swimming, and boating.

Nurses need to disseminate the safety education needs of school-age children, as follows:

1. Teach school-age children safe ways to use the stove, garden tools, and other equipment.
2. Teach them traffic rules for bicycling.
3. Teach them safety rules for swimming, boating, skateboarding, and other recreations.
4. Supervise them when they use saws, or electric appliances and tools, and other potentially dangerous equipment.
5. Teach them not to play with fireworks, gunpowder, and firearms.

Adolescents

Adolescents spend much of their time away from home with their peer groups. However, they still need guidance from parents. The accident rate among adolescents is high, and the major cause is automobiles. In addition, adolescents are at risk of injury when riding motorcycles, snowmobiles, and minibikes. Firearms and drowning are other causes of deaths among adolescents.

To prevent accidents, adolescents need to follow these safety measures:

1. Develop the discipline necessary for safe driving.
2. Wear safety helmets when riding motorcycles and similar vehicles.
3. Wear seat belts when driving.
4. Learn to swim and understand water safety.
5. If using firearms, learn how to use these competently.
6. Understand the dangers of drugs and alcohol.

Adults

Accidents rank fourth as the cause of death among middle-aged adults. Alcohol is a significant factor in many of these accidents. Consequently, adults need to learn not to drink if they are driving motor vehicles, boating, or swimming.

Accident prevention starts with education about precautions such as these:

1. Store combustibles and corrosives, for example, oily rags and lye, in appropriate places.
2. Ensure that electrical plugs, wires, and appliances are in good repair.
3. Anchor small rugs securely.
4. Clean up litter or spills on the floor immediately.
5. Keep stairs and walkways free from obstructions, snow, and ice.
6. Avoid using unsteady ladders or chairs.
7. Screen fires and heaters.
8. Avoid wearing plastic aprons or loose clothing around open flames.
9. Do not smoke in bed.
10. Put nonskid material in bathtubs and shower stalls.
11. Ensure that automobiles are mechanically sound.
12. Wear safety belts when driving, and make sure that windshields, side mirrors, and rearview mirrors are clean.

Elderly people are particularly prone to accidents. They require education in how to make living environments safe. Sturdy handrails on stairways and in bathrooms are essential. Small rugs must be safely tacked down. Dishes and other frequently used supplies should be in easy reach. Hallways, stairways, and closets must be adequately lit.

Modifying the Environment

The living environment may need to be modified to prevent falls and self-inflicted injury, fire, burns, injury due to electricity, poisoning, asphyxiation, and radiation. In addition, people often require special protective measures against communicable diseases.

Falls and self-inflicted injuries

Falls are common not only among the very young and among elderly people but also occur frequently among the ill or injured, who are weakened and frequently lose their balance.

In hospitals and homes, nurses need to be very much aware of patients who may fall. These safeguards are generally taken to prevent falls:

1. Bedside tables and overbed tables are placed near the bed or chair so that patients do not need to overreach and consequently lose their balance.
2. Patients who have had surgery or have been in bed for some time are advised to accept assistance when first getting out of bed.
3. Footstools have nonskid rubber feet and wheelchairs have wheel locks.
4. Floors have nonslip surfaces; rugs and carpeting are fixed securely. In some hospitals, special nonskid flooring is used in the halls and stairs, and special mats are placed in bathtubs.
5. The environment is kept tidy so that people do not trip over light cords or misplaced furniture.
6. Some hospitals have railings along corridors and in bathrooms.

In addition to the above measures, special safety devices, such as side rails and restraints, protect patients.

In some agencies, agency policy determines when these devices are used; in others, they are used at the order of the physician or at the nurse's discretion. It is very important that patients understand why these devices are being employed and what is expected of them. For example, a patient in a bed with side rails should be told not to leave the bed without assistance from the nurse. Some weakened patients climb over side rails with surprising agility and risk dangerous falls simply because they do not understand they should obtain assistance.

Side rails Side rails are attached to the side of the bed, and when elevated, help prevent a patient from falling out of bed. Side rails, however, are unlikely to stop the adult patient determined to get out of bed.

Side rails are frequently used on beds of unconscious, confused, or sedated patients. In addition, in some hospitals side rails are applied to the beds of all patients over 70 years of age, particularly at night. In other settings, side rails are used for all patients at night, regardless of age.

It is usual for nurses to take down the side rail on the side of the bed where they are working. It is important, however, to elevate the rail when leaving the bedside. Although an unconscious patient or child may appear quiet and unlikely to move, he or she may suddenly move and fall out of bed if the side rail is not in place.

Although some patients find side rails embarrassing, many others find they provide a sense of security. This is particularly true because hospital beds, which are at a fixed height, are higher and narrower than the usual bed at home. See Chapter 21 for additional information.

Restraints Recently, there has been a shift toward means other than restraints to protect patients. Restrained patients often become restless and anxious as a result of the loss of self-control. In many instances, however, restraints are necessary to prevent injury or interruption of therapy. Restraints are essential for the patient who tries to pull out a urinary or intravenous catheter or the infant who wants to scratch eczematous skin lesions.

Restraints have the following purposes:

1. To prevent falls from beds, stretchers, or chairs
2. To prevent the interruption of selected therapy, e.g., an intravenous infusion
3. To protect a patient from self-inflicted injury, for example, by pulling out a urinary catheter
4. To prevent a patient from injuring others

Legal implications of restraints Because restraints restrict an individual's ability to move freely, their use has legal implications. In some settings, the decision to use a restraint is the nurse's; in others, the decision must be made by a physician. Often a nurse can apply a restraint in an emergency; however, the physician must order the restraint if it is used subsequently. It is important to know the agency practices and the state or provincial laws about restraining patients.

Before restraining a patient, a nurse needs to try (and document) other nursing interventions, e.g., reorienting the patient to reality. The nurse needs to describe in the record what patient behavior led to the decision to use restraints. This information documents the fact that restraints were applied for the patient's safety, not for the nurse's convenience.

Additionally, the nurse must document the type of restraint used, the exact times the restraints were applied and removed, the patient's behavior before and with the restraints, the care given while the restraint was applied, and the notification of the physician. It is important to explain the need for the restraint both to the patient and to support persons; the nurse also should document the substance of these explanations.

Guidelines for use of restraints The nurse who applies a restraint should keep these guidelines in mind:

1. Explain the restraint and the need for it to the patient and the patient's support persons. Often hospital visitors are very disturbed to find a restrained friend or relative. A simple explanation and assurance that the restraint is not a punishment but a temporary measure to protect the patient is usually sufficient. A restraint must never be applied either as punishment or for the nurse's convenience.
2. Apply the restraint so that the patient can move as freely as possible without defeating the purpose of the

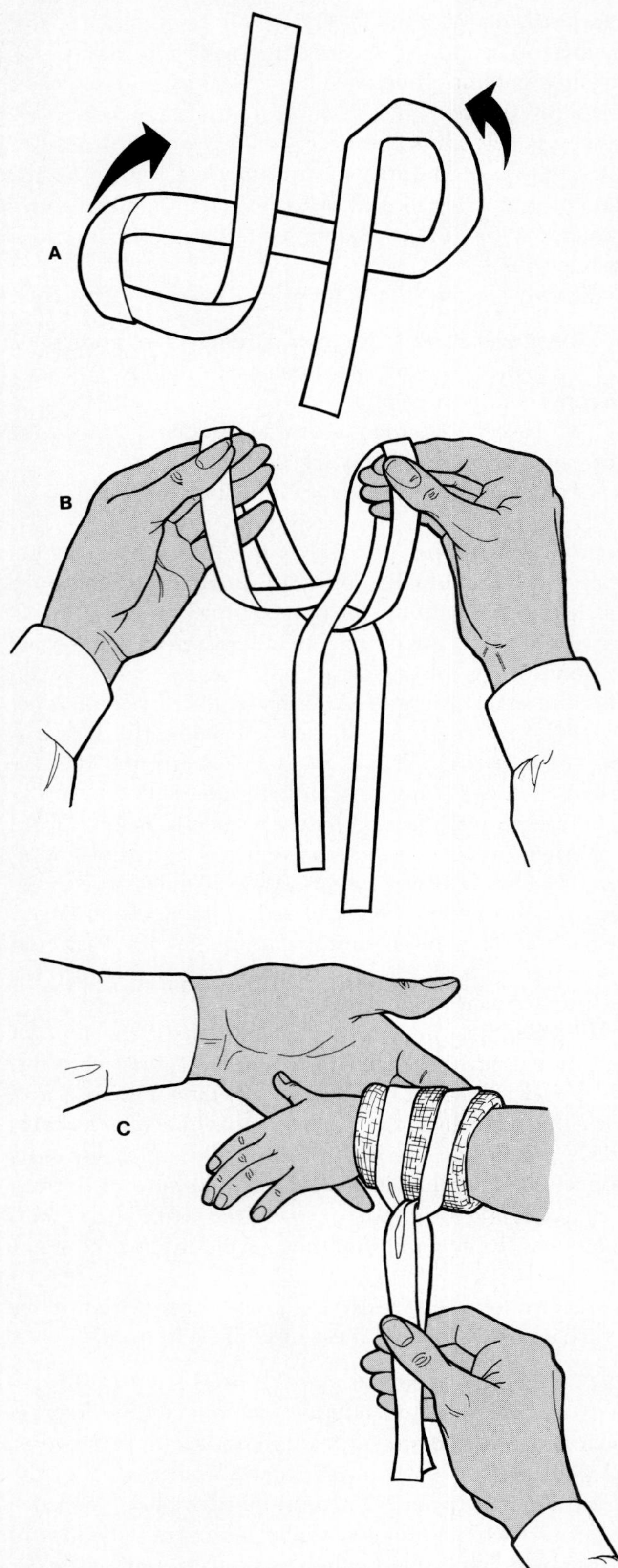

Figure 22–1 To make a clove hitch: **A,** Make a figure-eight; **B,** pick up the loops; **C,** put the limb through the loops and secure it.

restraint. For example, a jacket restraint need not pin the patient against the bed. It should permit some movement, such as bending forward or turning slightly to one side, yet still restrain the patient safely in bed.

3. Ensure that limb restraints are applied securely but not so tightly that they impede blood circulation to any body area or extremity.

4. Pad bony prominences (e.g., wrists and ankles) before applying a restraint over them. Without padding, such restraints can quickly abrade the skin.

5. Always tie a limb restraint with a knot that will not tighten when pulled. For example, a clove hitch applied to a wrist will stay secure, while a simple knot will tighten with pulling. A clove hitch is shown in Figure 22–1.

6. Tie the ends of a body restraint to the part of the bed that moves when the head rest is elevated. Never tie the ends to a side rail or to the fixed frame of the bed if the bed position is to be changed. The patient could be injured if the restraint is pulled tight when the bed moves.

7. Remove most limb restraints at least every 4 hours, and provide range-of-motion exercises (see Chapter 24) and skin care (see Chapter 21). Remove restraints on elderly patients more often, e.g., every 2 hours, to maintain blood circulation and mobility of the joints.

8. Do not leave the patient unattended when a restraint is temporarily removed.

9. Immediately report any persistent reddened or broken skin areas under the restraint to the responsible nurse and record them on the patient's chart.

10. At the first indication of cyanosis or pallid and cold skin, or if the patient complains of a tingling sensation, pain, or numbness, loosen the restraint and have the patient exercise the limb. Impaired blood circulation can cause these symptoms.

11. Apply a restraint so that it can be released quickly in an emergency. For example, secure a body restraint to an easily accessible place on the bed.

12 Apply a restraint so that the patient can assume a normal anatomic position; for example, with the elbow slightly flexed.

13. Provide emotional support by touching and talking to the patient. Some patients become very anxious when restrained and exhaust themselves fighting the restraint. Stay with the patient as required.

Selecting a restraint When selecting a restraint, the nurse must understand clearly the purpose of the restraint and choose a restraint that best meets the patient's needs. The following guidelines can help nurses select a restraint.

1. The restraint should restrict the patient's movement only as much as necessary. If a patient needs a restraint only on one arm, the nurse need not restrain the entire body.

2. The restraint should be as inconspicuous as possible. Both patients and visitors are often embarrassed by restraints. Even when patients and visitors understand why a restraint is necessary, they feel more comfortable if it is not obvious. A crossover jacket restraint can be less conspicuous than arm and leg restraints.

3. Restraints should not interfere with the patient's treatment or exacerbate a health problem. If a patient has poor blood circulation to the hands, the nurse should apply a restraint that does not aggravate that circulatory problem.

4. The restraint should be easy to change. Restraints need to be changed frequently, and whenever they become soiled. Keeping other guidelines in mind, the nurse chooses a restraint that can be changed with minimal disturbance to the patient.

5. It should be safe for the patient. For example, a physically active child could be injured trying to climb out of the crib if one wrist is tied to the side of the crib. A jacket restraint is safer for such a patient.

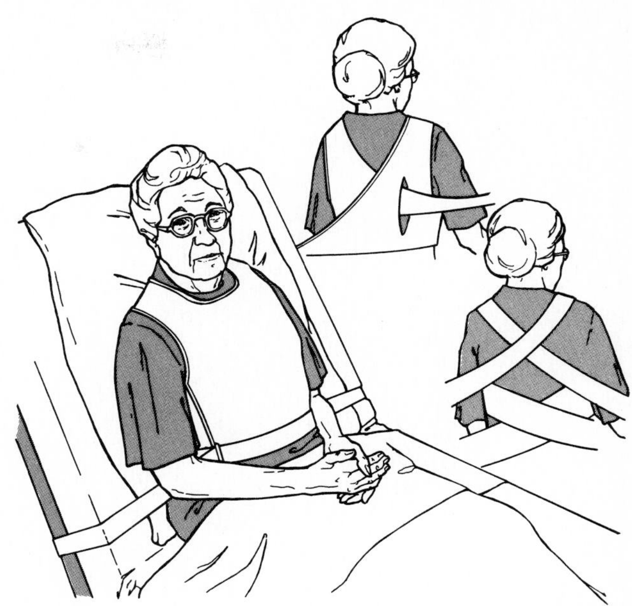

Figure 22–2 Jacket restraints (note various styles).

Types of restraints *Hand and foot restraints* are used to keep a limb relatively immobilized, for instance, to facilitate an intravenous infusion or to prevent a confused patient from removing a urinary catheter or nasal tube.

The wrist or ankle is padded with a thick gauze dressing or special felt pads. The cloth restraint is then tied on the body using a clove hitch, which will not tighten with pulling. See Figure 22–1. The ends are tied to the bed frame under the mattress.

Jacket restraints are used for both children and adults. The nurse usually ties the jacket at the back, but in some situations ties it at the front. See Figure 22–2. The straps from the jacket are then tied to the movable bed frame under the mattress or to the legs of a chair.

The mummy restraint and the papoose board are appropriate for small children. The *mummy restraint* is a special folding of a blanket or sheet around the child to prevent movement during a procedure such as gastric washing, eye irrigation, or collection of a blood specimen. The child lies supine on a blanket with the upper edge of the blanket slightly above the shoulders and the lower edge at least 10 to 12 inches below the feet. The child's right arm is placed at his or her side, then one side of the blanket is brought over the body and between the left arm and body and tucked under the body. Then the left arm is placed in anatomical position, and the other side of the blanket is brought over the length of the body and tucked under the child. The long end of the sheet is then brought over and tucked in beneath the child.

A *papoose board* restrains children for periods of time varying from 15 minutes to several hours. This restraint is useful during intravenous infusions, for circumcisions, and for other minor local surgical procedures. The board flaps are extended, and the board is padded with a blanket. The child lies face up on the board, and the wrists are placed through the loops on the board. The center strap is brought over the arms and body and fastened securely. Next, the chest strap is fastened, and last, the leg strap is brought over the thighs and lower legs.

Safety belts are used on older children and adults. The belt, which goes around the patient's waist, is attached to a longer belt, which is fastened in turn at each end to the bed frame under the mattress.

An *elbow restraint* (Figure 22–3) is used on occasion for small children. This is a piece of cloth with either rigid supports or slots into which tongue blades fit. The restraint is wrapped around the elbow and tied at the ends. The ties on the upper edge are then pinned to the baby's shirt to prevent the restraint from sliding down the arm. Elbow restraints are commonly used to prevent small children from touching an incision or scratching.

Mitt restraints are used to prevent confused patients from using their hands or fingers to injure themselves. With mitts on, patients are unable to remove a urinary catheter or pull off surgical dressings yet are able to move their arms freely. Mitts are convenient for ambulatory patients, since other types of restraints confine them to a bed or chair.

Commercially prepared mitts are available (Figure 22–4), or the nurse can make them using large dressings and stockinette. The nurse asks the patient to grasp a small pad, so that the hand assumes a natural position. The patient's wrist is padded with large dressings to prevent skin abrasions, and all skin surfaces are care-

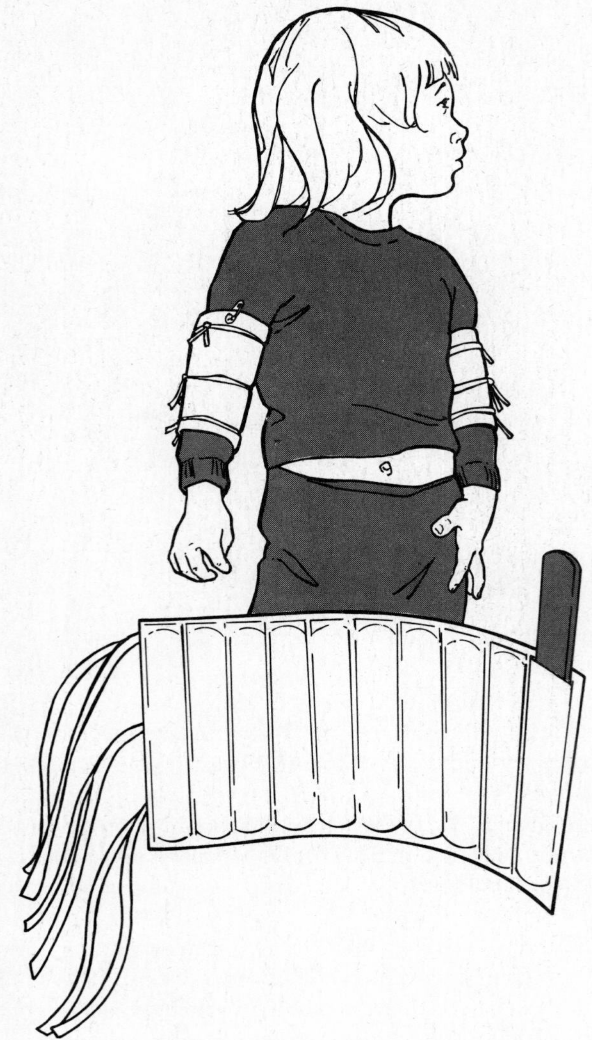

Figure 22–3 An elbow restraint for a young child.

Figure 22–4 A commercially made mitt restraint.

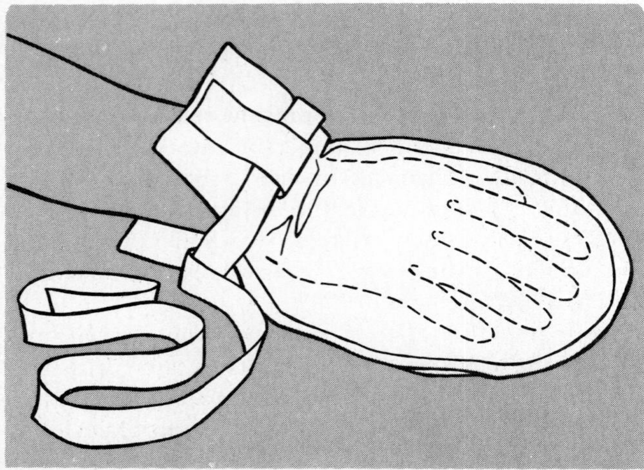

fully separated, also to prevent abrasions. The nurse then places two large dressings over the hand, one from side to side and the other from the ventral surface to the dorsal surface. The dressings are secured with gauze bandage in a recurrent pattern and adhesive tape. See the section on bandaging turns in Chapter 40. Stockinette is then put over the hand and secured just above the wrist pad with adhesive tape.

Mittens need to be removed at least once in 24 hours to permit the patient to wash and exercise the hands. If the patient reports discomfort, the nurse needs to take off the mitten and check the circulation to the hand.

Fire

Fire is a constant danger in any environment, including the hospital. Statistics show that electrical fires, usually due to faulty electrical equipment, are the most common type of fire in homes and hospitals. The second most common cause of fire in hospitals is smoking in bed. Hospital fires are especially dangerous because patients are often incapacitated and unable to leave the building without assistance.

These simple guidelines help the nurse if there is a fire:

1. Know the location of fire exits.
2. Know the location of fire extinguishers and learn to operate them.
3. Be familiar with the practices of the hospital and with the alarm system.

Most hospitals have procedures to be followed during a fire. Nurses should carry these out regardless of how small the fire is initially. A small fire in a wastebasket can quickly become a large fire. Some hospitals post the following procedures:

1. Remove any patients who are in immediate danger.
2. Activate the fire alarm if there is one nearby.
3. Notify the hospital switchboard of the location of the fire.
4. Use the fire extinguisher on the fire.
5. Close windows and doors to reduce ventilation.
6. Turn off oxygen and any electrical appliances in the vicinity of the fire.
7. Clear fire exits, if necessary.

If the fire is on the other side of a door, it is advisable to contain the smoke by placing damp cloths or blankets around the edges of the door.

Kinds of fires There are generally three kinds of fires: paper and wood fires (class A); flammable liquid fires, such as grease and anesthetics (class B); and electrical fires (class C).

All fires require three elements: sufficient heat to start

the fire, a combustible material, and sufficient oxygen to support the fire.

Types of fire extinguishers Five types of fire extinguishers are in general use today:

1. *Carbon dioxide extinguisher.* This extinguisher is effective against grease fires and electrical fires (classes B and C). The nurse directs the nozzle toward the fire and pulls the trigger, thereby releasing carbon dioxide, which cuts off the oxygen supply.
2. *Soda and acid extinguisher.* This is a water extinguisher, which puts out paper and rubbish fires (class A). The acid and soda in the extinguisher mix when it is turned upside down. These produce carbon dioxide, which permits the water to be released under pressure. To stop the flow from the extinguisher, the operator turns the extinguisher rightside up. This type of extinguisher is not effective against either electrical or grease fires because water conducts electricity and causes grease to splatter, thus possibly spreading the fire.
3. *Dry chemical extinguisher.* This extinguisher blankets a fire with a foamlike material, which excludes oxygen from the fire. The extinguisher contains chemicals, sodium bicarbonate, and carbon dioxide. It is used for both rubbish and electric fires (classes A and C). The operator pulls a pin, either opens a valve or presses a lever on the extinguisher, and squeezes the nozzle valve.
4. *Water pump extinguisher.* This extinguisher, used only for class A fires, contains water, which is pumped by hand. The operator pumps the handle while directing the nozzle toward the fire.
5. *Antifreeze or water extinguisher.* Water or antifreeze is stored under pressure in this extinguisher. A pressure gauge on the outside of the can indicates pressure and readiness for use. To use this type of extinguisher, the operator pulls a pin and then pulls the handle of the extinguisher. It is effective against class A and B fires.

Evacuating patients There are four methods of carrying persons from the scene of a fire. Generally, nurses use these carries for patients when they cannot wheel out bedridden patients in their beds or carry them out on stretchers.

1. *Swing carry.* The swing is a two-person carry. The patient, in a sitting position, places the arms around each nurse's shoulders. Each nurse holds the patient's wrists, which are over each nurse's shoulders, to support the patient. Each nurse then reaches behind the patient and grasps the other nurse's shoulder or upper arm. The nurses then release the patient's wrists, reach under the patient's thighs, and grasp each other's wrists. They lift and carry the patient in this sitting position. See Figure 22–5.

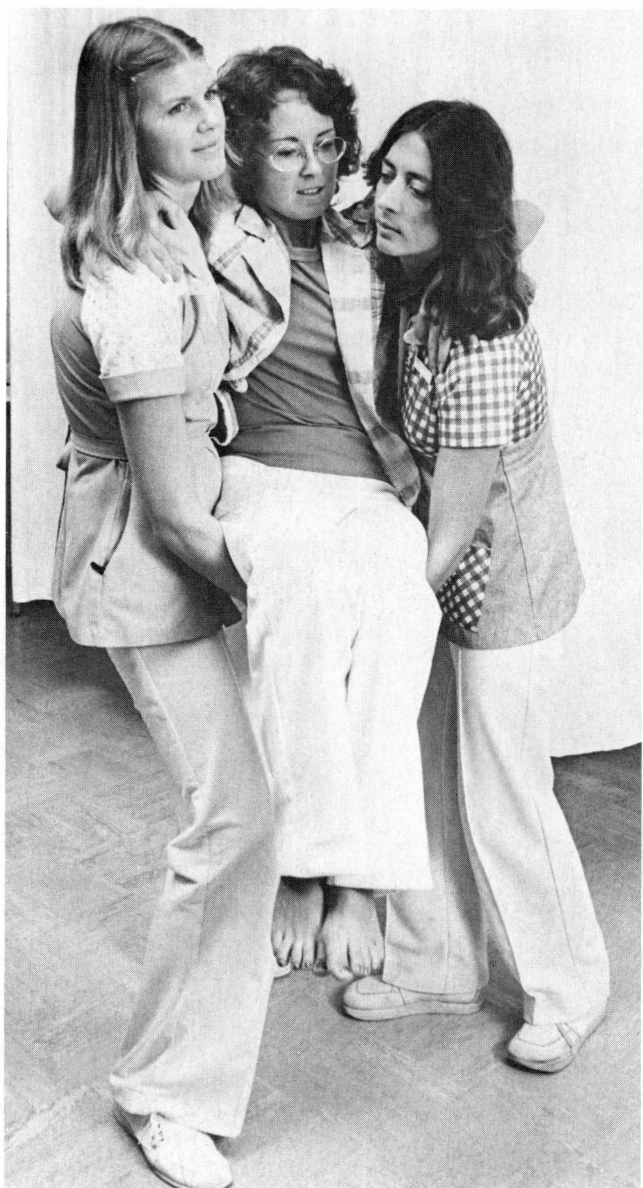

Figure 22–5 The swing carry.

2. *Pack strap carry.* The pack strap is a one-person carry. The nurse faces the seated patient and grasps the wrists. The nurse's right hand grasps the patient's left wrist; the left hand grasps the patient's right wrist. The nurse then pivots and slips under one of the patient's arms so that the nurse's back is to the patient and the patient's arms are crossed in front of the nurse. The nurse assumes a broad stance, one leg in front of the other, and rolls the patient onto her or his back. See Figure 22–6.
3. *Hip carry.* The patient lies laterally at the side of the bed facing the nurse. The nurse faces the head of the

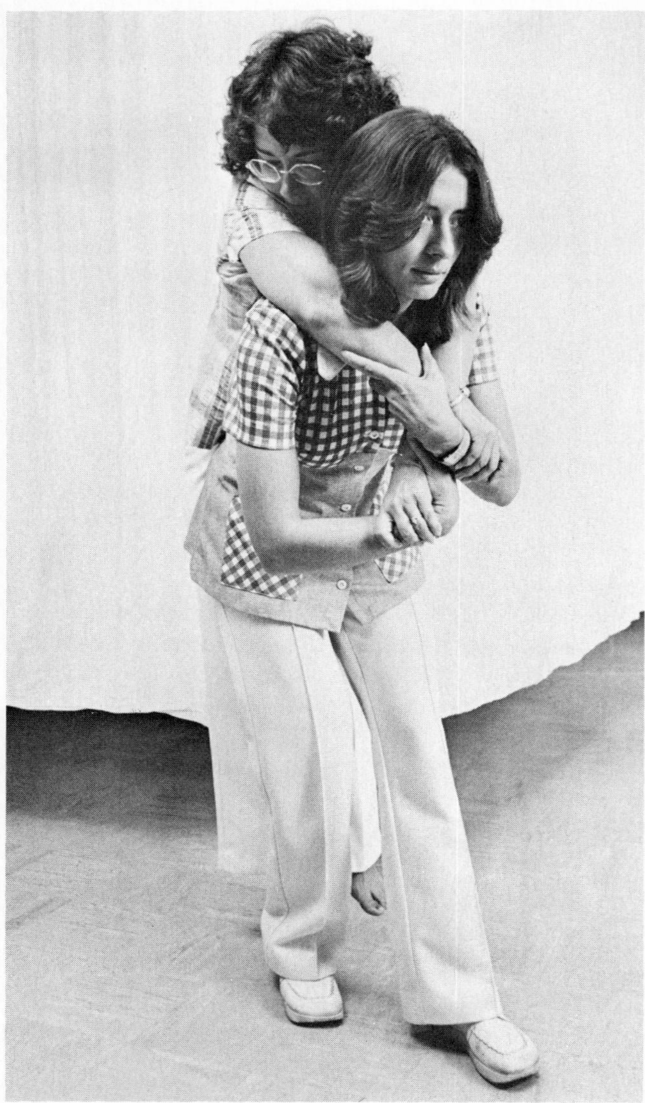

Figure 22–6 The pack strap carry.

bed. The nurse places the arm nearest the patient over the patient's back and under the lower axilla. The nurse then turns away from the patient and places the second arm around and under the thighs. Assuming a broad stance for balance, the nurse then draws the patient onto the nurse's hips so that the patient's abdomen is over the nurse's hips. See Figure 22–7.

4. *Three-person carry.* See the instructions for lifting a patient between a bed and a stretcher, Chapter 23.

Burns

Fires are not the only cause of burns, for example, a heat lamp too close to the skin can burn a patient. Patients who are ill may be unaware that they are being burned. Also, people can be accustomed to a degree of heat that is injurious to tissues. The use of heat as a therapeutic measure is discussed in Chapter 40. It is important to assess the degree to which patients can protect themselves and what special precautions, if any, the nurse needs to take.

Hospital equipment is often unfamiliar to patients, and they usually need warnings not to touch equipment that becomes very hot. Such equipment should be out of the reach of small children, who learn by touching and whose curiosity may be awakened by warnings and explanations.

Electricity

Electricity is used extensively in health care. Most machines used in patient care are electric, and most diagnostic equipment uses electricity in some way. Part of nursing intervention is keeping patients safe from electric hazards in health care and other settings.

There are two types of electricity: *dynamic* (moving electric charges) and *static* (stationary electric charges). Dynamic electricity poses a danger in that a current can pass through the body to the ground, giving the individual a shock or a macroshock. Nurses need to use electric equipment that is properly *grounded* (that transmits an electric current from an object or surface to the ground). In modern buildings, electric outlets are normally grounded to prevent shocks by a third wire.

Dynamic electricity operates most equipment. If the equipment is faulty, e.g., if a cord is frayed, there is a danger of electric shock. Also, faulty electric equipment can start fires. For example, an electric spark near certain anesthetic gases or a high concentration of oxygen may cause a serious fire.

If an individual receives a macroshock, it is important not to touch that person until the electricity is shut off and the person is safely away from the electric current. A macroshock can cause both superficial and deep burns, muscle contractions, and cardiac and respiratory arrest. Macroshock is prevented by using machines in good repair, wearing shoes with rubber soles, standing on a nonconductive floor, and using nonconductive gloves.

Static electricity builds up on the surface of the body and of certain materials. It is caused by the transfer of *electrons* (negatively charged electric particles) from one surface to another. Lightning is the most powerful form of static electricity.

Static electricity is a danger in hospital operating rooms, where the building up and sparking of static charges near anesthetic agents could cause an explosion. To prevent explosions, nylon, dacron and other materials that tend to build up static charges are not used. Because dry air is conducive to the buildup of static electric charges, the air is humidified and antistatic sprays are used in areas where explosion is a danger.

Poisoning

Ingestion of toxic agents is very common in children 5 years or younger, particularly in 2-year-olds, whose curiosity and independence prompts them to investigate objects, often by tasting them. Almost all nonfood substances, including many house plants, are potentially harmful to children. The major reasons for poisoning in children are inadequate supervision and improper storage of the many toxic substances (over 500, on average) in the home.

Ways to prevent poisoning include:

1. Place potentially toxic agents out of reach of crawling infants.
2. Put all drugs (prescription and nonprescription) in a locked cabinet. Even though legislation mandates child-guard tops on prescription drugs, many 4-year-olds can manipulate these.
3. Lock cleaning agents in a cupboard or attach special plastic hooks to the inside of cabinet doors to keep them securely closed. Unlatching these hooks, obtainable at most hardware stores, requires firmer thumb pressure than small children can usually exert.
4. Avoid keeping a large surplus of cleaning agents, laundry additives, furniture polish, insecticides, paints, and solvents.
5. Avoid storing toxic liquids or solids in food containers, such as soft drink bottles, peanut butter jars, or milk cartons. Even though the containers are well labeled, the child who cannot read associates them with food.
6. Do not remove container labels or reuse empty containers to store different substances. Laws mandate that the labels of all poisons specify antidotes. Removing labels or changing the contents thus negates this safety measure.
7. When children are old enough to learn, teach them the difference between food and those substances that must never be ingested or tasted.
8. Place poison warning stickers designed for children on containers of bleach, lye, kerosene, solvent, and other toxic substances.

People need to be prepared to deal with poisoning in the event it occurs. Nurses can intervene by educating the public in measures to take in the event of poisoning. Recommended information and actions include:

1. Identify the specific poison by searching for an opened container, empty bottle, or other evidence.
2. Know the location of the poison control center and contact it in the event of suspected poisoning. Try to indicate the exact quantity of poison the person ingested, and state the person's age and apparent symptoms.
3. Induce vomiting or neutralize the poison as appropriate. See the section immediately following.
4. If indicated by the poison control center, transport the victim to the hospital as soon as possible. All evidence of the poison, such as urine, vomitus, substance container, etc., should be taken.
5. Keep the victim as quiet as possible and position the victim on one side or with head placed between the legs to prevent aspiration of vomitus.

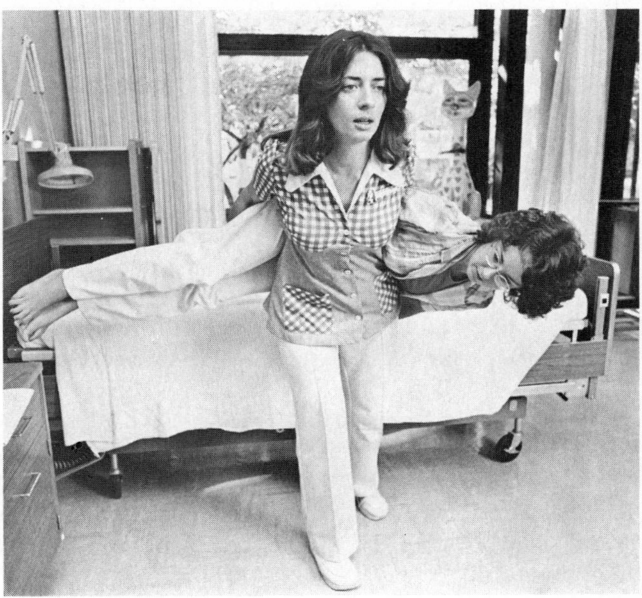

Figure 22–7 The hip carry.

When not to induce vomiting Inducing vomiting is contraindicated when the victim is unconscious or convulsing or when the poison is one of the following:

1. A strong corrosive (acid or alkali), such as lye (drain or oven cleaners), chlorine bleach, electric dishwasher granules, and household ammonia
2. A petroleum distillate, such as kerosene, turpentine, cleaning fluid, lighter fluid, furniture polish, metal polish, and some insecticides

To induce vomiting

1. Administer *syrup of ipecac*, a nonprescription emetic available in single-dose 15 ml vials in all drugstores. This emetic should be on hand in all households. The usual dose for a child over 1 year of age is 10 to 15 ml (2 or 3 tsp) with one or two cups of water or other liquid. Liquid ensures vomiting rather than retching if the stomach is empty. If emesis does not occur in 20 minutes, administer a second dose. Proper use and dose of ipecac syrup is essential. Overdoses have occurred due to multiple doses of syrup or to the use of fluid extract of ipecac, 14 times more potent than the syrup.

2. Do not administer syrup of ipecac to infants under 1 year of age. If the victim is an infant, administer a large glass of water and tickle the back of the victim's throat with a spoon or other blunt instrument.

3. Alternatively, administer large amounts of water or milk: 120 to 240 ml (1 to 2 cups) for children between ages 2 and 5; 1 liter (1 quart) for children over age 5.

To neutralize a corrosive poison Administer 45 ml (2 Tbsp) of lemon juice or vinegar in 2 glasses of water to neutralize an alkali. Milk helps neutralize an acid. Also administer a soothing, bland agent such as egg white or oil to coat the gastrointestinal tract. Do not induce vomiting.

To stop absorption of a petroleum distillate Administer mineral oil, cooking oil, or activated charcoal to reduce absorption of a petroleum distillate. Again, do not induce vomiting.

Asphyxiation

Asphyxiation, or suffocation, is lack of oxygen due to interrupted breathing. Asphyxiation can occur if the air source is cut off; for example, if the victim is under water or has a plastic bag around the head. Asphyxiation can also occur when there is a barrier in the upper respiratory tract to the movement of air into and from the lungs. Two examples are the inspiration of a piece of food into the trachea and acute swelling of the pharyngeal tissues.

If the victim does not obtain immediate relief, interrupted breathing leads to respiratory and cardiac arrest and subsequent death. However, most incidents of asphyxiation in the community and hospital are preventable. Education of the public about accident prevention is important. The following are some aspects of such a prevention program.

1. Encourage people to remove doors from old refrigerators, freezers, etc., so that children cannot close themselves inside.

2. Encourage people to lock freezers and similar containers if young children play around them.

3. Teach the public to keep plastic away from infants and young children and to avoid using plastic in cribs.

4. Teach children and adults to take suitable safety precautions, such as wearing life jackets when boating, fishing, etc.

5. Encourage children to learn to swim. Educate adults not to leave young children unsupervised near pools or at beaches.

6. Encourage the use of nonskid surfaces in bathtubs, particularly those used by elderly people.

7. In hospitals, always supervise tub baths for patients at risk, e.g., those who have epilepsy, hypertension, brain tumors, etc.

8. Maintain suction equipment at the bedsides of patients who might choke, such as patients who have difficulty swallowing.

If a person begins to suffocate, any obstruction to the air passages must be removed immediately and cardiopulmonary resuscitation (CPR) established if cardiac or respiratory arrests have occurred. See Chapter 29 for information about the Heimlich maneuver (used to expel foreign objects in the airway), CPR, and suctioning techniques.

Radiation

Radiation as a health hazard is a recent source of concern. Nurses are concerned specifically with those radioactive materials used in diagnostic and therapeutic practices. Radiation injury can occur from overexposure or from exposure to radiation that treats specific tissues and at the same time injures other tissues.

Radioactive materials are used in diagnostic procedures such as radiography, fluoroscopy, and nuclear medicine. In nuclear medicine, radioactive isotopes that have an affinity for specific tissues are given by mouth or intravenously. Isotopes of these elements are used: calcium, which has an affinity for bones; iodine, which is attracted to the thyroid gland; and phosphorus, which is attracted to blood.

Radioactive materials are provided in sealed sources and unsealed liquid sources. For example, cobalt implants are sealed; iodine 131 and phosphorus 32 are unsealed liquids.

Principles governing the degree of exposure to radiation are as follows:

1. The longer the time in the presence of radiation, the greater the exposure

2. The closer a person is to the radioactive source, the greater the exposure

3. The more extensive the use of lead and other radiation shields, the greater the protection against radiation.

Assisting patients receiving radioactive materials Often nurses help care for patients treated or diagnosed with radioactive substances.

The patient diagnosed through radiography or fluoroscopy generally receives minimal exposure, and few precautions are necessary. The nurse restraining a small child during radiography needs to wear a lead apron. Patients with radioactive implants are a source of radiation to the immediate environment. The nurse who is in close contact with such patients also needs to wear a lead apron.

It is important to deal with any radioactive body discharges in a safe manner. Nurses wear rubber gloves and in some instances may place excreta in containers for special disposal. It is also important that the nurse's gloved hands be washed well before the gloves are moved and that contaminated materials be placed in a special container for disposal.

Hospitals in which radioactive materials are used usually have a radioisotope committee. This committee establishes policies and procedures to be used in the care of patients who receive radioactive materials. It is important that nurses be cognizant of these policies.

One important aspect of caring for patients receiving radiation treatment is making sure they understand the treatment and the precautions they need to take. Often such patients are restricted to bed or to a confined area to protect others. Like patients who are on protective asepsis, these patients need emotional support to deal with the precautions. They accept treatments and precautions better when they know what will happen, when, and why.

Immunization

Immunity is the body's resistance to the effects of harmful agents, such as pathogens or their toxins. The various types of immunity—natural or acquired, and passive or active—are described in Chapter 9, page 190.

Immunity is acquired through antigen-antibody reactions that occur whenever a foreign agent or its product enters the bloodstream. An *antigen* is a protein or protein-polysaccharide capable of producing antibodies in the body. Most antigens are considered foreign to the body and, when taken into the body, stimulate the production of antibodies. However, there is recent evidence that some antigenic substances react to antibodies or cells but cannot induce the formation of antibodies. They are called *haptens*. An *antibody* is a protein substance (an adapted plasma globulin) formed by body cells; antibodies have the capacity of neutralizing or reacting with antigens.

The goal of *immunization*, the process of becoming immune or rendering someone immune, is to protect people from *communicable diseases*, which spread from one person to another. Modes of transmission include (a) direct contact, such as contact with body excreta or discharges from open sores; (b) indirect contact, such as contact with contaminated drinking glasses, clothing, toys, or other objects, and; (c) *vectors* (carriers), such as flies, mosquitoes, or other animals that spread the disease. Infections and infection control are discussed in Chapter 19. Common communicable diseases and their incidence are cited in Table 22–4.

Epidemiology is the study of the occurrence and distribution of disease as it occurs in humans. *Epidemic* describes the occurrence of disease in many people at the same time or in rapid succession in an area. *Pandemic* describes widespread occurrence of a disease in many parts of the world at the same time.

Immunization needs Immunization against communicable diseases is a preventive health measure advocated by government agencies in the United States and Canada.

Newborn infants have limited ability to produce antibodies until they are about 3 months of age. However, during the last few months of pregnancy certain maternal antibodies pass through the placenta, thus providing the baby with some passive immunity. This immunity is temporary; so it is vital to practice good hygiene around infants, sterilize their formulas, and separate them from people who have infections.

At 2 or 3 months of age, children should receive their first immunizations. Antigens in the form of *vaccines* (living or dead microorganisms) or *toxoids* (detoxified toxins) are administered to induce active immunity. Tables 22–5 and 22–6 show the immunizations advised in the United States and Canada. In addition, rubella (German measles) vaccine is recommended for (a) all susceptible children between the ages of 15 months and 12 years and (b) female adolescents and women of

Table 22–4 Incidence (Reported Cases) of the Eight Leading Communicable Diseases in the United States, 1969 and 1976

Disease	1969	1976
Gonorrhea	534,872	1,001,994
Syphilis	92,162	71,761
Measles (rubeola)	25,826	41,126
Infectious hepatitis	48,416	33,288
Tuberculosis	39,120	32,105
Salmonellosis (excluding typhoid fever)	18,419	22,937
Bacillary dysentery	11,946	13,140
Rubella (German measles)	57,686	12,491

From U.S. Department of Health, Education, and Welfare, *Facts of life and death* (Hyattsville, Md.: Department of Health, Education, and Welfare, 1978), pp. 14–15.

Table 22–5 Recommended Schedule for Active Immunization of Normal Infants and Children

Recommended age	Vaccine(s)	Comments
2 months	DTP,[1] OPV[2]	Can be initiated earlier in areas of high endemicity
4 months	DTP, OPV	2-month interval desired for OPV to avoid interference
6 months	DTP (OPV)	OPV optional for areas where polio might be imported (e.g., some areas of Southwest United States)
12 months	Tuberculin test[3]	May be given simultaneously with MMR at 15 months
15 months	Measles, mumps, rubella (MMR)[4]	MMR preferred
18 months	DTP, OPV	Consider as part of primary series—DTP essential
4–6 years[5]	DTP, OPV	
14–16 years	Td[6]	Repeat every 10 years for lifetime

[1]DTP—diphtheria and tetanus toxoids with pertussis vaccine.

[2]OPV—oral, attenuated poliovirus vaccine contains poliovirus types 1, 2, and 3.

[3]Tuberculin test—Mantoux (intradermal PPD) preferred. Frequency of tests depends on local epidemiology. The Committee on Infectious Diseases, American Academy of Pediatrics, recommends annual or biennial testing unless local circumstances dictate less frequent or no testing.

[4]MMR—live measles, mumps, and rubella viruses in a combined vaccine.

[5]Up to the 7th birthday.

[6]Td—adult tetanus toxoid (full dose) and diphtheria toxoid (reduced dose) in combination.

For all products used, consult manufacturer's brochure for instructions for storage, handling, and administration. Biologics prepared by different manufacturers may vary, and those of the same manufacturer may change from time to time. The package insert should be followed for a specific product.

From American Academy of Pediatrics, *Report of the committee on infectious diseases*, 19th ed. (Evanston, Ill.: American Academy of Pediatrics, 1982).

childbearing age who are not protected against the disease. Rubella contracted during the first trimester of pregnancy poses the threat of birth defects of the eyes, heart, and brain.

Immunizations are normally not given to persons with elevated temperatures, but mild infections, such as a cold without a fever, do not contraindicate immunizations. The most frequent reaction to an immunization is slightly elevated temperature; occasionally a reaction can be more severe—high temperature, sleepiness, or even convulsions. Physicians need to be consulted if the immunized person has a severe reaction or continues to feel ill 48 hours after the immunization.

Tests for immunity It is sometimes advisable for the nurse to test patients for antibodies to a disease before giving the toxoid or vaccine. Examples of tests for immunity are:

1. Schick test for diphtheria. A specified amount of diphtheria toxin is given intracutaneously. Reddening at the site of inoculation, and *induration* (hardness) of 10 mm or more in diameter in 24 to 48 hours signals a positive reaction and lack of immunity (i.e., no antitoxin is present). A negative reaction indicates previous exposure to diphtheria, neutralization of the toxin, and thus immunity.

2. Moloney test for diphtheria. A specified amount of diphtheria toxoid is given by intradermal injection (see Chapter 37, page 974). A positive reaction (an area redness with induration of 10 mm or more in diameter) in 12 to 24 hours indicates previous exposure and immunity to diphtheria and contraindicates further use of the toxoid. A negative reaction indicates absence of antibodies (antitoxoid) and no immunity.

3. Dick test for scarlet fever. A specified amount of group A beta hemolytic streptococcus toxin is injected intracutaneously. A positive reaction (redness of 1 cm or more in diameter at the inoculation site) indicates absence of antitoxin and no immunity; a negative reaction indicates previous exposure, neutralization of the toxin, and immunity.

4. Tuberculin test for tuberculosis. A specified amount of tuberculin purified protein derivative (PPD) is given intracutaneously. A positive reaction (area of redness) indicates previous exposure to the disease.

Summary

The provision of a safe external environment is a constant concern of the nurse. Physical factors in the environment and psychologic and physiologic abilities of the individual person need to be considered. General characteristics of a safe environment include comfortable temperature and humidity, appropriate lighting, noise levels below 120 decibels, freedom from pathogens, and absence of fire, radiation, and electric and chemical hazards.

Sanitation is important to health. Areas of concern include water purification, environmental pollution, disposal of human wastes, milk pasteurization, food sanitation, and the control of insects and rodents.

Accidents are a major cause of death among individuals of all ages in the United States and Canada. The eight major causes of accidental deaths in the United States are motor vehicle accidents, falls, fires and flames, drowning, poisoning, suffocation, surgical and medical complications, and firearms. Most accidents are due to negligence and are preventable.

Nursing assessment of the patients at risk includes assessment of age, life-style, sensory-perceptual alterations, impaired level of awareness, impaired mobility, extreme emotional states, language barriers, history of previous accidents, and knowledge and use of safety precautions.

Nursing diagnoses for patients at risk for accidental injury can be categorized as potential for trauma, for poisoning, and for suffocation.

Nursing intervention must include education in accident prevention and modification of the environment to make it safe. Protective measures for infants include guard rails at the top and bottom of stairs, covered electrical wall outlets, large soft toys that do not have parts infants can remove and swallow, cribs with closely spaced rungs, and constant observation during feeding and bathing. Toddlers are curious and must be protected from such hazards as medicines, sharp tools, and cleaning solutions. Fences should enclose pools or ditches and the play area. Teaching toddlers that *no* and *don't* are spoken at times of risk is essential. Preschoolers can be taught to observe and to act safely. They should be taught to observe traffic safety, to play in safe areas, to swim, and to keep toys from underfoot. Preschoolers imitate the behavior of parents, who can use this trait to teach safe behavior. School-age children prefer grown-up equipment to toys and need instruction in safe use of such equipment. Adolescents need water safety instruction and information about the hazards of motor vehicles, firearms, and drugs and alcohol. Elderly people need home safety devices that counteract their diminished sensory acuity and balance.

Table 22–6 Recommended Routine Immunization Schedules—Canada

Age	Agent	Description
2 months	DPT 0.5 ml	Combined diphtheria toxoid, pertussis vaccine, and tetanus toxoid
	TOPV (Sabin) 3 gtt	Trivalent oral polio vaccine
4 months	DPT 0.5 ml TOPV 3 gtt	
6 months	DPT 0.5 ml TOPV 3 gtt	
12 months	MMR 0.5 ml	Combined measles, mumps, and rubella vaccine (see alternative for rubella vaccine at age 12)*
18 months	DPT 0.5 ml TOPV 3 gtt	
4–6 years	DPT 0.5 ml TOPV 3 gtt	
11–12 years	Rubella (for girls) 0.5 ml	
14–16 years	Td 0.5 ml	Combined diphtheria and tetanus toxoid (weaker than DT, the diphtheria and tetanus toxoid used for the very young) given to persons 7 years and older
Adults	Tetanus toxoid every 10 years	

*Rubella vaccine may be given at or after age 1 year or may be given to prepubertal girls at about age 12.

From National Committee on Immunization, *A guide to immunization for Canadians—1980*, Catalog no. H49-8/1980 (Ottawa: Minister of Supply and Services, Canada Health Protection Branch, Laboratory Centre for Disease Control, March 1979), pp. 16, 63.

Nurses are concerned with falls, fires, and other accidents that endanger the health and lives of patients outside and inside a hospital. Side rails and handrails protect patients from falls, and restraints keep patients from inflicting injuries on themselves and others. Because restraints restrict a patient's basic freedom to move, careful assessment and accurate, complete documentation is important when restraints are used. When a fire occurs in an agency, nurses must safeguard patients as well as deal with the fire. Most agencies have established procedures in the event of fire. Nurses must learn to carry patients from the scene of a fire.

Faulty electric equipment and improper grounding pose health hazards. Poisoning can usually be prevented. Any interruption to breathing is a serious health threat that calls for immediate measures to prevent death from asphyxiation. In hospitals, radioactive substances are used for both diagnostic and treatment purposes. Agency policy should be followed to safeguard patients and staff from inadvertent exposure.

Immunizations combat communicable diseases. Certain routine immunizations are recommended. In some cases, patients should be tested for immunity prior to an immunization.

Suggested Activities

1. Assess the safety of your own living environment.
2. Visit the home of a family with growing children or an elderly couple and assess what safety education is required.
3. Visit a school nurse and identify the safety education programs offered to children in grades 1 to 6, 7 to 10, and to adolescents.
4. Determine the immunization schedules recommended in your community.
5. Invite a community health worker to your school to discuss the environmental sanitation measures used in your community.

Suggested Readings

Feycock, M. W. January 1975. A do-it-yourself restraint that works. *Nursing 75* 5:18.

This article describes how to make a restraint that can be used to elevate a limb.

Lynn, F. H. June 1980. Incidents—need they be accidents? *American Journal of Nursing* 80:1098–1101.

A study of the accidents in one hospital describes when accidents occurred, what type of patients had accidents, and how they can be prevented.

Mylrea, K. C., and O'Neal, L. B. January 1976. Electricity and electrical safety in the hospital. *Nursing 76* 6:52–59.

The authors describe the basics of electricity, discuss electric hazards, and give pointers on how to prevent problems. Explanations of voltage, current, resistance, alternating current, and capacitance are included.

Selected References

Bauer, J. D.; Ackerman, P. G.; and Toro, G. 1974. *Clinical laboratory methods*. 8th ed. St. Louis: C. V. Mosby Co.

Boeker, E. H. April 1965. Radiation safety. *American Journal of Nursing* 65:111–15. Reprinted in Meyers, M. E., editor. 1967. *Nursing fundamentals*. Dubuque, Iowa: William C. Brown Co.

Breeding, M. A., and Wollin, M. May 1976. Working safely around implanted radiation sources. *Nursing 76* 6:58–63.

Carmack, B. J. August 1981. Fighting fire: Your role in hospital fire safety. *Nursing 81* 11:61–63.

Cooper, S. July-August 1981. Accidents and older adults. *Geriatric Nursing* 2:287–90.

Hillman, H. May 1973. The optimum human environment. *Nursing Times* 69:692–95.

Kukuk, H. M. May, June 1976. Safety precautions: Protecting your patients and yourself. Part 1. *Nursing 76* (May) 6:45–51. Part 2. *Nursing 76* (June) 6:49–52.

Kummer, S. B., and Kummer, J. M. February 1963. Pointers to preventing accidents. *American Journal of Nursing* 63:118–19.

Long, B. C., and Buergin, P. S. June 1977. The pivot transfer. *American Journal of Nursing* 77:980–82.

MacDonald, S. G. G., and Burns, D. M. 1975. *Physics for the life ana health sciences*. Menlo Park, Calif.: Addison-Wesley Publishing Co.

Maslow, A. H. 1968. *Toward a psychology of being*. 2nd ed. New York: Van Nostrand Reinhold Co.

Meth, I. M. July 1980. Electrical safety in the hospital. *American Journal of Nursing* 80:1344–48.

Misik, I. August 1981. About using restraints—with restraint. *Nursing 81* 11:50–55.

Morris, E. M. July 1968. In case of fire emergencies. *American Journal of Nursing* 68:1496–99.

O'Grady, R., and Dolan, T. January 1976. Whooping cough in infancy. *American Journal of Nursing* 76:114–17.

Phegley, D., and Obst, J. July 1976. Improving fire safety with posted procedures. *Nursing 76* 6:18–19.

Rantz, M., and Courtial, D. 1981. *Lifting, moving and transferring patients: A manual*. 2nd ed. St. Louis: C. V. Mosby Co.

Rumack, B. H. October 1980. The poison control center: Answers not antidotes. *Hospital Practice* 15:123–29.

Scheffler, G. L. October 1962. The nurse's role in hospital safety. *Nursing Outlook*. 10:680–82. Reprinted in Meyers, M. E., editor. 1967. *Nursing fundamentals*. Dubuque, Iowa: William C. Brown Co.

Statistics Canada. 1981. *Canada year book 1980–81*. Ottawa: Minister of Supplies and Services.

U.S. Department of Health, Education, and Welfare. 1978. *Facts of life and death*. DHEW Publication no. (PHS) 79-1222. Hyattsville, Md.: Department of Health, Education, and Welfare.

Chapter 23

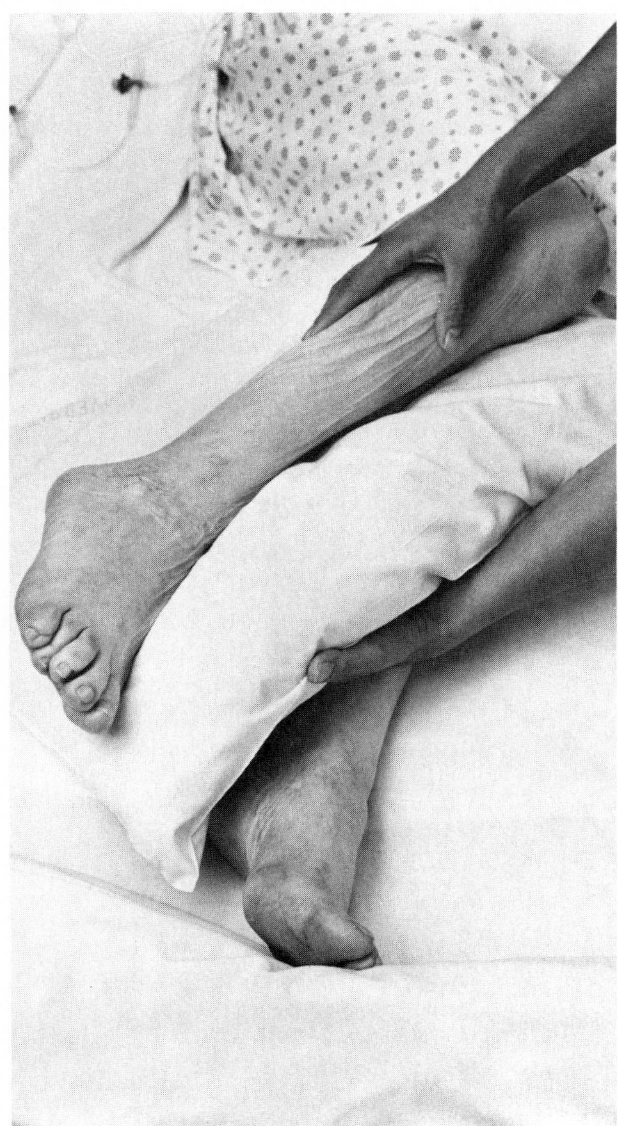

Body Alignment

CONTENTS

Objectives

1. Know essential terms and facts about body movement and body mechanics

- **1.1** Define selected terms
- **1.2** Identify the functions of bones, ligaments, cartilage, and tendons
- **1.3** Describe the neuromuscular process involved in body movement
- **1.4** List the three basic elements of body mechanics
- **1.5** State the purpose of good body alignment
- **1.6** List three factors essential to body balance
- **1.7** List three physical forces involved in moving objects
- **1.8** Outline the major muscle groups involved in lifting and moving objects
- **1.9** Identify specific concepts and principles basic to body mechanics

2. Know information required to assess body alignment

- **2.1** Identify criteria essential for assessing alignment
- **2.2** Identify factors that influence body alignment
- **2.3** Identify postural variations according to development and age

3. Understand essential facts about nursing measures to maintain, promote, and/or restore normal body alignment

- **3.1** Identify goals for nursing intervention for the patient with poor body alignment
- **3.2** Identify guidelines for positioning patients
- **3.3** Identify essential supportive devices to maintain patient alignment in various bed positions
- **3.4** Relate problems to be prevented to each supportive device used for various positions assumed by patients

4. Understand essential steps of procedures to assist patients to move in bed

- **4.1** Outline essential steps of procedures
- **4.2** Give the rationale for various steps of procedures

5. Apply the nursing process when positioning and moving patients

- **5.1** Obtain necessary assessment data
- **5.2** Analyze and relate assessment data
- **5.3** Write relevant nursing diagnoses
- **5.4** Write relevant nursing goals
- **5.5** Plan appropriate nursing interventions
- **5.6** Implement appropriate nursing interventions
- **5.7** State the outcome criteria essential for evaluating the nursing interventions

6. Perform techniques used to position and move patients effectively

- **6.1** Position patients effectively in bed lying and bed sitting positions
- **6.2** Assist patients to move: (a) up in bed, (b) to the side of the bed, (c) to a lateral position in bed, (d) to a sitting position in bed or on the edge of the bed, (e) from a bed to a chair
- **6.3** Assist patients to raise the buttocks while in bed

Terms

abductor muscle
alignment
antagonist muscle
balance
body mechanics
concave
convex
cupula
dorsal recumbent position
extensor muscle
femoral anteversion
flexor muscle
foot drop
Fowler's position
friction
genu valgum
genu varum
gravity
high Fowler's position
hyperphosphatemia
hypocalcemia
hypophosphatemia
insertion (of muscle)
kyphosis
lateral position
lever
lordosis
metatarsus adductus
origin (of muscle)
osteomalacia
pronation
prone position
rickets
scoliosis
semi-Fowler's position
Sims's position
supine position
talipes equinovarus
tonus
torticollis
trochanter roll

Many people who are ill are able to move relatively easily, much as they would when well. They may move a little more slowly than usual and perhaps less steadily; however, with the presence of a nurse and the consequent reassurance that help is available if required, walking and turning over in bed, for example, are not major problems to these patients.

There are patients, however, for whom even moving in bed can be a major problem. For patients who have difficulty moving or a complete inability to move, skillful nursing assistance is extremely important. There are a number of patients for whom nurses can anticipate that assistance to move will be required. Some of these are:

1. Patients who are unconscious or paralyzed
2. Patients who are in weakened states, e.g., because of surgery, prolonged periods in bed, or recent injury
3. Very young or elderly patients
4. Patients who have certain disease conditions, such as multiple sclerosis
5. Patients who require rest and who must not exert themselves, such as those who have recently had myocardial infarctions

The degree of assistance that patients require from a nurse will depend upon their own ability to move and the amount of exertion they can safely expend. In most instances, the nurse needs to be sensitive to the needs of patients both to function independently and to obtain assistance to move. Frequently, explanations from the nurse about the reason for the assistance at the particular time, together with reassurance regarding future independent functioning if this is possible, will help people to accept assistance.

This chapter includes the principles and techniques that can be used by both patients and nurses to assist patients to move in bed, to move between a bed and a stretcher or chair, and to ambulate.

Physiology of Body Movement

Body movement involves the function of the bony skeleton, the muscles, and the nervous system. The skeleton is made up of bones, which are joined together by ligaments, cartilage, and muscles. The skeleton serves three main purposes:

1. It protects the soft tissues of the body that lie under it.
2. It provides a lever system for movement. A *lever* is a rigid bar that revolves around a fixed point.
3. It provides a structural framework for the body.

In the body, bone is continually being formed and torn down. In a state of homeostasis, a balance is maintained between these two processes. Bone is composed of organic substances, which provide it with pliability, and inorganic substances such as calcium salts, which give it hardness. The amount of inorganic substances increases with age; thus the bones of a 2-year-old child are normally more pliable than those of an adult, and the bones of an elderly person are less pliable than those of a middle-aged person.

The bones of the skeleton are linked together at joints by ligaments, cartilage, and muscles. Ligaments are broad fibrous bands that hold two or more bones together. Cartilage, a firm substance, is found in many places, such as between the vertebrae (fibrous cartilage), in the auricle of the external ear (elastic cartilage), and as a precursor of bone (hyaline cartilage). The fibrous cartilage between bones provides a smooth surface over which the bones can glide. It can also absorb shocks from blows or sudden falls. Tendons are fibrous cords that attach muscles to bones. One of the best known is the Achilles tendon, which attaches the gastrocnemius muscle (calf muscle) to the calcaneus (heel bone).

In movement of the body, the bones act as levers that vary both in size and in rigidity. The bones are attached to muscles. The fixed or less movable attachment of a muscle to a bone is called the *origin* of the muscle. The *insertion* is the more movable point of attachment of the muscle.

Muscles contract and relax. When a muscle contracts, it becomes shorter, bringing the bones to which it is attached closer. At the same time, muscles on the other side of the joint relax or lengthen, to permit the movement. Each muscle normally has an *antagonist muscle*, which acts in the opposite manner. For example, the hamstring muscles flex the leg (bend the knee) and the quadriceps femoris muscles extend the leg (straighten the knee). Skeletal muscles are normally in a state of slight contraction or *tonus*. In body mechanics, the large muscles of the abdomen and the legs are frequently used.

Body movements are brought about through the action of muscles. As a result of neuroelectrical factors and complex chemical processes within the muscle fibers, involving glucose and phosphocreatine, the muscles contract, and thus their fibers shorten and thicken. In effect, chemical energy is converted to mechanical energy in muscles.

Muscular activity is controlled by the nervous system, with centers chiefly in the cerebral cortex, the brainstem, the cerebellum, and the spinal cord. When a person wants to use a muscle, a stimulus originates in the cerebral cortex and is transmitted by the motor pathways to the medulla. There the majority of the nerve tracts cross over and enter the spinal cord. Stimuli pass along the motor fibers in several tracts of the cord. They synapse (join) with lower motor neurons in the anterior horns, and the individual muscles are innervated by the spinal nerves, which leave the anterior horns and travel to the muscles. The nerve fiber transmits an electrical impulse that activates the sacroplasmic reticulum of the muscle to release calcium. The calcium triggers chemical changes within the muscle that bring about contraction of the muscle fiber. This is how chemical energy is converted into mechanical energy.

Body Mechanics

Body mechanics refer to the movement and coordination of the body in response to stimuli and the body's coordinated efforts to maintain its balance while responding to these stimuli. The coordinated body movement of a barefoot person trying to maintain balance after stepping on a piece of jagged glass on a beach can be described as body mechanics.

In a restricted sense, the term *body mechanics* is commonly used to describe efficient body movements used by people to move other persons or objects. However, body mechanics are operant in periods of rest as well as activity, such as when standing, sitting, or lying. Good posture while standing, for example, involves the synergistic action of muscle groups enabling balance and stability. The major purpose of good body mechanics is to facilitate safe and efficient use of appropriate groups of muscles.

The use of good body mechanics is not restricted to the health-illness environment. Good posture is one criterion of beauty and enhances health. Conversely, poor posture detracts from beauty and can affect normal body functioning. In this context, *body alignment* and *good body posture* are used as synonymous terms. *Alignment* refers to the position of the body that facilitates body function.

Body mechanics, therefore, involve three basic elements:

1. Body alignment (posture)
2. Balance (stability)
3. Coordinated body movement

Good body mechanics are essential to nurses to prevent strain and injury. They also prevent fatigue, because a minimum amount of energy is expended.

Body Alignment

When the body is well aligned, undue strain is not placed on the joints, muscles, tendons, or ligaments to maintain balance. Muscles are usually in a state of slight tension (tonus) when the body is healthy and well aligned. This state requires minimal muscular force and yet maintains adequate support for the body's internal framework and organs.

Posture and body alignment are often considered in terms of the standing and sitting positions of the healthy human. See page 558 for some criteria of the well-aligned person in a standing and a sitting position. However, when a person is ill and confined to bed, body alignment in several sitting and lying positions is of extreme importance.

Balance

Good body alignment is essential to body balance. When there is poor alignment, the body can become unbalanced, so that the pull of gravity overcomes it, and the person tips and falls.

It is difficult to separate body balance from body alignment, although balance is the result of proper alignment. Both depend on the same three factors:

1. A base of support that stabilizes the body
2. A center of gravity that lies within the base of support
3. A line of gravity that runs from the center of gravity through the base of support

Whenever the line of gravity and the center of gravity lie outside the base of support, the body becomes unbalanced and strained. See Figure 23-1. A body in balance or equilibrium is stable, secure, and unlikely to tip or fall. *Balance* is described as a state of equipoise in which opposing forces counteract each other.

To maintain balance, the body responds to changes of position through information received by the cerebellum from receptors in the ampullae of the three semicircular ducts of the inner ear. Each duct contains endolymph, and the three are arranged at right angles to one another. Any body movement is relayed by the endolymph in these ducts to sensory hair cells imbedded in a gelatinous, dome-shaped structure called the *cupula*. Stimulation of the hair cells produces nerve impulses that flow along the nerve fibers of the vestibular division of the vestibulocochlear nerve to the brain. See Figure 23-2.

Body balance can be greatly enhanced by altering two of the three factors governing it: widening the base of support and lowering the center of gravity, bringing it closer to the base of support. The base of support is easily widened by spreading the feet further apart. The center of gravity is readily lowered by flexing the hips and knees until a squatting position is achieved. The importance of these alterations cannot be overemphasized for nurses. The practice of good body mechanics is basic to all techniques that assist patients to move and that require lifting and transporting objects.

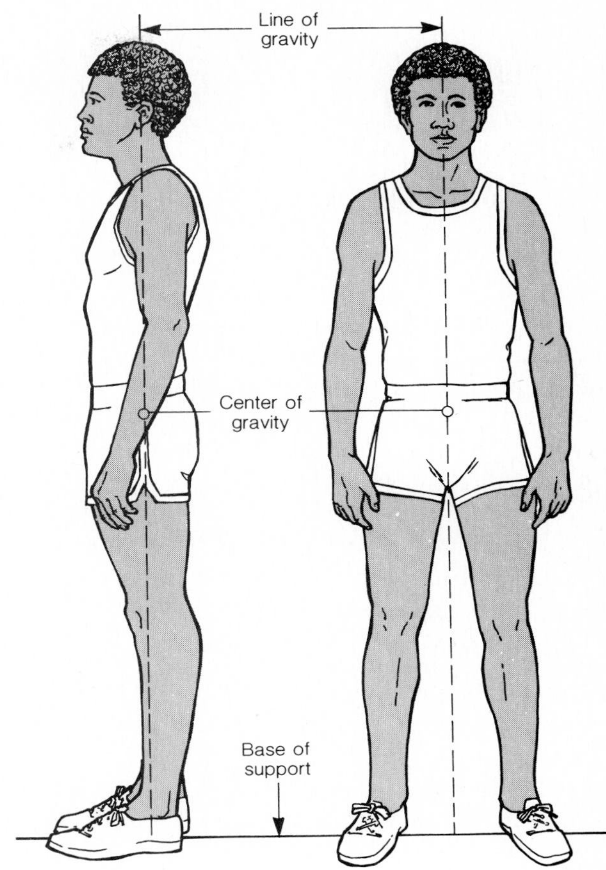

Figure 23-1 Body alignment.

Coordinated Body Movement

Every nursing care activity uses the musculoskeletal system, either to stand, walk, sit, or squat or to carry,

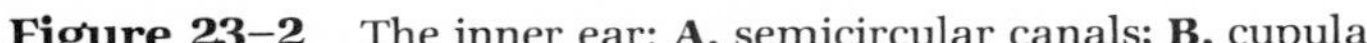

Figure 23-2 The inner ear: **A,** semicircular canals; **B,** cupula.

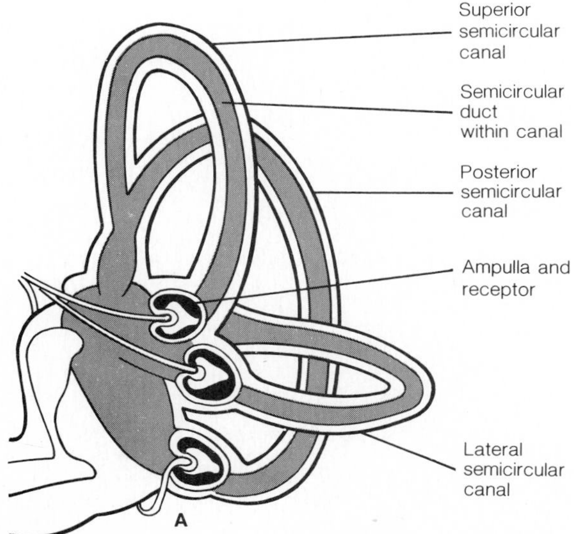

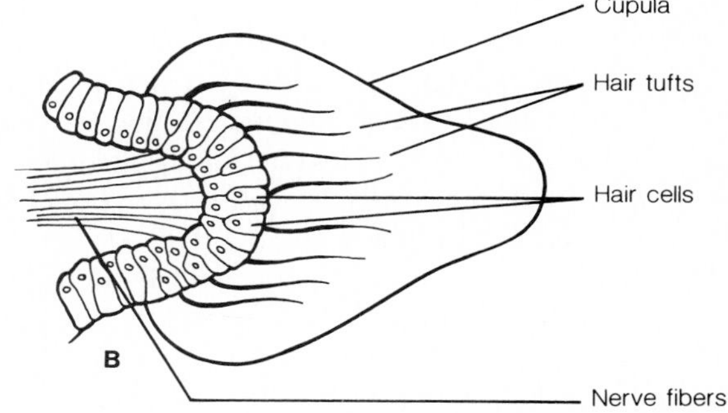

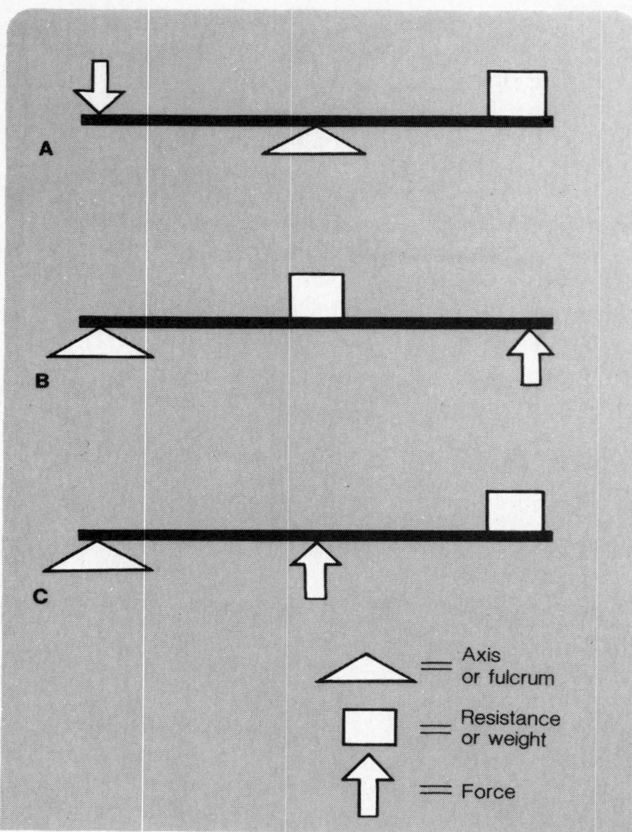

Figure 23–3 Types of levers: **A,** fulcrum between weight and force; **B,** weight between fulcrum and force; **C,** force between fulcrum and weight.

lift, push, or pull objects. When the body is used effectively, muscle strain, fatigue, and injury are avoided. To move the body effectively, the nurse works with the physical forces of friction, leverage, and gravity.

Friction increases the amount of effort required to move an object. It can be reduced by using a smooth, dry, clean surface in contrast to a rough, wet, or soiled surface. To reduce friction when moving (sliding) a patient up in bed, for example, the nurse provides a smooth, dry, firm bed foundation.

Leverage is a force that can be used by nurses to increase their lifting power and to make lifting easier. There are three basic types of levers. See Figure 23–3. The simplest example of the lever shown in Figure 23–3, *A*, is a seesaw (teeter-totter), on which a child can lift a heavier person. Nurses frequently use this type of leverage to lift objects. The resisting force or weight is held in the hands or on the forearms, the fulcrum is the elbow, and the force is applied by contraction of the biceps (flexor) muscles of the arm. The lifting power is increased when the elbow (fulcrum) is supported on a bed surface or a countertop.

Table 23–1 Major Muscles and Their Functions

Body part	Muscles	Function
Forearm	Biceps brachii	Flexes forearm
	Triceps brachii	Extends forearm
Upper arm	Deltoideus	Abducts upper arm; assists in flexion and extension of upper arm
	Pectoralis major	Flexes upper arm upward
	Latissimus dorsi	Extends upper arm downward
Thigh	*Gluteal group*	
	1. Gluteus maximus	Extends and rotates thigh outward
	2. Gluteus medius	Abducts thigh and rotates it outward
	3. Gluteus minimus	Abducts thigh and rotates it inward
	Iliopsoas	Flexes thigh
	Rectus femoris	Flexes thigh and extends lower leg
Lower leg	*Quadriceps femoris group*	
	1. Rectus femoris	Flexes thigh and extends leg
	2. Vastus lateralis	Extends leg
	3. Vastus medialis	Extends leg
	4. Vastus intermedius	Extends leg
	Hamstring group	
	Biceps femoris	Flexes leg and extends thigh
Abdomen	Obliquus externus abdominis Obliquus internus abdominis Transversus abdominis Rectus abdominis	All compress abdomen, pull front of pelvis upward, and flatten lumbar curvature
Pelvic floor	Levator ani Coccygeus	Both support floor of pelvic cavity

The force of gravity frequently has to be overcome when the nurse lifts and moves objects or patients. *Gravity* (weight) is the pull toward the center of the earth. The center of gravity of a person is normally considered to be on the midline halfway between the umbilicus and the symphysis pubis. To work effectively against gravity, the nurse needs to use major muscle groups rather than weaker ones. These major muscle groups include:

1. Flexors, extensors, and abductors of the thighs
2. Flexors and extensors of the knees
3. Flexors and extensors of the upper and lower arms
4. Flexors of the abdominal cavity and the pelvic floor

For the specific muscles used and their functions, see Table 23–1.

A *flexor muscle* acts to bend a joint, decreasing the angle between two bones. An *extensor muscle* acts to straighten a joint, increasing the angle between two bones. An *abductor muscle* draws bones away from a center or median line. See Chapter 24 for further information.

Guidelines for Good Body Mechanics

The following are specific concepts and principles basic to good body mechanics:

1. Start any body movement with proper alignment and balance. Increase the body's stability as necessary, by enlarging the base of support and/or lowering the center of gravity toward the base of support.

2. Adjust the working area to waist level, and keep the body close to the area. Elevate adjustable beds and overbed tables or lower the side rails of beds to prevent stretching and reaching. Stretching creates unnecessary muscle fatigue and strain and places the line of gravity outside the base of support, resulting in instability.

3. Use major muscle groups rather than smaller muscles. For example, to lift a heavy object, use the gluteal and femoral muscles rather than the sacrospinal muscles of the back. The former are employed by flexing the knees and hips to grasp an object and lift it rather than by bending from the waist. For the major muscle groups used in movement, see Table 23–1.

4. Use a wide base of support (a wide stance) with the center of gravity in the middle, to maintain balance.

5. Prepare the muscles in the pelvic area before bringing them into action. This has two aspects: "putting on the internal girdle" and "making a long midriff." The internal girdle is made by contracting the abdominal muscles upward and the gluteal muscles (buttocks) downward. The long midriff is made by stretching the muscles at the waist. Preparation of these muscles stabilizes the pelvis and supports the abdomen. As a result, all of these muscles can assist the muscles of the arms and legs in activities such as lifting and pushing.

6. Use your own weight to counteract an object's or patient's weight when you push or pull, thereby requiring less energy.

7. Avoid working against gravity. Because of the gravitational pull, more force is required to lift an object than to push or pull an object. Pushing and pulling do not involve directly overcoming the gravitational pull.

8. Use the least amount of effort required. To accomplish this:

a. Make the body movements smooth and rhythmical.

b. When lifting or carrying heavy objects, hold the objects as close to the body as possible.

c. Push or pull objects along a surface rather than lifting, if possible. In many instances, patients can assist by pushing or pulling themselves. This uses the body's own weight as well as muscle power to counteract the object's weight.

d. When moving a heavy object, directly face the direction of the force. For example, when a nurse assists a patient toward the head of the bed, the nurse's body should face the head of the bed. This avoids torsion (twisting) of the spine.

e. To pivot, place one foot ahead of the other, raise the heels very slightly, and put the body weight on the balls of the feet. When the weight is off the heels, the frictional surface is decreased, and the knees are not twisted when turning. Keeping the body aligned, turn (pivot) about 90° in the desired direction. The foot that was forward will now be behind.

f. When lifting heavy objects, squat rather than stoop. Bending from the waist (stooping) to lift a heavy load is a major cause of back strain, since it forces the relatively small sacrospinal muscles to pull the body upright and to lift the weight. The squatting position uses the larger and stronger gluteal and femoral muscles of the buttocks and thighs. In the squatting position, the abdominal muscles are also tensed, supporting the internal organs and preventing inguinal herniation. Better balance is maintained by the squatting position, since the center of gravity is lower than in the stooping position and the line of gravity falls within the base of support. When squatting, place one foot ahead of the other, to distribute the body weight on the front foot and the ball of the back foot. Lower the body by flexing the knees, and keep the back straight. When returning to the standing position, lift the body using the muscles of the thighs and hips.

9. Reduce friction to reduce the effort required to move an object, by using a smooth surface rather than a rough surface. Nurses can apply this principle by ensuring a firm, smooth foundation for a bed before moving a patient in bed.

10. Prevent muscle fatigue by interspersing rest periods with periods of muscle use. Continuous muscular exertion can result in muscle strain, the overstretching or overexertion of muscles.

11. Use the palmar grip when grasping and lifting objects. Extend the fingers and the hand around the object. Fingers alone have little power; the strength of the entire hand should be used for safety and to avoid muscle fatigue.

12. Use other persons or mechanical aids as required. Some objects are too heavy to be moved without assistance. Mechanical devices can assist nurses to move patients, thereby avoiding muscle strain. These devices are discussed later in this chapter.

Assessment

Inspection of Body Alignment

A general inspection of the individual will provide information about body alignment. By viewing the patient standing, walking, sitting, or lying down the nurse can assess body alignment. See the earlier discussion on body alignment and the discussion of alignment in various bed positions later in this chapter. Alignment criteria in standing and sitting positions are presented next.

Well-aligned adult standing position

1. A vertical line from the body's center of gravity (located on the midline halfway between the umbilicus and the symphysis pubis) falls between the feet (the body's base of support).

2. The toes are pointed forward.

3. The ankles are flexed to maintain the feet at right angles to the lower leg.

4. The knees are slightly flexed. A line drawn through the patella and the middle of the ankle ends at the second or third toe.

5. The hips are straight.

6. The hands are positioned midway between pronation and supination, with the fingers slightly flexed. The wrists are neither flexed nor extended.

7. The arms fall at the sides with the elbows slightly flexed.

8. The head is erect, with the neck neither flexed forward nor extended backward nor flexed laterally, and with the chin held in.

9. The vertebral curves are normal. In infants, the primary vertebral curve is posteriorly convex. *Convex* means rounded and elevated from the surface of an organ or other structure, in contrast to *concave*, which means rounded and depressed or hollowed-out from the surface of an organ. After children can hold up their heads, stand, and walk, the following three vertebral curves are present:

- **a.** The lumbar curve is anteriorly convex.
- **b.** The thoracic curve is posteriorly convex.
- **c.** The cervical curve is anteriorly convex.

These normal curves may differ among individuals as a result of variations in walking, prolonged changes in posture, and pregnancy.

10. The main body weight is borne well forward on the outer sides of the feet.

11. The lower abdomen is pulled in and up.

12. The person appears to be stretched fully but is relaxed and poised with minimal muscle strain. See Figure 23–1 earlier in this chapter.

Anatomic position is a term used to describe a position of normal alignment and also serves as a reference for the three body planes: transverse, frontal, and sagittal. In anatomic position, a person stands with:

1. Arms at the side

2. Thumbs adducted, hands pronated, and fingers slightly flexed

3. Head erect, neither flexed nor hyperextended

4. Feet directed ahead with ankles in normal flexion

5. Knees slightly flexed

6. Hips straight

Well-aligned adult sitting position

1. The head is erect, neither flexed forward nor extended backward.

2. There is normal alignment of the vertebral column.

3. The weight of the body from the head to the buttocks is centered on the buttocks and thighs.

4. Both feet are on the floor with normal flexion of the ankle joints as in the standing body alignment position.

One foot may be placed slightly ahead of the other for comfort.

5. The popliteal spaces are at least 2.5 cm (1 in) away from the edge of the chair to avoid pressure on the blood circulation and the nerves of the legs.

6. The thighs are in a horizontal position.

7. The forearms are supported on the lap or armrests or a table in front.

For information on the assessment of muscle function, see Chapter 14. For information on gait and the range of motion of the joints, see Chapter 24.

Factors that Influence Body Alignment

A number of factors influence an individual's body alignment: physical growth and development, fatigue, joint mobility, life-style, attitudes or values, and pain or disease processes.

Physical growth and development

Body alignment or posture changes significantly during growth and with age. An understanding of the normal variations is helpful for the nurse in promoting good posture and in assessing and assisting people to correct postural faults. The following sections describe normal developmental postural variations.

Newborns and infants In the newborn, the neck is short and straight. The head moves freely from side to side and flexes and extends easily. The spine is straight, but it can be flexed. Shoulders, scapulae, and iliac crests are on the same plane. All extremities are generally flexed, but they can be passively moved through a full range of motion. For example, in the upper extremities, the fists are clenched; the wrists flex more than 90° and extend slightly less than 90°; the arms can be extended, but they promptly return to a state of flexion. In the lower extremities, the feet appear flat, due to a fat pad in the position of the transverse arch. They may normally turn inward (inversion); they can be passively turned outward (eversion). The lower legs flex toward the thighs and the knees extend but do not hyperextend. The range of motion of the hip joint is normally about 110–120° in flexion and extension, and the thighs, when flexed at the hip, abduct to an angle of 45–50° each. The abdomen is rounded and prominent but not overextended.

Having the toes point in, or being pigeon-toed, is normal in early infancy. This is due to internal tibial torsion or inward rotation of the lower legs. However, if the lower legs are straight and toeing-in occurs in early infancy, it can be due to an abnormal congenital condition called *metatarsus adductus*, which warrants treatment. Toeing-in can also be caused by an internal rotation of the hip, which rotates the entire limb. When the internal hip rotation extends beyond the normal position of the hip, it is called *femoral anteversion.*

The appearance of flat-footedness due to a fat pad in the instep is normal in infants and may occur in toddlers with knock-knees to a mild degree. In most cases tibial torsion, femoral anteversion, and mild metatarsus adductus tend to disappear without treatment as the child grows.

When infants learn to stand at about one year of age, they stand with feet far apart, toes turned outward, and knees locked. The head and upper part of the trunk are carried forward. Their balance is rather precarious, and, when they fall, they usually fall backward.

Toddlers The posture of the toddler reveals a marked lumbar *lordosis* (swayback or marked anterior concavity in the lumbar spinal curvature) with a protruding abdomen. The pelvis tilts forward, and there is only a slight convex curvature of the thoracic spine. Some toeing-out and a wide stance may occur normally in 2-year-olds due to a slight outward rotation of the hips. The feet are typically everted. Growth, with its functional stresses, eventually produces an inward rotation of the hips, which results in disappearance of the foot eversion.

Children In early childhood children become slimmer, taller, and more solid looking. They assume the so called little adult appearance, as the protrusion of the abdomen decreases and the length of arms and legs increases. By the time children are 3 years old, they are more steady and evenly balanced on their feet. They walk erect, can stand on one foot, and can go upstairs alternating their feet. They begin to swing their arms in an alternating pattern similar to the adult's and no longer widely abduct their arms for balance.

By age 5, children are even more closely knit and in greater control. Their arms are held near the body, and their stance is even more narrow. In late childhood, from ages 9 to 11, all body parts increase in size and function. Muscles and ligaments become firmer and stronger, and thus body posture is improved over that of the young child. Both body stance and balance are efficient for erectness.

Adolescents Significant changes in body proportions and contours occur during adolescence. In early adolescence, a boy's form is characterized by straight leg lines, narrow hips, wide shoulders, a broad chest, and noticeable muscular development in the shoulders, arms, and thighs. In contrast, a young adolescent girl has curved leg lines; her hips become wider, and her breasts develop. In the buttocks, thighs, and upper arms, fat is deposited.

Motor awkwardness is common at this age because of the rapid and uneven growth of the muscles and bones. For example, when the bones grow more quickly than the muscles, the muscles become tight and respond in quick, jerky motions. If, on the other hand, the muscles grow more quickly than the bones, the muscles are loose and sluggish, resulting in a clumsy performance. This awkwardness of leg and arm movements disappears once growth of the bones and muscles is stabilized.

Postural problems often occur at this age because of the discrepancies in weight and height between girls and boys. Because the growth spurt in girls occurs between 8½ and 11½ years of age, while for boys it happens from 10½ to 14½ years of age, it is not uncommon for girls to hover above their male partners on a dance floor. Posture may suffer as a consequence. By late adolescence, the gawky look and awkward movements of early adolescence disappear.

Adults Body alignment and posture of adults are described earlier in this chapter.

Pregnant women During pregnancy, both gait and posture change due to the increasing weight of the growing fetus and uterus, a changing center of gravity, stretching of the abdominal muscles, and relaxation of pelvic muscles and ligaments as a result of hormonal influences. In the typical pregnant stance, a woman leans backward to counterbalance the weight of the enlarged uterus. This produces a progressive spinal lordosis and the common complaint of backache. Improper shoes with high heels can aggravate this balance, adding strain to the lower back and pelvic muscles.

Back discomfort and body alignment in pregnancy can be significantly improved by emphasizing good posture and body mechanics in daily activities. The woman needs to learn to pull her abdomen up and in and to align her head, shoulders, and spine as if against a wall. See Figure 23–4. She may also need a reminder to stand as tall as possible without being rigid and to distribute her weight on the outer borders of her feet. Better balance can be achieved by encouraging the pregnant woman to broaden her base of support by standing with feet separated and one leg slightly forward.

Abdominal, pelvic, and back exercises such as abdominal contraction, pelvic floor contraction, and pelvic tilting are advised. See Chapter 24. Use of firm, supporting, low-heeled shoes, avoidance of stooping, and use of the leg muscles to spare the back, for example, when lifting objects or climbing stairs, are recommended. To avoid leaning forward when climbing stairs, the woman should place the entire sole of her foot on the stairs and use her leg muscles to raise herself from step to step. All activities during pregnancy may need to be of shorter duration than usual. Periods of standing, walking, and sitting should be varied frequently. Rest periods with the feet elevated need to be interspersed with activities.

Figure 23–4 Body alignment during pregnancy.

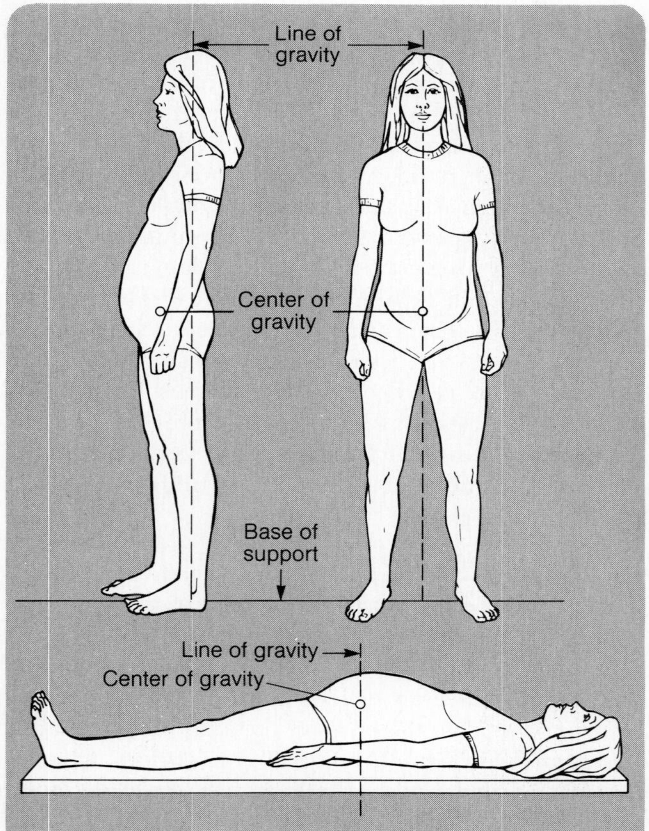

Older adults The typical posture of older adults is one of flexion. The head and neck are flexed slightly forward with eyes turned downward. The spinal column is flexed in the thoracic and lumbar areas, producing a mild dorsal *kyphosis* (humpback or marked posterior convexity in the thoracic spinal curvature) and loss of the normal lumbar lordosis. The hips and the knees are slightly flexed. During ambulation, the speed of gait is slowed in response to this flexed posture. Small shuffling steps are taken, and the ability to balance without the strength of the hip and knee extensor muscles is reduced.

Fatigue

The degree of fatigue (psychological or physical) can influence body alignment. The fatigued adult often assumes a more flexed position while standing or sitting. The shoulders are depressed, and the thoracic curvature is accentuated as the neck is flexed. In a supine position the legs are externally rotated as the person uses the bed rather than the muscles to support his or her limbs.

Joint mobility

Joint mobility can often affect the positions the body can assume. A person who has a rigid right elbow due to arthritis will be unable to change the relative positions of the lower and upper arm. Normal joint mobility is discussed in Chapter 24.

Life-style

An individual's life-style can affect posture. Postures repeatedly assumed during work can result in permanent postural defects; for example, a mail carrier may walk for years leaning to one side from carrying a heavy bag, or an assembly line worker may sit for hours hunched over a bench. Repeated physical activity, for example by a weight lifter, can produce muscle hypertrophy and concomitant alignment changes to accommodate the hypertrophy. A child who has a diet low in calcium may develop malformations of the bones, such as rickets.

Attitudes and values

Personal values about body alignment are important influences. The tall adolescent may slouch because he or she does not value being taller than peers. Some people value good posture and intentionally try to maintain body alignment for reasons of health, appearance, etc.

Pain and disease processes

A patient's ability to assume and/or maintain a body position is often influenced by pain or disease processes. The person with abdominal pain often will assume only a position with knees and hips flexed, to help relieve the pain. Patients with a large amount of fluid in the abdominal cavity may prefer a Sims's position for comfort. The disease process often determines the amount of assistance required to move to and maintain a position. For example, a patient who is emaciated due to an advanced malignancy may require assistance for every movement and supportive measures to maintain the body in alignment.

Diagnostic Tests

Diagnostic tests chiefly used in relation to body alignment involve roentgenography (x-ray examination). Because the skeleton has a high tissue density, it blocks the electromagnetic waves being transmitted to a photographic film, and the bones are thus outlined on the film. The size, location, and shape of the bones show on the film as well as areas of variable density. For example an area of less dense bone will appear darker in comparison to the rest of the bone, because it has permitted more of the waves to pass through to the film.

It is important that the nurse explain roentgenography procedures to the patient and support persons. The explanation needs to include the positions the patient will assume, the length of time the examination will take, any special preparation, and when the results will be known. Following the x-ray filming, the patient is assisted to a comfortable position and the plan of care is adjusted as required.

Blood tests for levels of serum calcium are carried out to determine some types of bone pathology. Normal serum calcium is 4.3–5.3 mEq/liter (Byrne 1981:139). Calcium deficiency can result in the decalcification of bone; it is called *rickets* when found in children and *osteomalacia* in adults. Serum phosphate (PO_4^{3-}) and inorganic phosphorus (P) levels (normal adult, 1.8–2.6 mEq/liter; child, as high as 4.1 mEq/liter) have a function in maintaining serum calcium concentrations. Phosphate is needed for the generation of bone. Phosphate levels are always in inverse proportion to calcium levels in the blood.

Increased phosphorus levels (*hyperphosphatemia*) are often found with kidney dysfunction. They are also associated with bone tumors and *hypocalcemia* (calcium deficiency). Phosphorus deficiency (*hypophosphatemia*) is found in rickets and osteomalacia.

Nursing Diagnoses

Problems related to the neuromusculoskeletal systems include improper body alignment (postural deviations), impaired balance, and impaired coordination. This section focuses on improper body alignment. Impaired balance and coordination affect a person's mobility, and these are discussed in Chapter 24.

Impairments in body alignment are generally caused by congenital abnormalities, developmental variants, abnormal intrauterine positions, or harmful postures during the growing years. For a description of specific postural deviations, their causes, and their treatment, see Table 23–2.

Table 23–2 Postural Deviations

Deviation	Description	Cause	Treatment
Torticollis (twisted or wry neck)	Limitation of the range of motion of the neck, with inclination and rotation of the head away from the midline of the body	Congenital muscular contraction of the sternocleidomastoid muscle due to birth injury or vascular insufficiency	Daily stretching of the involved muscle is effective in most situations; surgical release of one of the muscle attachments is occasionally needed
Scoliosis	Lateral curvature of the spine, which increases during active growth periods	May be secondary to other deformities, such as a discrepancy in leg lengths, or defects of spinal supporting tissues (a functional scoliosis); the most common cause of structural scoliosis is heredity, which produces an idiopathic structural scoliosis, a condition occurring five times more often in females than males, between the ages of 8 and 15	Treatment of underlying cause or application of a brace or cast from occiput to pelvis; surgical fusion of the spinal vertebrae may be necessary
Kyphosis (roundback or humpback)	A fixed flexion deformity of the thoracic spine	The cause is unknown	Exercises to extend the thoracic spine; sleeping without a pillow; occasionally bracing or spinal fusion may be required
Lordosis (swayback)	A fixed extension deformity of the lumbar spine	Most often secondary to other abnormalities such as kyphosis or muscular dystrophy	The underlying disease is treated
Hip dislocation	A bilateral or unilateral instability of the hip in infants, with an adduction contracture and limited abduction of the hip; after walking starts, the foot may be externally rotated and the thigh shortened due to proximal dislocation of the head of the femur; the knee joint is higher on the affected side, and the inguinal and gluteal creases may be asymmetrical	Congenital abnormality; breech deliveries	Treatment varies with age; infants are double diapered to abduct the hips, or abduction splints may be used; in young children a closed reduction and casting may be necessary; in older children, open reduction (surgery) may be required
Genu valgum (knock-knees)	The medial aspects of the knees touch each other in the standing position, and the feet remain apart; normal between 3 and 4 years of age	Usually a developmental variant, if not due to rickets or a congenital bone disorder	Corrected by growth; in some cases knee braces are used if knee ligaments become stretched
Genu varum (bowlegs)	The feet are held together but the knees remain apart; normal until 2 to 2½ years of age	Same as for genu valgum	Corrected by growth; measurement of the distance between the knees when the inner ankles are held together gauges the process

Table 23–2 continued

Deviation	Description	Cause	Treatment
Pronation (flat feet)	The medial longitudinal arch of the foot is relaxed, and weight is borne on the medial side of the foot; in most infants and toddlers, what appears to be flat-footedness is normal; fat pads create a fullness suggestive of a flat foot	Familial occurrence	Young children are taught to stand on tiptoes 5 to 10 minutes daily; older children are taught to walk pigeon-toed 5 to 10 minutes daily, with weight thrown on the lateral border of the foot; mechanical supports for the arch, such as medial heel wedges or shoe inserts, may be necessary
Talipes equinovarus (clubfoot)	The foot is malpositioned in plantar flexion (equinus) at the ankle with adduction and inversion of the heel and forefoot	Males are affected twice as often as females; the cause is unknown; it is thought to be partly due to heredity and partly due to an abnormal intrauterine position	Application of casts and splints, such as the Denis Browne splint; surgical correction may be needed in difficult cases
Toeing-in (pigeon-toes)	The entire foot or only the forefoot is rotated inward; some degree of toeing-in is common in all infants, due to their intrauterine position	Three common causes are:	
		1. Metatarsus adductus (adduction of the forefoot with no deformity of the hind part of the foot), a congenital disorder	**1.** Passive stretching, reversed shoes, or casts and wedging started as early as possible
		2. Inward tibial torsion, which is always associated with a tibial bow; this can be aggravated by infants' sleeping on their knees with feet turned inward or sitting on top of in-turned feet	**2.** Growth corrects tibial torsion; children are trained to avoid harmful postures; wearing reversed shoes for a time may be helpful
		3. Inward femoral torsion	**3.** No treatment is required; correction does not occur with growth, but the development of an outward tibial torsion compensates for the defect

Examples of nursing diagnoses for a patient with, e.g., bowlegs are:

1. Impaired body alignment (bowlegs) related to vitamin D deficiency
2. Risk of calcium and phosphorus imbalance related to vitamin D deficiency
3. Risk of increasing deformity related to inadequate bone calcification and stress of bearing weight
4. Risk of injury (greenstick fractures) related to softened, weakened bones

Planning and Intervention

Nursing Goals

The overall nursing goal for patients with potential or actual postural deviations is to maintain or restore good body alignment. Subgoals include:

1. Prevention of deformities
2. Prevention of muscle strain and fatigue
3. Prevention of pressure sores

Planning

Good body alignment and special positions for the patient are planned based on the assessment data obtained and the nursing diagnoses established. The nurse also needs to consider the factors influencing body alignment and the patient's need for assistance in assuming and maintaining body alignment in particular positions.

A nurse's intervention is frequently required in the following situations:

1. When a patient needs to assume a specific position for therapeutic reasons. For example, a patient may need to assume a specific side-lying position to facilitate drainage from a wound, or a patient with respiratory distress may need to rest in an upright position.
2. When a patient is weak or paralyzed and unable to move independently.
3. When a patient is in discomfort and requires assistance to find a comfortable position.

In some situations, a physician orders a specific position for a patient. However, assisting the patient with problems about positions is usually a nursing function. Generally patients are most comfortable when they closely approximate good body alignment. Many bed patients, however, require supports such as pillows and sandbags. A firm mattress is essential to good alignment and a basic requirement for all positions that patients assume in bed. If the mattress is not firm, the use of a bed board under the mattress is essential.

Planning also involves the establishment of outcome criteria. For suggestions, see Evaluation later in this chapter.

Guidelines for Positioning Patients

Although each patient has personal needs and a plan of care, there are certain general guidelines that the nurse can use to assist in planning care related to body positions.

1. A pillow beneath the head, unless contraindicated, should be of sufficient thickness to support the patient's head in an aligned position, neither flexing, hyperextending, nor laterally flexing the neck.
2. Feet need to be supported with a footboard, sandbags, or rolls in a dorsal flexion position, if the patient is to remain in bed for a prolonged period or is unable to move the feet freely.
3. Extremities should be in positions in which they can move freely, whenever possible. For example, the top bedclothes need to be loose enough so that the patient can move the feet.
4. Elbows, hips, and knees should be slightly flexed.
5. Uppermost shoulder and hip should be supported away from the body in side-lying positions to prevent adduction and pressure on underlying parts of the body.
6. The patient should change position fairly frequently, at least every 2 hours.
7. Joints need exercise, either active or passive, regularly—generally, at least once a day. See Chapter 24.
8. Pressure areas of the body need special care with each change of position. See Chapter 21.
9. See Table 23–2 for care required for specific postural deviations.

Bed Sitting Positions

Fowler's position

In *Fowler's position* (semisitting position), the head of the bed is raised to at least 45°. This position is frequently assumed by patients in bed for both comfort and therapeutic purposes. It is convenient for eating in bed, and it is a comfortable position from which to see visitors, to read, or to watch television. If it is not therapeutically contraindicated, it is a refreshing change for a person from any lying position.

In this position, the knees may or may not be flexed: Nurses need to clarify the criteria of Fowler's position in a particular agency, because in some hospitals Fowler's position refers to elevation of the upper part of the body without knee flexion, and the term *semi-Fowler's* is used to refer to the sitting position with knee flexion. In other agencies, semi-Fowler's has the meaning discussed later in this section.

In Fowler's position, the main weight of the body is borne by the buttocks, that is, the inferior aspects of the pelvis and the ischium, which is the inferior aspect of the ilium bone. Other areas that bear less weight are the heels, the sacrum, and the scapulae.

There are two adaptations of Fowler's position: high Fowler's and semi-Fowler's positions. *High Fowler's* is a position in which the head of the bed is elevated to 90°, that is, at a right angle to the foundation of the bed. This position is the one most analogous to sitting in a chair, where the back of the chair is at an upright angle. In this position, patients in bed can be supported by an overbed table placed in front of them. The patient then puts his or her arms on pillows placed on the table. This permits the patient to maintain body alignment and allows maximum chest expansion. High Fowler's is particularly helpful to patients who have problems exhaling, because they can press the lower part of the chest against the table.

Semi-Fowler's position usually refers to elevation of the head of the bed to about 30°. This is a particularly comfortable position for patients who must remain in bed. It also provides some chest elevation and is thus often indicated for patients who have cardiac and respiratory problems.

Table 23–3 Fowler's Position

Unsupported position	Problem to be prevented	Corrective measure
Bed sitting position with upper part of body elevated 30° to 90° commencing at hips; head rests on bed surface	Posterior convexity of lumbar curvature	Pillow at lower back (lumbar region); second pillow to support upper back, shoulders, and head
Legs lie flat and straight on lower bed surface	Hyperextension of knees	Small pillow under patient's thighs to flex knees
Legs are externally rotated	External rotation of hips	Trochanter roll lateral to femur
Heels rest on bed surface	Pressure on heels	Pillow or roll under lower legs
Feet are in plantar flexion	Plantar flexion of feet	Footboard to provide support for dorsal flexion
Arms fall at sides	Shoulder muscle strain, possible dislocation of shoulders, edema of hands and arms with flaccid paralysis; flexion contracture of hand at wrist	Pillows to support arms and hands if patient does not have normal use of them

Patients who assume any of the Fowler's positions usually require some supportive pillows to maintain normal alignment (see Table 23–3):

1. A pillow is placed at the patient's lower back to support the lumbar spinal curve.
2. A second pillow is placed above this pillow to support the upper area of the back including the head. With good body alignment the patient's head should be upright, with the neck neither flexed nor hyperextended. If the patient is very thin, a third pillow may be needed to support the back and head.
3. A small pillow can be placed under the patient's thighs. See Figure 23–5. This will provide slight flexion of the knees. Supports should be used with great care under the popliteal spaces. The popliteal artery, which supplies blood to the lower leg and foot, can be occluded with continual pressure, thus inhibiting circulation of blood and delivery of oxygen and nutrients to the cells in those areas.

Figure 23–5 Fowler's position (supported).

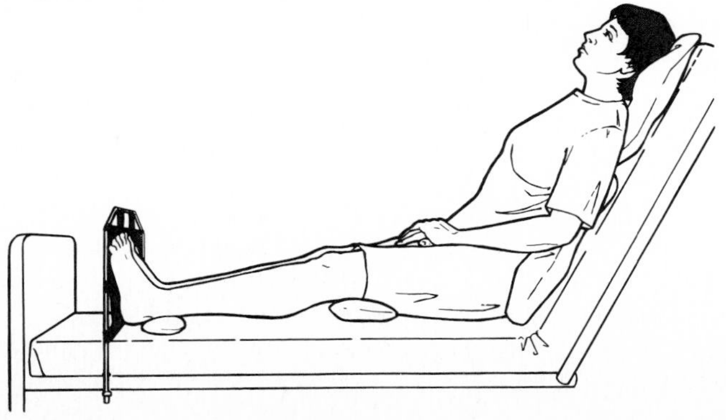

4. A small pillow or a roll can be used to support the ankles, thus raising the heels and reducing pressure on them from the bed. This measure is particularly important when a patient cannot move the legs or when the heels have become irritated from prolonged pressure. A footboard will support the feet in the dorsal flexion position.
5. A towel support, referred to as a *trochanter roll*, is placed firmly against the hips to prevent external rotation of the lower limb. A trochanter roll can be prepared as shown in Figure 23–6. Once in place, the roll is tightened securely until the thigh is well aligned.
6. If a patient does not have movement or use of the arms, pillows at each side will support them effectively. If the arms are permitted to hang downward for a length of time, frequently the return flow of blood is inhibited. In paralyzed patients, continual pulling on the shoulders by the weight of the arms can eventually result in dislocation of the joints and limited functioning.

Bed Lying Positions

Dorsal recumbent position (supine position)

In the *dorsal recumbent position*, a person lies on his or her back; the head and shoulders are usually slightly elevated with the support of a small pillow. In the dorsal position referred to as the *supine position*, the head and shoulders are not elevated. These positions are usually required by patients after surgery on the spinal vertebrae or after a spinal anesthetic.

In the dorsal recumbent position the following supports are provided (see Table 23–4):

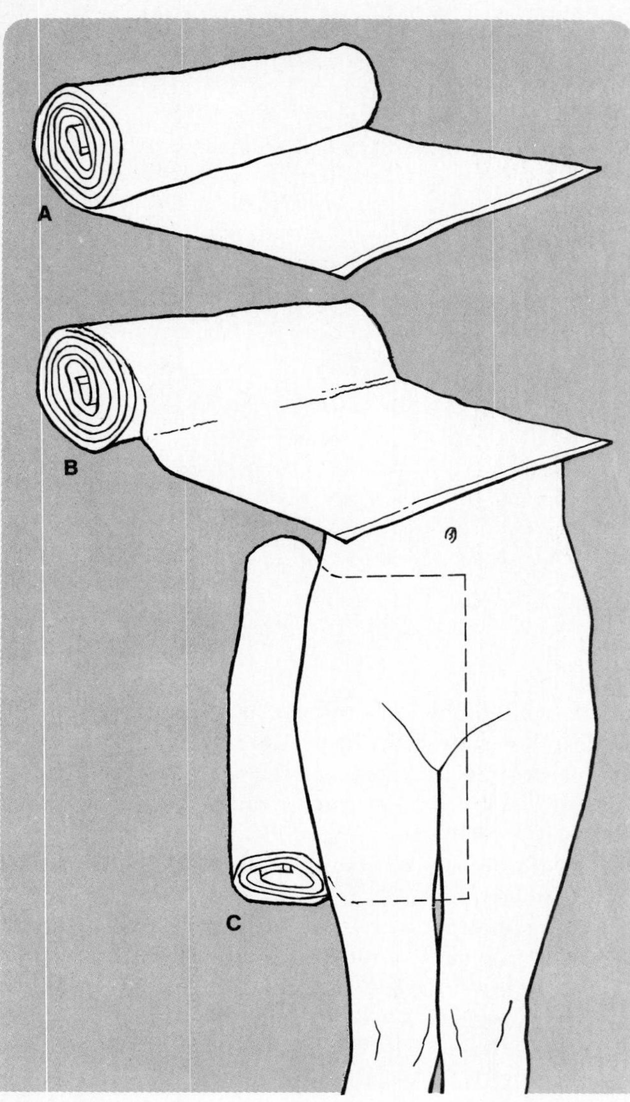

Figure 23–6 Making a trochanter roll: **A,** roll a towel, folded lengthwise, to 30 cm (12 in) from one end; **B,** turn the towel over so that the roll is underneath; **C,** place the unrolled portion of the towel under the patient's hip and buttock, and tighten the roll against the patient's hip.

1. The patient's head is erect or the neck is slightly flexed. It is not hyperextended with the support of a pillow. In the supine position, the head is slightly hyperextended, particularly for persons who have thick chests. Although slight flexion of the cervical vertebrae helps the patient to see and eat while lying on the back, prolonged lying in this position can result in a permanent flexion of the cervical vertebrae and limited movement of the head.

2. The lumbar curvature is usually apparent. It generally requires the support of a small pillow over a firm mattress. A firm mattress will not yield to the weight of the patient and provides good support.

3. Normally, the patient's thighs rotate externally. Placing a roll at the lateral aspect of each thigh opposite the femoral trochanter will keep the patient's legs in alignment.

4. In good body alignment, the knees are normally slightly flexed. To attain this and thus support a comfortable position, small pads or pillows are placed under the thighs superior to the popliteal spaces. See Figure 23–7. As explained earlier, direct pressure on these spaces is avoided.

5. Without support, the feet normally assume a plantar flexion position. If this is maintained for a prolonged period, the gastrocnemius and soleus muscles of the lower legs become involuntarily contracted, resulting in a condition known as *foot drop.* With this condition a person is unable to put the heel of the foot on the floor

Table 23–4 Dorsal Recumbent Position

Unsupported position	Problem to be prevented	Corrective measure
Head is flat on bed surface; neck may be slightly hyperextended in thick-chested person	Hyperextension of neck and flexion of neck	Pillow of suitable thickness under head and under shoulders if necessary for alignment
Lumbar curvature of spine is apparent	Flexion of lumbar curvature	Roll or small pillow under lumbar curvature
Legs are externally rotated	External rotation of legs	Roll or sandbag placed laterally to trochanter of femur
Legs are extended	Hyperextension of knees	Small pillow under thigh to flex knee slightly
Feet assume plantar flexion position	Plantar flexion and foot drop	Footboard or rolled pillow to support feet in dorsal flexion
Heels on bed surface	Pressure on heels	Pillow or roll under lower legs

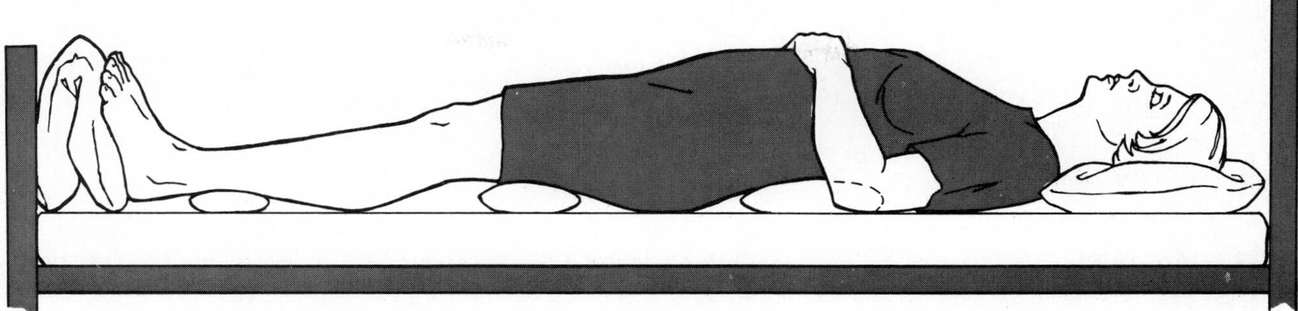

Figure 23–7 Dorsal recumbent position (supported).

and thus is unable to walk properly. To prevent foot drop, the feet are supported off the surface of the bed by a roll or pillow under the lower leg.

Prone position

In the *prone position* a person lies on his or her abdomen, legs extended and head turned to the side. This position is often used by children and adults as a comfortable sleeping position. Some people flex one or both arms over their heads. This is the only position other than the supine position in which the patient does not have the hips flexed. For this reason it is recommended as an alternative position for patients on prolonged bed rest since it maintains normal alignment of the hips.

In the prone position the following supports are needed (see Table 23–5):

1. The patient's head is turned to the side and rests either on the flat surface of the bed or on a small pillow. A thick pillow would hyperextend the neck.
2. A small pillow under the patient's abdomen just below the diaphragm supports the lumbar curvature of the spine, eases breathing, and takes some of the weight of the body off the breasts of a woman. See Figure 23–8. To prevent the toes from resting on the bed surface and to avoid plantar flexion, the patient is positioned so that the feet fall naturally over the end of the mattress.

Lateral position (side-lying position)

In the *lateral position*, the patient lies on his or her side, and most of the body weight is borne by the lateral aspect of the lower scapula and the lateral aspect of the lower ilium. This position is comfortable for most people and a welcome change for the patient who spends a good deal of time in the dorsal recumbent position. The advantages of this position are that (a) pressure is taken off the back of the head, scapulae, sacrum, and heels, and (b) the legs and feet are in flexion without support, rather than in extension as they are in the supine position. The major disadvantage is the tendency for the upper shoulder and upper thigh to rotate inward unless adequately supported.

Support is provided in the following ways (see Table 23-6 and Figure 23–9):

1. A pillow under the head supports the head in good alignment and prevents lateral flexion of the neck and fatigue of the sternocleidomastoid muscles.

Table 23–5 Prone Position

Unsupported position	Problem to be prevented	Corrective measure
Head is turned to side and neck is slightly flexed	Flexion or hyperextension of neck	Small pillow under head unless contraindicated because of promotion of mucus drainage from mouth
Body lies flat on abdomen accentuating lumbar curvature	Hyperextension of lumbar curvature; difficulty breathing; pressure on breasts for women	Small pillow or roll under abdomen just below diaphragm
Toes rest on bed surface; feet are in plantar flexion	Plantar flexion of feet	Allow feet to fall naturally over end of mattress

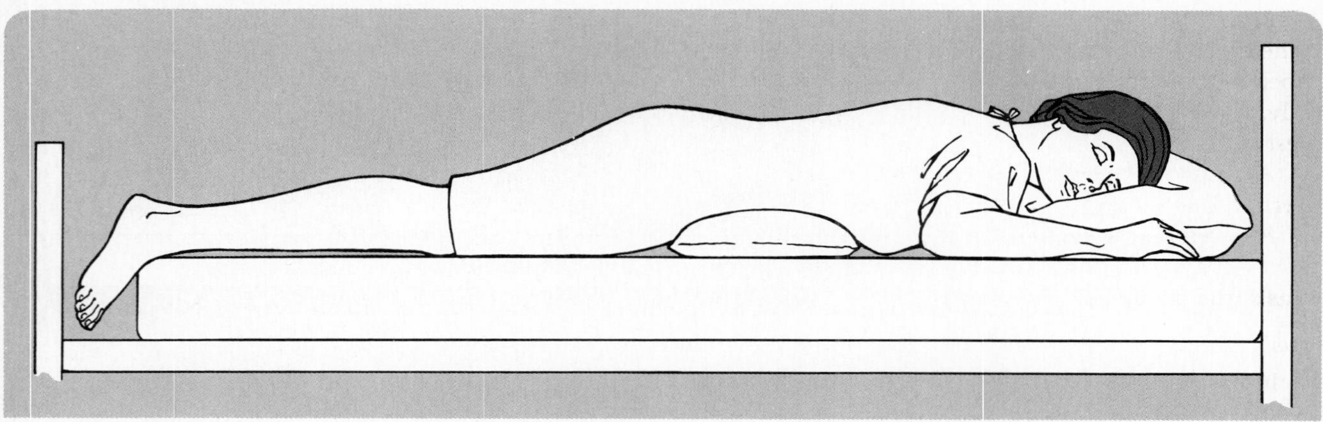

Figure 23–8 Prone position (supported).

Table 23–6 Lateral Position

Unsupported position	Problem to be prevented	Corrective measure
Body is turned to side, both arms in front of body, weight resting primarily on lateral aspects of scapula and ilium	Lateral flexion and fatigue of sterno-cleidomastoid muscles	Pillow under head to provide good alignment
Upper arm and shoulder are rotated internally and adducted	Internal rotation and adduction of shoulder and subsequent limited function	Pillow under arm to place it in good alignment
Upper thigh and leg are rotated internally and adducted	Internal rotation and adduction of thigh and subsequent limited function	Pillow under leg and thigh to place them in good alignment

Figure 23–9 Lateral (side-lying) position (supported).

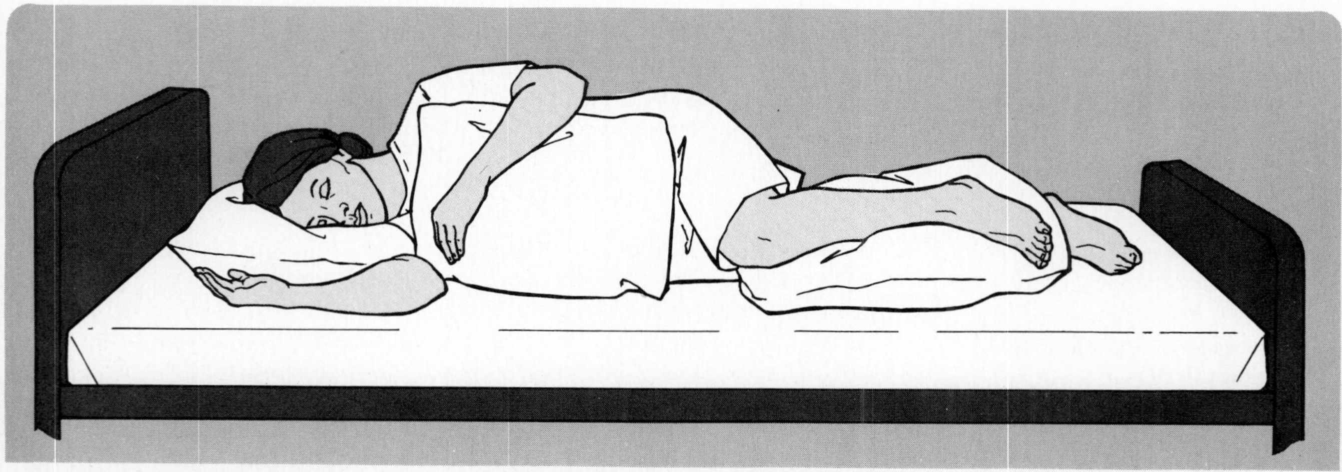

2. Both arms are in a slightly flexed position in front of the body. A pillow is generally needed to support the upper arm and shoulder, which tend to rotate internally. Supporting the shoulder and arm also permits the chest to expand more easily, thus facilitating breathing.
3. A pillow is placed under the upper leg to prevent internal rotation and adduction of the hip.
4. A rolled pillow is placed at the patient's back.

Sims's position (semiprone position)

Sims's position is similar to the lateral position in that the patient lies on his or her side, but in Sims's the patient's weight is borne by the anterior aspects of the ilium and the humerus and clavicle rather than the lateral aspects of the ilium and the scapula. Therefore, in Sims's position, the points of pressure of the body differ from those in the lateral, Fowler's, dorsal recumbent, and prone positions.

Sims's position is frequently used for patients who are unconscious, because it facilitates the drainage of mucus from the mouth. It is a comfortable position for many other people, including women in the last trimester of pregnancy.

In Sims's position, the patient's lower arm is behind him or her, and the upper arm is flexed at both the shoulder and the elbow. Both legs are also flexed in front of the patient. The upper one is more acutely flexed at the hip and the knee than the lower one.

Support is provided in the following ways (see Table 23-7 and Figure 23-10):

1. A pillow under the patient's head keeps the head in good alignment, preventing lateral flexion of the head

Table 23-7 Sims's Position (Semiprone Position)

Unsupported position	Problem to be prevented	Corrective measure
Head rests on bed surface, weight is borne by lateral aspects of cranial and facial bones	Lateral flexion of neck and head	Pillow supports head, maintaining it in good alignment
Upper shoulder and arm are internally rotated	Internal rotation of shoulder and arm; pressure on chest, restricting expansion during breathing	Pillow under arm places it in alignment
Upper leg and thigh are adducted and internally rotated	Internal rotation and adduction of hip and leg	Pillow under leg to support it in alignment
Feet assume plantar flexion	Foot drop if position is maintained for prolonged period	Sandbags to support feet in dorsal flexion

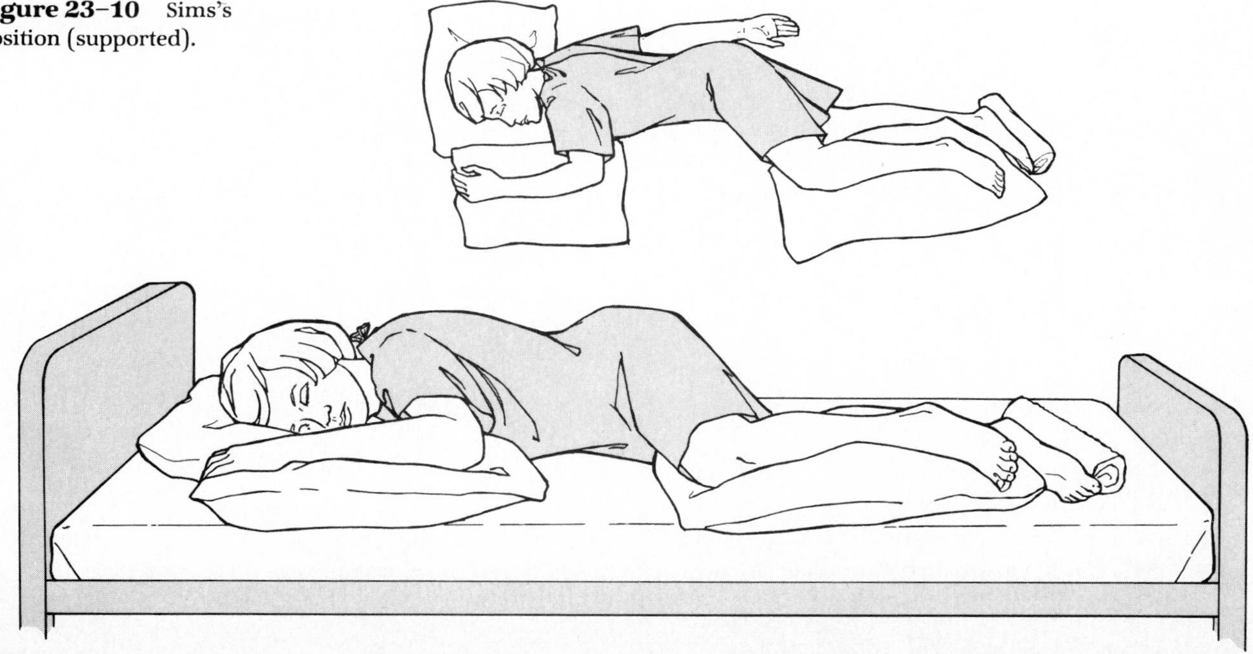

Figure 23-10 Sims's position (supported).

and neck. This is generally indicated unless mucus drainage from the mouth is to be facilitated by the laterally flexed position.

2. A pillow under the patient's upper arm reduces internal rotation of the shoulder and arm and permits the chest expansion necessary for breathing.

3. A pillow under the upper leg prevents adduction and internal rotation of the hip and leg.

4. The feet normally assume a plantar flexed position. If Sims's position is to be maintained for a prolonged period, supports to keep the feet in dorsal flexion are indicated. Sandbags are frequently used for this purpose.

Assisting Patients to Move in Bed

Patients require varying degrees of assistance to move while they are in bed. Some are completely helpless and require the assistance of nurses to make the smallest change in position. Those who are weak or very ill frequently require assistance from a nurse, although they may be able to help themselves a little.

Before nurses assist any patient to move, they need to be aware of the following information:

1. The degree to which patients can exert themselves, specifically considering their physical condition. For example, it may be that patients who have cardiac pathologic conditions should not exert themselves in the slightest even though they feel well enough to help. Although a patient wants to be helpful, it may be contraindicated at that particular time.

2. The position that the patient needs to assume and the degree to which the patient can tolerate another position. The patient who has a respiratory pathologic condition may require a Fowler's sitting position while in bed to be able to breathe satisfactorily. This patient may or may not be able to tolerate lying flat on the back even for a few minutes.

3. The discomfort the patient experiences when moving or assuming a particular position. For example, a patient with an advanced malignancy may find any movement painful. Nurses can help move such a patient at a time when the analgesic is most effective, for example, half an hour after an injection of morphine, to minimize discomfort.

4. Any special problems the patient might have, such as particularly fragile skin, bones, or blood vessels. Patients with some diseases may have specific problems. For example, in some conditions even normal, gentle handling by a nurse can cause a bone to fracture or blood vessels to break. In these instances, soft pads can be used by the nurse to provide less pressure on a specific area of the skin and to provide broader support when helping the patient turn in bed.

Procedure 23–1 Assisting a Patient to Move Up in Bed

Moving a patient up toward the head of the bed is facilitated if the patient can safely tolerate having the head of the bed lowered to a flat position and the head pillow removed for a few minutes. If this is not possible, the nurse would be wise to obtain the assistance of a second person to help from the other side of the bed. With the additional assistance, the patient will experience less exertion and less discomfort. The steps presented here are followed by either one or two nurses.

Goals

1. To improve the patient's body alignment.
2. To promote comfort.

Preparation

1. Explain to the patient what you plan to do, and gain the patient's assistance if possible.
2. Wash hands to avoid transmitting microorganisms to the patient.
3. Adjust the head of the bed to a flat position or make it as low as the patient can tolerate.
4. Remove all pillows; then place one at the head of the bed to pad the patient's head and protect it from inadvertent injury against the top of the bed.

Intervention

1. Facing the head of the bed, assume a broad stance with the foot nearest the bed behind the other foot.

   Rationale A broad stance increases balance. Proper foot placement prevents unnecessary twisting of the body when the patient is moved.

2. Ask the patient to flex both knees, bringing both heels up to the buttocks, and to flex the neck so that the chin is tilted toward the chest.

Procedure 23–1, continued

Rationale Flexed knees ensure that the patient uses the femoral muscles when subsequently asked to push. The chin pulled toward the chest prevents hyperextension of the neck as the head resists moving against the bed surface.

3. If the patient is able to assist, have him or her:
   a. Grasp the bed head with both hands,
      or
   b. Grasp the trapeze bar,
      or
   c. Push with the hands on the bed surface by flexing the elbows and hyperextending the shoulder joints.

   Rationale Patient assistance provides additional power to overcome friction when the move is made.

4. If the patient cannot assist, place his or her arms across the chest.

   Rationale Placing the arms across the chest prevents them from dragging on the bed surface and thus decreases friction.

5. Flex your knees and hips to bring your forearms to the level of the bed.

   Rationale Flexed knees and hips allow the nurse to use the major muscle groups of the thighs and legs to move the patient and also brings the nurse's center of gravity closer to the patient's.

6. Place one arm under the patient's shoulders and the other arm under the patient's thighs. See Figure 23–11.

   Rationale This placement of the arms distributes the patient's weight and supports the heaviest part of the body (the buttocks).

7. Tighten your gluteal and abdominal muscles.

   Rationale These muscles assist other large muscle groups to lift and push; they are less likely to be injured if tightened.

8. Rock from the back leg to the front leg and back again; then shift weight to the front leg as the patient pushes with the heels and pulls with the arms.

   Rationale Rocking helps to attain a balanced, smooth motion and to overcome inertia. The nurse's weight shift helps counteract the patient's weight.

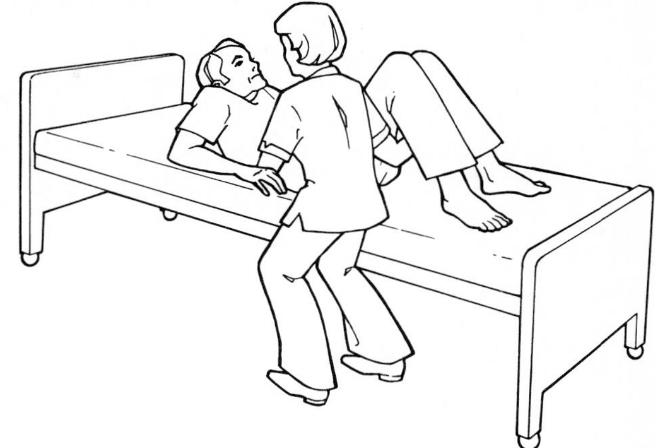

Figure 23–11

9. Provide appropriate supportive devices for the patient's new position. See the earlier discussion of the supine position or Fowler's position.

Variation: Two Nurses Using a Hand-Forearm Interlock

Two people are required to move a patient who is unable to assist because of his or her condition or weight. Using the technique described above, with the second nurse on the opposite side of the bed, the two nurses interlock their forearms under the patient's thighs and shoulders. See Figure 23–12.

Figure 23–12

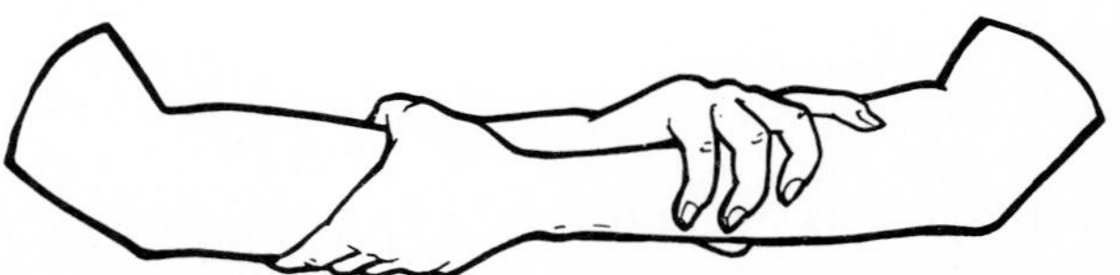

Procedure 23–2 Moving a Patient to the Side of the Bed in Segments

Occasionally a patient who must remain on his or her back needs to be moved to the side of the bed. This may be necessary when changing a bed or carrying out some treatment for the patient within easy reach. In this movement, the nurse's weight is used to counteract the patient's weight; the nurse's arms serve as connecting bars between the patient and the nurse.

Goal

To move the patient closer to the nurse safely and comfortably.

Preparation

See Procedure 23–1, steps 1–3, on page 570.

Intervention

1. Position yourself at the side of the bed toward which the patient will move and opposite the part of the body to be moved.

   Rationale This position reassures the patient that he or she cannot fall and avoids the need for the nurse to reach.

2. Place the patient's near arm across his or her chest.

   Rationale Placing the patient's arm across the chest avoids resistance to the patient's movement and prevents injury to the arm.

3. Assume a broad stance, with one foot in front of the other, and flex your knees.

   Rationale The broad stance provides balance. Flexing the knees lowers the center of gravity (increasing stability) and ensures use of the large muscle groups in the legs during movement.

4. Place your arm nearest the head of the bed under the patient's far shoulder so that the patient's head rests on your forearm and elbow crease. Place your other arm under the patient's lumbar curvature.

   Rationale The arm under the patient's shoulder securely supports the head and shoulders. The other arm supports the trunk.

5. Tighten your gluteal and abdominal muscles.

   Rationale Tensing these muscles prepares them for use and protects the internal organs against injury.

6. Pull the patient's head, shoulders, and thorax to the near side of the bed by rocking backward and shifting your weight to the rear foot.

   Rationale Pulling avoids lifting against gravity. Rocking backward uses the nurse's body weight in the direction of the pull.

7. To move the patient's buttocks, place one arm under the patient's waist, the other under the thighs. Repeat steps 5 and 6, pulling the buttocks.

   Rationale Placement of the arms under the waist and thighs centers the weight of the buttocks.

8. To move the patient's legs and feet, place one arm under the thighs, the other under the calves. Repeat steps 5 and 6, pulling the legs.

9. Elevate the side rail next to the patient.

   Rationale The side rail must be up to prevent the patient from falling off the edge of the bed.

Procedure 23–3 Assisting a Patient to a Lateral Position in Bed

This movement is most easily accomplished if the patient is lying on a flat bed; however, it can be accomplished if the head or the foot of the bed is raised. It is easiest if the patient is in a supine position. Before moving a patient to a lateral (side-lying) position, the patient is moved closer to the side of the bed opposite the side he or she will face when turned. See Procedure 23–2. This ensures that the patient will be positioned safely in the center of the bed after turning.

Goals

1. To relieve potential pressure areas from the previous position (e.g., a supine position).
2. To provide comfort.

Procedure 23–3, continued

Preparation

See Procedure 23–1, steps 1–3, on page 570.

Intervention

1. Elevate the side rail on the side nearest the patient.
2. Position yourself opposite the patient's abdomen on the side of the bed toward which the patient will turn.

   Rationale Taking a position opposite the patient's abdomen prevents spinal torsion by the nurse when moving the patient and centers the nurse's weight opposite the patient's central weight.
3. Assume a broad stance with one foot ahead of the other.

   Rationale A broad stance enhances balance.
4. Place the patient's arm nearest you away from his or her body.

   Rationale Pulling the patient's arm away from the body prevents the patient from rolling onto this arm.
5. Flex the patient's far arm over the chest; place the far leg over the near leg. See Figure 23–13.

   Rationale Pulling the far arm and leg forward facilitates forward turning by the patient.
6. Tighten your gluteal and abdominal muscles, and flex your knees.

   Rationale Tensing the muscles prepares them for use and prevents injury. Flexing the knees lowers the center of gravity (increasing stability) and ensures use of the large muscle groups in the legs during movement.
7. Place one hand on the patient's far hip and the other hand on the far shoulder.

   Rationale This placement of the hands distributes the patient's weight and supports the heaviest part of the body.
8. Roll the patient toward you:
   a. Rock backward and shift your weight to the rear foot.
   b. Increase your knee flexion and lower your pelvis. See Figure 23–14.

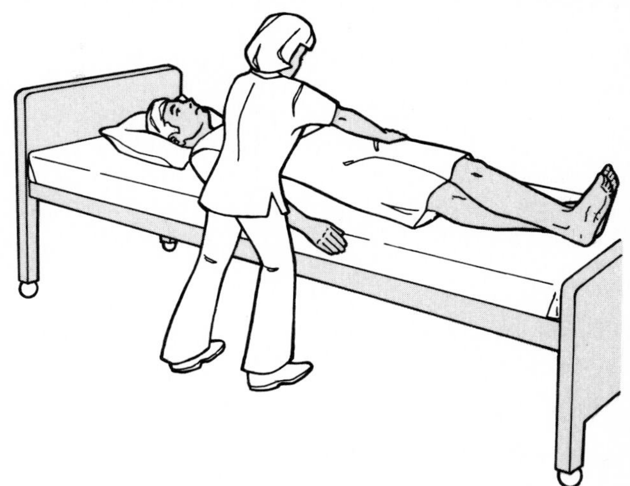

Figure 23–13

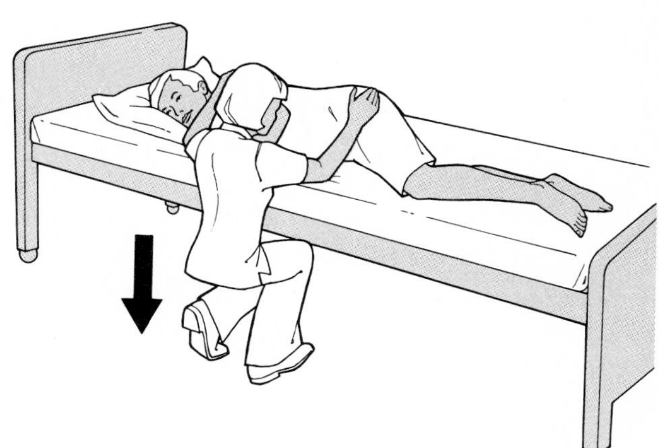

Figure 23–14

   Rationale Rocking backward makes use of the nurse's body weight in the direction of the movement. Increased knee flexion lowers the nurse's center of gravity, enhancing stability.
9. Align the patient appropriately. See the earlier discussion of the lateral position.

Procedure 23–4 Assisting a Patient to a Sitting Position in Bed

Patients may need assistance to sit in bed while pillows are rearranged or, in some instances, for back care. The degree of assistance required depends on the patient's condition. When assisting patients to a sitting position the nurse's weight is again used to counteract the patient's weight, and in one method the nurse's arm serves as a lever, with the elbow as the fulcrum.

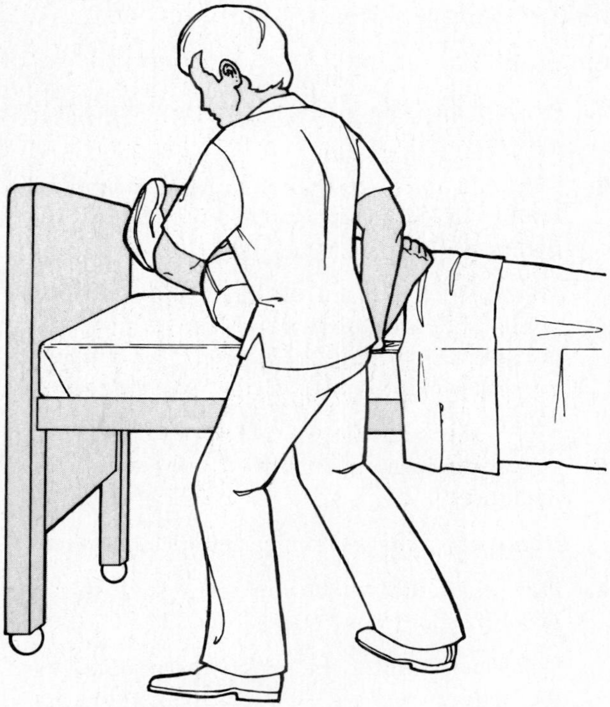

Goal

To move the patient to a sitting position safely and comfortably.

Preparation

1. See Procedure 23–1, steps 1–2, on page 570.
2. Assist the patient to a supine position.
3. Adjust the bed to a flat or low Fowler's position as tolerated by the patient.

Intervention

1. Ask the patient to place his or her arms at the sides with the palms of the hands against the surface of the bed.

   Rationale The patient can push against the bed surface to assist the nurse.

2. Facing the head of the bed, stand at the side of the bed and opposite the patient's buttocks. Assume a broad stance with the foot nearest the bed behind the other foot.

   Rationale Facing the head of the bed prevents twisting of the nurse's body in the motion that follows. A broad stance provides balance.

3. If the patient is helpless, place your hand farthest from the patient over his or her near shoulder at a point between the shoulder blades. Place the hand of your free arm on the bed surface. See Figure 23–15.

   Rationale This hand placement is designed to lift the patient's upper trunk evenly. The resting hand provides balance and leverage.

Figure 23–15

4. If the patient can assist, ask the patient to flex the knees. Then the patient and the nurse grasp the back of each other's arms. The nurse's elbow rests on the bed surface when lifting the patient. See Figure 23–16.

   Rationale Having the patient flex the knees facilitates upward movement of the trunk against gravity. The nurse's elbow is the fulcrum for the lever action of the arm.

5. Raise the patient to a sitting position by shifting your weight to the back leg and flexing your knees to bring your hips downward. At the same time have the patient push with the arm that is not grasping your arm.

   Rationale The nurse uses her or his own weight to counteract the patient's weight.

Figure 23–16

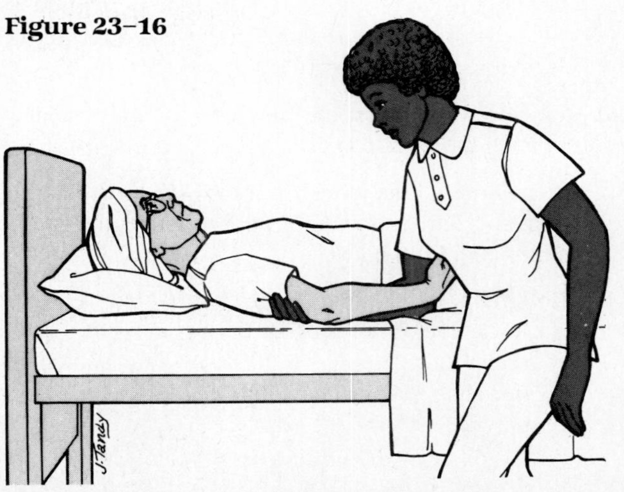

Procedure 23–5 Assisting a Patient to a Sitting Position on the Edge of the Bed

In this movement the nurse's weight is again used to counterbalance the patient's weight. It is crucial that the nurse's balance be maintained while shifting weight from the front leg to the rear one.

Goal

To move the patient safely and comfortably to a sitting position on the edge of the bed.

Preparation

1. See Procedure 23–1, steps 1–2, on page 570.
2. Assist the patient to a lateral position facing the nurse. See Procedure 23–3.
3. Raise the head of the bed to about 60° to decrease the distance that the patient needs to move to sit up.

Intervention

1. Facing the patient and the far bottom corner of the bed, stand opposite the patient's hips. Assume a broad stance, placing the foot nearest the bottom of the bed to the rear.

   Rationale This position enhances balance and prevents twisting the nurse's body.

2. Place the patient's feet and lower legs just over the edge of the bed.

   Rationale This position prevents the feet from resisting the sitting up movement.

3. Place one arm under the shoulders of the patient and the other arm over the far thigh with the hand resting on the posterior aspect of the thigh. See Figure 23–17.

   Rationale This hand placement prevents the patient from falling backward when sitting up.

4. Pivot toward the rear leg so that the patient's legs swing downward and the nurse's weight shifts to the rear leg. See Figure 23–18.

   Rationale The nurse's weight counteracts the patient's weight.

5. Maintain support of the patient until he or she is balanced and comfortable.

   Rationale This movement may cause some patients to feel faint.

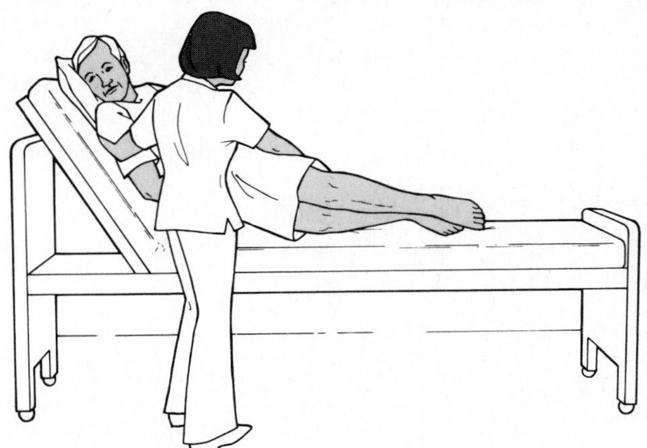

Figure 23–17

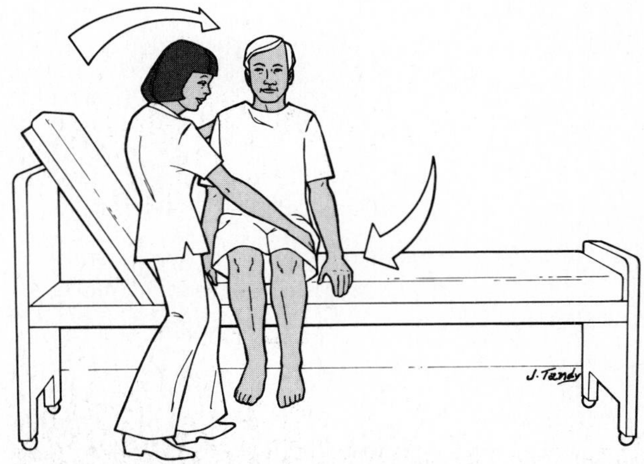

Figure 23–18

Procedure 23–6 Assisting a Patient to Move from a Bed to a Chair

For this movement, the bed should be in the low position so that the patient can step easily to the floor. If the bed is not adjustable in this way, then a broad-based and stable footstool can be used; the patient needs to understand that he or she will step initially onto the stool and next step down to the floor.

Goal

To move the patient from a bed to a chair safely and comfortably.

Preparation

1. See Procedure 23–1, steps 1–2, on page 570.
2. Obtain a dressing gown and slippers or shoes for the patient. The slippers or shoes should have nonskid soles.
3. Assist the patient to a sitting position on the side of the bed. See Procedure 23–5.
4. Assist the patient to put on the dressing gown and slippers or shoes.
5. Lower the bed to the low level or obtain a broad-based, stable footstool.

Intervention

1. Assume a broad stance facing the patient, with your foot that is nearest the chair forward.

   Rationale The broad stance provides stability and a smooth, balanced movement when turning; it also prevents twisting of the body.

2. Flex your knees and hips.

   Rationale This ensures use of major muscle groups of the thighs and legs if the patient requires lifting or holding up.

3. Have the patient place his or her hands on your shoulders and put your hands on either side of the patient's waist.

   Rationale This hand placement provides balance and support for the patient.

4. When the patient steps to the floor or the footstool, brace your front knee against the patient's knee.

   Rationale This prevents the patient's knee from buckling and keeps the patient from falling.

5. After the patient feels steady, step back with your forward leg and guide the patient forward until the back of his or her legs are against the chair.
6. Keep your knee against the patient's knee.
7. Assist the patient to lower into the chair by flexing your knees and hips as the patient flexes his or her knees and hips.

   Rationale Flexing the knees and hips prevents strain to the arm and back muscles.

8. Align the patient appropriately in the chair.

Variation: Two-Nurse Assist from a Bed to a Chair

Another method of assisting a patient from a bed to a chair requires two nurses. In this method, the bed is left in the raised position.

The patient is assisted to a sitting position on the side of the bed and suitably attired for sitting out of bed. The chair for the patient is placed at the side of the bed with its back toward the foot of the bed, about 30 to 60 cm (1 to 2 ft) away from the bed.

The nurses assume a broad stance with knees flexed on opposite sides of the patient. Each nurse places an arm under the patient's near axilla reaching from front to back, with the nurse's arm extending behind the back of the patient to the far axilla. The nurses can either hold the patient on his or her back just below the far axilla or grasp each other's forearms. Each nurse's other arm is placed under the patient's thighs, where the nurses grasp each other's forearms.

The patient places his or her arms around the nurses' shoulders if possible. The nurses together extend their knees to lift the patient and then move the patient to the chair with coordinated movements. The nurse nearer the chair sidesteps in front of the chair to the side farther from the bed, while the other nurse moves forward to the side of the chair near the bed. The patient is now over the chair. Each nurse flexes the knees to lower the patient into the chair.

Procedure 23–7 Assisting a Patient in Bed to Raise the Buttocks

This position is frequently used to assist the patient onto a bedpan. In this movement, the nurse's arm acts as a lever, with the elbow on the bed surface as the fulcrum. The nurse's body weight is the force applied to the lever and hence to the patient.

Goal

To assist the patient onto a bedpan safely and comfortably, or to massage the patient's sacrum.

Preparation

1. See Procedure 23–1, steps 1–3, on page 570.
2. Place the bedpan or other required supplies within easy reach.

Intervention

1. Assume a broad stance at the patient's side opposite the buttocks.

   Rationale A broad stance provides stability because the center of gravity falls between the feet.
2. Have the patient flex the knees to bring the feet close to the buttocks.

   Rationale This allows the patient to use his or her femoral and gluteal muscles to raise the buttocks.
3. Have the patient place arms at sides, with elbows slightly bent, and palms facing down against the bed ready to push. See Figure 23–19. For patients who are on restricted bed rest, a trapeze may be helpful and require less effort.

   Rationale Patient assistance lessens the energy required by the nurse.
4. Place your forearm and hand (palm upward) that are near the head of the bed under the patient's sacrum. Rest your elbow on the mattress.

   Rationale The elbow serves as a fulcrum and the forearm as a lever.

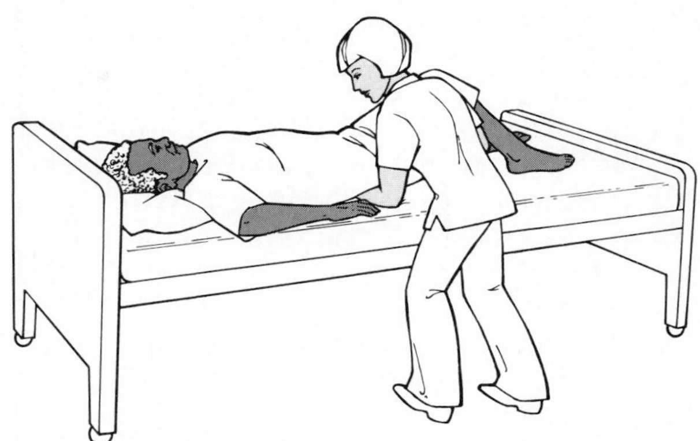

Figure 23–19

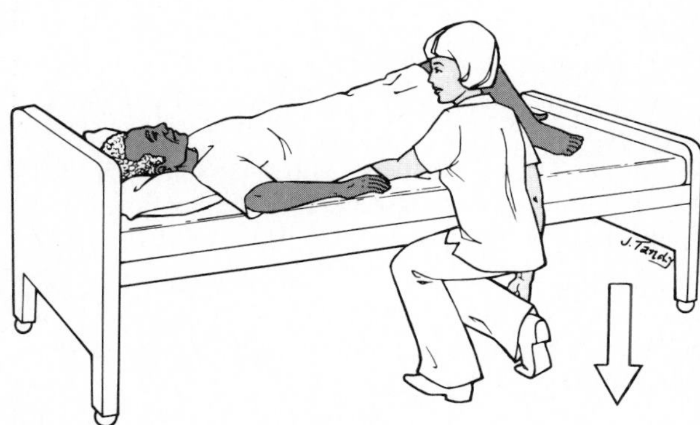

Figure 23–20

5. Flex your knees and lower your buttocks at the same time as the patient pushes to elevate his or her buttocks. See Figure 23–20.
6. With your free hand, put the bedpan in place or massage the sacral area.
7. Lower the patient and assist him or her to a comfortable position.

Lifting a Patient between a Bed and a Stretcher

Lifting and carrying the average adult from a bed to a stretcher or to another bed and at the same time maintaining the patient's horizontal position generally requires three people. A child, on the other hand, may be more easily moved by just two persons, and a baby by one person safely.

The stretcher or bed to which the patient needs to move is best placed at right angles to the patient's bed with the head near the foot of the bed. The wheels of both stretcher and bed should be locked, so that they will not slip out from under the patient.

In the three-person lift for adult patients, the tallest nurse takes the upper part of the patient. This nurse probably has the longest reach and can thus best support the patient's head and shoulders. The strongest nurse stands opposite the patient's hips. This second nurse will support the middle third of the patient, which is usually the heaviest portion. The third nurse will support the patient's legs and feet. The first and third nurses place their arms close to the second nurse's arms in order to assist with the heaviest weight. If two nurses are moving a child, the first supports the head, shoulders, and waist, and the second supports the hips and legs.

For the three or two nurses to coordinate their movements, the nurse at the patient's head calls the numbers by which they all move.

1. The three nurses face the side of the patient's bed. Each assumes a broad stance with the foot closer to the stretcher forward, that is, if the stretcher is to the nurse's right, the right foot of each nurse is placed in front of the left foot.
2. If the patient cannot move his or her arms, they are placed across the chest to avoid injury to them during the move.
3. The nurses flex their knees and then slip their arms under the patient. The first nurse's arms are positioned under the patient's neck and shoulders and under the waist. The second nurse's arms are placed under the patient's waist and hips. The third nurse puts one arm under the patient's hips and the other arm under the patient's lower legs. See Figure 23–21.
4. At the count of "one," the patient is moved to the side of the bed toward the nurses.
5. At the count of "two," the nurses tilt the patient slightly toward them with their elbows resting on the bed, until the patient lies against them.
6. At the count of "three," each nurse rises and steps back with the forward foot; then they walk in unison to the receiving bed or stretcher.
7. At the count of "four," the nurses flex their knees and rest their elbows on the second bed.
8. At the count of "five," the nurses extend their forearms, thus permitting the patient to roll gently and slowly to his or her back.
9. At the count of "six," the nurses withdraw their arms from beneath the patient.

Devices Used to Assist Patients to Move

The hydraulic lifter

The hydraulic lifter is also known as a patient lifter or by the name of the particular model, such as a Hoyer lift. Each model has its own instructions regarding use, and the nurse should become aware of these in the individual setting. Rachet lifters are also available.

Some models have canvas straps, which fit under the patient in a lying position or under the buttocks and around the back of a patient in a sitting position. See Figure 23–22. Two nurses are generally required when using a patient lifter; one nurse guides the patient while the other operates the lifter.

Lifters are used chiefly for patients who cannot help themselves, particularly those who are too heavy for others to lift. Transfers are commonly made from a bed to a stretcher and from a wheelchair to a bathtub.

To use a hydraulic lifter to move a patient from a bed to a wheelchair:

Figure 23–21 The three-person carry. Note the positions of the lifters' arms.

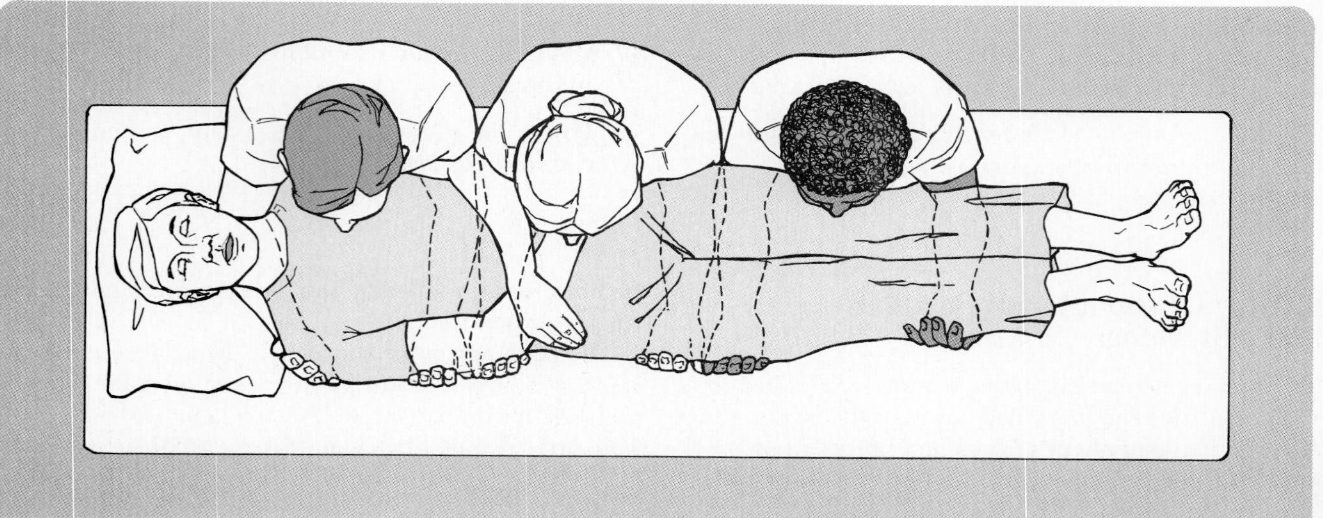

1. The nurses place the wheelchair nearby, allowing enough room for the lifter to be turned. The wheelchair brakes are then set.
2. The lifter is wheeled to the bed and placed so that the wheel base is under the bed and at right angles to the bed. The nurses adjust the height of the lifting bar so that the canvas straps can fit under the patient.
3. One nurse closes the hydraulic pressure valve to hold the lifting bar in place.
4. Both nurses place the canvas straps under the patient, one strap under the buttocks and upper thighs and the other strap under the patient's back just below the axillae.
5. The nurses fasten the canvas straps to the appropriate hooks on the lifting bar.
6. One nurse releases the hydraulic pressure valve and pumps the lever. The lifter will then lift the patient. When the patient is clear of the bed, the nurse closes the hydraulic pressure valve.
7. One nurse rolls the lifter to the wheelchair; the other nurse steadies the patient and guides him or her to a position over the wheelchair.
8. One nurse releases the hydraulic pressure valve, and the patient is lowered into the wheelchair. The nurses unhook the straps from the lifting bar and remove them from beneath the patient.

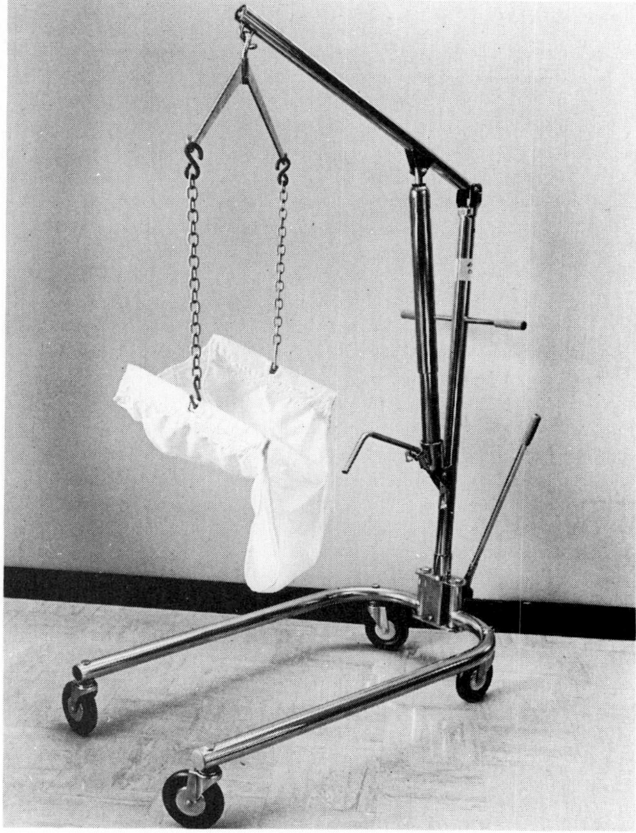

Figure 23–22 A rachet lifter used to lift and move patients.

Drawsheet

A drawsheet can also be used to assist a patient to move in bed.

To assist a patient to move up in bed, two nurses are required:

1. The nurses check that the drawsheet extends from the patient's shoulders to the thighs.
2. The nurses stand on opposites sides of the bed. Each nurse flexes the knees and grasps the drawsheet.
3. The nurses then extend their knees and transfer their weight from the foot nearer the foot of the bed to the other foot, moving the patient up toward the head of the bed.

One nurse can assist a patient to turn on his or her side using a drawsheet:

1. The patient lies on his or her back, the arm nearer the nurse over the chest or slightly away from the patient's body.
2. The nurse loosens the drawsheet on the far side of the bed.
3. Standing at the side of the bed to which the patient will turn, the nurse grasps the far side of the drawsheet and pulls it over the patient in a manner that will roll the patient over toward the nurse.
4. The nurse places her or his elbows on the bed surface edge to stop the patient's turn and prevent falling if the patient is too near the edge of the bed.

Evaluation

Examples of outcome criteria for patients with body alignment problems are:

1. The patient's posture reflects good body alignment in a standing or sitting position.
2. There is absence of muscle strain and fatigue.
3. The position of the hands is similar to that used to grasp a ball.
4. The feet are in dorsal flexion.
5. Pressure points of the body (points on which body weight rests), such as the sacrum, appear healthy; that is, they have the same color as other parts of the skin, are intact and free of abrasions, are warm to the touch, and convey a normal sense of feeling to the patient.
6. The joints move through their normal ranges of motion.

Summary

For patients who are ill, moving even a little in bed can be a major challenge. Some patients are completely unable to move and rely on nursing personnel to change their positions. A knowledge of body mechanics will assist nurses to help patients without injuring themselves or the patients.

Good posture is essential to normal physiologic functioning. There are specific characteristics of the well-aligned child and adult, both standing and sitting. The pregnant woman also needs to maintain correct body alignment. The postural changes of pregnancy begin in the second trimester. Correct posture is important in preventing strain on the spinal muscles and joints. Characteristically posture also changes with age. It is important to know normal posture to assess abnormal alignment.

Patients assume a variety of positions in bed for both comfort and therapeutic reasons. Nursing intervention often involves assisting a patient to assume a position and providing the required support. Once a patient has assumed a position, nurses need to provide care in terms of exercise, skin care, and change of position.

Specific guidelines can be applied to assist a patient to move. By following the guidelines nurses can assist patients in various ways in bed and out of bed. Two devices that are used to assist patients to move are the hydraulic lifter and the drawsheet. The use of these often decreases the effort required by the patient and the nurse.

Suggested Activities

1. Observe the normal posture of individuals in each of the seven age groups: newborns or infants, toddlers, children, adolescents, adults, pregnant women, and older adults. Note similarities and differences.

2. In a hospital, note the bed positions assumed by patients. Assess the positions in terms of body alignment. Draw up a plan to correct any poorly aligned position.

3. Using a student as a patient, assist the patient to move in bed as described in this chapter. Ask another student to observe your body mechanics while you are doing this.

Suggested Readings

Howden, L. July/August 1981. Basic back care: It doesn't have to hurt. *Canadian Nurse* 77:46–50.
The author describes the anatomical structure of the spine, the physiology of back pain, assessment of pain, and treatment modalities. The proper mechanics of lifting are described, as well as measures to avoid back strain.

Owen, B. D. May 1980. How to avoid that aching back. *American Journal of Nursing* 80:894–97.
This illustrated article discusses how to reduce the risk of straining the back while lifting objects by using a new technique. It also explains exercises that can strengthen the back.

Selected References

American Rehabilitation Foundation. 1962. *Rehabilitative nursing techniques: 1, Bed positioning and transfer procedures for the hemiplegic.* Minneapolis: American Rehabilitation Foundation.

Bilger, A. J., and Greene, E. H., editors. 1973. *Winters' protective body mechanics.* New York: Springer Publishing Co.

Byrne, C. J.; Saxton, D. F.; Pelikan, P. K.; and Nugent, P. M. 1981. *Laboratory tests: Implications for nurses and allied health professionals.* Menlo Park, Calif.: Addison-Wesley Publishing Co.

Clausen, J. P., et al. 1973. *Maternity nursing today.* New York: McGraw-Hill Book Co.

Dickason, E. J., and Schult, M. O., editors. 1975. *Maternal and infant care: A text for nurses.* New York: McGraw-Hill Book Co.

Drapeau, J. September 1975. Getting back into good posture: How to erase your lumbar aches. *Nursing 75* 5:63–65.

Ford, J. R., and Duckworth, B. January 1976. Moving a dependent patient safely, comfortably. Part 1: Positioning. *Nursing 76* 6:27–36.

———. February 1976. Moving a dependent patient safely, comfortably. Part 2: Transferring. *Nursing 76* 6:58–65.

Helms, D. B., and Turner, J. S. 1976. *Exploring child behavior.* Philadelphia: W. B. Saunders Co.

Mitchell, J. J. 1973. *Human life: The first ten years.* Toronto: Holt, Rinehart and Winston of Canada.

Nordmark, M. T., and Rohweder, A. W. 1975. *Scientific foundations of nursing.* 3rd ed. Philadelphia: J. B. Lippincott Co.

Nursing 74. October 1974. How to negotiate the ups and downs, ins and outs of body alignment. *Nursing 74* 4:46–51.

Rantz, M. J., and Courtial, D. 1981. *Lifting, moving and transferring patients: A manual.* 2nd ed. St. Louis: C. V. Mosby Co.

Smith, D. W., and Bierman, E. L. 1973. *The biologic ages of man: From conception through old age.* Philadelphia: W. B. Saunders Co.

Stevens, C. B. 1974. *Special needs of long-term patients.* Philadelphia: J. B. Lippincott Co.

Chapter 24

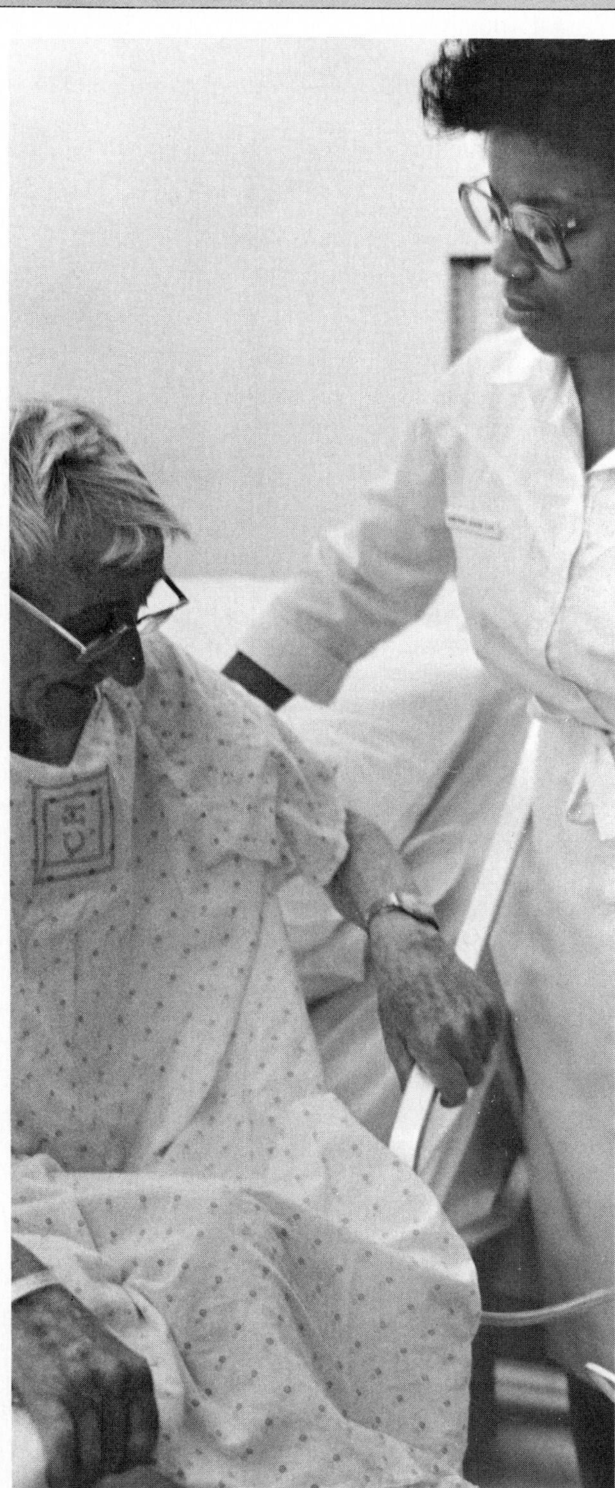

Exercise and Ambulation

CONTENTS

Objectives

1. Know essential facts about mobility
   1.1 Name five essential aspects of mobility
   1.2 List five types of synovial joints
   1.3 Identify thirteen synovial joint movements
   1.4 Describe the mechanics of walking
   1.5 List four purposes of exercise
   1.6 Identify positive effects of exercise
   1.7 Identify five kinds of exercise
2. Know information necessary to assess a patient's mobility
   2.1 Identify the ranges of motion of body joints
   2.2 Identify the essentials of an appropriate station and gait
   2.3 Identify factors influencing mobility
   2.4 Identify variations in mobility for different age groups
   2.5 Identify indices used to assess activity tolerance
3. Understand essential facts about immobility
   3.1 Identify four kinds of immobility
   3.2 Identify common problems of immobility
   3.3 Explain the reasons for problems related to immobility
4. Understand facts about nursing measures required to maintain, promote, and restore mobility of patients
   4.1 Identify measures required to prevent immobility
   4.2 Identify measures required to maintain joint mobility
   4.3 Identify measures required to maintain muscle strength and endurance
5. Apply the nursing process when providing care to selected patients to meet their mobility needs
   5.1 Obtain necessary assessment data
   5.2 Analyze and relate assessment data
   5.3 Write relevant nursing diagnoses
   5.4 Write relevant nursing goals
   5.5 Plan appropriate nursing interventions
   5.6 Implement appropriate nursing interventions
   5.7 State outcome criteria for evaluating the effectiveness of nursing interventions
6. Safely perform techniques to assist patients to ambulate and exercise
   6.1 Assist patients to ambulate effectively without mechanical aids
   6.2 Assist patients to ambulate effectively with mechanical aids
   6.3 Provide passive exercises appropriately

Terms

abduction
active-assistive exercise
active (isotonic) exercise
activity
adduction
ambulation
ankylosis
anorexia
atony
atrophy
catabolism
circumduction
contracture
coronal plane
demineralization
dyspepsia
eversion
extension
flaccid
flexion
gait
hypercalciuria
hyperextension
hypertonicity
hypertrophy
hypostatic
hypotonicity
inversion
isometric (static) exercise
ligament
orthostatic hypotension
osteoporosis
pace
passive exercise
pronation
protraction
resistive exercise
retraction
rigidity
rotation
sagittal plane
spastic
station
supination
synovial joint
thrombus
tonus
transverse plane

Activity has been described as energetic action or being in a state of movement. Being mobile, able to move freely, is essential and normal for most people. Loss of mobility, even for a short time, generally requires tremendous adjustments by the patient and support persons.

This chapter discusses the need for mobility and activity by people of all ages and conversely the effects that rest in bed (immobility) and inactivity can have on people. A description of the physically fit person will assist nursing students to identify problems that people may have when they exercise inadequately. The kinds of exercise are described, together with guidelines for nurses when they assist patients to meet their exercise needs. The six different types of joints and the types of movements that are normally possible are described. Specific exercises for special situations are also included.

Because many sick people spend more time in bed

than they would normally, ambulation can become a major problem to them. Helping patients retain or regain their ambulatory skills can be an important nursing function. Not only does ambulation usually mean to patients that they are closer to resuming their normal activities but it also can indicate that many problems connected with immobility are likely to be avoided.

Although most physical activity also serves as a stimulus to the mind, diversional activities are chiefly directed to this end. They not only help patients pass the time but also meet needs for accomplishment and serve as vehicles for socializing for people who may otherwise have few common interests. These stimulation needs are discussed further in Chapter 35. This chapter notes that physical activity is a basic need of people, and nurses are frequently called on to assist patients with it.

Mobility

Being mobile—that is, being able to move about freely—is a basic human need. To be able to carry out most of life's activities a person needs to be able to move. However, movement is not limited to moving the body from place to place; a person's gestures, facial expressions, and mannerisms also depend on the ability to move.

A number of aspects of mobility are of particular relevance in health care: joint mobility, station and gait, exercise, and activity tolerance.

Joint Mobility

A joint is the functional unit of the musculoskeletal system. It is where the bones of the skeleton articulate. Most of the skeletal muscles attach to the two bones at the joint. These muscles are categorized according to the type of joint movement they produce upon contraction. Muscles are therefore called *flexors, extensors, internal rotators,* etc. The flexor muscles are stronger than the extensor muscles. Thus, when a person is inactive, the joints are pulled into a flexed (bent) position. If this is not counteracted with exercise and position changes, permanent shortening of the muscles develops, and the joint becomes fixed in a flexed position.

Range of motion

The range of motion of a joint is the maximum movement that is possible for that joint. Not all people possess a similar range of motion. Each person's range of motion is determined by genetic inheritance, developmental patterns, the presence or absence of disease, and the amount of physical activity in which the person normally engages.

Types of synovial joints

The body has six types of synovial joints and certain specific movements that are normally possible for each type. A *synovial joint* is freely movable and characteristically has a cavity enclosed by a capsule. Within this capsule is a lining of synovial membrane, which secretes synovial fluid to lubricate the joint. Cartilage of a joint provides a smooth surface upon which a bone can glide during movement. Thick bands of collagenous fibers extending from one bone to another are called *ligaments*; these provide strength for the joint, and they are usually stretched tautly when the joint is in the position of greatest stability. The muscles surrounding the joint provide the most stability for the joint. Synovial joints of the body serve primarily to bear weight and to provide for movement.

Ball and socket In ball and socket joints, the ball-shaped head of one bone fits into the concave socket of another bone or bones. This type of joint provides for the greatest movement in all planes. Examples are the hip and shoulder joints.

Hinge In the hinge joint, a bone with a convex surface fits into one with a concave surface. The motion of this type of joint is limited to flexion and extension. Examples are the elbow and knee joints.

Pivot The pivot joint is made up of a process that rotates within a bony fossa around a longitudinal axis. The motion of this joint is limited to rotation. Examples are the axis and atlas joints of the vertebral column.

Condyloid In the condyloid joint, an oval-shaped bony projection fits into an elliptical cavity. This kind of joint does not permit rotation; it permits movement in only two planes. An example is the wrist, which permits flexion, extension, and hyperextension in one plane, and abduction and adduction in the second plane, but not rotation.

Saddle In the saddle joint, each bony surface has a convex and a concave surface so that the two bones fit together. This kind of joint does not permit rotation, but movement is possible in the two planes at right angles to each other. For example, the carpometacarpal joint of the thumb and the hand permits flexion and extension, abduction and adduction.

Gliding The gliding joint is formed when the two bone surfaces are flat or when one is slightly convex and the other is slightly concave, so that they glide over each other. Examples are the joint between the tibia and fibula and the intervertebral joints.

Synovial joint movements

Each type of synovial joint has specific movements of which it is capable. These movements are described in relation to the anatomic body position and the three body planes: sagittal, transverse, and coronal. The *sagittal plane* is a vertical line or plane dividing the body or its parts into right and left portions. The *transverse plane* is a horizontal line or plane dividing the body or its parts into superior and inferior portions. The *coronal plane* is any plane dividing the body into anterior (ventral) and posterior (dorsal) portions at right angles to the sagittal plane.

The following are movements of synovial joints:

1. *Flexion*—decreasing the angle between two bones, that is, bending the joint (for example, bending the arm at the elbow joint).
2. *Extension*—increasing the angle between two bones, that is, straightening the joint (for example, straightening the arm at the elbow joint).
3. *Hyperextension*—further extension between two bones or stretching out a joint (for example, bending the head backward).
4. *Abduction*—movement of the bone away from the midline of the body (for example, raising the arm at the shoulder joint laterally).
5. *Adduction*—movement of the bone toward the midline of the body (for example, lowering the arm held laterally toward the side of the body).
6. *Rotation*—movement of the bone around its central axis (for example, turning the head as if to look over the shoulder). Internal rotation is turning toward the midline, external rotation is turning away from the midline. An example of these kinds of rotation occurs at the hip joint. In the back-lying position, a person's leg normally rotates externally at the the hip.
7. *Circumduction*—movement of the distal part of the bone in a circle while the proximal end remains fixed (for example, describing a circle with the arm, moving the shoulder joint).
8. *Eversion*—turning the sole of the foot outward by moving the ankle joint.
9. *Inversion*—turning the sole of the foot inward by moving the ankle joint.
10. *Pronation*—moving the bones of the forearm so that the palm of the hand is moved from anterior to posterior in anatomic position or turning the hand face downward when held in front of the person.
11. *Supination*—moving the bones of the forearm so that the palm of the hand is moved from posterior to anterior in anatomic position or turning the hand face upward when held in front of the person.
12. *Protraction*—moving a part of the body forward in the same plane parallel to the ground (for example, pushing the lower jaw outward).
13. *Retraction*—moving a part of the body backward in the same plane parallel to the ground (for example, pulling the lower jaw inward).

Table 24–1 Muscles Used in Walking

Muscle	Action
Psoas major	Flexes the thigh
Biceps femoris	Flexes the knee
Gluteus maximus	Extends the thigh
Quadriceps femoris	Extends the knee, flexes the thigh
Tibialis anterior	Dorsiflexes the foot
Gastrocnemius	Plantar flexes the foot
Soleus	Plantar flexes the foot

Station and Gait

Station, or stance, is the way a person stands; *gait* is the way a person walks or ambulates. The desirable station of a person provides good body alignment. However, because of postural habits or disease processes, a poor stance can develop. Poor body alignment causes the individual to place undue strain on some of the muscles and bones of the body. See Chapter 23, page 558, for descriptions of the well-aligned adult sitting and standing positions, and page 559 for postural variations according to age. The chief muscles used in walking are the muscles of the thighs and legs. Table 24–1 lists some of these muscles and their actions.

The mechanics of walking take place in two phases: the swing phase and the weight-bearing phase. From a standing or a double-stance position (both feet bearing weight), the individual starts the swing phase by shifting the body weight to one foot while lifting the other foot and bringing it forward. The foot that is brought forward is dorsiflexed. See Figure 24–1. During the swing phase the body turns slightly, but balance is maintained by moving the arm on the opposite side. The heel of the forward foot is then placed on the ground, completing the swing phase.

The weight-bearing phase includes shifting the body weight to the forward heel, moving the weight along the outer edge of the foot to the ball of the foot, and then moving the weight to the toes, from which the individual starts the next step.

When walking, the well-aligned person appears as follows:

1. The head is erect.
2. The vertebral column is normally straight.
3. The toes point forward.
4. The patellas (kneecaps) point forward.
5. The elbows are slightly flexed.

Pace is the distance covered in a step or the number of steps per minute. The normal walking pace of an adult is 70–100 steps per minute. A fast pace is 120 steps per minute. An elderly person often has a slow pace, perhaps 40 steps per minute. Children have a slower pace, depending on their age.

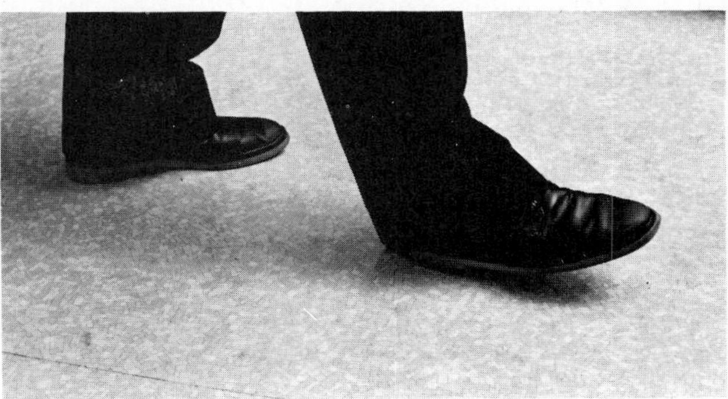

Figure 24–1 When a person walks, the foot that is brought forward is dorsiflexed.

Exercise

Exercise has a number of purposes: (a) to restore, maintain, or increase the tone and strength of the muscles, (b) to maintain or increase the flexibility of the joints, (c) to maintain or promote the growth of bones through the application of physical stressors, and (d) to improve the functioning of other body systems.

Effects of exercise

Exercise has a number of positive effects and can prevent a number of health problems. The latter benefit is of particular importance to patients who are ill and need to avoid further health complications. Effects on each of the body systems are discussed in turn.

Musculoskeletal system Since use of an organ tends to maintain its normal state, exercise maintains the tone and strength of muscles. *Tonus*, the continual slight contraction of muscles, is a normal state of muscles. Healthy muscles have good tone. A muscle with no tone is referred to as an *atonic muscle*, or one in a state of *atony*. *Hypertonicity* refers to excessive muscle tone and *hypotonicity* to inadequate muscle tone.

Muscle size changes in proportion to use; an unused muscle will atrophy, whereas an overused muscle will hypertrophy. *Atrophy* means a wasting away or decrease in size, and it can refer to a cell, tissue, or other organ of the body as well as to a muscle. *Hypertrophy* is an increase in size of an organ or tissue, e.g., muscle tissue. It is due to an increase in size of the cells. People confined to bed tend to develop atrophy of their muscles as a result of disuse. Athletes, on the other hand, often develop hypertrophied muscles from continual use; for example, distance runners may have hypertrophied femoral muscles and boxers hypertrophy of the biceps muscles.

Exercise also maintains joint mobility. Joints that lose their normal range of motion may develop problems such as ankylosis and contractures. *Ankylosis* refers to a stiffening of a joint. This is generally caused by scar tissue or bony growth, and it can result in complete immobility of the joint or in some cases deformity. *Contracture* is permanent shortening (contraction) of a muscle. See page 600 for further information.

Because bone density is maintained through weight bearing, it too is aided by exercise and activity.

Cardiovascular system The blood circulation, especially venous flow, is improved with exercise. The cardiac rate is increased, and blood vessels in the working muscles dilate to deliver needed nutrients to the muscles. The increased blood flow also assists in elimination of waste products from the muscles and in delivery of oxygen and nutrients to the tissues. As muscles contract, superficial veins are milked or compressed, thus assisting the return flow of blood against gravity to the heart. This muscular action in the lower extremities is often likened to a pump and thus is referred to as the second pump of the body (the heart being the prime pump). The increased cardiac rate also helps to increase the strength of the cardiac muscle.

Metabolism Exercise increases the metabolic rate, as energy is required for muscle function. It also stimulates the appetite.

Respiratory system The ventilation rate and depth are increased with exercise, as the body requires more oxygen in response to the increased metabolic rate. The increased respiration supplies oxygen to the active muscles and eliminates carbon dioxide so that it does not accumulate in the blood, which would increase the acidity of the blood.

Gastrointestinal system Appetite is improved and the muscle tone of the gastrointestinal tract is increased by exercise. As a result, elimination of feces and flatus is facilitated.

Psychoneurologic system Exercise assists in restoring a sense of relaxation and equilibrium. People perceive an increase in their energy and a sense of well-being with regular exercise.

Urinary system Exercise promotes urinary function by improving the blood flow to and from the kidneys. Thus body wastes are excreted more effectively.

Kinds of exercises

There are a number of kinds of exercise. The choice appropriate to the individual patient depends on the health and strength of the person and the purpose to be accomplished.

Active or *isotonic exercises* are carried out by the patient, who supplies the energy to move the body parts. This type of exercise serves both to increase and to maintain muscle tone, to maintain joint mobility, and to provide the other effects discussed earlier.

Passive exercises are those in which the energy required to move the body part is provided by a nurse, by mechanical equipment, or by the patient to an impaired extremity. These exercises maintain joint mobility only; because the muscles do not contract, muscular atrophy is not prevented.

Active-assistive exercises are carried out by the patient with some assistance from a nurse. The patient moves the body part as far as personally possible, and then the nurse moves it through the remainder of the normal range of motion. These exercises encourage normal muscle function.

In *isometric* or *static exercises* no joint movement occurs, and the length of the muscle is unchanged. The patient consciously increases the tension of the muscles without moving joints, by holding the tension for several seconds, then relaxing. These exercises maintain muscle strength, thus preventing significant atrophy, but they do not affect joint mobility. Patients who have casts frequently require these exercises.

Resistive exercises consist of contraction of a muscle against an opposing force. The force may be manual or mechanical (for example, lifting a weight). Resistive exercises increase muscle size, strength, and power and involve some joint mobility.

Activity Tolerance

Activity tolerance or endurance is the ability to withstand activity in terms of duration. It generally increases with repeated activity over a period of time. Tolerance is affected by a number of factors: pain, physical strength, cardiopulmonary status, age, lifestyle, and emotional state.

The individual who experiences pain with activity will normally tolerate the activity for a shorter time than the person who experiences no pain. Physical strength is directly proportional to activity tolerance; the weaker the person, the greater the energy required to carry out the activity, and the sooner muscle fatigue is experienced. Impaired functioning of the cardiopulmonary systems can limit the flow of oxygen and nutrients to the exercising muscles, decreasing activity tolerance. The elderly often tolerate exercise less well than younger persons. With increasing age the body's muscle mass, and thus the person's strength, is reduced. People with a less active life-style tire sooner with exercise than those who have good muscle tone. A positive attitude and the desire to carry out an activity also increase an individual's tolerance. The depressed person often tires sooner than an emotionally healthy person.

Assessment

Activity and mobility are highly individual. They depend to a large degree upon habits developed throughout life and the importance the individual attaches to activity as a means of maintaining health. Four major areas of assessment related to activity are: factors influencing mobility and activity; joint movements; station and gait; and activity tolerance.

Factors Influencing Mobility and Activity

Life-style

People learn early in life, often from their families, the value of activity in relation to health. Some children are encouraged to play actively out of doors, while others spend much of their time in front of the television set. Some people participate in physical activity regularly in an effort to maintain or improve their health.

Other life-style factors include the use of alcohol or tobacco. These can affect the individual's activity pattern. For example, the person who drinks alcohol during an evening is not likely to go jogging or swimming; a heavy smoker is likely to become short of breath quickly with physical exertion.

Disease process or injury

To be mobile and active, an individual needs to have functioning musculoskeletal and nervous systems. Disease processes such as multiple sclerosis and injuries to the spinal cord can seriously affect an individual's mobility and subsequent activity.

Mobility can also be limited because of fear and/or pain. A patient who has recently undergone surgery may be reluctant to move for fear of opening the incision or because of the pain experienced with movement.

A person who has a disease or is injured is often restricted in activity by the physician. Bed rest is commonly advised in illness. It usually has two purposes: (a) to conserve the body's energy, so that a diseased or injured part of the body will heal, and (b) to prevent further damage to a body part. A person who has had a myocardial infarction usually requires bed rest for both purposes. A person with a fractured hip may be confined to bed with the leg in traction until adequate healing has taken place. Whatever the cause, when people enter the hospital their activity is generally restricted by regulations of the institution.

Culture

Some cultures place greater stress on physical activity than others. The boy who lives in a small town in France walks to and from school each day, while the North American boy living in a middle-class suburb rides to and from school. Adults in North America often watch sports activities, while adults in less industrialized nations often participate in their own activities.

Individual energy level

Energy levels vary greatly among individuals and within a person. Sometimes people voluntarily restrict their activity, without always knowing why or without feeling ill. The reason is generally that the person requires withdrawal from physical and psychologic stressors to maintain physical and psychologic equilibrium. A student, after final examinations, may want only to go to bed and sleep, to regain energy and stability.

Age and developmental status

Age greatly affects activity levels. For example, the average person of middle age and older "slows down" from earlier activity levels. Assessment information for developmental levels from birth to age 5 is presented in the sections that follow.

Neonates (birth to 28 days) The functioning of the central nervous system is immature for some time after birth. Control of neonates' motor activity thus lacks coordination. Their extremities move in a random fashion, and they cannot direct their movements toward any purpose. However, their muscles are firm, and, when an extremity is extended passively, the flexor muscles offer assistance. Many of the newborn's activities are reflexive. These are:

1. Coughing and sneezing
2. Yawning
3. Hiccupping
4. Blinking
5. Withdrawing from pain
6. Crying when uncomfortable
7. Sucking
8. Rooting (turning the head to the side on which the cheek is touched)
9. Swallowing, gagging, and vomiting
10. The grasp reflex
11. The stepping reflex
12. The Moro reflex
13. The tonic neck reflex

These reflexes are discussed in Chapter 11 on page 243.

Infants (28 days to 1 year)

Movement of the head When placed in a prone position, newborns can turn the head readily from side to side. By 4 weeks of age, infants can lift the head off the surface.

At 3 months of age, infants can lift the head and chest from the surface with arms extended in front, and at 4 months they can raise the head to the vertical position and turn it easily from side to side. By 7 months, infants in the prone position can pivot when pursuing an object.

In the supine position, infants lie with the head turned to one side. In this position at 6 months they can lift the head up and spend much time showing interest in their legs.

Head control is lacking when infants are placed in a sitting position or an upright position until about 5 months of age. In the first 2 months, the head falls backward when an infant is pulled from a supine to a sitting position, and it bobs around without control in the upright position. For this reason, when picking up or holding an infant under 3 months old, the nurse must support the head and back (which bows forward).

By 3 months of age, some head control is evident when infants hold the head forward in the upright position. At 4 months, they can hold the head fairly erect in the sitting position but tilt the head slightly forward in the upright position. By 5 months, the head is held steadily in the erect position.

Movements of the hands The grasp reflex (curling of the fingers around an object placed in the palm) continues for about two months until eye and hand coordination develops sufficiently for an active grasp to become possible. At 3 months of age, infants attempt to hold an offered object briefly and can purposefully move the hand to the mouth to satisfy sucking needs. At 4 months, infants can grasp objects of moderate size and move them to the mouth for exploration. Small objects are not properly visualized. By 6 months, they can extend a hand toward a desired large object such as a rattle, grasp it, and transfer it from hand to hand. By 7 months, they can visualize small objects and may pursue these with raking motions of the fingers, but they are unable to pick them up.

After 6 months, the hand movements primarily involve the radial side. At first the thumb is used in conjunction with the palm of the hand. Between 6 and 9 months, the movements are more clearly refined into pincer motions of the thumb and forefinger. At 9 months, the index finger is used to poke at objects. At that age an infant might release an object upon request if another person grasps the object. By 1 year, most infants will independently release an object into an offered hand.

Sitting By 4 to 5 months of age, infants enjoy being in a sitting position but must be supported. Not until after 6 months are infants able to sit alone as they lean forward on their hands. By 8 to 9 months, they can assume a sitting position from the supine position without help.

Standing, creeping, and walking At 5 to 6 months, infants support their weight on extended legs when pulled from a sitting to a standing position. By 8 months, they are able to stand steadily for a short while, if their hands are held. By 9 to 10 months, most infants have mastered creeping or crawling and can walk a few steps if both hands are held.

Ages 1 to 5 During the second year, children begin to reveal a high degree of locomotor control, progressing from an awkward upright stance to taking a few steps with assistance. Children develop the ability to walk alone by about 15 months. The skill of running is acquired at about 18 months although the motion at first appears awkward and stiff. Between 18 and 24 months, children are very active and run about, often into dangerous environments unless safeguarded. This is the age that has been so aptly called the "terrible twos," in which children actively and vigorously explore all objects in their environment. Everything within reach is grasped and examined; wastebaskets, drawers, and shelves will all be emptied. Motor control of the hand is also refined. For example, children will place small objects into small containers, balance building blocks one on top of the other, and scribble on paper, eventually producing some vertical, horizontal, and circular lines.

The ability to climb stairs begins at the age of 18 months, when children can ascend one step at a time with one hand held. Going downstairs in the same manner soon follows. By 3 years of age, children can alternate feet when ascending stairs, and they can descend in that manner by age 4. Standing on one foot is mastered by most children at the age of 3, and by age 5 most can hop on one foot and skip. See Table 24–2 for a summary of motor skills up to 5 years.

Joint Movements

The joints of the body have normal ranges of motion. When there is any indication or danger of restricted joint movement (for example, with prolonged bed rest), it is important to assess the range of motion of the patient's joints. The following sections describe normal joint movements and their ranges of motion.

Neck—pivot joint

1. Flex the neck by bringing the chin to rest on the chest. Range: 45°. Primary muscle: sternocleidomastoideus. See Figure 24–2.
2. Extend the neck by returning the head to an upright position. Range: 45°. Primary muscle: trapezius. See Figure 24–3.
3. Hyperextend the neck by bending the head back as far as possible. Range: 10°. Primary muscle: trapezius. See Figure 24–4.

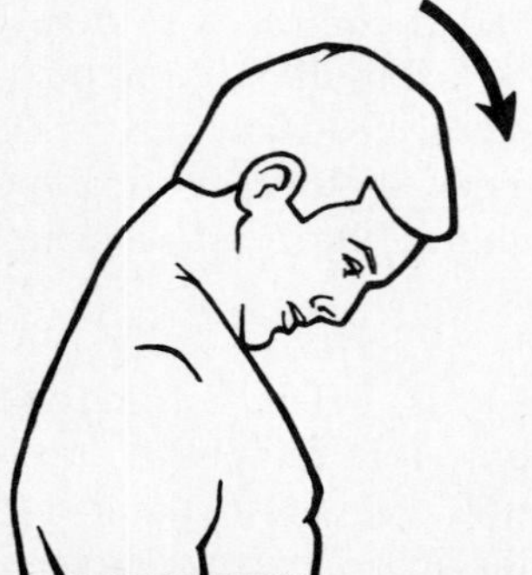

Figure 24–2 Neck flexion.

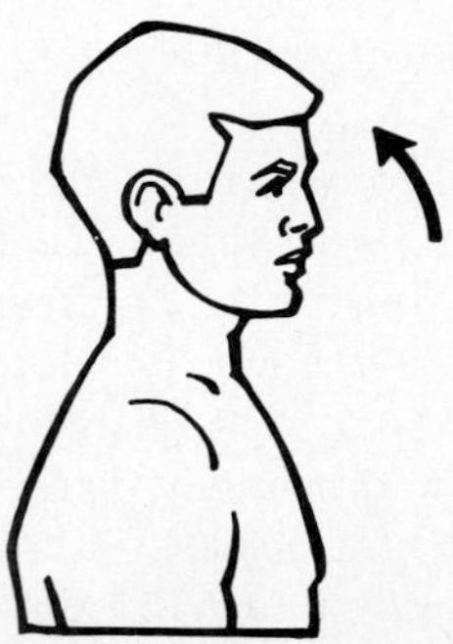

Figure 24–3 Neck extension.

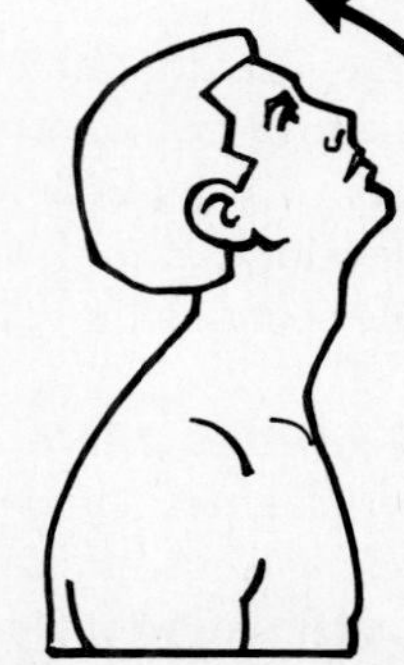

Figure 24–4 Neck hyperextension.

Table 24–2 Summary of Motor Skills from Birth to 5 Years of Age

Age level	Motor skills
First month	Prone: lies in flexed position; turns head from side to side Supine: generally flexed and somewhat stiff Active reflexes: Moro response; grasp reflex; stepping reflex; tonic neck reflex
At 1 month	Prone: holds chin up; turns head; lies with legs more extended Supine: tonic neck posture is predominant; body is more relaxed and supple; head falls backward when infant pulled to sitting position
At 2 months	Prone: raises head farther; active infant may roll over Supine: same as at 1 month
At 3 months	Prone: arches back, lifts head and chest with arms extended forward; makes crawling movements with legs Supine: tonic neck posture still predominant; reaches toward but misses objects; indicates preference for prone or supine position Sitting: head lag partially controlled on pull to sitting position; back is rounded Manual: clutching and scratching movements Active reflexes: Moro response is absent; makes some defensive withdrawal reactions
At 4 to 6 months	Prone: lifts head and chest; head is held in a nearly vertical axis; legs are extended; intentional rolling over by 4 months Supine: symmetrical posture predominates; reaches and grasps objects; brings objects to mouth Sitting: head is held erect, steady, and forward on pull to sitting position; enjoys sitting with spinal and head support Standing: pushes with feet when held upright Manual: arms and hands progress to coordinated reaching and grasping; picks up objects at 4 months; intentionally releases them at 6 months
At 7 months	Prone: can pivot and roll over Supine: lifts head; rolls over; squirms Sitting: sits briefly, leaning forward on hands; spine is rounded from head to buttocks Standing: may support most of weight and bounces Manual: reaches and grasps large objects with thumb to palm; transfers items from hand to hand; rakes at small objects
At 10 months	Sitting: sits up alone without support; spine is straight Standing: pulls to standing position Moving: creeps or crawls
At 12 months	Walks with one hand held or by holding onto furniture
At 15 months	Walks alone; crawls upstairs
At 18 months	Runs awkwardly; sits on small chair; walks upstairs with one hand held, one step at a time; explores all objects in reach
At 24 months	Runs well; walks up and down stairs with one hand held, one step at a time; climbs on furniture; opens doors; can tower building blocks; can scribble in circular manner
At 30 months	Jumps
At 36 months	Goes up stairs alternating feet; rides tricycle; stands on one foot
At 48 months	Hops on one foot; throws ball; climbs well; manipulates scissors; goes down stairs alternating feet
At 60 months	Skips

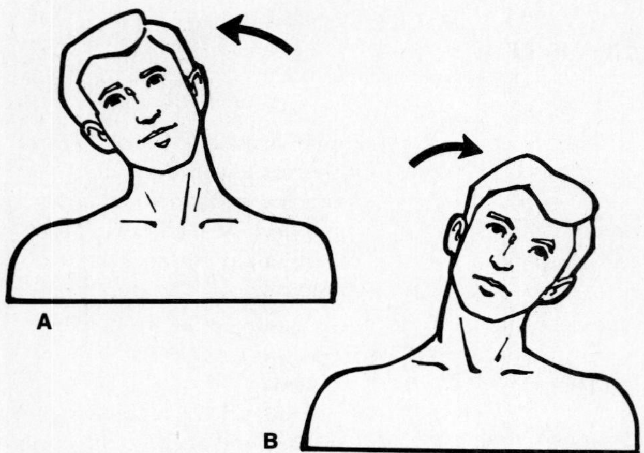

Figure 24–5 Neck lateral flexion: **A,** to the right; **B,** to the left.

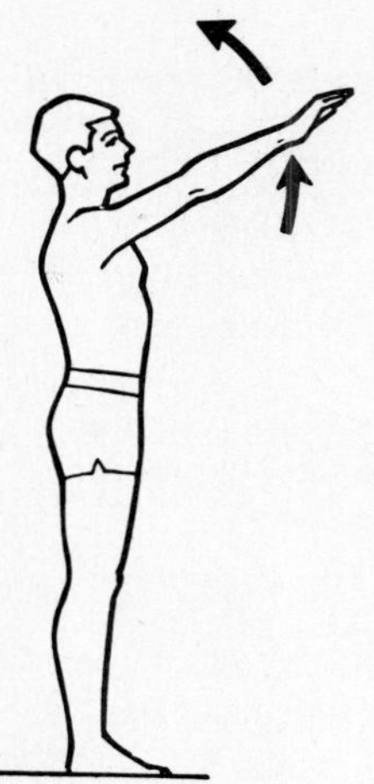

Figure 24–7 Shoulder flexion.

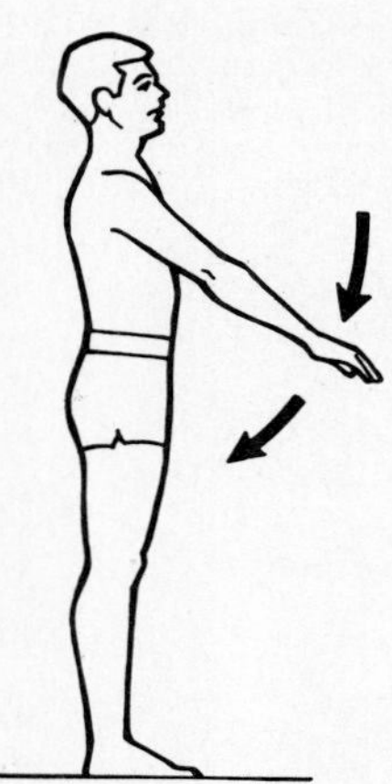

Figure 24–8 Shoulder extension.

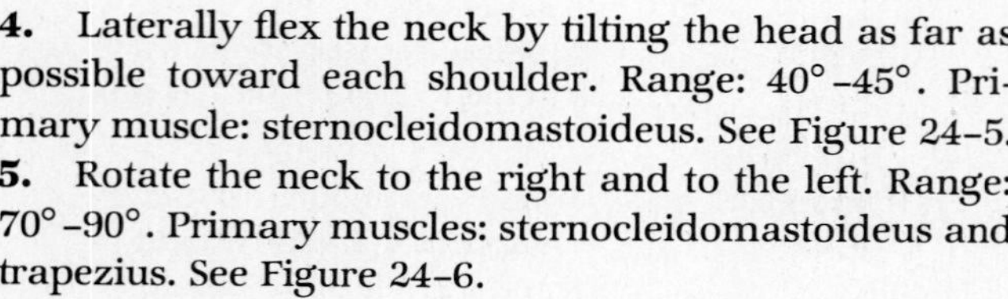

4. Laterally flex the neck by tilting the head as far as possible toward each shoulder. Range: 40°–45°. Primary muscle: sternocleidomastoideus. See Figure 24–5.
5. Rotate the neck to the right and to the left. Range: 70°–90°. Primary muscles: sternocleidomastoideus and trapezius. See Figure 24–6.

Shoulder—ball and socket joint

1. Flex the shoulder by raising the arm from the side position forward to a position above the head, palm facing forward (also called *forward elevation*). Range: 180°. Primary muscles: deltoideus, coracobrachialis. See Figure 24–7.

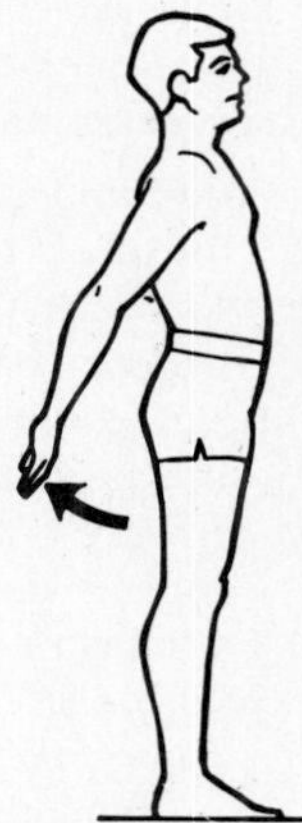

Figure 24–9 Shoulder hyperextension.

2. Extend the shoulder by returning the arm to a position at the side of the body. Range: 180°. Primary muscles: latissimus dorsi, teres major, deltoideus. See Figure 24–8.
3. Hyperextend the shoulder by moving the arm behind the body. Range: 50°–60°. Primary muscles: latissimus dorsi, teres major, deltoideus. See Figure 24–9.
4. Horizontally flex the shoulder by moving the arm, with the elbow extended, through a horizontal plane from a side position to as far across in front of the body as possible. Range: 130°–135°. Primary muscle: pectoralis major. See Figure 24–10.
5. Horizontally extend the shoulder by moving the arm, with the elbow extended, through the horizontal plane from a side position to as far across in back of the body as possible. Range: 45°. Primary muscles: latissimus dorsi, teres major, deltoideus. See Figure 24–11.
6. Circumduct the shoulder by moving the arm in a full circle. Range: 360°. Primary muscles: deltoideus, coracobrachialis, latissimus dorsi, teres major. See Figure 24–12.

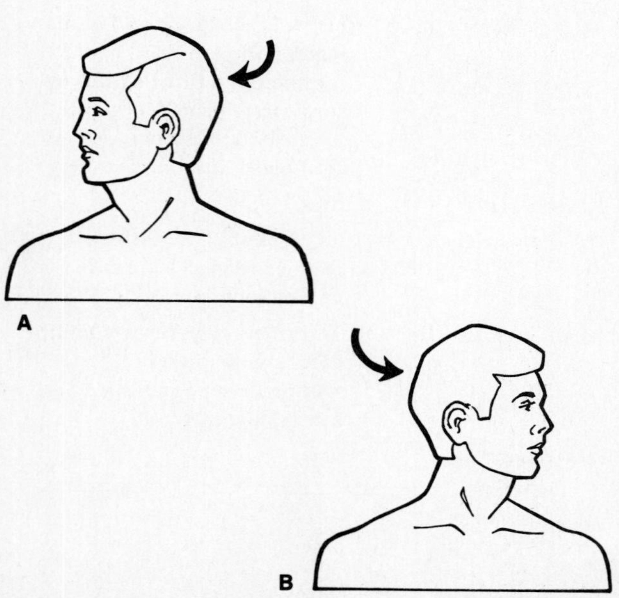

Figure 24–6 Neck rotation: **A,** to the right; **B,** to the left.

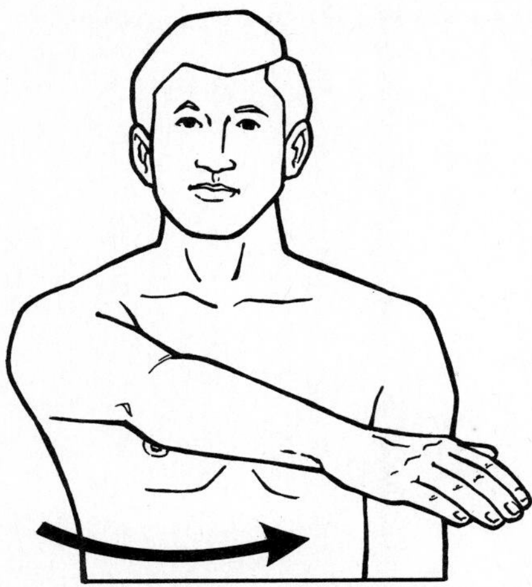

Figure 24–10 Horizontal shoulder flexion or horizontal adduction.

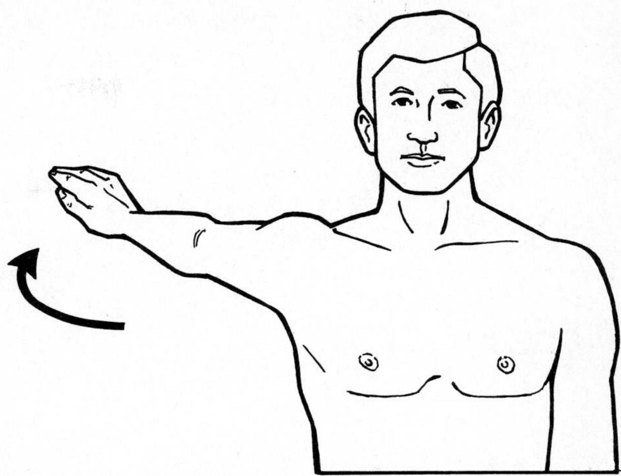

Figure 24–11 Horizontal shoulder extension or horizontal abduction.

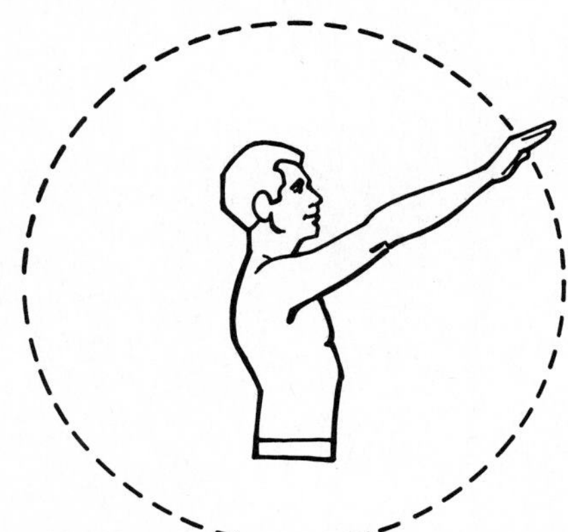

Figure 24–12 Shoulder circumduction.

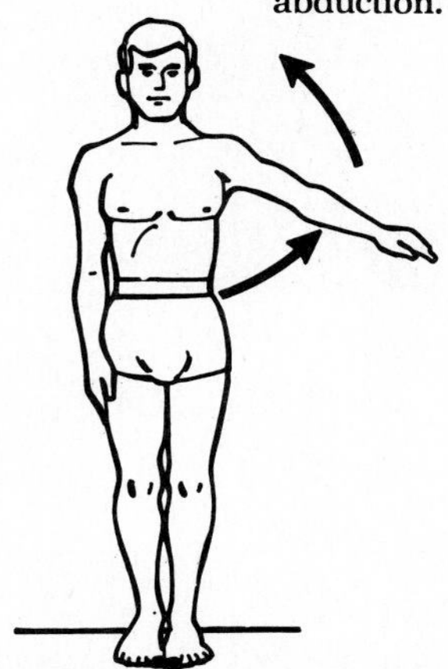

Figure 24–13 Shoulder abduction.

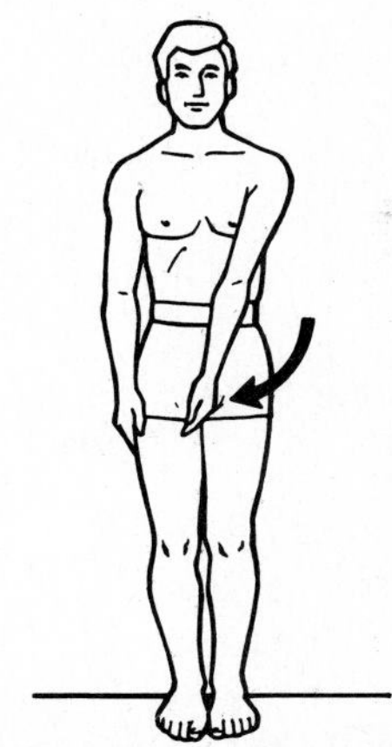

Figure 24–14 Shoulder adduction.

7. Abduct the shoulder by raising the arm to the side until it is above the head, palm facing away from the head. Range: 180°. Primary muscles: deltoideus, supraspinatus. See Figure 24–13.

8. Adduct the shoulder by lowering the arm sideways and across the body as far as possible. Range: 230°. Primary muscle: pectoralis minor. See Figure 24–14.

9. Externally rotate the shoulder by moving the arm until the thumb is lateral to the head. Range: 90°. Primary muscles: infraspinatus, teres minor. See Figure 24–15.

10. Internally rotate the shoulder by moving the arm until the thumb is turned inward and to the back. Range: 90°. Primary muscles: subscapularis, pectoralis major, latissimus dorsi, teres major. See Figure 24–16.

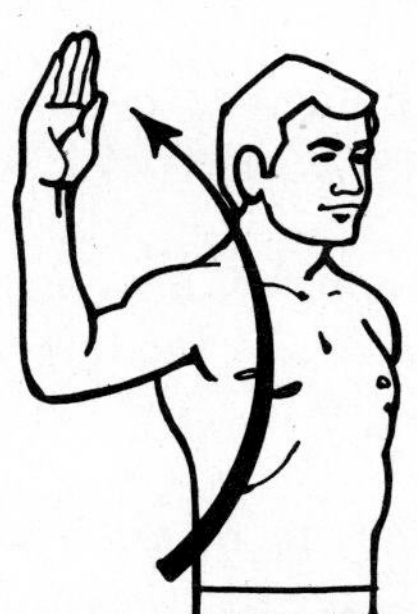

Figure 24–15 External rotation of the shoulder.

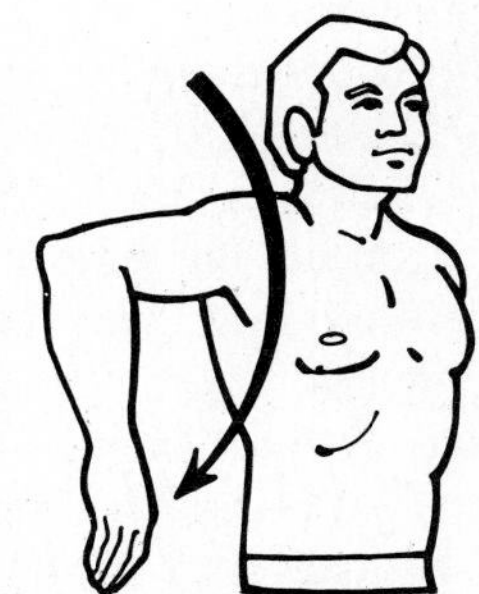

Figure 24–16 Internal rotation of the shoulder.

Elbow—hinge joint

1. Flex the elbow by bending the lower arm so that the hand is at the shoulder. Range: 150°. Primary muscles: biceps brachii, brachialis, brachioradialis. See Figure 24–17.

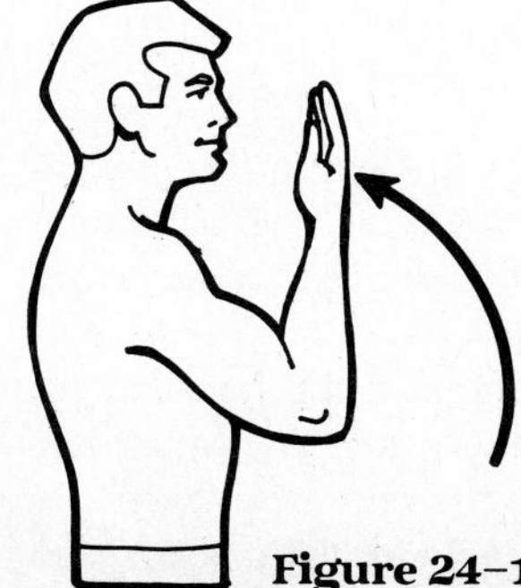

Figure 24–17 Elbow flexion.

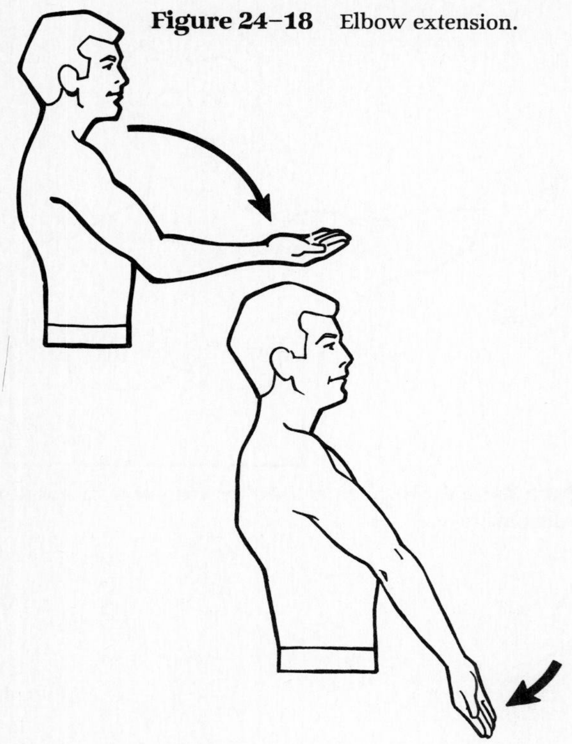

Figure 24–18 Elbow extension.

Figure 24–19 Elbow hyperextension.

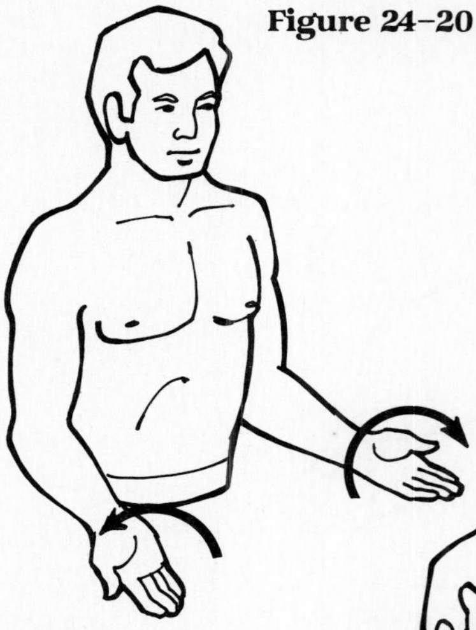

Figure 24–20 Elbow supination.

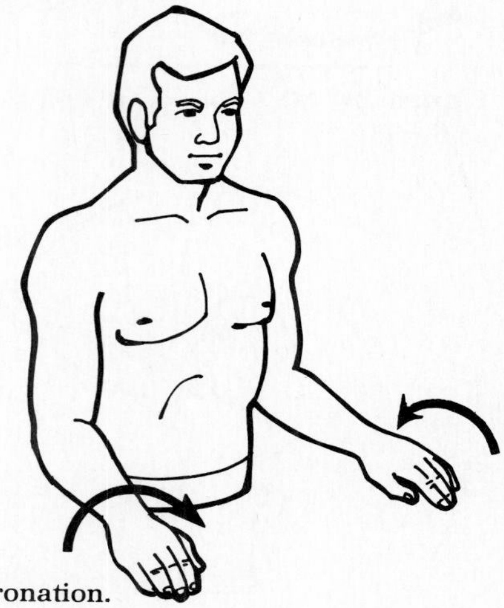

Figure 24–21 Elbow pronation.

2. Extend the elbow by straightening the lower arm. Range: 150°. Primary muscle: triceps brachii. See Figure 24–18.
3. Hyperextend the elbow by bending the lower arm back. Range: 0°–15°. Primary muscle: triceps brachii. See Figure 24–19.
4. Rotate the elbow for supination by turning the hand and lower arm so that the palm is facing upward. Range: 70°–90°. Primary muscles: biceps brachii, supinator. See Figure 24–20.
5. Rotate the elbow for pronation by turning the hand and lower arm so that the palm is facing downward. Range: 70°–90°. Primary muscles: pronator teres, pronator quadratus. See Figure 24–21.

Wrist—condyloid joint

1. Flex the wrist by bringing the fingers toward the inner aspect of the forearm. Range: 80°–90°. Primary muscles: flexor carpi radialis, flexor carpi ulnaris. See Figure 24–22.
2. Extend the wrist by straightening the hand to the same plane as the arm. Range: 80°–90°. Primary muscles: extensor carpi radialis longus, extensor carpi radialis brevis, extensor carpi ulnaris. See Figure 24–23.
3. Hyperextend the wrist by bringing the fingers back as far as possible. Range: 70°–90°. Primary muscles: extensor carpi radialis longus, extensor carpi radialis brevis, extensor carpi ulnaris. See Figure 24–24.
4. Abduct the wrist (ulnar flexion) by bending it laterally toward the fifth finger. The wrist is pronated. Range: 30°–50°. Primary muscle: extensor carpi radialis longus. See Figure 24–25.
5. Adduct the wrist (radial flexion) by bending it laterally toward the thumb. The wrist is pronated. Range: 0°–20°. Primary muscle: extensor carpi ulnaris. See Figure 24–26.

Hand, fingers, and thumb: metacarpophalangeal joints—condyloid; interphalangeal joints—hinge

See Figure 24–27.

1. Flex the hand and fingers by making a fist. Range: 90°. Primary muscles: flexor pollicis brevis, flexor pollicis longus. See Figure 24–28.
2. Extend the hand and fingers by straightening them. Range: 90°. Primary muscles: extensor pollicis brevis, extensor pollicis longus. See Figure 24–29.
3. Hyperextend the hand by bending the metacarpophalangeal joints backward. Range: 30°–90°. Primary

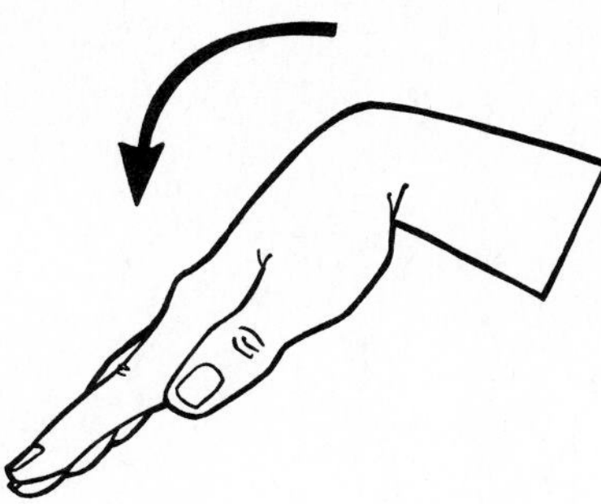

Figure 24–22 Wrist flexion.

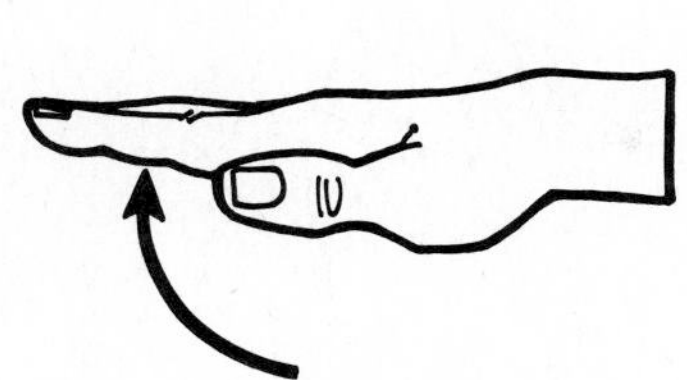

Figure 24–23 Wrist extension.

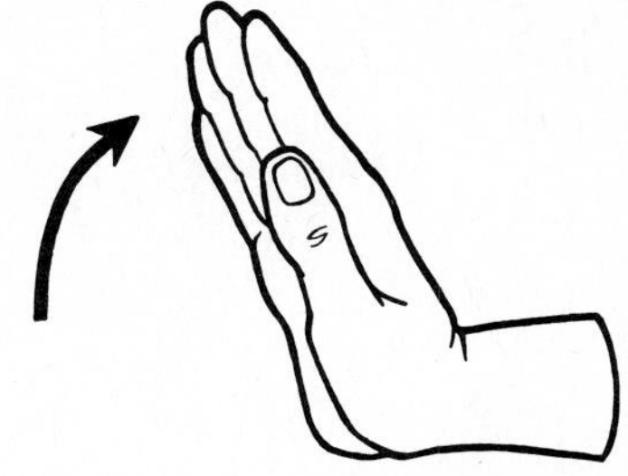

Figure 24–24 Wrist hyperextension.

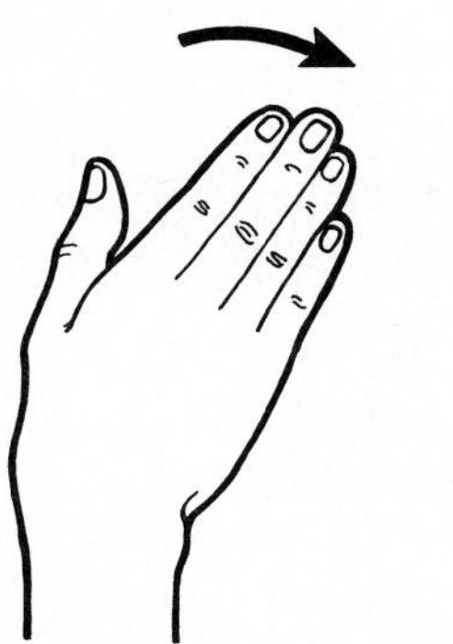

Figure 24–25 Wrist abduction.

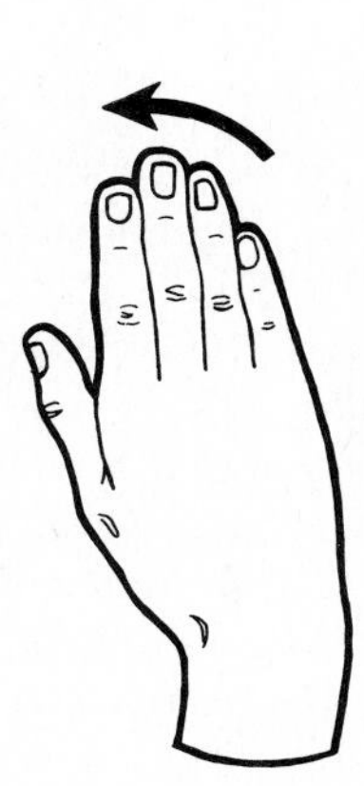

Figure 24–26 Wrist adduction.

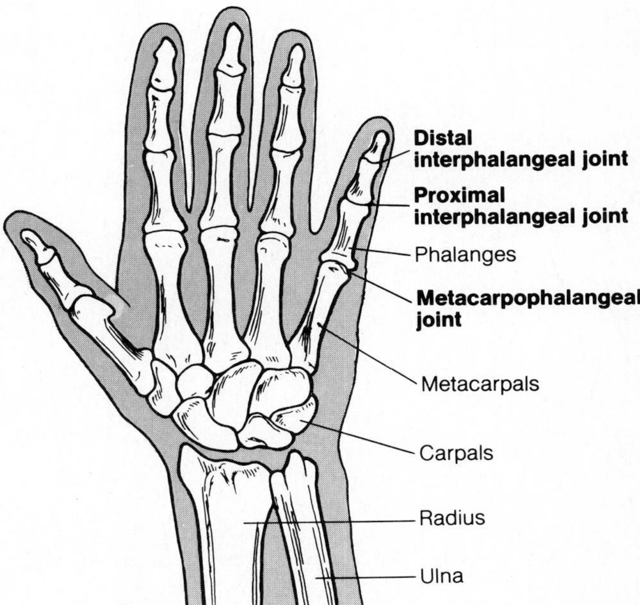

Figure 24–27 Joints of the hand.

muscles: extensor pollicis brevis, extensor pollicis longus. See Figure 24-30.

4. Abduct the fingers by spreading the fingers and thumb. Range: 20° between fingers. Primary muscles: abductor pollicis longus, abductor pollicis brevis, interossei dorsales manus, abductor digiti minimi manus. See Figure 24-31.

5. Adduct the fingers by bringing them together. Range: 20° between fingers. Primary muscles: adductor pollicis caput obliquum, adductor pollicis caput transversum, interossei palmares. See Figure 24-32.

6. Oppose the thumb by touching the tip of each finger. The thumb joint movements involved are: abduction, rotation, and flexion. Primary muscles: opponens pollicis, opponens digiti minimi. See Figure 24-33.

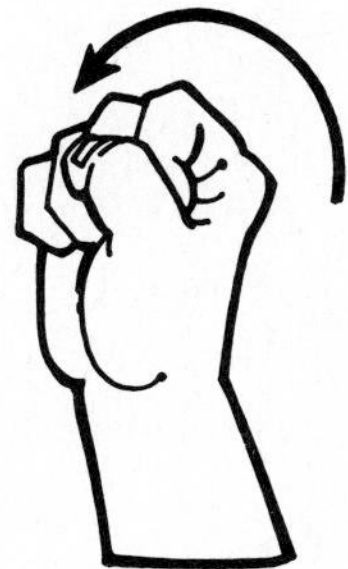

Figure 24–28 Flexion of the hand and fingers.

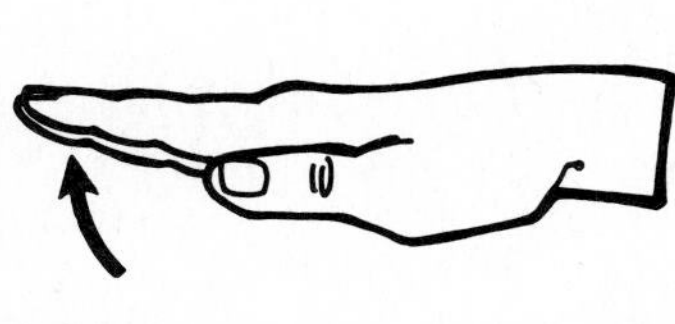

Figure 24–29 Extension of the hand and fingers.

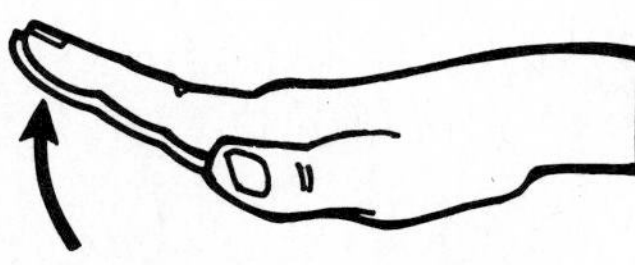

Figure 24–30 Hyperextension of the hand and fingers.

Hip—ball and socket joint

1. Flex the hip by moving the leg forward and up. Range: knee straight, 90° or less; knee flexed, 110°–120°. Primary muscles: psoas major, iliacus. See Figure 24-34.

2. Extend the hip by moving the leg back down beside the other leg. Range: knee straight, 90° or less; knee

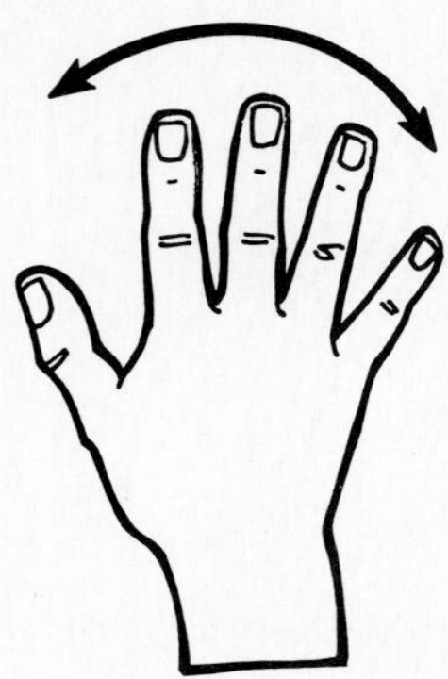

Figure 24–31 Abduction of the fingers and thumb.

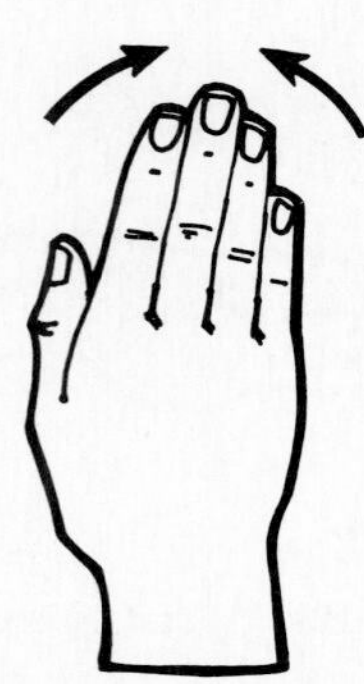

Figure 24–32 Adduction of the fingers and thumb.

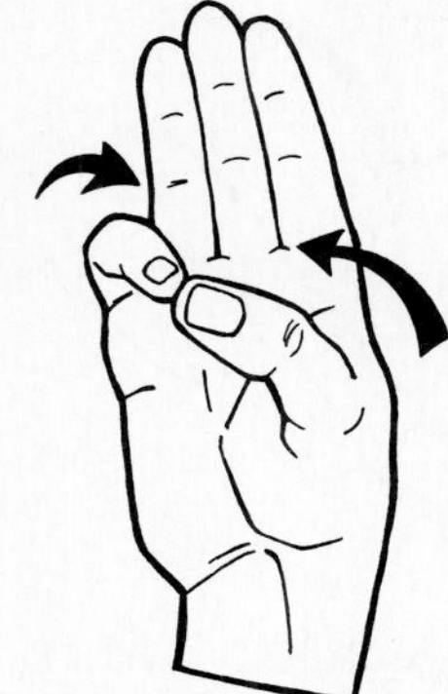

Figure 24–33 Opposition of the thumb.

flexed, 110°–120°. Primary muscles: gluteus maximus, semitendinosus, semimembranosus, biceps femoris. See Figure 24–35.

3. Hyperextend the hip by moving the leg behind the body. Range: 30°–50°. Primary muscles: gluteus maximus, semitendinosus, semimembranosus, biceps femoris. See Figure 24–36.

4. Abduct the hip by moving the leg out to the side. Range: 45°–50°. Primary muscle: gluteus medius. See Figure 24–37.

5. Adduct the hip by moving the leg to the other leg and beyond it. Range: 20°–30° beyond the other leg. Primary muscles: adductor magnus, adductor brevis, adductor longus, pectineus. See Figure 24–38.

6. Circumduct the hip by moving the leg in a circle. Range: 360°. Primary muscles: psoas major, gluteus maximus, adductor magnus, gluteus medius. See Figure 24–39.

7. Inwardly rotate the hip by turning the foot and leg so that the toes are turned as far as possible toward the other leg. Range: 90°. Major muscles: gluteus minimus, tensor fasciae latae. See Figure 24–40.

8. Outwardly rotate the hip by turning the foot and leg so that the toes are turned as far as possible away from the other leg. Range: 90°. Major muscles: obturator externus, obturator internus, quadratus femoris. See Figure 24–41.

Knee—hinge joint

1. Flex the knee by bending the leg, bringing the heel toward the back of the thigh. Range: 120°–130°. Primary muscles: biceps femoris, semitendinosus, semimembranosus. See Figure 24–42.

2. Extend the knee by straightening the leg. Range: 120°–130°. Primary muscles: rectus femoris, vastus intermedius, vastus medialis, vastus lateralis. See Figure 24–43.

3. In some people the knee can also be hyperextended 10°.

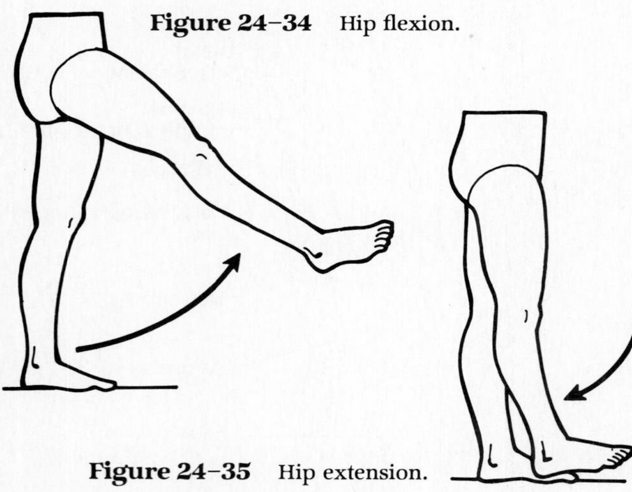

Figure 24–34 Hip flexion.

Figure 24–35 Hip extension.

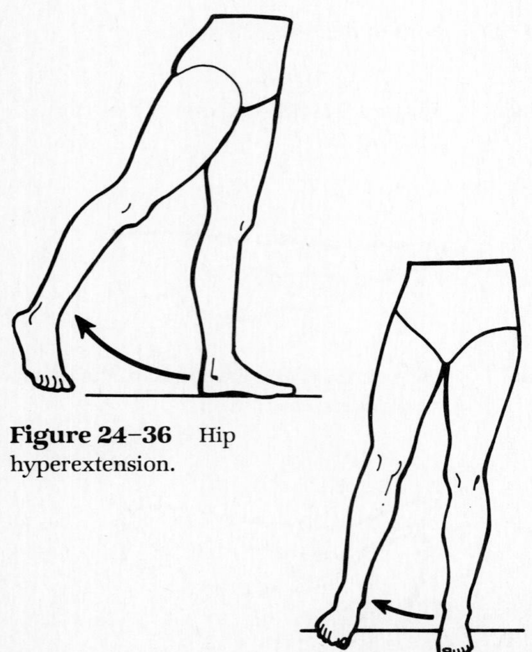

Figure 24–36 Hip hyperextension.

Figure 24–37 Hip abduction.

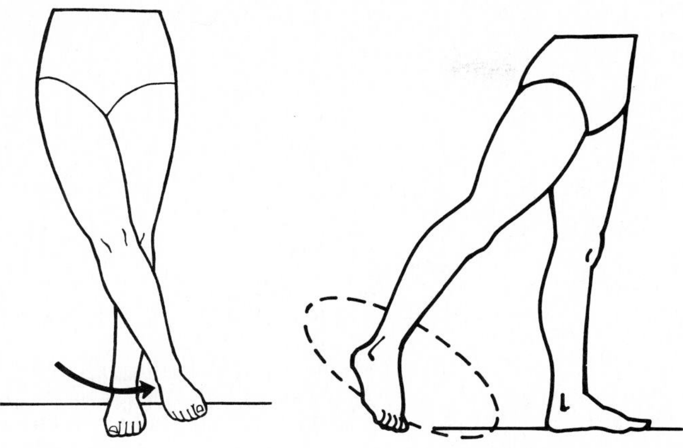

Figure 24–38
Hip adduction.

Figure 24–39
Hip circumduction.

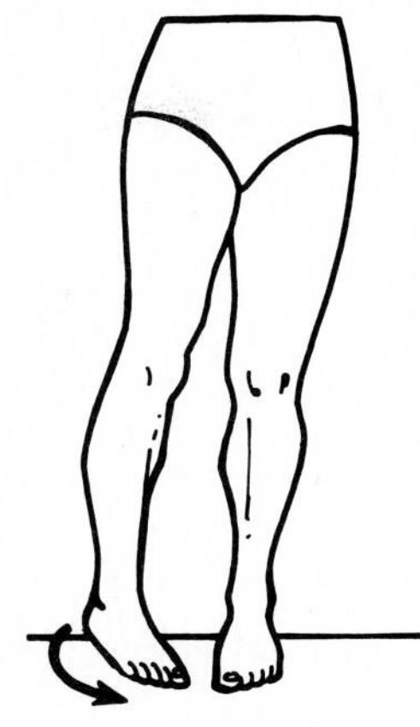

Figure 24–40
Internal rotation of the hip.

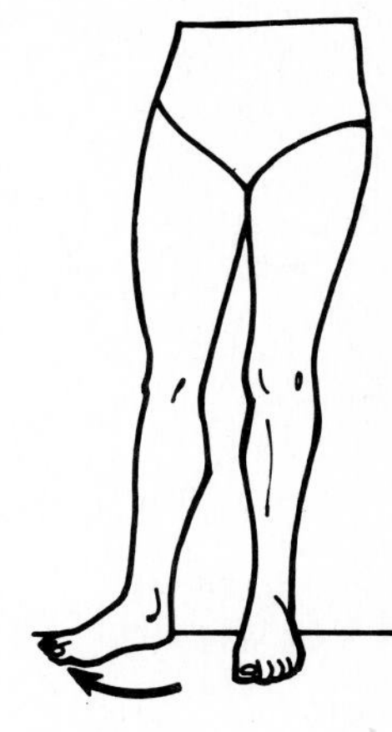

Figure 24–41
External rotation of the hip.

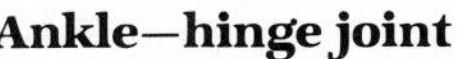

Ankle—hinge joint

1. Move the ankle to plantar flexion (flexion) so that the toes are pointed down. Range: 45°–50°. Primary muscles: gastrocnemius, soleus. See Figure 24–44.
2. Move the ankle to dorsal flexion (dorsiflexion, extension) so that the toes point up toward the knee. Range: 20°. Primary muscle: tibialis anterior. See Figure 24–45.

Foot and toes: interphalangeal joint—hinge; metatarsophalangeal joint—hinge

See Figure 24–46.

1. Evert the foot joints by turning the sole of the foot laterally. Range: 5°. Primary muscles: peroneus longus, peroneus brevis. See Figure 24–47.

Figure 24–46 Joints of the foot.

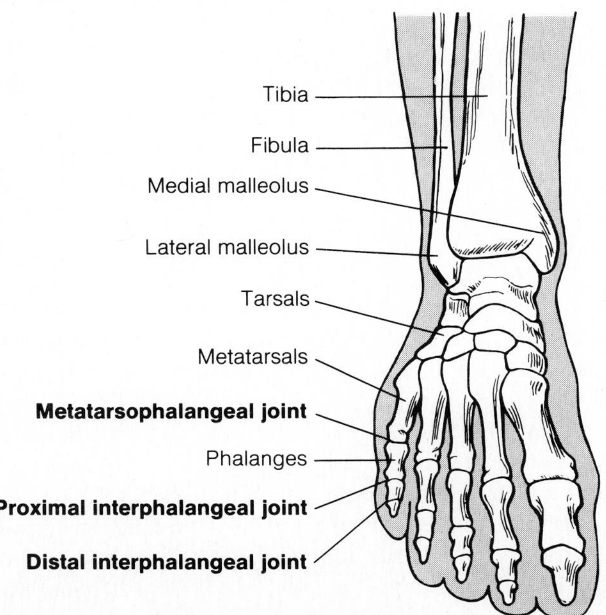

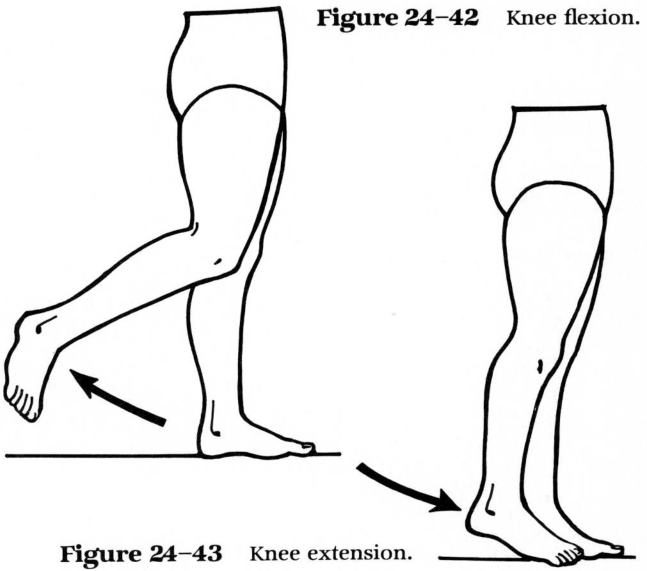

Figure 24–42 Knee flexion.

Figure 24–43 Knee extension.

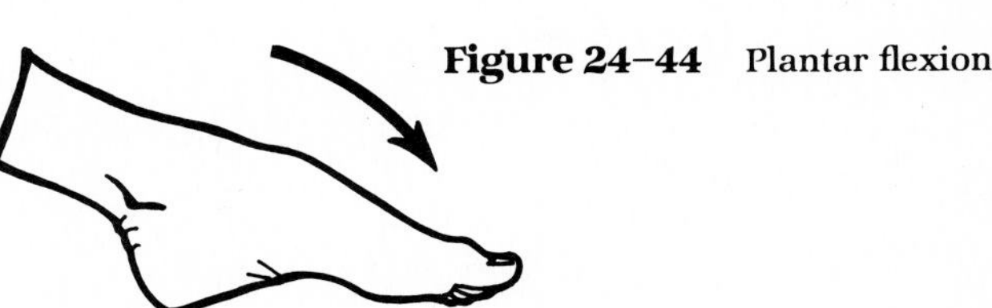

Figure 24–44 Plantar flexion.

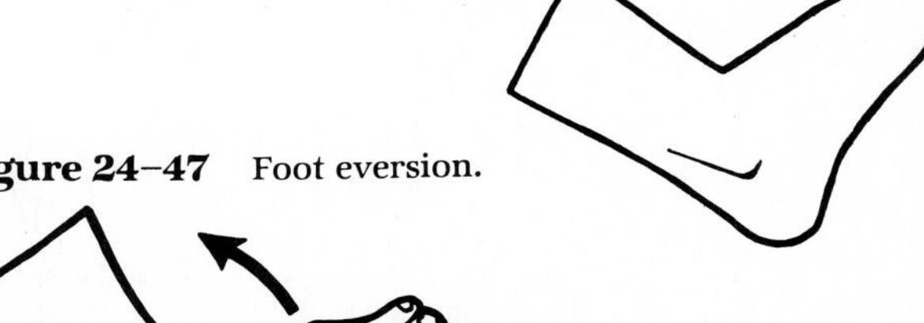

Figure 24–45 Dorsal flexion.

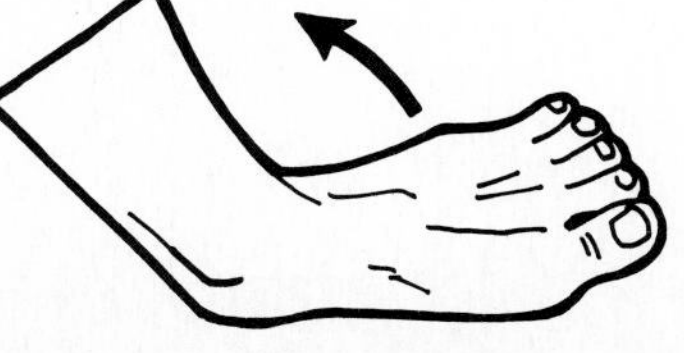

Figure 24–47 Foot eversion.

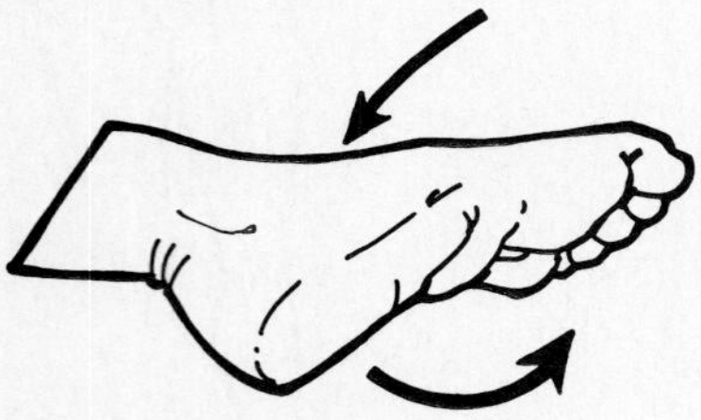

Figure 24–48 Foot inversion.

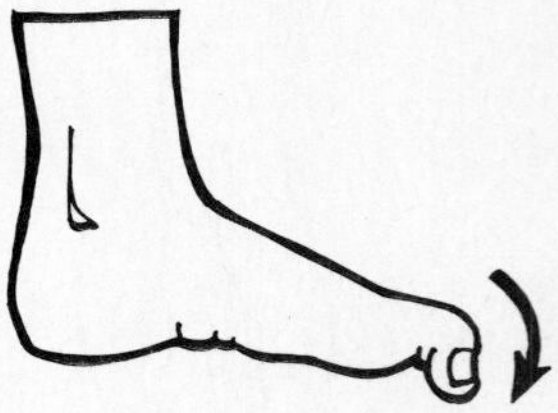

Figure 24–49 Toe flexion.

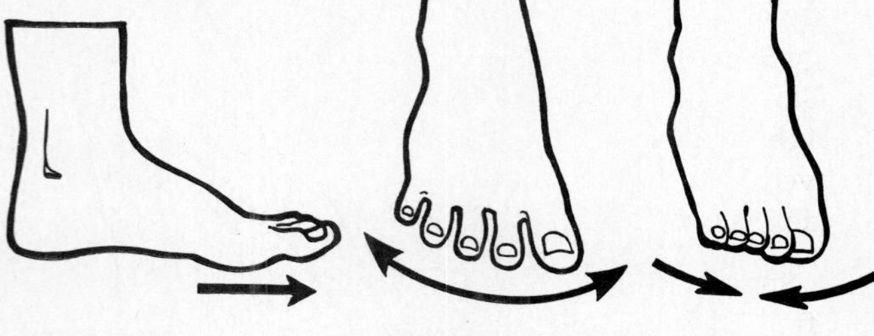

Figure 24–50 Toe extension.

Figure 24–51 Toe abduction.

Figure 24–52 Toe adduction.

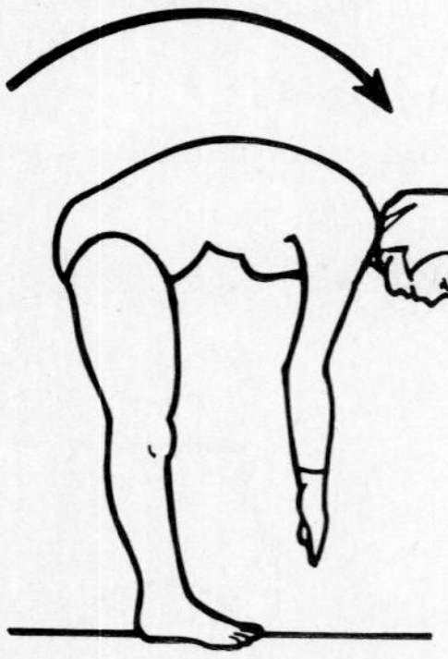

Figure 24–53 Trunk flexion.

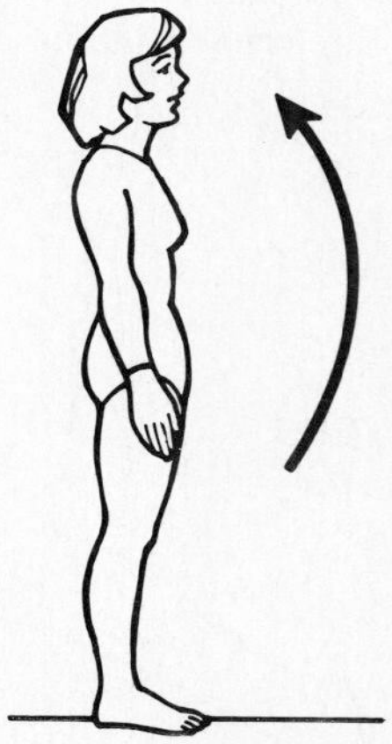

Figure 24–54 Trunk extension.

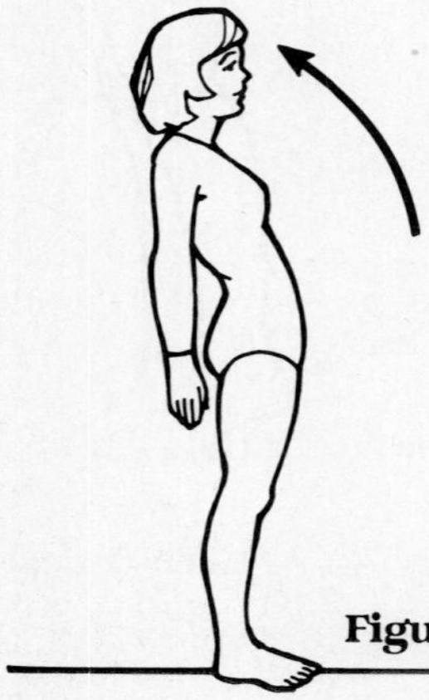

Figure 24–55 Trunk hyperextension.

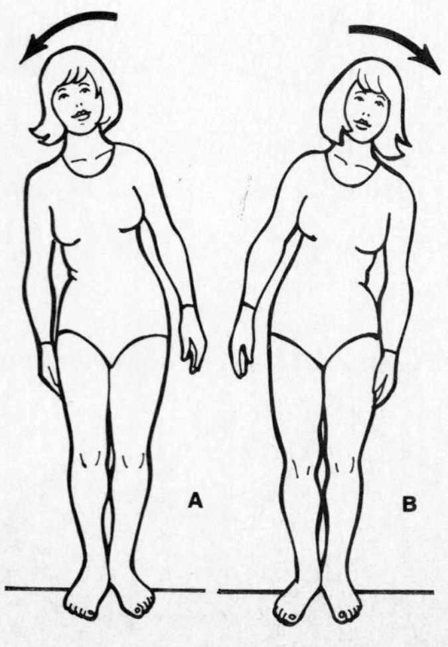

Figure 24–56 Trunk lateral flexion: **A,** to the right; **B,** to the left.

2. Invert the foot joints by turning the sole of the foot medially. Range: 5°. Primary muscle: tibialis posterior. See Figure 24–48.

3. Flex the toe joints by curling them downward. Range: 35°–60°. Primary muscles: flexor hallucis brevis, lumbricales pedis, flexor digitorum brevis. See Figure 24–49.

4. Extend the toes by straightening them. Range: 35°–60°. Primary muscles: extensor digitorum longus, extensor digitorum brevis. See Figure 24–50.

5. Abduct the toes by spreading them apart. Range: variable, 0°–15°. Primary muscles: interossei dorsales pedis, abductor hallucis. See Figure 24–51.

6. Adduct the toes by bringing them together. Range: variable, 0°–15°. Primary muscles: adductor hallucis, interossei plantares. See Figure 24–52.

Trunk—gliding joint

1. Flex the vertebral joints by bending the trunk toward the toes. Range: 70°–90°. Primary muscle: rectus abdominis. See Figure 24–53.

2. Extend the vertebral joints by straightening the trunk. Range: 70°–90°. Primary muscles: longissimus thoracis, iliocostalis thoracis, spinalis thoracis, iliocostalis lumborum, quadratus lumborum. See Figure 24–54.

3. Hyperextend the vertebral joints by bending the trunk backward. Range: 20°–30°. Primary muscles: longissimus thoracis, iliocostalis thoracis, spinalis thoracis, iliocostalis lumborum, quadratus lumborum. See Figure 24–55.

4. Laterally flex the trunk by bending it to the right and left sides. Range: 35° on each side. Primary muscle: quadratus lumborum. See Figure 24–56.

5. Rotate the vertebral joints by turning the upper part of the body from side to side. Range: 30°–45° on each side. Primary muscle: sacrospinalis. See Figure 24–57.

Station and Gait

The station of an individual is assessed by observing the body alignment in a standing position. See Chapter 23, page 558, for adult alignment in a standing position.

Gait is assessed in both the swing phase and the weight-bearing or stance phase. The phases are observed for rhythm and smoothness. A description of the patient's gait should include:

1. Shifting of the pelvis and trunk: normally very little shift
2. Distance between the heels: normally 5 to 10 cm (2 to 4 in)
3. Stride length (length of the swing) and symmetry
4. Cadence: symmetry and rhythm
5. Trunk posture
6. Pelvic posture
7. Arm swing: symmetry and length of swing

In particular, any limping or shuffling is observed and any pain associated with the gait noted. The pain is described relative to the phase of the gait.

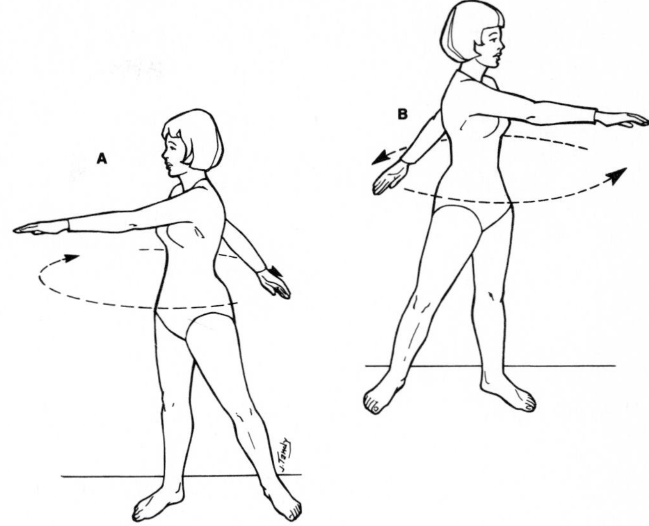

Figure 24–57 Trunk rotation: **A,** to the right; **B,** to the left.

Activity Tolerance

Assessment of activity tolerance is particularly important in planning exercise schedules for persons with cardiac or respiratory disease. This assessment is also advantageous, however, in planning range-of-motion exercise programs to prevent the complications of immobility or planning activity programs to provide psychologic benefits to patients.

Preactivity assessment

Before selecting appropriate activities for patients, it is necessary to assess the patient's preactivity status. Activity expenditure guides, such as that provided by Zohman and Tobis (1970), are useful for this purpose. In lieu of a guide or along with a guide, the nurse needs to consider the following factors about the patient (Gordon 1976:73):

1. Cardiovascular-respiratory status
2. Other physical impairments, e.g., disease, recent surgery, low hemoglobin level, elevated hematocrit, electrolyte and acid-base imbalances
3. Baseline (sleeping or before-exercise) vital signs, i.e., heart rate and rhythm, blood pressure, and respiratory rate, rhythm, and depth
4. Comfort level (e.g., pain)
5. Age and sex
6. Weight
7. Time lapse since food or drugs were last taken, particularly tranquilizers, stimulants, sedatives, coffee, and tobacco
8. Emotional and motivational state
9. Preillness activity level

Assessment indices

Ten indices (physiologic responses) used to measure activity tolerance are (Gordon 1976):

1. Heart rate (apical or radial pulse)
2. Heart rhythm (radial pulse)
3. Pulse strength
4. Blood pressure
5. Respiratory rate, depth, and rhythm
6. Skin color
7. Skin temperature and moistness
8. Posture and equilibrium
9. Activity rate
10. Emotional state

When supervising patients in a new activity, e.g., a cardiac patient undertaking exercise for the first time, measurements are required at three different times: (a) before the activity, (b) during the activity, if the activity takes a relatively long time to perform, and (c) following cessation of the activity. The choice of measurements used for each patient depends on the patient's level of illness, the opportunity to take measurements, and knowledge of the patient's response patterns. Specific assessment guidelines for each index are outlined in Table 24–3.

Table 24–3 Assessing Activity Tolerance

Index	Expected outcome	Unexpected outcomes and actions
Heart rate (apical or radial pulse)	For patients on bed rest or postcardiac precautions, a 20 beat/minute increase during or immediately after activity. Within 5 minutes postactivity, heart rate should return to baseline.	If preactivity tachycardia is present, notify the physician to prescribe a specific expected outcome, e.g., a maximum heart rate permitted or whether exercise is advisable. If the heart rate decreases or exceeds the expected outcome, terminate the activity. If the postactivity recovery extends beyond 5 minutes, the activity was too strenuous or prolonged.
Heart rhythm (radial pulse)	Rhythm remains regular.	If the rhythm becomes irregular, terminate the activity.
Pulse strength	Strength remains similar or increases.	If pulse becomes weak, stop the activity.
Blood pressure (used for patients with cardiac pathology or hypertension)	Slight rise in systolic pressure with strenuous activity; no change with less strenuous activity. Slight increase or no change in diastolic pressure.	If systolic pressure *drops* more than 20 mm Hg, cardiac output or vascular dilation is decreased, and termination of the activity is indicated.
Respiratory rate, depth, rhythm (of particular importance for patients with lung disease or surgery)	Increase in rate and depth; rhythm remains steady.	If irregular rhythm, dyspnea, or a decrease in rate occurs, terminate the activity.
Skin color	No change or slight flush in cheeks, lips, and nail beds. Light-skinned persons may show marked flushing.	If extreme redness, cyanosis, or pallor appears, terminate the activity.
Skin temperature and moistness	Increased warmth and perspiration.	If the skin becomes cool, this indicates vascular constriction and impending shock; terminate the activity.
Posture and equilibrium	No change.	If the patient manifests muscle fatigue, by leaning against objects for support, drooping the head and shoulders, or complaining of dizziness or fatigue, this indicates lack of tolerance.
Activity rate	Maintenance of performance rate throughout activity. No physical discomfort.	If there is progressive slowing, taking frequent rest periods, or reduced dexterity, this indicates lack of tolerance. If tightness, heaviness, or pain occurs in the chest or legs, immediately terminate the activity.
Emotional state	No change or positive response.	If the patient manifests a worried expression, grimacing, muscle tension or tremors, irritability, or sighing, this indicates anxiety, fear, or boredom.

Adapted from M. Gordon, Assessing activity tolerance, *American Journal of Nursing*, January 1976, 76:72–75.

Immobility

The concept of immobility is relative rather than absolute. It does not necessarily mean complete lack of movement; it refers to a decrease in activity from that normally carried out. It has been described as "the prescribed or unavoidable restriction of movement in any area of the patient's life" (Carnevali and Brueckner

1970:1502). The areas of immobility have been described as physical, intellectual, emotional, and social (ibid., pp. 1503–6).

Physical Immobility

Immobility in which the patient is physically restricted is frequently seen. Either the patient or factors in the environment may cause this immobility. It may be a limitation in physical movement or a limitation of physiologic processes, such as breathing.

Intellectual Immobility

Immobility can be due to a lack of knowledge of how to function. As a result the person is constrained from acting. People who have brain damage due to a disease process or injury may be unable to act or to learn how to act appropriately in a given setting. Mentally retarded people who have a limited capacity to learn may be immobilized for that reason.

Emotional Immobility

People who are highly stressed, perhaps because of impending surgery or the loss of a loved one, may become immobilized emotionally and sometimes even physically. This can happen as a result of a sudden change that has not permitted the person time to adjust to and cope with the situation. Nurses frequently see this in the hospital when a patient learns, for example, of a terminal malignancy.

Social Immobility

Social immobility refers to changes in social interaction, which often occur as a result of illness. Patients who are admitted to the hospital may experience decreased interactions when separated from their families. Even elderly persons who live alone find that their normal interaction is decreased in these circumstances.

Nursing Diagnoses

A person who is immobilized for a prolonged period is faced with a number of stressors (psychologic, social, and physical), each of which may produce various problems identified in nursing diagnoses.

Psychologic and Social Problems

1. Motivation to learn is decreased; learning ability and retention of material are decreased.
2. Motivation to solve problems is decreased, including a loss in the ability to receive sufficient content to discriminate among alternatives. For example, a patient may hear only a few of the nurse's statements and may be unable to differentiate between important and unimportant matters.
3. Drives such as hunger are generally diminished, and emotions are expressed in a variety of ways, including apathy, withdrawal, and aggression.
4. The person's body image and self-concept as a whole person and worthwhile being change.
5. Immobility can produce exaggerated emotional reactions that are often inappropriate to a situation and not normal for that particular person. For example, a patient may express sudden anger over an error in the dinner, a reaction the person normally would not have.

Because of immobility, people receive a reduced quality and quantity of sensory stimuli. The male patient in a hospital bed for months may see only nurses, patients, and a few visitors. He no longer meets with people at work and friends on Saturdays. His life is much narrower, and the variety of stimuli is decreased. As a result, his perception of time intervals may deteriorate. For example, he may think he waited for his lunch a long time (hours), when in effect it was only 15 minutes. The ability to estimate time intervals is largely related to a person's attitudes. Often "time flies" when people are busy and happy.

Another psychologic change for this immobilized patient occurs in his role activities. As a father, he normally attended his son's baseball games, but he now is unable to do so; as a husband, he contributed to household income and decision making, but he cannot do these activities; as an employee, he earned a salary and produced work, but he is not doing so now. All of these changes can be stressors and may bring out feelings of fear, anxiety, and worthlessness. For further information, see Chapter 32.

Physical Problems

Physical problems from immobilization can result even in body systems that were healthy before the inactive period. Just as exercise can be good for all parts of the body of a healthy person, immobility can affect every organ and system of the body. The physical effects of immobility can be categorized as musculoskeletal, urinary, metabolic, gastrointestinal, respiratory, and cardiovascular (Olson 1967).

Musculoskeletal problems

Deterioration of muscles and bone function due to inactivity can result in a number of problems:

1. Demineralization of the bones (*osteoporosis*)
2. Stiffness and pain in the joints
3. Atrophy of the muscles
4. Contracture of the muscles
5. Skin breakdown

Demineralization of bones, that is, a depletion chiefly of calcium, which gives bones their strength and solidity, results from immobility. In the healthy person, bone is continually being built and at the same time being broken down at similar rates. With inactivity, the building process is hampered but the breakdown process continues. This is because the osteoblasts, which form the bony matrix, require the stress and strain of weight-bearing activity and muscular pull against the bone to function.

Continual demineralization causes bones to become spongy, and they may gradually deform or compress and fracture easily. Regardless of the amount of calcium in the person's diet, this demineralization process takes place with immobility. The unneeded calcium is simply excreted or deposited in the muscles, the joints, and the kidney pelvis. Deposits of calcium in the joints contribute to the stiffness and pain in these areas. Excessive excretion of calcium through the kidneys and urinary tract (*hypercalciuria*) may contribute to stone formation, especially in the presence of urinary stagnation in the kidney pelvis (see the later discussion of urinary problems).

Muscle atrophy as a result of disuse tends to develop in people who are confined to bed, since muscle fibers that are not contracted for some time gradually diminish in size. When the muscles are exercised, the fibers increase in size again.

Contracture is a permanent shortening (contraction) of a muscle that eventually involves the soft tissue structures around the joint, such as the tendons, ligaments, and capsule of the joint. It occurs when joints are not moved frequently through their full range of motion. The most common contractures are flexion contractures of the hip, knee, shoulder, elbow, wrist, and ankle. They occur in situations where a patient's flexor muscles are contracted for prolonged periods of time and the extensors are not used. For example, the patient confined to a wheelchair does not extend the hips, knees, and elbows; the patient confined to a bed with tight bedcovers may develop plantar flexion contractures. Eventually in these situations the flexor muscles contract permanently (are unable to lengthen), and the joints become permanently flexed unless corrected by surgical intervention.

Skin breakdown and the occurrence of decubitus ulcers may also result from inactivity. Muscle activity is required for normal venous and arterial blood circulation. The impeded circulation that can result from immobilization and the prolonged pressure on the skin impede nourishment to specific areas, resulting in the formation of decubitus ulcers. See Chapter 21 for common pressure areas.

Urinary problems

The urinary system functions best when a person is in the upright position. Back-lying positions and immobility predispose patients to such problems as (a) stasis of urine in the kidney pelvis, (b) calculi (stones), (c) urinary infection, and (d) urinary retention and incontinence.

In the back-lying position, the patient's kidney pelvis does not empty completely. Normal emptying depends on the force of gravity in the upright position and the peristaltic action of the ureters. Stasis of urine occurs in the kidney pelvis after just a few days in the supine position.

This stagnation of urine is accompanied by increased levels of minerals (see the earlier discussion of musculoskeletal problems) and can result in the formation of calculi, which are often composed of calcium salts. The pH of the urine is elevated due to increased alkalinity from calcium excretion, and this can produce urinary infections. Normally urine is slightly acid (pH of 4.5 to 7.5).

With lack of activity, urinary control is diminished, and urinary retention and incontinence may occur. Normal urination is reflexively dependent on effective contraction of the bladder (by the detrusor muscle of the bladder wall), which increases the pressure within the bladder and relaxes the bladder sphincters so that urination occurs. However, in immobilized patients, this sequence of events is suppressed by reduced muscle tone of the bladder and inability to relax the perineal muscles for the bladder to empty. Urine is retained in the bladder, which then becomes distended. Increasing distention leads to urinary incontinence. See Chapter 28, page 716.

Gastrointestinal problems

Bed rest and immobility affect all three chief functions of the gastrointestinal tract (ingestion, digestion, and elimination), resulting in (a) anorexia, (b) diarrhea, and (c) constipation.

Patients who are immobilized are in a state of negative nitrogen balance due to the accelerated catabolic process. *Catabolism* is a breakdown process by which complex substances (e.g., proteins) are converted into simpler compounds. See Chapter 26, page 657. As a result of accelerated catabolism, immobilized patients frequently experience *anorexia* (lack of appetite). When the anorexic patient fails to eat, malnutrition can result, which can hinder the healing of a disease. The prolonged stress of immobility also stimulates the parasympathetic nervous system, which produces symptoms such as anorexia, *dyspepsia* (indigestion), and diarrhea or constipation. These states can further lessen the patient's appetite and subsequent intake and digestion of food.

Elimination from the bowel is also affected. The immobilized patient may lose the defecation reflex and/or fecal expulsive power, due to interference with the skeletal muscle activity and the visceral reflex patterns used in defecation. The patient then is likely to become constipated because of the weakened muscles and a pattern of ignoring the defecation reflex. A supine position for defecation interferes with this reflex and with the muscles normally used in the defecation process. See Chapter 27.

Constipation is frequently accompanied by the symptoms of headache, anorexia, abdominal distention, malaise, and vertigo. All of these symptoms can interfere with the person's ability to ingest and digest food.

Respiratory problems

The immobilized person is vulnerable to potential respiratory problems of three basic types:

1. Decreased respiratory movement
2. Accumulation of secretions in the respiratory tract
3. Imbalance in the oxygen/carbon dioxide ratio

The patient's chest may be restricted in its movement by loss of muscle coordination, perhaps due to muscle disuse, and by certain pharmacologic agents, such as sedatives and anesthetics.

Chest expansion can be further limited by the sitting or lying position of the patient. For example, Sims's position without shoulder or upper arm support can compress the lateral part of one side of the chest. Chest movement can also be limited by abdominal distention, due to indigestion or other causes, which puts upward pressure on the diaphragm, or by the use of tight chest or abdominal binders.

Secretions may accumulate in the respiratory tract and further interfere with respiration when a patient is immobile. Normally secretions are moved by coughing or by changing position or posture. In patients who find it uncomfortable to cough and who do not change position, these secretions may well accumulate, leading to lung congestion and *hypostatic* pneumonia (pneumonia resulting from poor circulation or stagnant secretions). With lack of fluid intake, these secretions may become thickened and even more difficult to cough up.

Oxygen/carbon dioxide imbalance is the third type of respiratory problem. Where there is decreased respiratory movement, there may be decreased intake of oxygen and decreased output of carbon dioxide. Although increased carbon dioxide in the blood and decreased oxygen initially stimulate respiration, eventually they depress respiration. See Chapter 29. Accumulation of secretions in the lungs further inhibits respiration and aggravates the oxygen/carbon dioxide imbalance.

Cardiovascular problems

Immobility has three major effects on the cardiovascular system: (a) orthostatic hypotension, (b) increased workload on the heart, and (c) thrombus formation.

When a person has been in a lying position for a prolonged period, the autonomic nervous system is unable to equalize the blood supply to the body when the person gets up. This results in a condition known as *orthostatic hypotension* (low blood pressure in the standing position). Two factors underlying this condition are generalized loss of muscle tone and decreased ability of the blood vessels to contract reflexively to reduce and distribute the blood volume. Normally, active muscle action of the body exerts pressure on the veins and assists in the return of venous blood to the heart. When there is poor muscle tone, this blood tends to pool in the dependent areas of the body, that is, areas lower than the heart, such as the feet and legs in a standing position.

When a person is immobilized for a period of time in a supine position, the heart needs to work harder than when the person is active in the erect position (Olson 1967:781). Changes in the vascular resistance and the hydrostatic pressure are associated with the altered distribution of the blood that occurs in the supine position. Because of the decreased gravity pull, more of the blood leaves the legs to be distributed in other parts of the body. This increases the volume of circulating blood which must be pumped by the heart. The heart rate is increased, and the stroke volume (the amount of blood ejected from the heart with each ventricular contraction) is increased.

Another factor affecting the heart that nurses need to monitor closely is Valsalva's maneuver. When patients in bed use their arms and upper trunk muscles, either to move up in bed or to sit on a bedpan, they tend to hold their breath. This builds up pressure, interfering with the blood entering the large thoracic veins, and reduces the heart rate. When they then release the breath, the blood suddenly flows to the heart, and the heart rate increases. This can result in serious cardiac problems for certain patients.

Thrombus formation is the third problem faced by immobilized patients. A *thrombus* is a solid mass of blood constituents, which forms in the heart or blood vessels. The tendency to form thrombi may be due to pooling of the blood in the veins from inactivity, possible increased viscosity of the blood due to dehydration, or external pressure on the veins, exerted by the knee gatch of the hospital bed.

Examples of Nursing Diagnoses

Nursing diagnoses for immobilized patients may include the following actual or potential problems:

1. Altered self-concept related to dependence
2. Sensory deprivation related to confinement to bed
3. Decreased ability to solve problems related to sensory deprivation
4. Risk of muscle atrophy, contracture, and osteoporosis related to inactivity
5. Risk of skin breakdown related to inability to change position
6. Risk of urinary stasis and infection related to confinement to supine position
7. Risk of impaired O_2/CO_2 exchange related to accumulation of secretions
8. Risk of injury related to dizziness with position change
9. Risk of venous stasis in the legs related to inactivity

Planning and Intervention Related to Immobility

Planning

The overall nursing goal for the immobilized patient is to prevent the hazards of immobility. Subgoals may include:

1. To reduce the extent of immobilization
2. To promote the patient's ability to cope with unavoidable immobility

Planning also involves establishing outcome criteria. For suggestions, see Evaluation later in this chapter.

Guidelines for Nursing Intervention

Many of the hazards of immobility can be prevented by planning and implementing the following measures:

1. *Exercise.* A planned schedule of exercise needs to be implemented to prevent musculoskeletal, cardiovascular, respiratory, and metabolic problems.
   a. *Joints and muscles.* The plan might include passive or active joint range-of-motion exercises (see page 588), isometric exercises (see page 610), and self-care activities (e.g., eating, bathing, dressing) in amounts allowed by the patient's condition. Exercises maintain muscle tone and size, prevent bone demineralization, maintain joint ranges of motion, and promote the return flow of blood to the heart by exerting muscular pressure on the veins. They also increase the energy demands of the patient's body cells, thus increasing the metabolic rate and reducing catabolic processes.
   b. *Breathing and coughing.* Regular breathing exercises are also essential to facilitate adequate lung expansion, oxygen/carbon dioxide exchange, and movement of respiratory secretions. Patients need to be taught how to breathe deeply and prolong exhalation, using the abdominal muscles, diaphragm, and intercostal muscles. If secretions are present, coughing should be encouraged with deep breathing exercises. Postural drainage with percussion and vibration may also be necessary. See Chapter 29, page 754.
2. *Position changes.* Changing the patient's position every hour helps prevent skin breakdown, contractures, postural hypotension, urinary stasis, and respiratory problems. If possible, a positioning schedule needs to include standing, sitting, supine, prone, and lateral positions. See Chapter 23. The standing and sitting positions are particularly helpful in preventing postural hypotension and urinary stasis; the prone and supine positions prevent hip and knee flexion contractures. For patients unable to stand, a CircOlectric bed (see page 526) or tilt table (see Figure 24–58) may be used to place the patient in an upright position.

   Patients who are able to move themselves need to be taught effective ways to move and relieve pressure on supporting body parts. Normally a person changes position every few minutes. Persons confined to a bed can be taught to shift their position for at least 60 seconds every 15 or 30 minutes. The patient in a supine position can shift weight from the back to the side. The patient in a sitting position can shift weight off the buttocks by using an overhead trapeze bar, by pushing up with both arms to elevate the buttocks, or by shifting weight from one buttock to the other. For patients unable to move themselves, sheepskin pads and alternating pressure mattresses need to be used. One type of mattress (Cloud Nine) consists of two plastic bags that are alternately inflated by an air pump at 5-minute intervals, thus shifting the pressure from one side to the other.
3. *Skin care.* Position changes and use of special pressure mattresses do not obviate the need for constant skin care to susceptible pressure areas. Keeping the skin

lubricated, clean, and dry and protecting damaged skin are essential. See Chapter 21, page 490.

4. *Food and fluids.* Adequate intake of food and fluids prevents protein catabolism, skin breakdown, constipation, and urinary stasis. For essential foods and nutrients, see Chapter 26; for adequate volumes of fluid, see Chapter 30. Sufficient amounts of carbohydrates are necessary to prevent protein catabolism. To maintain skin integrity and prevent tissue breakdown, a sufficient protein and vitamin intake is necessary. High-fiber foods and sufficient amounts of fluids can prevent constipation. See Chapter 27. High intakes of fluid can also prevent urinary stasis, with its risk of infection and calculi formation. When the urine is kept dilute, urinary stasis is less likely to occur and calcium particles are less likely to precipitate. The patient's fluid intake and output are monitored to ensure a sufficient fluid intake and urinary output.

5. *Bowel and bladder routine.* A bowel and bladder routine can prevent urinary incontinence and constipation. By scheduling bowel evacuation at the same time every day, such as after breakfast, bowel regularity can be established. See Chapter 27, page 693, for further information. Urinary incontinence can be avoided largely by providing appropriate assistance without delay. See Chapter 28, page 720.

6. *Extended area of confinement.* The nurse needs to be creative in planning measures to reduce the psychologic effects of being confined in a restricted area. Placing the patient's bed by a window facing a garden, changing the assigned room periodically to provide different views, and taking the patient to a rooftop solarium or a lounge are examples of ways to extend the patient's area.

7. *Social interaction.* To prevent social immobility, measures need to be planned that help the patient achieve sufficient interactions with persons meaningful to him or her. Such measures may include providing access to a telephone and having friends and family members arrange a visiting schedule so that social contacts are regular and frequent.

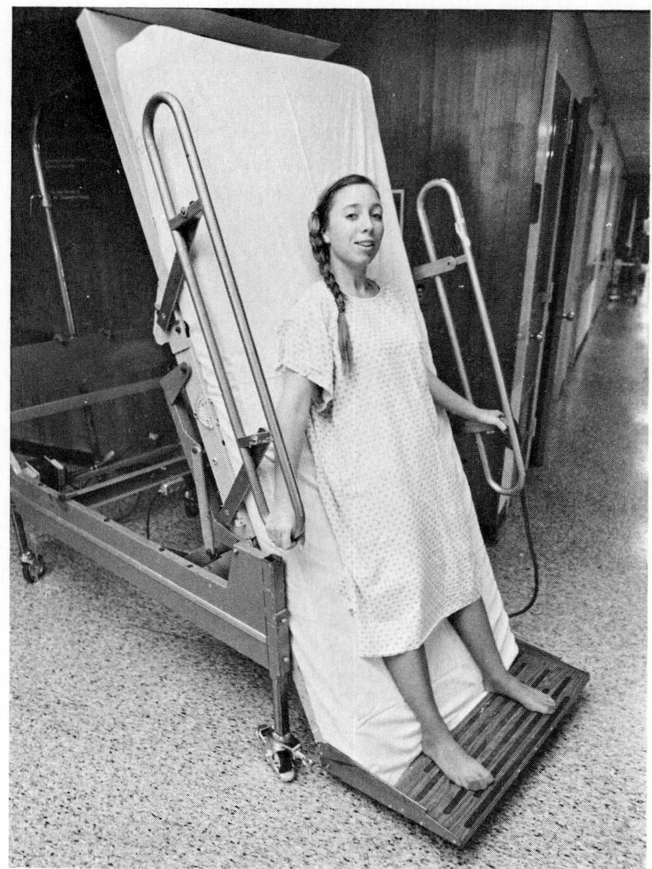

Figure 24–58 A tilt table.

8. *Decision making.* Intellectual and emotional immobility can be minimized by encouraging the patient to collaborate in and make decisions about his or her plans of care. When decisions are made for the patient, frustration, anger, and withdrawal result. Independence of thought and action and a feeling of control need to be supported.

Planning and Intervention Related to Mobility

The overall nursing goal related to meeting mobility needs of patients is to promote mobility to the maximum degree possible for the patient. Subgoals may include:

1. To maintain, restore, or increase the tone and strength of muscles

2. To maintain, restore, or increase the range of motion of joints

3. To prevent the problems associated with immobility

Nursing interventions include a wide range of activities discussed subsequently: assisting the patient to ambulate with or without mechanical aids (canes, crutches, or walkers), meeting specific exercise needs, and, in the case of healthy individuals, maintaining or promoting physical fitness. Planning also involves establishing outcome criteria. For suggestions, see Evaluation later in this chapter.

Ambulation

Ambulation is the act of walking. Most people who are ill require only a brief period of bed rest, and then can walk about and gradually increase their activity. The more physically fit a person is before becoming ill, the quicker the person's return to health is likely to be. This is particularly true for the elderly who have fewer reserves to call upon at a time of illness.

Even a day or two in bed can make a person feel weak and unsteady. Remaining in bed for a few days because of a cold can weaken muscles sufficiently so that a person feels shaky when first getting up. A patient who has had surgery or a fever is likely to feel more pronounced weakness. The elderly person is likely to experience some joint stiffness in addition, as a result of immobility. There is no question that the potential problems of bed rest and immobility are less likely to occur when a patient becomes ambulatory as soon as possible.

Because of age, general physical condition, or length of time spent in bed, a patient may need to prepare for ambulation by doing conditioning exercises to improve muscle tone, muscle strength, and joint flexibility.

Exercises Preparatory to Ambulation

Hip flexion and extension

Lying on the bed in the supine position, the patient extends one leg in front, then flexes the knee and brings it to the chest, pointing the toes upward in a dorsal flexion position. When the knee is as close to the chest as possible, the knee is extended (straightened), then the leg is returned to the fully extended position. This exercise is repeated with the other leg.

Hip rotation

1. With both the knee and the ankle extended, the patient rolls one leg inward and then outward from the hip. This is repeated with the other leg.
2. With both legs extended at the knee and the ankle, the patient turns both legs inward until the toes touch and then outward until the heels touch.

Abduction and adduction of the hips

With the leg extended at the knee and with the toes in dorsal flexion, the patient moves one leg over to the near side of the bed, then to the far side of the bed over the other leg. This exercise is repeated for the other leg.

Knee extensions

With the leg extended, the patient pushes the back of the knee against the bed surface and raises the heel off the bed as far as possible. This is repeated for the other leg.

Ankle flexion, inversion, and eversion

The patient rotates the foot in a circular motion clockwise and counterclockwise. This is repeated with the other foot.

Toe flexion and extension

The patient flexes and extends the toes upward and downward.

Strengthening muscles of the abdomen, buttocks, and thighs

1. The patient tightens the muscles of the abdomen, then relaxes them.
2. The patient breathes deeply to tighten the abdominal muscles.
3. The patient tightens the buttocks and then elevates the hips while lying in the supine position.

These exercises should not be done long enough to tire the patient. As a rough guide, a patient may be able to carry each out three times in a row, twice or three times a day.

In addition to these specific exercises, some of the activities that patients carry out while they are in bed can be used for preparation for ambulation. One example is the bath patients give themselves.

Assisting a Patient to Walk

Normally when people walk they move their arms and legs alternately; that is, the right arm swings forward as the left leg moves forward, and conversely the left arm moves with the right leg. Techniques that will support a patient and facilitate this normal body movement are usually best. This is particularly true for patients who have sufficient muscle and bone development and strength in both legs to stand and move themselves.

One-nurse methods

After the patient is assisted from bed and has balance, the nurse goes beside the patient, supporting the patient at the waist with both hands. The nurse may wrap a towel folded lengthwise around the patient's waist or use a walking belt (see Figure 24–59), which fits around the patient's waist. The advantage of this position is that the patient is assisted to maintain a center of gravity in the middle of the base of support (between the feet); that is, the patient is not encouraged to lean to one side or the other.

The patient should take only a few steps at first, to assess steadiness and ability to balance. If the patient feels confident about continuing, the nurse follows beside, supporting the patient at the waist.

If the patient feels faint or thinks he or she may fall, the nurse assumes a broad stance, one foot in front of the other, so that the patient is supported by the nurse's body. The patient can then be gently lowered to the floor without harm if additional assistance is not available to provide support.

If the patient feels unsteady and has a weakness in one leg (a common condition, for example, after a stroke), the nurse may find it advantageous to assume a position at the affected side. In this position the nurse's near arm goes under the patient's near arm, and the nurse's hand grasps the inferior aspect of the patient's near upper arm. The nurse can then grasp the patient's near lower arm or hand with the other hand. In this position the nurse can assist the patient in a fall by sliding the near arm up to the patient's near axilla and then, after taking a broad stance, supporting the patient's body against the nurse's body with much of the weight against the nurse's hip. Again the patient can be gently lowered to the floor if additional assistance is not available.

Another position that a nurse can assume to assist a patient to walk is particularly effective when the patient has a distinct body weakness. In this position the nurse goes to the patient's unaffected side and places the near arm around the patient's waist. The patient's near arm goes over the nurse's far shoulder, and the nurse grasps this with the free hand. The patient and nurse then step forward together on their inside feet. As the patient advances the weak far leg forward, the nurse's opposite leg is advanced to provide as wide a base of support as possible.

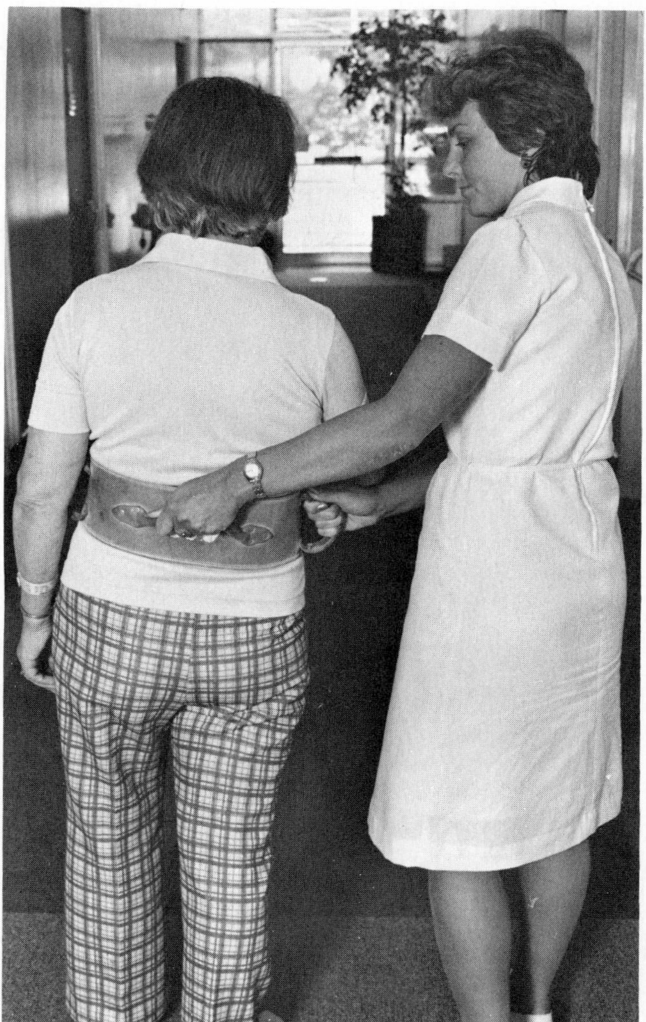

Figure 24–59 A walking belt.

Two-nurse methods

Each nurse stands at one side of the patient and grasps the inferior aspect of the patient's upper arm with the nearest hand and the patient's lower arm or hand with the other hand. The two nurses and the patient then walk in unison. Again the nurses can slide their hands up to the patient's axillae to give additional support if required. This technique provides more support than can be given by one nurse.

A two-nurse position that provides even more support again has the nurses stand at each side of the patient, but in this case they slip their near arms under the patient's arms to the back and grasp each other's arms. The patient's arms are placed over the nurses' far shoulders, and the nurses grasp the patient's hands with their free hands. For this technique to be effective, both nurses and the patient need to be about the same height.

Mechanical Aids for Walking

Cane

Three types of canes may be used to aid walking: the single, straight-legged cane; the tripod (crab) cane, which has three prongs; and the quad cane, which has four prongs and provides the most support. A patient who requires a cane should hold it with the hand on the stronger side of the body. This provides maximum support and appropriate body alignment when walking. The tip of the cane is positioned about 15 cm (6 in) to the side of the foot.

When *maximum support* is required, the patient (a) moves the cane forward about 30 cm (12 in) while the body weight is borne by both legs, (b) moves the weak leg forward to the cane while the weight is borne by the cane and stronger leg, (c) moves the stronger leg forward ahead of the cane and weak leg while the weight is borne by the cane and weak leg, and (d) repeats steps (a)–(c). This pattern of moving provides at least two points of support on the floor at all times.

As the patient becomes stronger and *less support* is required, the patient can (a) move the cane and weak leg forward at the same time, while the weight is borne by the stronger leg, and (b) move the stronger leg forward, while the weight is borne by the cane and the weak leg.

Walker

A walker is a mechanical device with four legs for support. It has bars at the top that go in front of and around the sides of the patient, providing a feeling of security as well as assisting with balance. It is usually made of a lightweight metal such as aluminum, so it can be easily lifted and moved.

The patient holds the upper bar of the walker at each side, moves the walker forward, and then steps into it. The disadvantage of using a walker is that normal body alignment and walking motion are not encouraged, since the patient must bend forward to move the walker.

Braces

Sometimes patients are provided with braces for their weak legs. These are generally made of a lightweight metal with leather straps that attach the brace to the leg. Some braces support the ankle and lower leg; others extend to the upper leg, offering support to the knee. Patients who have braces usually learn to put them on and take them off themselves.

Crutches

Sometimes it is necessary for a patient to use crutches for a period of time. Although there are several types of crutches, two of the most commonly used types are the underarm and the forearm support crutches.

Measuring for crutches Nurses may need to assist patients in measuring for underarm crutches. This can be done with the patient either in a supine position in bed or standing. The nurse measures from the anterior fold of the patient's axilla either (a) to a point 15 cm (6 in) lateral to the patient's heel, or (b) to the heel and adds 5 cm (2 in). See Figure 24–60.

Appropriate length of crutches When the patient is standing erect with correctly measured crutches, the top of the crutch is 5 cm (2 inches) below the axilla and the tip of each crutch is 15 cm (6 in) in front of the foot at the side. Weight should not be borne by the axillae. Prolonged pressure on the axillae can damage the underlying nerves, producing what is called a *crutch paralysis*. The axilla is protected poorly by a layer of fat, which does not support it against pressure.

The hand grips need to be placed so that when the patient is holding them the elbows are slightly flexed.

Guidelines for using crutches Patients who use long (underarm) crutches need to understand why pressure on the axillae is to be avoided. Because the person's hands carry most or all of the patient's weight, the hand bars may be padded. It is important that padding not rotate or slip. When a patient initially obtains crutches, the axillary bar should not be padded, because padding encourages the patient to lean on it while walking, thus increasing the danger of pressure on the brachial nerve plexus. However, after patients have learned to walk with crutches, they may like a small pad on the bar that does not touch the axilla when they

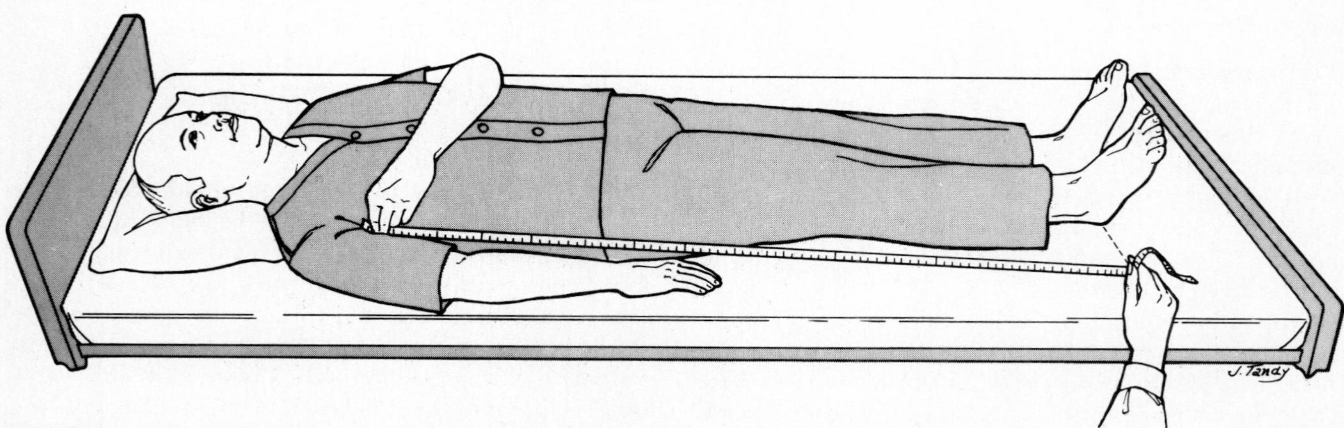

Figure 24–60 Measuring for crutches.

move but that offers a little softer support when they lean on the crutches briefly while standing.

Before using crutches, the patient who has been in bed may well need to do exercises to strengthen the shoulder and upper arm muscles. In particular, the triceps, trapezius, and latissimus muscles are used in crutch walking. Simple exercises that a patient can do in bed to strengthen these muscles are:

1. Push-ups from a sitting position—the patient places both arms at the sides, palms flat on the bed surface, and raises the buttocks. This exercise is excellent for developing the triceps muscles.
2. Raising the body off the bed by grasping a trapeze attached to a Balkan frame. This develops the arm and shoulder muscles.

The legs also need strengthening for standing and walking. For balance and posture the abdominal and back muscles need to have good tone.

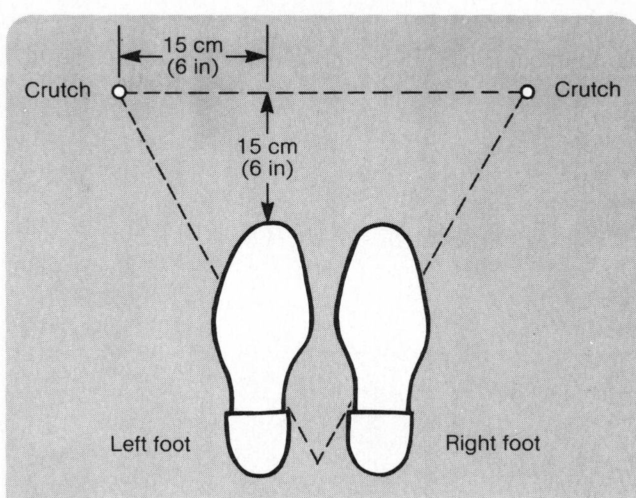

Figure 24–61 Tripod position.

Crutch stance (tripod position)

Before crutch walking is attempted, posture and balance are of utmost importance. The proper standing position with crutches is called the *tripod (triangle) position.* See Figure 24–61. The crutches are placed about 15 cm (6 in) in front of the feet and out laterally about 15 cm (6 in), creating a wide base of support. The feet are slightly apart. A greater height requires a broader base to provide stability. Thus a tall person requires a wider base than a short person. Hips and knees are extended, the back is straight, and the head is held straight and high. There should be no hunch to the shoulders and thus no weight borne by the axillae. The palms are positioned lateral to the feet, and the elbows are extended sufficiently to allow weight bearing on the hands.

Sometimes patients are discouraged when crutch walking commences, because the limitations with crutches become apparent. Weakness that was not apparent in bed can become prominent when standing or walking. Patients realize that balance can no longer be taken for granted with the weight of a heavy cast or a paralyzed limb. Frequently, progress may be slower than the patient anticipated. Thus encouragement from the nurse and the setting of realistic goals are especially important.

Crutch gaits

There are four standard crutch gaits, which all begin with the tripod position. Physiotherapists usually teach crutch walking, and they will teach the gait or gaits particularly suitable for the patient. However, in situations where there is no physiotherapist (for example, in a small hospital in a rural setting), nurses teach crutch walking.

Four-point alternate gait The four-point alternate gait is used by patients who can bear partial weight on both feet—for example, arthritic or cerebral palsy patients. It is a particularly safe gait, in that there are three points of support on the floor at all times. The gait has the following foot sequence: right crutch, left foot, left crutch, right foot. See Figure 24–62. This gait provides a normal walking pattern and makes some use of the muscles of the lower extremities.

Three-point alternate gait For the three-point alternate gait the patient must be able to bear the total body weight on one foot; the affected foot or leg is either partially or totally non-weight-bearing. In this gait the two crutches are moved forward together with the injured leg while the weight is being borne by the patient's hands on the crutches. The unaffected leg is then advanced forward. See Figure 24–63.

Two-point gait If the patient can bear partial weight on both feet, the two-point gait may be used. With practice, patients can frequently move relatively quickly. The left crutch and the right foot move forward simultaneously as in normal walking. Then the right crutch and the left foot advance forward. See Figure 24–64.

Swing gaits There are two main swing gaits: the swing-to-crutch and the swing-through gaits. They do not use the quadriceps and other lower extremity muscles a great deal, because they do not simulate the nor-

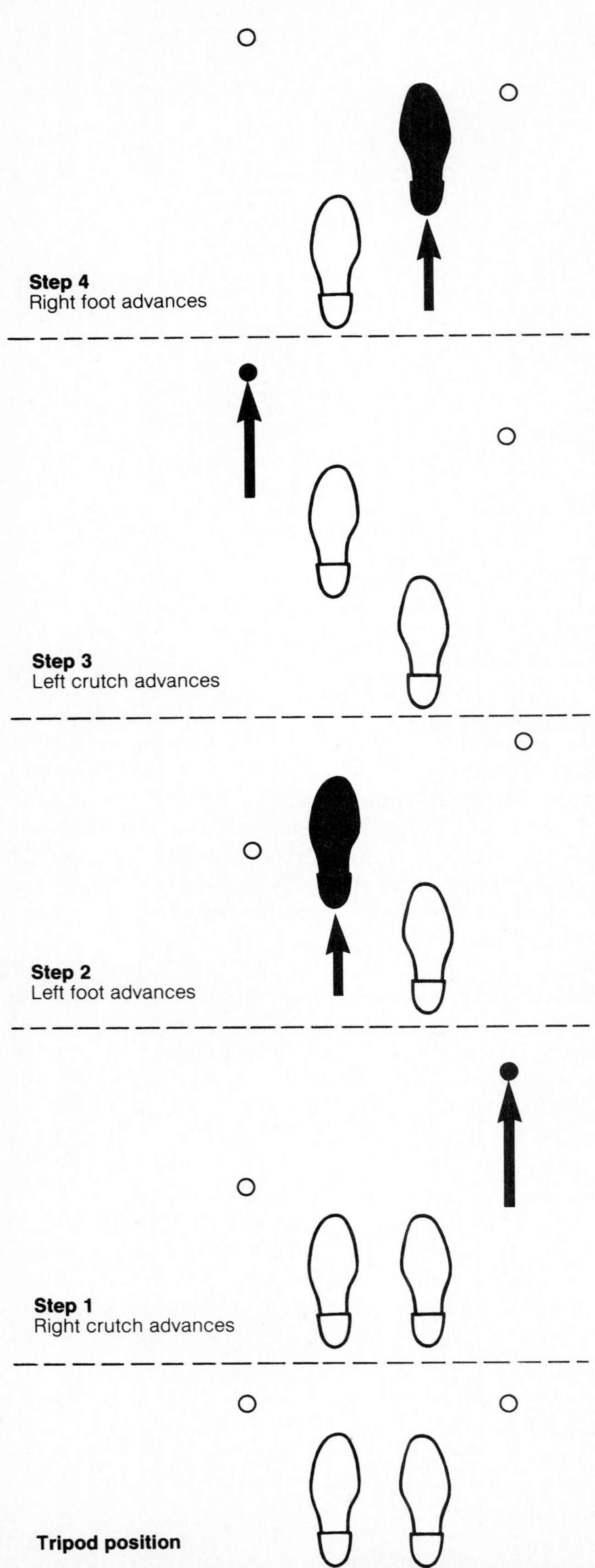

Figure 24–62 (Left) Four-point alternate crutch gait diagramed from bottom to top.

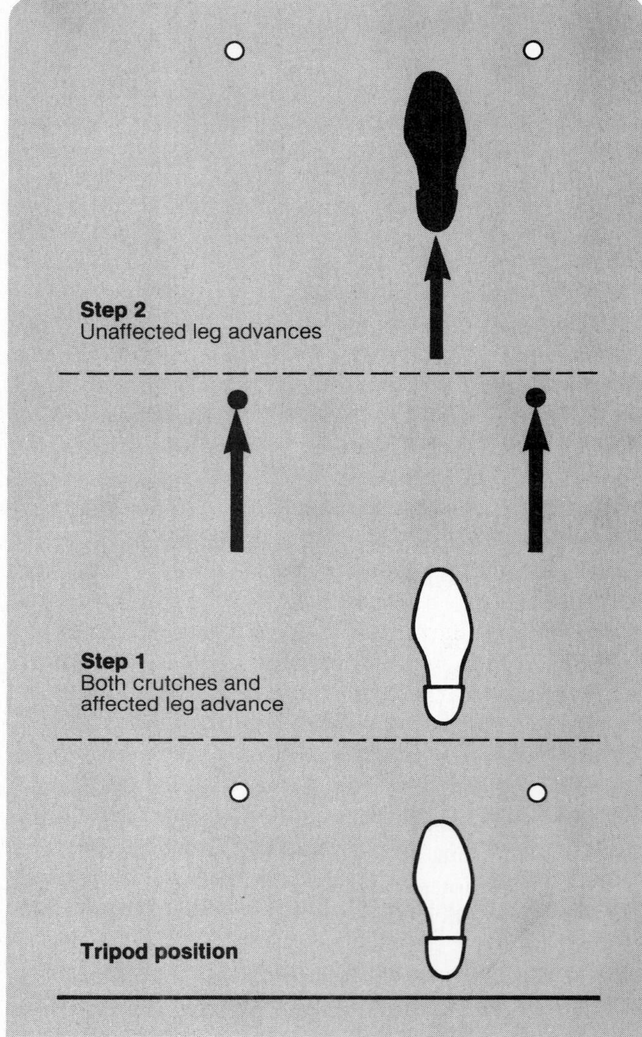

Figure 24–63 Three-point alternate crutch gait diagramed from bottom to top.

mal walking motion. They are indicated when a patient is paralyzed or cannot move the lower extremities, although the patient may be able to bear weight. Prolonged use of these gaits results in atrophy of the unused muscles. The advantage of these gaits is that they allow rapid movement.

In the *swing-to-crutch gait*, both crutches are placed forward, and then the patient swings forward to the crutches. See Figure 24–65. This action is repeated for

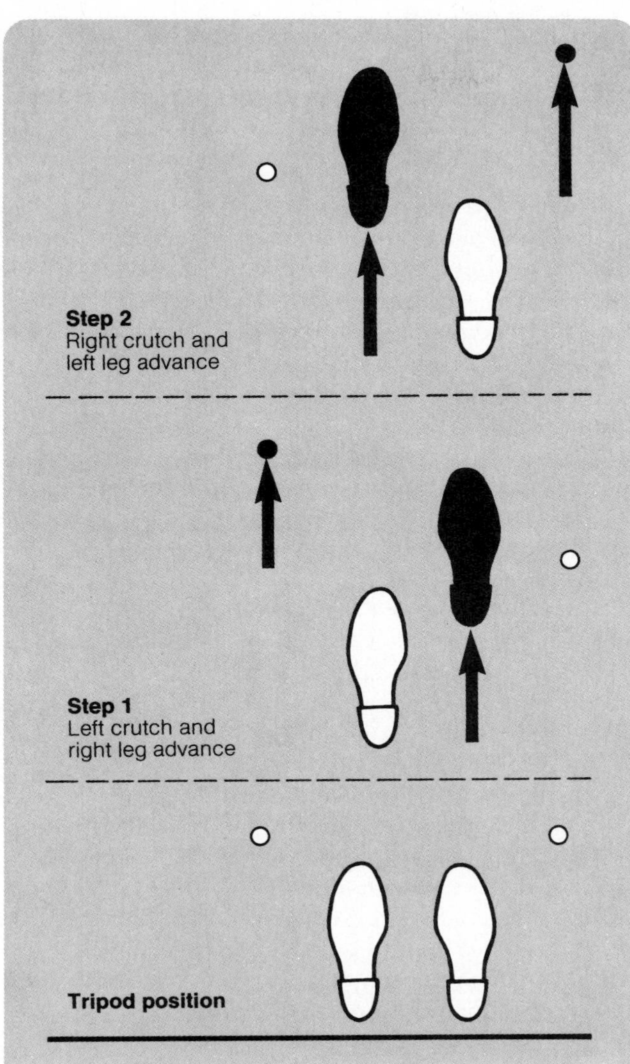

Figure 24–64 Two-point crutch gait diagramed from bottom to top.

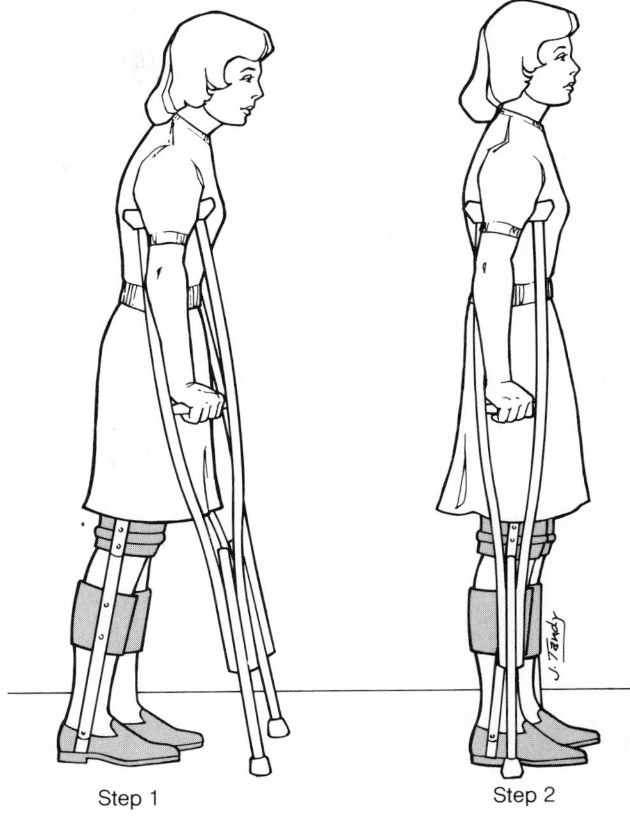

Figure 24–65 Swing-to-crutch gait.

each move forward. The gait is similar in motion to the three-point alternate gait, except that equal weight can be borne by both feet in the swing gait.

For the *swing-through gait*, the crutches are placed ahead of the patient, and the patient then swings to the crutches and beyond to a position in front of them. See Figure 24–66. Weight is shifted from the palms of the hands to the feet. This process is then repeated.

Exercise

Promoting exercise is an essential nursing activity to maintain the patient's muscle tone and joint mobility. Unless contraindicated, active, active-assistive, or passive range-of-motion (ROM) exercises need to be done regularly. These can be provided through both the activities of daily living and a planned exercise program. The act of dressing involves many valuable motions of the joints. For example, to put on a shirt requires several head, shoulder, arm, and trunk movements. The nurse needs to be selective in choosing ROM exercises for each patient, since not all exercises are required for every patient.

Passive Exercises

Passive exercises are normally done to correct the patient's specific muscle problems; if the patient's leg rolls outward, emphasis is placed on rolling the leg inward. For passive exercises, the patient assumes a position that will permit free movement of the joint to be moved. Often a supine position is advised, if the patient can tolerate it.

There are three major factors in providing passive exercises: (a) the range of motion of the joint being exercised, (b) support for the joint against gravity and

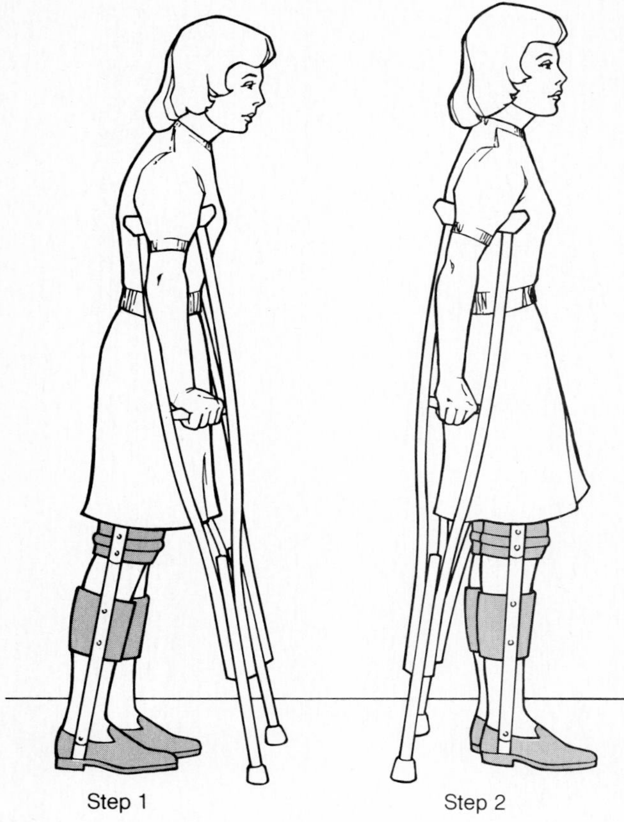

Figure 24–66 Swing-through crutch gait.

unwanted movement, and (c) the movement provided by the other person's hands to exert effort and control. Normally a joint is supported both above and below. See Figure 24–67.

Guidelines for providing passive exercises

1. Ensure that the patient understands the reason for doing ROM exercises.

Figure 24–67 Supporting a limb above and below the joint for passive exercise.

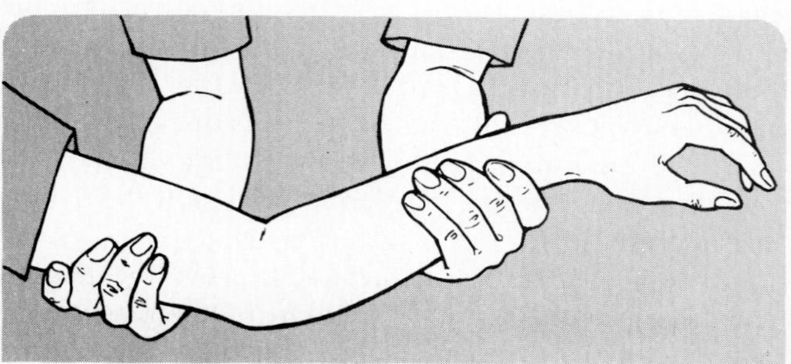

2. Use good body mechanics when providing ROM exercises, to avoid muscle strain or injury to both nurse and patient.

3. Expose only the limb being exercised, to avoid embarrassing the patient.

4. Support the patient's joints and limbs as needed to prevent muscle strain or injury. This is done by cupping a joint in the palm of the hand (see Figure 24–68, *A*) or cradling a limb along the forearm (see Figure 24–68, *B*). If a patient's joint is painful (e.g., in an arthritic person), the limb is supported in the muscular areas above and below the joint.

5. Use a firm, comfortable grip when handling the limb.

6. Move the body parts smoothly, slowly, and rhythmically. Jerky movements cause discomfort and possible injury. Fast movements can cause *spasticity* (spasms) or *rigidity* (stiffness or inflexibility) in some patients.

7. Avoid moving or forcing a body part beyond the patient's existing range of motion. Muscle strain, pain, and injury can result. This is of particular importance for patients with a *flaccid* (weak or lax) paralysis, whose muscles can be stretched and joints dislocated without the patient's awareness.

8. If spasticity of a muscle occurs during movements, stop the movement temporarily but continue to apply slow, gentle pressure on the part until the muscle relaxes; then proceed with the motion.

9. If a contracture is present, apply slow, firm pressure without causing pain to stretch the muscle fibers.

10. If rigidity occurs, apply pressure against the rigidity and continue the exercise slowly.

Isometric Exercises

For patients who are unable to move specific joints (e.g., the patient who has a cast on the leg and is unable to move the knee joint), isometric exercise is essential to maintain muscle strength and size. Isometric exercises attempt to use the whole muscle as a unit. All skeletal muscles can be exercised isometrically in a short time and without special equipment. With maximum effort all fibers in a muscle will shorten.

Isometric exercises increase muscle strength, and they require very little time. They should be used in conjunction with other exercises. The technique is to maintain tension in a muscle for a given period of time. Maximum muscular effort for 6 seconds once a day is recommended. In the breaking-in period, two methods are suggested: a three-quarter effort for 6 seconds or a full effort for 2 to 4 seconds. The exercise is carried out once a day to avoid fatigue. All muscles should be exercised for general conditioning, which takes less than 2 minutes.

Prenatal Exercises

During pregnancy a woman needs to learn Kegel's exercises to strengthen her pubococcygeal muscle. This muscle is the master sphincter of the bladder, bowel function, and vaginal perception and response during intercourse. The exercise consists of three aspects: (a) contracting the anal sphincter, (b) contracting the introitus, and (c) contracting the meatal sphincter, then holding for a count of 10 before relaxing. This exercise is done three or four times per day.

Pelvic rocking can be done prenatally to relieve low backache. The woman assumes a hands-and-knees position, a standing position, or a supine position. The abdominal wall is tightened and the buttocks tucked in. This rocks the pelvis upward, flattening the lower back. The abdomen and buttocks are then slowly relaxed; this allows the hollow to return in the back. See Figure 24–69. The exercise is repeated four to six times.

Tailor sitting is done prenatally to stretch the thigh and pelvic floor muscles. The woman sits with her knees flexed in front and feet drawn toward her. The knees are comfortably lowered toward the floor. See Figure 24–70. This position needs to be assumed as often as possible.

Postnatal Exercises

Postnatal exercises serve to trim the woman's figure and improve muscle tone. If the delivery was uncomplicated, these can be started two or three days postpartum. It is usual to start with simple exercises and progress to more strenuous ones. The exercises should not be tiring. The following postpartum exercises are often practiced:

1. Deep breathing. The woman takes a deep breath, then lets it all out, relaxing all the muscles of the body. This exercise is designed to promote relaxation to prepare for exercises.
2. Abdominal tightening. The woman takes a deep breath, lets it out, tightens the abdominal muscles, pulling in and up, holds to a count of 3, and then relaxes.
3. Chin lift. Lying on her back, the woman tightens the abdominal muscles, lifts the head so that the chin is on the chest, then relaxes, and lets the head return to the pillow.
4. Pelvic tilting. Lying in the supine position with knees flexed, the woman inhales and, while exhaling, flattens the back against the bed. While doing this, she tightens the muscles of the abdomen and buttocks. See Figure 24–71.
5. Leg raising (modified). Lying on her back, the woman tightens the abdominal muscles, presses the lower back into the bed, raises the right leg and foot until they rest on the left toes, then relaxes and lowers the leg. This is repeated with the left leg.

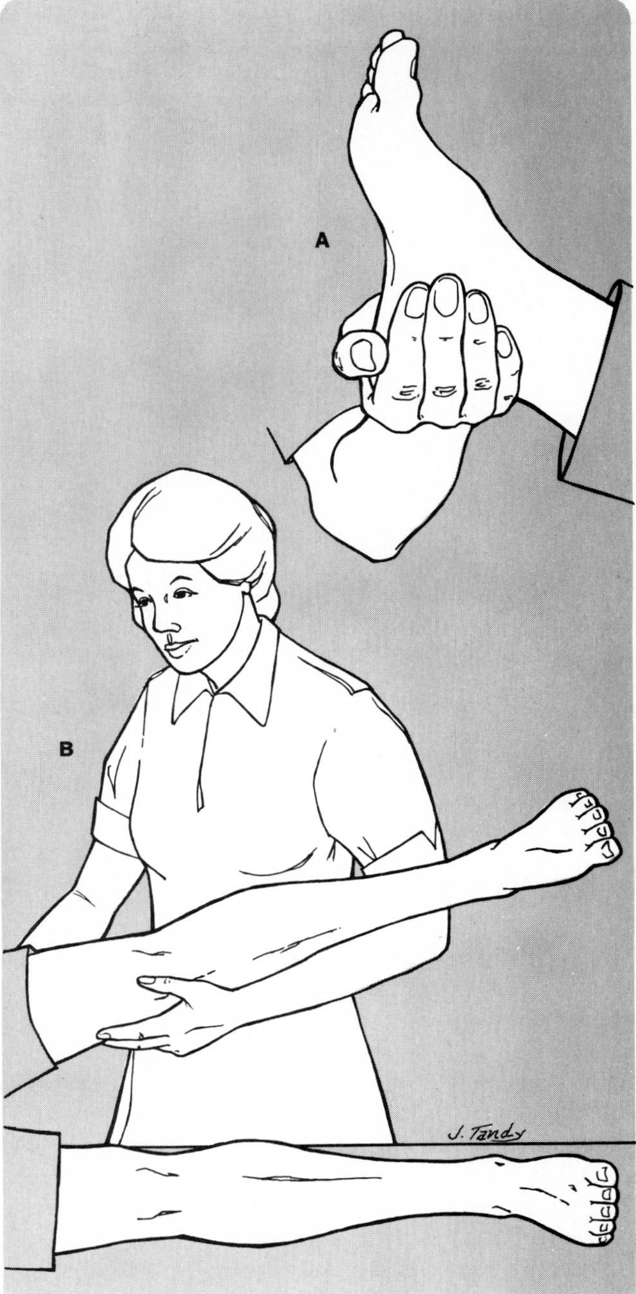

Figure 24–68 Holding limbs for support during passive exercise: **A,** cupping; **B,** cradling.

Kegel's exercises are also done, to strengthen the pubococcygeal muscle postnatally. A postpartum exercise schedule calls for gradual increased exercise. The following schedule is used in some areas:

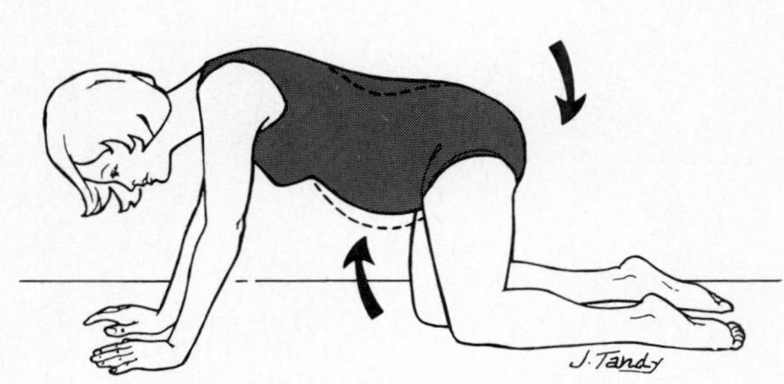

Figure 24–69 Pelvic rocking exercise.

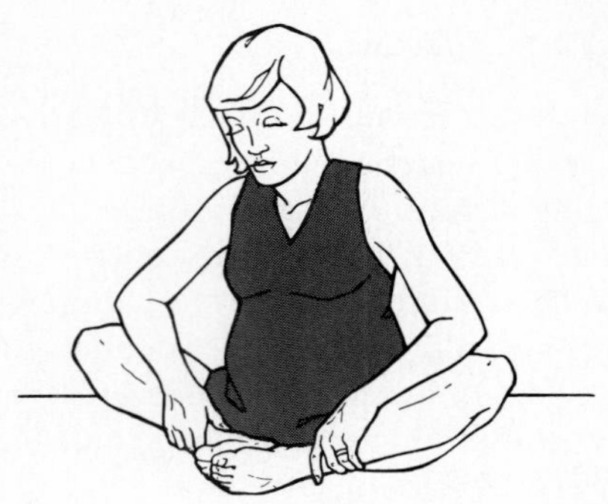

Figure 24–70 Tailor sitting.

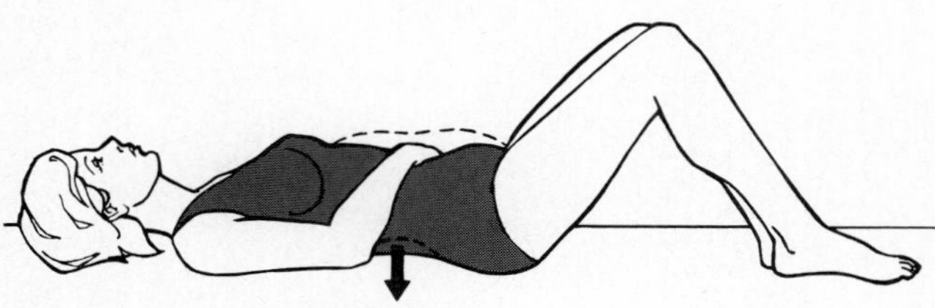

Figure 24–71 Pelvic tilting.

1. Delivery day
   a. Deep breathing
   b. Abdominal tightening
2. First day postpartum
   a. Repeat of above
   b. Chin lift
3. Second day postpartum
   a. Repeat of above
   b. Pelvic tilt
4. Third day postpartum
   a. Repeat of above
   b. Leg raising (modified)

Maintaining Physical Fitness

Regular exercise is necessary for a person to maintain good health. Physical fitness in daily life encompasses both caloric balance and functional fitness. The former is concerned with balancing the number of calories taken in daily with the number of calories expended. See Table 24–4.

Functional physical fitness has three aspects: joint flexibility, muscle tone, and endurance. A purposeful program of exercises can be designed to maintain each of these aspects. To assist patients to maintain physical fitness, nurses may teach the following exercises; nurses too may benefit from such a program.

Joint Flexibility Exercises

1. Circumduction of the shoulder joints. Standing with a broad stance, the person makes full circles with both arms to the front, the rear, and across the body. See Figure 24–72.

2. Rotation of the hips. Standing with feet apart, the person rotates the hips through a full circle while the feet stay on the ground and the knees are slightly flexed. See Figure 24–73.

3. Twisting the trunk. With a semibroad stance and arms extended at the sides, the person slowly twists around to each side, following the leading hand with the eyes. Feet remain fully on the floor, knees slightly flexed. See Figure 24–74. Movement should be slow and smooth, not sudden.

4. Rotating the head and neck. The person rotates the head slowly through a full circle and repeats in the opposite direction. See Figure 24–75.

5. Flexing and hyperextending the shoulder and hip joints. Standing on the left leg, the person supports the body with the left hand and swings the right arm and leg backward and forward in opposite directions. See Figure 24–76. This is then repeated swinging the left arm and leg.

6. Flexing the back. Sitting with legs extended and spread apart, the person places hands on the floor, palms down, between the thighs, then slowly bends forward, sliding the hands along the floor toward the feet. Movement is made smoothly without bouncing. Then the person returns to the sitting position. See Figure 24–77.

7. Hyperextending the shoulders, neck, and hips. Lying on the stomach, the person puts arms at the sides or

Table 24–4 Balance of Calorie Intake and Output

To take in 100 calories (one of the following)		To burn up 100 calories (one of the following)		
			Time	
Food/liquid	*Amount*	*Activity*	*Female*	*Male*
Apple	1¼	Clean windows	30 min	25 min
Banana	1	Bicycle 8 km/h (5 mph)	20 min	19 min
Ice cream	100 ml (2/5 cup)	Play table tennis	30 min	24 min
Raw carrot stick	5	Run 15 km/h (9 mph)	9 min	6 min
Celery stick	20	Run (in place) 140 counts/min	5 min	4 min
Whole milk	155 ml (⅝ cup)	Swim crawl 20 m/min	25 min	20 min
Skim milk	240 ml (1 cup)	Dance (moderate)	30 min	23 min
Ground beef	70 g (2½ oz)	Walk (fast)	19 min	14 min
Hot dog	⅓	Play tennis (moderate)	16 min	13 min
French fried potato	8 pieces			
Baked potato	1			
Cheddar cheese	28 g (1 oz)			
Fried egg	1 small			
Bacon	2 slices			
Bread	1¼ slices			
Beer	240 ml (8 oz)			
Tea or coffee with milk	475 ml (2 cups)			
and sugar	240 ml (1 cup)			

Note: To lose 1 kg (2.2 lb), approximately 3500 calories must be burned.

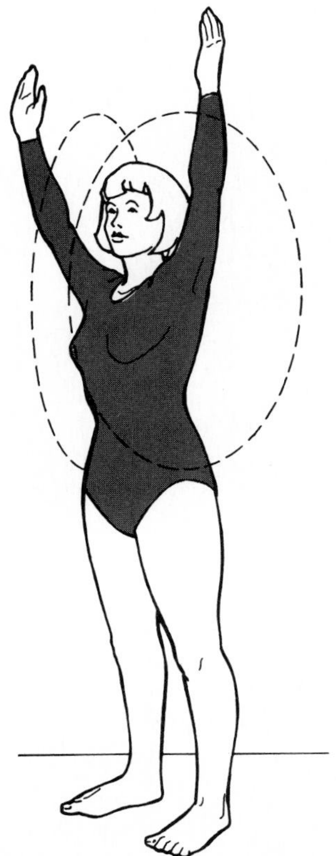
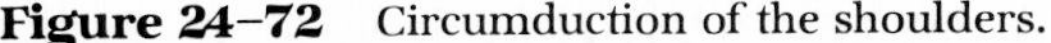

Figure 24–72 Circumduction of the shoulders.

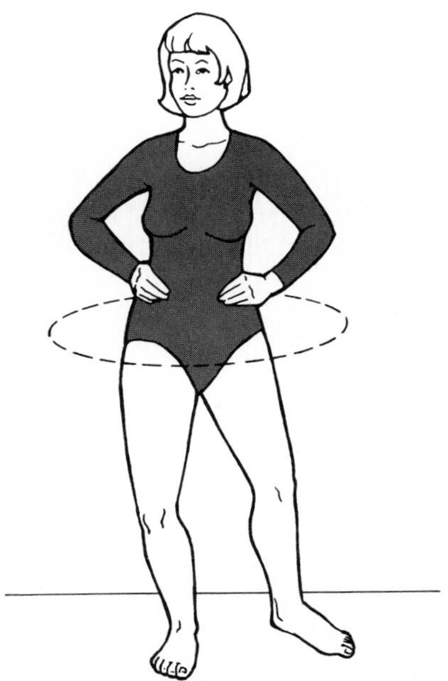

Figure 24–73 Rotation of the hips.

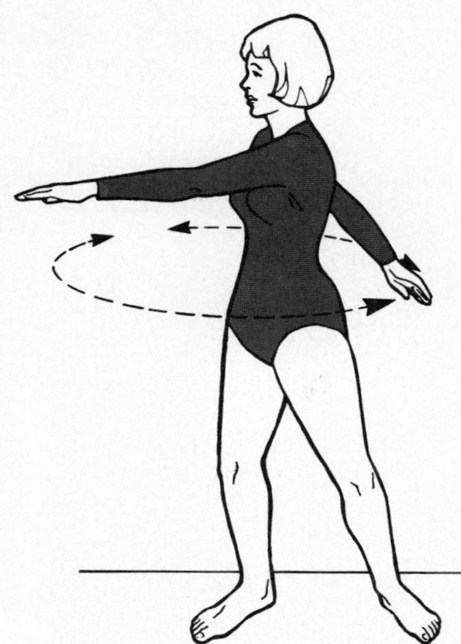

Figure 24–74 Twisting the trunk.

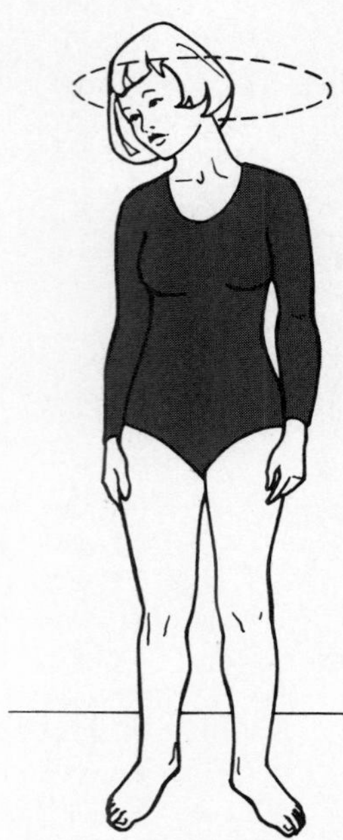

Figure 24–75 Rotating the head and neck.

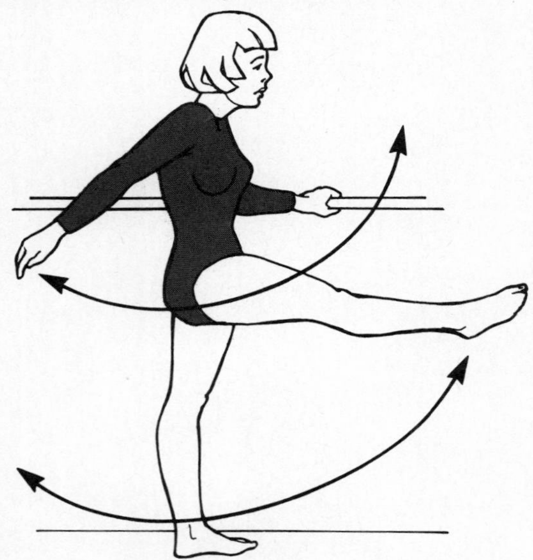

Figure 24–76 Flexing and hyperextending the shoulder and hip joints.

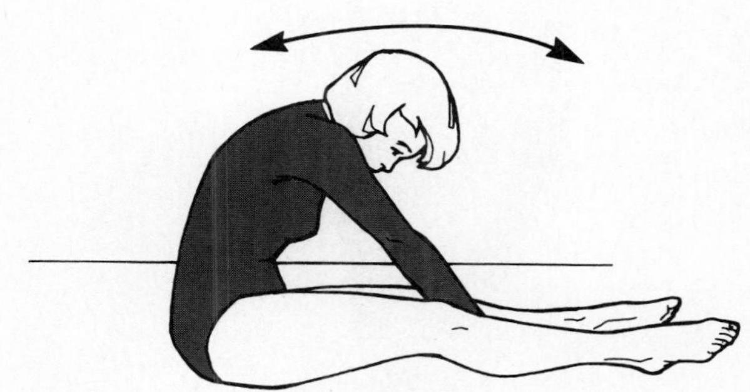

Figure 24–77 Flexing the back.

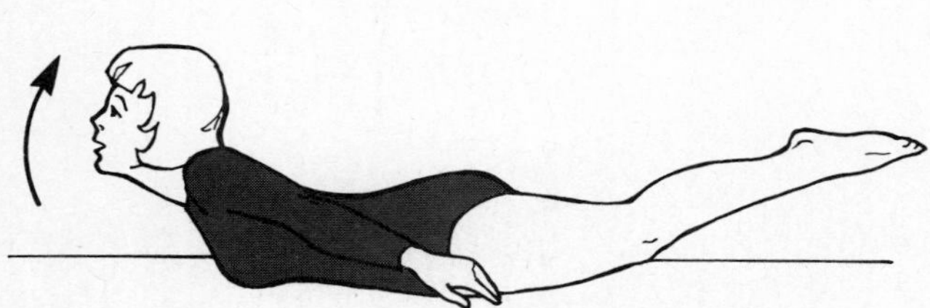

Figure 24–78 Hyperextending the shoulders, neck, and hips.

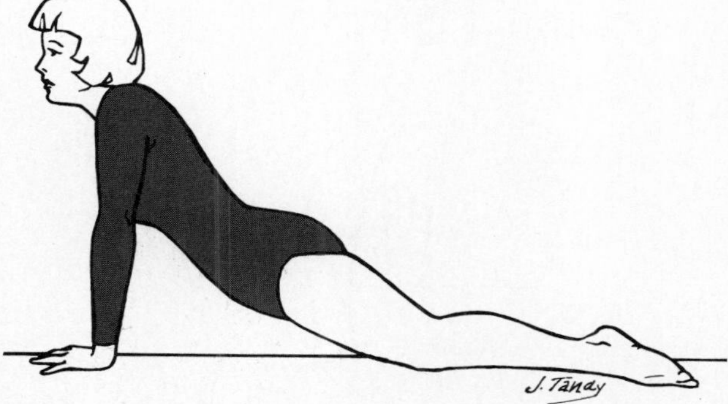

Figure 24–79 Push-ups.

stretches them outward, and tightens the back muscles so that the legs and upper body are lifted from the floor at the same time. See Figure 24–78.

Muscle Tone Exercises

1. Push-ups. The person lies on the stomach, placing hands beneath the shoulders, palms down. The arms are pushed up until straight, then flexed to lower the body to the floor. Beginners may keep the knees on the floor; advanced exercisers may pivot at the toes keeping the entire length of body straight. See Figure 24–79.
2. Sit-ups. The person sits on the floor with knees bent and feet supported (feet may be placed under the edge of a sofa). The person then lies down and sits up. See Figure 24–80. When individual ability improves, hands can be interlocked behind the head while lying and sitting.

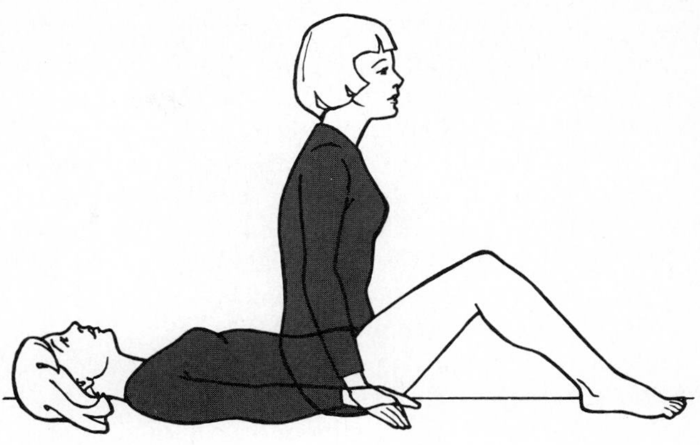

Figure 24–80 Sit-ups.

Endurance Exercises

Endurance exercises are activities such as walking, cycling, or jogging that are done for an extended time period. The person attempts to keep moving for at least 15 minutes, even if it is necessary to slow down. The goal is to work up to and sustain a target heart rate, based on the person's age, during the exercise. For suggested rates, see Table 24–5. One of the simplest methods of assessing this is to take the pulse.

To cool down after the exercise, the person keeps moving with light activity for at least another 5 minutes. The exercise should be done three to five times per week (Collis 1974). As the fitness level improves, the person can elect either to go on to higher heart rates or to continue for longer times at the same rate.

Table 24–5 Suggested Heart Rates for Endurance Exercises

Age (both sexes)	Target heart rate/minute
20–29 years	133
30–39 years	127
40–49 years	125
50–59 years	120
60–69 years	115

From M. Collis, Prescription for fitness, *British Columbia Medical Journal*, September 1974, 16:262.

Evaluation

Outcome criteria to evaluate the effectiveness of nursing interventions depend on the specific nursing goals set for each patient and the nursing diagnoses. Examples of outcome criteria for patients with mobility problems are:

1. Stands erect when walking
2. Walks from bed to nursing station independently three times a day
3. Performs range-of-motion exercises independently two times per day
4. Absence of pain or stiffness in joints
5. Absence of contractures
6. Absence of muscle atrophy
7. Performs scheduled exercise activity without evidence of fatigue

Summary

Mobility and exercise are essential to human health. Mobility allows for movement from place to place and the ability to carry out most of life's daily activities. Even gestures and facial expressions rely on the ability to move body parts. Factors influencing a person's mobility include life-style, disease process or injury, culture, individual energy level, age, and developmental status. Developmental variations in body movement are notable in the first five years of life.

Mobility depends on adequate movement of the body joints. There are six types of joints in the body: ball and socket, hinge, pivot, condyloid, saddle, and gliding. Each has a normal range of motion. Thirteen joint movements are described in relation to the anatomic body position. Examples are flexion, extension, rotation, abduction, and adduction.

Exercise has many positive effects. For example, it maintains the muscle tone of the skeletal muscles and internal organs, facilitates blood circulation, increases metabolism and appetite, aids excretion of body wastes, and provides a sense of mental equilibrium.

Various kinds of exercise may be used in accordance with an individual person's health and strength: active (isotonic), passive, active-assistive, isometric, and resistive exercises. The purposes and indications for use vary for each of these. The normal major range of motion exercises of each body joint are described and illustrated. The nurse's role in providing passive exercises and the value of isometric, prenatal, and postnatal exercises are emphasized.

Limitations in mobility vary in degree but are generally described as immobility even though there is not complete lack of mobility. Broadly speaking, immobility includes physical, intellectual, emotional, and social aspects. Many problems ensue with prolonged immobility. Included are decreased ability to learn, decreased motivation to solve problems, exaggerated emotional reactions, osteoporosis, muscle atrophy, urinary calculi, constipation, accumulation of respiratory secretions, and orthostatic hypotension.

The nurse's role in meeting the mobility needs of patients includes: (a) assessment of individual factors influencing mobility, joint range of motion, station, gait, and activity tolerance, (b) establishing a nursing diagnosis, (c) planning goals, (d) planning appropriate interventions such as ambulation or exercise, and (e) establishing outcome criteria to evaluate the effectiveness of nursing interventions.

Ambulation requires movement of the joints and muscles of the hip and lower extremities. Muscles of the abdomen and buttocks also assist in maintaining balance. When patients are bedridden, these muscles weaken, and exercises preparatory to ambulation are necessary.

When assisting patients to walk, the nurse needs to employ good body mechanics. Various positions and methods may be used to offer security and balance to the patient. Mechanical aids, such as canes, walkers, limb braces, and crutches, offer the patient independence of movement without the nurse's assistance. Four different gaits can be achieved with crutches for varying degrees of mobility.

Physical fitness requires regular exercise in balance with daily caloric intake. Three aspects of functional physical fitness include joint flexibility, muscle tone, and endurance. There are specific exercises for each and suggested target heart rates for endurance exercises.

Suggested Activities

1. Observe a 2-year-old and a 5-year-old. Compare their motor development.
2. Assess your physical fitness in the areas of joint flexibility, muscle tone, and endurance.
3. Observe a physiotherapist with a patient. Identify the kind and purpose of exercises being carried out.
4. Identify patients who require passive exercises. Carry out the appropriate exercises for one patient.
5. Visit a setting where people need assistance with their ambulation. Identify specific problems the patients encounter and the measures taken to assist these patients.

Suggested Readings

Gordon, M. January 1976. Assessing activity tolerance. *American Journal of Nursing* 76:72–75.
The author discusses how to determine an individual's appropriate exercise level. Assessment includes heart rate; heart rhythm; pulse strength; blood pressure; respiratory rate, depth, and rhythm; skin temperature and moistness; posture and equilibrium; activity rate; and emotional state.

Milazzo, V. October 1981. An exercise class for patients in traction. *American Journal of Nursing* 81:1842–44.
This article with photographs explains exercise sessions for patients in traction. Included is a description of particular exercises and the reasons for their inclusion.

Sivarajan, E. S., and Halpenny, C. J. December 1979. Exercise testing. *American Journal of Nursing* 79:2162–70.
The authors describe the physiologic changes in the pulmonary and cardiovascular systems as a result of exercise. They describe three tests, the common responses of patients to these tests, and the information that nurses need to give patients who will be participating in exercise programs.

Selected References

Carnevali, D., and Brueckner, S. July 1970. Immobilization—reassessment of a concept. *American Journal of Nursing* 70:1502–7.

Cohen, S. April 1981. Programmed instruction patient assessment: Examining joints of the upper and lower extremities. *American Journal of Nursing* 81:763–86.

Collis, M. September 1974. Prescription for fitness. *British Columbia Medical Journal* 16:262.

Dehn, M. M. March 1980. Rehabilitation of the cardiac patient: The effects of exercise. *American Journal of Nursing* 80:435–40.

Drapeau, J., et al. September 1975. Getting back into good posture: How to erase your lumbar aches. *Nursing 75* 5:63–65.

Frankel, L. J. December 1977. Exercises to help the elderly—to live longer, stay healthier, and be happier. *Nursing 77* 7:58–63.

Gordon, M. January 1976. Assessing activity tolerance. *American Journal of Nursing* 76:72–75.

Hirschberg, G. G.; Lewis, L.; and Vaughan, P. May 1977. Promoting patient mobility and other ways to prevent secondary disabilities. *Nursing 77* 7:42–46.

Martin, N.; Holt, N.; and Hicks, D. 1981. *Comprehensive rehabilitation nursing*. New York: McGraw-Hill Book Co.

Olson, E. V. April 1967. The hazards of immobility. *American Journal of Nursing* 67:780–97.

Pratt, M. A. September/October 1978. Physical exercise: A special need in long term care. *Journal of Gerontological Nursing* 4:38–42.

Ranalls, J. December 1972. Crutches and walkers. *Nursing 72* 2:21–24.

Russek, A. S., et al. 1964. *Isometric exercises for physical fitness*. Rehabilitation Monograph no. 25. New York: Institute of Rehabilitation Medicine, New York University Medical Center.

Snyder, M., and Baum, R. July 1974. Assessing station and gait. *American Journal of Nursing* 74:1256–57.

Toohey, P., et al. 1968. *Range of motion exercise: Key to joint mobility*. Rehabilitation Publication no. 703. Minneapolis: American Rehabilitation Foundation.

Wiggins, J. D. S. 1979. *Childbearing: Physiology, experiences, needs*. St. Louis: C. V. Mosby Co.

Winslow, E. H., and Weber, T. M. March 1980. Rehabilitation of the cardiac patient: Progressive exercise to combat the hazards of bed rest. *American Journal of Nursing* 80:440–45.

Wolanin, H. T., and Putt, A. M. May/June 1980. The long road back from stroke. *Geriatric Nursing* 1:34–36.

Zohman, L. R., and Tobis, J. S. 1970. *Cardiac rehabilitation*. New York: Grune and Stratton.

Chapter 25

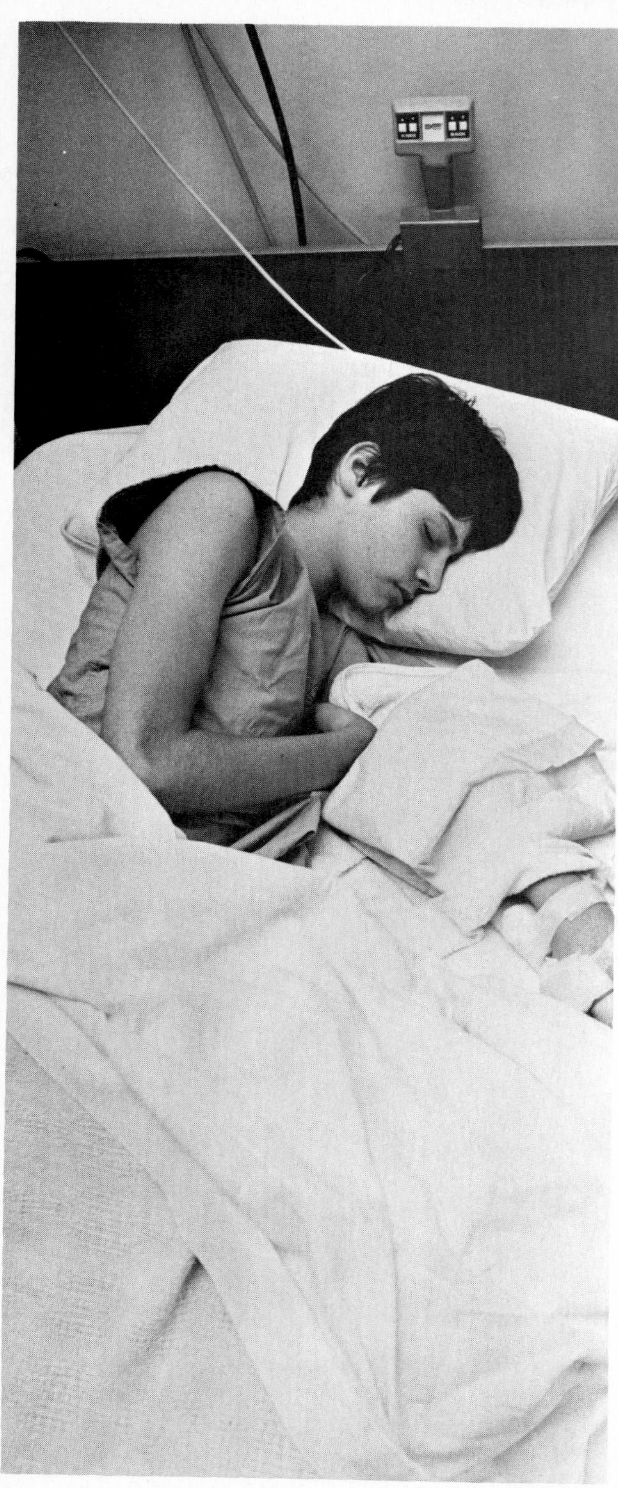

Rest, Sleep, and Relief from Pain

CONTENTS

(Continued on next page)

Objectives

1. Understand essential facts about rest and sleep
  1.1 Define selected terms
  1.2 Identify six conditions necessary to promote rest
  1.3 Compare three common human biorhythmic cycles
  1.4 Identify characteristics of NREM and REM sleep
  1.5 Identify four stages of NREM sleep

2. Know information required to assess a person's sleep and rest patterns
  2.1 Identify required information to assess sleep habits
  2.2 Identify clinical signs and symptoms indicative of insufficient rest and sleep
  2.3 Identify developmental variations in rest and sleep patterns
  2.4 Identify factors influencing rest and sleep

3. Know essential facts about common rest and sleep disorders and nursing diagnoses
  3.1 Define terms related to common rest and sleep disorders
  3.2 Identify three types of insomnia
  3.3 Identify factors contributing to selected sleep disorders
  3.4 Identify data indicative of common rest and sleep disorders
  3.5 Give examples of nursing diagnoses related to sleep disorders

4. Understand facts about nursing interventions required to maintain, promote, and restore normal rest and sleep patterns
  4.1 Identify interventions that promote sleep and rest in newborns and infants, toddlers, preschoolers, school-aged children, adolescents, and adults
  4.2 State the rationale for selected interventions to promote sleep
  4.3 Identify interventions to restore appropriate sleep and rest patterns for selected disorders

5. Apply the nursing process to promote rest and sleep in selected patients
  5.1 Obtain necessary assessment data
  5.2 Analyze and relate assessment data
  5.3 Write relevant nursing diagnoses
  5.4 Write relevant nursing goals
  5.5 Plan appropriate nursing interventions
  5.6 Implement appropriate nursing interventions
  5.7 State outcome criteria against which to evaluate the patient's response

6. Know essential facts about pain physiology, perception, and reaction
  6.1 Identify various types of pain
  6.2 Identify three types of pain receptors
  6.3 Identify two types of nerve pain fibers
  6.4 Describe pain pathways to the brain
  6.5 Describe the gate control theory of pain perception
  6.6 Describe the relationship of endorphins to pain perception
  6.7 Contrast pain threshold and pain tolerance
  6.8 Identify physiological manifestations of four kinds of response to pain

7. Know information required to assess a patient's pain
  7.1 Identify characteristics by which pain is assessed
  7.2 Identify essential facts to obtain for a pain history
  7.3 Identify factors influencing the experience of pain

8. Understand essential facts about interventions to relieve pain
  8.1 Explain how distraction relieves pain
  8.2 Identify five methods of distraction
  8.3 Identify situations in which relaxation techniques can relieve pain effectively
  8.4 Identify essential steps of one relaxation technique
  8.5 Explain essential aspects of the conscious suggestion technique
  8.6 Identify selected skin stimulation techniques used to relieve pain
  8.7 Identify major types of analgesics
  8.8 Identify the rationale for using placebos and four ways of maximizing a positive response to them

8.9 Identify two drugs commonly used to control intractable cancer pain

8.10 Outline essential guidelines for pain management

8.11 Identify selected medical interventions to control pain

9. Apply the nursing process when providing care to selected patients experiencing pain

9.1 Obtain necessary assessment data

9.2 Analyze and relate assessment data

9.3 Write relevant nursing diagnoses

9.4 Write relevant nursing goals

9.5 Plan appropriate nursing interventions

9.6 Implement appropriate nursing interventions

9.7 State outcome criteria by which to evaluate the patient's progress

Terms

aching pain
acupuncture
analgesic
biorhythmology
burning pain
cataplexy
chemosensitive pain receptors
circadian rhythm
circa dies
cordotomy
distraction
dorsal column stimulator
endogenous
endorphin
enkephalin
hypersomnia
hypnosis
infradian rhythm
insomnia
intractable pain
mechanosensitive pain receptors
narcolepsy
narcotic
narcotic agonist-antagonist
nerve block
neurectomy
night terrors
nocturnal enuresis
NREM (non-REM) sleep
pain
pain threshold
pain tolerance
parasomnia
pavor nocturnus
pericutaneous electric stimulation
peripheral nerve implant
phantom pain
pricking pain
psychogenic (functional) pain
referred pain
REM sleep
rest
rhizotomy
sleep
sleep apnea
somatogenic (organic) pain
somnambulism
substantia gelatinosa
sudden infant death syndrome
sympathectomy
thermosensitive pain receptors
transcutaneous electric stimulation
ultradian rhythm

Rest, sleep, and comfort are all essential for health. Everyone needs rest and sleep to function at an optimal level. During sleep, the body repairs itself for the next day. People who are ill frequently require more rest and sleep than normal. Often, debilitated people expend unusual amounts of energy just to maintain the activities of daily living. As a result, such people experience increased and frequent fatigue and thus need more rest and sleep than usual. In addition, the ill person's normal sleep schedule is usually changed, and nursing intervention may be needed to promote the sleep required.

Comfort has both physical and emotional components. Physical comfort includes freedom from pain and harmony with the environment. For example, people in very hot environments experience physical discomfort. Emotional comfort is freedom from mental distress, such as anxiety or depression.

In this chapter, comfort is considered as it relates to pain and freedom from pain. Pain is frequently a problem for patients and challenges the nurse to provide measures that give relief.

Rest

The ill and injured need rest. Rest, however, is not merely inactivity, and distraught patients may find rest difficult. *Rest* implies calmness, relaxation without emotional stress, and freedom from anxiety. Therefore, rest does not always imply inactivity; in fact, certain people find some activities restful. For example, a student studying for examinations may find it restful to walk in the fresh air. The meaning of rest and the need for rest vary among individuals. Providing a restful environment for patients is an important function of nurses. To assess the patient's need for rest and to evaluate how effectively this need is met, nurses need to consider conditions that promote rest.

Narrow (1967:1645) outlines six characteristics most people associate with rest. These summarize the meaning of rest and guide the nurse in assessing and promoting rest for patients.

Most people can rest when they:

1. Feel that things are under control
2. Feel accepted
3. Feel that they understand what is going on
4. Are free from irritation and discomfort
5. Have a satisfying amount of purposeful activity
6. Know that they will receive help when it is needed

To rest, the patient needs to feel both that his or her personal life is under control and that he or she is receiving competent health care. By providing competent care, the nurse gives peace of mind and allows the patient to relax. A nurse often can promote rest by listening carefully to patients' personal concerns and alleviating them when possible. For example, a man taken to an emergency ward may be unable to relax until a nurse telephones his wife to inform her. A busy lawyer who suffers a heart attack may be more worried about whether certain papers were delivered to a client than about pain and discomfort.

Even when the person comes prepared for hospitalization, the nurse must consider the patient's personal concerns and worries. For example, if a patient admitted for elective diagnostic cystoscopy is also recovering successfully from a fractured hip and routinely walks prescribed distances each day, the patient may worry that recovery from the fracture will be slowed by this interruption in exercise. Many patients experience discomfort or anxiety when well-established routines are interrupted. The routine might be reading oneself to sleep, drinking hot milk each evening, or following certain religious practices. Children often have security rituals before sleeping. Patients hospitalized for long periods may need the routine of sleeping in on a Saturday or Sunday morning or scheduled daily quiet or privacy. Most people need some time to themselves.

Rest is impossible for patients who do not feel accepted. Patients need to feel acceptable to themselves and to others. Grooming is often one important aspect of self-acceptance. Women may be concerned about the growth of body hair on their legs or the need for a shampoo or manicure; men may be concerned about an untrimmed beard or mustache. The nurse needs to be sensitive to and attend to these aspects of care. Acceptance by the staff is also important to the patient. Acceptance can be conveyed, for instance, by recognizing both the patient's limitations and progress and recognizing individual differences.

Understanding what is happening is another condition essential for rest. The unknown generates varying degrees of anxiety and interferes with rest. The nurse can help by offering explanations about diagnostic tests, surgery, agency policies or routines, and the patient's progress. When information is given freely, patients do not feel the tension associated with having to ask questions.

Irritation and discomfort have both physical and emotional aspects. Generally, the nurse can easily detect physical discomforts, such as pain, insufficient supports for body positions, damp bedclothes, or loud noise. Emotional discomforts include having too many or too few visitors, feeling a lack of privacy, being hurried, having to wait long periods, being alone, or being concerned about the life problems of self or others.

Purposeful activity can be relaxing and often provides a sense of self-worth. The grandparent who knits a scarf for a grandchild, the person who helps make the bed, the adolescent who makes a wallet for her father, or the child who makes a toy puppet generally have a sense of contentment and accomplishment. Such activity often promotes rest throughout the day and undisturbed sleep at night.

The last prerequisite for rest is the security of knowing help is available when needed. The patient who feels isolated and helpless cannot rest properly. Friends and family members can promote rest by helping the patient with daily tasks and difficult decisions. Nurses can help by anticipating and meeting patients' needs. Knowing that the call bell will be answered, for example, can be exceedingly important to the patient. Also, the support and understanding of the nurse can help patients facing major decisions, such as "Shall I place the baby for adoption?" or "Shall I move to a nursing home?" Although such decisions are the patient's alone, nurses can be instrumental in helping the patient clarify issues, for example, by offering additional information about referral agencies or by helping the patient express feelings.

Sleep

Sleep, a basic physiologic need, is defined as a state of unconsciousness from which a person can be aroused by appropriate sensory or other stimuli (Guyton 1981:679). Sleep is characterized by minimal physical activity, variable levels of consciousness, changes in the body's physiologic processes, and decreased responsiveness to external stimuli.

The purpose of sleep is not clearly known, but it appears to be both integrative and restorative. It is believed necessary for mental and emotional equilibrium and well-being. Theorists believe that during sleep the day's events are reviewed, processed, and filed for future use and that sleep restores the balance among different parts of the central nervous system. Sleep is believed to mediate stress, anxiety, and tension and to help the person regain energy for concentrating, coping, and maintaining interest in daily activities.

Sleep does not appear to be necessary to recharge energy lost during the day. If that were the case, the relative durations of wakefulness and sleep would remain constant, and they do not. For example, when people are deliberately kept awake for 3 to 10 days, they sleep for less than a day after the enforced wakefulness. Conversely, when people are immobilized for long periods, they still sleep and apparently need to. Sleep is also not necessary for body organ function, although physiologic changes occur during sleep. Sympathetic activity decreases, occasionally parasympathetic activity increases, and muscle tone becomes almost nil. Consequently, arterial blood pressure falls, pulse rate decreases, gastrointestinal tract activity sometimes increases, muscles become completely relaxed, and the basal metabolic rate decreases (Guyton 1981:682).

Biorhythms

Biorhythmology, the study of the biologic rhythms of the body, is receiving increasing attention from biologists and health professionals. Rhythmic biologic clocks (biorhythms) exist in plants, animals, and humans. In humans, these are controlled from within the body and synchronized with environmental factors, such as light and darkness, gravity, or electromagnetic stimuli. Human rhythms are demonstrated biologically and behaviorally. Examples of biologic rhythms in humans are the repetitive rhythmic contractions of the heart muscle, the waking and sleeping cycles, and regular temperature fluctuations. Each biorhythmic cycle has peaks and troughs. These cycles vary somewhat among individuals. For example, most adults sleep at night, and most sleep about 8 hours. However, some people, referred to as "night owls," seem to be more alert during the late evening hours and retire late. Others, referred to as "early birds," prefer to retire early and perform well in the early hours of the morning. Some people need only 4 hours of sleep daily.

Biorhythms are classified according to the length of the cycle. The most common cycle is the *circadian rhythm*, a 1-day cycle. The term *circadian* is from the Latin *circa dies*, meaning "about a day." A second rhythm is the *infradian rhythm*, a monthly cycle. An example is the menstrual cycle. A third rhythm is the *ultradian rhythm*, consisting of cycles completed in minutes or hours. An example is the rapid eye movement (REM) cycle of sleep. Biorhythms are not altered by changes in the environment. They are *endogenous*, arising from within the human body and persisting regardless of environmental influences (Deters 1980:250).

Circadian regularity approaching that of adults begins by the 3rd week of life and may be inherited. Babies are awake most often in the early morning and the late afternoon. After 4 months of age, babies enter a 24-hour cycle, in which they sleep mostly during the night. By the end of the 5th or 6th month, babies' sleep-wakefulness patterns are almost like those of adults.

Kinds of Sleep

Electroencephalograms (EEGs) provide a good picture of what occurs during sleep. Electrodes are placed on various parts of the sleeper's scalp. The electrodes transmit electric energy from the cerebral cortex to pens, which record the fluctuations in energy (brain waves) on graph paper. Each pen of the electroencephalogram corresponds to an electrode and moves up when the electric charge is negative and down when it is positive.

There are two kinds of sleep: REM (rapid eye movement) sleep and NREM (non-REM sleep). REM sleep is not a passive, but a relatively active state; so *REM sleep* is also referred to as *paradoxical sleep*. Its characteristics include:

1. Vivid (colorful and busy) dreaming
2. Profound muscle relaxation
3. Irregular, often faster, heart and respiratory rates
4. Variable blood pressure
5. Irregular muscle movements, e.g., muscle twitches
6. Frequent bursts of rapid eye movement
7. Release of steroids in small bursts
8. Increased gastric secretion
9. Penile erections in males of all ages

The sympathetic nervous system dominates during REM sleep. REM sleep is thought to restore a person mentally—that is, for learning, psychologic adaptation, and memory (Hayter 1980:458). During REM sleep, the sleeper reviews the day's events and processes and stores the information. The sleeper gains perspective on problems and may resolve some problems. Thus, there is wisdom in the traditional advice to "sleep on" a problem or big decision.

NREM sleep is also referred to as deep, restful sleep or *slow wave sleep* because the brain waves of a sleeper during NREM sleep are slower than the alpha and beta waves of a person who is awake or alert. See Figure 25–1. Characteristics of NREM sleep include:

1. Dreamlessness
2. Profound restfulness
3. Decreased blood pressure
4. Decreased respiratory rate
5. Decreased metabolic rate
6. Slow and rolling eye movements

Stages of NREM Sleep

NREM sleep has four distinct stages, each of which is characterized by distinct brain wave patterns.

Stage I

Stage I is a transition stage, lasting about 5 minutes, during which the person drifts off from wakefulness to sleep. The person feels drowsy and relaxed. The eyes roll slightly from side to side, and the heart and respiratory rates drop slightly. The alpha waves of wakefulness are replaced by slower theta waves. See Figure 25–1. A person can be readily awakened from stage I.

Stage II

During stage II, there is light sleep, and body processes continue to slow down. The eyes are generally still, heart and respiratory rates decrease slightly, and body temperature and metabolic rate fall. The brain waves of stage II are characterized by sleep spindles and K complexes. Stage II is short, lasting 10 to 15 minutes.

Stage III

During stage III, the heart and respiratory rates as well as other body processes slow further, due to domination of the parasympathetic nervous system. The sleeper becomes more difficult to arouse. The brain waves become more regular. Slow delta waves are added to the stage II pattern.

Stage IV

Stage IV signals deep sleep, during which delta waves predominate and become even slower. Sleepers' heart and respiratory rates drop 20% to 30% below those they exhibit during waking hours. The sleeper is very relaxed, rarely moves, and is difficult to arouse. Stage IV is thought to restore the body physically. Physical exercise, if it occurs 2 hours before bedtime, promotes stage IV sleep (Hayter 1980:457).

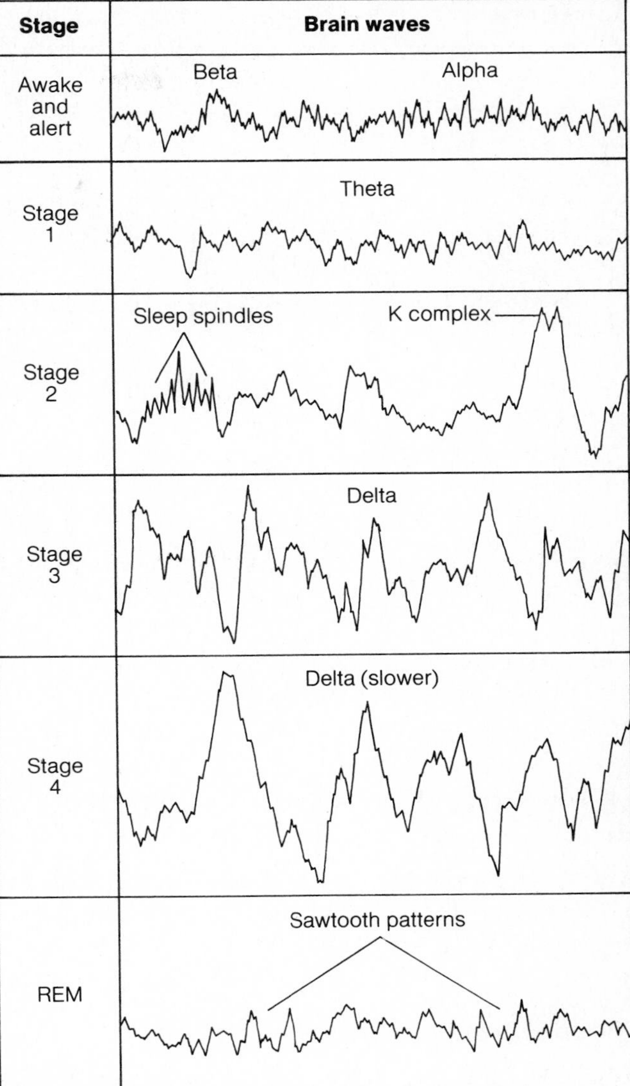

Figure 25–1 Stages of sleep. (Adapted from W. F. Ganong, *Review of medical physiology*, 10th ed. [Los Altos, Calif.: Lang Medical Publications, 1981], pp. 151–53; M. Clark, M. Gosnell, D. Shapiro, and M. Hager, The mystery of sleep, *Newsweek* July 13, 1981, pp. 48–51; and data from the Sleep-Wake Disorders Center, Montefiore Hospital, New York.)

Sleep Cycle

Sleep is cyclic. The usual sleeper experiences four to six cycles of sleep during 7 to 8 hours. Each cycle lasts about 90 minutes. The cycle is made up of most if not all stages of NREM sleep and the final stage—REM sleep. See Figure 25–2. A sleeper passes from stage I NREM sleep through stages II and III to stage IV in about 20 to 30 minutes. Stage IV may last about 30 minutes. The process is then reversed, and the sleeper ascends through stages III and II, after which REM sleep occurs. REM sleep completes the first cycle, and then the cycle repeats. The sleeper who is awakened during any stage must begin anew at stage I NREM sleep and proceed through all the stages to REM sleep.

The duration of NREM stages and REM sleep varies throughout the 8-hour sleep period. As the night progresses, the sleeper becomes less tired and spends less time in stages III and IV of NREM sleep. REM sleep increases, and dreams tend to lengthen. See Figure 25–2. If the sleeper is very tired, REM cycles are often short—for example, 5 minutes instead of 20—during the early portion of sleep. Before sleep ends, periods of near wakefulness occur, and stages I and II NREM sleep and REM sleep predominate.

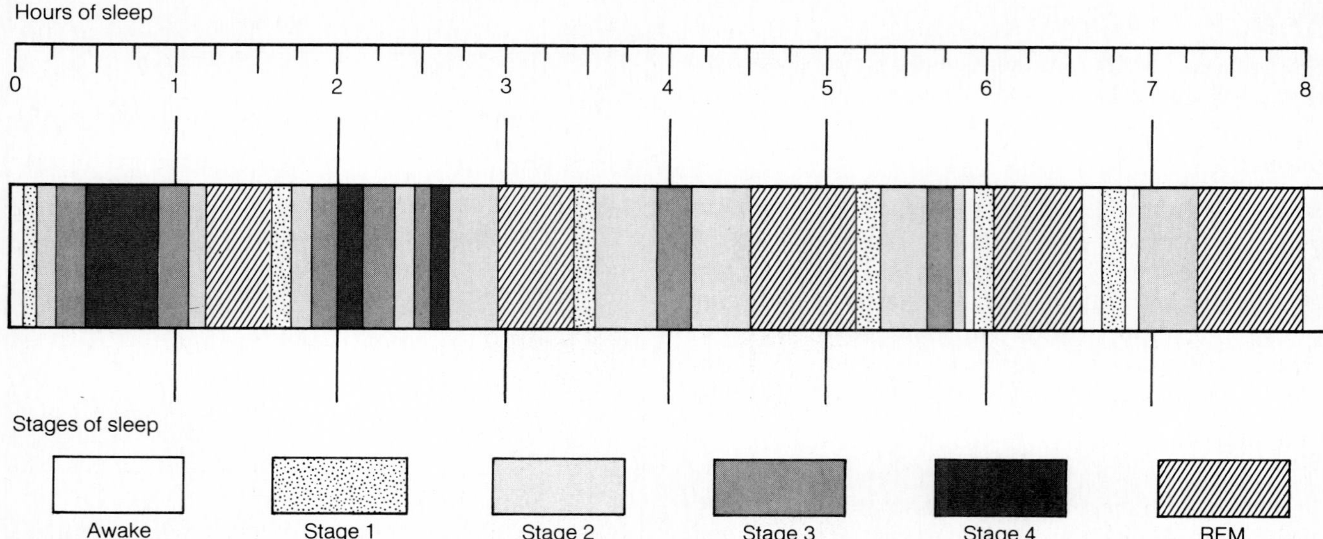

Figure 25–2 Sleep cycles. (Adapted from data from the Sleep-Wake Disorders Center, Montefiore Hospital, New York, and M. Clark, M. Gosnell, D. Shapiro, and M. Hager, The mystery of sleep, *Newsweek*, July 13, 1981, pp. 48–55.)

The ratio of NREM to REM sleep varies with age (see the section on developmental changes, below) and with other factors. Psychological stress creates a need for more REM sleep. As a result, the person awakens with the feeling that sleep was not restful and that he or she dreamt more than usual.

Assessing the Need for Rest and Sleep

The nurse assesses (a) sleep habits, (b) clinical signs and symptoms of the need for sleep, (c) developmental changes, and (d) factors influencing rest and sleep.

Sleep Habits

When assessing an individual's sleeping habits, the nurse must consider:

1. Patient's usual amount of sleep
2. Patient's usual practices prior to sleeping, such as reading
3. Patient's usual hours for sleeping
4. Time it takes the patient to fall asleep
5. Number of times the patient awakens during sleep and the reasons
6. Medications taken by the patient and how they affect sleep
7. Patient's usual sleep environment
8. Patient's perceptions of the need for sleep
9. Accustomed position during sleep

Clinical Signs

People's reaction to insufficient rest and sleep are highly individual. Some early clinical signs and symptoms of insufficient rest and sleep are:

1. Expression of a feeling of fatigue
2. Irritability and restlessness
3. Lassitude and apathy
4. Darkened areas around the eyes, puffy eyelids, reddened conjunctivas, and burning eyes
5. Marked periods of inattention
6. Headache
7. Nausea

Sleep deprivation or prolonged loss of sleep triggers certain biochemical changes in the body. Sleeplessness lowers the seizure threshold. Consequently, people with epilepsy should not go without sleep for prolonged periods. Some of the clinical signs of sleep deprivation are:

1. Behavior and personality changes, such as aggressiveness, withdrawal, or depression
2. Increased restlessness
3. Distorted perceptions
4. Visual or auditory hallucinations
5. Confusion and disorientation to time and place
6. Decreased coordination
7. Slurred speech or inappropriate speech and tone

Developmental Changes

The amount of sleep individuals require decreases not only with age but also as the growth rate decreases. See Table 25–1.

Newborns and infants

The newborn, regardless of gestational age or type of delivery, is awake, alert, and active during the transition from intrauterine to extrauterine life. This activity lasts only for about 90 minutes, however, and a sleep of 4 to 8 hours follows, depending on the stresses of birth. After this initial phase, periods of wakefulness stabilize, occurring every 3 or 4 hours. For the first few weeks, the infant's wakefulness is dictated largely by hunger. Later, the need to socialize affects wakefulness. On the average, newborns sleep 17 hours daily, and by the end of the 1st month, the periods of wakefulness gradually increase. For example, some may stay awake during the day from one feeding to another and sleep longer at night. Sounds in the environment seem to have minimal, if any, effect on the newborn's sleep. This fact can be observed in nurseries, where often one newborn cries loudly in one crib and another newborn sleeps soundly in an adjacent crib.

Newborns usually can be aroused easily from sleep, and they return to sleep just as easily, provided they are comfortable. Frequent body movements and facial grimaces are normal during sleep and indicate REM sleep. When newborns do not sleep well and cry or fuss for long periods, they are usually hungry, wet, hot, or cold. If comfort measures offer no relief, illness may be the cause.

In infants of 2 months, the observer may note a preference for one sleeping position, but this preference may have been present at birth. By 3 months, the infant exhibits routines before sleeping, such as crying, sucking on fingers or toys, or shifting positions repeatedly. By 4 months, most infants sleep through the night and have a scheduled pattern of daytime naps that varies with individuals during the day. They generally awaken early in the morning, however. At the end of the 1st year, an infant usually has one or two naps per day and sleeps about 14 of every 24 hours. The infant also begins to show fear of being left alone.

Table 25–1 Sleep Patterns According to Age

Developmental level	Normal sleep pattern
Newborn	Sleeps 14 to 18 hours/day Regular breathing, little body movement 50% REM sleep Sleep cycles 45 to 60 minutes
Infant	Sleeps 12 to 14 hours/day 20 to 30% REM sleep May sleep through the night
Toddler	Sleeps about 11 to 12 hours/day 25% REM sleep Sleeps during the night and takes naps
Preschooler	Sleeps about 11 hours/day 20% REM sleep
School-aged child	Sleeps about 10 hours/day 18.5% REM sleep
Adolescent	Sleeps about 8.5 hours/day 20% REM sleep
Young adult	Most sleep 7 to 8 hours/day 20 to 25% REM sleep
Middle-aged adult	Sleeps about 7 hours/day About 20% REM sleep May have insomnia (difficulty falling asleep)
Elderly adult	Sleeps about 6 hours/day 20 to 25% REM sleep May have insomnia (difficulty staying asleep)

Adapted from L. Malasanos, V. Barkauskas, M. Moss, and K. Stoltenberg-Allen. *Health assessment* (St. Louis: C. V. Mosby Co., 1977), pp. 80–81 and from L. F. Whaley and D. L. Wong, *Nursing care of infants and children* (St. Louis: C. V. Mosby Co., 1979), pp. 66–67.

Toddlers

The sleep requirements of toddlers (1 to 3 years) decrease to 10 to 14 hours per day. Most toddlers still need an afternoon nap, but the necessity for midmorning naps gradually decreases. However, toddlers may have problems going to sleep. Frequently parents of toddlers seek guidance to handle their children's difficulty in going to sleep. During toddlerhood, dreams and nightmares are common.

At bedtime, toddlers frequently resist sleep, feel tense, may be irritable, may cry, and may not want to leave the company of adults or older siblings. It is normal for toddlers to assert independence by refusing to take a nap or go to sleep at predesignated times. This behavior reflects the toddler's growing independence, self-control, curiosity, and endless vigor for exploration. However, toddlers like rituals and insist on them. A typical ritual takes this form: the parent helps the child into bedclothes, tells the child that bedtime is in half an hour, and tells the child a story. The child gives others a goodnight hug; and the parent gives the child a security toy and glass of juice, draws the shades, and dims the lights. Firm adherence to such rituals is essential. Consistency is more important than the form of the ritual.

Toddlers often develop their own ways of going to sleep. They may talk to themselves for awhile, roll their heads, rock in bed, or play with a toy. These behaviors are normal and relieve tension. Similar behavior is observed before daytime naps; prenap rituals also should be consistent. Often, mothers of toddlers require an afternoon nap that can be scheduled to coincide with the toddler's.

Preschoolers

Preschoolers (3 to 6 years), like toddlers, are not aware that they need rest or sleep. Preschoolers are more interested in what is happening around them and also may resist sleep. The difference is that the preschooler requires more privacy, not only for sleep but also for fantasy, sexual explorations, enjoyment of possessions, or for intervals to deal with disappointments and hurts. Preschoolers need a room or portion of a room to themselves for these private activities.

Three-year-olds frequently have nightmares associated with real or imagined fears. Sometimes it is difficult for them to differentiate between what is real and what is not. It is not unusual for preschoolers to wander into their parents' bedroom and want to sleep with them. Children who have difficulty sleeping at night may become less restless if they have naps during the day. Sleeping near older siblings or parents can also be comforting.

At age 4 or 5, children resist daytime sleep. Children who cannot sleep during the day often need a rest period. Parents can promote rest by darkening a room and providing restful or quiet activities. Day-care centers and kindergartens commonly schedule such rest periods. By age 5, children usually sleep restfully through the night but may require occasional daytime naps if activities are overly stimulating. Nightmares may persist but are to be expected.

School-age children

A peaceful night's sleep is often not possible for school-age children. Although the sleep requirements are less (9 to 13 hours), the child may have nightmares, often associated with fears of death, a concept the child is beginning to understand. Parents can expect questions, discussions, and confidences from children of this age.

Growing children increasingly want a say about the time they go to bed. Parental judgment is still required, however. Parents need to set limitations on the child's activities and schedule specific bedtimes to ensure sufficient rest. More flexibility in schedules is possible with older children.

Adolescents

Adolescents usually sleep from 8 to 10 hours per day. Because adolescents are very active, they need rest and sleep. Sometimes adolescents are unaware of their needs, and adults must set limits so that teenagers can obtain the necessary rest and sleep. Reading and other restful activity help the adolescent avoid fatigue. Adolescents seldom wake spontaneously in the night.

Young adults

Young adults' need for sleep is largely determined by such factors as emotional and physical health, amount of activity, pregnancy, and personality. Although most young adults require 7 to 8 hours, it is also normal for adults to sleep less than 6 and more than 9 hours.

Sometimes young adults find their sleep disturbed by young children. Sleeping a few hours at a time produces the same effect as sleeping less, even though the total time is the same. Stage IV sleep is most often disturbed, and the sleeper obtains little REM sleep. When such a young adult gets the opportunity to sleep undisturbed, he or she gets more REM sleep than usual. *Insomnia* (inability to get enough sleep) in young adults is an increasing problem. Commonly, the difficulty is getting to sleep rather than waking midsleep.

Middle-aged adults

Middle-aged adults normally sleep on an average of 7 hours a day. Middle-aged adults get more non-REM (deep and restful) sleep than young adults. The 90-minute REM cycle remains relatively constant; however, there is marked decrease in the amount of stage IV sleep.

Elderly adults

People 60 and older take longer to go to sleep and tend to awaken earlier. Older adults also experience changes in sleep patterns. The amount of stage IV sleep decreases by about 15% to 30% (Hayter 1980:460). Elderly people wake more often during the night. The number of times adults awaken during the night increases from once in young adulthood to 6 per night at age 60 (ibid., p. 460). It is also believed that women's sleep patterns change about 10 years later than men's.

Factors Influencing Sleep

Both the quality and the quantity of sleep are affected by several factors. *Quality* describes the individual's ability to stay asleep and to get appropriate amounts of REM and non-REM sleep. Sleep stages can be differentiated and measured only in a laboratory. The quantity of sleep is the total time the individual sleeps.

A number of factors can affect the quality and quantity of sleep adversely. Some of the most common are illness, environment, fatigue, emotions, medications, and alcohol. See Table 25–2.

Illness

People who are ill require more sleep than normal, and the normal rhythm of sleep and wakefulness is also disturbed. People deprived of REM sleep subsequently spend more sleeping time in this stage than normal. Pain also can affect sleep. Pain can prevent sleep or awaken the sleeper.

Environment

Environment can promote or hinder sleep. People usually become accustomed to the sleeping environments in their homes, and any change in the environment—e.g., a change in the noise level—can inhibit sleep. People often become accustomed to certain noises, lights, etc., and the absence of these or the presence of strange stimuli can keep them from sleeping. A nurse may hear a patient say, "I can't sleep here; it is too quiet" or "I can't sleep because of the bell that rings every hour."

Fatigue

Fatigue also affects the sleep pattern—the more tired the person, the shorter the first period of paradoxical (REM) sleep. As the person rests, the REM periods become longer.

Anxiety

Anxiety and other emotional upsets affect a person's ability to sleep. An anxious patient is often preoccupied with problems that do not allow relaxation prior to sleep.

Medications

Medications, especially hypnotics and sedatives, affect the sleep pattern. Hypnotics and barbiturates decrease REM sleep even though they may increase the total sleep time. Amphetamines and antidepressants decrease REM sleep abnormally. Long-term use of amphetamines can produce abnormal behavior, which can be attributed to long-term REM deprivation.

Table 25–2 Factors Influencing Sleep

Factor	Effect
Liver failure	Day-night reversal
Encephalitis	Day-night reversal
Hypothyroidism	Decreases stage IV sleep
Antidepressant	Decreases REM sleep
Amphetamine	Decreases REM sleep
Alcohol	Speeds onset of sleep but decreases REM sleep and disrupts other stages
Depression	Decreases or increases REM sleep
Sedative-hypnotic drugs	Suppresses REM sleep and decreases stages III and IV. On withdrawal causes rebound REM sleep with vivid dreams and increased awakening
Tranquilizer	Interferes with REM sleep
Bedtime snacks of protein foods	Induce and maintain sleep

A patient withdrawing from any of these drugs gets much more REM sleep than usual and as a result may experience upsetting nightmares. Nurses need to be aware of this possibility and give the patient support.

Alcohol

Alcohol depresses the normal REM stage of sleep. While making up for this lost REM sleep after withdrawal from alcohol, patients also experience terrible nightmares. Tolerance to alcohol can result in insomnia and subsequent irritability.

Nursing Diagnoses

Common Sleep Disorders

The two most common sleep disorders are insomnia in adults and parasomnias in children. Less usual sleep disorders are hypersomnia, narcolepsy, sleep apnea, and sudden infant death syndrome.

Insomnia

Insomnia is the inability to obtain sufficient quality or quantity of sleep. It is not the total lack of sleep; in fact, people with insomnia often obtain more sleep than they realize. There are three types of insomnia: inability to fall asleep (initial insomnia), inability to stay asleep because of frequent waking (intermittent insomnia), and early awakening and subsequent inability to go back to sleep (terminal insomnia). Terminal insomnia is characteristic of depressed patients. Insomniacs do not feel refreshed on arising.

Insomnia can result from physical discomfort but more often is a result of mental overstimulation due to anxiety. People sometimes become anxious because they think they might not be able to sleep. People who become habituated to drugs or who drink large quantities of alcohol are likely to have insomnia.

Treatment for insomnia frequently requires the patient to develop new behavior patterns that induce sleep. The usefulness of sleeping medications is questionable. Such medications do not deal with the cause of the problem, and their prolonged use creates drug dependencies.

Nurses need to encourage insomniacs to develop an effective sleep/rest and exercise routine. Insomniacs should (a) get adequate exercise during the day; (b) avoid excitement during the evening; (c) establish a relaxing pastime before sleep, such as reading, playing solitaire, etc.; (d) go to bed only when sleepy, not when the time seems appropriate; (e) when unable to sleep at night, get up and pursue some relaxing activity until they feel drowsy (or if unable to sleep in the early morning, get up and pursue some activity that provides a sense of accomplishment).

Hypersomnia

The opposite of insomnia, *hypersomnia*, is excessive sleep of more than 9 hours at night. The afflicted person often sleeps until noon and takes many naps during the day. Hypersomnia is generally related to psychophysiologic problems, such as psychiatric disorders (depression or anxiety), central nervous system damage, and some kidney, liver, or metabolic disorders.

Parasomnias

Parasomnias refer to a cluster of disorders that interfere with children's sleep, such as *somnambulism* (sleepwalking), *night terrors (pavor nocturnus)*, and *nocturnal enuresis* (bedwetting). These disorders often appear together in the same child, run in families, and tend to occur during stages III and IV of NREM sleep.

Somnambulism is not uncommon in children and is normally outgrown without incident. The main concern is to protect the somnambulist from injury. Usually the sleepwalker can be awakened and quietly led back to bed.

Night terrors are frightening to both parents and the child. Children 6 and younger are most often afflicted. After having slept for a few hours, the child bolts upright in bed, shakes and screams, appears pale and terrified, but is difficult to arouse. In contrast to nightmares, night terrors are not remembered the next morning.

Nocturnal enuresis can occur in preadolescent children. Its cause is unknown, although in preschool children it may be due to training that is too severe or too early, or to overtraining (Marlow 1977:619). If the child is 3 or 4 years, environmental factors, such as a dark hall, may contribute to the child's reluctance to go to the bathroom. In the schoolchild, enuresis may be caused by inadequate bladder capacity or jealousy over a new brother or sister. Parents should rule out physical abnormalities first and provide an environment in which the child feels loved. Restricting fluids before bedtime may reduce the incidence of bedwetting but does not address the cause of the problem.

Narcolepsy

Narcolepsy, from the Greek words *narco* meaning "numbness" and *lepsis* meaning "seizure," is a sudden wave of overwhelming sleepiness that occurs during the day; thus it is referred to as a "sleep attack." Its cause is unknown, although it is believed to be a genetic defect of the central nervous system in which the REM period cannot be controlled. In narcoleptic attacks, sleep starts with the REM phase. Even though they sleep well at night, narcoleptics nod off several times during a day.

Many narcoleptics have bouts of *cataplexy*, partial or complete muscle paralysis. Sometimes the person's jaw slackens or the head falls to the chest. These cataplectic bouts are often preceded by moments of exertion or strong emotion, such as laughing or crying.

Narcoleptics are often accused of laziness, disinterest in life and work, and even drunkenness. Their handicap, however, is life threatening in a world fraught with many potential hazards. Drug therapy is used with some success to treat narcolepsy. Stimulants such as amphetamines or methylphenidate hydrochloride (Ritalin) prevent attacks; and antidepressants, such as imipramine hydrochloride (Tofranil), prevent the muscle weakness and paralysis of cataplexy. Narcoleptics should avoid liquor, which increases drowsiness.

Sleep apnea

Sleep apnea is the periodic cessation of breathing during sleep. This disorder needs to be assessed by a sleep expert, but it is often suspected when the person has obstructive snoring, excessive daytime sleepiness, and sometimes insomnia. The periods of apnea, which last from 10 seconds to 3 minutes, occur during REM or NREM sleep. Frequency of episodes ranges from 50 to 600 per night. These apneic episodes drain the person of energy and lead to excessive daytime sleepiness.

Obstructive apnea is caused by defects—for instance, an excessively thick palate, enlarged tonsils, or a jaw deformity—that temporarily obstruct the air passages and deplete the supply of oxygen to the lungs. Central apnea is caused by defects in the respiratory centers of the brain. These defects cause a transient diaphragmatic arrest, and the lungs stop moving. When the level of carbon dioxide in the blood reaches a certain level, the person is jolted to near wakefulness (e.g., may sit up with a sudden start) but does not regain consciousness.

Sleep apnea profoundly affects a person's work or

school performance. In addition, prolonged sleep apnea can cause a sharp rise in blood pressure and may also lead to cardiac arrest. Over time, apneic episodes can cause pulmonary hypertension and subsequent left-sided heart failure.

The treatment of sleep apnea depends on the cause. Central apnea is sometimes treated with powerful tranquilizers, while some obstructive types are treated by a tracheostomy, a permanent, surgical opening of the trachea. The opening is uncapped during sleep but capped during the day to allow normal breathing.

Sudden infant death syndrome

Sudden infant death syndrome, which afflicts children during their first 12 months, is also referred to as SIDS or crib death. Its cause is unknown, although some attribute it to an immature nervous system or to sleep apnea. Others believe it is a defect in the infant's sleep pattern, since most crib deaths occur in infants of 2 to 4 months, an age when the infant's REM sleep decreases. When the infant is awake, external sights and sounds stimulate a part of the brain (reticular formation) that plays a key role in respiration. When the infant sleeps, this stimulation is replaced to some degree by REM sleep. Thus when REM sleep decreases, the reticular formation is stimulated less.

Examples of Diagnoses

Nursing diagnoses for patients with rest or sleep problems may be categorized broadly as sleep pattern disturbances or may be stated more specifically as insomnia, hypersomnia, sleep deficit (deprivation), etc. Sleep is a complex phenomenon influenced by many factors. To complete the nursing diagnosis, the nurse needs to determine the specific contributing factor. Some examples of nursing diagnoses associated with sleep disorders are:

1. Insomnia related to:
   a. Situational stress, such as bereavement, marital problems, business pressures, etc.
   b. Pain or discomfort from a medical condition, e.g., arthritis
   c. Withdrawal from mood-altering drugs, such as alcohol, sedatives, or stimulants
   d. Inadequate exercise and boredom
2. Sleep deprivation related to:
   a. 24-hour intensive care (noise and frequent interruptions)
   b. Sleep apnea
3. Altered behavior related to sleep deprivation
4. Lowered self-esteem related to nocturnal enuresis
5. Potential for injury related to somnambulism
6. Hypersomnia related to liver disease

Planning and Intervention to Promote Rest and Sleep

The overall nursing goal is to promote a satisfactory rest-sleep pattern. Nursing subgoals are:

1. To prevent fatigue
2. To balance activity and rest appropriately
3. To restore physical energy
4. To restore mental and emotional well-being

Plans

Planning includes consideration of the patient's environment and comfort, and the timing and scheduling of tests, treatments, etc. The environment should be conducive to sleep. The nurse works to minimize disturbing stimuli. Comfort includes freedom from pain, proper positioning, a clean, dry bed, etc. The nurse needs to involve the patient in planning the times for the sleep. Perhaps the patient expects visitors or wants to see a certain television program. Sleep should be scheduled to not interfere with these events. Because visits from health team personnel or trips to hospital departments can interrupt sleep, these should be scheduled to interfere with sleep as little as possible. Planning also involves establishing outcome criteria. For suggestions see the outcome criteria on page 631.

Interventions

Nursing interventions should be responsive to the sleep patterns and needs of individual patients. Some general measures, for patients categorized by age, follow.

Newborns and infants

Measures to promote sleep and rest in infants also include some safety and security measures. The nurse needs to:

1. Provide a firm mattress covered with thick plastic material that cannot be pulled over the face and cause suffocation. A flat surface provides the best alignment for bone development.

2. Avoid pillows. They, too, can cause accidental suffocation.

3. Position the infant appropriately according to age. Newborns should not be placed on their abdomens unless they are observed very closely. They are unable to turn their heads from side to side and may suffocate if their noses press down firmly against the mattress. The side-lying position is safe, but the infant must be shifted from one side to the other every 2 to 3 hours. See Figure 25–3. Alternating the infant's position prevents flattening of the bones of the skull. The back-lying position is also avoided for newborns and young infants, because of the danger the child may aspirate fluids if he or she vomits. When able to turn the head from side to side, the infant may be positioned on the back, abdomen, or side. It is recommended that various positions be used.

4. Ensure that the room temperature is comfortable, approximately 18 to 21 C (65 to 70 F) in the daytime and 15.5 to 18 C (60 to 65 F) at night. The nurse should place the child away from drafts and tuck blankets under the mattress to minimize danger of suffocation.

5. Provide soft lighting directed away from the eyes. Sleeping infants dislike both darkness and bright light and like to face a dim light. One way to reposition a sleeping child and still have the child face a stationary light is to place the child's head alternately at the foot and head of the crib instead of turning the child from left to right.

6. Ensure that the infant is dry and comfortable. Provide dry diapers and warm, soft clothing.

7. Provide quieting activities before putting the infant to bed, such as cuddling or rocking the infant, talking in soothing tones, and establishing consistent routines and a quiet environment.

Toddlers

To promote sleep in toddlers, nurses need to:

1. Provide consistent bedtime or naptime rituals.

2. Adhere firmly to sleeping schedules.

3. Encourage quieting activities before sleep.

4. Support tension-reducing activities, such as head-rolling or talking. Nurses should give the child only one toy at bedtime. Too many toys create too much stimulation.

5. Avoid putting the toddler to bed as a disciplinary measure at any time.

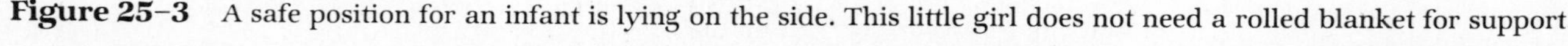

Figure 25–3 A safe position for an infant is lying on the side. This little girl does not need a rolled blanket for support.

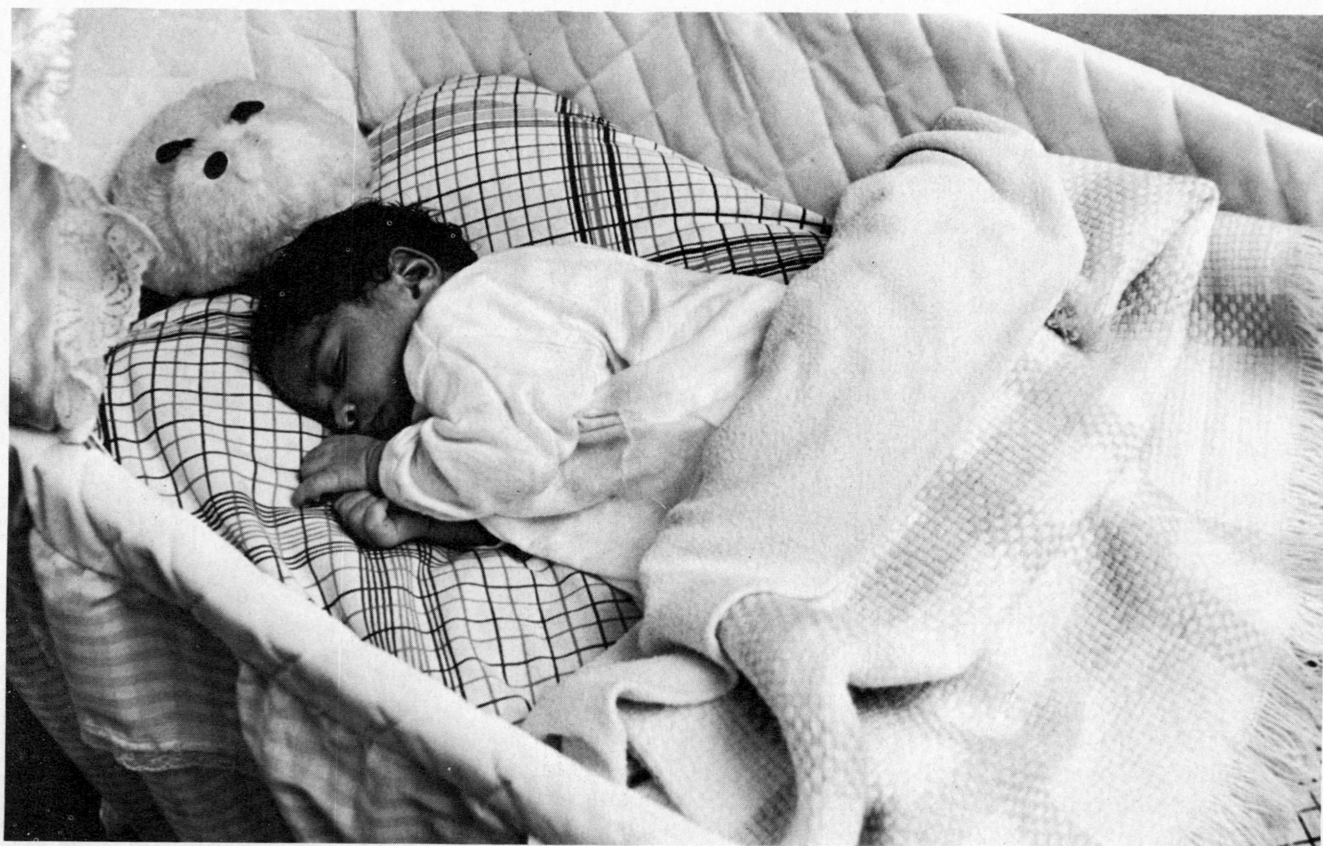

Preschoolers

Measures to promote sleep and rest in preschoolers are similar to those for toddlers. Toddlers show increasing independence during the presleep ritual, but must be encouraged to express fears, which also increase at this age. The nurse usually can reassure the child by listening to the child's fears and making it clear that nurses will be nearby.

Sometimes preschoolers have difficulty getting to sleep because they are so highly stimulated. They often need a time to settle down before sleep, for example, a quiet time during which the nurse reads bedtime stories.

If children fear going to sleep, reassurance that others are nearby will help allay fears. Some children feel less afraid when there is a night light in the room.

School-age children

Children in this age group still require considerable rest; however, they often want to stay up longer than is wise. As children grow, they should have greater say in the decision of when to go to bed.

Adolescents

The nurse must sometimes set limits so that hospitalized or ill adolescents get enough rest and sleep. The adolescent often needs time before sleeping to tend to grooming and personal hygiene, frequent preoccupations of adolescents.

Adults (young, middle-aged, elderly)

The following measures frequently help promote the sleep of adults (and in some instances children). The nurse can:

1. Help the patient relax before sleep. The nurse helps the patient relax, for instance, by providing diversions, pain relief, a clean, comfortable bed, and an odor-free room.
2. Help the patient maintain usual before-sleep routines. Some people like a tub bath before a night's sleep, others like to read or listen to quiet music. Sometimes, a patient's sleeplessness is related to a disrupted routine. For example, a patient may find it difficult to sleep if unable to follow the lifelong habit of brushing teeth before retiring. It is usually helpful for the hospitalized sick person to adhere to routines unless they are contraindicated for health reasons.
3. Eliminate unnecessary noise, such as loud laughter, while patients are asleep.
4. Provide an environment in which patients feel safe and assured that help is nearby even when they sleep.
5. Provide sufficient covers so that the patient does not feel cold. Elderly people often need additional covers because normal body temperature drops as people age.
6. Encourage progressive relaxation exercises. These are helpful particularly for persons who have mild or moderate insomnia. See the relaxation techniques described on page 641.
7. Provide a light snack or glass of warm milk before the patient sleeps. Milk and most protein foods as well as some vegetables contain an amino acid (L-tryptophan) that is a precursor of the neurotransmitter serotonin. Serotonin is thought to induce and maintain sleep.
8. Provide a hypnotic or sedative if it is ordered by the physician and needed by the patient. If the patient also requires an analgesic, administer the analgesic before the sedative so the patient feels comfortable when becoming sleepy.
9. Assist a patient to his or her normal position for sleeping if this is possible.
10. Give the patient a backrub to promote emotional and muscular relaxation.

Evaluating Rest and Sleep Interventions

The outcome criteria for patients who have sleep problems (actual or potential) depend on the nursing diagnosis. Some suggested criteria are:

1. Slept 8 hours without awakening
2. Has restored strength and energy to walk to the end of the hall and back unaided
3. Demonstrates mental and emotional well-being by decreased confusion and irritability

Pain

Pain is a highly unpleasant and very personal sensation that cannot be shared with others. It can occupy all of one's thinking, direct one's activities, and change one's life. Pain is an important sign that there is something physiologically wrong. As such, pain is useful because it prompts the patient to seek help for a health problem that might otherwise go unnoticed. Pain is usually accompanied by other bodily sensations such as pressure, heat, or perhaps cold. Engel (1970:45) defines pain as "a basically unpleasant sensation referred to the body which represents the suffering induced by the psychic perception of real, threatened, or phantasied injury."

McCaffery (1979:11) defines pain as "whatever the experiencing person says it is, existing whenever he says it does." Basic to this definition is the caregiver's willingness to believe the patient's pain.

Types of Pain

Pain can be described as either acute or chronic. *Acute pain* is generally of relatively short duration, such as the pain of a fracture or abdominal surgery. A patient with acute pain normally exhibits one or two of the following clinical signs: increased perspiration, increased cardiac rate or blood pressure, and pallor. Patients may respond to acute pain by crying, moaning, or rubbing the painful area, although the absence of these behaviors does not mean a patient is not experiencing pain. *Chronic pain* develops more slowly and lasts much longer than acute pain, and sufferers may find it difficult to remember when such pain first started. Patients with chronic pain may present few if any clinical signs of pain. Some patients find a way to handle the pain or are so accustomed to it that their reaction is minimal.

Pain has also been described as somatogenic or psychogenic. *Somatogenic* or *organic pain* has a physical origin, whereas *psychogenic* or *functional pain* has a psychic or mental origin. Most people with localized pain experience a combination of somatogenic and psychogenic pain. Acute pain is frequently associated with anxiety, whereas chronic pain is associated with reactive depression (McCaffery 1979:16). Anxiety and depression generally exacerbate pain.

Intractable pain is resistant to cure or relief. An example is the pain of arthritis, for which narcotic analgesics are contraindicated because of the long duration of the disease and the danger of addiction. Behavior modification is used in some cases of intractable pain. Behavior that is not pain oriented is rewarded, and pain-oriented behavior is ignored. The aim of this technique is to change behavior so that the patient can live more comfortably and productively.

Guyton (1982:376) classifies pain into three major types: pricking, burning, and aching pain. *Pricking pain* is like the pain of a knife piercing the skin, and *burning pain* is like the pain of a burn. *Aching pain* is a deep pain of varying degrees of intensity.

Sometimes a patient feels pain in an area other than the site of the source of the pain. This is called *referred pain*. For example, cardiac pain may be felt radiating to the left shoulder and down the left arm, or the pain from an inflamed appendix may be felt throughout the abdomen. Referred pain is the result of a synapse formed between nerve fibers that carry the pain impulses in the spinal cord and neurons that carry pain impulses from the skin. Thus the individual has the perception that the pain originates in the skin or internal tissues.

Phantom pain is felt in a part of the body that is no longer present, such as an amputated foot. Phantom pain is thought to occur because of stimulation of the severed dendrite rather than stimulation of the usual receptor. Thus, the individual perceives the pain in the removed part.

Pain has three components: (a) initiation of the pain impulse, (b) perception of the pain, and (c) response to the pain. These are discussed subsequently.

Physiology of Pain

The skin and other body tissues have pain receptors. The skin, certain internal tissues such as the periosteum, and the arterial walls have many receptors, whereas most other tissues have fewer pain receptors. The alveoli of the lungs have no pain receptors.

Basically, three types of stimuli excite pain receptors: mechanical, thermal, and chemical. Some pain receptors are stimulated almost exclusively by mechanical stimuli; they are called *mechanosensitive pain receptors*. Others are sensitive to heat and cold and are called *thermosensitive pain receptors*. Receptors sensitive to chemicals are called *chemosensitive pain receptors*. Certain chemicals, including bradykinin, serotonin, potassium ions, acids, and acetylcholine, stimulate chemosensitive receptors.

Pain signals are transmitted along two types of fibers: delta type A fibers and type C fibers. Type A fibers transmit the signal relatively quickly, i.e., between 6 and 30 meters per second. It is thought type A fibers chiefly transmit pricking pain. Type C fibers transmit signals more slowly, i.e., 0.5 to 2 meters per second, and it is believed they transmit burning and aching pain. Therefore, a sudden pain can give a double sensation: a pricking pain sensation followed by a slow burning sensation. The latter tends to become more painful over time (Guyton 1982:378).

Pain fibers enter the spinal cord through the dorsal roots. From there they ascend or descend one or two cord segments to terminate in neurons in the dorsal horns of the gray matter called the *substantia gelatinosa*. Type A fibers terminate in the gray matter of laminae I and V, type C fibers in that of laminae II and III. Most signals pass through one or more neurons before reaching long-fibered neurons that cross to the opposite side of the cord. The stimulus then passes upward via the anterolateral spinothalamic tract to the brain.

In the brain, the pain pathways divide into two: the pricking pain pathway (type A delta fibers) and the burning pain pathway (type C fibers). The pricking pain pathway terminates in the ventrobasal complex of the thalamus. See Figure 25–4. From that point, signals are transmitted to other parts of the thalamus and to the somatic and sensory cortex of the brain. The burning pain fibers terminate in the reticular area of the brain stem and in the intralaminar nuclei of the thalamus. The reticular area and the intralaminar nuclei are part of the reticular activating system, which transmits signals to most parts of the brain. These signals then activate most of the nervous system, creating in the person a sense of urgency about the pain. Through stimulation of the cortical areas, the individual interprets the *quality* of the pain.

Pricking pain can be localized within 10 to 20 cm of the stimulated area, whereas burning or aching pain can be localized only generally, for example, in the abdomen or an arm.

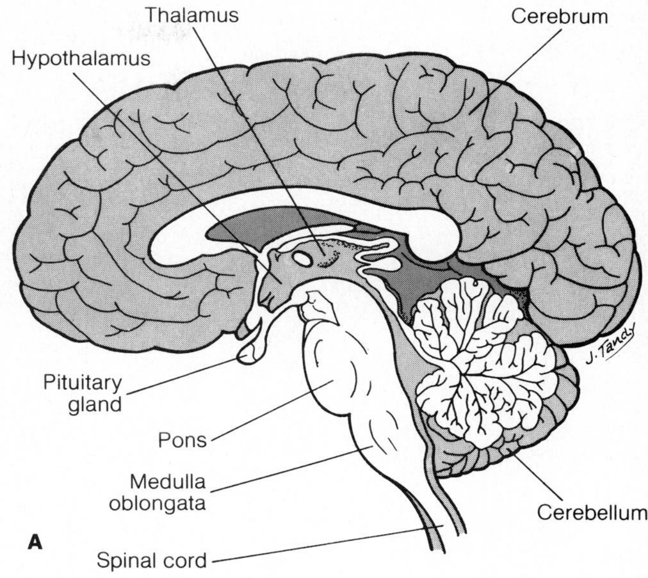

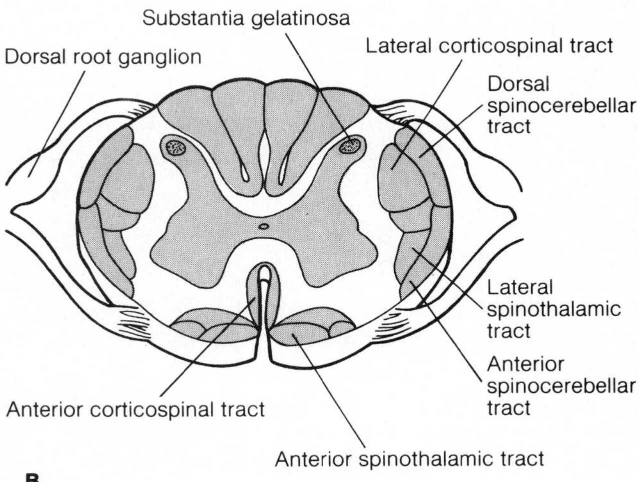

Figure 25–4 **A,** Midsagittal section of the brain; **B,** transverse section of the spinal cord.

Pain Perception

Individuals vary widely in their perception of pain; some perceive a cut finger as exceedingly painful, whereas others hardly notice the cut. In 1965, Melzack and Wall proposed the gate control theory. According to this theory, the synapses in the dorsal horns act as gates that close to keep impulses from reaching the brain or open to permit impulses to ascend to the brain. Melzack and Wall further hypothesize that when there are a great number of impulses along the thick nerve fibers, which carry impulses of heat, cold, touch, etc., the gates close to the pain impulses on the thinner fibers, thus blocking the pain. (Pain impulses are thought to travel along these thinner fibers). Only when the synaptic gates are open, as when impulses on the pain fibers predominate, does the patient feel pain.

Subsequent research uncovered enkephalins and endorphins. These endogenous compounds, which are chemically similar to opiates, are polypeptides. Endorphins have been found throughout the body, including the pituitary gland, gastrointestinal tract, and the central nervous system. In the central nervous system, they are found in abundance in the hypothalamus, parts of the limbic system, and the substantia gelatinosa. One theory is that these compounds are located in the synapse between the nerve fibers and that they have the capacity to transmit, alter, or inhibit painful impulses. They may also be able to relieve pain, thus explaining the variable individual perceptions of pain. Researchers have found that people who feel less pain than would be expected have high endorphin levels. (Endorphin, in this context, is used to refer to all the opiatelike polypeptides.) It is further thought that the release of endorphins is essential to the effectiveness of pain relievers and that endorphins may reduce anxiety, which increases the perception of pain.

Researchers agree that the brain plays an important function in mediating and even inhibiting pain impulses (West 1981:51). It is also known that the stimulation of tactile receptors in the skin depresses the transmission of pain impulses. This fact explains why rubbing the skin with liniments often relieves pain. The *pain threshold* refers to the amount of stimulation a person requires before feeling pain. Pain thresholds are generally fairly uniform in people, although they can be dramatically altered by a person's state of consciousness. An anesthetized patient does not feel pain; an

Table 25–3 Initial Responses to Pain

Sympatho-adrenal responses	Muscular responses	Emotional responses
Increased pulse rate	Increased muscle tension or rigidity	Excitement
Increased systolic blood pressure	Writhing	Irritability
Increased respiratory rate	Restlessness	Behavior change
Excessive perspiration	Knees drawn up to abdomen or other unusual postures	Extreme quietness
Nausea and vomiting due to blood flow shift from viscera to muscles of the lungs, heart, and striated body muscles	Rubbing	Groaning
Pallor	Scratching	Crying
	Immobility	Increased alertness

unconscious patient may or may not react to suborbital pressure, that is, pain on the lower aspect of the eye. Reaction to suborbital pressure is one way of testing the level of consciousness.

Pain tolerance is the maximum amount and duration of pain that an individual is willing to endure. Some patients are unwilling to tolerate even the slightest pain, while others are willing to endure severe pain rather than be treated for it.

Response to Pain

Physiologic responses to pain vary with the degree of anxiety that accompanies the pain. Pain without anxiety involves slight increases in pulse rate, respiratory depth, and palmar sweating. However, most acute pain is accompanied by anxiety, and the responses reflect both the pain and the anxiety.

The individual's physiologic responses to pain also depend on the severity and the duration of the pain. The reaction to sudden intense pain is almost immediate. The sympathetic nervous system is dominant. Among the prominent physiologic manifestations are increased pulse and respiratory rates, pallor, and dilated pupils. See Table 25–3 for additional responses. When the original pain sensation is intense but of short duration, a brief parasympathetic response may occur. Responses include slower pulse rate, lower blood pressure, constricted pupils, nausea, and vomiting.

When the pain is long-lasting, the physiologic response is adaptation, i.e., a decreased sympathetic response. Perhaps adaptation is due to endorphin counteracting the pain; see the section on pain perception immediately preceding. The body experiences a general adaptive reaction when the pain lasts for many hours or days. See the section on the general adaptation syndrome, Chapter 9, and Figure 9–2 for current concepts of physiologic reactions to stress.

Changes in body chemistry due to pain influence a person's behavior. The secretion of excessive norepinephrine causes the individual to feel powerful, in control, confident, and excited. However, when norepinephrine is depleted, for example, when the pain is prolonged, the individual may feel helpless, worthless, and lethargic. Stimulation of the inhibitory system increases the production of serotonin. This reaction is seen in patients after they meditate or take narcotics. The individual feels secure, serene, and safe. Depleted serotonin levels, seen in patients with chronic pain, produce tension, agitation, anxiety, hypersensitivity, and a variety of sleep disorders (Booker 1982:49). Patients with depleted levels of both norepinephrine and serotonin may demonstrate agitated depression. In addition, depression may be aggravated by narcotics, which block the norepinephrine and serotonin receptor sites in the central nervous system (ibid., p. 49).

Assessing Pain

Because pain is such a personal experience, nurses must rely on the patient's ability to communicate verbally about pain. In addition, nonverbal actions can convey information about the pain. Pain is assessed by its location, intensity, time, duration, and quality as well as by the nonverbal behavior of the patient and precipitating factors. In addition, an assessment needs to include a pain history and consideration of factors influencing the pain.

Characteristics

Location

Superficial pain usually can be located accurately by a patient; however, pain arising from the viscera is perceived more generally. Nurses need to ascertain where the patient experiences pain. The various abdominal sections, which the nurse can use when describing the location of abdominal pain, are shown in Chapter 14. In addition, the nurse needs to use such terms as *proximal, distal, medial,* and *lateral* when describing the location of pain. See Chapter 24. The term *diffuse* refers to pain perceived over a large area.

When assessing the location of a child's pain, the nurse needs to understand the child's vocabulary. For example, *tummy* might refer to the abdomen or part of the chest. It is wise for a nurse to ask a child to point to the pain rather than to rely on the child's description, which may be highly idiosyncratic. Parents can help nurses interpret the meaning of a child's words. Observation of when a smaller child or baby cries in response to movement can help the nurse establish the location of a baby's pain.

Intensity

The intensity or severity of pain is also important. Although this value is subjective, it is also true that certain tissues are more sensitive than others. Several factors affect the perception of intensity. One is distraction, or the patient's concentration on another event; a second is the patient's state of consciousness, and a third is the person's expectations.

Pain may be described as slight, mild, medium, severe, or excruciating. It is very important to note and report any change in intensity described by the patient. This change may indicate a change in the patient's pathologic condition. For example, the abrupt cessation of acute abdominal pain may indicate a ruptured appendix.

Reports of pain by a patient must be considered in relation to the patient's ability and need to report. The elderly or confused patient may distort the intensity of the pain, while a child may minimize pain to avoid admission to the hospital or unpleasant tests.

Time and duration

The nurse needs to record when the pain began; how long the pain lasts; whether it recurs and, if so, the interval without pain; and when the pain last occurred.

The interval between pains can be very important. For example, the intervals between labor contractions help the maternity nurse assess the patient's progress in labor. As the birth becomes more imminent, the labor pains become more frequent and more severe.

Quality

Descriptive adjectives help people communicate the quality of pain. Patients use the terms they know: A headache may be described as "hammerlike" or an abdominal pain as "piercing like a knife." Sometimes patients have difficulty describing pain because they have never experienced any sensation like it. This is particularly true of children and of adults who have pain originating within the nervous system. Following is a list of some of the terms used to describe pain.

Aching
Burning
Constant
Cramping
Crushing
Cutting
Diffuse
Dull
Excruciating
Gnawing
Hammering
Heavy
Intermittent (spasmodic)
Irritating
Jabbing
Knifelike
Knotting
Lancing
Piercing
Pinching
Pounding
Prickly
Radiating
Searing
Sharp
Shifting
Squeezing
Stabbing
Tearing
Throbbing
Tingling
Viselike

Nurses need to record the exact words patients use to describe pain. A patient's words are more accurate and descriptive than a nurse's interpretation in the nurse's words.

Nonverbal behavior

Nonverbal behavior is of particular importance in assessing pain experienced by patients unable to communicate verbally. The very young, the aphasic, and confused or disoriented persons often communicate their experience of pain only nonverbally. Several types of nonverbal behavior are sources of data.

Facial expression is often the first indication of pain and may be the only one. Clenched teeth, tightly shut eyes, open somber eyes, biting of the lower lip, and other facial grimaces are indicative of pain.

Body movement can help the nurse assess pain. Immobilization of the body or a part of the body may indicate pain. The patient with chest pain often holds the left arm across the chest. A person with abdominal pain may assume the position of greatest comfort, often with the knees and hips flexed, and moves reluctantly. Even babies flex their hips and legs when experiencing abdominal pain, although they do not tend to remain in that position.

Purposeless body movements can also indicate pain. The person may toss and turn in bed or fling the arms about. Involuntary movements, such as a reflexive jerking away from a needle inserted through the skin, indicate pain. An adult may be able to control this reflex; however, a child may be unable or unwilling to control this response.

Rhythmic body movements or rubbing may indicate pain. The teething baby likes to chew on an object; an adult or child may assume a fetal position and rock back and forth when experiencing abdominal pain. During labor the woman may massage her abdomen rhythmically with her hands.

Patients' speech and vocal pitch can help the nurse assess pain. Rapid speech and elevated pitch reflect anxiety, while slow speech and monotonous tone can signal intense pain. For additional information on nonverbal behavior see Chapter 15.

Precipitating factors

The nurse needs to report factors, if any, that precipitate pain. Certain activities sometimes precede pain; for example, physical exertion may precede chest pain, or abdominal pain may occur after the patient eats. These observations are helpful not only in preventing the pain but also in determining the cause of the pain.

Environmental factors can increase pain in people who are well or ill. Extreme cold and extremes in humidity can affect some types of pain. Sudden exercise on a hot day can cause muscle spasm. In addition, physical and emotional stressors can precipitate pain. Emotional tension frequently brings on a migraine headache. Intense fear or physical exertion can cause angina.

Pain History

It is important for nurses to obtain from the patient a history of pain experienced previously. The history should include location, intensity, duration, etc., of previous pain. During discussion with the patient, the nurse can establish how long the patient has experienced pain; what effects the pain had on normal activity; how the pain occurred, e.g., quickly or slowly; and what events precipitated it. The history should also include a description of measures employed to relieve the pain.

Factors Influencing Pain

In addition, the nurse should consider factors that influence the individual's experience of pain. Some of these are environment, age, fatigue, past experience, coping mechanisms, religious beliefs, culture, and the presence of support persons.

Environment

Pain is often aggravated by extremes in environmental stimuli. Loud noises and bright lights can increase the intensity of pain. When environmental stimulation is inadequate, patients sometimes perceive pain as more severe. For example, a patient alone in a room at night or an immobilized patient may feel pain more acutely. The solitary person, undistracted by conversation, is more likely to dwell on pain. The immobilized person may feel helpless, and this is an emotion that can intensify pain.

Age

As people grow older, their pain tolerance generally increases. In addition, the ability to understand and control pain often develops with age. An infant does not understand that keeping a leg still, for example, will eliminate pain.

Children often fear pain because they do not understand what is happening to them. One study examined what pain means to 10- and 11-year-old children and found that their fear of bodily damage was exaggerated (Schultz 1971:672). Children of this age view pain as a deterrent to the gratification of their needs and desires. The meaning of pain for these children is exemplified by two common responses: "It hurts" and "I can't play football."

Fatigue

Fatigue not only intensifies pain but also decreases normal coping abilities. Therefore, a patient often experiences less pain after restful sleep than at the end of the day.

Past experience

A patient's past experience with pain can alter the experience of pain later. Coping mechanisms learned previously may or may not be effective in another situation.

Coping mechanisms

Patients sometimes learn highly effective ways of coping with pain. These methods may modify the pain to such a degree that assessment of pain will be incomplete unless the nurse is aware of them. For example, a patient may tell a nurse that his abdominal pain lasted only a few minutes and neglect to say that he took an antacid when the pain started.

Religious beliefs

Religious beliefs can influence how individuals deal with pain. An individual may believe that pain is deserved punishment and consequently bear the pain stoically because it resolves his or her guilt. Another person may consider pain unjust and react angrily, intensifying the pain.

Culture

Response to pain is in part culturally determined. The meaning of pain and the expected interventions vary among cultures. Some groups, such as Native American Indians and Chinese people, respond stoically to pain. Other groups, such as Italians and Jews, tend to react more expressively (Blaylock 1968:270).

It is important that nurses recognize the wide variety of learned responses considered appropriate by different cultural groups. The stoical response is largely accepted in North American society; however, because many ethnic groups live in North America, nurses observe various responses to pain. Nurses need to avoid judging any response to pain as good or bad. It is also important to realize that a stoical person probably will not tell the nurse when he or she is in pain; thus, nonverbal clues are important during assessment.

Support persons

The presence of support persons often increases a patient's ability to handle pain. Toddlers tolerate pain more readily when supportive parents or nurses are near. Adults, too, handle pain better when supportive, trusted people are present.

McGill and Melzack (Meissner 1980:51) devised a pain questionnaire in 1975. This questionnaire provides a way to measure pain, in particular chronic pain. The patient answers the questionnaire both before and after health personnel attempt to relieve the pain. The nurse uses the patient's responses to the second questionnaire to assess how effective pain relief measures have been (Meissner 1980:50). A number of other pain assessment tools have been developed to help nurses gather data about a patient's pain. For an example, see McGuire (1981:49).

Nursing Diagnoses

Common Problems

Headache

Barrett-Griesemer et al. (1981:50–53) isolate three types of headaches: psychogenic, vascular, and miscellaneous (associated with various medical disorders). *Psychogenic* headaches include tension headaches, the most common type, and neurotic headaches. *Vascular* headaches include migraine, cluster, and hypertension headaches. *Miscellaneous* headaches include those associated with sinusitis, eye strain, trigeminal neuralgia, temporomandibular joint (TMJ) dysfunction, and cranial disorders (e.g., brain tumor, postconcussion, and subarachnoid hemorrhage). Each type of headache has unique etiology and signs and symptoms and therefore requires different management. See Table 25-4.

Low back pain

Low back pain is a common complaint of pregnant women and adults suffering from degenerative joint disease of the spine or following injury (e.g., a ruptured intervertebral disc). The pain may be aggravated by flexion of the trunk, coughing, or sneezing. It may also be accompanied by sciatic pain radiating down the leg.

Unless there are major neurological defects, low back pain is generally treated conservatively. The patient is instructed to rest on a firm mattress, either in a lateral position or supine position, with the head slightly elevated and the knees flexed. Also, the patient is advised to maintain good spinal alignment when standing and sitting and to use good body mechanics when moving or lifting objects. See Chapter 23. If the pain is accompanied by severe muscle spasm, heating pads, analgesics, and antispasmodics may be helpful. In some situations, physical therapy in the form of heat, massage, and active and passive muscle exercises performed in warm water is recommended.

Intractable cancer pain

In terminal stages of cancer, patients often suffer intractable pain that requires special measures for relief,

Table 25–4 Causes, Manifestations, and Management of Various Types of Headaches

Type of headache	Cause and incidence	Signs and symptoms	Management
Psychogenic			
Tension	Anxiety Excessive contractions of head and neck muscles	Steady pain, rather than sharp or pulsating, starts at base of skull and radiates bilaterally toward the front Tense and tender cervical muscles	Encouragement to express emotions and relieve tension Teach muscle relaxation Aspirin Acetaminophen Tranquilizer, e.g., diazepam (Valium)
Neurotic	Possible indulging anxiety or depression	Constant, around-the-clock headache Possible early morning insomnia Tendency to cry when asked if he or she is having any problems	Psychotherapy with antidepressant medications, e.g., imipramine (Tofranil), amitriptyline (Elavil)
Vascular			
Migraine	Usually in family history Occurs most in women (60%) May start in childhood but most often before age 30 Cause is intracranial vasoconstriction and subsequent vasodilation of cerebral arteries Possible involvement of vasoactive substances such as serotonin	*Classic symptoms* Initial visual aura, e.g., flashing lights, blind spots, visual hallucinations Severe, throbbing, unilateral pain Nausea and vomiting Fatigue and tension before headache *Common symptoms* Nondescript aura Headache for 12 to 72 hours Sensitivity to loud noises Weakness and fatigue Possible increase in intensity of symptoms by alcohol ingestion, stress, menstruation, oral contraceptives, and tyramine-containing foods, e.g., chicken liver, aged cheese, pickled herring	Ergot alkaloids, e.g., ergotamine tartrate (Cafergot, Wigraine), which constrict extracranial blood vessels, need to be taken at first sign of headache Tranquilizer, e.g., phenobarbital, to reduce anxiety Prophylactic medications such as propanolol (Inderal) for persons suffering more than two migraines per month
Cluster	Usually affects young men	Severe, unilateral eye pain Intense, stabbing, knifelike pain Occurs daily at same time and may last up to 10 days Tearing and redness of affected eye Runny nose Perspiration on affected side of face Eyelids may droop or constrict	As for migraine
Hypertension	Diastolic blood pressure exceeding 120 mm Hg	Severe, throbbing pain	Measures to reduce blood pressure

Table 25–4 continued

Type of headache	Cause and incidence	Signs and symptoms	Management
Miscellaneous			
Associated with sinusitis	Congestion of sinuses	Facial pain near frontal and maxillary sinuses Accompanied by runny nose and fever Sinuses are sensitive to touch	Antibiotics Antihistamines
Associated with eye strain	Prolonged, demanding use of eyes	Pain around eyes at end of day after arduous visual tasks	Rest the eyes
Associated with trigeminal neuralgia	Unknown	Electriclike facial pain lasting 20 to 30 seconds Avoidance of touching trigger zone that causes attack, e.g., avoids washing face, shaving, or chewing·	
Associated with temporomandibular joint dysfunction	Poor jaw alignment, incorrect bite, muscular stress	Headache and neckache Dizziness Ringing in ears Sore jaw, face, or neck muscles Grinding or clenching of teeth Clicking of the jaw joint	Dental referral and therapy
Associated with cranial disorders	Brain tumor, subarachnoid hemorrhage, or postconcussion	*Brain tumor* Pain in same site each morning Accompanied by nausea, vomiting, seizures, dizziness Increased intensity with coughing, stooping, or exertion	Neurologic therapy or surgery
		Subarachnoid hemorrhage Sudden, severe headache Nausea and vomiting Decreased level of consciousness	Neurosurgery
		Postconcussion Long-lasting headache (1 to 30 days) following trauma Dizziness and blurred vision	Rest for 24 hours or until feeling better Aspirin or acetaminophen If headache persists or becomes more intense, notify physician

From P. Barrett-Griesemer, S. Meisel, and R. Rate, A guide to headaches—and how to relieve their pain, *Nursing 81*, April 1981, 11:50–57.

such as injectable analgesics or narcotic infusions. Specific methods are discussed on page 643.

Chest pain

Chest pain of cardiac origin is a serious problem that needs to be appropriately assessed and differentiated from noncardiac pain. In addition, angina must be differentiated from the pain of a myocardial infarction. For pertinent signs and symptoms of cardiac pain see Tannenbaum et al. (1981) and Frank-Stromborg and Stromborg (1981), listed in the Suggested Readings at the end of the chapter.

Leg pain

Leg pain is often associated with vascular dysfunction. See Doyle (1981), listed in Suggested Readings, for information about assessing arterial insufficiency.

Examples of Diagnoses

Nursing diagnoses for patients in pain take one of two forms. In the first, the pain component is the first part of the nursing diagnosis, i.e., the statement of the patient's response. Alternately, the pain may be the second part of the diagnosis, i.e., the contributing factor. Some examples of pain-related nursing diagnoses follow. The first three list the pain as the primary diagnosis; the fourth and fifth list the pain as a contributing factor.

1. Pain (or alterations in comfort) related to:
   a. Abdominal surgery
   b. Impaired circulation to the feet
   c. Uterine contractions of early labor
   d. Lack of knowledge about preventive measures
   e. Lack of knowledge about effective methods to manage the pain
   f. Fear of taking analgesics
2. Increased pain perception related to:
   a. Anxiety
   b. Fatigue
   c. Situational stress
   d. Previous experience
   e. Disturbing environmental stimuli
   f. Insufficient environmental stimuli
   g. Depression
3. Headache related to:
   a. Depression
   b. Anxiety
   c. Tension
   d. Brain tumor
4. Impaired mobility related to painful knee joint
5. Inability to work related to back pain

Planning and Intervention for Pain

The overall nursing goal is to maintain the patient's comfort. Nursing subgoals are:

1. To enhance the individual's sense of comfort and security
2. To enhance the individual's ability to perform physical activities necessary for recovery (e.g., coughing and deep breathing, ambulation)
3. To prevent sleep deprivation

Plans

When planning to prevent pain or modify existing pain, the nurse needs to consider the patient's learning needs, schedule measures that promote pain relief, and determine which measures are appropriate for the patient. For example, a patient scheduled for surgery may need to learn that postoperative pain will be relieved. Lack of understanding about pain and doubt about whether it will be relieved increase anxiety, which in turn increases pain. Stress increases production of norepinephrine, which increases pain. Also, a patient may need to learn not to use excessive caffeine, nicotine, or alcohol, which may increase pain and interfere with substances that help control pain (Booker 1982:49).

Scheduling measures to prevent pain is far more supportive of the patient than trying to deal with pain when the patient feels it. Many postoperative patients need regularly administered analgesics as well as other nursing measures. In this way, the patient's pain is anticipated and avoided, and recovery often hastened. When planning, nurses need to choose pain relief measures appropriate for the patient. Heat stimulates serotonin; cold, norepinephrine. One of these may be appropriate if not contraindicated for another reason. The nurse may need a physician's order before applying heat or cold.

Planning also requires establishing outcome criteria. See the suggested outcome criteria on page 646.

Interventions

Nursing intervention to relieve pain can take many forms, depending on the individual patient and the pathologic condition. In some situations, removal of the pain stimulus is a highly effective and often long-lasting method of relieving pain. Removing a wet, irritating dressing, smoothing a wrinkled bed, and loosening a bandage that restricts circulation are all examples of removing the pain stimulus. Sometimes medications are also used in this manner; for example, antispasmodic drugs can relieve muscle spasm. The application of heat to a body area can increase circulation and thus relieve localized ischemia. In other instances, the stimulus can be removed by a change in activity. The patient with cardiac pain, for example, may prevent pain by limiting physical activity. The person with a gastric ulcer can often prevent pain by drinking milk regularly. Pain upon voiding after a prostatectomy can often be eliminated by drinking more fluids.

Sometimes the reaction of pain receptors can be reduced. Local anesthetics prevent the transmission of pain at the receptors of the skin. Another example is padding a bony prominence before applying a bandage to prevent irritation and pain from the bandage.

In many situations, the patient's perception and interpretation of pain can be altered. Narcotic analgesics change a patient's interpretation of and response to pain. Hypnotics such as phenobarbital, when given in small doses, tend to change pain interpretation and decrease sensitivity to pain. For example, a patient may still perceive pain but may no longer regard it as important or disturbing.

Interaction between the nurse and the patient can

change the interpretation of the pain. Specific methods used to alleviate pain follow.

Distraction

Distraction draws the person's attention away from the pain and lessens the perception of pain. In some instances, distraction can make a patient completely unaware of pain. For example, a patient recovering from surgery may feel no pain while watching a football game on television, yet feel pain again when the game is over. The way in which distraction decreases pain can be explained by the gate control theory. In the spinal cord, the receptor cells receiving the peripheral pain stimuli are inhibited by stimuli from other peripheral nerve fibers carrying different stimuli. Because pain messages are slower than diversional messages, the spinal cord gate, which controls the amount of input to the brain, closes and the patient feels less pain (Cummings 1981:62). Distraction is most effective when pain is mild or moderate, but intense concentration on other subjects can also relieve acute pain. An example of the latter is an adolescent who feels pain from a fractured foot bone only after she finishes playing a basketball game. A person who is anxious, lonely, or bored feels pain more intensely. In addition, disturbing stimuli such as loud noises, bright lights, unpleasant odors, or an argumentative visitor can increase pain perception. Therefore, the nurse needs to reduce disturbing stimuli.

Some distraction techniques include (McCaffery 1980b:56):

1. *Slow, rhythmic breathing.* The nurse has the patient stare at an object; inhale slowly through the nose while the nurse counts 1, 2, 3, 4; and exhale slowly through the mouth while the nurse counts 1, 2, 3, 4. The nurse encourages the patient to concentrate on the sensation of breathing and to picture a restful scene. This process is continued until a rhythmic pattern is established. When the patient feels comfortable, he or she can count silently and perform this technique independently.
2. *Massage and slow, rhythmic breathing.* The patient breathes rhythmically as in step 1 but at the same time massages a part of the body with stroking or circular movements.
3. *Rhythmic singing and tapping.* The patient selects a well-liked song and concentrates all attention on its words and rhythm. The nurse encourages the patient to mouth or sing the words and tap a finger or foot. Loud, fast songs are best for intense pain.
4. *Active listening.* The patient listens to music and concentrates on the rhythm by tapping a finger or foot.
5. *Guided imagery.* The nurse asks the patient to close the eyes and imagine and describe something pleasurable. As the patient describes the image, the nurse asks about the sights, sounds, and smells imagined.

Relaxation

Relaxation techniques are effective primarily for chronic pain and provide many benefits:

1. Relaxation reduces anxiety related to pain or stress.
2. It eases muscle tension pain.
3. It helps the person dissociate from pain.
4. It promotes maximum benefits from rest and sleep periods.
5. It enhances the effectiveness of other pain therapies.
6. It relieves hopelessness and depression associated with pain.

For many years, maternity nurses have encouraged women in labor to relax and breathe rhythmically. These techniques, however, can be useful for any patient in pain.

Three requisites to relaxation are correct posture, a mind at rest, and a quiet environment. The patient must be positioned comfortably with all body parts supported (e.g., pillow supporting neck), joints slightly flexed, and no strain or pull on muscles (e.g., arms and legs should not be crossed). To rest the mind, the patient is asked to gaze slowly around the room, i.e., across the ceiling, down the wall, along a window curtain, around the fabric pattern, back up the wall, etc. This exercise focuses the mind outside of the body (away from the pain) and creates a second center of concentration. To relax the face, the patient is encouraged to smile slightly or let the lower jaw sag.

Stewart (1976:959) describes this relaxation technique:

1. The patient takes a deep breath and fills the lungs with air.
2. The patient slowly hisses out the air while letting the body go limp and concentrating on how good this feels.
3. The patient breathes in natural rhythm a few times.
4. The patient takes another deep breath and releases it slowly, this time letting only the legs and feet go limp. The nurse asks the patient to concentrate on how each leg feels—loose, heavy, and warm.
5. The patient repeats step 4, concentrating on the arms, abdomen, back, and other muscle groups.
6. After the patient is relaxed, slow, rhythmic breathing is added. Either abdominal or chest breathing may be used. If pain becomes intense, the patient can use a more rapid, shallow breathing pattern.

There are several relaxation methods. Some recommend that separate muscle groups (e.g., neck, shoulder, back, arm, leg, etc.) be first tensed and then relaxed. After all muscle groups are tensed and relaxed, the whole body is tensed and then relaxed.

Others suggest a stretching form of relaxation. The patient lies supine, points the toes toward the knees, presses the back of the knees against the mattress or floor, flattens the hollow of the back and neck as much as possible, holds this position for several minutes, and then relaxes completely for several minutes.

Conscious suggestion by the nurse can help an anxious, frightened patient in pain to relax. It involves skillful use of the voice, body language, and word choice. A calm, soft but distinct voice makes the patient listen and gives a sense of security. Bending near the patient, establishing eye contact, and placing a hand on the patient's shoulder communicates the nurse's concern and calmness to the patient. Positive, affirmative words help to convey the suggestion of relaxation to the patient. During the session, the nurse, after calming and reassuring the patient, might make this suggestion: "You will allow yourself to relax as the doctors and nurses treat you." For further information see Holderby (1981), cited in the Suggested Readings at the end of the chapter.

Skin stimulation

Stimulation of the skin by cold packs, analgesic ointments, counterirritants, and contralateral stimulation can reduce pain:

1. *Cold packs* slow the conduction of pain impulses to the brain and of motor impulses to muscles in the painful area. They provide quicker and longer-lasting pain relief than hot packs (McCaffery 1980b:57). Cold packs help relieve headaches, muscle strains, joint pain, muscle spasm, and back pain during childbirth.

2. *Analgesic ointments* containing menthol relieve pain, but the analgesic mechanism is unknown. These ointments produce immediate sensations of warmth that last for several hours, and even longer if the body part is wrapped in plastic. They are very commonly used to relieve joint or muscle pain. However, menthol ointment rubbed into the neck, scalp, or forehead sometimes relieves tension headaches, and some cultures (e.g., Filipino) use it on the abdomen to relieve gas pains or on the abdomen or lower back to relieve the pain of labor or delivery (McCaffery 1980b:57).

3. *Counterirritants*, such as mustard plasters, flaxseed poultices, and liniments, relieve the aching joint pain of rheumatoid arthritis and osteoarthritis. Counterirritants are thought to relieve pain by increasing circulation to the painful area. Increased circulation removes trapped tissue metabolites, lessens muscle spasm, and improves joint mobility.

4. *Contralateral stimulation* is stimulation of the skin in an area opposite to the painful area (e.g., stimulating the left knee if the pain is in the right knee). The contralateral area is scratched for itching, massaged for cramps, or treated with cold packs or analgesic ointments. This method is useful when the painful area cannot be touched because it is hypersensitive, because it is made inaccessible by a cast or bandages, or because the pain is felt in a missing part (phantom pain) (McCaffery 1980b:57).

Analgesics

Analgesics alter perception and interpretation of pain by depressing the central nervous system at the thalamus and cerebral cortex. Analgesics are more effective when given before the patient feels severe pain than when given after the pain is severe. For this reason, analgesics are given at regular intervals, such as every 4 hours (q.4h.) after surgery.

Types There are two major classifications of analgesics: narcotic (strong analgesics) and nonnarcotic (mild analgesics). *Narcotic analgesics* include opiate derivatives, such as morphine and codeine. Narcotics relieve pain largely by altering the emotional aspect of the pain experience (i.e., pain perception). Changes in mood and attitude and feelings of well-being make the person feel more comfortable even though the pain persists. *Nonnarcotic analgesics* include derivatives of salicylic acid such as aspirin; para-aminophenols such as phenacetin (Empirin); and pyrazolon derivatives such as phenylbutazone (Butazolidin). In addition, several combinations of analgesic drugs are available, e.g., a combination of a strong analgesic and a mild analgesic. An example is Tylenol #3, which combines acetaminophen, a nonnarcotic, with codeine, 30 mg. The specific way in which nonnarcotic analgesics relieve pain is unknown. It is thought that their primary site of action is the peripheral nervous system (PNS), where sensitization of the pain receptors is prevented.

A newer type of injectable analgesic is the *narcotic agonist-antagonist*. This type has *agonistic* properties in that it acts like a narcotic and relieves severe pain, but it also has *antagonistic* properties in that it also acts against a narcotic. When given to a patient who has taken a pure narcotic, these drugs reverse its effects; when given to a narcotic-free patient, they have a narcotic effect. Examples are butorphanol (Stadol), nalbuphine (Nubain), and pentazocine (Talwin, Fortal).

Choice of analgesic When choosing an analgesic, the health team member considers the quality and intensity of the pain and the specific actions of each analgesic. Narcotics should not be given when nonnarcotics will suffice but must be used when potent analgesia is required. Some nurses hesitate administering narcotics even when warranted because they fear causing addiction. See the section on guidelines, page 644. Narcotics are essential in such situations as acute heart attack, renal or biliary colic, vascular occlusion anywhere in the body, fractures, burns, postoperative pain, and terminal malignancies. It is essential that the nurse review the side effects. For example, narcotic analgesics depress respiration and must be used cautiously in patients with respiratory problems. Nonnarcotics such as aspirin, however, may aggravate gastrointestinal bleeding and therefore are contraindicated in patients with peptic ulcers.

Placebos

A placebo is any form of treatment, e.g., medication or nursing intervention, that produces an effect in the patient because of its intent rather than its physical or chemical properties (McCaffery 1982:22). A medication that contains no analgesic properties (e.g., sugar, normal saline, or water) but is intended to relieve pain is a placebo. Years ago, the patient who claimed the placebo gave relief was assumed to be malingering or falsely claiming pain. These assumptions have been proved wrong. Placebos do provide pain relief. Thirty-six percent of patients in a study of 446 patients with severe postoperative pain reported relief after taking a placebo (Goodwin et al. 1982:25). Placebos may help patients return to health and do have a physiologic effect; in some instances, they cause the body to release endorphins, which are powerful analgesics (McCaffery 1982:23–24).

Before administering a placebo, nurses must have a physician's order. Just because there are no active chemical ingredients in a placebo does not mean that nurses can administer them independently. It is important that nurses know why a placebo is being given before they give it. Placebos should not be used to punish a "difficult" patient. Nor can they be used to prove that a patient does not really have pain. Since it is legal to administer placebos, nurses must also examine their own values relative to the ethics of giving placebos. Nurses have at least four choices:

1. They can deceive the patient by giving the placebo and saying it is another medicine.
2. They can refuse to give the placebo.
3. They can inform the patient about the placebo and obtain his or her consent to use it.
4. They can set up a double-blind technique. Neither the nurse nor the patient knows whether a placebo or an active drug is being administered, because both have been packaged to this end by the pharmacist. The nurse can explain the double blind to the patient and request his or her consent.

McCaffery (1982) suggests that there is greater probability of a positive response to a placebo if:

1. The treatment makes sense to the patient and includes stimuli that convince him or her that the pain will be relieved. For example, intravenous administration is more likely than oral to elicit a positive placebo response.
2. The treatment is administered by an expert whom the patient trusts.
3. There is a focus on the patient's pain—thorough pain assessment and explanations that the treatment will relieve the pain.
4. The intent of the measure is explained to the patient (e.g., "This is another way to relieve your pain").

Management of intractable cancer pain

The management of intractable cancer pain presents a challenge to nurses. Drugs commonly used are methadone, Brompton's mixture, and continuous morphine infusion.

Methadone is advantageous because it is effective orally, has a long duration of action, has a cumulative effect that can maintain steady analgesic levels, and does not substantially alter the patient's mood (Maxwell 1980:1606). See the Suggested Readings for further information.

Brompton's mixture, developed in the 1930s at Brompton's Hospital, London, was originally used as an oral analgesic for postoperative patients. This medication was valued because it relieves pain without clouding the patient's mind. Several different preparations are called Brompton's mixture, since these mixtures are prepared in hospice and hospital pharmacies. The original mixture contained heroin (narcotic analgesic), cocaine (CNS stimulant to counteract the sedation and respiratory depression of the narcotic), alcohol (flavor enhancer), and syrup and chloroform water to improve the taste and texture (Gever 1980:57). In many places in North America, morphine or methadone is substituted for heroin, and amphetamine is used in place of cocaine, since cocaine is poorly absorbed and its importation is curtailed. The alcohol component may be ethanol, gin, or brandy. Fruit-flavored syrups are used to improve the flavor. In some hospitals, an antiemetic is also added for its tranquilizing effect.

Brompton's mixture is prescribed every 3 to 4 hours if it contains morphine or every 6 to 8 hours if it contains methadone, which has a longer action. It is given on schedule rather than as needed (p.r.n.) to prevent, not relieve, pain. Because Brompton's mixture is stable for only 2 weeks, the nurse needs to check the preparation date before administering the mixture. Because the narcotic depresses respiration, the nurse must monitor the respirations of patients receiving Brompton's mixture.

Continuous morphine infusion is used for patients with end-stage terminal illness who are suffering extreme pain, who have built up a tolerance to other pain medication, who have difficulty taking anything orally, and who cannot tolerate repeated injections. The goals of this method of pain control are (a) to provide continuous pain relief, (b) to allow the patient limited functional capacity, (c) to make the patient as comfortable as possible as long as he or she survives, and (d) to support the desire to die with dignity (O'Donnell and Papciak 1981:69–71).

Morphine infusions are administered through an infusion control pump with a microdrip infusion set and usually through a secondary intravenous line, although a primary line may be used. See Chapter 31, page 812, for a description of this equipment. A physician's order for dosage and infusion rate is essential. Starting dosages are based on the patient's previous pain medication, the patient's level of tolerance, and the severity of the pain. Generally, morphine is mixed in solutions of 5% dextrose in water (D5W), but it can be mixed with any intravenous solution. If other medications are being infused, drug incompatibilities must be ascertained. Some incompatible drugs are heparin, aminophylline, and sodium bicarbonate. Dosages may range from 4 to 40 mg of morphine in 100 ml of solution; 8 to 80 mg in 200 ml of solution; and 10 to 100 mg of morphine in 250 ml of solution (ibid., p. 72). Nurses need to follow agency policies and guidelines for use of continuous morphine infusions. Policy statements and guidelines should include (ibid., pp. 69, 72):

1. *Which patients are selected for the procedure.* For example, a patient may be eligible only if he or she has intractable pain and requires injectable narcotics.
2. *What responsibilities the attending physician has.* For example, the physician (a) records the terminal nature of the patient's illness and justifies the intravenous morphine infusion on the patient's progress notes, (b) discusses the potential side effects with the patient or support persons, (c) supplies a written signed request specifying the dosage and rate of infusion to the pharmacist, and (d) supplies a daily written order for the infusion.
3. *Who prepares the infusion.* In some agencies, the pharmacist or nurse prepares the infusion solution.
4. *How the infusion is to be administered.* For example, it may be administered by microdrip infusion set and infusion control pump.
5. *What responsibilities the nurse has, with emphasis on measures to prevent an overdose.* For example, the nurse (a) records a baseline blood pressure reading and respiratory rate prior to the infusion, (b) initiates the infusion, and (c) monitors blood pressure and respiration rates at specified intervals, such as every 30 minutes for the first 2 or 3 hours and then as nursing assessments warrant.
6. *What changes in rates of blood pressure and respiration during infusion are acceptable and what actions to take when unacceptable changes occur.* For example, if the respiratory rate falls below 14, the infusion rate may be slowed by 50% and the respiration rate monitored every 10 or 15 minutes. The infusion is discontinued with continued decreases in respiratory rate.
7. *How respiratory depression is managed, should it occur.* Naloxone hydrochloride (Narcan), a narcotic antagonist, should be available at the nursing station for administration by the physician, or nurse, if ordered, in the event of respiratory depression.

Guidelines for Pain Management

Nurses need to:

1. Determine the cause of pain and try other palliative measures before administering drugs or use palliative measures as well as administer analgesics. For example, proper positioning, massage, relief of anxiety, or heat can often negate the need for analgesics or can enhance their effects in patients with muscle spasm.
2. Involve the patient and support persons in planning, carrying out, and evaluating the pain management program. It is obvious that participation and cooperation of the patient is essential for distraction and relaxation techniques and for evaluation of the selected intervention. They also need information about the effects of certain therapies and need to be involved in planning what best suits them. Support persons may need education in helping the patient continue selected therapies at home, e.g., education in guided imagery or distraction techniques.
3. Use nonnarcotic analgesics rather than narcotics if the pain is mild to moderate, since these drugs do not have the adverse side effects of narcotics—sedation, res-

piratory depression, constipation, and increased tolerance to the drug by the patient (reduced effectiveness over time).

4. Learn not to avoid using narcotics for fear of causing addiction. Studies show that less than 1% to 3% of patients become addicted, and people stop taking narcotics when pain stops (McCaffery 1980a:38). Narcotics are essential for management of severe pain.

5. Assess the patient's response to analgesics and note the degree and duration of pain relief and side effects. If pain is not relieved within an hour after administration or if the patient is in too much pain to perform activities required for recovery, such as coughing, deep breathing, and ambulation, the dosage is insufficient. If the patient complains of pain before the next dose is scheduled, the interval between doses may be too long. If the patient experiences significant respiratory depression (e.g., a drop from 18 to 12) or is overly sedated, the dosage is excessive. *Before* administering narcotics, the nurse needs to assess a patient's respiratory rate and level of alertness for baseline data. The nurse also needs to note other side effects, such as nausea or vomiting.

6. Give analgesics at regular, scheduled intervals rather than as needed (p.r.n.). This is particularly essential for oral analgesics, which may take 1 hour to act. The patient on an inadequate schedule could be in pain a substantially long time before feeling relief.

7. Give analgesics *before* the patient feels pain or *as soon as* pain starts to return. Higher doses are needed to alleviate severe pain than to prevent it. Patients often need to be encouraged to inform nurses before pain becomes too severe.

8. Individualize the drug and the dosage for each patient. This is normally done by the physician. Patients vary considerably in the amount of analgesic they require. No two persons have the same intensity of pain, nor is the absorption, metabolism, or excretion of the drug identical in any two patients.

9. Beware of so-called potentiators of analgesia. Most potentiators sedate the patient. Commonly prescribed *potentiators* (drugs that are said to increase the effectiveness of analgesics or the duration of pain relief) are hydroxyzine (Vistaril and Atarax) and promethazine (Phenergan). Neither of these drugs potentiates narcotic analgesia (McCaffery 1980a:39).

10. Keep in mind the patient's disease process and allergies when administering analgesics. Patients with certain respiratory diseases are at increased risk from respiratory depression induced by narcotics, and patients with bleeding gastrointestinal ulcers need to avoid aspirin. Patients with liver or kidney disease may not metabolize or excrete drugs appropriately. Patients with intestinal problems may not absorb oral medications appropriately. Thus, the nurse always needs to bear in mind the side effects of analgesics in relation to the patient's disease.

11. Schedule required activities, such as physical therapy, ambulation, or diagnostic procedures, at times when analgesics are having their fullest effect.

12. When possible, stay with patients who are in pain unless they prefer to be left alone. Some patients with migraine headaches desire minimal stimulation, and others may fear loss of control or be embarrassed about sharing their coping methods of cursing or shouting. Usually, however, the nurse's presence comforts patients and may distract them and help them focus attention externally rather than internally.

Medical Intervention

Nerve Blocks

A *nerve block* is chemical interruption of a nerve pathway, effected by injecting a local anesthetic—e.g., lidocaine (Xylocaine) or procaine (Novocain) into the nerve. Nerve blocks are widely used during dental work: The injected drug blocks nerve pathways from the painful tooth, thus stopping the transmission of pain impulses to the brain. Nerve blocks are often used to relieve the pain of whiplash injury, low back disorders, bursitis, and cancer. Sometimes alcohol blocks are used. These, however, destroy nerve fibers and as a result are usually used for peripheral blocks, since peripheral nerve fibers regenerate.

Electric Stimulation

Electric stimulation is sometimes used to combat certain intractable pain. There are several methods. In *transcutaneous electric stimulation*, electrodes are placed on the surface of the skin over the painful area and over peripheral nerve pathways. In *pericutaneous stimulation*, needles are inserted near a major peripheral nerve (e.g., the sciatic nerve). In both methods, an electric charge blocks the pain impulse by stimulating the gate control mechanism. The pericutaneous method is used primarily to determine whether a patient should consider having a permanent implant inserted.

Two implantable devices are the *peripheral nerve implant* and the *dorsal column stimulator.* The peripheral implant is an electrode attached to a major sensory nerve. The column stimulator is an electrode attached to the dorsal column of the spinal cord. Both devices have a transmitter that the patient wears externally. The transmitter sends an impulse that blocks the transmission of the pain impulse (Gaumer 1974:504–05). The blocking of pain impulses is generally within the scope of a physician's practice only. However, some nurses functioning in expanded roles may have responsibility for such procedures.

Acupuncture

Acupuncture has been practiced for centuries in China and is receiving increasing attention in North America. It is currently being used selectively in North America to treat chronic pain. The acupuncturist inserts long, slender needles into the body at various sites, which are not necessarily near the body parts to be treated. The needles can be heated, attached to a mild electric current, or twirled continuously with the hand.

Traditional acupuncturists believe acupuncture corrects a disharmony between the life forces of yin and yang. See Chapter 10. Western scientists, puzzled by the effectiveness of acupuncture, theorize that it closes the gate mechanism to pain or stimulates sites near pain fibers leading to the brain, thereby blocking the perception of pain. It is also possible that there are neurologic links between body sites. Stimulation of one site may affect pain at another. This idea is supported by the fact that organic pain is often referred to a distant body part. Cardiac pain, for example, is often referred to the shoulder, back, or lower jaw.

Hypnosis

Hypnosis has been used to treat psychogenic pain, to achieve anesthesia, and to enhance the effectiveness of medications given for pain aggravated by tension. The susceptible person accepts positive suggestions, which tend to alter perceptions. The success of hypnosis depends to a large degree on the person's openness to suggestion, emotional readiness, and faith in the effectiveness of the hypnosis (American Journal of Nursing 1974a:515).

Surgery

Pain conduction pathways can be interrupted surgically. Because this disruption is permanent, surgery is performed only as a last resort, generally for intractable pain. Several surgical procedures may be performed:

1. In *cordotomy*, the spinothalamic portion of the anterolateral tract is severed. This procedure obliterates pain and temperature sensation below the level severed, and is usually done for pain in the legs and trunk.
2. In *rhizotomy*, the anterior or posterior nerve root between the ganglion and the cord is interrupted. Interruption of anterior *motor* nerve roots stops spasmodic movements that accompany paraplegia. Interruption of posterior *sensory* nerve roots eliminates pain in areas innervated by that specific nerve root. Rhizotomies are generally performed on cervical nerve roots to alleviate pain of the head and neck from cancer or neuralgia.
3. In *neurectomy*, peripheral or cranial nerves are interrupted to alleviate localized pain, such as pain in the lower leg or foot arising from a vascular occlusion.
4. In a *sympathectomy*, pathways of the sympathetic division of the autonomic nervous system are severed. This procedure eliminates vasospasm, improves peripheral blood supply, and thus is effective in treating painful vascular disorders such as angina and Raynaud's disease.

Biofeedback

Biofeedback is a method of controlling certain physiologic functions by providing information normally unavailable to an individual. In the past, most physiologic processes were considered involuntary. However, it has been discovered that many of these processes are partially subject to voluntary control. Studies show that muscle tension, heart beat, blood flow, and pain, for example, can be controlled voluntarily. The feedback is usually provided through auditory or visual means, e.g., the patient sees an electromyogram that shows the electric potential created by the contraction of muscles.

Biofeedback allows the patient to be fully involved in his or her treatment. The responsibility in biofeedback training lies primarily with the patient. The patient may require months or even years of training before the optimum level of response is reached. Therefore, patients must usually be highly motivated to participate in biofeedback programs.

Evaluating Interventions for Pain

The outcome criteria for patients who have pain (actual or potential) depend on the nursing diagnosis. Some suggested criteria are:

1. Feels no postoperative abdominal pain
2. Does deep breathing exercises and coughs without severe pain

3. Performs work activities without back pain
4. Walks to end of hall and back without undue discomfort
5. Performs relaxation exercises as scheduled
6. Has relaxed head and neck muscles

Summary

A common nursing responsibility is helping patients meet their needs for rest and sleep. Although rest is necessary and frequently prescribed, it is not always easy for patients to rest. To rest, a patient must feel that the illness and personal concerns are under control, feel acceptable to self and to others, feel knowledgeable about what is happening, be free of physical and emotional discomfort, have purposeful activity, and know that help is available when needed.

Sleep is thought necessary for mental and emotional equilibrium and well-being. It is also thought to mediate stress and anxiety. Sleep patterns and requirements vary with the individual, with age, and with circadian biorhythms. Sleep cycles have been measured by electroencephalograms. There are two types of sleep: non-REM (NREM or slow wave) sleep and paradoxical (REM) sleep. There are four stages of NREM sleep; each stage has associated alpha and delta brain wave changes, changes in vital signs, and different levels of arousability. These four stages occur in cycles of about 90 minutes throughout sleep.

Assessing rest and sleep requires assessment of sleeping habits, clinical signs of the need for sleep, developmental changes, and factors influencing rest and sleep. Several factors affect sleep. Age determines the amount of sleep required; the relative duration of REM sleep decreases with age. Fatigue shortens the first period of REM sleep. Illness often increases the time needed for sleep and alters the person's normal sleep patterns. Emotional problems can result in insomnia. Hypnotics and sedatives increase sleeping time but decrease REM sleep. Overuse of sedatives can lead to REM deprivation.

The need for sleep is evident when a person expresses a feeling of fatigue or exhibits periods of depression, apathy, irritability, aggressiveness, and inattention. Confusion and hallucinations can result from marked sleep deprivation.

Nursing interventions to promote sleep need to be adapted to the individual patient. Some general measures nurses can take are providing a relaxing environment, helping the patient maintain bedtime routines, eliminating noise, attending to safety and security needs, providing adequate warmth, and administering hypnotics or sedatives as prescribed. Three common sleep problems are insomnia, enuresis, and somnambulism. These require additional nursing measures.

Pain is probably the most common symptom of disease that nurses encounter. Regardless of whether it is acute, chronic, or intractable, pain is a highly personal sensation that only the patient can describe. The experience of pain includes pain perception and pain reaction. The neurophysiology of pain is complex: Pain receptors are distributed unevenly among body tissues. Pain signals travel along type A and type C fibers to the spinal cord through the dorsal roots. From there they ascend or descend to terminate in neurons in the substantia gelatinosa or the dorsal horns. Signals then cross to the opposite side of the cord and ascend through the anteriolateral spinothalamic tract to the thalamus of the brain. In the brain, pain pathways divide in two, and types A and C fibers differentiate.

Pain is sometimes perceived to be in an area other than its source. Examples are referred pain and phantom pain. The perception of pain is also sometimes blocked or altered. The gate control theory and theories of other control systems in the thalamus and cerebral cortex provide some explanations for these alterations. Endorphins are endogenous compounds that block and otherwise alter the perception of pain.

When assessing pain, nurses rely heavily on explicit data from the patient. Data collected need to include the location of the pain, its intensity, the time of its onset and its duration, its quality or description, and associated nonverbal behavior. Previous experiences with the pain and any precipitating factors also need to be described. Assessment also includes taking a pain history and considering factors that influence the pain.

Nursing intervention may include removing the pain stimulus or altering the patient's perception and interpretation of the pain. Specific methods are distraction, relaxation, skin stimulation, administration of analgesics and placebos. Intractable, severe pain may call for strong analgesics, such as methadone and Brompton's mixture. The nurse treating patients in pain can follow certain guidelines. Medical intervention for pain includes nerve blocks, electric stimulation, acupuncture, hypnosis, surgery, and biofeedback. The nurse can evaluate the effectiveness of interventions for pain by gauging changes in the patient against previously determined criteria.

Suggested Activities

1. Interview a 5- or 6-year-old, an adolescent, a young adult, and an elderly adult. Collect the following information, take it back to a student group, and compare data and assess differences by age group.
   a. How much sleep does the person need?
   b. When does the person go to bed?
   c. What rituals, if any, help the person sleep?
   d. Does the person ever have difficulty sleeping? If so, what helps the person get to sleep?

2. Help two patients in a hospital setting get ready for sleep. With a group of other students, discuss how each patient was helped to prepare and how this preparation could have been improved.
3. Talk to a patient who has had pain recently. How was the pain relieved? Which nursing activities helped relieve the pain and which did not? How did the patient describe the pain?
4. Using the guidelines in this chapter, perform a complete assessment of a patient in pain. Compare your findings with those of your teacher or another nurse. Record your findings on the patient's chart.

Suggested Readings

Rest and sleep

Fabijan, L., and Gosselin, M. D. April 1982. How to recognize sleep deprivation in your ICU patient and what to do about it. *The Canadian Nurse* 78:20–23.
These authors discuss the key signs of sleep deprivation and make eight related recommendations to incorporate in an intensive care patient's nursing care plan.

Hayter, J. March 1980. The rhythm of sleep. *American Journal of Nursing* 80:457–61.
Hayter describes the five stages of sleep, diseases that alter sleep rhythm, and factors related to REM deprivation.

Martin, I. C. June 8, 1978. Twitch and between, Part 1. Aspects of the relaxation technique. *Nursing Times* 74:953–55.
Progressive relaxation techniques promote sleep.

Pain

Dolan, M. B. January 1982. Controlling pain in a personal way. *Nursing 82* 12:68.
Palliative measures such as positioning, massage, and "guided imagery" need to be implemented before administering analgesics. Thirteen rules for pain management are stated.

Doyle, J. E. April 1981. If your patient's legs hurt the reason may be arterial insufficiency. *Nursing 81* 11:74–78.
The author provides a guide for assessing peripheral arterial insufficiency. Physical examination of the feet is discussed, and color photographs of some of the signs of arterial insufficiency, such as gangrene, ulcers, and atrophic skin, are included. Pulse evaluation is also discussed.

Fagerhaugh, S. Y., and Strauss, A. February 1980. How to manage your patient's pain . . . and how not to. *Nursing 80* 10:44–47.
These authors, after surveying 20 hospital units, discovered that each nurse follows his or her own pain philosophy. The result is confusion among patients. They recommend clearly defined drug policies and suggest ways in which nurses can build pain management into a surgical unit's patient care system.

Frank-Stromborg, M., and Stromborg, P. August 1981. Test your knowledge of chest pain. *Nursing 81* 11:21–30.
This article is a series of multiple-choice questions that test knowledge of chest pain, chest pain management, and medications for chest pain. Answers are provided at the end of the article.

Holderby, R. A. May 1981. Conscious suggestion: Using talk to manage pain. *Nursing 81* 11:44–46.
This chaplain and crisis counselor discusses essential aspects of the conscious suggestion technique used to manage pain.

McCaffery, M. September 1980. Understanding your patient's pain. *Nursing 80* 10:26–31.
The author defines pain and describes the signs of acute pain. The causes of pain are discussed together with descriptions of psychogenic and somatogenic pain. Duration, severity, and patient tolerance are considered.

———. November 1980. How to relieve your patients' pain fast and effectively . . . with oral analgesics. *Nursing 80* 10:58–63.
The author outlines guidelines that help nurses choose and administer oral analgesics effectively. Equianalgesic lists are provided for commonly used oral analgesics.

———. June 1981. When your patient's still in pain don't just do something: Sit there. *Nursing 81* 11:58–61.
This article outlines the advantages of staying with patients in pain, tells when not to be there, and describes problems the nurse may encounter by being there.

Maxwell, M. B. September 1980. How to use methadone for the cancer patient's pain. *American Journal of Nursing* 80:1606–9.
This author, who directs a nurse-practitioner chemotherapy clinic, describes in detail dosage regimens for patients on methadone.

Tannenbaum, R. P.; Sohn, C. A.; Cantwell, R.; Rogers, M.; and Hollis, R. September 1981. Pain: Angina pectoris—how to recognize it; how to manage it. *Nursing 81* 11:44–51.
Angina and myocardial infarction pain are compared. The types of angina are described together with the palliative action of the nitrates. Also included are the teaching aspects of nursing, including the precautions to be taken by patients.

Wright, Z. July 1981. From I.V. to P.O. Titrating your patient's pain medication. *Nursing 81* 11:39–43.
This oncology clinical nurse specialist describes the plan used to switch a patient's narcotic analgesic (Dilaudid) from the intravenous route used in hospitals, to the oral route for home care. An equianalgesic list is provided for commonly used narcotics.

Selected References

Rest and sleep

Binzley, V. January 1977. State: Overlooked factor in newborn nursing. *American Journal of Nursing* 77:102–3.

Deters, G. E. July-August 1980. Circadian rhythm phenomenon. *Maternal Child Nursing* 5:249–51.

Diekelmann, N. L. August 1976. The young adult; the choice is health or illness. *American Journal of Nursing* 76:1274–77.

Fass, G. December 1971. Sleep, drugs, and dreams. *American Journal of Nursing* 71:2316–20.

Grant, D. A., and Klell, C. November 1974. For goodness sake—let your patients sleep. *Nursing 74* 4:54–57.

Guyton, A. C. 1981. *Textbook of medical physiology.* 6th ed. Philadelphia: W. B. Saunders Co.

Harvey, A. Mc.; Johns, R. J.; McKusick, V. A.; Owens, A. H.; and Ross, R. S. 1980. *The principles and practice of medicine.* 20th ed. New York: Appleton-Century-Crofts.

Hayter, J. March 1980. The rhythm of sleep. *American Journal of Nursing* 80:457–61.

McFadden, E. H., and Giblin, E. C. May-June 1971. Sleep deprivation in patients having open heart surgery. *Nursing Research* 20:249–54.

Marlow, D. R. 1977. *Textbook of pediatric nursing.* 5th ed. Philadelphia: W. B. Saunders Co.

Milne, B. April 1982. Sleep-wake disorders and what we can do about them. *The Canadian Nurse* 78:24–27.

Murray, R. B., and Zentner, J. P. 1979. *Nursing assessment and health promotion through the life span.* 2nd ed. Englewood Cliffs, N.J.: Prentice-Hall.

Narrow, B. W. August 1967. Rest is . . . *American Journal of Nursing* 67:1646–49.

Oswald, I. March 13, 1980. Sleep: No place for the worried. *Nursing Mirror* 150:34–35.

Whaley, L. F., and Wong, D. L. 1979. *Nursing care of infants and children.* St. Louis: C. V. Mosby Co.

Woods, N. F., and Falk, S. A. March-April 1974. Noise stimuli in the acute care area. *Nursing Research* 23:144–50.

Pain

American Journal of Nursing. March 1974a. Hypnotic suggestion. *American Journal of Nursing* 74:515.

———. March 1974b. Chemical and surgical intervention. *American Journal of Nursing* 74:511.

Barrett-Griesemer, P.; Meisel, S.; and Rate, R. April 1981. A guide to headaches—and how to relieve their pain. *Nursing 81* 11:50–57.

Beyerman, K. February 1982. Flawed perceptions about pain. *American Journal of Nursing* 82:302–4.

Blaylock, J. 1968. The psychological and cultural influences on the reaction to pain: A review of literature. *Nursing Forum* 7(3):262–74.

Booker, J. E. March 1982. Pain: It's all in your patient's head (or is it?) *Nursing 82* 12:46–51.

Breeden, S. A., and Kondo, C. November 1975. Using biofeedback to reduce tension. *American Journal of Nursing* 75:2010–12.

Copp, L. A. March 1974. The spectrum of suffering. *American Journal of Nursing* 74:491–95.

Cummings, D. January 1981. Stopping chronic pain before it starts. *Nursing 81* 11:60–62.

Davitz, L. J.; Sameshima, Y.; and Davitz, J. August 1976. Suffering as viewed in six different cultures. *American Journal of Nursing* 76:1296–97.

Drakontides, A. B. March 1974. Drugs to treat pain. *American Journal of Nursing* 74:508–13.

Engel, G. L. 1970. Pain. In MacBryde, C. M., and Blacklow, R. S., editors. *Signs and symptoms: Applied physiologic physiology and clinical interpretation.* 5th ed. Philadelphia: B. Lippincott Co.

Gaumer, W. R. March 1974. Electrical stimulation in chronic pain. *American Journal of Nursing* 74:504–5.

Gever, L. N. May 1980. Brompton's mixture. How it relieves the pain of terminal cancer. *Nursing 80* 10:57.

Goloskov, J., and LeRoy, P. March 1974. Use of the dorsal column stimulator. *American Journal of Nursing* 74:506–7.

Goodwin, J. S.; Goodwin, J. M.; and Vogel, A. V. February 1982. Placebo misuse. *Nursing 82* 12:24–25.

Guyton, A. C. 1982. *Human physiology and mechanisms of disease.* 3rd ed. Philadelphia: W. B. Saunders Company.

Jacox, A. K. May 1979. Assessing pain. *American Journal of Nursing* 79:895–900.

Lewis, K. P. August 1980. Pain cocktails. *Nurses' Drug Alert* 4(10):76.

McCaffery, M. 1979. *Nursing management of the patient with pain.* 2nd ed. Philadelphia: J. B. Lippincott Co.

———. October 1980a. Patients shouldn't have to suffer: How to relieve pain with injectable narcotics. *Nursing 80* 10:34–39.

———. December 1980b. Relieving pain with noninvasive techniques. *Nursing 80* 10:55–57.

———. February 1982. Would you administer placebos for pain? These facts can help you decide. *Nursing 82* 12:22–27.

McGuire, L. March 1981. A short, simple tool for assessing your patient's pain. *Nursing 81* 11:48–49.

McLachlan, E. March 1974. Recognizing pain. *American Journal of Nursing* 74:496–97.

McMahon, M. A., and Miller, P. 1978. Pain response: The influence of psycho-social cultural factors. *Nursing Forum* 17(1):58–71.

Mastrovito, R. C. March 1974. Psychogenic pain. *American Journal of Nursing* 74:514–19.

Meissner, J. E. January 1980. McGill-Melzack pain questionnaire. *Nursing 80* 10:50–51.

Melzack, R., and Wall, P. D. 19 November 1965. Pain mechanisms: A new theory. *Science* 150:971–79.

O'Donnell, L., and Papciak, B. August 1981. When all else fails: Continuous morphine infusion for controlling intractable pain. *Nursing 81* 11:69–72.

Perry, S. W., and Heidrich, G. April 1981. Placebo response: Myth and matter. *American Journal of Nursing* 81:720–25.

Putt, A. M. January 1979. A biofeedback service by nurses. *American Journal of Nursing* 79:88–89.

Ryan, B. J. 1979. Biofeedback training: The voluntary control of mind over body and mind. *Nursing Forum* 14(1):48–55.

Schultz, N. V. October 1971. How children perceive pain. *Nursing Outlook* 19:670–73.

Siegele, D. S. March 1974. The gate control theory. *American Journal of Nursing* 74:498–502.

Silman, J. January 1979. The management of pain. *American Journal of Nursing* 79:74–78.

Sterman, L. T. November 1975. Clinical biofeedback. *American Journal of Nursing* 75:2006–9.

Stewart, E. June 1976. To lessen pain: Relaxation and rhythmic breathing. *American Journal of Nursing* 76:958–59.

West, B. A. February 1981. Understanding endorphins: Our natural pain relief system. *Nursing 81* 11:50–53.

Wilson, R. W., and Elmassian, B. J. April 1981. Endorphins. *American Journal of Nursing* 81:722–25.

Chapter 26

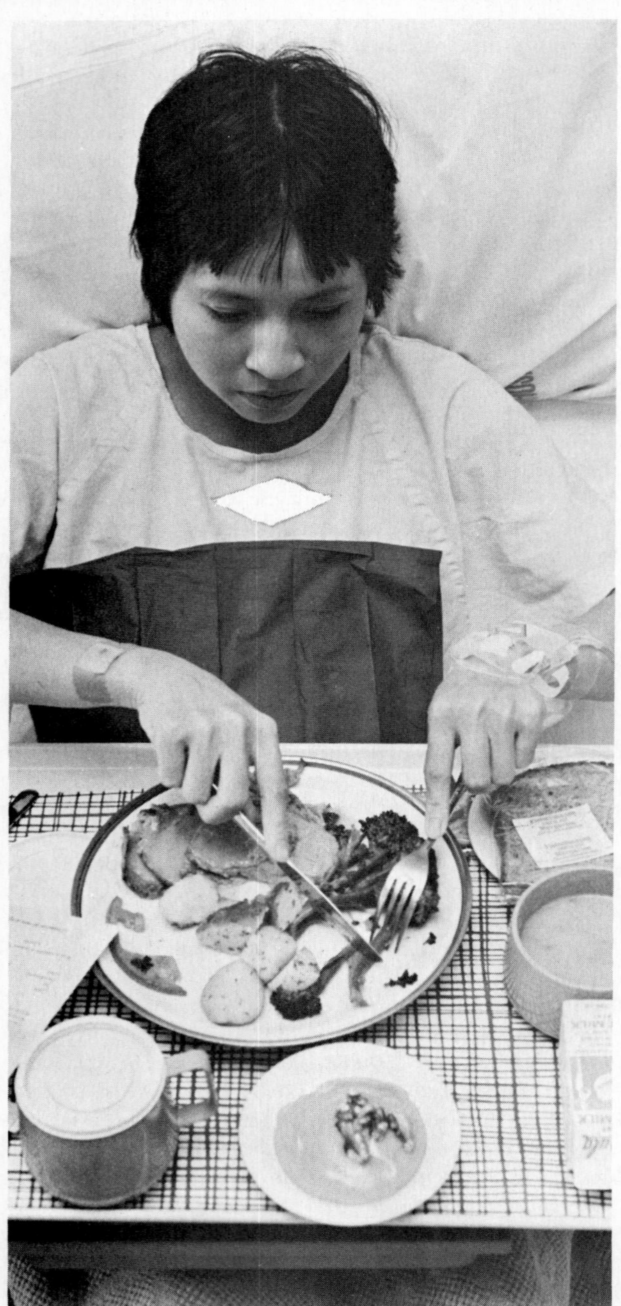

Nutrition

CONTENTS

Objectives

1. Know essential facts about required nutrients
   - **1.1** Define selected terms
   - **1.2** Identify ways nutrients are classified
   - **1.3** Identify good sources of required nutrients
   - **1.4** Identify mechanisms involved in the digestion of nutrients
   - **1.5** Describe mechanisms involved in the absorption of nutrients
   - **1.6** Describe how nutrients are stored in the body
   - **1.7** Identify essential mechanisms involved in the metabolism of nutrients
2. Know essential facts about balanced nutritious diets
   - **2.1** Outline essential aspects of daily food guides recommended by governments
   - **2.2** Identify types of vegetarian diets
   - **2.3** Describe the prudent diet
   - **2.4** Describe the concept of energy-balanced diets
   - **2.5** Identify variables in dietary needs according to age
3. Know essential information and methods required to assess nutritional status
   - **3.1** Describe anthropometric techniques
   - **3.2** Identify factors that influence a person's eating patterns
   - **3.3** Identify clinical signs of inadequate nutritional status
4. Understand essential facts about common nutritional problems
   - **4.1** Differentiate among common nutritional problems
   - **4.2** Identify factors contributing to nutritional problems
   - **4.3** Identify indicators of common nutritional problems
5. Understand facts about nursing measures that maintain, promote, and restore good nutrition
   - **5.1** Identify measures to stimulate a patient's appetite
   - **5.2** Identify the essentials of various hospital diets
   - **5.3** Identify measures that help patients obtain nourishment
   - **5.4** Identify essential steps in administering nasogastric or gastrostomy feedings
6. Apply the nursing process when providing care to patients with nutritional problems
   - **6.1** Obtain necessary assessment data
   - **6.2** Analyze and relate assessment data
   - **6.3** Write relevant nursing diagnoses
   - **6.4** Write relevant nursing goals
   - **6.5** Plan appropriate nursing interventions
   - **6.6** Implement appropriate nursing interventions
   - **6.7** State outcome criteria against which to evaluate the patient's progress

Terms

adenosine triphosphate (ATP)
amino acid
anabolism
anorexia
anorexia nervosa
anthropometric measurement
antrum
basal metabolic rate (BMR)
cachexia
caloric density
caloric value
calorie (small calorie)
carbohydrate
catabolism
cholesterol
chyme
citric acid cycle (Krebs cycle)
deamination
diet
disaccharide
dysphagia
emaciation
emulsification
enteric feeding
enzyme
ester
fad
fat
fatty acids
fiber
gastrostomy
gavage
gluconeogenesis
glycogen
glycogenesis
glycogenolysis
glycolysis
hydrolysis
hyperalimentation
ketogenesis
kilocalorie (Calorie, large calorie)
lipids
mastication
micronutrient
monosaccharide
nausea
negative nitrogen balance
nitrogen balance
nutrient
nutrition
nutritional deficit
nutritive value
obesity
overweight
peristalsis
phosphorylation
polysaccharide
positive nitrogen balance
protein
prudent diet
segmentation contractions
sodium cotransport theory
special (therapeutic) diet
triglyceride
vitamin

Nutrition education is making North Americans more aware of the importance of a healthy diet. Unfortunately, however, advice about nutrition is often conflicting, and people end up confused about which food choices are best. Many people worry that certain foods may be unsafe, especially since commonly used additives (e.g., cyclamates and saccharin) have been linked with cancer and birth defects and banned by the Food and Drug Administration (FDA). As a result, growing numbers of individuals, believing that "natural" and "organic" foods are the safest foods to eat, are shopping in health food stores. In addition, the public is being given the message that overconsumption of fats, cholesterol, and sugar is unhealthy and shortens lives. For example, people are learning to cut down on major sources of cholesterol (e.g., eggs), calories, and fat and to use vegetable oils (polyunsaturated fats) rather than animal fats (saturated fats) to prevent cardiovascular diseases such as heart disease, cerebrovascular accidents, and high blood pressure.

Health professionals have a major role in promoting health by helping people make informed food choices. Effective education emphasizes an understanding of not only essential nutrients but also of methods to change eating habits. To be an effective promoter of health and to effect beneficial changes in eating behaviors, the nurse must consider the many factors (e.g., emotions, culture, life-style, and financial resources) that affect a person's food choices.

Essential Nutrients

Nutrition is what a person eats and how the body uses it. People require essential nutrients for the growth and maintenance of all body tissues and the normal functioning of all body processes. *Nutrients* are the organic and inorganic chemicals found in foods and required for proper body functioning. An adequate food intake consists of a balance of essential nutrients, which include carbohydrates, proteins, fats, vitamins, minerals, and water. Foods differ greatly in their *nutritive value* (the nutrient content of a specified amount of food), and no one food provides all essential nutrients.

Nutrients have one or more of the following functions (Suitor and Hunter 1980:4):

1. To provide energy for body processes and exercise
2. To provide structural material for body tissues, e.g., bones and muscles
3. To regulate body processes

The most basic nutrient need is water. It is the most abundant compound in the body and vital to all body processes. Fortunately, people are impelled by thirst to drink water long before the body's water levels are too low. Chapters 30 and 31 provide detailed information about this nutrient.

Because every cell requires a continuous supply of fuel, the body's most urgent nutritional need, after water, is for nutrients that provide fuel, or energy. The energy-providing nutrients are carbohydrates, fats, and proteins. Hunger impels people to eat enough energy-providing nutrients to satisfy their energy needs. The amount of energy that nutrients or foods supply to the body is their *caloric value*. A *calorie* is a unit of heat energy. A *small calorie* is the amount of heat required to raise the temperature of 1 g of water 1 degree C. A *large calorie* (Calorie, kilocalorie, or kcal) is the amount of heat required to raise the temperature of 1 kg of water 1 degree C and is the unit used in nutrition. The energy liberated from each gram of carbohydrate and protein after it is metabolized is about 4 kcal; that liberated from each gram of fat, about 8 kcal. The average North American receives approximately 45% of energy from carbohydrates, 40% from fat, and 15% from protein (Guyton 1982:558). In most other parts of the world, people derive far more energy from carbohydrates than from fats and proteins. People in Mongolia, for example, derive 80 to 85% of energy from carbohydrates (Guyton 1982:558). See the section on energy balance, page 664, for further information.

No clear-cut body signals lead a person to ingest certain vitamins or minerals, both of which are often referred to as *micronutrients*. Lack of such signals, however, does not mean that people do not need these nutrients. Micronutrients are essential for vital structures and regulatory functions of the body.

Carbohydrates

Definition and description

Carbohydrates are composed of the elements carbon, hydrogen, and oxygen and are of two basic kinds: sugars (simple carbohydrates) and starches (complex carbohydrates). The sugars may be *monosaccharides* (single molecules), which include glucose, fructose, and galactose, or *disaccharides* (double molecules), which include sucrose or table sugar (a combination of glucose and fructose), maltose or grain sugar (two glucose molecules), and lactose or milk sugar (a combination of glucose and galactose). Starches are *polysaccharides* because they are composed of branched chains of dozens of molecules of glucose. Nearly all carbohydrates (with the exception of those in milk and milk products, which contain the disaccharide lactose) are derived from plants.

Carbohydrates are also categorized as natural (those found in foods as they come from the earth, e.g., fruits, vegetables, wheat) and refined or processed (those extracted from their natural sources and added to foods, e.g., cookies, candy, cakes, and pies). The natural carbohydrates supply vital nutrients such as protein, vitamins, and minerals and an important nonnutrient, dietary fiber. *Fiber*, a carbohydrate derived from plants, cannot be digested by humans and has few or no calories but supplies roughage or bulk to the diet. This bulk not only satisfies appetite but also helps the digestive tract function effectively and eliminate wastes. Refined carbohydrates are relatively low in nutrients in relation to the large number of calories they contain and thus are often referred to as empty calories.

Digestion

Ingested food must be altered physically and chemically before the body can absorb it from the gastrointestinal tract.

Physical alterations include mechanical breakdown, mixing, and emulsification:

1. Mechanical breakdown results from the *mastication* (chewing) of food, which breaks cell walls, releases their nutrients, and increases the surface area of food, thus facilitating chemical digestion.
2. Mixing of food with secretions occurs in the mouth, stomach, and intestines. Initial mixing of food with saliva in the mouth begins the chemical digestion of carbohydrates and aids the passage of all swallowed food to the stomach. Mixing waves usually start at the midpoint of the stomach but are very vigorous in the *antrum* (portion of the stomach between the fundus or body and the pylorus). Food is churned with gastric secretions. In the intestine, mixing of *chyme* (mixture of food and secretions passing from the stomach into the duodenum) is continued by *segmentation* (local) *contractions* and to a lesser degree by *peristalsis*. These contractions mix the chyme with digestive secretions and bring the chyme into contact with the intestinal mucosa, thus facilitating absorption of nutrients.
3. *Emulsification* is the process by which *lipids* (fats and other fat-soluble substances that are insoluble in water) are broken up and evenly dispersed in an aqueous medium. Emulsification occurs in the small intestine, where bile salts are mixed with the chyme. See the section on the digestion of fat, page 659, for further information.

Chemical alterations include the digestive processes that convert food nutrients to a form the body can absorb. Energy nutrients (carbohydrates, fats, and proteins) and vitamins are altered chemically by *hydrolysis*, a process that involves the splitting of a molecule in the presence of particular digestive enzymes with the addition of water. (*Enzymes* are biologic catalysts that speed up chemical reactions.) Very large molecules can be hydrolyzed hundreds of times to much smaller molecules suitable for absorption. Digestive enzymes, which break down nutrients chemically into smaller compounds by hydrolysis, are categorized according to the types of nutrients on which they act. See Table 26–1.

The desired end products of carbohydrate digestion are monosaccharides (glucose, fructose, and galactose). Some simple sugars, therefore, require no digestion. Of the three monosaccharides, glucose is by far the most abundant. Major enzymes of carbohydrate metabolism include ptyalin (salivary amylase), pancreatic amylase, and the disaccharidases: maltase, sucrase, and lactase.

Absorption and transport

The small intestine provides an extremely large mucosal surface area, since it is covered with tiny projections (villi) that in turn have smaller projections (microvilli), referred to as the brush border. These projections increase the surface area of the mucosa enormously, making possible the absorption of large amounts of nutrients.

In healthy persons, essentially all digested carbohydrate is absorbed by the small intestine. The precise mechanism by which monosaccharides are absorbed is not known. It is thought that a carrier for transport of glucose and some other monosaccharides (e.g., galactose) is present in the brush border of the epithelial cells. This carrier, however, will not transport the glucose in the absence of the transport of sodium. (See the section on active transport of sodium, Chapter 30, page 782.) Thus it is thought that the carrier has receptor sites for both a glucose molecule and a sodium ion and will not transport glucose to the inside of cells unless the receptor site for sodium is simultaneously filled (Guyton 1982:516). This hypothesized carrier mechanism for glucose transport is the basis of the *sodium cotransport theory*.

Monosaccharides are absorbed into the portal blood and, after passing through the liver, are transported everywhere in the body by the circulatory system. Fructose and galactose undergo chemical changes in the liver, which converts them into glucose. Thus, essentially all of the monosaccharides that circulate in the blood are glucose.

Transport of glucose through the cell membrane into

Table 26–1 Actions of Major Digestive Enzymes

Name	Source	Site of action	Agents acted upon	Resulting products
Carbohydrate enzymes				
Ptyalin (salivary amylase)	Saliva (secretions from parotid and submaxillary glands)	Mouth; some in body of stomach	Starch, e.g., grains, potatoes, legumes	Dextrins, maltose, glucose
Pancreatic amylase	Pancreatic secretions	Small intestine	Starch Dextrins	As above Maltose, glucose
Disaccharidases	Small intestine	Brush border of small intestine	Disaccharides	Monosaccharides
a. Lactase			Lactose in milk	Glucose and galactose
b. Maltase			Maltose in corn syrup	Glucose
c. Sucrase			Sucrose in table sugar, fruits	Glucose and fructose
Protein enzymes				
Pepsin	Peptic cells of stomach; inactive proenzyme pepsinogen is activated to pepsin by hydrochloric acid	Stomach	Large protein molecules	Proteoses, peptones, and large polypeptides
Rennin (in infants only)	Gastric mucosa	Stomach; calcium is necessary for activity	Casein in milk	Coagulated milk
Trypsin	Pancreatic cells; inactive proenzyme trypsinogen activated to trypsin by enterokinase (hormone produced in duodenal wall)	Lumen of small intestine	Whole and partially digested proteins, e.g., proteoses, peptones	Smaller polypeptides and dipeptides
Chymotrypsin	Pancreatic cells; inactive proenzyme chymotrypsinogen is activated to chymotrypsin by trypsin	Lumen of small intestine	Same as trypsin	Same as trypsin; also coagulates milk
Carboxypeptidase	Pancreatic cells; inactive proenzyme procarboxypeptidase is activated to carboxypeptidase by trypsin	Lumen of small intestine	Same as trypsin	Same as trypsin plus some amino acids
Aminopeptidase	Glands in intestinal wall	Brush border of small intestine	Polypeptides	Short chain peptides and amino acids
Dipeptidase	Glands in intestinal wall	Brush border of small intestine	Dipeptides	Amino acids
Fat enzymes				
Pancreatic-lipase	Pancreas	Small intestine	Triglycerides, diglycerides	Diglycerides, monoglycerides, fatty acids

the tissue cells occurs by facilitated diffusion. Because glucose is too large a molecule to diffuse through cell membranes, it first combines with a carrier substance (thought to be a protein of small molecular weight) that makes glucose soluble in the cell membrane and able to diffuse readily to the cell interior. After passage through the cell membrane, glucose is dissociated from the carrier.

The rate of glucose transport through the cell membrane is greatly increased by insulin. In the absence of insulin, the amount of glucose that diffuses to the cell interior is far too little to supply normal requirements for energy (with the exception of the liver and brain cells). Glucose metabolism is therefore controlled by the rate at which insulin is available from the pancreas.

After entry into the cells, glucose combines with phosphate by an irreversible process called *phosphorylation*. This process captures the glucose in the cell; i.e., once in the cell, glucose cannot diffuse back out. Three exceptions to this irreversible process are liver, renal tubular epithelial, and intestinal epithelial cells, where specific enzymes (phosphatases) are available to reverse the reaction. Once in the cell, glucose is either used for immediate release of energy or stored.

Storage

Glucose is stored in cells in the form of *glycogen* (a large polymer of glucose). Although all cells of the body are capable of storing some glycogen, certain cells—liver and muscle—can store large amounts. The process of glycogen formation is called *glycogenesis*, and the breakdown of glycogen to re-form glucose is called *glycogenolysis*. Two hormones activate glycogenolysis: glucagon from the alpha cells of the pancreas, and epinephrine from the adrenal medulla. Glucagon is secreted when blood glucose concentrations fall to low levels; glucagon stimulates glycogenolysis mainly in the liver. The liver delivers large amounts of glucose into the blood stream, thus elevating the blood glucose. Epinephrine is released whenever the sympathetic nervous system is stimulated. Epinephrine stimulates glycogenolysis in both liver and muscle cells, thereby releasing energy needed by the body for action during sympathetic stimulation. Most of the glucose formed in the liver as a result of glycogenolysis passes directly into the blood stream; thus liver glycogenolysis always causes an increase in the blood glucose concentration. In most other cells of the body, however, particularly muscle cells, the glucose from glycogenolysis is used inside that cell and does not enter the bloodstream.

When the body's stores of carbohydrates fall below normal, certain quantities of glucose are formed from protein (amino acids) and fat reserves by *gluconeogenesis*, a process that occurs in the liver. Up to 60% of the amino acids in the body's protein can be converted into glucose. Some types of amino acids cannot be converted. During periods of starvation, the body depletes its fat first and later its protein reserves.

Metabolism

Once in the cells, glucose undergoes a series of reactions to produce energy for the body's varied demands. There are two major pathways for breaking down glucose into the end products of carbon dioxide and water, thus producing energy:

1. Glycolysis and the formation of pyruvic acid (Embden-Meyerhof glycolytic pathway)
2. Citric acid cycle (Krebs cycle or tricarboxylic acid cycle)

Glycolysis is the release of energy through the *catabolism* (breaking down) of a glucose molecule into two molecules of pyruvic acid. This is a complex process involving 10 successive steps of chemical reactions, each of which is catalyzed by specific enzymes. During the process, the end-products of glycolysis are oxidized, and energy is released in small packets to form *adenosine triphosphate* (ATP). ATP is a compound with high energy bonds that stores the energy produced during glucose oxidation. Not all of the energy is stored, however. Some of it is lost in the form of heat. Because of the formation of ATP, the body's energy supply is conserved rather than dissipated all at once. During the cycle, two ATP molecules are formed from one glucose molecule (Guyton 1982:528). The formation of pyruvic acid ends this glycolytic pathway; however, pyruvic acid provides the gateway to the next pathway, the citric acid cycle. The pyruvic acid is first broken down into two molecules of acetyl coenzyme A (acetyl-CoA).

The *citric acid cycle* is a complex series of chemical reactions by which the acetyl portion of acetyl-CoA is broken down to carbon dioxide and hydrogen atoms. The hydrogen atoms are subsequently oxidized, thus releasing more energy to form ATP. In the initial stage of the citric acid cycle, acetyl-CoA combines with oxaloacetic acid to form citric acid, which gives this cycle its name. For each molecule of glucose metabolized in the citric acid cycle, two molecules of ATP are formed (Guyton 1982:530).

Proteins

Definition and description

Proteins are organic substances that upon hydrolysis or digestion yield their constituent building blocks—amino acids (Williams 1981:51). Like carbohydrates, proteins are composed of carbon, hydrogen, and oxygen, but proteins also contain nitrogen. Every cell in the body contains some protein, and about three-quarters of body solids are proteins. Protein is part of muscle, bone, cartilage, skin, blood, and lymph. Many hormones and all enzymes are proteins. The only body substances normally lacking protein are urine and bile.

Proteins can be categorized by chemical structure as simple or compound.

Simple proteins contain only amino acids or their derivatives. *Amino acids* are nitrogen containing chemicals, the building blocks of protein. Examples of simple proteins are (Williams 1981:52):

1. Albumin, e.g., lactalbumin in milk and serum albumin in blood
2. Albuminoid, e.g., keratin in hair and skin, and gelatin
3. Globulin, e.g., ovoglobulin in egg and serum globulin in blood
4. Glutelin, e.g., gluten in wheat
5. Prolamin, e.g., zein in corn and gliadin in wheat

Compound proteins are composites of simple protein and another nonprotein group. Examples are (ibid., p. 52):

1. Chromoproteins composed of a protein and a chromorphic or pigmented group, e.g., hemoglobin
2. Glycoproteins and mucoproteins composed of a protein and carbohydrate, e.g., mucin found in mucous membrane secretions
3. Lipoproteins composed of a triglyceride or other lipid, e.g., cholesterol or phospholipid
4. Nucleoproteins composed of one or more proteins and nucleic acid, e.g., purines found in glandular tissue

Amino acids are categorized as essential or nonessential. Essential amino acids are those that cannot be manufactured in the body and must be supplied in their final form as part of the protein ingested in the diet. They are essential for tissue growth and maintenance. Ten essential amino acids are threonine, leucine, isoleucine, valine, lysine, methionine, phenylalanine, tryptophan, histadine, and arginine. Histadine and arginine are necessary during growth but not during adulthood (Brody 1981:36 and Williams 1981:53).

Nonessential amino acids are those that the body can manufacture. The body takes apart amino acids derived from the diet and reconstructs new ones from their basic elements (carbohydrates and nitrogen). Nonessential amino acids include glycine, alanine, aspartic acid, glutamic acid, proline, hydroxyproline, cystine, tyrosine, and serine (Williams 1981:53).

Proteins are also categorized as complete or incomplete. Complete proteins contain all of the essential amino acids plus many nonessential ones. Most animal proteins, including meats, poultry, fish, dairy products, and eggs, are complete proteins. Some animal proteins, however, contain less than the required amount of one or more essential amino acids and therefore alone cannot support continued growth. These proteins are sometimes referred to as partially complete proteins. Examples are some fish, which have small amounts of methionine, and the milk protein casein, which has little arginine.

Incomplete proteins are deficient in one or more essential amino acids and include those derived from vegetables. Incomplete proteins are most commonly deficient in lysine, methionine, or tryptophan. If, however, an appropriate mixture of plant proteins is provided in the diet, a balanced ration of essential amino acids can be created. Because protein is not stored, these mixtures must be eaten at the same meal. For example, a combination of corn (low in tryptophan and lysine) and beans (low in methionine) is a complete protein. Such combinations of two or more vegetables are called complementary proteins.

Another way to take full advantage of vegetable proteins is to eat them with a small amount of animal protein. Examples are spaghetti with cheese, rice with pork, noodles with tuna, cereal with milk, etc.

Digestion

Physical alterations Like carbohydrates, protein foods are altered physically by mechanical breakdown in the mouth and mixing with secretions in the stomach and intestine.

Chemical alterations Chemical digestion of protein begins in the stomach by three agents present in gastric secretions: pepsin, hydrochloric acid, and rennin. Pepsin is the main gastric enzyme specific for proteins. It is formed inside the peptic cells as pepsinogen, which has no digestive action. When, however, pepsinogen comes in contact with hydrochloric acid, it immediately forms active pepsin. This active pepsin then breaks the protein down into proteoses, peptones, and large polypeptides, smaller but still relatively large protein derivatives. Complete digestion of proteins to amino acids (the desired end products of protein digestion) could occur in the stomach if protein were held in the stomach longer. However, because the stomach normally empties in a relatively short time, only the beginning stages of protein breakdown are activated by pepsin. Protein breaks down into successively smaller molecules in this sequence: proteins, proteoses, peptones, polypeptides, dipeptides, and finally amino acids.

Hydrochloric acid, which converts inactive pepsinogen to the active enzyme pepsin, is secreted by the parietal cells and is an essential catalyst for protein digestion.

Rennin is a gastric enzyme necessary for infants to digest milk. Rennin is lacking in the gastric secretions of adults. Rennin and calcium act on the casein in milk, coagulate it, and delay its passage from the stomach.

Chemical digestion of protein continues in the intestine, where proteolytic enzymes from pancreatic and intestinal secretions break down large complex proteins into progressively smaller peptide chains and ultimately into the end products of water-soluble amino acids. Pancreatic enzymes include trypsin, chymotrypsin, and carboxypeptidase. Intestinal enzymes include aminopeptidase and dipeptidase. See Table 26–1 on page 654.

Absorption and transport

Amino acids are absorbed from the small intestine directly into the portal blood. It is thought that amino acids are absorbed by the same sodium cotransport system that facilitates carbohydrate diffusion (Guyton 1982:516).

Amino acids are transported into the cells only by active transport or facilitated diffusion through carrier mechanisms. The nature of these carrier mechanisms is still poorly understood.

Storage

Soon after entry into the cells, amino acids are converted by intracellular enzymes into cellular protein. Thus, amino acids are not stored in the cells as amino acids but as actual proteins. Many of these intracellular proteins, however, can be decomposed again into amino acids and transported back out of the cell into the blood when blood levels fall below normal. Some tissues decompose stored protein more than others; for example, the liver, kidney, and intestinal mucosa reverse protein storage more readily than muscle, brain, and skin tissues.

Several hormones regulate the balance of amino acids in the cells (tissues) and the amino acid concentration of plasma. Insulin and growth hormone increase the formation of tissue proteins (*anabolism*); adrenocortical glucocorticoid hormones and thyroxine increase the concentration of plasma amino acids (catabolism).

The plasma proteins (albumin, globulin, and fibrinogen) are produced primarily in the liver and can be used for the rapid replacement of tissue proteins. Whole plasma proteins can be transferred (under the influence of the reticuloendothelial system) into the tissue cells, where they are split into amino acids, transported back into the blood, and used throughout the body to build cellular proteins. Plasma proteins therefore act as a labile protein storage medium.

Metabolism

Metabolic activities of protein can be categorized into three broad divisions of anabolism (building tissue), catabolism (breakdown of tissue), and balance (Williams 1981:58).

Anabolism Proteins are synthesized in all cells of the body provided the appropriate amino acids are present. The types of proteins formed depend on the functional characteristics of each cell and are controlled basically by the genes of the cells.

Breakdown of tissue Because there is a limit to the amount of protein that can accumulate in a cell, additional amino acids are degraded and used for energy or stored as fat. This degradation occurs primarily in the liver and begins with the process of *deamination*—the removal of the amino (NH_2) groups by hydrolysis from the amino acids. Ammonia (NH_3) is a toxic byproduct of this process. Ammonia is removed from the blood almost entirely by the liver, which converts ammonia to urea. Urea is then excreted by the kidney.

After deamination, keto-acid products are released. These acids may be oxidized to release energy for metabolism. Because some of the deaminated amino acids are similar to the breakdown products of glucose and fat metabolism, they may also be converted to glucose or fatty acids. For example, deaminated alinine is pyruvic acid, which can be converted into glucose or glycogen (gluconeogenesis) or converted into acetyl-CoA. Acetyl-CoA can then be converted into fatty acids by a process called *ketogenesis*.

An obligatory loss of proteins occurs daily if a person eats no proteins. Certain proportions of body proteins (20 to 30 g) continue to be degraded into amino acids, then deaminated and oxidized. Thus to prevent a net loss of protein, a person must ingest at least 20 to 30 g of protein each day (Guyton 1982:544).

Balance All body protein is in a dynamic state of breakdown and renewal. Free amino acids present in the liver and plasma comprise an amino acid pool. This pool is a supply of essential and nonessential amino acids that can be used for protein synthesis in any part of the body. The supply of amino acids in the pool is maintained by dietary intake of protein and by catabolism of body proteins.

The state of protein nutrition is usually referred to as the state of *nitrogen balance*, since nitrogen is the element that distinguishes protein from carbohydrate and fat. Almost all nitrogen ingested is in the form of protein. However, most of the nitrogen lost from the body is in the form of nonprotein nitrogen compounds, i.e., the end products of protein catabolism. These end products include urea, creatinine, uric acid, and ammonia salts.

The state of nitrogen balance is the net result of intake and loss of nitrogen. When intake of nitrogen equals output, a state of nitrogen balance exists. Nurses can assume that a person is in nitrogen balance if he or she is (Suitor and Hunter 1980:175):

1. Ambulatory and healthy
2. Not growing or replenishing body tissue
3. Consuming a diet adequate in essential amino acids, calories, and micronutrients

Positive nitrogen balance exists when nitrogen input exceeds output; in other words, when the total anabolism of protein and other nitrogenous substances exceeds catabolism and loss. Nurses can assume that a state of positive nitrogen balance exists (ibid., p. 175):

1. During periods of growth, such as:
   a. During childhood and adolescence, when there are increases of height and lean body mass
   b. During pregnancy, when there are increases in maternal and fetal tissues
   c. During phases of physical exercise, when there are increases in muscle growth
2. During periods of tissue replacement, such as:
   a. During convalescence from an illness that caused protein depletion, when body tissues are regenerated
   b. After fasting or inadequate intake of protein and calories, when body tissues are regenerated

Eating more protein than is necessary to meet body needs does *not* result in an increase in positive nitrogen balance or lean body mass in healthy adults. However, excess protein intake can lead to weight gain (positive caloric balance). Generally, a surplus of nitrogen intake is balanced by increased excretion of nitrogen as urea.

Negative nitrogen balance exists when nitrogen output exceeds intake (when catabolism exceeds anabolism). This state occurs when (ibid., p. 175):

1. The diet is inadequate in essential amino acids and calories.
2. A person is immobilized.
3. A person is exposed to unusual stress as a result of trauma (e.g., surgery or disease).

Fats

Definition and description

Fats are groups of organic substances (fats, oils, waxes, and related compounds) that are greasy and insoluble in water but soluble in alcohol or ether (Williams 1981: 34). These organic substances are *lipids*. Fats have the same elements (carbon, hydrogen, and oxygen) as carbohydrates, but the hydrogen content of fats is higher. Fats are actual or potential esters of fatty acids, which are used in metabolism. *Fatty acids* are the basic structural units of fats. *Esters* are compounds of an alcohol and an acid.

Fats can be classified as simple lipids or compound lipids. Simple lipids or neutral fats are known also as *triglycerides*, since they are esters of fatty acids with glycerol in the ratio of three fatty acids to each glycerol base. Neutral fat is found in food of both animal and plant origin. Compound lipids are various combinations of neutral fat with other components. Three compound lipids important in nutrition are:

1. Phospholipids, which are compounds of neutral fat, phosphoric acid, and a nitrogen base.
2. Glycolipids, which are compounds of fatty acids combined with carbohydrates and nitrogen. Because these are found mainly in brain tissue they are also referred to as cerebrosides.
3. Lipoproteins, which are compounds of various lipids with protein. They contain mixtures of triglycerides, phospholipids, cholesterol, and protein. There are three major classes of lipoproteins:
   a. Very low density lipoproteins contain high concentrations of triglycerides and moderate concentrations of phospholipids and cholesterol.
   b. Low density lipoproteins contain few triglycerides but very high concentrations of cholesterol.
   c. High density lipoproteins contain small concentrations of lipids but high concentrations of protein (about 50%).

Cholesterol is also classified as a lipid. Although cholesterol does not contain fatty acid, it does have many of the physical and chemical properties of other lipids and is capable of forming esters with fatty acids. Large quantities of cholesterol and phospholipids are present in cell membranes and are essential for the structural elements of cells. Exogenous cholesterol is ingested in the diet and absorbed; endogenous cholesterol is formed in the body's cells, principally in liver cells.

Fatty acids are described as saturated or unsaturated. The degree of saturation is determined by the relative number of hydrogen atoms in the fatty acid. Saturated fatty acids are saturated with hydrogen. All carbon atoms are filled to capacity with hydrogen. An example of a saturated fatty acid is butyric acid found in butter. Unsaturated fatty acids have less hydrogen attached to the available carbon atoms. When several carbon atoms in a fatty acid are not bonded to a hydrogen atom, the fatty acid is polyunsaturated. An example of a polyunsaturated fatty acid is linoleic acid found in vegetable oil.

Williams (1981:37) gives a list of food fats, with the most saturated first:

Saturated (animal fat)	*Unsaturated (plant fat)*
beef suet	olives, olive oil
mutton tallow	vegetable oils (peanut, soybean, cottonseed, corn, safflower)
red meats	
poultry	
seafood	
egg yolk	
dairy fat	

Digestion

Physical alterations Like carbohydrates and proteins, fats are altered physically by mechanical breakdown in the mouth and mixing with secretions in the stomach and intestine. In addition, fats are emulsified in the small intestine by bile salts, which are produced in the liver and released in bile. Bile salts promote the breakdown of fat globules into minute particles by lowering the surface tension of the globules. Emulsification greatly increases the surface area of lipids, thus enhancing their digestion and absorption. Bile is released from the gall bladder whenever fats are present in the duodenum. Fats in the duodenum stimulate the secretion of cholecystokinin from glands in the intestine. Cholecystokinin stimulates the gallbladder to contract and secrete bile via the common bile duct into the duodenum.

Chemical alterations Although chemical digestion of fats begins in the stomach, fats are digested mainly in the small intestine. Enzymes that break down fats include lipase, a pancreatic enzyme, and enteric lipase, an intestinal enzyme. Most chemical digestion is facilitated by pancreatic lipase. See Table 26–1 on page 654. The desired end products of chemical digestion of fats are monoglycerides, fatty acids, and glycerol.

Absorption

Some end products of fat digestion (e.g., glycerol and some free fatty acids) are absorbed into the portal blood system and carried to the liver. Other end products (e.g., monoglycerides and cholesterol) are absorbed into the abdominal lacteals and transported through the lymphatic system to the thoracic duct, where they enter the blood through the left subclavian vein.

Storage

Large quantities of fat are stored in two major tissues: adipose tissue and the liver. Adipose tissue, referred to as the fat depot, stores triglycerides until they are needed for energy. Adipose tissue also has the subsidiary function of providing body insulation.

Metabolism

Large quantities of lipases are present in adipose tissue. Some lipases facilitate the deposition of triglycerides; others cause splitting of the triglycerides to release fatty acids into the blood.

The liver functions in lipid metabolism are (a) to degrade fatty acids into smaller compounds that can be used for energy, (b) to synthesize triglycerides from carbohydrates and to a lesser extent from proteins, and (c) to synthesize other lipids from fatty acids, such as cholesterol and phospholipids (Guyton 1982:536). Triglycerides are used for energy. More than half of all the energy used by the cells is supplied by fatty acids derived from triglycerides or indirectly from carbohydrates. Oxidation of fatty acids produces acetyl-CoA, which enters the citric acid cycle discussed earlier.

Release of fatty acids from fat tissue is facilitated by the stress hormones epinephrine and norepinephrine from the adrenal medulla, corticotropin from the anterior pituitary gland, and glucocorticoids from the adrenal cortex. In addition, growth hormone and thyroid hormone cause rapid mobilization of fat.

Vitamins

Definition and description

A *vitamin* is an organic compound that cannot be manufactured by the body and is needed in small quantities for normal metabolism. Thus, when vitamins are lacking in the diet, metabolic deficits result.

Vitamins are generally classified as fat soluble or water soluble. *Fat-soluble* vitamins include A, D, E, and K; *water-soluble* vitamins include C and the B-complex vitamins. The body cannot store water-soluble vitamins, thus people must get a daily supply in the diet. The body can store fat-soluble vitamins, although there is a limit to the amounts of vitamins E and K the body can store. A daily supply of fat-soluble vitamins is therefore not absolutely necessary.

Daily requirements

Table 26–2 indicates the usually recommended daily requirement of vitamins. These requirements, however, vary considerably, as follows (Guyton 1982:563):

1. The greater a person's size, the greater the vitamin requirement.
2. Growing persons require greater quantities.
3. Exercise increases vitamin requirements.
4. Disease and fever increase vitamin requirements.
5. Pregnancy and lactation increase the requirement for vitamin D.

Table 26–2 Vitamins: Requirements, Functions, Food Sources, and Signs of Deficiency

Name	Recommended daily requirements	Selected functions	Major food sources	Signs of deficiency
Vitamin A	500 IU (international units)	Assists normal vision, maintains skin and mucous membranes, promotes normal growth of most cells	Liver, carrots, sweet potato, spinach, broccoli, cantaloupe, squash, apricots, pumpkin	Scaliness of skin, failure of growth, and corneal opacity and blindness
B-Complex vitamins				
B_1 (thiamine)	1.5 mg	Needed for metabolism of carbohydrates and many amino acids	Pork, liver, whole grains, milk, legumes	*Clinical syndrome called beriberi:* • Impaired central nervous system function due to decreased use of glucose by nervous tissue, which depends almost entirely on glucose for energy • Degeneration of peripheral nerves resulting in polyneuritis and, if severe, paralysis • Weakening of heart muscle leading to cardiac failure • Impaired gastrointestinal function due to inadequate glucose for energy resulting in indigestion, constipation, anorexia, gastric atony, and reduced HCl acid
B_2 (riboflavin)	1.8 mg	Necessary for oxidative processes in cells and for normal tissue maintenance; lengthens lives of red blood cells; protects protein of eye lenses	Milk, organ meats (liver, heart, kidney), broccoli, wild rice, brewer's yeast, almonds, cheese (Brie, Camembert, and Roquefort)	*Mild:* • Inflammation and cracking at angles of mouth • Dermatitis at angles of nares • Keratitis of corneas *Severe:* • Muscular spasticity and weakness • Vomiting and diarrhea • Coma • Declining body temperature
B_3 (niacin or nicotinic acid)	20 mg	Necessary for oxidative processes in cells (assists in hydrogen ion transfer) and synthesizes fats and proteins	Meat, poultry, fish, liver, whole grains	*Clinical syndrome called pellagra*: • Primarily gastrointestinal symptoms • Neurological symptoms • Dermatitis (cracked, pigmented scaliness in skin areas exposed to irritation) • Inflammation of oral and gastrointestinal mucous membranes resulting in digestive abnormalities

Table 26–2 continued

Name	Recommended daily requirements	Selected functions	Major food sources	Signs of deficiency
B_6 (pyridoxine)	2 mg	Protein metabolism, acts in transport of some amino acids across cell membranes, converts tryptophan to niacin	Wheat germ, yeast, fish, liver, pork, lentils	Convulsions, dermatitis, gastrointestinal disturbances (nausea and vomiting)
B_9 (Folic acid, pteroylglutamic acid)	0.4 mg	Promotion of growth, reproduction of cellular genes, maturation of red blood cells	Green leafy vegetables, liver, meats, fish, whole grains, nuts	Specific types of anemia (megaloblastic and macrocytic anemia)
B_{12} (Cobalamin)	3 mg	Promotion of growth, maturation of red blood cells, synthesis of RNA and DNA	Liver, kidney, fresh green leafy vegetables, asparagus	Pernicious anemia, loss of peripheral sensation and paralysis
Pantothenic acid	Unknown	Assists in formation of acetyl-CoA from pyruvic acid, therefore aids carbohydrate and fat metabolism	Liver, egg yolk, yeast, whole grains	Depression of carbohydrate and fat metabolism; no definite deficiency syndrome due to its wide occurrence in foods and because small amounts can be synthesized in body
Vitamin C (ascorbic acid)	45 mg	Aids in metabolism of certain amino acids; aids collagen formation for healing; enhances iron absorption	Citrus fruits, cantaloupe, strawberries, tomatoes	*Clinical syndrome called scurvy:* • Failure of wounds to heal • Cessation of bone growth • Extremely fragile blood vessels • Lesions of gums • Loosening of teeth • Mouth infections • Hemorrhage, e.g., hematemesis, bloody stools, cerebral
Vitamin D	400 IU	Increases calcium absorption from gastrointestinal tract; helps control calcium deposition in bones	Fortified milk and fish liver oils; is synthesized in skin on exposure to sunlight	*Clinical syndrome called rickets:* • Abnormal size and shape of bones, e.g., bowlegs and knock-knees
Vitamin E	15 IU	Aids in protection of cell structure and in formation of red blood cells	Wheat germ, green leafy vegetables, vegetable oils	Rare; causes male sterility in lower animals, therefore called "antisterility vitamin"
Vitamin K	None	Necessary for formation of prothrombin in liver; prothrombin is essential for blood clotting	Green leafy vegetables, liver, soybean oil	Not applicable; is synthesized by bacteria in the colon

Recommended requirements from A. C. Guyton, *Human physiology and mehanisms of disease*, 3rd ed. (Philadelphia: W. B. Saunders Company, 1982), p. 563.

6. Greater than normal metabolism of carbohydrates increases the requirement for B vitamins, e.g., thiamine and other B-complex vitamins.

In addition, some medications interfere with vitamin absorption (e.g., aspirin interferes with vitamin C absorption).

Food sources and functions

A balanced diet of carbohydrate, fat, and protein contains the necessary vitamins. See Table 26-2 for food sources, functions, and signs of deficiencies of major vitamins.

Minerals

Minerals are found in organic compounds, as inorganic compounds, and as free ions. Upon oxidation, minerals leave an ash, which can be acid or alkaline. Calcium and phosphorus make up 80% of all the mineral elements in the body. There are two categories of minerals: minerals found in the body in relatively large amounts and trace elements (micronutrients), present in minute amounts. The former group includes calcium, phosphorus, potassium, chlorine, sodium, sulfur, and magnesium. The latter group includes iron, copper, iodine, and manganese. Minerals play a part in many body processes, including the regulation of the acid-base balance of the body. For further information, see Chapter 31. A common mineral deficiency among women is iron deficiency.

Food sources of minerals include green leafy vegetables, milk and milk products, eggs, and organ meats. Liver is an excellent source of iron. Whole-grain cereals and brown rice are also good sources. Iodized salt is a major source of iodine.

Balanced Nutrition

Four approaches to balanced nutrition are reflected by daily food guides, vegetarian diets, energy balance, and prudent diets.

Daily Food Guides

Both the United States and Canadian governments publish recommended daily food guides. See Table 26-3. These food guides separate foods into four main groups and recommend daily amounts from each group. The four groups are milk and milk products, meats, vegetables and fruits, and breads and cereals.

Some foods do not belong to any of the four groups. The major ingredients of these foods are fats, sugar, starch, and unenriched refined grains. Examples are butter, jelly, carbonated beverages, bacon, and white flour. Most of these foods are high in calories and low in nutrients.

The daily food guides do not include convenience foods such as hamburgers, milk shakes, pizzas, etc., which have become so much a part of the North American diet. The food guides also do not address caloric intake, a particularly important aspect of nutrition in both the United States and Canada. Users of the guides should pay attention to adequate iodine intake. In areas of the country where the iodine content of food is low, iodized salt should be used. Unless there is an adequate supply in drinking water, fluoride, too, should be supplemented. Also, it is possible to follow the food guides yet still eat insufficient fiber, found in raw fruits, vegetables, and whole grains.

Vegetarian Diets

In the United States and Canada, there are increasing numbers of vegetarians. There are two basic vegetarian diets: those that allow only plant foods and those that include milk, eggs, and dairy products. Some people, not strictly vegetarians, eat fish and poultry but not beef, lamb, or pork; others eat only fresh fruit, juices, and nuts; and still others eat plant foods and dairy products but not eggs. See Table 26-4.

People may become vegetarians for economic, health, religious, ethical, and ecologic reasons. Increased meat prices during the last decade have forced some people to become vegetarians or eat meat infrequently. Some people avoid meat because they believe it is healthy to do so. They cite as evidence that vegetarians tend to be less obese than others and that blood cholesterol levels of vegetarians tend to be lower, two factors that reduce the probability of heart disease. Among those who practice vegetarianism for religious reasons are Seventh-Day Adventists and followers of certain Oriental religious philosophies. Some people are vegetarians for ethical reasons: They object to the killing of animals or the way they are raised. People who follow vegetarian diets for ecological reasons point out the wastefulness of eating animals that consume a large part of the world's supply of grain when this grain could be better used for people.

Vegetarian diets can be nutritionally sound if they include a wide variety of legumes, grains, fruits, vegetables, nuts, milk, and milk products. Vegans and fruit-

Table 26–3 Recommended Daily Food Guides

United States	Canada
Milk group Children: 3 or more glasses; smaller glasses for some children under 8 years Adolescents: 4 or more glasses Adults: 2 or more glasses Cheese, ice cream, and other foods made from milk can supply part of the milk	*Milk and milk products* Children (up to 11 years): 2–3 servings Adolescents: 3–4 servings Pregnant and nursing women: 3–4 servings Adults: 2 servings Examples of 1 serving: 250 ml (1 cup) milk, yogurt, cottage cheese 45 g (1½ oz) cheddar or processed cheese A vitamin D supplement is recommended when the milk consumed does not contain added vitamin D
Meat group 2 or more servings of meats, fish, poultry, eggs, or cheese with dry beans, peas, nuts as alternatives	*Meat and alternatives* Two servings Examples of 1 serving: 60 to 90 g (2–3 oz) lean cooked meat, poultry, liver, or fish 60 ml (4 Tbsp) peanut butter 250 ml (1 cup) cooked dried peas, beans, or lentils 80 to 250 ml (⅓–1 cup) nuts or seeds 60 g (2 oz) cheddar, processed, or cottage cheese 2 eggs
Fruit-vegetable group 4 or more servings; include dark green or yellow vegetables, citrus fruits, or tomatoes	*Fruits and vegetables* 4–5 servings (include at least 2 yellow or green leafy vegetables) Examples of 1 serving: 125 ml (½ cup) vegetables, fruits, or juice 1 medium potato, carrot, tomato, peach, apple, orange, or banana
Grain group 4 or more servings, enriched or whole grain; added milk improves nutritional values	*Breads and cereals* 3–5 servings whole grain or enriched (whole grain products are recommended) Examples of 1 serving: 1 slice bread 125 to 250 ml (½–1 cup) cooked or ready-to-eat cereal 1 roll or muffin 125 to 200 ml (½–¾ cup) cooked rice, macaroni, spaghetti

From National Dairy Council, *A guide to good eating* (Washington, D.C.: National Dairy Council) and Canada, Department of Health and Welfare, *Canada's food guide* (Ottawa: Department of Health and Welfare).

arians may have insufficient complete protein and require, for example, additional rice, beans, and tacos to provide the protein. In addition, they should ensure that they get sufficient calories, vitamins (particularly B_{12}, D, and riboflavin), and minerals (especially calcium.

Jane Brody (1981:37) suggests the following ways to combine vegetable proteins in the same meal to get the protein equivalents of meat and other animal foods:

1. Rice with:
   a. wheat, or
   b. legumes (soybeans, peanuts, black-eyed peas, kidney beans, chick peas, navy beans, pinto beans, and lima beans), or
   c. sesame seeds
2. Wheat with:
   a. legumes, or
   b. soybeans and peanuts, or

Table 26–4 Types of Vegetarian Diets

Kind	Description
Vegans (some Seventh-Day Adventists)	Strict vegetarians, use no animal or milk products
Lacto-ovo-vegetarians (Some American yoga sects, Seventh-Day Adventists)	Drink milk and eat eggs but eat no other products of animals
Lacto-vegetarians (Hare Krishnas [American Hindu sect], Sikhs, some American Moslem sects)	Drink milk but do not eat eggs or other products of animals
Ovo-vegetarians	Eat eggs but do not drink milk or eat other meat products
Pesco-vegetarians	Eat fish but no other meat products
Partial vegetarians (semivegetarians)	Eat chicken and fish but do not eat red meat
Fruitarians	Eat only fresh (raw) fruits, juices, and nuts

Table 26–5 Caloric Intake by Age

Age	Weight kg	Weight lb	Energy (kcal)
Newborn to 6 months	6	14	kg × 117
6 months to 1 year	9	20	kg × 108
1 to 3 years	13	28	1300
4 to 6 years	20	44	1800
7 to 10 years	30	66	2400
Males			
11 to 14 years	44	97	2800
15 to 18 years	61	134	3000
19 to 22 years	67	147	3000
23 to 50 years	70	154	2700
51 years and over	70	154	2400
Females			
11 to 14 years	44	97	2400
15 to 18 years	54	119	2100
19 to 22 years	58	128	2100
23 to 50 years	58	128	2000
51 years and over	58	128	1800
Pregnancy			+300
Lactation			+500

Adapted from Food and Nutrition Board, National Research Council, Academy of Sciences, *Recommended dietary allowances* (Washington, D.C., 1974).

   c. soybeans and sesame seeds, or
   d. rice and soybeans

3. Legumes with:
   a. corn, or
   b. rice, or
   c. wheat, or
   d. sesame seeds, or
   e. barley, or
   f. oats

Lacto-vegetarians and lacto-ovo-vegetarians can use the daily food guides, with a few adaptations, when planning diets. They should:

1. Use whole grains (including nuts and seeds) as the basic food in the diet.
2. Eat one serving of legumes, lentils, meat substitutes (e.g., vegetarian wieners), eggs, or extra milk each day.
3. Drink the recommended milk or milk equivalents for the age of the individual. Fortified skim milk or fortified low-fat milk are recommended.
4. Limit foods that are high in calories and have little nutrient value.
5. Eat a variety of fruits and vegetables daily, including one serving of a dark leafy green vegetable, such as spinach.

Energy Balance

A person's weight depends on calories taken in and energy expended. To maintain a specific weight, a person needs to balance caloric (energy) intake and energy output. See Tables 14–1 and 14–2, pages 325–26, for recommended weights. There is a higher incidence of diabetes mellitus, gallbladder disease, and cardiovascular disease among overweight people. Obesity decreases life expectancy and may negatively affect the quality of life. As a result, health authorities in recent years have stressed maintaining normal weight as a preventive health measure.

The energy in food, expressed as Calories (kcal), maintains the basal metabolic rate of the body and provides energy for activities such as running and walking. The *basal metabolic rate* (BMR) is the rate at which the body metabolizes food to maintain body functions, such as breathing at rest. The caloric requirements of individuals vary with age and growth, sex, climate, health, sleep, food, and activity.

Age and growth

During periods of growth, the body uses more energy. Rapid growth during the first 2 years of life, adolescence, and pregnancy demands more calories than normal. For example, an active adolescent body may need 3600 kcal, whereas a 70-year-old woman may require only 1800 kcal or less. See Table 26–5 for caloric intake variables by age.

Sex

Men usually have higher basal metabolic rates than women, a fact largely explained by the greater proportion of muscle in men's bodies. Pregnant women also have higher basal metabolic rates than normal.

Climate

Climate affects heat production. People in cold climates have a higher (about 20%, on average) metabolic rate than people in hot climates. This fact may be due to increased thyroxine levels in people who live in cold climates.

Health

Some illnesses, such as those accompanied by high temperature or infection, increase metabolic rate. In malnourished people, however, the metabolic rate is lowered.

Sleep

People need less energy during sleep, when the muscles are relaxed and physiologic processes are slowed. The metabolic rate drops about 10% to 15% during sleep (Boykin 1975:204).

Food

The body's metabolism is stimulated by all foods, but by some more than others. Proteins increase heat production about 30%, carbohydrates and fats about 5%.

Activity

Muscular activity affects metabolic rate more than any other factor; the more strenuous the activity, the greater the stimulation. Mental activity, which requires only about 4 kcal per hour, provides very little stimulation.

Overnutrition or obesity is a serious problem in the United States and Canada. People become obese by eating too much food or eating too many foods of high caloric density. *Caloric density* describes the number of kilocalories per unit weight of food. Fats and oils have the highest caloric density, whereas vegetables such as celery and lettuce have low densities. Energy expenditure is also a factor in weight control. By increasing activity, the individual increases energy expenditure and often decreases weight. See Table 24–4, page 613, for activities required to burn 100 kcal.

Prudent Diets

Increasingly, overabundant diets are being associated with cancer, heart disease, hypertension, diabetes mellitus, dental caries, diverticulosis, and cirrhosis of the liver. Because these diseases have been associated with the life-styles and diets in certain developed countries, they have been called the "diseases of overabundance." Some physicians and nutritionists suggest that certain prudent changes in diet benefit the individual, even though it cannot be said at this point that such a diet prevents disease. In December 1977, the Senate Select Committee on Nutrition and Human Needs released the second edition of *Dietary Goals for the United States*, which recommends the following (U.S. Senate Select Committee on Nutrition and Human Needs 1977:4):

1. Increased intake of vegetables, fruits, and whole grains
2. Decreased intake of processed and refined sugars and foods high in sugars
3. Decreased intake of foods high in fat and partial substitution of saturated vegetable and animal fats with polyunsaturated fats
4. Decreased intake of animal fat and the selection of meats and poultry that have less saturated fat
5. Use of low-fat and nonfat milk instead of whole milk and of low-fat dairy products instead of high-fat dairy products, except for young children
6. Decreased intake of butterfat, eggs, and other foods high in cholesterol
7. Decreased intake of salt and foods high in salt, e.g., potato chips and processed cheese

Dietary Variables According to Age

Infants

Breastfeeding and bottle feeding

Breastfeeding usually begins within 1 hour of the infant's birth, when bonding between the mother and the infant occurs. To start the baby feeding, the mother expresses a little milk onto the baby's lips and strokes the cheek nearest the nipple to encourage the child to turn the mouth toward the breast. Some infants obtain sufficient nourishment from one breast; others need to feed from the other breast as well. At the next feeding, the baby feeds first from the fuller breast, the one used less during the previous feeding.

During breastfeeding, the mother should assume a

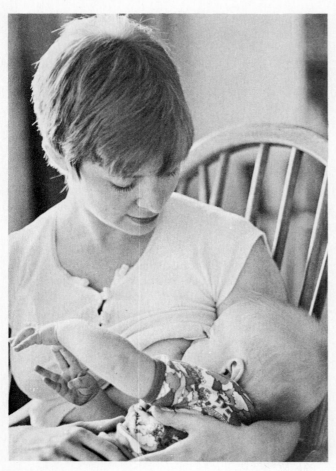

Figure 26–1 Both mother and infant are comfortable during breast feeding.

comfortable position and hold the baby so that he or she can swallow easily. Some mothers prefer a side-lying position; other prefer to sit in a chair and cradle the infant in the arms. The latter position can also be used for bottle feeding. See Figure 26–1.

Infants normally establish their own feeding schedules. A very young infant may require 10 to 12 feedings every 24 hours; however, before long the infant establishes intervals, usually of 3 to 4 hours, between feedings. If a child cries within 3 hours after a feeding, the child may be receiving insufficient nourishment or may have swallowed too much air during the previous feeding. By the age of 2 months, most infants sleep through the night without a feeding, and by the 4th or 5th month they no longer require a late evening feeding.

Bottle-fed babies usually drink commercially prepared formulas. Some formulas require dilution with an equal volume of water. Some of these come in disposable bottles; others are measured into a bottle. Formulas can be prepared in the home; however, it is important to prepare them under sanitary conditions, thus not contaminating the formula or the bottles. Formulas usually contain milk (often evaporated milk), sugar, and water. Bottle formulas are warmed to body temperature. The baby is held in much the same way as for breastfeeding, with the nipple touching the lips. The nipple should be full of formula to minimize the air swallowed by the baby.

Whether breastfed or bottle fed, babies need to burp to release swallowed air. To help the baby burp, the adult places the baby over one shoulder or holds the baby in sitting position and supports the baby's chin with one hand. Often patting or gently rubbing the baby's back makes the baby burp.

Human milk from healthy lactating women offers an infant many nutritional benefits. The composition of human milk varies with what the mother eats and how long she breastfeeds. Generally, the protein in human milk accounts for 7% of its calories, whereas the protein in cow's milk accounts for 20%. The carbohydrate lactose in human milk supplies 42% of its calories; in cow's milk, 30%. The percentage of calories supplied by fat and the amount of water are similar in both milks.

Infants normally require about 52 calories per pound of body weight per day during the first 3 months. Cow's milk and breast milk provide adequate amounts of vitamins A and B. Human milk, however, is also a good source of vitamin C, whereas cow's milk contains very little. Human milk supplies more vitamin E and less vitamin K than cow's milk. Cow's milk contains more minerals (calcium and phosphorus), but human milk has adequate quantities of vitamin D as well as antibodies and enzymes that help protect the infant from infection. Some physicians, however, recommend a daily supplement of vitamin D for breastfeeding infants.

However, the nutritional needs of bottle-fed babies can be met by cow's milk or several types of commercially prepared formulas. These are usually fortified with essential nutrients, including iron. Because of the higher protein content in cow's milk and some commercially prepared formulas, bottle-fed babies gain weight faster than breastfed babies. Skim milk is not advised for children under 2 years of age since it has excessive protein and is inadequate in calories, fat, and fatty acids. Milk allergies are more common among bottle-fed babies than breastfed babies. In such instances, special formulas are prescribed.

Most infants need supplementary fluoride, particularly where the community drinking water has inadequate fluoride. Sodium fluoride drops are often added to the infant's water. See Chapter 21, page 511.

Infants normally have copious iron stores, and opinions vary as to the need for iron supplements. Breastfed babies are able to absorb the small amount of iron in breast milk, and some authorities recommend against iron supplements.

However, some formulas are fortified with iron, and some authorities recommend them during the 1st year. Iron-enriched formulas can cause constipation. Parents, therefore, need to know how to alleviate this problem. By about 4 months, most babies deplete their iron stores, and pediatricians generally prescribe iron supplements for infants 4 months or older.

Newborns usually get between-meal feedings of boiled water since they need more fluid than is supplied in breast milk or formulas. The infant's thirst determines the amount given. If the water supply in the community is safe, the infant can drink unboiled water at about 4 months or when prescribed by the pediatrician.

Introduction of solid foods

Infants are generally introduced to solid foods at 4 months, but the decision of when to introduce solid foods and which foods to introduce first is an individual one. Cereal, because of its iron content, is a traditional first food (infants begin to lose iron stores at 4 months). When they are older than 4 months, infants generally have caloric requirements that cannot be met by milk alone. Also, at this time the extrusion reflex begins to diminish. This reflex causes young infants to spit out solids rather than swallow them. A common sequence for introducing solid foods is cereals first, followed by fruits, vegetables, and then meat. See Table 26–6. The sequence can vary, e.g., vegetables can be introduced first, followed by meat, fruits, and then cereals.

New foods are introduced one at a time and in small amounts. The adult places 2 ml (¼ tsp) of food well back on the infant's tongue without exerting pressure that would cause the infant to gag. New foods are offered when the infant is hungry and before the formula or food to which the baby is accustomed. No sweetener or medications should be added. Initially, the foods need to be soft and smooth (strained or pureed) and at moderate temperatures. When their teeth begin to erupt, infants prefer foods that they can chew, e.g., teething biscuits or chopped cooked vegetables. The shift from pureed to chopped foods needs to be gradual. The amount of solids is gradually increased from 8 ml (1 tsp) per day to about 24 to 40 ml (3 to 5 Tbsp) per day.

Common allergens, such as orange juice and egg white, are introduced with caution. Small amounts of well-cooked mashed egg yolk are often given when the infant is first given solid food, but whole eggs are generally not given until the end of the 1st year. Traditionally, infants were given orange juice early (e.g., at 2 months), although the juice was diluted with water at the outset. The recent trend is not to introduce orange juice until after the 1st year because of the possibility of allergy.

Infants start to drink from a cup at about 5 months; at that age weaning from the bottle or breast to more solid food can also begin. By 1 year, the infant can hold and drink from a cup with assistance.

Table 26–6 Introduction of Solid Foods

Age (in months)	Foods introduced
1	
2	Milk feeding (most important food in first year)
3	
4	Cereals: 15–60 ml (1–4 Tbsp)
5	Vegetables: 15–60 ml (1–4 Tbsp) carrot, squash, potato Fruits: 15–60 ml (1–4 Tbsp)
6 (introduce any time between 6 and 8 months)	Meat, poultry, fish: 15–60 ml (1–4 Tbsp) Dairy products: 15–60 ml (1–4 Tbsp)
7	Finger foods: rusks, pieces of cooked vegetables
8	Egg yolk: 2 ml (¼ tsp) to 1 yolk
9	Other vegetables: cauliflower, broccoli
10	Baked beans, lentils, peas
11	Egg whites: 2 ml (¼ tsp) to 1 whole egg white
12	Whole egg

From Ministry of Health, Province of British Columbia, *Infant nutrition: Guide to the introduction of solids* (Health Promotion Programs, Division of Nutrition and Health Education). Adapted from Metropolitan Health Service of Greater Vancouver.

Toddlers and Preschoolers

More teeth erupt when the infant is 2 years old. By age 3, when most of the deciduous teeth have emerged, the child is able to bite and chew adult table foods well. Manipulative skills are sufficiently developed for self-feeding, although the child still needs some adult assistance and small utensils. Children should be taught table manners only after they master manipulative skills. The average toddler or preschooler generally requires (Scipien 1975:223):

1. The milk group: four servings per day (one serving equals ½ to ¾ cup)
2. The meat group: two or more servings per day (one serving equals 3 to 4 Tbsp)
3. Cereals and breads: four or more servings per day (one serving equals ½ to 1 slice of bread or ½ to ¾ cup of dried or cooked cereal)
4. Vegetables and fruits: four or more servings per day, to include at least one or more servings of citrus fruit and one or more servings of green or yellow vegetables (one serving equals 3 to 4 Tbsp)

It is important that children develop good food habits early. They should be seated comfortably. Appetite will vary from one meal to the next, so it is better to serve less than more of what they will eat. Overly large servings can discourage children from eating. Children need forks and spoons they can handle; fork tines should be blunt to prevent harm.

Children should be served new foods at the beginning of a meal along with well-liked foods. If a child refuses a food, it is best to remove it without discussion. Children quickly learn to attract attention by not eating.

School-Age Children

Children of school age need the same number of servings per day of the four basic food groups as preschoolers, but in larger amounts to meet growth needs. For example, one serving of milk is 1 cup; one serving of meat is 6 to 8 Tbsp; one serving of vegetable or fruit is ⅓ to ½ cup; and one serving of bread and cereal equals 1 to 2 slices or ½ to 1 cup.

Adolescents

Teenage boys and girls have high energy requirements due to their rapid growth and need a diet plentiful in milk, meats, and green and yellow vegetables. Adults should encourage teenagers to eat nutritious snacks, e.g., fresh fruit and vegetables. Food fads are common among teenagers, some of which may be extreme and a cause for concern. For information about anorexia nervosa, a problem of some adolescents, see page 673.

The pregnant adolescent often requires special counseling about nutrition and related issues. Worthington-Roberts et al. (1981:135–37.) outline these issues as follows: (a) acceptance of pregnancy, (b) body image, (c) living conditions, (d) relationship with the father, (e) peer acceptance, (f) nutritional state, (g) prenatal care, (h) nutrition attitudes and knowledge, (i) food resources, (j) previous reproductive experience/contraceptives, and (k) preparation for child feeding.

Pregnant adolescents may need to learn to eat regular, well-balanced meals. Their energy requirements are usually very high because of their own growth needs as well as those of the fetus. They also need extra protein, iron, and calcium.

Young Adults

Young adults require balanced diets and caloric intakes appropriate to energy output. Of special consideration, however, is the pregnant and lactating woman. In addition to the basic diet for an adult, the pregnant woman needs:

1. Increased protein because of the growth of the fetus and accessory tissues of the woman
2. Double the usual calcium and phosphorus requirements
3. An additional 150 mg of magnesium daily
4. Iron to build sufficient hemoglobin and provide iron for the fetus
5. Iodine (175 mg), found commonly in iodized salt, seafood, and milk
6. Zinc (5 mg above the normal daily requirement) to meet the needs of newly forming maternal and fetal tissue

Some physicians also recommend folic acid supplements; however, the need for general vitamin supplements is questionable unless the woman is at nutritional risk.

Middle-Aged Adults

Both men and women in the middle years need to reduce their caloric intakes primarily because metabolic rates decrease, growth is complete, and activity slackens. Therefore, middle-aged adults need to eat less or increase activity to prevent obesity.

People in their middle years need to choose their foods from the four food groups and at the same time adhere to a prudent diet (Howard and Herbold 1982:35). The latter includes more low-fat milk products, poultry, fish, and beans and limits eggs to three times per week. Vegetables, fruit, cereals, and whole-grain breads are recommended for their fiber and protein content.

Elderly Adults

The metabolic rate decreases with age; therefore, elderly people require fewer calories than previously. Whole-grain breads and cereals are recommended for their fiber, commonly lacking in the diets of elderly people. Protein requirements for older adults are the same as for younger adults, but elderly people may need to decrease fat consumption because of their decreased ability to synthesize and excrete lipids and because reduction in fat intake lessens the risk of coronary artery disease and obesity. Many elderly people are deficient in iron, often because their diets are low in iron-rich proteins. The use of mineral oil as a laxative by elderly people can impede the absorption of vitamins A, D, E, and K. Many elderly people also have a lactose intolerance and must obtain protein and calcium from sources other than milk, such as dark green vegetables, nuts, and beans.

The sense of taste of the older adult may be altered, often because of a decrease in the number of taste buds or because of ill-fitting dentures. Also, some elderly people who live alone do not want to cook for themselves or eat alone. As a result, the elderly person may adopt poor dietary habits and is at risk of malnourishment.

Those who provide meals for elderly people can promote good nutrition by:

1. Serving food attractively, providing color contrast for visual appeal
2. Cooking food well so that it can be easily chewed by denture wearers
3. Serving essential foods first and providing sweet foods (carbohydrates) in moderation afterward
4. Noting foods that cause indigestion and not serving them again
5. Serving the heaviest meal at noon to those who have difficulty sleeping at night after a heavy meal
6. Not serving tea, coffee, or other stimulants in the evening to those who have difficulty sleeping

Assessing Nutritional Status

Nutritional status is determined by what and how much the individual eats, by his or her body's ability to use nutrients, and by the state of the person as a result of the intake of nutrients. The nurse considers the following when assessing nutritional status:

1. Anthropometric measurements
2. Dietary history
3. Clinical signs of poor nutrition
4. Energy level
5. Factors that influence eating

Anthropometric Measurements

Anthropometric measurements are measurements of the size and composition of the body. They include height, weight, skin fold, and arm circumference measurements. Assessment of height and weight is discussed in Chapter 14. Normal weight ranges by age, sex, and frame for adults are given in Tables 14–1 and 14–2. An inadequately nourished person can be underweight, overweight, or obese: in every case his or her caloric intake is not in balance with expenditure of energy.

The mid-upper arm circumference (MUAC) provides information about the individual's muscle mass. To obtain this measurement, the nurse asks the patient to let the nondominant arm hang freely in a dependent position. The midpoint is between the tip of the olecranon process and the acromial process of the scapula. The nurse uses a tape measure to find the circumference of the arm at this point (see Figure 26–2) and compares the measurement against a standard to determine whether the skeletal muscle mass for an adult is normal. For example, a standard of 29.3 cm (11.5 in) is a normal muscle mass for a male (Keithley 1979:71).

A skin fold measurement of the triceps or subscapular folds indicates the amount of body fat. See Figure 26–3. Special calipers are used for these measurements. The triceps skin fold measurement is taken at the midpoint of the upper arm. The subscapular measurement is taken just below and lateral to the angle of the scapula. To take the triceps measurement, the nurse grasps the skin on the back of the forearm along the long axis of the humerus and uses the calipers to measure the thickness of the fold about 1 cm below the nurse's fingers. See Figure 26–4. To measure the subscapular fold, the nurse picks up the skin below the scapula so that three fingers are on top of the fold just below the

Figure 26–2 Measuring the upper arm circumference to assess muscle mass.

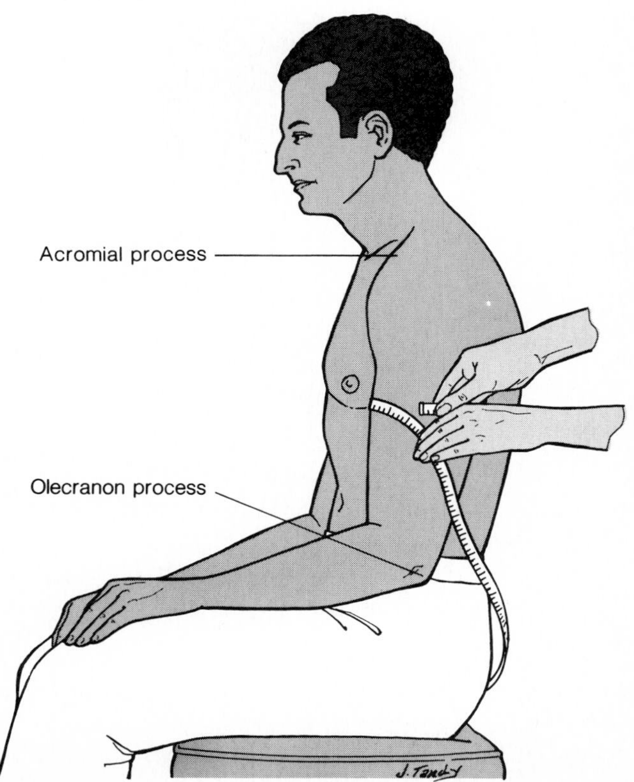

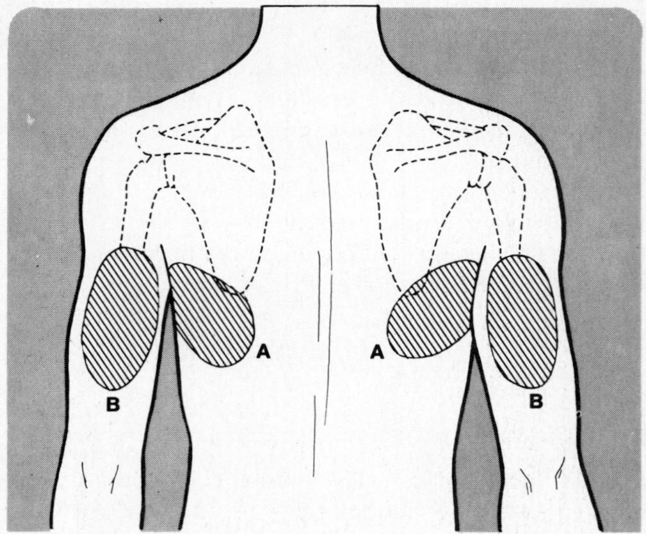

Figure 26–3 Body areas used to measure the skin fold for assessing the amount of adipose tissue: **A,** subscapular; **B,** triceps.

scapula, with the thumb below the fold and the forefinger at the lower tip of the scapula. See Figure 26–5. The skin fold should be at a 45° angle from the horizontal so that it goes upward medially and downward laterally (Caly 1977:1608). The calipers are used in the same manner. The nurse compares the measurements with a standard accepted by the agency.

Dietary History

A record of a person's food intake is usually taken over a 3-day period. This record provides information about types and amount of food eaten, types and amount of liquids taken, and food allergies and idiosyncracies. If eating habits vary on a weekend, the dietary history should also be taken during a weekend.

Clinical Signs

Examination often reveals signs of good or poor nutrition. Dryness of the cornea and conjunctiva and corneal opacity are often associated with vitamin A deficiency. Infiltration by the blood vessels into the cornea may signal vitamin B_2 deficiency. Cracks or fissures on the

Figure 26–4 Using calipers to measure the triceps skin fold.

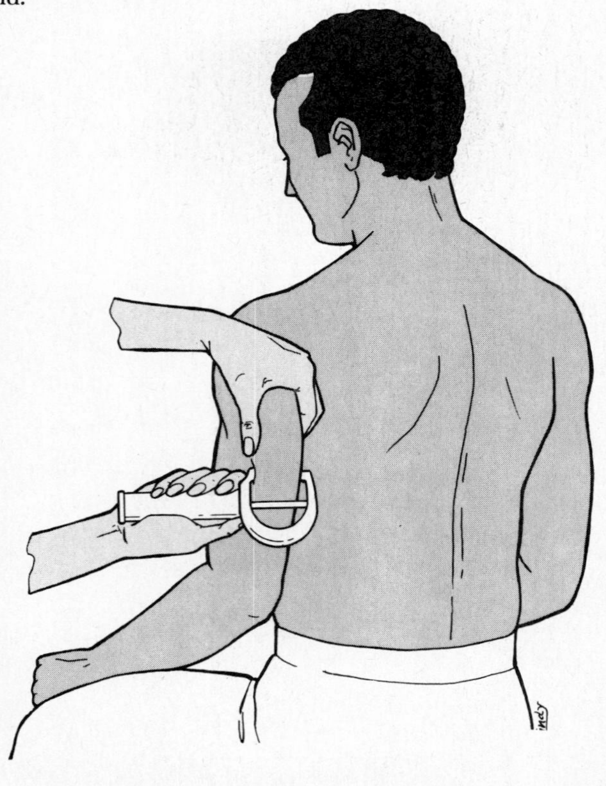

Figure 26–5 Measuring the subscapular skin fold.

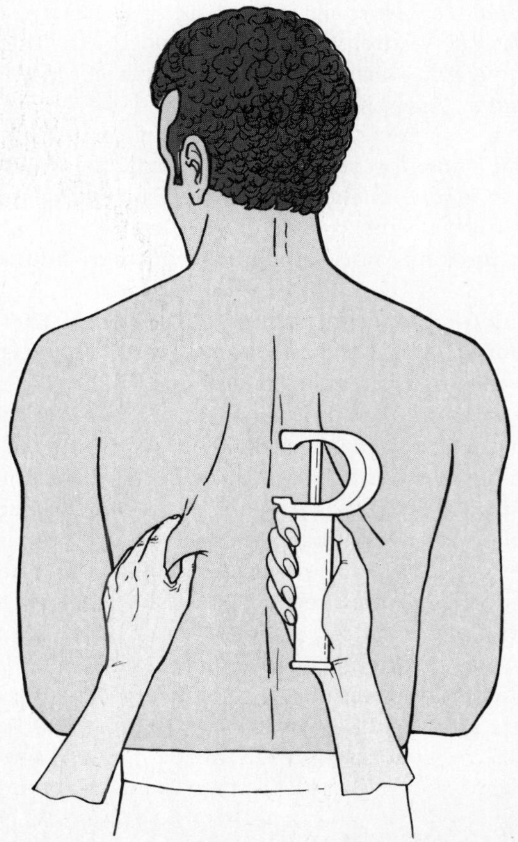

Table 26-7 Selected Signs of Nutritional Deficiency

Body part or system	Clinical sign	Possible deficiency
General appearance	Underweight, lethargic	Calories
	Dehydrated, thirsty	Water
	Growth failure	Vitamin A
Hair	Lacks luster, depigmented, decreased diameter of hairs	Protein
Skin	Dermatitis	Niacin, riboflavin, biotin
	Dermatoses in infants	Fat
	Petechial hemorrhages	Ascorbic acid
	Eczema	Pyridoxine
Eyes	Photophobia	Riboflavin
	Night blindness	Vitamin A
Mouth	Stomatitis, glossitis	Riboflavin
	Glossitis	Niacin, folic acid, vitamin B_{12}, or iron
Teeth	Dental caries	Fluorine
Neuromuscular	Tetany	Vitamin D
	Muscle weakness	Potassium
Bones	Rickets	Vitamin D
Gastrointestinal	Anorexia	Thiamine
	Anorexia, nausea and/or vomiting	Salt (NaCl)
Endocrine	Simple goiter	Iodine
Cardiovascular	Hemorrhages, decreased prothrombin time	Vitamin K
	Cardiac disease	Thiamine
	Anemia	Iron
		Pyridoxine
Nervous system	Mental changes and peripheral neuropathy	Vitamin B_{12}

mouth or redness of the lips may reflect riboflavin deficiency. Dull, depigmented hair may be due to protein deficiency, and enlargement of the thyroid gland can indicate insufficient iodine.

The neuromuscular and skeletal function can reflect extended nutritional problems. Tenderness of the calf muscles and cramps in the legs may reflect a calcium imbalance. Impaired muscle coordination and peripheral neuritis can result from deficiencies in thiamine and pantothenic acid. Forgetfulness may be a result of vitamin B_{12} and niacin deficiencies. Changes in the senses of smell and taste can occur with vitamin B_6 deficiency, and bone pain can occur with the intake of excessive amounts of vitamin A over a period of time. For further information, see Tables 26-2 and 26-7.

Clinical study of a patient's urine and blood can give information about nutritional status. The urine of an individual who is starving or in metabolic or respiratory acidosis is highly acidic. Vegetarians tend to have alkaline urine. Ketone bodies often appear in the urine of a starving person or a person whose diet is very high in fats and low in carbohydrates.

Blood tests can identify iron deficiency anemia. Lowered hemoglobin levels occur with abnormally low iron intake or absorption and with the loss of blood. Blood tests also show cholesterol levels. Increased cholesterol is associated with coronary artery disease.

Energy Level

An adequately nourished person has sufficient energy for the usual daily activities of a person that age. A poorly nourished person may be underweight or overweight, but his or her energy quickly dissipates, making it difficult to carry out normal activities.

Fatigue and lethargy can indicate inadequate nourishment. The person may not show specific signs of deficiency diseases but may complain of lethargy and fatigue. Such a person is considered marginally undernourished.

Factors Influencing Eating Patterns

It is important to determine the factors that affect an individual's eating habits. Some of these are culture, religion, socioeconomic status, personal preference, emotions, hunger, appetite, satiety, and health.

Culture

Ethnicity often determines food preferences. The diversity of cultures in the United States bears out this fact. Traditional foods—for example, rice for Orientals, pasta for Italians, curry for Indians—are eaten long after other traditional customs are abandoned. Geography also affects food preferences. For instance, seafood is popular along the North American coasts, and the regional cooking of the southern United States emphasizes fried foods.

Religion

Religion also affects diet. Both Orthodox Judaism and Islam prohibit pork. Orthodox Jews observe kosher customs, eating certain foods only if they are inspected by a rabbi and prepared according to dietary laws. Roman Catholics avoid meat on certain days, and some Protestant faiths prohibit tea, coffee, or alcohol. The nurse must be sensitive to such religious dietary practices. See Chapter 34 for further information.

Socioeconomic status

What, how much, and how often a person eats are frequently affected by social and economic status. Poor and elderly people may not be able to afford beef and vegetables. Limited income may restrict their diets to tinned fish and bread. Social groups also affect food habits. Pâté and snails are popular foods in some groups; others may prefer hamburgers and beans.

Personal preference

What an individual likes and dislikes significantly affects eating habits. People often carry childhood preferences into adulthood. Father dislikes curry, thus does his son; mother loves oysters, and so does her daughter. People also develop likes and dislikes based on associations with a typical food. A child who loves to visit his grandparents may love pickled crabapples because they are served in the grandparents' home. Another child who dislikes a very strict aunt grows up to dislike the chicken casserole she often prepares. Individual likes and dislikes can also be related to familiarity, particularly for children. Children often say they dislike a food before they sample it. Certain foods—onions and cabbage are common offenders—cause indigestion in certain people and as a result are disliked.

Emotions

Sometimes people associate certain foods with specific emotions, which often originate in childhood. Desired food that was withheld as a punishment may be associated with feelings of guilt. Food used as a reward may elicit pleasant feelings. If a parent becomes angry during a meal, a child may associate specific foods with this anger and reject them. Certain people associate food with love or comfort and eat when they are depressed or lonely.

Hunger, appetite, and satiety

Hunger is largely an unpleasant sensation due to the deprivation of food. Appetite, by contrast, is pleasant; the person desires food and anticipates it. An appetite can be general, or it may focus on specific foods.

Satiety is the feeling of fullness that results from satisfying one's desire for food. Hunger, appetite, and satiety are controlled by the central nervous system, including the hypothalamus, and by hormones and gastric secretions. When these mechanisms are faulty, the person may never experience satiety and thus overeat, becoming obese. The lack of appetite is known as *anorexia*. Prolonged anorexia can prevent a person from eating needed food, resulting in body *emaciation* (excessive thinness). *Cachexia* is a state of weakness, emaciation, and malnutrition often seen in wasting diseases such as terminal malignancies.

Health

An individual's health greatly affects his or her eating habits. A sore mouth or the absence of teeth often mean an individual will choose soft foods. People who have difficulty feeding themselves may give up trying even though they are hungry.

Nursing Diagnoses

Nursing diagnoses for patients with nutritional problems may be broadly stated as alterations in nutrition and further categorized as:

1. Less than body requirements or *nutritional deficit* (insufficient intake)
2. More than body requirements or *obesity* (excessive intake)

3. Potential for more than body requirements, or potential for obesity (Kim and Moritz 1982:300–1; Gordon 1982:64–70)
4. Potential for less than body requirements, or potential for nutritional deficit

Nutritional Deficit

Nutritional deficit is insufficient intake of one or more nutrients required to meet metabolic needs (Gordon 1982:68). When possible, the nurse should state the specific deficit, e.g., inadequate protein, iron, or vitamin C intake. Indications of nutritional deficits of specific vitamins are outlined in Table 26–2. The following signs may indicate other generalized deficits:

1. Weight 20% or more under the ideal for height and frame
2. Loss of weight with adequate food intake
3. Food intake less than that recommended by food guides or evidence of lack of food
4. Eating difficulties
5. Gastrointestinal signs, such as abdominal pain, cramping, diarrhea, and hyperactive bowel sounds
6. Muscle weakness and reduced energy level
7. Excessive loss of hair
8. Pallor of skin, mucous membranes, and conjunctiva

A very severe protein deficit results in kwashiorkor, a disease seen in many Eastern undernourished populations. It is characterized by retarded growth and development; mental apathy; extreme muscular wasting, which may be masked by edema; depigmentation of the hair and skin; and scaly changes in skin texture.

The factors that contribute to nutritional deficits are discussed in the sections that follow.

Economics

The high cost of nutritious foods, especially proteins, is a major reason for malnutrition. For this reason, nutritional deficits are widespread among the poor.

Education

Lack of knowledge about nourishment and nutritious foods contributes to malnutrition. People with minimal or no education are frequently unaware of nutritional needs and the foods that best supply nourishment.

Social and class values

People often eat foods eaten by others of the same social class. Immigrants in the United States and Canada usually follow the eating customs of their native countries. Indigenous diets, evolved slowly over centuries, are with few exceptions well balanced. Nurses must be sensitive to culturally determined food preferences and allow them whenever possible. Immigrants are at nutritional risk when they abandon traditional diets for highly refined North American foods. Social influences on eating habits are also evident among teenagers, who may forgo a well-balanced meal in favor of chips and beer consumed while socializing with peers. Teenagers' food fads can, over time, lead to nutritional deficits.

Anatomic and physiologic factors

Before food taken into the body can be used, the body must digest and absorb it. Many physiologic factors can impair this process. The lack of teeth, ill-fitting teeth, or a sore mouth make the mastication of food difficult. Difficulty swallowing (*dysphagia*) due to a painfully inflamed throat or a stricture of the esophagus can discourage a person from obtaining adequate nourishment.

Impaired digestion in the stomach and gastrointestinal tract may have a variety of causes. Pathologic processes such as tumors or ulcers are not uncommon. Restricted flow of digestive juices can also affect digestion. Gallstones, which can block the flow of bile, are a common cause of impaired digestion of fat.

People who take certain medications may have impaired digestion. Iron in some forms taken orally is a common cause of indigestion, *nausea* (the urge to vomit), and even vomiting. Anorexia and nausea can affect a person's eating habits and nutritional status adversely.

Persons receiving antineoplastic agents for cancer are at risk of nutritional deficits. Normal tissue cells, such as those of the bone marrow and the gastrointestinal mucosa, are naturally very active and particularly susceptible to these agents. Oral ulcers, intestinal bleeding, or diarrhea resulting from the toxicity of antineoplastics can diminish a person's nutritional status seriously.

Psychologic factors

Anorexia and weight loss can indicate depression. Although some people overeat when depressed or lonely, others eat very little under the same conditions. *Anorexia nervosa* is a condition seen most frequently in female adolescents; the afflicted person refuses to eat, loses weight, and in some instances starves to death.

Food fads

Food fads involve nontraditional food practices. A *fad* is a widespread but short-lived interest or a practice followed with considerable zeal. Often the truth about a food is exaggerated or used out of context to support the rationale behind the fad. A fad may be based either on the belief that certain foods have special curative powers or on the notion that certain foods are harmful.

Food fads appeal, for example, to the individual seeking a miracle cure for a disease or the person who desires superior health and wants to delay aging. Food fads also appeal to people who follow fashion and to people who distrust the medical profession. The latter group hope that the diet will allow them to avoid medical treatment.

Some fad diets are harmless, but others are potentially dangerous. An example that has received considerable publicity is the liquid protein diet, which has been linked to several deaths. It is important for the nurse to consider what needs the fad diet fills for the patient. The nurse can then both support these psychologic needs and suggest a more nutritious diet.

Nurses have these further responsibilities to patients who are considering or following food fads:

1. If a patient is thinking about following some advertised practice, it is the nurse's responsibility to suggest that the patient discuss it with the physician.
2. Fads that are contrary to accepted nutritional practice need to be investigated further, perhaps with a nutritionist or nurse.
3. Fads that promise improbable results need to be considered in light of the advice of a physician, nutritionist, or nurse.
4. People who believe in fads based on false statements require correct information. For example, some people believe that taking large amounts of vitamin E or yogurt will retard aging. Such people need information on the possibly toxic effects of taking very large doses of certain vitamins and education on the importance of balanced diet to health.

Obesity

Obesity is the result of calorie intake that exceeds metabolic need. Obesity is evidenced by weight 20% greater than the ideal for height and frame and by triceps skin folds greater than 15 mm in men and 25 mm in women (Kim and Moritz 1982:300). *Overweight* refers to weight 10% greater than the ideal for height and frame (White and Schroeder 1981:550). Obesity is currently one of the most prevalent health problems in North America. It is associated with hypertension, cardiovascular diseases, and diabetes. Factors contributing to obesity include:

1. Sedentary habits (low activity level)
2. Inappropriate eating patterns (e.g., eating large amounts of carbohydrates and saturated fats)
3. Depression or anxiety (often accompanied by stressors such as a death in the family or a change in marital or work status)
4. Eating the largest meal at the end of the day

Factors placing a person at risk for obesity may include sedentary habits, genetic predisposition, obesity in one or both parents, and a pattern of excessive food intake in early infancy and childhood.

Examples of Nursing Diagnoses

Examples of nursing diagnoses for patients with nutritional problems include:

1. Potential nutritional deficit related to lack of awareness about:
   a. Increased requirements during pregnancy
   b. Necessary requirements for growth
   c. Ways to get essential proteins on vegetarian diets
2. Nutritional deficit related to improper nutritional management or more specifically:
   a. Iron deficiency related to excessive intake of junk foods
   b. Vitamin C deficiency related to inadequate ingestion of citrus fruits
3. Nutritional deficit (potential or actual) related to disease process or its effects or therapy such as:
   a. Esophageal stricture
   b. Malabsorption syndrome
   c. Inadequate production of digestive enzymes (specify)
   d. Inadequate amounts of regulating hormones (e.g., insulin)
   e. Prolonged nausea and vomiting
4. Obesity related to:
   a. Excessive intake of carbohydrates
   b. Sedentary habits
   c. Compulsive overeating

Planning and Intervention for Nutrition

The overall nursing goal is to maintain good nutrition. Nursing subgoals are:

1. To prevent nutritional problems
2. To restore good nutrition
3. To improve the present nutritional status of the patient
4. To make eating enjoyable and comfortable

When planning measures to meet the patient's nutrition needs, the nurse needs to consider the learning needs of the person and to implement measures to help him or her obtain nourishment. A patient may need to learn information about diet and even new skills for eating. For example, the patient with limited ability to move the arms may need to learn to eat with a spoon with a long handle.

Planning also involves establishing outcome criteria. For suggestions see the section on evaluation, page 678, later in this chapter.

Stimulating Appetite

Anorexia frequently accompanies illness. Some reasons for anorexia are:

1. An accompanying physical illness
2. Unfamiliar food or food the patient finds unpalatable
3. Environmental factors such as unpleasant odors or an elevated room temperature
4. Psychologic factors such as anxiety or depression
5. Physical discomfort or pain

Lowered food intake of a few days' duration is not often a problem for adults; however, a prolonged decreased food intake leads to weight loss, decreased strength and stamina, and subsequent nutritional problems. Decreased food intake is often accompanied by decreased fluid intake, which may cause fluid and electrolyte problems. See Chapter 31 for further information.

Increasing a person's appetite requires determining the reason for the lack of appetite and then dealing with the problem. Some nursing interventions that may improve patients' appetites are:

1. Relieving illness symptoms that deaden appetite prior to meal time, for instance, giving an analgesic for pain or an antipyretic for a fever or allowing rest for fatigue.
2. Providing food that the person likes and with which the patient is familiar. Often the relatives of patients are pleased to bring food from home but may need some guidance about special diet requirements. It is also important to present the food in sufficiently small quantities so as not to discourage the anorexic patient.
3. Making the environment conducive to eating. It needs to be fresh and free of unpleasant odors. Unpleasant or uncomfortable treatments should not be carried out immediately before or after a meal. A tidy, clean environment that is free of unpleasant sights is also important. A soiled dressing, a used bedpan, an uncovered irrigation set, or even used dishes can destroy appetite.
4. Reducing psychologic stress. A lack of understanding of therapy, the anticipation of an operation, and fear of the unknown can cause anorexia. Often, the nurse can help by discussing feelings with the patient, giving information and assistance, and allaying fears.

Counseling about Nutrition

People frequently need nutrition counseling. Nurses need to know the special nutritional needs of different age groups and sources of nutrients, especially inexpensive sources.

Nurses may also be asked about common problems, such as feeding problems of babies and children and nutritional needs of pregnant and lactating women. Although most patients know that proper diet promotes healing, the nurse may need to explain the relationship of nutrition to health in terms that are meaningful to the individual.

Teaching about Special Diets

Assisting patients and support persons with special diets is a function of nurses. Nurses must understand the relationship between the patient's problems and the components of the diet.

Physicians order special diets for patients who cannot eat the usual foods. A *diet* is the food and fluid regularly consumed by an individual each day. A *special* or *therapeutic diet* is one in which the amount of food, the kind of food, or the frequency of eating is prescribed. Special diets are used for one or more of the following reasons:

1. To treat a disease process, e.g., a low-salt diet for high blood pressure
2. To prepare for a special examination or surgery
3. To promote health, e.g., a low-calorie diet for an overweight patient

Some diets are temporary, observed perhaps for one meal or one week, but some patients must follow certain diets (e.g., the diabetic diet) for a lifetime. If the diet is long term, the patient must not only understand the diet but also develop a healthy, positive attitude toward it. The patient needs to know that failure to follow the diet for even one day, perhaps because of anger, could result in acute illness.

The following are some common special diets. Diets are often unique to institutions, and nurses need to be familiar with the diets prescribed in their agencies.

Regular diet

Patients who do not have special needs eat the regular or general diet, whose quantity and content are designed to meet the needs of most patients. Some hospitals offer patients a daily menu from which to select their meals for the next day. Other hospitals provide standard meals to each patient on a general diet. Certain foods (e.g., cabbage, which tends to produce flatus, and highly seasoned and fried foods, which are difficult for some people to digest) are usually omitted from the regular diet.

Light diet

A variation of the regular diet is the light diet, designed for postoperative and other patients who are not ready for the regular diet. Foods in the light diet are plainly cooked. Foods containing large amounts of fat are usually omitted, as are bran and foods containing a great deal of fiber. Not all agencies provide a light diet.

Soft diet

A soft diet is easily chewed and digested. It is often ordered for patients who have difficulty chewing and swallowing (dysphagia). A soft diet is a lightly seasoned, low-residue (low-fiber) diet.

Full liquid diet

A full liquid diet contains only liquids or semisolid foods (foods that turn to liquid at room temperature, such as ice cream). Full liquid diets are eaten by patients who have gastrointestinal disturbances or are otherwise unable to tolerate solid food.

Clear liquid diet

The clear liquid diet is often limited to water, tea, coffee, clear broths, ginger ale or other carbonated beverages, apple juice, and plain gelatin. It does not permit milk. This diet provides the patient with fluid and carbohydrate (in the form of sugar), but it does not supply adequate protein, fat, vitamins, and minerals. It is usually a short-term diet for patients who are seriously ill or is given immediately after certain surgery.

Other special diets

There are many other special diets, sometimes especially devised for individual patients:

1. A reducing diet provides a limited number of calories so that the patient will lose weight.
2. A diabetic diet provides protein, fat, and carbohydrate in accordance with the individual's ability to produce insulin.
3. A low salt (NaCl) or sodium-restricted diet is designed to limit the patient's sodium (Na) intake. Some low salt diets merely limit the salt added to food during cooking or eating. Others restrict certain foods because they are naturally high in sodium. These diets are usually prescribed for patients with certain cardiovascular diseases.
4. Allergy diets omit the particular foods to which a patient is allergic. Some foods that commonly produce allergic reactions are cow's milk, wheat, and eggs.

Patients often need assistance adapting their diets to their cultural, religious, ethnic, and economic patterns. Helping the patient adapt the diet to food habits is of great importance. Most diets in North America are devised for the Anglo-American taste and omit many otherwise acceptable ethnic foods. Such a diet may be unfamiliar or unpalatable to the ethnic patient. Nutritionists and dietitians can often assist nurses to adapt a diet to suit a person's life-style.

Another important aspect is adapting a diet to a person's economic status. Often less costly foods can substitute for recommended foods, such as powdered milk for fresh milk.

Motivation is highly important for the success of a dieter. If a patient does not accept the need for a diet, she or he will probably not adhere to it, and its therapeutic value is lost. Understanding is also important. A patient may understand that sugar in coffee is not allowed on a low-calorie diet, but may not understand that bread also contains sugar and is also restricted. A teenager may understand that a diet applies to what is eaten at meals, but may not understand that it also applies to between-meal snacks. An elderly patient may understand that she is not to add salt to foods when cooking but salts her food at the table. This patient does not really understand the importance or the reason for salt restriction.

Helping Patients Obtain Nourishment

Nurses need to help the very young or very ill obtain nourishment. When people are ill, they usually have little energy and often need more time than usual to eat. Very weak children and adults may need to be supported in their usual eating positions. Sometimes small children are best held on the nurse's knee, or the nurse can place pillows in the high chair or crib when positioning the child for eating. People usually like to assume the normal sitting position while eating. If they are unable to sit in a chair even with the support of pillows, the nurse can raise the head of the bed, approximating the eating position as closely as possible. See Figure 26–6. It is difficult for most people to eat while in the supine position. If they cannot assume a sitting position, the next best position is a lateral one. In this position the patient is less likely to choke, and swallowing is facilitated.

All patients except infants are usually accustomed to feeding themselves. The nurse must be sensitive to feelings of embarrassment, resentment, and loss of autonomy in patients who cannot feed themselves. Young children who have learned to feed themselves only recently and are proud of their new accomplishment may be especially resentful of the need for help. Whenever possible, the nurse should help incapacitated patients feed themselves rather than feed them.

Special utensils can assist a patient to eat. Straws help many people who have difficulty drinking from a cup or glass. Straws often permit the patient to obtain liquids with less effort and with less spillage, which can be embarrassing to many patients. Other special utensils are weighted cups and glasses, which are easier to handle, and forks and spoons with wide handles, which are more easily gripped than usual utensils. Special drinking cups are also available. One model has a spout; another is especially designed to permit drinking with less tipping of the cup than is normally required.

A nurse who is helping to feed a patient should ask the patient which food she or he wants first; if the patient is blind, the food should be described. Nurses can help blind patients who can feed themselves by orienting them to where the food is on the plate. For instance, the nurse may say, "The potatoes are at six o'clock." If the blind patient is a child, the nurse may say, "Think of the plate as a face. The potatoes are where the mouth would be."

Hospitalized patients are often served meals on trays. Food frequently is prepared and dished out in central locations and then delivered to a nursing unit to be served. When a tray is delivered to a patient, the nurse needs to check the following:

1. The name on the tray card should correspond to the patient's.
2. The patient should have received the food requested if menu service is provided.
3. Hot foods should be hot and cold foods should be cold.
4. Liquids should not have been spilled.
5. The tray should be attractively and conveniently arranged.

There are alternative feeding methods for the unconscious and patients who are unable to eat for other reasons.

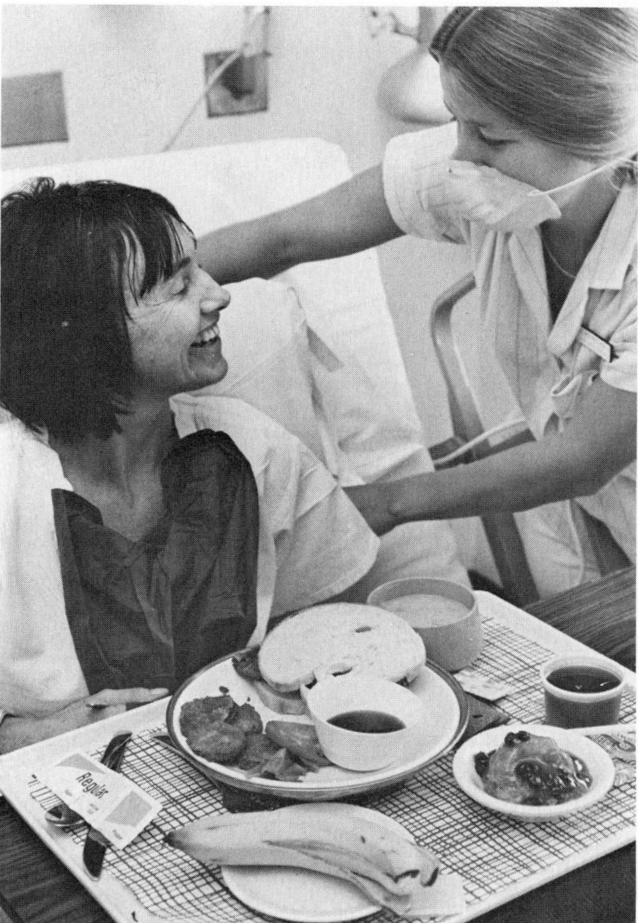

Figure 26–6 A supported sitting position contributes to a patient's comfort while eating.

Nasogastric feeding

A feeding administered through a nasogastric tube (e.g., Levin, Entriflex) is referred to as a gastric *gavage*. A gastrostomy feeding is the instillation of liquid nourishment through a tube that enters a surgically made opening through the abdomen into the stomach (*gastrostomy*). In some instances the tube is inserted past the stomach into the small intestine for *enteric feedings* (intestinal feedings). The tube is usually long, narrow, and made of flexible plastic. The tube is initially lubricated with water and then inserted through an unobstructed nostril and passed through the nose and nasopharynx into the esophagus, terminating in the stomach. In some instances the tube is passed through the mouth and pharynx into the esophagus and stomach, although this route may be more uncomfortable for the adult patient and cause gagging. This approach is often used for infants who are obligatory nose breathers (who must breathe through the nose) and premature infants who have no gag reflex.

The nurse inserts a nasogastric tube only if a physician orders it. The procedure requires considerable skill because the nurse must ensure that the tube does not inadvertently terminate in the patient's lungs. A nasogastric feeding must never be administered until the nurse confirms that the tube is in the stomach. The safest way to confirm this fact is by withdrawing some stomach contents with a syringe. See Table 26–8 for ways of determining whether the tube is in the stomach or in the lungs. See Chapter 39 for a description of how to insert a Levin tube.

Feeding mixtures to be administered nasogastrically are available commercially or may be prepared by the dietary department in accordance with the physician's orders. The preparations are liquid and contain a variety of nutrients, depending on the physician's order. The frequency of feedings and amounts to be administered are also ordered by the physician. An adult often requires 300 to 500 ml of mixture per feeding. The

Table 26–8 Methods of Determining Placement of a Nasogastric Tube

Nurse's action	If tube is in stomach	If tube is in lungs
Attach distal end of tube to a syringe and withdraw plunger*	Some gastric contents will fill tube	No fluid will be in tube
Ask the conscious patient to talk and hum	Patient will be able to talk or hum	Patient will be unable to talk or hum and will cough and/or choke
Note the unconscious patient's color	Color will be normal	Patient will be cyanotic
Using a stethoscope, listen over the epigastric area of the abdomen while injecting 10 ml of air into the tube	Air will make a rushing sound	There will be no sound
Listen to the distal end of the tube	There will be no sound	There will be a crackling sound

*The surest way to confirm correct placement

standard solution contains 1 calorie per milliliter of solution with protein, fat, carbohydrate, minerals, and vitamins in specified proportions. The foods commonly included are milk, sugar, water, eggs, and vegetable oil. The nurse first ensures appropriate placement of the tube in the stomach, next instills 10 to 15 ml of water through the tube to ensure the tube is patent (open), and then regulates the clamp and administers the mixture slowly. The feeding mixture should be at room temperature because hot or cold fluids can irritate the mucosa of the stomach. It is important that the feeding not be administered with undue pressure, which can cause flatus and reflex vomiting. For this reason, the nurse usually attaches the tube to a container placed about 1 foot above the patient's head and allows the liquid to enter the stomach slowly by gravity. The nurse needs to insert the gavage fluid by syringe slowly and with minimal pressure.

Following the feeding, the nurse administers 15 to 30 ml of water if the tube is to remain in the patient. The water cleans out the lumen and prevents future blockages. Some agencies recommend clamping the tube to prevent air from entering the stomach; other agencies recommend leaving the tube unclamped. The end of the tube is covered with gauze held by an elastic band. The tube is attached to the patient's gown. See Figure 26–7.

Hyperalimentation

A more recently developed method of administering nutrients to a patient is *hyperalimentation* (total parenteral nutrition). See Chapter 31 for a discussion of parenteral hyperalimentation.

Evaluation

The outcome criteria for patients with nutritional problems depends on the nursing diagnoses. Some suggested criteria are:

1. Will feed self independently
2. Will have sufficient energy to stay awake until 2000 hours
3. Will lose 2 kg (4 lb) in 14 days
4. Will gain 2 kg (4 lb) in 7 days
5. Will tolerate entire meal without feeling nauseated
6. Will plan a balanced meal using the diet information provided

Summary

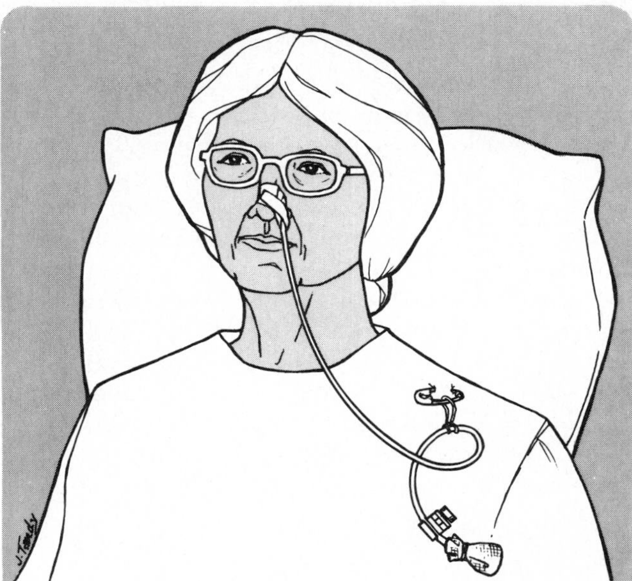

Figure 26–7 Pinning a nasogastric tube safely to the patient's gown.

People are becoming increasingly aware of the importance of a healthy diet. Nurses and other health professionals play an important role by helping people make informed food choices.

Essential nutrients required for health are water, carbohydrates, proteins, fats, vitamins, and minerals. Carbohydrates—sugars and starches—are abundant in grain products, fruits, and vegetables, and are the major source of energy for the body. Fiber is an essential nonnutritive carbohydrate. Proteins are essential for growth and repair of body tissues. Major sources are dairy products and meat. Fats, in addition to meeting energy needs, are essential as a vehicle of transport for fat-soluble vitamins. These vitamins, A, D, E, and K, have important functions, respectively, maintenance of healthy skin, hair, eyes, and mucous membranes; skeletal and tooth development; protection of cell structure and manufacture of red boood cells; and blood clotting. The water-soluble vitamins B and C require daily replenishment, since they are not stored in the body. The B vitamins include thiamine (B_1), riboflavin (B_2), niacin (B_3), pyridoxine (B_6), and cobalamin (B_{12}) and are essential for metabolism and red blood cell development (B_{12}). Vitamin C is essential for the metabolism of amino acids and enhances iron absorption. The major minerals required include calcium, phosphorus, potassium, sodium, chlorine, sulfur, and magnesium. Micronutrient minerals include iron, iodine, copper, and manganese.

Four approaches to balanced nutrition are reflected by daily food guides, vegetarian diets, energy balance theory, and prudent diets.

Daily food requirements are recommended by both the United States and Canadian governments. These guides give minimum requirements and must be adjusted to individual requirements. Increasing numbers of people in the United States and Canada are following vegetarian diets. There are seven types of vegetarian diets; most vegetarian diets can be nutritionally sound if a wide variety of legumes, grains, fruits, vegetables, nuts, milk and milk products are eaten. Vegetarians should pay close attention to meeting requirements for protein, calories, vitamins (B_{12}, D, and riboflavin), and minerals.

Energy balance is another approach to diet. Weight depends on the relation between calorie (kcal) intake and energy expenditure. The caloric needs of people vary according to age, sex, climate, health, sleep, food, and activity. Prudent diets include measures that are generally thought to promote health such as increased vegetable, fruit, and grain intakes; decreased sugar and fat intakes; and decreased intake of salt, butterfat, eggs, and foods high in cholesterol.

Breastfed infants require supplements of fluoride if the water supply is not fluoridated. Formulas often include vitamin D, but bottle-fed infants may also require fluoride. Infants generally establish their own feeding schedules, which vary from every 2 to 3 hours initially to every 4 hours with progressively fewer night feedings. Pediatricians make varying recommendations about which foods to introduce first and when. Iron-fortified cereal is often the first food started at about 4 months, when infant iron stores are depleted.

The toddler and preschooler require well-balanced diets to meet their growth needs. A recommended menu, which can be adjusted to the child's needs, includes all of the essential foods. Teenagers have increased energy and growth requirements and need meat, milk, and vegetables at regular meals. Snacks are often necessary but should be nutritious. Menstruating females may need additional iron.

To meet their own growth demands and those of the fetus, pregnant and lactating women require increased amounts of several nutrients, including protein, calcium, phosphorus, iron, magnesium, iodine, and vitamins A, B, C, and E. Middle-aged adults need to reduce their caloric intake and follow a prudent diet.

The elderly person requires fewer calories than the adult but needs the same amounts of protein, minerals, and vitamins. Elderly people must reduce carbohydrate and fat intake but should maintain or increase fiber intake.

To assess nutritional status, the nurse must take anthropometric measurements and a diet history, assess clinical signs of poor nutrition, assess energy level, and consider factors that influence eating. Anthropometric measurements include height, weight, mid-upper arm circumference (MUAC), and skin fold measurements.

Many factors, including culture, religion, socioeconomic status, personal preference, emotions, hunger or appetite, and health affect a person's eating habits.

Nursing diagnoses for patients with nutritional problems are broadly categorized as nutritional deficits, excessive food intake (obesity), and potential for less or more than the body requirements. Obesity is a common nutritional problem of people in the United States and Canada.

Nursing plans and interventions include motivating patients to eat, counseling patients about nutrition, teaching about special diets, and helping patients obtain nourishment (including giving nasogastric feedings). Outcome criteria for nutrition interventions relate to nursing diagnoses. One example is "will feed self independently."

Suggested Activities

1. List your own dietary intake over a 3-day period. Analyze it for caloric and nutrient value. Compare your intake with the food intake recommended by the government.

2. In a laboratory setting, select a partner and take turns feeding each other. Also practice the following:

- **a.** While supine, eat solids and drink liquids through a straw
- **b.** With eyes closed, eat solids and drink from a glass
- **c.** Use a feeder cup
- **d.** Eat solids from a fork and then from a spoon

After each activity, have the "patient" comment on ways in which the "nurse" made the experience as pleasant as possible.

3. In a clinical setting, observe an adult patient being fed, an infant being bottle fed, and an infant being fed solid foods. Note what the nurse did to help each patient and what improvements you would make, if any.

4. In a clinical setting, observe a group of patients who are eating a meal. Identify factors that encouraged and factors that inhibited eating.

5. In a clinical setting, select a patient who requires assistance with a meal. After assisting the patient, identify the problems you and the patient encountered.

Suggested Readings

American Journal of Nursing. March 1981. Overeaters Anonymous: A self-help group. *American Journal of Nursing* 81:560–63.
Hyperphagia (compulsive overeating) is a chronic illness. Overeaters Anonymous provides a plan that includes 12 steps and 6 tools to control the problem for the rest of one's life.

Caghan, S. B. October 1975. The adolescent process and the problem of nutrition. *American Journal of Nursing* 75:1728–31.
The development of the adolescent personality and the use of food as a defense is discussed. Also included are recommendations for helping adolescents be well nourished.

Glaser, S. September-October 1981. How to improve the first stage of digestion. *Geriatric Nursing* 2:350–53.
The author describes ways to help ill, elderly people eat. Included is a discussion of how to serve the food and how to assess cough, gag, bite, and suck reflexes as well as neck and jaw control.

Kornguth, M. L. March 1981. When your client has a weight problem: Nursing management. *American Journal of Nursing* 81:553–54.
This article includes realistic weekly weight loss goals, nutrition education information, and general tips for dieters.

Kroog, E. April 1975. Helping people stretch their grocery dollars. *American Journal of Nursing* 75:646–48.
A family can buy nourishing food and still stretch their dollars. Best buys among milk products, meats, fruits, vegetables, and cereals are discussed.

Miller, B. K. March 1981. Jejunoileal bypass: A drastic weight control measure. *American Journal of Nursing* 81:564–68.
This article describes this surgery, and ways to prevent postoperative complications.

Mojzisik, C. M., and Martin, E. W. March 1981. Gastric partitioning: The latest surgical means to control morbid obesity. *American Journal of Nursing* 81:569–72.
This article describes the selection of patients for this procedure, the procedure itself, preoperative and postoperative care, and the benefits of this procedure.

Rubin, R. Spring 1967. Food and feeding: A matrix of relationships. *Nursing Forum* 6:195–205.
The role of food in early learning and early socialization, responses to offered food, and the social meanings of offering food are discussed.

White, J. H., and Schroeder, M. A. March 1981. When your client has a weight problem: Nursing assessment. *American Journal of Nursing* 81:550–52.
These authors are consultants who work with overweight clients in the community. Guidelines for an assessment interview are outlined along with a concise assessment tool.

Yen, P. K. May-June 1980. What is an adequate diet for the older adult? *Geriatric Nursing* 1:64, 71, 73.
This article describes the Recommended Dietary Allowances (RDA) for elderly people including energy, protein, vitamin, and mineral requirements. These are related to the physiological changes of the elderly person. The authors give nurses six suggestions for promoting good nutrition in elderly people.

Selected References

Barckley, V. May-June 1980. How to eat on $1.18 per day. *Geriatric Nursing* 1:50–51.

Bass, L. February 1977. More fiber—less constipation. *American Journal of Nursing* 77:254–55.

Bechtel, S. November 1981. B_{12} for healthy nerves and blood. *Prevention* 33:63–67.

———. May 1982. Look to nutrition for sharper vision. *Prevention* 34:103–7.

Bowen, E., and Mondshein, N. November-December 1980. Give your patients a portion of good nutrition education. *Journal of Practical Nursing* 30:23–24, 65.

Boykin, L. S. 1975. *Nutrition in nursing.* New York: Medical Examination Publishing Co.

Brody, J. E. 1981. *Jane Brody's nutrition book.* New York: W. W. Norton and Co.

Buckley, J. E.; Addicks, C. L.; and Maniglia, J. 1976. Feeding patients with dysphagia. *Nursing Forum* 15:69–85.

Caly, J. C. October 1977. Helping people eat for health: Assessing adult's nutrition. *American Journal of Nursing* 77:1605–10.

Carbary, L. J. April 1980. Fiber is a factor. *Journal of Practical Nursing* 24:23–24, 37.

Crim, S. R. September 1969. Nutritional problems of the poor. *Nursing Outlook* 17:65–67.

Crow, R. A. March 1977. An ethological study of the development of infant feeding. *Journal of Advanced Nursing* 2:99–109.

Dansky, K. H. October 1977. Assessing children's nutrition. *American Journal of Nursing* 77:1610–11.

Endres, J. B., and Rockwell, R. E. 1980. *Food, nutrition, and the young child.* St. Louis: C. V. Mosby Co.

Fulmer, T. October 1977. On vitamins, calories, and help for the elderly. *American Journal of Nursing* 77:1614–15.

Gordon, M. 1982. *Manual of nursing diagnosis.* New York: McGraw-Hill Book Co.

Grall, E. September-October 1981. It was easier, but . . . benefits of congregate eating far outweigh the drawbacks. *Geriatric Nursing* 2:353–54.

Grenby, M. April 1977. Living to eat: Nutrition for senior citizens. *The Canadian Nurse* 73:42–44.

Griggs, B. A., and Hoppe, M. C. March 1979. Update—nasogastric tube feeding. *American Journal of Nursing* 79:481–85.

Guyton, A. C. 1982. *Human physiology and mechanisms of disease.* 3rd ed. Philadelphia: W. B. Saunders Co.

Hayter, J. January-February 1981. Diabetes and the older person. *Geriatric Nursing* 2:32–36.

Hill, M. May 1979. Helping the hypertensive patient control sodium intake. *American Journal of Nursing* 79:906–9.

Howard, R. B., and Herbold, N. H. 1982. *Nutrition in clinical care.* 2nd ed. New York: McGraw-Hill Book Co.

Keithley, J. C. February 1979. Proper nutritional assessment can prevent hospital malnutrition. *Nursing 79* 9:68–72.

Kim, M. J., and Moritz, D. A., editors. 1982. *Classification of nursing diagnoses: Proceedings of the third and fourth national conferences.* New York: McGraw-Hill Book Co.

Lambert, M. L. March 1975. Drug and diet interactions. *American Journal of Nursing* 75:402–6.

Langford, R. W. March 1981. Teenagers and obesity. *American Journal of Nursing* 81:556–59.

Lavine, R. L. April 1979. How to recognize . . . and what to do about . . . hypoglycemia. *Nursing 79* 9:52–55.

Maclean, G. D. March 1977. An appraisal of the concepts of infant feedings and their application in practice. *Journal of Advanced Nursing* 2:111–26.

Malasanos, L.; Barkauskas, V.; Moss, M.; and Stoltenberg-Allen, K. 1981. *Health assessment.* 2nd ed. St. Louis: C. V. Mosby Co.

Mallison, M. October 1978. Updating the cholesterol controversy: Verdict—diet does count. *American Journal of Nursing* 78:1681.

Manning, M. L. April 1965. The psychodynamics of dietetics. *Nursing Outlook* 13:55–59. Reprinted in Meyers, M. E., editor. 1967. *Nursing fundamentals,* pp. 174–81. Dubuque, Iowa: William C. Brown Co.

Markesbery, B. A., and Wong, W. M. October 1977. Helping people eat for health: Points for maternity patients. *American Journal of Nursing* 77:1612–14.

Mazer, E. March 1982. Vitamin A—good health insurance. *Prevention* 34:18, 22–24.

Mead, Johnson and Company. 1980. *How to feed your baby . . . the first year: A valuable guidebook for baby's nutritional needs.* Evansville, Ind.: Mead, Johnson and Company.

Olds, S. B.; London, M. L.; Ladewig, P. A.; and Davidson, S. V. 1980. *Obstetric nursing.* Menlo Park: Addison-Wesley Publishing Co.

Pechter, K. March 1982. Riboflavin is ready to help. *Prevention* 34:107–12.

Pipes, P. L. 1981. *Nutrition in infancy and childhood.* 2nd ed. St. Louis: C. V. Mosby Co.

Rose, J. C. July 1978. Nutritional problems in radiotherapy patients. *American Journal of Nursing* 78:1194–96.

Scipien, G. M., et al. 1975. *Comprehensive pediatric nursing.* New York: McGraw-Hill Book Co.

Suitor, C. W., and Hunter, M. F. 1980. *Nutrition: Principles and application in health promotion.* Philadelphia: J. B. Lippincott Co.

Todd, B. September-October 1981. When the patient has a potassium deficiency. *Geriatric Nursing* 2:373.

U.S. Senate Select Committee on Nutrition and Human Needs. 1977. *Dietary goals for the United States.* 2nd ed. Washington, D.C.: Government Printing Office.

White, J. H., and Schroeder, M. A. March 1981. When your client has a weight problem: Nursing assessment. *American Journal of Nursing* 81:550–52.

Williams, E. R. December 1975. Making vegetarian diets nutritious. *American Journal of Nursing* 75:2168–73.

Williams, S. R. 1981. *Nutrition and diet therapy.* 4th ed. St. Louis: C. V. Mosby Co.

Worthington-Roberts, B. S.; Vermeersch, J.; and Williams, S. R. 1981. *Nutrition in pregnancy and lactation.* 2nd ed. St. Louis: C. V. Mosby Co.

Chapter 27

Fecal Elimination

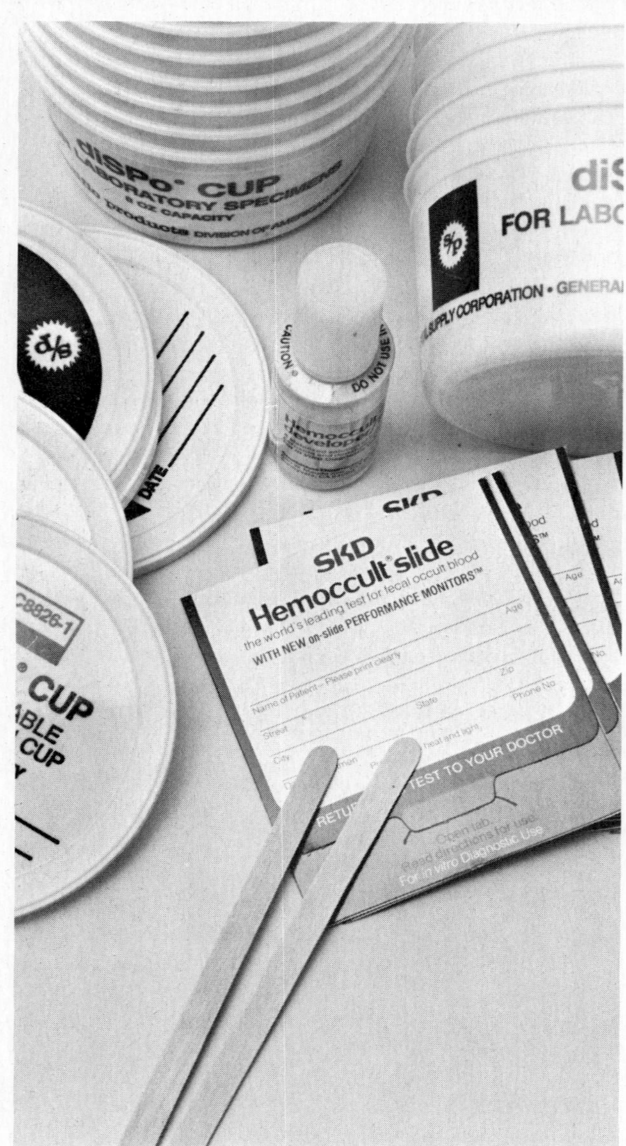

CONTENTS

Objectives

1. Know essential facts about the lower intestinal tract and the development of bowel control

- **1.1** Define selected terms
- **1.2** Identify the anatomy of the lower intestinal tract
- **1.3** Describe the process of stool formation
- **1.4** Identify the age at which bowel control is achieved
- **1.5** List measures that promote the development of bowel control

2. Know essential information and methods required to assess a person's fecal elimination status

- **2.1** Identify factors that influence fecal elimination
- **2.2** Identify factors that influence patterns of defecation
- **2.3** Identify normal characteristics and constituents of feces
- **2.4** Identify abnormal characteristics and constituents of feces
- **2.5** Describe methods used to assess the intestinal tract

3. Understand essential facts about common fecal elimination problems and nursing diagnoses

- **3.1** Differentiate among specific common fecal elimination problems
- **3.2** Identify common causes and effects of selected fecal elimination problems
- **3.3** Identify assessment data indicative of common fecal elimination problems

4. Understand facts about nursing interventions required to maintain, promote, and restore normal functioning of the lower intestinal tract

- **4.1** Identify measures that maintain normal fecal elimination patterns
- **4.2** Relate common interventions to specific fecal elimination problems
- **4.3** Give reasons for selected nursing interventions

5. Apply the nursing process when providing care to patients with fecal elimination problems

- **5.1** Obtain necessary assessment data
- **5.2** Analyze and relate assessment data
- **5.3** Write relevant nursing diagnoses
- **5.4** Write relevant nursing goals
- **5.5** Plan appropriate nursing interventions
- **5.6** Implement appropriate nursing interventions
- **5.7** State outcome criteria essential for evaluating the patient's progress

6. Perform selected fecal elimination techniques safely

- **6.1** Administer an enema effectively
- **6.2** Siphon an enema effectively
- **6.3** Obtain a stool specimen
- **6.4** Digitally remove a fecal impaction

Terms

acholic
adsorbent
astringent
atony
bilirubin
borborygmi
carminative
cathartic
chyme
constipation
defecation
demulcent
diarrhea
enema
eructation
flatulence
flatus
hemorrhoids
impaction (fecal)
incontinence (fecal)
ingestion
laxative
stool (feces)
tympanites

The elimination of feces is a prominent topic in North America. Laxative advertisements, describing such feelings as tiredness due to irregularity, keep the subject in the public consciousness. Some elderly people are preoccupied with their bowels. Often elimination is a matter of great concern to them when they are hospitalized. For people who believe they have had a bowel movement once a day for 75 years, missing 1 day can be seen as a serious problem, even though they may not have eaten anything for 2 days and thus have little fecal matter to eliminate.

In this chapter the physiology of *defecation* (the discharge of feces from the bowels) is discussed. Interventions to promote defecation are outlined. To assist the nurse in health teaching, factors that affect normal defecation are indicated.

Nurses frequently are consulted or involved in assisting patients with elimination problems. These problems are often embarrassing and can cause considerable discomfort. An understanding, competent nurse can provide information and assistance, thereby relieving discomfort.

Physiology of Defecation

Essential to health is elimination of the waste products of digestion from the body. These excreted waste products are referred to as *stool* or *feces*.

Large Intestine

The large intestine extends from the ileocecal (ileocolic) valve, which lies between the small and large intestines, to the anus. The colon (large intestine) in the adult is generally about 125 to 150 cm (50 to 60 in) long. It has seven parts: the cecum; ascending, transverse, and descending colons; sigmoid colon; rectum; and anus or external orifice. See Figure 27–1.

The waste products leaving the stomach through the small intestine and then passing through the ileocecal valve are called *chyme*. Usually about 450 ml of chyme enters the adult cecum each 24 hours. Of this amount only about 100 ml remains for excretion by the time it reaches the rectum; the remainder is reabsorbed into the capillaries of the large intestine (Nordmark and Rohweder 1975:145).

The contents of the colon normally represent foods ingested over the previous 4 days, although most of the waste products are excreted within 48 hours of *ingestion* (the act of taking food).

The colon has two kinds of movement: a mixing movement and a movement that propels the chyme along the digestive tract. The mixing movement helps absorption take place. Water, sodium, and chloride ions are normally absorbed from the colon, whereas potassium and bicarbonate ions are normally excreted into the chyme. The peristaltic waves are mass movements, and they normally occur only a few times a day. Mass peristaltic waves in the colon are caused by the gastrocolic and duodenocolic reflexes, which are initiated when the stomach and duodenum fill with food.

Figure 27–1 The large intestine and rectum.

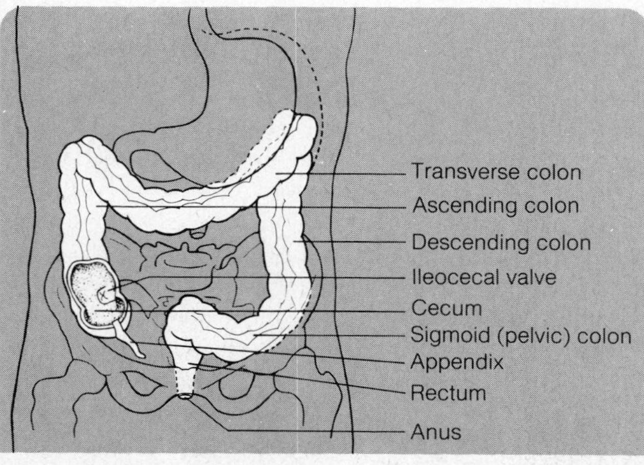

The muscles of the colon are innervated by the autonomic nervous system. The parasympathetic nervous system stimulates movement, and the sympathetic system inhibits movement.

Peristaltic waves occur in the large intestine anywhere from one to four times during 24 hours. With these waves the mass of feces moves along the colon to the sigmoid colon and rectum, where it stays until defecation. Most feces remain in the sigmoid colon until just prior to defecation.

Rectum and Anal Canal

The rectum in the adult is usually 10 to 15 cm (4 to 6 in) long; the most distal portion, 2.5 to 5 cm (1 to 2 in), is the anal canal. Variations in the length of the rectum according to age groups are (King, Wieck, and Dyer 1981:505):

1. Infant: 2.5 to 3.8 cm (1 to 1.5 in)
2. Toddler: 4 cm (2 in)
3. Preschooler: 7.6 cm (3 in)
4. School-age child: 10 cm (4 in)

In the rectum there are three folds of tissue that extend across the rectum and several folds that extend vertically. Each of the vertical folds contains a vein and an artery. It is believed that these folds help retain feces within the rectum. When the veins become distended, as can occur with repeated pressure, a condition known as *hemorrhoids* occurs.

The anal canal is bound by an internal and an external sphincter muscle. See Figure 27–2. The internal sphincter is under involuntary control, and the external sphincter normally is voluntarily controlled. The external sphincter's action is augmented by the levator ani muscle of the pelvic floor. The internal sphincter muscle is innervated by the autonomic nervous system; the external sphincter is innervated by the somatic nervous system.

Defecation

Defecation normally takes place from several times per day to only two or three times per week. There is a wide range in the frequency of defecation in normal, healthy individuals.

Defecation can be described in a number of steps.

1. Feces move into the rectum from the sigmoid colon. The sensory nerves in the rectum are stimulated as a result of the presence of the feces, and impulses travel by the nerves to the spinal cord and from there to the sacral nerves. Other impulses travel to the brain by the spinothalamic tract. They arouse the person's perception of the need to defecate.

2. The internal sphincter muscle relaxes, and at the same time more feces move from the sigmoid colon to the rectum.

3. The person becomes aware of the need to defecate, finds a toilet or bedpan, and voluntarily relaxes the external sphincter. Additional pressure is exerted to expel the feces by contraction of the abdominal muscles and the diaphragm, which increases the abdominal pressure. Contraction of the levator ani muscles in the pelvic floor lifts the anal canal over the feces in the canal. The feces are expelled.

Normal defecation can be facilitated by (a) thigh flexion, which places pressure on the abdomen, and (b) a sitting position, which increases the downward pressure on the rectum.

If the defecation reflex is ignored or if defecation is consciously inhibited by contraction of the external sphincter muscle, the reflex generally disappears for a few hours before occurring again. After age 4, most people have sufficient neuromuscular development and control to delay defecation; however, irregular bowel habits can lead to constipation.

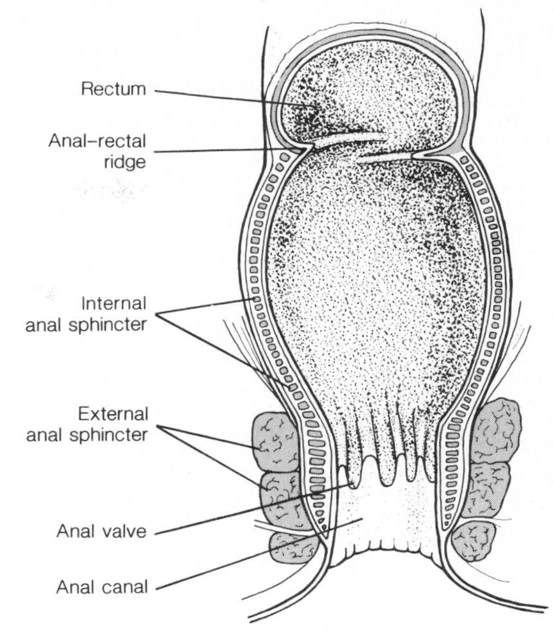

Figure 27–2 Interior view of the rectum and anal canal.

Bowel Training

Bowel training usually can begin after children learn to walk at about age 1½ to 2. At this age, they can ask to go to the toilet during the day when they feel the need. At this age, too, their nervous and muscular systems are sufficiently well developed to give them some degree of control.

Guidelines for Bowel Training Children

When children are being toilet trained, it is important for them to be as independent as possible in this function. The following measures are helpful:

1. They need pants they can remove easily themselves.

2. They need an easily accessible training toilet. See Figure 27-3. This may be a portable toilet or a special seat on the toilet with steps up to it so that the toddler can reach it.

When children are admitted to the hospital, it is important that the nurse learn from the parents the children's stage of toilet training. In particular, it is important to know what words the children use to indicate

Figure 27–3 A toddler being toilet trained on a potty.

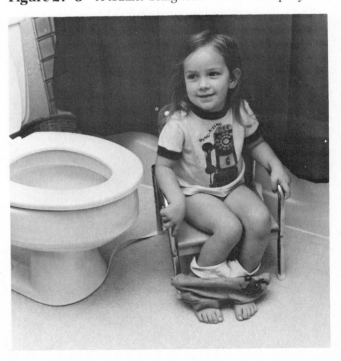

their needs and their usual routine for defecation. It is best if children continue the habits established at home. If the child is not trained, training is usually not begun in the hospital for two reasons: A sick and anxious child will not readily tolerate the stress of learning new habits, and the child's mother or a significant person is not present in the hospital. Pleasing the significant person motivates children during toilet training.

Stages of Bowel Training

1. Awareness of the discomfort created by an incontinent bowel movement.
2. Identification of elimination as the reason for the discomfort.
3. Awareness of the body sensation that indicates the need to defecate.
4. Desire to avoid the discomfort caused by involuntary defecation. This discomfort can be physical and sociologic. The latter is demonstrated by the disapproval expressed by others and the social isolation sometimes suffered by an incontinent child. *Incontinence* in this context is the inability to control defecation.

The methods used to accomplish toilet training vary; usually they must incorporate five aspects:

1. Involvement of a significant person—a person the child wishes to please
2. Sufficient time and a consistent pattern
3. Meaningful communication between the child and the significant person
4. Praise and reinforcement of successful behavior
5. Lack of punishment or disapproval when the child is unsuccessful so that the situation does not become too stressful

If any of these is absent, the child may have difficulty during training. Daytime bowel control is normally attained by the age of 30 months.

Assessment

Each individual has a unique pattern of fecal elimination. These patterns are learned in childhood largely through the family's influence. Bowel training techniques vary considerably among individuals and among different groups within society. During this early training, individuals develop attitudes and habits about fecal elimination. Some people learn to provide regular time for defecation, while others ignore the first urge to defecate and retain the feces until a later time.

Assessment of an individual's fecal elimination includes:

1. Factors that influence fecal elimination
2. The pattern of defecation
3. Assessment of feces
4. Physical assessment of the intestinal tract

Factors That Influence Fecal Elimination

Age

Age affects not only the character of fecal elimination but also its control. The very young are unable to control elimination until the neuromuscular system is developed. This development occurs between the ages of 2 and 3 years. The elderly also experience changes that can affect bowel evacuation. Two of these are *atony* (lack of normal muscle tone) of the smooth muscle of the colon, which can result in a slower peristalsis and thus hardened (drier) feces, and decreased tone of the abdominal muscles, which also decreases the pressure that can be exerted during bowel evacuation. Some elderly people also have decreased control of the anal sphincter muscles, which can result in an urgency to defecate.

Diet

Food is a major factor affecting fecal elimination. Sufficient bulk (cellulose, fiber) in the diet is necessary to provide fecal volume. Certain foods are difficult or impossible for some people to digest. This inability results in digestive upsets and, in some instances, the passage of watery stools. Eating at regular times affects defecation; irregular eating can impair regular defecation. Individuals who eat at the same times every day have a regularly timed, physiologic response to the food intake and a regular pattern of peristaltic activity in the colon.

Fluid

Fluid intake also affects fecal elimination. When fluid intake is inadequate or output (urine or vomitus, for example) is excessive for some reason, the body continues to reabsorb fluid from the chyme as it passes along the colon. As a result the chyme becomes drier than normal, resulting in hard feces.

Exercise

Exercise programs help people of all ages to maintain muscle tone. Well-toned abdominal and pelvic muscles and the diaphragm are important in defecation. Activity also stimulates peristalsis, thus facilitating the movement of chyme along the colon. Conversely, immobility depresses colonic motility.

Psychologic stressors

Excessive stress can affect fecal elimination. When anxious, afraid, or angry, some people experience increased peristaltic activity and subsequent diarrhea, whereas others experience constipation. Constipation is most likely when the person is depressed.

Life-style

The individual's life-style influences fecal elimination in a number of ways. Early bowel training may establish the habit of defecating at regular times, such as daily after breakfast, or it may lead to an irregular pattern of defecation. The availability of toilet facilities, embarrassment about odors, and the need for privacy also affect fecal elimination patterns. A patient who shares a room in a hospital may be unwilling to use a bedpan because of the lack of privacy and embarrassment about odors.

Constipation is a common problem in North America. People can promote regular and complete defecation by establishing a regular time and heeding the defecation reflex.

Medications

Some drugs have side effects that can interfere with normal elimination. Some cause diarrhea; others, such as large doses of some tranquilizers and repeated administration of morphine and codeine, cause constipation.

Some medications directly affect elimination. *Laxatives* are medications that stimulate bowel activity and so assist fecal elimination. There are medications that soften stool, facilitating defecation. Certain medications such as dicyclomine hydrochloride (Bentyl), suppress peristaltic activity and sometimes are used to treat diarrhea.

Pattern of Defecation

The time of defecation and the amount of feces expelled are as individual as the frequency of defecation. Some people normally defecate once a day; others defecate only three or four times a week. Some defecate after breakfast; others do so in the evening. Often the patterns individuals follow depend largely on early training and on convenience. Most people develop the habit of defecating after breakfast, when the gastrocolic and duodenocolic reflexes cause mass movements in the large intestine.

The amount of feces depends on the amount of food intake, in particular on the amount of bulk and fluid in the diet. In the average adult, about 450 ml of chyme enters the cecum daily, and all but 100 ml is reabsorbed in the large intestine (Nordmark and Rohweder 1975:145). This remaining amount is eliminated as feces. The amount of feces passed at one time is generally described as large, moderate or medium, or small.

Flatus is air or gas in the gastrointestinal tract. Three primary causes of flatus are: (a) action of bacteria on the chyme in the large intestine, (b) swallowed air, (c) gas that diffuses from the bloodstream into the intestine. Normally all but 0.5 liter of this gas is absorbed into the intestinal capillaries.

Assessment of Feces

Normal feces are brown. The color is due to the bilirubin derivatives stercobilin and urobilin, and to the action of the normal bacteria within the intestine. *Bilirubin* is a yellow pigment in the bile.

Feces may have other colors, especially when there are abnormal constituents. For example, black, tarry feces may indicate the presence of blood from the stomach or small intestine; clay-colored (*acholic*) feces usually indicate the absence of bile; and green or orange stools may indicate the presence of an intestinal infection. Food may also affect the color of feces: beets can color stool red or sometimes green. Medications, too, can alter the color of feces. Iron, for example, can make stool black.

Consistency

Normally feces are formed but soft and contain about 75% water if the person has an adequate fluid intake. The other 25% is solid materials. See Table 27–1.

Watery feces contain more than the normal 75% water. The stool has moved more quickly than is normal through the intestine, thus less water and fewer ions were reabsorbed into the body.

Hard stool contains less water than normal and in some instances may be difficult and painful to excrete. Some people, in particular babies and young children, may pass stool containing undigested food.

Shape

Feces are normally the shape of the rectum. Abnormalities in the shape must be noted. A stringlike stool may indicate a pathologic condition of the rectum.

Table 27–1 Composition of Normal Feces

Constituent	Percentage of feces	Percentage of solid constituents
Water	75	
Solid materials	25	
Dead bacteria		30
Fat		10 to 20
Inorganic matter		10 to 20
Protein		2 to 3
Undigested roughage and dried constituents of digestive juices (e.g., bile pigment and sloughed epithelial cells)		30

Adapted from A. C. Guyton, *Human physiology and mechanisms of disease*, 3rd ed (Philadelphia: W. B. Saunders Co., 1982), p. 517.

Odor

The odor of feces results from the action of bacteria in the intestine, and it normally varies somewhat from person to person. It is important for the nurse to note any changes in odor that the patient notices. A putrid (rotten, distasteful) odor may indicate a digestive disorder.

Blood

Blood in feces is abnormal. The blood may be frank and bright red; this blood colored the feces late in the eliminative process. Black, tarry feces may mean that blood entered the chyme in the stomach or small intestine. Some medications and foods, however, can make feces red or black; therefore, the presence of blood should be confirmed by a test. Blood in the stool need not be visible. Such blood is referred to as *occult* (hidden).

Tests for presence of blood in feces are routinely performed in clinical areas. There are several tests available commercially. The Hematest uses reagent tablets, whereas the Guaiac and Hemoccult tests use reagent solutions. Every test calls for a stool specimen (see the section on obtaining samples later in this chapter). The Guaiac test is commonly used: A thin layer of feces is applied to a filter paper or paper towel. The reagent is then applied and the color noted; blue indicates the presence of blood. The manufacturer's directions should be followed for each test.

Abnormal constituents

Sometimes feces contain foreign objects that have been ingested accidentally; accidental ingestion of foreign objects is most common in young children. Other abnormal constituents include pus, mucus, parasites, fat in large quantities, and pathogenic bacteria. Tests for the presence of any of these are usually performed in a laboratory.

Physical Assessment of the Intestinal Tract

Intestine

During assessment of the intestines, the patient assumes a supine position and is draped so that only the abdomen is exposed. This assessment can be conducted as part of a general assessment of the abdomen as described in Chapter 14 or with specific reference to the intestinal tract.

Inspection Nurses observe the abdominal wall for visible waves indicating peristalsis. Except in exceedingly thin people peristalsis is not normally observable. When the waves can be seen, they often start in the upper left quadrant and move inferiorly and medially over the abdomen. Observable peristalsis may indicate an intestinal obstruction.

Auscultation Bowel sounds are assessed with a stethoscope. Bowel sounds chiefly reflect small intestine peristalsis; they are described according to intensity, pitch, and frequency or degree of activity. Intensity indicates the force of the sounds or the rate of peristalsis. Pitch is the vibration of the intestinal wall as a result of the peristaltic waves; with intestinal distention there may be an increased pitch. The degree of activity or frequency of the bowel sounds is also assessed. Bowel sounds normally occur every 5 to 15 seconds (Malasanos 1977:244). They occur irregularly, and each sound may last anywhere from less than one second to several seconds. Bowel sounds become more frequent after eating.

Bowel sounds are normally relatively high pitched, gurgling, and soft. They must be heard over each of the four quadrants of the abdomen and in the epigastrium (see Figures 14–20 and 14–21, page 343). They are usually described as audible, hyperactive, hypoactive, or inaudible. Before concluding that bowel sounds are absent—that peristalsis has decreased or ceased—the nurse listens for 5 minutes. Cessation or decreased peristalsis can occur for several reasons: extensive handling of the intestines during surgery; electrolyte disorders, such as abnormally low serum potassium levels; and peritonitis. Abnormally intense and frequent bowel sounds (*borborygmi*) occur in enteritis and with obstructions of the small intestine.

Percussion The abdomen is percussed to detect fluid in the abdominal cavity, distention of the intestines due to flatus, and masses such as an enlarged spleen or liver.

The entire abdomen is percussed, first in the upper right quadrant and clockwise from there. Flatus produces resonance (tympany), whereas fluid and masses produce a dull sound.

When abdominal fluid is present, percussion produces dullness below the fluid level. When the patient lies on one side, the ascitic fluid flows to that side. Percussion reveals a line of demarcation between dullness and tympany; this line indicates the level of the fluid. A line drawn on the abdomen lets the nurse gauge if fluid is increasing or decreasing when the abdomen is next percussed.

Palpation Both light and deep palpations are carried out, usually to detect and explore any tender areas and masses. The four quadrants of the abdomen are palpated. See Chapter 14. Palpation of the spleen and liver is discussed in Chapter 14.

Rectum and anus

The rectum and anus are usually examined by a nurse practitioner. The nurse places the patient in either a left Sims's position or a genupectoral position. A female patient can also assume a lithotomy position or a dorsal recumbent position with knees flexed. See Figure 14–25, page 347.

Inspection The perianal region is inspected for discolorations, inflammations, scars, lesions, fissures, fistulas, and hemorrhoids. The color, size, location, and consistency of any lesion is noted.

Palpation A gloved finger is inserted through the anus to palpate the anal canal, anal sphincters, and rectal canal. About 6 to 10 cm (2 to 4 in) can be palpated during this examination.

Adult female To palpate the anus and rectum, the nurse puts on a glove and lubricates the index finger. The patient is asked to bear down, and the nurse slips the lubricated finger through the anus into the anal canal. The muscle around the anus will tighten, but this should not be painful to the patient. The nurse palpates both the anterior and the posterior walls of the rectum and in particular feels for masses. See Figure 27–4. If a mass is palpated, its location, size, firmness, mobility, smoothness, tenderness, and regularity are described. On the anterior wall of the rectum, the cervix is palpated. It should feel smooth, round, firm, and movable and not be tender to palpation. During pregnancy the cervix becomes larger and softer, and during labor the opening of the cervix dilates in readiness for passage of the baby. After the rectal examination, the nurse removes the glove, washes hands, and records the observations.

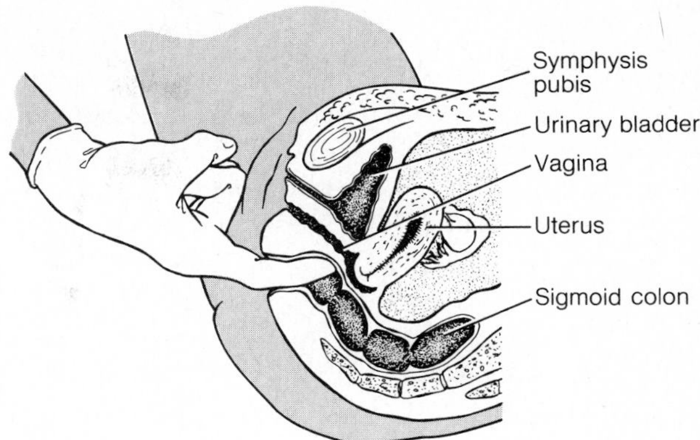

Figure 27–4 Palpating the rectum of a female.

Adult male The nurse inserts a lubricated, gloved finger into the rectum. The prostate gland can be palpated on the anterior wall of the rectum. See Figure 27–5. Each lobe of this gland is felt for masses, consistency of size of the two lobes, firmness, and tenderness. It is also important to examine the rectal wall of a male for nodules or masses.

Figure 27–5 Palpating the rectum of a male.

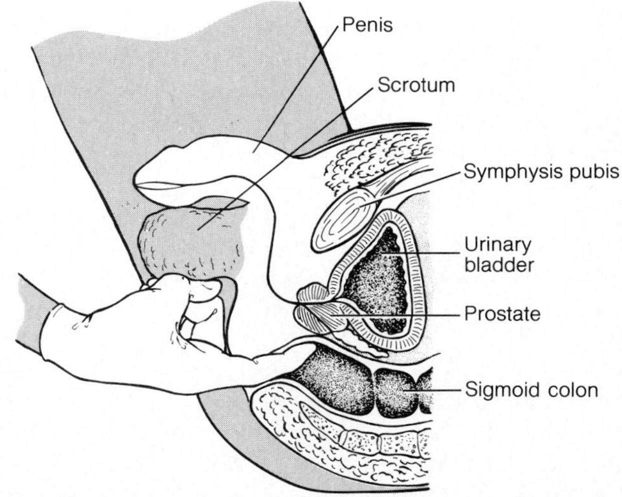

Diagnostic Tests

Direct viewing

Direct viewing techniques include anoscopy, the viewing of the anal canal; proctoscopy, the viewing of the rectum; and proctosigmoidoscopy, the viewing of the rectum and sigmoid colon. These tests are discussed further in Chapter 38, page 988.

Roentgenography

Roentgenography of the large intestine requires the introduction into the colon of barium, a radiopaque substance. Barium permits the viewing of the outline of the colon by either fluoroscopy or roentgenography. For further discussion, see Chapter 38, page 996.

Nursing Diagnoses

The most frequent problems related to bowel elimination are constipation, fecal impaction, diarrhea, fecal incontinence, and flatulence leading to intestinal distention. Examples of nursing diagnoses are included with the discussion of each problem.

Constipation

Constipation refers to the passage of small, dry, hard stool or the passage of no stool for a period of time. It occurs when the movement of feces through the large intestine is slow, thus allowing time for additional reabsorption of fluid from the large intestine. Associated with constipation are difficult evacuation of stool and increased effort or straining of the voluntary muscles of defecation. It is important to define constipation in relation to the person's regular elimination pattern. Some people normally defecate only a few times a week and therefore are not necessarily constipated when they miss a day or two. Other people defecate more than once a day, and to them a movement only once a day can indicate constipation. Careful assessment of the person's habits is necessary before a diagnosis of constipation is made.

There are many causes for constipation:

1. *Irregular bowel habits.* One of the most frequent causes of constipation is irregular bowel habits. When the normal defecation reflexes are inhibited or ignored, these conditioned reflexes tend to be progressively weakened. When habitually ignored, the urge to defecate is ultimately lost. Children at play may ignore these reflexes; adults ignore them because of the pressures of time or work. Hospitalized patients may suppress the urge because of embarrassment about using a bedpan or because defecation is too uncomfortable. Change of routine and diet can also contribute to constipation. The best way to prevent constipation is to establish regular bowel habits throughout life.

2. *Overuse of laxatives.* Laxatives are used frequently to relieve bowel irregularity. Overusing laxatives has the same effect as ignoring the urge to defecate; natural defecation reflexes are inhibited. The habitual user of laxatives eventually requires larger or stronger doses of laxatives, since they have a progressively reduced effect with continual use.

3. *Increased psychologic stress.* Strong emotion is thought to cause constipation by inhibiting intestinal peristalsis through the action of epinephrine and the sympathetic nervous system. Stress can also cause a spastic bowel (spastic or hypertonic constipation or an irritable colon). Associated with this type of constipation are abdominal cramps, increased mucus, and alternating periods of constipation and diarrhea.

4. *Inappropriate diet.* Bland diets and low-roughage diets are lacking in bulk and therefore create insufficient residue of waste products to stimulate the reflex for defecation. Low-residue foods such as rice, eggs, or lean meats move more slowly through the intestinal tract. Increasing the fluid intake with these foods increases their rate of movement.

5. *Medications.* Many drugs have side effects that cause constipation. Some of these, such as morphine or codeine as well as adrenergic and anticholinergic drugs, slow the motility of the colon through their action on the central nervous system, thus causing constipation. Others, such as iron tablets, have an astringent effect and act more locally on the bowel mucosa to cause constipation. Iron also has an irritating effect and can cause diarrhea in some people.

6. *Insufficient exercise.* The effects of lack of exercise were discussed in Chapter 24. In patients on prolonged bed rest, generalized muscle weakness extends to the muscles of the abdomen, diaphragm, and pelvic floor, which are used in defecation. Indirectly associated with lack of exercise is the lack of appetite and possible subsequent lack of roughage, which is necessary to stimulate defecation reflexes.

7. *Age.* The muscle weakness and poor sphincter tone that occur in elderly people contribute to constipation.

8. *Disease processes.* Several disease conditions of the bowel can produce constipation. Among these are bowel obstruction; painful defecation due to hemorrhoids, which makes the person avoid defecation; paralysis, which inhibits the patient's ability to bear down; or pelvic inflammatory conditions, which create paralysis or atony of the bowel.

Examples of nursing diagnoses related to constipation are:

1. Constipation related to low fluid intake, low fiber intake, and inactivity
2. Risk of nutritional deficits related to inadequate intake of fruits and vegetables
3. Risk of overuse of *cathartics* (laxatives or purgatives) related to discomfort from constipation

Fecal Impaction

Fecal impaction can be defined as a mass or collection of hardened, puttylike feces in the folds of the rectum. Impaction results from prolonged retention and accumulation of fecal material. In severe conditions the feces accumulate and extend well up into the sigmoid colon and beyond. Fecal impaction is recognized by the passage of liquid fecal seepage (diarrhea) and no normal stool. The liquid portion of the feces seeps out around the impacted mass. Impaction can also be assessed by digital examination of the rectum during which the hardened mass can often be palpated.

Along with fecal seepage and constipation, symptoms include frequent but nonproductive desire to defecate and rectal pain. A generalized feeling of illness results; the patient becomes anorexic, the abdomen becomes distended, and nausea and vomiting may occur.

The causes of fecal impaction are usually poor defecation habits and constipation. Certain medications (see page 690) also contribute to impactions. The barium used in radiologic examinations of the upper and lower gastrointestinal tracts can be a causative factor. Therefore, after these examinations, measures are taken to ensure removal of the barium. In the elderly, a combination of factors contribute to impactions: poor fluid intake, insufficient bulk in the diet, lack of activity, and weakened muscle tone. In some people, impactions tend to occur regardless of the measures taken to prevent them.

Examples of nursing diagnoses for the patient with fecal impaction are:

1. Fecal impaction related to inactivity and prolonged use of codeine
2. Risk of recurring constipation related to life-style

Diarrhea

Diarrhea refers to the passage of liquid feces and an increased frequency of defecation. It is the opposite of constipation and results from rapid movement of fecal contents through the large intestine. Rapid passage of chyme reduces the time available for the large intestine to reabsorb water and electrolytes. Some people pass stool with increased frequency, but diarrhea is not present unless the stool is relatively unformed and excessively liquid. The person with diarrhea finds it difficult or impossible to control for very long the urge to defecate. Diarrhea and the threat of incontinence are a source of concern and embarrassment. Often spasmodic, piercing abdominal cramps are associated with diarrhea. Sometimes the patient passes blood and excessive mucus; nausea and vomiting may also occur. With persistent diarrhea, irritation of the anal region extending to the perineum and buttocks generally results. Fatigue, weakness, malaise, and emaciation are the results of prolonged diarrhea.

When the cause of diarrhea is irritants in the intestinal tract, diarrhea is thought to be a protective flushing mechanism. It can create serious fluid and electrolyte losses in the body, however. These can develop within frighteningly short periods of time, particularly in infants and small children. See Chapter 30 for further information concerning fluid and electrolyte losses in the body.

Among the numerous reasons for the development of diarrhea are:

1. *Intestinal infection (enteritis).* Infectious diarrhea can be caused by either bacteria or viruses. Generally, the distal end of the ileum and the large intestine are involved in the infectious process. When the bowel becomes exceedingly irritated, both the rate of secretion of ileal juices and motility are increased substantially. The increased fluid flushes the infectious agent toward the anus. Flushing is promoted by the strong propulsive movements of the colon.
2. *Increased stress.* Probably everyone has experienced diarrhea associated with periods of increased emotional tension, such as prior to final examinations. This emotional or psychogenic diarrhea results from excessive stimulation of the parasympathetic nervous system, which increases both the motility and secretions of the distal colon. Alternating bouts of constipation and diarrhea often characterize prolonged anxiety states.
3. *Dietary indiscretions.* People vary in their tolerance of some foods and fluids. Temporary diarrhea may occur after the ingestion of rich pastries, coffee, alcoholic beverages, or strong seasonings. People with allergies to certain foods may respond with diarrhea to the allergen.
4. *Abuse of cathartics.* Excessive irritation of the colon from overuse of cathartics leads to diarrhea. The person who has irregular bowel habits and becomes constipated may be inclined to overuse laxatives periodically.

5. *Medications.* Some medications are irritating to the gastrointestinal tract and can cause diarrhea as a side effect. A few examples are the antibiotic tetracycline; the iron preparation ferrous sulfate; and the antihypertensive drug reserpine.

6. *Other disease conditions.* Malabsorption syndromes, such as congenital celiac disease or ulcerative colitis, interfere with the bowel's ability to reabsorb water, thus creating diarrhea. Other diseases, such as electrolyte imbalances and neuromuscular disorders, can also cause diarrhea.

Examples of nursing diagnoses for the patient with diarrhea are:

1. Diarrhea related to intestinal infection
2. Risk of dehydration and serum potassium deficit related to excessive fluid losses
3. Risk of perianal skin excoriation associated with irritating liquid feces

Fecal Incontinence

Incontinence refers to loss of voluntary ability to control the fecal and gaseous discharges through the anal sphincter. The incontinence may occur at specific times, such as after meals, or it may occur irregularly.

Fecal incontinence is generally associated with impaired functioning of the anal sphincter or its nerve supply, such as in some neuromuscular diseases, spinal cord trauma, and tumors of the external anal sphincter muscle.

Fecal incontinence is an emotionally distressing problem that can ultimately lead to social isolation. Afflicted persons withdraw into their homes or, if in the hospital, the confines of their room to minimize the embarrassment associated with soiling. Such people may come to prefer easily washable night garments to street clothes. Skin irritation and excoriation around the anal region can become a serious problem, which warrants preventive measures.

Examples of nursing diagnoses for the incontinent patient are:

1. Fecal incontinence related to impaired perception of the need to defecate
2. Risk of low self-esteem and social isolation related to lack of anal control
3. Risk of perianal skin excoriation associated with irritating effects of feces

Flatulence Leading to Intestinal Distention

Flatulence is the presence of excessive amounts of gases (flatus) in the intestines and leads to stretching and inflation of the intestines (intestinal distention). This condition is also referred to as *tympanites.* Large amounts of air and other gases can accumulate in the stomach, resulting in gastric distention.

A certain amount of gas in the gastrointestinal system is normal. Sources of intestinal gas are swallowed air, gas from the bacterial decomposition of food residue, and gas diffused from the bloodstream. Swallowed air accounts for approximately two-thirds of normal flatus, and bacterial decomposition and diffusion from the bloodstream account for the remaining third. Normally the gas is propelled by peristalsis along the tract and is absorbed. The swallowed air is usually *eructated* (belched).

Flatus may be expelled orally or anally, relieving the distention, or it may be retained. With increasing distention the abdomen becomes progressively swollen, and the patient may complain of cramps, pain, and shortness of breath. The last occurs when the diaphragm is elevated as a result of intraabdominal pressure.

Common causes of flatulence and distention are constipation; codeine, barbiturates, and other medications that decrease intestinal motility; and anxiety states during which large amounts of air are swallowed. Most people have experienced some flatulence and distention after eating such gas-forming foods as beans or cabbage. Postoperative distention after abdominal surgery is commonly seen in hospitals. This type of distention generally occurs on about the third postoperative day and is caused by the effects of anesthetics, narcotics, dietary changes, and reduction in activity. See Chapter 39.

Examples of nursing diagnoses for the patient with flatulence are:

1. Flatulence and intestinal distention related to abdominal surgery and effects of narcotics
2. Abdominal pain associated with distention
3. Risk of inactivity, nausea, and subsequent inadequate food and fluid intake associated with abdominal discomfort

Planning and Intervention for Fecal Elimination

Nursing plans are designed to promote, maintain, or restore the patient's anticipated pattern of defecation. Such plans are based on the assessment data obtained and the nursing diagnoses established. It is also essential that the nurse consider factors influencing the patient's normal fecal elimination.

The overall nursing goal is to restore the patient's normal defecation pattern. Subgoals may include:

1. To prevent constipation or its recurrence
2. To prevent fluid and electrolyte imbalance in patients who have diarrhea
3. To prevent perianal skin excoriation in patients who have diarrhea
4. To reduce or prevent flatulence in patients who have excessive gas

Because people's elimination patterns vary, there can be no comprehensive list of interventions that promote normal defecation. Some people stimulate the gastrocolic reflex in highly individual ways and may be unable to defecate, for example, unless they first drink hot lemonade. Nonetheless, it is possible to list some general measures that promote regular defecation:

1. A balanced diet that contains adequate bulk (fiber content)
2. Adequate fluid intake
3. Regular meals
4. A regular time for defecation and adequate time to defecate
5. Regular exercise
6. Privacy for defecation
7. Rectal suppositories, enemas, or laxatives when necessary

Constipation

A nurse who seeks to relieve a patient's constipation first assesses the factors contributing to the constipation. If there are no pathologic causes, such as bowel obstruction, the nurse and patient can together establish a plan of action. Some suggestions follow:

1. Increase the patient's daily fluid intake, or have the patient take a hot drink when arising.
2. Include bulk in the diet by having the patient eat prunes, raw fruit, bran products, and the like
3. Increase the person's physical activity by planning ambulation periods if possible.
4. Provide a regular time for fecal evacuation, such as after breakfast each day or at the person's usual time.
5. Provide for privacy and comfort. Offer a warm bedpan to bedridden patients, and assist them to assume a high Fowler's position with knees flexed. Curtain off the area, and allow them privacy and time to relax.
6. Promote measures to relieve tension, and try to prevent factors that make the patient suppress the urge to defecate.

Other measures, such as the administration of cathartics and enemas, are sometimes necessary.

Cathartics

Cathartics are drugs that induce defecation. They vary in their degree and method of action. Cathartics can have a laxative effect or a purgative effect; a laxative effect is mild in comparison to a purgative effect, which produces frequent movements of the bowel, soft liquid stools, and sometimes abdominal cramps. Different cathartics have different effects, but even the same cathartic may have either a purgative or laxative effect depending on the dosage taken. A large dose of a cathartic may have a purgative effect, while a small dose of the same cathartic may have a laxative effect and produce a normal bowel movement.

Cathartics induce defecation in several ways:

1. *Bulk-forming cathartics* act by increasing the fluid, gaseous, or solid bulk of the intestinal content. The increased bulk stimulates peristalsis, and defecation occurs. Fluids must be taken with this type of cathartic. An example is psyllium hydrophilic mucilloid (Metamucil).
2. *Emollient cathartics*, such as liquid petrolatum, act to soften and delay the drying of the fecal mass. Prolonged use of liquid petrolatum is contraindicated, since it inhibits the absorption of some fat-soluble vitamins.
3. *Chemical irritants* irritate the bowel mucosa and cause rapid propulsion of the contents from the small intestine. Considerable fluid is passed with the stool because of the rapid movement of the feces, which does not allow the normal absorption of fluid from the bowel. Castor oil is an example of a chemically irritating cathartic. It causes complete evacuation of the bowel, and no movements may occur for a day or two after its administration. Another example is cascara, although its irritant effect occurs primarily in the large intestine.
4. *Moistening or wetting agents* act by lowering the surface tension of the fecal matter, thus allowing water to penetrate and become well mixed with the feces. A soft, formed stool is the result. An example is Colace.
5. *Saline cathartics* are soluble salts, which are not absorbed or only slightly absorbed in the intestine. The fluid bulk is increased because water absorption is decreased when the salt solution is in the large intestine. Examples of these are magnesium hydroxide (milk of magnesia) and magnesium sulfate (Epsom salts).

The administration of cathartics is prescribed with caution and in many instances is ordered by the physician. Constipation is not the only reason for prescribing cathartics. For example, cathartics are prescribed in preparation for radiologic examinations or surgery, for which the bowel must be evacuated.

The nurse's function with constipated patients is to teach them not to abuse cathartics, but to use them effectively. Some patients come to rely on cathartics and need help to learn how to change this habit. Others may need to take cathartics regularly or periodically. An example is elderly persons who have difficulty increasing the bulk in their diet because they are edentulous or who do not have the physical health to carry out appropriate exercise.

Before administering cathartics, the nurse also needs to be aware of any other pathologic condition the patient may have. The classic example is the person who has an inflamed appendix. Giving this person a cathartic can rupture the appendix as a result of the increased peristaltic action of the bowel brought about by the cathartic. Some other contraindications are ulcerative conditions of the intestine, pathologic obstructions, or severe debilitation from electrolyte imbalances.

Suppositories

Some cathartics are given in the form of suppositories. These act in various ways: by softening the feces, by releasing gases such as carbon dioxide to distend the rectum, or by stimulating the nerve endings in the rectal mucosa. Suppositories need to be inserted beyond the internal anal sphincter. A finger cot or disposable glove is worn by the nurse, and the suppository is well lubricated prior to insertion, to prevent friction and tissue damage. The suppository is inserted gently 7.5 or 10 cm (3 or 4 in), or the length of the nurse's index finger, for an adult and less for a child or baby. The patient is instructed to breathe through the mouth, because mouth breathing may relax the anal sphincter. To be effective, the suppository needs to be placed along the wall of the rectum rather than lodged in the feces. Immediately after inserting the suppository, the nurse can help dispel any urge the patient has to expel the suppository by pressing the patient's buttocks together for a few seconds. After the procedure, the nurse removes the glove or finger cot by turning it inside out and discards it. Nondisposable gloves are washed in soap and water. See Chapter 37 for rectal insertion.

Generally, suppositories are effective within 30 minutes. The best results can be obtained by inserting the suppository 30 minutes before the patient's usual defecation time or when the peristaltic action is greatest, such as after breakfast.

Enemas

A cleansing or oil retention enema may be necessary to relieve constipation. These are discussed on page 696.

Fecal Impaction

Ideally, fecal impaction can be prevented. However, therapeutic measures are sometimes necessary to remove an impaction.

Enemas

Often an oil retention enema is given, followed by a cleansing enema 2 to 4 hours later. Daily follow-up with additional cleansing enemas, suppositories, or laxatives is sometimes indicated.

The technique for giving an oil retention enema is similar to that for giving a cleansing enema (see Procedure 27–1). Because small amounts of oil are administered, the oil is usually placed in a small pitcher and then administered directly through the rectal tube with an Asepto syringe or through a small funnel that is attached by a connecting tube to the rectal catheter.

Digital removal

Digital removal of the fecal impaction is sometimes necessary. The nurse breaks up the fecal mass digitally and then removes portions of it. This procedure is distressing and uncomfortable, and patients may desire the presence of another nurse or family member for support. Care must be taken to avoid injuring the bowel mucosa and thus to prevent bleeding. For this reason, agency policies vary about who may break up impactions digitally. After disimpaction, follow-up measures to encourage normal defecation, such as administering enemas or suppositories, are implemented for a few days.

The procedure for digital removal of a fecal impaction is:

1. Help the patient assume a side-lying position, with the knees flexed and the back toward you. Although some patients may prefer to stand by a toilet, the bed position is advised because disimpaction can be exhausting.
2. Place a waterproof bedpad under the patient's buttocks and a bedpan nearby to receive stool.
3. Put on a pair of plastic or rubber gloves and liberally lubricate the index finger to be inserted.
4. Gently insert the index finger into the rectum and move the finger toward the patient's umbilicus, moving along the length of the rectum.
5. Loosen and dislodge stool by gently massaging around it. Break up stool by working the finger into the hardened mass. Take care to avoid injury to the mucosa of the rectum.
6. Work stool downward to the end of the rectum and remove it in small pieces. Continue to remove as much fecal material as possible. Periodically assess the patient for signs of fatigue, such as facial pallor, diaphoresis, or change in pulse rate.
7. Following disimpaction, assist the patient to clean the anal area and buttocks. Then assist the patient onto a bedpan or commode for a short time, because digital stimulation of the rectum often induces the urge to defecate.

8. Wash hands and record the amount and characteristics of the fecal material.

Diarrhea

Nursing interventions for diarrhea vary according to its contributing factors and its severity. When there is excessive fluid and electrolyte loss, a major nursing responsibility is to replace the fluid and electrolytes. In some instances, intravenous therapy is prescribed. When possible, oral intake of fluids and food is encouraged. Because ingestion of foods and fluids stimulates the gastrocolic and duodenocolic reflexes, thus inducing more stool, the patient may be reluctant to eat or drink. Eating small amounts of bland foods can be helpful, since they are more easily absorbed. Potassium losses may be great with diarrhea, and the ingestion of food or fluids containing potassium should be encouraged. See the discussion of hypokalemia in Chapter 31. Excessively hot or cold fluids should be avoided because they stimulate peristalsis.

Because the patient with diarrhea has difficulty controlling the urge to defecate, a bedpan or commode must be placed in a convenient place. Liquid feces are often malodorous and therefore can be embarrassing to patients. These patients need rooms that can be well ventilated, if possible, and prompt emptying of their bedpans. Skin excoriation around the anal region can be prevented by using soft tissues and by cleaning and drying the area properly after defecation. Protective creams such as petroleum jelly and zinc oxide or nonirritating powders are also used.

In some instances the patient may accidentally soil the bed or clothing. The nurse needs to provide linen changes and convey understanding of and support during the patient's distress or embarrassment. Adequate rest and reduced physical activity are also helpful in lessening bowel activity.

If the cause of the diarrhea is sustained anxiety, the nurse may assist by helping the patient to talk about those stressful life situations and consider ways to reduce stress. Referral for psychiatric counseling may be indicated.

The nurse will also be involved in medical therapies to treat the cause of the diarrhea. Antidiarrhetics may be ordered by the physician. Some of these mechanically coat the irritated bowel and act as protectives (*demulcents*). Others absorb gas or toxic substances from the bowel (*adsorbents*) or shrink swollen and inflamed tissues (*astringents*). In certain situations, sedatives and antispasmodics may be ordered.

Fecal Incontinence

Many incontinent patients can be helped to regain bowel control with a planned program of bowel retraining. This plan is usually initiated by the physician, who determines the possibility of success in accordance with the underlying causes. The measures used will vary with the patient, but can include the following:

1. Determining with the patient the time of day for evacuation, such as after breakfast. After breakfast the gastrocolic reflex is stimulated, and defecation may be induced.
2. Arranging to have the patient on the commode or toilet at the specified time, since defecation is facilitated by gravity and by the more efficient muscular contraction this position affords.
3. Providing a drink of hot coffee or tea in the early morning to stimulate peristalsis.
4. Administering oral stool softeners daily or a laxative suppository 30 minutes prior to the prescribed defecation time. These stimulate the rectal mucosa.
5. Teaching the patient to lean forward at the hips while on the toilet, to apply pressure on the abdomen with the hands, and to bear down as is normally done. These measures increase the pressure on the large colon and help achieve the best possible results. Straining should be discouraged, however, because hemorrhoids may result.
6. Providing privacy and a time limit for defecation. Some patients find that reading a book helps them to relax. A suggested time limit is 20 minutes.
7. Ensuring that the patient's diet has sufficient roughage and that permitted exercise is encouraged.

Bowel retraining requires patience by the patient. The nurse needs to offer praise for the patient's efforts and encouragement to pursue the program consistently.

Flatulence Leading to Intestinal Distention

Several nursing measures can be employed to relieve flatus and abdominal distention, depending on their causes. Minimizing the amount of swallowed air may be necessary. The patient who is anxious, hyperventilating, and swallowing large amounts of air may need to learn appropriate breathing patterns and to plan ways to reduce anxiety. Limiting carbonated beverages, not using straws to drink, and not chewing gum will also reduce the amount of air ingested. After some abdominal surgeries, nasogastric tubes are used. In addition to removing fluid, these tubes enhance the passage of gas from the upper gastrointestinal tract. Ambulation or movement in bed will facilitate even more efficient removal of flatus.

Insertion of a rectal tube

The insertion of a rectal tube can provide temporary relief from flatulence. This measure is usually implemented when others fail. Rectal tube insertion may require a physician's order and is not carried out following rectal surgery. Standard size rectal tubes are used (# 22 to # 30 French for adults, # 16 to # 24 for children). The rectal tube is lubricated prior to insertion to reduce resistance during its passage through the anal sphincters. It can be inserted deeper than recommended for enemas, since fluid will not be administered. For adults, insertion to 15 cm (6 in) is recommended; for infants and small children, 5 to 10 cm (2 to 4 in), depending on age. An absorbent pad should be placed under the patient's buttocks before the tube is inserted.

After the rectal tube is inserted, the patient lies quietly in bed in the lateral position so that the tube is not dislodged. If necessary the tube may be taped to one buttock. The open end of the tube is then placed in a folded or rolled absorbent pad or towel to catch any seepage of liquid fecal material. Some agencies advocate attaching the open end of the rectal tube to some connecting tubing, which is in turn inserted in a receptacle containing water. The passage of flatus is then shown by gas bubbles in the water. The end of the connecting tubing must be below the level of the water for bubbles to be noted.

Prolonged use of rectal tubes can reduce the responsiveness of the anal sphincters and irritate the rectal mucosa. It is recommended that rectal tubes remain inserted for no longer than 30 minutes and be reinserted as needed every 2 to 3 hours.

After removing the rectal tube, the nurse notes the patient's response. If no flatus is expelled and the patient is still distended after several attempts, the physician is notified.

Administration of a carminative or return flow enema

Carminative or return flow enemas can be effective in removing flatus. See the discussion of enemas next.

Enemas

An *enema* is a solution introduced into the rectum and sigmoid colon. Its function is to remove feces and/or flatus.

Types of Enemas

Enemas can be classified according to their action or purpose:

1. *Cleansing enemas* act primarily by stimulating peristalsis through irritation of the colon and rectum and through distention by volume. A volume of 1000 ml is administered to adults. Infants normally receive no more than 250 ml. Some agencies differentiate between high and low cleansing enemas. A high enema is given to clean as much of the large bowel as possible. Usually about 1000 ml of solution is administered. It is administered at a higher pressure than other enemas, and the patient changes from the left lateral position to the dorsal recumbent position and then to the right lateral position during the administration so that the fluid can flow through the large intestine. A low enema is used to clean only the rectum and sigmoid colon. About 500 ml of solution is administered at a lower pressure.

2. *Carminative enemas* are given primarily to expel flatus, and they act by releasing gas that distends the sigmoid colon and rectum. Usually 180 to 240 ml of fluid is instilled into the rectum and colon.

3. *Oil retention enemas* lubricate the rectum and sigmoid colon and soften feces, making defecation easier. About 150 to 200 ml of oil is administered to adults. For small children, 75 to 150 ml is considered suitable.

4. *Return flow enemas.* A return flow enema is sometimes referred to as a *Harris flush* or *colonic irrigation* and is used to expel flatus. It is a repetitive instillation of fluid into and drainage of fluid from the rectum. First a solution (100 to 200 ml for an adult) is instilled into the patient's rectum and sigmoid colon. Then the solution container is lowered so that the fluid flows back out through the rectal tube into the container. This alternating flow of fluid into and out of the large intestine stimulates peristalsis and the expulsion of flatus. The inflow-outflow process is repeated five or six times, until gas bubbles cease or abdominal distention and discomfort is relieved. The solution may need to be replaced several times during the procedure if it becomes thick with feces. Because the solution is replaced, a total of about 1000 ml is usually used for an adult.

5. *Medicated enemas.* Medicated enemas are administered for various reasons. A neomycin enema, for example, may be given to clean the colon prior to surgery. Other substances act locally, e.g., to soothe and treat an irritated bowel mucosa or to stop hemorrhage.

6. *Cooling enemas.* Solutions as cool as 35 C (95 F) were traditionally given to reduce fever. When the cool solution reaches the vascular system of the bowel, heat is transferred to the solution and the body temperature is lowered.

Preparation of Solutions

Enemas for adults and children are commercially prepared, or they can be made up in the home and hospital. Tap water is commonly used for adults but should not be used for infants because of the danger of electrolyte imbalance. The colon absorbs water, and repeated tap water enemas can result in cardiovascular overload and subsequent electrolyte imbalance. The symptoms of this overload include dizziness, pallor, sweating, and vomiting.

Soap suds and physiologic saline are used in cleansing enemas. Too strong a solution or repeated use can irritate the lining of the colon and damage the mucous membrane.

If a commercially prepared product is used, the strength should not be greater than 5 ml of soap per 1000 ml of water. If the soap to be used is already in solution form, it is more difficult to gauge the strength of the solution. Only bland, white soap should be used. Common household detergents are too strong for the colon and rectum. Bar soap in enema solutions must be previously unused; enemas made with previously used soap can introduce pathogenic microorganisms into the patient. Castile soap packets are available commercially. They are convenient and permit accurate measurement of the strength of the enema.

Physiologic saline distends the colon and rectum, thus stimulating peristalsis. One problem with repeated saline enemas is the absorption of fluid and electrolytes into the bloodstream. Most agencies have a policy regarding the strength of saline enemas. One guide is 9 ml of sodium chloride to 1000 ml of water.

Some commercially prepared disposable enemas come as hypertonic solutions. They distend the colon and rectum and irritate the mucous membrane, thus stimulating peristalsis. The amount of solution instilled is about 120 ml. Hypertonic solutions draw fluid into the bowel from the circulation, thus increasing the fluid volume in the colon and rectum. A hypertonic solution is usually left for 5 to 7 minutes before the patient defecates. This time allows the fluid volume within the colon to increase sufficiently to stimulate defecation.

Hypertonic enemas are contraindicated for dehydrated persons because they cannot tolerate a fluid transfer from the circulation to the bowel. In the well-hydrated person, the loss of fluid from the bloodstream is quickly replaced by fluid from other reservoirs in the body. In the dehydrated person, fluid reservoirs are depleted, and a fluid loss from the circulation can induce shock.

For oil retention enemas, salad oil or liquid petrolatum is commonly used at a temperature of 33 C (91 F). There are also commercially prepared retention enemas. Once the oil has been administered (adults usually receive about 180 ml of oil), it is retained for from 1 to 3 hours before it is expelled.

There are number of carminative enemas, and many agencies have a preferred type. Three commonly used types are the 1–2–3 enema, the milk and molasses enema, and the Mayo enema.

The 1–2–3 enema, also referred to as the MGW enema, contains 30 ml (1 oz) of magnesium sulfate, 60 ml (2 oz) of glycerine, and 90 ml (3 oz) of warm water.

The milk and molasses enema contain equal amounts of milk and molasses. The amounts vary from 180 ml to 240 ml.

The Mayo enema contains 240 ml of water, 60 ml of white sugar, and 30 ml of sodium bicarbonate. The last ingredient is added immediately before the enema is administered so that the solution is bubbling during administration.

Guidelines for Administering Enemas

1. The appropriate size rectal tube needs to be used. For adults this is usually # 22 to # 30 French. Children use a smaller tube, such as a # 12 French for an infant and a #14 to #18 French for the toddler and school-age child.

2. Rectal tubes must be smooth and flexible with one or two openings at the end through which the solution flows. They are usually made of rubber or plastic. Any tube with a sharp or ragged edge should not be used because of the possibility of damaging the mucous membrane of the rectum. The rectal tube is lubricated with a water-soluble lubricant to facilitate insertion and decrease irritation of the rectal mucosa.

3. The temperature of the enema solution is normally 40.5 to 43 C (105 to 110 F). High temperatures can be injurious to the bowel mucosa; cold temperatures are uncomfortable for the patient and may create spasm of the sphincter muscles.

4. The amount of solution to be administered depends on the kind of enema and the age and size of the person.

- **a.** Infant: 250 ml or less
- **b.** Toddler, preschooler: 250 to 350 ml or less
- **c.** School-age child: 300 to 500 ml
- **d.** Adolescent: 500 to 750 ml
- **e.** Adult: 750 to 1000 ml

5. When an enema is administered, the patient usually assumes the left lateral position (see Figure 27–6) so that the sigmoid colon is below the rectum, thus facilitating instillation of the fluid. During a high cleansing enema, the patient changes position from left lateral to dorsal recumbent and then to right lateral. In this way the entire colon is reached by the fluid.

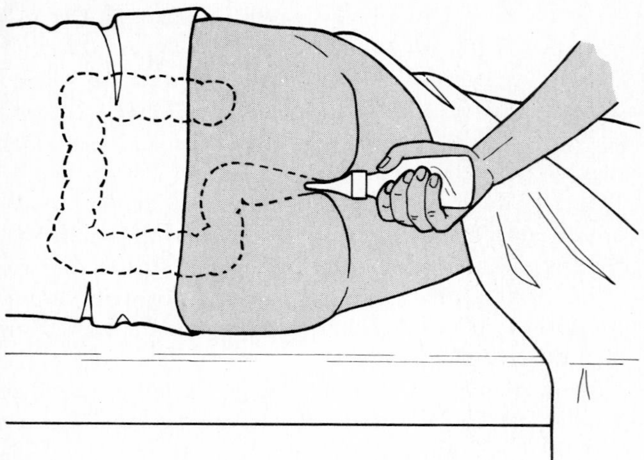

Figure 27–6 The left lateral position is assumed for an enema. Note the commercially prepared enema.

6. The distance to which the tube is inserted depends on the age and size of the patient. In adults, it is normally inserted 7.5 to 10 cm (3 to 4 in). In children it is inserted 5 to 7.5 cm (2 to 3 in) and in infants only 2.5 to 3.75 cm (1 to 1.5 in). If any obstruction is encountered when the tube is inserted, the tube should be withdrawn and the obstruction reported.

7. The force of flow of the solution is governed by (a) height of the solution container, (b) size of the tubing, (c) viscosity of the fluid, and (d) resistance of the rectum. The higher the solution container is held above the rectum, the faster the flow and the greater the force (pressure) in the rectum. During most adult enemas, the solution container should be no higher than 30 cm (12 in) above the rectum. During a high cleansing enema, the solution container is usually held 30 to 45 cm (12 to 18 in) above the rectum, because the fluid is instilled farther to clean the entire bowel. For an infant, the solution container is held no more than 7.5 cm (3 in) above the rectum.

8. Prepackaged enemas have their own instructions, which are followed unless there are other instructions from the physician or the agency.

9. The time it takes to administer an enema largely depends on the amount of fluid to be instilled. Large volumes such as 1000 ml may take 10 to 15 minutes to instill; small volumes require less time.

10. The length of time that the enema solution is retained depends on the purpose of the enema and the ability of the patient to contract the external sphincter to retain the solution. Oil retention enemas are usually retained 2 to 3 hours. Other enemas are normally retained 5 to 10 minutes. To assist an incontinent person to retain the solution, the nurse can press the buttocks together, providing pressure over the anal area.

11. While the enema solution is in the body, the patient may have a feeling of fullness and some abdominal discomfort.

12. When it is time for the patient to defecate, the nurse may assist him or her to a commode or toilet, depending upon the patient's preference and physical condition.

Procedure 27–1 Administering an Enema

Goals

1. To stimulate peristalsis and remove feces or flatus
2. To soften feces and lubricate the rectum and colon
3. To clean the rectum and colon in preparation for an examination
4. To remove feces prior to a surgical procedure or a delivery, thereby preventing inadvertent defecation and subsequent contamination of a wound
5. To reduce body temperature
6. To relieve a specific problem by administering a medication rectally

Equipment

1. A disposable enema unit (see Figure 27–7)

   or

   An enema set containing:

   a. A container to hold the solution.

   b. Tubing to connect the container to the rectal tube.

   c. A clamp to compress the tubing, to control the flow of solution into the patient.

   d. A rectal tube of the correct size. See guideline 1 on page 697.

   e. Lubricant to apply to the rectal tube before it is inserted.

   f. A bath thermometer to check the temperature of the solution.

   g. Soap, salt, or other ingredients as required.

Procedure 27–1, continued

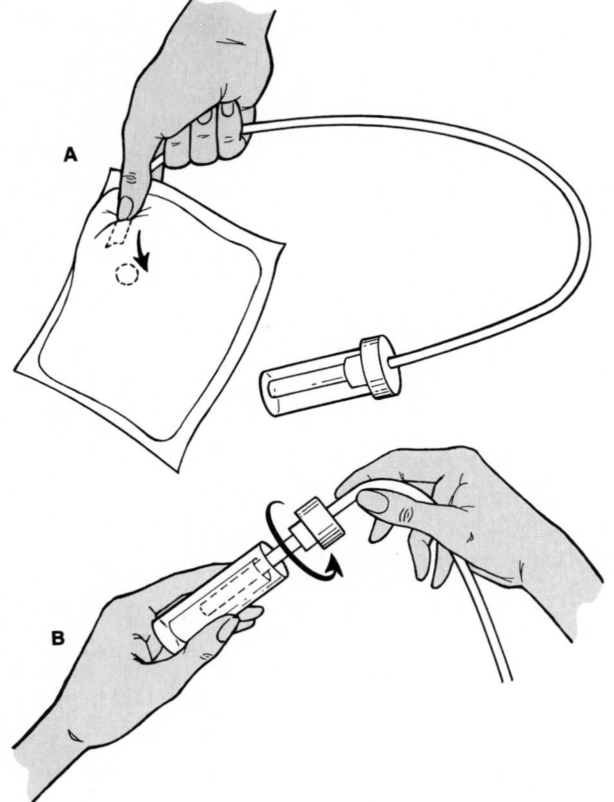

Figure 27–7 One type of commercially prepared disposable enema: **A,** the bead that seals the tube is expelled from the tube into the bag so that the solution can flow through the tubing; **B,** the protector cover of the insertion tip is rotated to distribute the lubricant on the tip before the cover is removed; **C,** after the tube has been inserted, the bag is inverted and compressed.

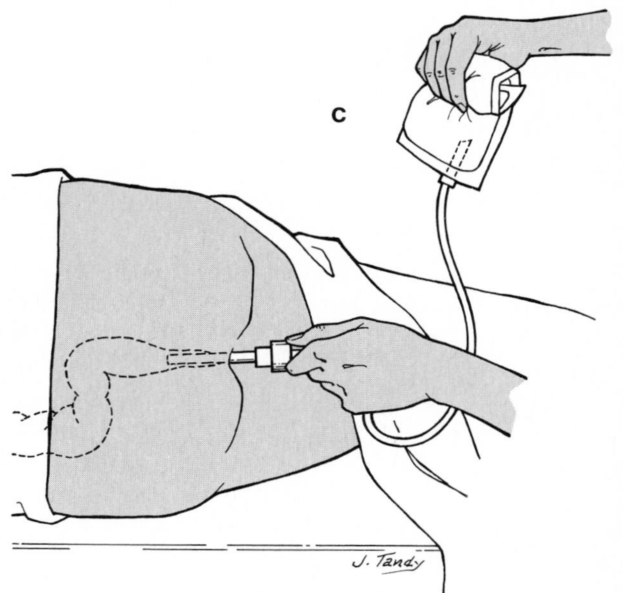

   h. The prescribed amount of solution at the correct temperature. The nurse places the solution in the container, checks that the temperature and the amount of solution are correct, and then adds the soap, salt, and other ingredients as needed.

2. A bath blanket to drape the patient.

3. A waterproof absorbent pad to protect the bed.

4. Tissue wipes.

5. A bedpan or commode if the patient is unable to reach the bathroom.

Preparation

1. Explain the procedure to the patient. Indicate that the patient may experience a feeling of fullness while the solution is being administered.

2. Provide for privacy, since exposure of the buttocks may embarrass the patient.

3. Elevate the bed to a working height, and lower the side rail on the near side.

4. Assist adult and school-aged patients to a left lateral position, with the right leg acutely flexed, and drape them with the bath blanket. This position facilitates the flow of solution by gravity into the sigmoid and descending colon, which are on the left side. See Figure 27–6 earlier in this chapter. Having the right leg acutely flexed provides for adequate exposure of the anus. For infants and small children the dorsal recumbent position is frequently used. Position them on a small padded bedpan with support for the back and head. Secure the legs by placing a diaper under the bedpan and pinning it around the thighs.

5. Place the waterproof pad under the patient's buttocks to protect the bed linen.

Procedure 27–1, continued

Intervention

1. Lubricate 5 cm (2 in) of the rectal tube if the enema is for an adult and 2.5 cm (1 in) if it is for a child. Some commercially prepared enema sets already have lubricated nozzles.

   Rationale Lubrication facilitates insertion through the sphincters and minimizes trauma.

2. Open the clamp, and run some solution through the connecting tubing and the rectal tube; then close the clamp.

   Rationale The tubes are filled with solution to expel any air in them. Air instilled into the rectum causes unnecessary distention.

3. Insert the rectal tube smoothly and slowly into the rectum, directing it toward the umbilicus. Insert the tube 7.5 to 10 cm (3 to 4 in) for an adult, 5 to 7.5 cm (2 to 3 in) for a child, and 2.5 to 3.75 cm (1 to 1.5 in) for an infant.

   Rationale Inserting the tube toward the umbilicus guides the tube along the length of the rectum. The rectum of the average adult is 10 to 20 cm (4 to 6 in) long but the size varies with age. See the description of the rectum and anal canal on page 684. The rectal tube is inserted beyond the internal sphincter.

4. If resistance is encountered at the internal sphincter, ask the patient to take a deep breath, and run a small amount of solution through the tube. If the resistance persists, withdraw the tube and report the resistance to the responsible nurse.

   Rationale Deep breathing and inserting a small amount of solution may relax the sphincter.

5. Open the clamp, and raise the solution container to the appropriate height above the rectum: 30 to 45 cm (12 to 18 in) for an adult; 7.5 cm (3 in) for an infant.
   or
   Compress a pliable commercial container by hand.

   Rationale At this height, the solution does not exert enough pressure to damage the lining of the rectum.

6. Administer the fluid slowly, use the clamp to stop the flow for 30 seconds if the patient complains of fullness or pain, and then restart the flow at a slower rate. Roll up a plastic commercial container as the fluid is instilled.

   Rationale Administering the enema slowly and stopping the flow momentarily decreases the likelihood of intestinal spasm and premature ejection of the solution. Rolling up the container prevents subsequent suctioning of the solution.

7. After all the solution has been instilled, or when the patient cannot hold any more and wants to defecate, close the clamp, and remove the rectal tube from the anus.

   Rationale The urge to defecate usually indicates that sufficient fluid has been administered.

8. Apply firm pressure over the anus with tissue wipes, or press the buttocks together, to assist retention of the enema. Have the patient remain lying down. Encourage the patient to hold the enema.

   Rationale Some enemas are more effective if they are retained from 5 to 10 minutes. The time depends on the type of enema. It is easier for the patient to retain the enema when lying down than when sitting or standing because gravity promotes drainage and peristalsis.

9. Assist the patient to a sitting position on the bedpan, commode, or toilet. If a specimen of feces is required, have the patient use a bedpan or commode.

   Rationale A sitting position is preferred because it promotes defecation.

10. Ask the patient not to flush the toilet if he or she is using one.

    Rationale The nurse needs to observe the feces.

11. Collect and remove the equipment.

12. Wash hands.

13. Record administration of the enema; the amount, color, and consistency of returns; and the relief of flatus and abdominal distention.

Special Enema Administration Problems

Administering an enema to an incontinent patient

Occasionally a nurse may need to administer an enema to a patient who is unable to contract the external sphincter muscle and retain the solution inside the body. Some elderly people have this problem. In this instance the patient sits on a bedpan during administration of the enema. The head of the bed can be raised to a 30° angle and pillows positioned to support the patient's lumbar region and head.

The nurse wears a glove on the hand that holds the rectal tube in place because the solution and feces will be expelled over the hand into the bedpan while the solution is being administered.

This technique is also used when administering an enema to a baby or small child. The infant-size bedpan is usually padded to prevent injury to the skin of the child.

Siphoning an enema

In some instances a patient may be unable to expel the solution after administration of an enema. The solution must then be siphoned off. In siphoning, the nurse uses the force of gravity to draw the fluid out of the rectum and colon.

The equipment required is a bedpan, a funnel and rectal tube, lubricant, and a container of water at 40 C (105 F). During siphoning, the patient asumes a right side-lying position so that the sigmoid colon is uppermost, thus facilitating drainage of the solution from the rectum and the colon. The patient lies on the bed with hips close to the side of the bed. The nurse places a bedpan on a chair at the side of the bed near the patient's hips. The chair must be lower than the bed. The rectal tube is lubricated and attached to the funnel. The tube and half of the funnel are filled with solution, then the tube is pinched and gently inserted into the rectum as for an enema. The nurse holds the funnel about 10 cm (4 in) above the anus, releases the pinched rectal tube, and quickly lowers the funnel over the bedpan. This action should draw the fluid from the colon and rectum, permitting it to flow through the rectal tube and funnel into the bedpan. The nurse then notes the amount of fluid siphoned off as well as the color, odor, and presence of any feces or abnormal constituents, such as blood or mucus.

Obtaining Stool Specimens

Stool specimens are frequently required for laboratory analysis. Agencies usually provide special containers in which to place a fecal sample. It is important that the nurse know why the specimen is being obtained and that the correct container be used. Sometimes containers hold preservatives specific to the tests to be performed. Attached to or written on the container may be special directions, which need to be followed when obtaining the specimen.

Often a patient can obtain the specimen if given adequate information. The feces should not be mixed with urine or water, thus the patient defecates in a bedpan or a commode.

A wooden or plastic tongue depressor is used to transfer the specimen, and about 2.5 cm (1 in) is placed into the container. If the stool is liquid, 15 ml to 30 ml is collected. The container is then closed securely, and the appropriate requisitions are completed. The fact that the specimen has been obtained is entered on the patient's chart.

For certain tests, fresh stool samples are needed. If so, the specimen is taken immediately to the laboratory. A stool specimen should not be left at room temperature for long because bacteriologic changes take place. Specimen containers usually have directions for storage; these should be followed if the specimen cannot be delivered immediately to the laboratory. In some instances refrigeration is indicated.

To secure a stool specimen from a baby or young child who is not toilet trained, a specimen is taken from newly passed feces. When the stool is being cultured for microorganisms, it is transferred to the container with a sterile applicator.

Evaluation

The outcome criteria for patients with fecal elimination problems depend on the specific nursing diagnosis and stated nursing goals. Examples are:

Constipation and/or fecal impaction

1. Decreased incidence of constipation
2. Intake of 3000 ml of fluid daily

3. Walks 30 minutes three times per day
4. Takes 4 servings of fruit and vegetables daily

Diarrhea
1. Decreased incidence of diarrhea
2. Fluid intake in balance with fluid output
3. Absence of signs of potassium depletion (see the discussion of hypokalemia, page 803)
4. Intact perianal skin
5. Refrains from eating high-fiber foods as instructed

Fecal incontinence
1. Decreased incidence of fecal incontinence
2. Intact perianal skin
3. Increased sense of self-esteem, manifested by self-confidence and talking about accomplishments and activities

Flatulence leading to intestinal distention
1. Increased expulsion of flatus
2. Decreased abdominal distention
3. Absence of abdominal pain and nausea
4. Ambulates without encouragement
5. Eats appropriate food and fluids as instructed

Summary

Elimination of the waste products of digestion is essential to health. Although patterns of fecal elimination vary, regularity is important to most people. When any irregularity occurs, the person may become preoccupied about reestablishing regularity and may use laxatives. Nurses are frequently involved in assisting patients with bowel problems brought about by illness, age, or such factors as dietary changes and diagnostic tests.

Adequate elimination of the body's waste products requires proper functioning of the small and large intestines. As chyme moves through the small intestine, many nutrients are absorbed, and the waste products pass through the ileocecal valve to the large intestine. Absorption of substances (water and electrolytes) continues in the large intestine until a firm stool is formed and retained in the rectum. The act of defecation is facilitated by the gastrocolic reflex and by a sitting position. It is consciously controlled and learned by about the age of 2 years. Effective bowel training requires sufficient time, a consistent pattern, and praise to the child being trained from a parent or other significant person.

Factors that influence defecation include age, diet, fluid intake, exercise, psychologic stressors, life-style, and medications. The pattern of defecation is highly individual. The time and frequency of defecation vary, as does the amount of feces. Feces are described by their color, consistency, odor, and the presence of blood and other abnormal constituents.

Common problems of fecal elimination include constipation, fecal impaction, diarrhea, fecal incontinence, and flatulence leading to intestinal distention. The causes for each of these and the specific nursing intervention required are outlined. Some of the interventions include the administration of cathartics, antidiarrhetics, and suppositories; digital removal of impactions; bowel retraining programs; insertion of rectal tubes; and enemas.

Enemas are given for a variety of reasons and are classified according to their action: cleansing, oil, and carminative. Solutions of soap and normal saline are commonly used for cleansing enemas in amounts that distend the bowel (500 to 1000 ml) and stimulate peristalsis. Oil enemas of 100 to 200 ml lubricate the rectum and soften feces; they need to be retained for a few hours. Carminative enemas are used primarily to expel flatus. Commonly used types are the 1–2–3, the milk and molasses, and the Mayo enema. Guidelines for the nurse administering an enema and proper technique are outlined. Siphoning an enema is occasionally necessary for those who are unable to expel the solution.

Suggested Activities

1. Interview a young mother and a grandmother about the bowel training methods they used with their children. Compare the methods.
2. Visit a clinical setting. Note the methods used to maintain regular bowel function in elderly patients. Discuss and compare your findings with a group of classmates.
3. For a patient who has a specific elimination problem, outline a nursing care plan that reflects the health instruction required.

Suggested Readings

Blackwell, A. K., and Blackwell, W. January 1975. Relieving gas pains. *American Journal of Nursing* 75:66–67.

The authors describe five positions patients can assume to relieve their gas pains; these positions facilitate the expulsion of flatus through the rectum.

Corman, M. L.; Veidenheimer, M. C.; and Coller, J. A. February 1975. Cathartics. *American Journal of Nursing* 75:273–79.

The authors discuss the use of different cathartics and make recommendations for improving bowel function. Over-the-counter laxatives are listed, together with sites of action.

Habeeb, M. C., and Kallstrom, M. D. April 1976. Bowel program for institutionalized adults. *American Journal of Nursing* 76:606–8.
This article describes a program by which incontinent patients can achieve fecal continence. The program includes low residue diet, medications, rectal examinations, and enemas when needed.

Selected References

Aman, R. A. September 1980. Treating the patient, not the constipation. *American Journal of Nursing* 80:1634–35.

Bass, L. February 1977. More fibre—less constipation. *American Journal of Nursing* 77:254–55.

Copeland, L. March 1977. Chronic diarrhea in infancy. *American Journal of Nursing* 77:461–63.

Currie, J. E. J. September 13, 1979. Whole gut irrigation. *Nursing Times* 75:1570–71.

Gillies, D. A., and Alyn, I. B. 1976. *Patient assessment and management by the nurse practitioner.* Philadelphia: W. B. Saunders Co.

Keusch, G. June 1973. Bacterial diarrheas. *American Journal of Nursing* 73:1028–32.

King, E. M.; Wieck, L.; and Dyer, M. 1981. *Illustrated manual of nursing techniques.* 2nd ed. Philadelphia: J. B. Lippincott Co.

Kozier, B., and Erb, G. 1982. *Techniques in clinical nursing: A comprehensive approach.* Menlo Park, Calif.: Addison-Wesley Publishing Co.

Lewin, D. March 25, 1976. Care of the constipated patient. *Nursing Times* 72:444–46.

Malasanos, L.; Barkauskas, V.; Moss, M.; and Stoltenberg-Allen, K. 1981. *Health assessment.* 2nd ed. St. Louis: C. V. Mosby Co.

Nordmark, M. T., and Rohweder, A. W. 1975. *Scientific foundations of nursing.* 3rd ed. Philadelphia: J. B. Lippincott Co.

Sheridan, J. L. March 1975. Obstructions of the intestinal tract. *Nursing Clinics of North America* 10:147–55.

Smith, I., et al. September 1980. Constipation . . . in children . . . in the elderly . . . in the terminally ill. *Nursing (Oxford): The Add-On Journal of Clinical Nursing* 1:751–55.

Whaley, L., and Wong, D. 1979. *Nursing care of infants and children.* St. Louis: C. V. Mosby Co.

Chapter 28

Urinary Elimination

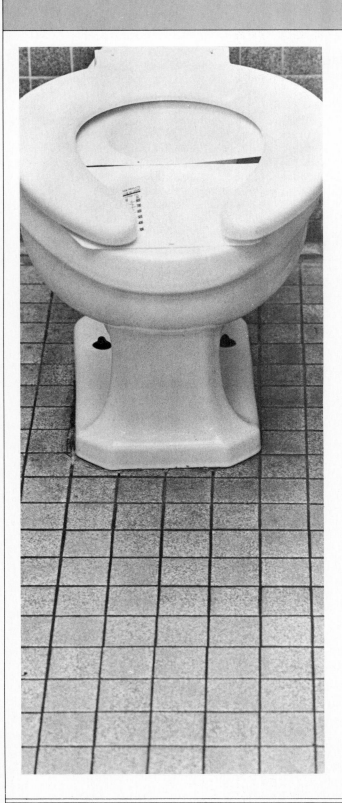

CONTENTS

Objectives

1. Know essential facts about the urinary tract and the development of bladder control
   - **1.1** Identify specific structures of the urinary tract
   - **1.2** Describe the process of urine formation
   - **1.3** Describe the process of micturition
   - **1.4** Identify the ages at which bladder control is achieved
   - **1.5** List measures that promote the development of bladder control
2. Know essential information and methods to assess a person's urinary status
   - **2.1** Identify factors that influence urinary habits
   - **2.2** Identify factors that influence patterns of urination
   - **2.3** Describe methods used to assess the kidneys, bladder, and urethral orifice
   - **2.4** Identify normal characteristics and constituents of urine
   - **2.5** Identify abnormal characteristics and constituents of urine
   - **2.6** Describe diagnostic measures to assess kidney function or urinary tract abnormalities
3. Understand essential facts about common urinary problems
   - **3.1** Differentiate among specific urinary problems
   - **3.2** Identify common causes and effects of selected urinary problems
   - **3.3** Identify indications of common urinary problems
4. Understand facts about nursing measures to maintain, promote, and restore normal functioning of the urinary system
   - **4.1** Identify measures to maintain normal voiding patterns of adults and children
   - **4.2** Outline common interventions for specific urinary problems
   - **4.3** Give reasons for selected nursing interventions
5. Apply the nursing process when providing care to selected patients with urinary problems
   - **5.1** Obtain necessary assessment data
   - **5.2** Analyze and relate assessment data
   - **5.3** Write relevant nursing diagnoses
   - **5.4** Write relevant nursing goals
   - **5.5** Plan appropriate nursing interventions
   - **5.6** Implement appropriate nursing interventions
   - **5.7** State outcome criteria essential for evaluating the patient's progress
6. Perform selected urinary techniques safely
   - **6.1** Assist patients to use bedpans and urinals
   - **6.2** Perform a urinary catheterization for a male or female patient
   - **6.3** Obtain a sterile specimen from a retention catheter
   - **6.4** Apply a condom device and drainage apparatus
   - **6.5** Collect urine specimens
   - **6.6** Perform urinary catheter and bladder irrigations

Terms

albuminuria
anuria
calculus
catheter
condom
costovertebral
Credé's maneuver
cystitis
dermatitis
detrusor muscle
dysuria
enuresis
flaccidity
frequency
glomerular filtrate
glomerulus
glycosuria
hematuria
hesitancy
hydrometer
incontinence
meatus
micturition (voiding, urination)
nephron
nocturia
oliguria
polydipsia
polyuria (diuresis)
proteinuria
pyuria
reflux
renal pelvis
residual urine
retention
retroperitoneal
Skene's glands
specific gravity
sphincter
stasis
stricture
suppression
trigone
urethritis
urgency
urinalysis

Although bowel habits are discussed in various advertising media in relation to the sale of laxatives, urinary elimination is seldom discussed. Elimination from the urinary tract is generally taken for granted by most people. It is only when a problem arises that people usually become aware of their urinary habits and any adjunctive symptoms.

A person's urinary habits depend on both social culture and personal habit. In North America, most people are accustomed to privacy and clean (even decorative) surroundings while they urinate. The lack of privacy that is normal in many European and Far Eastern countries surprises and frequently disturbs North Americans traveling there.

Personal habits regarding urination are affected by the social propriety of leaving to urinate, the availability of a private clean facility, and initial bladder training. Urinary elimination is essential to health, and voiding can be postponed for only so long before the urge normally becomes too great to control.

Physiology of the Urinary System

For an adult, the desire to void is normally experienced when the bladder contains between 250 and 450 ml of urine. Normal output of urine for an adult is about 1500 ml/day. A person's age, however, also affects urinary output. See Table 28–1.

Urinary Tract

The urinary tract is lined with mucous membrane, which extends from the meatus of the urethra to the kidneys. Although microorganisms are normally not present in the tract beyond the lower urethra, this continuous mucous membrane provides an excellent growth medium for some pathogens and for the spread of infection. Women are particularly prone to urinary tract infections because of the shortness of their urethras.

The urinary tract is only one route through which body wastes are eliminated. Urination eliminates the following products:

1. Water, 96%.
2. Solutes, 4%.
   a. Organic solutes include urea, ammonia, creatinine, and uric acid. Urea is the chief organic solute.
   b. Inorganic solutes include sodium, chloride, potassium, sulfate, magnesium, and phosphorus. Sodium chloride is the most abundant inorganic salt.

Table 28–1 Average Daily Excretion of Urine

Age	Amount
First and second days of life	15 to 60 ml
Third to tenth days	100 to 300 ml
Tenth day to age 2 months	250 to 450 ml
2 months to 1 year	400 to 500 ml
1 to 3 years	500 to 600 ml
3 to 5 years	600 to 700 ml
5 to 8 years	700 to 1000 ml
8 to 14 years	800 to 1400 ml
14 years through adulthood	1500 ml
Older adulthood	1500 ml or less

For the constituents of wastes eliminated by other routes, see Table 27–1, page 688, and Table 30–4, page 785.

Urine is formed in the kidneys, which are situated in the *retroperitoneal* space within the body (behind the peritoneum). The kidneys filter from the blood any products for which the body has no use. It is estimated that, in the average adult, 1200 ml of blood passes through the kidneys every minute. This figure represents about 21% of the cardiac output (5600 ml per minute). From this blood, the functional unit of the kidney, the *nephron* (see Figure 28–1), forms a fluid called *glomerular filtrate* (about 180 liters per day). The *glomerulus* is a tuft or cluster of blood vessels surrounded by Bowman's capsule. Because the glomerular membrane is relatively porous, water and all of the dissolved constituents of plasma (the fluid portion of the blood) except proteins filter through to the Bowman's capsule. Thus, the glomerular filtrate is almost the same as plasma except that it has only minute quantities of protein (0.03%) compared to plasma (7%). After the filtrate enters the Bowman's capsule, it passes into the tubular system where about 99% of this filtrate is reabsorbed into the bloodstream. The remainder (about 1 liter) forms the urine to be excreted from the body (Guyton 1982:253).

Once the urine is formed in the kidneys, it enters the ureters via collecting ducts and then passes on to the bladder. See Figure 28–2. The ureters are from 25 to 30 cm (10 to 12 in) long in the adult and about 1.25 cm (0.5 in) in diameter. The upper end of each ureter is funnel shaped as it enters the kidney, forming what is referred to as the *renal pelvis*. The lower ends of the ureters enter the bladder at the posterior corners of the floor of the bladder. At this junction between the ureter and the bladder there is a fold of mucous membrane which acts as a valve to prevent the backflow (*reflux*) of urine up the ureters to the kidneys.

The bladder is a reservoir for urine and the organ of excretion. The body of the bladder is made up of three layers of muscle, which collectively are called the *detrusor muscle*. The base of the bladder is called the *trigone*, a triangular area marked by the ureter openings at the posterior corners forming the base and the opening of the urethra at the anterior inferior corner forming the apex. Urine exits from the bladder through the urethra. The amount of urine normally stored in the bladder varies to some degree among individuals and with age.

During pregnancy the growing fetus puts pressure on the bladder, causing increased sensitivity and reduced storage capacity. This often causes urgency and frequency (see the discussion of these problems later in this chapter). The bladder is normally a convex organ; however, due to pressure of the uterus it becomes concave.

The urethra extends from the bladder to the urinary *meatus* (opening or passage) and is the exit passage for the urine. It is lined with mucous membrane. In the adult male the urethra is about 20 cm (8 in) in length. It is divided into three parts: the prostatic urethra, which starts at the bladder and extends through the prostate gland; the membranous urethra, which extends from the prostatic section to the third section; and the cavernous urethra, which extends from the triangular ligament to the urethral orifice. See Figure 28–3.

In the adult female the urethra is about 3.7 cm (1.5 inches) in length. See Figure 28–4. Because of its shortness it is particularly prone to bacterial invasion.

The urethra has two sphincter muscles, which control retention and excretion of urine. A *sphincter* is a ringlike band of muscle fibers that closes a natural orifice or constricts a passage. The *internal* sphincter is located at the base of the bladder and is under involuntary control. It is innervated by the autonomic nervous system. The *external* sphincter muscle is under voluntary control, thus enabling the person to retain or eliminate urine consciously. In the male this muscle is situated distal to the prostatic urethra. In the female it is situated at about the midpoint of the urethra. Normally both sphincters remain contracted until the person needs to urinate.

Urination

Micturition, voiding, and *urination* all mean the process of emptying the urinary bladder. Urine collects in the bladder until pressure stimulates special sensory nerve endings in the bladder wall called *stretch receptors.* This occurs when the adult bladder contains between 250 and 450 ml of urine. In children, a considerably smaller volume, 50 to 200 ml, stimulates these nerves.

Once excited, the stretch receptors transmit impulses to the spinal cord, specifically to the voiding reflex center located at the level of the second to fourth sacral vertebrae. Some impulses continue up the spinal cord to the voiding control center in the cerebral cortex. If the time is appropriate to void, the brain then sends impulses through the spinal cord to the motor neurons in the sacral area, causing stimulation of the parasympathetic nerves. The parasympathetic nervous system innervates the detrusor muscle and the internal urethral

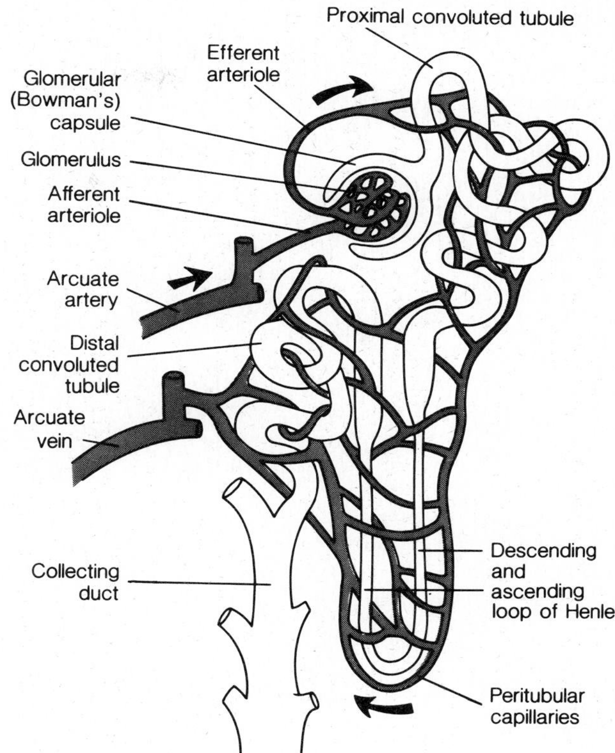

Figure 28–1 The nephron of the kidney.

Figure 28–2 Anatomic structures of the urinary tract.

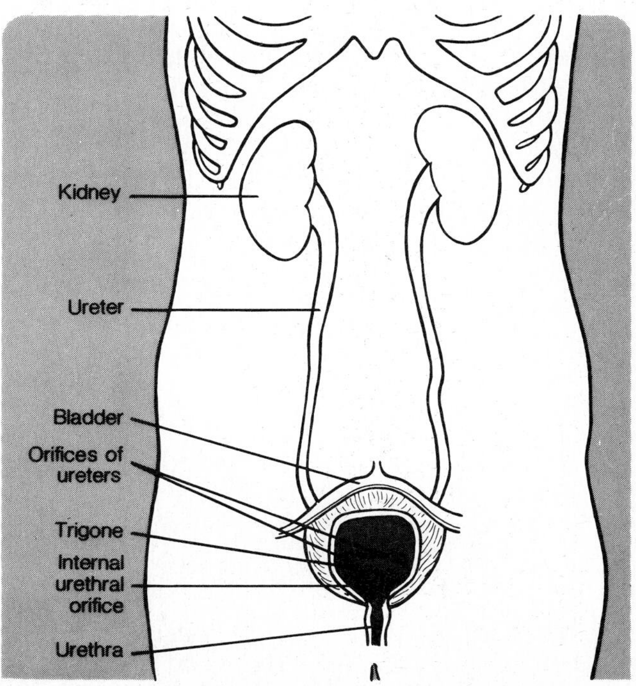

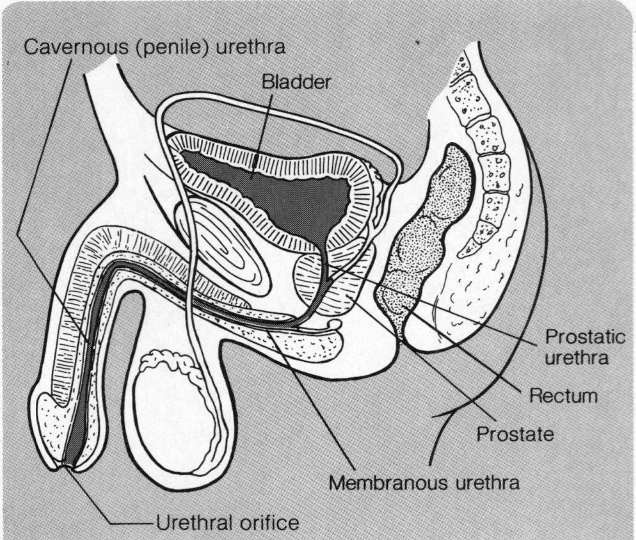

Figure 28–3 The male urogenital system.

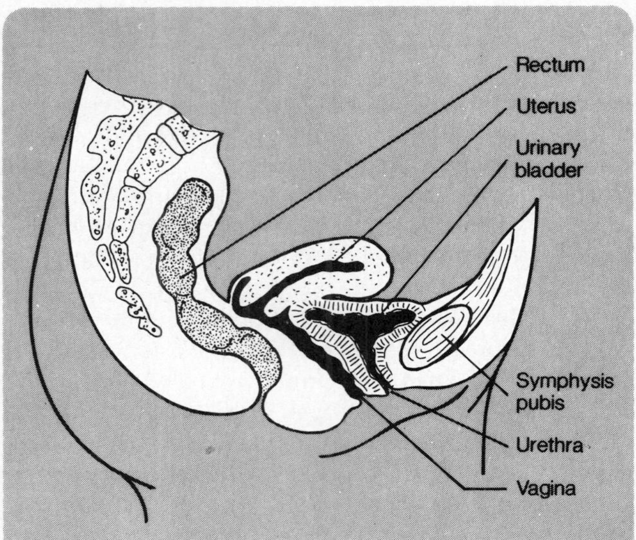

Figure 28–4 The female urogenital system.

sphincter muscle, producing (a) contraction of the detrusor muscle, and (b) relaxation of the internal sphincter muscle. As a result, urine can be released from the bladder, but it is still impeded by the external urinary sphincter. If the time and place are appropriate for urination, the conscious portion of the brain relaxes the external urethral sphincter muscle, and urination takes place. If the time and place are inappropriate, the micturition reflex usually subsides until the bladder becomes more filled and the reflex is stimulated again.

The sympathetic nervous system also innervates the bladder, causing it to relax. However these nerves do not normally enter into micturition control.

Development of Bladder Control (Toilet Training)

Babies are born without urinary control; however, children learn during the second year that it is essential to gain bladder as well as bowel control to obtain parental approval.

Toddlers must be sufficiently mature physiologically before they can learn this control. Usually it is started after bowel control has begun and when the child is able to hold the urine for 2 hours. Children generally communicate when they are ready to begin bladder training, perhaps by pointing or gesturing before they begin urinating.

The age at which control is achieved varies but is usually between 2 and 4½ years. Boys are slower than girls in gaining control. Most children are able to control their urination during the daytime by the time they are 2 years old. Nighttime control might not be learned until 3 or 4 years of age.

Control is considered to be learned in four steps:

1. Children first become aware that they have already urinated and will point to their diapers.

2. They learn to hold their urine for a brief period beyond the urge to void and will warn their parents of the urge to void.

3. Children acquire daytime control, which usually becomes well established by 2 years of age.

4. They acquire nighttime control by 3 to 4 years of age. At this point all involved muscle groups are coordinated, and the child can urinate at almost any degree of bladder fullness.

Training for bladder control needs to be a gradual process, starting when children are physically mature enough and have a desire to learn. Toddlers learn to control their urination, like their bowel movements (see Chapter 27), in response to their parents' approval. Trusting relationships developed between the child and the parents thus facilitate the motivation to succeed. Older siblings can also be an influence. A young child may see older children using the toilet and want to mimic their behavior or the siblings may laugh at the toddler's puddles on the floor. As young children become more active they also find wet clothing increasingly uncomfortable.

Praise should be offered when the child first shows awareness of having urinated. However, a period of time must pass before the child will indicate the need to void prior to urinating. Specific words will be used to communicate what is expected, such as "pee" or "wee-wee." When the child has been dry for a few hours, he or she needs to be put on the toilet. The ability to stay dry for this amount of time generally occurs at about 18 months of age. Parents who say their children are trained before this age have probably trained themselves to catch the child's urination at regular times. The child can be helped to keep dry during the day by observing the usual times of urination and by taking the child to the toilet at these times, for example, before or after meals, before or after naps, before or after going outside, and before bedtime. It is not necessary for the child to remain on the toilet longer than a few minutes. The bladder will empty relatively quickly, since it is just starting to fill up to near capacity.

Training pants during the day and suitable clothing also assist the child. Changing the pants when they are even slightly wet helps the child to become accustomed to being dry, and being out of diapers can make him or her feel more grown up. A sense of independence is achieved with the use of pull-down trousers that the child can manage alone. Steps to enable the child to climb up to the adult toilet and an attachable child's seat may be helpful. Little boys first learn to urinate sitting down and learn to stand up to urinate by watching other males. Thus the age at which boys stand to urinate varies with their contact with older males. Little girls may also want to urinate in the standing position but soon realize the problems this creates.

A casual, patient, matter-of-fact attitude is required by parents for bladder training their children. This skill is learned more slowly than bowel training, and it has periods of success alternating with periods of failure or accidents. Growing children are active and busy, and, although they may have learned the signals of a full bladder, these signs may go unnoticed during play until an accident occurs. They then generally run to their parents to tell them about it, an indication that some responsibility about urinating has been learned. Wetting may also occur when children are excited.

Each time a child urinates in the toilet or training chair, praise and cuddling should be given. When the child fails to do so, it is best not to display disapproval or disappointment, or the child may develop feelings of fear or inferiority.

Nighttime bladder control takes even more time than daytime control. It is recommended that this not be hurried. Some advise that the child's intake of fluids be restricted in the late afternoon and evening; however, the child may then cry of thirst during the night. Getting the child up to urinate between 2200 and 2400 hours may help, but it is not advised if the child is antagonized by being wakened or has long periods of sleeplessness following. Increasing maturity generally brings nighttime control. Even when the child has acquired good control, there normally may be lapses in control when the child is too fatigued or is suffering emotionally.

Assessment

Patterns of Urination

People's patterns of urination are highly individual. Most people take their normal pattern for granted, but they are quick to recognize any abnormalities; people who normally sleep through the night without the need to urinate are sharply aware when they must arise twice for that purpose. The pattern and frequency of micturition depends on many of the factors discussed in the next section.

Frequency

It is not unusual to void five or more times a day depending on individual habits and opportunities. Most people void about 70% of their daily urine during the waking hours and do not need to void during the night. People usually void when they first awake in the morning, before they go to bed, and around meal times. The urine voided upon wakening is the most concentrated urine excreted during the 24 hours.

Volume

The volume of urine excreted varies because of a number of factors, which are discussed next. See also Table 28–1, page 706. For an adult a volume of under 500 ml or over 3000 ml in a 24-hour period is unusual and needs to be reported.

Factors Influencing Urinary Habits

Each person has unique urinary habits. Many of these are learned in childhood, others are learned later in life. Toilet training often establishes attitudes toward urinary function. Parents who set rigid schedules often produce inflexible patterns in their children. Parents who convey distaste for or punish urinary incontinence by their children often help the children form rigid attitudes and beliefs about "good" or "bad" related to urinary function.

To assess the individual in relation to urinary function, the following areas need to be considered:

1. *Diet and fluid intake.* The amount and type of food are major factors that influence the output of urine. Some foods, such as beets, change the urine color to red. Other foods, in particular those containing protein and sodium, affect the amount of urine formed. Coffee, for example, increases urine formation.

The amount of fluid intake also affects the amount of fluid output. Fluid intakes much greater than the body's needs result in high fluid outputs.

2. *Response to the initial urge to void.* Some people habitually ignore the initial urge to void and void only later when the urge is stronger. As a result they retain urine in their bladders for a longer time and void a greater amount at a time. These people may have a larger than normal bladder capacity.

3. *Life-style.* Many facets of life-style affect a person's practices regarding urine elimination. The availability of toilet facilities or a bedpan can markedly affect frequency of elimination. A family's practices regarding elimination can also influence behavior. Children who are punished for bedwetting may, from fear, develop the habit of making several trips to the bathroom during the night, and this habit might carry through into adulthood. In some families time is taken to urinate when the urge occurs; in others it is usual to defer to a more convenient time. In some households privacy is provided and is important. For a person from such a family, urinating where there is not complete privacy can prove difficult and distressful.

4. *Psychologic stressors.* During a time of increased stress, individuals may perceive the need for increased frequency of urination. This may be due to increased sensitivity to the urge to void and/or to an increase in the amount of urine produced. Most people are familiar with the increased need to void just before an important date or before a school examination.

5. *Activity level.* Physical activity is necessary to maintain good muscle tone. The elimination of urine requires good bladder muscle tone as well as functioning internal and external sphincter muscles. Loss of bladder muscle tone occurs in people who have draining indwelling catheters for long periods of time. Because the urine is continually flowing out of the bladder, the bladder muscle is never stretched and can become nonfunctional.

Activity also affects the amount of urine produced by the kidneys. The greater the activity, the greater the body's metabolism and resulting urine production.

6. *Developmental level.* The level of growth and development also affects the pattern of urination. The development of bladder control was discussed earlier in this chapter. Table 28–1, page 706, provides guides to the average amount of urine produced according to age. In addition, pregnant women usually experience a change in pattern of urination. As the fetus grows in size, it places pressure on the bladder so that bladder capacity may be decreased and the urge to void is experienced more frequently.

7. *Pathologic conditions.* A wide variety of conditions can increase or decrease urination. Fever and heavy perspiration may decrease urine production because of the excessive loss of fluid via the skin. Inflammatory conditions and irritation of the urinary organs can promote retention of urine in the bladder.

8. *Medications.* Some medications can cause changes in the production of urine, in both amount and character. For example, diuretics increase urine output, whereas some analgesics cause urinary retention. Other medications cause urine to change in color.

Physical Assessment of the Urinary Tract

For a physical assessment of the urinary tract, the patient assumes a supine position and is draped appropriately. The kidneys and urinary bladder are usually palpated as part of the assessment of the abdomen. The urinary meatus is examined at the time the external genitals are assessed. The female patient assumes a lithotomy position for this part of the examination.

Kidneys

The upper lobes of both kidneys touch the diaphragm, and the kidneys descend upon inhalation. The right kidney is normally more easily palpated than the left because the right one lies a little lower than the left one. The right kidney lies in line with the 12th rib and the left kidney with the 11th rib. See Figure 28–5.

The adult kidney is normally smooth, solid, firm, and shaped like a lima bean. It is generally 11.4 cm (4.5 in) in length, 5 to 7.6 cm (2 to 3 in) in width, and 2.5 cm (1 in) in thickness. Kidneys are not usually tender unless an inflammatory process is present.

Palpation To palpate the right kidney, the nurse stands to the right of the supine patient and places the left hand under the patient's flank to elevate it. The right hand is put on the anterior abdominal wall at the midclavicular line and at the inferior edge of the costal margin. To palpate the left kidney, the nurse reaches

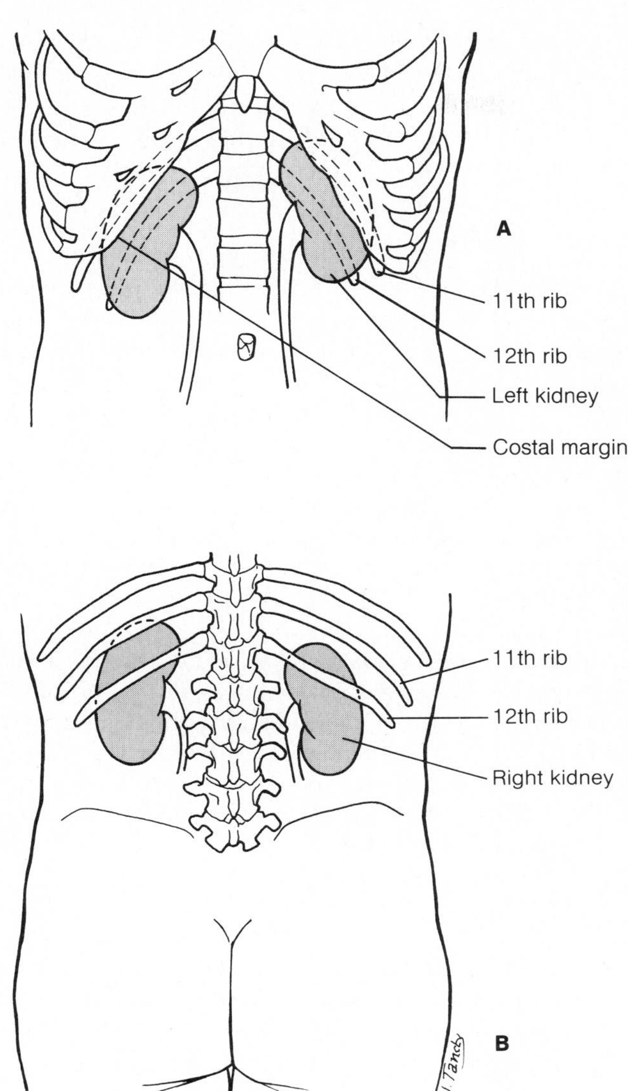

Figure 28–5 Location of the kidneys: **A,** anterior view; **B,** posterior view.

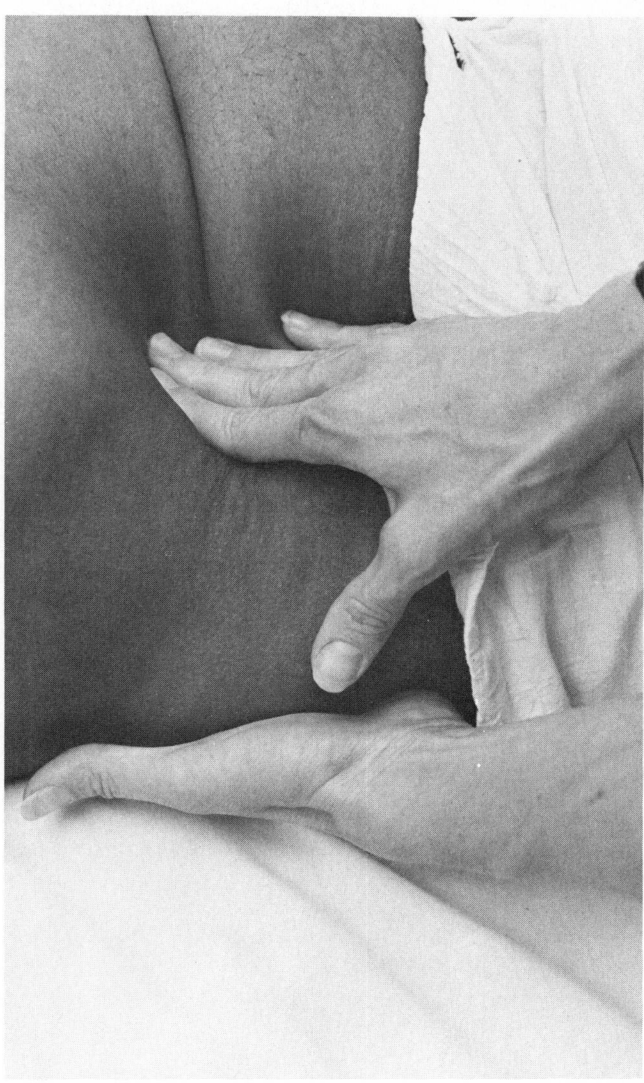

Figure 28–6 Palpating the right kidney. The patient is lying on the back. The nurse's left hand is under the patient's flank, while the right hand palpates the abdominal wall.

across the patient to place the left hand under the patient's flank. See Figure 28–6. As the patient inhales deeply, the nurse applies pressure with the right hand against the abdominal wall, pressing more deeply with each inhalation until maximum palpation depth is reached. When the patient inhales again the nurse palpates the kidney as it moves down. Normally the lower aspect of the right kidney is palpable but the left kidney may be palpable only in very thin people or those with poor abdominal musculature.

In some instances, it may be impossible to palpate the kidneys, particularly those of obese people or people with very firm abdominal muscles. If so, the nurse may try to "capture" the kidney: As the patient exhales, the nurse increases the pressure of both hands slightly, so as to hold the kidney; then the nurse releases it slowly and it slips upward as the patient continues exhalation.

The nurse checks the kidney for contour (shape), size, tenderness, and lumps. The examination is repeated for the left kidney.

Jarring the costovertebral angle If the kidney cannot be palpated, it may be possible to detect tenderness over the *costovertebral* angle (the angle formed by the 12th rib and the spine). The patient assumes a sitting position, and the nurse's left palm is

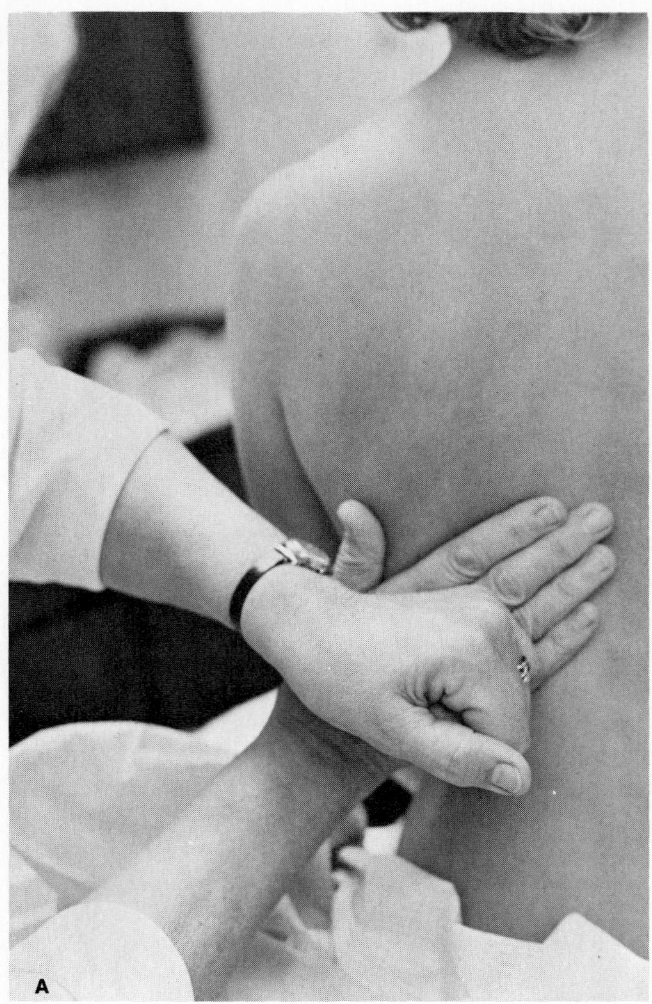

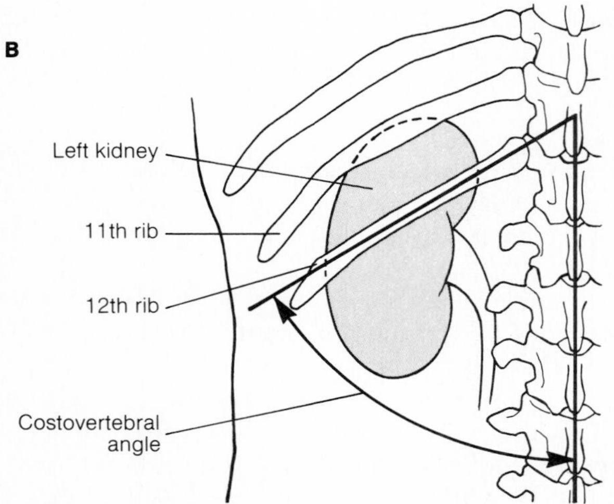

Figure 28–7 Assessing kidney tenderness over the left costovertebral angle: **A,** position of the nurse's hands; **B,** position of the kidney in relation to the costovertebral angle.

placed on the patient's back over the costovertebral angle. The nurse sharply strikes the back of that hand with the other fist. See Figure 28–7. Normally the patient will perceive a jar but not pain unless a kidney infection is present.

Urinary bladder

Normally the urinary bladder cannot be percussed or palpated when it is empty. When it is distended with urine, however, it can be both percussed and palpated. When it is greatly distended, swelling can be observed on the abdominal wall above the symphysis pubis.

Percussion The nurse percusses the area over the symphysis pubis. See Figure 5–8, page 131, for percussion technique. If the bladder is empty, the percussion sound will be tympanic (resonant); if it contains urine, the sound will be dull.

Palpation With one or two hands, the nurse palpates the area above the symphysis pubis. See Figure 28–8. When the bladder is distended, it can be felt as a smooth, firm mass. The edge of the bladder may extend as far as the umbilicus. The nurse measures in centimeters how far the upper edge of the bladder extends above the symphysis pubis.

Urethral orifice

In males, the urethral orifice is normally situated at the tip of the penis. In females, it is normally inferior to the clitoris and superior to the vaginal orifice. See Figure 28–12, on page 724. It is usually in the midline of the vestibule; however, in women who have had vaginal surgery, it may be to one side.

The nurse observes the area for the presence of ulcers, abnormal exudate, inflammation, and tumors. If any such condition is present, it is described, including size or amount, color, odor, and discomfort.

The urethral orifice is normally slitlike and the same color as the tissue surrounding it. There should be no discharge from this area, and the openings of the Skene's glands should not be visible unless they are infected. (*Skene's glands* are paraurethral glands that open into the urethra just within the external urinary meatus.)

Assessment of Urine

It is often a nursing function to perform certain tests on urine. Collecting urine specimens is discussed later in this chapter. Assessments are commonly made for color, odor, specific gravity, clarity, pH, protein, blood, glucose, ketone bodies, and other abnormal constituents. See Table 28–2 for the characteristics of normal urine.

Color

Normal urine is straw colored or amber colored. The latter is most likely early in the morning when it is most concentrated. The color of urine can be altered by certain drugs, such as phenazopyridine hydrochloride (Pyridium), which turns urine a dark orange color. Any abnormal color needs to be reported. Red, brown, or orange urine may be indicative of disease processes; red or brown may indicate the presence of blood in the urine.

Odor

Normal urine has a characteristic faint aromatic odor. A strong odor may be indicative of some problem, such as an infection, or the ingestion of certain medications.

Specific gravity

Specific gravity is the weight or degree of concentration of a substance compared with that of an equal volume of another, such as distilled water, taken as a standard. Specific gravity is a particularly important characteristic of urine, since an abnormal specific gravity can indicate kidney dysfunction. The specific gravity of distilled water is 1.00 g/ml (in other words, 1 ml of water weighs 1 gram). The normal range for specific gravity of urine is 1.010 to 1.025 (French 1980:27).

To measure specific gravity, a *hydrometer* is placed in a tube of urine. This instrument is made of glass and has a mercury bulb at the bottom and a specific gravity scale at the top. The amount of urine displaced measures its concentration in comparison to water. See Figure 28–9. The more concentrated the urine, the higher the instrument rises in it. The nurse then reads the scale at the level of the urine.

Table 28–2 Characteristics of Normal Urine

Factor	Normal characteristics
Color	Straw or amber; transparent
Odor	Faint aromatic
pH	4.5 to 7.5
Specific gravity	1.010 to 1.025
Amount (adult)	1200 to 1500 ml/day
Consistency	Clear liquid
Sterility	Free of microorganisms

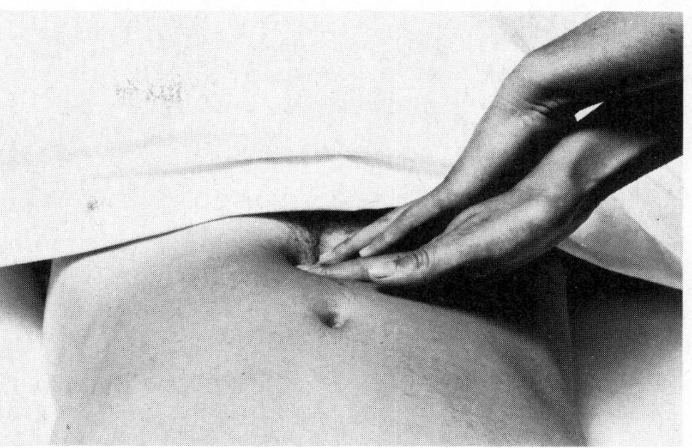

Figure 28–8 Palpating the bladder using two hands.

Figure 28–9 A hydrometer used to measure the specific gravity of urine.

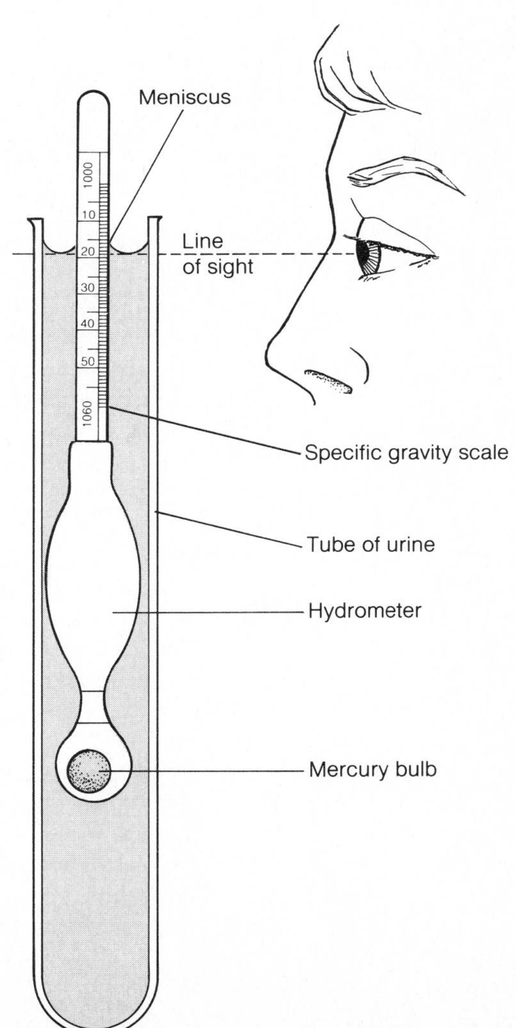

Clarity

Normal urine is clear or transparent. Urine may become cloudy due to the presence of mucus or pus.

pH

Normal urine is slightly acid, with a pH ranging from 4.5 (greater acidity) to 7.5 (lesser acidity). This can be tested by dipping a reagent paper, such as Nitrazine, in the urine. The paper stick will change color reflecting the pH. See Table 28-2 for normal values.

Urine that is left at room temperature for several hours will gradually become alkaline because of bacterial action. Vegetarians normally excrete a slightly alkaline urine.

Protein

The presence of protein in the urine, often albumin, can be tested with a reagent strip. Normally, large protein molecules such as albumin, fibrinogen, and globulin are not filtered through the kidneys into the urine. However, in cases of damaged kidneys, albumin, the smallest molecule of the three, can filter into the urine from the blood. The presence of protein in the urine is called *proteinuria*; the presence of albumin is referred to as *albuminuria*.

Blood

Blood in the urine may be clearly visible or not visible (occult). To test for bleeding, commercially available reagent strips (Hemastix) are dipped into the urine and their color change is compared to a color chart. The presence of blood in the urine is called *hematuria*.

Glucose

Normally, the amount of glucose in the urine is negligible, although if a person has recently ingested large amounts of sugar some glucose may be present. Glucose testing is usually done to detect diabetes mellitus or to follow the progress of a person known to have diabetes. The presence of glucose in the urine is called *glycosuria* or *glucosuria*.

There are a number of commercial products available to test for the presence of glucose. Commonly used are Clinitest tablets, Clinistix, Diastix, and Testape reagent strips. Each uses a color scale to measure the amount of glucose present. It is important to note that the scales of different products are not interchangeable. A freshly voided specimen is used, and often a second-voided specimen is required because it more closely reflects the current condition of the patient. Urine that has accumulated in the bladder (e.g., overnight) reflects the condition of the body at the time the urine was produced. Therefore, the nurse obtains a specimen from urine voided 30 minutes after the initial voiding.

The manufacturer's directions are followed for the test and the results are usually stated: negative, trace, one plus (1+ or +), two plus (2+ or ++), three plus (3+ or +++), etc. Each of these grades reflects a percentage of glucose, which varies from one product to another.

Ketone bodies

A test for the presence of ketone bodies is also referred to as testing for acetone. These ketone bodies are actually products of incomplete fat metabolism, and acetone is the most common ketone. They are present in the urine in instances of uncontrolled diabetes mellitus, starvation, and pernicious vomiting.

To test for ketone bodies, either (a) one or two drops of urine are placed on a reagent tablet (e.g., an Acetest tablet), or (b) a reagent test strip (e.g., Ketostix) is dipped into the urine. Color changes indicate the presence of the ketone bodies; there is a color chart for each product. The results are graded: negative, small, moderate, or large amounts of ketones; or negative, positive, or strongly positive.

Other abnormal constituents

Other abnormal constituents of urine include large amounts of mucus, crystals, pus (*pyuria*), epithelial cells, and red and white blood cells. A few of these in the urine may be normal, but large numbers are generally indicative of a pathologic process such as *calculi* (solidified masses of mineral salts or stones), tumors, and infections.

Tests for these constituents are usually made with a microscope. The urine is centrifuged to separate the sediment from the liquid. The sediment is placed on a slide and examined under a microscope. While these tests are usually carried out in a laboratory, nurses are frequently responsible for collecting the urine specimen. Collection of urine specimens is discussed later in this chapter.

Diagnostic Tests

A number of diagnostic tests and procedures are carried out to determine urinary tract pathology. Two blood tests commonly conducted to examine renal function are the blood urea nitrogen (BUN) clearance test and the creatinine clearance test. These measure how effectively the kidneys are excreting the respective substances. A normal range of BUN is 8 to 28 mg/100 ml of blood. The normal range for creatinine is 0.5 to 1.2 mg/100 ml of blood. A former blood test for kidney function was the nonprotein nitrogen (NPN) test. Nonprotein nitrogen compounds are small molecule crystaloids of body fluids. They are normally present in the blood at levels of 10 to 40 mg/100 ml of blood. This test has been largely replaced by more specific tests of the constituent compounds, such as creatinine, urea nitrogen, and uric acid.

Other diagnostic procedures involving the urinary tract include cystoscopy, intravenous pyelogram, and retrograde pyelogram. These are discussed in Chapter 38. X-ray films of the kidneys, ureters, and bladder (KUB) are also frequently taken to investigate the presence of tumors and distortions in the shapes of the organs.

Nursing Diagnoses

Common urinary problems are urinary retention, urinary incontinence, enuresis, and other altered urinary patterns such as frequency, urgency, polyuria, and urinary suppression. Examples of nursing diagnoses are included with the discussion of each problem in the sections that follow.

Common causes of these problems include: (a) obstruction, (b) abnormal tissue growth, (c) calculi, (d) infection, and (e) systemic problems.

An *obstruction* can occur almost anywhere in the urinary tract—the kidneys, ureters, bladder, or urethra. The cause of the obstruction can be abnormal cell growth (tumor), swelling as a result of an inflammatory process or local trauma, and calculi (stones), which are discussed later.

Abnormal tissue growth can also occur without producing an obstruction. A tumor of the bladder may, for example, occupy part of the bladder space and yet not impede the flow of urine.

Calculi are stones that form in the urine and may either be passed when voiding or lie in a space in the urinary system such as the kidney pelvis or the bladder. Occasionally a calculus may be lodged in a ureter, causing an obstruction.

An *infection* of the urinary tract may be secondary to one of the other problems mentioned or occur alone. An infection in any part of the urinary tract can readily spread to other parts because of the continuous mucous membrane lining of the tract.

Systemic problems such as heart disease and central nervous system disturbances can also present urinary problems. In particular, they can interfere with the formation and/or excretion of urine.

Retention

Urinary retention is the accumulation of urine in the bladder and inability of the bladder to empty itself. Because urine production continues, retention results in distention of the bladder. An adult urinary bladder normally holds 250 to 450 ml of urine when the micturition reflex is initiated. With urinary retention, some adult bladders may distend to hold 3000 to 4000 ml of urine.

Occasionally a patient will have *urinary retention with overflow*. In this situation, the bladder is holding urine, and only the overflow urine is excreted when the pressure of the urine becomes too great for sphincter control. The patient then voids small amounts of urine frequently or dribbles urine, while the bladder remains distended.

Retention can be identified by several clinical signs: discomfort in the pubic area, bladder distention, inability to void or frequent voiding of small volumes (25 to 50 ml), a disproportionately small amount of fluid output in relation to intake, and increasing restlessness and need to void. Bladder distention can be assessed by palpation and percussion above the symphysis pubis (see Figure 28–8, page 713).

There are several causes of urinary retention. It is often seen postoperatively, particularly in patients who have had surgery involving the lower abdomen, pelvis, bladder, and/or urethra. Retention is also commonly associated with urethral obstructive conditions such as an enlarged prostate gland that occludes the urethra. Urethral strictures and swelling of the urethral meatus and surrounding tissues from the trauma of childbirth can also produce urinary retention. Permanent retention problems may be caused by injuries to the spinal cord. Prolonged retention leads to *stasis* (a slowing of the flow of urine) and stagnation of urine, which increase the possibility of urinary tract infection.

Examples of nursing diagnoses for patients with urinary retention are:

1. Urinary retention related to enlarged prostate gland
2. Risk of urinary tract infection related to urinary stasis

Incontinence

Urinary incontinence is a temporary or permanent inability of the external sphincter muscles to control the flow of urine from the bladder. It is the opposite of retention. If the bladder is totally emptied during incontinence it is referred to as *complete incontinence*; if not totally emptied it is referred to as *partial incontinence* (e.g., dribbling).

Incontinence is commonly seen in elderly patients as part of the aging process. It is also seen in patients who have enlarged prostate glands, spinal cord injuries, urinary tract infections, bladder spasms, or loss of consciousness, or who are taking medications that interfere with sphincter control, e.g., narcotics and sedatives.

Two specific kinds of incontinence are distinguished:

1. *Stress incontinence* is the inability to control urine flow at a time when the intraabdominal pressure increases, for example, when coughing, sneezing, or even laughing. It is generally caused by inability of the external sphincter muscle to close. It is seen in children who have not learned to control the external sphincter and in adults who have a disease process interfering with the sphincter action.
2. *Urge incontinence* occurs when the patient's need to void is so urgent that he or she cannot get to the toilet in time. This kind of incontinence is commonly caused by lower urinary tract infections or bladder spasms.

Incontinence is physically and emotionally distressing to patients, because it is considered socially unacceptable. Often the patient is embarrassed about dribbling or about having an accident and may restrict normal activities for this reason. Emotional support and understanding need to be provided as well as measures to keep the patient dry and clean. Bed linens and clothes saturated with urine irritate and excoriate the skin. Prolonged skin dampness leads to *dermatitis* (inflammation of the skin) and subsequent decubitus ulcer formation.

Examples of nursing diagnoses for patients with urinary incontinence are:

1. Urinary incontinence related to spinal cord injury
2. Risk of skin breakdown related to irritating effects of urine
3. Embarrassment related to inability to control urine

Enuresis

Enuresis (bedwetting) occurs most often in children. When wetting occurs in a child over the age of 4, it generally occurs at night and is referred to as *nocturnal enuresis*. It may happen once or several times during the night. Some children may wet in the daytime during periods of excitement or when absorbed with play, particularly on cold, damp days. Still others may not yet have learned to be dry. In school-age children, wetting rarely occurs during the school hours but sometimes does occur during play hours at recess, during the lunch hour, or after school. Because of absorption in play, the child does not realize the need to urinate until it is too late to reach a toilet. It is estimated that 15% to 20% of school-age children are bedwetters, with a definite male predominance (de Castro et al. 1972:91).

Children who are bedwetters need understanding help. Generally, wetting is corrected relatively easily with the appropriate steps.

The most common cause of persistent bedwetting is too early and too vigorous training before the child is physiologically ready. As a result, enuresis may express an unconscious desire to regress and to receive the attention and care the child had when younger. It may also be an expression of resentment toward the parent.

Many other explanations for nocturnal enuresis have been proposed, and no doubt there are several causes or contributing factors in each individual situation. Some of these are:

1. The bladder capacity is smaller than normal.
2. The child is a sound sleeper, and signals from the bladder indicating the need to urinate go unnoticed until it is too late for the child to get out of bed and to the bathroom.
3. The bladder is irritable and thus unable to hold large quantities of urine.
4. An unpleasant emotional climate in the home results in a revenge type of enuresis for lack of love (for example, sibling rivalry and quarrelsome parents).
5. Parents who have the idea that the child will outgrow the habit without help do not train the child.
6. Infections of the urinary tract or physical or neurologic defects of the urinary system are causing enuresis.
7. Foods that are too rich in salts and minerals or spicy foods, such as pickles and relishes, are irritating the urinary system.
8. The child fears walking down a dark corridor to the bathroom at night.

Examples of nursing diagnoses for the child with enuresis are:

1. Enuresis related to insecurity
2. Feelings of rejection related to enuresis

Other Altered Urinary Patterns

Frequency

Frequency is generally considered voiding at frequent intervals, that is, more often than usual. Normally there is some increase in the frequency with which a person voids with an increase in fluids. Frequency without an increase in fluid intake may be the result of *cystitis* (an acutely inflamed bladder), stress, or pressure on the bladder, for example, because of pregnancy.

With frequency, the total amount of urine voided may be normal, since the amounts voided each time are small, such as 50 to 100 ml.

Nocturia or *nycturia* is increased frequency at night that is not a result of an increased fluid intake. Like frequency, it is usually expressed in terms of the number of times the person gets out of bed to void, for example, "nocturia × 4."

Examples of nursing diagnoses for the patient with frequency are:

1. Frequency related to cystitis
2. Risk of upper urinary tract infection related to cystitis

Urgency

Urgency is the feeling that the person *must* void. There may or may not be a great deal of urine in the bladder, but the person feels a need to void immediately. Often the person hurries to the toilet with the fear of being incontinent if he or she does not urinate. Urgency accompanies psychologic stress and irritation of the trigone and urethra. It is also common in young children who have poor external sphincter control.

Dysuria

Dysuria means either painful or difficult voiding. It can accompany a *stricture* (decrease in caliber) of the urethra, urinary infections, and injury to the bladder and/or urethra. Often patients will say that they have to push to void or that burning accompanies or follows voiding. Burning during micturition is often due to an irritated urethra; burning following urination may be the result of a bladder infection when the irritated rugae (ridges) of the trigone rub together. The burning may be described as severe, like a hot poker, or more subdued, like a sunburn.

Other signs that may accompany dysuria include *hesitancy* (delay and difficulty in initiating voiding), hematuria, pyuria and frequency.

Examples of nursing diagnoses for the patient with dysuria are:

1. Dysuria related to urethral infection
2. Risk of upper urinary tract infection related to urethral infection

Polyuria

Polyuria or *diuresis* refers to the production of abnormally large amounts of urine by the kidneys, such as 2500 ml/day, without an increased fluid intake. This can happen as a result of diabetes mellitus, hormone imbalances (e.g., deficiency of antidiuretic hormone, or ADH), and chronic kidney disease. Other signs often associated with diuresis are *polydipsia* (intense thirst), dehydration, and weight loss.

Examples of nursing diagnoses for the patient with polyuria are:

1. Polyuria related to diabetes insipidus (deficiency of ADH)
2. Risk of fluid and electrolyte imbalance related to ADH deficiency

Urinary suppression

Suppression is the sudden stoppage of urine production. Normally the kidneys produce urine continuously at the rate of 60 to 120 ml/hour (720 to 1440 ml/day) in the adult. Newborns need to start micturition within 24 to 36 hours after birth.

A situation in which the kidneys are producing no urine, or less than 100 ml/day, is *anuria*. The terms *complete kidney shutdown* or *renal failure* have the same meaning. *Oliguria* is the production of abnormally small amounts of urine by the kidneys, for example, 100 to 500 ml/day.

Both anuria and oliguria can occur as a result of kidney disease, severe heart failure, burns, and shock. These signs can be fatal if some other means, such as an artificial kidney, is not used to remove the body wastes.

Other critical signs of renal failure are the presence of uremic frost (urea crystals) on the skin, an elevated BUN, an aromatic odor to the skin, and signs of fluid and electrolyte imbalances (see Chapter 31).

Examples of nursing diagnoses for the patient with urinary suppression are:

1. Urinary suppression related to chronic kidney disease
2. Risk of elevated blood urea related to oliguria
3. Risk of fluid overload and peripheral and pulmonary edema related to oliguria
4. Risk of hyperkalemia (elevated serum potassium) related to oliguria

Planning and Intervention

The overall nursing goal for patients with potential or actual urinary elimination problems is to maintain or restore the patient's normal urinary elimination pattern. Nursing subgoals may include:

1. To provide an appropriate fluid intake
2. To ensure a balanced fluid intake and output
3. To prevent fluid and electrolyte imbalance
4. To prevent urinary tract infection or its recurrence

5. To prevent skin breakdown (in situations of incontinence)
6. To restore the patient's self-esteem or prevent emotional distress (in situations of incontinence)
7. For young children, to promote urinary control and self-esteem

Planning also involves the establishment of outcome criteria. For suggestions, see Evaluation later in this chapter.

General Measures

Appropriate fluid intake

Patients who have urinary problems often have their amount of daily fluid intake prescribed by the physician. The fluid may be taken orally or it may include intravenous fluids.

When patients have urinary infections, fluids are often increased. The adult patient usually needs an intake of 3000 to 4000 ml over a 24-hour period. The exact amount is frequently ordered by the physician or specified by agency policy. Occasionally fluids may be restricted, for example, when the kidneys are being rested or when a patient has a large amount of edema.

Measurement of fluid intake and output

If a male patient is able to go to the bathroom, he needs to void into a urinal rather than the toilet and then save the urine to be measured. For the female patient a bedpan is used instead of the toilet to collect the urine. Some agencies provide a collecting "hat" that fits into the toilet, for female patients to use.

Many patients can measure and record their own fluid intakes. For those who are unable to do so, it is important that the nurse record the intake volumes in milliliters accurately. See Measurement of Fluid Intake and Output in Chapter 30.

Assistance to maintain normal voiding patterns

Some patients need assistance to maintain their usual voiding habits. Nurses can help in a number of ways:

1. Assist the patient to his or her normal position for voiding. Male patients may find it easier to void when standing rather than sitting or lying down; standing at the side of the bed with a urinal may be helpful. A female patient may find it easier to void using a commode at the side of the bed, if feasible, rather than a bedpan in bed.
2. Provide privacy for the patient. Even children may be accustomed to privacy and may be unable to void in the presence of another person.
3. Provide any assistance required when the patient first feels the need to void. If the patient waits, the desire to void may pass, and difficulty starting to void can result.
4. If a bedpan or urinal is used, make sure that it is warm. A cold bedpan may prompt contraction of the perineal muscles of the female patient and inhibit voiding.
5. For patients using a bedpan, elevate the head of the bed to Fowler's position and place a small pillow or rolled towel at the small of the back to increase physical support and comfort.
6. Pour warm water over the perineum, if required, to encourage voiding. If the urine volume is to be measured, the amount of water to be poured must first be measured.
7. Turn on running water within hearing distance of the patient or provide water in which the patient's fingers can be dangled to encourage voiding.
8. Provide medications as necessary to relieve pain and foster muscle relaxation. Local application of heat to the perineum of a woman or a hot water bottle to the lower abdomen of both men and women may also foster muscle relaxation.
9. Place gentle downward pressure on the bladder as necessary to facilitate voiding.
10. Set aside sufficient time to help the patient.
11. Be reassuring to the patient and avoid producing anxiety. With emotional support, the patient is more likely to be relaxed and able to void.

Hygienic measures

Hygienic measures are taken to maintain the cleanliness of the genital area. Good hygiene is essential for two main reasons: to promote the patient's comfort and to prevent infection. A patient with a urinary tract problem may have a discharge or urine that has an unpleasant odor and that may be irritating to surrounding mucous membranes and skin. Normally the genital area is cleaned several times a day or more often if indicated. See Perineal and Genital Care in Chapter 21.

Keeping the genital area clean can also help to prevent microorganisms from entering the urinary meatus, which subsequently can cause a urinary infection. Because of the continuous mucous membrane lining, an infection of the urethra can extend into the kidney pelvis.

Assisting the Hospitalized Child to Urinate

Children who are hospitalized and separated from their parents may regress in their ability to control the bladder and may wet occasionally. On the child's admission to the hospital, the nurse records the child's stage of development and determines the methods of training that were or are being used. For example, the nurse finds out what equipment is being used, what words the child uses about urinating, and the times the child habitually urinates in the toilet each day. The child's customary methods of urinating should be continued in the hospital as much as possible. However, some children will have to use bedpans or urinals for a period of time. This equipment is best shown to the child in the parents' presence, with the hope that their approval will encourage the child to cooperate in using it.

Even children who are toilet trained have accidents. Children who wet accidentally in the hospital generally are upset and need understanding help and acceptance from the nurse. It is important that nurses examine their own feelings about children who wet or soil their beds or clothing. Feelings of repugnance need to be controlled.

If children are not toilet trained, it is advised that toilet training not be started while they are in the hospital, unless they are to have an extended stay. When young children are hospitalized, they feel abandoned by their parents and suffer enough emotional strain without adding the stress of toilet training. During a prolonged hospitalization, toilet training is planned and carried out by the parents and preferably by a nurse who is liked by the child.

A few children in the hospital use soiling as a means of gaining attention or getting even with their parents for abandoning them. In these instances the nurse needs to avoid censuring the child, accept this behavior in a matter-of-fact fashion, and determine the reason for the behavior. Together the nurse and the child need to work out a way to meet the child's love and attention needs more appropriately.

Bedpans and Urinals

Bedpans and urinals are receptacles used to collect urine and feces from patients who cannot go to the bathroom or whose urine output is to be measured. Bedpans are used for both urine and feces from female patients and for feces from male patients. Urinals are used for urine from male patients.

Bedpans are made of metal and of nylon resins. Stainless steel bedpans are frequently used today. Metal bedpans feel cold and therefore should be warmed under running warm water before being given to a patient. There are two basic types of bedpans, one that is about 5 cm (2 in) deep all around and one called a *slipper pan* or *fracture pan* that slips more easily under a patient because it is no deeper than 1.3 cm (0.5 in) at the upper end (the end that fits under the patient's sacrum).

It is easier for a patient to use a bedpan in bed if the head of the bed is slightly elevated, thus providing a more normal position in which to urinate. From this position it is also easier for the patient to lift himself or herself onto the pan. If for any reason this exertion is contraindicated, the nurse can assist by placing one hand under the patient's sacrum and using that arm as a lever. See Procedure 23-7 in Chapter 23. Some patients can help to lift themselves up by using a trapeze attached to a bar above the bed.

When providing a patient with a bedpan, the nurse need not expose the patient. Usually it is satisfactory just to turn back a corner of the top bedclothes and then slip the bedpan under the bedclothes and the patient. The bedpan is placed in such a manner that the curved smooth edge fits under the patient and the sharper edge is toward the foot of the bed.

After the bedpan is in place, the toilet paper is left near the patient and the signal cord is placed within reach. The patient is then left in privacy. When the patient signals that he or she is through with the bedpan, the nurse removes it. If patients cannot wipe themselves, the nurse needs to do this. For removing the bedpan, the patient raises the hips, and the nurse slips the pan out. If the patient is unable to raise the hips, he or she can roll to a lateral position away from the nurse, while the nurse holds the bedpan. The patient is then in a suitable position for wiping and cleaning, if required. The toilet paper roll is put away, and the patient is provided with a moistened cloth to wipe the hands.

For male patients a urinal is easier to use than a bedpan. Often a sitting position facilitates its use; the patient may sit or stand at the side of the bed if this is possible.

For female patients who are in body casts and completely unable to move, some agencies have female urinals. These fit against the female perineum, permitting the patient to urinate without moving.

If a patient is able to use a bathroom, the nurse must make sure that the patient is safe. Often patients feel well enough while in bed to walk to the bathroom, but after getting up they do not feel as strong as they believed they were. If the patient is weak or at all unsteady, he or she is walked by the nurse to the bathroom and assisted to the toilet. Often the nurse remains just outside the bathroom and reenters when the patient indicates readiness to return to bed.

The frequency with which a bedpan or urinal needs to be offered depends on the individual patient and the situation. Nurses need to offer a bedpan often enough to prevent problems for the patient such as discomfort or bedwetting. Because these are uncomfortable and embarrassing to patients, some may make extraordinary efforts to get to the bathroom even though this is contraindicated by their conditions. Most nurses can recall at least one incident of the "weak little old lady who climbed over the bedside rails to go to the bathroom and then climbed back"!

Measures for Specific Urinary Problems

Retention

Measures that assist the patient to maintain a normal voiding pattern, discussed on page 718, are applicable when dealing with urinary retention. If retention occurs postoperatively, ensure that prescribed analgesics are given as directed. Voiding difficulties often occur because of pain in the incision area. Urinary catheterization (see page 721) or administration of bethanecol chloride (Urecholine) may be necessary as directed if measures to facilitate voiding fail. Bethanecol chloride is a parasympathomimetic agent that stimulates micturition.

Incontinence

The following bladder training program can be used to reduce the problem of incontinence:

1. Establish a regular voiding schedule and help the patient to maintain it, for example, every 1 or 2 hours, whether feeling the urge or not. Often when the patient finds that voiding can be controlled this way, the intervals between voiding can be lengthened slightly without loss of continence. The stretching-relaxing sequence of such a schedule tends to increase bladder muscle tone and promote more voluntary control.
2. Regulate fluid intake, particularly before the patient retires, to reduce the need to void during the night. Fluids may be encouraged about half an hour before the voiding time, while at other times they are carefully regulated. Large amounts of fruit juices and carbonated beverages are avoided, since they alkalize the urine and cause bladder irritation respectively. A sufficient daily fluid intake (at least 2000 ml) is essential.
3. Increase physical activity, to improve muscle tone and blood circulation, thus helping the patient to control voiding.
4. Make sure that toilets and bedpans are within reach. Being able to get to a bedpan or toilet quickly helps the incontinent patient gradually gain control and develop confidence in the ability to control voiding.
5. Encourage perineal exercises, to increase the tone of muscles concerned with micturition, in particular the perineal and abdominal muscles. Periodic tightening of the perineal muscles and intentionally stopping and restarting of the urine stream can also assist a patient in gaining voiding control.
6. As a protective measure, apply protector pads to keep the bed linen dry and provide specially made waterproof underwear to contain the urine and decrease the patient's embarrassment. These need to be changed whenever wet to keep the skin dry. Clean and dry the skin at changing time to prevent skin breakdown.
7. For patients who have *bladder flaccidity* (weak, soft, and lax bladder muscles), manual exertion of pressure on the bladder may be necessary to force urine out. This is known as *Credé's maneuver* or *method.* It is not advised without the order of a physician and is used only for patients who have lost and are not expected to regain voluntary bladder control. For patients who are expected to regain control, this maneuver does not promote increased bladder muscle tone and may cause damage to the urethral sphincters.
8. For ambulatory or bedridden male patients whose incontinence cannot be controlled, application of a condom and catheter to the penis permits collection of the urine in a bag. See page 731.

Enuresis

The complexity of enuresis is obvious; therefore a comprehensive history with physical and psychologic assessment is warranted in determining the cause. The child's feelings about bedwetting need to be explored carefully. Some may think they have a weak bladder and feel totally disinterested in seeking control. Others may be interested in their problem but feel utterly hopeless about it and react by fearing to go to sleep. Professional counseling may be necessary, and a referral by the physician is then indicated.

A *urinalysis* (physical, chemical, or microscopic examination of urine) is usually performed initially, and subsequent tests, such as culture and sensitivity, are often carried out. Other urologic examinations are done when abnormalities are found, to rule out infection or structural problems. In the majority of situations the cause is psychologic; thus the goal of therapy is to help the child and family find a comfortable way to cope with the situation.

Some practical methods include: providing a waterproof pad on the bed to prevent soiling of the mattress and prevent worry and conflict for both parents and child; restricting fluids at bedtime, and arranging a time for the child to be awakened to urinate. These methods frequently achieve the best results when the child is involved in the plans and encouraged to assume some responsibility for them. It is recommended that no punishment be imposed. Praise for success is the most effective reward. If something is upsetting the child emotionally, such as a change to a new neighborhood or excessive expectations from the parents about manners or neatness, this needs to be considered. It is important to convey to the child the idea that he or she can be helped.

Other therapies include a conditioning program to increase the child's bladder capacity. This is accomplished by increasing the child's fluid intake during the daytime and then encouraging the child to suppress the desire to void for as long as possible. Sometimes medications such as tranquilizers or belladonna derivatives are prescribed, although their effectiveness is questionable. In many situations, continued family counseling is warranted.

Frequency, urgency, and dysuria

A comprehensive history that includes physical and psychologic assessment is required to determine the cause of the problem and plan appropriate interventions. If the cause is stress, for example, relaxation techniques may be implemented to help the patient cope with or prevent stressful situations. The most common cause is lower urinary tract infection, and measures to reduce the bacterial infection are implemented. Such measures may include:

1. *Increased fluid intake.* Adequate hydration promotes dilution of infected urine and its subsequent removal by frequent emptying of the bladder. Fluid intake and output are monitored.
2. *Instruction about perineal hygiene.* Female patients are particularly prone to bladder infections because the female urethra is short and in close proximity to the vagina and the anus. Bacteria from the anus or vagina migrate to the periurethral area and ascend through the urethra to the bladder. Females therefore need instruction about careful cleaning of the perianal region with soap and water after defecation and after intercourse.
3. *Control of the urinary pH.* Normally urine is slightly acid. By changing the composition of the diet the urine can be made either acid or alkaline. Most vegetables and fruits yield an alkaline urine, while meat, fish, fowl, eggs, and cereals yield an acid urine. Alkalinization of the urine may be warranted to soothe an irritated bladder. Acidification of the urine may be required to inhibit the growth of certain bacteria.
4. *Hot sitz baths.* Sitz baths may be particularly helpful in relieving discomfort associated with *urethritis* (inflammation of the urethra).
5. *Administration of medications as directed.* Urinary tract infections may be treated with antimicrobials (e.g., antibiotics or sulfonamides), antispasmodics (e.g., atropine), or urinary analgesics (e.g., phenazopyridine hydrochloride).

Polyuria

Measures to correct polyuria depend largely on the cause. If the cause is a deficiency of antidiuretic hormone, this hormone may be administered as directed, intramuscularly or topically as a nasal spray. If the cause is diabetes mellitus, insulin may be required. Nursing interventions are directed largely to monitoring the patient's fluid intake and output, ensuring an adequate fluid intake, assessing for signs of fluid or electrolyte loss (see Chapter 31), and instructing the patient about the medications.

Urinary suppression

Urinary suppression is a serious problem with life-threatening consequences. The nursing intervention is complex and beyond the scope of this book.

Urinary Catheterization

Urinary catheterization is the introduction of a tube (a *catheter*) through the urethra into the urinary bladder. This is usually performed only when absolutely necessary, since certain hazards are involved. Because the urinary structures are normally sterile except at the end of the urethra, the danger exists of introducing microorganisms into the bladder. This hazard is greatest for patients who have lowered resistance due to disease processes. Once an infection is introduced into the bladder, it can ascend the ureters and eventually involve the kidneys. Even after the catheter has been inserted and left in place for a time, the hazard of infection remains, since pathogens can be introduced through the catheter lumen. Thus, strict sterile technique is used for catheterizations.

Another hazard is trauma, particularly in the male patient, whose urethra is longer and more tortuous. It is important to insert a catheter along the normal contour of the urethra. Damage to the urethra can occur if the catheter is forced through strictures or at an incorrect angle. For females, the urethra lies posteriorly, then takes a slightly anterior direction toward the bladder. See Figure 28-10. For males, the urethra is normally curved (see Figure 28-3 on page 708), but it can be straightened by elevating the penis to a position perpendicular to the body.

Types of Catheters

Catheters are commonly made of rubber or plastic. Some agencies have catheters made of woven silk or metal. Catheters are often categorized as straight catheters or retention (Foley) catheters. The straight catheter is a single-lumen tube with a small eye or opening

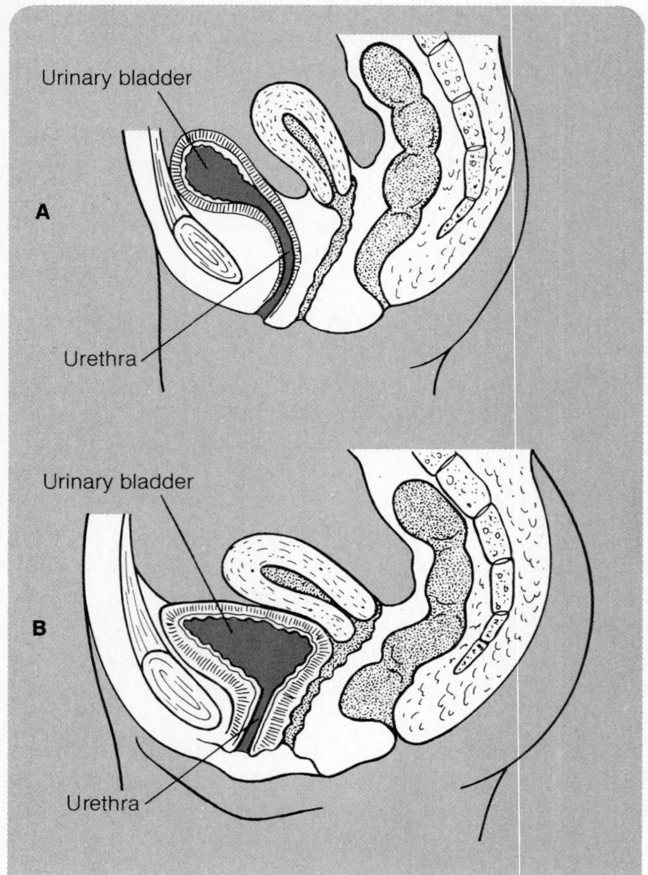

Figure 28–10 Position of the female bladder and urethra: **A,** in a young child; **B,** in an adult. Note how the angle of the urethra changes.

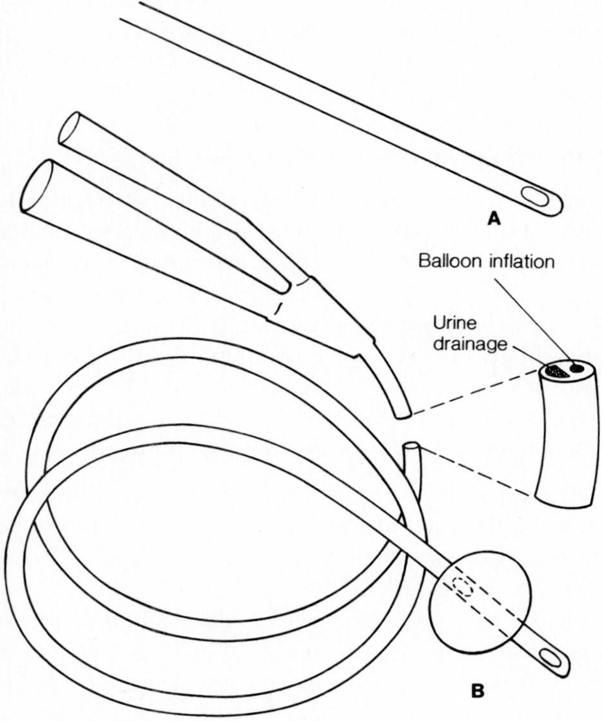

Figure 28–11 **A,** a straight catheter; **B,** a two-way Foley (retention) catheter.

about 1.3 cm (0.5 in) from the insertion tip. The retention catheter contains a second, smaller tube throughout its length on the inside. This tube connects to an inflatable balloon near the insertion tip. After insertion, the balloon is inflated and holds the tube in place within the bladder. The opposite end of the retention catheter is bifurcated, that is, it has two openings, one to drain the urine, the other to inflate the balloon. See Figure 28–11.

The size of a catheter is the diameter of the lumen, which is graded according to a French scale of numbers; the larger the number, the larger the lumen. For children, small sizes are used, such as # 8 or # 10. For adults, # 14, # 16, and # 18 are commonly used. Only even numbers are available.

Purposes of Catheterization

Patients are catheterized for a variety of reasons:

1. To obtain a sterile urine specimen for diagnostic reasons
2. To measure the amount of *residual urine* (the amount of urine remaining in the bladder after voiding) when the bladder is being incompletely emptied
3. To empty the bladder prior to surgery involving adjacent organs, such as the rectum or vagina, to prevent inadvertent injury to the bladder
4. To prevent bladder distention postoperatively or to provide gradual decompression of an overdistended bladder when all other measures to facilitate voiding have failed
5. To manage incontinence when all other measures to prevent skin breakdown have failed
6. To provide for intermittent or continuous bladder drainage and irrigation
7. To prevent urine from contacting an incision after perineal surgery

A straight or single-lumen catheter is usually used, except for purposes 4–7 above or as ordered by the physician.

Procedure 28–1 Female Urinary Catheterization

Goals

1. To relieve discomfort due to bladder distention and to provide gradual decompression of an overdistended bladder
2. To assess the amount of residual urine if the bladder is emptied incompletely
3. To obtain a urine specimen to assess the presence of abnormal constituents and the characteristics of the urine
4. To empty the bladder completely prior to surgery, so as to prevent inadvertent injury to adjacent organs such as the rectum or vagina

Equipment

1. A sterile catheterization kit containing:
   - **a.** Gloves.
   - **b.** Drapes to protect the bed and to provide a sterile field.
   - **c.** A fenestrated drape (optional) to place over the perineum.
   - **d.** An antiseptic solution recommended by agency policy, e.g., aqueous benzalkonium chloride (Zephiran Chloride) 1:750, to clean the labia and the urinary meatus.
   - **e.** Cotton balls or gauze squares to apply the antiseptic.
   - **f.** Forceps to apply the antiseptic.
   - **g.** A water-soluble lubricant to lubricate the insertion tip of the catheter for easy insertion and to reduce the chance of trauma to the mucous membrane lining the urethra.
   - **h.** A catheter of appropriate size (see page 722).
   - **i.** A receptacle for the urine. Often the base of the kit serves this purpose.
   - **j.** A specimen container if a specimen is to be acquired.
2. A bag or receptacle for disposal of the cotton balls
3. A flashlight or lamp to provide light on the genital area
4. A mask, clean gown, and cap, if required by agency policy

Preparation

1. Obtain assistance if the patient requires help to maintain the required position.
2. Explain the technique to the patient and provide support as needed. Some patients fear pain and need to learn that they will experience no pain, only a slight sensation of pressure.
3. Provide privacy. Exposure of the genitals is embarrassing to most patients. Relieving the patient's tension can facilitate insertion of the catheter, because the urinary sphincters are more likely to be relaxed.
4. Assist the patient to a supine position with knees flexed and thighs externally rotated. Pillows can be used to support the knees and elevate the buttocks. Raising the patient's pelvis gives the nurse a better view of the urinary meatus.
5. Drape the patient. Use a bath blanket to cover the patient's chest and abdomen. Pull the patient's gown up over her hips. Cover her legs and feet with the bed sheet or another blanket. Place it diagonally on the patient with a corner around each foot.
6. Wash the perineal-genital area with warm water and soap; rinse and dry. Disposable gloves may be used. Cleanliness reduces the possibility of introducing microorganisms with the catheter. Appropriate rinsing removes soap that could inhibit the action of the antiseptic used later.
7. Adjust the light for vision of the urinary meatus. It may be necessary to use a flashlight or to place a gooseneck lamp at the foot of the bed so that it focuses on the perineal area.
8. Put on a mask if required by agency policy. Some agencies also advocate the use of a clean gown and a surgical cap if the nurse's hair is long.
9. Wash hands using a surgical aseptic wash. This is done before the sterile equipment is opened.

Intervention

1. Open the sterile kit at the patient's bedside and don the sterile gloves (see Chapter 20, page 477). The kit can be placed between the patient's thighs.
2. Drape the patient with the sterile drapes, being careful to protect the sterility of your gloves. Use the first drape as an underpad and place it under the buttocks. Keep the underpad edges cuffed over your gloves to prevent contamina-

Procedure 28–1, continued

tion of the gloves against the patient's buttocks. If the other drape is fenestrated, place it over the perineal area exposing only the labia. Place thigh drapes from the side farthest to the side nearest you. If an underpad is not available, place the two thigh drapes so that they overlap between the patient's thighs.

3. Pour the antiseptic solution over the cotton balls, if they are not already prepared.

4. Lubricate the insertion tip of the catheter liberally. Place it aside in the sterile container ready for use.

   Rationale Water-soluble lubricant facilitates insertion of the catheter by reducing friction. It is important to lubricate at this point, because the nurse will subsequently have only one sterile hand available.

5. Clean the labia majora on each side using forceps and cotton balls or swabs. Use a swab only once, and move downward from the pubic area to the anus.

   Rationale This cleans from the area of least contamination to the area of greatest contamination.

6. Separate the labia majora with the thumb and fourth finger and clean the labia minora on each side. Then separate the labia minora with the index and middle fingers, still using the same hand.

   Rationale The hand that touches the patient becomes contaminated. It remains in position exposing the urinary meatus while the other hand remains sterile holding the sterile forceps.

7. Expose the urinary meatus and clean first from the meatus downward and then on either side. Be sure to expose the urinary meatus adequately by retracting the tissue of the labia minora in an upward (anterior) direction. See Figure 28–12. Once the meatus is cleaned, do not allow the labia to close over it.

   Rationale Keeping the labia apart prevents the risk of contaminating the urinary meatus.

8. Place the drainage end of the catheter in the urine receptacle. Then pick up the insertion end of the catheter with your uncontaminated, sterile, gloved hand, holding it approximately 5 to 8 cm (2 to 3 in) from the insertion tip for an adult and 2 to 3 cm (1 in) for a baby or small child. If agency policy requires, use forceps to pick up the catheter.

   Rationale The adult female urethra is approximately 4 cm (1.5 in) long. The nurse holds the catheter far enough from the end to allow full insertion into the bladder and to maintain control of the tip of the catheter so it will not accidentally become contaminated.

9. Gently insert the catheter into the urinary meatus about 5 cm (2 in) for an adult, 2.5 cm (1 in) for a small child, or until urine flows. Insert the catheter in the direction of the urethra. If the catheter meets resistance during insertion, do not force it. Ask the patient to take deep breaths. If this does not relieve the resistance, discontinue the procedure, and report the problem to the responsible nurse. Exercise caution to prevent the catheter tip from be-

Figure 28–12

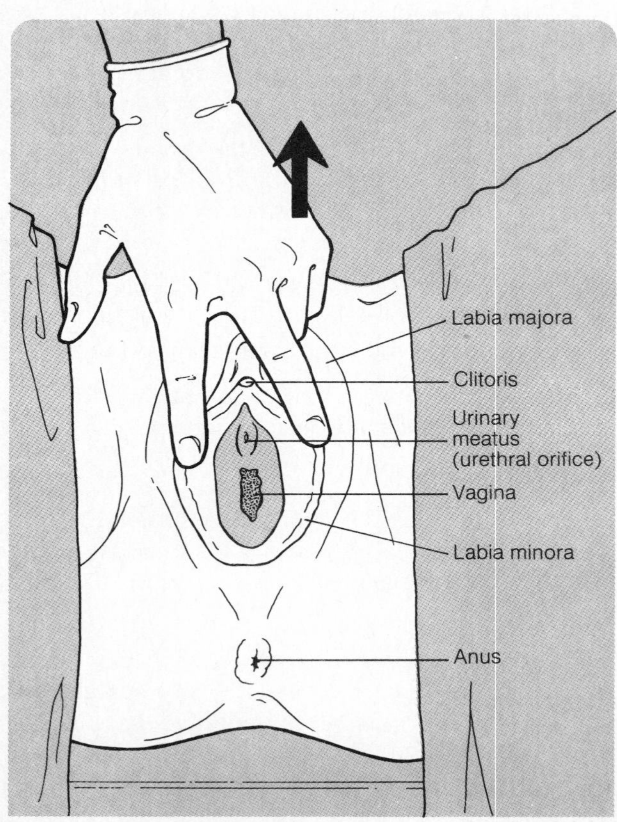

Procedure 28–1, continued

coming contaminated. If it becomes contaminated, discard it.

Rationale Forceful pressure exerted against the urethra can produce trauma. Deep breaths by the patient may relax the external sphincter.

10. When the urine flows, transfer your hand from the labia to the catheter to hold it in place at the meatus.

11. Collect a urine specimen, if required, after the urine has flowed for a few seconds. Pinch the catheter before transferring the drainage end of it into the sterile specimen bottle. Usually 30 ml of urine is sufficient for a specimen.

12. Empty the bladder and remove the catheter slowly. For adult patients experiencing urinary retention, it is recommended that no more than 750 ml be removed at one time.

    Rationale Removing large amounts of urine too quickly can induce engorgement of the pelvic blood vessels and hypovolemic shock. Usually the physician prescribes the amount to be removed and times at which the remaining urine is to be withdrawn.

13. Dry the patient's perineum with a towel or drape.

14. Remove the equipment. Assist the patient to a comfortable position, and leave the room in order.

15. Record the reason for catheterization and any other pertinent observations, such as the color and amount of the urine.

16. Send the specimen to the laboratory.

Procedure 28–2 Male Urinary Catheterization

Goals

See Procedure 28–1 on page 723.

Equipment

See Procedure 28–1 on page 723. A #16 or #18 catheter is usually used for an adult.

Preparation

1. Follow Procedure 28–1, steps 1–3.

2. Assist the patient to a supine position with the knees slightly flexed and the thighs slightly apart. This allows greater relaxation of the abdominal and perineal muscles and permits easier insertion of the catheter.

3. Drape the patient by folding the top bedclothes down so that the penis is exposed and the thighs are covered. Use a bath blanket to cover the patient's chest and abdomen.

4. Follow Procedure 28–1, steps 6–9.

Intervention

1. Open the sterile tray and don the sterile gloves (see Chapter 20, page 477). Place the tray directly on the patient's thighs, if he is not restless.

2. Place a drape under the penis and a second drape above the penis over the pubic area. If a fenestrated drape is available, place it over the penis and pubic area, exposing only the penis.

3. Pour the antiseptic solution over the cotton balls if they are not already prepared.

4. Lubricate the insertion tip of the catheter liberally for about 5 to 7 cm (2 to 3 in). Place it aside on the sterile tray ready for insertion.

   Rationale Water-soluble lubricant facilitates insertion of the catheter by reducing friction. It is important to do this step before cleaning, since the nurse will subsequently have only one sterile hand available.

5. Clean the meatus by grasping the penis firmly behind the glans and spreading the urinary meatus between the thumb and forefinger. Retract the foreskin of an uncircumcised male. Clean the meatus first, and then wipe the tissue surrounding the meatus in a circular fashion.

Procedure 28–2, continued

Use forceps to hold the swabs, and discard each swab after only one wipe.

Rationale To avoid stimulating an erection, firm pressure rather than light pressure is used to grasp the penis. The gloved hand holding the penis is now considered contaminated. Using forceps in the other hand maintains the sterility of the nurse's glove.

6. Place the drainage end of the catheter in the urine receptacle. Then pick up the insertion end of the catheter with the uncontaminated, sterile, gloved hand, holding it about 8 to 10 cm (3 to 4 in) from the insertion tip for an adult or about 2.5 cm (1 in) for a baby or small boy. In some agencies the catheter is picked up with forceps.

Rationale The male urethra is approximately 20 cm (8 in) long. The nurse holds the catheter far enough from the end to maintain control of the tip of the catheter so it will not accidentally become contaminated.

Figure 28–13

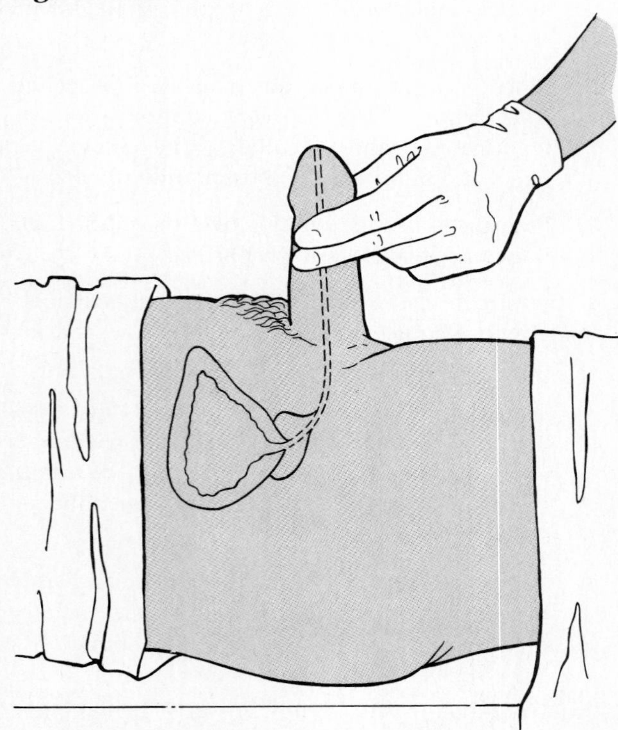

7. To insert the catheter, lift the penis to a position perpendicular to the body (90° angle) and exert slight traction (pulling or tension). See Figure 28–13. Insert the catheter steadily about 20 cm (8 in) or until urine begins to flow. To bypass slight resistance at the sphincters, twist the catheter or wait until the sphincter relaxes. Have the patient take deep breaths or try to void. If difficult resistance is met, discontinue the procedure and report the problem to the responsible nurse.

Rationale Lifting the penis to a position perpendicular to the body straightens the downward curvature of the cavernous urethra. Slight resistance is normally encountered at the external and internal urethral sphincters. Taking deep breaths can help to relax the external sphincter. Forceful pressure exerted against a major resistance can traumatize the urethra.

8. While the urine flows, lower the penis and transfer your hand to hold the catheter in place at the meatus.

9. Collect a urine specimen (if required) after the urine has flowed for a few seconds. Pinch the catheter before transferring the drainage end of the catheter into the sterile specimen bottle. Usually 30 ml of urine is sufficient for a specimen.

10. Empty the bladder and remove the catheter slowly. For adult patients experiencing urinary retention, it is recommended that no more than 750 ml be removed at one time.

Rationale Removing larger amounts of urine too quickly can induce engorgement of the pelvic blood vessels and hypovolemic shock. Usually the physician prescribes the amount to be removed and times at which the remaining urine is to be withdrawn.

11. Dry the patient's penis with a towel or drape.

12. Follow Procedure 28–1, steps 14–16.

Catheterization of Infants and Children

Catheterization is rarely performed on young children because of the danger of introducing an infection. When catheterization is necessary, the presence of a second nurse is recommended to restrain and support the very young child or to support the cooperative older child. The procedure is almost identical to that described for the adult except that a small catheter size is used, such as #8 or #10. One other difference relates to the position of the bladder: In the infant it is located more anteriorly and higher than in the adult, as shown in Figure 28–10, *A*, on page 722. Note the C-shaped curve of the urethra. During the first 3 years of life the bladder descends relatively rapidly and then changes position gradually until the adult position is reached in late adolescence. Thus, for a female infant, the catheter should be directed posteriorly on insertion even more than it is for an adult female.

Retention Catheterization

Insertion

An indwelling or retention catheter is used when the catheter is to remain in place for a period of time. Commonly the Foley catheter is used. Insertion of a retention catheter differs from the basic catheterization technique only after the catheter is inserted.

Equipment In addition to the equipment used for a straight catheterization, the following equipment is needed:

1. A retention catheter, size #16 or #18 for an adult, with a 5 ml balloon unless a larger size is ordered by the physician or has been used previously. Balloon sizes vary from 5 to 30 ml and are indicated in writing on each catheter along with the French size, for example, "Foley #14, 5 ml."
2. A 10 ml syringe with an adapter or needle, to inflate the balloon.
3. Sterile water or sterile normal saline, to inflate the balloon.
4. A drainage bag and tubing to collect the urine.
5. Adhesive tape to attach the tubing to the female patient's thigh or the male patient's abdomen.

Some disposable retention catheter sets include all of the necessary equipment; others do not include the drainage bag and tubing. Agency equipment thus needs to be checked when preparing for this procedure.

Testing the balloon Before inserting a retention catheter it is important to test the balloon. This is done using sterile technique. The nurse fills the syringe with the prescribed amount of sterile water or normal saline, injects it into the lumen of the catheter that fills the balloon, and leaves it in for a few seconds. If a leak is present, another catheter is selected and tested. When the nurse is assured that there is no leak, the fluid is withdrawn, the catheter is detached from the syringe, and the syringe is set aside on the sterile tray ready for use after the catheter is inserted. Whether an adapter or a needle is attached to the syringe to inflate the balloon depends upon the design of the catheter. Some have a self-sealing inlet so that a needle can be used; others need an adapter and then must be clamped or clipped in some manner.

Inflating the balloon After the catheter is inserted and the bladder has been emptied of urine (not exceeding 750 ml), the balloon is inflated in the bladder. Because the balloon is located behind the opening at the insertion tip, it is important to insert the catheter an additional 2.5 cm (1 in) after first obtaining urine. This ensures that the balloon is inflated in the bladder and not in the urethra. See Figure 28–14. If the patient complains of discomfort or pain during the balloon inflation, the nurse should withdraw the balloon fluid, insert the catheter a little further into the bladder, and then again inflate the balloon. After the balloon is safely inflated in the patient's bladder, the nurse applies slight tension on the catheter to ensure that it is anchored well in the bladder.

Establishing the drainage system Urinary drainage systems may be open or closed. The *open drainage system* is one that can be disconnected or opened between the catheter and tubing and between the tubing and the drainage bag. This system is becoming obsolete because of the danger of introducing pathogenic microorganisms and causing a urinary tract infection when the system is opened. As a result, the *closed drainage system* is now preferred. It is a continuous, sterile system including a disposable catheter, tubing, and a drainage bag that cannot be separated at any point. Some of these are equipped with special air filters in the drainage bag that allow the air to escape but prevent the entrance of microorganisms.

Urinary drainage systems for indwelling catheters operate on the principle of gravity and are often referred to as *straight drainages*. Commonly, disposable clear plastic equipment is used, but rubber tubing and a glass drainage bottle with a rubber stopper that allows air to escape can suffice. The drainage receptacle must always be kept below the level of the patient's bladder so that urine can flow with gravity and is prevented from flowing back to the bladder. When the patient is in bed, the receptacle is usually attached to the lower side of the bed, not to a side rail (see Figure 28–15); when the patient is ambulating, it is carried below hip level or

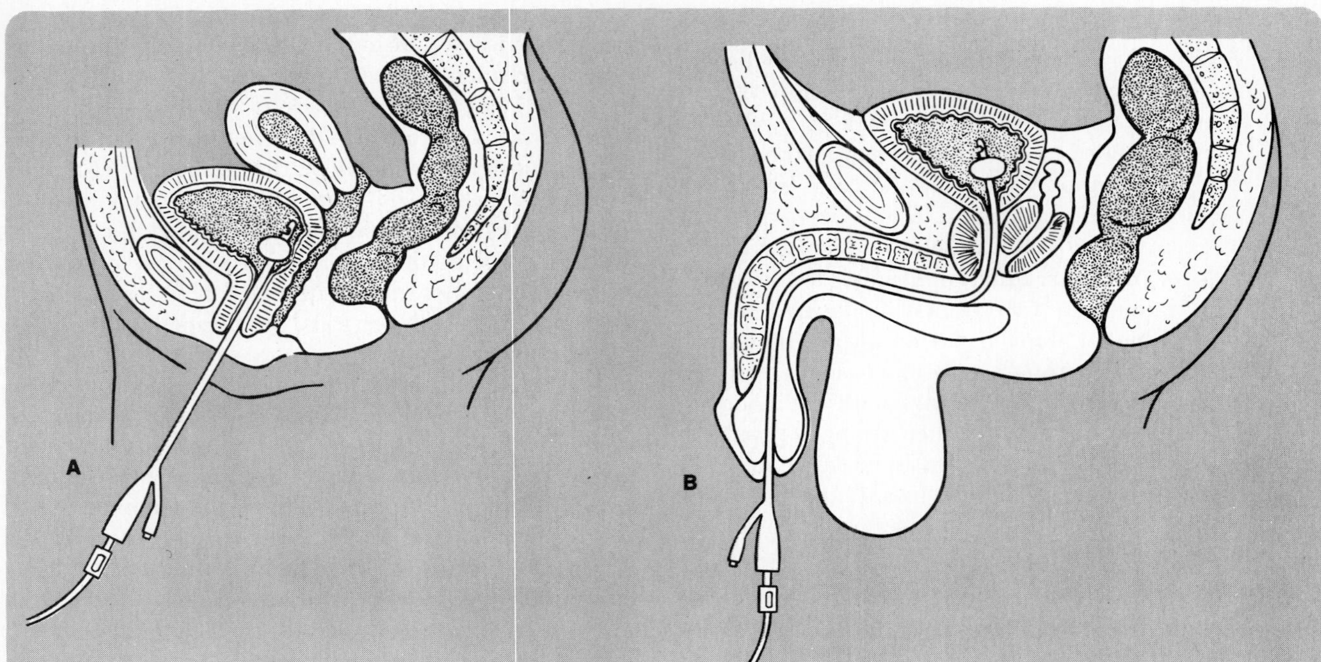

Figure 28–14 Retention catheters in place: **A,** female; **B,** male.

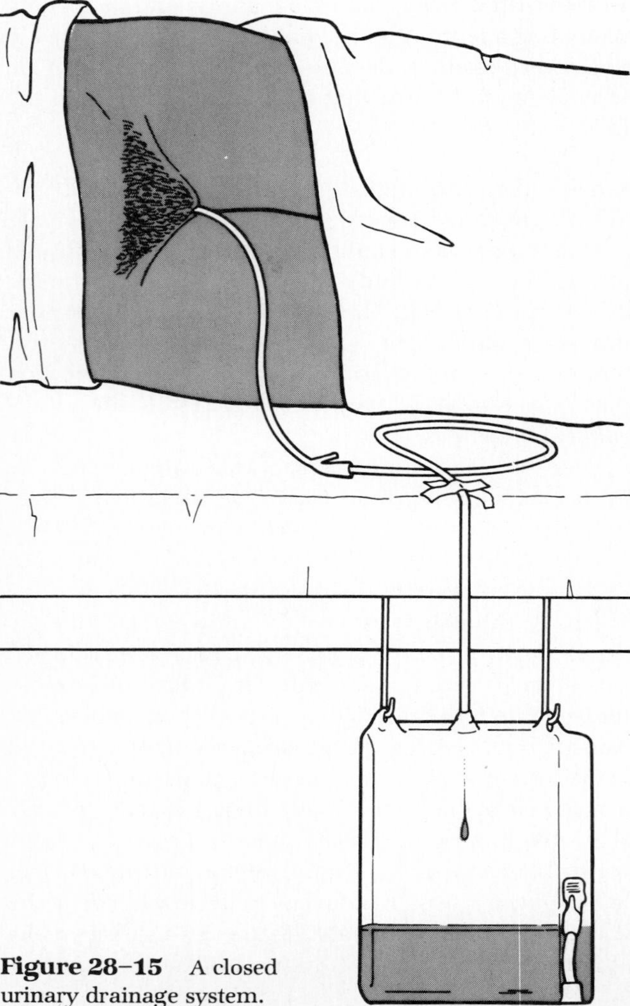

Figure 28–15 A closed urinary drainage system.

pinned to the dressing gown. When the patient is in a chair, it is often attached to the chair.

The drainage tubing must be of sufficient length to allow the patient freedom to move about in bed and elsewhere. Because it is longer than the distance between the catheter and the bag, the tubing needs to be coiled and pinned or taped in some manner to prevent kinks that obstruct the flow of urine or loops that fall below the drainage receptacle and thus require urine to flow against gravity, causing it to pool in the tubing. The tubing can be attached to the bedding in a number of ways.

1. By pinching a piece of sheet on either side of the tubing and then pinning the sides over the tubing, without puncturing the tubing.
2. By taping the tubing to the sheet with adhesive looped under and over the tubing to form a crisscross. This is the preferred method when safety pins cannot be used because of the danger of puncturing an alternating pressure mattress.
3. By looping an elastic band around the tubing and then pinning the elastic band to the bedclothes. This method allows even more freedom of movement, since any tension exerted on the catheter or tubing is absorbed by the elastic band, which stretches readily.
4. By using a special tubing clamp or clip provided with some disposable drainage sets.
5. By looping a piece of adhesive tape around the tubing and then pinning the tape to the bedclothes.

It is important not to pull the retention catheter, since pulling may create pressure on and trauma to the bladder and urethra. Commonly the catheter is taped with a nonallergenic tape to the patient's upper thigh. Some agencies advocate taping the catheter to the lower abdomen of a male patient, with the penis directed toward his head. See Figure 28–16. This is thought to prevent irritation and excoriation at the normal angle of the penis and scrotum.

The patient's position in bed can inhibit urinary drainage. When the patient is lying on the back, it is important that the tubing lie over the thigh, not under the thigh, so that it is not compressed by the patient's weight. When the patient is on the side facing the system, the tubing can rest on the bed in front of the patient and be unobstructed. However, when the patient's back is to the drainage receptacle, the tubing is best placed directly back between the patient's thighs rather than over the upper thigh, because otherwise the amount and pressure of urine in the bladder must increase significantly to force urine up into the tubing over the thigh for drainage to occur.

Urinary drainage receptacles that attach to the patient's thigh are available for ambulatory patients. They are made of plastic or rubber and are designed so that the catheter fits directly into the top of the receptacle. The bag is equipped with straps that fasten around the thigh. With this type of system the patient can be fully clothed, and the system is concealed from view.

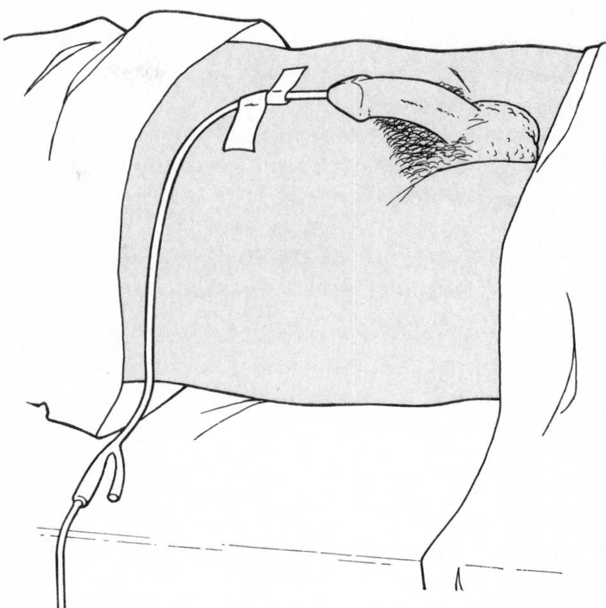

Figure 28–16 Taping the retention catheter to the lower abdomen of a male patient.

Nursing intervention for patients with retention catheters

Nursing care of the patient with an indwelling catheter and continuous drainage is largely directed toward preventing infection of the urinary tract and encouraging urinary flow through the drainage system. It includes encouraging large amounts of fluid intake, accurate recording of the fluid intake and output, providing perineal-genital care, changing the retention catheter and tubing, maintaining the patency of the drainage system, preventing contamination of the drainage system, and teaching these measures to the patient. The first two measures are discussed in Chapter 30.

Perineal-genital care Perineal-genital care is recommended at least twice daily for the patient with an indwelling catheter. It is considered one of the most significant measures to reduce the incidence of infection. Any secretions or encrustations that accumulate at the urethral orifice provide an excellent medium for pathogens, which can ascend the tract. Most agencies recommend specific cleaning methods. Some advocate routine perineal-genital care with warm water and soap. For the uncircumcised male patient, the foreskin is retracted to clean well under it. Any encrustations on the catheter are also removed. Then an antiseptic solution or aerosol is applied around the urinary meatus and around the catheter adjacent to the meatus. After this, an antibiotic ointment, such as a neomycin-hydrocortisone preparation, is sometimes also applied with sterile cotton balls or applicators around both the meatus and the adjacent catheter. Disposable gloves are used during this nursing care.

Changing the catheter and tubing Agency policies may specify the frequency of catheter and tubing changes. Some agencies advocate that both be changed weekly; others advocate more frequent changes for the tubing and drainage bag, such as every 24 to 48 hours. Recommendations for changes are made on the basis of reducing the incidence of infection and preventing unpleasant odors. Some authorities recommend that catheters be changed as infrequently as posible.

During tubing changes, strict sterile technique is essential to prevent contamination of the distal lumen of the catheter. The nurse acquires a new sterile drainage bag and tubing, a sterile towel or sterile gauzes, and a clamp. The steps involved are:

1. Wash hands using surgical aseptic technique.
2. Open the sterile towel or sterile gauze.
3. Open the new drainage and tubing package.
4. Remove the protective cap from the drainage tube, and place the open end of the tubing on the sterile towel or gauze.
5. Clamp the catheter above the tubing connector, and disconnect the catheter from the old tubing, being careful to not contaminate the end of the catheter.

6. Connect the catheter to the new tubing.
7. Unclamp the catheter, and establish drainage by securing the tubing and drainage receptacle to the bed at an appropriate level.
8. Apply waterproof tape around the connection site of the catheter and the tubing, if recommended, to ensure a closed drainage system.

Maintaining patency of the drainage system To ensure continual patency of the system, nurses need to:

1. Check that there are no obstructions in the drainage, for example, that there are no kinks in the tubing, that the patient is not lying on the tubing, and that the tubing is not clogged with mucus or blood (if the patient is bleeding or passing pus).
2. Check that there is no tension on the catheter or tubing, that the catheter is taped to the patient's thigh or abdomen, and that the tubing is fastened appropriately to the bedclothes.
3. Check that gravity drainage is facilitated, for example, that there are no loops in the tubing before entry to the drainage receptacle.
4. Check that the drainage system is well sealed or is closed, for example, that no leaks are detectable at the connection sites in open systems.

Preventing contamination of the drainage system Some agencies recommend instillation of a 37% formaldehyde solution in the drainage bag. Although this solution has an unpleasant odor, it is germicidal against all forms of microorganisms and viruses and is not affected by organic matter. Agency policies vary, however.

When emptying the drainage bag, the nurse must maintain surgical aseptic technique. The bag is emptied usually at the end of each shift of duty, and the tube at the bottom of the bag is used to drain the bag. The amount of drainage is noted in accordance with calibrations on the bag, or a graduated pitcher is brought to the bedside to assess the output. It is important for the nurse not to contaminate the end of the tubing and to reattach it appropriately when the bag is emptied.

Figure 28–17 Obtaining a urine specimen: **A,** from a retention catheter; **B,** from a drainage port.

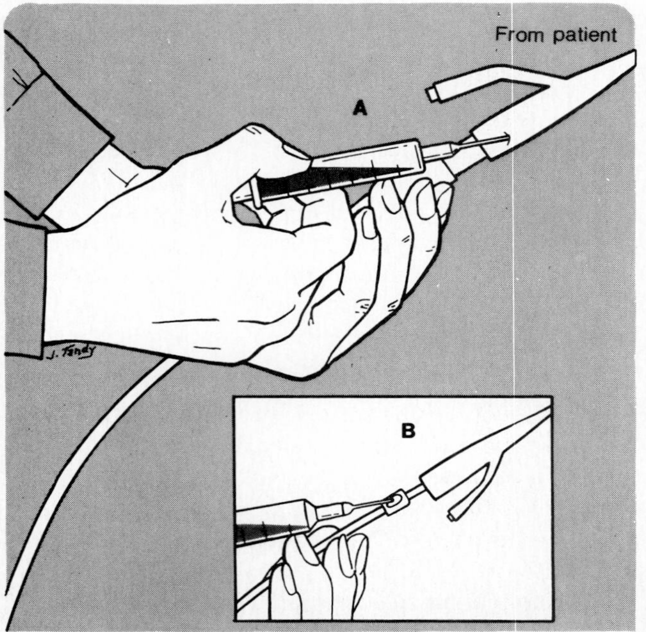

Patient learning Usually nurses need to teach the patient some principles about the gravity drainage system and the importance of maintaining a closed system. The patient has to understand that the drainage tubing and drainage bag need to be kept lower than the bladder at all times. The patient also needs to know how to prevent tension on the catheter tubing, to prevent loops or kinks in the drainage tubing, and to avoid lying on the tubing. Understanding how to manipulate the system when ambulating can give the patient a sense of independence.

Obtaining a sterile specimen from a retention catheter

To obtain a sterile specimen from a retention catheter connected to a closed drainage system, a nurse requires a sterile #21 to #25 gauge needle, a 3 ml syringe, and a cotton swab with a disinfectant. The needle can be inserted in catheters with seal-sealing rubber (not Silastic, plastic, or silicone catheters). The sealing area (distal area) is wiped with the disinfectant, and then the needle is inserted at an angle into the catheter lumen. See Figure 28–17, *A*. Care is taken not to puncture the lumen leading to the balloon. Some urine bags have special sampling ports in the tubing. See Figure 28–17, *B*.

If the urine does not flow into the syringe, the nurse lifts the distal tubing slightly to return a little urine from the tubing to the area. Caution is exercised not to return the urine to the bladder. Another way to secure urine is to kink the tubing about 7.5 cm (3 in) distal to the catheter and hold it with a rubber band until urine is visible.

After the urine has been drawn into the syringe, it is transferred to a sterile container. Sterile technique is maintained at this time also. The container is closed, labeled, and sent to the laboratory.

Catheter removal

To remove an indwelling catheter the nurse requires a receptacle for the catheter and a sterile syringe with which to remove the sterile water from the balloon. The nurse first checks the label on the catheter to ascertain how much fluid is in the balloon (5 to 30 ml). All the fluid is then withdrawn, and the catheter is gently withdrawn from the urethra. If the catheter does not come out readily, it is not forced. The nurse discontinues removal and notifies the physician.

A patient who has had a retention catheter in for weeks or months may well experience some frequency after its removal while the bladder regains its muscle tone. Encouraging the patient to drink fluids will assist in developing bladder muscle tone and at the same time flush out any microorganisms that may be present. Occasionally the urethra has become irritated by the catheter, and as a result the patient may experience burning when voiding. This usually passes in a few days and is helped by maintaining a dilute urine with a high fluid intake. Patients are sometimes reluctant to take fluids because of the burning upon urination, and thus an explanation by the nurse is important.

After removal of a retention cathether, the patient's intake and output are usually measured until any problems are over. It is also important to assess how often the patient is voiding, the amount of urine, and any unusual symptoms such as pain.

Application of a Condom

The *condom* or *condom catheter* is a device that can be applied externally to the penis as a means of catching urine and directing it to a drainage bag. It can sometimes be used to replace the indwelling catheter, which presents the risks of trauma to the urethra and allowing microorganisms to enter the bladder. The condom is usually made of soft, pliable plastic or rubberized material and fits snugly high up over the penis. When the patient is ambulating, the condom is often connected to a bag that is attached to the patient's thigh; when the patient is in bed, the condom is connected to the straight drainage bag used for an indwelling catheter.

Assembling a Condom Appliance

Condom appliances are available in commercially prepared packages, or they may be assembled by connecting a condom to a piece of rubber tubing 7.5 to 10 cm (3 to 4 in) in length and about 1.3 cm (0.5 in) in diameter. The two are attached by means of adhesive tape, elastic bands, or thin rubber rings that are cut from the piece of rubber tubing. A method for assembling a condom appliance using rubber rings is presented in Figure 28–18.

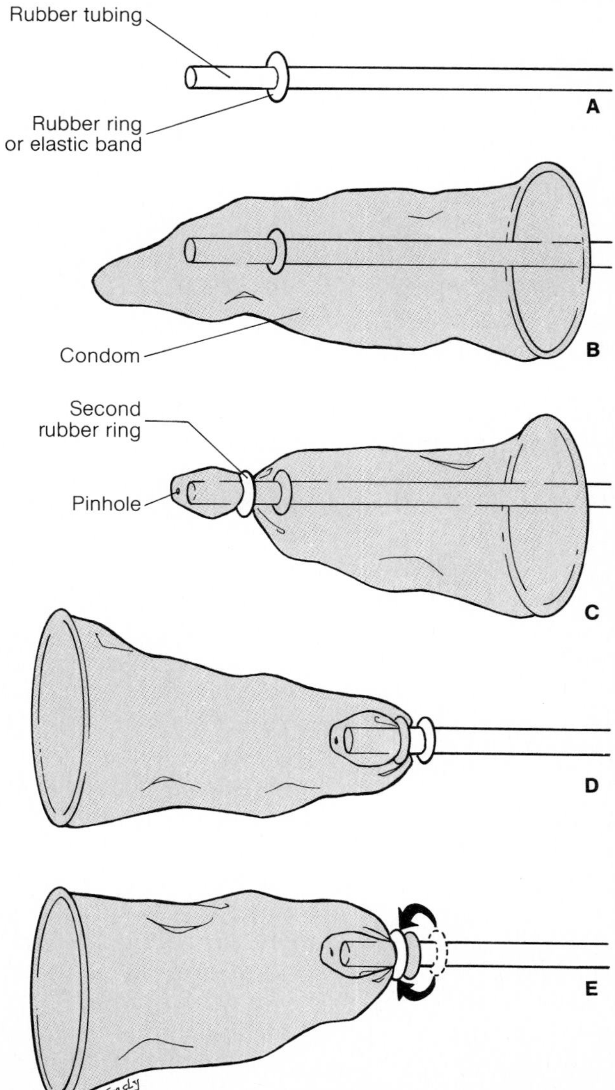

Figure 28–18 Assembling a condom appliance: **A,** put one rubber ring around the rubber tubing midway along its length; **B,** with the rolled edge of the condom in the inside, put the condom over the end of the tubing and over the rubber ring; **C,** place a second rubber ring over the end of the condom, attaching it firmly to the rubber tube about 2.5 cm (1 in) from the end; make a pinhole through the condom covering the lumen of the tube to allow for drainage; **D,** pull the condom back over the second ring; the condom will now have the rolled edge on the outside; **E,** to further secure the condom to the tubing, draw the first rubber ring over the second rubber ring.

Applying the Condom

Generally, condoms are applied by male nurses and orderlies, although in some instances female nurses may be required to apply them.

Before the condom is applied, the genital area is thoroughly washed and dried. Methods of attaching the condom vary. In some agencies a thin layer of tincture of benzoin is applied and allowed to dry well; then surgical cement is applied around the foreskin of the penis. The condom is rolled up over the entire penis, making sure that the tip of the tubing is kept about 2.5 to 5 cm (1 to 2 in) beyond the tip of the penis. This prevents irritation of the glans penis. In addition, some agencies secure the condom by applying a strip of elastic adhesive around the condom and penis. This adhesive needs to be applied snugly but not so tightly as to cause constriction of the blood supply. The nurse is advised to check agency policy about other methods that may be used.

Nursing Interventions for Patients with Condom Appliances

Skin excoriation is a possible problem with the use of a condom appliance. Generally, the condom can be applied for about 48 hours before it is changed. At each change, the skin is cleaned with soap and water, dried well, and inspected for signs of irritation. This is best done when the patient is bathed. The condom is removed before a bath and a new one applied after the bath.

Maintaining free urinary drainage is important. Because the condom is pliable, it sometimes becomes twisted at the tip of the penis, obstructing urinary flow. The nurse needs to check the patient's condom for this at periodic intervals throughout the day. Leaks sometimes occur also and require a change of the condom.

Urinary Bladder and Catheter Irrigations

A bladder irrigation is carried out on a physician's order, usually to wash out the bladder and/or apply an antiseptic solution to the bladder lining. Sterile technique is used. Catheter irrigations are usually carried out to maintain or restore the potency of a catheter. A physician's order may or may not be required, depending on agency policy.

In some instances a continuous bladder irrigation is set up using a three-way Foley catheter. In this type of catheter, one lumen permits the drainage of urine, a second leads to the balloon that is inflated to retain the catheter in place in the bladder, and the third lumen permits the passage of irrigating fluid into the bladder. The first lumen of the catheter is connected to a drainage tube that leads to a closed drainage bag. In this way the system is entirely closed to the air, to prevent the entry of microorganisms into the bladder.

In the usual bladder irrigation, either a two-way Foley catheter is already in place or a straight catheter is inserted for the irrigation. For a bladder irrigation, the frequency of irrigations and type of solution to be used are ordered by the physician. It is not unusual to prepare about 1000 ml of irrigating solution at room temperature for an adult and to administer 180 to 240 ml at one time. For a catheter irrigation, 200 ml of solution is usually required, and 30 to 40 ml is instilled into the catheter each time.

In a catheter or bladder irrigation where a closed drainage system is being employed, the following sterile equipment is required: a container for the irrigating solution, a container and solution such as benzalkonium chloride (Zephiran Chloride) to clean the catheter, a receptacle for the returned solution, absorbent balls, a moisture-resistant drape, a tubing clamp, and a syringe and needle. A 30 or 50 ml syringe and #18 or #19 needle are frequently used.

The nurse washes hands and sets up the equipment before taking it to the patient. If a mask is required, it is donned before washing. The patient is draped appropriately, and the moisture-resistant drape is placed on the bed beside the patient's hips under the end of the catheter. The tubing below the catheter is clamped for a bladder irrigation and left unclamped for a catheter irrigation. The sterile set is opened, the sterile solution is drawn up into the syringe, and the needle is attached. The tubing port or the place on the catheter over the lumen in which the solution is to be instilled is wiped with disinfectant. The needle is then inserted, and the solution is gently introduced into the catheter. When the prescribed amount has been instilled, the needle is removed. In a catheter irrigation, the catheter tube is lowered so that the solution returns down the tubing. For a bladder irrigation the tubing is unclamped. This procedure is repeated until the total amount of solution has been used or, if the catheter or tubing was occluded, until the solution drains freely.

In recording the irrigation, it is important to include the time of treatment, the type and strength of solution used, and the character of the return flow.

On irrigating an open drainage system, see Kozier and Erb (1982:816). If a catheterization is required prior to the bladder irrigation, see Procedures 28–1 and 28–2.

Measuring Residual Urine

The physician usually prescribes the measurement of residual urine, although it may be routinely done at the nurse's discretion in specific situations and in accordance with agency policy. Normally, residual urine in adults is nil or only a few milliliters. Large amounts of residual urine can occur in situations of bladder outlet obstruction, for example, in prostatic hypertrophy or in loss of bladder muscle tone. The latter can result from disorders affecting the nervous system's control of the bladder or after surgery or indwelling catheterization of the bladder. Incomplete emptying of the bladder is generally suspected when small amounts of urine are voided frequently, for example, 100 ml during one voiding in the adult. The ultimate consequence of residual urine is a urinary infection.

To determine the amount of residual urine, the bladder is first emptied by natural voiding, and then the patient is catheterized. Both the amount of urine voided and the amount of residual urine are noted and recorded. If the amount of residual urine exceeds 50 ml, the physician may order that an indwelling catheter be inserted for a period of time.

Residual urine is also frequently measured for patients with suprapubic catheters. This type of catheter is inserted through the abdominal wall above the pubic area into the bladder. To ascertain the residual urine the suprapubic catheter is first closed with a clamp for 2 to 4 hours. The patient then voids by the normal route, emptying the bladder as completely as possible. After this the residual urine is obtained by releasing the suprapubic catheter and allowing any remaining urine to drain. Both the amount of urine voided and the amount of residual urine are measured. It is important to follow sterile technique when handling the suprapubic catheter.

Collecting Urine Specimens

Kinds of Specimens

Several kinds of urine specimens are often needed for analysis. Four of these are (a) the early morning specimen, (b) the sterile specimen, (c) the sterile voided (midstream or clean-catch) specimen, and (d) the 24-hour specimen.

Early morning specimen

An early morning specimen is taken when the patient first arises in the morning. This specimen usually contains the most concentrated urine of the day and is the one generally used for routine urinalysis. It is put in a clean but not sterile container, and thus it is not suitable for bacteriologic study.

Sterile specimen

A sterile specimen is one required for bacteriologic study. To obtain this sample, the patient is catheterized (see Procedures 28-1 and 28-2), unless a catheter is already in place, and the urine is drained into a sterile container.

Sterile voided (midstream or clean-catch) specimen

A sterile voided specimen is also referred to as a *midstream* or *clean-catch* specimen. The purpose is to obtain a specimen that is free of any microorganisms that may be at the urinary meatus.

For both male and female patients, the area around the urinary meatus is thoroughly cleaned with soap and water. For the female patient it is important to wipe from the urinary meatus toward the rectum, that is, from the area of least contamination to the area of greatest contamination. The patient then starts to void; the first part of the urine stream is discarded, and the sample is taken from the midstream or the middle portion of the voiding. The sample is voided directly into a sterile bottle or test tube, which is immediately covered with a sterile top. The last portion of the urine stream is also discarded.

Once the urine specimen has been obtained, it is immediately delivered to the laboratory for testing. Permitting the urine to stand for a time fosters the growth of any bacteria in the urine and the breakdown of the urea component, changing the urine to a more alkaline pH.

24-hour specimen

A 24-hour urine specimen is needed for some diagnostic studies, for example, assessment of the corticosteroid levels excreted in certain adrenal or pituitary diseases or assessment of the fluid and electrolyte excretion in infants. Adult patients need to know that all their urine is to be collected during a specified 24-hour period such as 0700 hours one day to 0700 hours the following day. A reminder that the urine is to be kept separate from the stool can be helpful. Usually the first specimen is taken and discarded; then all urine is kept after this initial voiding. Because the reasons for 24-hour urine collections vary, it is important for the nurse to understand the specific test involved. Sometimes the urine is collected in one large receptacle; at other times, individual receptacles are provided for each voiding and labeled according to sequence and time. Refrigeration of the urine is generally warranted to prevent decomposition of the urine; in some situations, preservatives are added to the containers. For certain tests a 24-hour urine specimen is first taken for control purposes. The patient is then given a medication at specified times, and a second 24-hour specimen is collected a day or so later. The second sample is compared to the control sample.

Specimens from Infants and Children

A urine specimen is routinely collected from children, like adults, on admission to the hospital. For children who have not yet acquired bladder control, plastic disposable collection bags are available in various designs. These bags generally have nonallergenic adhesive tape around the opening, which is attached securely around the genitals, and some have a drainage tab that can be removed to drain the bag after the specimen is collected.

Prior to applying the bag, the nurse cleans, rinses, and dries the child's perineal-genital area. Cotton swabs are used for this. For girls the area is wiped from the clitoris to the anus using one cotton swab for each stroke. For boys the foreskin is retracted, if necessary, and the penis is wiped in a circular motion from the tip to the scrotum.

Two nurses may be needed for this procedure, one to comfort and restrain the child, the other to apply the collecting device. The infant is positioned on the back; the hips are externally rotated and abducted, and the knees are flexed. The collecting device is then taped to the perineum. The device is generally applied starting at the perineum between the rectum and vagina for girls and working upward. For boys the bag is fitted over the penis, and the flaps are pressed firmly all around the perineum. It is important that the adhesive be applied without puckers to prevent leakage. A diaper may be put on over the bag to prevent the child from tampering with it. To assist urine drainage by gravity, the head of the crib can be elevated.

After the infant has voided, the bag is removed carefully to prevent skin injury. Depending upon the design of the collection device, the specimen is either transferred through the drainage tab to another collection container, or the adhesive surfaces are closed and the specimen is sent in the plastic bag to the laboratory. The child's perineum is inspected and cleaned prior to rediapering.

Routine urine specimens can readily be obtained from preschool or school-age children. The genitals are cleaned first. Then the female child is placed on a training chair and voids into a container or bedpan placed beneath. The male child uses a urinal. It is more difficult to collect a midstream or clean-catch specimen from a child than a routine specimen. The child needs careful explanations and encouragement to first void a small amount into an unsterile container and then void the rest into a sterile container.

When continuous collections of urine are required from small children during certain illnesses, procedures vary in accordance with the equipment available. Some agencies have specially designed cribs for infants up to 2 years of age that allow the urine to flow through a mesh hammock into a collecting bottle below. The advantage of this system is that the infant does not need to be restrained. In other agencies, plastic devices similar to the one described for routine urine specimen collection are used. These devices are then attached to a collecting bottle beneath the crib. In this situation the nurse needs to check frequently to prevent leakage of urine and skin excoriation.

Evaluation

Examples of outcome criteria for patients with urinary elimination problems are:

Retention

1. Urinary output in balance with fluid intake
2. Absence of urinary infection (e.g., negative urine culture)

Incontinence

1. Decrease in frequency of incontinence
2. Intact perineal skin
3. Increased self-esteem

Enuresis

1. Decreased incidence of nocturnal enuresis
2. Increased self-esteem and sense of security

Frequency, urgency, dysuria

1. Decreased incidence of frequency and urgency
2. Absence of dysuria

3. Urinary pH of less than 5.5
4. Negative urine culture
5. Urine output in balance with fluid intake

Polyuria
1. Decreased incidence of polyuria
2. Balanced fluid intake and output
3. Absence of signs of fluid or electrolyte imbalance

Urinary suppression
1. Urinary output of at least 2000 ml/day
2. Electrolyte balance (e.g., potassium range of 3 to 6 mEq/liter and sodium range of 125 to 145 mEq/liter)
3. Blood urea nitrogen below 28 mg/100 ml of blood
4. Absence of urinary infection

Summary

Urinary elimination is a need taken for granted by most people until a health problem occurs. The volume of urine eliminated each day varies according to age and other factors. Urine has certain characteristics that need to be recognized by the nurse. Urinary control is a learned response that occurs after bowel control is established. Daytime control is generally achieved by the age of 2 years, but nighttime control may not be achieved until age 4. Four steps are involved in learning bladder control and nurses can facilitate this learning process.

The normal process of micturition includes sufficient accumulation of urine in the bladder to stimulate the sensory stretch nerves in the bladder wall. In the adult, micturition generally occurs after 250 to 450 ml of urine have collected in the bladder, but in children the amounts are smaller (50 to 200 ml). Impulses from these stretch receptors then travel to the spinal cord to the voiding reflex center and to the voiding control center in the cerebral cortex, where conscious control of micturition is regulated.

Many factors influence a person's urinary elimination. Increased amounts of urine may be excreted when large amounts of fluid are ingested, during stress, when activity is increased, or when diuretics are prescribed. Pathologic conditions may increase or decrease the amount of urine eliminated. When assessing a person's urinary function, the nurse needs to consider systematically (a) patterns of urination, such as frequency of voiding and volume, (b) characteristics of the urine, such as color and odor, and (c) problems that the patient is experiencing, such as retention, incontinence, frequency, or dysuria. From the assessment data obtained, the nurse establishes the nursing diagnoses, sets nursing goals, and plans nursing interventions.

Nursing interventions related to urination are generally directed toward facilitating the normal functioning of the urinary system or toward assisting the patient with particular problems. Interventions include (a) assisting the patient to maintain an appropriate fluid intake, (b) assisting the patient to maintain normal voiding patterns, (c) monitoring the patient's daily fluid intake and output, and (d) maintaining cleanliness of the genital area. Nurses may also have to assist hospitalized children to urinate. Frequently bedridden patients need to use bedpans and urinals. Factors to consider in their use include type of container, bed position, patient position, privacy, and level of assistance needed.

Specific nursing interventions are required for patients experiencing urinary incontinence, urinary retention, childhood nocturnal enuresis, and other altered urinary frequency, urgency patterns (e.g., dysuria, polyuria, and urinary suppression).

Urinary catheterization is frequently required for patients with urinary problems. Nurses often perform this technique. Sterile technique is essential to prevent ascending urinary infections. Catheterization technique differs between male and female and between child and adult patients.

Urinary retention catheters require additional interventions by the nurse. Prior to insertion the nurse needs to test the balloon. After insertion the balloon must be safely inflated and a drainage system attached and maintained. Care of patients with indwelling catheters is directed toward preventing infection of the urinary tract and encouraging urinary flow through the drainage system. Measures include accurate recording of fluid intake and output, providing perineal-genital care, changing the catheter and tubing in accordance with agency policies, maintaining the patency of the drainage system, and preventing contamination of the system. Frequently the patient can be taught to assist with these measures. After removal of a retention catheter, the nurse needs to monitor the patient's ability to void and to measure intake and output until these are satisfactory.

In lieu of a retention catheter, a condom appliance is frequently used for male patients. It may be assembled with rubber tubing and two rubber rings. After applying the condom, the nurse needs to observe the patient frequently for signs of skin excoriation, leakage, and obstruction of the patency of the system. Other techniques related to urinary elimination include bladder irrigation, measuring residual urine, and the collection of urine specimens.

Specific outcome criteria are used to evaluate nursing interventions for patients with diagnoses of urinary retention, incontinence, enuresis, frequency, urgency, dysuria, polyuria, and suppression.

Suggested Activities

1. In a clinical setting, select a patient with a urinary problem. Compare the patient's urinary output in relation to fluid intake. Assess the characteristics of the urine compared to normal, and take into account whether the patient's customary urinary habits have been altered.
2. In a hospital setting, note the policies and practices in regard to patients who have indwelling catheters. Justify the reasons for these.
3. In a laboratory setting, assemble a condom appliance.
4. Interview a mother who has a 3- or 4-year-old child. Determine how the child was or is being bladder trained.
5. Investigate why urine specimens are collected in a specific agency. Relate the method of collection to the reason for the specimen.

Suggested Readings

Baum, M. E. February 1978. "I want to be dry": The (almost) carefree way to conquer urinary incontinence. *Nursing 78* 8:75–76, 78.
The author describes setting up a urinary training program for an incontinent child. Two external urinary appliances are described, with instructions on fitting the appliance and caring for the appliance and the patient's skin.

DeGroot, J. December 1976. Urethral catheterization: Observing "niceties" prevents infections. *Nursing 76* 6:51–55.
This article provides step-by-step descriptions of inserting and taping a catheter; obtaining a urine specimen; cleaning, irrigating, and flushing a catheter; and positioning a drainage bag. It is illustrated with many photographs.

Demmerle, B., and Bartol, M. A. November/December 1980. Nursing care for the incontinent person. *Geriatric Nursing* 1:246–50.
The authors describe nursing care of the incontinent elderly person directed at reversing or controlling incontinence and preventing the secondary problems that can result from incontinence.

McGuckin, M. B. January 1981. Getting better urine specimens with the clean-catch midstream technique. *Nursing 81* 1:24–25.
A specimen collection system is described, including a patient teaching plan for men and for women to assist them to provide a good midstream specimen.

Selected References

Beaumont, E. January 1974. Urinary drainage systems. *Nursing 74* 4:52–60.

Beber, R. March 1980. Freedom for the incontinent. *American Journal of Nursing* 80:482–84.

Byrne, E. J., et al. 1981. *Laboratory tests: Implications for nurses and allied health professions.* Menlo Park, Calif.: Addison-Wesley Publishing Co.

Clark, R.; Creamer, L.; Lawson, E.; and Tracey, P. December 1978. Infection control: A team approach that really works. *Canadian Nurse* 74:16–19.

deCastro, F. J., et al. 1972. *The pediatric nurse practitioner.* St. Louis: C. V. Mosby Co.

DeGroot, J. August 1976. Catheter-induced urinary tract infections: How can we prevent them? *Nursing 76* 6:34–37.

DeGroot, J., and Kunin, C. M. March 1975. Indwelling catheters. *American Journal of Nursing* 75:448–49.

French, R. M. 1980. *Guide to diagnostic procedures.* 5th ed. New York: McGraw-Hill Book Co.

Garner, J. February 1974. Urinary catheter care: Doing it better. *Nursing 74* 4:54–56.

Guyton, A. C. 1982. *Human physiology and mechanisms of disease.* 3rd ed. Philadelphia: W. B. Saunders Co.

Kinney, A. B.; Blount, M.; and Dowell, M. November/December 1980. Urethral catheterization: Pros and cons of an invasive but sometimes essential procedure. *Geriatric Nursing* 1:258–63.

Kozier, B., and Erb, G. 1982. *Techniques in clinical nursing: A comprehensive approach.* Menlo Park, Calif.: Addison-Wesley Publishing Co.

Tudor, L. L. November 1970. Bladder and bowel retraining. *American Journal of Nursing* 70:2391–94.

Wells, T., and Brink, C. November/December 1980. Helpful equipment: What's available to make life pleasanter for patients and staff. *Geriatric Nursing* 1:264–69.

Chapter 29

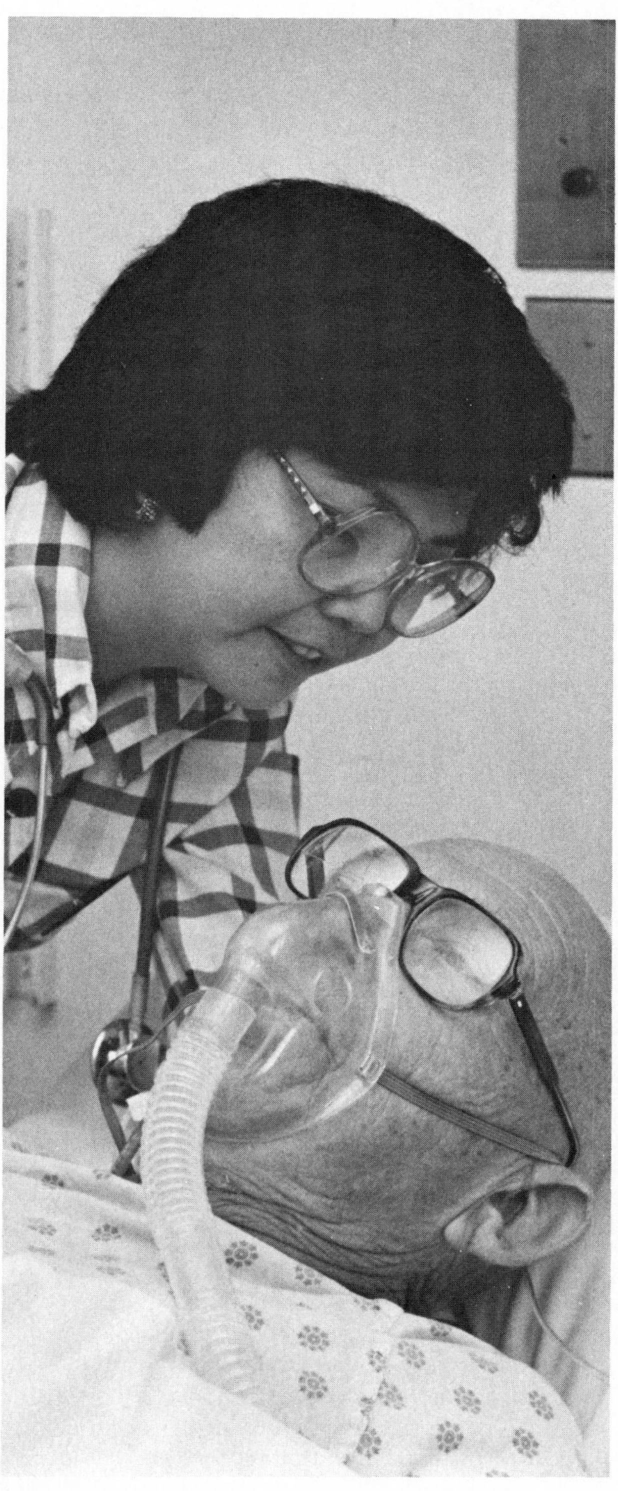

Oxygen

CONTENTS

Objectives

1. Know essential terms and facts about the physiology of respiration

1.1 Define selected terms

1.2 Name three phases of respiration

1.3 Describe the basic mechanics of breathing

1.4 Identify four pulmonary volumes

1.5 Identify four pulmonary capacities

1.6 Identify two pulmonary pressures

1.7 Relate changes in the pulmonary pressures to the act of breathing

1.8 Identify four requirements for adequate ventilation

1.9 Identify mechanisms regulating the respiratory process

1.10 Identify four factors that influence the rate of diffusion of gases through the respiratory membrane and give examples of each

1.11 Describe how oxygen is transported to and carbon dioxide is transported from the tissues

1.12 Identify major factors influencing oxygen transport

2. Know information and methods required to assess a person's respiratory and circulatory status

2.1 Identify terms used to describe respiratory and circulatory status

2.2 Identify factors influencing respiratory and circulatory function

2.3 Identify clinical signs of hypoxia

2.4 Describe diagnostic measures performed to assess respiratory function

3. Know essential facts about nursing diagnoses related to respiratory and circulatory function

3.1 Identify four patient responses to alterations in respiratory and circulatory status

3.2 Identify manifestations of and factors contributing to ineffective airway clearance

3.3 Identify manifestations of and factors contributing to ineffective breathing patterns

3.4 Identify manifestations of and factors contributing to decreased cardiac output

4. Understand facts about nursing intervention required to maintain, promote, and restore normal respiratory and circulatory function

4.1 Identify interventions to maintain normal respirations

4.2 Explain two common breathing exercises

4.3 Explain the purpose of incentive respiratory devices

4.4 Identify indications for intermittent positive pressure breathing (IPPB) therapy and ways to assist patients with this therapy

4.5 State the purposes of postural drainage and the accompanying techniques of percussion and vibration

4.6 Identify positions used to drain specific lung segments by gravity

4.7 Identify areas to percuss (or vibrate) during postural drainage of various lung segments

4.8 Identify various types of humidifiers and their purposes

4.9 Identify the main parts of a nebulizer and the indications for its use

4.10 Identify purposes of oropharyngeal and nasopharyngeal suctioning

4.11 Give reasons for essential steps in the suctioning procedure

4.12 List safety precautions to take when oxygen is administered

4.13 Describe various methods to administer oxygen

4.14 Give reasons for essential steps in administering oxygen therapy by nasal cannula, nasal catheter, face mask, and Croupette

4.15 Describe essential steps in oral resuscitation

4.16 Describe essential steps in cardiopulmonary resuscitation

5. Apply the nursing process when providing care to patients with respiratory and circulatory problems

5.1 Obtain necessary assessment data

5.2 Analyze and relate assessment data

5.3 Write relevant nursing diagnoses

5.4 Write relevant nursing goals

5.5 Plan appropriate nursing interventions

5.6 Implement appropriate nursing interventions

5.7 State outcome criteria against which to evaluate the patient's progress

6. Perform selected respiratory and resuscitation techniques safely

6.1 Assist patients with deep breathing and coughing exercises

6.2 Assist patients with IPPB therapy

6.3 Provide postural drainage, percussion, and vibration

6.4 Assist patients with nebulization therapy

6.5 Use various types of humidifiers

6.6 Apply suction to oropharyngeal and nasopharyngeal passages

6.7 Administer oxygen by nasal cannula, nasal catheter, face mask, and Croupette tent

6.8 Provide oral resuscitation

6.9 Provide cardiopulmonary resuscitation

Terms

anoxia
apnea
artificial respiration
atelectasis
bradycardia
bradypnea
bubbling
carbaminohemoglobin
carbonic acid
cardiac arrest
cardiac output
cardiopulmonary resuscitation (CPR)
carina
chemoreceptors
Cheyne-Stokes breathing
cilia
creps (crepitation)
cyanosis
cytology
diffusion
diffusion coefficient
dyspnea
erythrocytes
erythropoiesis
eupnea
expiration
expiratory reserve volume
external cardiac massage
flail chest
functional residual capacity
hematocrit
hemoglobin
hemoptysis
Hering-Breuer reflex
hypertension
hyperventilation
hypotension
hypoventilation
hypoxemia
hypoxia
inhalation (aerosol) therapy
inspiration
inspiratory capacity
inspiratory reserve volume
intercostal retraction
intermittent positive pressure breathing (IPPB)
intrapleural pressure
intrapulmonic pressure
lingula
lung compliance
lung recoil
morphology
nebulizer
nonproductive cough
orthopnea
oxyhemoglobin
$Pa{CO_2}$
$Pa{O_2}$
paradoxical breathing
partial pressure
$P{CO_2}$
pleural rub (friction rub)
$P{O_2}$
postural drainage
pressoreceptors (baroreceptors)
productive cough
proprioceptors
pulmonary capacities
pulse deficit
rales
reduced hemoglobin
residual volume
respiration
respiratory acidosis
respiratory alkalosis
respiratory membrane
resuscitation
rhonchi
spirometry
stertor
stretch receptors
stridor
substernal retraction
suctioning
supraclavicular retraction
suprasternal retraction
surfactant
tachycardia
tachypnea
tidal volume
total lung capacity
tracheal tug
transudation
ventilation
vital capacity
wheeze

Physiology of Respiration

Respiration is the transport of oxygen from the atmosphere to the body cells and the transport of carbon dioxide from the cells back to the atmosphere. The process has three parts:

1. Pulmonary ventilation, or the inflow and outflow of air between the atmosphere and the alveoli
2. Diffusion of gases (oxygen and carbon dioxide) between the alveoli and pulmonary capillaries
3. Transport of oxygen and carbon dioxide between the blood and tissue cells

Pulmonary Ventilation

Ventilation of the lungs includes the basic mechanics or act of breathing (inspiration and expiration). The degree of chest expansion during ventilation is minimal with normal breathing but can reach maximum capacities during strenuous activity. These normal pulmonary volumes and capacities are described and considered in this section. The relationship of the pulmonary pressures to inspiration and expiration is also included. Many factors are essential for adequate ventilation: adequate atmospheric oxygen, clear air passages, adequate pulmonary compliance, and regulation of respiration.

Mechanisms of breathing

The act of breathing is like the working of a bellows. Breathing consists of *inspiration*, the inflow of air from the atmosphere to the lungs, and *expiration*, the outflow of air from the lungs to the atmosphere. Inspiration lasts normally 1 to 1.5 seconds, and expiration lasts 2 to 3 seconds, including a short resting phase. *Eupnea* (normal breathing) is silent and effortless. It is accomplished largely by movement of the diaphragm. The diaphragm contracts or flattens on inspiration, thus lengthening and pulling the lower chest cavity downward. On expiration, the diaphragm simply relaxes or moves upward. This upward movement of the diaphragm is enhanced by contraction of the abdominal muscles. These muscles push the abdominal organs up against the bottom of the diaphragm. See Figure 29–1.

Breathing during strenuous exercises or illness requires greater chest expansion and effort. The greater chest expansion of heavy breathing is accomplished by intercostal and other muscles that elevate or depress the rib cage. During inspiration, the ribcage is pulled upward by the action of the anterior neck muscles and contraction of the external intercostals. During expiration, the ribcage is pulled downward by the anterior abdominal muscles. Active use of these muscles and noticeable effort in breathing are seen in patients with obstructive respiratory disease. See the section on inspecting the shape and symmetry of the chest, Chapter 14, p. 335. The changes in thoracic diameters during ventilation are associated with changes in pulmonary volumes and pulmonary pressures.

Pulmonary volumes The volume to which the lungs expand during ventilation depends on whether breathing is normal and whether maximum inspiration and expiration occur. In the young male adult, the volume of air inspired and expired during a normal breath is about 500 ml. This volume is about 20% to 25% less in the female. Volumes may be smaller in small persons or greater in large or athletic persons. Volumes discussed subsequently also characterize the adult male, and in all cases the female volumes should be considered 20% to 25% smaller. This normal volume of air inspired and expired is referred to as the *tidal volume*. See Figure 29–2. Three other volumes are classified, which, when added to the tidal volume, produce the maximum volume to which the lungs can be expanded. These are as follows:

1. *Inspiratory reserve volume* approximates 3000 to 3300 ml and refers to the additional volume of air that can be inspired beyond the normal tidal volume.
2. *Expiratory reserve volume* approximates 1000 to 1200 ml and is the amount of air that can be forcefully expired after the normal tidal volume.
3. *Residual volume* averages about 1200 ml and refers to the amount of air remaining in the lungs after exhalation of both the tidal and the expiratory reserve volumes. Residual air is important because it allows continuous exchange of gases between the alveoli and the pulmonary capillaries between breaths. Thus the concentrations of oxygen and carbon dioxide do not rise or fall drastically.

These three volumes added to the tidal volume (500 ml) average about 5700 to 6200 ml and are referred to as the *total lung capacity* (the maximum volume to which the lungs can be expanded).

Figure 29–1 Movement of the diaphragm during inspiration and expiration.

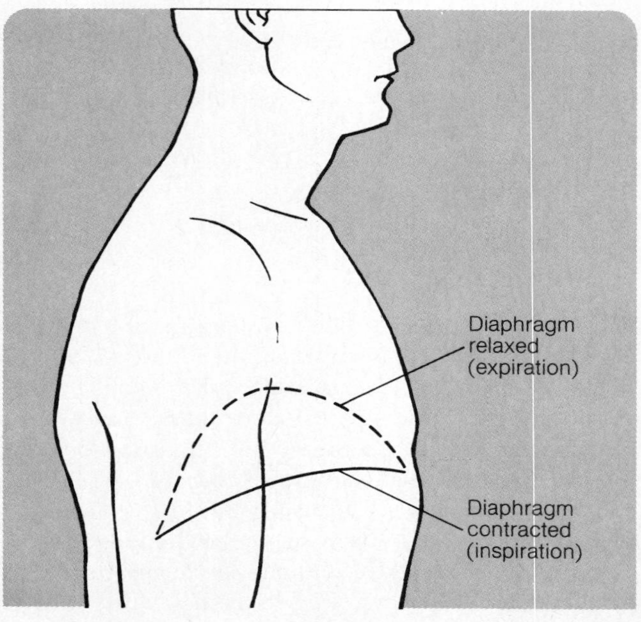

Pulmonary capacities Pulmonary volumes are often grouped in combinations of two or more. These combined volumes are referred to as the *pulmonary capacities* and include total lung capacity plus:

1. *Inspiratory capacity*, which comprises the tidal volume (500 ml) and the inspiratory reserve volume (3000–3300 ml).
2. *Vital capacity*, which comprises the tidal volume (500 ml) plus the inspiratory reserve volume (3000–3300 ml) plus the expiratory reserve volume (1000–1200 ml) or, in other words, all pulmonary volumes except the residual volume. The vital capacity of individual persons varies with (a) anatomical build, (b) position, (c) strength of the respiratory muscles, and (d) distensibility of the lungs and thorax. Vital capacity is normally about 4500 to 5000 ml. A tall, thin person has a higher capacity than an obese person. Athletes may develop vital capacities up to 7000 ml. Standing increases vital capacity, whereas lying down reduces it. In the person who is lying down, the abdominal organs tend to push against the diaphragm and the volume of pulmonary blood increases, both of which reduce pulmonary space and air. Weakness or paralysis of respiratory muscles, such as occurs in quadriplegics, can decrease the vital capacity to a point that is just ade-

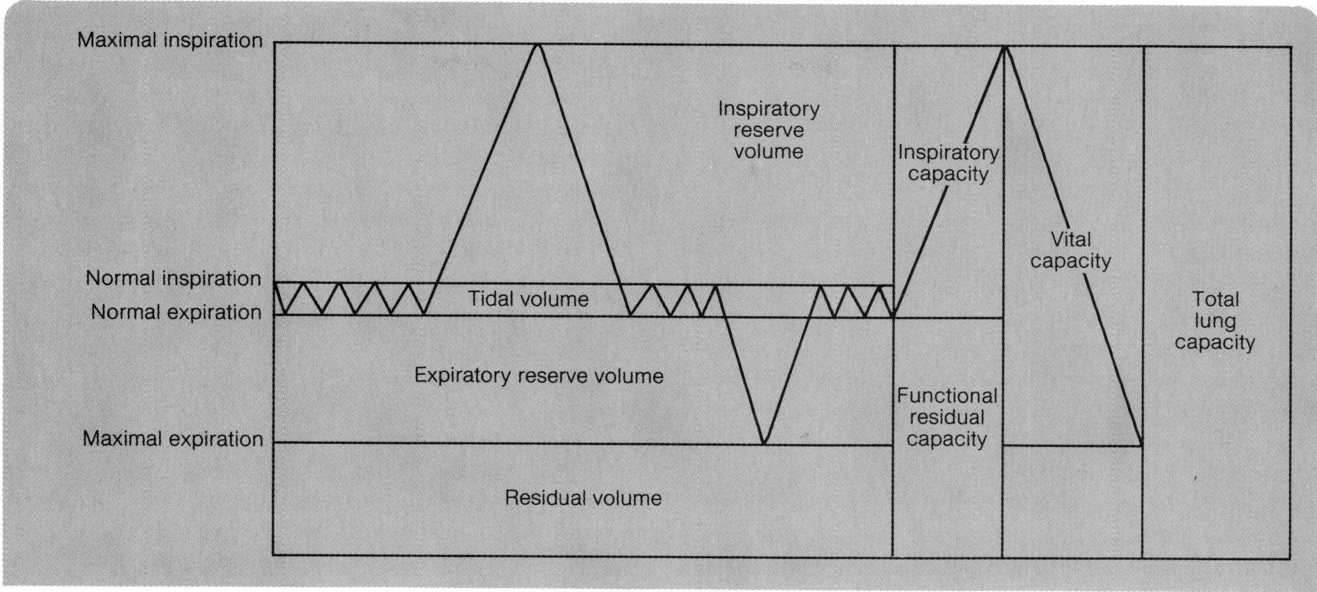

Figure 29–2 Pulmonary volumes and capacities.

quate to sustain life or lower (500 to 1000 ml). Diseases that impair lung distensibility, such as pulmonary edema or lung cancer, seriously reduce vital capacity.

3. *Functional residual capacity*, which comprises the expiratory reserve volume (1000–1200 ml) and the residual volume (1200 ml), is the total amount of air left in the lungs after normal expiration (2200–2400 ml).

Measurement of the pulmonary volumes and capacities is frequently done by *spirometry*. The patient breathes a mixture of air and oxygen through a mouthpiece from a drum suspended over a chamber of water. As the patient breathes in and out, the gas drum rises and falls in the water, and a recording is made on another drum (spirogram). All lung volumes and capacities can be measured by spirometry except for the residual volume and thus the functional residual capacity and total vital capacity, which include the residual volume. See Figure 29–2.

Pulmonary pressure Breathing causes pressure changes within the lungs (*intrapulmonic*) and outside or around the lungs (*intrapleural*). These pressure changes are related to the changes in the lung volumes in accordance with Boyle's Law, which states that the volume of a gas varies inversely with its pressure as long as the temperature of the gas remains constant. In other words, as the volume increases the pressure decreases, and vice versa.

Boyle's Law applies to respiration in this way: On inspiration the volume of the lungs increases, and thus the intrapulmonic pressure decreases. This decreased pressure allows atmospheric air to enter, since its pressure is greater. Conversely, on expiration the volume of the lungs decreases, and the intrapulmonic pressure increases. This allows the air to escape to the atmosphere, whose pressure is now lower than the lungs'. At sea level the atmospheric pressure is about 760 mm Hg. Only very small pressure changes are required to move air in and out of the lungs. On inspiration, the intrapulmonic pressure drops less than 1 mm Hg below the atmospheric pressure, whereas on expiration it rises to +1 mm Hg above the atmospheric pressure (Guyton 1982:295).

The intrapleural pressure is always negative unless the chest cavity is damaged or opened. This negative pressure is essential because it creates the suction that holds the visceral pleura and the parietal pleura together as the chest cage expands and contracts. The recoil tendency of the lungs is a major factor responsible for this negative pressure. The fluid in the intrapleural space, however, provides even more negative pressure. Intrapleural fluid causes the pleura to adhere, much as a film of water can cause two glass slides to adhere.

Essential requirements for ventilation

Ventilation of the lungs depends on (a) adequate atmospheric oxygen, (b) clear air passages, (c) adequate pulmonary compliance and recoil, and (d) regulation of respiration.

Adequate atmospheric oxygen The presence of oxygen in the atmosphere in adequate concentration is basic to adequate respirations. Concentrations of oxygen are lower at high altitudes than at sea level. In some instances people at very high altitudes need supplementary oxygen.

Clear air passages During inspiration, air passes through the nose, pharynx, larynx, trachea, bronchi, and bronchioles to the alveoli, and expiration reverses that course. The nose performs three important functions. It warms, moistens, and filters the air. These functions are appreciated by people required to breathe directly through a tube into the trachea (tracheostomy); dry, unfiltered air can lead to infections of the lung. Large particles in the air are filtered by the hairs at the entrance of the nares, and smaller particles are filtered by nasal turbulence. Each time air contacts the nasal turbinates or the septum it must change direction, and in the process small particles are precipitated.

Air passages are cleared by the mucous membrane lining, which contains *cilia* (hairlike projections of the respiratory mucous membrane). Mucus entraps organisms or other small foreign material while the cilia move the material from the trachea, for example, toward the pharynx. Material can be moved as much as 1 cm per minute along the trachea (Guyton 1982:301). The cough reflex and the sneeze reflex are also essential cleaning mechanisms. The cough reflex is triggered by irritants that send nerve impulses through the vagus nerve to the medulla. Any foreign matter in the larynx, trachea, or bronchi initiates the cough reflex. A particularly sensitive area is the *carina*, the ridge or junction where the main bronchi meet at the trachea. The sneeze reflex is to the nasal passages as the cough is to lower respiratory passages. Sneezing is initiated when irritating impulses pass by way of the fifth cranial nerve to the medulla.

Adequate pulmonary compliance and recoil *Compliance* is expansibility or stretchability. It generally includes expansibility of both the lungs and the thorax but sometimes denotes compliance of the lungs alone. Compliance can be measured by noting the increase in lung volume produced by units of increased intraalveolar pressure. Expansibility is obviously essential to adequate inspiration.

Inadequate compliance can be caused by any condition that destroys lung tissue, such as edema or tumors, or any condition that inhibits thoracic expansion, such as paralysis or kyphosis.

In contrast to lung compliance is *lung recoil*. The lungs have a continual tendency to collapse away from the chest wall. Two factors are responsible for this recoil tendency: (a) elastic fibers present in lung tissue and (b) surface tension of the fluid lining the alveoli. The latter accounts for two-thirds of the recoil phenomenon. Counterbalancing this surface tension in the alveoli is a lipoprotein mixture called *surfactant*. When surfactant is absent, lung expansion is exceedingly difficult, and the lungs collapse. Normally, the secretion of surfactant by the alveoli is stimulated several times each hour by yawning, sighing, or deep breaths. Surfactant stimulation is important for patients on automatic ventilation. The alveoli must be stretched several times every hour by a sigh mechanism on the respirator.

Regulation of respiration Several factors regulate the respiratory process. The primary regulator is the respiratory center in the medulla oblongata. This area maintains the normal smooth rhythm of respiration by mechanisms not fully understood. It is thought that two alternating circuits operate: one for inspiration and one for expiration. Each inhibits the other in an oscillating fashion; thus when one is active, the other is inactive.

Other specialized receptors throughout the body transmit impulses to the respiratory center to bring about changes in respiration. Included are stretch receptors, chemoreceptors, pressoreceptors, and proprioceptors. The *stretch receptors*, located in the walls of the bronchi and bronchioles, are activated when the lungs become overly inflated. Impulses are transmitted through the vagus nerves to the brainstem and from there to the respiratory center. Inspiration is then inhibited, and overdistention of the lungs is prevented. This protective mechanism, commonly called the *Hering-Breuer reflex*, prevents excess inflation of the lungs. It is thought that the walls of the alveoli contain compression receptors that control lung deflation. They inhibit expiration much as stretch receptors inhibit inspiration.

Chemoreceptors (chemical receptors) that affect respiration are present in the respiratory center, along the arch of the aorta, and in carotid sinuses slightly above the bifurcation of the common carotid arteries. These receptors respond to changes in the chemical composition of the blood and tissue fluids, specifically to the changes in oxygen, carbon dioxide, or hydrogen ion concentrations. Changes in carbon dioxide and hydrogen ion concentrations stimulate receptors directly in the respiratory center. When the levels of carbon dioxide and hydrogen ions increase, the respiratory center is greatly stimulated. Changes in arterial oxygen concentrations do not have a direct effect on the respiratory center; instead, changes in oxygen concentrations stimulate the chemoreceptors in the aortic and carotid bodies. A low level of oxygen stimulates these chemoreceptors, which in turn stimulate the respiratory center to increase ventilation. Of the three factors that stimulate chemoreceptors (relative concentrations of carbon dioxide, hydrogen ions, and oxygen in the blood), carbon dioxide concentrations stimulate respiration most strongly. However, in patients with certain lung ailments, such as pneumonia and emphysema, oxygen concentrations, not carbon dioxide concentrations, play the major role in regulating respiration.

Pressoreceptors (or *baroreceptors*) are stretch receptors located in large arteries such as the internal carotid arteries, in the carotid sinus, and in the arch of the aorta. These control daily variations in arterial blood pressure. Baroreceptors are stimulated by pressures above 60 mm Hg, causing vasodilation, and decreased heart rate. Low blood pressure has the opposite effect: accelerated heart rate and vasoconstriction (Guyton 1982:172–73).

Proprioceptors in the muscles and tendons of movable joints are stimulated by passive body movements and vigorous exercise. These receptors transmit impulses to the respiratory center and stimulate increased or intense respiration. This explains why an increase in ventilation occurs at the beginning of an exercise period. It was formerly believed that hypoxia of the muscles during and after exercise initiated increased respiration (Guyton 1981:524).

Diffusion of Gases

After the alveoli are ventilated, the second phase of the respiratory process—the diffusion of oxygen from the alveoli into the pulmonary blood vessels—begins. (*Diffusion* is the movement of gases or other particles from an area of greater pressure or concentration to an area of lower pressure or concentration.) In the opposite direction, carbon dioxide diffuses from the pulmonary blood vessels into the alveoli. Because the alveolar walls are very thin and are surrounded by a closely intertwined network of blood capillaries, these membranes are together often referred to as the *respiratory membrane.*

Four factors influence the rate of diffuson of gases through the respiratory membrane. These are (a) thickness of the membrane, (b) surface area of the membrane, (c) diffusion coefficient of the gas, and (d) pressure difference on each side of the membrane (Guyton 1981:498).

The thickness of the respiratory membrane increases in patients with pulmonary edema and certain other pulmonary diseases. Any increase in the thickness of this membrane can seriously decrease gaseous diffusion. The surface area of the membrane can also be altered. Conditions such as emphysema, in which alveoli coalesce, or lobectomy, the surgical removal of a portion of the lung, impede gaseous exchange. In patients at rest, the loss of some surface area is not a serious deficit. However, a loss of more than 25% is serious. Also, when for some reason (e.g., exercise and certain diseases) there is increased pulmonary demand, a loss of less than 25% can be a serious deficit.

The *diffusion coefficient* of oxygen and carbon dioxide is also a significant factor. This coefficient depends on the molecular weight and solubility of the gases in the membrane. Carbon dioxide diffuses about 20 times more rapidly than oxygen. Thus, in some situations an oxygen lack is seen without a carbon dioxide build-up. Carbon monoxide diffuses 200 times more rapidly than oxygen, which accounts for the rapidity of fatality by carbon monoxide poisoning.

Pressure differences in the gases on each side of the respiratory membrane obviously affect diffusion. When the pressure of oxygen is greater in the alveoli than in the blood, oxygen diffuses into the blood. The reverse happens with carbon dioxide. Normally the oxygen pressure gradient between the alveoli and the blood entering the pulmonary capillaries is about 40 mm Hg. The *partial pressure* (the pressure exerted by each individual gas in a mixture according to its concentration in the mixture) of oxygen (Po_2) in the alveoli is about 100 mm Hg, whereas the Po_2 in the entering venous blood of the pulmonary arteries is about 60 mm Hg. These pressures equalize very rapidly, however, so that the arterial pressure (Pao_2) also becomes about 100 mm Hg. By contrast, carbon dioxide in the venous blood entering the pulmonary capillaries has a partial pressure of about 45 mm Hg, whereas that in the alveoli has about 40 mm Hg. These partial pressures are used frequently diagnostically to assess deficiencies or excesses of oxygen and carbon dioxide levels in persons with pulmonary disease.

The partial pressure of oxygen in arterial blood is abbreviated as Pao_2. The partial pressure of oxygen in the air or in venous blood is written as Po_2. Pco_2 and $Paco_2$ denote pressures of carbon dioxide in venous and arterial blood, respectively.

Transport of Oxygen and Carbon Dioxide

The third part of the respiratory process involves the transport of respiratory gases. Oxygen needs to be transported from the lungs to the tissues, and carbon dioxide must be transported from the tissues back to the lungs.

Oxygen transport

Normally most of the oxygen (97%) combines loosely with the hemoglobin in the red blood cells and is carried to the tissues as *oxyhemoglobin* (the compound of oxygen and hemoglobin). The remaining oxygen is dissolved and transported in the fluid of plasma and cells. The amount of oxygen that the blood will absorb before it is fully saturated is about 20 ml per 100 ml of blood. This ratio is expressed as 20 vol%. As the hemoglobin releases oxygen to the tissues, it is referred to as *reduced hemoglobin.* Normally, only about 25% or 5 ml (¼ of 20 ml) of oxygen per 100 ml of blood, is diffused to the tissues (utilization coefficient). However, this rate of release can be increased to 75% during periods of stress or increased exercise, since more oxygen is utilized by the cells. In situations of extreme oxygen lack in the tissues caused by a sluggish blood flow or a very high metabolic rate, the tissues can remove all (100%) of the oxygen from the blood.

Influencing factors

Several factors affect the rate of oxygen transport from the lungs to the tissues. The major factors are: (a) cardiac output, (b) number of erythrocytes, (c) exercise, and (d) blood hematocrit.

The normal *cardiac output* (amount of blood pumped by the heart) is approximately 5 liters per minute. In the person at rest, 250 ml of oxygen is transported per minute. Any pathologic condition that decreases cardiac output diminishes the amount of oxygen delivered to the tissues. Disease such as myocardial infarction (heart attack) weakens the pumping motion of the heart and thus inhibits the transport of oxygen. Hemorrhage or dehydration can significantly reduce the blood volume and subsequently the cardiac output. The backlog of blood in the venous system for any reason prevents adequate return of blood to the heart. These all reduce cardiac output and thus diminish oxygen transport. Generally, the heart compensates for inadequate output by increasing its pumping rate. Normally, compensatory cardiac output can increase the oxygen transport fivefold, but when disease conditions exist, this is not possible.

The second factor influencing oxygen transport is the number of *erythrocytes* (red blood cells or RBC). The normal number of circulating erythrocytes in men is about 5 million per cubic milliliter of blood, and in women it is about 4½ million per cubic milliliter. Reductions in these normal values can be brought about by anemia of any cause.

Exercise also has a direct influence on oxygen transport. In well-trained athletes, oxygen transport can be increased up to 20 times the normal. This increase is due in part to an increased cardiac output and to increased utilization of oxygen by the cells (utilization coefficient).

The *blood hematocrit* is the percent of the blood that is erythrocytes. It is also referred to as the packed cell volume per 100 ml. Normally this ratio is about 40% to 50% in men and 35% to 45% in women. Excessive increases in the blood hematocrit increase the blood viscosity, reduce the cardiac output, and therefore reduce oxygen transport. Excessive reductions in the blood hematocrit, such as occur in anemia, also reduce the oxygen transport. It is interesting to note that persons who develop elevated hematocrits when acclimatizing to high altitudes do not often have oxygen transport problems. This is thought to be due to an associated increase in the numbers and sizes of peripheral blood vessels, thus preventing a fall in cardiac output.

Carbon dioxide transport

On the return trip to the lungs the hemoglobin, having released its oxygen, carries carbon dioxide. (Hemoglobin has the ability to combine with carbon dioxide as *carbaminohemoglobin.*) However, only a moderate amount (30%) of carbon dioxide is transported this way. The largest amount of CO_2 (about 65%) is carried in the form of bicarbonate (HCO_3^-) inside the red blood cells. Smaller amounts (5%) are transported in solution in the plasma and as *carbonic acid* (the compound formed when CO_2 combines with water). In the normal resting person, about 4 ml of CO_2 in each 100 ml of blood is transported from the tissues to the lungs. Carbon dioxide is an important factor in the acid-base balance of the body. This function is discussed in Chapter 30.

Assessment

When assessing respiratory and circulatory function, the nurse must consider:

1. Vital signs
2. Factors influencing respiratory and circulatory function
3. The condition of the thorax, lungs, and heart
4. Clinical signs of hypoxia
5. Diagnostic tests

Vital Signs

Methods to assess respiratory rate, rhythm, and character and blood pressure are described in Chapter 13. See also Table 13–1 on page 300.

Terms used to describe respiratory status

The terms used to describe respiratory status can be considered in the following categories: (a) breathing patterns, (b) breath sounds, (c) chest movements, and (d) secretions and coughing.

Breathing patterns Breathing patterns relate to rate, volume, rhythm, and relative ease or effort of respiration.

1. Rates
   Eupnea—normal respiration that is quiet, rhythmical, and effortless. Variations in rates according to age are discussed in Chapter 13.
   Tachypnea—rapid respiration marked by quick, shallow breaths.
   Bradypnea—abnormally slow breathing.
   Apnea—cessation of breathing.
2. Volumes
   Hyperventilation—an increase in the amount of air in the lungs characterized by prolonged and deep breaths; associated with anxiety.
   Hypoventilation—a reduction in the amount of air in the lungs; characterized by shallow respirations.
3. Rhythm
   Cheyne-Stokes breathing—rhythmic waxing and waning of respirations from very deep breathing to very shallow breathing and temporary apnea; often associated with cardiac failure, increased intracranial pressure, or brain damage.
4. Ease or effort
   Dyspnea—difficult and labored breathing during which the patient has a persistent unsatisfied need for air and feels distressed.
   Orthopnea—ability to breathe only in upright sitting or standing positions.

Breath sounds Breath sounds include those that are audible without amplification and those that are best heard with a stethoscope:

1. Sounds audible without amplification
   Stridor—a shrill, harsh sound heard during inspiration with laryngeal obstruction.
   Stertor—snoring or sonorous respiration, usually due to a partial obstruction of the upper airway.
   Wheeze—whistling respiratory sound on expiration that usually indicates some narrowing of the bronchial tree.
   Bubbling—gurgling sounds as air passes through moist secretions in the respiratory tract.
2. Sounds audible by stethoscope
   Rales—rattling or bubbling sounds generally heard on inspiration as air moves through accumulated moist secretions.
   Rhonchi—coarse, dry, wheezy, or whistling sound more audible during expiration as the air moves through tenacious mucus or a narrowed bronchi.
   Creps (crepitation)—a dry crackling sound like crumpled cellophane produced by air in the subcutaneous tissue or by air moving through fluid in the alveoli.
   Pleural rub—coarse, leathery, or grating sound produced by the rubbing together of the pleura; also called *friction rub.*

The nurse needs to note the absence of normal breath sounds or abnormally quiet breath sounds over certain areas of the chest auscultated by stethoscope. These findings indicate inadequate ventilation or expansion.

Chest movements

1. Retractions
   Intercostal—indrawing between the ribs.
   Substernal—indrawing beneath the breast bone.
   Suprasternal—indrawing above the breast bone.
   Supraclavicular—indrawing above the clavicles.
   Tracheal tug—indrawing and downward pull of the trachea during inspiration.
2. *Flail chest* is the ballooning out of the chest wall through injured rib spaces. It results in *paradoxical breathing*, during which the chest wall balloons during expiration but is depressed or sucked inward on inspiration.

Secretions and coughing

1. Secretions
   Hemoptysis—the presence of blood in the sputum. The nurse needs to determine amount, kind, color, and odor; for example, thick, frothy, pink, rusty.
2. Cough
   Productive—a cough accompanied by expectorated secretions.
   Nonproductive—a dry, harsh cough without secretions.

Terms used to describe circulatory status

1. Heart rate
   Tachycardia—excessively rapid heart rate, over 100 beats per minute in the adult.
   Bradycardia—abnormal slowness of the heart rate, below 60 beats per minute in the adult.
   Pulse deficit—the difference between the apical and radial pulse.
2. Blood pressure
   Hypertension—elevated arterial blood pressure.
   Hypotension—abnormally low arterial blood pressure.
3. Oxygenation
   Anoxia—systematic absence or reduction of oxygen below physiologic levels in body tissues. Anoxia is frequently accompanied by increased pulse rate, rapid or deep respirations, cyanosis, restlessness, anxiety, dizziness (vertigo), or faintness (syncope).

Hypoxemia—deficient oxygenation of the blood as measured by laboratory tests.
Hypoxia—diminished availability of oxygen for body tissues due to internal or external causes.
Cyanosis—bluish color of mucous membrane, nail beds, or skin due to excessive deoxygenation of hemoglobin.

Factors Influencing Respiratory and Circulatory Function

Respiratory function

Factors that influence respiratory function include altitude, environment, emotions, exercise, health, and life-style.

Altitude The higher the altitude, the lower the pressure of the oxygen (Po_2) which an individual breathes. Consequently, the arterial blood has a lower Pao_2. As a result, the person at high altitudes has increased respiratory and cardiac rates and increased respiratory depth, which are usually most apparent to the individual upon exercise.

Environment The need for oxygen is also affected by the environment. In response to heat, the peripheral blood vessels dilate; consequently, blood flows to the skin, increasing the amount of heat lost from the body surface. Also, because of vasodilation, the lumens of blood vessels enlarge, thus decreasing the resistance to the blood flow. In response, the heart increases output to maintain the individual's blood pressure. The increased cardiac output requires additional oxygen, thus the rate and depth of breathing increase.

By contrast, in a cold environment the peripheral blood vessels constrict, raising the blood pressure. As a consequence, cardiac action decreases, reducing the oxygen need.

Emotions An accelerated heart rate is one body response to emotions such as fear, anxiety, and anger. It is thought that cardiac action is influenced by impulses from the higher centers in the cerebrum by way of the hypothalamus, which stimulates the cardiac centers (cardioinhibitory and cardioaccelerator) in the medulla of the brain. Motor fibers from those centers carry the impulses to the parasympathetic and sympathetic neurons, which then transmit the impulses to the heart. For further information on stress reactions, see Chapter 9, page 194.

Exercise Physical exercise or activity increases respirations and hence the supply of oxygen in the body. The mechanism underlying this effect is not completely known; however, it is thought that a number of factors, including chemical, neural, and temperature changes, are involved.

Health In the healthy person, the cardiovascular and respiratory systems can normally provide the oxygen the body needs. However, diseases of the cardiovascular system often affect the delivery of oxygen to the cells of the body. In addition, diseases of the respiratory system can affect the oxygenation of the blood adversely. In both these instances, hypoxemia can result.

Life-style It is important to assess the life-style of the person with special oxygen needs. Data about smoking and the inhalation of polluted air can provide some indication of the condition of the patient's lungs. Certain occupations predispose to lung disease. For example, silicosis is seen more often in sandstone blasters and potters than in the rest of the population; asbestosis in asbestos workers; anthracosis in coal miners; and organic dust disease in farmers and agricultural employees who work with moldy hay.

Circulatory function

Factors influencing pulse rate and blood pressure are discussed in Chapter 13, pages 308 and 315.

Physical Assessment

Physical assessment of the thorax, lungs, and heart are discussed in Chapter 14, pages 335 and 340. Included are inspection of the thorax for posture, shape and symmetry of expansion, percussion of the lungs, chest auscultation for normal and abnormal breath and voice sounds, inspection and palpation of the heart, and auscultation of the heart.

Clinical Signs of Hypoxia

Hypoxia may be acute or chronic. Early clinical signs of hypoxia are increased pulse rate, increased rate and depth of respirations, and slight increase in systolic blood pressure. Later signs include a slower pulse rate and lower systolic blood pressure, dyspnea, cough, and hemoptysis. Cyanosis may be present; however, a patient can be hypoxic without exhibiting cyanosis. Cyanosis of the skin and mucous membranes requires these two conditions: (a) the blood must contain about 5 g or more of unoxygenated hemoglobin per 100 ml of blood, and (b) the surface blood capillaries must be dilated. Any factors that interfere with either of these conditions, e.g., severe anemia or the administration of adrenaline, will eliminate cyanosis as a sign even if the patient is experiencing hypoxia.

Other clinical signs of acute hypoxia are nausea, vomiting, oliguria, and possibly anuria. Hypoxia can affect the central nervous system, resulting in headache, apathy, dizziness, irritability, and memory loss. The cerebral cortex can tolerate hypoxia for only 3 to 5 minutes before permanent damage occurs.

The face of the acutely hypoxic person usually appears anxious, tired, and drawn. Such a person usually assumes a sitting position, often leaning forward slightly to permit greater expansion of the thoracic cavity. The hypoxic patient may or may not experience pain upon breathing. Although lung tissue does not have pain receptors, pain can come from the pleura, chest wall, or upper respiratory tract.

In long-term hypoxia, the patient often appears fatigued. He or she is lethargic. The body often adapts to the lack of oxygen in the following manner: (a) pulmonary ventilation increases, (b) the red blood cell count increases, and (c) the hemoglobin concentration increases. The patient's fingers are often clubbed as a result of long-term lack of oxygen in the arterial blood supply to the fingers. With clubbing, the base of the nail becomes swollen and the ends of the fingers and toes increase in size. The angle between the nail and the base of the nail increases to more than 160°. See Figure 29-3.

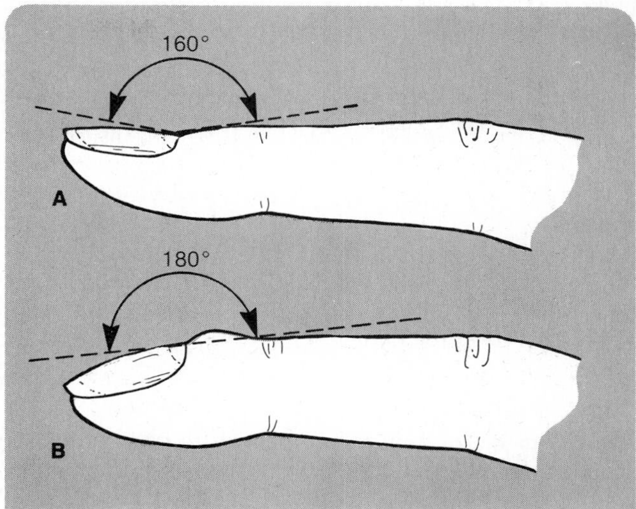

Figure 29–3 Normal and clubbed fingers: **A,** the normal angle between the nail and the base of the nail is 160°, and the nail is firm; **B,** in late clubbing the angle exceeds 180°, and the base of the nail is swollen and springy.

Diagnostic Tests

Many diagnostic tests can reveal information about respiratory function. Types of examinations include:

1. Sputum tests
2. Throat culture
3. Venous blood tests
4. Arterial blood tests
5. Visualization procedures—roentgenography, fluoroscopy, lung scan, bronchoscopy
6. Pulmonary function tests
7. Thoracocentesis (see Chapter 38, page 992)

Nurses are usually responsible for preparing the patient for the test, collecting a specimen when indicated, and looking after the patient following the test. These tests are normally ordered by a physician, although nurses with special preparation may order them in some situations.

Sputum

Sputum is mucus secreted from the lungs, bronchi, and trachea. It is important to differentiate sputum from saliva, which is clear liquid secreted by the salivary glands in the mouth. Healthy individuals do not produce sputum. If a sputum specimen is needed, patients cough to bring sputum up from the lungs, bronchi, and trachea into the mouth and then expectorate it into the collecting container.

Sputum specimens are normally examined for the following reasons:

1. To aid in the diagnosis and treatment of the respiratory illness. The microorganisms or cells present in the sputum are identified. If a pathogen is cultured, the antibiotics to which it is sensitive are also identified.
2. To confirm the presence or absence of the tuberculosis bacillus, sometimes referred to as acid-fast bacilli (AFB), in the sputum.
3. To assess the effectiveness of therapeutic measures.
4. For cytology; i.e., to identify the presence of any abnormal cells. (*Cytology* is the examination of the origin, structure, function, and pathology of cells.)

Sputum specimens are often collected in the morning. Upon awakening, the patient can cough up the secretions that have accumulated during the night. The patient rinses his or her mouth with water but does not eat or drink until the sputum has been expectorated (spit out). Sometimes specimens are collected during postural drainage, when the patient can usually produce sputum. When a patient cannot cough, the nurse must sometimes use pharyngeal suctioning to obtain a specimen.

Sputum containers need to have a wide mouth and a tightly fitting lid. The usual sputum specimen is about 15 to 30 ml (1 to 2 Tbsp or 4 to 8 fluid drams). After obtaining the specimen, the nurse closes the container tightly to prevent contamination of the outside of the container and contamination of the sputum by microorganisms in the air. After giving the specimen, the patient may need a mouthwash to remove any unpleasant taste. Sputum is usually described by amount, color, odor, consistency (thick, tenacious, watery, etc.) and the presence of blood (hemoptysis). For more information on collecting sputum specimens, see Kozier and Erb (1982:545–49).

Throat culture

A specimen is collected from the mucosa of the throat and then cultured and examined for the presence of pathogens. (To culture is to cultivate microorganisms or cells in a special growth medium.) Sometimes a culture is tested for sensitivity. (Sensitivity in this context refers to the response of cultured microorganisms to an antibiotic or other drug.)

Figure 29–4 The tonsils and the oropharynx are sites commonly used for taking throat specimens.

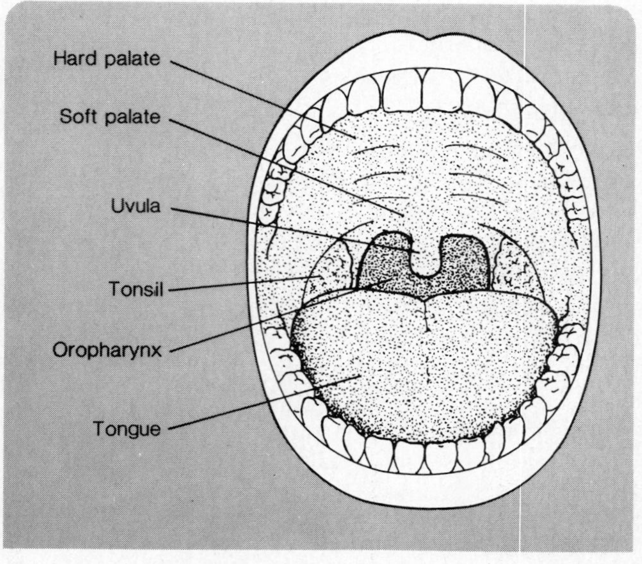

Throat specimens are usually collected for one of the following reasons:

1. To identify the presence of pathogenic microorganisms and the antibiotics to which they are sensitive
2. To evaluate the effectiveness of therapy, e.g., treatment with penicillin

The equipment required for obtaining a throat specimen includes sterile swabs or applicators, a tongue blade, and sterile containers for the specimen. Usually, glass tubes with secure caps are used. Some agencies use special tubes that contain about 2 ml of broth, which keeps the air in the tube moist so that the specimen does not dry out. The swab is suspended so that it does not touch the broth.

A sitting position is most comfortable for the patient and lets the nurse see the pharynx clearly. The patient opens the mouth, extends the tongue, and says "ah." If the nurse cannot see the posterior oropharynx, she or he uses the tongue blade to depress the tongue. The nurse then inserts the swab and passes it lightly along the tonsils, along any erythematous (reddened) areas, or along areas that have an exudate. See Figure 29–4. The nurse places the swab in the sterile container and caps it. A second specimen is often taken in the same manner. When recording, the nurse includes the appearance of the mucosa of the pharynx and tonsils and the color, extensiveness, and consistency of any exudate. If the patient felt discomfort during the procedure, the nurse also records this fact. See Kozier and Erb (1982:570–75) for more information.

Venous blood

Specimens of venous blood are taken for a complete blood count (CBC). A complete blood count includes hemoglobin and hematocrit measurements, erythrocyte (RBC) count, leukocyte (WBC) count, and a differential red cell and white cell count. For the venipuncture technique, see Chapter 31, page 815, and Kozier and Erb (1982:584–93).

Hemoglobin is a protein and the chief component of red blood cells. The transportation of oxygen to the body cells depends to a great degree on the hemoglobin level. See Table 29–1 for normal values.

The hematocrit is the packed cell volume. It denotes the percent of a given volume of whole blood occupied by erythrocytes (RBCs). Therefore, a hematocrit level of 25% indicates that erythrocytes make up 25% of the

Table 29–1 Normal Values of a Complete Blood Count

	Hemoglobin g/dL*	Hematocrit %	RBC million/μL†	WBC /μL‡
Newborn	14–20	42–62	4.0–6.3	9,000–30,000
1 year	11.2–14	29–54	3.6–5.0	6,000–18,000
3 years	11.2–12.5	29–41		
10 years	12.5–13	36–40	3.9–5.2	4,500–13,500
Adult men	14–18	40–54	4.5–6.2	4,500–11,000
Adult women	12–16	37–47	4.0–5.5	4,500–11,000

*g/dL = grams per deciliter (1/100 L, metric equivalent)

†million/μL = million per microliter (10^{-3} mL; metric equivalent)

‡/μL = per microliter (10^{-3} mL, metric equivalent)

From C. J. Byrne, D. F. Saxton, P. K. Pellikan, and P. M. Nugent, *Laboratory tests: Implications for nurses and allied health professionals* (Menlo Park, Calif.: Addison-Wesley Publishing Co., 1981), p. 353.

total volume of whole blood. Hematocrit levels are usually related to hemoglobin values.

Erythrocyte counts show the number of red blood cells in 1 ml or 1 ml^3 of whole blood. The level of red blood cells is regulated by their rate of formation in the bone marrow. The rate of red blood cell formation normally remains relatively constant; however, in patients with hypoxia, *erythropoiesis* (the formation of red blood cells) is stimulated.

A white blood cell count determines the number of circulating leukocytes (white blood cells) in 1 ml or 1 ml^3 of whole blood. Above normal WBC counts indicate increased production of leukocytes by the bone marrow, often in response to the presence of bacterial pathogens in the body. Decreased WBC levels, by contrast, are due to decreased production of leukocytes, often due to the presence of viruses or toxic chemicals in the body.

Differential leukocyte and erythrocyte counts enumerate the different kinds of white and red blood cells in the blood specimen. A number of white blood cells are identified and classified according to their *morphology* (their form and structure). The percentage distribution of the different kinds of white blood cells can assist in diagnosis because characteristic patterns of distribution are consistent with certain disorders. Red blood cells are examined for their size, shape, color, maturation, and content.

Arterial blood

Specimens of arterial blood are normally taken by nurses in specialty areas or medical technicians. Tests performed on arterial blood can indicate a patient's respiratory status: Arterial blood is often tested for partial pressure of oxygen (Pa_{O_2}), partial pressure of carbon dioxide (Pa_{CO_2}), oxygen saturation (S_{O_2} or O_2Sat), hydrogen ion concentration (pH), and the amount of bicarbonate (HCO_3^-) and base excess (BE). For further information about these tests, see Chapter 31.

Blood for these tests is taken from the radial, brachial, or femoral arteries. Because of the relatively great pressure of the blood in these arteries, it is important to prevent hemorrhaging by applying pressure to the puncture site for about 5 minutes after removing the needle.

Visualization procedures

A number of procedures help medical personnel view parts of the respiratory tract: roentgenography, fluoroscopy, lung scan, and bronchoscopy. For further information about these procedures and the nursing responsibilities involved, see Chapter 38.

Pulmonary function tests

Pulmonary function tests measure many of the lung functions discussed earlier in this chapter. Pulmonary function tests do not require an anesthetic and are usually carried out by a respiratory technologist in a laboratory. The patient breathes into a machine. The tests are painless, but the patient's cooperation is essential. Nurses need to explain the tests to patients beforehand and help them get rest afterward, because the tests are often tiring.

Nursing Diagnoses

Patient's responses to alterations in respiratory or circulatory status may be stated as: ineffective airway clearance, ineffective breathing patterns, impaired gas exchange, and decreased cardiac output (Kim and Moritz 1982:283–84, 292). When the latter three diagnoses are made, the patient must be referred for medical evaluation.

Ineffective Airway Clearance

Inability to effectively clear secretions or an obstruction in the respiratory tract may be manifested by abnormal breath sounds audible to the ear alone or by stethoscope, a productive cough with excessive secretions, a nonproductive cough, cyanosis, dyspnea, and changes in respiratory rate or depth (ibid., p. 283).

Factors contributing to ineffective airway clearance include:

1. Excessive, tenacious secretions or foreign objects that obstruct respiratory passages
2. Accidental or intentional trauma, such as tracheostomy, that hinders coughing
3. Abdominal or chest pain that interferes with proper chest expansion and coughing
4. Medications that depress the cough reflex and respiratory center (e.g., morphine)
5. Loss of consciousness from anesthesia or a disease process that interferes with the ability to cough, expectorate secretions, and maintain an open airway
6. Inadequate hydration, which contributes to the formation of thick, tenacious secretions that are difficult to expectorate
7. Immobility or chronic lung disease, which promote accumulation of secretions

Ineffective Breathing Patterns

This patient response refers to respiration that is insufficient to maintain an oxygen supply adequate for cellular demands. It may be manifested by dyspnea, increased respiratory rate, very shallow respirations, chest retractions, cough, flaring of the nares, pursed lip breathing with a prolonged expiratory phase, increase in the anterior-posterior chest diameter (barrel chest), cyanosis, flail chest, orthopnea, abnormal arterial blood gases (see Chapter 31), fremitus, and asymmetry of chest expansion.

Factors contributing to ineffective breathing patterns include:

1. Inadequate chest expansion from immobility, obesity, or pain
2. Neuromuscular impairments, such as those associated with quadriplegia, head injuries, certain drugs, and anesthetics
3. Musculoskeletal impairments, such as those associated with fractured ribs, or injuries leading to collapse of the lung
4. Chronic lung diseases, such as emphysema, that obstruct bronchial airflow and distend the alveoli
5. Hyperventilation associated with periods of high anxiety
6. Obstruction of airways, which accompanies, for example, acute infections or allergic reactions that create bronchial spasm or edema
7. Reduction in elimination of carbon dioxide associated with certain lung diseases (see the section on respiratory acidosis, in Chapter 31, page 805)

Impaired Gas Exchange

Changes in the acidity or alkalinity of the blood may lead to *respiratory acidosis* (insufficient exhalation of carbon dioxide) or *respiratory alkalosis* (excessive exhalation of carbon dioxide). Patient responses and contributing factors are discussed in detail in Chapter 31, page 805.

Decreased Cardiac Output

This response may be manifested by cardiac arrhythmias, variations in blood pressure readings, tachycardia or bradycardia, pallor or cyanosis of the skin and mucous membranes, cold and clammy skin, restlessness, fatigue, jugular vein distention, reduced urine output, edema, and respiratory problems (e.g., orthopnea, dyspnea, shortness of breath, rales, cough, and frothy sputum).

Factors contributing to decreased cardiac output include:

1. Cardiac dysfunctions associated with coronary artery disease, valvular heart disease, structural abnormalities, conduction failures, etc.
2. Reduced blood volume due to hemorrhage, severe dehydration, severe allergic reactions, or burns
3. Cardiac arrest due to electrocution, heart attack, acute respiratory failure, etc.
4. Specific electrolyte imbalances, such as excessive blood potassium

Nursing Interventions to Maintain Normal Respirations

Positioning

Normally, adequate ventilation is maintained by frequent changes of position, ambulation, and exercise. When persons become ill, however, their respiratory functions may be inhibited for a variety of reasons. A common reason is immobility induced by surgery or medical therapy. Lying too long in one position compresses the thorax, limits chest expansion, and thus inhibits the movement of air through the lungs. Sitting in a slumped position also inhibits chest expansion, since the abdominal contents are pushed up against the diaphragm. Another frequent cause of limited chest expansion is abdominal pain or chest pain. The patient often voluntarily limits chest movements to relieve the pain. Shallow respirations inhibit both diaphragmatic excursion and lung distensibility. The result of inadequate chest expansion is stasis and pooling of respiratory secretions, which ultimately harbor microorganisms and promote infection. This situation is often compounded in the hospitalized patient who receives narcotics for pain because narcotics further depress the rate and depth of respiration.

Interventions by the nurse to maintain the normal respirations of patients include (a) positioning the patient to allow for maximum chest expansion, (b) encouraging or providing frequent changes in position for bed patients, (c) encouraging ambulation, and (d) implementing measures that promote comfort, such as giving pain medications. The semi-Fowler's or high Fowler's position encourages maximum chest expansion in bed patients, particularly dyspneic patients. The nurse needs to encourage patients unable to assume this position to turn from side to side frequently, so that alternate sides of the chest are permitted maximum expansion.

Deep Breathing and Coughing

In addition to positioning patients, the nurse can facilitate respiratory functioning by encouraging deep breathing exercises and coughing to remove secretions. The nurse can demonstrate such exercises. The nurse places the hands palm down on the border of the rib cage and inhales slowly and evenly until the greatest chest expansion is achieved, holds the breath for a few seconds, and exhales slowly through the mouth. Exhalation continues until maximum chest contraction is achieved. As the patient breathes deeply, the nurse may place his or her hands on the border of the patient's chest.

The number of breaths and the frequency of exercises vary with the patient's condition. Patients on bedrest or recovering from abdominal or chest surgery need deep breathing exercises at least three or four times daily. At each session, the patient should take a minimum of five deep breaths. Patients who are prone to pulmonary problems may need deep breathing exercises every hour. Patients with chronic respiratory disease need special breathing exercises, including pursed-lip breathing and abdominal breathing exercises.

Voluntary coughing in conjunction with deep breathing facilitates the movement and expectoration of respiratory tract secretions. Frequently, deep breathing exercises initiate the cough reflex. Voluntary coughing, however, is encouraged for patients who are susceptible to accumulating respiratory secretions. An example is the postoperative patient. Medications administered preoperatively and general anesthesia depress the action of the cilia and the respiratory center. Secretions then accumulate and may become tenacious and thick, eventually obstructing some airways. The nurse should encourage and help such patients to cough, particularly those with chest or abdominal incisions.

Coughing is most effective when the patient is sitting. After a deep inhalation, the patient coughs forcefully, using the abdominal and other accessory respiratory muscles. If the patient has an incision, the nurse can support it by placing the palms of the hands on either side of the incision as the patient coughs. Patients with abdominal incisions can be instructed to support (splint) the incision with a firmly rolled pillow.

Adequate Hydration

Adequate hydration maintains the moisture of the respiratory mucous membranes. Normally respiratory tract secretions are thin and therefore moved readily by ciliary action. However, when the patient is dehydrated or when the environment has a low humidity, the respiratory secretions can become thick and tenacious. The mucous membranes then become irritated and prone to infection. Nursing measures to increase and monitor fluid intake are discussed in Chapter 30. If the air lacks humidity, humidifiers may be necessary. See the discussion of humidifiers later in this chapter.

Promoting Health Practices and a Healthy Environment

The effects of cigarette smoking and air pollution on health are well known. Chronic bronchitis associated with both can progress to disabling breathlessness and prolonged respiratory and cardiovascular ailments. Smoking is associated with (a) increased incidence of lung cancer, (b) prevalence of bronchitis and emphysema with recurrent episodes of respiratory infection, (c) development of premature coronary heart disease, (d) birth of babies with a lower than average birth weight, and (e) higher rates of cancer of the larynx, pharynx, oral cavity, esophagus, pancreas, and urinary bladder (World Health Organization 1975:8). The nurse can be instrumental in providing health instruction to individual patients and the public. Many communities now offer supportive programs to help people stop smoking. When young people stop smoking, pulmonary functions may return to normal. In persons with moderately severe obstructive lung impairments, the return of normal function may never occur. However, dyspnea and cough can be significantly reduced.

Nursing Interventions to Relieve Respiratory Impairment

Lung Inflation Techniques

Breathing exercises

Special breathing exercises are carried out primarily to promote the exchange of gases in the lungs, to strengthen the muscles used for breathing, and to increase breathing efficiency. Breathing exercises are frequently indicated for patients with restricted chest expansion, i.e., people with chronic lung disease (COPD) or patients recovering from thoracic surgery. Breathing exercises stress exhalation rather than inhalation. Two commonly employed breathing exercises are pursed-lip breathing and abdominal (diaphragmatic) breathing.

Figure 29–5 Triflow bottles expand the alveoli and strengthen muscles of expiration.

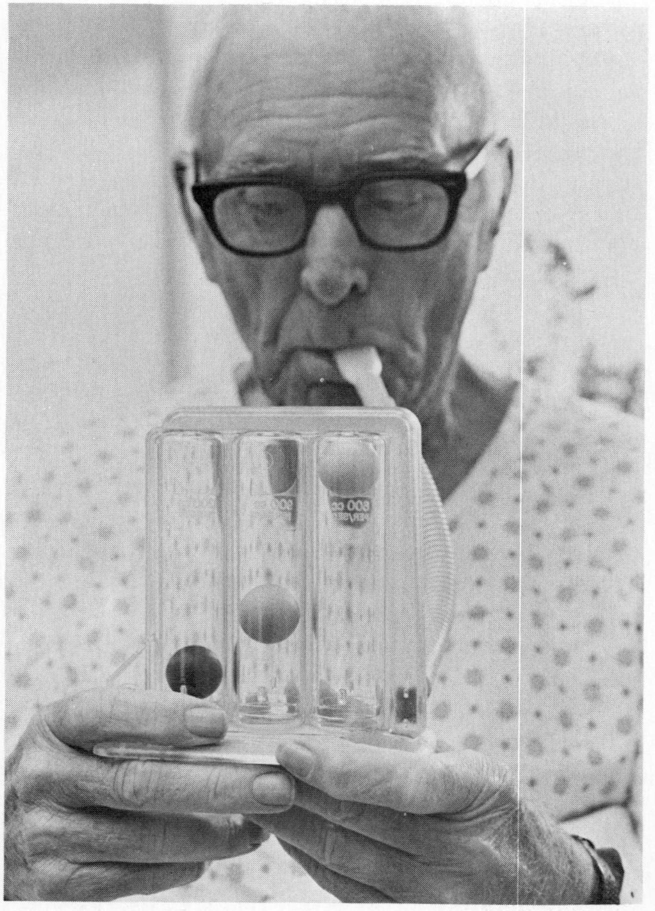

Pursed-lip breathing is a controlled breathing pattern patients can use when they experience shortness of breath. Once learned, pursed-lip breathing can become automatic. It slows the respiratory rate, promotes deep breaths, and facilitates expiration. It is therefore particularly useful during activities that normally cause dyspnea and an increased respiratory rate.

After a normal inspiration through the nose, the individual purses (puckers) the lips and gradually exhales. Some advise exhaling to a count of seven. Putting pressure on the abdominal muscles by bending forward slightly or holding a pillow against the abdomen facilitates expiration.

Abdominal breathing is best learned in the supine position. The patient learns to augment normal abdominal breathing. With one hand on the chest and one on the abdomen, the patient inhales deeply through the nose while elevating the abdomen. This action lowers the diaphragm further, thus increasing lung capacity. The patient then exhales slowly while pressing the abdomen inward and upward, expiring all but the residual volume. This sequence is repeated as tolerated by the patient. Once the patient learns augmented abdominal breathing in the supine position, the patient can progress to breathe similarly in sitting and then standing positions.

Blow bottles

Blow bottles are two bottles half filled with water and connected by tubing. The person moves the water from one bottle to the other by blowing into a short tube connected to the first bottle. Triflow bottles are used in some agencies. See Figure 29–5. The pressure in the bottle increases as the water displaces the air. When using blow bottles, the patient increases the pressure of the alveolar air because of the prolonged exhalation against pressure. This is believed to expand collapsed alveoli and strengthen the muscles of expiration.

When using blow bottles, the patient needs to seal the lips tightly around the tubing so that the exhaled air does not leak from the tubing. The goal of the adult patient is to move about 100 ml of water with each exhalation. The nurse should determine the amount of water moved with each exhalation and the response of the patient to the technique.

Incentive respiratory spirometry

There are many incentive respiratory devices designed to improve the volume of inspiration. The spirometer is one. The patient seals the lips tightly around the mouthpiece, takes as deep an inspiration as possible, holds it for a few seconds, and then exhales slowly. If the volume of the inspiration reaches a predetermined level (up to 5000 ml), the machine provides feedback, for example a light may come on when the predetermined volume is reached.

Intermittent positive pressure breathing therapy

Intermittent positive pressure breathing (IPPB) is a breathing pattern established by inflating the lungs with positive (above atmospheric) pressure during inspiration and by releasing the pressure so that expiration occurs passively. Some IPPB machines can exert pressure during expiration, and the abbreviations IPPB/I (inspiratory) and IPPB/E (expiratory) are sometimes used to differentiate the two methods. Generally, however, the term *IPPB* refers to positive pressure therapy administered during inspiration, a safer and more common practice.

As with most oxygen equipment, various types of IPPB machines are marketed. Two commonly used ones are the Bird Respirator and the Bennett Respirator. See Figure 29–6. Usually, IPPB treatments are given by respiratory technicians or by nurses who have had special training. However, the general nurse needs to understand the reason for IPPB therapy and its principles to assist patients as needed in the absence of special technicians. The nurse must also observe the patient's progress and response to such therapy. This discussion is limited to IPPB therapy that is patient activated and given on an intermittent basis. Controlled or time-cycled continuous therapy is used for patients unable to initiate inspiration. The breathing of such patients is maintained entirely by machine.

Indications for IPPB IPPB therapy is frequently prescribed in 15- to 20-minute periods three or four

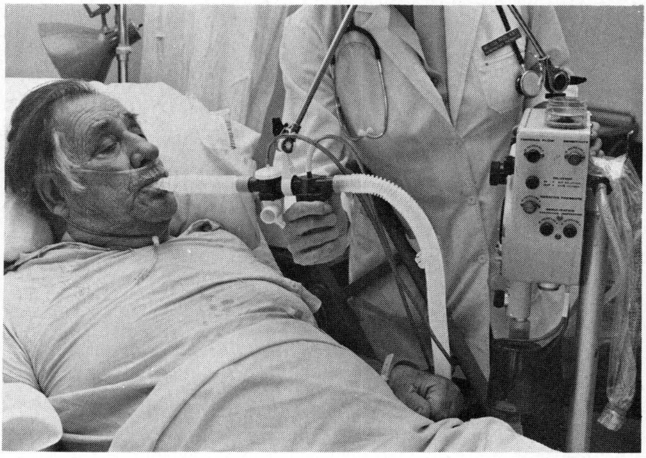

Figure 29–6 IPPB machines are effective in delivering aerosol medications to the lung and increasing the depth of respiration. As a result, infection and the accumulation of secretions are prevented.

times a day. The purposes of therapy include one or more of the following:

1. To deliver aerosol medications, such as antibiotics, bronchodilators, detergents, or mucolytics
2. To increase the depth of respiration periodically and prevent accumulation of secretions that may result in infections or *atelectasis* (lung collapse)
3. To facilitate the clearing of bronchial secretions in patients who have difficulty coughing or inspiring deeply
4. To orient patients preoperatively to the IPPB therapy that may be used postoperatively
5. To provide moisture to the respiratory mucous membranes

Assisting patients with IPPB Patients receiving IPPB therapy need to be upright, preferably in a chair or in the high Fowler's position. The upright position provides the most adequate ventilation of the lungs. The patient also needs to be taught to breathe through the mouth and not the nose. Nose clips are available but are not usually necessary if the patient receives appropriate instruction. The patient needs to practice with a mouthpiece prior to therapy. The mouthpiece must be completely sealed by the lips and made airtight for the IPPB system to operate efficiently.

Encouraging the patient to breathe normally is also helpful. Some patients have a tendency to force their respiration or to struggle with the apparatus. When advised not to force breaths, to relax, to breathe slowly, and to allow time for expiration (which takes longer than inspiration), these patients normally adjust to the therapy readily. The nurse should remind patients that they control the respirator: Each time patients breathe in, they start the machine; each time patients breathe out, they stop the machine. Extra effort is not required because the machine does not dictate breathing. The machine will not start until the patient breathes in. However, it is often necessary to encourage the patient to allow the pressure to reach its peak before exhaling. The patient should try not to breathe out until the positive pressure respirator fills the lungs.

The nurse needs to observe the patient's lung expansion during therapy and the efficacy of the therapy. The degree of lung expansion can be visually observed; however, the gauges on the respirator can be more reliable measures. If the needle gauge on the respirator reaches the preset pressure levels as the patient inhales, then respiration is satisfactory. However, if there is inadequate or no deflection of the needle gauges, the nurse needs to assess the problem. Is the system airtight? Perhaps the patient has not sealed the lips around the mouthpiece adequately. Is the patient relaxed? Perhaps the patient is not breathing normally or is blowing back into the mouthpiece before the lungs are filled. Is the machine triggering? Perhaps the patient does not have sufficient inspiratory effort to start the machine, in which case the sensitivity gauge needs to be adjusted. Perhaps the patient is sucking or using too much inspiratory effort, so that the needle deflection is too negative. By staying with the patient during IPPB therapy, the nurse can provide constructive assistance and instruction.

Postural Drainage

Postural drainage is the use of specific positions to drain, by gravity, secretions from various lung segments. It is used (a) to remove secretions that have accumulated in patients with chronic lung disease or other respiratory problems, and (b) to prevent the accumulation of secretions in patients who are unconscious or receiving mechanical ventilation. Retained secretions promote bacterial growth and subsequent infection and can obstruct small airways. Secretions in the major airways, such as the trachea and the right and left main bronchi, are usually coughed out or can be removed by suctioning. See the section on oropharyngeal and nasopharyngeal suctioning in this chapter. However, the peripheral lung segments cannot drain into these main airways unless postural techniques are used.

The physician or nurse determines which positions to use by assessing which areas need draining. Assessment of the areas involved is determined by auscultation, percussion, or roentgenograms. Abnormal breath sounds such as rales can be heard on auscultation; dullness or flatness can be determined by percussion.

Supportive techniques

Prior to postural drainage, the patient may be given bronchodilator medications or nebulization therapy to promote drainage and expectoration of secretions. The nurse needs to tell the patient to use abdominal breathing throughout the drainage session. During postural drainage, the nurse or physiotherapist can facilitate the loosening or dislodgment of dry or tenacious secretions by using percussion (cupping) and vibration techniques.

Percussion is the technique of using cupped hands to strike forcefully the chest wall over the congested area. The nurse holds the fingers and thumb together and slightly flexed to form a cup, such as one forms when scooping water with the hands. With the hands in this position, the nurse loosely and rapidly flexes and extends the wrists to slap the thoracic cage. It is important to keep the hands cupped to maintain an air-cushioned impact and avoid hurting the patient. During percussion, the nurse should avoid striking the spinal column, the breasts, or the kidneys. Percussion usually lasts 1 or 2 minutes and is usually confined to the most congested areas.

Vibration is a vigorous quivering. This technique is used after percussion and over the same areas, but only while the patient exhales. The nurse places one hand flat on the chest wall and the other hand on top of the first. Using mainly the heel of the hand, the nurse tenses all hand and arm muscles and then presses downward and vibrates the chest wall. The nurse relaxes the pressure as the patient inhales. The nurse vibrates each area four or five times during one session.

Periodically during postural drainage, percussion, and vibration, the nurse encourages the patient to cough up secretions. Tissues and a paper bag must be provided for this purpose. After postural drainage, the nurse gives the patient mouthwash to refresh and clean the mouth. The nurse records the effectiveness of the therapy, noting the color, character, and amount of sputum expectorated and the reaction of the patient to therapy. Many patients may require instruction to use these techniques at home.

Scheduling postural drainage

Frequently, postural drainage treatments are scheduled two or three times daily, depending on how congested the patient is. The best times include before breakfast, before lunch, in the late afternoon, or before bedtime. It is best to avoid hours shortly after meals because postural drainage at these times can tire the patient and induce vomiting.

The length of treatments must also be considered. Usually, the entire treatment, including preparatory nebulization and deep breathing as well as all postures, takes 30 minutes. Some patients can tolerate long, relatively infrequent treatments. Others require shorter, more frequent treatments. The nurse needs to evaluate the patient's tolerance of these treatments by observing the stability of the patient's vital signs, particularly the pulse and respiratory rates, and by noting signs of intolerance, such as pallor, diaphoresis, dyspnea, or fatigue.

Some patients do not react well to certain drainage positions, and the nurse must make appropriate adjustments. For example, some become dyspneic in the Trendelenburg positions and require only a moderate tilt or a shorter time in those positions.

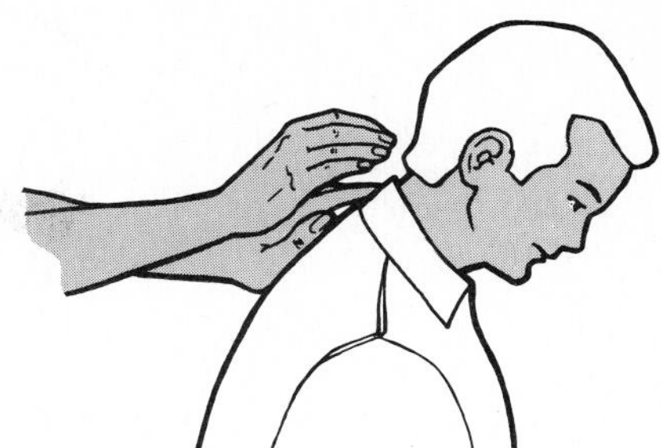

Figure 29–7 Position for drainage of apical segments of the upper lobes.

Positions for postural drainage

Positions for adults are described below. Positions for small children are given in Kozier and Erb (1982: 1182–90). There are three broad categories of positions:

1. Positions that drain the upper lung segments or upper lobes.
2. Positions that drain the middle lung segments. Note that only the right lung has a middle lobe.
3. Positions that drain the basal lung segments or lower lobes.

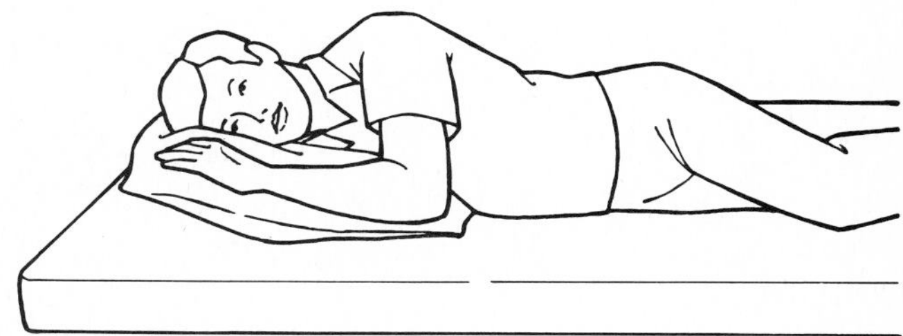

Figure 29–8 Position for drainage of posterior segments of the upper lobes.

Drainage of the upper lobes The upper lobes consist of three segments: the apical or uppermost segments and the anterior and posterior segments, which lie below the apical segments.

1. To drain the apical segments, the patient sits upright in a chair with the head bent slightly forward. See Figure 29–7. The nurse percusses the area between the clavicle (collarbone) and the scapulae (shoulder blades).
2. To drain the posterior segments, the patient lies partly on the side and partly on the abdomen, with a pillow under the head, chest, and arm. The bed should be flat while the *right* posterior segment drains; the nurse elevates the head of the bed about 15° while the *left* posterior segment drains. See Figure 29–8. The nurse percusses the upper back on both sides between the scapulae.
3. To drain the anterior segments, the patient lies on a flat bed with pillows under the knees to flex them while the nurse percusses the upper chest below the clavicle down to the nipple line, except for women. The breasts of women are not percussed to avoid causing pain. See Figure 29–9.

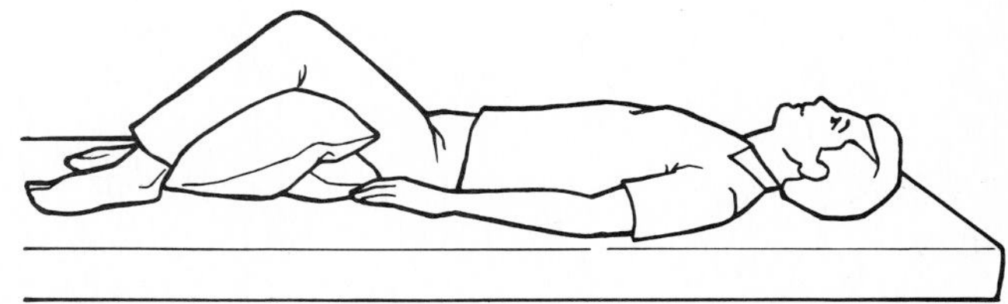

Figure 29–9 Position for drainage of anterior segments of the upper lobes.

Drainage of the right middle lobe and left middle segments Only the right lung has a middle lobe, which has two segments (lateral and medial). The left lung has superior and inferior segments at the lower half of its longer upper lobe, which is called the *lingula* of that lobe.

1. To drain the *left lingular segments*, the nurse elevates the foot of the bed about 40 cm (15 in) and the patient lies on the right side. The nurse helps the patient lean back slightly (about a quarter turn) against pillows extending from the shoulder to the hip. See Figure 29–10. If the patient is male, the nurse percusses over the left side of the chest at the level of the nipple between the fourth and sixth ribs. If the patient is female, the nurse, with the heel of the hand toward the armpit and the cupped fingers extending forward beneath the breast, percusses beneath the breast.
2. To drain the *right middle lobe*, the nurse elevates the foot of the bed about 40 cm (15 in) and the patient

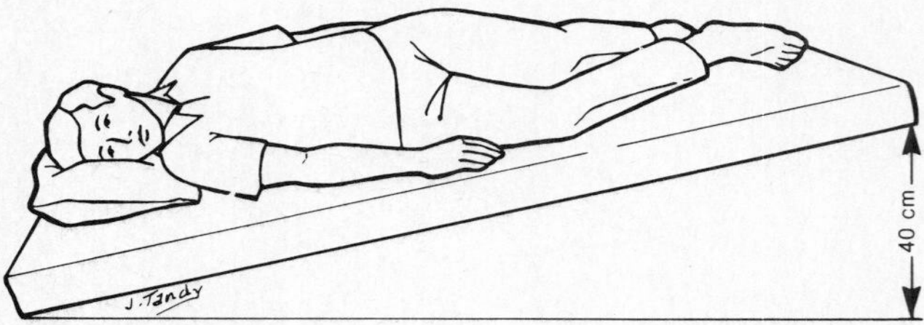

Figure 29–10 Position for drainage of the left lingular segments.

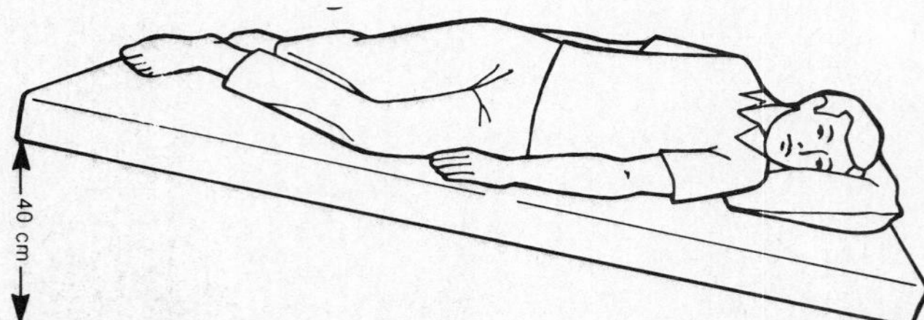

Figure 29–11 Position for drainage of the lateral and medial segments of the right middle lobe.

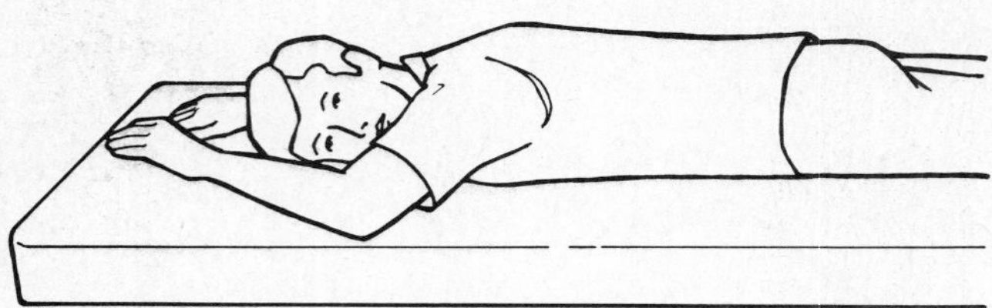

Figure 29–12 Position for drainage of the superior segments of the lower lobes.

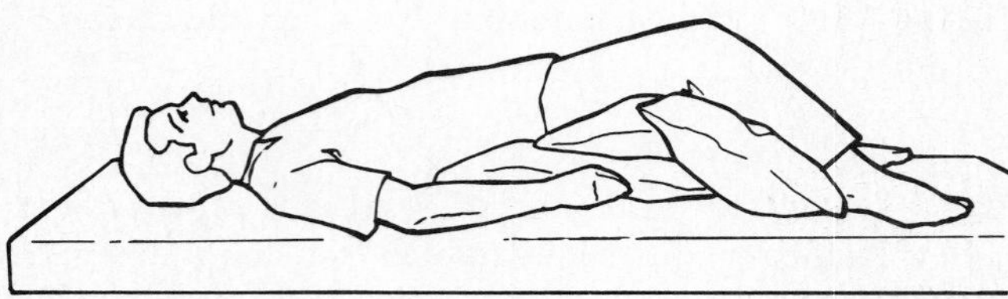

Figure 29–13 Position for drainage of the anterior basal segments of the lower lobes.

assumes the position opposite to that described above, i.e., lying on the left side. The nurse percusses the right side of the chest. See Figure 29–11.

Drainage of the lower lobes The lower lung lobes have four segments: a superior segment and three basal (lowermost) segments, i.e., anterior basal, lateral basal, and posterior basal.

1. To drain the *superior segments*, the patient lies on the abdomen on a flat bed. The nurse percusses the middle area of the back (below the scapulae) on both sides of the spine. See Figure 29–12.
2. To drain the *anterior basal segments*, the patient lies on the back. The nurse elevates the foot of the bed about 45 cm (18 in) or to the height tolerated by the patient *or* uses two or three pillows to elevate the patient's hips so that they are higher than the shoulders. See Figure 29–13. The nurse percusses both sides of the chest over the lower ribs, avoiding the stomach.
3. To drain the *lateral basal segments*, the patient lies partly on the side and partly on the abdomen. The nurse elevates the foot of the bed about 45 cm (18 in) or elevates the patient's hips with pillows. See Figure 29–14. The nurse percusses the uppermost side of the lower ribs. To drain the left lateral basal segment, the patient lies on the right side; to drain the right lateral segment, the patient lies on the left side.
4. To drain the *posterior basal segments*, the patient lies prone. The nurse elevates the foot of the bed about 45 cm (18 in) or elevates the hips on three or four pillows to produce a jackknife position from the knees to the shoulders. See Figure 29–15. The nurse percusses over the lower ribs on both sides close to the spine, but not directly over the spine or the flanks, under which the kidneys lie.

Humidifiers

The provision of moisture for the respiratory mucous membranes is a common therapy for persons with respiratory problems. Humidification is offered in a variety of ways and often is a necessary adjunct to other

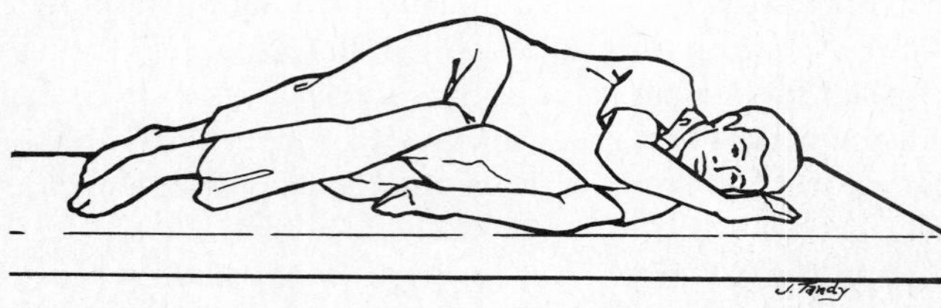

Figure 29–14 Position for drainage of the lateral basal segments of the lower lobes.

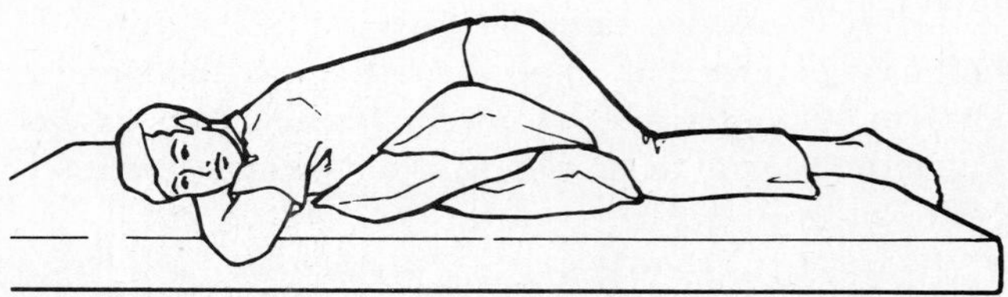

Figure 29–15 Position for drainage of the posterior basal segments of the lower lobes.

therapies such as oxygen inhalation and nebulization. Hot steam inhalators and Croupette humidity tents are two widely used humidifiers.

Hot steam inhalators

Several types of steam inhalators are manufactured commercially. In the home, however, an ordinary electric kettle may be used. When inhaled, steam provides warmth and moisture to the mucous membrane. Both facilitate the expectoration of secretions. The warmth increases the blood supply and hydration of the respiratory membranes by transudation. *Transudation* is the passage of body fluid through a membrane or tissue surface. Warmth also relaxes the smooth muscles of the respiratory passages. The moisture liquefies secretions and decreases irritation. For optimal effectiveness, steam must be inhaled deeply, slowly, and as directly as possible. Precautions are necessary, however, to avoid burns to the patient's face or elsewhere by accidental contact with the equipment. For continuous steam inhalations, such as for bedridden patients, the nurse directs the nozzle of the steam inhalator so that steam surrounds the patient's head. The steam should not, however, flow directly toward the patient's face. Drafts need to be prevented or minimized, and damp linen needs to be changed to avoid chills. The nurse should encourage the patient to expectorate and provide tissues and a disposal container. For intermittent inhalations, the patient may sit close to the inhalator and breathe deeply.

Steam inhalation may be prescribed as a vehicle to administer medications. A common home remedy is tincture of benzoin. The steam may be directed over the medication, or the medication may be mixed with the water.

Croupette humidity tent

The Croupette humidity tent, a rectangular, clear plastic tent, is often used for infants and young children with respiratory problems. See Figure 29–16. It provides

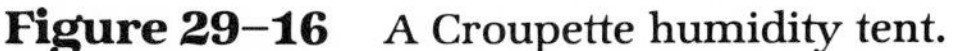

Figure 29–16 A Croupette humidity tent.

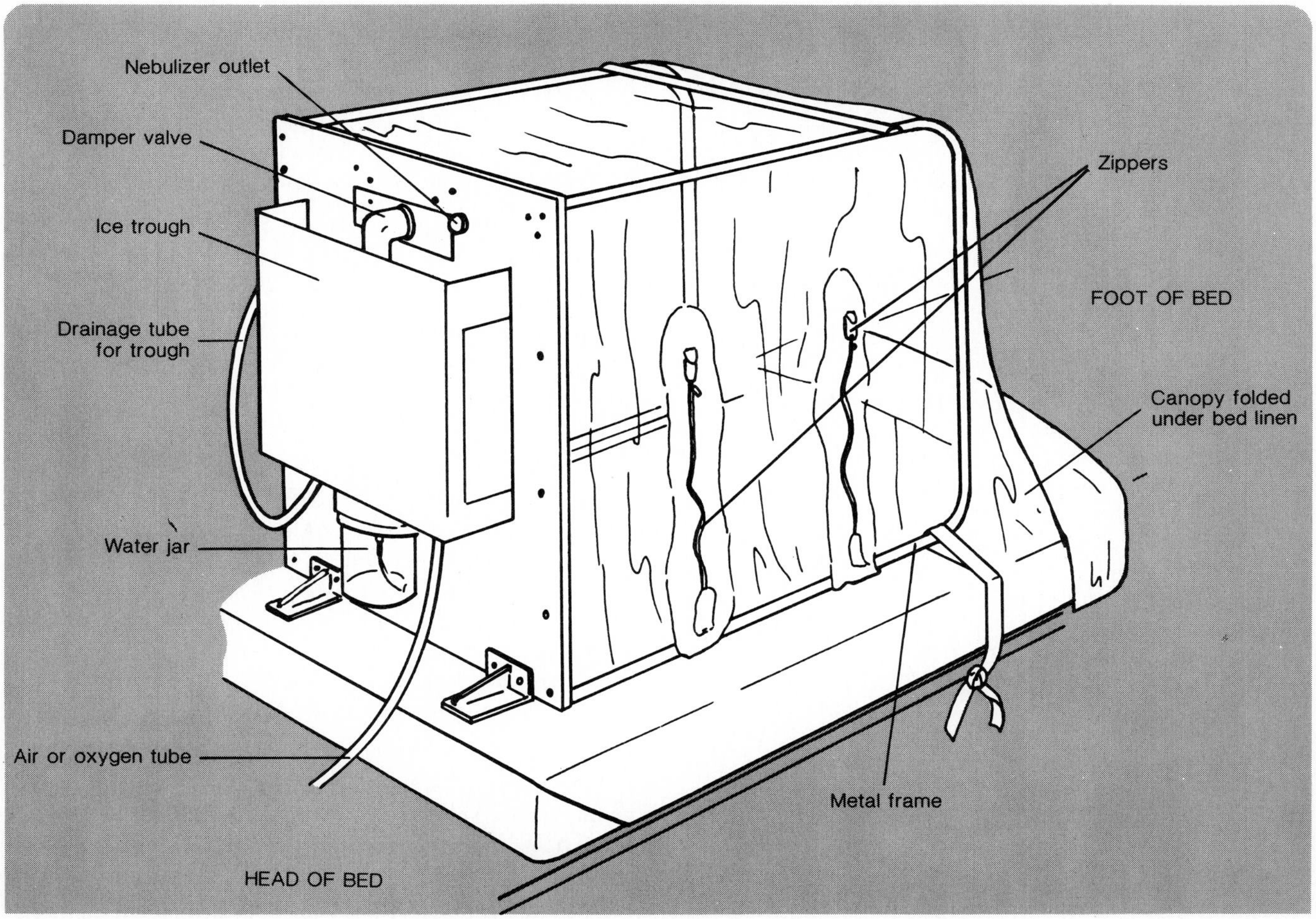

high humidity and can increase the percentage of oxygen in the air breathed to 40% to 60%. The cooling and moisturizing effects help reduce fevers accompanying respiratory infections and also help liquefy respiratory secretions. The temperature is maintained at 20 to 21 C (68 to 70 F). It is checked by placing a bath thermometer inside the canopy. The canopy of the tent is supported by a metal frame, which is usually tied with gauze strips to the upper third of the bedsprings. The tent has one or two zippers on each side that allow the nurse to care for the infant or child yet keep the humidity and oxygen levels in the tent relatively constant. At the end of the tent, which lies against the head of the bed, are the various mechanical parts, which provide humidity and oxygenation. The largest container is the trough, which is filled with ice to the depth (about 10 in) indicated by a line on the trough. A drainage tube connected to the trough is kept in an elevated notch or opening until drainage is desired, at which time it is detached and lowered into a receptacle below. A damper valve, located on the large tube between the trough and the tent, is opened periodically and then closed to minimize condensation or adjusted for continuous operation in accordance with doctor's orders. Another tube beneath the trough connects to the air or oxygen source. Before placing the infant in the tent, the nurse floods the tent with air and oxygen if ordered. The flowmeter is then adjusted to deliver the required amount of oxygen. (See the section on oxygen therapy for further information.) Alongside the air tube is a jar with a screw cap. This jar is filled with distilled water to a mark indicated by a black line. Its purpose is to moisturize the air or oxygen entering the Croupette, and it must be refilled at least every 8 hours to maintain this level. In addition, a nebulizer outlet is provided to supply aerosol antibiotics or other aerosols as required. This outlet is attached to additional tubing and a secondary air or oxygen source. The front part of the canopy is fan-folded well into the bedclothes or into an additional overlying drawsheet to ensure closure of the tent. All sides of the canopy must be well tucked under the mattress.

The child in a Croupette needs physical protection and frequent observation. The nurse needs to protect the child from chilling and from the dampness of condensation. Additional gowns or a cotton blanket can be used. Some agencies provide gowns with hoods, or the nurse may wrap a small towel around the infant's head. The bed linen and clothing needs to be changed frequently. A small pillow or rolled towel placed at the head of the Croupette can keep the child from bruising or bumping the head. This padding also absorbs the excess, condensed moisture. When administering care, the nurse must maintain humidity and oxygen therapy. This can be accomplished by moving the canopy up around the infant's head and neck and securing it under a pillow when providing care. The nurse also needs to provide emotional support to the child, particularly to preschoolers, who can be exceedingly anxious.

Maintenance of the equipment is essential. The water needs to be drained and the ice in the trough replenished as necessary. The distilled water in the screw-cap bottle must also be maintained. The air and oxygen flow must also be monitored frequently to maintain appropriate concentrations. All connections should be airtight.

Figure 29–17 The basic parts of the nebulizer include: **A,** cylindrical chamber for aerosol; **B,** opening into chamber used to insert aerosol and closed by a cork or cap when filled; **C,** wide, open end that attaches to a patient's mouth piece or a Croupette humidity tent; and **D,** narrow, open end that attaches to a pressure source, such as a hand pump.

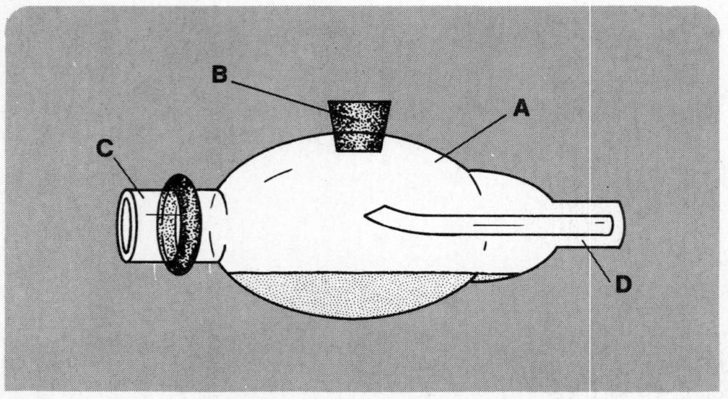

Nebulization

A *nebulizer* is an atomizer or sprayer. These come in various designs and materials but in essence have four main parts. See Figure 29–17.

1. A cylindrical chamber, *A*, which holds the prescribed amount of aerosol.
2. An opening at the top of the chamber, *B*, into which the aerosol is inserted. A small syringe with or without a needle needs to be used to inject the aerosol into the chamber of some nebulizers.
3. A wide, open end, *C*, that may be affixed to a Croupette humidity tent or to a mouthpiece through which the patient inhales.
4. A smaller, open end, *D*, containing a tube that is attached to a pressure source such as oxygen or a hand pressure pump.

Nebulization therapy is also referred to as *inhalation* or *aerosol therapy*. Frequently medications such as bronchodilators or mucolytic agents are administered by nebulization. These are inhaled directly from various commercially prepared aerosol containers or may be administered in conjunction with oxygen or compressed air or through respirators (see the earlier section on intermittent positive pressure breathing). The latter method is useful when aerosol treatments need to be administered for 10- or 15-minute periods. Nebulization in conjunction with IPPB equipment is especially effective for reaching lower respiratory passages. The IPPB equipment promotes slow, deep breathing and delivers a very fine mist, both of which help the aerosol penetrate into the lower respiratory passages. Hand atomizers, by contrast, deliver larger droplets and are more effective for the upper respiratory passages.

Artificial Oropharyngeal Airways

The oropharyngeal airway is the simplest type of artificial airway. It is a curved rubber or plastic device used to bypass the obstruction of the tongue lying against the posterior pharynx in unconscious patients. This airway is available in a variety of sizes for children and adults. To determine the appropriate size for a person, the nurse places the airway along the side of the external cheek. When the flange of the airway is parallel to the front teeth, the airway should extend back to the angle of the jaw. Placement of too large an airway forces the epiglottis down onto the laryngeal opening, obstructing it.

Insertion of the airway is achieved by gently placing it over the tongue and first pointing it toward the cheek. Once it has passed over the back of the tongue, the nurse gently turns the airway so that it points toward the patient's feet. When the flange of the airway is external to the teeth and the curved tip lies at the level of the epiglottis, the airway is correctly placed.

This type of airway is commonly used for patients recovering from anesthesia postoperatively. Upon regaining consciousness, the patient automatically dislodges the mouth piece. Suctioning of the airway may be necessary to maintain its patency.

Oropharyngeal and Nasopharyngeal Suctioning

The nurse must sometimes apply suction to the oropharynx and nasal passages of patients who have difficulty swallowing or expectorating secretions. *Suctioning* is the aspiration of secretions often through a rubber or polyethylene catheter connected to a suction machine or wall outlet. Catheters used for suctioning vary in size from 14 to 18 French for adults and from 8 to 18 French for children. The tip of a suction catheter has several openings along the sides. These openings distribute the negative pressure of the suction over a wide area, thus preventing excessive irritation to any one area of the respiratory mucous membrane. The suction apparatus includes a collection bottle, a tubing system connected to the suction catheter, and a gauge that registers the degree of suction. These gauges are either portable or wall mounted.

Suctioning of the upper respiratory airways is indicated when the patient (a) is unable to cough, (b) is unable to swallow, and (c) makes light bubbling or rattling breath sounds that signal the accumulation of secretions.

Procedure 29–1 Suctioning Oropharyngeal and Nasal Passages

Goals

1. To remove secretions that obstruct the airway and to facilitate respiratory ventilation
2. To obtain secretions for diagnostic purposes
3. To prevent infection that may result from accumulated secretions

Equipment

1. Portable suction machine or gauge to attach to wall suction
2. Sterile suction catheter
3. Y-connector to facilitate opening and closing of the suction system if the catheter does not have a thumb port
4. Container of sterile water or sterile normal saline to lubricate and flush the catheter
5. Sterile gloves
6. Sterile gauze to wipe the catheter and the patient's mouth or nose
7. Moisture-resistant bag to discard disposable catheters and gloves
8. Towel to protect the patient's gown and pillows

Preparation

1. Wash hands using surgical aseptic technique.

   Rationale Aseptic technique prevents the transfer of microorganisms to the sterile equipment and the patient.

Procedure 29–1, continued

2. Explain the procedure to the patient. Mention that the procedure is painless but may stimulate the cough, gag, or sneeze reflexes.

   Rationale Knowing that the procedure will relieve breathing problems often reassures the patient and enlists his or her cooperation.

3. Position a conscious patient who has a functional gag reflex in the semi-Fowler's position with the patient's head turned to one side for oral suctioning and neck hyperextended for nasal suctioning.

   Rationale These positions facilitate the insertion of the catheter and help prevent aspiration of secretions.

4. Position an unconscious patient in the lateral position, facing the nurse.

   Rationale This position allows the patient's tongue to fall forward, thus preventing obstruction to the catheter on insertion. It also facilitates drainage of secretions from the pharynx and prevents the possibility of aspiration.

5. Place the towel over the pillow or under the patient's chin.

Intervention

1. Set the pressure on the suction gauge and turn on the suction. For wall units the pressure is set at:
   a. 115 to 150 mm Hg for adults
   b. 95 to 115 mm Hg for children
   c. 50 to 95 mm Hg for infants
   For portable units, use:
   a. 10 to 15 in Hg for adults
   b. 5 to 10 in Hg for children
   c. 2 to 5 in Hg for infants

2. Don the sterile gloves. One sterile glove for holding the catheter is usually sufficient.

3. Pick up the catheter with the sterile gloved hand and attach it to the suction unit.

4. Make an approximate measure for the insertion. Mark the position on the tube with the fingers of the gloved hand. An appropriate measure is the distance between the tip of the nose and the ear lobe, or about 13 cm (5 in) for an adult.

5. Moisten the catheter tip by dipping it in the container of sterile water or saline.

   Rationale Moistening the catheter reduces friction and eases insertion.

6. For a nasopharyngeal suction, insert the catheter gently through one nostril with your thumb away from the suction control (i.e., not applying suction). Direct the catheter along the floor of the nasal cavity. If one nostril is not patent, try the other. Never force the catheter against an obstruction.

   or

   For an oropharyngeal suction, insert the catheter through the mouth along one side into the oropharynx.

   Rationale Gentle insertion and not applying suction during insertion prevent trauma to the mucous membrane. Directing the catheter along the floor of the nasal cavity avoids the nasal turbinates. Directing the catheter along one side of the mouth prevents gagging.

7. Apply your finger to the suction control port and gently rotate the catheter. Apply suction for 5 to 10 seconds, then remove the finger from the control and remove the catheter. It may be necessary during oropharyngeal suctioning to apply suction to secretions that collect in the vestibule of the mouth and beneath the tongue. A suction attempt should last only 15 seconds. During this time the catheter is inserted, the suction applied and discontinued, and the catheter removed.

   Rationale Placing the finger over the suction (thumb) control port starts the suction. Gentle rotation of the catheter ensures that all surfaces are reached and also prevents trauma to any one area of the respiratory mucosa due to prolonged suction.

8. Wipe off the catheter with sterile gauze, flush it with sterile water or saline, lubricate it, and repeat steps 6 and 7 until the air passage is clear, but do not apply suction for more than 3 to 5 minutes in total.

   Rationale Applying suction for too long can decrease the patient's oxygen supply.

Procedure 29–1 continued

9. Encourage the patient to breathe deeply and cough between suctions.

   Rationale Coughing and breathing help carry secretions from the trachea and bronchi into the pharynx, where they can be reached with the suction catheter.

10. When the catheter has been removed, rinse the catheter by flushing it with water.

    Rationale Rinsing the catheter removes secretions from the tubing.

11. Dispose of the catheter, glove, water, and container.

12. Ensure that equipment is available for the next suctioning. Change suction collection bottles and tubing daily or more frequently as necessary.

13. Record the amount, consistency, color, and odor of secretions and observe the patient's breathing status. For example; foamy, white mucus; thick, green-tinged mucus, or blood-flecked mucus.

Oxygen Therapy

Additional oxygen is indicated for numerous patients who have *hypoxemia* (poor blood oxygenation). Many conditions produce hypoxemia. Examples are lung congestion from any cause that reduces the diffusion of oxygen through the respiratory membrane, heart failure leading to inadequate transport of oxygen, substantial loss of lung tissue due to tumors or surgery, and airways narrowed or obstructed by infections or other disease processes. In most situations, oxygen therapy is prescribed by the physician, who specifies the specific concentration, method, and liter flow per minute. The concentration is of more importance than the liter flow per minute.

When the administration of oxygen is an emergency measure, the nurse may initiate the therapy after assessing the clinical signs of acute hypoxemia. These signs generally include, in order of occurrence:

1. Increased rapid pulse
2. Rapid, shallow respirations and dyspnea
3. Increased restlessness or lightheadedness
4. Flaring of the nares
5. Substernal or intercostal retractions
6. Cyanosis

Difficult breathing creates apprehension and panic. The nurse, therefore, needs to be competent in providing support and appropriate therapy.

Safety precautions during oxygen therapy

Oxygen will not by itself burn or explode, but it does facilitate combustion. For example, a bed sheet ordinarily burns slowly when ignited in the normal atmosphere; however, if saturated with free-flowing oxygen, it will burn rapidly and explosively when ignited by a spark. The greater the concentration of oxygen, the more rapidly fires start and burn. Extinguishing such fires can be difficult. Because oxygen is colorless, odorless, and tasteless, people are often unaware of the presence of oxygen and need reminding. The staff, the patient, and visitors must all take safety precautions. The nurse ensures safety by:

1. Placing cautionary "No smoking: Oxygen in Use" signs on the patient's door, at the foot or head of the bed, and on the oxygen equipment.
2. Removing matches and cigarette lighters from the bedside.
3. Requesting other patients in the room and visitors to smoke in areas provided elsewhere in the hospital.
4. Removing or storing electrical equipment, such as razors, hearing aids, radios, televisions, and heating pads, in case short-circuit sparks occur.
5. Avoiding materials that generate static electricity, such as woolen blankets or synthetic fabrics. Cotton blankets are provided, and nurses are advised to wear cotton fabrics.
6. Avoiding the use of volatile, flammable materials, such as oils, greases, alcohol, or ether, near patients receiving oxygen. Lip ointments, if required, should have a water-soluble base such as K-Y Jelly or glycerine. Alcohol back rubs are avoided, and nail polish removers or the like should be removed from the immediate vicinity.
7. Grounding electrical monitoring equipment, suction machines, and portable diagnostic machines. Oxygen therapy should be discontinued temporarily if portable radiographic equipment is required. Monitoring and suction equipment needs to be placed on the bedside opposite the oxygen source.

8. Making known the location of fire extinguishers and making sure personnel are trained in their use.

Supply of oxygen

Oxygen can be supplied from steel cylinders (oxygen tanks) that store 244 cubic feet of oxygen or smaller portable tanks designed for emergency or home use. The oxygen is stored under a pressure of 2200 psi (pounds per square inch). Many hospitals now provide piped-in oxygen from wall outlets next to each bed. Piped-in oxygen is usually stored under low pressure, about 50 to 60 psi.

Using oxygen tanks Oxygen tanks are generally encased in wheeled metal carriers whose broad, flat base allows the tanks to be placed upright at the bedside. A cap on the top protects the valves and outlets. Oxygen tanks should be placed beside the bedhead away from traffic and heaters. When in use, oxygen tanks must have regulators and humidifiers. The regulator has two parts: a flowmeter and a cylinder contents gauge. The purpose of the regulator is to reduce the pressure of the oxygen to a level safer than that in the cylinder. The flowmeter regulates the gas flow in liters per minute. Two types of regulators are shown in Figure 29–18. To assemble the oxygen tank for use, the nurse needs to:

1. Remove the protector cap.
2. Remove any dust in the outlets by slightly opening the handwheel at the top of the tank slowly and then closing it quickly. This is referred to as "cracking the tank." People can be frightened if not forewarned that there will be a loud, forceful hissing when the tank is opened. To open the tank, the nurse turns the handwheel clockwise.
3. Connect the flow regulator gauge to the tank output, shown in Figure 29–19, and tighten the inlet nut with a wrench, ensuring that the regulator is held firmly.
4. Stand at the side of the cylinder and open the cylinder valve very slowly until the needle on the cylinder gauge stops moving.
5. Regulate the flowmeter to the desired rate of flow in liters per minute. The rate of flow of the Thorpe regulator is adjusted by turning the flow-adjusting valve. The Bourdon is adjusted by turning the flow-adjusting handle slowly to the right.
6. Fill the humidifier bottle with distilled water to the mark indicated, and attach it below the flowmeter (see the next section).
7. Attach oxygen tubing and equipment specifically prescribed for the patient, for example, a nasal catheter, a nasal cannula, or a face mask.

Using piped-in oxygen To tap into a piped-in oxygen supply, the nurse uses only a flowmeter and a humidifier. The nurse must:

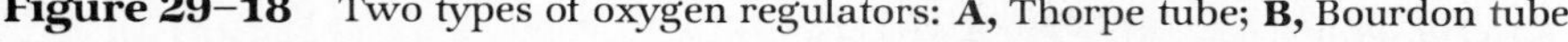

Figure 29–18 Two types of oxygen regulators: **A,** Thorpe tube; **B,** Bourdon tube.

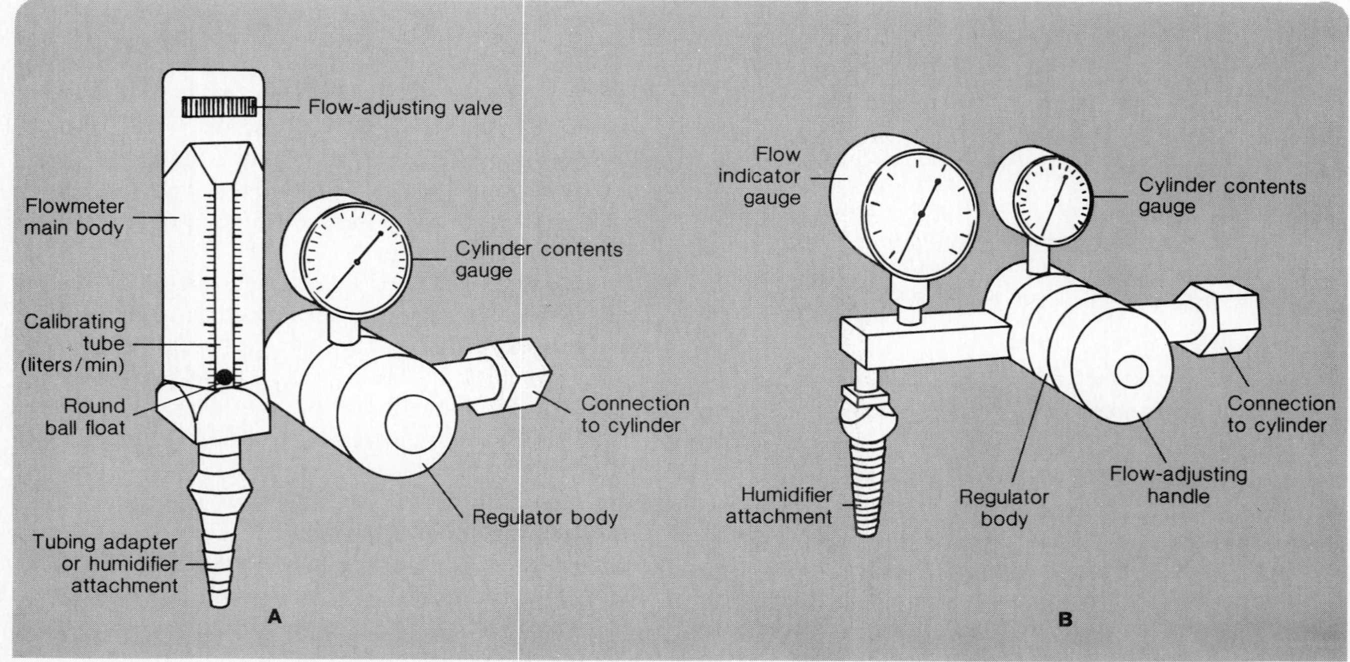

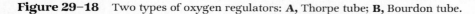

1. Attach the flowmeter to the wall outlet, exerting firm pressure. The flowmeter should be in the *off* position.
2. Fill the humidifier bottle with distilled water (this can be done before reaching the bedside).
3. Attach the humidifier bottle to the base of the flowmeter.
4. Attach oxygen tubing and the prescribed oxygen device.
5. Regulate the flowmeter to the desired level.

Oxygen humidifying devices

Oxygen administered from cylinders or pipeline systems is dry. Dry gases dehydrate the respiratory mucous membranes of patients. Thus, humidifying devices are an essential adjunct to oxygen therapy. See Figure 29–20. All humidifiers employ the simple method of passing the gas through sterile water so that the gas picks up water vapor before it reaches the patient; the more bubbles created, the more water vapor produced.

Methods of Oxygen Administration

Oxygen can be administered by nasal cannulae, nasal catheters, oxygen masks, Croupette and other oxygen tents, incubators, and respirators. Each method has different advantages and indications.

Nasal cannula

The nasal cannula (nasal prongs) is a relatively simple and comfortable method of supplying oxygen of low concentrations (22% to 30%) at flow rates of 1 to 5 liters per minute. The physician generally specifies the flow rate desired. The cannula does not interfere with the patient's ability to eat and does not bypass the natural respiratory functions of the nose. The patient wearing a cannula has freedom to move about in bed or from the bed to an adjacent chair.

The cannula consists of a rubber or plastic tube that extends from each cheekbone and has 0.6 to 1.3 cm (0.25 to 0.5 in) curved prongs that fit into the nostrils. It is held in place by an elasticized band that can be easily adjusted to fit around the patient's head. See Figure 29–21. Although it is not usually necessary to tape the cannula in place, the cannula may be taped to each side of the face of a confused or particularly active patient. The cannula is connected to oxygen tubing and an oxygen supply.

Relatively high concentration and flow rates can be administered by nasal cannula; however, when the flow rate is above 8 liters per minute, the patient has a tendency to swallow air and the nasal or pharyngeal

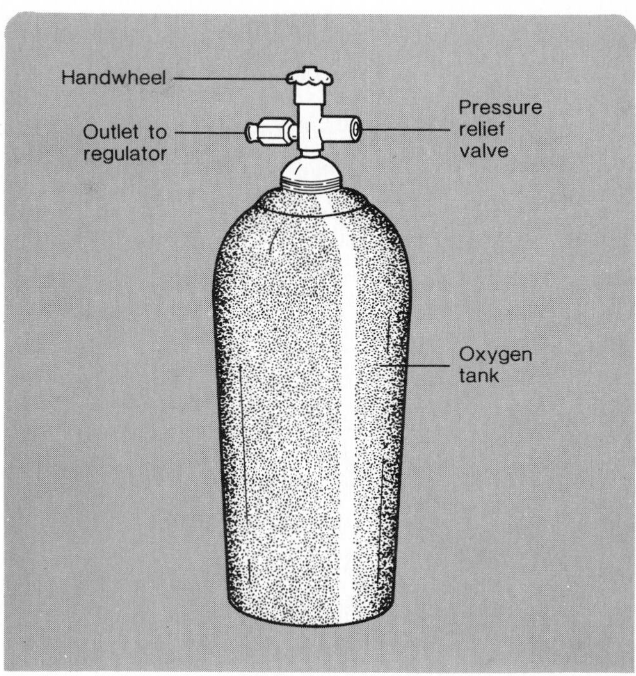

Figure 29–19 Basic parts of an oxygen tank.

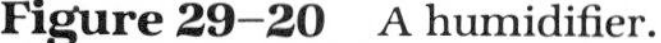

Figure 29–20 A humidifier.

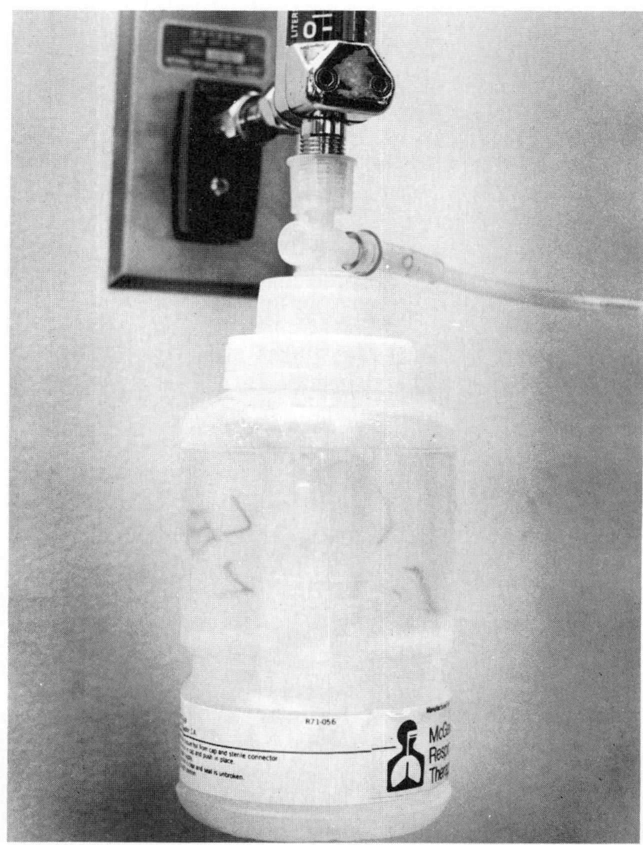

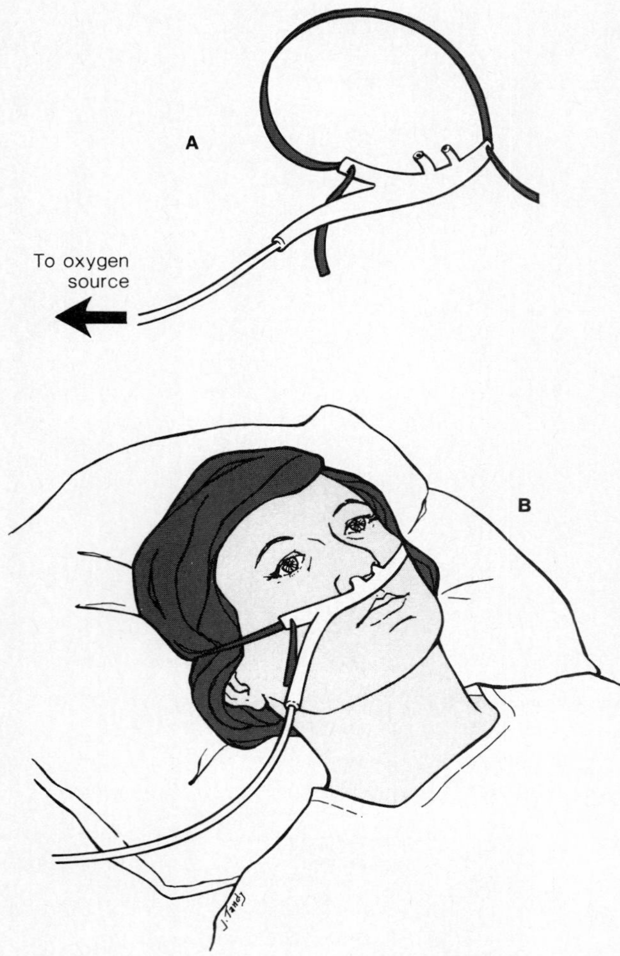

Figure 29–21 A nasal cannula: **A,** unattached; **B,** attached to patient.

Figure 29–22 A nasal catheter used for oxygen therapy.

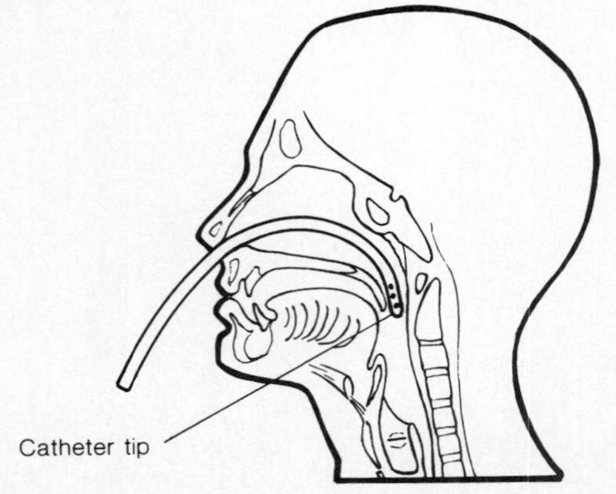

mucosa may become irritated. Primary responsibilities of the nurse caring for a patient with a nasal cannula include the following:

1. Assembling the equipment, including the humidifier.
2. Orienting the patient to this therapy and instructing the patient to breathe through the nose. Mouth breathing dilutes the oxygen concentration received.
3. Teaching the patient about safety precautions required during oxygen therapy.
4. Changing the cannula every 8 hours or as dictated by agency policy.
5. Inspecting the nares for encrustations or irritation and applying a water-soluble lubricant to the nares when necessary (e.g., every 4 hours).
6. Inspecting the skin for signs of irritation if tape is used to hold the cannula in place.
7. Maintaining the flow rate and the level of the distilled water in the humidifier bottle.
8. Maintaining the patient in a position that promotes lung expansion and encouraging turning and deep breathing exercises every 2 to 4 hours.
9. Assessing the patient's vital signs and breathing patterns periodically to determine the patient's response to therapy.

Nasal catheter

The nasal catheter is also used to administer low to moderate oxygen concentrations but can deliver higher concentrations of oxygen than the nasal cannula. At flows of 1 to 5 liters per minute, concentrations of 30% to 35% can be achieved. Catheters are used more frequently than nasal cannulae in some agencies. Catheters are effective, allow the patient the same mobility as cannulae, and are accepted without fear by most patients. See Figure 29–22.

Major problems associated with the nasal catheter are laryngeal ulceration from the constant flow of oxygen into the larynx and gastric distention caused by air and oxygen entering the stomach. Gastric distention can be relieved by inserting a nasogastric tube. See Chapter 39. Laryngeal ulceration may be prevented by moving the catheter from one nostril to the other every 8 hours (Fuchs 1980:39). Agency policy should be followed.

Nursing responsibilities toward patients with nasal catheters are similar to those toward patients with a nasal cannulae. The nurse must change the nasal catheter every 8 hours and insert it alternately in one naris and then the other. This prevents the development of encrustations and irritation of the respiratory mucosa.

Procedure 29–2 Inserting a Nasal Catheter

Goals

1. To deliver a low concentration of oxygen
2. To prevent irritation of the mucosa of the nares and the larynx

Equipment

1. Nasal catheter of appropriate size—8 or 10 French for children; 10 or 12 French for women; 12 or 14 French for men
2. Oxygen tubing
3. Flowmeter for piped-in oxygen; regulator for oxygen cylinder
4. Humidifier filled with sterile distilled water to moisten and vaporize the oxygen
5. "No smoking" signs
6. Water-soluble lubricating jelly and a gauze square to facilitate catheter insertion
7. Adhesive tape (nonallergic preferred) to secure catheter to the patient's face
8. Flashlight and tongue depressor to help assess correct placement of the catheter
9. Glass of water to test the oxygen flow

Preparation

1. Check the physician's order to determine the desired rate of flow of oxygen.
2. Teach the patient about the therapy and the safety precautions required. Answer questions and allay anxiety if necessary.
3. Put up the "No smoking" signs.
4. Help the patient assume the best position. A patient who requires oxygen is often best positioned in a semi-Fowler's position that eases breathing by allowing for maximum expansion of the chest.
5. Wash hands thoroughly.
6. Attach the flowmeter to the wall outlet or the regulator to the oxygen tank after cracking the tank.
7. Attach the humidifier to the flowmeter.
8. Attach the oxygen tubing to the humidifier and to the catheter.
9. Test the oxygen flow by turning on the oxygen flowmeter to 3 liters per minute and inserting the tip of the catheter into the glass of water. Bubbling indicates that oxygen is flowing.

Intervention

1. Determine how deeply to insert the catheter by placing the end of the catheter in a straight line between the tip of the patient's nose and the ear lobe. This distance can be marked with tape. See Figure 29–23.

   Rationale This external distance approximates the distance from the nares to the oropharynx.

2. Lubricate the tip of the catheter with water-soluble jelly. The lubricant can be squeezed into a square gauze and the catheter rotated over it. Do not use mineral oil or petroleum jelly, since, if aspirated, these can cause severe lung irritations or lipoid pneumonia.

   Rationale Lubrication facilitates insertion and prevents injury to the nasal mucous membrane.

3. Start the flow of oxygen at about 3 liters per minute prior to inserting the tube.

   Rationale The flow of oxygen prevents the catheter from becoming plugged by secretions during insertion.

Figure 29–23

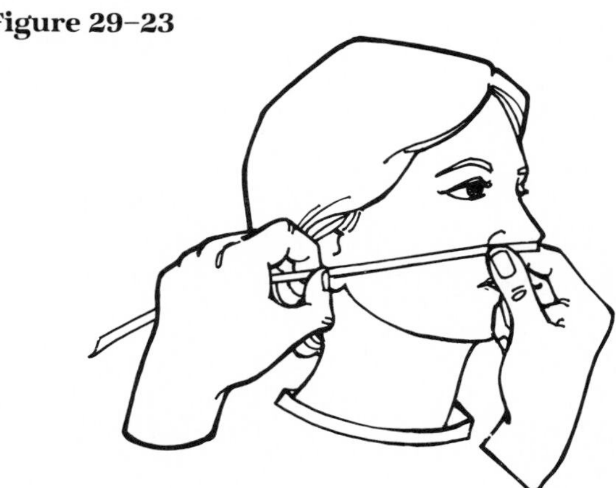

Procedure 29–2, continued

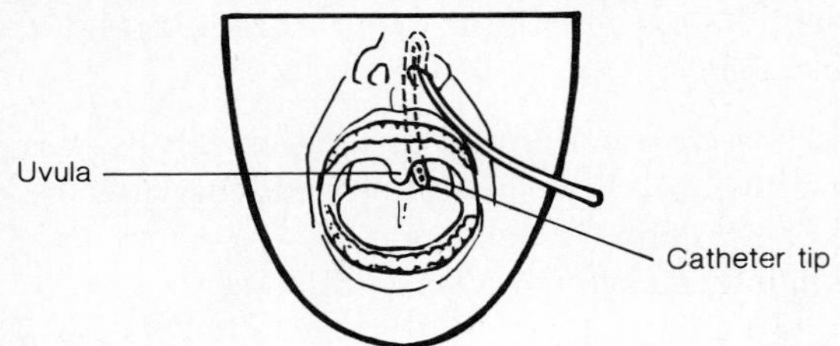

Figure 29–24

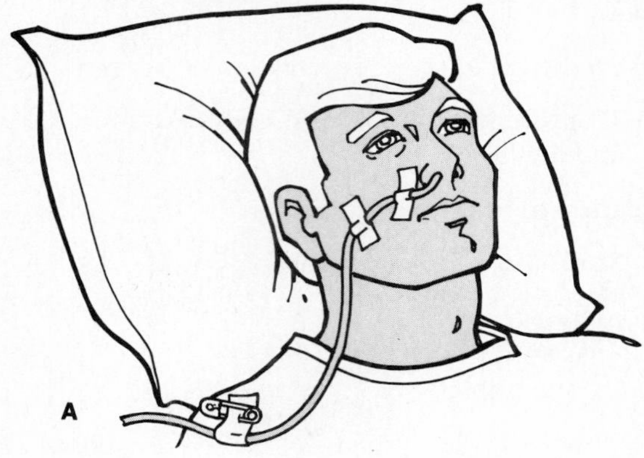

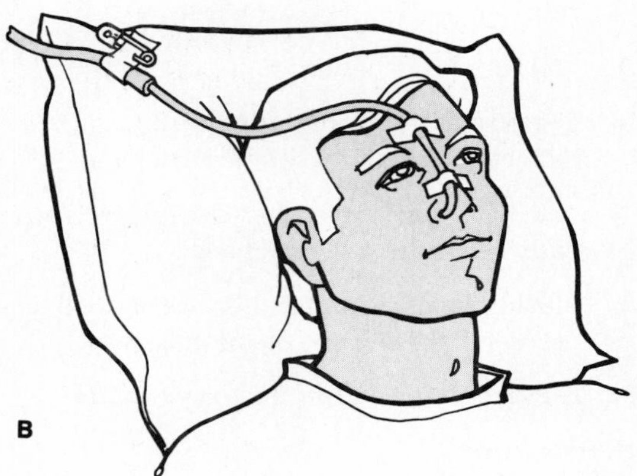

Figure 29–25

4. Introduce the catheter slowly through one nostril until the tip is at the entrance to the oropharynx (the marked distance). See Figure 29-24. The tip of the catheter will be visible through the mouth beside the uvula.

5. Withdraw the tip slightly so that it can no longer be seen.

   Rationale When the catheter is in this position, the patient is less likely to swallow oxygen.

6. Tape the catheter to the patient's face at the side of the nose and cheek (Figure 29-25, *A*) or tape the catheter to the tip of the nose and the forehead (Figure 29-25, *B*).

   Rationale If taped, the catheter will not be displaced when the patient moves.

7. Adjust the flow to the prescribed rate.

8. Assess the patient's immediate response to the oxygen and provide support to the patient as he or she adjusts to the catheter.

9. Secure the connecting tube to the bed or to the patient's gown with tape or an elastic band and a safety pin. Leave slack in the tubing.

   Rationale Sufficient slack allows the patient to move without pulling on the tubing.

10. Record the initiation of the procedure and the patient's response to therapy, including time, method, and flow rate.

Oxygen face mask

A variety of oxygen face masks that cover the patient's nose and mouth are marketed. See Figure 29-26. Oxygen concentrations delivered through masks generally range from about 25% to 60% at flow rates of 8 to 12 liters per minute. A few, e.g., the non-rebreather mask (Figure 29-26, *C*) are designed to deliver 90% concentrations. However, concentrations above 60% are rarely prescribed because of the danger of oxygen toxicity. Oxygen face masks are advantageous for patients who are unable to breathe solely through their nose. Most masks are made of clear pliable plastic or rubber that can be molded to fit the face snugly. Some have a metal clip that can be bent over the bridge of the nose for a snug fit. They also have several holes in the sides (exhalation ports) to allow the escape of exhaled carbon dioxide. The masks are fastened to the patient's head with elasticized bands. Some masks have reservoir bags attached. These are also referred to as partial rebreath-

Figure 29–26 Three types of oxygen masks: **A,** a simple plastic mask; **B,** a mask with a partial rebreathing bag (note that it has fewer exhalation ports at the side than A); **C,** a Venturi mask.

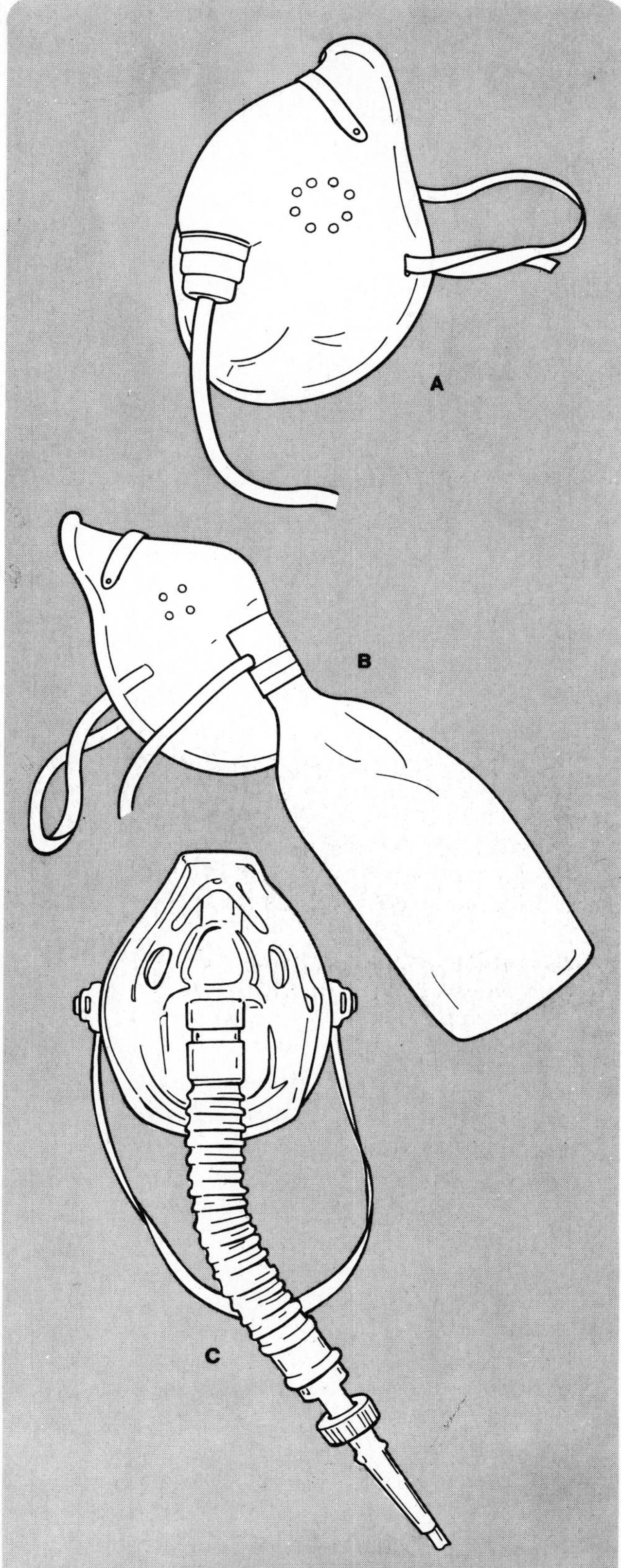

ing bags. See Figure 29–26, *B*. They provide for higher oxygen concentrations to the patient because a portion of the patient's expired air is directed into the bag and rebreathed. Because this air does not take part in gaseous exchange, its oxygen concentration remains high. Thus, when this air is added to the inflow from the oxygen source, an increased oxygen concentration is provided.

To initiate oxygen therapy by a face mask, the nurse follows most of the same steps as when giving oxygen by nasal cannula and nasal catheter, except that the nurse must find a mask of appropriate size. Smaller sizes are available for children. When fitting a patient with a face mask, the nurse needs to:

1. Familiarize the patient with the mask when possible. Allow the patient to hold the mask, guide it toward the face, and get used to the sensation of the mask covering the nose and mouth. Instruct the patient to put on the mask from the nose downward during expiration.
2. Turn on the oxygen to the prescribed rate of flow and allow the patient to adjust to the flow of the oxygen. When the mask has a reservoir bag, the nurse should first flush the mask with oxygen until it is partially inflated.
3. Gradually fit the mask to the contours of the face, and encourage the patient to breathe normally. The mask should be molded to prevent oxygen escaping upward into the patient's eyes or around the cheeks or chin. If the mask has a reservoir bag, the nurse must adjust the oxygen flow so that the bag does not collapse when the patient inhales deeply.
4. Secure the elasticized band around the patient's head, and adjust it for a comfortable but snug fit. See Figure 29–27.
5. See that the patient is positioned comfortably in the semi-Fowler's or high Fowler's position.
6. Stay until the patient is at ease. Some patients respond with panic, restlessness, and fear of suffocation.
7. Tell the patient how frequently you will return to check her or his progress. The nurse times visits according to the patient's needs. In the beginning, visits should be frequent—every 10 to 15 minutes. The call signal should be in easy reach of the patient.
8. Assess the patient's pulse rate and breathing rates and patterns.
9. Record the initiation of therapy and the patient's response.

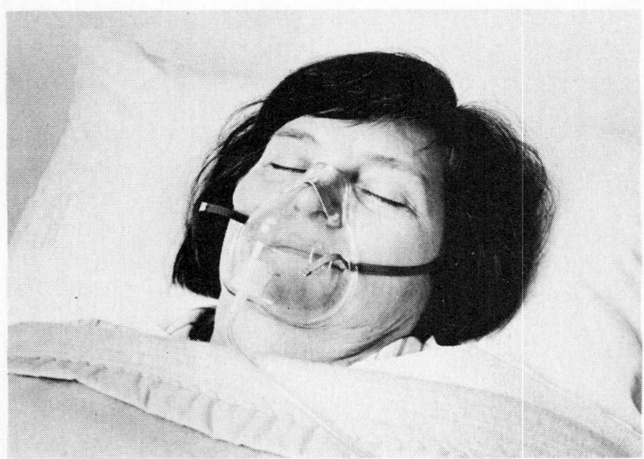

Figure 29–27 An oxygen mask should fit snugly.

To maintain oxygen therapy by face mask, the nurse observes the same procedures as for maintaining therapy by nasal catheter or cannula; that is, (a) maintaining the flow rate, (b) maintaining the level of distilled water in the humidifier bottle, (c) positioning the patient appropriately, (d) encouraging adequate hydration, movement, and deep breathing exercises, (e) observing safety precautions, and (f) noting the patient's progress. In addition, the nurse needs to remove the face mask periodically (every 2 hours) to observe the skin. Condensation occurs, and the patient's face needs to be sponged and dried. Lubrication of oral mucous membranes is also essential, since mouth breathing has a drying effect. For more information on administering oxygen by mask, see Kozier and Erb (1982:1215–18).

Oxygen tent

Traditionally, the oxygen tent was a clear plastic canopy placed over the upper half of a bed. Attached to it was a motor unit that circulated oxygen in the tent. These tents are seldom used today, perhaps because of the high volumes of oxygen required to maintain desired concentrations.

An adaptation of the oxygen tent is the face tent: clear plastic molded to fit under the chin and in front of the mouth and nose. The face tent has many of the advantages of a nasal cannula and catheter and can supply high humidity with the oxygen. A face tent can supply 30% to 55% oxygen concentration with a flow rate of 4 to 8 liters per minute. When caring for patients using face tents, nurses need to pay special attention to care of the patients' facial skin.

Resuscitation

Resuscitation includes all measures to revive patients who have stopped breathing due to either respiratory or cardiac failure. *Artificial respiration* is used when the patient's breathing has stopped while the heart continues to beat. *External cardiac massage* is used when both the heartbeat and breathing have stopped. In such an instance, both artificial respiration and external cardiac massage are applied at the same time. These combined measures are often called *cardiopulmonary resuscitation* (CPR). Other measures include administration of oxygen and use of mechanical resuscitators such as the Ambu-resuscitator.

Artificial Respiration

The purpose of artificial respiration is to force air into and out of the lungs. This is achieved in two ways: (a) oral resuscitation, for instance, mouth-to-mouth or mouth-to-nose resuscitation and (b) hand compressible breathing bags. The Ambu-resuscitator, frequently supplied in hospitals or ambulances, is the preferred breathing bag.

Oral resuscitation

Mouth-to-mouth resuscitation depends on the large amount of air that a normal person can inspire and therefore breathe into the victim's lungs. Although the oxygen content of expired air is slightly reduced, it is sufficient for revival.

Procedure 29–3 Oral Resuscitation

Goals

1. To prevent irreversible brain damage from anoxia
2. To restore normal breathing pattern

Preparation

1. Using the index finger in a sweeping motion, clear the patient's mouth and the back of the throat of any obstructive material. Remove fluids by turning the patient's head to the side or face down.

   Rationale Clearing the airway prior to resuscitation permits air to move freely in and out of the respiratory passages.

2. Place the patient in the supine position on a hard surface if possible and place a coat or pillow under the victim's shoulders.

   Rationale A pillow under the victim's shoulders helps the nurse to tilt the patient's head.

3. Tilt the patient's head back as far as possible by pressing one hand palm downwards on the patient's forehead while lifting the patient's neck with the other hand placed palm upwards under the neck. See Figure 29–28. An infant's head is tilted backward only *slightly* since an infant's breathing passages are more pliable and may be obstructed by forceful extension. See Figure 29–29.

   Rationale This position ensures an open airway since the tongue is prevented from falling back to obstruct the airway. See Figure 29–30. When the patient's neck is *not* hyperextended, the tongue obstructs the pharynx. When the neck is hyperextended, the tongue does not obstruct the airway. Spontaneous breathing may occur as soon as the airway is opened.

Figure 29–28

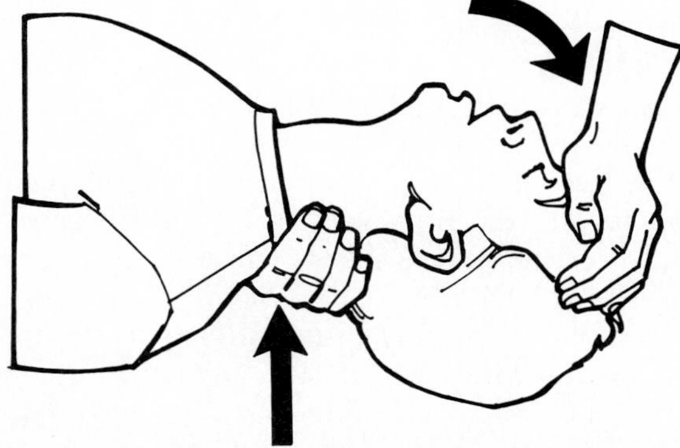

Figure 29–29

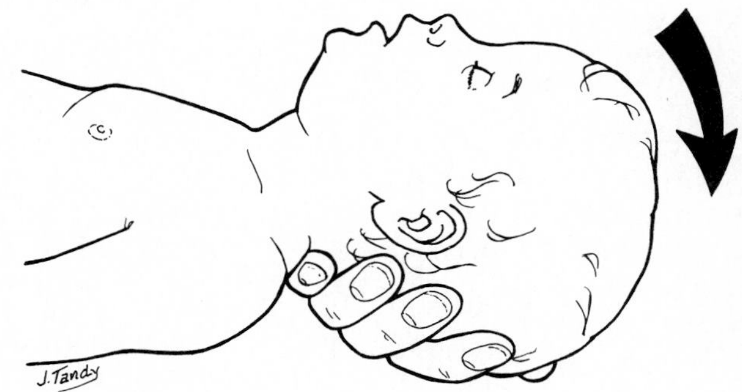

Figure 29–30

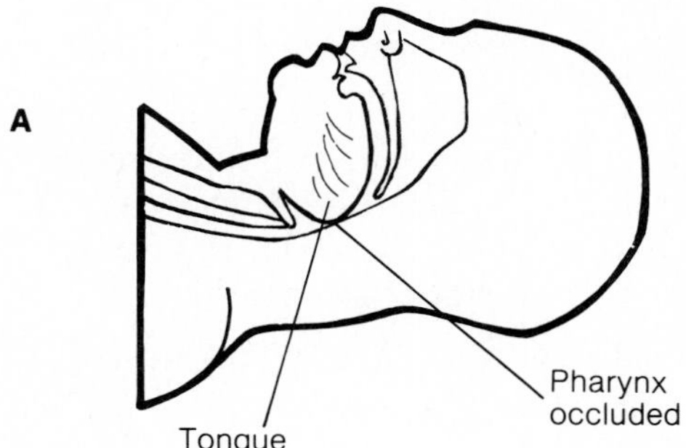

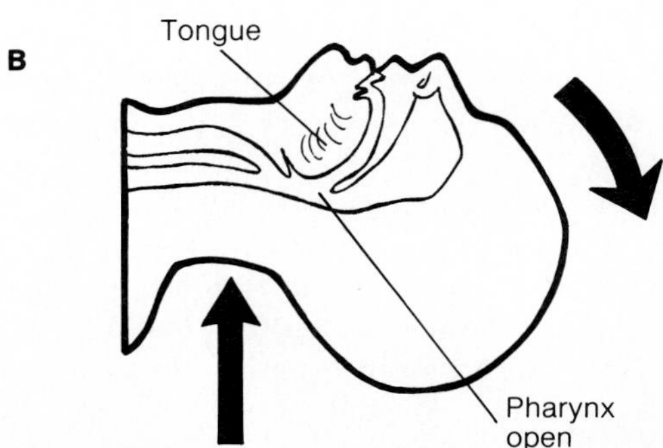

Procedure 29–3, continued

Intervention

1. Check the patient's breathing by placing your ear close to the patient's mouth and nose:
   a. Listen for air escaping during exhalation.
   b. Feel for air escaping against your cheek.
   c. Observe the chest and abdomen for rising and falling movements.

2. If breathing is not restored, begin artificial respiration.

3. Pinch the patient's nostrils with the index finger and thumb of your hand on the patient's forehead.

   Rationale Pinching closes the nostrils and prevents air blown in from escaping through them.

4. Take a deep breath and place your mouth, opened widely, around the patient's mouth. Ensure an airtight seal. See Figure 29–31.

5. Blow four quick, full breaths into the patient's mouth. At this stage, do not allow the patient's lungs to deflate between breaths.

6. Check to see if the patient's breathing is restored by placing your ear close to the patient's mouth. Listen and feel for the escape of air and watch the chest for rising and falling.

7. Check the patient's carotid pulse by palpating the common carotid artery. To feel the carotid artery, first locate the larynx and slide your fingers alongside it into the groove between the larynx and the neck muscles.

8. If you feel a carotid pulse, but breathing is not restored, repeat steps 3 and 4 and inflate the patient's lungs at the rate of 12 breaths per minute (1 breath every 5 seconds). Blow forcibly enough to make the patient's chest rise. If chest expansion fails to occur, ensure that the head is hyperextended and the jaw lifted upward, or check again for the presence of obstructive material, fluid, or vomitus.

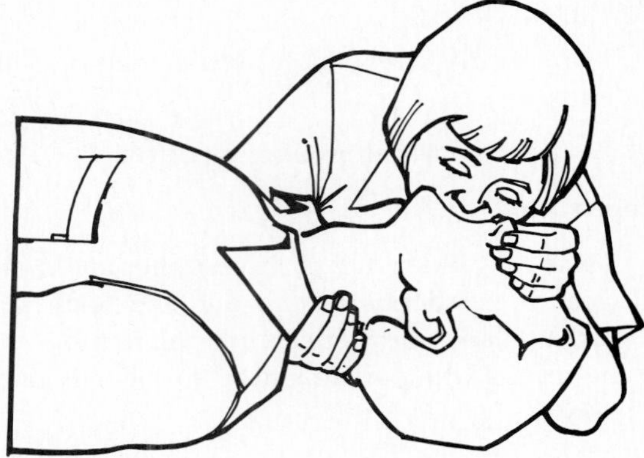

Figure 29–31

9. After each inflation, move your mouth away from the patient's mouth by turning your head toward the patient's chest.

   Rationale This movement allows the air to escape when the patient exhales. It also gives the nurse time to inhale and to watch for chest expansion.

10. Recheck the carotid pulse after every 12 inflations (after 1 minute). If you cannot locate the pulse, the patient's heart has stopped, and artificial circulation also needs to be provided. See Procedure 29–4.

Mouth-to-nose or mouth-to-mouth-and-nose methods

Artificial respiration can also be given by the mouth-to-nose method and the mouth-to-mouth-and-nose method. When using these methods, the nurse takes the same preliminary measures as for the mouth-to-mouth method—clearing the airway and positioning the patient properly.

The *mouth-to-nose* method can be used when there is an injury to the mouth or jaw or when the patient is edentulous (toothless), making it difficult to achieve a tight seal over the mouth. The nurse closes the patient's mouth by pressing the thumb over the lips. After taking a deep breath, the nurse places the mouth (opened widely) over the patient's nose, ensuring a tight seal against the cheeks around the patient's nose. The resuscitator presses the cheek against the patient's lips.

The *mouth-to-mouth-and-nose* method is used for infants and children. See Figure 29–32. After taking a breath, the nurse places the mouth tightly over the patient's nose and mouth and puffs gently from the cheeks only once every 3 seconds. Forceful breathing overinflates the infant's lungs and may also cause gastric distention. To relieve gastric distention, the nurse turns the infant on the side and applies gentle pressure to the epigastrium. The lateral position prevents aspiration of vomitus.

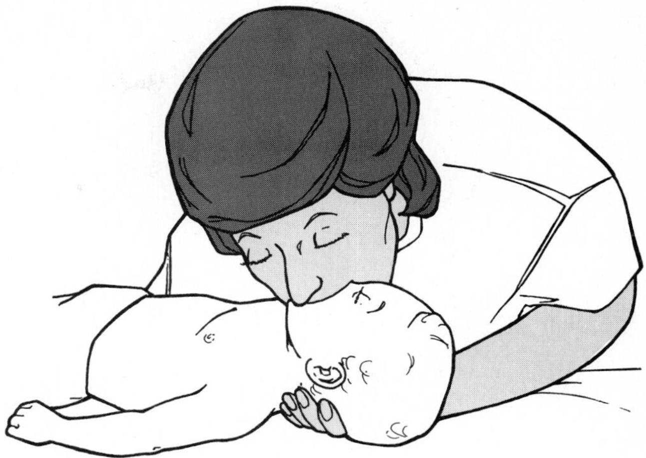

Figure 29–32 The nurse places the mouth tightly over the infant's mouth and nose.

Hand-compressible breathing bags

Many agencies use rubberized breathing bags attached to face masks for respiratory resuscitation. A common one is the Ambu-bag. They are easily applied and used. The bags are compressed by hand to deliver air into the mask and rapidly self-inflate after compression. The exhaled air of the patient is released through an exhaust valve to prevent its entry back into the bag. One significant advantage of the breathing bag is that supplemental oxygen can be attached.

This method of resuscitation incorporates the same measures as other ventilation methods. The patient is positioned on the back with the shoulders elevated, head hyperextended, and jaw upward. The resuscitator stands at the patient's head and nose. One hand is used to secure the mask at the top and bottom as well as hold the jaw forward. See Figure 29–33. The other hand is used to alternately squeeze and release the bag. The compression on the bag is released when sufficient elevation of the patient's chest is observed. Ventilation is repeated 12 times per minute. The standard preliminary actions of clearing the mouth and throat are essential before this procedure or when there is insufficient lung expansion.

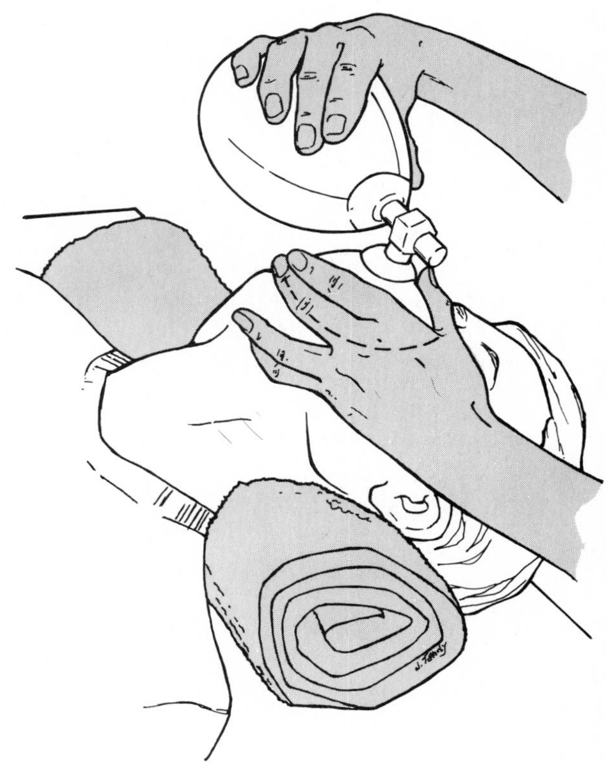

Figure 29–33 An Ambu-resuscitator in use. One hand secures the mask and supports the jaw while the other hand compresses and releases the bag.

Cardiopulmonary Resuscitation

Cardiac arrest is a sudden state of apnea and circulatory failure. It is a dramatic event that requires instant respiratory resuscitation and cardiac stimulation and massage. Within only 4 to 6 minutes after cardiac arrest, lack of oxygen can cause permanent brain and heart damage. Causes of cardiac arrest are many and include electrocution, myocardial infarction (heart attack), respiratory failure, extensive hemorrhage, and brain injury. The three cardinal signs of cardiac arrest are (a) apnea, (b) absence of a carotid or femoral pulse, and (c) dilated pupils.

The victim's skin appears pale or grayish and feels cool. Cyanosis is evident when respiratory function fails prior to heart failure. The three cardinal signs must be assessed prior to resuscitation.

The ABCs of cardiopulmonary resuscitation (CPR) are as follows:

A: clear the *airways*.
B: initiate artificial *breathing* (oral resuscitation).
C: initiate *cardiac* compression or artificial *circulation*.

This sequence is recommended because spontaneous breathing may occur after any one action, such as after the airway is opened or after a few artificial respirations are provided. For the steps used to clear the airway and initiate breathing, see Procedure 29–3.

External cardiac compression

The purpose of external cardiac compression is to provide *artificial circulation.* Compression reproduces the normal intermittent heart contractions that pump blood through the body. *External cardiac compression* is manual, intermittent, rhythmical compression to the patient's sternum by the heel of the nurse's hand. The heart is squeezed between the sternum and the vertebrae lying posteriorly. Cardiac resuscitation is ineffective unless there is simultaneous artificial respiration to oxygenate the bloodstream. External cardiac compression should never be practiced on a person with a functioning heart because it could interfere with the normal cardiac contractions.

Procedure 29–4 External Cardiac Compression

Goals

1. To maintain blood circulation and prevent irreversible brain damage from anoxia
2. To restore normal cardiac function

Intervention

One resuscitator

1. Position an *adult* or *child* on the back on a flat, firm surface. Place a cardiac board, if available, under the back of a bed patient. If necessary, place the patient on the floor. If the patient is an infant, support the back either by:
   a. Placing one hand under the back or
   b. Encircling the chest with both hands and compressing the sternum with the thumbs (see Figure 29–34)
2. Kneel beside the patient's chest. If the patient is in bed, you may have to kneel on the patient's bed.
3. Locate the lower end of the sternum (the xiphoid process), by following the lower edge of the near ribs to the notch where the ribs and the sternum join.
4. If the patient is an adult, measure upward about 4 to 5 cm (1.5 to 2 in) from the lower point of the xiphoid process. You will apply pressure at that location above the xiphoid process.

   Rationale Proper positioning of the hands during cardiac compression prevents injury to underlying organs and the ribs.
5. Place the heel of one hand on the chest at the point indicated in step 4, and place the heel of the other hand on top of the first hand. The hands should be parallel, with the fingers directed away from the nurse. The fingers should not be against the chest. It may be easier to interlock the fingers. See Figure 29–35.

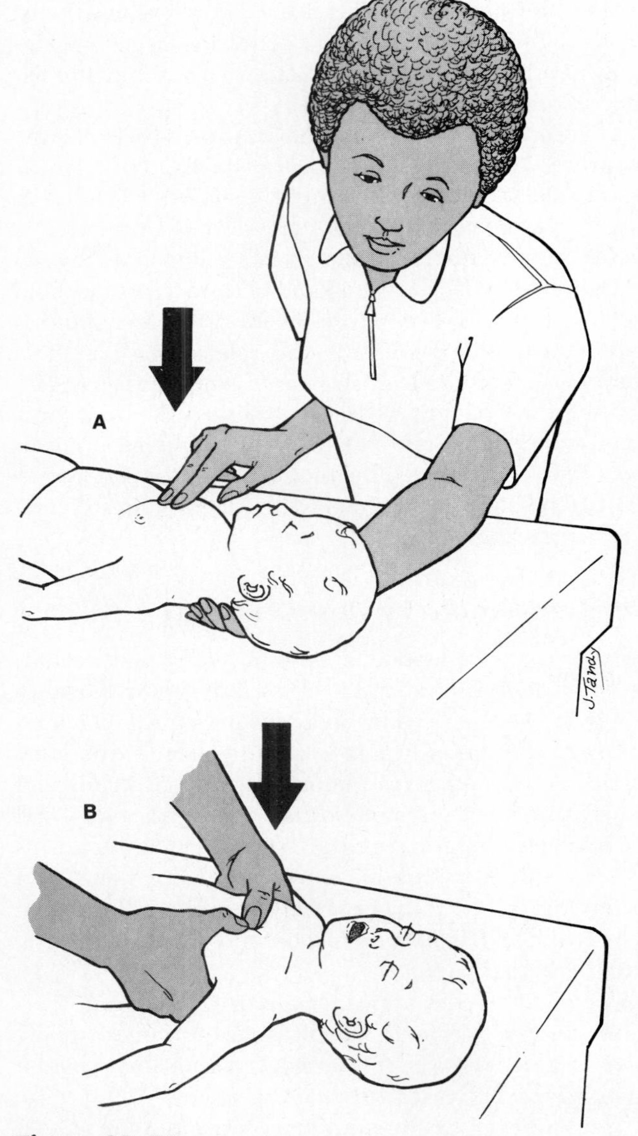

Figure 29–34

Procedure 29–4, continued

Rationale Compression occurs only on the sternum through the heel of the hands. The muscle force of both arms is needed for adequate compression of adults.

6. Lean forward so that your shoulders are directly above the adult patient's chest with arms extended and elbows firmly locked.

   Rationale The weight of the shoulders and trunk supplies power for compression. Extension of the elbows ensures an adequate and even force throughout compression.

7. Using your own weight, press down on the adult patient's chest so that the sternum depresses about 4 to 5 cm (1.5 to 2 in).

   a. For children, compress the middle of the sternum about 2 to 3.5 cm (0.75 to 1.5 in), using the heel of only one hand.
   b. For *infants*, depress the mid-sternum 1.2 to 2 cm (0.5 to 0.75 in) with both thumbs while you support the back by encircling the chest with both hands. If the back is well supported, depress the sternum with the tips of the index and middle fingers of one hand. See Figure 29–36.

   Rationale The pressure compresses the heart between the sternum and the vertebral column and squeezes blood out of the chambers of the heart. Less pressure is required for children and infants.

8. Release all pressure, but do not remove your hands. Establish a rhythmic motion, using a rate of 80 compressions per minute for adults. For both infants and children, use a rate of 80 to 100 compressions per minute. Maintain the rhythm by counting "one one thousand, two one thousand," etc.

   Rationale Releasing the pressure allows the sternum to return to its normal position and allows the heart chambers to fill with blood.

9. Continue until the patient revives or until someone relieves you.
   a. If you do not have help, give two quick lung inflations after every 15 chest compressions.
   b. For infants and young children, give one lung inflation after every 5 chest compressions.

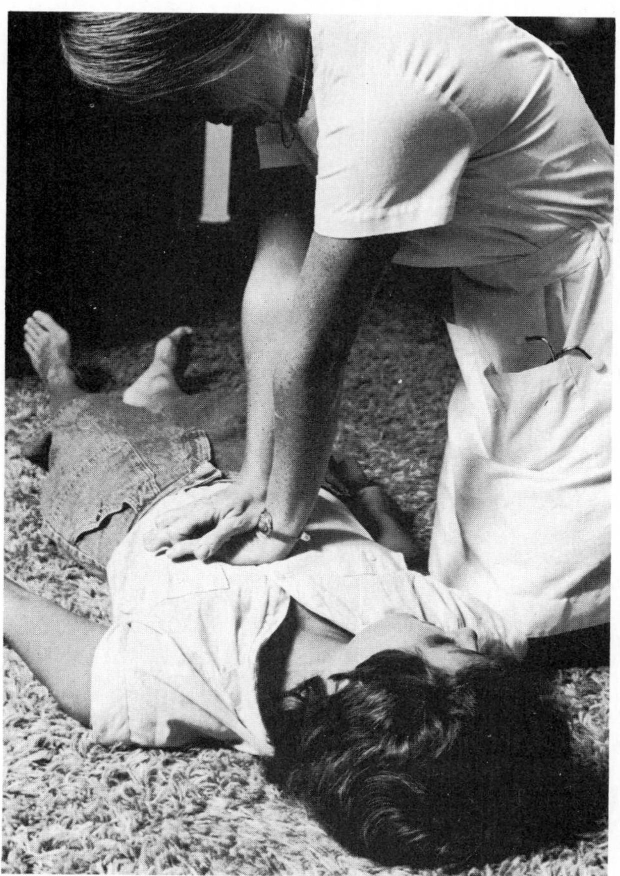

Figure 29–35

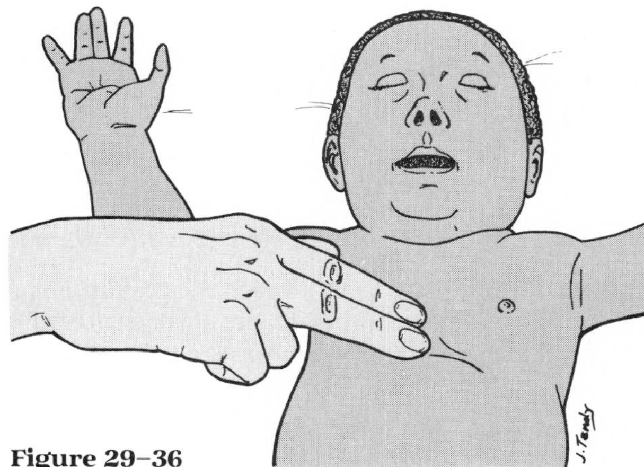

Figure 29–36

10. Check the patient's carotid pulse after inflating the lungs and after 1 minute of cardiac massage.

Procedure 29–4, continued

Two resuscitators

When there are two people to provide cardiopulmonary resuscitation, one person can provide external cardiac massage and the other pulmonary resuscitation. If the patient is an adult, compress the chest 60 times per minute and inflate the lungs once for every five chest compressions. If the two people need to exchange positions, e.g., because of fatigue, make the change at the count of five when person A, who is providing pulmonary resuscitation, gives one lung inflation and then moves person B's hands from the chest to take over cardiac massage. Person B is then ready to provide lung inflation at the next count of five and may check the carotid pulse before transferring.

Terminating CPR

CPR is terminated when one of the following events occurs:

1. Specially trained personnel arrive to take over.
2. The heartbeat and breathing are reestablished.
3. A physician states that the individual is dead and CPR is to be discontinued.
4. The person providing CPR becomes exhausted, and there is no one to take over.

Evaluation

Examples of outcome criteria for patients with altered respiratory and circulatory function include:

1. Increased respiratory ventilation (or vital capacity)
2. Loosened secretions
3. Full lung expansion during deep breathing exercises
4. Decreased respiratory rate
5. More efficient and relaxed respirations
6. Reaches preset volume level when using incentive spirometer
7. Absence of shortness of breath
8. Absence of gurgling breath sounds
9. More productive coughing
10. Absence of cough
11. Clear breath sounds on auscultation (absence of rales)
12. Arterial Pa_{O_2} and Pa_{CO_2} within normal range
13. Increased breathing efficiency and comfort
14. Absence of chest retractions
15. Pulse rate within normal range
16. Healthy skin color
17. Blood pressure within normal range

Summary

Respiration is vital to the body's functioning and survival. Normally, respiration is effortless and accomplished without conscious awareness. However, during strenuous exercise or when respiratory disease is present, a person becomes acutely aware of the mechanics of inspiration and expiration. Respiration has three phases: pulmonary ventilation, diffusion of oxygen and carbon dioxide, and transportation of these respiratory gases to and from the cells.

Ventilation includes the processes of inspiration and expiration, both of which are associated with changes in pulmonary volumes and pressures. The pulmonary volumes include the total volume, the inspiratory and expiratory reserve volumes, and the residual volume. All of these volumes added together are the total lung capacity. When two or more of the pulmonary volumes are considered in combination, they are referred to as pulmonary capacities (inspiratory, vital, and functional residual). These capacities are frequently assessed by spirometry to determine the degree of lung impairment in persons with respiratory disease. Changes in pulmonary pressures also occur during ventilation. These pressure changes are indirectly related to the volume changes and account for the movement of air into and out of the lungs. Four requirements for adequate ventilation are (a) adequate atmospheric oxygen, (b) patency of the air passages, (c) sufficient pulmonary compliance and recoil, and (d) satisfactory regulatory mechanisms.

Diffusion of the respiratory gases through the respiratory membrane is the second phase of respiration. Four major factors influence the rate of this diffusion. These are the thickness of the membrane, the surface area of the membrane, the diffusion coefficient of the gas, and the pressure difference on each side of the membrane. Disease conditions can affect any or all of these four factors and seriously impair this phase of respiration. Examples are pulmonary edema, carbon monoxide poisoning, and emphysema. In clinical situations, the pressure gradients of oxygen and carbon dioxide are frequently measured to assess deficiencies or excesses.

The third phase of respiration is the transport of oxygen to the cells and the transport of carbon dioxide from the cells. The rate of oxygen transport to the cells is influenced largely by the cardiac output, the number of circulating erythrocytes, exercise, and the blood hematocrit.

Assessment of the respiratory and circulatory status of patients is a frequent and essential function of the nurse. The methods used to assess the chest cage, lungs, heart, pulse, and respirations are discussed in Chapters 13 and 14. Emphasized in this chapter are clinical signs of oxygen impairment (hypoxia) and the terms used to describe breathing patterns, breath sounds, chest movements, secretions, coughing, and circulatory status. Factors influencing respiratory and circulatory status include altitude, environment, emotions, exercise, health and life-style, and age.

Nursing diagnoses for patients with respiratory or cardiac problems include: ineffective airway clearance, ineffective breathing patterns, impaired gas exchange, and decreased cardiac output. Signs indicative of these patient responses and the many factors contributing to them are outlined.

Four general nursing interventions to maintain normal respirations are positioning patients to facilitate maximum lung expansion, encouraging frequent deep breathing exercises and coughing, providing adequate hydration to moisten the respiratory membranes, and promoting individual health practices and a healthy environment.

Persons who suffer respiratory impairment may require additional therapy. Lung inflation techniques such as breathing exercises (pursed-lip and abdominal breathing), blow bottles, incentive respiratory spirometry, and intermittent positive pressure breathing (IPPB) therapy are effective means of increasing respiratory efficiency. Postural drainage along with percussion and vibration are implemented when secretions accumulate and are retained in various lung segments. Humidification may be provided by hot steam inhalators or by the Croupette humidity tent for infants and young children. Nebulization therapy is an effective means of delivering required medications to the respiratory membrane. Artificial oropharyngeal airways and oropharyngeal and nasopharyngeal suctioning may be needed to maintain airway patency in unconscious patients or in patients who have difficulty swallowing or expectorating secretions.

Additional oxygen is indicated for patients with hypoxemia. A variety of methods are used to administer oxygen. These include the nasal cannula, the nasal catheter, the face mask, and the oxygen tent. Since oxygen supports combustion, safety precautions are taken during oxygen therapy.

Nurses must be skilled in resuscitation techniques. Resuscitation techniques include oral resuscitation, use of hand compressible breathing bags, and external cardiac compression. Nurses need to become skilled in performing cardiopulmonary resuscitation as a single rescuer and in partnership with another person.

Suggested Activities

1. Assess and compare the respiratory and the pulse rates of an infant, toddler, school-age child, adult, and elderly person.

2. In a clinical setting, determine what methods of administering oxygen are used most frequently and why.

3. Observe a nurse or a physiotherapist helping a patient learn postural drainage, deep breathing, and effective coughing. Identify the points of emphasis.

4. In a laboratory, set up an oxygen mask and outline nursing intervention required.

5. Practice resuscitation techniques on a mannequin in a laboratory setting.

6. In a clinical setting, identify patients receiving IPPB. Determine the purpose and evaluate the effectiveness of this therapy.

Suggested Readings

American Journal of Nursing. February 1978. Techniques of cardiopulmonary resuscitation in infants. *American Journal of Nursing* 78:265.

This one-page article lists and illustrates the steps for cardiopulmonary resuscitation of infants.

Foley, M.; Tomashefski, J.; and Underwood, E., Jr. September 1977. Pulmonary function screening tests in industry. *American Journal of Nursing* 77:1480–84.

Screening tests help detect early signs of pulmonary disease. However, individual variations need to be considered in calculating the test results. The tests are reviewed, and the steps are given for interpreting results.

Manzi, C. C. March 1978. Cardiac emergency! How to use drugs and CPR to save lives. *Nursing 78* 8:30–39.

In addition to the ABCs of life support, this article emphasizes the D step for life support: definite treatment (diagnosis, drugs, and defibrillation). The rationale for giving drugs and the nurse's role in CPR are included.

Rau, J., and Rau, M. April 1977. To breathe or be breathed: Understanding IPPB. *American Journal of Nursing* 77: 613–17.

This article outlines principles of IPPB, its treatment goals, some hazards of IPPB, and a procedure for administering this treatment. The Bird and Bennett respirators are compared.

Sandham, G., and Reid, B. October 1977. Some Q's and A's about suctioning with an illustrated guide to better techniques. *Nursing 77* 7:60–65.

A series of questions and answers about suctioning equipment, preparation for suctioning, and suctioning. Photographs illustrate the steps.

Waterson, M. March 1978. Teaching your patients postural drainage. *Nursing 78* 8:51–53.

This article includes a patient teaching aid showing six commonly prescribed positions. Patient reminders are outlined in a Do and Don't format.

Selected References

Allcock, M., and Wilson, S. November 1975. "Code 66!" From anxious "amateurs" to smooth-working code team. *Nursing 75* 5:17–20.

Canadian Heart Foundation. August 1976. Cardiopulmonary resuscitation (CPR). Part I. Recommended standards for basic life support. Ottawa: Canadian Heart Foundation.

Chrisman, M. April 1974. Dyspnea. *American Journal of Nursing* 74:643–46.

Ellmyer, P., and Thomas, N. J. January 1982. A guide to your patient's safe home use of oxygen. *Nursing 82* 12:56–57.

Felton, C. L. January 1978. Hypoxemia and oral temperatures. *American Journal of Nursing* 78:56–57.

Flatter, P. A. January 1968. Hazards of oxygen therapy. *American Journal of Nursing* 68:80–84.

Fuchs, P. L. December 1979. Understanding continuous mechanical ventilation. *Nursing 79* 9:26–33.

———. December 1980. Getting the best out of oxygen delivery systems. *Nursing 80* 10:34–43.

Garvey, J. April 1975. Infant respiratory distress syndrome. *American Journal of Nursing* 75:614–17.

Glover, D. W., and Glover, M. M. 1978. *Respiratory therapy basics for nursing and allied health professions.* St. Louis: C. V. Mosby Co.

Graas, S. October 1974. Thermometer sites and oxygen. *American Journal of Nursing* 74(10):1862–63.

Guyton, A. C. 1981. *Textbook of medical physiology.* 6th ed. Philadelphia: W. B. Saunders Co.

———. 1982. *Human physiology and mechanisms of disease.* 3rd ed. Philadelphia: W. B. Saunders Co.

Kim, M. J., and Moritz, D. A. 1982. *Classification of nursing diagnoses: Proceedings of the third and fourth national conferences.* New York: McGraw-Hill Book Co.

Kirilloff, L. H., and Maszkiewicz, R. C. November 1979. Guide to respiratory care in critically ill adults. *American Journal of Nursing* 79:2005–12.

Kozier, B., and Erb, G. 1982. *Techniques in clinical nursing: A comprehensive approach.* Menlo Park, Calif.: Addison-Wesley Publishing Co.

LeFort, S. February 1978. Cardiopulmonary resuscitation (CPR): Step-by-step. *The Canadian Nurse* 74:38–47.

Nielsen, L. December 1980. Mechanical ventilation: Patient assessment and nursing care. *American Journal of Nursing* 80:2191–2217.

Nussbaum, G. B., and Fisher, J. G. January 1978. A crash cart that works. *American Journal of Nursing* 78:45–48.

Promisloff, R. A. October 1980. Administering oxygen safely: When, why, how. *Nursing 80* 10:54–56.

Razzell, M. September 1975. No thanks, I've quit smoking. *The Canadian Nurse* 71:23–25.

Rifas, E. M. June 1980. How you—and your patient—can manage dyspnea. *Nursing 80* 10:34–41.

Ryan, M. A. August 1974. Helping the family cope with cardiac arrest. *Nursing 74* 4:80–81.

Wade, J. F. 1981. *Respiratory nursing care physiology and technique.* 3rd ed. St. Louis: C. V. Mosby Co.

Waldron, M. W. February 1979. Oxygen transport. *American Journal of Nursing* 79:272–75.

Weaver, T. E. February 1981. New life for lungs through incentive spirometers. *Nursing 81* 11:54–58.

World Health Organization. 1975. *Smoking and its effects on health.* Geneva. WHO Tech. rep. no. 568.

Chapter 30

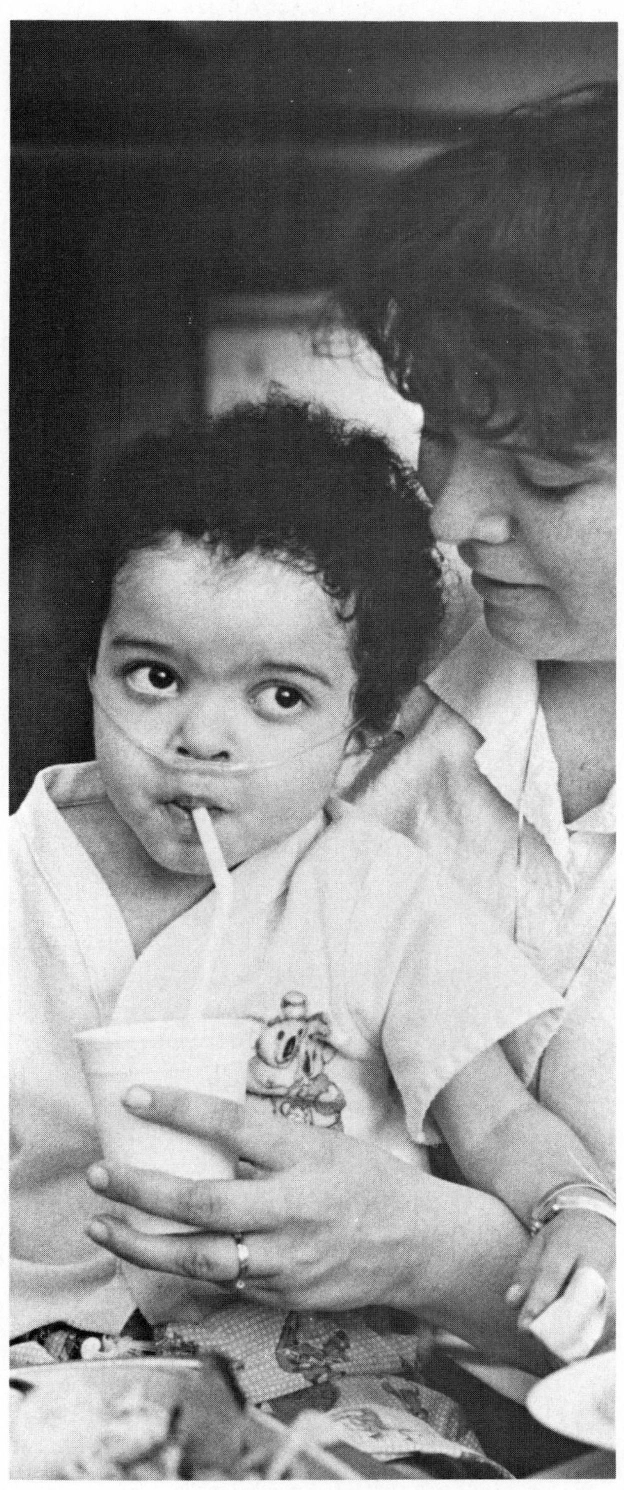

Fluid and Electrolytes: Part I

CONTENTS

Objectives

1. Know essential terms and facts about body fluid and fluid, electrolyte, and acid-base balance

- **1.1** Define selected terms
- **1.2** Describe factors affecting the proportion of body weight that is fluid
- **1.3** Name the body's fluid compartments
- **1.4** Identify major constituents (electrolytes) of intracellular and extracellular fluid compartments and body secretions
- **1.5** Describe ways in which fluids and electrolytes move through the body
- **1.6** Identify ways in which osmotic and hydrostatic pressures influence movement of fluid through membranes
- **1.7** Identify mechanisms that regulate the body's fluid and electrolyte volume
- **1.8** Describe how these mechanisms regulate fluid and electrolyte balance
- **1.9** Identify the role of the kidneys and lungs in regulating acid-base balance
- **1.10** Identify three major sources of body fluid
- **1.11** Identify sources of fluid output
- **1.12** Identify normal fluid intakes and outputs

2. Know information and methods required to assess a person's fluid, electrolyte, and acid-base balance

- **2.1** Identify essential information to obtain in a health history
- **2.2** Identify ways in which selected factors influence fluid and electrolyte needs
- **2.3** Describe clinical signs of the well-hydrated person
- **2.4** Identify essential steps in measuring a person's fluid intake and output
- **2.5** Identify essential diagnostic tests and their significance

Terms

acidosis
active transport
alkalosis
anion
cation
colloids
crystalloids
dialyzing membranes
diaphoresis
diffusion
electrolyte
excretion
extracellular fluid (ECF)
hydrostatic pressure
hypertonic
hypotonic
interstitial
interstitial fluid
intracellular (cellular) fluid (ICF)
intravascular
ion
isotonic
milliequivalent
millimol
mol
obligatory loss
osmolarity
osmosis
osmotic pressure
pH
plasma
secretion
solute
solvent

Fluids and electrolytes are necessary to maintain good health, and their relative amounts in the body must be maintained within a narrow range. The balance of fluids and electrolytes in the body is a part of homeostasis. See Chapter 8.

A great deal has been learned about the roles of fluids and electrolytes in both health and disease. This delicate balance is maintained in health by the body's physiologic processes. Almost every illness, however, threatens the balance. Even in normal daily living, excessive temperatures or excessive activity can disturb the balance if adequate water or salt intake is not maintained. Some therapeutic measures for patients, such as the use of diuretics, can also disturb the body's homeostasis unless replacement water and electrolytes are given.

This chapter emphasizes the normal aspects of body fluids and electrolytes. For nurses to appreciate the dangers of imbalances, they must first understand the amounts of fluid and electrolytes required to maintain health. The role of fluids in the body, their distribution, and variations in composition in the various compartments are discussed.

Proportions of Body Fluid

The proportion of the human body composed of fluid is surprisingly large, considering that the external appearance suggests mostly solid tissue such as muscle and bone. Fluid comprises about 57% of the average healthy adult man's weight. In health, this volume of body fluid remains relatively constant. In fact, a healthy person's weight varies less than 0.2 kg (0.5 lb) in 24 hours regardless of the amount of fluid ingested. In some diseases, serious excesses or deficiencies of body fluid occur. For example, a patient with heart failure can retain fluid in the tissues and may suffer a fluid excess. A patient with kidney disease may not be able to excrete the required amount of urine and also suffer a fluid excess. A patient with a mouth injury may not be able to drink and may suffer a fluid loss.

The percentage of total body fluid varies according to the individual's age, body fat, and sex. See Table 30–1. Humans begin life with the highest proportion of fluid, and as life progresses the proportion decreases. Body fat is essentially free of fluid; therefore, the amount of fat a person has alters the proportion of body fluid to body weight. In other words, the less body fat present, the greater the proportion of body fluid. For example, a thin man's body may be 70% fluid, whereas an obese man's may be only 55%. This variable, body fat, also accounts for the difference in total body fluid between the sexes. After adolescence, women have proportionately more fat than men. Thus, they have a smaller percentage of fluid in relation to total body weight than do men.

Table 30–1 Fluid Percentage of Body Weight by Age

Developmental stage	Percentage of water
Early human embryo	97
Newborn infant	75
Adult male	57
Adult female	55
Elderly adult	45 (approx.)

Note: As age increases, proportion of body water decreases.

Distribution of Body Fluid

The body's fluid is divided into two major reservoirs, intracellular and extracellular. The *intracellular fluid* (ICF), also referred to as the *cellular fluid*, is fluid found within the cells of the body. It comprises two-thirds to three-quarters of the total body fluid. The *extracellular fluid* (ECF) is fluid found outside the cells; it is subdivided into two compartments, *intravascular* (plasma) and *interstitial*. *Plasma* is fluid found within the vascular system; *interstitial fluid* is fluid that surrounds the cells, and it includes lymph. Extracellular fluids comprise one-third to one-fourth of the total body fluid.

Extracellular fluid is in constant motion throughout the body. Although it is the smaller of the two compartments, it serves as the transport system for nutrients and waste products to and from the cells. Plasma carries oxygen from the lungs and glucose from the gastrointestinal tract, for example, to the capillaries of the vascular system. From there, the oxygen and glucose move across the capillary membranes into the interstitial spaces and then across the cellular membranes into the cells. The opposite route is taken for waste products, such as carbon dioxide going from the cells to the lungs and metabolic acid wastes going eventually to the kidneys. Interstitial fluid transports wastes from the cells by way of the lymph system as well as directly into the blood plasma through capillaries. Lymph circulation ultimately enters the vascular circulation through the thoracic duct into the venous system.

Interstitial fluid comprises three-quarters of extracellular fluid. Normal body functioning requires that the volume of each fluid compartment remain relatively constant. Regulating mechanisms are discussed later in this chapter.

Secretions and excretions are also part of the body's total fluid volume and provide essential functions. They are part of the extracellular fluid. A *secretion* is the product of a gland, for example, the salivary glands. Some specific secretions are cerebrospinal fluid, synovial fluid, pericardial fluid, and alimentary secretions. An *excretion* is waste produced by the cells of the body. Just as balances exist between cellular and extracellular compartments, so do special balances occur between plasma and secretions and excretions. Alimentary secretions for an adult, for example, are estimated to be about 7200 ml per day. See Table 30–2.

Table 30–2 Secretions of the Adult Alimentary Tract

Secretion	Volume (ml/day)
Saliva	1200
Gastric secretion	2000
Pancreatic secretion	1200
Bile	700
Succus entericus	2000
Brunner's gland secretion	50
Large intestine secretion	60
Total	7210

Adapted from A. C. Guyton, *Textbook of medical physiology*, 6th ed. (Philadelphia: W. B. Saunders Co., 1981), p. 803.

Large volumes of fluid also carry dissolved waste materials through the kidneys and through the gastrointestinal tract. However, in both instances, most of this fluid is reabsorbed into the vascular spaces and reused in the body. For example, of 7200 ml produced in the alimentary tract, only 200 ml is usually excreted in the feces, just enough to keep the feces lubricated. Of 180 liters of glomerular filtrate that filters through the kidneys per day, only 1.5 liters are excreted from the body under normal conditions.

Nurses need to be aware of abnormal amounts of secretions and excretions. Excessive losses can seriously deplete first the extracellular fluid volume and then the intracellular fluid volume. Excessive or inadequate secretions interfere with a number of body processes such as digestion and elimination.

Body Electrolytes

Extracellular and intracellular fluids are similar in their content of electrolytes and other substances. These fluids contain oxygen from the lungs; dissolved nutrients from the gastrointestinal tract, including glucose, fatty acids, and amino acids; excretory products of metabolism, of which carbon dioxide is the most abundant; and particles called *ions*.

Many salts dissociate in water, that is, break up into electrically charged ions. The salt sodium chloride breaks up into one ion of sodium (Na^+) and one ion of chloride (Cl^-). These charged particles are called *electrolytes* because they are capable of conducting electricity. Ions that carry a positive charge are called *cations*, and ions carrying a negative charge are called *anions*. Examples of cations are sodium (Na^+), potassium (K^+), calcium (Ca^{2+}), and magnesium (Mg^{2+}). Anions include chloride (Cl^-), bicarbonate (HCO_3^-), monohydrogen phosphate (HPO_4^{2-}), and sulfate (SO_4^{2-}).

Electrolyte Composition of Body Fluids

The electrolyte composition of fluids varies from one compartment to another. Principal ions of extracellular fluid are sodium and chloride; principal ions of cellular fluid are potassium and phosphate. See Figure 30–1. The ion composition of the two extracellular fluid reservoirs (intravascular and interstitial) is similar; the main difference is that intravascular fluid (plasma) has a greater quantity of protein than interstitial fluid. This is because large particles of protein have difficulty passing through the vascular (capillary) membranes into the interstitial fluid. All other electrolytes move readily between these two extracellular compartments.

The higher quantity of protein in plasma plays a significant role in maintaining the intravascular fluid volume and blood pressure. When quantities of plasma protein are low in the body, the blood volume diminishes noticeably and results in a state of hypotension (low blood pressure). This is particularly manifest in people with diseases of the liver (the source of body plasma proteins), who are unable to produce sufficient quantities of plasma proteins.

Just as fluid volumes must be maintained within compartments, so must the electrolyte composition of the various compartments. Balances of electrolytes are maintained in proportion to the quantities of fluid in the compartments. Although the specific numbers of cations and anions may differ in the fluid compartments, in a state of homeostasis the total number of cations equals the number of anions within each compartment.

Body secretions and excretions also contain electrolytes. This is of particular concern when excretions are abnormally increased or decreased or when a secretion is lost from the body (for example, when gastric suction removes the gastric secretions). Fluid and electrolyte imbalance can result from prolonged loss through these routes. See Table 30–3 for the electrolyte composition of some body secretions and excretions.

Measurement of Electrolytes

Electrolytes are measured in milliequivalents per liter of water (mEq/liter) or milligrams per 100 milliliters (mg/100 ml). The term *milliequivalent* means one thousandth of an equivalent; equivalent refers to the *chemical combining power* of a substance or the power of cations to unite with anions to form molecules. This chemical combining activity is measured in relation to the chemical combining activity of the hydrogen ion (H^+). Sodium and chloride ions are equivalent, since they combine equally: 1 mEq of Na^+ equals 1 mEq of Cl^-. However, these cations and anions are not equal in weight: 1 mg of Na^+ does not equal 1 mg of Cl^-; rather, 3 mg of Na^- equals 2 mg of Cl^-.

Clinically, the milliequivalent system is commonly used. However, nurses need to be aware of the different systems of measurement when interpreting laboratory results. It is also important to realize that a laboratory examination usually indicates the findings of blood plasma, since intracellular fluid is not easily accessible for examination. Examination of extracellular fluid (plasma), can frequently reflect the state of the intracellular fluid though not always precisely.

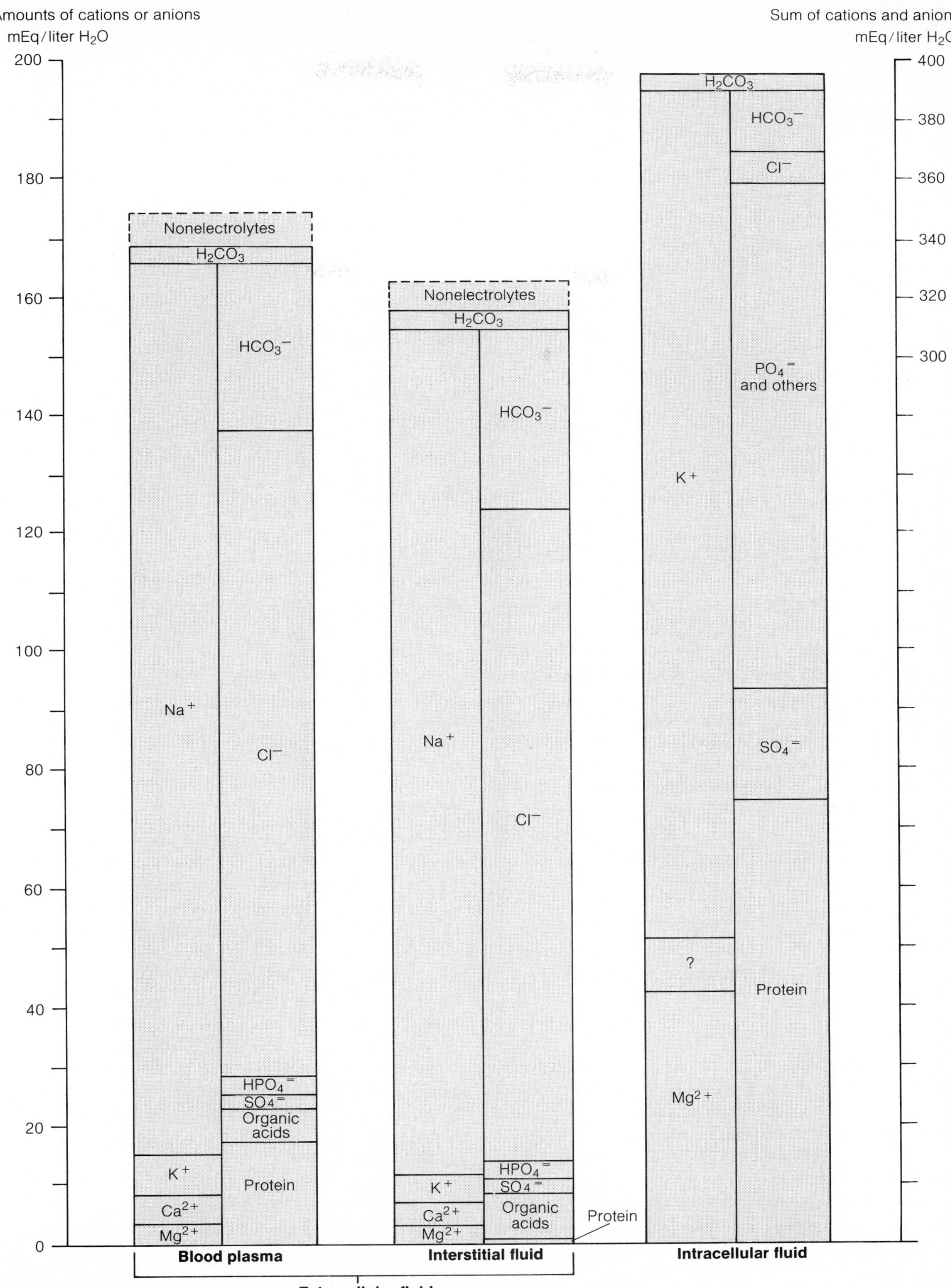

Figure 30–1 The composition of body fluids. (Courtesy of A. P. Spence and E. B. Mason, *Human anatomy and physiology* [Menlo Park, Calif.: Benjamin/Cummings Publishing Co., 1979], p. 737.)

Table 30–3 Electrolyte Composition of Secretions and Excretions Compared to Plasma

	Electrolyte (mEq/liter)			
Substance	*Sodium* (Na^+)	*Potassium* (K^+)	*Chloride* (Cl^-)	*Bicarbonate* (HCO_3^-)
Plasma	135–145	3.6–5.0	95–108	21–28
Gastric secretions	70	5+	140	5
Pancreatic juice	140+	5	35	115+
Hepatic duct bile	140+	5	100+	40
Jejunal secretions	140	5	135	30
Perspiration	80	5	85	—
Diarrhea in children	15	18	10	No method of determining; thought to be as high as K^+

Movement of Body Fluid and Electrolytes

Movement of fluid and transport of substances occur in three phases. First, blood plasma moves around the body within the circulatory system, and nutrients and fluids are picked up from the lungs and the gastrointestinal tract. Second, interstitial fluid and its components move between the blood capillaries and the cells. Third, fluid and substances then move from the interstitial fluid into the cells. In the reverse direction, fluid and its components move back from the cells to the interstitial spaces and then to the intravascular compartment. The intravascular fluid then flows to the kidneys where the metabolic by-products of the cells are excreted.

Methods of Movement

The methods by which body fluids and electrolytes move are: diffusion, osmosis, and active transport.

Diffusion

Diffusion is the continual intermingling of molecules in liquids, gases, or solids, brought about by the random movement of the molecules. For example, two gases become mixed by the incessant motion of their molecules. The process of diffusion occurs even when two substances are separated by a thin membrane. In the body, diffusion of water, electrolytes, and other substances occurs through the "slit pores" of capillary membranes.

The rate of diffusion of substances varies according to (a) size of the molecules, (b) concentration of the solution, and (c) temperature of the solution. Larger molecules move less quickly than smaller ones, since they require more energy to move about. Molecules move more rapidly from a solution of higher concentration to a solution of lower concentration. Increases in temperature increase the rate of motion of molecules and therefore the rate of diffusion.

Osmosis

The term *osmosis* refers to the movement of water across cell membranes. The direction of flow is from the less concentrated solution to the more concentrated solution. In other words, water goes where the most solute is. A *solute* is a substance dissolved in a solution. A *solvent* is the component of a solution that can dissolve a solute. In a salt solution, water is the solvent, and sodium chloride (NaCl) is the solute. The process of osmosis is important in maintaining proper balance in the volumes of extracellular and intracellular fluid.

Osmolarity is a measure of the concentration of a solution, expressed in a unit called the *osmol:* 1 osmol is the number of particles in 1 gram molecular weight of dissociated solute. Osmolarity is expressed in osmols per liter of solution.

Active transport

Substances can move across cell membranes from a less concentrated solution to a more concentrated one by *active transport*. This process differs from diffusion and osmosis in that metabolic energy is expended. In active transport, the substance combines with a carrier on the outside surface of the cell membrane. The combined carrier and substance then move to the inside surface. Once inside, they separate, and the substance is released to the inside of the cell. A specific carrier is required for each substance, and enzymes are required for active transport.

This process is of particular importance in maintaining the differences in sodium and potassium ion concentrations of extracellular and intracellular fluid. Under normal conditions, sodium concentrations are higher in the extracellular fluid, while potassium concentrations are higher inside the cells. To maintain this balance, the active transport mechanism (the *sodium-potassium* pump) is activated, moving sodium from the cells and potassium into the cells.

Fluid Pressures

A number of pressures are exerted as part of the movement of fluid and electrolytes from one compartment to another. Two of these are osmotic pressure and hydrostatic pressure, each of which can cause a flow of fluid through the capillary membranes.

Osmotic pressure

Osmotic pressure is the pressure exerted by a solution to stop osmosis. The osmotic pressure exerted by particles such as ions or molecules that cannot penetrate the membrane depends upon the number of particles per unit of volume, not the total mass of the particles. The reason is that each particle in a solution exerts the same amount of pressure upon the membrane regardless of its mass.

Osmotic pressure is the force exerted by solute particles drawing water across membranes. The solute particles may be *crystalloids* (salts that dissolve readily into true solutions) or *colloids* (substances such as large protein molecules that do not readily dissolve into true solutions). Normally, the net movement of fluid across cell membranes is nil; that is, the distribution of electrolytes on both sides of membranes is even. Should the concentration of the solute on one side of a membrane become greater, the osmotic pressure and attraction for water will increase on that side, and water will flow toward the solution of greater concentration until the concentration gradient disappears.

The principle of osmosis can be applied clinically in the administration of intravenous solutions. Usually, solutions are given that are *isotonic*, having the same concentration (osmolarity) as blood plasma. This prevents sudden shifts of fluids and electrolytes. In some cases, however, hypertonic or hypotonic solutions are infused. *Hypertonic* solutions have a greater concentration of solutes than plasma; *hypotonic* solutions have a lesser concentration of solutes. An example of a hypertonic solution is 50% glucose. It may be given to reduce cerebral edema. The high concentration of glucose temporarily draws fluid from interstitial spaces in the brain into the blood compartment. Use of hypotonic solutions is rare.

The osmotic pressure of plasma is greater than the osmotic pressure of interstitial fluid, for two reasons: (a) the protein concentration (solute) in plasma is greater than that in interstitial fluid; and (b) protein molecules are large, resemble colloids, and do not readily pass through capillary membranes. This greater colloid osmotic pressure of plasma is extremely important in maintaining the intravascular fluid volume.

Hydrostatic pressure

Counterbalancing the osmotic pressure of plasma, which attracts fluid, is the hydrostatic pressure of the blood flowing through the capillaries, which pushes fluid out of the vascular space. *Hydrostatic pressure* is the pressure exerted by a fluid within a closed system. Thus the hydrostatic pressure of blood is the force exerted by blood against the vascular walls such as the artery walls. It is also referred to as *filtration force*. The principle involved in hydrostatic pressure is that fluids move from the area of greater pressure to the area of less pressure. For this reason fluid moves out of blood vessels.

The net movement of water from plasma to tissue spaces thus depends on which force is greater: hydrostatic pressure, which forces fluid out of the blood vessels, or osmotic pressure, which draws fluid into the blood vessels. Normally, fluid moves out of capillaries at the arterial end where the intravascular hydrostatic pressure exceeds the colloid osmotic pressure. At the venous end of the capillaries, where the colloid osmotic pressure is greater, fluid is drawn from the interstitial compartment into the intravascular compartment.

Selective Permeability of Membranes

Capillary and cellular membranes in the body are described as selectively permeable, because not all substances move with the same ease across the membranes. Compounds such as proteins and glycogen do not readily cross capillary and cellular membranes. Organic compounds such as glucose and amino acids move freely across capillary walls, although they often require active transport. Certain membranes, called *dialyzing membranes*, allow water molecules and particles in true solution (crystalloids) to move through but not particles in colloid dispersion. Most of the membranes that surround cells are dialyzing membranes.

Cellular (not capillary) membranes are particularly selective in regard to sodium and potassium ions. Movement of potassium across cell membranes depends upon metabolic cellular activities. Administration of glucose or insulin accelerates the movement of potassium into the cells. Sodium enters in greater quantities when the cells lose potassium. Any factor that alters the properties of the cell membranes brings about changes in the distribution of sodium and potassium. Some of these factors are excitation of nerve and muscle cells, changes in pH, and anoxia.

Regulating Fluid Volume

Health is usually maintained as long as the fluid volume and chemical composition of the fluid compartments stay within narrow safe limits. Normally a person's fluid intake is counterbalanced by fluid loss. However, in illness this balance may be upset, so that the body has too little or too much fluid.

Fluid Intake

The average adult (assuming moderate activity at moderate temperature) drinks about 1500 ml per day but needs 2500 ml per day, an additional 1000 ml. This added volume is acquired from foods (referred to as preformed water) and from the oxidation of these foods during metabolic processes. Interestingly, the water content of food is relatively large, contributing about 750 ml per day. The water content of fresh vegetables is approximately 90%, of fresh fruits about 85%, and of lean meats around 60%.

Oxidative water, which is formed as a by-product of the body's oxidation of food, accounts for most of the remaining fluid volume required. For each 100 calories of protein, fat, and carbohydrate, metabolism produces 14 ml of water as an end product. A 2500-calorie diet produces 350 ml of water $([2500 \div 100] \times 14 = 350)$. The oxidation of hydrogen in the food accounts for the synthesis of a small amount (150 to 250 ml) per day (Guyton 1981:392).

The primary regulator of fluid intake is the body's thirst mechanism. The thirst center is situated in the supraoptic nuclei in the lateral preoptic area of the hypothalamus. A number of stimuli trigger this center: intracellular dehydration, excess angiotensin II (a hormone released into the blood in response to very low blood pressure) in the body fluids, hemorrhage, and low cardiac output resulting in lowered blood volume. Angiotensin II is a potent vasoconstrictor. It forms largely in the small blood vessels in the lungs, in response to release of renin to the bloodstream from the kidneys.

Dryness of the mouth is often associated with thirst but can occur independently (for example, when a person's salivary glands do not secrete saliva). Thirst is normally relieved immediately after drinking a small amount of fluid, even before it is absorbed from the gastrointestinal tract. However, this relief is only temporary, and the thirst returns in about 15 minutes. The thirst is again temporarily relieved after the ingested fluid distends the upper gastrointestinal tract. These mechanisms protect the individual from drinking too much, because it takes from one-half to one hour for the fluid to be absorbed and distributed throughout the body. If a person continued to drink during that time, the fluid ingested would overdilute the body fluids.

Fluid Output

Fluid losses counterbalance the adult's 2500 ml daily intake of water. The main channel of excretion is the kidneys, which are responsible for an output of about 1500 ml per day in the adult. This approximates the amount of fluid an adult drinks per day. Oral intake and kidney output are frequently and easily measured in nursing practice.

Three other routes of fluid output are:

1. Insensible loss through the skin as perspiration and through the lungs as water vapor in the expired air
2. Noticeable loss through the skin as sweat
3. Loss through the intestines in feces

See Table 30–4 for the average daily fluid output for an adult. The normal loss from skin and lungs accounts for about two-thirds of the urinary loss, whereas loss in the feces is minimal. It is important to remember that *daily intake equals daily output.*

Obligatory loss is the essential fluid loss required to maintain body functioning. Water lost as vapor in expired air and as vapor from the skin, a minimum volume of about 500 ml from the kidneys, and the fluid required to excrete the solid metabolic wastes produced daily are the obligatory losses, totaling about 1300 ml per day.

Since the vaporized losses are not readily measured, the measured obligatory kidney loss becomes of prime importance in critical illness. An adult hourly urine volume of less than 30 ml or daily volume under 500 ml is serious. Patients with inadequate output require immediate attention, and such a finding by the nurse must therefore be reported promptly. Although losses from the skin, lungs, and intestines in health account for approximately half of the daily loss, they can account for a much larger percentage of loss from a patient who has a fever or accelerated respiration. Increases in respiratory rate, fever, *diaphoresis* (sweating), and diarrhea can magnify fluid loss from the normal routes immensely. Other routes of loss, such as from the stomach through emesis or suction or from abnormal body openings such as fistulas or surgically implanted drainage tubes, often account for significant losses, all of which require intake replacements.

In health, the output volumes shown in Table 30–4 may vary noticeably from day to day and throughout one day. For example, sweat gland activity can increase when the environmental temperature increases. Urinary volume automatically increases as the amount of fluids ingested increases, e.g., on a hot summer day. If fluid loss from the skin is large, however, the urinary volume may decrease to maintain the fluid volumes in the body. Balance is maintained between the intake and output by the homeostatic mechanisms already discussed in this chapter.

Table 30–4 Average Daily Fluid Output for an Adult

Route	Amount
Urine	1400 to 1500 ml
Insensible losses:	
Lungs	350 to 400 ml
Skin	350 to 400 ml
Sweat	100 ml
Feces	100 to 200 ml
Total	2300 to 2600 ml

Urine

The formation of urine by the kidneys and its subsequent excretion from the urinary bladder is the major avenue of fluid output. The two kidneys each contain about 1,200,000 nephrons. The nephron was described in Chapter 28 on page 706. The glomerulus filters glomerular fluid into a long tubule where most of the fluid is reabsorbed into the bloodstream. The remainder of the fluid that is not absorbed becomes urine. The formation of urine and control of that process are highly complex. One of the major controls of urine formation is the blood volume of the individual. When the volume of circulating blood becomes excessive, the stretch receptors in the walls of the left and right atria are triggered to transmit impulses to the brain. The brain reacts by inhibiting sympathetic nervous impulses to the kidneys, reducing the secretion of antidiuretic hormone (ADH), and dilating the body's peripheral capillaries. As a result of these mechanisms, the rate of urine output is increased and excess blood volume filters temporarily into the tissue spaces.

Another control mechanism is the osmoreceptor of sodium and antidiuretic hormone system. This feedback system controls the concentration of sodium in the extracellular fluid, the fluid's osmolarity, and thus urine formation. An increase in the osmolarity (sodium concentration) of the extracellular fluid stimulates osmoreceptors, which are located in the supraoptic nuclei of the hypothalamus. These stimulate the production of antidiuretic hormone (ADH) by the hypothalamus and release of ADH by the posterior pituitary gland. ADH acts on the cells of the distal and collecting tubules of the glomeruli to make them more permeable to water. As a result, more fluid is reabsorbed into the bloodstream to dilute the sodium and other substances in the extracellular fluid, and less urine is formed. When the extracellular fluid becomes sufficiently diluted, the osmoreceptors respond to the decreased sodium concentration by reducing the production of ADH. Consequently, the antidiuretic effect ceases, and additional urine is produced.

Insensible losses

Insensible fluid loss occurs through the skin and lungs. It is called *insensible* because it is usually not noticeable. The insensible loss through the skin is by diffusion. It is normally controlled by the outer layer of the epidermis, the stratum corneum. However, when the skin layers are destroyed, by burns and abrasions, fluid loss can increase considerably.

Another type of insensible loss is the water in exhaled air. In an adult this is normally about 350 ml per day. With an accelerated respiratory rate, e.g., due to exercise or an elevated body temperature, this loss can increase.

Sweat

Sweating occurs when the body becomes overheated. The sweat glands secrete large quantities of sweat onto the surface of the body to provide cooling by evaporation. Sweating occurs in response to stimulation of the preoptic area in the anterior hypothalamus. Impulses are transmitted to the spinal cord and via the sympathetic nervous system to the skin.

The rate of flow of sweat can vary from none in a cold environment to 1.5 liters per hour in an adult acclimatized to a hot environment. Thus, a person could lose more than 1.3 kg (3 lb) of body weight per hour in sweat (Guyton 1982:552).

Large amounts of sweat contain large amounts of sodium chloride, whereas small amounts of sweat contain lower concentrations of sodium chloride. Sweat also contains urea, lactic acid, and potassium ions. The concentrations of these substances can be very high when the rate of sweat secretion is low and are lower when the rate of sweat secretion is high (Guyton 1981:889).

Feces

When chyme passes from the small intestine into the large intestine, it is composed of water and electrolytes. The volume of chyme that passes through the ileocecal valve in an adult is normally about 800 ml per day. Of this amount, all but about 80 to 150 ml is reabsorbed in the proximal half of the large intestine. Sodium and chloride ions are also actively absorbed, and bicarbonate ions are secreted by the mucosa of the large intestine. The bicarbonate helps to neutralize the acidic end products of bacterial action in the colon. For further information about the composition of feces, see Chapter 27, page 688.

Regulating Electrolytes

The major electrolytes of the body are the cations sodium, potassium, and calcium and the anion chloride.

Sodium

The sources of sodium for the body are largely table salt (NaCl) and foods high in sodium such as cheese, pork products, salted meats, bread, potato chips, and cereals.

Normal sodium concentrations in the extracellular fluid are regulated by ADH and aldosterone. Aldosterone, a hormone produced by the adrenal cortex, acts to maintain sodium concentrations, although its action can be overridden by ADH and the thirst mechanism described earlier. ADH regulates the amount of water absorbed into the blood from the renal tubules. Aldosterone regulates the amount of sodium reabsorbed into the blood. When aldosterone is secreted and increased sodium is reabsorbed, the sodium concentration in the extracellular fluid is increased. In a feedback mechanism, the increased extracellular sodium causes the adrenal cortex to decrease the secretion of aldosterone. If the body must conserve sodium for any reason, it can excrete sodium-free urine.

Sodium not only moves into and out of the body but also moves in careful balance among the three fluid compartments. It is found in most body secretions, for example, saliva, gastric and intestinal secretions, bile, and pancreatic fluid. Therefore, continuous excretion of any of these fluids, e.g., via intestinal suction, could result in a sodium deficit in the body.

The functions of sodium within the body are largely control and regulation of the body fluids. When sodium is reabsorbed into the blood from the tubules of the glomeruli, chloride is reabsorbed with it. The combined reabsorption increases the fluid held in the body. Sodium also helps maintain blood volume and interstitial fluid volume through this mechanism. With potassium, sodium helps maintain the electrolyte balance of intracellular and extracellular fluids by means of the active transport mechanism, the sodium-potassium pump.

Potassium

Potassium is the major cation of intracellular fluid (see Figure 30–1, earlier). Major sources of potassium are bananas, broccoli, canteloupe, citrus fruits, and potatoes.

Potassium balance is regulated in the kidneys by two mechanisms: exchange with sodium ions in the kidney tubules and secretion of aldosterone. Aldosterone is extremely important in controlling potassium concentrations in extracellular fluids. The aldosterone-potassium feedback system works in three steps:

1. Increased potassium concentration in extracellular fluid causes an increase in the production of aldosterone.
2. The increased aldosterone increases the amount of potassium excreted by the kidneys.
3. As increased potassium is excreted, the concentration of potassium in the extracellular fluid decreases, which decreases the aldosterone production.

Potassium is necessary for all types of neuromuscular activity. It also acts as part of the body's buffer system (see the discussion of acid-base balance later in this chapter).

Calcium

The richest sources of calcium are milk and milk products. Smaller amounts are found in grains, fruits, nuts, shellfish, and eggs. Drinking water in some parts of the country also contains an absorbable calcium.

Calcium functions in bone formation and in the transmission of nerve impulses, muscle contraction, blood coagulation, and activation of certain enzymes, such as pancreatic lipase and phospholipase.

Calcium is excreted in urine, feces, bile, digestive secretions, and sweat. The concentration of body calcium is controlled indirectly by the effect of parathyroid hormone on bone reabsorption. When extracellular fluid calcium falls too low, the parathyroid glands are stimulated to secrete increased parathyroid hormone (parahormone), which acts directly on the bones to increase the release of calcium into the blood. When the bones run out of calcium, parathyroid hormone acts on both the kidney tubules and the intestinal mucosa to increase the reabsorption of calcium from the kidneys and the intestine.

Chloride

Chloride is the major anion of extracellular fluid (see Figure 30–1, earlier). Chloride is found in blood, interstitial fluid, and lymph. A very small amount is found in intracellular fluid. It functions as sodium does to maintain the osmotic pressure of the blood. Its reabsorption in the kidney is secondary to that of sodium; that is, each sodium ion reabsorbed is accompanied by a chloride or bicarbonate ion. Aldosterone therefore indirectly controls the reabsorption of chloride by its control of sodium.

The chief dietary sources of chloride are dairy products and meat. Chloride is also found with sodium as salt (NaCl) in the foods described earlier.

Acid-Base Balance

The body's cellular activity requires an alkaline medium. Alkalinity and its opposite, acidity, are measured in terms of hydrogen ion concentration, expressed on a scale called *pH*. Body fluids are normally maintained at a pH of about 7.4. Alterations of pH of even a few tenths can be incompatible with cellular activity.

Opposing the body's alkalinity are cellular chemical processes that are constantly producing large amounts of acid as by-products of metabolism. Fortunately, precise control mechanisms maintain the pH of body fluids within a very narrow range. The pH is controlled by buffer systems in all body fluids and by respiratory and kidney regulatory systems.

Three major buffer systems of the body fluids are the bicarbonate buffer, the phosphate buffer, and the protein buffer. Discussion here is limited to the bicarbonate buffer system, since the phosphate and protein buffer systems operate in almost the same manner.

Bicarbonate Buffer System

The bicarbonate buffer system consists of sodium bicarbonate ($NaHCO_3$) or potassium bicarbonate ($KHCO_3$) and carbonic acid (H_2CO_3) in the same solution. Buffers do not neutralize; acid-base buffers decrease the effect of strong acids and strong bases, so that the pH of a body fluid falls or rises only slightly. For example, if a strong acid such as hydrochloric acid (HCl) is introduced to a glass of water, the pH of the fluid drops significantly to 1 or 2. However, if a bicarbonate buffer system is already present in the water, the HCl quickly combines with the buffer, producing a weaker acid (carbonic acid), and the pH drops only slightly. The reaction is:

$$HCl + NaHCO_3 \rightarrow H_2CO_3 + NaCl$$

(hydrochloric acid) (sodium bicarbonate) (carbonic acid) (sodium chloride)

A strong acid is a compound that completely dissociates its hydrogen ions; for example, HCl yields H^+ and Cl^-. A weak acid is one that frees only some of its hydrogen ions; for example, H_2CO_3 yields H^+ and HCO_3^-. One hydrogen ion is free, the other is not.

On the alkaline side, when a strong base such as sodium hydroxide is added to body fluids, it combines with carbonic acid to form a weaker base, sodium bicarbonate:

$$NaOH + H_2CO_3 \rightarrow NaHCO_3 + H_2O$$

(sodium hydroxide) (carbonic acid) (sodium bicarbonate) (water)

Although the bicarbonate buffer system is not the strongest buffer system in the body (the most powerful and plentiful one consists of the proteins of plasma and cells), it is important, because the concentration of sodium bicarbonate is regulated by the kidneys and the concentration of carbonic acid by the respiratory system.

Respiratory Regulation

Elimination of carbon dioxide by the lungs also regulates acid-base balance. The carbon dioxide that a person exhales comes from carbonic acid as follows:

$$H_2CO_3 \rightarrow CO_2 + H_2O$$

The more CO_2 exhaled, the more H_2CO_3 is removed from the blood, thus elevating the blood pH to a more alkaline level. Hyperventilation is an example of this shift. Increasing the ventilation rate raises the pH. On the other hand, holding one's breath, or hypoventilating, retains CO_2, which is then available to form carbonic acid, leading to a reduced or more acid pH. Significant changes in the pH of body fluids, therefore, are made by altering respiratory activity.

Renal Regulation

The kidney's role in maintaining acid-base balance is complex. To simplify, the kidneys excrete hydrogen ions and form bicarbonate ions in specific amounts as indicated by the pH of the blood. When the plasma pH drops (becomes more acidic), hydrogen ions (acid) are excreted, and bicarbonate ions (base) are formed and retained. Conversely, when the plasma pH rises (becomes more alkaline), hydrogen ions are retained in the body, and bicarbonate ions are excreted.

Imbalances

The normal pH range of extracellular fluid is 7.35 to 7.45. This precise balance is maintained as long as the ratio of 1 carbonic acid molecule to 20 bicarbonate ions is maintained in the extracellular fluid. The ratio, rather than the specific amount of each, is important.

Imbalances in pH can result in either *acidosis* or *alkalosis.* To simplify, acidosis occurs with increases in blood carbonic acid or with decreases in blood bicarbonate. Alkalosis occurs with increases in blood bicarbonate or decreases in blood carbonic acid. A patient will not become acidotic or alkalotic, however, unless the normal ratio of 1 carbonic acid molecule to 20 bicarbonate ions is altered. Compensatory (adaptive) mechanisms operate to maintain this balance. See the discussion of acid-base imbalances in Chapter 31.

Two adjectives describe the general cause or origin of a pH imbalance: metabolic and respiratory. *Metabolic acidosis* and *metabolic alkalosis* are imbalances brought about by changes in bicarbonate levels as a result of metabolic alterations. *Respiratory acidosis* and *respiratory alkalosis* are imbalances brought about by changes in carbonic acid levels as a result of respiratory alterations.

Assessing Fluid, Electrolyte, and Acid-Base Balance

Nursing History

A patient history relative to fluid and electrolyte balance should include information about usual and present fluid intake and output, usual and present nutritional intakes (see Chapter 26), usual body weight, acute changes in body weight, reasons for an insufficient or excessive fluid and/or food intake, specific losses, such as drainage from a wound or diarrhea, and any changes in urinary output.

Table 30–5 Average Daily Water Requirements by Age and Weight

Age	Water requirement *ml*	*ml/kg body weight*
3 days	250–300	80–100
1 year	1150–1300	120–135
2 years	1350–1500	115–125
4 years	1600–1800	100–110
10 years	2000–2500	70–85
18 years	2200–2700	40–50
Adult	2400–2600	20–30

Adapted from V. C. Vaughan et al., *Nelson textbook of pediatrics*, 11th ed. (Philadelphia: W. B. Saunders Co., 1979), p. 175; R. B. Howard and N. H. Herbold, *Nutrition in clinical care*, 2nd ed. (New York: McGraw-Hill Book Co., 1982), p. 153.

Factors Influencing Fluid and Electrolyte Needs

Age

Fluid intake requirements vary with age. Intake requirements have been determined for various ages in relation to body surface area, metabolic requirements, and body weight.

Infants and growing children have much greater fluid turnover than adults, that is, greater water needs and greater water losses. This is due to their greater metabolic rate, which increases fluid loss through the kidneys. Immature kidneys in infants are less efficient than adult kidneys, thereby increasing the loss of fluid through the kidneys. Infant losses from both the lungs and the skin are also greater in proportion to body weight, essentially because respirations are more rapid and the body surface area is proportionately greater. The more rapid turnover of fluid plus the losses produced by disease can create critical fluid imbalances in children much more rapidly than in adults. See Table 30–5 for approximate fluid requirements at different ages according to body weight. A 70 kg adult requires 20–30 × 70 = 1400–2100 ml of fluid per day, whereas a 1-year-old weighing 10 kg requires 120–135 × 10 = 1200–1350 ml daily; the infant requires more than four times the amount per kilogram of body weight of the adult.

Fluid requirements are determined most accurately from metabolic rate, that is, calories metabolized, or from surface area of the body, which varies directly with metabolic rate. Because neither of these is easily

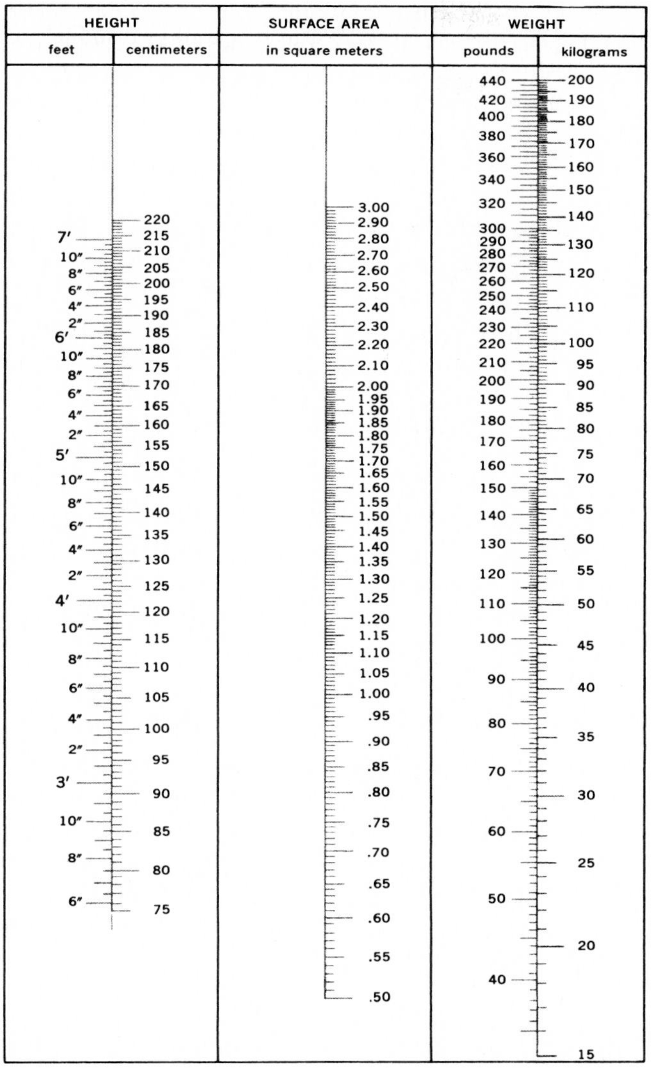

Figure 30–2 To determine the surface area of older children and adults, a straight line is drawn between the point on the left vertical scale representing the patient's height to the point on the right vertical scale showing the patient's weight. The point where the line crosses the middle vertical scale is the patient's surface area in square meters.

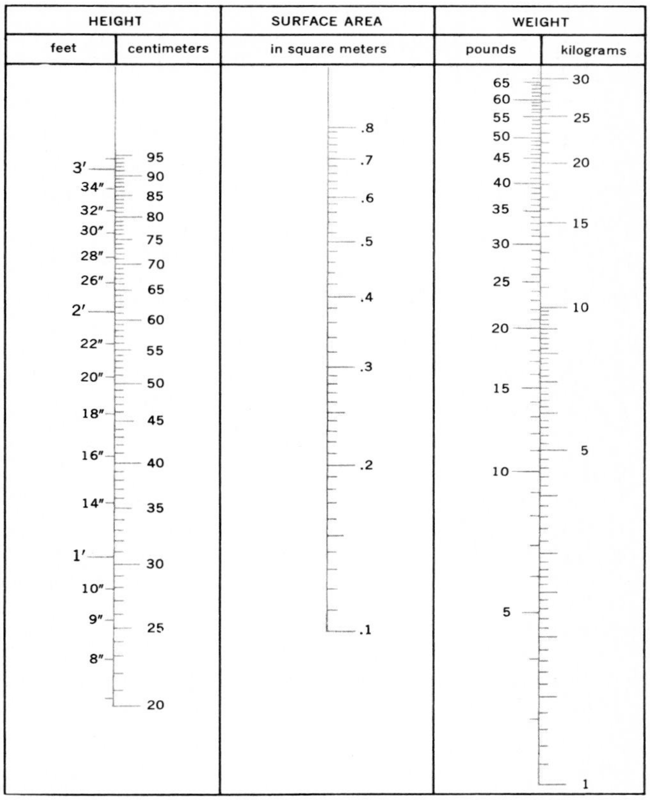

Figure 30–3 The surface area of infants and young children is determined in the same manner as for adults (see Figure 30–2).

measured clinically, tables have been produced that calculate the body surface area from the individual's height and weight. See Figures 30–2 and 30–3. Basic fluid requirements per square meter of surface area are generally the same for all people: 1500 ml/m^2.

Body fat

Because females tend to have more fat deposits than males, their percentage of body fluid is generally less, since fat is essentially free of fluid. For the same reason, obese people have a lower percentage of body water, sometimes as low as 45% in an adult (Guyton 1981:392).

Exercise

Exercise increases the loss of body water, primarily through water vapor exhaled at an increased respiratory rate and through excessive sweating. Sweating also increases the loss of sodium chloride, lactic acid, potassium, and urea from the body.

Environmental temperature

The environmental temperature also affects fluid and electrolyte loss from the body. Higher temperatures tend to increase sweating and consequent loss of the fluids and substances described above.

Stress

Prolonged stress can affect fluid and electrolyte balance. A stressor causes the hypothalamus in the brain to release corticotropin-releasing hormone (CRH), which stimulates the anterior pituitary gland to secrete increased adrenocorticotropic hormone (ACTH). ACTH stimulates the adrenal cortex to increase the secretion of aldosterone, which increases reabsorption of water and sodium from the kidney tubules. Stimulation of the posterior pituitary gland by impulses from the hypothalamus also causes increased secretion of antidiuretic hormone (ADH). ADH acts to increase water retention (decrease urine formation). The overall response of the body to stress is to increase the blood volume through these mechanisms. For further information, see Chapter 9 and Figure 9–2 on page 186.

Health

Fluid and electrolyte needs are affected by many disease processes and treatments, for example, burns, intestinal suction, and malignancies. In addition to causing abnormal fluid and electrolyte loss, some conditions affect fluid and electrolyte intake; for example, persistent vomiting can seriously impair a person's capacity to take in fluids or nourishment. For additional information, see Chapter 31, pages 796–809.

Physical Examination

The patient is examined for clinical signs of fluid, electrolyte, and acid-base imbalances. The nurse needs a knowledge of significant signs as well as the normal clinical picture presented by the patient. Specific assessments should include body weight and assessment of each body system. See Chapter 14, page 325. Table 31–3 on page 807 describes some common clinical signs related to fluid, electrolyte, and acid-base imbalances. For information on the assessment of urine, see Chapter 28, page 712.

The well-hydrated person shows the following signs:

1. Stable weight from day to day
2. Moist mucous membranes
3. An appropriate food intake
4. Straw-colored urine with a specific gravity of 1.010 to 1.030
5. Good tissue turgor
6. Mental orientation
7. No complaint of thirst
8. An appropriate amount of excreted urine in relation to fluid intake
9. No evidence of edema
10. No evidence of dehydration, such as depressed periorbital spaces

Table 30–6 Sample Metric Measurements for Fluid Containers

Container	Amount
Water glass	200 ml
Juice glass	120 ml
Cup	180 ml
Soup bowl (adult)	180 ml
Soup bowl (child)	100 ml
Teapot	240 ml
Creamer (large)	90 ml
Creamer (small)	30 ml
Water pitcher	1000 ml
Gelatin or custard dish	100 ml
Ice cream dish	120 ml
Paper cup (large)	200 ml
Paper cup (small)	120 ml

Measurement of Fluid Intake and Output

It is often the nurse's function to assess the oral fluid intake of patients. For those who have a fever or an infection, the nurse should advise additional fluid intake of up to 3000 ml per day. Recording fluid intake (I) and output (O) for the patient may be warranted, and a physician may prescribe the exact amount of fluid that the patient should have in a 24-hour period. In some situations, intake may be limited, for example, for a patient who has a pathologic condition of the kidney or heart. For dehydrated patients, fluids are frequently encouraged.

To measure oral intake, household measures must be converted to milliliters. See Table 30–6. Most agencies provide conversion tables, since the size of the dishes used is variable. Printed intake and output records are usually available. See Figure 30–4. Generally 8-hour records are kept at the patient's bedside and then converted to 24-hour records on the patient's chart. The nurse proceeds as follows:

1. Place an intake and output record at the patient's bedside at beginning of each shift and a 24-hour record on the patient's chart. Make sure of the equivalents used by the agency for measuring intake and output.
2. Explain to the patient the reasons for and importance of measuring and recording fluid intake and output. Emphasize that all fluids taken are to be measured, including oral, intravenous, and any other liquids pertinent to the patient's situation, such as gastric feedings. Instruct ambulatory patients to save their urine by

voiding in a bedpan or urinal. Encourage patients to keep track of their own intake if they so desire.

3. With the patient, make a plan for providing the prescribed fluid intake; for example, if the goal is 2000 ml in 24 hours, allocate an amount per shift:

Day shift, 900 ml
Evening shift, 900 ml
Night shift, 200 ml

Consider the patient's fluid preferences, and provide for these when possible.

4. Check and record the fluids taken at mealtimes and nourishment times. Often the patient will assist with this. When recording the intake of fluid, measure all obvious fluids plus such foods as ice cream, gelatin, sherbet, and Popsicles. Recording output when patients are incontinent of urine or feces presents problems of accuracy, but some assessment of amount should be recorded, for example, "half a drawsheet saturated with urine × 2" (twice).

5. Record 8-hour and daily intake and output volumes on the appropriate records.

6. Note other losses, such as vomiting, diarrhea, excessive perspiration, and losses from suctions, and measure and record these.

BEDSIDE INTAKE-OUTPUT RECORD

Name: Mary Brown   Room No.: 747-2   Date: 7/11

	INTAKE		OUTPUT		
Time	Liquids	Intravenous	Urine	Emesis	Drainage etc.
8–4	0900 Juice 120 Coffee 180 Cream 90 0930 Water 90 1200 Tea 180 Cream 90 Jello 50 1400 Juice 180		0700 - 250 1100 - 400 1500 - 350		
Total	980		1000		
4–12					
Total					
12–8					
Total					

Figure 30–4 A sample 24-hour bedside fluid intake and output record.

Diagnostic Tests

Electrolyte levels

Serum electrolyte levels are frequently tested to determine the acid-base and electrolyte balance of the body fluids. The most commonly ordered serum tests are for sodium, potassium, carbon dioxide (bicarbonate), and chloride. Serum sodium and potassium tests are done to determine changes in fluid and sodium balances in patients who have fluid imbalances, have endocrine disorders, or are receiving intravenous infusions with electrolytes. Variations in the serum chloride level usually occur with changes in sodium level. Elevated serum chloride is found in disorders such as prostatic obstruction and renal failure. Decreased chloride levels may be found in patients with congestive heart failure or burns.

The carbon dioxide content of plasma reflects the body's ability to control acid-base balance. The total carbon dioxide content of the blood consists of: dissolved carbon dioxide gas (CO_2), carbonic acid (HCO_3) and bicarbonate ions (HCO_3^-). In the past, carbon dioxide content was determined in terms of carbon dioxide combining power—that is, the amount of CO_2 gas that could be absorbed by a specimen of plasma. However, it is now thought that this is not an accurate measure, because the CO_2 is combined at a constant pressure of 40 mm Hg rather than at the varying pressures that exist in the patient (Byrne et al. 1981:135). Therefore, this test is being replaced by tests such as the bicarbonate ion concentration test. A normal plasma bicarbonate level is 21 to 28 mEq/liter.

Acid-base balance

Tests normally carried out to determine acid-base balance are called *blood-gas determinations* and routinely include: blood pH, $Paco_2$ (carbonic acid concentration), total CO_2 (bicarbonate ion plus carbonic acid), Pao_2, and O_2 saturation. Specimens of arterial blood are taken for these tests.

The pH measures the concentration of hydrogen ions, indicating the blood's acidity or alkalinity. Normally arterial blood has a pH of 7.35 to 7.45. Any variation from normal can reflect a problem in the bicarbonate and carbonic acid buffer system.

The $Paco_2$ measures the pressure exerted by carbon dioxide gas dissolved in the blood. The Pa stands for partial arterial pressure—here, the pressure exerted by CO_2 in the arterial blood. This pressure is regulated by the lungs and reflects the amount of carbonic acid available to the bicarbonate and carbonic acid buffer system. A normal $Paco_2$ is 35 to 45 mm Hg.

Total CO_2 content is the measure of both the bicarbonate ion and carbonic acid in the blood. It is expressed in millimols per liter (mmol/liter). A *mol* of a substance is a molar solution (a solution containing the molecular weight in grams of the solute per 1000 ml of solution). A *millimol* is 1/1000 of a mol. The total CO_2 measure provides an accurate guide to the functioning of the bicarbonate and carbonic acid buffer system. The combined measurement in arterial blood is normally 21 to 30 mmol/liter.

Partial pressure of oxygen (Pao_2) is the pressure exerted by the small amount of oxygen that is dissolved in the plasma. This oxygen is separate from the oxygen carried by the hemoglobin of the erythrocytes. Normal values of Pao_2 are 80 to 100 mm Hg in arterial blood.

Oxygen saturation (O_2 Sat) is the ratio of the oxygen in the blood to the maximum amount of oxygen the blood can carry. Normal values are 95% to 98% in arterial blood and 60% to 85% in venous blood. Oxygen saturation provides some indication of the functioning of the patient's lung ventilation.

Summary

A balance of both fluid and electrolytes is necessary for health and life. The total body fluid of an adult male comprises about 57% of his weight. The younger the person, the higher this proportion. Body fluid is distributed in two major reservoirs: intracellular (ICF) and extracellular (ECF). The extracellular is further subdivided into two compartments: intravascular (plasma) and interstitial. Extracellular fluid is about one-third to one-quarter of the total body fluid. The extracellular component is in constant motion and serves as the transport system for nutrients and wastes.

The body electrolytes (ions) are of two types: positively charged (cations) and negatively charged (anions). The principal ions of extracellular fluid are sodium and chloride, and the principal ions of intracellular fluid are potassium and phosphate. Electrolytes are measured in milliequivalents per liter of water (mEq/liter).

Fluid moves among the body compartments by diffusion, osmosis, and active transport. The major fluid pressures of the body are the osmotic or drawing pressure and the hydrostatic or pushing pressure. The membranes of the cells and capillaries are selectively permeable; that is, not all substances can pass through them.

Normal fluid intake for an adult is about 2500 ml per day, of which 1500 ml is liquid intake. Other sources of fluid are food and by-products of the oxidation of food. The amount of fluid required varies according to age. A 1-year-old requires about 1000 to 1500 ml per day. Fluid needs are calculated according to body surface area.

Body fluid volume depends on the balance of fluid intake and fluid output. Fluid intake is regulated by the body's thirst mechanism. Fluid output occurs through the urine, insensible vapor losses, sweat, and feces. The average adult needs to lose about 2500 ml per day for health. Urine is the major output vehicle for fluids and electrolytes. It is controlled by a complex mechanism involving circulating blood volume, osmoreceptors of sodium, and antidiuretic hormone.

Electrolytes are also regulated by complex systems often involving hormones. Sodium, potassium, calcium, and chloride are the major electrolytes of the body. The acid-base balance of the body is controlled by three buffer systems: bicarbonate, phosphate, and protein buffers. These buffers decrease the effects of strong acids and strong bases. The respiratory system and the kidneys also help to regulate acid-base balance.

Nursing assessment relative to fluids, electrolytes, and acid-base balance includes: a health history; consideration of factors that influence fluid, electrolyte, and acid-base balance; physical assessment of the patient; measuring intake and output; and diagnostic tests.

Suggested Activities

1. Assess the daily fluid intake of a healthy adult, an infant, and a preschooler. Compare the results.

2. In a clinical setting, survey the intake and output records used. With a group of classmates from different clinical settings, note the similarities and differences in these records.

3. In a nursing laboratory, measure the amount of fluid contained in each of the following:

- **a.** Soup bowl
- **b.** Small glass
- **c.** Paper cup
- **d.** Cup
- **e.** Water glass
- **f.** Water pitcher
- **g.** Bedpan
- **h.** Urinal
- **i.** Kidney (emesis) basin

4. Using the I & O form of a hospital in which you practice, keep an I & O record on yourself for 24 hours. A previously measured paper cup can be used to measure your urine. Looking at your calculations, are you in fluid balance?

Suggested Readings

Lane, G., and Peirce, A. G. January 1982. When persistence pays off: Resolving the mystery of an unexplained electrolyte imbalance. *Nursing 82* 12:44–47.
A patient is admitted to hospital; her serum sodium level is 125 mEq/liter, potassium level 3 mEq/liter, and chloride level 85 mEq/liter. The article describes the course of this patient's illness and her therapy.

Sharer, J. E. June 1975. Reviewing acid-base balance. *American Journal of Nursing* 75:980–83.
An overview of acid-base balance is presented, including acid-base control systems (buffers, respiratory mechanism, and renal mechanism). Acid-base imbalances are explained with illustrations to clarify the content.

Twombly, M. June 1978. The shift into third space. *Nursing 78* 8:38–41.
This article describes when fluid shifts into the interstitial fluid compartment, a process called *third spacing*, the physiologic changes that occur during two phases, and the nursing intervention.

Selected References

Burke, S. R. 1980. *The composition and function of body fluids.* 3rd ed. St. Louis: C. V. Mosby Co.

Byrne, C. J.; Saxton, D. F.; Pelikan, P. K.; and Nugent, P. M. 1981. *Laboratory tests: Implications for nurses and allied health professionals.* Menlo Park, Calif.: Addison-Wesley Publishing Co.

Fenton, M. May 1969. What to do about thirst. *American Journal of Nursing* 69:1014–17.

Grant, M. M., and Kubo, W. M. August 1975. Assessing a patient's hydration status. *American Journal of Nursing* 75:1306–11.

Guyton, A. C. 1981. *Textbook of medical physiology.* 6th ed. Philadelphia: W. B. Saunders Co.

———. 1982. *Human physiology and mechanisms of disease.* 3rd ed. Philadelphia: W. B. Saunders Co.

Keithley, J. K., and Fraulini, K. E. March 1982. What's behind that I.V. line? *Nursing 82* 12:32–45.

Metheny, N. A. March 1975. Water and electrolyte balance in the postoperative patient. *Nursing Clinics of North America* 10:49–57.

Reed, G. M. March 1974. Confused about potassium? Here's a clear concise guide. *Nursing 74* 4:20–28.

Urrows, S. T. September 1980. Symposium on fluid, electrolyte, and acid-base balance: Physiology of body fluids. *Nursing Clinics of North America* 15:537–47.

Vaughan, V. C., III; McKay, R. J.; and Behrman, R. E. 1979. *Nelson textbook of pediatrics.* 11th ed. Philadelphia: W. B. Saunders Co.

Weldy, N. J. 1980. *Body fluids and electrolytes: A programmed presentation.* 3rd ed. St. Louis: C. V. Mosby Co.

Chapter 31

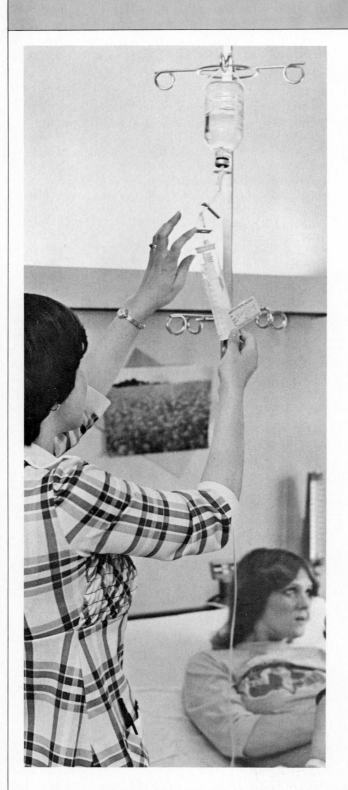

Fluid and Electrolytes: Part II

CONTENTS

Objectives

1. Understand essential facts about nursing diagnoses (common patient problems) related to fluid, electrolyte, and acid-base imbalances

1.1 Identify four types of fluid imbalances

1.2 Identify causes of water deficits and excesses

1.3 Compare effects of water deficits and excesses

1.4 Identify causes of extracellular fluid deficits and excesses

1.5 Compare effects of extracellular fluid deficits and excesses

1.6 Contrast clinical signs and laboratory findings of all types of fluid imbalances

1.7 Contrast medical therapies required for all types of fluid imbalances

1.8 Identify causes of specific electrolyte deficits and excesses

1.9 Identify clinical signs and laboratory findings of specific electrolyte imbalances

1.10 Identify medical therapies prescribed for specific electrolyte deficits and excesses

1.11 Identify four acid-base disturbances

1.12 Compare respiratory acidosis and alkalosis with metabolic acidosis and alkalosis

1.13 Compare clinical and laboratory findings of four acid-base disturbances

1.14 Give examples of nursing diagnoses related to fluid, electrolyte, and acid-base imbalances

2. Understand essential facts about intravenous fluid therapy, blood transfusions, and total parenteral nutrition

2.1 Identify objectives of IV therapy

2.2 Identify various IV solutions

2.3 Identify essential parts of IV infusion equipment

2.4 Identify common sites for venipuncture

2.5 Identify essential steps of venipuncture

2.6 Give reasons for selected steps in the venipuncture procedure

2.7 Identify four main human blood groups

2.8 Explain why various blood groups are incompatible

2.9 Explain when and why an Rh-positive fetus can present problems for an Rh-negative mother

2.10 Explain the differences in purpose and technique of TPN and IV therapy

2.11 Identify various solutions used in TPN

3. Understand facts about nursing interventions to maintain, promote, and restore fluid and electrolyte balance

3.1 Identify measures required to maintain IV therapy

3.2 Identify potential problems of IV therapy

3.3 Explain methods of calculating infusion flow rates

3.4 Identify factors influencing infusion flow rates

3.5 Identify essential steps in changing intravenous containers and tubing

3.6 Identify essential steps in discontinuing an IV infusion

3.7 Identify potential problems and risks of blood transfusions

3.8 Identify essential guidelines for assisting with blood transfusions

3.9 Identify essential nursing responsibilities associated with TPN

4. Apply the nursing process when providing care to selected patients with actual or potential fluid and electrolyte problems

4.1 Obtain necessary assessment data

4.2 Analyze and relate assessment data

4.3 Write relevant nursing diagnoses

4.4 Write relevant nursing goals

4.5 Plan appropriate nursing interventions

4.6 Implement appropriate nursing interventions

4.7 State outcome criteria essential for evaluating the patient's progress

5. Perform selected IV therapy techniques

5.1 Perform a venipuncture using a butterfly needle (in a laboratory setting only)

5.2 Set up an IV infusion

5.3 Change IV infusion containers

5.4 Change IV infusion tubing

5.5 Monitor and maintain an IV infusion

5.6 Discontinue an IV

5.7 Monitor and maintain a blood transfusion

5.8 Monitor and maintain TPN

Terms

acidosis (acidemia)
agglutination
agglutinins
agglutinogen
alkalosis (alkalemia)
anabolism
anasarca
anastomose
anuria
ascites
circulatory overload
colloids

dependent edema
dextrose
edema
emboli
erythroblastosis fetalis
hemolysis
hemosiderosis
hydrolysates
hyperalimentation
hypercalcemia
hyperkalemia
hypernatremia
hypervolemia
hypoalbuminemia
hypocalcemia
hypodermoclysis
hypofibrinogenemia
hypokalemia
hyponatremia
hypovolemia
infiltration
Intralipid
Kussmaul breathing
lactate
normal saline solution
oliguria
osmolarity (osmolality)
parenteral
phlebitis
pitting edema
Rh factor
tetany
thrombi
thrombocytopenia
total parenteral nutrition (TPN)
transfusion
universal donor
universal recipient
Valsalva maneuver

Fluid and electrolyte imbalances are produced by factors that affect the intake, output, or distribution of water and electrolytes. These imbalances may be the primary cause of illness but more commonly are the result of other physiologic disorders (e.g., cardiovascular or renal disorders). Thus, to understand fluid and electrolyte imbalance and to make an accurate assessment of the patient's problems, the nurse often needs to consider these disorders in the context of other pathologic conditions. Nurses are best able to assess existing and potential fluid and electrolyte needs when they have a complete picture of patients' health problems.

This chapter covers fluid imbalances, electrolyte imbalances, and acid-base imbalances. Each disturbance is discussed separately, but the student should be aware that imbalances are interrelated and rarely occur alone. Often, however, one imbalance requires immediate correction, and it is thus important to understand the general principles of each type of imbalance. From a nurse's standpoint, most electrolyte disturbances are diagnosed after laboratory examination of blood plasma rather than by observable signs and symptoms. These laboratory values apply to extracellular fluid rather than to intracellular fluid, which is not readily available for study.

Nursing Diagnoses

Fluid imbalances are categorized as:

1. Water deficit
2. Water excess
3. Extracellular fluid deficit (both sodium and water)
4. Extracellular fluid excess (both sodium and water)

Electrolyte imbalances are categorized as:

1. Sodium deficit or excess
2. Potassium deficit or excess
3. Calcium deficit or excess

Acid-base imbalances are categorized as:

1. Acidosis
2. Alkalosis

Any of these problems may be actual or potential.

Water Deficit (Dehydration)

Causes of dehydration

An isolated water deficit refers to a loss of water proportionately greater than the loss of solute. Isolated water deficits may occur because of insufficient water intake, excessive solute intake, profuse and prolonged sweating, and certain disorders creating large renal fluid losses (Harvey et al. 1980:53–54).

Insufficient intake Dehydration due to insufficient intake of water is confined to the very young, the very old, and persons too debilitated to satisfy their own water needs. Insufficient intake is especially likely during hot weather, when there are increased rates of loss through the skin. When the greatest fluid loss is through perspiration, the sweating person may also lose significant amounts of sodium, resulting in a coexisting sodium deficit.

Excess solute intake Excess solute intake is most commonly seen in ill, elderly patients who receive nasogastric tube feedings, which have high protein and sodium chloride contents (e.g., 120 g of protein and 10 g of salt). Such solute intakes result in obligatory excretion of urine in volumes between 1200 and 1500 ml per day (Harvey et al. 1980:54). Urine volumes may exceed 2000 to 2500 ml per day in elderly people, who often have significant impairments in renal concentrating ability. Thus, a greatly increased water intake (e.g., up to 3 or 4 liters per day) may be required to meet the demand created by a high solute intake.

Prolonged sweating Profuse, prolonged sweating can rapidly lead to fluid deficits (and moderate sodium deficits) if the sweating person does not drink sufficient fluids. Work in extremely hot environments, vigorous sports in hot weather, and prolonged exposure to sunlight may all produce profuse sweating and large water losses (e.g., up to 8 liters per day).

Disorders creating renal loss Normally, water deficits by renal loss are rare since antidiuretic hormone (ADH) acts promptly to decrease the rate of loss when any significant water deficit elevates the *osmolarity* (concentration of solutes in solution) of plasma. However, certain disorders of the hypothalamus, posterior pituitary gland, and kidney can lead to excessive fluid loss through the kidneys. These are:

1. Diabetes insipidus, a disorder of inadequate production of ADH by the hypothalamus or inadequate release of ADH by the posterior pituitary gland. Without sufficient ADH, the body excretes large quantities of dilute urine, resulting in a fluid deficit. Persons with diabetes insipidus may excrete more than 3000 ml of urine with a specific gravity less than 1.010 and a solute concentration (osmolarity) of less than 300 mOsm/kg. The healthy person excretes an average of 600 mOsm/kg of solutes daily, although this amount is determined largely by the quantity of solute intake.
2. Diseases that impair renal concentrating ability. For example, sickle cell anemia, *hypercalcemia* (excessive blood calcium levels), and *hypokalemia* (low blood potassium levels) are all characterized by pathology of the kidney that leads to impaired renal concentrating ability. These conditions result in only moderate increases in urine output because in these disorders the kidney is able to excrete urine that is at least isotonic to plasma. However, when dehydration occurs together with these diseases, the kidneys are ineffective in conserving water.
3. Nephrogenic diabetes insipidus, a hereditary kidney disorder associated with marked water loss via the kidney that is unresponsive to ADH.

The above discussion has centered on isolated water deficiency. In actual practice, however, health personnel often face mixed disturbances in which losses of both solute and water occur in varying proportions.

Many illnesses are characterized by excessive losses of gastrointestinal fluids. Fluid loss accompanies vomiting, diarrhea, fistulas, tube drainages, and bowel obstructions (in which fluids are not reabsorbed). With such losses, varying amounts of solutes are also lost. Urine and sweat losses also create deficits in electrolytes. For practical purposes, it is wise to assume that in other than mild dehydration, the body also loses sodium, chloride, and potassium.

Effects of dehydration

The effects of dehydration depend on the rate and volume of loss. Dehydration can be categorized as mild, moderate, severe, or very severe. See Table 31–1. Losses that exceed 20% of body weight are fatal. In young, elderly, or generally debilitated patients, the effects are more acute. A baby who takes in no water will, in 5 days, lose a volume of fluid equal to his or her extracellular fluid volume, whereas it takes an adult 10 days to lose the same proportion of fluid (MacBryde and Blacklow 1970:749). People who have a low proportion of water to body weight are also vulnerable to more rapid depletion.

Changes brought about by dehydration of the extracellular fluid compartment are: (a) reduced extracellular fluid (ECF) volume and (b) hypertonicity or a hyperosmolar fluid imbalance. These changes occur because with dehydration there is more solute in proportion to fluid. When the body is deprived of water, the extracellular fluid compartment, including interstitial fluid, is reduced. However, water passes into plasma immediately. The water gained passes by osmosis from the intracellular compartments through interstitial fluid to the plasma. This transfer of water tends to preserve the circulating blood plasma volume. If the kidneys are functioning normally, they will attempt to retain water and salt by reducing the excretion of sodium chloride and water to minimal amounts. As dehydration progresses, the concentrations of the sodium ion (Na^+) and the chloride ion (Cl^-) in plasma rise, thus increasing blood concentration (increased serum osmolality).

Patients go into shock when intravascular fluid compartments become greatly depleted. Shock indicates that the deficits are so great that the regulatory mechanisms of the body can no longer maintain the plasma volume. This blood volume reduction, called *hypovolemia*, is responsible for such manifestations as a rapid weak pulse, fall in blood pressure, and increased concentration of blood solutes. Since the kidneys rely on sufficient arterial blood pressure to produce urine, hypovolemia results in *oliguria* (decreased urine output). Oliguria progresses to *anuria* (absence of urine). As a consequence, metabolic wastes accumulate, the patient quickly becomes disoriented and comatose, and death ensues due to the effects of the acid waste products on the cells.

The electrolyte changes that accompany dehydration vary greatly. The nature of these changes depends on many factors, including:

Table 31–1 Severity of Fluid Deficit and Excess

Severity	Magnitude of deficit or excess (liters)	% of body water deficit or excess	Serum Na* (mEq/liter)	Serum osmolality* (mOsm/kg)
Fluid deficit				
Mild	1.5–2	3–4.5	149–151	294–298
Moderate	2–4	4.5–10	152–158	299–313
Severe	4–6	10–15	159–166	314–329
Very severe	>6	>15	>166	>330
Fluid excess				
Mild	1.5–4	3–8	139–132	275–261
Moderate	4–6	8–13	131–127	262–251
Severe	6–10	13–22	126–118	250–233
Very severe	>10	>22	<118	<233

*Normal serum Na is 144 mEq/liter and normal serum osmolality is 285 mOsm/kg.

From A. M. Harvey, R. J. Johns, V. A. McKusick, A. H. Owens, and R. S. Ross, *The principles and practice of medicine*, 20th ed. (New York: Appleton-Century-Crofts, 1980), pp. 53, 57.

1. Volume and composition of the fluid lost. In vomiting due to pyloric obstruction, large amounts of chloride may be lost, whereas in severe diarrhea, large amounts of sodium and potassium can be lost.
2. Renal function. The function of the kidneys may be impaired as a result of dehydration or other underlying disease, thus altering the plasma electrolyte concentrations.
3. Underlying disease processes and water and electrolyte intakes. For example, patients with diabetes mellitus lose large amounts of sodium, chloride, and water with the diuresis associated with the disease. In addition, large amounts of water may be lost by vaporization from the lungs due to hyperventilation associated with diabetes. Also, large amounts of potassium may be lost from the intracellular compartment. These losses are magnified when the intake is also reduced.
4. Proportionate loss of electrolytes as compared to the water loss. Fluids and electrolytes are not necessarily lost in the same proportions. Any one of the following may take place:

- **a.** Electrolyte loss exceeds proportionate fluid loss.
- **b.** Electrolyte loss is proportional to fluid loss.
- **c.** Electrolyte loss is proportionately less than fluid loss.

Clinical signs of dehydration

People who are dehydrated manifest certain signs and symptoms. The nurse should be able to assess the initial signs and symptoms of dehydration as well as symptoms indicating more advanced dehydration:

1. Low fluid intake, or disproportionately high fluid output
2. Complaints of thirst (early sign)
3. Dry skin, which may be flaky
4. Dry, sticky mucous membrane
5. Decreased urine output
6. Amber urine
7. Sudden weight loss
8. Lethargy and complaints of weakness
9. Loss of skin turgor
10. Sunken eyeballs; depressed fontanelles in children
11. Low blood pressure or postural hypotension (late sign)
12. Mental disorientation (late sign; may be manifested earlier in elderly patients)
13. Coma (late sign)

Laboratory findings of dehydration

1. A serum sodium level of 144 mEq/liter is normal. Higher levels indicate dehydration. In mild fluid deficits, the serum sodium level may be about 150 mEq/liter; in a very severe fluid deficit, the serum sodium may exceed 166 mgEq/liter.
2. Serum osmolality of 285 mOsm/kg is normal. In mild fluid deficits, the serum osmolality may rise to 295 mOsm/kg; in very severe fluid deficits, it may exceed 330 mOsm/kg (Harvey et al. 1980:53). See Table 31–1.

Medical therapy for dehydration

Therapy for water deficit is adequate water replacement by fluids administered orally, if possible, or intravenously. Intravenous solutions used to correct water deficits include:

1. A solution of 5% dextrose in distilled water for moderate deficits. The dextrose is metabolized to glycogen, making solute-free water available for replenishing the deficit.
2. A solution of 2.5% dextrose in distilled water, used when (a) the patient is diabetic and has difficulty metabolizing glucose or (b) when large volumes must be administered.

Water Excess (Overhydration)

Causes of overhydration

Water excess (overhydration or water intoxication) occurs when the body accumulates water in excess of solutes. The following may be causes of overhydration (Harvey et al. 1980:57).

Iatrogenic water administration Excessive fluid administered to patients with continued ADH secretions can lead to water intoxication. Patients are especially vulnerable to such overhydration following surgery or trauma (stress), following injections of morphine sulphate, and following anesthesia.

Kidney impairment Both acute renal failure with oliguria and chronic renal failure impair the kidneys' ability to excrete water excesses and result in the accumulation of fluid.

Congestive heart failure A fluid excess often occurs with severe congestive failure since there is decreased blood flow to the kidneys and decreased glomerular filtration, resulting in inadequate urine outputs.

Cirrhosis of the liver Cirrhosis leads to *ascites* (accumulation of serous fluid in the abdomen). Water retention accompanying this condition is extreme.

Effects of overhydration

Changes brought about by overhydration of the extracellular fluid (ECF) compartment are (a) expanded ECF volume and (b) hypotonicity or a hypo-osmolar imbalance, since there is insufficient solute in proportion to fluid. This hypotonic water excess quickly becomes an *intra*cellular water excess. Because extracellular osmotic pressure decreases, water moves into the cells to equalize the concentration gradient on both sides of the cell membrane. The cells, as a result, become swollen. Because brain cells are particularly sensitive to increases in intracellular fluid, changes in mental status can be a sign of water intoxication. See the clinical signs listed immediately following. Also see Table 31–1 for categories of fluid excess according to severity.

Clinical signs of overhydration

People who are overhydrated exhibit the following signs and symptoms:

1. Sudden weight gain
2. Decreased fluid output in comparison to intake
3. Headache (early sign)
4. Blurred vision
5. Drowsiness, weakness
6. Muscle cramps and twitches
7. Disorientation
8. Slight peripheral edema but no pitting edema (see page 801.
9. Stupor (late sign)
10. Coma (late sign)
11. Convulsions (late sign)

Laboratory findings of overhydration

1. A serum sodium level of 144 mEq/liter is normal. In mild water excesses, the serum sodium may fall to 132 mEq/liter. In very severe water excesses, the serum sodium level may fall to 118 mEq/liter or below.
2. Serum osmolality of 285 mOsm/kg is normal. In mild water excesses, the serum osmolality may fall to 261 mOsm/kg. In very severe water excesses, the serum osmolality may fall to less than 233 mOsm/kg. See Table 31–1.

Medical therapy for overhydration

Reduction in excess body water is achieved by:

1. Reduction in fluid intake to 500 ml per day. This process is difficult and slow and also requires alterations in diet. Because the average daily diet contains 700 ml of water, the diet must be altered to ensure that food contains no more than 200 ml of water. The patient may drink the remaining 300 ml of fluid.
2. Use of osmotic agents such as urea, mannitol, or hypertonic sodium solution (e.g., 3% sodium chloride solution). These agents accelerate water loss by stimulating the kidneys to excrete proportionately more water than sodium, restoring the osmolality of body fluids to normal. This therapy is given with caution to

cardiac patients who are susceptible to volume overloads.

Extracellular Fluid Deficit (ECF Depletion)

Causes of ECF depletion

Losses of sodium and water together are referred to as *isotonic volume deficits* or *extracellular fluid deficits* (ECF depletion). Extracellular deficits are characterized by acute sodium loss accompanied by water loss in isotonic proportions. ECF is lost primarily from the gastrointestinal tract or skin. Sources of loss include:

1. Diarrhea (most common cause)
2. Vomiting
3. Profuse sweating
4. Bowel obstruction or paralytic ileus
5. Draining fistulas
6. Ileostomy and cecostomy drainage
7. Extensive burns
8. Hemorrhage

Effects of ECF depletion

Changes brought about by extracellular fluid losses are (a) reduced ECF volume (hypovolemia) and (b) elevated hematocrit. Because of the isotonic loss of both water and sodium, serum sodium concentration and serum osmolality remain normal, i.e., isotonic. However, the hematocrit is elevated because the volume of ECF is reduced. In early stages, there is no shift of fluid from the intracellular fluid (ICF) spaces because the body osmolality remains the same. When the condition persists longer than several days, urea nitrogen and creatinine are also elevated, and the body draws water from intracellular fluids to restore the blood volume. Long-term extracellular fluid loss, then, results in depletion of intracellular fluid as well.

Clinical signs of ECF depletion

Persons who suffer ECF losses manifest signs and symptoms of hypovolemia:

1. Postural hypotension (early sign); significant if pressure of supine patient drops 10 mm Hg or more when patient assumes upright position
2. No complaints of thirst
3. Complaints of weakness, faintness, or dizziness on standing
4. Nausea and anorexia
5. Weight loss
6. Low blood pressure
7. Oliguria
8. Shock (late sign)

Laboratory findings of ECF depletion

1. Hematocrit increased over normal (42)
2. Normal serum sodium
3. Normal serum osmolality
4. Normal or increased serum urea nitrogen
5. Increased specific gravity of urine

Medical therapy for ECF depletion

Restoration of the ECF volume is achieved by:

1. Control of underlying cause; for example:
   a. Control of hemorrhage
   b. Control of vomiting by antiemetics
   c. Control of diarrhea by antidiarrheal drugs
2. Increased salt intake for patients who can tolerate oral foods and fluids
3. Intravenous administration of isotonic fluids, e.g., normal saline solution

Extracellular Fluid Excess (ECF Excess)

Causes of ECF excess

Retention of sodium and water in isotonic proportions is referred to as *isotonic volume excess, extracellular fluid excess* (ECF excess), or *circulatory overload*. Extracellular fluid excesses are most commonly associated with:

1. Cardiac failure
2. Cirrhosis of the liver
3. Kidney failure
4. Toxemia of pregnancy
5. Iatrogenic causes, such as cortisone therapy or rapid, intravenous administration of too much saline solution

Effects of ECF excess

Excesses of extracellular fluid lead to (a) *hypervolemia* (increased blood volume) and (b) *edema* (excess fluid in the interstitial compartment). Normally, the interstitial fluid compartment is not bogged with water but compact, elastic, and expandable, with just enough fluid to fill the crevices between tissues. This compact state facilitates diffusion of nutrients from the plasma to the intracellular fluid (ICF) and diffusion of metabolic wastes from the cells to the plasma. Edema increases the distance between the blood capillaries and the cells and thus hinders cell nutrition. See Figure 31–1.

Overloading of the vascular fluid compartment increases blood hydrostatic pressure, which forces fluid into the interstitial spaces. *Anasarca* (edema that is generalized throughout the body) is the result. Greatly increased hydrostatic pressure forces large amounts of fluid through the alveolar-capillary membrane into the alveoli of the lungs, causing pulmonary edema, a serious problem that can result in death by suffocation. Manifestations of pulmonary edema are frothy sputum, dyspnea, cough, and gurgling sounds on respiration. The most common cause of pulmonary edema is left-sided heart failure, with resulting increases in the pressure of the pulmonary blood capillaries and the interstitial spaces of the lung tissue.

The nurse needs to exercise caution when administering intravenous fluids to patients with cardiac problems because of the danger of overload of the lung capillaries. Caution is also necessary with infants and elderly persons. Infants, because of their small lungs and small extravascular reserves, cannot handle large amounts of fluid. Elderly people have inelastic blood vessels and tolerate only small increases in blood volume before the hydrostatic pressure is substantially increased.

Because there is no change in the tonicity of body fluids in ECF volume excess, fluid does not move into the ICF compartment. Thus, patients with ECF excess do not develop cerebral signs as do patients with isolated water excess. The serum sodium level and serum osmolality also remain normal. The hematocrit may be normal or decreased. In persistent ECF excesses associated with heart failure or cirrhosis, the patient's hematocrit is usually normal. In acute ECF excesses, however, the hematocrit decreases in proportion to the severity of the problem.

When fluid moves from the vascular compartment into the interstitial spaces, the blood volume drops. As a response, the body releases antidiuretic hormone (ADH) and aldosterone, which stimulate the kidneys to retain fluid and sodium. This response adds to the existing problem because the retained fluid can also move into the interstitial spaces, thus augmenting the edema. Therefore, generalized edema is a self-perpetuating condition.

Clinical signs of ECF excess

Persons who suffer ECF volume excesses manifest the following signs and symptoms:

1. Sudden weight gain. A person can accumulate up to 4.5 kg (10 lb) of fluid before its presence is apparent.
2. *Dependent edema* (edema of the lowest or most dependent parts of the body, where hydrostatic pressure is greatest). If a person is ambulatory, this edema may first be evident in the feet and ankles. If the person is confined to bed, the edema is more likely to occur in the sacral region.
3. *Pitting edema* (edema that leaves a small depression or pit after finger pressure is applied to the swollen area). The pit is caused by movement of fluid to adjacent tissue, away from the point of pressure. Within 10 to 30 seconds, the pit normally disappears. Pitting edema is never seen in patients with a pure water excess (Harvey et al. 1980:56). (In *nonpitting edema* the fluid in edematous tissues cannot be moved to adjacent spaces by finger pressure. Nonpitting edema is not a sign of ECF excess but often accompanies infections and traumas that cause fluid to collect and coagulate in tissue spaces. The coagulation prevents displacement of fluid to other areas by pressure.)

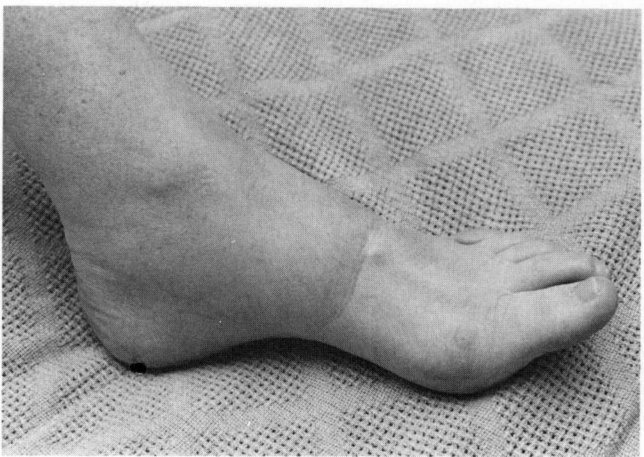

Figure 31–1 The movement of fluid, electrolytes, and nutrients to and from the tissues is impaired by edema, a result of an isotonic sodium and fluid excess.

4. Decreased fluid output in comparison to intake.
5. Increased central venous pressure.
6. Neck vein engorgement.
7. Signs of pulmonary edema. See above.

Laboratory findings of ECF excess

1. Normal or decreased hematocrit
2. Normal serum sodium level
3. Normal serum osmolality

Medical therapy for ECF excess

1. Control of underlying cause; for example, giving cardiotonic drugs (e.g., digitalis) for cardiac failure
2. Diuretics
3. Sodium and fluid restriction

Electrolyte Imbalances

Electrolyte imbalances are usually determined through laboratory assessment of electrolyte levels in blood plasma. Because blood plasma has a composition and concentration of electrolytes similar to those of interstitial fluid, plasma is used to measure the composition of extracellular fluids. The one difference is that plasma contains plasma proteins called *colloids*, which interstitial tissue fluid does not contain. At this time, scientists are unable to measure precisely the electrolyte concentrations of intracellular fluid.

Imbalances can be described as excesses or deficits in electrolytes. Electrolyte imbalances of sodium, potassium, and calcium will be described. The bicarbonate imbalances are discussed with acid-base imbalances.

Sodium deficit or excess

The sodium ion (Na^+), referred to in this section as sodium, plays a major role in the body's fluid balance and in therapy for fluid disturbances. The major source of sodium for most people is table salt (NaCl) used in cooking and added to foods as a condiment.

Sodium is the major cation (Na^+) of the extracellular fluids, that is, of blood plasma and interstitial fluid. The sodium ion moves rapidly between the plasma and the interstitial fluid. This movement is closely related to the movement of fluid between the two spaces. Under normal conditions, the body loses very little sodium; sodium excretion is regulated chiefly by the kidneys. When sodium levels fall, the pituitary gland stimulates the adrenal cortex to produce aldosterone, which acts on the kidney tubules to increase reabsorption of sodium.

Profuse sweating can cause sodium loss. Also, ill persons can lose abnormally large amounts of sodium through the gastrointestinal tract. The sodium content of pancreatic secretions and gastric mucus is especially high. Severe, prolonged diarrhea or a draining pancreatic fistula can result in abnormally high sodium loss, just as can gastric suction, which withdraws gastric mucus along with other gastric fluids.

Hypernatremia is an elevated level of sodium in the blood plasma. *Hyponatremia* is a lowered sodium level in the blood plasma. Hypernatremia occurs with dehydration, while hyponatremia occurs with overhydration.

Hyponatremia Two situations can precede a sodium deficit:

1. Sodium loss that exceeds corresponding water loss, such as in prolonged, excessive sweating or with the prolonged use of strong diuretics
2. Intake of water that exceeds corresponding intake of sodium, as by drinking excessive quantities of water

Clinical signs Nurses may observe some or all of the following signs in the hyponatremic patient:

1. Feelings of apprehension and impending doom
2. Abdominal cramps and diarrhea
3. Convulsions in extreme hyponatremia, which can cause death

Laboratory findings

1. Sodium level of plasma below 135 mEq/liter, as low as 20 mEq/liter
2. Specific gravity of urine below 1.010

Medical therapy Sodium chloride tablets are provided to patients whose excessive losses are caused by increased sweating, such as to persons working in high environmental temperatures. In other situations, the underlying cause, such as a draining fistula, is treated. Saline infusions may be necessary if the patient cannot ingest salt tablets.

Hypernatremia Hypernatremia can occur when:

1. Sodium intake greatly exceeds water intake, as when a person mistakenly ingests a large number of sodium chloride tablets.
2. Water loss exceeds sodium loss. For example, a patient may lose more water than sodium through a draining intestinal wound and as a result become hypernatremic. Nurses may also see hypernatremia about the 5th or 6th day after the onset of untreated diarrhea.

Clinical signs Nurses may observe some or all of the following signs in a hypernatremic patient:

1. Oliguria
2. Agitated behavior, which can lead to gross hyperactivity (mania) or convulsions
3. Firm, rubbery skin turgor
4. Dry, sticky mucous membrane
5. High body temperature

Laboratory findings

1. Sodium level of plasma above 145 mEq/liter
2. Specific gravity of urine above 1.030

Medical therapy Treatment has two main objectives: first, to treat the reason for the excess sodium, that is, the diarrhea or the draining wound; and second, to administer fluids. If the sodium excess is not too severe, oral administration of fluids may be all that is necessary, but if the excess is extreme, an intravenous infusion of, for example, water with 5% glucose is frequently given.

Depending on her or his condition, the patient may need a low-sodium diet. Often, not adding salt during cooking or at the table is sufficient. Patients on such diets need to buy unsalted foods, such as unsalted butter.

Potassium deficit or excess

Potassium (K^+) is the principal cation of the intracellular fluids. Potassium is significant in maintaining the body's fluid and electrolyte balance, particularly that of the intracellular fluid. Just as with sodium, the body normally balances the intake and output of potassium. The average adult's diet meets the daily need for potassium (about 2 to 4 g).

Potassium affects the functions of most of the body systems, such as the cardiovascular system, the gastrointestinal system, the neuromuscular system, and the respiratory system. Of particular importance is potassium's role in transmitting electrical impulses to muscles such as the heart, to lung tissues, and to intestinal tissues. Most of the body's potassium is found inside the cells. A small amount is found in the plasma and interstitial fluids.

Potassium is usually excreted by the kidneys. However, the kidneys do not regulate potassium excretion as effectively as sodium excretion. Therefore, an acute potassium deficiency can develop rapidly. Of the body's secretions, the gastrointestinal secretions are high in potassium.

As is true of the other electrolytes, potassium is continually moving in and out of the cells. This movement from the interstitial fluid, which has less potassium, to the intracellular fluid, which has a greater concentration, is influenced by the adrenal steroids, testosterone, pH changes, glycogen formation, and hyponatremia. If tissues are damaged, the body can lose potassium quickly. It has been estimated that about a third of all hospital patients show signs indicating a deficiency in potassium. People receiving diuretics are frequently deficient in potassium if their intake does not reach 30 to 45 mEq daily (Abbott Laboratories Ltd. 1970:19). *Hyperkalemia* is an excess of potassium, and *hypokalemia* is a deficit of potassium in the body.

Hypokalemia Potassium deficits are not uncommon. Potassium can be lost rapidly as a result of diarrhea, vomiting, some kidney diseases, diuretic therapy, and increased stress.

Clinical signs The following observations may indicate hypokalemia:

1. Muscle weakness, including weakened skeletal, intestinal, and respiratory muscles
2. Arrhythmias of the heart (variations in normal heart rhythm), which can be reflected in irregular pulse rhythms
3. Anorexia and abdominal distention

Laboratory findings

1. Potassium level of the blood plasma is repeatedly below 3.6 mEq/liter.
2. Electrocardiogram may show flattening of the T waves and depression of the S-T segment. (See the normal cardiogram shown in Figure 38–3.)

Medical therapy The therapy frequently prescribed is the administration of potassium by intravenous infusion or in some cases by mouth. Potassium must be administered slowly to elderly patients to avoid the risk of cardiac arrest.

Hyperkalemia An excess of potassium is usually a result of leakage of potassium out of the cells. It can also occur as a result of renal failure or administration of excessive potassium by intravenous infusion.

Clinical signs The following signs may indicate hyperkalemia:

1. Intestinal colic
2. Oliguria, which may progress to anuria
3. Diarrhea
4. Heart muscle weakness, which may be reflected by an irregular pulse

Laboratory findings

1. Potassium of the blood plasma is repeatedly above 5.0 mEq/liter.
2. Electrocardiogram first shows high T waves and depressed S-T segments and in later stages no T waves and heart block.

Medical therapy The major objective in hyperkalemia therapy is to reduce the level of the serum potassium. Reduced serum potassium levels can usually be brought about by:

1. Increasing the output of potassium by the kidneys. It may be necessary only to increase fluid intake. Sometimes peritoneal dialysis is needed.
2. Reducing the intake of potassium by eliminating all foods or intravenous infusions that contain potassium.

Calcium deficit or excess

More than 90% of the body calcium is contained in bones. If the serum calcium level falls below normal (normal range is 4.3 to 5.3 mEq/liter), the body withdraws calcium from the bones to make up the deficit in the blood serum. *Hypocalcemia* is a calcium deficit, and *hypercalcemia* is an excess of calcium.

Hypocalcemia Two common causes of hypocalcemia are removal of the parathyroid glands and excessive loss of intestinal secretions, which contain a great deal of calcium.

Clinical signs The following signs may indicate hypocalcemia:

1. Complaints of muscle cramps
2. Complaints of tingling in the fingers
3. *Tetany* (muscle spasms, sharp flexion of the wrists and ankles, cramps), which may lead to convulsions

Laboratory findings

1. Plasma calcium is below 4.3 mEq/liter.
2. Electrocardiogram shows a prolonged Q-T interval.

Medical therapy The therapy includes the provision of calcium orally, intramuscularly, or intravenously. Calcium is seldom administered intravenously because of the reservoir of calcium in bone and because an intravenous infusion does not prevent the decalcification of bone.

Hypercalcemia The major reason for hypercalcemia is overactivity of the parathyroid glands. It may also be seen in malignant disease of the bone and in hyperthyroidism.

Clinical signs Hypercalcemia tends to affect nearly all the systems of the body. Some signs are:

1. Relaxed muscles
2. Pain in the flank as a result of kidney stones
3. Deep pain in the thighs due to the honeycombing of the bones
4. Pathologic fractures of bones
5. Nausea, vomiting, and eventually stupor and coma due to cardiac arrest from calcium crisis

Laboratory findings

1. Serum calcium level is above 5.3 mEq/liter.
2. Electrocardiogram reflects neuromuscular changes.

Medical therapy The therapy not only treats the reason for the excess calcium but also reduces the intake of calcium. Persons who consume large amounts of milk may experience some symptoms of hypercalcemia, which readily disappear when they reduce the milk intake. Patients who have hyperfunctioning parathyroid glands because of a tumor or enlarged glands generally undergo surgery.

Figure 31–2 The pH of body fluids is maintained at a slightly alkaline state between the precise range of 7.35 and 7.45.

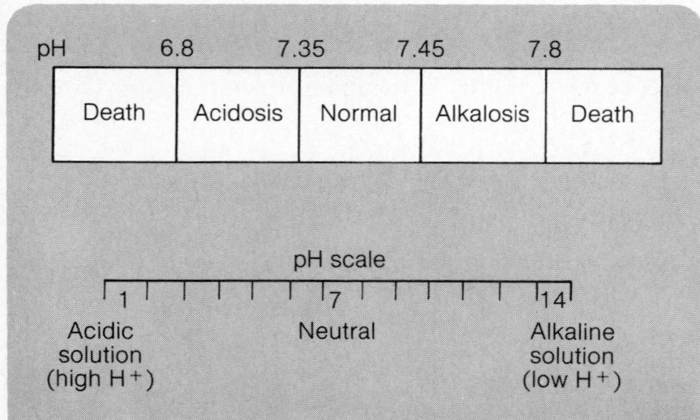

Acid-Base Imbalances

Body fluids are maintained within a precise pH range of 7.35 and 7.45 (a slightly alkaline state, since neutrality is 7.0). The pH reflects the hydrogen ion concentration of body fluids. Normally, the ratio of carbonic acid to bicarbonate is 1 to 20.

Normal metabolic processes continually introduce acids into the body fluids. For instance, carbonic acid (H_2CO_3) is formed from water (H_2O) and carbon dioxide (CO_2), a chief end product of metabolism. Carbonic acid is sometimes considered a respiratory acid, since the lungs excrete it as carbon dioxide and water. Other acids produced as waste products of metabolism are sulfuric, phosphoric, and lactic acids, all of which enter the bloodstream. The liver converts some of these acids to other acids (e.g., lactic becomes pyruvic acid) before the kidneys excrete them.

Imbalances in the pH of body fluid result in either acidosis or alkalosis. These are further subdivided into respiratory or metabolic imbalances. Thus, the four acid-base disturbances are (a) respiratory acidosis, (b) metabolic acidosis, (c) respiratory alkalosis, and (d) metabolic alkalosis.

The respiratory imbalances are brought about by changes in the blood carbonic acid, which is regulated by the lungs, whereas the metabolic imbalances are brought about by changes in the blood bicarbonate, which is regulated by the kidneys. Both respiratory and metabolic acidosis are more frequently encountered clinically than alkalotic conditions. Death can occur when the pH falls below 6.8 or rises above 7.8. See Figure 31–2.

The clinical signs of acid-base imbalance are not as specific as the laboratory signs. Major clinical signs include changes in respirations and in mental alertness.

The nurse needs to be alert to such signs as hypoventilation or hyperventilation and to signs of disorientation that progress to stupor and coma. These changes can occur rapidly or take several days.

The laboratory signs include the pH of plasma, the pH of urine, the $Paco_2$ level of plasma, which reflects the blood carbonic acid level, the bicarbonate level of plasma, and the base excess. The Pao_2 level of plasma is often taken in addition for patients with pulmonary problems. See Table 31–2 for laboratory indications of acid-base imbalances.

Acidosis

Acidosis, also referred to as *acidemia*, is a blood pH below 7.35.

Respiratory acidosis (carbonic acid excess) Respiratory acidosis occurs when exhalation of carbonic dioxide is inhibited, creating a carbonic acid excess in the body. Hypoventilation is its general cause. Two major conditions that cause hypoventilation are central nervous system depression and obstructive lung disease. Morphine poisoning or anesthesia are examples of central nervous system depression, whereas asthma and emphysema are obstructive lung diseases. Hypoventilation, whatever its cause, makes the body retain carbon dioxide and therefore carbonic acid. Thus, acidosis ensues.

Clinical signs Nursing observations that may indicate respiratory acidosis are:

1. Hypoventilation evidenced by shallow respirations, poor exhalation, or respiratory embarrassment
2. Loss of mental alertness and disorientation progressing to stupor, indicating central nervous system depression

Laboratory findings

1. Low plasma pH (below 7.35) or a normal pH if compensated (compensation discussed subsequently)
2. Low urine pH (below 6)
3. High $Paco_2$ (above 45 mm Hg)
4. Normal or high plasma bicarbonate (HCO_3^-)
  a. Above 28 mEq/liter in adults
  b. Above 25 mEq/liter in children
5. Base excess is 0 or positive (for example, +6) with chronic conditions that are compensated

Metabolic acidosis (base bicarbonate deficit) Metabolic acidosis occurs when levels of base bicarbonate are low in relation to carbonic acid blood levels. The kidneys normally retain bicarbonate (HCO_3^-) or excrete hydrogen ions (H^+) in response to altered blood pH. Starvation, renal impairment, and diabetes mellitus are among the conditions that deluge the plasma with acid metabolites. Prolonged diarrhea can decrease bicarbonate.

Table 31–2 Laboratory Indications of Acid-Base Imbalance

Sign	Normal	Interpretation
Plasma pH	7.35–7.45	Less than 7.35 → acidosis More than 7.45 → alkalosis
Urine pH	4.6–8.0	Below 6 → acidosis Above 7 → alkalosis
$Paco_2$	35–45 mm Hg	Less than 35 → respiratory alkalosis More than 45 → respiratory acidosis
Bicarbonate (HCO_3^-)	21–28 mEq/liter (about 25 mEq/liter)	Less than 21 → metabolic acidosis More than 28 → metabolic alkalosis
Base excess (BE)	Male: −3.3 to +1.2 Female: −2.4 to +2.3	Positive results → alkaline excess Negative results → alkaline deficit These values do not always indicate a state of acidosis or alkalosis but show deficits or excesses of base.
Pao_2	80 to 100 mm Hg	May be greater than 100 mm Hg if patient is on oxygen and less than 75 if there is a pulmonary problem.

Clinical signs Nursing observations that may indicate metabolic acidosis are:

1. *Kussmaul breathing* (deep rapid breathing), a compensatory mechanism, but is absent in infants
2. Weakness
3. Disorientation
4. Coma

Laboratory findings

1. Low plasma pH (below 7.35) or a normal pH if compensated
2. Low urine pH (below 6)
3. Normal $Paco_2$ or low if compensated (an attempt by the lungs to blow off more acid)
4. Low plasma bicarbonate
   a. Below 21 mEq/liter in adults
   b. Below 20 mEq/liter in children
5. Base excess with negative results (for example, –6)
6. Hyperkalemia usually associated with metabolic acidosis

Alkalosis

Alkalosis, also referred to as *alkalemia,* is a blood pH above 7.45.

Respiratory alkalosis (carbonic acid deficit) Respiratory alkalosis occurs when exhalation of carbonic dioxide is excessive, resulting in a carbonic acid deficit. Its cause is, broadly, hyperventilation, which can be due to fever, anxiety, or pulmonary infections. Hyperventilation blows off abundant carbon dioxide, resulting in lowered carbonic acid blood levels.

Clinical signs Nursing observations that may indicate respiratory alkalosis are:

1. Hyperventilation (deep and/or rapid breathing)
2. Unconsciousness

Laboratory findings

1. High plasma pH (above 7.45)
2. High urine pH (above 7)
3. Low plasma bicarbonate as a compensatory measure (body compensation depends upon the kidneys and is often slow.)
   a. Below 21 mEq/liter in adults
   b. Below 20 mEq/liter in children
4. Low $Paco_2$ (below 35 mm Hg)
5. Base excess: 0

Metabolic alkalosis (bicarbonate excess) Metabolic alkalosis occurs when the level of base bicarbonate is high. Metabolic alkalosis may be due to excess intake of baking soda and other alkalis, prolonged vomiting, and other conditions that flood plasma with the bicarbonate anion. Prolonged vomiting causes the body to lose chloride (Cl^-) and hydrogen (H^+) ions. Loss of chloride ions causes an increase of bicarbonate in the blood.

Clinical signs Nursing observations that may indicate metabolic acidosis are:

1. Depressed respiration (compensatory)
2. Hypertonic muscles
3. Tetany
4. Mental dullness

Laboratory findings

1. High plasma pH (above 7.45)
2. High urine pH (above 7)
3. High plasma bicarbonate
   a. Above 28 mEq/liter in adults
   b. Above 25 mEq/liter in children
4. Normal or high $Paco_2$ (above 45 mm Hg)—compensatory elevation
5. Base excess—positive results indicating an excess (for example, +8)
6. Low K^+

Compensation

In all acid-base imbalances, there is a corrective body response by both the kidneys and the lungs. Any given acid-base imbalance can be described as compensated until body reserves are used up. Then the condition is described as uncompensated.

In compensated acidosis or alkalosis, the kidneys and lungs are able to restore the altered ratio of one carbonic acid molecule to 20 bicarbonate molecules, thereby maintaining a normal pH. In respiratory acidosis, the plasma pH is maintained at normal even though there is an increase in the $Paco_2$ (carbonic acid) because the kidneys retain bicarbonate.

When the plasma pH is not maintained, the condition is uncompensated. In uncompensated respiratory acidosis, there is an increase in the $Paco_2$ (carbonic acid), the pH is lower (more acid) than normal, and the kidneys can no longer retain enough bicarbonate. See Table 31-3 for an overview of fluid and electrolyte data.

Table 31–3 Summary Data Regarding Fluid and Electrolytes

Clinical factor	Body normal	Predisposing conditions	Deficit symptoms	Excess symptoms	Food source
Extracellular fluid	Infant: 29% of body weight Adult: 15% of body weight	*Deficit:* Insufficient fluid intake, vomiting, diarrhea *Excess:* Excessive administration or intake of fluid with NaCl	Weight loss, dry skin and mucous membrane, thirst, oliguria, low blood pressure, plasma pH above 7.45, urine pH above 7.0	Weight gain, edema, puffy eyelids, high blood pressure	Meats, fruits, vegetables, liquids
Bicarbonate (HCO_3^-)	Plasma bicarbonates 21–29 mEq/liter, urine pH 4.6–8.0, plasma pH 7.35–7.45 (arterial blood)	*Deficit:* Uncontrolled diabetes mellitus, starvation, severe infectious disease, renal insufficiency *Excess:* Loss of Cl^- and H^+ through vomiting, gastric suction, hyperadrenalism, prolonged insertion of alkali	Metabolic acidosis, disorientation, weakness, shortness of breath, sweet fruity odor to breath, plasma pH below 7.35, HCO_3^- below 25 mEq/liter	Metabolic alkalosis, slow and shallow respirations, tetany, hypertonic muscles, plasma pH above 7.45, HCO_3^- above 30 mEq/liter	
Carbonic acid (H_2CO_3)	Pa_{CO_2} 35–45 mm Hg, plasma pH 7.35–7.45 (arterial blood)	*Deficit:* Oxygen lack, fever, anxiety, pulmonary infections, hyperventilation *Excess:* Hypoventilation, chronic asthma, emphysema, barbiturate poisoning	Respiratory alkalosis, deep and rapid breathing, unconsciousness, plasma pH above 7.45, low Pa_{CO_2}	Respiratory acidosis, disorientation, shallow respirations, plasma pH below 7.35, high Pa_{CO_2}	
Sodium (Na^+)	135–145 mEq/liter (plasma)	*Deficit:* Excessive perspiration, gastrointestinal suction, diarrhea *Excess:* Inadequate water intake	Apprehension, abdominal cramps, rapid and weak pulse, oliguria, plasma sodium below 135 mEq/liter	Dry and sticky mucous membranes, fever, thirst, firm rubbery tissue turgor, plasma sodium above 145 mEq/liter	Table salt (NaCl), cheese, butter and margarine, processed meat (ham, bacon, pork), canned vegetables, vegetable juice
Potassium (K^+)	3.6–5.0 mEq/liter (plasma)	*Deficit:* Diarrhea, vomiting, some kidney disease, diuretic therapy, increased stress *Excess:* Renal failure, burns, excessive administration	Muscle weakness, abnormal heart rhythm, anorexia, abdominal distention	Oliguria, intestinal colic, irritability, irregular pulse, diarrhea	Nuts, fruits, vegetables, poultry, fish

(Continued on next page)

Table 31–3 continued

Clinical factor	Body normal	Predisposing conditions	Deficit symptoms	Excess symptoms	Food source
Calcium (Ca^{2+})	4.3–5.3 mEq/liter (plasma)	*Deficit:* Removal of parathyroid glands, excessive loss of intestinal fluids, massive infections *Excess:* Overactive parathyroid gland, excessive ingestion of milk	Muscle cramps, tingling in the fingers, tetany, convulsions	Relaxed muscles, flank pain, kidney stones, deep bone pain	Dairy products, meat, fish, poultry, whole grain cereals, greens, beans
Chloride (Cl^-)	98–108 mEq/L	*Deficit:* Increased HCO_3^-, loss through vomiting, excessive ECF loss through intestinal fistula *Excess:* Increased Na^+, excessive fluid loss through kidneys, severe dehydration	*See* sodium	*See* sodium	Table salt, dairy products, meat

Clinical situations

When interpreting laboratory results, the nurse can find a systematic method helpful. To determine whether the patient has acidosis or alkalosis, the nurse looks first at the plasma pH. If it is high or low, the interpretation is straightforward. However, if the pH of the plasma is normal, the patient may still have a compensated acid-base imbalance. The nurse then needs to note the Pa_{CO_2}. Pa_{CO_2} values above or below normal indicate, respectively, a respiratory acidosis or alkalosis. If the Pa_{CO_2} is normal, the nurse needs to look at the plasma bicarbonate level. An elevation of this value indicates a metabolic alkalosis, whereas a deficit indicates a metabolic acidosis. The nurse also needs to be aware that chronic disease conditions are usually compensated. Therefore the Pa_{CO_2} and bicarbonate values may be altered accordingly. Examples follow:

Problem 1. Respiratory acidosis

Acute

pH = 7.25	(low)
Pa_{CO_2} = 60 mm Hg	(high)
HCO_3^- = 25 mEq/liter	(normal)
Base excess (BE) = 0	(normal)
Pa_{O_2} = 60 mm Hg	(low)

Chronic (compensated)

pH = 7.36	(normal)
Pa_{CO_2} = 70 mm Hg	(high)
HCO_3^- = 32 mEq/liter	(high)
BE = + 7	(excess)
Pa_{O_2} = 80 mm Hg	(normal)

Problem 2. Metabolic acidosis

Acute

pH = 7.30	(low)
$Paco_2$ = 40 mm Hg	(normal)
HCO_3^- = 19 mEq/liter	(low)
BE = −6	(deficit)
Pao_2 = 75 mm Hg	(low)

Chronic (compensated)

pH = 7.38	(normal)
$Paco_2$ = 31 mm Hg	(low)
HCO_3^- = 18 mEq/liter	(low)
BE = −6	(deficit)
Pao_2 = 80 mm Hg	(normal)

Problem 3. Respiratory alkalosis

Acute

pH = 7.52	(high)
$Paco_2$ = 31 mm Hg	(low)
HCO_3^- = 25 mEq/liter	(normal)
BE = 0	(normal)

Problem 4. Metabolic alkalosis

Acute

pH = 7.50	(high)
$Paco_2$ = 40 mm Hg	(normal)
HCO_3^- = 31 mEq/liter	(high)
BE = + 8	(excess)

Examples of Nursing Diagnoses

Some examples of nursing diagnoses for patients with fluid, electrolyte, and acid-base imbalances are:

1. Fluid deficit related to:
  a. Reduced intake
  b. Excess solute intake
  c. Prolonged sweating
  d. Excessive urination
  e. Diarrhea
  f. Vomiting
2. Fluid excess related to:
  a. Excessive fluid administration after surgery
  b. Kidney impairment
  c. Congestive heart failure
  d. Liver impairment
  e. Toxemia of pregnancy
3. Sodium deficit related to:
  a. Prolonged, excessive sweating
  b. Inadequate intake
4. Sodium excess related to diarrhea
5. Potassium deficit related to:
  a. Diarrhea
  b. Diuretic therapy
6. Potassium excess related to renal failure
7. Calcium deficit related to removal of parathyroid glands
8. Calcium excess related to hyperparathyroidism
9. Acidosis related to:
  a. Obstructive lung disease
  b. Renal impairment
  c. Diabetes mellitus
10. Alkalosis related to:
  a. Pulmonary infection and hyperventilation
  b. Prolonged vomiting

Intravenous Therapy

Fluid therapy can be administered by the normal oral route, by nasogastric tube, or by the *parenteral routes* (not through the alimentary canal) of intravenous infusion or subcutaneous infusion (*hypodermoclysis*). Oral fluid therapy was discussed in Chapter 30 and nasogastric feedings in Chapter 26. This chapter discusses the intravenous route.

Intravenous (IV) fluid therapy is a common practice in hospitals today. It is an efficient and effective method of supplying fluids directly into the extracellular fluid compartment, specifically the venous system. Hypodermoclysis is not as commonly used, but it is useful in the very young or elderly person whose veins are too small or difficult to enter. Parenteral fluid therapy is ordered by the physician. The nurse is responsible for administering and maintaining the therapy.

Objectives of Intravenous Therapy

1. To supply fluids when patients are unable to take adequate fluids by mouth. Therapy must provide for average daily needs and compensate for excessive losses. IV fluids are commonly available in 250, 500, and 1000 ml bottles or bags.

2. To provide salts needed to maintain electrolyte balance. Common solutions used are isotonic normal saline (0.9% NaCl) or multiple electrolyte solutions discussed subsequently. Sometimes electrolytes are added to normal saline solutions; for example, 20 mEq KCl.

3. To provide glucose (dextrose), the main fuel for metabolism. Although many nutrient solutions are available, 5% glucose solutions, commonly referred to as D-5-W (dextrose, 5% in water), are the most frequently used. Solution containing glucose and saline (⅔–⅓) may be used. A ⅔–⅓ solution consists of 3.3% glucose and 0.3% sodium chloride. Each liter of 5% dextrose solution provides about 200 calories. Patients require sufficient carbohydrate (a minimum of 450 calories per day) to prevent catabolism of body fats for energy, a condition that can result in metabolic acidosis.

4. To provide some water-soluble vitamins, such as vitamins B and C, or other drugs intravenously. Berocca-C and Vi-Cert are two vitamin preparations meant to be given intravenously. Several medications can be administered intravenously when rapid action is wanted or when the drugs are irritating to subcutaneous or intramuscular tissues. Intravenous administration of antibiotics is common.

Determining Volumes

Volumes of fluid required are determined by considering the following:

1. Daily maintenance requirements
2. Losses prior to therapy
3. Concurrent losses, such as losses from gastric suction, vomiting, or diarrhea during therapy

Adults usually need from 2500 ml of fluid per day (moderate dehydration) to 3000 ml per day (severe dehydration). The amounts required by children vary with size and metabolic requirements as well as with their specific losses.

Types of Solutions

IV solutions serve different functions. In most therapy situations, solutions of normal saline, glucose, or glucose in normal saline are used. Some special purpose solutions follow.

Nutrient solutions

The patient resting in bed has a daily caloric requirement of about 450 calories. Intravenous nutrient solutions supply these calories in the form of carbohydrate, nitrogen (as amino acids), and vitamins, all of which are essential to metabolism. Some commercial preparations contain ethyl alcohol to supply additional calories.

With the advent of hyperalimentation, lipids (fats) are available in some solutions. See the section on total parenteral nutrition later in this chapter. The caloric content of nutrient solutions varies from approximately 200 to 1500 calories per liter. Nutrient solutions may contain the following:

1. Carbohydrate and water
  a. Dextrose (glucose)
  b. Levulose (fructose)
  c. Invert sugar (half dextrose and half levulose)
  d. Ethyl alcohol
2. Amino acids, for example, Amigen, Aminosol, Travamin
3. Lipids, for example, Lipomul, Lyposyn

Electrolyte solutions

Electrolyte solutions are either saline solutions or multiple electrolyte solutions. Saline solutions are available in isotonic, hypotonic, and hypertonic concentrations. The isotonic concentration, called *normal saline*, is most frequently used. Many multiple electrolyte solutions are available, all with varying amounts of cations and anions. Some of these solutions are:

1. Ringer's solution containing Na^+, K^+, Cl^-, Ca^{2+}
2. Lactated Ringer's solution containing Na^+, K^+, Cl^-, Ca^{2+}, HCO_3^-
3. Butler's solution containing Na^+, K^+, Mg^{2+}, Cl^-, HCO_3^-

Normal saline solutions are used frequently as initial hydrating solutions. Multiple electrolyte solutions are either balanced (maintenance) solutions that approximate the ionic profile of plasma or special solutions that restore or correct imbalances. Ringer's solutions are balanced; Butler's solution is corrective.

Alkalinizing and acidifying solutions

Alkalinizing solutions correct acidosis; for example, acidosis resulting from cardiac arrest or diabetic coma. Examples of alkalinizing solutions are sodium lactate and sodium bicarbonate solutions. *Lactate* is a salt of a weak acid and can pick up hydrogen ions (H^+) in solution, thus reducing acidity. The hydrogen ions are derived from carbonic acid (H_2CO_3), which ionizes to HCO_3^- (bicarbonate) and H^+. The effectiveness of lactate depends on liver function.

Acidifying solutions correct alkalosis. An acidifying solution is ammonium chloride.

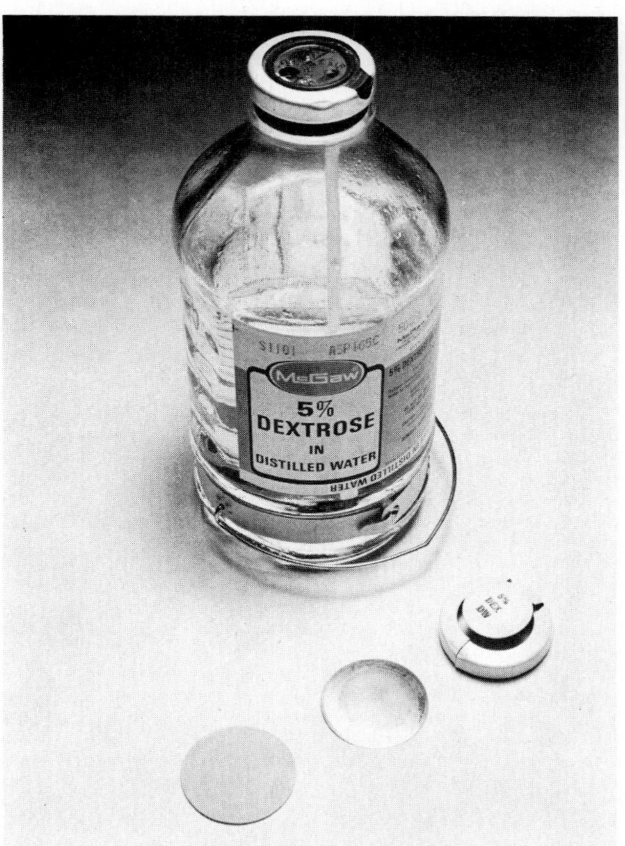

Figure 31–3 Intravenous bottles with sterile solutions are vacuum sealed. The tops are fitted with solid rubber stoppers. Bottles with indwelling vents are covered with a metal disk and rubber disk, then sealed with a metal cap.

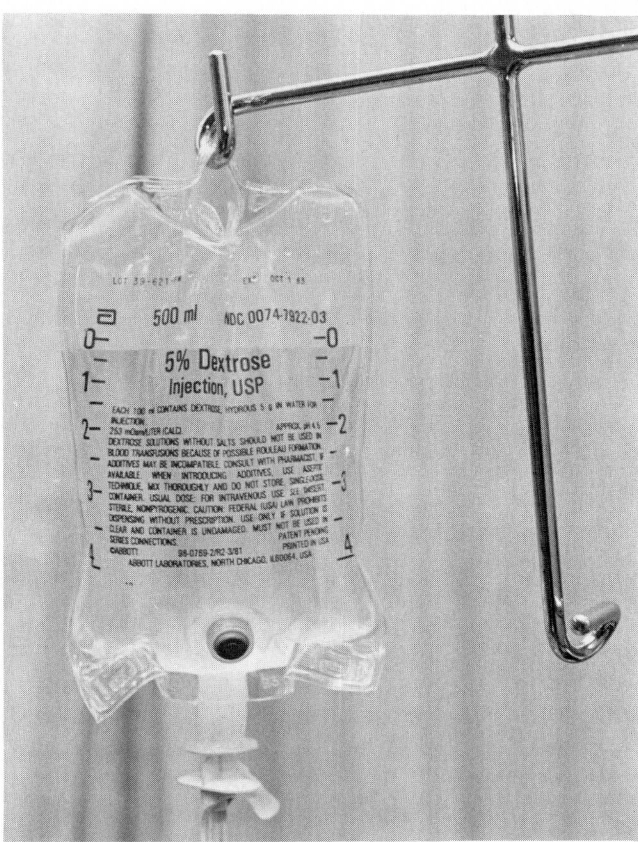

Figure 31–4 An intravenous solution bag.

Blood volume expanders

Blood volume expanders increase the volume of the vascular compartment after loss of blood or plasma. When whole blood is not available, the administration of plasma to severely hemorrhaging patients maintains the blood volume. In patients with severe burns, large amounts of fluid shift from the intravascular compartment to the burn site. Plasma is the preferred fluid to administer to burn victims. Other blood volume expanders are human serum albumin and dextran, which comes in various concentrations. Both of these have osmotic properties that directly increase the fluid volume of blood.

Intravenous Infusion Equipment

Commerical intravenous infusion sets vary. However, all of them work much alike. The solutions and equipment are sterile and ready for use. Many solutions are marketed, each labeled with the specific contents.

Intravenous solution containers

Intravenous solutions are supplied in glass bottles and plastic bags. See Figures 31–3 and 31–4.

Solution bottles are vacuum sealed with nonpyrogenic solutions. The tops of glass bottles are fitted with solid rubber stoppers and sealed with metal caps. Covering the rubber stopper is a metal disc that lies between the stopper and the metal cap. A marked circular area can be seen on the rubber stopper once it is exposed. The intravenous tubing is attached through this circular area. It is important to note that some types have two openings in the stopper, one to attach the tubing and the other to act as an air vent. The air vent is evident because a long tube extends from it to the bottom of the bottle. This latter type of bottle also has a rubber seal directly over the stopper. Before beginning the infusion, the nurse must remove the seal to open the air vent. As the solution runs out of the container, it is replaced with air.

Intravenous tubing

Intravenous tubing has an insertion spike at one end, a drip chamber, a clamp to regulate flow, and a connector at the end of the tubing, which is attached to the intravenous needle. See Figure 31-5. The sterility of each end of the tubing is maintained by protective plastic coverings. Insertion spikes may or may not need air vents, depending on whether the solution bottle is vented. The sizes of the openings into the drip chamber vary. The common sizes deliver 10, 15, or 20 drops per milliliter of solution. Each IV administration set has this information on the package.

In-line devices and secondary sets

Special volume control in-line devices are sometimes attached below the insertion spike. These are commonly referred to as *Volutrols* or *Pediatrols (Buretrols)*. They are designed to deliver minute quantities of fluid (60 drops per ml). They are particularly useful for administering precise volumes of fluid to infants and children and for administering medications in the intravenous solution. See Figure 31-6.

Figure 31-5 An intravenous administration set consists of an insertion spike, a drip chamber, plastic tubing with a control clamp, and a protective cap over the needle adaptor. Sets that have an air vent are used with nonvented bottles.

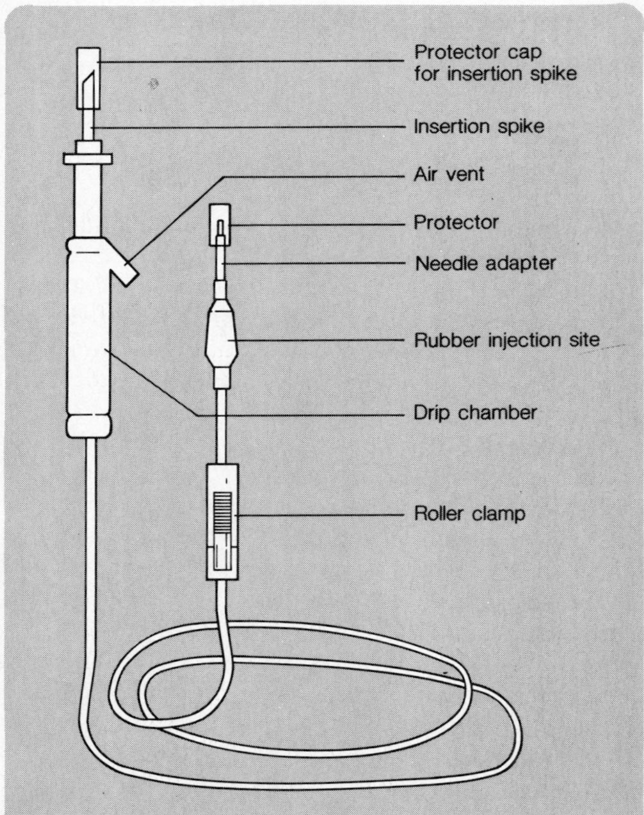

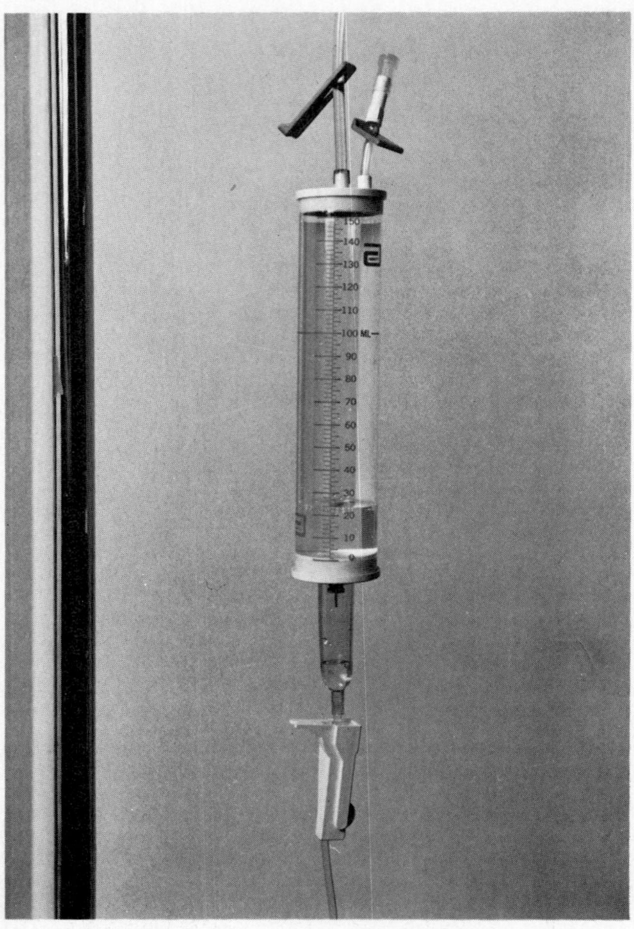

Figure 31-6 A volume control set above the drip chamber of an intravenous infusion.

Secondary sets and containers are used to administer two or more solutions at the same time or intermittently. These sets are attached in various ways (e.g., tandem or piggyback alignments). For information about the techniques for administering IV medications, see Kozier and Erb (1982:1109-23).

Intravenous needles and catheters

Needles for intravenous injections are usually packaged separately. Some are made of steel; others are plastic. The needle commonly used for intravenous infusions is a 21 gauge short bevel.

The age of the patient and the type of infusion determine the size of the needle. Blood transfusions require larger needles because of the thickness of the blood; also, larger veins receive the transfusion. Routine, short-term infusions require smaller butterfly or wing-tipped needles, which are put into smaller veins. Long-term therapy may require a catheter, a plastic tube that is inserted into a large vein. Some catheters fit over a needle during insertion, while others fit inside the needle. See Figure 31-7.

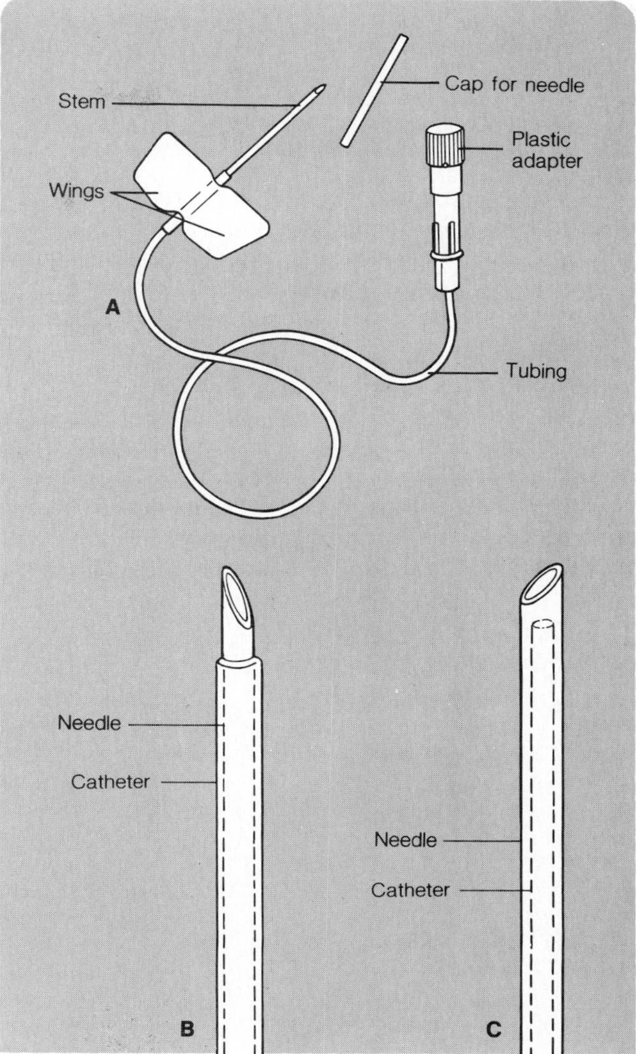

Figure 31-7 Intravenous needles and catheters: **A,** An intravenous butterfly needle; **B,** An over-the-needle catheter—after insertion in the vein, the needle is removed and the plastic catheter remains in place; **C,** An inside-the-needle catheter (intracatheter)—the plastic catheter is threaded through the needle after the venipuncture.

Venipuncture Sites

The type of infusion, duration of infusion, and age of the patient determine the location of the site.

Adults

The most convenient veins for venipuncture in the adult are the basilic and median cubital veins in the crease of the elbow (antecubital space). See Figure 31-8. Since these veins are large and superficial, they are frequently used by laboratory technicians to withdraw blood for examination. Unfortunately, use of these veins for prolonged infusions limits arm mobility because splints are needed to stabilize the elbow joint. Thus, for prolonged therapy other veins on the back of the hand and on the forearm are preferred. The metacarpal, basilic, and cephalic veins are commonly used. These sites are equipped with the natural splints of the ulna and radius and allow the patient more arm movement for activities such as eating. In right-handed patients, sites on the left arm allow more independence, and vice versa.

Ideally, for long-term therapy, sites at the distal end of the arm should be used first. If these veins have been used for prolonged periods or if veins are thrombosed (bruised), more proximal sites may be used. If arm veins are inaccessible, veins in the feet and legs may also be used.

Infants

Because infants do not have large veins in the antecubital fossa, blood specimens for examination are usually taken from the external jugular vein and femoral veins. If an infusion is to be maintained for long periods, veins are selected in the temporal region of the scalp or sometimes in the back of the hand or the dorsum of the foot.

Planning and Intervention for Fluid, Electrolyte, and Acid-Base Balance

The overall nursing goal is to maintain or restore a patient's fluid, electrolyte, and/or acid-base balance. Subgoals are:

1. To regulate fluid and electrolyte intake
2. To promote urinary output
3. To restore blood volume

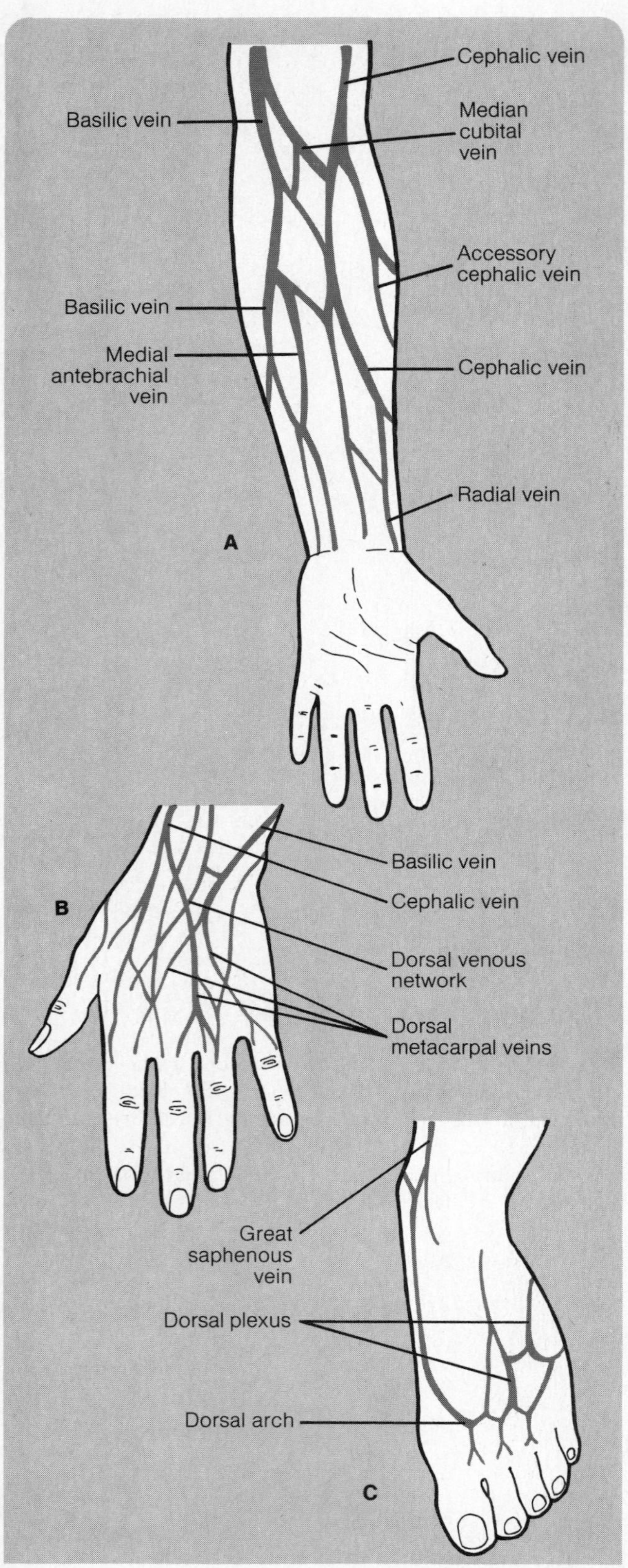

Figure 31–8 Commonly used venipuncture sites of the **A,** arm; **B,** hand; and **C,** foot.

Planning for fluid, electrolyte, and acid-base balance involves incorporating measures that maintain or restore balances while at the same time considering the patient's comfort, safety, nutrition, and therapy. It is also important to include measures for monitoring particular patients for imbalances (actual or potential). Some patients are more prone to imbalances than others. Patients especially at risk include those who have:

1. Alterations in their food and/or fluid intake
2. Alterations in their normal elimination
3. Abnormal fluid losses, e.g., draining wound, gastric suction, diarrhea
4. Excessively high body temperature
5. Disease conditions that directly affect fluid, electrolyte, and/or acid-base balance; e.g., malignancy or cardiac disease

Starting an Intravenous Infusion with a Butterfly Needle

Agency policy dictates which personnel perform arm venipunctures. In most agencies, laboratory technicians and nurses working in emergency or critical care areas customarily take blood samples from the veins in the antecubital space. Some agencies may require all registered nurses to perform venipunctures, regardless of the setting or the purpose of the venipuncture. Other hospitals have teams of specially trained nurses responsible for starting all IVs.

The following procedure describes venipuncture with a butterfly needle, but many of the steps apply just as well to venipuncture with a syringe and needle or with needles attached to catheters. The nurse observes strict sterile technique.

Procedure 31–1 Arm Venipuncture with a Butterfly Needle

Purpose

To start an infusion of fluid or blood

Equipment

1. Sterile butterfly (wing-tipped) needle; a 2.5 cm (1 in) needle, size #20 to #22 for most infusions; a size #18 or #19 needle for whole blood
2. Antiseptic swabs
3. Tourniquet
4. Receptacle for discarded fluid
5. Adhesive or nonallergic tape
6. Sterile parenteral solution (Discolored or cloudy solutions may be contaminated.)
7. An intravenous administration set
8. Intravenous stand (pole)
9. Towel or pad to place under the patient's arm
10. Arm splint, as required
11. Gauze squares or other appropriate dressing

Prepare the infusion equipment

1. Open the administration set and maintain the sterility of the ends of the tubing.
2. Slide the tubing clamp along the tubing until it is just below the drip chamber.
3. Close the clamp.
4. **a.** If using an intravenous bottle with a rubber stopper, remove the metal disc. Swab the protective stopper with disinfectant. Remove the cap from the tubing, then insert the spike firmly through the rubber stopper into the port, maintaining sterile technique.
   b. If using a bottle with an indwelling vent, remove the metal disc and the rubber seal, then insert the spike into the larger hole (the one without the vent). Listen for a hissing sound. If there is no hissing sound, discard the container because it was probably not sealed.
   c. To spike a plastic bag, read the manufacturer's directions. Some bags are first hung on the rod.
5. Hang the solution container on the rod, usually about 1 m (3 ft) above the patient's head.

   Rationale Sufficient height enables gravity to overcome venous pressure and facilitates flow of the solution into the vein.
6. If using a flexible drip chamber, squeeze gently until it is half full of solution. A firm drip chamber usually fills automatically.

   Rationale The drip chamber is partly filled with solution to prevent air from moving down the tubing.
7. To prime the tubing, remove the protective cap and hold the tubing over a cup or basin. Maintain the sterility of the end of the tubing and the cap. Release the clamp and let the fluid run through the tubing until all bubbles are removed. Tap the tubing with your fingers to help the bubbles move out.

   Rationale Air bubbles act as emboli if they are allowed to enter the bloodstream. They therefore have to be removed from the tubing by priming.
8. Reclamp the tubing.
9. Replace the tubing cap, maintaining sterile technique.
10. Hang the tubing on the stand.
11. Label the solution container, applying the label upside down on the container. Include the following information: the patient's name, identification number, bed number, dosage and absorption time, drip rate, the date, the time the container is hung, and the container number. The label is applied upside down so it can be readily read when the container is hanging up.
12. Apply a timing label on the solution container. An example of such a label is shown on page 819.
13. Label the IV tubing. Include the date, time of attachment, and your initials.

    Rationale Labeling helps ensure that the IV tubing is changed every 48 hours or more often as required by agency policy.

Procedure 31–1, continued

Intervention

Select and prepare the venipuncture site

1. Prepare strips of adhesive tape to stabilize the IV needle once it is inserted.
2. Select a site, starting at the distal end of the vein.

   Rationale Sclerosing of veins can result from the irritation of the infusion or the needle and interfere with venous flow. If sclerosing occurs, more proximal parts of the veins can be used.
3. If necessary, shave the skin where adhesive tape will be applied.

Dilate the vein

1. Place the extremity in a dependent position (lower than the patient's heart).

   Rationale Gravity slows venous return and distends the veins.
2. Apply a tourniquet firmly 6 to 8 inches above the venipuncture site. The tourniquet must be tight enough to obstruct venous flow but not too tight to occlude arterial flow.

   Rationale Obstructing arterial flow inhibits venous filling. If a radial pulse can be palpated, the arterial flow is not obstructed.
3. If the vein is not sufficiently dilated:
   a. Massage or stroke the vein distal to the site and in the direction of venous flow toward the heart.

      Rationale This action helps fill the vein.

   b. Encourage the patient to rapidly clench and unclench the fist.

      Rationale Contracting the muscles compresses the distal veins, forcing blood along the veins and distending them.

   c. Lightly tap the vein with your fingertips.

      Rationale Tapping may distend the vein.
4. If steps 1 to 3 fail to distend the vein, remove the tourniquet and apply heat to the entire extremity for 10 to 15 minutes. Then repeat steps 1 to 3.

   Rationale Heat dilates superficial blood vessels, causing them to fill.

Insert the needle

1. Clean the skin with an antiseptic swab at the site of entry.
2. Use one thumb to pull the skin taut below the entry site.

   Rationale This pulling stabilizes the vein and makes the skin taut for needle entry. It also makes initial tissue penetration less painful.
3. Hold the needle at a 30° angle with the bevel up and pierce the skin beside the vein about 1 cm (½ in) below the site planned for piercing the vein. See Figure 31–9.
4. Once the needle is through the skin, lower the needle so it is almost parallel with the skin. Follow the course of the vein and pierce the side of the vein.

   Rationale Lowering the needle reduces the chances of puncturing both sides of the vein.
5. When blood flows back into the needle tubing, insert the needle further up the vein (¾ to 1 in) or to the hub of the butterfly needle. Sudden lack of resistance can be felt as blood enters the needle.

Figure 31–9

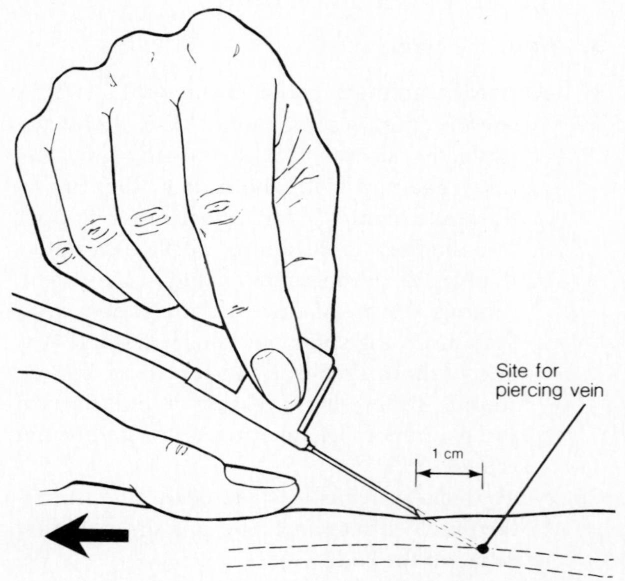

Procedure 31–1, continued

6. Release the tourniquet, attach the infusion, and initiate flow as quickly as possible.

Rationale Attaching the tubing quickly prevents the patient's blood from clotting and obstructing the needle.

7. Tape the needle securely by the H method (see Figure 31–10) or criss-cross method (see Figure 31–11). You may need to place a cotton ball or small gauze square under the needle to keep it in position in the vein.

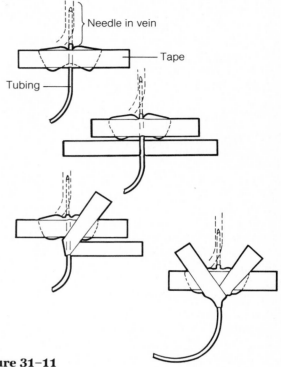

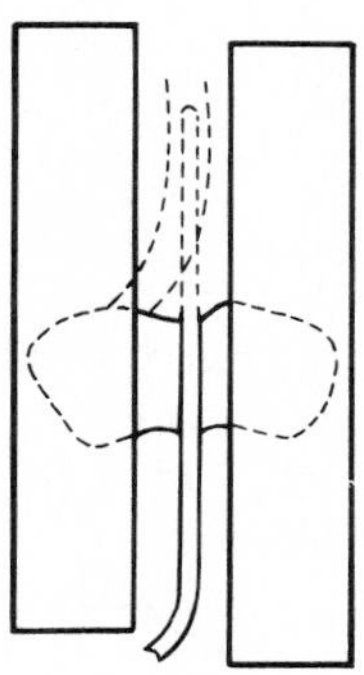

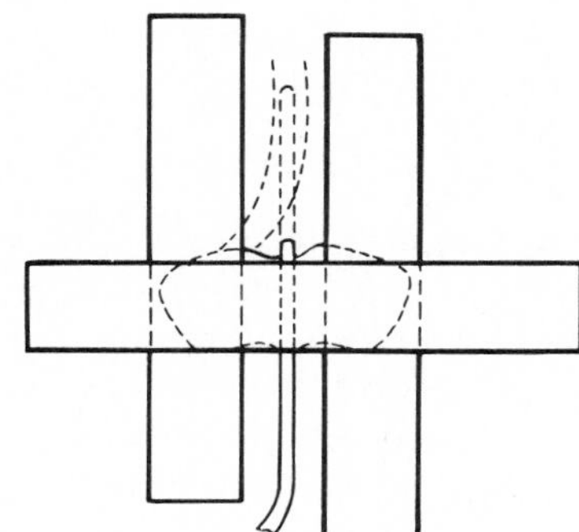

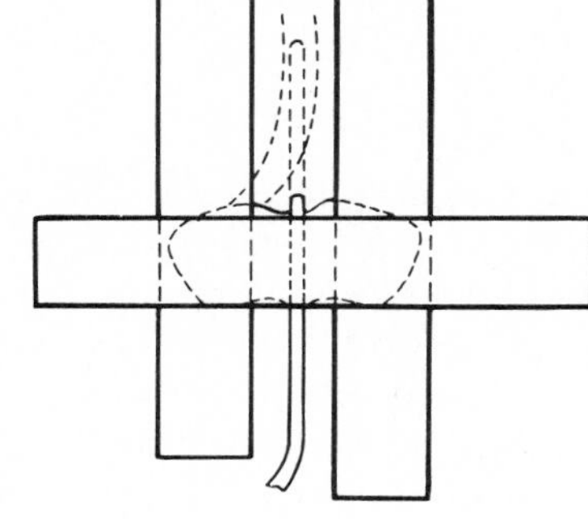

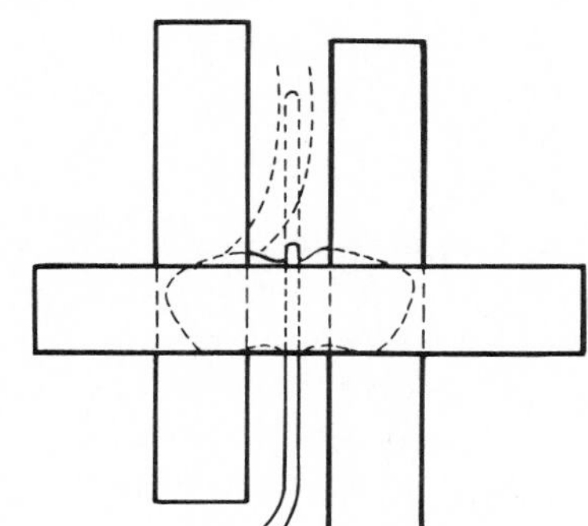

Figure 31–10

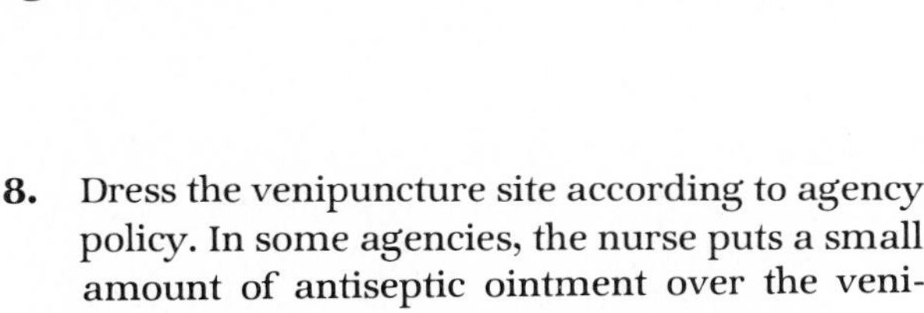

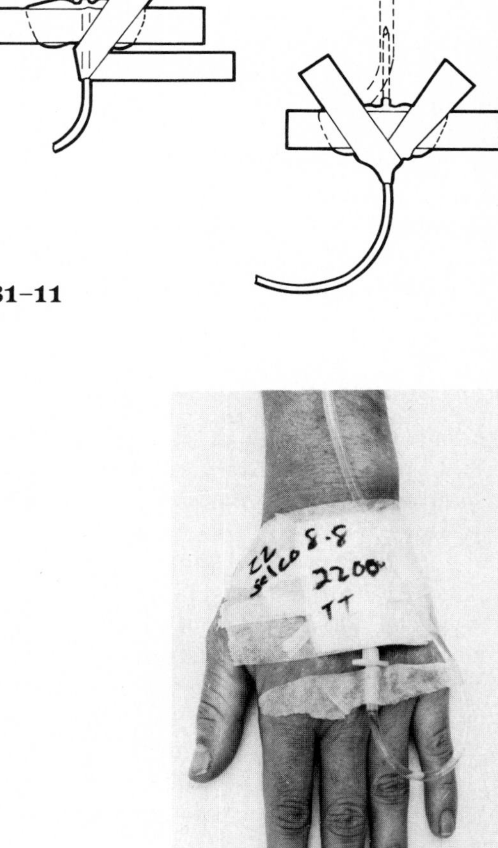

Figure 31–11

8. Dress the venipuncture site according to agency policy. In some agencies, the nurse puts a small amount of antiseptic ointment over the venipuncture site, then a gauze square.

9. Loop the tubing and secure it to the dressing with tape.

Rationale Securing the tubing to the dressing prevents the weight of the tubing or any movement from pulling on the needle.

10. Apply a padded armboard to splint the elbow or wrist joint if needed.

11. Adjust the rate of flow as ordered.

12. Label a piece of tape with the date and time of insertion, type and gauge of needle used, and the nurse's initials. Apply the tape label over the venipuncture dressing. See Figure 31–12.

Figure 31–12

Maintaining the Intravenous Infusion

A primary nursing function is to maintain intravenous therapy. This involves several important measures:

1. Explaining the procedures and equipment to the patient and teaching the patient
2. Giving comfort and assistance with activities of daily living throughout the therapy
3. Observing for possible complications
4. Regulating flow rates (discussed in the next section)

Explanation and education

Explanations can correct misconceptions, gain a person's cooperation, and give peace of mind. Using terms the person understands, the nurse explains the purpose of the infusion, the equipment, the time involved, how the patient can help, what activity is permitted, and how the nurse will help the patient meet his or her needs. Explanations need to be adjusted to each patient's own requirements and concerns. Individual or developmental variables are important. Some elderly people may equate intravenous therapy with death and need reassurance and correct information. Young children may see the IV as a punishment for not eating or drinking, and the very small child may be aware only of discomfort and fear.

Comfort and assistance for patients

Depending on the duration of infusion and placement of the needle, patients often require assistance with needs such as hygiene or ambulation. Often nurses need to help patients remove gowns. Most gowns allow the passage of an intravenous bottle. To remove a soiled gown, the nurse disengages it from the uninvolved arm first. Next, the nurse carefully slips the sleeve over the infusion site and tubing until it is off the patient's hand, removes the intravenous bottle from the stand, and lifts the gown over and off the bottle. Last, the nurse rehangs the bottle. To put on a new gown, the nurse reverses the order and puts the bottle and tubing through the sleeve of the new gown first. See Kozier and Erb (1982:403) for further information.

Restraints or splints should be removed periodically to check the skin and circulatory status of the extremity. Patients with infusions also require assistance to ambulate and to turn in bed. Portable intravenous stands make walking easier. The nurse may have to move intravenous equipment from one side of the bed to the other when helping to turn a patient in bed. When ambulating or turning patients, the nurse needs to avoid placing tension on the tubing so that the movement neither alters the flow rate nor injures the arm.

Observation for possible complications

The major complications of IV therapy are infiltration, phlebitis, circulatory overload, and bleeding. *Infiltration* is escape of fluid into subcutaneous tissue due to dislodgment of the needle. It is easily detected because the subcutaneous tissues swell, the skin becomes cold since the intravenous fluid is at room temperature rather than body temperature, and the patient may complain of pain at the site. Swelling can be checked by comparing the involved extremity with the other extremity. The earliest sign of infiltration can be a reduced rate of flow. Early recognition can prevent unnecessary discomfort. Some methods for identifying infiltration early are discussed later in this chapter (see the section on factors influencing flow rates).

Phlebitis is another potential complication of intravenous infusions caused by the mechanical trauma to the vein or the chemical irritation of infused substances, such as potassium chloride. Patients may complain of burning pain along the vein, or the nurse may notice redness and increased skin temperature over the vein. The venipuncture site needs to be changed and further use of the involved vein avoided. Phlebitis can lead to the formation of *thrombi* (blood clots) and *emboli* (clots that move through the bloodstream and lodge in smaller arterioles elsewhere in the body, causing obstruction).

Circulatory overload occurs when the intravascular fluid compartment contains more fluid than normal. Overload may be the result of overly rapid infusion rates and may lead to cardiac failure and pulmonary edema. See the section on extracellular fluid excess, page 800. Prevention is achieved by carefully monitoring flow rates so they do not exceed maximum volumes. Circulatory overload can occur if a nurse speeds up the flow rates for an infusion that is behind schedule. Overload is a particular threat to patients with cardiac or kidney disease because such patients cannot tolerate substantial increases in intravascular volume. The best way for the nurse to monitor such patients is to check their central venous pressure (CVP); it is the physician's responsibility, however, to insert the CVP line.

Bleeding at the site of an infusion can occur during the infusion but is more likely after the needle is removed from the vein. The site of the needle or catheter insertion should always be inspected for evidence of blood, particularly in patients who bleed readily; e.g., patients receiving heparin.

Regulating Infusion Flow Rates

Maintaining a constant rate of flow for infusions is a nurse's responsibility. Infusion rates that are too rapid overload the intravascular compartment, leading to serious cardiac and pulmonary complications. Infusion rates that are too slow replace fluids and electrolytes inefficiently. There are two methods of calculating flow rates: the number of milliliters per hour and the number of drops per minute. Since commercial brands of intravenous equipment differ, there are variations in the size of openings of drip chambers and thus in the number of drops per milliliter. Fortunately, drops per milliliter are indicated on the container boxes of intravenous infusion sets. Common drop factors are 10, 15, and 20 drops per milliliter for macrodrips and 60 drops per milliliter for microdrips.

Milliliters per hour

Hourly rates of infusion can be calculated by dividing the total infusion volume by the total infusion time in hours. For example, if 3000 ml is infused in 24 hours, the number of milliliters per hour is

$$\frac{3000 \text{ ml (total infusion volume)}}{24 \text{ hours (total time of infusion)}} = 125 \text{ ml/hour}$$

Nurses need to check infusions at least every 30 minutes to assure that the indicated milliliters per hour have infused. Some nurses add a strip of adhesive tape to the solution bottle marking the exact time and/or amount to be infused. See Figure 31-13. Some agencies make premarked labels available.

Drops per minute

When a nurse begins an infusion, he or she must regulate the drops per minute to ensure that the prescribed amounts of solution will infuse. Drops per minute are calculated by the following formula:

$$\text{Drops per minute} = \frac{\text{Total infusion volume} \times \text{drops/ml (or drip factor)}}{\text{Total time of infusion in } minutes}$$

If the requirements are 1000 ml in 8 hours (480 minutes) and the drip factor is 20 drops per ml, the drops per minute should be regulated as follows:

$$\frac{1000 \text{ ml (total infusion volume)} \times 20 \text{ drops/ml}}{480 \text{ minutes}} = 41 \text{ drops/minute}$$

Approximating this rate as 40 drops per minute, the nurse must then regulate the drops per minute by tightening or releasing the intravenous tubing clamp and counting the drops in much the same way as a pulse. Devices such as battery-operated rate meters and infusion pumps with alarm systems facilitate regulated flow.

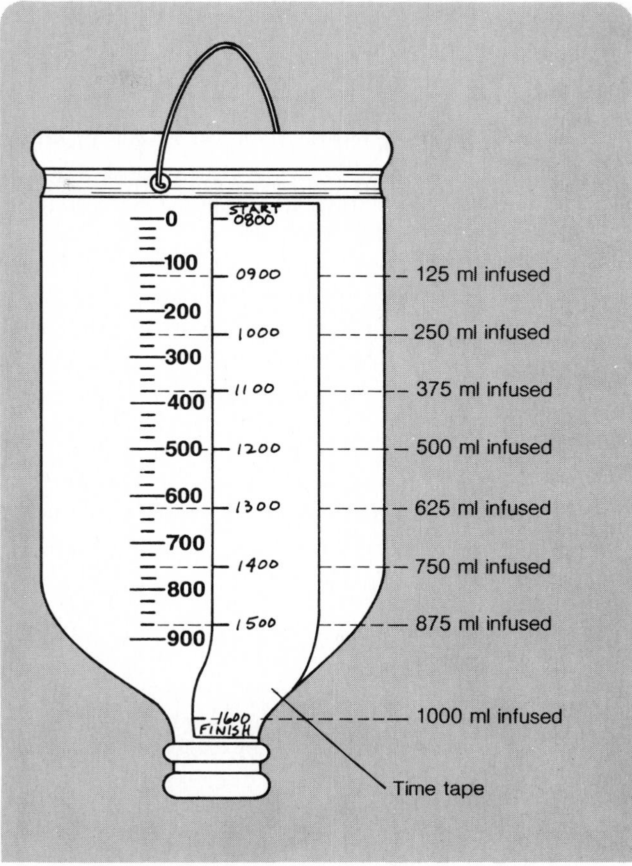

Figure 31-13 An adhesive marker placed on the solution container facilitates monitoring the flow rate. In this case, 125 ml of solution is to be infused hourly up to a total of 1000 ml. With a drip factor of 20, the solution is administered at 40 drops per minute (125 ml per hour) for 8 hours.

Factors influencing flow rates

No matter how often flow rates are regulated, several factors can change the rate of flow of IV infusions. If an infusion is too fast or too slow, the nurse needs to consider several factors:

1. *Position of the forearm.* Sometimes having the patient change the position of the arm increases flow. Slight pronation, supination, extension, or elevation of the forearm on a pillow can increase flow.
2. *Position and patency of the tubing.* Not infrequently, the tubing is obstructed by the patient's weight, by a kink, or by a clamp closed too tightly. The flow rate also diminishes when part of the tubing dangles below the puncture site.
3. *Height of the infusion bottle.* Elevating the height of the infusion bottle a few inches can speed the flow by creating more pressure.
4. Possibility of *infiltration or fluid leakage.* Swelling, a feeling of coldness, and tenderness at the venipuncture

site can indicate infiltration. If infiltration is not evident, the following measures can determine whether the needle is dislodged from the vein:

a. The nurse lowers the infusion bottle below the level of the venipuncture site to see if blood returns. Blood indicates that the intravenous needle is still in the vein, although this method is not foolproof because the needle may be penetrating the vein wall partially.

b. The nurse uses a sterile syringe of saline to withdraw fluid from the rubber at the end of the tubing. If blood does not return, the nurse discontinues the intravenous infusion.

c. The nurse tries to stop the flow by applying a tourniquet 4 to 6 inches above the insertion site and opening the roller clamp wide. If the infusion continues to flow slowly, the needle is in subcutaneous tissue (it has infiltrated).

Changing Intravenous Containers

Intravenous infusion containers need to be changed when a small amount of solution is in the neck of the bottle and fluid still remains in the drip chamber. The Center for Disease Control (CDC) recommends that no solution bottle hang for more than 24 hours. Sterile technique is essential when changing IV containers. To change an IV container, the nurse needs to:

1. Prepare the new container before the old one runs out.
2. Clamp the intravenous tubing. Clamping is not always necessary if the nurse acts quickly and efficiently.
3. Remove the spike from the old container and quickly insert it into the new one.
4. Hang up the new container.
5. Release the tubing clamp if it was closed, and reestablish the infusion with the prescribed rate of flow.
6. Label the solution container.
7. Follow agency policy when charting the amount and type of fluid infused and/or the amount and type of fluid added.

Changing Intravenous Tubing

The CDC recommends that tubing be changed every 48 hours to decrease the incidence of infection. However, nurses should follow agency policy dictating how often to change tubing. Tubing is changed most easily when a new container is added. To change tubing, the nurse needs to:

1. Prepare the new solution container.
2. Open the administration set and attach it to the container.
3. Tighten the tubing clamp and hang the container on the stand if it is not already up.
4. Remove the protective cap from the end of the tubing, prime the tubing (flush it with solution), clamp the tubing, and replace the protective cap.
5. Carefully remove the tape and the dressing from the needle, taking care not to dislodge the needle.
6. Holding the hub of the needle with the fingers of one hand, remove the tubing with the other hand using a twisting, pulling motion.
7. Continue to hold the needle and grasp the new tubing with the other hand, remove the protective cap, and, maintaining sterility, insert the tubing end tightly into the needle hub.
8. Open the clamp to start the solution flowing.
9. Clean the venipuncture site with antiseptic solution (e.g., iodine or ethyl alcohol). Clean from the insertion point outward in a circular manner.
10. Apply a sterile dressing and a labeled tape over the dressing. The label should show the date and time the dressing was applied as well as the date and time of the original venipuncture and the initials of the nurse who performed it.
11. Label the new tubing to show the date and time of the change and the initials of the nurse who changed the tubing.
12. Regulate the rate of flow of the solution according to the order on the chart.
13. Record the tubing change and the change of the solution container in the appropriate place on the patient's chart.

Discontinuing Intravenous Infusions

Intravenous infusions are terminated when the prescribed volume of fluid has infused or when infiltration occurs. To discontinue an infusion, the nurse needs to:

1. Loosen the tape at the venipuncture site while holding the needle firmly to prevent unnecessary trauma to the vein and discomfort to the patient. The tape does not need to be removed from the needle.
2. Clamp the infusion tubing to stop the flow of fluid and to prevent soiling the patient when the needle is removed.
3. Withdraw the needle by pulling on the needle hub in line with the vein while holding a dry sterile gauze or swab over the needle site.
4. As soon as the needle is withdrawn, apply firm pressure to the site with a dry swab or gauze for 2 to 3 minutes to stop the bleeding and prevent hematoma.
5. Apply a small sterile dressing over the needle site to stop further bleeding and prevent infection at the needle site. (This dressing can be removed the following day.)

6. Assist the patient to a comfortable position.
7. Discard the administration set and dispose of the equipment appropriately.
8. Wash hands.
9. On the intake record, note the amount of fluid infused, then enter the fact that the IV was discontinued on the patient's record.

Blood Transfusions

A *blood transfusion* is the introduction of whole blood or components of the blood, such as plasma, serum, erythrocytes, or platelets, into the venous circulation. See Table 31–4 for types of blood and blood products, and indications for use.

The reasons for blood transfusions are as follows:

1. To restore blood volume after severe hemorrhage
2. To restore the red blood cell level after severe and chronic anemias and to maintain blood hemoglobin levels
3. To provide plasma factors, such as antihemophilic factor (AHF), which controls bleeding

Blood Matching

Blood groups

Human blood is classified into four main groups (A, B, AB, and O) on the basis of polysaccharide antigens on the erythrocyte surface. These antigens, type A and type B, commonly cause antibody reactions and are called *agglutinogens.* In other words, Group A blood contains type A agglutinogen. Group B blood contains type B agglutinogen, Group AB blood contains both A and B agglutinogens, but Group O contains neither agglutinogen.

In addition to agglutinogens on the erythrocytes, *agglutinins* (antibodies) are present in the blood plasma. The agglutinins are referred to as *alpha (anti-A) agglutinins,* which agglutinate type A cells, and *beta (anti-B) agglutinins,* which agglutinate type B cells. No individual can have agglutinins and agglutinogens of the same type; that person's system would attack its own cells. Thus Group A blood does not contain agglutinin A but does contain agglutinin B. Group B blood does not contain agglutinin B but does contain agglutinin A. Group AB blood contains neither agglutinin, and Group O contains both anti-A and anti-B aggluti-

Table 31–4 Types of Blood and Blood Products and Indications for Use

Type	Indications
Whole blood (Type A, B, AB, O, and/or Rh positive or negative)	To treat blood volume deficiencies, for example in acute hemorrhage; not indicated for correction of chronic anemia
Plasma	To expand blood volume; to restore circulation and renal blood flow when plasma volume is decreased but the red cell mass is adequate, as in acute dehydration or burns; to replace deficient coagulation factors in bleeding disorders
Packed red cells (high hematocrit, since approximately 80% of the plasma is removed)	Used when blood volume is adequate but the red cell mass is inadequate, as in chronic anemia
Platelets	For patients with severe *thrombocytopenia* (reduced platelets); platelets plug small vascular leaks prior to clotting
Albumin	To expand the blood volume when blood volume is reduced in shock or burns; also to increase level of albumin in patients with *hypoalbuminemia*
Prothrombin complex (for example, Konyne, Proplex) contains factors VII, IX, and XI and prothrombin	Used for bleeding associated with deficiencies of those factors
Factor VIII fractions	For hemophiliacs
Fibrinogen preparations	Used particularly for bleeding associated with congenital *hypofibrinogenemia* (a deficiency of fibrinogen, a necessary factor for blood coagulation)

nins. The most common blood types are type A and type O. Twenty percent of the black population have type B blood, while only 9% of the white population have type B; however, almost 50% of both populations have type O blood. See Table 31–5.

Rhesus (Rh) groups

Rh antigens, also on the surface of erythrocytes, are present in about 85% of the population and can be a major cause of hemolytic reactions. Persons who possess the Rh factor are referred to as *Rh positive;* those who do not are referred to as *Rh negative.* Some other blood factors are the Hr, Kell, Lewis, M, N, and P factors. These latter factors rarely cause major reactions because their antigenic properties are poor. They have little effect on transfusions but may be important in forensic medicine. For example, it has been possible to determine disputed paternity by the presence of these factors. Usually, half of the factors in the child's blood are in the mother's blood and the other half in the father's.

The Rh factor differs from the A and B agglutinogens in that it cannot cause a hemolytic reaction on first exposure of mismatched blood. This is because the Rh antibody is *not* normally present in the plasma of persons who are Rh negative. Although a person with type O blood does not have either A or B agglutinogen but does have anti-A and anti-B agglutinins, the Rh-negative person has no anti-Rh antibodies. This person, however, can develop Rh antibodies if exposed to the Rh factor. When Rh-positive blood is given to an Rh-negative person, the individual produces Rh antibodies but does not manifest a reaction on first exposure. On second exposure, however, agglutination occurs.

Erythroblastosis fetalis is one of the major consequences of Rh incompatibility. This condition occurs in infants born to Rh-negative mothers and Rh-positive fathers. If the fetus inherits the Rh-positive factor from the father and thus has Rh antigen on its erythrocytes, some of these antigens can be passed to the mother through the placental membrane. This does not usually occur until parturition, when there is trauma and some mixing of blood. The mother then develops Rh antibodies, which may create problems for subsequent Rh-positive fetuses. Agglutination and destruction of the fetal red cells results. This process is fatal to many Rh-positive infants prior to birth. Those who survive birth need exchange transfusions. The Rh-positive infant is transfused with Rh-negative blood, and the Rh-positive blood is removed. The Rh antibodies in the infant's body fluids cannot destroy this Rh-negative blood. In approximately 1 month, the Rh antibodies are destroyed and the infant can produce blood safely.

Transfusion Reactions

Transfusion reactions can be categorized as hemolytic, febrile, and allergic. The *hemolytic reaction*, a fatal response, ocurs when agglutinins and agglutinogens of the same type come in contact; e.g., type A agglutinogen and anti-A agglutinin or type B agglutinogen and anti-B agglutinin. *Agglutination (clumping)* and *hemolysis* (rupture) of the red cells is the result of such contact. It is essential, therefore, to match the recipient's blood type to the donor's. Otherwise the agglutinins present in the recipient's plasma will agglutinate the red cells donated. Type A blood has anti-B agglutinins; therefore, if a person with type A blood is given type B, his or her anti-B agglutinins will agglutinate the type B blood cells donated. Because type O blood has neither A nor B agglutinogens, it can be donated to recipients with any of the four types of blood; it is called the *universal donor.* Type AB blood, because it has neither

Table 31–5 Survey of Information on Blood Groups

Blood type (red blood cell agglutinogens)	Agglutinins in plasma	Possible donors	Percentage of white population	Percentage of black population
A	Anti-B (beta)	Types A and O	41	30
B	Anti-A (alpha)	Types B and O	9	20
AB	None	Types AB, A, B, and O	3	3
O (no agglutinogen)	Anti-A and anti-B	Type O	47	47

anti-A nor anti-B agglutinins in plasma, is referred to as a *universal recipient*, being able to receive any of the four blood types.

In summary, similar agglutinins and agglutinogens react and produce agglutination and hemolysis of erythrocytes.

Type A (agglutinogen A)	+	Type B (anti-A agglutinin)	=	Hemolysis
Type B (agglutinogen B)	+	Type A (anti-B agglutinin)	=	Hemolysis

Table 31–5 shows compatibility among blood groups.

Febrile reactions (bacterial reactions) are rare. They occur as a result of contaminated blood or sensitivity to the donor's white blood cells. *Allergic reactions* are relatively common and are thought to be due to allergic substances or antibodies in the donor's plasma. See Table 31–6, which outlines the signs, symptoms, medical treatment, and nursing actions for each type of reaction.

Risks of Blood Transfusions

Although technologic advances have made blood transfusions a relatively safe procedure, some risks are involved; therefore transfusions are given only when absolutely necessary. It has been estimated that 1 in 2000 persons receiving a blood transfusion dies.

Mislabeling

Mislabeled containers can lead to fatal errors. Type B or type AB blood, incorrectly labeled as type A and given to a patient with type A blood, will cause a hemolytic reaction.

Transmission of diseases

Syphilis, malaria, and hepatitis can be transmitted by donors who are asymptomatic carriers. Although donors are screened, there is no foolproof method of detecting all carriers. The incidence of syphilis contracted through blood transfusions is rare now since the advent of serologic testing on all units of blood.

Hepatitis is not transmitted by albumin, which, unlike all other blood products, is subjected to heat in the preparation process. Heating frees albumin from all viral contaminants. However, hepatitis remains a risk in transfusion of all blood products except albumin. Recipients of infected blood have symptoms of the disease from 2 to 6 months after transfusion. The common signs are fever, jaundice, and lethargy.

Sensitivities

In most blood transfusions, the donor's red cells have some antigenic factor that the recipient's do not have. Uusually, these factors are poor antigens, but occasionally some can produce intense antibody formation. This creates a risk for the recipient when subsequent transfusions are given. Recipients can develop sensitivities to antigens of the donor's white cells, platelets, or some serum proteins.

Citrate toxicity

Citrate toxicity can occur when massive transfusions are required, such as six units of blood in less than 24 hours. Each unit of whole blood contains approximately 50 ml of acid-citrate dextrose (ACD) solution. Its purpose is to serve as an anticoagulant and to provide the red cells with sugar for metabolism.

Iron overload

Each unit (500 ml) of blood contains 250 mg of iron. Patients who have chronic anemia and who must have frequent transfusions develop hemosiderosis. *Hemosiderosis*, the deposition of iron in the skin, liver, spleen, and other organs, can interfere with normal physiologic function.

Assisting with Blood Transfusions

Hospitals usually have special practices and procedures governing the provision of blood. These are designed to protect the patient receiving blood and must be followed closely. The following guidelines are intended to help nurses care for patients who receive blood. Nurses need to:

1. Always use the correct administration set and follow the manufacturer's directions. Special administration sets, with a filter inside the drip chamber, are used for blood transfusions. See Figure 31–14.
2. Fill out blood requisitions carefully and accurately.
3. Identify the patient and ensure that the patient receives the correct blood. Some agencies require that two nurses carry out this procedure. The nurses make sure the identification number, blood group, and the complete patient name written on the blood match the patient's exactly.

Table 31–6 Survey of Information on Transfusion Reactions

Category and description	Incidence and cause	Signs and symptoms	Medical treatment	Nursing actions
Hemolytic reaction				
Agglutination (clumping) of erythrocytes occurs first; blockage of capillaries and eventually disintegration of RBC's occurs; then hemoglobin is released into the circulation; passes into the kidney tubules, becomes concentrated, precipitates, and plugs the tubules; death ensues from renal shutdown (1 to 2 weeks)	Incidence is 1 in 5000; cause is mismatched blood of ABO incompatibility or Rh incompatibility on second and subsequent exposures	Chills, fever, headache, back pain, hemoglobinemia, hemoglobinuria (red urine), oliguria, jaundice, dyspnea, cyanosis, chest pain, vascular collapse, hypotension	**1.** Large quantities of fluid (for example, D-5-W) to promote diuresis and prevent hemoglobin from precipitating **2.** Diuretics to increase flow of tubular fluids and prevent hemoglobin plugs (for example, mannitol) **3.** Administration of Leporin to combat intravascular coagulation **4.** Indwelling catheter to monitor urinary output **5.** Oxygen and epinephrine for wheezing and dyspnea **6.** Treatment of shock with matched blood and vasopressor drugs **7.** Sedation for restlessness	**1.** Observe patient closely for first 10 minutes of transfusion, since these reactions occur rapidly **2.** Discontinue blood immediately when reaction is assessed **3.** Notify physician of patient's symptoms and vital signs **4.** Notify laboratory to type and cross match blood and confirm diagnosis; the donor blood is sent back to the lab and a specimen of the recipient's blood is retested **5.** Maintain intravenous infusion with D-5-W or saline **6.** Monitor vital signs q.15 minutes to assess shock and temperature **7.** Record fluid intake and output to assess degree of kidney functioning **8.** Save first voided specimen for laboratory analysis **9.** Implement treatment as prescribed by the physician

Table 31–6 continued

Category and description	Incidence and cause	Signs and symptoms	Medical treatment	Nursing actions
Febrile reaction This is also referred to as bacterial reaction; the patient develops a fever and so-called red shock characterized by flushing of the skin due to massive peripheral dilatation	Incidence is rare with the advent of disposable plastic equipment and aseptic blood banking techniques; cause is: **1.** Contaminated blood, particularly of the gram-negative bacteria, which can produce 50% fatality rates **2.** Sensitivity to the donor's white cells or platelets, which is more common and less severe	Fever, shaking, chills, warm flushed skin, headache, backache, nausea, hematemesis, diarrhea, red shock, confusion or delirium	For acute reaction: **1.** Vasopressor drug to maintain systolic pressure over 100 mm Hg **2.** Corticosteroids to correct inflammation **3.** Antibiotics in high dosages to combat pyrogens **4.** Indwelling catheter to assess urinary output **5.** Intravenous fluids in accordance with output **6.** Antipyretics to abate fever For mild reaction: **1.** Antipyretics for fever **2.** Subsequent transfusions of leukocyte-poor blood	For acute reaction: **1.** Observe patient closely for the first 30 minutes of transfusion **2.** Stop the transfusion **3.** Maintain intravenous infusion with saline or D-5-W **4.** Monitor the patient's vital signs q.30 minutes **5.** Notify the physician **6.** Notify the lab to take a culture of patient's and transfusion blood **7.** Implement therapy as prescribed by physician **8.** Alcohol sponges may be given for fever
Allergic reaction Reactions are usually mild; rarely does anaphylactic shock occur	Incidence is 1% to 2% (relatively common); cause is thought to be allergenic substances (drugs or foods) or antibodies in the donor's plasma	Urticaria (hives), occasional wheezing, arthralgia, generalized itching, nasal congestion, bronchospasm, severe dyspnea, circulatory collapse	For mild reactions: **1.** Antihistamines **2.** Antipyretics For severe reactions: **1.** Epinephrine **2.** Corticosteroids **3.** Vasopressors	For mild reactions: **1.** Slow the transfusion **2.** Implement therapy as prescribed by physician For severe reactions: **1.** Stop the transfusion **2.** Notify physician immediately **3.** Maintain intravenous infusion with saline or D-5-W **4.** Monitor vital signs frequently

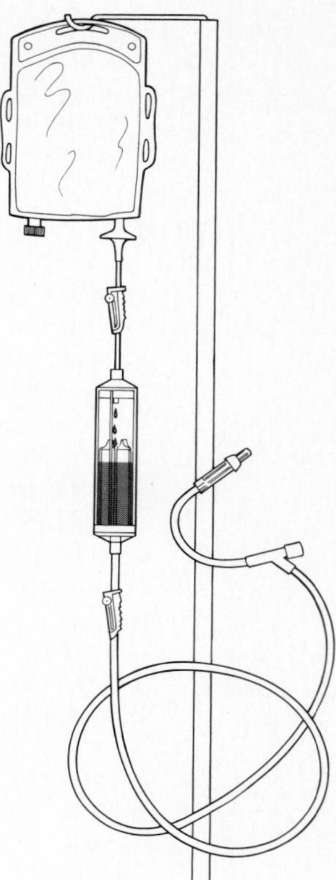

Figure 31–14 A blood container and blood administration set. The set contains a filter inside the drip chamber.

4. Observe a transfusion closely and regularly. In addition to assessing as for intravenous solutions, the nurse makes sure that the filter inside the drip chamber is submerged in blood.
5. Assess the site of the venipuncture for evidence of a hematoma, which, if evident, is reported to the responsible nurse. The transfusion may need to be terminated.
6. Assess the patient closely for any reactions to the transfusion. Untoward reactions can occur very soon after the transfusion begins and for up to 96 hours after it has terminated. Clinical signs; e.g., fever, chills, pain, nausea, vomiting, dyspnea, and shock, should be reported immediately to the responsible nurse. In some instances the transfusion is stopped and the vein is kept open with an infusion of normal saline.

Total Parenteral Nutrition

Total parenteral nutrition (TPN) is also referred to as *hyperalimentation*; it is the administration of hypertonic solutions of carbohydrate, protein, and fats (lipids) by indwelling intravenous catheters into the superior vena cava through the internal jugular and subclavian veins. Some solutions may be given through superficial veins, and if therapy is prolonged, external arteriovenous fistulas may be used. An arteriovenous fistula is created by a surgical procedure that *anastomoses* (joins) an artery in the arm to a vein in sideways fashion, thus making an opening between a large artery and a large vein. As the arterial blood flows directly into the large vein, it distends the vein and causes engorgement. The vein is therefore more easily punctured with larger needles such as 14 or 16 gauge.

The purposes of TPN are as follows:

1. To supply nutrients intravenously in amounts sufficient to achieve *anabolism* (positive nitrogen balance) and tissue synthesis in patients who are unable to eat or absorb nutrients normally. Routine intravenous solutions normally do not deliver sufficient calories to promote wound healing or weight gain in adults or normal growth in children. For example, 1 liter of 5% dextrose provides 200 calories, sufficient for only short-term maintenance therapy. Since the approximate minimum requirement of a normal resting adult is 450 calories, daily infusions of 2500 to 3000 ml can provide this minimum. However, caloric needs increase with wound healing, fevers, and certain disease conditions. If these are prolonged, daily needs can become greater than 3000 calories.
2. To permit rapid dilution of the hypertonic solution around the catheter tip, thus preventing phlebitis and thrombosis caused by concentrated solutions in superficial veins. The large volume of blood in the superior vena cava rapidly dilutes hypertonic solutions.
3. To free the extremities and permit more freedom for ambulation and activity. Use of the jugular vein restricts only the patient's neck mobility.
4. To allow for prolonged therapy, such as from 2 weeks to 3 months.
5. To protect the peripheral vascular epithelium from irritation during prolonged administration by administering Intralipid solution in conjunction with concentrated glucose solutions and amino acid mixtures.
6. To allow the gastrointestinal tract to rest and recover from certain diseases, such as ulcerative colitis and gastrointestinal fistulas. During TPN, activity of the gall bladder, pancreas, and intestines decreases.

Types of Fluids

Carbohydrates

Hypertonic solutions (10%, 20%, and 50%) of glucose can be given. The 10% solution is sometimes administered in superficial veins but only if given with Intralipid solution, which reduces irritation to the veins. One liter of 10% solution provides approximately 400 calories. Intralipid is the trade name for an intravenous fat emulsion used to correct or prevent deficiencies of essential fatty acids and to provide calories in high-density form.

Fats

Fats provide about twice the number of calories per gram as carbohydrates or proteins (9 calories as contrasted to 4); thus they are excellent sources of energy. One liter of 10% Intralipid solution provides 1100 calories, a large number of calories in a relatively small fluid volume. Intralipid solution can be given in superficial veins. It prevents irritation and sclerosing of blood vessels and is thus given in conjunction with concentrated glucose solutions and some amino acid solutions.

Amino acids

Several amino acid solutions are available. Some are categorized as protein hydrolysates, which are hydrolyzed proteins or amino acids; others are categorized as crystalline amino acids, which are more refined and more expensive. These solutions are frequently prepared in combination with dextrose and alcohol, thus providing additional calories per liter. A 5% solution of protein hydrolysate provides 170 calories per liter. Many solutions also have additives such as vitamins, electrolytes, and minerals.

Determining Dosages

The amount and type of solutions given vary with the patient's caloric requirements and proportions of carbohydrate, fat, and protein needed. The nurse regulates the flow in the same manner as for any intravenous solution, such as by milliliters per hour and drops per minute. All bottles should be taped and calibrated for milliliters per hour.

Nursing Intervention

Nursing responsibilities during TPN include the following measures:

1. Urine is checked regularly (q6h, every 6 hours) for glycosuria or acetone. If glycosuria (glucose in the urine) is found, the flow rate of the glucose solutions may be decreased, or insulin may be given on a sliding scale until the pancreas adjusts to accommodate the increased glucose supplied by the infusion.
2. Fluid intake and output is recorded accurately.
3. Weight is recorded daily to determine gain or loss.
4. Blood pressure is taken daily or more often.
5. Serum electrolyte levels are measured daily until regulated, and then measured on alternate days. Potassium is needed to transport glucose and amino acids across cell membranes. Commonly 40 mEq of potassium is added to each liter, but when the concentrations of protein and glucose are increased, the potassium must also be increased. It may be increased to 200 mEq/liter. Sodium chloride dosages are also determined by serum analysis.
6. An ambulation and exercise program is planned, since inactivity encourages catabolism.
7. The patient is assessed for complications (Table 31–7):
   a. Air embolism
   b. Infection at the site
   c. Circulatory overload
   d. Glycosuria, osmotic diuresis, hyperglycemia
   e. Brachial plexus injury
   f. Pleural puncture
8. The patient's psychologic needs are supported.
9. Mouth care is provided to moisten the mucous membranes and the lips.
10. Special dressing precautions are implemented to prevent infection. The nurse needs to check agency policies and practices.

Evaluation

Examples of outcome criteria for patients with fluid, electrolyte, or acid-base imbalances follow.

I. Fluid imbalances
  A. Fluid deficits
    1. Fluid intake of 3000 ml daily
    2. Fluid output in proportion to fluid intake
    3. Absence of thirst
    4. Moist oral mucous membranes
    5. Good skin turgor
    6. Weight gain of (specify)
    7. Mental alertness
    8. Normal serum sodium level
    9. Normal serum osmolality

Table 31–7 Potential Complications with Hyperalimentation

Complication	Cause	Signs and symptoms	Prevention	Treatment
Infection **A.** At entry site **B.** At catheter tip from blood-borne bacteria **C.** Through solution infusion	Poor technique		Rigid asepsis when starting infusion, changing bottles and tubing, preparing solutions, and changing dressings	
Hypoglycemia	Infusion rate that is too slow	Ketonuria, weakness, trembling, sweating	Check urine for acetone q6h and maintain flow rates	Contact physician
Hyperglycemia	Infusion rate that is too rapid; glucose cannot be metabolized	Extreme dehydration, nausea, headache, lassitude	Check urine for sugar q.6h. and maintain flow rates	Give insulin as ordered or slow infusion rate
Osmotic diuresis	Hyperglycemia; the body eliminates excess glucose, taking fluid with it, and thus produces dehydration	Glycosuria	As for hyperglycemia	
Air embolism	Air can be sucked into the intravenous system when the catheter is open and the patient takes in a deep breath (the pressure within the vena cava is decreased as thoracic pressure is reduced on inspiration)	Cyanosis, hypotension, rapid weak pulse, altered consciousness, restlessness	Have patient perform *Valsalva maneuver* (ask the patient to bear down with the mouth closed) during insertion of tubing and during tubing changes; check that all connections are secure	Clamp central venous line; have patient lie on left side to keep air in right ventricle and thus avoid pulmonary emboli
Acute fluid overload	Infusion rate that is too rapid, resulting in pulmonary edema and congestive heart failure	Shortness of breath, dyspnea, rapid and thready pulse, dyspnea, decreased urine output	Maintain flow rates; monitor central venous pressure	Slow infusion rate; contact physician

10. Normal hematocrit (with ECF deficit)
11. Absence of postural hypotension or normal blood pressure

B. Fluid excesses
1. Fluid output in proportion to fluid intake
2. Weight loss of (specify)
3. Absence of headache, drowsiness, weakness
4. Absence of muscle cramps or twitches
5. Mental alertness
6. Normal serum sodium level
7. Normal serum osmolality
8. Normal specific gravity of urine
9. Reduction of ankle edema or ascites (with ECF excess)
10. Clear breath sounds
11. Normal CVP

II. Electrolyte and acid-base imbalances

A. Electrolyte deficits or excesses
1. Fluid output in proportion to intake
2. Normal serum sodium level
3. Normal plasma potassium level
4. Normal plasma calcium level
5. Normal serum osmolality
6. Normal specific gravity of urine
7. Absence of signs of deficit or excess (specify)

B. Acid-base disturbances
1. Normal plasma pH
2. Normal urine pH
3. Normal $Paco_2$
4. Normal plasma bicarbonate level
5. Normal respiratory rate and depth

Summary

Fluid and electrolyte problems are often an integral part of other physiologic problems. Tests of body fluids such as blood, vomitus, and urine can reflect these problems. Fluid and electrolyte imbalances are discovered chiefly through laboratory examination of the blood plasma.

Four types of fluid imbalance are water deficit (dehydration), water excess (overhydration), isotonic sodium and water deficits, and isotonic sodium and water excesses. This chapter outlines the factors contributing to imbalances, their effects, their signs and symptoms, the clinical picture (laboratory findings) that these imbalances present, and the appropriate medical treatment for each.

The most common electrolyte imbalances are sodium, potassium, and calcium deficits or excesses. Acid-base imbalances occur when the pH of the body fluid is either higher or lower than the normal range of 7.35 to 7.45. There are two types of acid-base disturbances: respiratory and metabolic. With either type of disturbance, acidosis and alkalosis can occur. The kidneys or lungs respond to correct these acid-base imbalances.

Parenteral fluid therapy includes the intravenous administration of fluids and electrolytes. A wide variety of solutions are available for IV administration. Nursing intervention for patients receiving intravenous infusions includes the following:

1. Explanation and teaching
2. Comfort and assistance with activity as required
3. Maintenance of the intravenous infusion, which includes observing for possible complications, changing containers, regulating flow rates, and changing tubing

A number of venipuncture sites can be used. The choice usually depends on the type of infusion, the duration of the infusion, and the age of the patient. Blood transfusions are the intravenous introduction of whole blood or components of blood. The transfused blood needs to be matched with the patient's blood.

Total parenteral nutrition (hyperalimentation) is the administration of hypertonic solutions of carbohydrates, amino acids, and fats for nourishment. These are usually administered by intravenous catheter into the superior vena cava through the internal jugular and subclavian veins. Nursing intervention involves explanation and reassurance to the patient, maintenance of the infusion, record of intake and output, daily measurement of weight, daily blood pressure measurement, provision of exercise, urine analysis, and assessment for complications as well as mouth care.

Suggested Activities

In a laboratory setting:

1. Assemble the following equipment:
   a. IV solution containers: plastic containers (bags) and glass bottles with and without air vents
   b. Administration sets for each of the above containers
   c. IV pole
   d. Receptacle; e.g., a kidney basin
2. Set up an IV line in readiness for a venipuncture. First read the instructions on the package of the administration set. When spiking and priming the tubing, pay particular attention to maintaining sterile technique.
3. Regulate the drip rate. First check the drop factor on the administration package(s), place the tubing end into

a receptacle, and then regulate the flow for the following infusion orders:

- **a.** 1000 ml in 8 hours
- **b.** 2000 ml in 24 hours
- **c.** 100 ml per hour

4. Fill out a time label for a 1000 ml intravenous infusion that is to deliver 125 ml per hour and is to run from 0800 hours to 1600 hours. Place the label on the solution container and have another person check it for accuracy.

5. Change the fluid container, paying attention to maintaining sterile technique.

6. Attach the IV line to a venipuncture needle on a mannequin and change the fluid container, the IV tubing, and the venipuncture dressing.

In a clinical setting:

1. Select five patients who have had laboratory tests for blood electrolytes. Compare the results with the normal values. If any of the readings are abnormal, assess the patients for relevant clinical signs of deficits or excesses.

2. Review the records of several patients who are receiving IV therapy and note where and how the nurses recorded:

- **a.** An IV that was started
- **b.** A change of IV solution
- **c.** A change of IV tubing
- **d.** Discontinuance of an IV
- **e.** Measurement of the IV fluid on intake and output records

3. Determine the reasons why different patients are receiving IV therapy and the types of solutions used.

4. Observe a nurse perform a venipuncture on a patient.

Suggested Readings

Kurdi, W. J. November 1975. Refining your I.V. therapy techniques. *Nursing 75* 5:41–47.

Intravenous therapy procedures are outlined in a step-by-step format with accompanying photographs. Included are inserting the needle, taping needles and catheters, applying armboards, regulating flow rates, and changing bottles and tubing.

McGrath, B. J. January-February 1980. Fluids, electrolytes, and replacement therapy in pediatric nursing. *Maternal Child Nursing* 5:58–62.

After reviewing normal fluid and electrolyte levels, the author describes therapy for dehydration. Included are the nourishment required by infants, the administration of fluid to children of various ages, and IV therapy. Medication is discussed as a possible source of imbalance.

Scarlato, M. February 1978. Blood transfusions today: what you should know and do. *Nursing 78* 8:68–70, 72.

This article outlines the nurse's responsibilities and nursing guidelines for transfusions. Checklists are provided to help the nurse minimize the risks of transfusing whole blood, packed red blood cells, platelets, and plasma fractions.

Snively, W. D., Jr., and Roberts, K. T. 1973. The clinical picture as an aid to understanding body fluid disturbances. *Nursing Forum* 12(2):132–59.

A concise but comprehensive outline of 16 diagnostic classifications of body fluid disturbances. A resume of a few actual patients is included to emphasize the clinical picture approach to understanding the body fluid imbalance.

Selected References

Abbott Laboratories, Ltd. 1970. *Fluids and electrolytes.* Montreal: Abbott Laboratories.

Beaumont, E. July 1977. The new IV infusion pumps. *Nursing 77* 7:31–35.

Borgen, L. February 1978. Total parenteral nutrition in adults. *American Journal of Nursing* 78:224–28.

Burke, S. R. 1980. *The composition and function of body fluids.* 3rd ed. St. Louis: C. V. Mosby Co.

Byrne, C. J.; Saxton, D. F.; Pelikan, P. K.; and Nugent, P. M. 1981. *Laboratory tests implications for nurses and allied health professionals.* Menlo Park, Calif.: Addison-Wesley Publishing Co.

Dickens, M. L. 1974. *Fluid and electrolyte balance: A programmed text.* 3rd ed. Philadelphia: F. A. Davis Co.

Gahart, B. L. 1981. *Intravenous medications: A handbook for nurses and other allied health personnel.* St. Louis: C. V. Mosby Co.

Goldberg, P. B. September-October 1980. Medications that contain sodium. *Geriatric Nursing* 1:204–5.

Guyton, A. C. 1981. *Textbook of medical physiology.* 6th ed. Philadelphia: W. B. Saunders Co.

Harvey, A. M.; Johns, R. J.; McKusick, V. A.; Owens, A. H.; and Ross, R. S. 1980. *The principles and practice of medicine.* 20th ed. New York: Appleton-Century-Crofts.

Intermed Communications. 1981. *Monitoring fluid and electrolytes precisely.* Nursing Skillbook Series. Horsham, Pa.: Intermed Communications.

Kee, J. L., and Gregory, A. P. June 1974. The ABC's (and mEq's) of fluid balance in children. *Nursing 74* 4:28–36.

Keithley, J. K. March 1982. What's behind the IV line? *Nursing 82* 12:32–42.

Kozier, B., and Erb, G. 1982. *Techniques in clinical nursing: A comprehensive approach.* Menlo Park, Calif.: Addison-Wesley Publishing Co.

Kurdi, W. J. November 1975. Refining your I.V. therapy techniques. *Nursing 75* 5:41–47.

Lee, C. A.; Stroot, V. R.; and Schaper, C. A. August 1975. What to do when acid-base problems hang in the balance. *Nursing 75* 5:32–37.

MacBryde, C. M., and Blacklow, R. S. 1970. *Signs and symptoms: Applied pathologic physiology and clinical interpretation.* 5th ed. Philadelphia: J. B. Lippincott Co.

Reed, G. M. March 1974. Confused about potassium? Here's a clear concise guide. *Nursing 74* 4:21.

Sharer, J. E. June 1975. Reviewing acid-base balance. *American Journal of Nursing* 75:980–83.

Spence, A. P., and Mason, E. B. 1979. *Human anatomy and physiology.* Menlo Park, Calif.: Benjamin/Cummings Publishing Co.

Tripp, A. July 1976. Hyper and hypocalcemia. *American Journal of Nursing* 76:1142–45.

Ungvarski, P. J. December 1976. Parenteral therapy. *American Journal of Nursing* 76:1974–77.

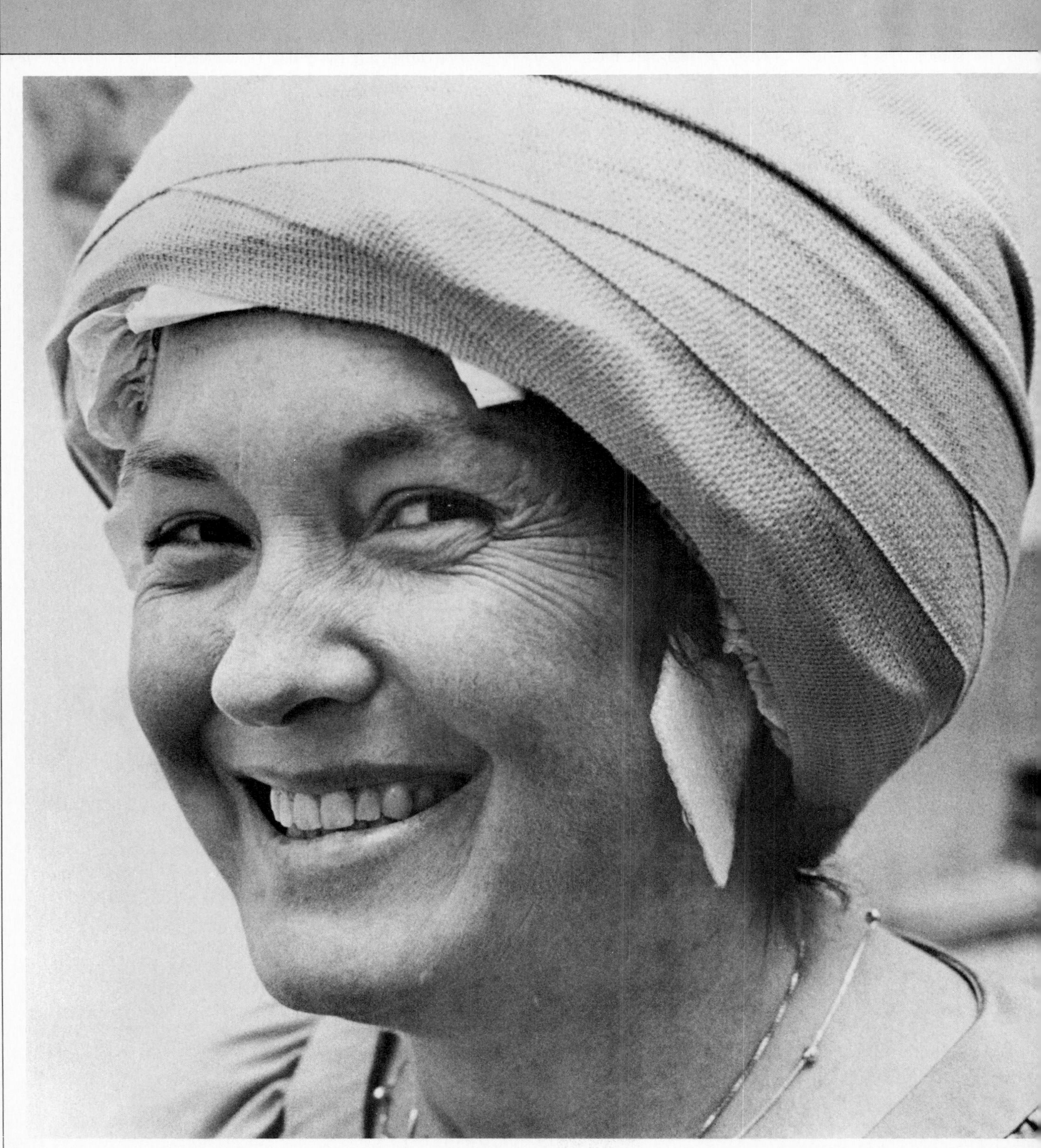

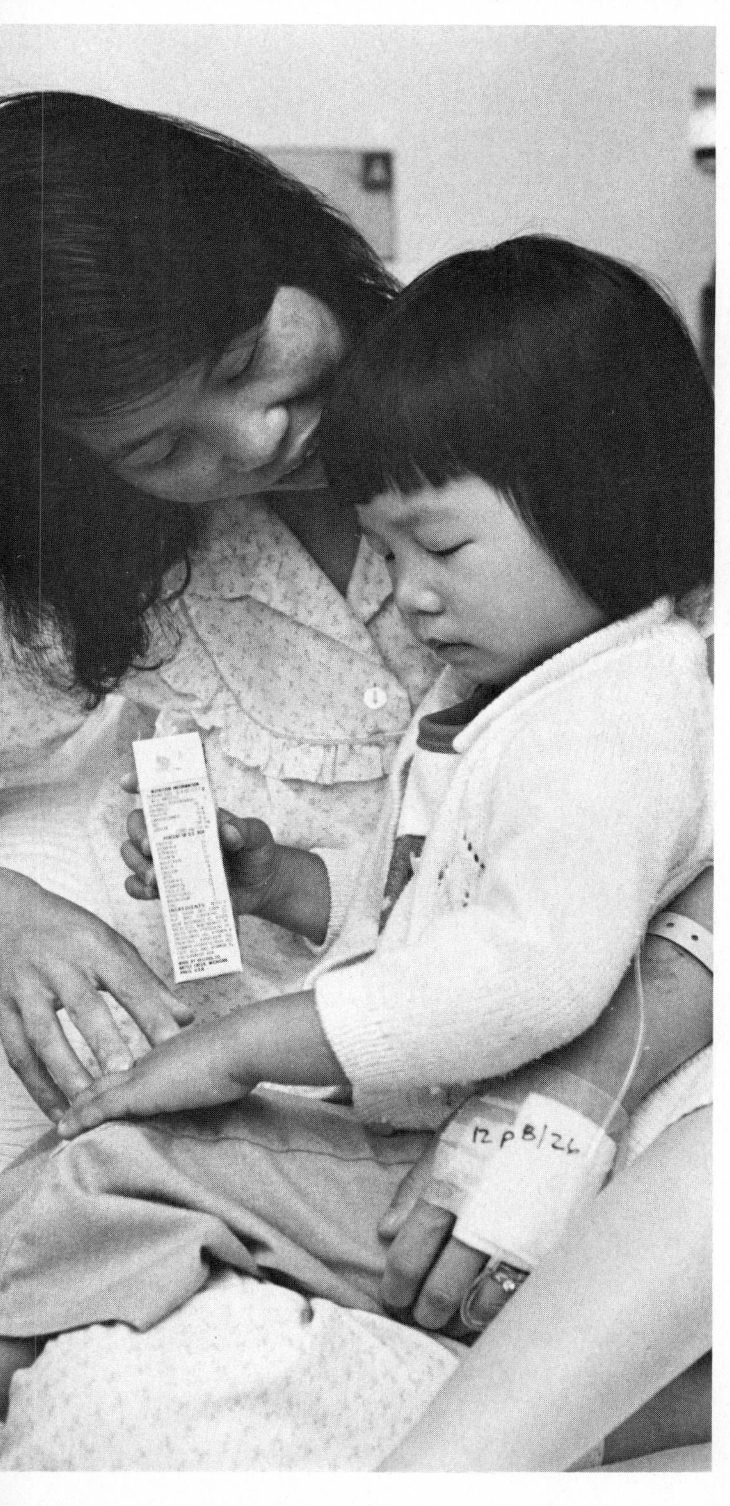

Unit VII

Psychosocial Needs of Patients

CONTENTS

Chapter 32

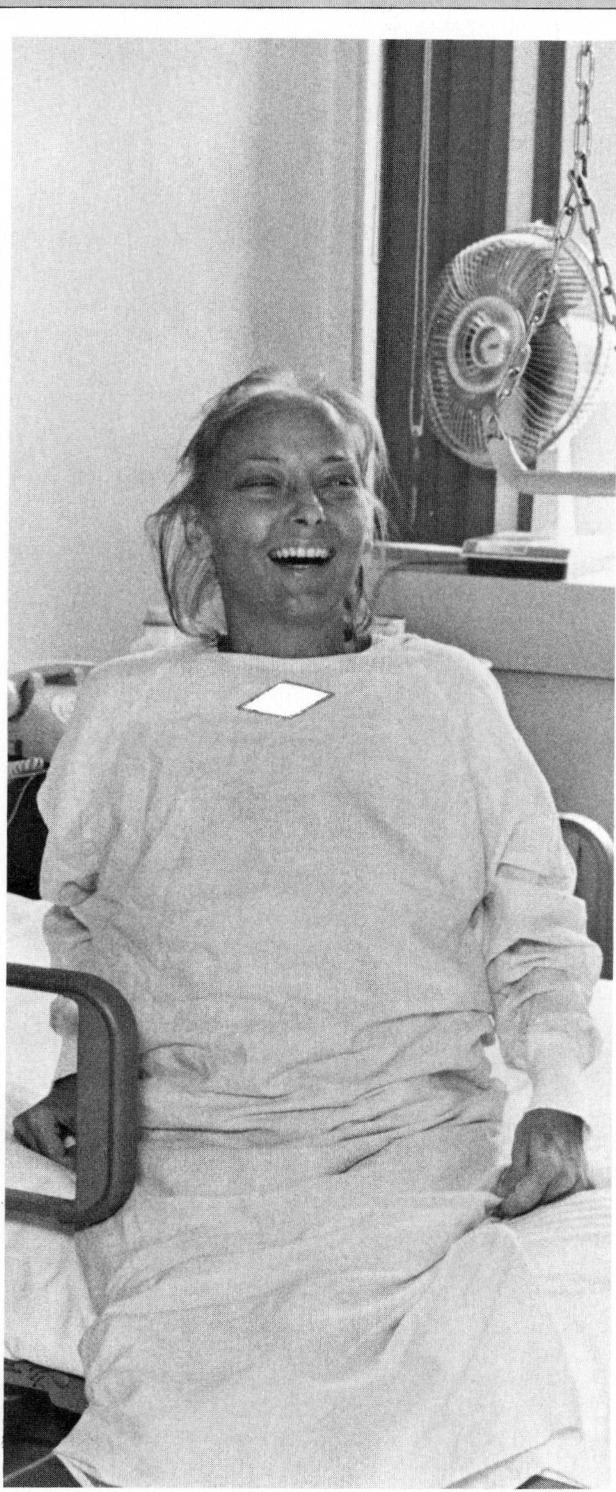

Healthy Self-Concept

CONTENTS

Objectives

1. Understand characteristics and components of self-concept
- **1.1** Define selected terms
- **1.2** Identify essential components of self-concept
- **1.3** Identify characteristics of self-concept
- **1.4** Identify essential aspects of the development of self-concept
- **1.5** Identify behaviors that indicate positive and negative self-concept
- **1.6** Identify factors that influence self-concept
- **1.7** Identify essential aspects of the concept of self-esteem
- **1.8** Identify essential aspects of the development of self-esteem

2. Know information and methods required to assess self-concept and its components
- **2.1** Identify essential information to obtain in a health history
- **2.2** Identify clinical signs and symptoms of behavior patterns such as anxiety, anger, guilt, powerlessness, overdependence, low self-esteem, and depression that indicate problems with self-concept

3. Know essential facts about nursing diagnoses and common problems related to self-concept
- **3.1** List common nursing diagnoses
- **3.2** Identify verbal and nonverbal cues indicating selected nursing diagnoses

4. Know essential facts about nursing measures to maintain, promote, and restore a patient's self-concept
- **4.1** Identify nursing goals
- **4.2** Identify general nursing guidelines
- **4.3** Identify specific interventions for anxiety, anger, guilt, powerlessness, dependence problems, low self-esteem, and body image disturbance

5. Apply the nursing process when providing care to selected patients with self-concept problems
- **5.1** Obtain necessary assessment data
- **5.2** Analyze and relate assessment data
- **5.3** Write relevant nursing diagnoses
- **5.4** Write relevant nursing goals
- **5.5** Plan appropriate nursing interventions
- **5.6** Implement appropriate nursing interventions
- **5.7** State outcome criteria for evaluating the patient's progress

Terms

aggression
anger
anxiety
behavior modification
body image
dependence
depression
ego integrity
fear
generativity
guilt
hostility
independence
interdependence
powerlessness
self-concept
self-consistency
self-esteem
self-expectancy
self-ideal
suicide
violence

Individuals derive their self-concepts from experiences and interactions, in particular with people they value highly. Body image is a part of self-concept that is of particular concern to nurses. After injury, a patient often must change his or her body image to conform to reality. Self-concept guides behavior and helps a person set goals.

Self-esteem (self-acceptance, self-worth), one aspect of self-concept, is an individual's feeling of personal value or worth. Self-esteem is a part of every feeling experienced by a person.

Sexuality is another part of self-concept. It is discussed in Chapter 33.

Self-Concept

Self-concept is the aggregate of beliefs and feelings one holds about oneself. It is the most complete description that an individual can give of himself or herself at any one time. It is also a person's frame of reference for experiencing and viewing the world. It has two major components:

1. The *body image* or physical self is an individual's perception of the shape, size, and mass of his or her body plus body functioning, sexuality, appearance, and state of health. An individual's body image may not conform to reality. For example, a man who has been thin for many years and gains weight in a relatively

short period may still think of himself as thin. Problems related to body image are usually connected with loss. The concept of loss is discussed in Chapter 36.

2. The *personal self* has three components (Driever 1976:175–76): the moral–ethical self, self-consistency, and self-ideal (or self-expectancy).

a. The moral-ethical self evaluates who the individual is. This component involves the values held by the individual (see Chapter 10 for additional information on values). It evaluates the relative desirability of perceptions and compares them to held values. When an individual's thoughts or behavior go against held values, the individual feels guilt—the result of conflict in the moral-ethical self.

b. *Self-consistency* is the component that strives to maintain a stable self-image. Therefore, self-image becomes a force in determining personality. Self-consistency explains why a man who loses an arm may think of himself as having two arms until he has had repeated experiences with one arm. Threats to self-consistency appear to cause anxiety.

c. *Self ideal* or *self-expectancy* relates to a person's expectations of being and doing; it is what the individual wants to become. Highly influential in determining the self-ideal are the expectations of significant others. In a close family group, parents influence their children's self-ideals about appearance, education, behavior, etc. When people have difficulty attaining their ideals, they may feel powerless, and this feeling can become a problem.

Self-concept possesses the following characteristics (Combs, Avila, and Purkey 1978:17–28):

1. It integrates the psychologic and physical self, i.e., body characteristics, attitudes, and values.
2. It acts as a screen between the individual and the environment.
3. It readily accepts experiences and perceptions that are in agreement with the self-concept; however, those not in agreement produce anxiety and discomfort.
4. It tends to support existing beliefs about the self. For example, a person who projects shyness will have difficulty making friends, which in turn will perpetuate the shyness.
5. It is stable and changes only with difficulty. For example, a patient who has always envisaged herself as extremely healthy may completely ignore the medications ordered for her heart.
6. It is developed from experiences and interactions with others. Significant others are particularly influential. If a young child learns that she is "stupid," this can remain in her self-perception all her life, unless a healthy self-concept is learned later.

Development of Self-Concept

In psychosocial development there are three major tasks: learning to live with tools, personal self-development, and learning to live with others (Driever 1976:183). Learning to live with tools includes acquiring skills appropriate for each stage of development. The tools can be the toys of a 2-year-old, the athletic skill of the adolescent, or the social skill of the executive in business. Personal self-development involves learning to live with oneself. It includes learning to live with one's impulses and drives and developing acceptable behaviors to deal with them. It also includes an awareness of one's strengths, feelings, and resources. Learning to live with others includes relating to people in a variety of roles and learning to accept and respect others.

Throughout life there are developmental stages. Erikson (1963) proposed eight stages in life that describe stresses on the maturational process (see Table 11–2, on page 235). The success with which a person copes with these stressors largely determines the development of the self-concept. Inability to cope results in self-concept problems both at the time and often later in life.

Trust versus Mistrust

During the first year of life the infant is entirely dependent upon others to meet needs—for nourishment, dryness, warmth, and safety that is positive and consistent. From experiences of having needs met, the infant develops trust in the external environment—a feeling of confidence in the sameness, continuity, and predictability of the environment (Driever 1976:185). From trust in the external environment the infant learns to trust himself or herself. When the infant is uncomfortable and cries, someone will come and assist him or her. The infant's cries can make something happen that will be satisfying.

If infants do not develop trust in the environment and themselves, mistrust can affect the remainder of their lives. They may be unable to trust or rely on themselves or others in future years. The development of trust is basic to the development of the personality, particularly the self-concept.

Behavior indicating trust

1. Requesting assistance and expecting to receive it
2. Expressing belief of another person
3. Sharing time, opinions, and experiences

Behavior indicating mistrust

1. Restricting conversation to superficialities
2. Refusing to provide a person with information
3. Being unable to accept assistance

Autonomy versus Shame and Doubt

An infant who has developed a sense of trust is ready to develop autonomy or a sense of "I." At this stage, the child will use words such as "no" and "I" a great deal. It is important that children have control over an area of living, such as putting toys away. When a child says "no," this needs to be respected by others; yet the child requires some environmental limits so that self-confidence can be maintained. It is important for children to appreciate their impulses as good and not be shamed into appropriate behavior.

Behavior indicating autonomy

1. Accepting the rules of a group but also expressing disagreement when it is felt
2. Expressing one's own opinion
3. Easily accepting deferment of a wish fulfillment

Behavior indicating shame and doubt

1. Failing to express needs
2. Not expressing one's own opinion when opposed
3. Overconcern about being clean

Initiative versus Guilt

With initiative a person develops plans and ideas and puts them into action. From 3 to 5 years most children undertake this developmental task. It is also an age of fantasy and imagination. Children question what they can do and be. It is important that they explore the world and live out various roles through play. Failure to achieve a sense of initiative can result in feelings of guilt. Some guilt feelings are normal, and they must be balanced by a sense of initiative. Also at this stage children start to develop a conscience. They attempt to sort out actions labeled "good" or "bad." Discipline that uses shame creates feelings of guilt and decreases feelings of self-worth.

Behavior indicating initiative

1. Starting projects eagerly
2. Expressing curiosity about many things
3. Demonstrating original thought

Behavior indicating guilt

1. Imitating others rather than developing independent ideas
2. Apologizing and being very embarrassed over small mistakes
3. Verbalizing fear about starting a new project

Industry versus Inferiority

After the development of initiative, the child has positive feelings about "I." At about age 5, the child is ready for school and the new experiences and routines associated with it. At this age, children begin to verbalize feelings about themselves and have both positive and negative judgments. They are heavily influenced by the judgments of significant others.

During this maturational stress period the focus is on learning to obtain recognition by producing things. The child learns to manipulate tools such as pencils and to concentrate on tasks. Completing the task is an objective that the child develops. At this time a child also learns to be active with others and to share.

Inadequacy can develop if children give up trying to handle tools and themselves in relation to given tasks. It is important that children receive guidance about how to succeed and obtain recognition for their successes.

Behavior indicating industry

1. Completing a task once it has been started
2. Working well with others
3. Using time effectively

Behavior indicating inferiority

1. Not completing tasks started
2. Not assisting with the work of others
3. Not organizing work

Identity versus Role Confusion

Adolescents seek answers to "Who and what am I?" At this stage they redefine trust, autonomy, initiative, and industry in terms of a new definition of self, including the sexual changes of adolescence and society's expectations of an adult. During adolescence, individuals reassess all their adaptive mechanisms. Because childhood responses are no longer appropriate, adolescents must change their past relationships, particularly with parents. Their new adult identity assists adolescents to cope with adult experiences and make adult decisions.

The person who is unable to form an adult identity will have role diffusion. Without a strong sense of self the person will feel confused and anxious and will find it difficult to respond to the demands of living in a realistic and stable way.

Behavior indicating identity

1. Establishing relationships with the same sex and then the opposite sex
2. Asserting independence
3. Planning realistically for future roles

Behavior indicating role confusion

1. Failing to assume responsibility for directing one's own behavior
2. Accepting the values of others without question
3. Failing to set goals in life

Intimacy versus Isolation

Achieving intimacy involves developing a close relationship with one special person. It includes committing the self to another person and abandonment of self in close relationships. Failure to achieve intimacy can lead a person to a sense of isolation and self-absorption. A person who is self-absorbed has difficulty perceiving feedback from others and subsequently developing a fuller sense of self.

Behavior indicating intimacy

1. Establishing a close, intense relationship with another person
2. Accepting sexual behavior as desirable
3. Making a commitment to that relationship even in times of stress and sacrifice

Behavior indicating isolation

1. Remaining alone
2. Avoiding close personal relationships with the opposite sex
3. Avoiding the sex role by mannerisms and dress

Generativity versus Stagnation

Generativity is concern with establishing and guiding the next generation. It includes both productivity and creativity. Generativity is not restricted to producing children; it can include producing something to be passed on to another generation such as writing, health, or ideas. When a person cannot pass along something, stagnation results; the person becomes chiefly concerned with self rather than others.

Behavior indicating generativity

1. Being willing to share with another person
2. Guiding others
3. Establishing a priority of needs, recognizing both self and others

Behavior indicating stagnation

1. Talking about oneself instead of listening to others
2. Showing concern for oneself in spite of the needs of others
3. Being unable to accept interdependence

Integrity versus Despair

This last stage in development is largely dependent on the previous stages. For the person who has a sense of trust, autonomy, initiative, industry, identity, intimacy, and generativity, the next developmental stressor is feeling satisfied with one's life and decisions. *Ego integrity* means feeling satisfied with one's life-style and accepting the inevitability of the life cycle.

The person who does not acquire integrity experiences despair and feels that the time left in life is too short to start another life.

Behavior indicating integrity

1. Using past experience to assist others
2. Maintaining productivity in some areas
3. Accepting limitations

Behavior indicating despair

1. Crying and being apathetic
2. Not accepting changes
3. Demanding unnecessary assistance and attention from others

Factors Influencing Self-Concept

A number of factors influence development of the self-concept. Driever (1976:189–90) lists nine factors in two groups: contextual (environmental or milieu) factors and residual factors (those held over from past experiences).

3. The person's present definition of the self-concept as a means of responding to stressors.
4. The person's learned coping mechanisms, such as methods of problem solving and handling feelings.
5. The competence an individual feels, especially in areas that he or she and others value.

Environmental Factors

1. Tools in the environment that a person can learn to use, such as a spoon for feeding oneself or a pencil for writing. When tools such as these are not available, the child will not learn to use them and his or her concept may reflect inability to learn or perform these activities.
2. Feedback, which assists people to learn who they are. Feedback comes from significant people, such as parents, and from all experiences in the environment, such as work or sports.

Past Experience Factors

1. Previous feedback the person has perceived about himself or herself from others, particularly from people considered significant.
2. Previous developmental and situational stressors and how the person coped with these.
3. The person's self-expectations and experiences with success and failure.
4. Particular experiences that either create or deny a sense of value and worth.

Self-Esteem

Self-esteem (self-acceptance, self-worth) is one's feeling of personal value. *Esteem* is worth; people need to value who and what they are. The need for self-esteem was discussed briefly in Chapter 8, on page 174. Maslow's hierarchy of needs presents self-esteem as a fifth-level need just below self-actualization. Kalish's adaptation of Maslow's hierarchy also presents esteem and self-esteem as fifth-level needs above love, belonging, and closeness and below self-actualization. See Figure 8–4 on page 170.

Self-esteem is closely related to self-concept. It is developed to a considerable degree as a result of feedback from others. Self-esteem is also closely related to the moral-ethical self, self-consistency, and the self-ideal (self-expectancy). If one's behavior is consistent with what one believes is moral and ethical, one sees oneself as "good" and valued; if one sees one's behavior as immoral or "bad," one's self-esteem is lowered. People also have a need to be consistent within a changing self-concept. See the discussion on self-concept earlier in this chapter. When consistency is threatened, people feel anxiety. The self-ideal is a person's set of self-expectations. Those who are unable to meet their expectations feel worthless, and their self-esteem is lowered.

Positive self-esteem is referred to as high self-esteem; the converse is low self-esteem or feelings of worthlessness. People who are emotionally healthy are relatively free of feelings of inadequacy and inferiority. Their self-confidence is based on an accurate assessment of themselves. They neither deny their limitations nor exaggerate their abilities (Wilson and Kneisl 1982:248). Problems of low self-esteem can result in depression.

Self-esteem is largely based on the individual's values. Some of these values may be relatively permanent, while others change. For example, at 18 years of age, a football player may value his physical strength and speed; later in life, he may value his family relationships and his work ability more than his strength and speed.

Development of Self-Esteem

Self-esteem is learned through interaction with others. Children with high self-esteem often come from families where the parents had high self-esteem, the children's accomplishments were valued and praised, there was a warm, affectionate relationship between children and parents, and yet fairly strict limits were set on the children's behavior (Bee 1975:285).

How a person learns to handle feelings of anger and

aggression affects self-esteem. People learn from others how to handle these feelings. For example, a little girl who loses a favorite doll may express her disappointment by angry, acting out behavior. Adults who wish the child to control her behavior may indicate that showing anger is bad. If the child is reprimanded not only for the behavior but for the feeling, and this is reinforced repeatedly, the child learns that to feel and express feelings is "bad." Because situations repeatedly arise when the girl has these feelings, she feels guilty for having "bad" feelings. She needs to deal with loss by not showing feelings of anger and sadness. She turns these feelings inward and feels less self-worth.

A second area in which children learn self-esteem is through the limitations placed on their behavior. Children who grow up within well-defined and enforced limits learn about reality because their behavior results in consequences. They learn to make decisions about their behavior and to obtain positive and negative reinforcement. The child who does not have limits set does not have the opportunity to obtain positive reinforcement and thus to attain high self-esteem. As an adult, this person will probably have low self-esteem and have more difficulty setting limits on both personal behavior and that of others.

Assessment of Self-Concept

Assessment of problems related to self-concept is normally indicated if (a) the patient and/or support persons present cues that could reflect problems, or (b) the patient's illness is one often associated with self-concept problems. Problems with self-concept are frequently manifested by expressions of anxiety, fear, anger, hostility, guilt, powerlessness, or low self-esteem. Behaviors reflecting excessive role conflict may also indicate the need for meaningful intervention by nurses.

The nursing assessment involves (a) health history, (b) examination for clinical signs, and (c) factors influencing self-concept.

Nursing History

Because this aspect of a nursing history is highly personal, it is important that the patient trust the nurse. Using Gordon's (1982:90–97) framework of health patterns in this context, the nurse assesses:

1. Self-perception–self-concept pattern
2. Role-relationship pattern
3. Sexuality-reproductive pattern (see Chapter 33)
4. Coping-stress-tolerance pattern
5. Value-belief pattern

Using Roy's (1976) organizational framework for self-concept, the nurse assesses:

1. Physical self
2. Personal self
    a. Moral-ethical self
    b. Self-consistency
    c. Self-ideal

After establishing the framework for collecting the data, the nurse asks specific questions; for example, to elicit information about the self-perception–self-concept pattern, "How would you describe yourself?" "Have you changed in the way you feel about youself?" "Do you find that some things frequently make you angry?" (Gordon 1982:18).

Clinical Examination

Clinical examination of the patient is both general and specific. General mental-emotional assessment was discussed in Chapter 14, on page 352. Specific assessments of the verbal and nonverbal behaviors that reflect manifestations of problems of self-concept (e.g., guilt) may also be required. Each patient presents a unique combination of clinical signs that may reflect an underlying problem. One patient who has low self-esteem may overeat, while another declines to eat.

Anxiety

Anxiety is mental uneasiness evidenced by an increased level of arousal due to an impending or anticipated threat to self or significant relationships. When a person's self-consistency is threatened, anxiety arises. Anxiety may be anticipatory or actual and may be mild, moderate, or severe. See Table 32–1 for signs of each degree. Anxiety is usually a precursor to fear.

Fear

Fear is a feeling of dread related to an *identifiable source* that the person validates (Kim and Moritz 1982:280). The identified source is perceived as a threat or danger to self. Contributing factors are a knowledge deficit and perceived or actual powerlessness (loss of control over events). Clinical signs of fear are similar to those of anxiety. See Table 32–1.

Table 32–1 Signs of Mild, Moderate, and Severe Anxiety

Sign	Mild	Moderate	Severe (panic)
Verbalization changes	Expresses feelings of increased arousal and concern Increased questioning or information seeking	Expresses feelings of tension, apprehension, nervousness, or concern Verbalizes expectation of danger Voice tremors and pitch changes Increased rate and quantity of verbalization	Expresses feelings of severe dread, apprehension, nervousness, concern, helplessness, and isolation Absence of verbalization Inappropriate verbalization, e.g., false cheerfulness or laughing while discussing a serious subject
Motor activity changes	Mild restlessness	Pacing Hand tremor or shakiness Increased muscle tension	Immobilization Purposeless activity Increased muscle tension Rigid posture
Perception and attention changes	Increased awareness Increased attending Ability to focus on most of what is really happening	Narrowed focus of attention Ability to focus on most of what is really happening	Fixed or scattered perceptual focus Intellectualizing about a subject, e.g., explaining the pathophysiology of leukemia rather than describing own feelings Intent and fearful watching of everything going on Inability to focus on what is really happening Inability to focus on reality, e.g., denial, saying "I don't want to talk about it"
Respiratory and circulatory changes	Nil	Rapid pulse Increased respiratory rate	Tachycardia Palpitations Hyperventilation
Other changes	Nil	Diaphoresis Sleep or eating disturbances, e.g., insomnia, somnolence, overeating, or anorexia Irritability	Diaphoresis Dilated pupils Pallor Clammy hands and skin Dry mouth Sullenness, withdrawal

Compiled from M. Gordon, *Manual of nursing diagnosis* (New York: McGraw-Hill Book Co., 1982), pp. 153–60; and Anxiety: Recognition and intervention (programmed instruction), *American Journal of Nursing*, September 1965, 65:129–52.

Anger

Anger is an emotional state consisting of a subjective feeling of animosity or strong displeasure. In North America the term is unfortunately often used to refer to physical attacks and violence; as a result, any expression of anger may be labeled bad. Many people feel guilty when they feel anger, because they have learned that to feel angry is wrong.

In fact, anger, hostility, violence, and aggression differ. Anger can be expressed in a nonalienating verbal manner; it is then considered a positive emotion and a sign of emotional maturity, since growth and beneficial interactions result from it.

Rothenberg (1971:454) defines the expression of anger as an assertive, altered communicative state that arises as an alternative to, and a defense against, anxiety. Anger is commonly manifested in (a) altered voice tone and (b) a communication to desist from some action or other. Verbal expression of anger can therefore be considered a signal to others of one's internal psychologic discomfort and a call for assistance to deal with perceived stress.

Hostility is usually marked by overt antagonism and harmful or destructive behavior. *Aggression* is usually defined as an unprovoked attack or a hostile, injurious, or destructive action or outlook. *Violence* is the exertion of physical force to injure or abuse. Verbally expressed anger differs from hostility, aggression, and violence, but it can lead to destructiveness and violence if the anger persists unabated.

The state of anger can be viewed as a communication process that involves a recurring sequence of events with several vicious cycles and means to achieve closure or completion. See Figure 32–1. The sequence of events, according to Rothenberg (1971:456), is:

1. A threat, need, or obstruction creates a stressful state, which causes anxiety. Anxiety is manifested by undirected, purposeless motor responses (e.g., pacing the floor) or avoidance or escape responses. Anxiety evokes feelings of helplessness and defenselessness.

2. Anxiety develops into anger when motor responses are directed at the real or imagined source of arousal. Anger provides a defense against anxiety and feelings of helplessness, because the person feels more powerful and in control when angry, unless the context makes the anger socially unacceptable. If anger is socially unacceptable, more anxiety is created. If in addition the person has destructive thoughts about the person or object causing the stressful state, guilt feelings often result, which further increase anxiety.

3. Tension is discharged and anger is prolonged or resolved by either:

a. Fight (attack) or flight responses coupled with noncommunication. These responses prolong tension and lead to potential hostility and violence.

b. Verbalizing internal experiences clearly or unclearly and avoiding physical attack. When anger is clearly communicated, tension is relieved and anger is dissipated; when it is not clearly communicated, i.e., the communication does not focus on the cause of the anger, the outcome is the same as when no communication has taken place.

People may fail to express anger verbally for several reasons (ibid.):

1. To be tactful or polite in social situations

2. To avoid loss of power and status or to avoid placing themselves at a disadvantage in conflict relationships

3. For fear of eliciting anger from others

4. For fear of revealing their needs and vulnerability to others in conflict relationships

5. For fear of evoking physical destructiveness in themselves or others

6. For fear of exposing their level of involvement in relationships, e.g., love relationships

7. Because of immediate recognition that they have made an error in perception

Clearly expressed verbal communication of anger is constructive. When the angry person tells the other person about the anger and carefully identifies the source, the anger is constructive. This clarity of communication gets the anger out into the open, so that the other person can deal with it and help to alleviate it. The angry person "gets it off his chest" and prevents an emotional buildup. Constructive expressions of anger have three elements: alerting, describing, and identifying (Duldt 1981:516). *Alerting* is the act of engaging another's attention. *Describing* is the process of delineating the source of the angry person's feelings, i.e., what has happened here and now. *Identifying* is the act of seeking a response and support from others. Examples of constructive anger are:

- "Damn it! (Alerting.) This electric drill makes me mad! It won't work. (Describing.) What am I doing wrong?" (Identifying.)
- "You SOB! (Alerting.) Your going to the football game this afternoon infuriates me. You said yesterday you'd clean the car for me before I have to drive my friends to the church social tonight. (Describing.) Now what am I going to do?" (Identifying.)

Unclear communication of anger is destructive. It is similar to constructive expressions only in the alerting behavior. Then the person fails to describe the source of the feelings adequately and denies any responsibility for the anger by blaming others or by generalizing to other people or past situations. Thus, those in the presence of the angry person are unable to respond helpfully. Examples of unclearly expressed anger are:

- "Damn it! (Alerting.) A woman can never win." (Generalizing.)
- "You SOB! (Alerting.) You're always leaving me in the lurch." (Generalizing, blaming.)

In assessing an individual's anger, the nurse notes verbal cues and any clinical signs presented by the person. Sometimes patients have difficulty expressing their anger directly because they are not aware of the feelings. The developmental stage of the individual is a

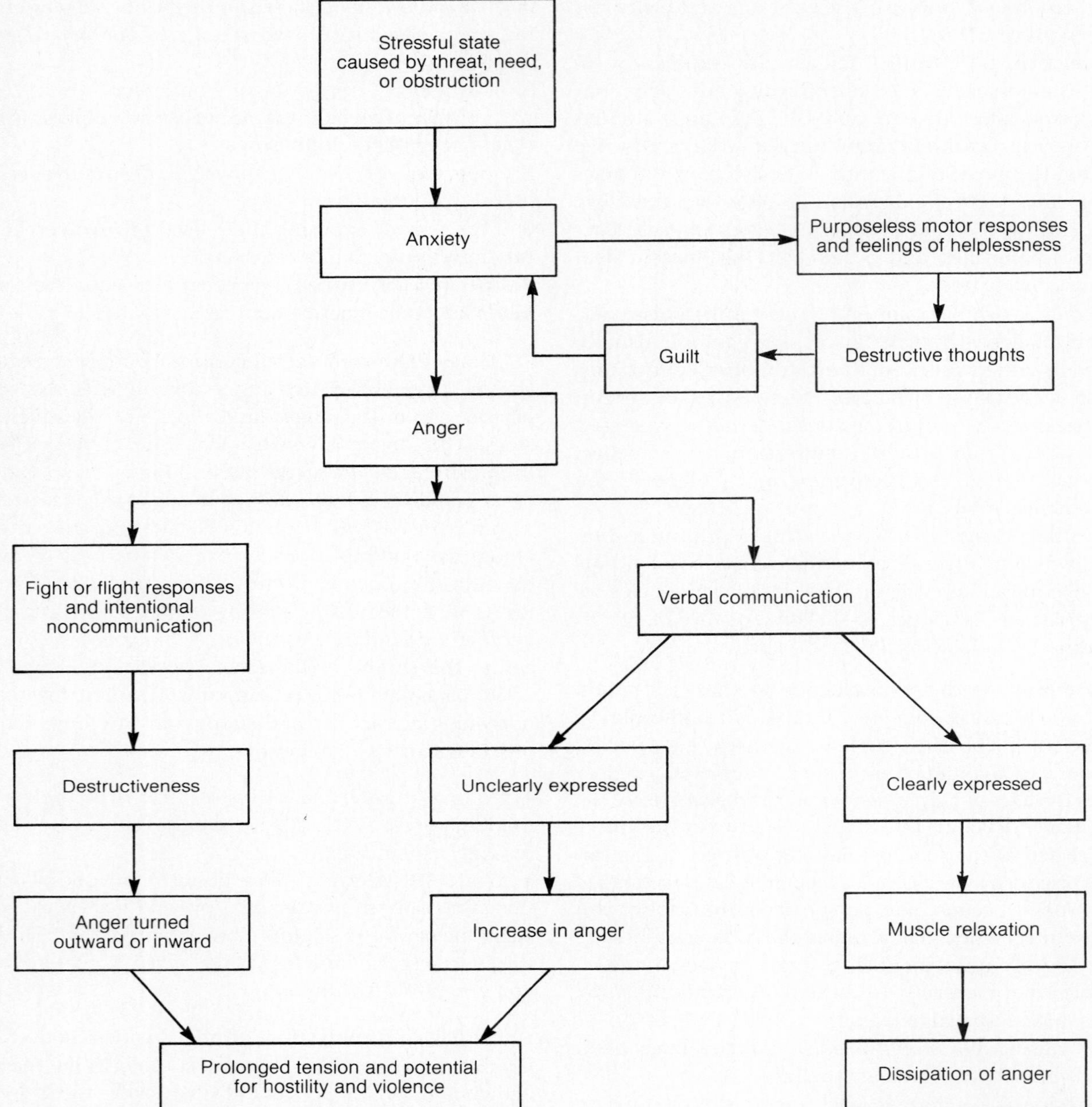

Figure 32–1 Model of anger as a communication process. (Adapted from B. W. Duldt, Anger: An occupational hazard for nurses, *Nursing Outlook*, September 1981, 29:514.)

factor in assessing the appropriateness of anger as a response. See Table 32–2.

Verbal cues

- "I really don't care what happens."
- "My family doesn't care."
- "I really gave him a good smack."
- "I am really furious underneath."
- "I feel like throwing that television out the window."

Clinical signs

- Excessive use of alcohol, drugs, smoking
- Refusal to follow medical advice
- Poor grooming, an unkempt appearance
- Flushed face and distended neck veins
- Pacing about, slamming doors, pounding a table with the fist
- Diaphoresis, continual motion of the hands or body
- Muscular tension and rigidity

Table 32–2 Normal Stimuli Producing Anger at Varying Developmental Stages

Age	Stimuli producing anger
Infant	Interference with movement or wishes
Toddler	Dependence on others to control internal and external environments
Adolescent	Perceived unfairness, sarcasm, teasing
	Interference with self-assertion
	Criticism, unwanted advice
Adult	Threat to self-esteem
	Frustration of plans or intentions

Guilt

Guilt is the painful feeling associated with transgression of a person's moral-ethical beliefs. The development of the superego (Freud's term) or conscience takes place after age 3. Persons usually internalize the norms of their culture, society, and religion and learn to control impulses contrary to these norms.

Verbal cues

- "I am to blame," "It's my fault."
- Apologizing frequently
- Encouraging reprimands from others to punish self
- Hypersensitivity to others
- Crying without obvious reason

Clinical signs

- Stooped posture and slow movement
- Decreased gastric functioning
- Stammering, flushing
- Insomnia

Powerlessness

Powerlessness is a person's perception of lack of control over events in a specific situation. The individual anticipates that he or she is unable to determine certain outcomes. Powerlessness results from a problem in the individual's self-ideal. To become what one desires and expects to be, one must have some control over events. For example, a young man who wants to become a lawyer may feel powerlessness because his father wants him to enter the family business and he feels he cannot act against his father's wishes.

Verbal cues

- "I'll do whatever anyone wants."
- "Whatever is destined will happen."
- "I can't make up my mind what to do."
- "I don't understand what's happening."
- "I feel depressed about all this."

Clinical signs

- Less than normal alertness to the environment
- Restlessness and sleeplessness
- Apathy
- Aimless wandering

Overdependence and overindependence

Dependence can be described as reliance on other people for satisfaction and reward. *Independence* is manifested by self-reliance and self-assertiveness. *Interdependence* is a balance of dependent and independent relationships (McIntier 1976:291).

In North America, interdependence is approved. Dependence is usually sanctioned during infancy, childhood, old age, and physical and mental illness. Traditionally, it was also sanctioned for females, but the women's movement of the 1970s has done a great deal to change this.

Overdependence and overindependence may be manifested by patients with self-concept difficulties.

Cues to overdependence

- Asks for physical assistance unnecessarily
- Seeks attention by speaking loudly, overcommunicating, and asking irrelevant questions
- Seeks affection by persistently touching another with the hands or whispering
- Seeks approval and praise, e.g., by asking for compliments or by giving gifts to gain recognition

Cues to overindependence

- Takes the initiative prematurely in a task
- Exhibits persistence and repeated effort in spite of obstacles, e.g., tries to eat repeatedly in spite of limitation to a supine position, fatigue, and difficulty reaching the food
- Shows stubbornness, e.g., refuses to take medications until the physician tells the patient personally that these are necessary
- Exhibits excessive firmness, e.g., refuses to allow relatives to arrange for the patient to enter a hospital even though the patient is ill

Low self-esteem

Levels of self-esteem range from high to low. A person who has high self-esteem deals actively with the environment, adapts effectively to change, and feels secure.

A person with low self-esteem sees the environment as negative and threatening (Driever 1976:233).

Verbal cues

- "I feel tired all the time."
- "I'm not interested in that."
- "Nobody really cares about me."
- "I can never tell her how she bothers me."
- "I'm just a burden to everyone."

Clinical signs

- Anorexia or overeating
- Constipation or diarrhea
- Insomnia
- Poor posture

Depression

Depression is an emotional condition experienced by most people at one time or another. It involves real or imagined loss of a particular function, capacity, object, dream, person, belief, or value to which the individual is "normally" or "inordinately" attached (Drake and Price 1975:163). Disruption of a "normal" attachment results in a sense of grief or loss that is usually self-limiting (see Chapter 36 for additional information on grief and loss). However, disruption of an "inordinate" attachment results in grief that leads to depression. "Inordinate" attachments occur when the lost relationship, ambition, or expectation is the basis of the person's feelings of self-esteem, competence, or security. Individuals whose self-concept is poor or whose self-esteem is low are highly vulnerable to a disruption or loss that leads to depression. The extent of a depressive reaction to loss is often determined by the nature and degree of the attachment.

Sources of disruption or loss The sources of a disruption can be internal or external. Internal sources include thoughts, attitudes, or actions that do not agree with the person's values, beliefs, or morals; and interpersonal conflicts that threaten the individual's self-consistency, self-esteem, or security (Drake and Price 1975:163–64). External sources include death of a significant other, job termination, illness, or loss of a body part.

Conceptual framework of depression A conceptual framework describing a significant disruption or loss leading to depression is shown in Figure 32–2. The stressor may be internal or external—for example, giving up a dream of living near a beloved daughter (internal), or failure to pass an examination (external). The meaning of the loss to the individual can stimulate other activities and subsequent resolution of the problem or stimulate feelings of helplessness, anger, and depression. The individual who has low self-esteem, ambivalent feelings, or unhealthy dependent relationships often denies his or her individuality and unique feelings; anger and aggressive activity are logical outcomes of this denial. If these are expressed outwardly in a constructive manner (for example, by confronting the instructor whose examination was failed and demanding an explanation of what the shortcomings were), then the problem may be resolved. If the anger is expressed destructively, however (for example, by swearing at or blaming the teacher or breaking windows in the school), anxiety and guilt are usually experienced subsequently. This guilt often leads to further feelings of helplessness. If the anger and aggression are turned inward, with the accompanying feelings of guilt, the person will acquire painful symptoms of depression to atone for the guilt. These symptoms can, in turn, cause disruption and loss, thus perpetuating the cycle.

The clinical signs and cues of depression may be overt or very subtle. Fatigue may be the most frequent indicator.

Verbal cues

- "I feel so tired all the time."
- "Nothing will help."
- "I'm not worth all that trouble."

Clinical signs

- Fatigue
- Insomnia
- Anorexia and weight loss or increased appetite and weight gain
- Constipation
- Dry skin
- Somatic complaints
- Inability to concentrate, loss of interest
- Ambivalance and indecisiveness

Suicidal tendencies

Suicide is taking one's own life. Many depressed people think about suicide at one time or another as a means of ending their suffering. People who present cues that reflect thinking about suicide should be taken seriously. Those who threaten suicide often follow up by doing it.

Verbal cues

- "When you're dead, there is nothing to worry about."
- "People who shoot themselves are smarter than those who take poison."

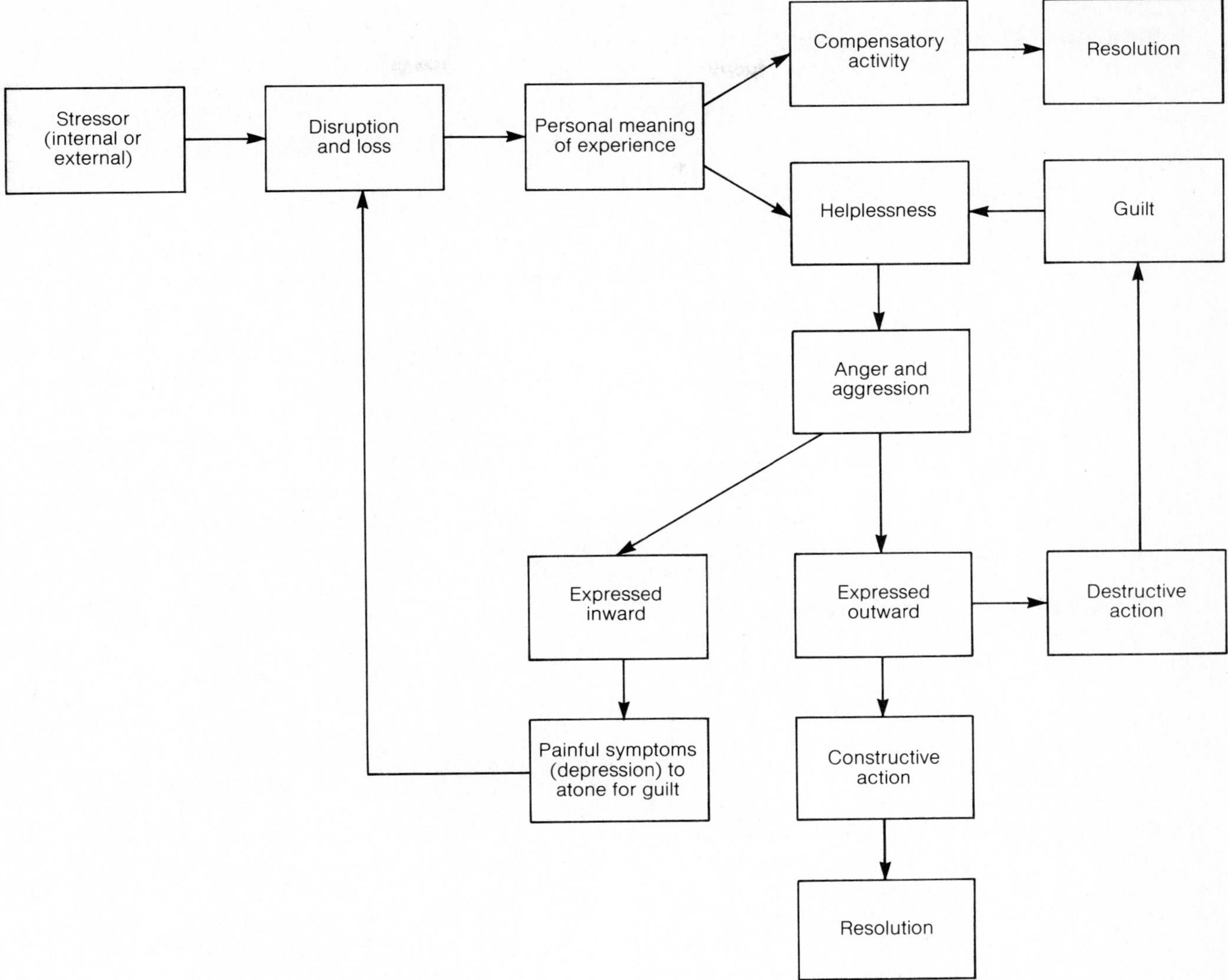

Figure 32–2 Process of disruption and loss leading to depression. (Adapted from R. E. Drake and J. L. Price, Depression: Adaptation to disruption and loss, *Perspectives in Psychiatric Care*, October/December 1975, 13:166.

Clinical signs

- Hiding supplies or equipment that can be used for suicide, e.g., tranquilizers or sedatives
- Abruptly changing mood from tense sadness to relaxed smiling; this often indicates that the patient has accepted the idea of suicide and made plans

Nursing Diagnoses

Nursing diagnoses for patients with problems related to self-concept include disturbances in body image, self-esteem, individual coping, and sexuality. Sexuality is discussed in Chapter 33.

Body image disturbance is defined as negative feelings or perceptions about characteristics, functions, or limits of the body or a body part (Gordon 1982:162). The patient's verbal or nonverbal cues indicating actual or perceived changes in body structure and function must be present before this diagnosis is made. Cues indicative of a body image disturbance are listed in Table 32–3.

Self-esteem disturbance is defined as negative feelings or conception of one's social self or capabilities (Ibid., p. 172). It is often related to unrealistic self-expectations or loss of significant roles. See Table 32–3 for verbal and nonverbal indications of a disturbance in self-esteem.

Table 32–3 Clinical Signs of Self-Concept Disturbances

Disturbance	Verbal cues (subjective data)	Nonverbal cues (objective data)
Body image disturbance	Fears reaction of others or rejection by others Has negative feelings about own body, e.g., that it is unsightly Feels powerless or hopeless Emphasizes previous appearance or function Talks excessively about loss or change Personalizes (gives name to) part or loss Depersonalizes (uses impersonal pronoun, such as "it" or "that" for) body part or loss	Does not look at body part Does not touch body part Hides body part Overexposes body part Changes social involvements or relationships
Self-esteem disturbance	Expresses shame or guilt, e.g., "I am to blame," apologizes excessively Evaluates self as unable to deal with situations	Avoids eye contact Stoops in posture Moves slowly Engages in self-destructive behavior, such as overindulgence in alcohol Does not follow through with activities Tends to be a listener rather than a participant Neglects appearance and care Is unable to accept compliments
Ineffective coping	Verbalizes inability to cope Expresses anxiety, fear, or anger	Manifests anxiety, fear, or anger Does not ask for help Cannot solve problems effectively Does not meet role expectations Does not meet own care needs Changes social participation Behaves destructively toward self and others Uses defense mechanisms inappropriately Has high accident and illness rate

Compiled from M. J. Kim and D. A. Moritz, *Classification of nursing diagnoses* (New York: McGraw-Hill Book Co., 1982); and M. Gordon, *Manual of nursing diagnosis* (New York: McGraw-Hill Book Co., 1982).

Ineffective coping is defined as impairment of a person's adaptive behaviors and problem-solving abilities to meet life's demands and roles (Kim and Moritz 1982:286). Contributing factors include (a) situational or maturational crises, (b) personal vulnerability, and (c) deficits in knowledge or problem-solving skills. See Table 32–3 for verbal and nonverbal cues indicating ineffective coping.

Examples of nursing diagnoses related to self-concept disturbances are:

1. Body image disturbance related to:
  a. Pregnancy
  b. Colostomy
  c. Obesity
  d. Chronic illness (e.g., arthritis, diabetes, or cerebrovascular accident)
  e. Amputation
  f. Mastectomy
  g. Massive scarring

2. Self-esteem disturbance related to:
   a. Unrealistic self-expectations
   b. Loss of role (specify)
   c. Unrealistic expectations by others
3. Ineffective coping related to:
   a. Divorce and change in financial status
   b. Death of mother
   c. Diagnosis of terminal illness
   d. Need for mutilating surgery
   e. Loss of job and income
   f. Inadequate personal resources and social support

Planning and Intervention for Self-Concept Problems

Planning

The *overall nursing goal* for patients who have self-concept problems is to help the patient develop a more positive self-concept. Subgoals may include:

1. To enhance the patient's body image
2. To enhance the patient's self-esteem
3. To assist the patient to develop satisfactory coping methods
4. To prevent the patient's feelings of powerlessness
5. To alleviate the patient's feelings of anxiety, fear, anger, and guilt
6. To assist the patient in developing his or her sexuality (see Chapter 33)

Planning also involves the establishment of outcome criteria based on the patient's nursing diagnosis. For examples of outcome criteria, see the section on evaluation later in this chapter.

General Guidelines for Nursing Intervention

1. Through purposeful communication and establishment of a trusting relationship with the patient, determine the patient's perception of the situation. What may be overt reality to the nurse is not always the patient's perception. To minimize the patient's anxiety and promote open communication, use open-ended questions, and observe the patient's overall behavior. Listen carefully to the patient's ideas, to learn his or her comprehension of the situation. Listen for hidden meanings of the conversation to determine incongruities or feelings. Note topics that the patient does and does not discuss.
2. Determine the patient's previous experiences with and ways of handling stress situations. If the patient's coping pattern is to withdraw or avoid verbal expression, devise ways to assist the patient to communicate and talk about feelings.
3. Determine the support persons and resources available to the patient and the responses of support persons. The responses of the nurse and support persons to the changes undergone by the patient influence the patient's acceptance of altered appearance or behavior.
4. Ascertain the role of the patient in the family, to determine any additional worries or fears this person has.
5. Arrange for the patient and support persons to have time and privacy to sort out feelings and thoughts. Provide them with a listening ear, interest, and concern rather than advice. People generally clarify problems and arrive at solutions themselves if they are permitted to express their thoughts and feelings.
6. Direct nursing intervention to the patient's or support person's presenting behavior. If, for example, the patient is denying the situation, do not argue or bluntly present reality. Raising questions in a doubtful voice, however, often suggests to the patient that he or she is being unrealistic. If a patient with a recent amputation says, "I'm going to walk right out of this hospital now," the nurse may respond matter-of-factly yet dubiously by saying, "You're going to walk right out of here—just like that?"
7. To the extent possible, follow the patient's suggestions for routines, the sequence of care, hygiene, handling of personal articles, etc., to give the patient a sense of control and reduce feelings of helplessness.
8. Accept the patient's anger, resentment, or feelings of inadequacy when they are displaced on you. Determine whether the remarks are justified, and act to correct justified criticisms. If remarks are not justified, simply listen and allow the patient to ventilate the feelings.
9. Ensure that consistency of care is provided, by communicating essential information to all health workers engaged in the patient's care.
10. Support the patient's family members or support persons so that they in turn can be supportive to the patient.
11. Provide the patient with adequate feedback through the use of touch and encouragement.

Guidelines for specific problems

Anxiety

One way to reduce or perhaps eliminate anxiety is to establish goals that are attainable. Often patients need the assistance of a nurse to do this.

First, patients have to recognize that they are anxious. This is achieved best in an atmosphere of warmth and trust. Sometimes patients who are anxious react negatively to nurses as a manifestation of their personal frustration. It is important for nurses to understand this and react to the behavior in a calm, accepting, and confident manner.

After patients realize that they are anxious, it is important to discuss all the possible reasons for their anxiety. Perley (1976:218) categorizes three underlying states of mind associated with anxiety:

1. *A sense of helplessness*, such as that in the person who has recently had a stroke and is unable to perform previous functions.
2. *A sense of isolation*, such as that in the person who believes no one understands how it really feels to have a chronic illness or an adolescent who fears rejection because of a venereal disease.
3. *A sense of insecurity*, such as that in a person who has had mutilating surgery and no longer feels sexually attractive to a partner or who is worried about being incapable of earning a living or paying medical bills.

When patients can identify the cause of their anxiety, they find it helpful to explore the cause, with the objective of learning better coping mechanisms. They may see that they have overestimated the threat or that they can reduce the threat by specific action (for example, asking a doctor whether a biopsy revealed cancer).

Anger

Self and Viau (1980) outline four steps for helping patients to deal with anger:

1. Identify the state of anger.
2. Let the patient know that you recognize and accept the anger. Appropriate responses by the nurse include: "You seem to be very upset," and "Many people feel angry when they are hospitalized." It is essential to avoid suppressing the anger by ignoring it, by trying to humor the patient out of it, or by smothering the patient with kindness.
3. Help the patient identify the source of the anger and express feelings. For example, has the patient's independence been overinhibited, has a support person disagreed with decisions made by the patient, or has information been withheld? Knowing the source helps the patient to gain some control over the situation. Expression of feelings reduces tension.
4. Help the patient to channel the anger constructively by providing increased independence, providing choices about health care as much as possible, and encouraging physical and social activities.

Occasionally, in some hospital settings (e.g., a psychiatric unit), nurses need to handle violent patients. Specific measures include (Anders 1977):

1. Allow some space between the patient and the staff and other patients. Ask other patients to leave the room.
2. Do not attempt to remove a weapon from the patient.
3. Help the patient identify the cause of the anger, and reassure the patient that he or she will not be allowed to lose control. The nurse may say, "You seem to be really upset about something, and I'm afraid you might injure someone if you do use that pitcher. I would like to help you control your behavior. I can't allow you to injure yourself or someone else."
4. Offer the patient alternatives to help regain some self-esteem. The nurse may suggest that the patient and the nurse sit down, talk it over, and have a cup of coffee. Generally this kind of intervention avoids the need for physical restraints. However, restraints must be used as a last resort. Specific steps for appropriate restraint of violent patients are presented in the articles by Anders and Pisarcik listed in Suggested Readings.

Guilt

Once the nurse has established that the patient's behaviors are indeed manifestations of guilt, the nurse may assist the patient to express feelings verbally and identify the factors influencing guilt. Has the patient violated a basic ethical code, such as "Thou shalt not lie," or has the patient experienced a forced transgression, such as a violation of independence by dependence imposed by illness, or violation of choice by placing a child for adoption. Exploring the situations producing guilt with the nurse may be an uncomfortable experience for the patient, and the nurse's emotional support and reassurance are important. During the discussion the patient may see that some of his or her thinking is irrational or expectations unreasonable. If unable to accept this, the patient may need psychiatric counseling to gain more realistic self-expectations or to change maladaptive behavior. Some patients, for example, continually commit transgressions to receive neurotic benefits from painful guilt feelings.

Powerlessness

The feeling of loss of control over events is not an uncommon one for patients in a hospital setting. Nurses can assist patients with this problem by including patients in the planning of their care. Nurses may encourage patients to schedule their visiting hours, choose their meals, and assist in setting the goals for their care.

When nurses personalize nursing care, patients feel

that they are important and do have some control. Calling patients by name, being interested in them, and demonstrating concern about matters that concern patients assist them to maintain a feeling of control over themselves and the events that affect them. If powerlessness is allowed to persist, a state of depression can result. See Chapter 36 for further information.

Dependence problems

Eliminating problems of dependence or independence usually requires patients to learn new ways of behaving. Patients can be encouraged to verbalize their feelings about a situation; identify the perceived and actual conflcts; and be reeducated through teaching, translation, interpretation, and extrapolation of perceptual data (Poush and Van Landingham (1976:318–19). The basic nursing intervention is creative listening and responding as means of establishing new behaviors.

Behavior modification, another method of changing behavior, elicits and rewards desired behavioral responses to reduce, modify, or extinguish ineffective coping responses (ibid., p. 320). One method is to provide the patient with a cue that tends to elicit a behavioral response. When a desired response is given, the patient is rewarded. For example, if a patient who does not want to eat is provided with a meal tray, accompanied by an encouraging statement from the nurse, and then eats the meal, the patient is rewarded in a manner that the patient values. A reward might be praise from the nurse and assistance with a crossword puzzle.

Low self-esteem

Patients who have low self-esteem need to explore the factors they interpret as negative in themselves and may need assistance seeing the positive aspects. Nurses can help patients to explore their expectations, how these can be met, and how reasonable they are. Patients may also need assistance in understanding how past experiences are influencing the present. They may have developed a maladaptive pattern of behavior and need to learn how to change this. With the assistance of the nurse, patients can often learn to see life experiences in a more positive manner. They can be helped to feel hope rather than despair. Patients can be assisted to identify both their feelings at a particular moment and how they want to feel. The nurse can assist patients to perceive themselves correctly and to choose activities that will help them to live up to their values.

An acute decrease in self-esteem is regarded as depression. Nursing intervention for this is discussed later in this chapter.

Body image disturbance

Nurses can intervene in a number of ways to assist patients who have problems related to body image:

1. Support the strengths of patients, and help them to recognize these. For example, a nurse may emphasize a man's ability to be an understanding father in spite of his physical disability.
2. Assist patients to look at themselves in totality rather than focusing on their limitations. This can be done by conveying interest in the patient rather than only the patient's disability.
3. Be alert to and support behavior indicating that patients are beginning to adapt to body alterations. Some of these indications include (Murray 1972b:702):
- **a.** Peeking at the dressing or surgical site or feeling the dressing or the stump of an amputation.
- **b.** Looking closely at the reactions of others (nurse, doctor, support persons) to the dressing or incision. This is done to learn others' feelings about the body changes.
- **c.** Beginning to talk about the real or imagined change in self and frequently repeating a perception of what has happened. This is an attempt to resolve personal feelings related to the body change.
- **d.** Expressing anger, rage, depression, or grief while talking about the body injury.
- **e.** Repeatedly asking questions about what has and is happening and what to anticipate in terms of healing, work, family relationships, etc.
- **f.** Becoming preoccupied with normal body functions, since these are less threatening than the impaired functions. This supports the patient's feeling of having control over something.

4. Recognize the difficulty patients have looking at and accepting their disfigurements. Allow patients to give the first cue, e.g., by talking about the injury and asking you how it looks. When this occurs, respond with matter-of-fact statements, such as "It is less red and swollen today," or "There is still some drainage." Such statements help to prepare patients for what they will see. It is also important to acknowledge the patient's hesitancy by saying, e.g., "It's not easy to get ready to look at the incision, is it?"
5. Provide kinesthetic feedback to patients with paralyzed limbs by telling them, e.g., "I am straightening your arm; now I am bending your arm."
6. Describe changes in functioning in realistic terms at a level appropriate to patients. By encouraging discussion, the nurse can uncover and correct misconceptions held by patients and their families. For example, a man who had a prostatectomy believed he was now sterile.
7. Encourage patients and their families to express their feelings and to understand them. Understanding

that these feelings are normal is often reassuring to people.

Depression

Nursing intervention for people who are depressed includes measures to improve their feelings of self-esteem and provide for their safety, nutrition, elimination, hygiene, rest, and activity.

Self-esteem The nurse should present an empathic presence so that the patient feels comfortable and accepted. Listening carefully and helping the patient to express negative feelings such as anger are also important. The nurse's accepting attitude helps to support the patient's self-esteem. Trying to "cheer up" the patient only increases feelings of guilt about not being cheerful and consequently lowers self-esteem.

Because depressed people often find it difficult to make decisions, scheduled activities should be arranged for the patient and the need for the patient to make decisions avoided. For example, when a walk is planned for 1400 hours, it is best for the nurse to say, "It is time for your walk; I will go with you," rather than, "Do you want to go for a walk with me?"

Safety If the patient is a suicide risk, nurses need to provide immediate safety measures to protect the patient. Appropriate counseling and arranging for a safe environment are important. If the patient has a history of attempting suicide by taking barbiturates, for example, intensive supervision of medications is needed.

Nutrition and elimination Some people who are acutely depressed do not want to eat and need encouragement and support to take adequate nourishment. Constipation is frequently a problem, and patients require increased fiber in their diets, increased fluid intake, and activity. Some patients may require laxatives or enemas to maintain fecal elimination.

Hygiene Sometimes depressed people forgo normal hygiene practices and become unkempt and dirty. This can lead to infections as well as lowering self-esteem further. These patients require assistance with hygienic practices. A firm approach is preferable to asking the patient to make a choice. For example, the nurse can say, "I will help you into the bathtub now, Mrs. Andriotti," not "Do you want your bath now?"

Rest and activity Depressed people may prefer to lie on their beds rather than participate in any activities. They often have difficulty sleeping, however, which is augmented with inactivity. Arranging a schedule that includes activities often improves the patient's sleep and appetite and directs the patient's thoughts to current activities or goals and away from past experiences.

Evaluation

Examples of outcome criteria for patients with self-concept disturbances are:

1. Verbalizes feelings of anger or sadness
2. Shows increased interest in participating in treatment plans and care
3. Assumes responsibility for self-care
4. Describes life as having meaning, hope, and choices
5. Absence of signs and symptoms of anxiety
6. Is able to focus attention and concentrate on things that must be done or decisions that must be made
7. Verbalizes perceived threats to well-being with minimal anxiety
8. Discusses options and alternatives when trying to solve problems
9. Expresses both feelings and thoughts about body changes

Summary

Self-concept has two major components: the body image and the personal self. Body image includes the person's physical attributes, body functioning, sexuality, appearance, and state of health. Subdivisions of personal self are the moral-ethical self, self-consistency, and the self-ideal. Self-concept is learned from significant others and experience.

The development of a self-concept is an important aspect of psychosocial development. Erikson describes eight stages of stresses in the maturational process:

1. Trust versus mistrust
2. Autonomy versus shame and doubt

3. Initiative versus guilt
4. Industry versus inferiority
5. Identity versus role confusion
6. Intimacy versus isolation
7. Generativity versus stagnation
8. Integrity versus despair

The success with which a person copes with these stressors largely determines the development of the self-concept.

Two groups of factors influence development of the self-concept: environmental factors and past experience factors. The first group includes objects in the environment, feedback, the person's present definition of self-concept, learned coping mechanisms, and the person's competence in valued areas. Experience factors include previous feedback, previous stressors, the person's self-expectations, and experiences that create or deny a sense of value.

The development of self-esteem affects how a person deals with the environment. An individual with high self-esteem deals more actively with the environment and feels secure. A person with low self-esteem sees the environment as threatening. Self-esteem is largely developed as a result of feedback from others. Learning to handle feelings is important in the development of self-esteem. Children also learn self-esteem from the limitations placed on their behavior.

Assessment of self-concept is normally indicated when the patient and/or support persons present cues that could reflect problems or when the patient's illness is likely to affect aspects of self-concept. To elicit essential data about self-concept, the nurse must develop a trusting relationship with the patient and be alert to verbal and nonverbal cues that suggest a problem. Self-concept disturbances may be manifested by clinical signs of anxiety, anger, fear, guilt, powerlessness, dependence problems, low self-esteem, and depression.

Common nursing diagnoses for patients with problems related to self-concept include body image disturbance, disturbance in self-esteem, and ineffective coping. Verbal and nonverbal cues indicate each diagnosis.

To plan and provide nursing interventions for patients with self-concept problems, the nurse first sets goals and outcome criteria and then selects appropriate interventions related to the stated nursing diagnosis. Both general and specific interventions may be used.

Suggested Activities

1. Observe people in each developmental stage described by Erikson. Identify behaviors that relate to developmental tasks associated with self-concept.
2. Interview an elderly person in a long-term care agency. Assess how this person perceives and values himself or herself.
3. Interview several pregnant women in their third trimester of pregnancy, and determine the body image and self-esteem of each. Compare your findings with those of students in your class.
4. In a clinical area, select a patient who has demonstrated one of the following behavior problems:
    a. Anxiety (moderate or acute) or fear
    b. Anger
    c. Powerlessness
    d. Guilt
    e. Low self-esteem

Explore this patient's nursing diagnoses related to self-concept, goals, outcome criteria, and planned nursing interventions. Discuss your findings with your classmates.

Suggested Readings

American Journal of Nursing. September 1965. Anxiety—recognition and intervention. *American Journal of Nursing* 65:129–52.

This programmed instruction can help students learn to recognize anxiety and provide appropriate responses.

Anders, R. L. July 1977. When a patient becomes violent. *American Journal of Nursing* 77:1144–48.

This author outlines specific steps for handling violent patients. Many photographs show how patients are restrained when this becomes necessary.

Hein, E., and Leavitt, M. May 1977. Providing emotional support. *Nursing 77* 7:38–41.

According to these authors, nurses can learn to be supportive just as they learn any other nursing technique. Concrete ways in which the nurse can provide support as a planned process are described.

Meissner, J. E. February 1980. Semantic differential scales for assessing patients' feelings. *Nursing 80* 10:70–71.

This article presents a semantic differential scale on which the patient is asked to check the boxes that most closely describe his or her feelings, e.g., "lonely," "nervous," "indifferent," "calm," and "dejected."

———. May 1980. Uncovering your patient's hidden psychological problems. *Nursing 80* 10:78–79.

The author provides a concise assessment tool for patients to answer so that nurses can plan helpful nursing interventions related to the patient's psychosocial needs.

Norris, C. M. October 1969. The work of getting well. *American Journal of Nursing* 69:2118–21.

This article about convalescence discusses the formidable tasks that patients must for the most part accomplish by themselves so that they do not say years later, "I never really got over my operation." It covers reintegration of body image, role failure, feelings about dependence, etc.

Piscarik, G. September 1981. Facing the violent patient. *Nursing 81* 11:62–65.
A psychiatric clinical specialist outlines the dos and don'ts for handling potentially violent patients.

Selected References

Anders, R. L. July 1977. When a patient becomes violent. *American Journal of Nursing* 77:1144–48.

Bee, H. 1975. *The developing child.* New York: Harper and Row.

Blaesing, S., and Brockhaus, J. December 1972. The development of body image in the child. *Nursing Clinics of North America* 7:597–607.

Cohen, S. June 1977. Helping depressed patients in general nursing practice: Programmed instruction. *American Journal of Nursing* 77:1007–38.

Cohn, L. December 1979. Coping with anxiety: A step-by-step guide. *Nursing 79* 9:34–37.

Combs, A. E.; Avila, D. L.; and Purkey, W. W. 1978. *Helping relationships: Basic concepts for the helping professions.* 2nd ed. Boston: Allyn and Bacon.

Craft, C. A. December 1972. Body image and obesity. *Nursing Clinics of North America* 7:677–85.

Cray, W. G., and Cray, G. C. March 1973. Depression. *American Journal of Nursing* 73:472, 474–75.

Dempsey, M. O. December 1972. The development of body image in the adolescent. *Nursing Clinics of North America* 7:609–15.

Drake, R. E., and Price, J. L. October/December 1975. Depression: Adaptation to disruption. *Perspectives in Psychiatric Care* 13:163–69.

Driever, M. J. 1976. Theory of self-concept and development of self-concept. In Roy, C. *Introduction to nursing: An adaptation model.* Englewood Cliffs, N.J.: Prentice-Hall.

Duldt, B. W. September 1981. Anger: An occupational hazard for nurses. *Nursing Outlook* 29:510–18.

Erikson, E. H. 1963. *Childhood and society.* 2nd ed. New York: W. W. Norton and Co.

Fujita, M. T. December 1972. The impact of illness or surgery on the body image of the child. *Nursing Clinics of North America* 7:641–49.

Gallagher, A. M. December 1972. Body image changes in the patient with a colostomy. *Nursing Clinics of North America* 7:669–76.

Gordon, M. 1982. *Manual of nursing diagnosis.* New York: McGraw-Hill Book Co.

Iffrig, M. C. December 1972. Body image in pregnancy: Its relation to nursing functions. *Nursing Clinics of North America* 7:631–39.

Johnson, D. E. April 1967. Powerlessness: A Significant determinant in patient behavior? *Jornal of Nursing Education* 6:39–44.

Kaluger, G., and Kaluger, M. F. 1979. *Human development: The span of life.* 2nd ed. St. Louis: C. V. Mosby Co.

Kerr, N. January/February 1978. Anxiety: Theoretical considerations. *Perspectives in Psychiatric Care* 16:36–40, 46.

Kim, M. J., and Moritz, D. A. 1982. *Classification of nursing diagnoses: Proceedings of the third and fourth national conferences.* New York: McGraw-Hill Book Co.

Knowles, R. D. January 1981a. Dealing with feelings: Managing anxiety. *American Journal of Nursing* 81:110–11.

———. September 1981b. Overcoming guilt and worry. *American Journal of Nursing* 81:1663.

———. February 1982. Managing angry feelings. *American Journal of Nursing* 82:299.

Lathrop, V. G. September/December 1978. Aggression as a response. *Persepctives in Psychiatric Care* 16:202–5.

Leonard, B. J. December 1972. Body image changes in chronic illness. *Nursing Clinics of North America* 7:687–95.

McIntier, T. M. 1976. Theory of interdependence. In Roy, C., *Introduction to nursing: An adaptation model.* Englewood Cliffs, N.J.: Prentice-Hall.

Malaznik, N. 1976. Theory of role function. In Roy, C., *Introduction to nursing: An adaptation model.* Englewood Cliffs, N.H.: Prentice-Hall.

Murray, R. L. E. December 1972a. Body image development in adulthood. *Nursing Clinics of North America* 7:617–29.

———. December 1972b. Principles of nursing intervention for the adult patient with body image changes. *Nursing Clinics of North America* 7:697–707.

Perley, N. Z. 1976. Problems in self-concistency: Anxiety. In Roy, C. *Introduction to nursing: An adaptation model.* Englewood Cliffs, N.J.: Prentice-Hall.

Poush, M., and Van Landingham, J. 1976. Problems of interdependence. In Roy, C. *Introduction to nursing: An adaptation model.* Englewood Cliffs, N.J.: Prentice-Hall.

Riddle, I. December 1972. Nursing intervention to promote body image: Integrity in children. *Nursing Clinics of North America* 7:651–61.

Riffee, D. March-April 1981. Self esteem changes in hospitalized school age children. *Nursing Research* 30:94–97.

Rothenberg, A. October 1971. On anger. *American Journal of Psychiatry* 128:454–60.

Roy, C., et al. 1976. *Introduction to nursing: An adaptation model.* Englewood Cliffs, N.J.: Prentice-Hall.

Self, P. R., and Viau, J. J. December 1980. 4 steps for helping a patient alleviate anger. *Nursing 80* 10:66.

Smith, C. A. December 1972. Body image changes after myocardial infarction. *Nursing Clinics of North America* 7:663–68.

Smitherman, C. October 1981. Your patient's anxious: What should you do? *Nursing 81* 11:72–73. (Canadian ed. 11:26–27).

Stewart, A. T. September/December 1978. Handling the aggressive patient. *Perspectives in Psychiatric Care* 16:228–32.

Swanson, A. R. April/June 1975. Communicating with depressed persons. *Perspectives in Psychiatric Care* 13:63–67.

Tyrer, P. November 1980. Anxiety states: Easy to recognize—difficult to diagnose—supportive and medical treatment. *Nursing Mirror* 151:36–37.

Walke, M. A. K. July 1977. When a patient needs to unburden his feelings. American Journal of Nursing 77:1164–66.

Wilson, H. S., and Kneisl, C. R. 1982. *Psychiatric Nursing.* 2nd ed. Menlo Park, Calif.: Addison-Wesley Publishing Co.

Chapter 33

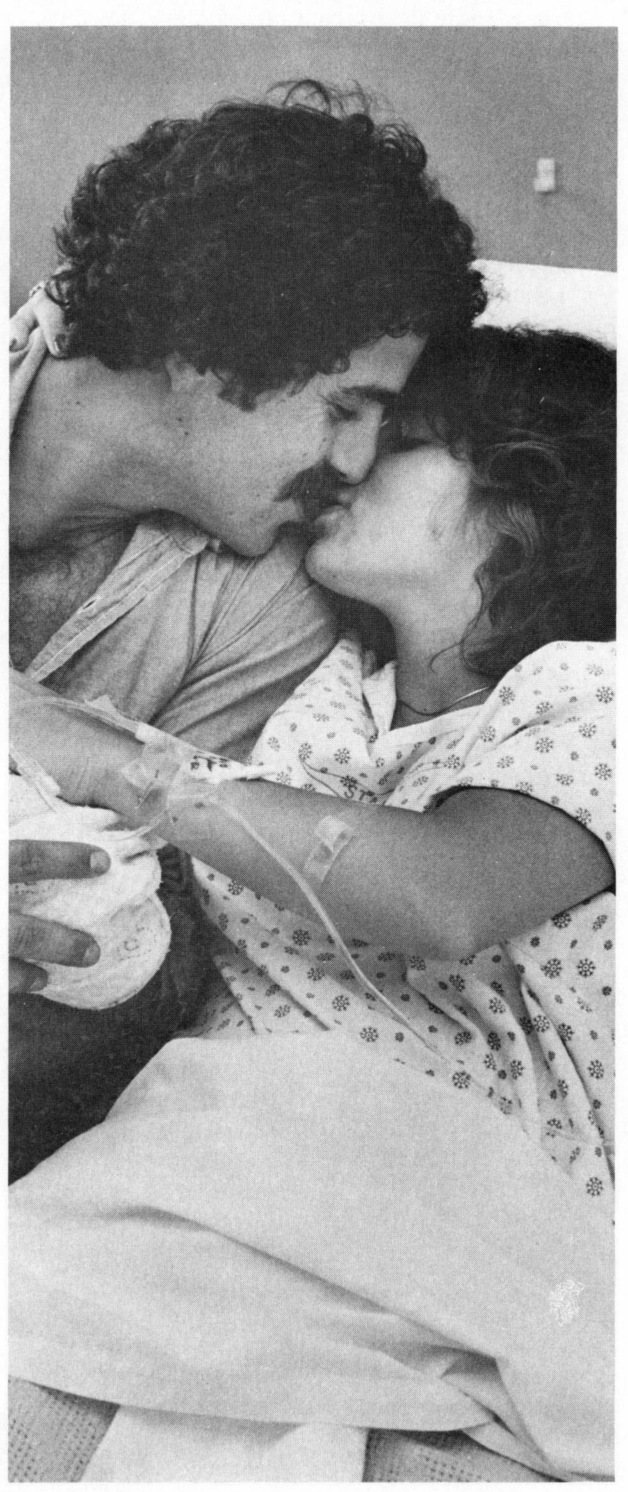

Sexuality

CONTENTS

Objectives

1. Know essential facts about sex and sexuality
   - **1.1** Define selected terms
   - **1.2** Describe the concept of sexuality
   - **1.3** Identify components of sexuality
   - **1.4** Identify essential aspects of the development of sexuality from the prenatal period to late adulthood
   - **1.5** Identify structure and function of male and female genitals
   - **1.6** Identify various physical and psychologic sexual stimulation patterns
   - **1.7** Identify Masters and Johnson's four phases of sexual response
   - **1.8** Identify physiologic changes that occur in males and females during each phase of the sexual response
2. Know essential information and methods required to assess sexuality
   - **2.1** Identify situations in which the nurse assesses sexual function
   - **2.2** Identify patient cues suggestive of a sexual problem
   - **2.3** Identify factors that affect an individual's sexual attitudes and behaviors
   - **2.4** Identify sexual aspects of a health history
   - **2.5** Identify essential aspects of breast and testicular examination
3. Know essential facts about nursing diagnoses and common problems related to sexuality
   - **3.1** Identify factors contributing to sexual dysfunction
   - **3.2** Identify factors that increase and decrease sexual motivation
   - **3.3** Identify common problems of intercourse and possible causes
   - **3.4** Identify common illnesses affecting sexuality
4. Understand facts about nursing interventions to promote sexual health
   - **4.1** Identify essential aspects of developing self-awareness about sexuality
   - **4.2** Identify two intervention models for sexual counseling
   - **4.3** Identify essentials of various contraceptive methods
5. Apply the nursing process when providing care to selected patients with sexual problems
   - **5.1** Obtain necessary assessment data
   - **5.2** Analyze and relate assessment data
   - **5.3** Write relevant nursing diagnoses
   - **5.4** Write relevant nursing goals
   - **5.5** Plan appropriate nursing interventions
   - **5.6** Implement appropriate nursing interventions
   - **5.7** State outcome criteria essential for evaluating the patient's progress

Terms

androsperm
anilingus
areola
atresia
basalis
biologic sex
bisexual
cervix
chromosomes
clitoris
coitus
condom
contraception
copulation
core-gender identity
cornification
corpus albicans
corpus luteum
cremaster
cryptorchidism
cunnilingus
detumescence
dildo
diploid number
dyspareunia
ectopic pregnancy
ejaculation
ejaculatory ducts
endometrium
epididymis
erection
fellatio
follicular (preovulatory) stage
foreplay (precoital stimulation)
foreskin (prepuce)
frenulum
frigidity
functionalis
gender behavior
gender identity
gender (sexual) role
glans clitoris
glans penis
Graafian follicle
granulosa cells
gynosperm
haploid number
homosexual
hymen
imperforate hymen
impotence
impregnation
interstitial cells of Leydig
intrauterine device (IUD)
labia majora
labia minora
libido
luteal (postovulatory) stage
mammary glands
masturbation
meiosis
menarche
menses
mitosis

mons pubis (mons veneris)
myometrium
orgasm
orgasmic dysfunction
ovulation
perimetrium
postovulatory stage
preovulatory stage
primordial follicles
proliferative (preovulatory) stage
reflexogenic erection
refractory period
rugae
scrotum
secretory (postovulatory) stage
semen
seminal plasma
seminiferous tubules
sex
sex behavior
sexual differentiation
sexual dimorphism
sexual dysfunction
sexual identity
sexuality
sexual role behavior
smegma
soixante-neuf
sperm
spermatogenesis
spermicide
testes
tubal ligation
tunica albuginea
tunica dartos
vaginal diaphragm
vaginal orifice
vaginal smear
vaginismus
vas deferens
vasectomy
vestibule
vulva (pudendum)
zygote

People's attitudes toward their bodies, including their perceptions of how others view their bodies, are important in health and illness. In addition, an individual's perception of his maleness or her femaleness also determines certain responses to illness and affects that person's health care needs. Sexual attitudes, values, and behaviors have changed in recent years, especially attitudes toward masturbation, premarital sex, homosexuality, and nudity.

Masturbation, or sexual self-stimulation, was traditionally considered wrong; negative attitudes toward masturbation exist even today. Most authorities do not consider masturbation harmful, but opinions vary as to whether it is helpful. Parents are advised not to punish children for masturbating, but to view this form of sexual expression as normal, though inappropriate in front of others. Premarital sexual relations are more frequent and more widely accepted today than previously. Alternate modes of sexual expression; e.g., homosexuality and bisexuality, are also receiving greater acceptance. A *homosexual* is one who is sexually attracted primarily to members of the same sex. A *bisexual* feels sexual attraction for, or has sexual contact with, people of both sexes. The American Psychiatric Association has officially recognized homosexuality and bisexuality as alternate forms of expression rather than illnesses. People's attitudes toward the body and toward nudity are also changing. Today's greater acceptance of nudity is reflected in movies, advertising, and daily life.

Greater acceptance, of course, does not mean universal acceptance. Many segments of North American society view changing sexual attitudes with disfavor. The nurse assisting patients with sexual problems needs to respect their attitudes yet at the same time assess those problems and correct misinformation.

Sex and Sexuality

Definition and Description

Sex denotes maleness or femaleness, but the term is commonly applied to sexual intercourse. *Sexuality* also denotes maleness or femaleness but in addition refers to individuals' sexual attitudes and activities. Sexuality, therefore, has a much broader meaning than sex. Sexuality includes physical, intellectual, emotional, social, and ethical aspects of sexual being and behavior.

Physical sexuality involves the reproductive organs, hormones, and sexual stimulation and response patterns, all of which are affected by health, disease processes, injury, and drugs. Emotional aspects of sexuality include feelings of love, sadness, joy, guilt, and desire. In the social context, sexuality usually means an intimate relationship with at least one other person. Social roles of males and females are also part of sexuality. Sexuality has ethical ramifications as well. People must make decisions about such issues as the morality of homosexuality, sperm banks, and nudism.

Sexuality, therefore, is highly complex, personal, and pervasive. An individual's sexual attitudes and activities are unique. As a result, sexuality is a major part of an individual's self-concept.

Components of Sexuality

Human sexuality is both inherited and learned. The inherited component is biological; the learned component comes through interaction with the social environment. However, every aspect of sexual behavior has both inherited and learned components. Lief (1975:4) identifies the following components:

1. Biologic sex
2. Sexual identity (core-gender identity)
3. Gender identity
4. Sexual role behavior
   a. Sex behavior
   b. Gender behavior

Biologic sex is genetically determined at conception by the XX or XY chromosomal combination. See this page. The embryo develops ovaries or testes, depending on genetic instructions. Normally, infants are born with clearly developed primary sex characteristics; people develop secondary sex characteristics at puberty. If primary sex characteristics are ambiguous at birth, the sex the parents assign to the child is a primary determinant of later sexual identity.

Sexual identity, also referred to as *core-gender identity*, is an individual's inner sense of maleness or femaleness. Children learn sexual identity when adults reinforce certain behaviors (e.g., verbal reinforcers such as "What a big, strong boy you are" or "What a sweet baby girl you are").

Sexual dimorphism describes the average differences between males and females. Males, for example, are generally taller, heavier, and physically stronger than females. However, these attributes are not always reliable indicators of sex; some women are taller, heavier, or stronger than some men.

Gender identity is an individual's sense of being masculine or feminine as distinct from being male or female. It is not uncommon for women to appear or feel masculine or men to appear or feel feminine. Traditionally, masculinity was associated with strength, aggression, stoicism, courage, rational thinking, intelligence, and career achievement. Femininity, by contrast, was associated with tenderness, nurturance, motherhood, dependence, passivity, and submission. These stereotypes, however, are changing. Gender identity is learned slowly through reinforcement by others. Self-doubts about gender identity are normal and common particularly during adolescence and middle age. Problems with gender identity can lead to poor sexual adjustments, promiscuity, excessive competitiveness in nonsexual pursuits, impotence, and lack of arousal and response.

Sexual role behavior has two components: *sex behavior* and *gender behavior. Sex behavior* is motivated by a desire for sexual pleasure. Sexual intercourse, physiologic responses to intercourse, and certain sexual dysfunctions can be part of sex behavior. *Gender behavior* is masculine or feminine behavior, reflected in sexual relationships and conforming to societal expectations. Sex behavior and gender behavior necessarily occur together and can be isolated only theoretically.

Development of Sexuality

From the beginning of life, the human is a sexual being.

Throughout life, the individual feels many biologic, psychosocial, and cultural influences that condition sexuality. From birth onward, humans are conditioned to behave in ways that conform to society's expectations of males or of females.

Prenatal Period and Infancy

Biologic components

All cells of the body have 23 pairs of chromosomes, referred to as the *diploid number*. These cells multiply by dividing in half and producing two new cells, each of which contain 23 pairs of chromosomes. Such cell division is called *mitosis*. Sperm cells (the male gametes or reproductive cells) and egg cells (the female gametes or reproductive cells), however, have only 23 single chromosomes, referred to as the *haploid number*. This number is the result of specialized cell division called *meiosis*. Thus when the sperm cell fertilizes the egg cell, the cell produced from their union has the required 23 pairs of chromosomes: 23 single ones from the female and 23 single ones from the male.

In the developing human, two of these chromosomes are the *sex chromosome pair*, which determine whether the gonads will develop as testes or ovaries. The female has two identical sex chromosomes, referred to as *XX*. The male has two different chromosomes designated as *XY*; thus one chromosome is the same as the female's (X) but the other is different (Y). Sperm are of two types. An X-bearing sperm is called a *gynosperm*, and a Y-bearing sperm is called an *androsperm*. If a gynosperm fertilizes the egg, the fetus develops into a female, but if an androsperm fertilizes the egg, the fetus will be male.

Androsperm are smaller, have longer tails, move or swim faster, and are more susceptible to vaginal pH and other changes in the environment than gynosperm. It is believed that for boys to be conceived, intercourse must occur very near or at the time of ovulation. At that time, androsperm move more quickly to the egg than gynosperm. Girls are thought to be conceived a few days before the egg is ready to be fertilized. Gynosperm are thought to move more slowly and withstand the relatively acid vaginal fluids secreted during this time and then unite with the egg once it is produced.

The gonads of a 4-to-6-week-old fetus are not recognizable as either ovaries or testes. Both chromosomal sex pairs (XX and XY) have two pairs of internal ducts that develop into reproductive organs. These are called the *müllerian* and *wolffian* ducts. The müllerian ducts are the genetic female pair, which eventually develop into the fallopian tubes, uterus, and upper one-third of the vagina. The wolffian ducts are the genetic male pair, which ultimately develop into the sperm ducts, seminal vesicles, and the epididymis. The external genitals of a fetus of either sex consist of a genital tubercle, genital folds, and genital swellings. The tubercles eventually develop into the clitoris or glans penis, the folds into the labia minora or shaft of the penis, and the swelling into the labia majora or the scrotum.

Sexual differentiation, or biologic sex, is fairly well determined by the 12th week of fetal life. The differentiation of these structures into male genitals requires two substances: a testicular inductor (androgens) and a müllerian inhibitor. The androgens stimulate the development of the internal and external male structures, while the inhibitor suppresses the development of the mullerian ducts, causing them to degenerate. When these hormones are absent, the fetus develops into a female. The wolffian ducts degenerate, and the female genitals develop.

Psychosocial differences during infancy

At birth, boys are generally larger, weigh more, and have greater musculatures than girls. Other sex differences have been noted by authorities:

1. Boys show greater motor activity and can raise their heads earlier.
2. Girls are more physically passive and are more irritable during physical examination.
3. Girls show greater sensitivity to tactile stimuli and pain.
4. At 6 months, girls have a longer attention span for visual stimuli such as a human face and show more responsiveness to social demands and parental wishes.
5. Boys have a longer attention span to a helix of light.
6. Boys prefer low-complexity stimuli.
7. Girls prefer highly complex stimuli.
8. Girls demonstrate earlier language development.
9. Boys spend more time away from their mothers and return less frequently.
10. Girls spend more time looking at and touching their mothers.
11. Boys are less frustrated with barriers in their path and attempt to get around them more often.
12. Girls prefer toys with faces and toys requiring more motor coordination.
13. Boys respond to objects that are not toys more than girls do and play with them longer.

The reasons for these differences are disputed. It is difficult to determine exactly where heredity ends and learning begins.

Early and Late Childhood

Psychosocial aspects

From the age of 2 years to the onset of puberty, children undergo several sexual developmental changes. Although genital development is slight compared to the rapid physical growth in every other body system, the child's sexual self-identity is established, and the child discovers sexual pleasure.

The establishment of sex identity is critical to children between the ages of 18 months and 4 years. It begins with an awareness, which is well established by age 4, that one belongs to one sex. At age 2, a child can distinguish between a male and female. By 3 years, children can correctly answer the question "Are you a little boy or a little girl?" By age 5 or 6 years, the child knows that a girl cannot be changed into a boy or vice versa.

Several factors influence the development of sexual identity. Some of these are communication, a sense of self, and imitation. Communication with parents gives children many clues about whether their behavior is appropriate for the sex role. Frequently, parents respond differently to girls than to boys beginning at birth. For example, parents may respond more to a baby girl's vocalizations than to a boy's. Nonverbal communication also may differ. Boys may be handled more roughly, whereas girls may be fondled and caressed. Girls may be allowed to cry while boys may not be. Even the choice of toys is significant. Many boys, for example, are discouraged from playing with dolls.

Learning appropriate *sex-typed behaviors* (those behaviors that typically elicit different rewards for one sex as distinct from the other) takes the child several years. Initially the child determines his or her biologic sex. Frequent use of the labels *boy* and *he* or *girl* and *she* and rewards to the child for correct self-labeling help the child learn. After learning biologic sex, the child learns the gender role by imitating an adult of the same sex. Freud referred to this process as identification.

The sense of self is another aspect of sexual identity. The sense of self is the ability to distinguish oneself from others. It begins during the first year of life as the child interacts with the parents. The establishment of trust, the primary task of the infant according to Erikson (see Table 11–2), is basic to the development of a sense of self. Not until infants gain a sense of trust can they relax, be alone, and allow their mothers out of sight. This feeling of trust eventually merges with an awareness and sense of self and ultimately with the feeling that one is an acceptable person.

During early childhood, children develop a sense of pride and pleasure in their bodies, including the genitals. When exploring their bodies, children derive pleasure from genital self-stimulation. Parents may perceive this activity as masturbation and may react negatively, conveying to children the notion that the act is "bad." Subsequently, children feel anxious, fearful, or guilty about such activity without knowing why. They may then associate pleasurable feelings with guilt.

Three- to 5-year-old children continue to be curious about their bodies. It is not uncommon for boys and girls to examine each other. Preschool children need to be allowed to observe sex differences at toilet or bathing time. This normal curiosity subsides by the time the child starts school. Parents and nurses need to accept exploratory behaviors. Often it is best to refrain from commenting, to answer the child's questions (if there are any) in a matter-of-fact manner, and to direct the child to the next activity, such as getting dressed and returning to play. This attitude conveys acceptance to the child.

At about 3½ years of age, children become interested in the roles, sleeping arrangements, and bathing arrangements of parents. The father emerges as a special love object for the female child and the mother for the male child.

Between the ages of 4 and 5 years, children indulge in fantasies. This is the stage of initiative versus guilt, according to Erikson, and the phallic stage, including the castration complex, according to Freud. At this time children fear punishment for dreams or fantasies about their genitals.

During the school-age years, children's curiosity about sexual behavior and reproductive processes is high. This accompanies their tremendous broadening of interests and social contacts. School-age children ask many questions about sex, such as, "Why do you have to go to the hospital to have a baby?" Another phenomenon of this age is social segregation of the sexes, which reaches its peak when children are about 12. This is often referred to as the homosexual stage of development, although there is no stage at which boys and girls do not show interest in each other. During this period, members of the same sex participate in mutual genital explorations. The idea that sex is evil can be reinforced during these experiences if parents happen to discover children and react in a horrified manner.

Puberty and Adolescence

Biologic changes

Physical changes in sexual anatomy and physiology are more profound during puberty than any other period. These changes are discussed in Chapter 11 on page 254 and in Chapter 12 on page 261.

Psychosocial aspects

Associated with these physical changes are profound psychologic changes. Included are the acceptance of altered body image, adjustment to different energy levels, the establishment of self-identity, and resolution of sexual conflicts.

Responses to altered body image among adolescents vary from anxiety to pleasure. Boys, for example, are often anxious about the size of their genitals, equating testicle and penis size with virility and potency. Girls are concerned about breast development and menstruation. Because the menstrual pattern during the 1st year is irregular, many girls become preoccupied with their menstrual timetables, particularly if they differ from their peers. Adolescents need to know that the size of the penis or breasts has no bearing on functional ability and that menstruation is normally irregular during the 1st year. Associated with these body changes is the adolescent's awareness of sexual feelings. These feelings also have to be incorporated into an acceptable image of self.

Sexual conflicts are a problem to adolescents. Although adolescents are recognized by Western society as physically mature adults, they may be denied the right to full adult sexual privileges. Thus, adolescence can be a stressful period. Adolescents experience and must control intense sexual impulses. During puberty, erotic play (masturbation) and genital examination with members of the same sex continues, particularly among boys. These activities are normal and largely an attempt to learn about growth patterns and physical reactions. Heterosexual activity among adolescents varies widely. It may include embracing, kissing, petting, or intercourse. Adolescents often associate such experiences with guilt. These feelings are frequently magnified by fears of pregnancy or venereal disease.

Adulthood and Middle Years

A number of sexual behavior patterns are seen among adults. These include heterosexual activities, masturbation, homosexual activities, and abstention. Typically, adulthood is seen as a time for marrying, parenting, and developing sexual intimacy with one partner. However, alternatives to marriage are gaining wider acceptance. Regardless of life-style, sexuality is usually a crucial component of interpersonal relationships. The capacity to give and receive gratification in a stable heterosexual relationship prevails as a societal task. This task encompasses not only the physiologic aspects of sexuality but also the concept of oneself as a sexual being with an associated sex role.

Biologic changes

Physical changes that accompany aging can threaten self-image and self-esteem, particularly in adults who value their youthful image. Wrinkles, a growing waistline, graying hair, and baldness are changes that many find difficult to accept. Fears about loss of femininity or masculinity are magnified by the media, which at times seem to glorify youth, especially in advertisements.

Middle-aged women experience a waning and finally a cessation of menses. The body stops producing estrogen, and the breasts and vagina atrophy. Vaginal lubrication is delayed, and the expansibility of the vaginal canal decreases. Estrogen therapy is often given to compensate for the changes. Males experience delay in attaining erections, a decrease in the expulsive force of ejaculation, and a decrease in the volume of semen ejaculated.

Psychosocial aspects

The sexuality of young adults is influenced by many factors. For instance, pregnancy may alter the woman's self-image as a sexual being. Throughout pregnancy, sexual desire of both partners vacillates. A newborn often focuses the spouses' attention away from each other. Growing children also may decrease opportunities and privacy for sexual interaction. The physical and emotional strain placed on adults by their work or careers often interferes with sexual desire. Also, many misunderstandings can arise because of the differences between the male and female sexual responses. In light of these factors, the more partners can learn about each other's unique responses and the more they can communicate their feelings, the greater their chance for a compatible sexual relationship.

Middle-aged adults may experience some decline in overall sexual interest and activity. However, sex continues to be important to middle-aged adults, and many enjoy intercourse at least once a week. It is thought that levels of sexual activity during youth and the older years are positively correlated. Another factor influencing sexual activity in the middle years is physical health. Disfiguring surgery or cardiac disease, for example, can alter sexual function.

Late Adulthood

Biologic changes

Contrary to popular belief, older people may desire sexual expression and intimacy well into their 70s and 80s, provided they maintain health and have an interesting partner. However, some common disease conditions, including prostatic and cardiac conditions, senile vaginitis, and diabetes, often make sexual adjustments necessary.

Due to changes in vaginal tissues following menopause, the aging woman takes longer to achieve vaginal lubrication. The sexual response pattern is characterized by less vaginal expansion, diminished orgasmic intensity, and a more rapid resolution. (See the section on sexual response patterns later in the chapter.) However, older women retain the capacity for multiple orgasms.

In the older male, sexual changes include lowered sperm production, reduction in the size and firmness of the testicles, and prostate gland difficulties. Older men take longer to achieve erection and reach orgasm but have greater ejaculatory control, which may enhance sexual relations for both the man and his partner. The sexual response pattern is characterized by less myotonia, reduced orgasm intensity, more rapid resolution, and longer refractory periods.

Psychosocial aspects

Aging persons find it necessary to nurture one another, and older adults may find that sexual relationships improve because they are free of the pressures of career and children. Sometimes, boredom with an unchanging sexual relationship and overindulgence in food or drink may decrease desire. On the other hand, a sexual routine and familiarity brings contentment to many couples. Regular intercourse and physical exercise often help maintain sexual functioning.

Older people who lose a mate may need a new outlet for sexual expression. Single older males and females may find masturbation a form of sexual release. Many form nonsexual unions that offer affectionate physical contact, intellectual stimulation, and opportunities to socialize.

Sexual Structure and Function

Male Genitals

The male genitals are a system for producing and transporting sperm. The organs of this system are two sperm-producing testes encased in the scrotum, a series of ducts (epididymis and vas deferens) that transport sperm, several glands that secrete fluid (semen) to protect sperm, and the penis to ejaculate the semen. See Figure 33–1.

Testes

The *testes*, or male gonads, are oval organs about 3.75 cm (1½ in) long and 2.5 cm (1 in) wide. Each testis is encased in a dense white fibrous capsule called the *tunica albuginea.* Inward extensions (septa) of this capsule divide the testis into 200 or more compartments (lobules). Each compartment contains several highly coiled tubules called *seminiferous tubules*, which manufacture sperm. Between the seminiferous tubules are clusters of cells called the *interstitial cells of Leydig*, which secrete male hormones. The two major functions of the testes are *spermatogenesis* (production of the sperm) and the production of sexual hormones.

A sperm consists of a head, neckpiece, midpiece, and tail. The sperm contains *chromosomes*, which transmit inherited characteristics. See page 858.

The second major function of the testes is the production of sexual hormones. The chief testicular hormone is *testosterone*, an androgen, which stimulates genital growth and the development of secondary sexual characteristics, such as a deeper voice, larger musculature, and hair on the face and chest. Additional hormones produced in the testes include estrogen and other androgens. Estrogen seems to control spermatogenesis and is also produced by the adrenal glands.

The male hormones are regulated by the hypothalamus. This organ secretes releasing factors that travel through the bloodstream to the pituitary gland. When stimulated by releasing factors, the pituitary gland secretes follicle stimulating hormone (FSH) and luteinizing hormone (LH). LH stimulates the secretion of testosterone, and FSH stimulates spermatogenesis. Both operate on the basis of a negative feedback system. See Chapter 8.

Scrotum

The testes are located outside of the body and are protected from injury by the *scrotum*, the sac that hangs behind the penis. The scrotal sacs of humans are located in the groin area and are outpouchings of the abdominal wall. The outer skin layer of the scrotum is wrinkled and relatively hairless. Beneath this layer of skin is a layer of smooth muscle and tough connective tissue called the *tunica dartos* and then another layer of striated muscle and connective tissue called the *cremaster.* Smooth muscles contract involuntarily, whereas striated muscles can contract voluntarily or involuntarily. Within these three layers of tissue the tes-

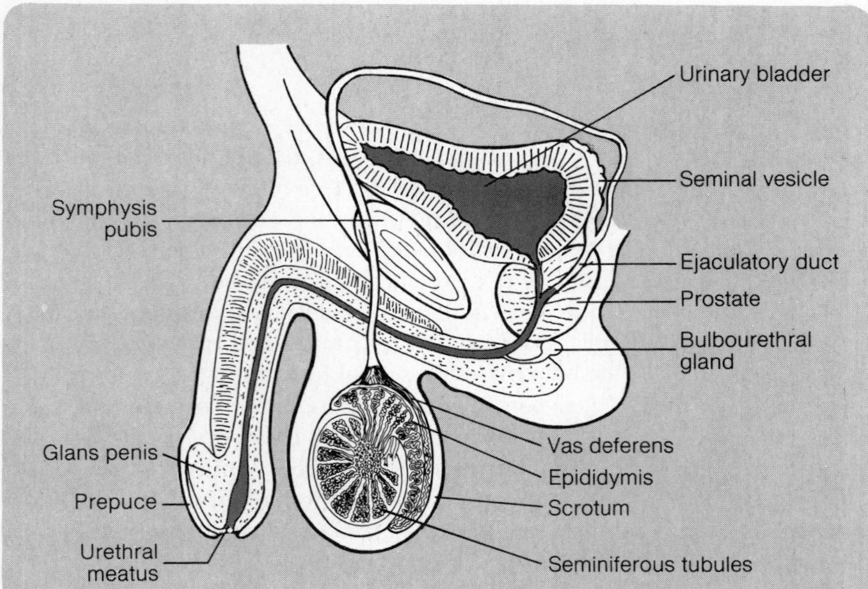

Figure 33–1 The male genitourinary system.

tes are protected. Usually the left testis hangs lower in the scrotal sac than the right.

In the fetus, the testes are located inside the abdominal cavity, but, before birth, male sexual hormones cause the testes to drop into the scrotal sacs. The testes descend through the inguinal canal in the groin, usually before birth.

Failure of one or both testes to descend is called *cryptorchidism* and in the majority of males is bilateral. During the 1st year of life, spontaneous descent of the testes may occur. If not, male hormonal therapy may be necessary during the ages of 1 to 4 years to stimulate descent. Surgical intervention is required to prevent damage to the testes and sterility if both testes fail to descend by age 5. Although males with undescended testicles produce the normal amounts of male sex hormones, they are usually infertile because the abdominal body temperature is too high for spermatogenesis.

Therefore, the scrotum not only protects the testes but also maintains an appropriate temperature for sperm. This cooler scrotal temperature is normally maintained as follows:

1. The thin scrotal skin, with little or minimal underlying fat, offers little insulation.
2. Many superficial small blood vessels in the scrotum dissipate heat as necessary.
3. Abundant sweat glands enhance cooling by evaporation.
4. Muscle receptors, particularly in the tunica dartos muscle, contract and push the testes up toward the groin to be warmed when temperatures are too cool.

Athletic supporters or tight garments that squeeze the scrotum up against the groin raise scrotal temperature. Prolonged wear of such garments can reduce sperm production. The cremaster muscle, though not largely involved in temperature regulation, also can influence scrotal temperature. Strong contractions of the cremaster muscle brought about by sexual excitement, fear, anxiety, or stimulation of the cremasteric reflex (a response to the stroking of the inner surface of the thighs) increase the blood flow from the testes back into the body, thereby increasing scrotal temperature. These contractions, however, are not sustained for long periods.

Epididymis, vas deferens, and ejaculatory ducts

The testes contain coiled seminiferous tubules that manufacture sperm. These tubules drain into a duct outside of the testis called the *epididymis*, a highly coiled duct. The epididymis then drains into the *vas deferens*, a long tube extending from the scrotum, curving around the urinary bladder, and emptying into *ejaculatory ducts*. The two ejaculatory ducts, one from each testis, are short, and both connect with the urethra. See Figure 33–1.

Sperm are transported to the epididymis by mechanisms not fully understood. Transport may be facilitated by contractions of the seminiferous tubules. Cilia, which line the tubules, also move the sperm toward the epididymis.

The epididymis has the following functions: (a) maturation of sperm prior to ejaculation, (b) transport from the testis to the exterior, and (c) secretion of small amounts of seminal fluid. The vas deferens serves as a holding tank for mature sperm between ejaculations. Both the vas deferens and ejaculating ducts serve as vehicles by which the sperm and semen are propelled into the urethra and then out of the body.

Seminal vesicles, prostate, and bulbourethral glands

These structures (see Figure 33–1) produce substances, collectively referred to as *seminal plasma*, which energize the sperm and enhance their transport but are not essential for mature sperm cells. The bulbourethral glands are also referred to as Cowper's glands. Seminal plasma combined with sperm is referred to as *semen*. Normal characteristics of semen are as follows:

1. Creamy texture
2. Gray or yellow
3. Ejaculate volume of 2 to 6 ml
4. 120 million sperm per milliliter of seminal plasma
5. Slightly alkaline pH (7.35 to 7.50)

Primary components of seminal plasma are:

1. Water to transport the sperm
2. Mucus to lubricate the ducts
3. Sugar (fructose) to energize the sperm
4. Salts to maintain isotonicity of the seminal plasma with body fluids
5. Base buffers to neutralize the acidity of the male urethra and subsequently the female vagina.
6. Coagulators to clot the semen in the vagina and prevent leakage of sperm from the vagina (Mann 1970:469–78).

Penis

The penis has two parts: the shaft and glans. In uncircumcised males, the skin of the shaft loosely encloses the glans. This is the *foreskin* (prepuce). *Smegma*, a cheesy material that is a mixture of the oil secretions of the glans and dead tissue cells, accumulates between the foreskin and the glans. Smegma must be cleaned from the glans at every washing.

Penis shapes and sizes vary considerably, not so much in circumference as in length. Males frequently feel concern about the penis size, relating size directly to their capabilities as lovers. Size, however, is unrelated to capability. Like breast size, penis length has little to do with function. Also, the vagina can stretch or contract to accommodate differences in penile circumferences.

The reproductive function of the penis is the transmission of semen to the female. This process includes erection of the penis and ejaculation of the semen, after which the penis returns to a flaccid state.

Erection is the lengthening, widening, and hardening of the penis as it becomes tumescent (congested) with blood. It is a spinal reflex that occurs when the erection center, located at the first to fourth sacral segments of the spinal cord, is stimulated. Erections commonly occur in response to erotic thoughts or other sexual stimuli or to the manipulation (touching) of the penis. However, occasionally erections occur without apparent sexual stimuli. These *reflexogenic erections* are often cause for embarrassment. For example, teenagers whose nervous systems are immature often experience unexpected erections when taking a shower after playing sports. It is not uncommon for nurses to encounter reflexogenic erections in nursing practice, for example, while removing the inguinal sutures of a young teenager. Erections upon awakening are also common among both men and boys. The reason for these erections is not fully understood; they may be due to the pressure of a full bladder, erotic dreams, friction against the sheets, or waking at the end of a paradoxical sleep phase.

Ejaculation is the propulsion of semen out of the penis. It is also a spinal reflex. However, the ejaculatory center is higher in the spinal cord than the erection center (from the third lumbar to the twelfth thoracic segment). Ejaculation has two stages: The semen is transported to the urethra (emission stage), and the semen is propelled out of the urethra (expulsion stage). The force of expulsion depends on degree of arousal, time lapse between ejaculations, age, and other factors. Semen may ooze out over the glans penis or may be projected a certain distance.

Sperm are concentrated in the first third of semen ejaculated. Sperm are also present in secretions from the seminal vesicles, prostate, and bulbourethral glands. These secretions collect at the urethral opening before ejaculation. Thus, pregnancy can occur without ejaculation. Couples who use withdrawal of the penis before ejaculation as a form of contraception need to know this fact.

After erection the penis returns to a flaccid state. This process is referred to as *detumescence* and occurs whether or not ejaculation has occurred. The penile arteries constrict, thus reducing the blood flow to the penis, and the venous outflow allows the engorged blood vessels to empty.

Female Genitals

The female genitals include two ovaries, two fallopian tubes, the uterus, the vagina, and the vulva. See Figure 33–2. These structures provide a system for receiving sperm, producing eggs, housing and nurturing the fertilized egg, and delivering the mature fetus. The mammary glands, although not part of the female genitals, are included in this discussion since they are necessary for suckling the young and give sexual pleasure.

Ovaries

The ovaries, or female gonads, are analogous to the testes in that they produce reproductive cells (ova, gametes) and secrete hormones, but they are located in the pelvic region of the abdominal cavity. Adult ovaries are oval and approximately 2.5 cm (1 in) long. The inner portion of the ovary is called the *medulla*, and the outer portion is called the *cortex*. The cortex develops the eggs and secretes the hormones. The medulla consists of spirals or coils of blood vessels and connective tissue.

The ovaries have two primary functions (a) production and expulsion of ova and (b) production of sexual hormones. In contrast to the testes, which produce sperm throughout life, the ovary contains all the primordial (primitive) ova at birth. These primordial ova originate on the outer surface (germinal layer) of the ovary but move from the outer layer of the cortex during fetal life into the main substance of the cortex. They then are surrounded by a single layer of *granulosa cells*. Once the ova are surrounded by these granulosa cells, they are referred to as *primordial follicles*. At birth about ¾ million primordial follicles are present in the two ovaries, but only about 450 of these follicles will develop sufficiently throughout the female reproductive life to expel their ova (Guyton 1981:1005). Primordial follicles degenerate throughout life. This degeneration is called *atresia*. By puberty only 400,000 follicles remain, and by menopause only a few remain (ibid., p. 1005).

Two female sex hormones are produced by the ovaries: estrogen and progesterone. In addition, some androgens are secreted. Estrogen has several effects, such as regulating fat distribution and breast development, and neutralizing vaginal pH during ovulation. Its primary control is exerted during the first half of the menstrual cycle. Progesterone controls the second half of the menstrual cycle but also influences breast devel-

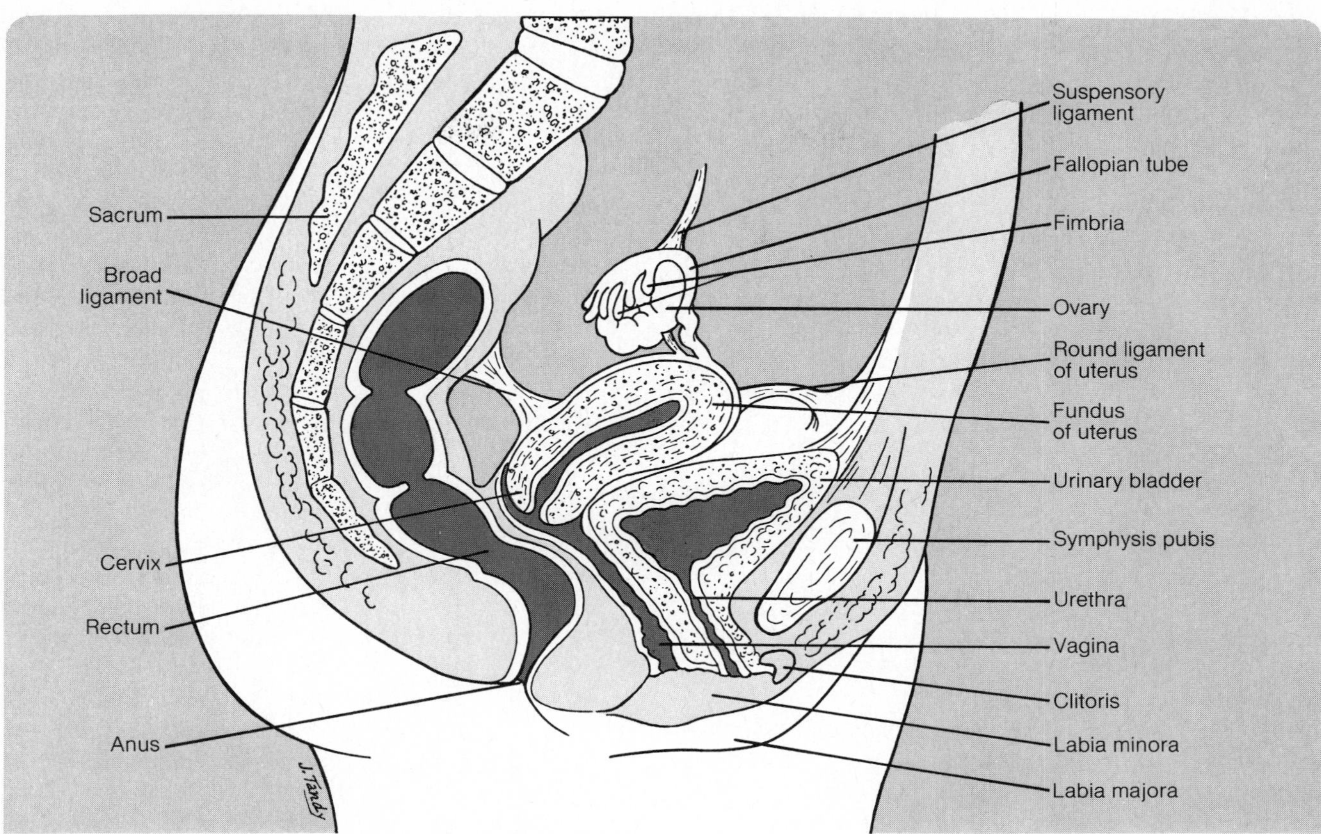

Figure 33–2 The female reproductive tract.

opment. It inhibits uterine muscle contractions during pregnancy. The androgens are thought to increase sexual motivation.

Like male hormones, female sexual hormones are controlled by homeostatic negative feedback systems, but they are produced cyclically (thus the female sexual cycle or the monthly menstrual cycle). These feedback systems also involve three different hierarchies of hormones: (a) releasing factors for FSH and LH from the hypothalamus, (b) the pituitary secretions of FSH and LH, and (c) the production of hormones (estrogen and progesterone) from the gonads (ovaries).

The duration of the female sexual cycle averages about 28 days, but can normally vary between 20 and 35 days. See Figure 33–3. This cycle can be considered in three stages.

Preovulatory stage The *preovulatory stage* lasts an average of 14 days (plus or minus 3 to 5 days), starting on the 1st day of menstrual flow and ending with *ovulation* (release of the ovum from the ovary). It is also referred to as the *proliferative* or *follicular stage*. On the 1st day of this stage, the follicles begin to grow spontaneously without hormonal control. Then the pituitary gland, stimulated by the hypothalmic FSH-releasing factor, produces FSH, which stimulates the follicles to enlarge further. One of these follicles, outgrowing the others, becomes large enough to ovulate. The other follicles undergo atresia. This enlarged follicle is called the *Graafian follicle* (maturing follicle). Estrogen secretion is then stimulated by this follicle under the influence of FSH. The effects of estrogen include the buildup of the endometrial lining of the uterus for anticipated conception and the final maturation of the Graafian follicle immediately before ovulation. Once estrogen reaches its peak level in the bloodstream, the production of FSH is decreased by negative feedback, but a sudden surge of LH is then released by the pituitary gland. This surge triggers ovulation.

Postovulatory stage The *postovulatory stage* of the female sexual cycle starts immediately after ovulation and averages about 13 days in the female whose cycle is 28 days. It ends when the woman begins her menstrual period. This phase is also referred to as the *secretory* or *luteal* stage. The term *secretory* is used because the lining of the uterus secretes a substance (carbohydrate glycogen) to provide nourishment for a fertilized ovum

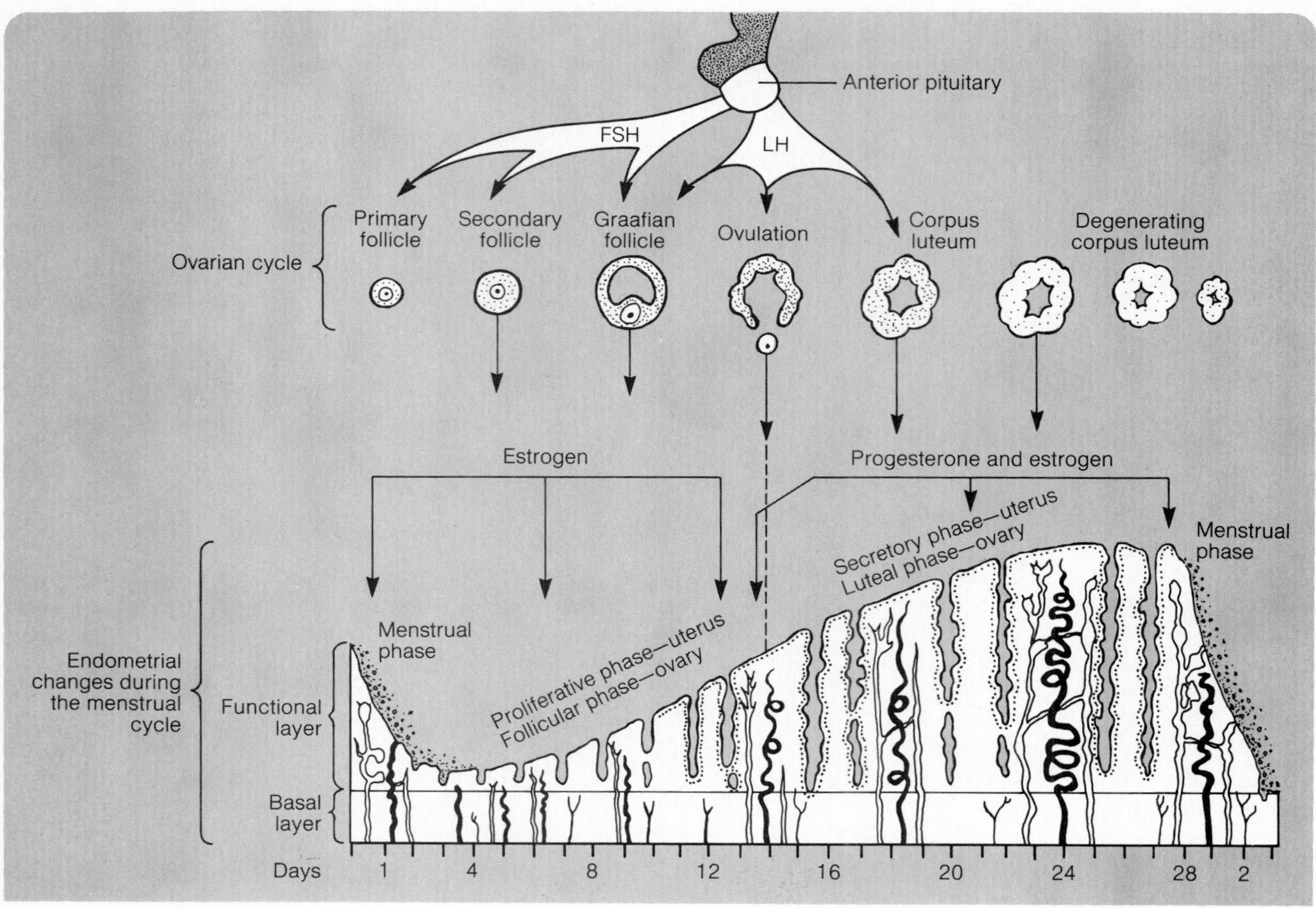

Figure 33–3 Changes in the endometrium and ovary during the menstrual cycle. (From S. B. Olds, M. L. London, P. A. Ladewig, and S. V. Davidson, *Obstetric nursing* [Menlo Park, Calif.: Addison-Wesley Publishing Co., 1980], p. 115.)

(*zygote*). The term *luteal* is used because the Graafian follicle undergoes changes, forming a yellowish mass in the ovary known as the *corpus luteum*. This occurs under the influence of LH. If the ovum is impregnated, the corpus luteum grows and persists for several months. It secretes the hormone progesterone as well as estrogen. Progesterone is responsible for maintaining the uterine lining for the reception and development of the zygote. The estrogen enhances the action of progesterone. By negative feedback, progesterone inhibits the production of LH, and estrogen inhibits the production of FSH. These luteal hormones maintain the implanted zygote for about 3 months until the placenta is developed. It then secretes these hormones. If fertilization does not occur, the corpus luteum gradually degenerates and becomes white and scarred. It is then referred to as the *corpus albicans*. Reductions in the production of progesterone and estrogen result, and menstrual flow is induced. The endometrium shrinks as the arteries collapse without hormonal stimulation. Deoxygenation of the endometrium results and the tissues die. Most of these dead tissues are sloughed off, and bleeding occurs through the weak, collapsed capillaries.

Menses *Menses* (menstruous flow) lasts for 3 to 7 days. Menstruation overlaps with the beginning of the preovulatory phase. The 1st day of flow is considered the 1st day of the sexual cycle. The amount of menstrual discharge varies among women and from cycle to cycle. The average discharge is about 90 ml (3 oz) but can range from 30 to 180 ml (1 to 6 oz). Women using the combination contraceptive pill tend to have less than the average discharge, whereas women with intrauterine devices (IUDs) often have heavier flows.

Menarche, the first menstrual period, occurs between the ages of 9 and 17 years. For the first few years, ovulation and menses may be somewhat erratic. Eventually a stable rhythm is established until menopause occurs. Menstrual cramps are common, particularly during the first few days of menstruation because of contractions of the uterus and cervix. The cause of these is undetermined. Moods also change before and during menstruation. A few days before, some women feel tense, anxious, irritable, depressed, or hostile. At menstruation, most of these feelings are eased or disappear. However, until the estrogen levels are elevated during the preovulatory stage, depression is common. By the time of ovulation, when the estrogen levels are at their peak, women tend to feel happy and self-confident.

Thus mood swings during the female sexual cycle are influenced by the hormonal changes that occur throughout the cycle; conversely, a woman's emotional state can also influence her hormonal levels. For example, a woman stressed by illness, a work crisis, or a family conflict, can experience altered hormonal levels that affect menstruation. Also, a woman may not menstruate during one cycle because of stress.

Fallopian tubes

The two fallopian tubes (oviducts) are about 10 cm (4 in) long and extend between the ovaries and uterus but are not attached to the ovaries. Their chief function is to provide an environment that is appropriate for the transport in opposite directions of the ova and sperm and thus for fertilization. Secretory cells in the mucosal lining of the tube are believed to nourish the ovum.

The mechanism by which the ova are transported from the ovaries into the fallopian tubes is not fully understood. Occasionally, because the two structures are unattached, an ovum is released into the abdominal cavity rather than into the fallopian tube. If this egg is fertilized and implanted in the abdominal cavity, the condition is referred to as an *ectopic pregnancy* (implantation of a zygote outside of the uterus). Ectopic pregnancies also occur occasionally in the fallopian tubes.

Fertilization of ova usually occurs in the middle third of a fallopian tube. The transport of the sperm is facilitated by muscle contractions of the tubes and by the sperm's active swimming movements. Transport of the zygote is facilitated by the motion of cilia in the tube, which sweep toward the uterus, and also by tubal muscle contractions. Generally, the zygote is transported to the uterus in about 3 days. However, this rate of transport is influenced by progesterone and estrogen: Progesterone retards the rate of transport, whereas estrogen accelerates it. Estrogen is therefore used to prevent implantation of the zygote. Large doses of estrogen administered after coitus accelerate the transport of the zygote before it is ready for implantation. Estrogen also alters the endometrial lining, making it inappropriate to receive the zygote.

Uterus

The uterus, one of the most changeable organs of the body, lies between the rectum and urinary bladder. It is thick walled and hollow. The three layers of the wall are the *perimetrium*, the thin outer layer of serous membrane; the *myometrium*, the middle thick layer of smooth muscle; and the *endometrium*, the inner mucous membrane lining. The perimetrium of the uterus covers all the uterus except the *cervix* (the neck of the uterus). The myometrium contains many muscle fibers that run in different directions. Contractions of these fibers occur during childbirth, nursing, sexual tension, and orgasm. During pregnancy the uterus enlarges, and the muscle fibers grow longer. Muscular contractions dilate the cervix and help expel the fetus.

The endometrium has two principal layers: the *functionalis*, the layer shed during menstruation, and the *basalis*, the layer closest to the myometrium. The basalis layer is maintained during menstruation and produces a new functionalis layer after menstruation. The endometrial lining is essential for the reception and maintenance of fertilized egg implants and for the development of the zygote. The uterine lining of the cervix has glands that produce mucus, which plug the opening into the uterus. During ovulation, when estrogen levels are high, the characteristics of this mucous plug change. The mucus becomes more copious, thinner, and thus more penetrable by sperm. Examination of the characteristics of the cervical mucous plug can help determine whether a woman is ovulating or infertile.

Vagina

The vagina has a threefold function. It serves as the lower part of the birth canal, the passageway for menstrual flow, and the receptacle for the penis during intercourse. The vagina, a muscular tubular organ lined with mucous membrane, is about 10 cm (4 in) long. The mucosa of the vagina is capable of a great deal of extension because it lies in a series of inwardly directed and transverse folds called *rugae*. The muscular layer of the vagina can also stretch considerably. This distensibility is important during delivery and intercourse.

Large amounts of glycogen (a type of carbohydrate) are produced in the vagina. Glycogen is decomposed into lactic acid by the normal bacteria of the vagina (Döderlein's bacilli). These acids create an environment with a low pH, which prevents many bacteria and yeasts from causing disease in the vagina. This acidity is also injurious to sperm cells, but the buffering action of semen ensures their survival. Döderlein's bacilli can be destroyed by antibiotics. Thus it is not uncommon for women taking antibiotics for other infections to get vaginal infections.

Changes in the vaginal mucosa occur in response to estrogen during the menstrual cycle and in response to sexual excitement. Normally, the cells of the vaginal mucosa continually slough off and are replaced by new ones. During the menstrual cycle these cells, under the influence of estrogen, undergo *cornification* (hardening). Such cells can be examined under a microscope. The cells are obtained from a vaginal swab and transferred to a glass slide. This examination is commonly called a *vaginal smear*. Examination of vaginal smears taken at the time of ovulation can help diagnose infertility. Estrogen levels at such times should usually be high.

During sexual excitement the numerous small blood vessels of the vagina become engorged with blood, and it develops a purplish hue. This congestion is also responsible for the lubrication of the vagina when a woman is sexually excited. Initially small droplets of fluid exude through the blood vessel walls. As sexual excitement increases, these droplets of fluid coalesce to form a shiny layer of lubricant over the mucosa.

At the *vaginal orifice* (the external opening of the vagina) there is a thin fold of vascularized mucous membrane called the *hymen*. It forms a border around the orifice and partially closes it. Sometimes the hymen is *imperforate*—it covers the orifice completely. This condition warrants medical intervention to permit the passage of menstrual flow.

Vulva

The external female genitals are collectively referred to as the *vulva*, or *pudendum*. The structures of the vulva include the mons pubis, two labia majora, two labia minora, the clitoris, and the vestibule.

The *mons pubis*, also referred to as the *mons veneris*, is a pillow of adipose tissue situated over the symphysis pubis and covered by coarse pubic hair. The mons pubis is highly sensitive and contains many touch receptors. Stimulation of the mons during intercourse or masturbation can lead to an orgasm.

The *labia majora* (large lips) are the two longitudinal folds of skin extending downward and backward from the mons pubis. They serve to protect the labia minora and the openings of the vagina and urethra. The labia majora are covered by hair on their upper outer surfaces and contain an abundance of adipose tissue and sebaceous and sweat glands. Usually the labia majora meet in a deep cleft. However, during periods of sexual excitement these lips separate and flatten against the inner thighs to expose the labia minora and vaginal opening.

The *labia minora* lie inside the labia majora. They are devoid of hair and have relatively few sweat glands; however, they do contain numerous sebaceous glands. The labia minora extend upward to unite and form the prepuce (foreskin) of the clitoris and downward to protect the vaginal opening. Because the small lips undergo vivid color changes during sexual excitement, they are often called the "sex skin." The color changes are due to increased influx of blood and vary in proportion to the level of arousal. Pregnancy also contributes to color changes. In nonpregnant women the labia minora are normally pale pink and become bright red when the woman is sexually excited. In pregnant women, the labia minora contain more blood vessels and thus are normally red in color. When a pregnant woman is sexually excited, the labia minora assume a deep wine color. These color changes are positive signs of approaching orgasm.

The *clitoris* is a small round mass of erectile tissue, blood vessels, and nerves located behind the junction of the labia minora (the prepuce). The exposed part of the clitoris is referred to as the *glans clitoris*. The clitoris is capable of enlargement when stimulated and is homologous to the penis. Its principal function is to receive and transmit erotic stimuli during sexual excitement. When a woman is aroused sexually, the glans becomes tumescent and is elevated upward so that it is hidden behind the prepuce.

The *vestibule* is the cleft between the labia and contains the vaginal orifice, urethral orifice, hymen, and openings of several ducts. The vaginal orifice occupies the major portion of the vestibule. Above the vaginal orifice and below the clitoris lies the urethral orifice. The ducts of glands that secrete mucus (the lesser vestibular glands) are located behind and on either side of the urethra. These lesser vestibular glands are homologous to the prostate. Larger glands (the greater vestibular glands) lie on either side of the vaginal orifice. Their ducts open into the space between the hymen and labia minora. These glands are homologous to the bulbourethral glands and produce a mucous secretion that acts as a lubricant during intercourse.

Mammary glands

The *mammary glands* (breasts) not only secrete milk but also respond to stimulation and give sexual pleasure. Each mammary gland consists of lobes (compartments) separated by adipose tissue, which is the primary factor determining the size of the breasts. Each lobe has smaller compartments called lobules. These contain milk-secreting cells called alveoli, which are clustered in grapelike arrangements. The milk from the alveoli is conveyed into a series of tubules and then into the mammary ducts, the ampullae (expanded sinuses where milk can be stored), and the lactiferous ducts, which terminate in the nipple. Each lactiferous duct conveys the milk from one of the lobes to the nipple. Surrounding the nipple is a circular pigmented area called the *areola*. It is bumpy or rough because it contains sebaceous glands.

The breasts begin to develop at puberty under the influence of estrogen produced by the ovaries, progesterone, growth hormone from the pituitary, prolactin from the pituitary, and thyroxine from the thyroid.

Women worry about the size and shape of breasts much as men worry about penis size and shape. The size and shape, however, do not affect functional abilities. Women also may worry about how pregnancy and nursing will affect breast size and shape. During pregnancy the breasts become heavier and some of the supporting ligaments may stretch, causing the breasts to hang slightly lower thereafter. However, nursing does not permanently alter breast size, shape, or "lift."

Sexual Stimulation and Response Patterns

Sexual Stimulation

Sexual stimulation may be physical or psychologic. Erotic stimuli (those that cause sexual arousal) may be real or symbolic. Imagination, sight, hearing, smell, or touch all contribute to sexual stimulation.

Physical stimulation

Physical stimulation occurs with touch, pressure, or bodily contact. Nerve receptors transfer these stimuli to the spinal cord and the brain. Kissing, breast stimulation, manual stimulation of the genitals, oral-genital stimulation, anal stimulation, and pain may all be sources of sexual pleasure. Physical contact or petting that increases sexual arousal prior to intercourse is called *foreplay*, or *precoital stimulation*. Wide variations exist in the amount and methods of foreplay among persons in North America.

Erogenous zones Certain areas of the body are richly supplied with nerve endings and give sexual pleasure when stimulated. Obviously the genitals of both sexes are highly erogenous. However, many other areas of the body, such as the mouth, ears, breast, back, buttocks, anus, neck, abdomen, and thighs, may give pleasure when stimulated and are thus also erogenous zones. The primary erogenous zones of males, other than the genitals, are the thighs, lips, and ears; erogenous zones of females are the breasts, thighs, and ears (Goldstein 1976:130). Erogenous zones adapt rapidly to continuous stimulation by becoming decreasingly responsive. Because touch and pressure receptors respond better to changes in stimulation, sexual arousal can be increased by alternating sites of stimulation rather than maintaining continuous contact with one or two areas.

Kissing Kissing is unique to humans as a source of erotic stimulation and varies from simple kissing to tongue kissing. It involves the senses of touch, taste, and smell. Kissing plays different roles in different cultures. Some cultures prefer oral-genital contact to kissing during foreplay.

Breast stimulation Oral or manual stimulation of the breasts can give sexual pleasure. Breast stimulation can cause pleasurable contractions in the pelvic region. Stimulation of the breasts is associated with the release of the pituitary hormone oxytocin, which produces milk secretion and causes smooth muscle contractions of the uterus and related structures. Thus, breast stimulation is often a source of sexual pleasure in women who are breast-feeding and can cause orgasm in some women. Breast stimulation during foreplay can maintain high sexual arousal levels and may be a significant source of satisfaction during intercourse.

Manual stimulation of the genitals This form of foreplay can by itself lead to orgasm. Manual stimulation may be reciprocal or may be *masturbation*, self-stimulation of the genitals or other body parts. Most males find the penis more sensitive to stimulation than the scrotum. The glans or the shaft of the penis can be stimulated by firm gripping and stroking, or the *frenulum* (the fold that connects the lower surface of the glans penis to the prepuce) can be lightly touched or tugged. When sexual excitement increases, manipulation becomes more rapid until ejaculation occurs. After ejaculation the glans penis is often hypersensitive to touch or pressure.

Manipulation of female genitals is more variable than manipulation male genitals. Direct stimulation of the glans clitoris is often considered the major erotic focus for females. However, this highly sensitive area rarely requires direct stimulation. Often it is sufficient to touch or tug the prepuce and labia lightly, which stimulates the clitoral shaft, or to apply pressure to the mons pubis or vulva.

Contrary to certain beliefs, masturbation is neither physically nor mentally harmful. The frequency of masturbation ranges from several times a day to several times a week. More than 80% of males and more than 50% of females masturbate. Most men masturbate earlier in life (often before the age of 20 years) than women, some of whom may not masturbate until age 40 or later. Sometimes genital substitutes are used during masturbation. Males sometimes use vaginal substitutes made of inflatable plastic. Women sometimes use *dildos* (artificial penises) or vibrators.

Oral-genital stimulation Cunnilingus, fellatio, and soixante-neuf are three types of oral-genital stimulation. *Cunnilingus* is the oral stimulation (kissing, licking, or sucking) of the clitoris and labia. Lubrication is provided by saliva. *Fellatio* is the oral stimulation of the penis. *Soixante-neuf,* the French term for "69," is simultaneous oral-genital stimulation by two persons. The acceptability of oral-genital contact is an individual and cultural matter. Some consider oral-genital stimulation a perversion, whereas others consider it highly desirable when performed voluntarily and privately.

Anal stimulation Oral-anal stimulation is *anilingus*. Anilingus is not anal intercourse. Anilingus is not a common method of precoital stimulation probably because of the association of the anus with feces. However, the anus is richly innervated and can be a source of sexual pleasure.

Pain Scratching, pinching, or biting can increase sexual arousal. For example, some people derive pleasure from having the ear lobes bitten, even to the point of drawing blood.

Psychologic stimulation

Erotic stimulation through smell, taste, hearing, sight, or fantasy is psychologic sexual stimulation. These stimuli often evoke pleasant past experiences or future hopes and desires.

1. *Odors.* Body odors can be sexually stimulating. Perfumes associated with a previous pleasurable sexual experience often produce a sexual response.
2. *Sights.* Certain sights can produce erotic responses. Individuals vary greatly in the sights they find erotic. Pictures of naked people, romantic photographs, inviting decor and colors, certain clothing, and changes in light can all be sexually stimulating.
3. *Sounds.* Sexual excitement is often enhanced by words or music. Again, people vary considerably in what words or music they find stimulating. Often, pleasing sounds relate to a previous positive sexual experience.

Sexual Response Patterns

Physiologic responses to sexual stimulation are basically the same for all individuals, male or female. However, the psychologic and sociologic aspects of the response to stimulation are highly variable. Variations occur between males and females, among members of the same sex, and even in the same person at different times.

Positions for sexual intercourse

Sexual intercourse (*coitus, copulation*) can be both physically and emotionally gratifying. There are many positions for sexual intercourse. Face-to-face, lying positions (with either the male or female on top) or side-by-side postures are common. Variations of these face-to-face positions include standing postures, which can allow more freedom of movement, and sitting-kneeling positions (the female sits on the edge of a bed or chair while the male kneels in front). In addition, several rear entry postures may be used. A couple's willingness to experiment with sexual positions depends on social influences, previous inhibitions, and their agility and imagination.

Because direct clitoral stimulation is important to the female during coitus, the side-lying positions and female-on-top positions are recommended (Masters and Johnson 1966:59). Although clitoral stimulation is also possible when the male is on top and high over his partner, it is thought that during intromission in this position the penis is directed more toward the posterior vaginal wall and rectum rather than into the canal.

Physiology of intercourse

Two primary physiologic changes occur during sexual intercourse: vasocongestion (congestion of the blood vessels) and myotonia (increased muscular tension). Physiologic changes during coitus occur in four phases: (a) excitement, (b) plateau, (c) orgasm, and (d) resolution (Masters and Johnson 1966:4).

The *excitement phase* develops from erotic stimuli and involves a gradual increase in the level of sexual arousal. Signs of this stage in the male include:

1. Erection
2. Tensing, thickening, and elevation of the scrotum
3. Enlarging of the testes with elevation toward the perineum as the spermatic cord shortens, signs due largely to vasocongestion and parasympathetic nervous system effects

In the female the signs of sexual excitement are:

1. Enlargement of the clitoral glans
2. Vaginal lubrication

3. Widening and lengthening of the vaginal barrel
4. Separation and flattening of the labia majora
5. Reddening of the labia minora and vaginal wall
6. Nipple erection, breast tumescence, and engorged areolae

Other signs during the excitement phase are common to both males and females. These are increases in heart rate and blood pressure in proportion to the level of arousal, involuntary tensing of the intercostal and abdominal muscles, and the appearance of the *sex flush*, a rashlike condition beginning on the abdomen and moving to the breasts, neck, face, and back. The sex flush is more common in females and increases with the level of arousal and high room temperatures.

The *plateau phase* is the period in which sexual tension intensifies to levels nearing orgasm, provided that adequate erotic stimulation is maintained. During this phase the influence of the sympathetic nervous system is evident in both sexes. Heart rates accelerate to 100 to 175 beats per minute; breathing rates increase up to 40 breaths per minute, particularly in the late stages of the plateau phase; and the systolic and diastolic blood pressures rise (20 to 80 mm Hg systolic and 10 to 40 mm Hg diastolic). Myotonia increases both voluntarily and involuntarily. Abdominal intercostal and facial muscles contract, and both males and females may voluntarily contract their anal sphincters to enhance stimulation.

In the male, changes during the plateau phase include:

1. Increase in the penile circumference at the coronal ridge and inconsistent deepening in color
2. 50% increase in testicular size and elevation closer to the perineum
3. Appearance of a few drops of mucoid secretions from the bulbourethral glands
4. Appearance of the sex flush late in the phase in some males

In the female, changes during the plateau phase include:

1. Retraction of the clitoris under the clitoral hood
2. Appearance of the orgasmic platform (an increase in size of the outer one-third of the vagina and labia minora due to congestion), which prevents leakage of semen after ejaculation and also increases friction on the penis
3. Further deepening and widening of the vaginal barrel
4. Further reddening of the labia minora
5. Appearance of a few drops of mucoid secretions from the greater vestibular glands, which correspond to the male bulbourethral gland secretions
6. Increasing engorgement of the labia majora
7. Increasing engorgement of the breast and nipples
8. Spread of the sex flush over the entire body

Orgasm is the involuntary climax of sexual tension, accompanied by physiologic and psychologic release. Although the total body is involved in orgasm, the pelvic area is perceived as the major focus. The orgasmic phase is short compared to the previous phases, lasting only a few seconds. This stage involves rhythmic, spasmodic contractions of the genitals. The heart rate, breathing rate, and blood pressure rise to peak levels during orgasm.

In the male, expulsive contractions of the penis occur, starting at less than 1-second intervals. After the first three or four contractions, the contractions are less frequent. Ejaculation has two stages. In the first stage, seminal fluid is expelled into the prostatic urethra. During the second stage, semen is expelled from the prostatic urethra to the urethral meatus. The force of ejaculation diminishes after the first few expulsive contractions. Secondary organs, such as the vas deferens, epididymis, seminal vesicles, and prostate, also contract during orgasm. During ejaculation the internal bladder sphincter closes to prevent retrograde passage of semen into the bladder. Many males report pleasure as the seminal fluid passes through the urethra.

Females experience approximately five to twelve contractions in the orgasmic platform during orgasm. The response is similar to the male response in that contractions initially occur at intervals of less than 1 second and then diminish in frequency and intensity. The muscles of the pelvic floor surrounding the lower one-third of the vagina and the uterine muscles also contract during orgasm. Sensations during orgasm are more varied for women than men. Common patterns of orgasm include (a) a minor orgasm in which the plateau phase fluctuates with only small surges toward orgasm, (b) multiple orgasms, and (c) a single orgasm comparable to the male's. Changes in orgasmic response patterns occur in females after many coital experiences. The factors causing these changes are unknown. Females seem to start with a minor orgasmic pattern and progress to either a multiple and then a single orgasmic response or to a single and then multiple orgasmic response.

The *resolution phase* is the return to the unaroused state. Usually this phase lasts about as long as the excitement phase. Many individuals perspire during this phase. Other responses include sleepiness, relaxation, or emotional outbursts such as crying or laughing. Immediately after orgasm, males undergo a physiologic *refractory period*, during which they cannot respond to continued sexual stimuli.

Assessment

Before starting an assessment, the nurse needs to recognize that sexuality is a highly personal subject. Patients' cooperation must never be assumed. Some people do not want to discuss their sexual attitudes, values, or behavior and will be offended when questioned.

Watts (1978) describes four levels of assessment and the professional competence required at each level. See Table 33–1. Even as part of a health history, screening for sexual function and dysfunction should be done only when:

1. The patient or support persons give verbal or behavioral cues to problems.
2. The patient's illness could cause sexual problems or concerns.

Cues to Sexual Problems

Patients and support persons may give the nurse verbal or behavioral cues to sexual problems. Questions such as "Will I be able to have sex after the operation?" or "Do you think my husband will want me?" offer the sensitive nurse an opportunity to explore the subject with the patient. Often such questions are simple requests for information, but they may be the patient's way to broach a more sensitive subject.

The following are some cues patients may present:

1. Asks questions about normal sexual activity
2. Refers to rigid upbringing in relation to sexual matters
3. Reflects judgmental attitudes; for instance, that sex is dirty or evil or that it is a necessary but unpleasant part of marriage
4. Expresses concern about sexual adequacy
5. Perceives self as unattractive
6. Reveals information about a previous rape, illegitimate birth, incest, homosexual experiences, or abortion
7. Refers to sexual partner in a negative manner
8. Shows lassitude, fatigue, and lack of interest in sexual matters after an illness

Certain behaviors can reflect a sexual problem; however, the nurse must interpret the behavior in light of the individual's culture, development, and current situation. Extreme embarrassment over exposure of the breasts may reflect a sexual problem; at the same time, such behavior may be normal in a particular social group. Certain other behaviors—for example, intentionally exposing the breasts or genitals or fondling a nurse suggestively—are clearer reflections of sexual problems.

Table 33–1 Levels for Sexual Assessment and Intervention

Competence level	Professional preparation	Appropriate assessment	Appropriate intervention
1	Professional nurse	Health history; screen for sexual function and dysfunction	Limited sex education; limited information about sexual feelings, behaviors, myths
2	Professional nurse plus training in sex education and counseling	Sexual history	Counseling on specific information about sex and sexuality; suggestions regarding sexual fears and adaptations to illness; anticipatory guidance
3	Professional nurse prepared as a trained sex therapist	Sexual problem history	Sex therapy; individuals and couple
4	Psychiatric nurse clinician with a master's degree and training in sex therapy	Psychiatric and psychosexual history	Intensive individual psychotherapy, sex therapy, and marital therapy

Adapted from R. J. Watts, Dimensions of sexual health, *American Journal of Nursing*, September 1979, 79:1570.

Effects of Illness

Certain disease conditions can create or augment sexual problems. Any condition that makes the patient less attractive or affects normal functioning may have sexual implications for the patient. Colostomy, disfigurement due to surgery or extensive burns, and paralysis of a limb from a stroke are only a few.

The extent of the assessment depends largely on the needs of the patient (i.e., actual problems and potential problems) and the competence of the nurse. A detailed assessment is usually necessary when the patient's illness directly affects sexual function. For example, following a spinal cord injury, the patient often needs to learn new methods of satisfying sexual needs. Detailed assessments are usually carried out by specially trained therapists. Other situations call for less extensive assessments; for instance, when a patient needs to know when he or she can resume sexual activity or when a patient recovering from a stroke or heart attack asks what precautions he or she need take during intercourse.

Attitudes toward Sexuality

One of the most important aspects of assessment is discovering the relevant attitudes of patients and their support persons. In some instances these attitudes can affect recuperation from an illness or a person's willingness to cooperate with care. For example, a woman might have attitudes or beliefs that make her unwilling to have a vaginal examination by a physician or give herself a douche. A man may be unwilling to have a prostatectomy because he believes he will be impotent following surgery.

Individual attitudes about sexuality derive largely from family, peer group, cultural, or religious influences; life experiences; and sexual orientation. A sensitive nurse can learn about these attitudes by carefully listening to and observing the patient and support persons. A patient's unwillingness to have a male physician examine her breasts should be recorded and reported to the physician.

Many factors affect an individual's sexual attitudes and sexual behavior. Some of these are development, culture, knowledge, and health.

Development

Sexual development is discussed earlier in this chapter. Changes that come with age may affect sexual behavior significantly. However, the precise relationship of these changes to sexual function is not directly known. The sexual responsiveness of older people appears to depend considerably on the nature of their relationships.

Culture

Culture affects sexual attitudes profoundly. Although many examples could be given, the Chinese illustrate the influence of culture on sexuality well. One study (Ellis, Ho 1982: 29) of Chinese living in Canada suggests that Chinese women, even those born in Canada, are embarrassed to discuss sex. Older women believed that women require yang (men) for health; that women without yang have yellow complexions, general weakness, and a tendency to depression and mood swings; and that men cannot live without yin (women) (ibid., p. 29). Therefore, the women believed that homosexuality was dangerous to health. The same study showed younger Chinese women's attitudes toward contraception differed from those of women born in China. Among the latter, abstinence was the most popular method of contraception, yet abortion was accepted. Elderly Chinese had negative feelings about contraception, while younger women valued family planning.

Knowledge

Knowledge about sexuality affects attitudes and beliefs. Also, attitudes may affect a person's ability to obtain and accept knowledge. Because sexuality is such a sensitive subject, people may resist or refuse to believe accurate information. Some common myths about sex are: Emotional illness develops when sexual needs are not met; all homosexuals molest children; and sexual desire normally disappears in old age. Lack of knowledge can create fears that affect behavior. A couple who believes that cancer is contagious may needlessly refrain from sexual activity long after the woman's cancerous uterus is removed.

Health

Health and illness affect an individual's sexual attitudes and activity. Also, sexual activity can be a cause of illness. Sexually transmitted disease can be passed on through intercourse with an infected person. Hospitalization can affect sexuality in several ways: Hospitalized persons lack privacy and may undergo changes in self-concept due to greater dependence. Patients requiring genital care or urinary catheterization may find these distressing and an invasion of their sexual privacy, perhaps indicating the need for further assessment by the nurse.

Illness can also affect sexuality directly if the patient has disease of breasts, penis, prostate, or uterus. Surgery on or radiation of these areas can threaten the patient's sexual image and function. In addition, certain treatments can have side effects that diminish sexual function. For example, reserpine and other antihypertensives can diminish libido and make a man unable to achieve or maintain an erection. Antihistamines can cause erectile dysfunction and vaginal dryness. Antidepressants can cause impotence.

Sexual Aspects of a Nursing History

The nurse elicits sexual information during a nursing history when problems are suspected or when the patient's illness could cause sexual problems. Privacy is essential during such an interview, whether the nurse asks only two questions about sex or obtains a complete sexual history. At level 1 (see Table 33–1), it is suggested that sex be explored during the review of systems (Watts 1979:1572). The nurse should know beforehand what information is required and ask only questions that elicit that information. See Chapter 5, page 127, for information on interviewing. See Table 33–2 for suggested questions.

Clinical Examination

The clinical examination of the female reproductive system and the male genitourinary system are described in Chapter 14, pages 346 and 347. Two additional examinations of particular importance are breast and testicular examination. Patients should learn to conduct these self-examinations at home. The goal of regular self-examination is early detection of cancer, which greatly improves the individual's chances of complete cure following treatment.

Breast self-examination

Of all cancers among women, cancer of the breast is the most frequent cause of death. Breast self-examination (BSE) should be conducted once a month. A regular time is best, such as immediately following menstrual flow or on the 1st day of the month.

Women who examine their breasts regularly become familiar with their shape and texture. Any changes must be reported immediately to a physician for accurate diagnosis. Before beginning to teach breast self-examination to a patient, the nurse needs to identify the patient's attitudes toward this procedure. Some patients are reluctant to conduct BSE because they fear what they might find. The nurse needs to explore these fears with the patient. Patients often offer these reasons for avoiding BSE: "I don't have time" and "I just don't think of doing it." The nurse also needs to explore

Table 33–2 Sample Questions for a Sexual Assessment during a Health History

Male	Female
Genitourinary system	*Reproductive system*
Do you presently have a genital infection or have you had one recently?	At what age did you start menstruating?
Do you have any discharge from your penis?	When was your last period?
Do you feel pain when urinating?	What was the duration of the flow?
How often do you urinate?	How heavy was the flow? How many pads did you use?
Do you need to urinate during the night?	Do you have pain with your periods?
Do you have difficulty starting to urinate?	Do you have any bleeding or discharge between periods?
What is the quality of your stream? Is it thin or forceful, for example?	How many children do you have? How many pregnancies, miscarriages?
	Do you practice contraception? What method do you use?
Sexual system	*Sexual system*
Do you have erections early in the morning?	Do you have sufficient vaginal lubrication prior to and during intercourse?
Are you able to achieve a firm erection when aroused?	Do you experience any pain during intercourse?
Have there been times when you have been unable to get an erection?	How often do you have intercourse?
Does your desire remain during sexual activity?	Is your desire for sex consistent or does it fluctuate?
Have you noticed any change in the volume of your ejaculate?	Are you able to achieve an orgasm?
Do you have any questions about sexual activity?	Do you get the best orgasm (climax) with masturbation or coitus?
	Are you satisfied with your sexual performance?
	Do you have any questions about sexual activity?

Adapted from R. J. Watts, Dimensions of sexual health, *American Journal of Nursing*, September 1979, 79:1569.

these reasons with the patient with particular reference to her self-esteem (see Chapter 32) and her need to spend time on herself.

Another reason for not conducting BSE is a reluctance to handle one's own breast. Manipulation may be associated with fondling and masturbation. This reason often goes unexpressed among older women and some religious and cultural groups. Changing such attitudes frequently requires in-depth counseling as well as accurate information about BSE. A patient may accept information only after attitudes have changed.

One technique for BSE is to stand in front of a mirror with hands first at one's sides and then clasped over the head. The woman observes each breast in both positions for:

1. Indentations, rippling, puckering, or dimpling
2. Asymmetry of the nipples; e.g., a nipple pulled to one side
3. Discoloration
4. Discharge from the nipple
5. Any change in the size or shape of the breasts

Figure 33–4 Palpating the right breast using the palmar surfaces of the first, second, third, and fourth fingers.

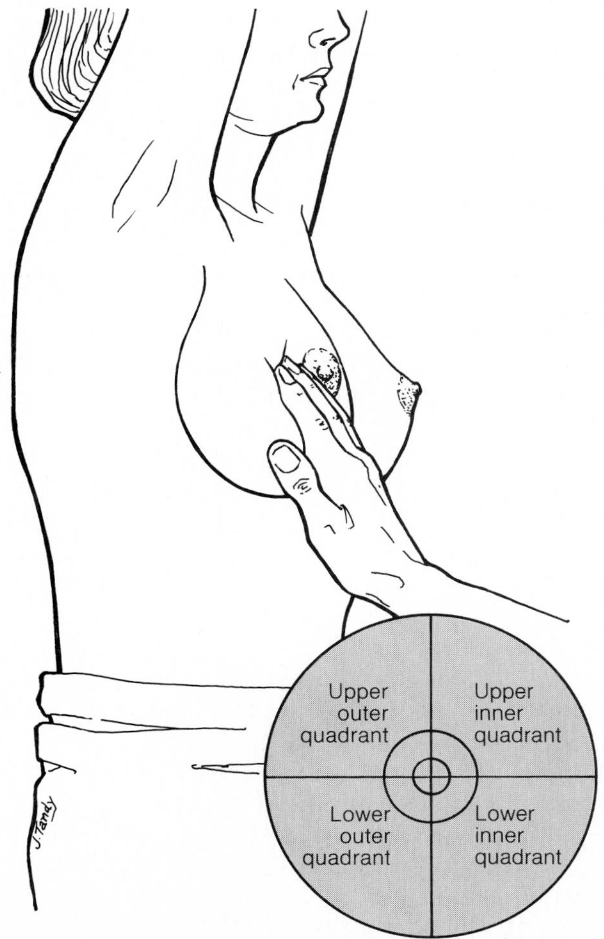

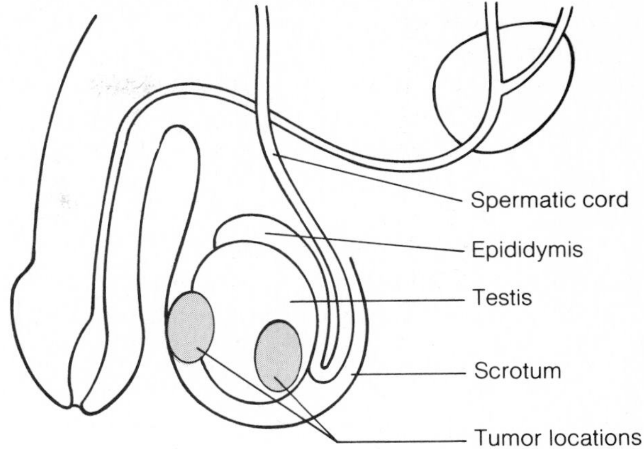

Figure 33–5 Common tumor locations of the testes.

The woman can observe symmetry of the breasts by bending over at the waist with the arms forward. She can continue the examination by lying on a bed with a pillow under the shoulders. To finish the examination, the woman must:

1. Place the left hand under the head and examine the left breast with the right hand. Press the palmar surfaces of the first, second, third, and fourth fingers down on the breast and move them in a slightly rotary motion, pressing the tissue against the chest wall. By dividing the breast into four imaginary quadrants, the woman has a reference point for recording any palpated masses. See Figure 33–4.
2. Place the left arm at the side and palpate the axilla for any lumps or enlarged lymph glands.
3. Repeat steps 1 and 2 for the right breast.

If the woman or nurse detects a mass, the following information is recorded:

1. Location of the mass in the breast, such as right inner quadrant, right breast
2. Shape of the mass; for example, nodules, round and smooth
3. Mobility; for instance, moves freely or is fixed
4. Discomfort; for example, appears painful to touch
5. Consistency; for example, hard, soft, rubbery

Testicular self-examination

Testicular self-examination is intended to detect changes in the testicles. Examinations should be conducted monthly. Testicular cancer is most commonly found on the anterior and lateral surfaces of the testes. See Figure 33–5. It accounts for approximately 1% of all the cancer in men and often occurs in men in their early thirties (Crooks and Baur 1980:89). This cancer is often serious and requires extensive surgery if in the later stages. In the early stages, the cancer is asymptomatic except for a mass within the testicle. The lump often feels hard and bumpy and can usually be differentiated from tissue around it. The patient may also experience a feeling of heaviness in the scrotum.

The man stands during testicular self-examination and uses both hands, one under the scrotum and the other over the scrotum. Using the thumb and fingers of both hands, the man palpates the testicle, which normally feels rubbery, smooth, and free of lumps. After palpating both testicles, the man compares the weights of the testicles and then palpates the epididymis, which is at the top of the testicle and extends behind it. It should feel soft and slightly tender (Murray and Wilcox 1978:2074). The man then locates the spermatic cord, which ascends from the epididymis behind the testicle. It normally feels firm and smooth.

Nursing Diagnoses

Nursing diagnoses for patients with sexual problems may be stated broadly as sexual dysfunction. *Sexual dysfunction* is defined as a perceived problem in achieving desired sexual satisfaction (Gordon 1982:210). The factors contributing to sexual dysfunction include (Kim and Moritz 1982:312):

1. Altered body structure or function due to disease or trauma, drugs, pregnancy or recent childbirth, or anatomic abnormalities of the genitals
2. Lack of knowledge or misinformation about sexuality
3. Physical abuse (e.g., rape)
4. Psychosocial abuse (e.g., destructive relationship)
5. Values conflict
6. Loss or lack of partner

Examples of nursing diagnoses for patients with sexual problems include:

1. Sexual dysfunction related to:
- **a.** Fear of effects of coitus following heart attack
- **b.** Spinal cord injury
- **c.** Neurologic changes due to diabetes mellitus
- **d.** Lowered body image following mastectomy
- **e.** Lack of knowledge about sexually transmitted disease
- **f.** Pregnancy and fear of harming fetus by coitus
- **g.** Excessive use of alcohol
- **h.** Guilt about enjoying sexual activities
- **i.** Traumatic rape experience
- **j.** Fear of inadequate sexual performance
- **k.** Lack of knowledge about conception
- **l.** Fear of pregnancy and lack of knowledge about contraception
- **m.** Painful intercourse from inadequate vaginal lubrication

Changes in Sexual Motivation

Libido (sexual motivation, sex drive) is the urge or desire for sexual activity. It fluctuates within each person and varies from person to person. Many factors, both biologic and social, affect sexual motivation.

Decreased sexual motivation

Factors that may contribute to decreased sexual motivation include:

1. *Drugs.* All central nervous system depressants, such as alcohol, barbiturates, and sedatives, may decrease libido. Morphine, heroin, and methadone (used in the rehabilitation of drug addicts) cause marked reduction of sexual desire. Other libido-inhibiting drugs include estrogens and adrenal steroids in large doses, certain psychotropic drugs, and some antihypertensive agents, e.g., reserpine (Serpasil) and methyldopa (Aldomet).
2. *Depression.* Depression slows all body functions and lowers libido. Depression in one partner can adversely affect the sexual functioning of the other. Libido generally returns when the depression is relieved.
3. *Disease.* Libido diminishes with general ill health and chronic diseases that cause debility, pain, and depression, such as arthritis and cancer. Any disorder that causes dyspareunia or brain damage also lowers libido. Examples are vaginitis, genital herpes, imperforate hymen, head trauma, and strokes.
4. *Pregnancy.* Sexual motivation may decrease during pregnancy because of physical discomfort, fear of injury to the fetus, and perceived loss of attractiveness. For about 4 weeks following delivery, libido is often reduced due to decreased vaginal lubrication, thinner vaginal walls, and a slower response to stimulation.

5. *Aging.* Older people vary greatly in their sexual motivation. It is not known whether decreased hormone production alters libido.

Increased sexual motivation

Factors contributing to increased sexual motivation include:

1. *Puberty and adolescence.* Both males and females experience increased sexual motivation during puberty and adolescence as a result of hormonal and body changes. This population is at risk of pregnancy and sexually transmitted disease if they do not receive appropriate sex education.
2. *Drugs.* Amphetamines and cocaine enhance sexual motivation for some people for short periods. Lysergic acid diethylamide (LSD) and marijuana increase libido in some but inhibit it in others.

Problems with Intercourse

It has been estimated that more than one half of married couples in North America have sexual problems. Common concerns are the woman's inability to achieve orgasm readily or the man's inability to maintain an erection or to delay ejaculation until his partner is satisfied (Goldstein 1976:161).

Impotence

The inability to achieve or maintain an erection sufficient for intercourse is referred to as *impotence.* Some men have spontaneous erections and erections while masturbating or during foreplay but lose the erection during various phases of sexual activity. Others always have erection problems during intercourse or may have erections with certain partners and not with other partners.

Impotence is classified as primary or secondary. A man with primary impotence has never been able to achieve an erection sufficient for intercourse. A man with secondary impotence functioned adequately for some time before he developed erectile dysfunction. Both types of impotence can be caused by physiologic or psychologic factors, but primary impotence is more often associated with psychologic factors. Physiologic factors include:

1. Neurologic disorders created by spinal cord injuries, injury to the genitals or perineal nerves, extensive surgery such as abdominal-perineal bowel resections, radical perineal prostatectomy, and diabetes mellitus
2. Prolonged use of drugs such as sedatives, heroin, antidepressants, or antipsychotics (phenothiazines)
3. Vascular diseases such as sickle cell anemia and leukemia
4. Endocrine disorders such as hypothyroidism and Addison's disease

Psychologic factors may include:

1. Doubts about one's ability to perform or about one's masculinity
2. Fatigue, anger, or stress caused by problems at work, in the family, and in interpersonal relationships
3. Traumatic early sexual experiences (e.g., rejection)
4. Pain, fear, or guilt associated with erection
5. Boredom associated with a specific female partner

The treatment for impotence depends largely on the cause. Penile implants have been used to treat physiologic impotence. Impotence of psychologic origin often requires a change in both partners' view of sexuality. Awareness of the cause of the condition and exercises designed to increase sensations are also used.

Premature ejaculation

Premature ejaculation occurs when a man cannot delay ejaculation from 30 seconds to 1 minute after penetration. Another definition is inability to delay ejaculation long enough to satisfy a partner. This condition may relate to early conditioning in which rapid orgasm was desirable.

Treatment advocated by Masters and Johnson includes increased sexual communication and responsiveness as well as decreased performance demands. The couple together practice sensate exercises (learning to enjoy the sensation of touch) and then work together to establish satisfying coitus.

Orgasmic dysfunction

Orgasmic dysfunction, the inability of a woman to achieve orgasm, is of two types: primary and situational. A woman with primary orgasmic dysfunction has never been able to achieve orgasm. A woman with situational dysfunction has experienced at least one orgasm but is at that time nonorgasmic. *Frigidity,* however, refers to a woman who has a low or nondetectable sex drive.

Orgasmic dysfunction can be caused by drugs, alcohol, aging, and anatomic abnormalities of the genitals. However, most cases have psychologic causes. Some of these can be hostility between partners, fear or guilt about enjoying the sexual act, or concern about performance. Therapy usually involves having both partners establish new attitudes about sex. Pelvic muscle exercises (Kegel's exercises) can also increase the capacity to achieve orgasm by increasing the strength of the pubococcygeal muscle. (See the section on postnatal exercises in Chapter 24.)

Vaginismus

Vaginismus is irregular and involuntary contraction of the muscles around the outer third of the vagina when coitus is attempted. The vagina closes before penetration. The cause can be severe sexual inhibition, often associated with early learning. Other causes can be rape, incest, and painful intercourse.

Treatment often involves sensate focus exercises and therapy to bring about psychologic changes. In some instances graduated vaginal dilators are used.

Dyspareunia

Dyspareunia is pain experienced by a woman during intercourse. It can occur as a result of inadequate lubrication, scarring, vaginal infection, or hormonal imbalance. Treatment, for instance, supplying additional lubrication before intercourse, corrects the underlying cause.

Common Illnesses Affecting Sexuality

Medical conditions

Heart disease and diabetes mellitus are two frequent long-term illnesses. Impotence can be a problem for diabetic men. This can be treated with hormones such as testosterone.

Following a myocardial infarction, some patients may fear sexual intercourse because of the increased heart and respiratory rates associated with sexual activity. Most patients can resume sexual activity 4 to 6 weeks after a myocardial infarction. The transient increases in heart and respiratory rates are generally within their capacities (Puksta 1977:602). A prescribed program of physical activity also improves the patient's tolerance for exercise and sexual activity. Postcoronary patients may find the bottom position during intercourse less stressful than the top position. Thus couples may need to adjust to a position of less strain, although some patients find accustomed positions less stressful than new positions.

Spinal cord injuries can present special sexual problems to patients. Some individuals with paraplegia are potent and fertile, depending on the location of injury. Some men are able to have erections with local stimulation; others can have erections with psychologic stimulation, and others are unable to have either reflexogenic or psychogenic erections. Sexual adjustments are one of many complex adjustments faced by these patients and families. Special rehabilitative programs and counseling are frequently indicated.

Surgical conditions

After certain surgical procedures such as a mastectomy, hysterectomy, or enterostomy, a person's concept of body image may be changed (see the discussion of body image in Chapter 32). The response of a loved one to any of these changes greatly affects the surgical patient's ability to reintegrate his or her self-image. Sexual relations can also be affected by the person's self-perceptions. The person who feels ugly and unloved may feel inadequate in a sexual relationship. This person may feel ashamed at having another see the body changes. Loss of reproductive organs can make a person feel sexually inadequate, even when the loss does not affect sexual function.

Accurate knowledge is important. Sometimes the couple requires assistance to express their feelings and to develop positive, constructive attitudes toward each other and the sexual relationship.

Women who undergo mastectomy often need counseling, especially if they equate a lost breast with lost femininity. Partners of such women may need assistance expressing their feelings about the loss of the breast. Some men may feel revolted at the sight of the scar; others may fear harming their wives if they have sexual intercourse. If the relationship is supportive, both partners find postoperative adjustment less difficult.

Planning and Intervention for Sexual Problems

The overall nursing goal for patients with sexual problems is to promote sexual health. Nursing subgoals include:

1. To develop awareness of one's own sexual attitudes, beliefs, and knowledge
2. To provide accurate sexual information and education to patients
3. To identify sexual problems and provide intervention as appropriate
4. To enhance the patient's body image and self-esteem

Planning also involves establishing outcome criteria. For suggestions see page 884.

Developing Self-Awareness

To be effective in helping clients with sexual problems, the nurse must first acquire accurate information about sexuality, identify and accept her or his own sexual values and behaviors and those of others, and be comfortable acquiring and disseminating information about sexuality. Results of a study conducted at the School of Nursing, University of Wisconsin, Madison, indicate that there was considerable misinformation and lack of information about sexual matters among graduate and undergraduate nursing students (Mims and Swenson 1978:122). Mims and Swenson reported the following misconceptions and their incidence:

1. Impotence in men over 70 is nearly universal (35%).
2. Certain mental and emotional instabilities are caused by masturbation (10%).
3. Women are not able to respond to further stimulation for a period of time following orgasm (24%).
4. A woman's chances to conceive are greatly enhanced if she has experienced orgasm (16%).
5. Most homosexuals have a distinguishing body build (27%).
6. Exhibitionists are latent homosexuals (32%).

Nurses who hold such misconceptions may be unable to give patients appropriate advice and assistance. Nurses need to become informed about the anatomy and physiology of sexual organs, psychosocial development of sexuality, psychosocial behaviors, sexual variations among people, and diseases and therapies that can alter sexual behavior.

Awareness of one's own attitudes (feelings, values, and beliefs) about sexuality is also essential. Before the nurse can understand patients' sexuality, he or she must develop an awareness and tolerance of his or her own sexuality. This kind of self-awareness can be acquired by values clarification exercises and discussions. Nurses need to consider some of their feelings about the following:

1. Masturbation
2. Unwanted pregnancy and abortion
3. Contraception
4. Homosexuality and other sexual variations
5. Nudity
6. Sterilization
7. Various modes of sexual stimulation
8. Sexually transmitted disease
9. Premarital intercourse
10. Unwed parents
11. Cohabitation

When the nurse clarifies her or his own attitudes, she or he gains a greater understanding and tolerance of sexuality in others.

Counseling and Referral

Frank (1981:64) suggests a three-part program for each sexual counseling session: (a) assessment, (b) information-sharing, and (c) discussion. The *assessment phase* involves asking the patient questions and evaluating his or her answers. Frank suggests that before asking the patient questions the nurse answer this question: "If I were in this patient's place, what questions would I ask?" This exercise helps the nurse devise a list of questions and think of ways to ask them. For example, the nurse might ask a patient who is recuperating from a heart attack the following questions:

1. "Now that you're recuperating and you've had some time to sort out your feelings, have you thought about how your heart attack might alter your sex life?"
2. "Have you and your wife discussed how you both feel about it?"

Information sharing and discussion should follow each question. In this case, information sharing means that the nurse gives the patient information on how his heart attack might affect his sex life. Such information might include the following:

1. "Your heart attack will not alter your capacity for sexual response. Most patients can resume intercourse in 4 to 6 weeks, but this should be confirmed by your doctor."
2. "Many postcoronary patients fear sexual intercourse because of increased heart and respiratory rates associated with it. However, your prescribed program of progressive physical activity will also increase your tolerance for sexual activity."

After information giving, the nurse should encourage discussion. If the nurse cannot answer the patient's questions, the nurse refers the patient to someone who can. The nurse may offer helpful suggestions during discussion, for example:

1. "A bottom position during intercourse is considered less strenuous than a top position, but some men find that assuming their usual position is less strenuous than a new position."
2. "Avoid intercourse after a heavy meal and when fatigued or intoxicated."

Another model, developed by Mims and Swenson (1978:123) to help nurses deliver sexual health care, outlines three levels of nursing intervention, all of which require use of the nursing process and communication skills. At the basic level, the nurse helps the patient develop awareness of sexuality, which involves his or her knowledge, attitudes, and perceptions. Mims and Swenson believe that all nurses, regardless of educational preparation, should function at this level.

The intermediate level includes permission giving and information giving. This level presupposes teaching skills by the nurse. Permission giving means that the nurse by attitude or word lets the patient know that sexual thoughts, fantasies, and behaviors between informed, consenting adults are sanctioned. Permission giving begins when the nurse acknowledges the patient's verbal and nonverbal sexual concerns. For example, an older male with a reduced libido may feel that he cannot discuss sex with the nurse unless the nurse broaches the subject. Other patients may need acknowledgment to feel comfortable about their virginity, homosexual activities, oral-genital sex, or masturbation. Often many sexual concerns are alleviated when the patient receives permission from the nurse to engage or not engage in certain sexual behaviors. Permission giving can be detrimental unless at the same time the nurse provides accurate information. Information given should include:

1. General information about sexuality including:
  a. Anatomy and physiology of sexual organs
  b. Stages of sexual development
  c. Sexual response cycles
  d. Coital positions

2. Information specific to the patient's needs, which may include:
  a. Alterations in sexuality made necessary by certain disease processes, medication, surgery, and therapies
  b. Alternative modes of sexual expression
  c. Contraception
  d. Sexually transmitted diseases
  e. Pregnancy
  f. Abortion
  g. Infertility

The third level of nursing intervention includes suggestion giving, which involves sexual therapy, educational programs, and research projects. For this level of functioning, the nurse requires advanced and specialized knowledge.

Teaching about Contraception

Contraception is the voluntary prevention of conception or *impregnation* (fertilizing or making pregnant). Contraceptive methods include the biologic or ovulation method, coitus interruptus, hormone therapy, and chemical, mechanical, and surgical procedures.

Biologic or ovulation method

The biologic method is preferred by people whose religious beliefs conflict with artificial birth control methods and by those who mistrust pharmacologic or mechanical birth control. Basic to this method is the identification of the days of the month when conception could take place and abstinence during that time. Women must learn the following signs of ovulation, since they can conceive when ovulating and must abstain during that time:

1. Changes in vaginal mucus. When the woman is not ovulating, her mucus is thick and yellow or sometimes cloudy. The mucus becomes clearer and thinner near the time of ovulation.

2. Breast tenderness.

3. Tenderness at either side of the lower abdomen.

4. Midcycle spotting of blood.

5. Rise in basal temperature. The temperature taken each morning upon arising drops about 0.2 C (0.3 F) 1 or 2 days prior to ovulation and then rises 0.4 to 0.5 C (0.7 to 0.8 F) 1 to 2 days after ovulation. The fertile period around ovulation extends from 1 to 2 days before ovulation to 2 days after.

Economy is one advantage of this method of contraception. Also, no drugs or mechanical devices that interfere with body physiology are used, and the method is readily learned. The disadvantages include abstinence from sexual activity for the period surrounding ovulation, and the fact that cooperation is required of both partners.

Coitus interruptus

This method of contraception involves the withdrawal of the penis prior to ejaculation. This method requires considerable self-control. It has two primary disadvantages. Some semen may escape into the vagina prior to ejaculation, and it may decrease sexual gratification.

Hormone therapy

Certain drugs (birth control pills) suppress ovulation and are used as contraceptives. Contraceptive pills usually contain synthetic estrogen and progesterone. Estrogen suppresses ovulation by inhibiting the release of LH and FSH. Progesterone produces changes in the cervical mucus, alters the tubal transport of the ovum, and renders the endometrium less suitable for implantation.

A pill is taken once a day for 20 or 21 days starting on the 5th day of the menstrual cycle. The pill is provided in two forms: combined or sequential. In the combined form, each pill contains both estrogen and progesterone. In the sequential form, estrogen only is contained in the first 15 pills and progesterone in the remaining 7 pills. Within 2 or 3 days of stopping the pills, the woman begins menstruation. After the 5th day of menstruation, she begins a new series of pills again. Some pharmaceutical companies manufacture 28-day packets that contain inert tablets for the "off" days. Using this packet, the woman takes a tablet each day. Tablet containers usually allow the woman to see at a glance how many pills she has taken.

Many pill users experience side effects. Minor side effects are nausea, weight gain, breast tenderness, headaches, decreased menstrual flow, spotting, missed periods, vaginal itching, yeast infections, and depression. If these persist, the patient should consult her physician. Other symptoms, such as severe headaches, severe abdominal pain, blurred vision, severe leg pain, and chest pain, are warnings of potentially serious problems. These symptoms must be reported to a physician. Birth control pills are contraindicated for patients with cardiac problems, circulatory problems (e.g., thrombophlebitis, thromboembolic disorders, and cerebrovascular disease), severe migraines, liver disease, diabetes mellitus, and known or suspected breast cancer.

Chemical methods

Chemical contraception is the insertion of foam, jelly, creams, or suppositories into the vagina before intercourse. These products, which were introduced in the 1950s, form a film of spermicide on the vagina. A *spermicide* destroys sperm.

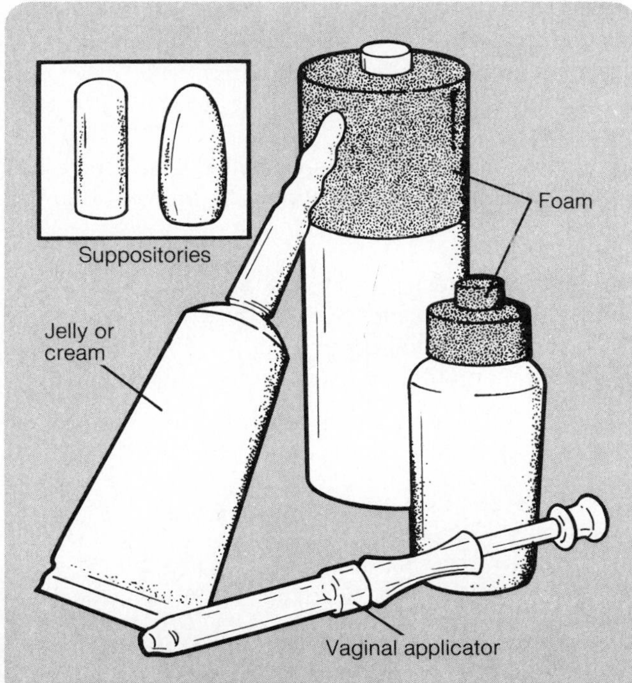

Figure 33–6 Types of spermicides. (From S. B. Olds, M. L. London, P. A. Ladewig, and S. V. Davidson, *Obstetric nursing* [Menlo Park, Calif.: Addison-Wesley Publishing Co., 1980], p. 175.)

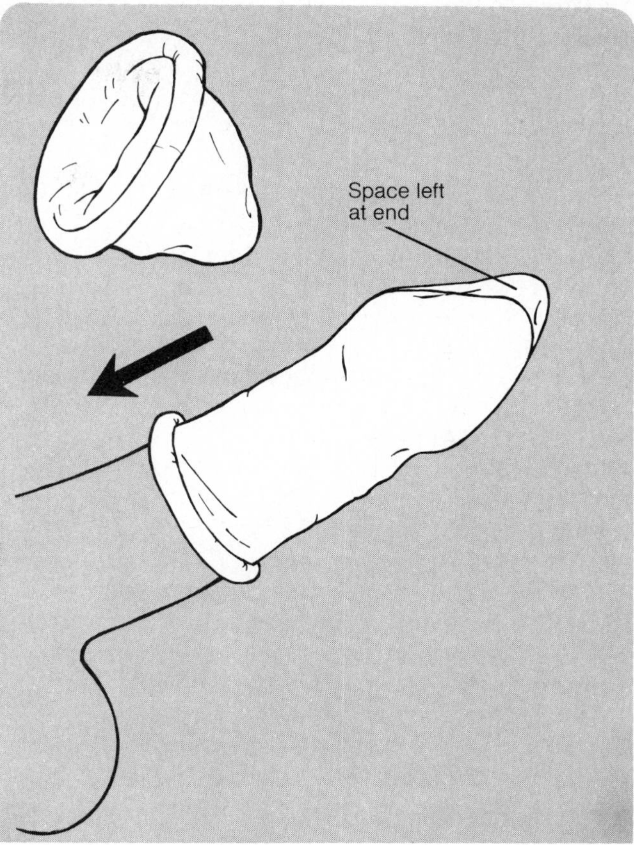

Figure 33–7 **A**, Condom; **B**, condom applied to penis with space left at end for collection of ejaculate. (From S. B. Olds, M. L. London, P. A. Ladewig, and S. V. Davidson, *Obstetric nursing* [Menlo Park, Calif.: Addison-Wesley Publishing Co., 1980], p. 172.)

These products are inserted with an applicator. See Figure 33–6. The woman fills the applicator, inserts it into the vagina, withdraws the applicator about 1¼ cm (½ in) and then depresses the plunger. The substance covers the cervical os (mouth or opening of the cervix), preventing sperm from entering the uterus.

Spermicides that effervesce in a moist environment have an immediate effect, and coitus may take place immediately after insertion. Suppositories do not offer protection until dissolved and may not dissolve for 30 minutes after insertion. The effectiveness of spermicides increases substantially when they are used with a diaphragm or condom. Their chief disadvantages are the difficulty some women have inserting the substance up to the cervical os and leakage from the vagina.

Mechanical devices

Condoms The *condom*, or sheath, is a covering placed over the penis prior to intercourse. See Figure 33–7. It must be inspected for holes. The ejaculate is

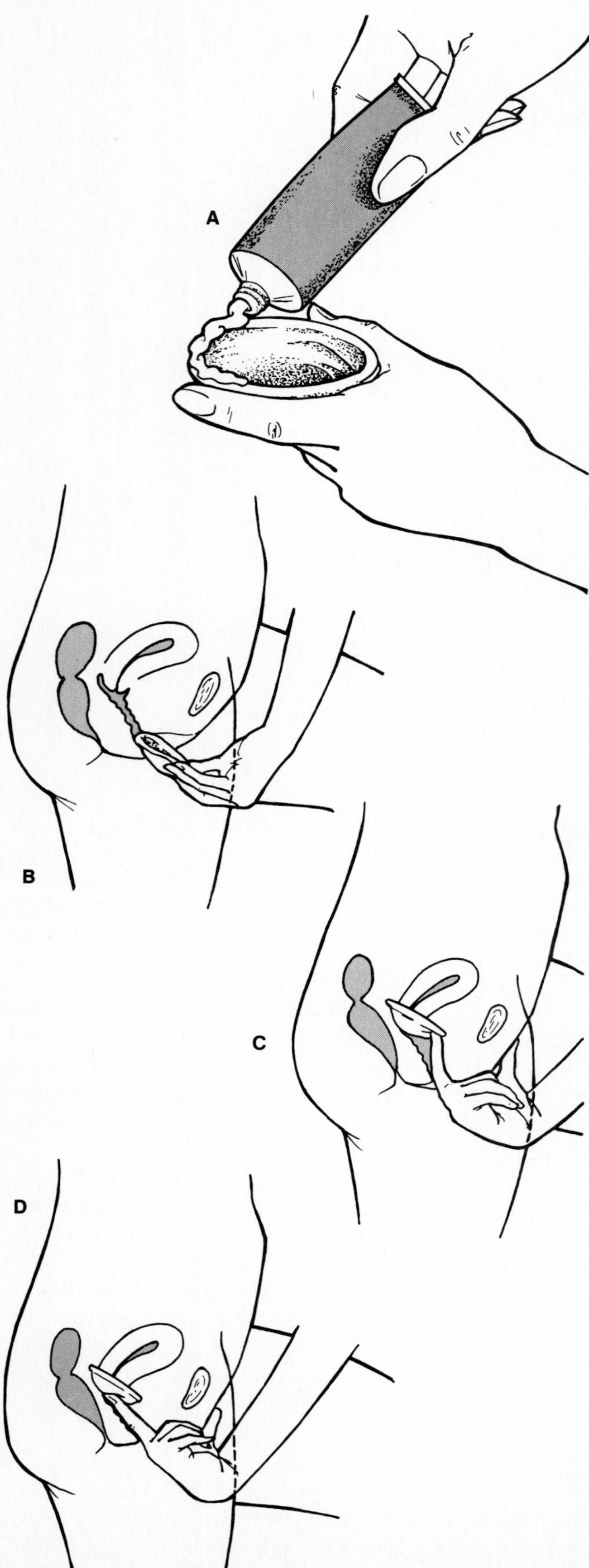

deposited in the condom rather than in the vagina. The man places the condom on the erect penis, rolling the sheath down from the tip to the end of the shaft and leaving a small space at the end of the condom for the ejaculate. This space prevents the condom from breaking at ejaculation. After intercourse, when the penis becomes flaccid, the man should hold the edge of the condom while withdrawing from the vagina to prevent the condom from slipping off and spilling semen. Condoms are not a foolproof method of contraception since they may split or be displaced during intercourse. Other disadvantages include expense and the fact that some couples feel condoms dull sexual sensations.

Vaginal diaphragms The *vaginal diaphragm* is a round rubber cup inserted into the vagina over the cervix. See Figure 33–8. It offers greater contraceptive protection than the condom especially when used with spermicide creams. Diaphragms must be properly fitted by trained personnel. They are then inserted by the woman prior to intercourse and must be left in place 6 hours after intercourse. Diaphragms need to be held up to a light and inspected periodically for holes or tears. Their fit must also be rechecked after each delivery and when there is a weight gain or loss of 20 pounds.

To insert the diaphragm, the woman is instructed to:

1. Apply spermicidal jelly to the diaphragm rim that will face the cervix.
2. Cup the diaphragm between the thumb and fingers and insert it into the vagina over the cervix.
3. Push the anterior rim of the diaphragm up under the symphysis pubis. (Some women report a popping sensation.)
4. Check its placement by touching the diaphragm with the index finger and feeling the cervix beneath. The cervix is a small rounded structure that feels somewhat like the tip of the nose. The diaphragm should be centered over the cervix.
5. If more than 4 hours elapse before intercourse additional spermicidal cream should be inserted into the vagina.

Some people feel that having to use a diaphragm inhibits the spontaneity of intercourse. Some women also find insertion and removal of the diaphragm, and the genital manipulation they require, offensive.

Figure 33–8 **A**, Diaphragm and gel; **B**, insertion of diaphragm; **C**, rim of diaphragm pushed up under the symphysis pubis; **D**, checking placement of diaphragm. The cervix should be felt through the diaphragm. (From S. B. Olds, M. L. London, P. A. Ladewig, S. V. Davidson, *Obstetric nursing* [Menlo Park, Calif.: Addison-Wesley Publishing Co., 1980], p. 172.)

Intrauterine devices *Intrauterine devices* (IUDs) inserted into the uterus are the most effective method of mechanical contraception. IUDs are second in reliability only to oral contraception. When inserted properly they are 95 to 99% effective (Huxall 1980:186). IUDs can be nonmedicated and medicated, but all of them, regardless of shape and consistency, create endometrial infiltration by leukocytes, which produces an endometrial exudate. IUDs are therefore thought to serve as a spermicide and inhibit implantation. They have no effect on ovulation, ovarian hormones, or gonadotropins. Nonmedicated IUDs, made of soft plastic, include the Lippes Loop and the Saf-T-Coil. See Figure 33–9. Medicated IUDs, slightly more effective than nonmedicated ones, include the Copper-7, the Copper-T, and Progestasert-T. See Figure 33–10. Copper IUDs have a fine copper wire wrapped around a plastic stem and release copper constantly into the endometrium. The Progestasert-T contains the natural hormone progesterone in the shaft of the T. The progesterone released has only a local effect on the endometrium, not a systemic one. IUDs must be inserted by competent trained personnel.

Contraindications to use of IUDs include a history of (a) recurrent or recent pelvic inflammatory disease (PID), (b) valvular heart disease, (c) a previous ectopic pregnancy if the woman desires a future pregnancy, (d) anemia, (e) uterine bleeding, (f) abnormal Pap smear, and (g) pregnancy. IUDs increase the risk of pelvic infections and subsequent loss of fertility.

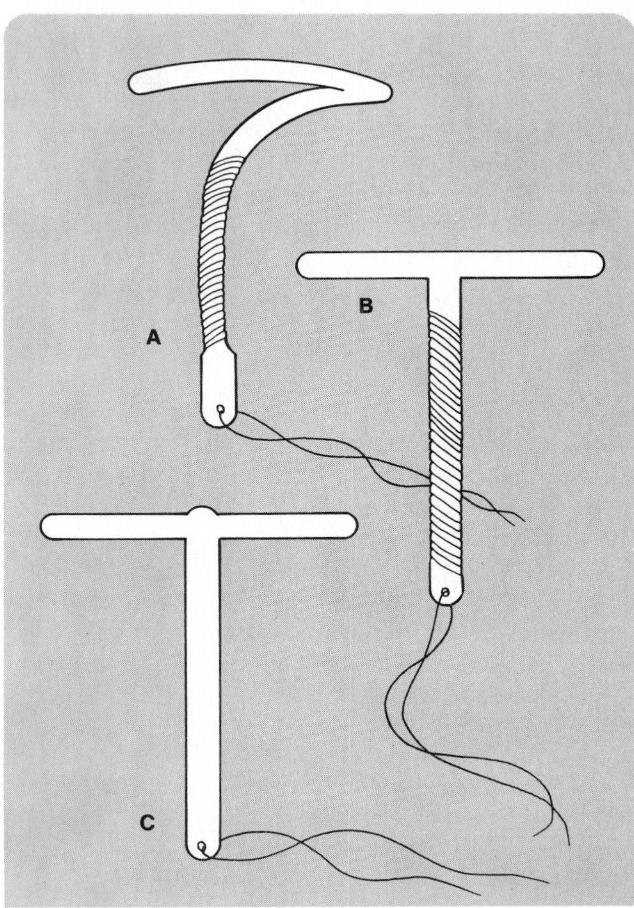

Figure 33–10 Medicated intrauterine devices: **A,** Copper-7; **B,** Copper-T; and **C,** Progestasert-T.

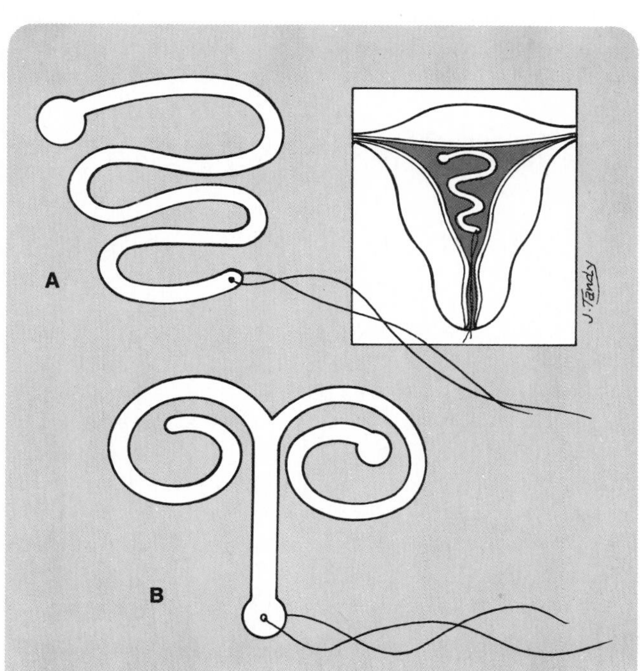

Figure 33–9 Nonmedicated intrauterine devices: **A,** Lippes Loop; **B,** Saf-T-Coil.

Side effects of IUDs include increased menstrual bleeding and cramping, intermenstrual spotting, and occasionally dyspareunia. Partial or complete expulsion of the device can also occur. Women need to be instructed to check the IUD strings regularly. If they are not detectable, if one string becomes longer than the other, or if the device protrudes through the cervix, she must notify her physician. She should also be alert to signs of pelvic infection such as abnormal vaginal discharge, fever, chills, pelvic or abdominal pain, dyspareunia, and development of a new menstrual disorder.

Although IUDs pose potential risks to users, their major advantages are contraceptive effectiveness, lack of systemic effects, and lack of interference with intercourse. They are also less expensive than oral contraceptives over time. Nonmedicated IUDs are less expensive than medicated ones and do not require periodic replacement. Medicated IUDs require replacement every 2 to 3 years.

Surgical methods

Surgical contraceptive methods include tubal ligation and vasectomy. A *tubal ligation* is the tying of the fallopian tubes to interrupt tubal continuity. A small abdominal incision is made below the umbilicus under local or general anesthetic.

A *vasectomy* is the ligation and cutting of the vas deferens on either side of the scrotum. The procedure is generally done under local anesthetic. Sperm are not cleared from the genitourinary system for 4 to 6 weeks and 6 to 36 ejaculations after vasectomy. Patients need to know that vasectomy affects fertility only, not potency, and that the procedure is usually permanent, although in some instances it can be reversed surgically.

Evaluation

The outcome criteria for patients with sexual problems (actual or potential) depend on nursing diagnoses. Some suggested criteria are:

1. States desired sexual satisfaction is achieved
2. Explains contraception method as instructed
3. Verbalizes desired conception control
4. Seeks confirmation of sexual desirability and attractiveness less frequently
5. Uses sexual terminology as taught
6. Expresses positive statements about alternate modes of sexual behavior

Summary

Sexuality is important in developing self-identity, interpersonal relationships, intimacy, and love. In its broad sense, sexuality involves physical, emotional, social, and ethical aspects of being and behaving. Sexuality has learned and inherited components.

An understanding of the structure and function of the male and female genitals is essential for nurses. The male genitals include the testes and scrotum, a series of ducts (epididymis and vas deferens) that transport the sperm, glands that secrete seminal plasma, and the penis. The female genitals include the ovaries, fallopian tubes, uterus, vagina, and vulva. The mammary glands, though not part of the female genitals, are a source of sexual pleasure.

The components that contribute to the development of sexuality are numerous. Both biologic and psychologic components exist at all ages. Biologic differences in the sexes are apparent at birth, but many behavioral differences are also notable throughout infancy and childhood.

The establishment of sexual self-identity and gender role are critical between the ages of 18 months to 4 years. The learning of sex-typed behaviors depends on communication from parents and on imitation of parental behavior. Learning appropriate sex-typed behaviors takes several years. Adolescents may have problems establishing sexual self-identity. Sexual conflicts are a major problem. Adults also often experience sexual problems. A major task of the adult is to develop an intimate relationship with a partner. During the middle and later years, there are physical changes in the genitals. However, the desire and ability to maintain satisfying sexual relationships can remain.

Assessing actual or potential sexual problems is conducted at four levels. This chapter deals with the first level only. Assessment should be carried out when patients or support persons present cues that problems exist or when an illness could cause sexual problems. Nurses assess attitudes toward sexuality, including factors that affect attitudes and behaviors. Part of assessment is taking a nursing history and clinical examination. Performing and teaching breast examination and testicular examination are both important nursing functions.

An understanding of sexual stimuli and response patterns can help individuals have satisfying sexual relationships. This understanding is also vital for nurses wishing to help patients with psychologic problems, such as feelings of inadequacy, or medical problems, such as spinal cord injuries or myocardial infarctions. Common sexual problems of healthy adults are changes in libido, impotence, premature ejaculation, orgasmic dysfunction, vaginismus, and dyspareunia. Illnesses that commonly affect sexuality are myocardial infarction and diabetes mellitus. Many surgical procedures also affect sexual abilities and sexual self-image. Some of these are mastectomy, hysterectomy, and enterostomy.

The nursing diagnosis for patients with sexual problems is “sexual dysfunction.” Many contributing factors exist. Some of these are altered body structure or function, lack of knowledge or misinformation about sexual matters, physical or psychologic abuse, values conflicts, and loss or lack of a partner.

Before assisting patients with sexual problems, the nurse must acquire accurate information about sexuality, identify and accept his or her own sexual values and behaviors as well as those of others, and be comfortable acquiring and disseminating information about sexuality. Nursing interventions include helping develop awareness of sexuality, permission giving, information giving, and, at an advanced level, suggestion giving.

Suggested Activities

1. Observe a group of children at play. Identify those activities related to sex role and sexual identity.
2. Interview the parents of a young child. Assess how they contribute to the development of the child's identity and role.
3. Discuss with an adolescent what he or she wants to know about sex. Find out where the adolescent obtains information about sex.
4. Interview a physician in the community and determine what sexual problems he or she encounters in the medical practice.

Suggested Readings

Allen, A. J. October 1975. All-American sexual myths. *American Journal of Nursing* 75:1770–71.
The article debunks 17 commonly believed myths about sex.

Boettcher, J. H., and Boettcher, K. July-August 1978. Sex education for fifth and sixth graders and their parents. *The American Journal of Maternal Child Nursing* 3:218–20.
Nurses, teachers, and parents can jointly sponsor father/son and mother/daughter nights to help parents communicate with their preteenagers.

Krozy, R. June 1978. Becoming comfortable with sexual assessment. *American Journal of Nursing* 78:1036–38.
This article lists characteristics of the sexually comfortable person and offers suggestions on how to approach the subject with patients.

Murray, B. L. S., and Wilcox, L. J. December 1978. Testicular self-examination. *American Journal of Nursing* 78:2074–75.
The technique for self-examination of the testicles and associated structures is described. Also included is information about diagnostic procedures and treatment.

Rybicki, L. L. May-June 1976. Preparing parents to teach their children about human sexuality. *The American Journal of Maternal Child Nursing* 1:182–85.
Nurses can help parents teach children about sex.

Spennrath, S. July-August 1982. Understanding the sexual needs of the older patient. *The Canadian Nurse* 78:25–29.
The nurse, as a patient advocate, has the responsibility of advising and counseling the elderly on health matters, including sex. The article includes facts about the elderly and sexuality, the effects of certain diseases on sexuality, and some problems of educating older people about sex.

Taylor, D. November-December 1976. A new approach to contraceptive teaching for teens. *The American Journal of Maternal Child Nursing* 1:378–83.
Lecturing teenagers about contraceptive methods is not an effective way to get them to use a form of birth control. A decision-making model is effective as a teaching strategy.

Wells, G. M. September-October 1977. Reducing the threat of a first pelvic exam. *The American Journal of Maternal Child Nursing* 2:304–6.
A woman's response to her first pelvic exam will in large part determine how conscientiously that woman will pursue her own health care. The first exam should be as constructive and comfortable as possible.

Zalar, M. K. May-June 1976. Sexual counseling for pregnant couples. *The American Journal of Maternal Child Nursing* 1:176–81.
Nurses can help parents-to-be recognize internal and external forces affecting sexual behavior and ways to cope with sexual concerns during this critical period.

Selected References

Adams, G. May-June 1976a. Recognizing the range of human sexual needs and behavior. *The American Journal of Maternal Child Nursing* 1:166–69.

———. May-June 1976b. The sexual health history as an integral part of the patient history. *The American Journal of Maternal Child Nursing* 1:170–75.

Comarr, A. E., and Gunderson, B. B. February 1975. Sexual function in traumatic paraplegia and quadriplegia. *American Journal of Nursing* 75:250–55.

Conklin, M., et al. December 1978. Should health teaching include self-examination of the testes? *American Journal of Nursing* 78:2073–75.

Contemporary Nursing Series. 1973. *Human sexuality: Nursing implications.* New York: The American Journal of Nursing.

Costello, M. K. August 1975. Sex, intimacy and aging. *American Jornal of Nursing* 75:1330–32.

Cowart, M., and Newton, D. W. June 1976. Oral contraceptives: How best to explain their effects to patients. *Nursing 76* 6:44–48.

Crooks, R., and Baur, K. 1980. *Our sexuality.* Menlo Park, Calif.: Benjamin/Cummings Publishing Co.

Duvall, E. M. 1977. *Marriage and family development.* 5th ed. New York: Harper and Row.

Easterbrook, B., and Rust, B. January 1977. Abortion counselling. *The Canadian Nurse* 73:28–30.

Ellis, D., and Ho, M. S. L. March 1982. Attitudes of Chinese women towards sexuality and birth control. *Canadian Nurse* 78:28–31.

Falk, G., and Falk, U. A. January 1980. Sexuality and the aged. *Nursing Outlook* 28:51–55.

Frank, D. I. January 1981. You don't have to be an expert to give sexual counseling to a mastectomy patient. *Nursing 81* 11:64–67.

Freedman, A. 1976. Drugs and sexual behavior. In Sadock, B.; Kaplan, H.; and Freedman, A.; editors. *The sexual experience.* Baltimore: Williams and Wilkins.

Friedeman, J. S. 1979. Sexuality in older persons: Implications for nursing practice. *Nursing Forum* 18(1): 92–101.

Goldstein, B. 1976. *Human sexuality.* New York: McGraw-Hill Book Co.

Gordon, M. 1982. *Manual of nursing diagnosis.* New York: McGraw-Hill Book Co.

Guyton, A. C. 1981. *Textbook of medical physiology.* 6th ed. Philadelphia: W. B. Saunders Co.

Hanlon, K. May 1975. Maintaining sexuality after spinal cord injury. *Nursing 75* 5:58–59, 61–62.

Huxall, L. K. November-December 1977. Today's pill and the individual woman. *The American Journal of Maternal Child Nursing* 2:359–63.

———. May-June 1980. Update on IUDs. *American Journal of Maternal Child Nursing.* 5:186–90.

Jensen, G. 1976. Adolescent sexuality. In Sadock, B.; Kaplan, H.; and Freedman, A.; editors. *The sexual experience.* Baltimore: Williams and Wilkins.

Kelley, G. F. 1980. *Sexuality: The human perspective.* Woodbury, N.Y.: Barron's Educational Series.

Kim, M. J., and Moritz, D. A., editors. 1982. *Classification of nursing diagnoses: Proceedings of the third and fourth national conferences.* New York: McGraw-Hill Book Co.

Lanahan, C. C. 1976. Homosexuality: A different sexual orientation. *Nursing Forum* 15(3):314–19.

Lief, H. I. 1975. Sexual counseling. In Romney, S. L., et al., editors. *Gynecology and obstetrics: The health care of women.* New York: McGraw-Hill Book Co.

Lief, H. I., and Payne, T. November 1975. Sexuality—knowledge and attitudes. *American Journal of Nursing* 75: 2026–29.

McCoy, N. L. 1976. Innate factors in sex differences. *Nursing Forum* 15 (3):277–89.

Mann, T. 1970. The biochemical characteristics of spermatozoa and seminal plasma. In Rosenberg, E., et al., editors. *The human testis.* New York: Plenum Press.

Marmor, J. 1976. Impotence and ejaculatory disturbance. In Sadock, B.; Kaplan, H.; and Freedman, A.; editors. *The sexual experience.* Baltimore: Williams and Wilkins.

Masters, W. H., and Johnson, V. E. 1966. *Human sexual response.* Boston: Little, Brown and Co.

———. 1970. *Human sexual inadequacy.* New York: Bantam Books.

Mims, F. H., and Swenson, M. February 1978. A model to promote sexual health care. *Nursing Outlook* 26:121–25.

Mims, F.; Yeaworth, R.; and Hornstein, S. May-June 1974. Effectiveness of an interdisciplinary course on human sexuality. *Nursing Research* 23:248–52.

Murray, B. L. S., and Wilcox, L. J. December 1978. Testicular self-examination. *American Journal of Nursing* 78:2074–75.

Puksta, N. S. April 1977. All about sex . . . after a coronary. *American Journal of Nursing* 77:602–5.

Rosen, R. A. H.; Werley, H. H.; Ager, J. W.; and Shea, F. P. May-June 1974. Some organizational correlates of nursing students' attitudes toward abortion. *Nursing Research* 23:253–58.

Schlesinger, B. October 1977. From A to Z with adolescent sexuality. *The Canadian Nurse* 73:34–37.

Smith, J., and Bullough, B. December 1975. Sexuality and the severely disabled person. *American Journal of Nursing* 75:2194–97.

Spence, A.P., and Mason, E. B. 1979. *Human anatomy and physiology.* Menlo Park, Calif.: Benjamin/Cummings Publishing Co.

Stanford, D. April 1977. All about sex . . . after middle age. *American Journal of Nursing* 77:608–11.

Stephens, G. T. January 1978. Creative contraries: A theory of sexuality. *American Journal of Nursing* 78:70–75.

Tanis, J. L. November-December 1977. Recognizing the reasons for contraceptive non-use and abuse. *The American Journal of Maternal Child Nursing* 2:364–69.

Timby, B. K. June 1976. Ovulation method of birth control. *American Journal of Nursing* 76:928–29.

Watts, R. J. 1978. The physiological interrelationships between depression, drugs, and sexuality. *Nursing Forum* 17(2):168–83.

———. September 1979. Dimensions of sexual health. *American Journal of Nursing* 79:1568–72.

Whaley, L. F., and Wong, D. L. 1979. *Nursing care of infants and children.* St. Louis: C. V. Mosby Co.

Woods, N. F. 1979. *Human sexuality in health and illness.* 2nd ed. St. Louis: C. V. Mosby Co.

Woods, N. F., and Mandetta, A. January-February 1975. Changes in students' knowledge and attitudes following a course in human sexuality: Report of a pilot study. *Nursing Research* 24:10–15.

Chapter 34

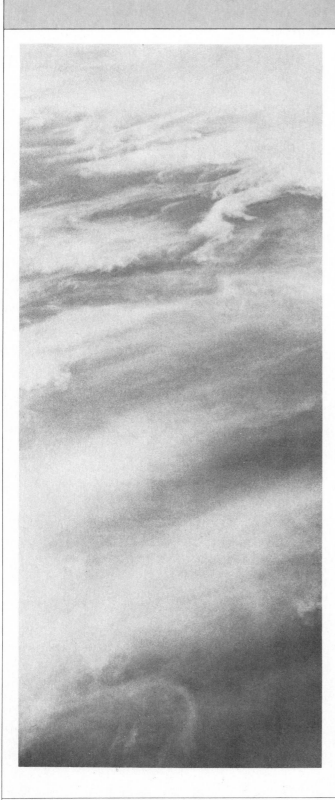

Spiritual Preference

CONTENTS

(Continued on next page)

Objectives

1. Know essential facts about spiritual beliefs and religious practices and doctrines related to health care

- **1.1** Define selected terms
- **1.2** Identify essential aspects of spiritual development from birth to older adulthood
- **1.3** Identify significant religious beliefs related to health care
- **1.4** Identify religious beliefs of selected groups that relate to health care

2. Know information required to assess and diagnose a patient's spiritual needs and problems

- **2.1** Identify patients who can benefit from pastoral care
- **2.2** Identify essential information to obtain in the nursing history
- **2.3** Identify clinical signs indicating a spiritual need
- **2.4** Identify essential aspects of nursing diagnoses related to spiritual concerns

3. Understand facts about nursing measures to support the patient's spiritual beliefs and religious practices

- **3.1** Identify nursing goals
- **3.2** Explain essential guidelines for nursing intervention related to spiritual needs

4. Apply the nursing process when providing care to selected patients with spiritual concerns

- **4.1** Obtain necessary assessment data
- **4.2** Analyze and relate assessment data
- **4.3** Write relevant nursing diagnoses
- **4.4** Write relevant nursing goals
- **4.5** Plan appropriate nursing interventions
- **4.6** Implement appropriate nursing interventions
- **4.7** State outcome criteria essential for evaluating the patient's progress

Terms

agnostic
atheist
clergy
Holy Communion
pastoral care
religion
spiritual belief
spiritual need

People generally desire to understand their relationship to the universe and the direction and meaning of life. Most people have some type of *spiritual belief* (belief in a higher power, creative force, divine being, or infinite source of energy), which may or may not be associated with a formal religion. A *religion* is an organized system of worship. Religions have central beliefs, rituals, and practices usually related to birth, death, marriage, and salvation. Spiritual and religious beliefs provide guidance to people about mores and ethical values. They also serve as an integrating force in society and give people inner strengths that are closely associated with emotional and physical health.

At a time of illness, many people look to spirituality for assistance and consolation, whether or not they profess to have a religious affiliation. Providing spiritual guidance is an aspect of treating the whole person: assisting the patient emotionally, physically, and spiritually.

Spiritual Development

Infants and Toddlers

Infants do not have a sense of right or wrong, spiritual beliefs, or convictions that guide their activities. Toddlers may follow certain rituals, such as saying their prayers at night, but they are only imitating to conform to the expectations of their parents. They may attend a church nursery school, but the emphasis of the teaching is typically on play and enhancing their positive self-image by having them accomplish simple tasks and telling them what they have accomplished.

Preschoolers

The greatest influence on preschoolers is their parents. Parental attitudes toward moral codes and religion convey to children what is considered good and bad. At this age children are imitators and tend to copy what they see rather than what they are told. If what they see and what they are told are contradictory, problems arise.

Preschoolers often ask questions about morality and religion, e.g., "Why is (some action or word) wrong?" and "What is heaven?" They think that their parents are like God: omnipotent. Two methods of spiritual education are used with preschool children: indoctrination and choosing their own way. Children will follow a religion at this age not because they understand it but because it is part of their daily life. Three-year-olds like prayers at night and before meals. Five-year-olds often make up prayers themselves.

Children 3 to 5 years old believe that God or actual human beings are responsible for natural events such as rain and wind. They may reason, "The rain is God crying; the wind is God blowing air out of His mouth." At this age children are old enough to go to church school and to participate in religious holidays. They ask many questions about the meaning of the holidays and need explanations about them. However, they are more occupied with the ideas such as Santa Claus coming at Christmas than with the reason behind the holiday. When children begin to question myths such as the Easter Bunny, they are ready for a more sophisticated explanation about Easter.

Superego (conscience) development is related to moral and religious development. Preschoolers identify with their parents and introject parental standards and values. Preschool children are exceedingly obedient and can be resentful if their parents do not live up to the child's superego demands. The superego continues to develop and, if it remains very strict, the child will grow up to be a self-righteous, intolerant adult. If the superego does not develop, the adult will be unable to follow society's ethical and moral standards and unable to form mature relationships. Such a person is referred to as a *sociopath* or one who has an antisocial personality.

School-Age Children

During the school years, children learn more about religion. Six-year-olds expect that their prayers will be answered, good rewarded, and bad punished. They have reverence for many thoughts and matters.

During the prepuberty stage, children become aware of spiritual disappointments. They realize that their prayers are not always answered on their own terms, and they begin to reason rather than accept a faith blindly. At this age some children drop or modify certain religious practices (e.g., praying for tangible benefits); others continue to follow religious practices because of dependence on their parents.

During adolescence, children compare the standards of their parents with others and determine which ones they want to incorporate into their own behavior. At this age parental standards may be kept. Adolescents also compare the scientific viewpoint with the religious viewpoint and try to bring the two together. By 16 years, many adolescents have decided whether to accept the family religion. They may experience personal religious awakenings, such as being saved or converted, either suddenly or gradually. Adolescents with parents of different faiths may choose one faith over the other or no faith. For some, a firm faith provides strength during these turbulent years.

Adults

Young adults who need to answer the religious questions of their own children may find that the teachings of their own early childhood are more acceptable to them now than during adolescence. During the middle years adults often find that they have more time for religious activities such as church groups since their children are older. Older adults who have developed religious values often endeavor to broaden them and to understand the newer values of younger people. They are comfortable with their own values but appreciate those of others. Elderly adults who do not have mature religious beliefs may experience a feeling of deprivation as activities such as employment are replaced with retirement. During these years, people face death—both their own and that of a spouse. This recognition may make them despondent. The development of a mature religious philosophy can often help older people face reality, participate in life, have feelings of self-worth, and accept death as inevitable.

Religious Beliefs Related to Health Care

Religious and spiritual beliefs often assist people during times of stress. Some people look to religion to answer why they are ill, others look on illness as a test of faith, and others see illness as punishment for sin, inflicted by some outside force. Patients and families at times use prayer, promise, and even penance to treat disease.

Sometimes religious beliefs can affect the course of an illness and how a person accepts the illness and therapy. Spiritual beliefs particularly affect birth, death, and medical procedures such as biopsies, abortions, amputations, autopsies, and transfusions.

Meeting the spiritual needs of patients and their families is part of the function of nurses as well as designated chaplains and other clergy. The *clergy* refers to priests, rabbis, ministers, church elders, deacons, and other spiritual advisers. Some religious groups, such as the Church of Latter-Day Saints and the Christian Scientists, do not have ordained clergy; they usually do have people whose role it is to minister to the ill, and these people must be recognized by nurses as having appropriate functions. In Christian Science, the role of ministering to the sick is carried out by a practitioner (reader).

Although nurses cannot expect to be well versed about the practices of all the religious groups in the United States or Canada, it is important to be familiar with the major religious groups of the community. Representatives of a religion are usually pleased to give nurses information required in the care of patients. Some of the larger religious groups are discussed briefly here. Other reference texts can supply greater detail and information not included in this summary.

American Indians

There are several hundred Native American Indian tribes in the United States and Canada, each with its own religious culture. Most have medicine men or shamans, who perform various actions against illness. Believers look to superhuman powers for protection from disease. Native American Indians have their own beliefs and practices with reference to death. For example, the Canadian coastal tribe at Bella Bella, British Columbia, places the body of the deceased in a casket and carries it out of the building through a window, not through a door, so that death will not reenter through the door.

Many Native American Indians today follow modern Christian religions; however, some follow traditional Indian beliefs, and some hold a combination of Christian and traditional beliefs.

Baha'is

People following the Baha'i faith use prayer at times of illness. Their beliefs permit use of alcohol and drugs only on a physician's order. It is written in the scriptures that ill persons are to seek competent medical assistance.

Baptists

Baptists believe in the possibility of cure of illness by the "laying on of hands." Although some believe in faith healing to the exclusion of medical therapy, most seek competent medical help. Generally no restrictions are placed on the use of drugs, blood, or vaccines; biopsies or amputation of limbs; transplants; autopsies; or burial or cremation. Birth control, sterilization, and abortion (therapeutic or demand) are left to individual choice. When patients are clearly terminally ill, artificial prolongation of life is discouraged. Full-term stillborn babies are buried; less than full-term fetuses are not. Infant baptism is not practiced.

Some Baptists do not drink coffee or tea, and many Baptists do not take alcohol. The clergy ministers to patients and families at times of illness.

Black Muslims (Nation of Islam)

The Black Muslim religion is a separate religion from Islam, although their beliefs are similar. Members emphasize black independence and are encouraged to obtain health care provided by the black community.

Black Muslims have a special procedure for washing and shrouding the dead and special funeral rites. Dietary considerations include prohibitions against alcoholic beverages and pork. Personal cleanliness is emphasized.

Buddhists

The doctrine of avoidance of extremes is practiced by Buddhists and applied to the use of drugs, blood, or vaccines. Buddhism does not condone the taking of lives in any form, but, if a patient is beyond recovery and can no longer strive toward "enlightenment," euthanasia *may* be permitted. Likewise, certain circumstances may warrant abortion. Buddhists approve either burial or cremation. Last rite chanting is frequently practiced at the bedside of the deceased.

Christian Scientists

Members of the Church of Christ, Scientist oppose human intervention to cure illness, seeing it as God's will. Sickness and sin are errors of the human mind and can be changed by altering thoughts rather than by medicine. People who strictly follow this religion will not accept a physician's consultation or medical treatment and rarely, if ever, enter a hospital. Christian Scientists do not permit psychotherapy, because in this process the mind is altered by others. A Christian Science "practitioner" can be called to minister to the sick, and spiritual healing is practiced. Doctors and midwives may be used during childbirth, however.

Drugs and blood transfusions are not used, and biopsies and physical examinations are not sought. Tobacco, alcohol, and coffee are considered drugs and not used. Vaccines are accepted as required by law. Christian Scientists do not have strictly defined policies about birth control, sterilization, or abortion. Autopsy is discouraged, and Christian Scientists are unlikely to seek or donate organs for transplant. Whether a person wishes to rely completely upon Christian Science is up to the individual. In some areas the church operates nursing homes in which there is complete reliance on church doctrine.

Eastern Orthodox Christians

There are a number of Eastern Orthodox denominations, including Greek Orthodox and Russian Orthodox. Most believe in infant baptism by immersion. The last rites are obligatory if death is impending. Dietary restrictions depend on the particular sect. Eastern Orthodox beliefs and practices generally do not restrict medical science; however, the Russian Orthodox church discourages autopsy as well as donation of body parts.

The Greek Orthodox church considers baptism important, and it is usually done at least 40 days after birth. The church advocates confession. The last rites include administration of *Holy Communion* (also referred to as the *Eucharist* or the *Lord's Supper*), a memorial sacrament in which the worshipper receives consecrated bread (or a thin wafer), representing the body of Jesus Christ, and wine or grape juice, representing the blood of Jesus. The church advocates fasting, usually on Wednesdays, Fridays, and during Lent; The church encourages prolonging life even for terminally ill patients. Abortion is prohibited.

Episcopalians (Anglicans)

The Episcopal or Anglican faith places no restrictions on the use of drugs, blood, or vaccines; biopsies; or amputations or transplants for saving life. It permits birth control and sterilization, autopsy, therapeutic abortion as a life-saving measure, burial or cremation, and genetic counseling. Abortion on demand, however, is regarded as unacceptable. Anglicans celebrate Holy Communion. Some members of this church fast before receiving Communion and abstain from meat on Fridays. Infant baptism is mandatory, but aborted fetuses are not baptized. The church advocates confession. The rite for anointing of the sick may be performed but is not mandatory. For information about anointing see page 893.

Hindus

Hindus practice special rites at death. The priest pours water into the mouth of the corpse and ties a thread around the wrist or neck to indicate blessing. This thread must not be removed. The body undergoes cremation, and the ashes are disposed of in holy rivers. Some injuries, such as loss of a limb, are considered signs of wrongdoing in a previous life, although the afflicted person is not an outcast from society. Hindus do believe there is a natural division among people, so that little mixing occurs among the classes.

Hindus have many dietary restrictions. Veal and beef and their derivatives are not eaten, and some Hindus are strict vegetarians. Alcohol may be consumed at western social functions. Most Hindus accept modern medical practices; artificial insemination is rejected, however, because sterility reflects divine will. When giving a Hindu medications, the nurse avoids touching the patient's lips, if possible.

Jehovah's Witnesses

Jehovah's Witnesses are opposed to blood transfusions, although some individuals do agree to them in a crisis. When parents refuse to have an infant transfused, a court order may be sought transferring custody to the courts or to an official of the hospital.

Members of the church eat meat that has been drained of blood. Some oppose modern medicine. Infant baptism is not practiced.

Jehovah's Witnesses generally have a neutral attitude toward birth control, believing it is a matter of individual conscience, but sterilization is condemned and prohibited. Both therapeutic and demand abortions are forbidden. Practices such as masturbation and homosexuality are condemned. Both burial and cremation are approved. Autopsy is approved only as required by law, and no parts of the body are to be removed. This restriction has implications for donor transplants.

Jews

There are three Jewish groups: the Orthodox is the most strict; the Conservative and Reform groups are less strict. Jewish law demands that Jews seek competent medical care. Use of drugs, blood, and vaccines, biopsies, and amputations are permitted. Some Orthodox Jews believe that the entire God-given body must be returned to the earth, and they require any body tissue to be buried. Donor transplants may therefore not be acceptable to Orthodox Jews. The nurse must ensure that amputated limbs or organs are made available to such Orthodox families for burial. Cremation is discouraged. Autopsy may be permitted in less strict groups as long as parts of the body are not removed. Bodies, even those of fetuses, are washed by the ritual burial society and buried as soon as possible after death.

Therapeutic abortion is permissible if the mother's physical or psychologic health is threatened. Demand abortion is prohibited. Vasectomy is not permitted.

Orthodox and Conservative Jews observe kosher dietary laws, which prohibit pork, shellfish, and other foods and the eating of milk products and meat products in the same meal. Reform Jews usually do not observe kosher dietary regulations.

Circumcision of male babies is performed by Orthodox and Conservative Jews on the eighth day of life, although it may be delayed if medically contraindicated. The rabbi and male synagogue members may be present, and a mohel (ritual circumciser acquainted with Jewish law and hygienic medical technique) performs the circumcision. Special arrangements generally need to be made for the ceremony and the physician's approval obtained.

Orthodox and some Conservative Jews observe the Sabbath from sundown Friday to sundown Saturday and may resist hospital admission or medical procedures during that period or during major Jewish festivals, unless the treatment is necessary to preserve life.

Lutherans

The Lutheran church imposes no restrictions on medical procedures, including autopsies and therapeutic abortions, and no dietary restrictions. Abortion on demand is not approved, however. Marriage and procreation are discouraged when offspring are likely to inherit severe physical or mental deficits. Birth control and sterilization are left to the individual's conscience. Members are baptized 6 to 8 weeks after birth, and those who wish may be anointed and blessed before death. Burial rites are generally performed on infants born after 6 to 7 months' gestation who do not survive.

Mennonites

Members of the Mennonite church are baptized in their middle teens. The church advocates no special dietary restrictions, although some congregations require abstinence from alcohol. No restrictions are placed on medical procedures, although demand abortion is not approved in some sects of the church; in others, it is left to individual conscience.

Mormons (Church of Jesus Christ of Latter-Day Saints)

Some Mormons believe in cure by the "laying on of hands"; however, there is no prohibition of medical therapy—in fact, the church operates health facilities. Alcohol, tobacco, tea, and coffee are prohibited, and meat is eaten sparingly. Some members of the church wear a special undergarment at all times. Mormon patients in the hospital may request the Sacrament of the Lord's Supper by a church priesthood holder.

Muslims/Moslems (Islam)

Islam is a major religion of North Africa and the Near East. There are over 70 sects of the Islamic faith. It emphasizes strict rituals and prayers.

All pork products are prohibited, and alcoholic beverages are disapproved except for medicinal purposes. There is a fasting period in the ninth month of the Mohammedan year (Ramadan), but people who are ill are exempt from it.

If a fetus is aborted 130 days or more after conception, it is treated as a fully developed human being. Before that time it is looked upon as discarded tissue.

The dying person must confess sins and beg forgiveness. Only relatives and family can touch the body after death. They wash and prepare it and turn it toward Mecca. Islam encourages prolonging life, even for the terminally ill.

Pentecostalists (Assembly of God, Foursquare Church)

The Pentecostal church has no doctrine against modern medical science, including blood transfusions. Members are encouraged to abstain from use of alcohol and tobacco and from eating strangled animals. Some members do not eat pork. Members may pray for divine healing, and in some congregations anointing with oil is practiced.

Roman Catholics

It is a Catholic belief that an infant has a soul from the moment of conception; therefore, a fetus must be baptized unless it is obviously dead, and so must all babies whose health or life is endangered. Baptism may be performed by any person (e.g., a physician or nurse in the absence of a priest) who does what the church requires. A valid baptism requires pouring water on the baby's head while repeating the prescribed Trinitarian invocation: "I baptize you in the name of the Father, and of the Son, and of the Holy Spirit." When performed by a nurse or physician, the baptism should be recorded on the infant's chart and the family and chaplain informed.

The Roman Catholic church encourages anointing of the sick. The sacrament of anointing is now considered both a source of strength or healing and a preparation for death. The priest anoints several areas of the body with oil. Before changes were instituted by the Second Vatican Council in 1963, this Catholic sacrament was administered to persons only when death was imminent and was referred to as *extreme unction* or the *last rites*, since it was one of the last rites of the church. Today, possibility of death may still be a reason for this sacrament, but death need not be the immediate concern. Catholics can now be anointed more than once. Many older Catholics, however, may respond to this sacrament with fear or dread, considering it a sign of imminent death. Thus, before a reluctant patient is anointed, the nurse or priest should interpret its current meaning to the patient, to minimize apprehension. Anointing of the sick may be preceded by confession and Holy Communion. These sacraments are also performed by a priest or other commissioned person. Receiving viaticum (Holy Communion) as a last rite before death is considered an obligation but anointing is not.

The Roman Catholic belief in the "principle of totality" underlies a general acceptance of medical procedures. A donor transplant is accepted as long as loss of the organ does not deprive the donor of life or functional integrity of the body. Biopsies and amputations are accepted in the same light, but some dioceses require burial of the amputated limb. Autopsy is also accepted; again, all major parts of the body (those retaining human quality) must be given an appropriate burial or cremation.

Strict laws govern birth control, sterilization, and abortion. The only approved method of birth control is abstinence; artificial means are illicit. Sterilization is forbidden unless there is a sound medical indication for it. Both demand and therapeutic abortions are prohibited, even to save the mother's life.

Some Catholics observe certain dietary and fasting practices but are excused from otherwise obligatory fasting or abstaining from meat on Ash Wednesday and Good Friday when in the hospital.

Salvationists

The Salvation Army places no restrictions on medical procedures including transplants and autopsies. Birth control and sterilization are acceptable within marriage. Demand abortions are opposed, but therapeutic ones are approved.

Seventh-Day Adventists (Church of God, Advent Christian Church)

The Adventist church is opposed to infant baptism but conducts baptism of adults by immersion. In dietary matters, it prohibits alcohol, tobacco, narcotics, and stimulants, and some members advocate ovolactovegetarian diets. Some sects practice divine healing and anointing with oil. Saturday is considered the Sabbath by some.

Adventists are encouraged to avoid drugs, but they recognize that blood transfusions, vaccines, and drugs are sometimes necessary. Birth control and sterilization are left to individual conscience. Abortion is approved if the mother's life is endangered or if pregnancy is due to rape or incest. The use of hypnotism is opposed.

Sikhs

Sikhism is a relatively new religion that opposes the caste system in India. Sikhs hold weekly religious services at their temple, from Friday morning through Sunday, in which each member in turn reads the holy scripture (the Granth Sahib) for 2-hour periods until the entire scripture is read.

Baptized male Sikhs wear unshorn hair and turbans, which symbolize dedication and group consciousness. A steel bracelet on the right wrist symbolizes restraint, a reminder not to do wrong. No significant dietary restrictions are imposed by the Sikh faith, but many Sikhs are vegetarians. Use of tobacco and alcohol is discouraged.

Unitarian/Universalists

Unitarian/Universalists emphasize reason, knowledge, individual responsibility, and personally established values. There are no dietary restrictions or official sacraments in the church, and no medical practices are prohibited. The Unitarian/Universalist church encourages its members to donate parts of their bodies to research and to medical banks such as the eye bank.

Assessing Spiritual Needs

A *spiritual need* is that which is needed by a person to maintain, increase, or restore his or her beliefs and faith, and to fulfill religious obligations. It is often the nurse who identifies a patient's spiritual needs and obtains the desired help. Sometimes patients ask directly for a visit from the hospital chaplain or their own clergyman. Others want to discuss their concerns with the nurse and ask about the nurse's beliefs as a way of seeking an empathic listener. Some people are embarrassed to ask for spiritual counsel, but they may hint at their concern by statements such as, "I've been wondering what really will happen to me when I die," or "Do you go to a church?" The nurse may also obtain clues about a patient's concerns through observation. Does the patient read a prayer book or the Bible each day? Does he or she wear or use religious medals, medallions, or symbols?

In a hospital, the admission record and the nursing history usually record the patient's religion. The nurse also can ask if the patient follows any religious practices and if the patient would like a visit from the appropriate clergy. It is important to ask the patient before obtaining assistance. Some people profess to have no religious beliefs and may be angered if the nurse makes arrangements for a chaplain to visit. The nurse needs to respect the patient's wishes and not make a judgment of right or wrong, good or bad.

Candidates for Pastoral Care

Pastoral care is an interpersonal relationship that focuses on the spiritual component of a person's life during an experience of distress. Provision of pastoral care is not limited to the clergy, although special or particular functions are provided by that group. The following list identifies groups of people who may benefit from pastoral care (the list is only a guide for nurses and should not replace individual assessment):

1. Patients who appear lonely and have few visitors.
2. Patients who express fear and anxiety.
3. Patients whose illness is related to the emotions or to religious attitudes.
4. Patients who face surgery.
5. Patients who must change their life-style as a result of illness or injury.
6. Patients who are preoccupied about the relationship of their religion and health.
7. Patients who are unable to have their pastor visit or who would not normally receive pastoral care.
8. Patients whose illness has social implications.
9. Patients who are dying.

The nurse should not restrict assessment of spiritual needs to the patient. At times of illness, families are stressed and often want spiritual assistance. The patient facing death may have accepted this fate, but the family may not have. Often relatives are grateful for spiritual support by a nurse or pastor. Assisting them with support may indirectly assist the patient.

Nursing History

The nurse may elicit data about the patient's spiritual beliefs and practices, ideally in response to the patient's verbal and nonverbal cues indicating spiritual concerns and after a sound relationship is established. Examples of questions are:

1. Are any particular religious practices important to you? If so, could you please tell me about them?
2. Will being here interfere with your religious practices?
3. Do you feel your faith is helpful to you? In what ways is it important to you right now?
4. In what ways can I help you to carry out your faith? For example, would you like me to read your prayer book to you?
5. Would you like a visit from your spiritual counselor or the hospital chaplain?
6. What are your hopes and your sources of strength right now?

Clinical Signs

The nurse observes the patient for the following cues to a spiritual need (Fish and Shelley 1978:61; Kim and Moritz 1982:314):

1. *Affect and attitude.* Does the patient appear lonely, depressed, angry, anxious, agitated, apathetic, or preoccupied?
2. *Behavior.* Does the patient appear to pray before meals or at other times? Does the patient read religious

literature? Does the patient complain frequently, need unusually high doses of sedation, pace the halls at night, joke inappropriately, have nightmares and sleep disturbances, or express anger at religious representatives or a deity?

3. *Verbalization.* Does the patient mention God, prayer, faith, the church, or religious topics (even briefly)? Does the patient ask about a visit from the clergy? Does the patient express fear of death, concern with the meaning of life, inner conflict about religious beliefs, concern about a relationship with the deity, questions about the meaning of existence, the meaning of suffering, or the moral/ethical implications of therapy?

4. *Interpersonal relationships.* Who visits? How does the patient respond to visitors? Does a minister come? How does the patient relate to other patients and nursing personnel?

5. *Environment.* Does the patient have a Bible, prayer book, devotional literature, religious medals, a rosary, or religious get-well cards in the room? Does a church send altar flowers or Sunday bulletins?

Nursing Diagnoses

The nursing diagnoses for patients with spiritual concerns may be stated as:

1. Spiritual distress related to separation from religious and cultural ties.
2. Spiritual distress related to challenge of the patient's belief and value system by:
- **a.** Intense suffering
- **b.** The moral/ethical implications of therapy

Because spiritual beliefs and religious practices are closely allied to a person's moral/ethical self, which is an important component of self-concept (discussed in Chapter 32), spiritual concerns may also contribute to problems with self-concept. Thus, nursing diagnoses for patients with spiritual concerns may include: Lowered self-esteem related to (a) violation of religious doctrine and feelings of guilt, or (b) broken relationship with deity.

Planning and Intervention Related to Spiritual Needs

Planning

The overall nursing goal for patients experiencing spiritual distress is to support the patient's spiritual beliefs and religious practices. Subgoals may include:

1. To provide spiritual resources otherwise unavailable
2. To help the patient fulfill religious obligations
3. To help the patient draw on and use inner resources more effectively to meet the present situation
4. To help the patient maintain or establish a dynamic, personal relationship with the deity in the face of unpleasant circumstances
5. To help the patient find meaning in existence and the present situation

Planning also involves establishing outcome criteria. For suggestions, see Evaluation later in this chapter.

Guidelines for Nursing Intervention

1. Examine and clarify the personal spiritual or religious convictions and beliefs that may influence your interactions with patients. Ask yourself:
- **a.** Are all religions and beliefs equally valid for the persons holding them, or is there only one true religion?
- **b.** What do I believe about life after death, euthanasia, birth control, sterilization, therapeutic and demand abortion, prolonging life, autopsy, burial or cremation, nonmedical modes of healing, donation of body parts, care of excised body tissue, and amputated limbs?
- **c.** Do I see any relationship among sin, punishment, suffering, and illness?
- **d.** How often have I read a Bible to or prayed with a person, and how comfortable would I be doing so with a patient? Would I feel frightened, uneasy, ambivalent, sure, or comfortable?
- **e.** If there is conflict between medical practice and religious doctrine, which should take preference?
- **f.** How will I respond if patients try to convert me to their beliefs and practices?
- **g.** How will I respond if a patient's beliefs and practices conflict with my own or are unacceptable to me?

2. Focus attention on the patient's perception of his or her spiritual needs rather than the practices or beliefs of the religious affiliation stated on the patient's record. The spiritual beliefs of a given church may vary greatly among members. People join religious groups for many reasons, e.g., to have a place of worship, to find an avenue for social action such as helping the poor or homeless, to gain friends for recreational purposes, or to have a place for important life events such as weddings and funerals. There are often different sects within a religious denomination—for example, among Jews there are Orthodox, Conservative, and Reform sects—with varying practices.

3. Do not assume that a patient has no spiritual needs because the patient's record states no religious affiliation or specifies atheist or agnostic. An *atheist* is a person who denies the existence of any god, while an *agnostic* is a person who believes that the existence of God is unknown.

4. Acknowledge and respond to the patient's nonverbal cues about spiritual need, such as visible devotional materials, religious articles, or visits from the clergy. Your interest in and questions about religious objects show that you care about the patient's religious concerns.

5. Respond to the patient's verbal cues with brief, specific, factual answers. Responding involves:

- **a.** Active listening: attempting to enter into the other person's frame of reference so as to understand more fully his or her feelings and experiences.
- **b.** Support: accepting the person, even though his or her beliefs may not agree with yours, by being there, showing genuine concern, asking questions, providing information, reflecting feelings, acknowledging strengths, etc.
- **c.** Awareness: being sensitive to what the patient is saying and not saying and to the patient's emotional tone.
- **d.** Empathy: understanding and experiencing the patient's feelings.
- **e.** Nonjudgmental understanding: accepting and understanding the person without approving or disapproving.

6. Determine the meaning the patient attributes to the situation. Such meanings can influence the patient's response to an illness or condition and may either hinder nursing intervention or provide hope, courage, and strength. For example, a person who believes that illness is God's punishment may feel powerless and demonstrate little interest in therapy designed to prevent illness.

7. Help the patient meet religious obligations:

- **a.** Prepare the patient and the environment for visits by the clergy.
- **b.** Ensure privacy for prayer and meditation.
- **c.** Greet the clergy when they enter the nursing unit and assist them as required.
- **d.** Protect the patient's religious objects from loss or damage.
- **e.** Help the patient meet religious dietary obligations.
- **f.** Allow helpless patients to say grace, if desired, before feeding them.
- **g.** Arrange for appropriate care of the body after death.

8. Inform patients about the services provided by the hospital to meet spiritual needs, and arrange for patients to participate in these as they are able. Many large hospitals have full-time chaplains who assist patients, family, and staff with spiritual needs. Chaplains of several faiths usually participate, including a rabbi, a Roman Catholic priest, and Protestant ministers, from denominations such as Episcopalian, Methodist, Lutheran, Baptist, and Presbyterian. For smaller hospitals that do not have chaplains, clergy in the community usually provide this service. Many nursing units have a list of clergy who are on-call when needed.

The chaplain functions in a variety of ways. Usually a newly admitted patient is visited, and spiritual needs are assessed. The chaplain then may read spiritual literature aloud, conduct special sacraments, or simply visit—whatever is appropriate for the person.

Some agencies have a chapel, where regular religious services are held for patients, families, and staff. Most hospitals also have quiet rooms that can be used by patients, families, and staff for meditation, counsel, and even worship services. Sometimes a patient prefers to meet the chaplain in a quiet room where there is privacy. This is particularly true when a patient is sharing a room.

A hospital may hold nondenominational religious services or several services for different denominations. If a patient expresses a desire to attend services, the nurse needs to help organize the patient's care so that this is possible.

9. Determine whether the patient wishes to receive Holy Communion. Communion is celebrated by most Christian churches (Protestant and Catholic), but practices and underlying theologic concepts vary considerably from denomination to denomination. When a hospitalized patient is to receive Holy Communion, determine what preparations are necessary. Some patients fast for several hours prior to this sacrament, but fasting is not required during periods of ill health. Medications are allowed if needed. Some agencies supply communion sets containing a white tablecloth, a candle, a spoon, and a small glass. Many clergy carry small communion sets with them.

10. Determine whether the patient wants a visit from religious groups that visit hospitals. If the patient does not want such a visit, respect this wish and communicate it tactfully to visitors.

11. In some instances, members of religious groups

will chant or wail at the patient's bedside during times of grief. If this is disturbing to others, intervene tactfully. It may be possible to move roommates temporarily to another room or provide a private place for the patient and visitors.

12. If you feel uncomfortable assisting the patient spiritually (e.g., reading devotional material to the patient or praying with the patient on request) verbalize this discomfort, and offer to obtain assistance for the patient. It is important to respect the patient's beliefs and maintain a supportive relationship. It is equally important not to feel guilty about your discomfort.

13. If a patient attempts to convert you to his or her beliefs and practices, tell the patient honestly that you have other beliefs and feel uncomfortable with this request. At the same time, acknowledge respect for the patient's beliefs, to maintain your relationship with the patient.

Evaluation

Examples of outcome criteria for patients with spiritual distress are:

1. Is able to rest calmly.
2. States acceptance of moral/ethical decision.
3. Expresses comfort with relationship with deity.
4. Demonstrates warm and open relationship with clergy.
5. Displays positive affect or absence of feelings of anger, guilt, or anxiety.
6. Displays more positive behavior or absence of agitation and inappropriate joking.
7. Expresses positive meaning to present situation and existence.

Summary

The spiritual needs of patients and their families often come into focus at a time of illness, when a patient has time to think of spirituality and when life may be threatened. Some patients profess to have no religious beliefs. Nurses must respect the right of people to believe in certain religions or to have no religious beliefs.

Spiritual development begins in early childhood. Preschoolers imitate certain religious rituals to conform to parental expectations. They learn what is good and bad from the moral code and religion of their parents. From this learning, the person's superego develops. School-age children learn more about religion and develop a reverence for many thoughts and matters. By prepuberty, children begin to reason rather than accept faith blindly. During adolescence, children compare parental religious standards with those of others, and by 16 years of age most adolescents have decided whether to accept the family religion. During adulthood, people develop a religious philosophy that helps them participate in life and face reality.

Many religions in the United States and Canada have particular practices or beliefs that relate to health and illness, birth, death, and medical procedures. It is important for the nurse to be aware of various religious groups in the community and to have some knowledge of the beliefs and practices that affect health care. Most patients or families when questioned will tell a nurse about religious practices they wish to observe, such as following special diet or receiving Holy Communion. Nurses need to be aware of these and to assist the patient by arranging nursing care so that the practices can be carried out.

Part of the nurse's function is to assist patients and families to meet their spiritual needs. Nurses may assess spiritual needs from the nursing history and clinical signs. Certain patients are particular candidates for pastoral care. Nurses may intervene directly to meet spiritual needs by being attentive, supportive, empathic, understanding, and nonjudgmental. They may also facilitate clergy to meet patients' needs. It is important that nurses feel comfortable when participating in a religious activity with a patient; otherwise they should suggest that another nurse or a chaplain do so.

Suggested Activities

1. In a group of 10 or 12 students, each choose a specific religion to study. Visit the local clergy of the religion you have chosen, and obtain information regarding its beliefs and practices pertinent to health and illness. Share your findings with the group.
2. Visit a local hospital, and find out what special arrangements are made to meet patients' spiritual

needs. Does the agency have a chapel, chaplain services, and means of accommodating religious dietary rules?

3. In the clinical agency to which you are assigned, note the assessment tool used to determine a patient's spiritual needs. Compare your findings with those of students from other clinical agencies.

Suggested Readings

Carson, V. January-February 1980. Meeting the spiritual needs of hospitalized psychiatric patients. *Perspectives in Psychiatric Care* 18:17–20.

This author describes how a prayer group for psychiatric patients promoted such benefits as increased support among members for each other.

Demsteegt, D. August 1975. Pastoral roles in presurgical visits. *American Journal of Nursing* 75:1336–37.

A pastor reveals how he felt about visiting hospitalized patients. He describes his role as alternating between clown and priest.

Morris, K. L., and Foerster, J. D. December 1972. Team work: Nurse and chaplain. *American Journal of Nursing* 72:2197–99.

The authors describe a program in which nurses and clergy worked together and the benefits to both patients and personnel.

Piepgras, R. December 1968. The other dimension: Spiritual help. *American Journal of Nursing* 68:2610–13.

This article suggests that little emphasis is placed on spiritual needs of patients, yet some patients need this help the most. Five manifestations of the need for spiritual help are outlined, and patient examples are included.

Selected References

Berkowitz, P., and Berkowitz, N. S. November 1967. The Jewish patient in hospital. *American Journal of Nursing* 67:2335–37.

Dickinson, C. October 1975. The search for spiritual meaning. *American Journal of Nursing* 75:1789–93.

Drakulic, L., and Tanaka, W. March 1981. The East Indian family in Canada. *Canadian Nurse* 77:24–26.

Ellis, D. September 1980. What happened to the spiritual dimension? *Canadian Nurse* 76:42–43.

Fish, S., and Shelley, J. A. 1978. *Spiritual care: The nurse's role.* Downers Grove, Ill.: Inter Varsity Press.

Gordon, M. 1982. *Manual of nursing diagnosis.* New York: McGraw-Hill Book Co.

Kelsey, M. T. 1973. *Healing and Christianity.* Toronto: Fitzhenry and Whiteside, Ltd.

Kim, M. J., and Moritz, D. A., editors. 1982. *Classification of nursing diagnoses: Proceedings of the third and fourth national conferences.* New York: McGraw-Hill Book Co.

Maslow, A. H. 1970. *Religious values and peak experiences.* Markham, Ont.: Penguin Books.

Naiman, H. L. November 1970. Nursing in Jewish law. *American Journal of Nursing* 70:2378–79.

Perk, D. 1975. *Man's quest for meaning, faith, identity.* Johannesburg: Aegis Press.

Pumphrey, J. B. December 1977. Recognizing your patient's spiritual needs. *Nursing 77* 7:64–69.

Stoll, R. T. September 1979. Guidelines for spiritual assessment. *American Journal of Nursing* 79:1574–77.

VanKaam, A. 1976a. *Dynamics of spiritual direction.* Denville, N.J.: Dimension Books.

———. 1976b. *In search of spiritual identity.* Denville, N.J.: Dimension Books.

———. 1976c. *Spirituality and the gentle life.* Denville, N.J.: Dimension Books.

Chapter 35

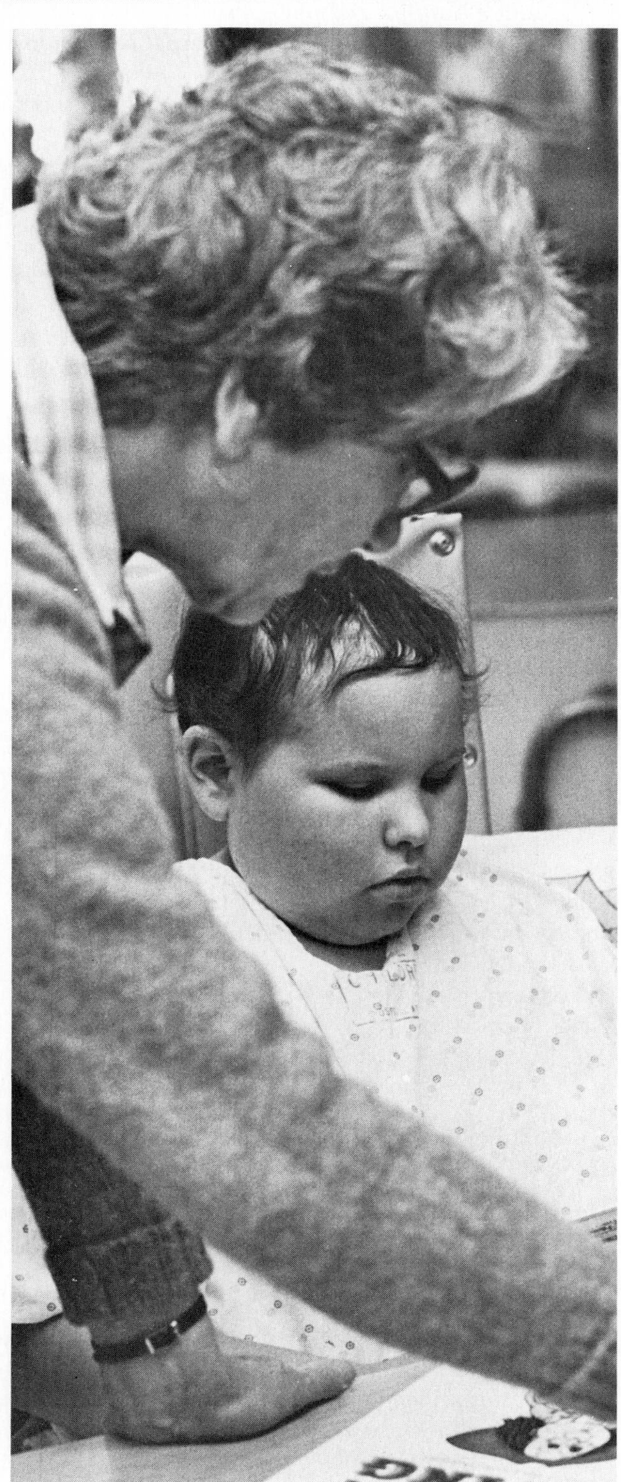

Stimulation

CONTENTS

Objectives

1. Know essential facts about sensory stimulation and the sensory-perceptual process

- **1.1** Define selected terms
- **1.2** Identify stages of awareness and consciousness
- **1.3** Identify structural and physiological elements of the sensory-perceptual process
- **1.4** Identify various types of sensation
- **1.5** Identify causes and signs of three kinds of sensory disturbance

2. Know information and methods required to assess and diagnose sensory-perceptual status

- **2.1** Identify patients susceptible to sensory disturbances
- **2.2** Identify data to obtain in the health history
- **2.3** Identify factors influencing sensory function
- **2.4** Identify physical examinations that assess sensory function
- **2.5** Identify clinical signs of sensory dysfunction
- **2.6** Identify nursing diagnoses of sensory disturbances

3. Know facts about nursing interventions to maintain and promote optimal sensory stimulation

- **3.1** Identify appropriate nursing goals
- **3.2** Identify measures to maintain sensory stimulation of hospitalized patients of all ages
- **3.3** Identify measures to counteract sensory overload
- **3.4** Identify measures to counteract sensory deprivation
- **3.5** Identify measures to assist patients with selected sensory deficits

4. Apply the nursing process when providing care to selected patients with sensory disturbances

- **4.1** Obtain necessary assessment data
- **4.2** Analyze and relate assessment data
- **4.3** Write relevant nursing diagnoses
- **4.4** Write relevant nursing goals
- **4.5** Plan appropriate nursing interventions
- **4.6** Implement appropriate nursing interventions
- **4.7** State outcome criteria against which to evaluate the patient's progress

Terms

auditory
awareness
comatose
consciousness
decussate
gustatory
hallucination
illusion
kinesthetic
lethargic
obtunded
olfactory
semicomatose
sensoristasis
sensorium
sensory adaptation
sensory deficit
sensory deprivation (input deficit)
sensory overload
stuporous
tactile
visceral
visual

Children need sensory stimulation to develop normally, and in recent years, sensory stimulation has been recognized as a basic need of all people. The public is becoming increasingly aware of positive and negative stimuli in the environment—noise levels, the relative beauty of surroundings, etc.

Problems in the perception of sensation affect thinking, behavior, and awareness. For example, the blind often develop other senses more than is normal in an effort to compensate for the loss of sight. Chronically ill and elderly people, who may be socially isolated and relatively immobile, suffer another form of sensory deprivation. Helping to meet needs for sensory stimulation is part of the nurse's function.

The amount of sensory stimulation people need for optimal functioning is highly individual. A hospitalized adult who normally lives alone may find several visitors overly stimulating; a mother of six children may find an empty house lacks the level of stimulation she needs.

States of awareness vary greatly with health and illness. Ability to respond to the environment is largely affected by state of awareness.

States of Awareness

Awareness is the ability to perceive environmental stimuli and body reactions and to respond appropriately through thought and action. The normal, alert person can assimilate many kinds of information at one time. The restaurant patron who dines with friends appreciates odors, tastes, conversation, and company at the same time. The normal person perceives reality accurately and acts on those perceptions. Part of this process is separating necessary stimuli from extraneous ones and reaching logical conclusions by correlating information. Most people do this with little or no awareness of the mental processes involved. Occasionally, normal persons exhibit abnormalities of thought; they become absent minded, lose their sense of direction, and so on. Often these episodes are due to intense concentration on one subject to the exclusion of others.

Consciousness is awareness of environment, self, and others. Illness and age can affect consciousness, as can hospitalization. Mildly confused hospitalized patients may momentarily forget they are not at home, wander from their rooms, misplace personal belongings, and so forth. Severely confused (disoriented) persons may not know family members or may think the nurse is a relative. Such persons may act atypically: Confused, normally docile people may become combative with nurses and others. Severely confused people do not know where they are or what time of day or day of the week it is.

Level of consciousness also affects awareness. See Table 35–1 for levels of consciousness.

Table 35–1 Levels of Consciousness

Level	Behavior
Alert	Awake and aware of environment without stimulation Oriented to time, place, and person Responds briskly and appropriately to minimal visual, auditory, and tactile stimuli
Lethargic	Sleeps much of the time when not stimulated Is easily aroused and when aroused is oriented Speech may be slow or hesitant
Obtunded	Difficult to arouse from sleep (e.g., must be shaken or given a painful stimulus) Responds verbally when awakened but response is confined to a few words that do not make sense Quickly returns to sleeping state when stimulation removed
Stuporous	Aroused only by painful stimuli (e.g., when the nurse presses a fingernail into the patient's nailbed or pinches the patient's Achilles tendon) No verbal response to painful stimuli Is never fully wakened
Semi-comatose	Reflex movement elicited by painful stimuli Gag reflex present (checked by holding tongue down with tongue blade and touching oropharynx with cotton-tipped applicator) Corneal (blink) reflex present (checked by lightly touching the cornea with a wisp of cotton Decorticate or decerebrate posturing may be present*
Comatose	No response to maximal painful stimuli Reflexes absent Absence of muscle tone in extremities

**Decerebrate posturing* (indicating midbrain damage) is recognized by extension, adduction, and internal rotation of the arms; extension of the legs with feet in plantar flexion; and arching of the back. *Decortical posturing* (indicating damage to the internal capsule and corticospinal tracts above the brain stem) is recognized by flexion and adduction of fingers, wrists, and shoulders; extension and internal rotation of legs and feet; and rigidity of all extremities.

Adapted from A. Ladyshewsky, Increased intracranial pressure: When assessment counts, *The Canadian Nurse*, October 1980, 76:34.

Sensory Perception

Sensory perception starts with a stimulus that triggers a receptor. The stimulus travels along a neuron (sensory neuron I) to the central nervous system. From the spinal cord or brain stem, the impulses travel along sensory neuron II to the thalamus. These neurons synapse with sensory neurons III, which conduct the impulses from the thalamus to the somatosensory area of the postcentral gyrus of the parietal lobe of the brain, also called the primary sensory area. See Figure 35–1. In most instances sensory pathways *decussate* (cross over) and register sensations from the opposite side of the body. Usually, decussation takes place at the level of sensory neuron II.

Figure 35–1 The lateral spinothalamic tract relays impulses of crude touch, pain, and temperature from receptors up the spinal cord to the thalamus. The thalamocortical tract relays the impulses from the thalamus to the somatic sensory area of the cortex (postcentral gyrus).

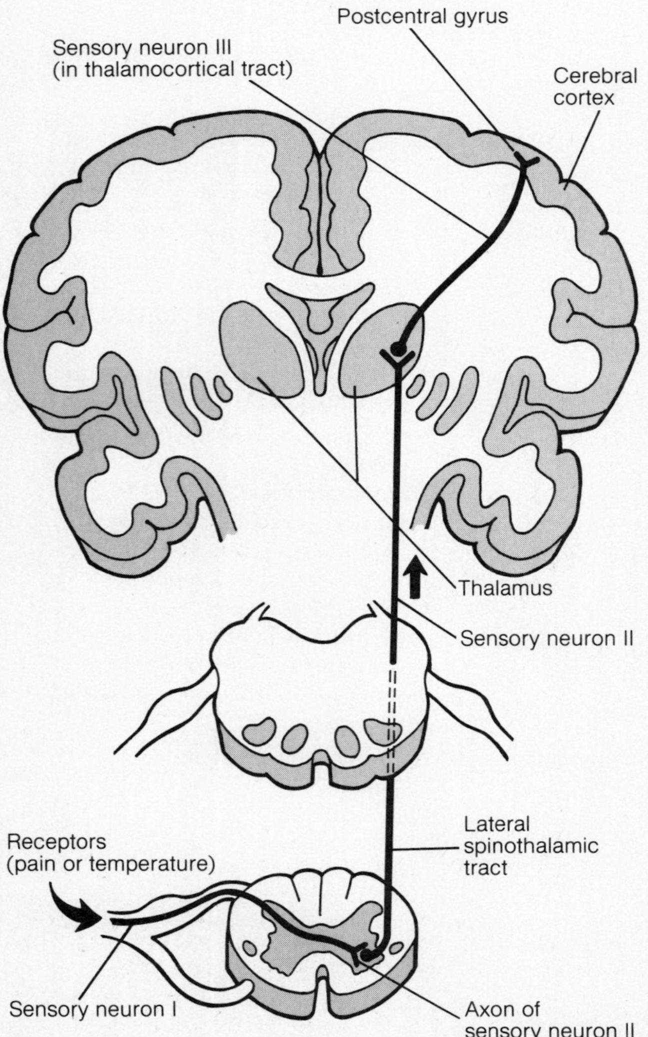

Sensory pathways carry information about heat, cold, touch, and pressure. Stereognosis (awareness of an object's size, shape, and texture), kinesthesia (ability to perceive muscle movement), vibratory sense, and two-point and weight discrimination are also sensory abilities that terminate in the primary sensory area. See Figure 35–2. Other special sensory areas are: visual, auditory, and olfactory association areas. The gustatory area is located in the parietal lobe deep in the lateral fissure.

Consciousness requires continuous stimulation of cortical neurons by impulses conducted through a relay of neurons called the reticular activating system. This system consists of centers in the brain stem that receive impulses from the spinal cord and relay them to the thalamus and from there to all parts of the cerebral cortex.

The need for sensory stimulation is called *sensoristasis*. Humans need constant and varied sensory stimuli. Insufficient stimuli cause sensory deprivation. Overstimulation at any one site causes *sensory adaptation*, a result of the ability of sensory receptors to adapt partially or completely to a repeated stimulus. At first, receptors respond at a very high impulse rate; with continued stimulation, the receptors respond less rapidly and finally many do not respond at all. For this reason, the brain ceases to perceive the repeated stimulus. Extreme concentration produces a similar effect: The brain does not perceive extraneous stimuli.

Sensory stimuli are either external or internal. External stimuli arise from outside of the person. They are *visual* (sight), *auditory* (hearing), *olfactory* (smell), *tactile* (touch), and *gustatory* (taste). Gustatory stimuli can be internal as well. Internal stimuli are kinesthetic or visceral. *Kinesthetic* refers to awareness of the position and movement of body parts. *Visceral* refers to any large organ in the body's interior.

Certain pathologic conditions create sensations that do not arise from normal external or internal stimuli. For example, a patient with a pathologic condition of the auditory nerve hears sounds that correspond to no external stimulus. *Hallucinations* (perceptions of external stimuli in the absence of such stimuli) are a result of pathology or hallucinogenic drugs. *Illusions* are misinterpretations of external stimuli. For example, a patient may interpret a shadow cast by a lamp as a person.

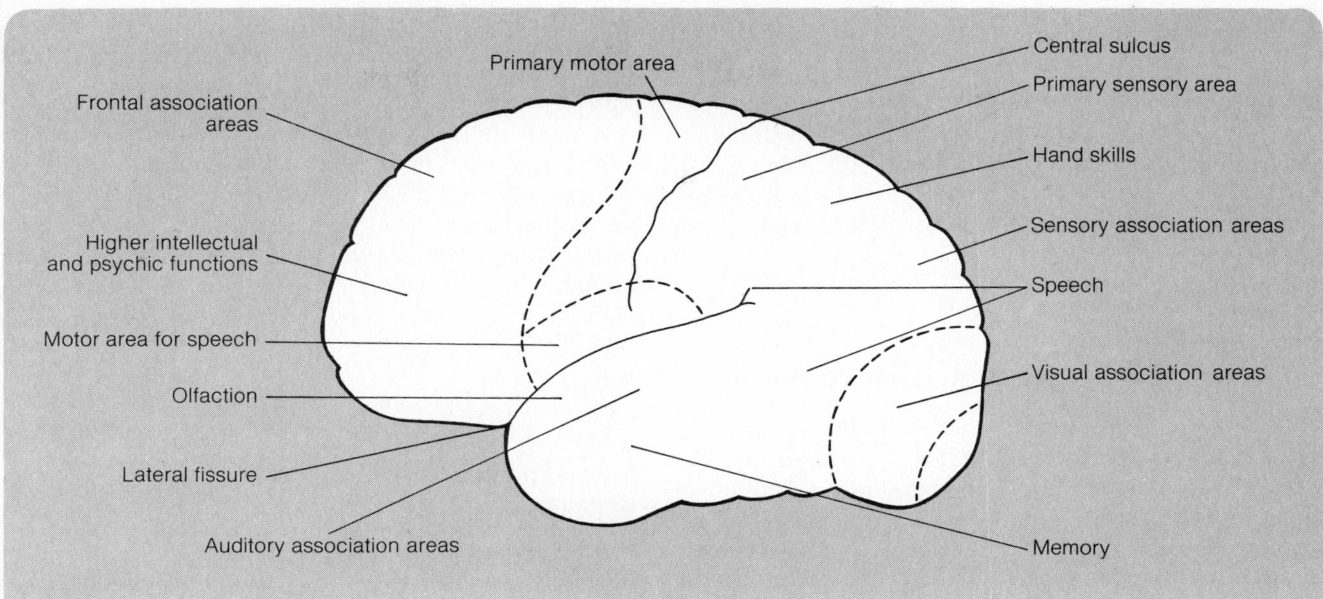

Figure 35–2 The lateral aspect of the functional areas of the left cerebral cortex.

Sensory Disturbances

Sensory Deprivation

Sensory deprivation describes a level of sensory input too low to allow normal functioning. Persons who were experimentally isolated from stimulation changed the content of their thought; they were alternately irritable and easily amused (Heron 1971:355–56). In a similar study, subjects had these symptoms: physical discomfort, space and time disorientation, sensory distortion, difficulty concentrating, and even hallucinations (Downs 1974:434–38).

Because of the increasing awareness of sensory deprivation, health agencies are recognizing the value of colorful, attractive surroundings for patients. Some agencies also provide background music or radios and television to give patients auditory stimulation.

There are three main causes of sensory deprivation: inadequate stimulation (e.g., isolation in a barren environment), impairment of a sensory organ (e.g., deafness), and impairment of brain centers that process sensory stimuli. The last occurs, for example, in patients with brain damage from cerebrovascular accidents (strokes).

Sensory Overload

Sensory overload is more sensory stimulation in a given period than one can tolerate. Hospitalized patients, exposed to bright lights, noise, unfamiliar machinery, and too many visits from friends and health personnel, may suffer sensory overload. A continuous barrage of stimuli can produce in patients many of the symptoms of sensory deprivation. The person may appear fatigued, agitated, and confused and may have hallucinations.

Sensory Deficit

A *sensory deficit* is impaired functioning of a sensory or perceptual process. Blindness and deafness are sensory deficits. When only one sense is affected, other senses may become more acute to compensate for the loss. However, sudden loss of eyesight can result in total disorientation.

When there is gradual loss of sensory function, individuals often develop behavioral alterations to compensate for the loss; sometimes the behaviors are unconscious. For example, a person with gradual hearing loss in the right ear may unconsciously turn the left ear toward a speaker. When the loss is sudden, compensatory behaviors take days or weeks to develop.

Some neurologic diseases cause changes in kinesthetic sense and tactile perceptions. Pathology of the inner ear, for example, can cause loss of kinesthetic sense. Spinal cord injuries and cerebrovascular accidents cause paralysis and loss of tactile perception.

Assessment

When assessing sensory-perceptual alterations and sensory deficits, the nurse needs to identify patients susceptible to sensory disturbances, take health histories, consider factors influencing sensory function, conduct a physical examination, and identify significant clinical signs.

Susceptibility to Sensory Disturbances

Nurses need to be aware of those patients who are particularly susceptible to sensory disturbances. By anticipating possible problems, the nurse can often implement measures to prevent them. The following circumstances may predispose to sensory disturbances.

Nonstimulating environments

People who normally live alone and have little contact with others may experience sensory overload when they are hospitalized. This is particularly true of the elderly and of people who work at home alone. In their homes, these persons are at risk of sensory deprivation. People who live in institutions with unchanging social and perceptual stimuli are also at risk of sensory deprivations.

Therapeutic isolation

Therapeutic isolation, either in the hospital or at home, can predispose to sensory disturbance. Patients on protective asepsis are often confined to a room, and their primary social contacts are with gowned, masked personnel. Immobile patients confined to bed, even though in rooms with other patients and allowed visitors, are also prone to sensory deprivation.

Medically intensive environments

Patients in constantly staffed environments are often overloaded with stimuli. Patients in intensive care and coronary care units are never left alone. The noises, machines, and lights of such environments further the risk of sensory overload.

Sensory deficits

Patients with sensory deficits are at risk of both sensory deprivation and sensory overload. Persons with visual problems may be unable to read, watch television, or recognize nurses by sight. An unfamiliar environment can add to their confusion. The blind often have highly structured home environments, and the diversity and unfamiliarity of the hospital environment can create sensory overload. At the same time, impaired vision often means inability to move around readily or socialize with others. Deaf persons who cannot lip-read also may feel isolated.

Special personality and developmental characteristics

Some people tolerate sensory deprivation and sensory overload better than others. People whose developmental levels are characterized by short attention spans, need for physical activity, and dependence on others for amusement are more susceptible to sensory deprivation than people who are more self-reliant and contemplative (Mitchell and Loustau 1981:326). Likewise, persons who are stressed and anxious have more difficulty coping with sensory deprivation. Certain drugs such as narcotics decrease awareness of the environment, and people taking such drugs may be susceptible to sensory deprivation. People tolerate sensory overload differently. For example a mother accustomed to six active, noisy children may hardly notice the noise of her environment, whereas another person would find the noise bothersome.

Nursing History

The nursing history includes not only the patient's present sensory perceptions but also his or her usual functioning. What is normal for one patient may be abnormal for another. In some instances, significant others can provide data the patient cannot. For example, a wife may observe her husband's hearing loss long before her husband is aware of it.

The nursing history should include the *sensorium* (consciousness or mental clarity), the sensory realm, and the affective realm. See Table 35-2. The nurse must also consider the sensory-perceptual environment. Obviously changes in environment affect sensory input. The elderly woman who moves from her daughter's busy home to a room in a boarding house experiences a change in level of sensory input. This change may affect cerebral functioning.

Table 35–2 Perceptual-Sensory History Outline

Sensorium
Consciousness (awareness of internal and external stimuli)
Orientation (person, place, time)
Attention span
Memory (recent and remote)
Cognitive skills (ability to learn, abstract, compute, etc.)

Sensory
Visual changes
Auditory changes
Gustatory changes
Tactile changes
Olfactory changes
Kinesthetic changes

Affective
Reaction to change
Decision making
Illusions or delusions

Factors Influencing Sensory-Perceptual Function

Developmental status

Perception of sensation is critical to the intellectual, social, and physical development of infants and children. As children grow, they learn that certain sensations provide cues for behavior already learned, such as stopping and looking both ways before crossing a street. Adults have many learned responses to sensory cues. Loss or impairment of any sense, therefore, has profound effects on both the child and young adult. The gradual diminishing of sensory perception that comes with age does not have as profound an effect.

Vision, hearing, and touch decline with age. Sight usually declines after age 45. Vision accuracy (both near and far perception), adaptation to light and dark, color discrimination, adaptation to glare, and visual acuity all diminish (Crandall 1980:142). Hearing begins to decline at about 25 years. Generally, elderly people experience loss of volume perception and loss of pitch perception. At about 55 years, people become less sensitive to changes in touch, temperature, and pain. Loss of sensitivity usually begins on the lower half of the body and spreads upward (ibid., p. 145). Taste and smell do not seem to change with age. It is thought that changes are more probably due to disease or to chronic smoking.

Illness and medical therapy

Certain illnesses affect sensory function. Atherosclerosis, arteriosclerosis, and similar disorders restrict blood flow to the receptor organ or the brain, decreasing awareness and slowing responses. Uncontrolled diabetes mellitus can impair vision. Central nervous system disease causes varying degrees of paralysis and sensory loss.

Narcotics, sedatives, and certain other medications affect cerebral functioning and therefore affect sensory input indirectly. Other drugs, such as central nervous system stimulants (amphetamines) can cause sensory overload.

Environment

Certain environments pose the risk of trauma to sensory organs. Foundry workers, for example, are exposed to constant, loud noise and may eventually have hearing loss unless they wear protective ear covers.

Cognitive and emotional resources

Individuals' cognitive and emotional resources also affect their capacity to deal with sensory deprivation and sensory overload. Mitchell and Loustau (1981:317) found that intelligent and creative people can cope with sensory deprivation better than others.

Physical Examination

Vision, hearing, as well as olfactory, gustatory, tactile, and kinesthetic status are examined. Some examiners also test vocal status (voice quality). See Chapter 14 for additional information about these examinations.

Clinical Signs

To assess sensory deprivation or overload, the nurse needs to know the level of sensory input the person is accustomed to and tolerates best. This level is highly individual. The child who has five brothers and sisters may be accustomed to a different level of sensory input than the only child.

Sensory deprivation

A person experiencing sensory deprivation may manifest boredom, inactivity, slowness of thought, daydreaming, increased sleeping, thought disorganization, anxiety, panic, or hallucinations (Cameron et al. 1972:33).

Both activity and inactivity can signal boredom. If active, the bored person occupies time with unimportant matters. The bored person may ask for assistance unnecessarily. An inactive person may appear apathetic and withdrawn. This person may also be irritable and exhibit childish emotional responses (Heron 1971:358).

Slowness of thought is demonstrated by difficulty grasping ideas and slowness in communicating. Reaction time is slow, and the person may appear clumsy.

Persons who are daydreaming appear absorbed in their own thoughts and may talk and laugh to themselves. It may be difficult to engage such a person in conversation. These persons may confuse a daydream with reality and imagine a conversation that did not take place. Increased sleeping is another manifestation of sensory deprivation. The person who lacks external stimulation may have difficulty staying awake and may sleep to pass time.

Difficulty remembering what one was saying may be evidence of thought disorganization. The person may start a sentence on one subject and end it with an unrelated subject. Thought disorganization may also be reflected in confusion about the time of day or the day of the week. The person may react inappropriately, for instance, by laughing at bad news, or experience sensory distortions, such as mistaking the smell of food for the smell of smoke.

Anxiety and panic are similar. Panic is severe anxiety. See the signs of increased stress listed in Chapter 9. Hallucinations can also be a result of sensory deprivation. The person may hear nonexistent voices or see nonexistent sights. The patient may misinterpret stimuli and, for example, see a shadow as a man with a knife. These misinterpreted stimuli are called illusions.

Sensory overload

Sensory overload may have the same symptoms as sensory deprivation. In addition, the patient may appear agitated and restless. If symptoms worsen when the patient's social contacts increase, sensory overload is probable.

Sensory deficits

Sensory deficits are generally assessed during initial health assessment. In addition, nurses need to observe and note behaviors that may reflect impairment of any of the senses.

Auditory

Is the person able to locate the direction of sounds? (Persons with hearing aids often have difficulties locating the direction.)

Can the person distinguish and differentiate voices?

Does the person report a humming, ringing, or buzzing in the ears?

Does the person speak loudly or shout?

Visual

Is the person able to see objects or persons nearby and at a distance?

Does the person hold the reading material close or far away?

Does the person report unusual distortions in vision?

Does the person have a full field of vision? Does the person see objects only directly in his or her line of vision?

Does the person report seeing spots, colored areas, or halos around objects?

Gustatory

Does the person report persistent, unusual tastes, such as bitterness or metallic tastes?

Can the person differentiate between sweet, sour, salt, and bitter tastes?

Olfactory

Can the person distinguish foods by their odors?

Does the person report nonexistent odors, such as smoke when nothing is burning?

Tactile

Does the person discriminate between dull and sharp?

Does the person perceive heat, cold, and pain?

Does the person perceive unusual sensations such as pins and needles?

Kinesthetic

Is the person aware of the position of the parts of his or her body?

Visceral

Does the person report unusual internal sensations, such as pain or pressure?

Nursing Diagnoses

Nursing diagnoses for patients with sensory-perceptual alterations may be specifically stated as sensory deprivation (input deficit), sensory overload (input excess), and sensory deficit. Isolation is the major cause of sensory deprivation, and a highly complex environment is the major cause of sensory overload. Sensory deficit has many causes. These sensory conditions are highly complex. To complete a nursing diagnosis, the nurse must find the specific contributing factor. Examples of nursing diagnoses associated with sensory disturbances are:

1. Actual or potential sensory-perceptual overload related to:
- **a.** 24-hour intensive care in the coronary care unit
- **b.** Removal of eye patches

2. Actual or potential sensory-perceptual deprivation related to:
- **a.** Isolation for protective asepsis
- **b.** Isolation because of inability to communicate in language other than Hungarian

3. Actual or potential sensory deficit related to:
- **a.** Administration of narcotics
- **b.** Brain tumor

Planning and Intervention for Optimum Sensory Function

The overall nursing goal is to promote optimal sensory stimulation. Subgoals for sensory-perceptual overload include:

1. Reduce environmental stimuli.
2. Establish an appropriate rest-sleep pattern for the patient.
3. Prevent excessive fatigue.

Subgoals for sensory-perceptual deprivation include:

1. Increase environmental stimuli.
2. Provide diversional activities.

Subgoals for sensory deficit include:

1. Protect the patient from accident or injury.
2. Teach the patient compensatory skills.
3. Prevent sensory deprivation.

Nursing intervention in this area has two functions: preventing sensory disturbances and managing existing sensory disturbances. Prevention includes educating others about sensory needs and implementing preventive measures for those susceptible to sensory disturbances.

During Growth and Development

Children require tactile, auditory, and visual stimulation. Nurses need to teach parents the importance of these stimuli. When infants and children are hospitalized, these needs are met largely by nurses, although in some settings volunteers play with children. Some agencies have playrooms where a play therapist helps meet children's play and stimulation needs.

The following provide stimulation:

1. Holding, talking to, and playing with infants who are not asleep, rather than leaving them alone in cribs
2. Placing bright objects of varied design near infants' cribs and giving children stimulating toys of different textures, sizes, and colors
3. Changing infants' environments by taking them for walks or scheduling play in a variety of settings
4. Providing music and auditory stimuli at suitable intervals
5. Providing foods with a variety of tastes, textures, and colors

Constant sensory stimulation without adequate sleep and rest periods can result in sensory overload. A child needs to rest in a quiet, dark, odor-free room. Sensory stimulation needs do not end when the infant or child is hospitalized or confined to bed at home.

Sensory-Perceptual Overload

When a patient is overstimulated, the nurse can counteract sensory overload by blocking stimuli, helping the patient organize the stimuli, and helping the patient alter responses to the stimuli.

Blocking stimuli

There are many ways of blocking stimuli. Dark glasses can partially block light rays and a sun screen or a drape over a window can reduce visual stimulation. Ear plugs reduce auditory stimuli, as do soft background music and earphones. Odors, too, can contribute to sensory overload. Odors from a draining wound are an unpleasant, constant stimulus. The odor can often be minimized by keeping the dressing dry and clean and applying a liquid deodorant on a gauze near the wound.

Another method of reducing sensory overload is to establish daily routines that reduce novelty and surprise. These routines should provide long rest intervals free of interruptions. Sometimes the number of visitors and the length of visits must be restricted. A nurse can organize care so that the patient has long periods of little stimulation. If the nurse carries out several nursing measures together, the patient can have a scheduled quiet period before the next activity.

Organizing stimuli

If the nurse explains the sounds in the environment, the patient can organize them mentally: A bell signals a change of shift; a buzzer, a change of IV. When patients understand their meaning, stimuli are frequently less confusing and more easily ignored.

Altering responses

Patients can learn to alter their responses to stimuli. Patients can employ relaxation techniques to reduce anxiety and stress despite continual sensory stimulation.

Sensory-Perceptual Deprivation

The nurse needs to determine the reasons for sensory deprivation before planning nursing intervention. Deprivation is usually due to inadequate stimuli, inability to receive stimuli, or inability to process stimuli.

Inadequate stimuli can mean insufficient stimuli. Stimuli are also inadequate when they are monotonous, infrequent, or too weak. A patient confined to bed in a private room without television or radio and receiving visitors only once a week is inadequately stimulated. After a month, this patient may experience sensory deprivation. The nurse could anticipate and prevent deprivation by arranging for visits from other patients or personnel, a radio or television, a variety of foods for meals, and books and magazines.

Acute sensory deprivation indicates a need for more interaction with nursing staff and health personnel as well as other stimuli such as television. When the patient is hallucinating, the nurse must first acknowledge the emotional component of the patient's experience: "I recognize that you are afraid." The nurse might then explain that there is nothing present to cause the fear: "There is only a clothes hamper in the corner, not an animal."

The understimulated patient usually benefits from being touched by nurses and others. The elderly patient, in particular, might suffer from touch deprivation. Most patients are reassured by this gesture of warmth, but some people dislike being touched. The nurse needs to observe each patient's tolerance of being touched.

Many hospitals for adults, particularly in long-term care facilities, have libraries and occupational or recreational facilities that provide stimulation for the inactive or underactive patient.

Sensory Deficits

Nursing intervention for patients with sensory deficits includes protecting the patient, helping the patient develop compensatory skills, and preventing sensory deprivation.

Impaired vision

The following nursing interventions may help patients with impaired vision:

1. Arrange suitable lighting including night lights for the patient.
2. Encourage the patient to have his or her eyes examined.
3. Obtain books with large printing and "reading tapes"—recorded books—for the patient.
4. Arrange furniture and other objects so that the patient will not trip and then explain the location of objects.
5. Provide written instructions in print large enough for the patient to read.
6. Leave bedside articles as the patient arranges them or explain if they must be moved.
7. Support the patient in any decision that gives mobility and independence, e.g., using a white cane or acquiring a seeing-eye dog.
8. Encourage the patient to develop other senses. For example, provide objects that are pleasant to touch. Many people obtain great joy from holding and stroking a pet.

Impaired hearing

Patients may or may not tell others when their hearing begins to fail. The loss may not always be evident, but the patient begins to feel isolated as he or she has difficulty conversing, using the telephone, and listening to television. As a result, the person with impaired hearing can withdraw and become depressed. Significant others should be involved in planning for the patient.

The following interventions are appropriate:

1. Obtain the patient's attention before speaking.
2. Speak distinctly while facing the patient.
3. Assume a position so that the person can see your face clearly, i.e., do not stand against the light or far away.
4. Rephrase your message if the patient does not understand it the first time.
5. Encourage the patient to have hearing tests and to obtain a hearing aid if one will be helpful.
6. Keep conversational groups small; the hearing-impaired find it difficult to follow conversation in large groups.

Decreased gustatory or olfactory senses

The following measures may assist patients with gustatory or olfactory impairment:

1. Serve hot food hot and cold food cold.
2. Serve well-seasoned, not bland, foods.
3. Serve meals that offer a variety of smells, tastes, and textures.

Altered Level of Consciousness

Nursing intervention for the patient with altered level of consciousness has four main objectives:

1. To provide emotional support to the patient and support persons
2. To alleviate the underlying injury or pathology
3. To provide a safe environment and otherwise ensure the patient's safety
4. To provide assistance with daily activities the patient cannot accomplish alone

Emotional support

Altered levels of consciousness can be frightening to both patients and their support persons. Often patients know that something is wrong and that they need help. The following interventions may help patients and support persons:

1. Reorient the confused patient to self, time, and place.
2. Listen carefully to the patient's and support persons' concerns. Often they simply want to express them.
3. Maintain the same schedule each day. Routine gives the patient a sense of security and sometimes decreases confusion.
4. Touch and stroke the unconscious patient.
5. Explain what is happening to the support persons and encourage them to talk to and touch the patient as if he or she were conscious. This auditory and tactile stimulation supports the patient and may restore some degree of consciousness.

Underlying pathology

Nursing intervention should facilitate the physician's diagnosis and treatment of the underlying disorder. Diagnostic tests, preparation for tests, etc., are discussed in Chapter 38.

Safety

The patient whose level of consciousness is altered needs protection. Side rails to prevent falls, restraints, appropriate positioning in bed, appropriate lighting, and reduced noise level are all common safety measures.

Activities of daily living

The patient whose level of consciousness is altered may need assistance with activities of daily living. If the patient is unconscious, necessary nursing interventions include bathing, giving skin care, feeding, and meeting elimination needs. If the patient is disoriented but conscious, the nurse may need to give instructions on how to perform these activities. Unless the patient is totally incapacitated, it is preferable to foster independence and feelings of self-worth by helping the patient care for himself or herself than to give complete care to a passive patient.

Evaluation

The outcome criteria for patients who have actual or potential sensory problems depend on the nursing diagnoses. Some suggested criteria are:

Sensory-perceptual overload

1. Slept for 6 hours without awakening
2. Indicates feelings of well-being and reacts less irritably

Sensory-perceptual deprivation

1. Knew day of the month, year, and place when questioned
2. Expressed interest in watching television

Sensory deficit

1. Read for 1 hour using new glasses
2. Communicated while using new hearing aid

Summary

Awareness is the ability to perceive environmental stimuli and body reactions and to respond appropriately. The need for sensory stimulation is sensoristasis. Perception requires constant and varied sensory stimuli. Stimuli can be visual, auditory, olfactory, tactile, gustatory, kinesthetic, and visceral. The major sensory disturbances are sensory deprivation, sensory overload, and sensory deficit. Sensory deprivation is a level of stimulation too low to allow normal functioning. Sensory overload is more sensory stimulation than one can tolerate. Sensory deficit is an impairment in the functioning of the sensory or perceptual processes. Sensory deficit can contribute to both deprivation and overload.

Certain patients, such as those on protective asepsis or those with a sensory deficit, are susceptible to sensory disturbances. Assessing sensory disturbance is a function of nurses. Patients who seem bored or who daydream or sleep excessively may have sensory deprivation. Sensory overload can produce in patients some of the symptoms of sensory deprivation. In addition, the patient may appear agitated and restless. Sensory deficit can be assessed systematically.

The goal of nursing intervention is to promote optimal sensory stimulation. The nurse must consider not only developmental stimulation needs but also needs arising from sensory-perceptual overload, sensory-perceptual deprivation, and sensory deficit. Patients whose level of consciousness is altered also need nursing intervention.

Suggested Activities

1. In a laboratory setting, plan to provide a meal to a blindfolded classmate. Provide food on a tray. Interview the classmate and find out how he or she felt during the exercise. What other stimuli assumed importance?

2. Visit a long-term care facility. Interview a patient and assess for symptoms of sensory disturbances. What activities does the agency offer to provide stimulation?

Suggested Readings

Bolin, R. H. 1974. Sensory deprivation: An overview. *Nursing Forum* 13(3):240–58.
The author provides a theoretical framework for concepts of sensory deprivation. Also included are an overview of clinical records of deprivation and the nursing implications.

Brozian, M. W., and Clark, H. M. March 1980. Counteracting sensory changes in the aging. *American Journal of Nursing* 80:473–76.
Aging causes changes in hearing; vision and depth perception; position sense; and response to temperature, smell, taste, light touch, vibration, and deep pressure. Nursing measures can help patients adjust to these changes.

Lindenmuth, J. E.; Breu, C. S.; and Malooley, J. A. August 1980. Sensory overload. *American Journal of Nursing* 80:1456–58.
This study of sensory overload in a coronary care unit found the three major patient problems were potential for disorientation, potential for physical discomfort, and loss of privacy. Nursing interventions for each of these patient problems are given.

Selected References

Amacher, N. J. May 1973. Touch is a way of caring and a way of communicating with an aphasic patient. *American Journal of Nursing* 73:852–54.

Brown, J., and Hepler, R. April 1976. Stimulation—a corollary to physical care. *American Journal of Nursing* 76:578–81.

Burnside, I. M. December 1973. Touching is talking. *American Journal of Nursing* 73:2060–63.

Cameron, C. F., et al. November 1972. When sensory deprivation occurs. *The Canadian Nurse* 68:32–34.

Chodil, J., and Williams, B. 1970. The concept of sensory deprivation. *Nursing Clinics of North America* 5(3):544–48.

Cohen, S. October 1981. Programmed instruction: Sensory changes in the elderly. *American Journal of Nursing* 81:1851–80.

Crandall, R. C. 1980. *Gerontology: A behavioral science approach.* Reading, Mass.: Addison-Wesley Publishing Co.

DeForest, J., and Porter, A. July-August 1981. Cuddlers: A volunteer infant stimulation program. *Canadian Nurse* 77:38–40.

Downs, F. S. March 1974. Bed rest and sensory disturbances. *American Journal of Nursing* 74:434–38.

Gordon, M. 1982. *Manual of nursing diagnosis.* New York: McGraw-Hill Book Co.

Heron, W. 1971. The pathology of boredom. In *Readings from Scientific American: Physiological psychology.* San Francisco: W. H. Freeman and Co.

Kim, M. J., and Moritz, D. A., editors. 1982. *Classification of nursing diagnoses: Proceedings of the third and fourth national conferences.* New York: McGraw-Hill Book Co.

Krieger, D. May 1975. Therapeutic touch: The imprimatur of nursing. *American Journal of Nursing* 75:784–87.

Krieger, D.; Peper, E.; and Ancoli, S. April 1979. Therapeutic touch: Searching for evidence of physiological change. *American Journal of Nursing* 79:660–62.

Ladyshewsky, A. October 1980. Increased intracranial pressure: When assessment counts. *The Canadian Nurse* 76:34.

McCorkie, R. March-April 1974. Effects of touch on seriously ill patients. *Nursing Research* 23:125–32.

Macrae, J. April 1979. Therapeutic touch in practice. *American Journal of Nursing* 79:664–65.

Mitchell, P. H., and Loustau, A. 1981. *Concepts basic to nursing.* 3rd ed. New York: McGraw-Hill Book Co.

Perron, D. M. June 1974. Deprived of sound. *American Journal of Nursing* 74:1057–59.

Smith, M. J. March-April 1975. Changes in judgment of duration with different patterns of auditory information for individuals confined to bed. *Nursing Research* 24:93–98.

Thomson, L. R. February 1973. Sensory deprivation: A personal experience. *American Journal of Nursing* 73:266–68.

Watson, C. A., and Wyatt, N. N. 1981. Altered levels of awareness. In Hart, L. K.; Reese, J. L.; and Fearing, M. O.; editors. *Concepts common to acute illness: Identification and management.* St. Louis: C. V. Mosby Co.

Wolanin, M. O., and Phillips, L. R. F. 1981. *Confusion: prevention and care.* St. Louis: C. V. Mosby Co.

Chapter 36

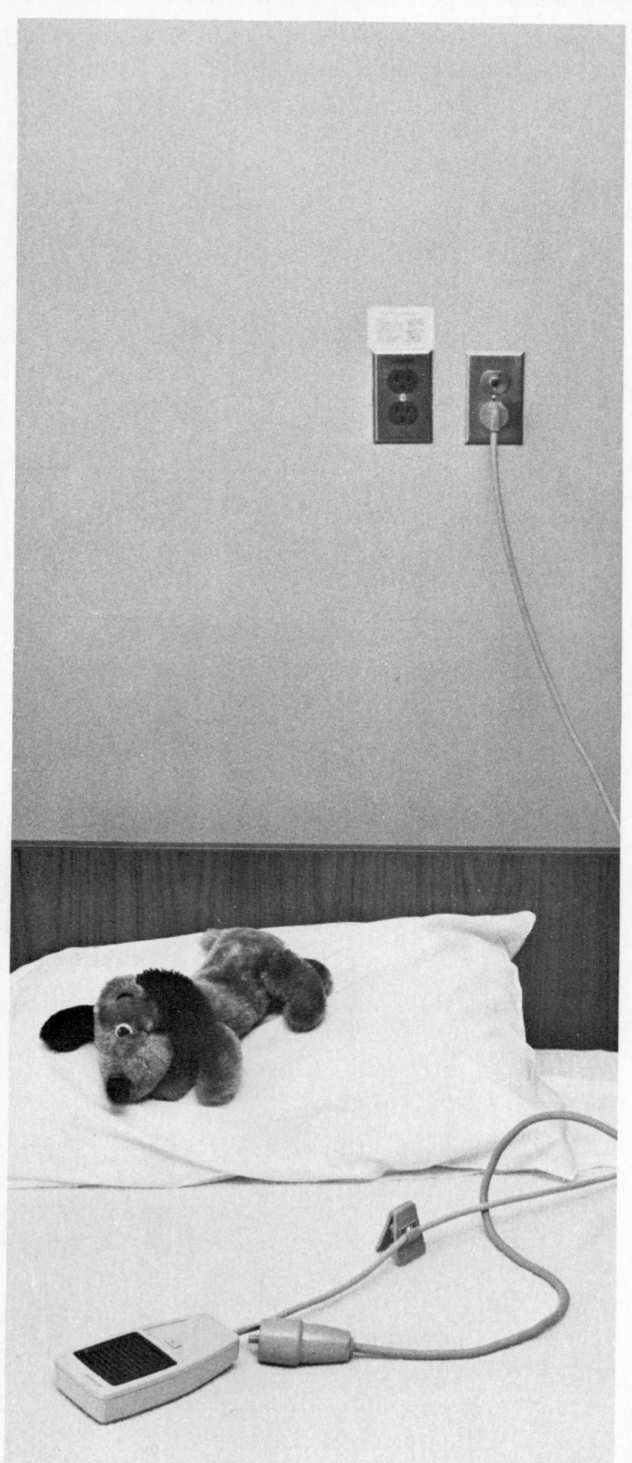

Accepting Loss and Death

CONTENTS

Objectives

1. Know essential facts about loss, grief, dying, and death
- **1.1** Define selected terms
- **1.2** Identify types of loss
- **1.3** Identify characteristics of grief
- **1.4** Identify Engel's and Shulz's stages of grieving
- **1.5** Identify Kübler-Ross's stages of dying
- **1.6** Identify legal implications of death

2. Know information and methods required to assess dying and grieving patients
- **2.1** Identify the dying patient's level of awareness
- **2.2** Identify clinical signs of impending and imminent death
- **2.3** Identify clinical signs of death
- **2.4** Identify clinical symptoms of grief
- **2.5** Identify factors affecting a loss reaction

3. Understand essential facts about nursing diagnoses for patients with problems related to dying and grief
- **3.1** Identify common fears associated with dying
- **3.2** Identify types of grief
- **3.3** Identify factors contributing to unresolved grief

4. Understand facts about nursing measures required to assist people with dying, grief, and care of the body after death
- **4.1** Identify the significance of developing self-awareness about death and dying
- **4.2** Identify essential aspects of helping patients to die with dignity
- **4.3** Identify measures to meet the emotional needs of patients in various stages of dying
- **4.4** Identify physiologic needs of dying patients
- **4.5** Identify special needs of infants, children, and adolescents who are dying
- **4.6** Identify measures that facilitate the grieving process
- **4.7** Identify changes that occur in the body after death
- **4.8** Identify essential nursing measures for care of the body after death

5. Apply the nursing process when providing care to selected patients experiencing loss or dying
- **5.1** Obtain necessary assessment data
- **5.2** Analyze and relate assessment data
- **5.3** Write relevant nursing diagnoses
- **5.4** Write relevant nursing goals
- **5.5** Plan appropriate nursing interventions
- **5.6** Implement appropriate nursing interventions
- **5.7** State outcome criteria essential for evaluating the patient's progress

Terms

active euthanasia
actual loss
algor mortis
anticipatory loss
autopsy (postmortem examination)
bereavement
cerebral death
coroner
euthanasia
grief
inquest
living will
livor mortis
loss
medical examiner
mortician (undertaker)
mourning
passive euthanasia
perceived loss
rigor mortis
shroud

For all people, death is inevitable and a loss. *Loss* is an actual or potential situation in which a valued object, person, etc., is inaccessible or changed so that it is no longer perceived as valuable. All people have some concern about death, and this is often expressed in terms of concern about health.

Other losses that people experience include loss of body image, a significant other, a sense of well-being, a job, personal possessions, beliefs, and a sense of self. Illness can threaten to produce a number of losses. The nurse's function in dealing with loss is to assess the needs of the patient and the family and to provide support to them.

Death is a lonely experience, which everyone ultimately faces alone. Yet even death, like any loss, can stimulate people to grow both in perception of themselves and others and in acceptance of reality.

Types of Loss

There are two general types of loss: actual and perceived. An *actual loss* can be identified by others. It may arise in response to or in anticipation of a situation. For example, a woman whose husband is dying may experience actual loss in anticipation of his death. A *perceived loss* is experienced by one person but cannot be verified by others. Psychologic losses are often perceived losses, in that they are not verifiable directly. For example, a woman who leaves her employment to care for her children at home may perceive a loss of independence and freedom. Like an actual loss, a perceived loss may be anticipatory. An *anticipatory loss* is experienced before the loss really occurs.

There are many sources of loss:

1. Loss of an aspect of oneself—a body part, a physiologic function, or a psychologic attribute
2. Loss of an object external to oneself
3. Loss of a loved or valued person
4. Separation from an accustomed environment

The loss of an aspect of self changes a person's body image even though the loss may not be obvious to others. A face scarred from a burn is generally obvious to people; loss of part of the stomach or loss of ability to feel emotion may not be as obvious. The degree to which these losses affect a person largely depends on the integrity of the person's body image (part of self-concept). Sometimes changes in self-image affect a person in terms of social roles, such as employee or father and husband. Any change that is perceived by the person as negative in the way he or she relates to the environment can be considered a loss of self.

Another aspect of loss of self occurs as a result of growth and development. See the discussion of development of the self-concept in Chapter 32. Failure to develop a normal self-concept can occur for many reasons. At each stage of growth lack of essential conditions for development can impair the self-concept. An infant learns to distinguish self from the environment by experience with tactile and auditory stimuli. Parents provide touch by holding, feeding, and bathing the infant; auditory stimuli come from talking and other environmental sounds. The toddler needs to learn about body parts through feeling them and requires an accepting attitude rather than a judgmental one. Schoolchildren need contact and feedback from peers that they are normal. Failure to receive this reassurance can result in formation of a negative or uncertain self-image.

In adulthood losses such as divorce can also have considerable impact on people. A divorce may mean loss of financial security, a home, daily routines, etc. Therefore, even when the divorce was desired, the sense of loss can last for some time following it.

Old age is another time when dramatic changes occur in physical and mental capabilities. Again the self-image is vulnerable, and support and reassurance are important. Old age is when people usually experience many losses: of employment, of usual activities, of independence, of health, of friends, of family, etc.

Loss of external objects includes (a) loss of inanimate objects that have importance to the person, such as the loss of money for a person not able financially to absorb it easily or the burning down of a family's house, and (b) loss of animate objects such as pets that provide love and companionship.

The loss of a loved one or a valued person through illness, separation, or death can be very disturbing. In illness such as brain damage from a viral infection or stroke, a person may undergo personality changes that result in a loss of that person to friends and family.

Separation from an environment and people who provide security can also result in a sense of loss. The 6-year-old who has had the protection of home and family is likely to feel loss when faced with first attending school and relating to more people. The university student who leaves home for the first time to live at school also experiences a sense of loss.

Loss through death is a permanent and complete loss. In primitive societies, death was considered a normal, natural event, and life was seldom prolonged. Grief was greatest for young men who died rather than for women, children, or elderly people. In contemporary North American society, death is considered unacceptable and usually does not occur in public unless there is an accident. It often happens in a hospital or in a home in the presence of immediate family members. There is a tendency to prolong and preserve life. The culture reveres youthfulness; although people expect to live to old age, this is not considered as attractive as youth.

Reaction to Loss: Grieving

Grief is the normal response to loss; it is a subjective emotional response. *Bereavement* is the state of a person who has experienced loss of a significant other through death. *Mourning* is a process through which grief is eventually resolved or altered; it is normally associated with death. Grieving in response to loss is essential for good mental health. It permits the individual to cope with the loss gradually and to accept it as part of reality. Grief is a social process, in that it is best shared and carried out with the assistance of others. Six characteristics of grief have been identified by Burgess and Lazare (1976b:421–22):

1. The bereaved person has a reaction of shock and disbelief.
2. The person feels sadness and emptiness when the lost person is recalled.
3. The person's discomfort is often accompanied by weeping, tightness in the chest, choking, shortness of breath, and sighing.
4. The person is preoccupied with the image of the deceased.
5. The person may experience feelings of guilt early in the grief, thinking, e.g., "Maybe there is something I could have done."
6. The person tends to be irritable and angry.

Sometimes people are unable to experience normal grief. The intensity or duration of their grief is greater than a normal response. Such people can become deeply depressed. On depression, see Chapter 32, page 846.

Stages of Grieving

Engel (1964:94–96) has identified six stages of grieving: shock and disbelief, developing awareness, restitution, resolving the loss, idealization, and outcome. See Table 36–1.

Schulz (1978:143–49) has divided the grief process into three phases: initial, intermediate, and recovery.

Initial Phase

The first phase begins with the loss, e.g., the death, and continues for several weeks. The grieving person reacts with shock and disbelief, perhaps feeling cold, numb, and confused. This usually lasts for several days. It then

Table 36–1 Engel's Stages of Grieving

Stage	Behavioral responses
Shock and disbelief	Refusal to accept loss Stunned feelings Intellectual acceptance but emotional denial
Developing awareness	Reality of loss begins to penetrate consciousness Anger may be directed at hospital, nurses, etc. Crying and self-blame
Restitution	Rituals of mourning, e.g., funeral
Resolving the loss	Attempts to deal with painful void Inability to accept new love object yet to replace lost person May accept more dependent relationship with support person Thinks over and talks about memories of the dead person
Idealization	Produces image of dead person that is almost devoid of undesirable features Represses all negative and hostile feelings toward deceased May feel guilty and remorseful about past inconsiderate or unkind acts to deceased Unconsciously internalizes admired qualities of deceased Reminders of deceased evoke fewer feelings of sadness Reinvests feelings in others
Outcome	Behavior influenced by several factors, such as: importance of lost object as source of support, degree of dependence on relationship, degree of ambivalence toward deceased, number and nature of other relationships, and number and nature of previous grief experiences (which tend to be cumulative)

From G. L. Engel, Grief and grieving, *American Journal of Nursing*, September 1964, 64:93–98.

is replaced with a feeling of overwhelming sorrow, and the individual may experience a conflict between expressing feelings by crying and appearing composed. The bereaved also has to deal with anxiety and fear.

Intermediate Phase

The second phase starts about 3 weeks after the death and extends to about 1 year later. It has three behavior patterns: (a) obsessional behavior, (b) a search for meaning for the death, (c) a search for the deceased. Obsessional behavior often involves repeated thinking about scenes associated with the death: "If only I had been driving," or "If only I had insisted he go to the doctor sooner." In the search for meaning, the bereaved person wants to understand why: "Why did this happen?" or "What did she do to deserve this fate?" The search for the deceased involves carrying out activities previously shared with the deceased person and feeling that he or she is present.

Recovery Phase

After about a year the grieving individual starts the recovery phase. Often the person decides not to dwell in the past and adopts the view that "life must go on." One sign is more active social participation.

Stages of Dying

Kübler-Ross (1969:34–121) describes five stages of dying: denial, anger, bargaining, depression, and acceptance. These stages are similar to Engel's. They are separate emotional states, but they overlap. In the normal process, the first stage is denial and the last is acceptance, but the order of the others varies considerably. The stages may be experienced for loss (e.g., of a body part or attribute) as well as for knowledge of impending death.

Denial

During the first stage, nonacceptance, the person thinks, "This is not happening to me" or "There must be some mistake." At this time the person is not ready to deal with any related problems, such as acquiring a prosthesis after the loss of a leg.

Some people react with artificial cheerfulness and prolong this stage. This is not always healthy, because the person is denying reality and not coping with it. In some instances, if denial continues and inhibits the person's progress, psychiatric counseling may be indicated.

Anger

The anger stage is expressed in many ways. The patient may appear angry at the hospital staff or friends for some reason. In reality the patient's anger is not directed specifically at these people but is general anger that "this has happened to me." The patient's family may also express anger about matters that normally would not bother them. For both patient and family this is a normal reaction and indicates they are responding characteristically to the anticipated loss.

Bargaining

The bargaining stage is learned in childhood. Children are taught that if they are good they will be rewarded: "If you eat your vegetables, you can have your dessert." The dying person seeks to bargain for a different outcome. Patients often say, "I will do anything to change this."

Depression

During the stage of depression the dying person grieves over what has happened and what cannot be. The man who loses an arm may be depressed about changing employment or loss of ability to play games with his children. A woman who has terminal cancer will be depressed about her death and the years of living she will lose. During this stage some people talk freely, but others withdraw and reject other people.

Acceptance

This is the last stage in the response to loss or death. Acceptance gradually develops as the person comes to terms with the changed body image or changed circumstances in life. At this stage it is helpful for the person to talk about personal reactions and to make any plans that are indicated. For the dying person this may necessitate a will; for the woman who has lost a breast it can mean a fitting for her prosthesis and discussion with her husband about his feelings.

Legal Implications of Death

Dying Patients' Wishes

A dying patient often must make many plans for self and family members, including a will, funeral arrangements, organ or body donation, and visits with significant others. It is important for patients to receive support from nurses to carry out the functions they wish.

Some patients have a *living will*—a statement that the patient desires not to be kept alive by artificial means or "heroic measures." Although living wills are not recognized as legal documents in all jurisdictions, they are considered statements of persons' wishes. California recognizes a living will as a legal document provided it was prepared while the patient was in relatively good health and free from any stress that would have impaired judgment. A living will should be discussed with the patient's physician, lawyer, and significant others well ahead of any problem. Family members often need time to accept the implications of a living will.

Some patients express a wish that CPR not be initiated once the heart fails. These patients are often designated "no heroics" or "no code" patients by the physician, meaning that no resuscitation measures are to be taken. For most patients, however, the nurse is expected to initiate CPR and maintain it until the patient recovers or the physician pronounces the patient dead. It is preferable to discuss a patient's "no heroics" request with the physician and family members prior to the illness.

Organ Transplants

Use of organ transplants is increasing. Kidneys, eyes, hearts, and other organs may be transplanted from a dead body (the donor) to a living patient (the recipient). For some transplants to be effective, they must be done within hours of the donor's death.

Some people carry donor cards, usually with their driver's license, indicating their wishes to make organ donations. See Figure 36-1. A nurse who is told of or finds a donor card should notify the physician immediately, so that arrangements can be made for the transplant. Often bereaved relatives and friends obtain considerable comfort from knowing that the patient's wishes are being carried out and that someone will be helped because of the death.

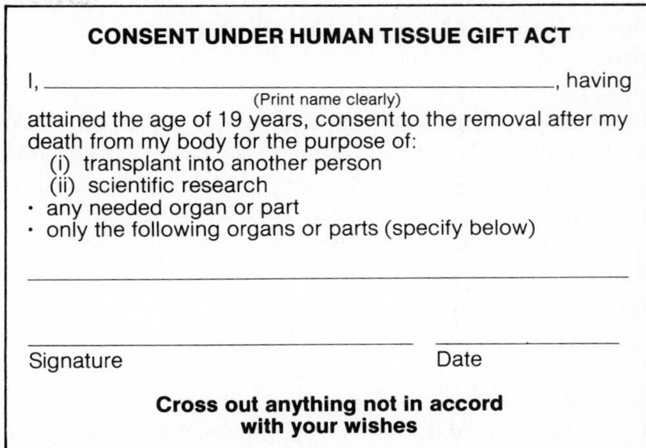

CONSENT UNDER HUMAN TISSUE GIFT ACT

I, ______________________________, having
(Print name clearly)
attained the age of 19 years, consent to the removal after my death from my body for the purpose of:
(i) transplant into another person
(ii) scientific research
· any needed organ or part
· only the following organs or parts (specify below)

____

______________________ ____________
Signature Date

Cross out anything not in accord with your wishes

Figure 36–1 An example of an organ transplant donor card.

Euthanasia

Euthanasia is derived from the Latin *eu* meaning good, and *thanasia* meaning death. It is the act or practice of killing for reasons of mercy. There are two types of euthanasia: passive and active. In *passive euthanasia* a person is allowed to die; measures to maintain life or prevent death are withheld or withdrawn. For example, a terminal cancer patient who is in acute pain and acquires pneumonia may die if the pneumonia is left untreated. Lack of therapy for the pneumonia is passive euthanasia. In *active euthanasia* acts are performed to shorten life. Active euthanasia is carried out by veterinarians when an animal is suffering and cannot be cured. A fast-acting medication that causes death is often administered intravenously. Active euthanasia for humans is a controversial issue. At present it is illegal.

Assessment

Assessing Dying Patients

Patient's level of awareness

People who are dying possess varying degrees of awareness. The amount of awareness of the patient and family is a factor in determining the nurse's role. Three types of awareness that have been described are closed awareness, mutual pretense, and open awareness (Strauss et al. 1970:300).

Closed awareness In closed awareness the patient and family are unaware of impending death. They may not completely understand why the patient is ill, and they believe he or she will recover. The physician may believe it is best not to communicate a diagnosis or prognosis to the patient or family. Nursing personnel are confronted with an ethical problem in this situation, and they have several choices. One course is to provide evasive or incorrect responses to questions, but ultimately the patient and family will know the truth, and at that time they may recognize that information given them earlier was incorrect. See Chapter 3, page 91, for further information.

Mutual pretense During mutual pretense, the patient, family, and health personnel know that the prognosis is terminal. They do not talk about this and make an effort not to raise the subject. Sometimes the patient refrains from discussing death to protect the family from distress. The patient may also sense discomfort on the part of health personnel and therefore not bring up the subject. Mutual pretense permits the patient a degree of privacy and dignity, but it places a heavy burden on the dying person, who then has no one to whom to confide fears.

Open awareness In open awareness, the patient and people around the patient know about the impending death and feel comfortable about discussing it, even though it is difficult. This awareness provides the patient with an opportunity to finalize affairs and even participate in planning funeral arrangements.

Not all people can handle open awareness. For example, a 45-year-old man who knows he is dying may be unable to discuss his forthcoming death without becoming angry with people around him.

Whether to inform dying patients of their terminality is a difficult issue for physicians. Some authorities believe that terminal patients acquire knowledge of their condition even if they are not directly informed. Others believe that many patients remain unaware of their condition until the end. It is difficult, however, to distinguish what a patient knows from what he or she is willing to accept. A study by Cappon (1969) asked groups of healthy nonpatients, physically ill patients, psychiatric patients, and dying patients whether they would like to know if a serious illness were terminal. The majority responded yes; however, of the four groups, the dying patients least desired this information (33% did not want to be told). Cappon concluded that physicians should be cautious and not give more information than the patient wants.

Clinical signs of impending death

Certain physical signs are indicative of impending death, in addition to signs related to the patient's specific pathology:

1. Loss of muscle tone, which results in:
   a. Relaxation of the facial muscles (e.g., the jaw may sag)
   b. Difficulty speaking
   c. Difficulty swallowing and gradual loss of the gag reflex
   d. Decreased activity of the gastrointestinal tract, with subsequent nausea, accumulation of flatus, abdominal distention, and retention of feces, especially if narcotics or tranquilizers are being administered
   e. Possible urinary and rectal incontinence due to decreased sphincter control
   f. Diminished body movement
2. Slowing of the circulation, which results in:
   a. Diminished sensation
   b. Mottling and cyanosis of the extremities
   c. Cold skin, first in the feet and later in the hands, ears, and nose (the patient, however, may feel warm due to elevated temperature)
3. Changes in vital signs:
   a. Decelerated and weaker pulse
   b. Decreased blood pressure
   c. Rapid, shallow, irregular, or abnormally slow respirations; mouth breathing, which leads to dry oral mucous membranes
4. Sensory impairment:
   a. Blurred vision
   b. Impaired taste and smell senses

Various levels of consciousness are seen just before death. Some patients are alert, while others are drowsy, stuporous, or comatose. Hearing is thought to be the last sense lost.

Clinical signs of imminent death

1. Dilated, fixed pupils
2. Inability to move
3. Loss of reflexes
4. Faster, weaker pulse
5. Cheyne-Stokes respirations
6. Noisy breathing, referred to as the *death rattle*, due to collection of mucus in the throat
7. Lowered blood pressure

Eyes may be partly open or closed.

Clinical signs of death

The traditional clinical signs of death were cessation of the apical pulse, respirations, and blood pressure. However, since the advent of artificial means to maintain respirations and blood circulation, identifying death is more difficult. In 1968 the World Medical Assembly adopted the following guidelines for physicians as indications of death:

1. Total lack of response to external stimuli
2. No muscular movement, especially breathing
3. No reflexes
4. Flat encephalogram (Benton 1978:18)

A committee of the Harvard Medical School in 1968 also published criteria indicating death:

1. Unreceptivity and unresponsivity
2. No movement or breathing
3. No reflexes
4. Flat encephalogram (ibid., p. 18)

The Harvard committee stated that, in instances of artificial support, absence of electric currents from the brain (measured by an electroencephalogram) for at least 24 hours is an indication of death. Only a physician can pronounce death, and only after this pronouncement can life support systems be shut off.

Another definition of death is *cerebral death*, which occurs when the higher brain center, the cerebral cortex, is irreversibly destroyed. The patient may still be able to breathe but is irreversibly unconscious. People who support this definition of death believe the cerebral cortex, which holds the capacity for thought, voluntary action, and movement, is the individual (Schulz 1978:92).

Assessing Grieving Patients

Reaction to the loss

The nurse assesses the grieving patient and/or family members following a loss to determine the phase or stage of grieving. The following clinical symptoms of grief are described by Schulz (1978:142–43):

1. Repeated somatic distress
2. Tightness in the chest
3. Choking or shortness of breath
4. Sighing
5. Empty feeling in the abdomen
6. Loss of muscular power
7. Intense subjective distress

The six characteristics of grief noted by Burgess and Lazare (1976b) (see page 915) are also assessed.

Physiologically, the body responds to a loss or anticipated loss with a stress reaction. The nurse can assess the clinical signs of this response (see Chapter 9, page 185).

Factors influencing a loss reaction

Significance of the loss The significance of a loss depends on the perceptions of the individual experiencing the loss. One person may experience a great sense of loss because of a divorce; another may find it only mildly disrupting. A number of factors affect the significance of the loss: the age of the person; the value placed on the lost person, body part, etc.; the degree of change required because of the loss; and the person's beliefs and values.

Expectations can also greatly affect significance. For elderly people who have encountered many losses already (e.g., family, health, independence), a loss such as their own death may not be important; they may be apathetic about it instead of reactive. Some may fear loss of control or becoming a burden more than death (Charmaz 1980:77).

Age Age affects a person's understanding of and reaction to loss. With experience, people increase their understanding and acceptance of life, loss, and death. See Table 36–2 for development of concepts about death.

Culture Culture influences an individual's reaction to loss. How grief is expressed is often determined according to the customs of the culture. It has been suggested that Protestant ethic values—individualism, self-reliance, independence, and hard work—lead to the practice of handling grief with significant others only, not a larger community (Charmaz 1980:284). In the United States and Canada, unless an extended family structure exists, grief is handled by the nuclear family, which, because of its small size, emphasizes self-reliance and independence.

Many Americans appear to have internalized the belief that grief is a private matter to be endured internally. Therefore, feelings tend to be repressed and may remain unidentified. People who have been socialized to "be strong" and "make the best of the situation" may not express deep feelings or personal concerns when they experience a serious loss.

Some cultural groups value social support and the expression of loss. In certain black churches the expression of emotion plays a prominent part. In Hispanic American groups where strong kinship ties are maintained, support and assistance are provided by family members, and the free expression of grief is encouraged.

Table 36–2 Development of the Concept of Death

Age	Beliefs and attitudes
Infancy to 5 years	Does not understand concept of death Believes death is reversible, a temporary departure or sleep
5 to 9 years	Understands death is final Believes personal death can be avoided
9 to 12 years	Understands death is the end of life and inevitable Expresses ideas gathered from parents and other adults about death
12 to 18 years	Fears a lingering death Seldom thinks about death but views it in religious and philosophic terms
18 to 45 years	Has attitude toward death influenced by religious and cultural beliefs
45 to 65 years	Accepts own mortality Encounters death of parents and some peers Experiences death anxiety peaks
65 years and older	Fears prolonged illness Encounters death of family members and peers Sees death as having many meanings, e.g., freedom from pain, reunion with predeceased family members

Spiritual beliefs Spiritual beliefs and practices greatly influence a person's reaction to loss and subsequent behavior. Most religious groups have practices related to dying, and these are often important to the patient and support persons. For additional information, see Chapter 34. To provide support at a time of death it is important for nurses to understand the particular beliefs and practices.

Sex roles The sex roles into which many people are socialized in the United States and Canada also affect their reactions at times of loss. Men are frequently expected to "be strong" and show very little emotion during grief, whereas it is acceptable for women to show grief by crying etc. Often when a wife dies the husband, who is the chief mourner, is expected to repress his own emotions and comfort sons and daughters in their grieving.

Sex roles also affect the significance to patients of body image changes. A man might consider a facial scar to be "macho" but a woman might consider it ugly. Thus, the man would not see it as a loss but the woman would.

Socioeconomic status The socioeconomic status of an individual often affects the support system available at the time of a loss. A pension plan or insurance, for example, can offer a widowed or disabled person choices of ways to deal with a loss: A woman who loses a hand and can no longer do her previous work may be able to pursue vocational reeducation; a man whose wife has died can afford to take a cruise or visit relatives in Europe. Conversely, a person who is confronted by severe loss and economic hardship at the same time may not be able to cope with either.

Nursing Diagnoses

Dying Patients

Many fears are associated with death, and the nurse needs to determine a patient's specific fears. Williams (1976:27) states that, in her experience, dying patients have three levels of fear: fear of pain, of loneliness, and of meaning less. Fear of pain and fear of loneliness are more easily alleviated by the nurse than fear of meaning less.

Schulz (1978:27) outlines the following fears related to a person's own death: pain, body misfunction, humiliation, rejection or abandonment, nonbeing, punishment, interruption of goals, and negative impact on survivors (e.g., psychologic suffering, economic hardship).

Sheehy (1981:27–62) in his discussion about common fears of dying includes fear of pain, loneliness, dependence, the moment of death, and annihilation. Although there is no pain at the moment of death and the transition from life to death seems easy, many people fear this moment. Sheehy believes that fear of the moment of death is the result of the emotional sting and pain experienced during the death of a parent. People remember this previous pain and, therefore, believe that dying is painful. Fear of annihilation or being reduced to nothingness after death and questions about immortality need to be faced. Does immortality rest in what the individual achieved in this life or does the soul survive after death? Whatever a person believes about life after death, both body and mind may be viewed as reentering the universe and becoming part of it in some form of energy.

Grieving Patients

Grief may be anticipatory, actual, or unresolved (dysfunctional). *Anticipatory grief* is experienced in advance of the event. The wife who grieves before her husband dies is anticipating the loss. Because dying often occurs over a long period, this type of grief is frequently encountered by nurses. In terms of other losses, a beauty queen may grieve in advance of an operation that will leave a scar on her body.

People experiencing anticipatory or actual grief may feel guilt, anger, or sorrow. They often have alterations in libido, concentration, and patterns of eating, sleeping, activity, and communication.

Unresolved grief is grief that is extended in length or severity. Persons experiencing unresolved grief manifest the same signs as those with anticipatory or actual grief but, in addition, have difficulty expressing their loss, deny the loss, or grieve beyond the expected time. Burgess and Lazare (1976a:100) refer to this unresolved grief as *pathologic*. They state that the diagnosis of pathologic grief may be inferred from the following data or observations:

1. The patient fails to grieve following the death of a loved one, e.g., a husband does not cry or absents himself from his wife's funeral.
2. The patient becomes recurrently symptomatic on the anniversary of a loss or during holidays (especially Thanksgiving and Christmas).
3. The patient avoids visiting the grave and refuses to participate in religious memorial services of a loved one although these practices are a part of the patient's culture.
4. The patient develops persistent guilt and lowered self-esteem.
5. The patient continues to search for the lost person after a prolonged period. Some patients make the search while in fugue states. Others may wander from town to town or act as if they were expecting the deceased to return. Some may consider suicide to effect the reunion.
6. A relatively minor event triggers symptoms of grief.
7. The patient is unable to discuss the deceased with relative equanimity after a period of time, e.g., the patient's voice cracks and quivers and the eyes become moist.
8. An interview of the patient is characterized by themes of loss.
9. The patient experiences physical symptoms similar to those of the dead person after the normal period of grief.
10. The patient's relationships with friends and relatives worsen following the death.

Many factors contribute to unresolved grief. Some of these are (ibid., pp. 97–100):

1. Ambivalence (intense feelings of love and hate) toward the lost person. The bereaved is often afraid to grieve for fear of discovering unacceptable negative feelings.
2. A perceived need to be brave and in control; fear of losing control in front of others.
3. Endurance of multiple losses, such as the loss of an entire family, which the bereaved finds too overwhelming to contemplate.
4. Extremely high emotional value (overcathexis) invested in the dead person. Failure to grieve in this instance helps the bereaved avoid the reality of the loss.
5. Uncertainty about the loss, for example, when a loved one is "missing in action."
6. Lack of support persons.
7. Subjection to a socially unacceptable loss that cannot be spoken about, e.g., suicide, abortion, or giving a child up for adoption.

Planning and Intervention

Planning

Dying patients

The overall nursing goal for patients who are dying is to assist the patient to a peaceful death. Subgoals include:

1. To provide relief from loneliness, fear, and depression
2. To maintain the patient's sense of security, self-confidence, dignity, and self-worth
3. To maintain hope
4. To help the patient accept his or her losses
5. To provide physical comfort

People facing death need help to face the fact that they will have to depend on others. Some dying patients require only minimal care and can be cared for at home; others need continuous attention and the services of a hospital and its staff. People need help to plan for the period of dependence well in advance of death.

They need to consider what will happen and how and where they would like to die.

Planning also involves the establishment of outcome criteria based on the patient's nursing diagnosis. For examples of outcome criteria, see Evaluation later in this chapter.

Grieving patients

The overall nursing goal for grieving patients is to assist in the effective resolution of the grief. Subgoals include:

1. To assist the patient to verbalize feelings of sorrow, anger, or loss
2. To help the patient verbalize understanding of feelings
3. To support the patient in resuming usual activities
4. To help the patient establish new relationships

Developing Self-Awareness about Death

People in North America are socialized to think of death as the worst occurrence in life. They therefore do their best to avoid thinking or talking about death—especially their own. Death is thought about rarely and almost exclusively in negative terms. Nurses are not immune to such attitudes. They need to take time to analyze their own feelings about death before they can effectively help others with a terminal illness. Nurses who are unconsciously uncomfortable with dying patients tend to impede the patients' attempts to discuss dying and death by:

1. Changing the subject, e.g., "Let's think of something more cheerful," or "You shouldn't say things like that"
2. Offering reassurance, e.g., "You are doing very well"
3. Denying what is happening, e.g., "You don't really mean that" or "You're going to live until you are a hundred"
4. Being fatalistic, e.g., "Everyone dies sooner or later" or "God will take you when He wants you"
5. Blocking discussion, e.g., "I don't think things are really that bad," conveying an attitude that stops further discussion of the subject begun by the patient
6. Being aloof and distant or avoiding the patient
7. "Managing" the patient's care and making the patient feel increasingly dependent and powerless

Many nursing schools and agencies provide special programs to help nurses explore the problems of direct contact with terminally ill patients and around-the-clock responsibility for their care. In such programs nurses learn not only their own attitudes and concerns but also ways to support and comfort each other when they experience feelings of anger and frustration in the grief process following the death of patients to whom they have become attached.

Helping Patients to Die with Dignity

Dignity may be defined as the ability to function as a significant and integrated person (Sheehy 1981:56). True dignity comes from within. Generally dependence on others and loss of control over oneself and interactions with the environment are associated with loss of dignity. When patients are dying they often feel that they have lost control over their lives and life itself. By introducing options that are available to the patient and significant others, nurses can restore and support feelings of control. Some choices patients can make are: the location of care, e.g., hospital, home, or hospice; times of appointments with health professionals; activity schedule; use of health resources; and times of visits from relatives and friends.

In the United States, hospice centers and in Canada palliative care units (PCUs) have been established to provide dying patients with the kind of care that allows them to concentrate on living right until the end—or "dying well." For additional information on hospice care, see Chapter 2, page 62.

Most patients who have been interviewed about dying indicate that they want to be able to manage the events preceding their death so that they can die peacefully. Nurses can help patients to find meaning and completeness and to determine their own physical, psychologic, and social priorities. Dying people often strive for self-fulfillment more than self-preservation and need to find meaning in suffering and continuing to live. Part of the nurse's challenge in helping patients find meaning in their lives is to maintain the patient's will and hope on a day-to-day basis.

Salter (1982:21) believes it is important for nurses and patients to focus not on the end but on three stages of living fully until death:

1. Developing and growing. In this stage the patient can be assisted to paint, sculpt, go to a library, visit an art gallery, etc. An occupational therapist can help patients do what they still can do and what is pleasurable.
2. Lying fallow. In this stage physiotherapy measures, such as breathing exercises and passive exercises, help the patient to relax and enhance self-esteem.
3. Letting go and becoming dependent. In this stage nursing intervention to meet both physical and psychologic needs is usually required.

Meeting Emotional Needs of Dying Patients

Stage of denial

The nurse needs to support the patient's denial, realizing that it serves a protective function and that the patient needs time before facing death. Yet the nurse has to be alert to cues that the phase is ending—for example, questions from the patient about his or her condition or prognosis. A common problem in meeting the patient's needs at this stage is that nurses themselves often feel comfortable not acknowledging that the patient is dying and prolong the stage. It is important, therefore, for nurses to examine their behavior and prevent avoidance of the next phase.

Stage of anger

The nurse is often the target of angry responses from the patient and/or support persons, who then may feel guilty and anxious because of their expressed anger. The nurse needs to help them understand that anger is a normal response to feelings of loss and powerlessness created by the impending death. The nurse may say, for example, "You seem very upset, and you have a right to be. I'd like to talk to you about it, so I can help. People in your situation often feel helpless and frustrated and can't help but get upset." Common unconstructive behaviors by nurses in this stage are withdrawal or retaliation with anger, both of which serve to isolate the patient or family further and increase guilt and anxiety. The nurse should not take such anger personally or label the patient or support persons as ungrateful or uncooperative. It may be helpful to the nurse to realize that anger is often directed at a trusted person with whom the patient feels safe and who will accept the anger and not cease to care. Nurses then can deal with some of the needs underlying the angry reaction. Providing structure and continuity in the patient's care can help to increase the patient's feelings of security. Allowing the patient as much control as possible over his or her life helps to decrease feelings of powerlessness.

Stage of bargaining

Bargaining may go unnoticed by nurses, since it is often done privately. When cues are presented, the nurse needs to listen attentively and encourage the patient to talk. For some patients, bargaining is based on guilt or fear of retribution for past sins, real or imagined. Talking can relieve guilt and irrational fears. In some situations, it may be advisable to refer the patient to a member of the clergy.

Stage of depression

Support persons often have difficulty coping with the stage of depression, since they feel uncomfortable and helpless being with a depressed person. It is often easier for them to avoid the patient or try to cheer the patient up. However, the patient has reason to be sad and must be allowed to express sadness. The nurse can assist depressed patients by being present and by listening when the patient wants to talk. Some patients review past losses, e.g., of money or a job, at this time and need a listening ear and support from the nurse. The most helpful nursing intervention during this phase is to communicate nonverbally, e.g., by sitting quietly and not expecting conversation, or conveying caring by touch. See also Chapter 15, page 375. The nurse needs to help the patient's support persons understand that being with the patient in silence is very important.

Stage of acceptance

During the acceptance phase, which is characterized by feelings of peace, quiet, and calmness, the patient's interest in surroundings and support persons often diminishes. Family and friends, therefore, need help to understand the patient's decreased interest in socializing and the need for short, quiet, uninterrupted visits. Nursing activities are directed toward maintaining the patient's self-worth and ensuring that the patient is not alone. To maintain self-worth, nurses encourage the patient to participate as much as possible in his or her treatment program. They spend time with the patient and convey caring to relieve the patient's feelings of loneliness or fear.

Meeting Physiologic Needs of Dying Patients

Physiologic needs are related to slowing of body processes and homeostatic imbalances. Interventions include personal hygiene measures, pain control, relief of respiratory difficulties, assistance with movement, nutrition, hydration, and elimination, and measures related to sensory changes.

Personal hygiene measures

Cleanliness of the skin, hair, and mouth is essential. Excessive diaphoresis may necessitate frequent baths and linen changes. Some patients wish to wear daytime clothes and should be encouraged to do so if comfortable. Secretions may gather in the eyes and require cleaning of the eyelids with absorbent cotton and saline.

Due to an elevated temperature, the patient's mouth may become dry, requiring mouth care.

Pain control

Many drugs have been used to control the pain associated with terminal illness: morphine, heroin, methadone, alcohol, marijuana, and LSD. In hospitals the most frequently used agents are morphine, methadone, and alcohol. See Chapter 25, page 643. Usually the physician determines the dosage the patient is to receive, but the patient's opinion should be considered; the patient is the one ultimately aware of personal pain tolerance and fluctuations of internal states. Because of decreased blood circulation, analgesics may be administered by intravenous infusion rather than subcutaneously or intramuscularly.

Relief of respiratory difficulty

Respiratory difficulties are likely to alarm support persons as well as the patient. For conscious patients, Fowler's position and throat suctioning are indicated. For unconscious patients, a semiprone position facilitates drainage of mucus from the mouth and throat. Oxygen therapy by cannula or mask may be necessary in some instances.

Movement

When possible, dying patients should be assisted out of bed periodically. Bedridden patients require regular changes of position to prevent decubitus ulcers. With progressive loss of muscle tone, the patient requires increasing support to maintain a comfortable position. Lateral positions are preferable to supine positions so that saliva, which cannot be swallowed, will drain from the mouth.

When patients are positioned in chairs, it is important to elevate the lower extremities to prevent pooling of blood due to reduced circulation.

Nutrition and hydration

Dying patients are often anorexic and nauseated, because of reduced peristalsis and accumulation of flatus. Antiemetics or alcoholic beverages may be given to control nausea and to stimulate appetite. High-calorie high-vitamin diets are indicated. Because of loss of muscle tone, the patient may be dysphagic and require semisolid or liquid foods or even intravenous infusions. To swallow effectively, the gag reflex must be present; the nurse, therefore, assesses the patient's gag reflex as required.

Elimination

Due to loss of muscle tone the patient may develop constipation, incontinence (fecal and urinary), or urinary retention. Laxatives may be necessary to prevent constipation. For skin irritation due to incontinence, a soothing ointment can be applied around the anus and perineum. A bedpan, urinal, or commode should be readily available for incontinent patients, or the nurse should assist or position the patient on the bedpan or urinal at scheduled intervals. Bed linens should be changed as often as necessary. If the patient is incontinent, absorbent pads are used and changed frequently. For urinary retention, catheterization may be necessary; in some cases, an indwelling catheter may be inserted. The environment needs to be kept free of unpleasant odors, using deodorants and adequate ventilation.

Measures related to sensory changes

As death approaches and the patient's vision becomes blurred, many prefer a lightened to a darkened room. The dying patient usually turns his or her head to the light. Although the sense of touch will be diminished, the patient will sense pressure. A dying patient may hear what people are saying after he or she can no longer see or respond. When talking to a dying patient, nurses and visitors need to take care to speak clearly and avoid whispering, since patients tend to become disturbed when unable to hear.

Special Needs of Dying Children

Infants

A dying infant requires comforting and care, as do both the parents. The grief of parents about their infant's death goes beyond comprehension. Often parents internalize their feelings of helplessness and act out these feelings in their social life and marriage (Kavanaugh 1976:44).

Parents can become obsessed with questions about genes, family heritage, and parental inadequacy, such as, "Did I really want the baby?" or "Did he die because I smoked during pregnancy?" Both parents require encouragement in verbalizing these feelings and in finding their own answers. Often parents vent their anger at nurses and the care the infant is receiving. It is important for nurses to accept this anger openly and then assist the parents to see beyond it.

The birth of a handicapped child, an infant who requires intensive care after birth, or a stillborn infant produces a grief reaction. Frequently parents ask themselves, "What have I done to have this happen?" Working through the grief is very important, and nurses can provide support to the parents while they do so. See the description of stages of grieving earlier in this chapter.

Children

Nursing intervention for the dying child needs to include the parents and siblings. Parents are generally exceedingly emotionally involved in the death of a child, more so than in the death of an elderly person.

It is important to listen carefully to a child's questions and to answer them truthfully. To a question such as, "Will I be home for Christmas?" nurses can truthfully answer, "I really don't know, but I hope so." Children may ask questions about death; often simple answers suffice, such as, "It means not living anymore."

Parents of a dying child may have guilt feelings and may need to talk out their feelings to help each other and the child (Northrup 1974:1068). Parents often fear that, as death nears, the child will suffer more. Honest reassurance that the child will not suffer unduly is important.

Part of a young child's fear of death is aloneness, being away from the parents. Parents should be encouraged to spend as much time as possible with their terminally ill child. This calms the child's fears and helps the family work through the tragedy (Williams 1976a:29).

Adolescents

Dying adolescents need to deal not only with the reality of dying but also with developmental tasks of their age. Because hospitalization imposes many restrictions on normal activity, adolescents are apt to feel frustrated and resentful. They need supportive understanding for their behavior. Like children, adolescents require honest answers to their questions, support in their thinking, and encouragement to accept the reality of death.

Helping the Bereaved

The resolution of grief involves three stages:

1. The bereaved person must separate self from the deceased by breaking the bond that holds them together.
2. The bereaved person must readjust to an environment from which the deceased is absent.
3. The bereaved person must form new relationships.

In most situations grief is resolved over time, but the process may take many months. The following measures can facilitate this process (Schulz 1978:157):

1. Encourage the person to express the pain of bereavement by verbalizing the sorrow, sense of loss, and feelings of guilt.
2. Ensure that the bereaved person has support persons.
3. Encourage the grieving person to maintain his or her usual life-style.
4. Encourage professional support from the clergy.
5. Encourage the bereaved person to continue in familiar roles and to accept new ones.
6. Avoid pushing the bereaved person into roles beyond his or her capabilities, since a failure only reinforces feelings of helplessness.
7. Ensure there is an "escape route" available to help the person regain control. An escape route may be a neighbor who says, "Drop by when things get tough," a job, or a tranquilizer or sedative.

Numerous national and local organizations have been created to aid the bereaved: Parents Without Partners, widow-widower clubs, Catholic Widow, women's fellowship groups, and bereavement clinics or programs associated with health care agencies.

Evaluation

Examples of outcome criteria for patients who are dying are:

1. Is free of pain
2. Participates in self-care activities
3. Verbalizes feelings of anger, sorrow, or loss
4. Participates in plans for therapy
5. Maintains open relationships with support persons and staff

Examples of outcome criteria for grieving persons are:

1. Verbalizes feelings of sorrow (or anger or loss)
2. Verbalizes understanding of feelings experienced
3. Has resumed usual activities
4. Has established new relationships

Care of the Body After Death

Body Changes

Rigor mortis

Rigor mortis is the stiffening of a body that occurs about 2 to 4 hours after death. It results from a lack of adenosine triphosphate (ATP), which is not synthesized because of a lack of glycogen in the body. ATP is necessary for muscle fiber relaxation. Its lack causes the muscles to contract, which in turn immobilizes the joints. Rigor mortis starts in the involuntary muscles (heart, bladder, etc.), then progresses to the head, neck, and trunk, and finally reaches the extremities.

Because the deceased's family members often want to view the body, and it is important that he or she appear natural and comfortable, nurses need to position the body, place dentures in the mouth, and close the eyes and mouth before rigor mortis occurs. Rigor mortis usually leaves the body about 96 hours after death.

Algor mortis

Algor mortis is the gradual decrease of the body's temperature after death. When blood circulation terminates and the hypothalamus ceases to function, the body temperature falls about 1 C (1.8 F) per hour until it reaches room temperature. At the same time, the skin loses its elasticity and can easily be broken when removing dressings and adhesive tape.

Postmortem decomposition

After blood circulation has ceased, the skin becomes discolored, because the red blood cells break down, releasing hemoglobin, which discolors the surrounding tissues. This discoloration, referred to as *livor mortis*, appears in the lowermost or dependent areas of the body, such as the buttocks in a sitting position.

Tissues after death become soft and eventually liquefied by bacterial fermentation. The hotter the temperature, the more rapid the change. Therefore, bodies are often stored in cool places to delay this process. Embalming reverses the process through injection of chemicals into the body to destroy the bacteria (Pennington 1978:847).

Legal Aspects of Death

Death must be certified by a physician. The nurse must accurately record the time of death and the name of the physician certifying it. The law may require that an autopsy take place. An *autopsy* is a postmortem examination of the body. Autopsies must be made when, for example, a person dies (a) within 24 hours of admission to hospital, (b) by suicide, (c) by homicide, or (d) from an unknown cause. In many instances the physician will ask next of kin to give permission for an autopsy even when one is not required by law, because autopsies contribute a great deal to medical knowledge. Specimens of organs are taken for study, and the organs are then incinerated, unless the family wishes them preserved for burial with the deceased. If the deceased is to be viewed following embalming, signs of an autopsy will not be noticeable. If family members have questions about an autopsy, nurses can give answers that may comfort them. Further discussion with the hospital chaplain or their clergyman may also be reassuring.

An *inquest* is a legal inquiry into the cause or manner of a death. When a death is the result of an accident, for example, an inquest will be held about the circumstances of the accident to determine any blame. This inquest is conducted under the jurisdiction of a coroner or medical examiner. A *coroner* is a public official appointed or elected to the position and does not need to be a physician. A *medical examiner* is a physician who usually has advanced education in pathology or forensic medicine. Agencies have policies about who is responsible for reporting deaths to the coroner or medical examiner.

Nursing Intervention

Nursing personnel may be responsible for care of a body after death. If the deceased's family or friends wish to view the body, it is important to make the environment as clean and pleasant as possible and to make the body appear natural and comfortable. All equipment and supplies should be removed from the bedside. Some agencies require that all tubes in the body be clamped and remain in place; in other agencies, tubes may be cut to within 2.5 cm (1 in) of the skin and taped in place. Soiled linen is removed so that the room is free from odors.

The body is normally placed in a supine position with the arms either at the sides, palms down, or across the abdomen. The wristband is left on unless it is too tight. One pillow is placed under the head and shoulders to prevent blood from discoloring the face by settling in it. The eyelids are closed and held in place for a few seconds so that they will remain closed. If they will not stay closed, a moistened cotton fluff will hold them in place. Dentures are usually inserted to help give the face a natural appearance. The mouth is then closed; a rolled towel under the chin will hold it closed.

Henry Lantz

Ⓡ hip

Knee chest (cracked pelvis)

Ø edema

Or external rotation

able to straiten

Mobile X Ray

leaves @ 4^{30}

Opal 5pm

ECAS to GGH 5pm 1/2°

Return 9am ī Tyl #3 >

ENTIAL	LTS	ABSOLUTE VALUES	2.00-7.00 $x10^3/cM$	2.00-7.00 $x10^3/cM$	0.00-1.00 $x10^3/cM$	1.10-4.00 $x10^3/cM$	0.20-0.80 $x10^3/cM$	0.0 x1

```
7-Jun-90  7:02 AM
Total reports:      1
Stats:              0
Originals:          1   Batch: 06/07/90  #(
Reprints:           0
Autodial Group:CRYSTAL
```

Soiled areas of the body are washed; however, a complete bath is not necessary, since the body will be washed by the *mortician* (also referred to as an *undertaker*), a person trained in care of the dead. Absorbent pads are placed under the buttocks to take up any feces and urine released because of relaxation of the sphincter muscles. A clean gown is placed on the patient and the hair is brushed and combed. All jewelry is removed, except a wedding band in some instances, which is taped to the finger. The top bed linens are adjusted neatly to cover the patient to the shoulders. Soft lighting and chairs are provided for the family. All the patient's valuables, including clothing, are listed and placed in a safe storage area for the family to take away.

After the body has been viewed by the family, additional identification tags are applied, one to the ankle and one to the wrist if the patient's wrist identification band was not left in place. The body is wrapped in a *shroud*, a large rectangular or square piece of plastic or cotton material used to enclose a body after death. Another identification band is then applied to the outside of the shroud. The body is taken to the morgue for cooling, if arrangements have not been made to have a mortician pick it up from the patient's room. Agencies vary in their policies about transporting bodies. Some close all patients' room doors before transporting a deceased patient through corridors, and service elevators are often used.

Summary

Nurses help patients dealing with four kinds of losses: loss of a body part or attribute, causing a change in self-concept (e.g., through scarring or amputation), loss of a valued external object, loss of a loved or valued person, and separation from an accustomed environment.

Loss through death is a permanent and complete loss. The manner in which death is dealt with depends largely upon the particular society. In North America, death is feared, while health and youth are revered.

Grief is the normal reaction to loss. Engel has identified six stages of grieving: shock and disbelief, developing awareness, restitution, resolving the loss, idealization, and outcome. Schulz divides the grief process into initial, intermediate, and recovery phases.

Kübler-Ross describes five stages of dying: denial, anger, bargaining, depression, and acceptance. Reaction to any loss can also be described in terms of these stages.

For nurses the legal implications of death involve the dying patients' wishes, the need for organ transplants, and the issue of euthanasia.

Nursing assessment related to death involves assessment of the dying person's level of awareness and observation of signs of impending or imminent death and death itself. Assessment of the grieving patient includes the person's reaction to loss and factors influencing the reaction to loss. Nursing diagnoses related to loss and dying include fears associated with death and anticipatory, actual, or unresolved grief.

To help people experiencing loss, nurses first need to analyze their own beliefs and attitudes toward death. Nursing interventions for dying patients are directed toward supporting the patient's level of awareness, helping patients die with dignity, and meeting the patient's emotional and physiologic needs. Nurses help the bereaved through three stages of resolving grief. In addition, nurses have specific responsibilities related to care of the body after death.

Suggested Activities

1. Interview a nurse who has assisted patients and their families during dying. What were identified as the patient's and family's needs? How did the nurse feel about providing this care?

2. Interview patients who have encountered some loss, such as loss of mobility due to a fractured hip. How did the patient perceive this loss? What were the patient's greatest needs?

3. With your instructor and a group of peers, discuss how you feel about giving care to a dying person and to the body after death.

Suggested Readings

Chaney, P. S., editor. 1976. How do you view death? In *Dealing with death and dying*, pp. 135–48. Nursing 77 Skillbook Series. Horsham, Pa.: Intermed Communications.

A set of 70 questions that have no right or wrong answers is provided to help nurses understand more about how they view death. (Responses can be compared with other nurses' responses by reading Chaney (1976a) in Selected References.)

French, J., and Schwartz, D. R. March 1973. Terminal care at home in two cultures. *American Journal of Nursing* 73:502–5.

The terminal care of a Navajo woman in Arizona is contrasted with that of an Italian man in Harlem. Cultural differences are noted, and values are pointed out.

Kavanaugh, R. E. May 1974. Helping patients who are facing death. *Nursing 74* 4:35–42.

This article describes the events and feelings surrounding a terminal illness. The actions of the physician, husband, and wife are revealed.

Mills, G. C. February 1979. Books to help children understand death. *American Journal of Nursing* 79:291–95.

An annotated list of books is recommended to assist children of various age groups understand death.

Rinear, E. E. March 1975. Helping the survivors of expected death. *Nursing 75* 5:60–65.

The ways in which nurses can assist surviving family members are described. Practical steps, such as summoning the family when death appears imminent, are discussed.

Salter, R. March 1982. The art of dying. *Canadian Nurse* 78:20–21.

This article describes the palliative care unit at Montreal's Royal Victoria Hospital and its integrated approach. Three stages of living to the very last are outlined.

Schultz, C. January/February 1980. Grieving children. *Journal of Emergency Nursing* 6:30–36.

This author believes that grief is often more traumatic for a child than for an adult. Too often parents try to shield and protect children from grief when the children need help to share fantasies, fears, and feelings.

Williams, J. C. March 1976. Understanding the feelings of the dying. *Nursing 76* 6:52–56.

This article describes the fears of dying patients and how nurses can assist patients and their families.

Wong, D. L. November/December 1980. Bereavement: The empty-mother syndrome. *American Journal of Maternal-Child Nursing* 5:385–89.

Following the death of a child, a mother must work through the long process of grieving to resolve her loss and feel alive again. This author outlines the process as: shock and disbelief, developing awareness, yearning (pining), estrangement, role seeking, and resolving grief.

Selected References

Benton, R. E. 1978. *Death and dying: Principles and practices in patient care.* New York: D. Van Nostrand Co.

Blake, S. L. 1976. Comforting each other. In *Dealing with death and dying*, pp. 97–105. Nursing 77 Skillbook Series. Horsham, Pa.: Intermed Communications.

Breu, C., and Dracup, K. January 1978. Helping the spouses of critically ill patients. *American Journal of Nursing* 78:50–53.

Brimigion, J. 1976. Living with dying. In *Dealing with Death and Dying*, pp. 91–96. Nursing Skillbook 77 Series. Horsham, Pa.: Intermed Communications.

Brown, I.; Molloy, S.; Burton, S.; and Wood, Y. February 1982. Four nurses talk about dying and death in a long-term care setting. *Canadian Nurse* 78:30–33.

Bunch, B., and Zahra, D. September 1976. Dealing with death: The unlearned role. *American Journal of Nursing* 76:1486–88.

Burgess, A. W., and Lazare, A. 1976a. *Community mental health: Target populations.* Englewood Cliffs, N.J.: Prentice-Hall.

———. 1976b. *Psychiatric nursing in the hospital and the community.* 2nd ed. Englewood Cliffs, N.J.: Prentice-Hall.

Cantor, R. C. 1978. *And a time to live.* New York: Harper and Row.

Cappon, D. February 1970. Attitudes towards death. *Coast Graduate Medicine* 47:257.

Chaney, P. S., editor. 1976a. How do others view death? In *Dealing with death and dying*, pp. 149–83. Nursing 77 Skillbook Series. Horsham, Pa.: Intermed Communications.

———, editor. 1976b. Surviving: Four patients talk. In *Dealing with death and dying*, pp. 111–34. Nursing 77 Skillbook Series. Horsham, Pa.: Intermed Communications.

Charmaz, K. 1980. *The social reality of death.* Reading, Mass.: Addison-Wesley Publishing Co.

Chee, C. M. March/April 1982. A child's right to die. *American Journal of Maternal-Child Nursing* 7:81–84, 88.

Davis, A. J. 1981. *Please see my need.* Charles City, Iowa: Satellite Continuing Education.

Decker, D. J. March 1978. Grief: In the valley of the shadow. *American Journal of Nursing* 78:417–18.

Engel, G. L. September 1964. Grief and grieving. *American Journal of Nursing* 64:93–98. Reprinted in Meyers, M. E., editor. 1967. *Nursing fundamentals*, pp. 88–100. Dubuque, Iowa: William C. Brown Co.

Garfield, C. A. 1979. *Stress and survival: The emotional realities of life-threatening illness.* St. Louis: C. V. Mosby Co.

Gordon, M. 1982. *Manual of nursing diagnosis.* New York: McGraw-Hill Book Co.

Gray, V. R. 1976a. Some physiological needs. In *Dealing with death and dying*, pp. 15–20. Nursing 77 Skillbook Series. Horsham, Pa.: Intermed Communications.

———. 1976b. The psychological response. In *Dealing with death and dying*, pp. 21–26. Nursing 77 Skillbook Series. Horsham, Pa.: Intermed Communications.

Grove, S. March 1978. Grief: I am a yellow ship. *American Journal of Nursing* 78:414.

Gyulay, J. E. March 1976. Care of the dying child. *Nursing Clinics of North America* 11:95–107.

———. 1977. *The dying child.* New York: McGraw-Hill Book Co.

Hampe, S. O. March-April 1975. Needs of the grieving spouse in a hospital setting. *Nursing Research* 24:113–19.

Kavanaugh, R. E. 1976. Children's special needs. In *Dealing with death and dying*, pp. 33–46. Nursing 77 Skillbook Series. Horsham, Pa.: Intermed Communications.

Kim, M. J., and Moritz, D. A. 1982. *Classification of nursing diagnoses.* New York: McGraw-Hill Book Co.

Klepser, M. J. March 1978. Grief: How long does grief go on? *American Journal of Nursing* 78:420–22.

Kovalesky, A. March 1978. Grief: That night in the neonate nursery. *American Journal of Nursing* 78:414–15.

Kowalsky, E. L. March 1978. Grief: A lost life-style. *American Journal of Nursing* 78:418–20.

Kübler-Ross, E. 1969. *On death and dying.* New York: Macmillan Publishing Co.

———. 1974. *Questions and answers on death and dying.* New York: Macmillan Publishing Co.

———. 1975. *Death: The final stage of growth.* Englewood Cliffs, N.J.: Prentice-Hall.

———. 1978. *To live until we say good-bye.* Englewood Cliffs, N.J.: Prentice-Hall.

LaCasse, C. M. March 1975. A dying adolescent. *American Journal of Nursing* 75:433–34.

LeRoux, R. S. 1977. Communicating with the dying patient. *Nursing Forum* 16(2):145–55.

McIver, V. September 1980. A time to be born. A time to die. *Canadian Nurse* 76:38–41.

McLaughlin, M. F. March 1978. Grief: Who helps the living? *American Journal of Nursing* 78:422–23.

Marks, M. J. B. September 1976. Dealing with death: The grieving patient and family. *American Journal of Nursing* 76:1488–91.

Mittler, J. May 1982. Tell me when you're ready, an open letter to the patient facing death. *Canadian Nurse* 78:20.

Northrup, F. C. June 1974. The dying child. *American Journal of Nursing* 74:1066–68.

Nursing 77. 1976. *Dealing with death and dying.* Nursing 77 Skillbook Series. Horsham, Pa.: Intermed Communications.

Pennington, E. A. May 1978. Postmortem care: More than ritual. *American Journal of Nursing* 78:846–47.

Prattes, O. 1976. Family support in action. In *Dealing with death and dying,* pp. 77–85. Nursing 77 Skillbook Series. Horsham, Pa.: Intermed Communications.

Ramsay, R. W., and Noorbergen, R. 1981. *Living with loss: A dramatic new breakthrough in grief therapy.* New York: William Morrow and Co.

Rinear, E. 1976. Confronting expected death. In *Dealing with death and dying,* pp. 63–72. Nursing 77 Skillbook Series. Horsham, Pa.: Intermed Communications.

Rossman, P. 1977. *A new approach to humane and dignified care for the dying: Hospice.* New York: Fawcett Columbine.

Salter, R. March 1982. The art of dying. *Canadian Nurse* 78:20–21.

Scholler, A. March 1978. Grief: Letter. *American Journal of Nursing* 78:424–25.

Schulz, R. 1978. *The psychology of death, dying and bereavement.* Reading, Mass.: Addison-Wesley Publishing Co.

Sheehy, P. F. 1981. *On dying with dignity.* New York: Pinnacle Books.

Sonstegard, L.; Hansen, N.; Zillman, L.; and Johnston, M. K. September 1976. Dealing with death: The grieving nurse. *American Journal of Nursing* 76:1490–92.

Strauss, A. L., et al. 1970. Awareness of dying. In Schoenberg, B., et al., editors. *Loss and grief.* New York: Columbia University Press.

U.S. Department of Health and Human Services. September 1980. *Coping with cancer: A resource for the health professional.* NIH Publication no. 80-2080. Bethesda, Md.: National Cancer Institute.

Waechter, E. H. June 1971. Children's awareness of fatal illness. *American Journal of Nursing* 71:1168–71.

Williams, J. C. 1976a. Allaying common fears. In *Dealing with death and dying,* pp. 27–32. Nursing 77 Skillbook Series. Horsham, Pa.: Intermed Communications.

———. 1976b. Stages in bereavement. In *Dealing with death and dying,* pp. 73–76. Nursing 77 Skillbook Series. Horsham, Pa.: Intermed Communications.

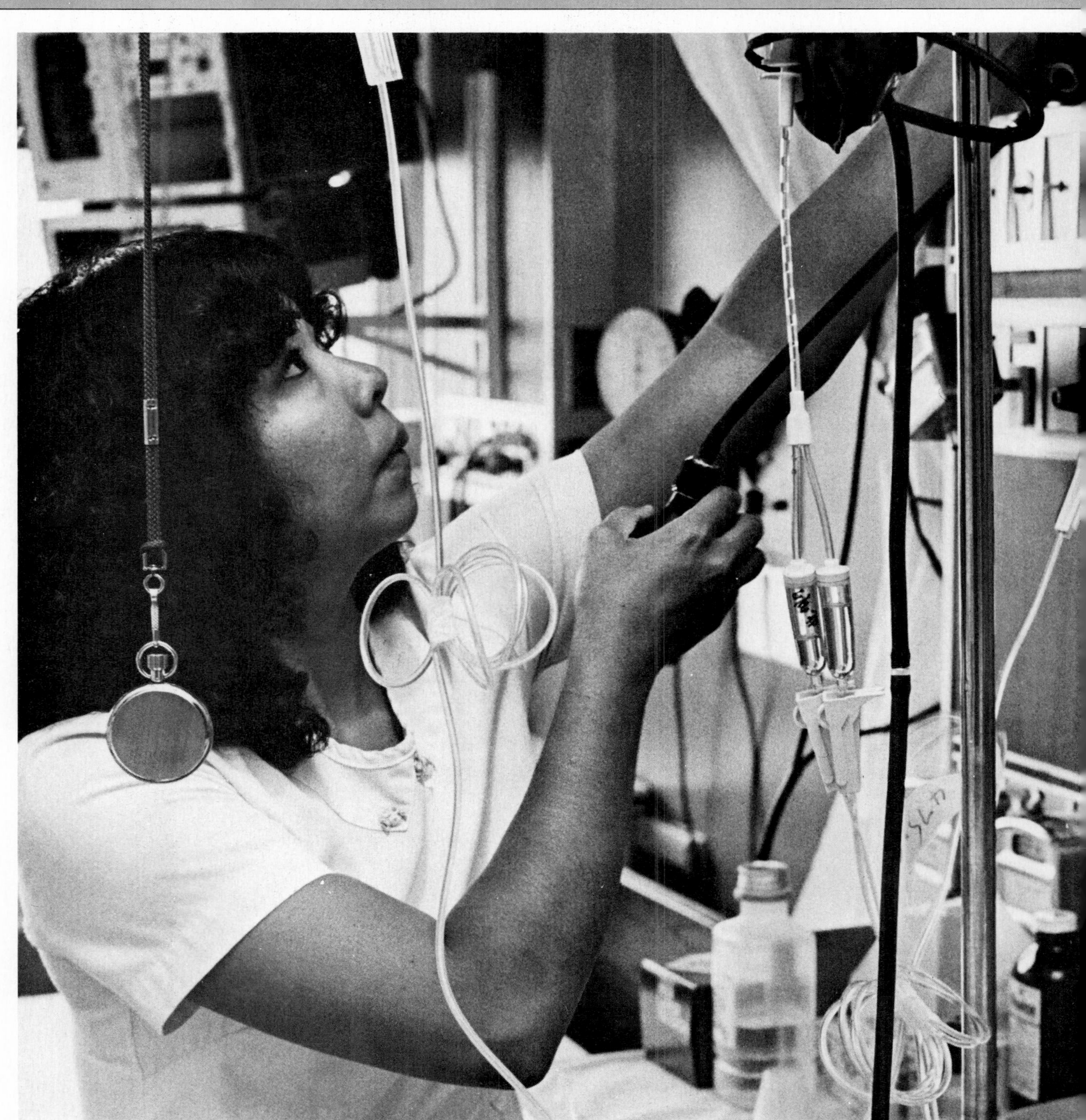

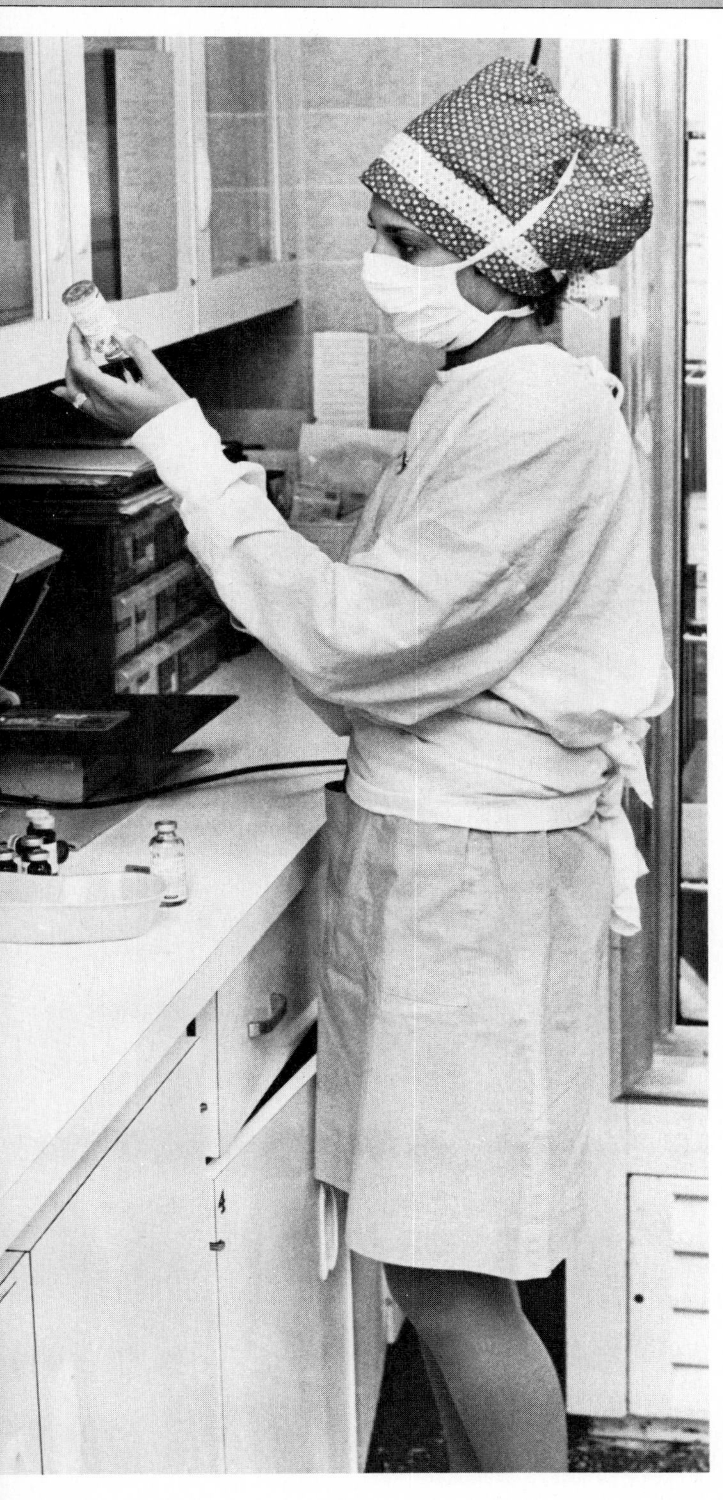

Unit VIII

Special Nursing Measures

CONTENTS

Chapter 37

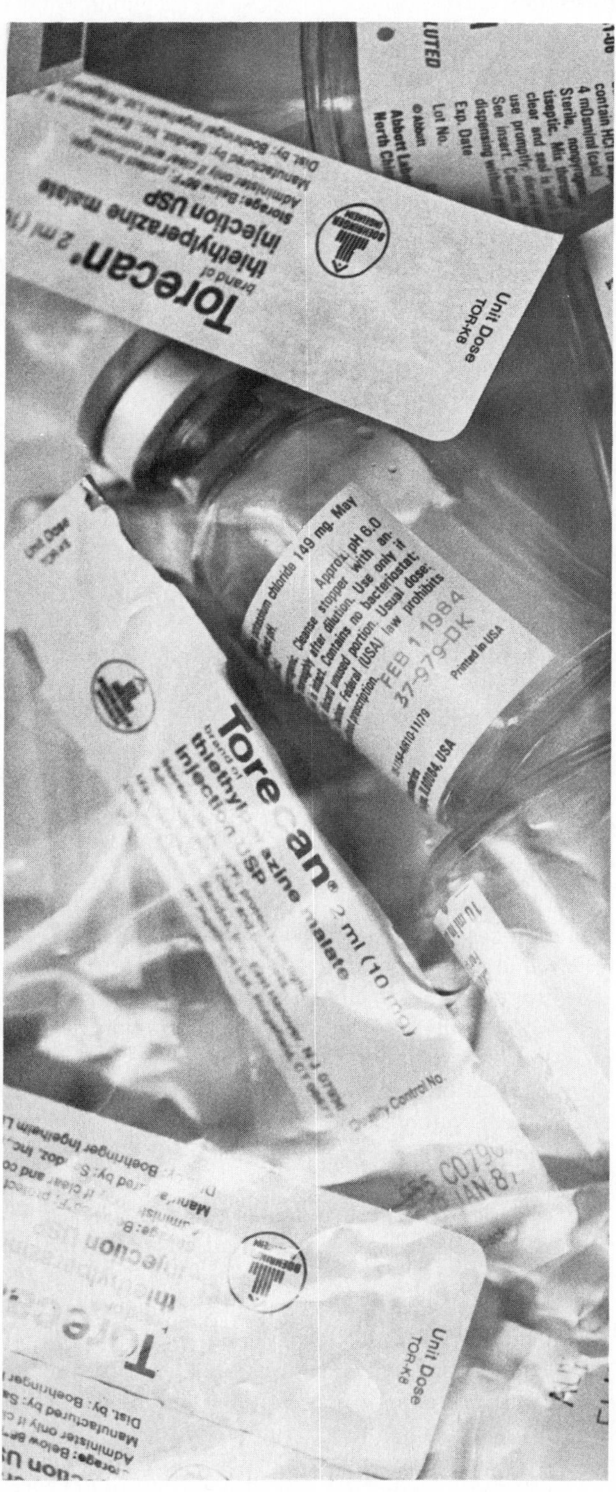

Medications

CONTENTS

(Continued on next page)

Calculating Fractional Dosages
Dosages for Children
Fractional Dosages from Stock Drugs

Assessment
Nursing Medication History
Clinical Signs

Administering Medications
Steps in Administering Medications
Guidelines for Administering Medications

Developmental Considerations in Administering Medications
Infants and Children
Elderly People

Oral Medications

Parenteral Medications
Equipment
Mixing Drugs
Preparing Powdered Drugs
Preparing Insulin

Subcutaneous Injections

Intramuscular Injections
Sites
Intramuscular Variation (Z-Track)

Intradermal Injections

Intravenous Medications

Topical Applications
Dermatologic Medications
Ophthalmic Instillations
Otic Instillations
Nasal Instillations
Vaginal Instillations
Rectal Instillations

Objectives

1. Know essential terms and facts about drugs

- **1.1** Define selected terms
- **1.2** Identify official drug listings
- **1.3** Identify major federal acts controlling drugs in the United States and Canada
- **1.4** Identify legal aspects of administering drugs
- **1.5** Identify drug preparations by type
- **1.6** Identify physiologic factors affecting drug action
- **1.7** Identify individual variables influencing drug action
- **1.8** Identify various adverse effects of drugs
- **1.9** Differentiate between noncompliance, drug misuse, and drug abuse
- **1.10** Identify three types of drug supply systems

2. Understand essential facts about the administration of medications

- **2.1** Identify various routes of drug administration
- **2.2** Identify various types of medication orders
- **2.3** Identify essential parts of a drug order
- **2.4** Identify abbreviations commonly used in medication orders
- **2.5** Identify basic units of weight and volume of the metric, apothecaries', and household systems
- **2.6** Identify approximate equivalents within each system of measurement and among systems
- **2.7** Calculate fractional dosages from stock drugs (tablets and vials or ampules)
- **2.8** Use body surface area and body weight to calculate fractional dosages of medications for infants and children

3. Know essential assessment information pertinent to medications and their administration

- **3.1** Identify essential data to obtain in the nursing history
- **3.2** Identify clinical data required to assess the patient receiving drugs

4. Know essential facts about administering medications by oral, parenteral, and topical routes

- **4.1** Identify five essential steps to follow when administering drugs
- **4.2** Identify essential guidelines for administering medications, including the five "rights"
- **4.3** Identify variations in methods of administering drugs to infants, children, and elderly persons
- **4.4** Identify physiologic changes in elderly persons that alter the effects of drugs
- **4.5** Outline steps required to administer oral medications safely
- **4.6** Identify equipment required for parenteral medications
- **4.7** Identify essential steps in mixing selected drugs from vials and ampules, and in preparing powdered drugs
- **4.8** Identify sites used for subcutaneous, intramuscular, and intradermal injections
- **4.9** Identify essential steps in safely administering a subcutaneous injection, an intramuscular injection, and an intradermal injection
- **4.10** Give reasons for steps in administering medications
- **4.11** Describe the Z-track technique

4.12 Identify essential steps in safely administering topical medications: dermatologic, ophthalmic, otic, nasal, vaginal, and rectal

5. Perform selected medication procedures safely

5.1 Administer oral medications

5.2 Give medications subcutaneously

5.3 Give medications intramuscularly

5.4 Give medications intradermally

5.5 Give an intramuscular injection by the Z-track method

5.6 Apply dermatologic medications

5.7 Instill ophthalmic drops and ointment

5.8 Instill otic drops

5.9 Instill nasal medications

5.10 Instill vaginal suppositories and creams

5.11 Instill rectal suppositories

Terms

ampule
anaphylactic reaction
anodyne
buccal
clinical pharmacist
compliance
cumulative effect (of drug)
dermatologic preparations
drug (medication)
drug abuse
drug allergy
drug dependence
drug habituation
drug interaction
drug misuse
drug tolerance
drug toxicity
emollient
formulary
iatrogenic disease
idiosyncratic effect
immunologic reaction
individual patient supply system
inhalation
instillation
intraarterial
intracardiac
intradermal
intramuscular
intraosseous
intrathecal (intraspinal)
intravenous
inunction
liniment
lotion
meniscus
minim
noncompliance
ointment
parenteral
paste
pharmacist
pharmacology
pharmacopoeia
pharmacy
pharmacy assistant
physiologic dependence
prescription
psychologic dependence
reconstitution
rubefacient
side effect
stock supply
subcutaneous
therapeutic effect
topical
unit dose system
vial

Medications have been known and used since antiquity. Crude drugs such as opium, castor oil, and vinegar were used in ancient times.

Knowledge about these drugs was relatively limited and pragmatic. Over the centuries the number of drugs available has increased greatly, and knowledge about these drugs has become correspondingly more accurate and detailed. It is estimated that some 25,000 drugs and drug products are available in North America today, and new ones are being added daily.

The nurse's role in administering drugs has become increasingly complex. The nurse is not only responsible for administering the correct drug and dosage by the correct route but also is responsible for recognizing incompatibilities when more than one drug is given, being aware of the legal responsibilities of those administering drugs, and being knowledgeable about the many drugs now used. Nurses need knowledge and skill to administer drugs without error. Drug administration is one of the nurse's most important responsibilities.

Drug Standards

Drugs may have plant, mineral, and animal (all natural) sources or they may be synthesized in the laboratory. For example, digitalis and opium are plant derived, iron and sodium chloride are minerals, insulin and vaccines have animal sources, and the sulfonamides and propoxyphene hydrochloride (the analgesic Darvon) are the products of laboratory synthesis. Early drugs were derived from the three natural sources. During the past 40 years, however, more and more drugs have been produced synthetically.

Drugs vary in strength and activity. Drugs that come from plants, for example, vary in strength according to the age of the plant, the variety, the place in which it is grown, and the method by which it is preserved. Drugs must be pure and of uniform strength if drug dosages are to be predictable in their effect. Drug standards have therefore been developed to ensure uniform quality.

In the United States, official drugs are those so designated by the Federal Food, Drug, and Cosmetic Act. These drugs are officially listed in the *United States Pharmacopeia (USP)* and described according to their source, physical and chemical properties, tests for purity and identity, method of storage, assay, category, and normal dosages. A *pharmacopoeia* is a book containing a list of products used in medicine with descriptions of the product, chemical tests for determining identity and purity, and formulas for certain mixtures. Two other publications, the *National Formulary* and the *Homeopathic Pharmacopoeia of the United States*, also list official drugs. In Canada the *British Pharmacopoeia* is used for the same purpose, although some drugs used in Canada conform to the *USP* because they are obtained from the United States.

Under the auspices of the World Health Organization, the *Pharmacopoeia Internationalis (Ph. I.)* is published in Spanish, French, and English. It has improved drug standards throughout the world.

A *formulary* is a collection of formulas and prescriptions. The United States *National Formulary* and the *Canadian Formulary* are published in North America. The *National Formulary* lists drugs and their therapeutic value and can include drugs that may still be used but not listed in the *USP*. The *Canadian Formulary* lists drugs used extensively in Canada but not necessarily listed in the *British Pharmacopoeia*.

Pharmacopoeias and formularies are invaluable reference sources for nurses and nursing students. Nurses not only administer thousands of medications but also are responsible for assessing their effectiveness and recognizing unfavorable reactions to drugs. Since it is impossible to commit to memory all pertinent information about a very large number of drugs, nurses must have a reliable reference readily available.

Significant Vocabulary

A *drug* (medication) is a substance administered to people or animals for the diagnosis, cure, treatment, mitigation (relief), or prevention of disease. In the health care context, the words *drug* and *medication* are generally used interchangeably. Lay people often use the term *drug* for illicitly obtained substances such as heroin, cocaine, or amphetamines. Lay people often refer to medications as medicines.

Pharmacology is the study of the effect of drugs on living organisms. Drugs are prepared by a *pharmacist*, a person licensed to prepare and dispense drugs and to make up prescriptions. A *clinical pharmacist* is a specialist who often guides the physician in prescribing drugs. A *pharmacy assistant* is a member of the health team who in some states administers drugs to patients. *Pharmacy* is the art of preparing, compounding, and dispensing drugs. The word also refers to the place where drugs are prepared and dispensed.

In the United States and Canada, drugs are usually dispensed on the order of physicians and dentists. In some states in the United States, nurse practitioners under a physician's license also prescribe drugs. The written direction for the preparation and administration of a drug is a *prescription*.

Legal Aspects of Drug Administration

The administration of drugs in both the United States and Canada is controlled by law. In the United States the major federal acts controlling drugs are the Food, Drug, and Cosmetic Act and its amendments and the Comprehensive Drug Abuse Prevention and Control Act (Controlled Substances Act). The Food, Drug, and Cosmetic Act was passed in 1938. The act and its amendments require proof of both safety and efficacy before a drug can be sold. The first federal narcotic act was the Harrison Narcotic Act of 1914; it was replaced by the Controlled Substances Act in 1970. This law was enacted to prevent drug abuse and drug dependence, to provide treatment and rehabilitation for drug users and drug dependent people, and to strengthen drug abuse laws. This act makes it illegal to possess a controlled substance without a valid prescription. Controlled substances such as narcotics, amphetamines, barbiturates, and tranquilizers are covered by this act. See Table 37-1 for additional information.

In Canada three federal acts control drugs: the Food and Drugs Act (1953), the Proprietary or Patent Medicine Act (1908) and the Narcotic Control Act (1961). The Food and Drugs Act controls the sale of food, drugs, and cosmetics. It also provides for appropriate labeling including expiration date and recommended single and daily adult dose, directions for use, etc. The Proprietary or Patent Medicine Act protects the public against unsafe or ineffective home remedies (over-the-counter medications). The dosage, efficiency, compatibility, directions for use, and claims of patent medicines such as cough syrups are controlled. The Canadian Narcotic Control Act governs the possession, sale, manufacture, production, and distribution of narcotics. This law applies to all narcotics including cocaine, morphine, opium, and marijuana. The Canadian Mounted Police enforce these laws. See Table 37–2 for additional information.

Nursing legislation also controls the administration of medications by nurses. Nurse practice acts describe legitimate nursing activity. The nurse practice acts of Alaska, Maine, New Mexico, Idaho, New Hampshire, North Carolina, Oregon, Tennessee, Vermont, and Washington include prescription writing as a nursing function, although in some states there must be a supervising physician. In other jurisdictions, prescription writing is the responsibility of the physician. A recent change in some agencies is the administration by nurses with the appropriate order of small volumes of intravenous medications by IV "push" or into IV tubing, a task previously carried out by physicians.

It is important for nurses to know how nursing acts in their areas define and limit their functions; it is equally important for them to recognize the limits of their own knowledge and skill. To function beyond the limits of nursing acts or one's ability is to endanger patients' lives and leave oneself open to malpractice suits.

Under the law, nurses are reponsible for their own actions regardless of whether there is a written order. If a physician writes an incorrect order, for example, Demerol 500 mg instead of Demerol 50 mg, a nurse who administers the written incorrect dosage is responsible for the error. Therefore, nurses should question an order that appears unreasonable or refuse to give the medication until the order is clarified.

Another aspect of nursing practice governed by law is the use of narcotics and barbiturates. In hospitals, narcotics are kept under double lock in a drawer or cupboard. Other medications, including barbiturates, are kept under single lock, although in some places barbiturates are kept with narcotics. Agencies have special forms for recording narcotics. The information required usually includes the name of the patient, date and time of administration, name of the drug, dosage, and signature of the person who prepared and gave the narcotic. The name of the physician who ordered the narcotic may also be part of the record.

Included on the record are narcotics wasted during preparation. In most agencies, narcotic and barbiturate counts are taken at the end of each shift. The count total should tally with the total at the end of the last shift minus the number used. If the totals do not tally, the discrepancy must be reported immediately.

Table 37–1 United States Drug Legislation

Legislation	Content
Food, Drug, and Cosmetic Act (1938)	Implemented by Food and Drug Administration (FDA). Requires that labels be accurate and that all drugs be tested for harmful effects.
Durkham-Humphrey Amendment (1952)	Differentiates clearly between drugs that can be sold with and without a prescription.
Kefauver Harris Amendment (1962)	Makes proof of safety and efficacy of a drug required for approval.
Comprehensive Drug Abuse Prevention and Control Act (1970) (Controlled Substances Act)	Categorizes controlled substances and limits how often a prescription can be filled.

The keys for drug and narcotic cupboards are carried by a nurse on duty. They should never be left in the lock, even if a nurse leaves the cupboard for only a minute.

Narcotics and barbiturates are closely controlled because they are highly addictive. The illegal sale of the opiate heroin receives much publicity. It is more potent than either morphine or codeine. Heroin, however, is

Table 37–2 Canadian Drug Legislation

Legislation	Content
Proprietary or Patent Medicine Act (1908)	Protects the public against unsafe and ineffective over-the-counter drugs.
Canada Food and Drugs Act (1953)	No food, drug, cosmetic, or device can be advertised as a cure for certain specified diseases. Sale of certain drugs is prohibited unless approved by the federal government.
Canadian Narcotic Control Act (1961)	Only authorized people can possess narcotics. Records about narcotics must be kept.

not used in health agencies because of the danger that a patient may become dependent on the drug. Related drugs such as morphine, meperidine hydrochloride (Demerol), hydromorphinone hydrochloride (Dilaudid), and codeine are more frequently used in hospitals and prescribed by physicians.

In the United States, drugs used in clinical areas should be officially listed in the *United States Pharmacopeia (USP)* or the *National Formulary*. Drugs used in Canadian agencies should be listed in the *British Pharmacopoeia*, the *USP*, or the *Canadian Formulary*. In the United States, a new drug must have investigational new drug exemption (IND) before it can be tested on people.

Names, Classifications, and Types of Medications

1. *Names.* One drug can have as many as four kinds of names: its generic name, official name, chemical name, and trademark or brand name. The generic name is given before a drug becomes official. The official name is the name under which it is listed in one of the official publications. The chemical name is the name by which a chemist knows it; this name describes the constituents of the drug precisely. The trademark or brand name is the name given by the drug manufacturer. Because one drug may be manufactured by several companies, it can have several trade names; for example, the drug hydrochlorothiazide (official name) is known by the trade names Esidrix, Diuril, Lexor, and Thiuretic.

2. *Classifications.* Drugs are classified according to their effect, their composition, and their purposes. Most classifications according to effect lack exactness because some drugs act on several systems of the body and may be used for different purposes for different people.

3. *Types of preparations.* Medications are differently prepared. The kind of preparation may determine the method of administration; an elixir, for example, is taken by mouth. It is important to administer the type of preparation specified in the order. See Table 37–3.

Table 37–3 Types of Drug Preparations

Type	Description
Aqueous solution	One or more drugs dissolved in water
Aqueous suspension	One or more drugs whose particles are mixed with but undissolved in a liquid such as water
Capsule	A gelatinous container around a drug in powder, liquid, or oil form
Elixir	A sweetened and aromatic solution of alcohol
Extract	A concentrated form of a drug from vegetables or animals
Fluid extract	An alcoholic solution of a drug from a vegetable source; the most concentrated of all fluid preparations
Liniment	An oily liquid used on the skin
Lotion	A drug in liquid suspension intended for external use
Lozenge (troche)	A flat, round, or oval preparation that dissolves in the mouth and releases a drug
Ointment	A semisolid preparation of one or more drugs
Paste	A preparation like an ointment but thicker and stiffer; it penetrates the skin less than an ointment
Pill	One or more drugs mixed with a cohesive material, in oval, round, or flattened shapes
Powder	A finely ground drug or drugs; some are used internally, others externally
Spirit	A concentrated alcoholic solution of a volatile substance
Suppository	One or several drugs mixed with a firm base such as gelatin and shaped for insertion into the body (rectum, vagina, urethra); the base dissolves gradually at body temperature, releasing the drug
Syrup	An aqueous solution of sugar often used to disguise unpleasant-tasting drugs and to soothe irritated membranes
Tablet	A powdered drug compressed into a hard small disc; some are readily broken along a scored line, others are enteric-coated to prevent them from dissolving in the stomach
Tincture	An alcoholic or hydroalcoholic solution prepared from drugs derived from plants

Actions of Medications

Drugs act on the body by either stimulating or inhibiting the function of certain cells or organisms. Tissues functioning abnormally can be stimulated or inhibited to function at normal levels; if functioning normally, they may be stimulated or inhibited to function at abnormal levels. For example, atropine is frequently given to patients preoperatively to inhibit the normal production of saliva, and epinephrine (Adrenalin) may be given to stimulate the functioning of an inadequate heart muscle and conduction system.

The action of a drug is the chemical interaction between the drug and the body cells. Most drugs are believed to interact with the cell membrane, the cell enzymes, or certain components of the cells. These interactions change the functioning of the cells, thus producing physiologic and biochemical body changes.

Physiologic Factors Affecting Drug Action

For a drug to act effectively, it must be present in the appropriate concentration at the site of the desired drug-cellular interaction. For example, before radioactive iodine can inhibit thyroid function, it must enter the thyroid gland in appropriate concentrations. Thus, if ingested, it needs to be absorbed into the bloodstream and then travel to the thyroid gland. Four factors that affect the action of a drug and hence its effects are (a) absorption of the drug, (b) movement of the drug in the body, (c) metabolism (biotransformation) of the drug, and (d) excretion of the drug metabolites.

Absorption of drugs

Absorption of a drug refers to the movement of the drug from the source of entry into the body to the bloodstream. For example, orally ingested iron is absorbed from the small intestine into the circulating systems. Except for topical drugs, all drugs must enter the bloodstream to be carried to their sites of action.

The rate of absorption is affected by five main factors. First is the route of administration (see the next section). Second is the solubility of the drug; for example, orally administered drugs in a solution are generally more rapidly absorbed than capsules and tablets. Third is the conditions at the site of administration; for example, good blood circulation to the site of an intramuscular injection speeds absorption, whereas poor circulation at the site inhibits it. The pH of the body fluid is the fourth consideration. The pH in the stomach is about 1.0 to 1.4 (acid); thus drugs such as barbiturates, which tend to stay in a nonionized state in the acid medium of the stomach, are more readily absorbed. The nonionized state means that the drug does not dissociate into acidic hydrogen ions (H^+) or basic hydroxyl ions (OH^-). Drugs that are acidic dissociate less in acid mediums such as the stomach, whereas drugs that are basic dissociate less in base mediums such as the small intestine. Drugs, such as morphine, that are slightly basic, therefore, tend to ionize into base ions in the stomach and are more poorly absorbed. In the small intestine the pH is higher, about 6 to 8 (alkaline), and morphine is absorbed more quickly there (Hahn, Barkin, and Oestreich 1982).

Movement of drugs in the body

After it is absorbed, the drug circulates in the blood and lymphatic systems. The drug then moves out of the circulation through cell membranes into certain tissues. Some drugs are restricted to special tissues and body solutions, whereas others, for example, ethyl alcohol, can be found in all fluids of the body. Some drugs are also attracted to certain tissues of the body, where they accumulate; for example, certain drugs have an affinity for body fat or for muscle. These drugs are then released when the blood level of the drug drops.

The movement of drugs to the appropriate tissue depends on the circulation of body fluids. Conditions that affect fluid circulation, such as fluid and electrolyte imbalances and cardiac pathologic conditions, can also affect the action of drugs in the body.

Metabolism

Once a drug circulates to the tissues where it interacts with the cells, it undergoes chemical alterations that convert it into a less active form, which is more easily excreted (biotransformation). These chemical alterations take place chiefly in the liver, although some occur in the blood plasma, the intestinal mucosa, and the kidneys. Most drugs are excreted in their less active forms. An exception is ether, which is excreted unchanged. For this reason, a nurse can usually detect the distinctive odor of ether for some time after it has been administered. Because the liver is the major organ metabolizing drugs, factors that affect liver physiology may also affect drug metabolism. For example, delayed drug metabolism as a result of hepatic diseases can result in a drug buildup in the body, whereas accelerated drug metabolism may cause lower serum levels.

Excretion of metabolites

After a drug is deactivated, its products need to be excreted from the body. The major routes for excretion are the kidneys (urine), the intestines (feces), and the lungs (exhaled air). Once the drug metabolites are formed in the liver, they are excreted from the liver in the bile, which is emptied into the intestine. Some of the products are excreted as feces; others are reabsorbed into the circulation and travel to the kidneys, finally leaving the body in the urine. The lungs excrete volatile substances such as anesthetics.

Variables Influencing Drug Action

Age and weight

Very young and elderly people are often highly responsive to drugs, requiring lower doses. Immature liver and kidney function as well as diminished renal functioning due to aging can both affect the action of a drug. See the section on developmental variables, page 954, later in this chapter. Body weight also directly affects drug action. The greater the body weight, the greater the dosage required.

Sex

Differences in the way men and women respond to drugs are chiefly due to two factors: differences in distribution of fat and water and hormonal differences. Because women usually weigh less than men, equal drug dosages are likely to affect women more than men. Women usually have more fatty pads than men, and men have more body fluid than women. Some drugs may be more soluble in fat, whereas others are more soluble in water. Thus, men absorb some drugs more easily than women and vice versa.

Genetic factors

Individuals may react differently to drugs as a result of genetic factors. A patient may be abnormally sensitive to a drug or may metabolize a drug differently than most people because of genetic influences. Sometimes these reactions are mistaken for allergic reactions.

Psychologic factors

How one feels about a drug and what one believes it can do influence its effect. A traditional example is the reaction of some people to a placebo, a substance (such as normal saline) often given to relieve pain. For some patients, the placebo has the same effect as an analgesic. See Chapter 25, page 643, for further information.

Illness and disease

Illness and disease can affect the action of drugs. For example, a person with chronic severe pain may require large quantities of morphine before feeling relief, yet there is little likelihood the patient will become psychologically dependent on it. The same amount of morphine given to a person who does not have this pain may produce a *psychologic dependence*, emotional reliance on a drug to maintain well-being. See the section on effects of drugs below. Another example is aspirin. Aspirin can reduce the body temperature of a patient with fever but has no effect on the body temperature of a patient without fever. Drug action is altered in patients with circulatory, liver, or kidney dysfunctions. Diabetics need larger doses of insulin than usual if the condition is complicated by fever or infection.

Time of administration

The time of administration of oral medications affects the relative speed with which they act. Orally administered medications are absorbed more quickly if the stomach is empty. Thus, oral medications taken 2 hours before meals act faster than those taken after meals. However, some medications irritate the gastrointestinal tract and need to be given after a meal, when they will be better tolerated. An example is iron (ferrous sulphate).

A patient's sleep-wake rhythm may affect the action of a drug. Circadian variations in urine output and blood circulation, for example, may affect a patient's response to a drug.

Environment

The patient's environment can affect the action of drugs, particularly those used to alter the behavior and mood of a patient. Therefore, nurses assessing the effects of a drug need to consider the drug itself as well as the patient's personality and mileu. An example of a drug that needs to be considered in this context is amitriptyline hydrochloride (Elavil).

The temperature of the environment may also affect drug activity. When environmental temperature is high, the peripheral blood vessels dilate, thus intensifying the action of vasodilators. On the other hand, a cold environment and consequent vasoconstriction inhibit the action of vasodilators but enhance the action of vasoconstrictors.

Effects of Drugs

Therapeutic and side effects

The *therapeutic effect* is the primary effect desired, or the reason a drug is prescribed. *Side effects* are unintended. Side effects are usually predictable and may be harmless or potentially harmful. For example, digitalis increases the strength of myocardial contractions, but it can have the side effect of inducing nausea and vomiting. Some side effects are tolerated for the drug's therapeutic effect; hazardous side effects justify the discontinuation of the drug.

Unexpected effects

Toxicity *Drug toxicity* (deleterious effects of a drug on an organism or tissue) results from overdosage, ingestion of a drug intended for external use, and buildup of the drug in the blood because of impaired metabolism or excretion (cumulative effect). Almost every drug can have toxic effects. Sometimes toxic effects are apparent immediately; sometimes they are not apparent for weeks or months. Fortunately most drug toxicity is avoidable if careful attention is paid to dosage and monitoring for toxicity.

Drug allergy A *drug allergy* is the immunologic reaction to a drug to which a person has already been sensitized. When a patient is first exposed to a foreign substance (antigen), the body may react by producing antibodies. This is called an *immunologic reaction.* See Chapter 9. A patient can react to a drug as to an antigen and thus develop symptoms of an allergic reaction.

Allergic reactions can be either mild or severe. A mild reaction has a variety of symptoms from skin rashes to diarrhea. See Table 37–4. It can occur anytime from a few hours to 2 weeks after the administration of the drug.

Table 37–4 Common Mild Allergic Responses

Symptom	Description/rationale
Skin rash	Either an intraepidermal vesicle rash or a rash typified by an urticarial wheal or macular eruption; rash is usually generalized over the body
Pruritus	Itching of the skin with or without a rash
Angioedema	Edema due to increased permeability of the blood capillaries
Rhinitis	Excessive watery discharge from the nose
Lacrimal tearing	Excessive tearing
Nausea, vomiting	Stimulation of these centers in the brain
Wheezing and dyspnea	Shortness of breath and wheezing upon inhalation and exhalation due to accumulated fluids and edema of the respiratory tissues
Diarrhea	Irritation of the mucosa of the large intestine

A severe allergic reaction usually occurs immediately after the administration of the drug; it is called an *anaphylactic reaction.* This response can be fatal if the symptoms are not noticed immediately and treatment is not obtained promptly. The earliest symptoms are acute shortness of breath, acute hypotension, and tachycardia.

Drug tolerance *Drug tolerance* exists in a person who has unusually low physiologic activity in response to a drug and who requires increases in the dosage to maintain a given therapeutic effect. Drugs that commonly produce tolerance are opiates, barbiturates, ethyl alcohol, and tobacco.

Cumulative effect A *cumulative effect* occurs when a person is unable to metabolize (break down) one dose of the drug before another dose is given. As a result, the amount of the drug builds up in the patient's body unless the dosage is adjusted. This can be to the patient's benefit unless it produces toxic effects.

Idiosyncratic effect *Idiosyncratic effects* are unexpected and individual. Underresponse and overresponse to a drug may be idiosyncratic. Also, the drug may have a completely different effect from the normal one or cause unpredictable and unexplainable symptoms in a particular patient.

Drug interaction A *drug interaction* occurs when administration of one drug before, at the time of, or after another drug, alters the effect of one or both drugs. The effect of one or both drugs may be either increased (potentiating effect) or decreased (inhibiting effect). Drug interactions may be beneficial or harmful. Combination drug therapy exploits beneficial drug interactions. For example, Probenecid, which blocks the excretion of penicillin, is often given with penicillin to increase blood levels of the drug for longer periods (potentiating effect). Two analgesics, such as aspirin and codeine, are often given together because together they provide greater pain relief (additive effect). Other drugs are used in combination to prevent or minimize certain side effects. For example, two diuretics may be administered together because one depletes the body's potassium levels while the other spares potassium.

Some drugs when given together, however, are antagonistic because the combination either exerts an inhibiting effect or increases toxicity. Changes in dosage or timing of one or both drugs can avoid the problem. One incompatible combination is tetracycline and certain antacids (in fact, any substance, such as milk, that is high in calcium). Calcium reduces the absorption of tetracycline, inhibiting its efficacy; thus, tetracycline should be given 1 hour before or 2 hours after products containing calcium. There are many incompatible combinations. The nurse needs to check incompatability charts or ask a clinical pharmacologist about such combinations when any new drug is added to the patient's regimen. Some drugs are incompatible with foods. For example, ampicillin and erythromycin should not be taken with fruit juices, and antihistamines should not be taken with alcohol.

Iatrogenic disease

Iatrogenic disease (disease caused unintentionally by medical therapy) can be due to drug therapy. Five major syndromes can be induced by drug therapy (Hahn et al. 1982:55):

1. Blood dyscrasias from bone marrow depression, resulting in anemia and thrombocytopenia
2. Hepatic toxicity resulting in biliary obstruction or hepatic necrosis
3. Renal damage, especially of the glomerulus
4. Dermatologic effects such as eczema, acne, and psoriasis
5. Malformations of the fetus as a result of drugs taken during pregnancy

Drug Use

Two terms describe how an individual follows the directions of drug therapy. *Compliance* is careful adherence to the prescribed drug therapy. The individual takes the correct drug and dosage at the times prescribed and follows other suggested measures, such as taking milk with the medication. *Noncompliance* is failure to follow the prescribed therapy. There are many reasons for noncompliance, although no reason should be assumed unless explicitly stated by the patient. Some reasons are:

1. Insufficient money to purchase the medications
2. Not understanding the medication order
3. Belief that the medication is not effective
4. Perception of wellness, i.e., lack of symptoms

Noncompliance should be explored with the patient.

Drug Misuse

Drug misuse is the improper use of common medications in ways that lead to acute and chronic toxicity (Rodman and Smith 1979:72). Drug misuse leads to problems such as gastrointestinal bleeding, kidney damage, or liver damage. Both over-the-counter drugs and prescription drugs may be misused. Some people who are stressed or ill take unprescribed medications in the hope of saving time and money or perhaps because they do not want to bother the physician. Self-medication poses the danger of masking symptoms but not treating the cause. As a result, problems can go undetected for prolonged periods.

Laxatives, antacids, vitamins, headache remedies, and cough and cold medications are often self-prescribed and overused. Most people suffer no harmful effects from these drugs, but some people do. A persistent cough may go undiagnosed until the underlying problem is serious and advanced. Persistent use of some of the over-the-counter or prescribed drugs can also damage body parts that were initially healthy. For example, prolonged use of headache remedies containing phenacetin can cause kidney damage and even death.

Drug Abuse

Drug abuse is inappropriate intake of a substance, either continually or periodically. By definition, drug use is abusive when society considers it abusive. For example, the intake of alcohol at work may be considered alcohol abuse, but intake at a social gathering may not. Frequently abused drugs are alcohol, amphetamines, caffeine, tobacco, sedatives, and tranquilizers.

Drug abuse in North America is growing. It has two main facets, drug dependence and habituation. *Drug dependence* is a person's reliance on or need to take a drug or substance. There are two types of dependence: physiologic and psychologic. They may occur separately or together. *Physiologic dependence* is due to biochemical changes in body tissues, especially of the nervous system. These tissues come to require the substance for normal functioning. When the person no longer takes the drug, he or she experiences withdrawal symptoms. Withdrawal symptoms vary with the drug used, the amount used, and the duration of use. The patient taking opiates may manifest elevated mood, relief of anxiety, and pinpoint pupils. On withdrawal, the patient may be restless, feel chilly, yawn, sneeze, and have increased nasal and lacrimal secretions, for example. Sometimes withdrawal is sufficiently severe to cause cardiovascular collapse.

Psychologic dependence is emotional reliance on a

drug to maintain a state of well-being, accompanied by feelings of need or cravings for that drug. There are varying degrees of psychologic dependence, ranging from mild desire to craving and compulsive use of the drug. In severe cases, the dependent person gives up other goals and satisfactions to satisfy his or her dependence. For example, a man highly dependent on tobacco may give up his job and increase a health problem rather than stop smoking.

Drug habituation denotes a mild form of psychologic dependence. The individual develops the habit of taking the substance and feels better after taking it. The habituated individual tends to continue the habit even though it may be injurious to his or her health. However, the average, emotionally stable person can deal with its discontinuance and does not seek out the substance compulsively or manifest other behaviors typical of the psychologically dependent person.

In regard to problems of dependence and substance habituation, nurses have these broad responsibilities:

1. To identify when a patient is becoming dependent and to report this
2. To observe for symptoms of habituation to or dependence on substances and to identify withdrawal symptoms
3. To make available information on drug habituation and to help patients develop healthy habits

Systems of Delivery

Systems to deliver medications to patients vary among health care agencies and with their facilities and equipment, supply systems, and procedural policies and practices. All systems are designed to ensure the safe storage and administration of medications.

Facilities and Equipment

Nursing units have at least one area designated for stocking drugs ready to dispense to patients. Many agencies have specially designed central medications rooms with locked cupboards containing the medications for all patients on the unit. Other agencies have locked wall cupboards near patients' rooms or mobile carts with locked drawers. In all facilities, narcotics are kept in a double-locked drawer, box, or cupboard.

Supply Systems

Procedures for delivering medications are based on three supply systems: the stock supply, the individual patient supply, and the unit dose systems.

In the *stock supply* system, medications are kept on the unit in relatively large quantities, from which individual doses are taken and administered by nursing personnel. For example, individual doses of a certain laxative or antibiotic are taken from a large stock supply bottle. Sedatives and narcotics are commonly provided as stock supply medications on each nursing unit.

In the *individual patient supply* system, the medications for each patient are supplied separately in specified doses and quantities for a specified period of time. For example, 20 250 mg tetracycline capsules are supplied in a separate container or envelope only for Mr. John Brown. This supply is not used for other patients.

The *unit dose* system is increasingly used since pharmacy personnel have begun to participate in administering medications to patients and in evaluating their effects. In this system, pharmacy personnel prepackage and label an individual dose, called the unit dose, for each patient. The unit dose is the ordered amount of medication the patient is to receive at a prescribed hour. Depending on agency practice, the medications are administered by pharmacy personnel or nursing personnel from the pharmacy or on the nursing unit. Many believe that the unit dose system makes error less likely and saves time for nursing personnel.

Policies and Practices

Dispensing medications is the responsibility of pharmacists. The pharmacist may dispense directly to the patient or to a person who will administer the drug. In some agencies, a senior nurse may be delegated the responsibility of dispensing drugs in the absence of a pharmacist, e.g., on the night shift or on a holiday.

In most agencies, graduate nurses are permitted to administer all types of medications (oral, topical, and parenteral), unless the unit dose system is used and pharmacy personnel are delegated this function. Agency practice determines who is permitted to administer intravenous medications; agency practices vary. Licensed vocational nurses are often permitted to administer oral medications only, while registered nurse students who have demonstrated competence are generally allowed to administer all types of medications. It is essential that the nursing student check agency policies and practices governing medications before administering them.

Routes of Administration

Pharmaceutical preparations are generally designed for one or two specific routes of administration. Normally, the route of administration is ordered when the drug is ordered. If a nurse is administering the drug, it is essential that the pharmaceutical preparation be appropriate to the route ordered. For example, phenobarbital is taken orally; phenobarbital sodium may be taken parenterally.

Oral

Most commonly, drugs are administered orally. Oral administration is usually least expensive and most convenient for most patients. It is also a safe method of administration in that the skin is not broken as it is for an injection.

The major disadvantages of oral administration are that the drugs may have an unpleasant taste, irritate the gastric mucosa, be absorbed irregularly from the gastrointestinal tract, be absorbed slowly, and, in some cases, harm the patient's teeth.

Sublingual

A drug may be placed under the tongue (sublingually), where it dissolves. See Figure 37–1. The drug is largely absorbed into the blood vessels on the underside of the tongue in a relatively short time. The medication should not be swallowed. Drugs such as nitroglycerine are commonly given in this manner.

Buccal

Buccal means pertaining to the cheek. In buccal administration, a medication (e.g., a tablet) is held in the mouth against the mucous membranes of the cheek until the drug dissolves. See Figure 37–2. The drug may act locally on the mucous membranes of the mouth or systemically when it is swallowed in the saliva.

Parenteral

Parenteral administration is administration other than through the alimentary tract, i.e., by needle. Some of the more common routes for parenteral administration are:

1. *Subcutaneous* (hypodermic): into the subcutaneous tissue, just below the skin
2. *Intramuscular:* into a muscle
3. *Intradermal:* under the epidermis (into the dermis)
4. *Intravenous:* into a vein

Some of the less commonly used routes for parenteral administration are *intraarterial* (into an artery), *intra-*

Figure 37–1 Sublingual administration of a tablet.

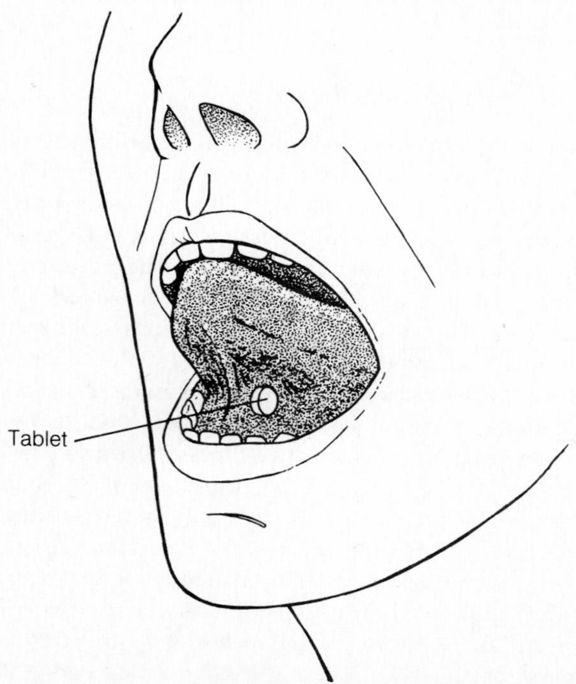

Figure 37–2 Buccal administration of a tablet.

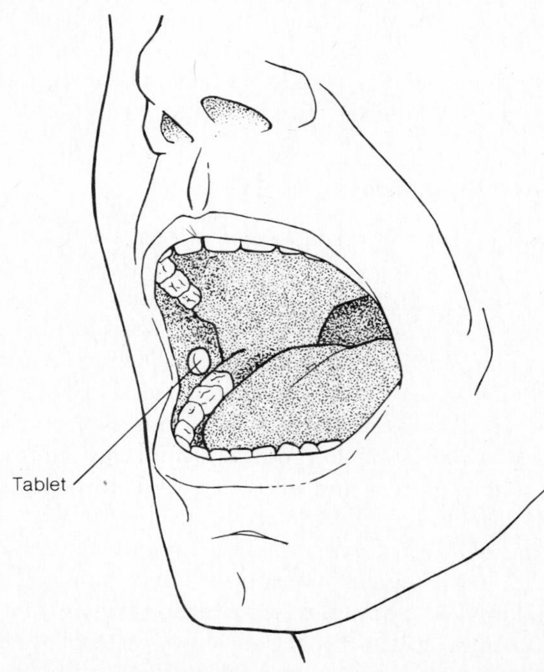

cardiac (into the heart muscle), *intraosseous* (into a bone), and *intrathecal* or *intraspinal* (into the spinal canal). These less common injections are normally carried out by physicians. All parenteral therapy utilizes sterile equipment and sterile drug solutions. Parenteral therapy has the primary advantage of fast absorption of a measured amount of drug.

Topical

Topical applications are those applied to a circumscribed surface area of the body. They affect only the area to which they are applied. Topical applications include:

1. *Dermatologic preparations*, medications applied to the skin.
2. *Instillations*, medications applied into body cavities or orifices such as the urinary bladder, eyes, ears, nose, rectum, or vagina.
3. *Inhalations*, medications administered into the respiratory tract by nebulizers or positive pressure breathing apparatuses. Air, oxygen, and vapor are generally used to carry the drug into the lungs. See Chapter 29.

Medication Orders

A physician is the person who usually determines the patients' medications needs and orders medications, although in some settings nurse practitioners now order some drugs. Usually, the order is written, although telephone and verbal orders are acceptable in a number of agencies. Nursing students need to know the agency policies about medication orders. In some hospitals, for example, only graduate nurses are permitted to accept telephone and verbal orders.

Types of Medication Orders

Four common medication orders are the stat order, the single order, the standing order, and the p.r.n. order.

1. A stat order indicates that the medication is to be given immediately and only once, e.g., Demerol 100 mg IM stat.
2. The single order is for a medication to be given once at a specified time, e.g., Seconal 100 mg h.s. before surgery.
3. The standing order may or may not have a termination date. A standing order may be carried out indefinitely (e.g., multiple vitamins daily) until an order is written to cancel it, or they may be carried out for a specified number of days (e.g., Demerol 100 mg IM q.4h. × 5 days). In some agencies, standing orders are automatically canceled after a specified number of days and must be reordered.
4. A p.r.n. order permits the nurse to give a medication when in her or his judgment the patient requires it, e.g., Amphojel 15 ml p.r.n. The nurse must use good judgment as to when the medication is needed and when it can be safely administered.

Policies about physicians' orders vary considerably from agency to agency. Generally, there is an order as to which medicines are to be given to a patient by nurses and which medications a patient can keep at the hospital bedside to self-administer. Hospitals also have varying policies regarding orders. It is not unusual for a patient's orders to be automatically canceled after surgery or an examination involving an anesthetic. New orders must then be written. This policy is a safety measure to ensure that physicians are aware of their patients' conditions, particularly at critical times. Most agencies also have lists of abbreviations officially accepted for use in the agency. Both nurses and physicians may need to refer to these lists if they have been working in a different agency. These abbreviations can be used on legal documents, such as patients' charts. See Appendix A for commonly used abbreviations.

Drug Order: Essential Parts

The drug order has six essential parts: (a) full name of the patient, (b) date the order is written, (c) name of the drug to be administered, (d) dosage of the drug, (e) method of administration, and (f) signature of the physician or nurse practitioner. In addition, unless it is a standing order, it should state the number of doses or the number of days the drug is to be administered.

Full name of the patient

A patient's full name, that is, the first and last names and middle initials or names, should always be used to avoid confusion between two patients who have the same last names. In some agencies the patient's admission number is put on the order as further identification.

Some hospitals imprint the patient's name and hospital number on all forms. This imprinter is on the nursing unit; it is much like the credit card imprinters used in shops.

Date

Shown on an order are the day, the month, and the year the order was written; some agencies also require that the time of day be written. Writing the time of day on the order can eliminate errors when nursing shifts change. Putting the time of day on the order also makes it clear when certain orders automatically terminate. For example, in some settings, narcotics can be ordered only for 48 hours after surgery. Therefore a drug that is ordered at 1600 hours February 1, 1983 is automatically canceled at 1600 hours February 3, 1983.

Many agencies use the 24-hour clock, which eliminates confusion between morning and afternoon times. Time with the 24-hour clock starts at midnight, which is 0000 hours. See Figure 18–6, page 435.

Name of the drug

The name of the drug ordered must be clearly written. In some settings only generic names are permitted; however, trade names are widely used in hospitals and health agencies. In most settings where drug orders are written, nurses and physicians can refer to the *Physician's Desk Reference*, the *Compendium of Pharmaceuticals and Specialties*, and similar sources. A nurse who is unsure about a drug that is ordered needs to look it up in a suitable reference before preparing or administering the drug. Some hospitals provide their own formulary listing all drugs stocked in the hospital.

In some situations, hospital patients may continue to take medications prescribed before they were admitted. To know what drug the patient is taking, the nurse needs to check the drug label or check with the physician or the pharmacy if the bottle is unlabeled.

Figure 37–3 A sample medication card containing essential information.

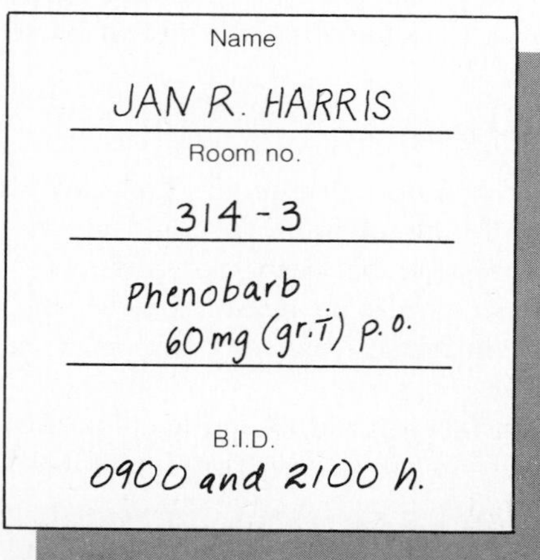

Dosage

The dosage of the drug includes the amount, the times or frequency of administration, and in many instances the strength; for example, tetracycline *250 mg* (amount) *four times a day* (frequency); hydrochloric acid *10%* (strength) *5 ml* (amount) *three times a day with meals* (time and frequency).

Dosages can be written in apothecaries' or metric systems, but the metric system is being used increasingly in North America.

Method of administration

Also included in the order is the method of administering the drug. This part of the order, like other parts, is frequently abbreviated. See Appendix A for abbreviations of routes of administration. It is not unusual for a drug to have several possible routes of administration; therefore, it is important that the route be included in the order. If the nurse believes the patient's condition makes the ordered route of administration inappropriate, the nurse must notify the physician to change the order. Changes in patients' conditions sometimes make it impossible to carry out a standing order. For example, if a patient becomes unconscious, a standing order for an oral medication must be changed.

Signature

The signature of the ordering physician or nurse makes the drug order a legal request. An unsigned order has no validity, and the ordering physician or nurse needs to be notified if his or her order is unsigned.

In agencies where telephone orders are taken, the nurse usually indicates the name of the person who phoned in the order. The nurse signs the order, but usually the person who ordered the drug must also sign at a later date. Some hospitals have policies that those who give orders by telephone must sign those orders within a certain time, for example, 48 hours after they have communicated the order.

Communicating a Medication Order

A drug order is usually written on the patient's chart or in a special book designed for that purpose. From there it is usually transcribed by a nurse or clerk to the Kardex and to a medication card (see Figure 37–3) or to a medication list.

Medication cards vary in form but include the patient's name, room and bed number, name of the drug, dose, times, and method of administration. In some agencies the date that the order was prescribed and the date the order expires are also included, along with the signature of the person transcribing the order. The responsibility for transcribing medication orders is the nurse's; however, it may be delegated to a clerk.

Problems with Orders

Although not usual, problems with medication orders can arise. Generally, the problems are of three types:

1. The nurse is unable to read the directions.
2. The drug or dosage appears unsuitable for the patient.
3. The patient is unable to take or to tolerate the drug.

Nurses must be able to read all orders and understand them completely. If unable to decipher or understand an order, the nurse must ask for clarification before proceeding. Often nurses read the order just after it is written so that they can ask questions immediately rather than spend time later locating the writer.

If in the nurse's judgment a drug seems unsuitable or a dosage not within the usual range, the nurse should ask questions. Such questions are usually welcomed. Often there is no error, and the nurse gains information about the drug therapy. Sometimes an error has been made, and the error can be corrected before the patient is involved. Questions from nurses protect both patients and health personnel from inadvertent error.

A patient may become unable to take an ordered medication because of a change in his or her condition, and it is the nurse's responsibility to notify the physician of this fact. The nurse has a similar responsibility when a patient cannot tolerate a certain drug and the physician does not know about this intolerance.

If a nurse questions an order and is not satisfied with the answer, still believing the order is incorrect, the next step is to notify the nurse in charge of the hospital unit or agency. It is the nurse's responsibility and right to refuse to administer any drug that in the nurse's judgment is unsafe for the patient.

Some agencies post lists of techniques and drugs that nurses and nursing students are not permitted to carry out or administer. For instance, in some agencies heparin can be administered intravenously only by physicians. It is the nurse's right and responsibility to decline to carry out techniques in violation of agency policy. The nurse in this situation should, however, convey this information to the nurse in charge.

Systems of Measurement

Three systems of measurement are used in North America: the metric system, the apothecaries' system, and the household system, which is similar to the apothecaries' system. It would be much simpler for everyone if one system were universally accepted; however, because all systems are in current use, it is necessary for nurses to become familiar with the three systems and to be able to convert from one to the other as it is necessary. In recent years Canada has officially adopted the metric system, and it is being used increasingly in the United States.

Metric System

The metric system, devised by the French in the latter part of the 18th century, is the system prescribed by law in most European countries. The metric system is very logically organized into units of ten; it is a decimal system. Basic units can be multiplied or divided by ten to form secondary units. Multiples are calculated by moving the decimal point to the right, and divisions by moving the decimal point to the left.

Basic units of measurement are the meter, the liter, and the gram. Prefixes derived from Latin designate subdivisions of the basic unit: deci (1/10 or 0.1), centi (1/100 or 0.01), and milli (1/1000 or 0.001). Multiples of the basic unit are designated by prefixes derived from Greek: deka (10), hecto (100), and kilo (1000). Only the measurements of volume (the liter) and of weight (the gram) are discussed in this chapter. These are the measures used in medication administration. See Figure 37–4. In medical and nursing practice the kilogram (kg) is the only multiple of the gram used, and the milligram (mg) and microgram (mcg) subdivisions.

Figure 37–4 Basic metric measurements of volume and weight.

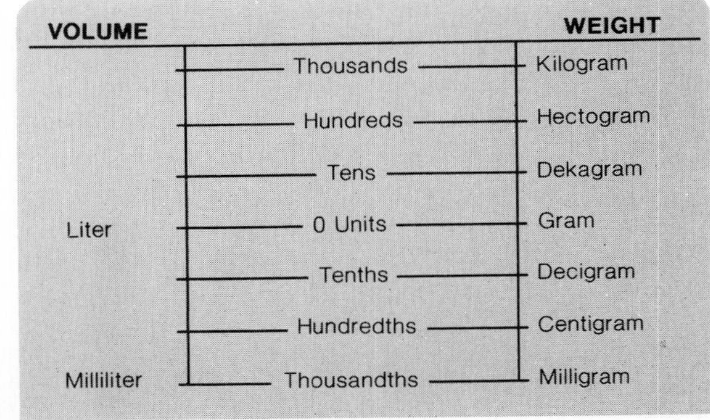

Fractional parts of the liter are usually expressed in milliliters (ml), for example, 600 ml, and multiples of the liter are usually expressed, for example, as 2.5 liters or 2500 ml.

Apothecaries' System

The apothecaries' system, older than the metric system, was brought to the United States from England during the colonial period. North Americans are familiar with most units of measure in the apothecaries' system, since they have been used in everyday life. For example, milk is bought in pints or quarts, gasoline is purchased by the gallon, people weigh themselves in pounds, and distances are measured in feet or inches and miles.

The basic unit of weight in the apothecaries' system is the grain, likened to a grain of wheat, and the basic unit of volume is the minim, a volume of water equal in weight to a grain of wheat. The word *minim* means "the least." In ascending order the other units of weight are the scruple, the dram, the ounce, and the pound. Today the scruple (scr) is seldom used. The units of volume are, in ascending order, the fluid dram, the fluid ounce, the pint, the quart, and the gallon.

Quantities in the apothecaries' system are often expressed by lowercase Roman numerals, particularly when the unit of measure is abbreviated. The Roman numeral follows rather than precedes the unit of measure. For example, a fluid ounce is abbreviated as f℥. Two fluid ounces are written as f℥ii, and 4 fluid ounces are written as f℥iv. One-half fluid ounce is written as f℥ss, and 1½ fluid ounces as f℥iss. See Appendices C and D.

Household System

Household measures may be used when more accurate systems of measure are not required. Included in household measures are drops, teaspoons, tablespoons, cups, and glasses. Although pints and quarts are often found in homes, they are defined as apothecaries' measures. Equivalent units of the household system are in Appendix D.

Converting Units of Weight and Measure

Sometimes drugs are dispensed from the pharmacy in grams when the order specifies milligrams, or they are dispensed in milligrams but ordered in grains. The nurse preparing a medicated irrigation may find that the order calls for quarts and that the solution is dispensed in liter containers. In all situations it is the nurse's responsibility to convert units of measure or weight, and thus nurses must be aware of approximate equivalents within each system of measurement and among systems.

Converting Weights within the Metric System

It is relatively simple to arrive at equivalent units of weight within the metric system, since the system is based on units of ten. Only three metric units of weight are used for drug dosages, the gram (g), milligram (mg), and microgram (mcg): 1000 mg or 1,000,000 mcg equals 1 g. Equivalents are computed by dividing or multiplying; e.g., to change milligrams to grams, milligrams are divided by 1000. The simplest way to divide by 1000 is to move the decimal point three places to the left.

1000 mg = 1 g
500 mg = 0.5 g

Conversely, to convert grams to milligrams, the grams are multiplied by 1000, or the decimal point is moved three places to the right.

0.006 g = 6 mg

Converting Weights and Measures among Systems

When preparing medications for patients, a nurse may find it necessary to convert weights or volumes from one system to another. As an example, the pharmacy may dispense milligrams or grams of chloral hydrate, yet the nurse must administer an order that reads chloral hydrate grains viiss. To prepare the correct dose for the patient, the nurse must convert from the apothecaries' to the metric system. The nurse may have to convert from the apothecaries' or metric system to the household system to give patients a useful, realistic measure to use at home. All conversions are approximate, that is, not precisely accurate.

Converting units of volume

It is advisable for a nurse to learn some commonly used approximate equivalents, such as those in Table 37–5.

Table 37–5 Equivalent Measures: Metric, Apothecaries', and Household

Metric		Apothecaries'		Household
1 ml	=	15 minims (min or m)	=	15 drops (gtt)
15 ml	=	4 fluid drams (f℥)	=	1 tablespoon (Tbsp)
30 ml	=	1 fluid ounce (f℥)	=	same
500 ml	=	1 pint (pt)	=	same
1000 ml	=	1 quart (qt)	=	same
4000 ml	=	1 gallon (gal)	=	same

Table 37–6 Approximate Weight Equivalents: Metric and Apothecaries' Systems

Metric	Apothecaries'
1 mg	= 1/60 grain
60 mg	= 1 grain
1 g	= 15 grains
4 g	= 1 dram
30 g	= 1 ounce
500 g	= 1.1 pound (lb)
1000 g (1 kg)	= 2.2 lb

By learning the equivalents in Table 37–5, the nurse can make many conversions readily. For example, 15 minims = approximately 15 drops; therefore 1 minim is approximately 1 drop. Similarly, 1 quart approximates 1000 ml, and 1 gallon approximates 4000 ml; therefore 4 quarts is approximately 1 gallon.

The following are some situations in which nurses need to apply a knowledge of volume conversion.

1. Milliliter dosages may need to be fractionalized. The nurse can fractionalize milliliter dosages by remembering that 1 ml contains 15 drops or minims.
2. Fluid drams and ounces are commonly used in prescribing liquid medications such as cough syrups, laxatives, antacids, and antibiotics for children. The fluid ounce is frequently converted to milliliters when measuring a patient's fluid intake or output.
3. Liters and milliliters are the volumes commonly used in preparing solutions for enemas, irrigating solutions for douches, bladder irrigations, and solutions for cleaning open wounds. In some situations, the nurse needs to convert the volumes of such solutions.

Converting units of weight

The units of weight most commonly used in nursing practice are the gram, milligram, and kilogram and the grain and the pound. Household units of weight are generally not applicable.

Table 37–6 shows metric and apothecaries' approximate equivalents. Learning these equivalents helps the nurse make weight conversions readily.

Nurses need to convert units of weight in the following situations:

1. Converting a person's body weight from kilograms to pounds and vice versa
2. Converting grams and milligrams to grains and vice versa, for example, when preparing medications

When converting units of weight from the metric system to the apothecaries' system, the nurse should keep in mind that a milligram is smaller than a grain (1 mg = 1/60 grain and 1 grain = 60 mg). The result of converting a smaller unit (milligram) to a larger unit (grain) is a smaller number. Thus, the nurse must divide (by 60 if converting from milligrams to grains). Conversely, when converting from a larger unit to a smaller unit, the nurse multiplies (by 60 if converting from grains to milligrams), and the product is a larger number. In other words:

Small units (mg) to large units (grains) = a smaller number

Large units (grains) to small units (mg) = a larger number

$$\frac{3000\text{ mg}}{60} = 50\text{ grains}$$

$$50\text{ grains} \times 60 = 3000\text{ mg}$$

When converting pounds to kilograms, the nurse applies the same rule. The pound is a smaller unit than the kilogram, and the nurse converts by dividing or multiplying by 2.2.

$$\frac{110\text{ lb}}{2.2} = 50\text{ kg}$$

$$50\text{ kg} \times 2.2 = 110\text{ lb}$$

The conversion of milligrams to grams was previously discussed. The decimal point is moved three spaces to the left.

$$3000\text{ mg} = 3\text{ g}$$

Calculating Fractional Dosages

The need to calculate fractional dosages from stock drugs arises chiefly when small dosages must be administered to infants and children. Such calculation may also be necessary in preparing preoperative medications, injectable analgesics, and intravenous medications for adult patients.

Dosages for Children

Although the dosage is stated in the medication order, nurses must understand something about the safe dosages for children. Unlike adult dosages, children's dosages are not always standard. There are several formulas to determine pediatric dosages using body surface area and weight. These formulas should be checked with a pharmacist or other staff members.

Body surface area

Body surface area is determined by using a normogram and the child's height and weight. See Figure 30–2, page 789, about the normogram. After obtaining the body surface area, the nurse can use one of two formulas:

$$\frac{\text{Body surface area of child}}{\text{Body surface area of adult}} \times \text{Adult dose} = \text{Estimated child's dose}$$

The second formula does not use the adult dose but requires information about the average dose per square meter (m^2) of body surface area:

$$\text{Surface area of child in m}^2 \times \text{Dose per m}^2 = \text{Estimated child's dose}$$

Body weight

Using Clark's rule, the nurse can use the child's body weight to calculate a child's dosage. Because weight is used, Clark's rule applies to children of all ages. An average adult weight of 150 pounds (approximately 68 kg) is used. The child's dose is obtained by creating a fraction of the child's weight over the adult's weight (150 lb) and multiplying by the adult dose:

$$\text{Child's dose} = \frac{\text{Weight of child in pounds}}{150} \times \text{Adult dose}$$

If the adult dose of a drug is 1/6 grain, the amount a child weighing 30 pounds should receive is:

$$\frac{30}{150} \times \frac{1}{6} = \frac{1}{30} \text{ grain}$$

Fractional Dosages from Stock Drugs

The stock drug problem arises chiefly when the nurse prepares an injectable drug by dissolving a tablet in water or when the nurse calculates how much solution of a certain concentration is required to achieve a certain dosage.

Tablets

Determining a smaller dose of a drug from a tablet In recent years injectable drugs have been packaged in individual-dose ampules or multidose vials, which have largely replaced tablets. However, it is still advisable for a nurse to learn how to calculate fractional dosages from tablets. Because it is impossible to divide a hypodermic tablet accurately, a whole tablet must be used and dissolved inside a syringe or sterile medicine glass. Sterile water or sterile normal saline from commercially prepared vials is used to dissolve the tablet, and then a fraction of the entire solution is used. How large a fraction to administer is determined by dividing the amount of the drug that is desired by the amount of drug on hand, as follows:

$$\frac{\text{D (amount desired)}}{\text{H (amount on hand)}} = \text{Fraction of tablet needed}$$

If morphine is available in 1/4 grain tablets but 1/6 grain is the dose ordered, the fraction of the tablet to be given would be:

$$\frac{1/6 \text{ grain}}{1/4 \text{ grain}} = \text{Fraction of tablet}$$

Invert the divisor and multiply:

$$\frac{1}{6} \times \frac{4}{1} = \frac{2}{3} \text{ tablet} = \frac{1}{6} \text{ grain}$$

Dissolving and preparing the dose After the proportion of the tablet to be used is determined, the nurse prepares the required amount in a syringe for injection. The nurse must dissolve the entire tablet, but in most cases does not inject all the solution. In the example just given, only two-thirds of the tablet is needed, so the nurse injects only two-thirds of the solution. The nurse now considers this question: What is the appropriate volume of solution in which to dissolve the tablet? The nurse keeps in mind these two factors:

1. The amount of solution that is acceptable for administration

2. The metric (milliliter) and apothecaries' (minim) calibrations on the syringe

The recommended minimum amount of solution for injections is 8 minims or ½ ml, and the maximum amount is about 32 to 40 minims or 2 to 2½ ml. The amount that should be administered depends on the route, the site of injection, and the size of the patient. A large muscular adult may safely absorb up to 5 ml intramuscularly, whereas an intradermal injection is normally about 0.2 ml.

Disposable syringes are usually available in a 3 ml size for medications.

Solution volume in the syringe can be determined by the metric calibrations (tenths) on one side of the syringe, or the minim calibrations (sixteenths) on the other side (16 minims approximate 1 ml). Thus if the tablet is dissolved in 1 ml and the dosage is two-thirds of a tablet, two-thirds of the solution (either 0.6 to 0.7 ml or 10 minims) is administered. In this case a third of the solution is discarded prior to administering the drug.

When preparing very small doses for children, it is frequently necessary to dilute the tablets further. For example, to prepare 1/30 grain from 1/6 grain (the dose calculated previously by Clark's rule) it is first necessary to calculate what fraction of the tablet to use:

$$\frac{\text{D (amount desired)}}{\text{H (amount on hand)}} = \frac{1/30}{1/6}\text{ grain} = \frac{1}{30} \times \frac{6}{1} = \frac{1}{5}$$

The volume to be injected would be too small to administer (only 1/5 ml) if the tablet were dissolved in 1 ml. It is necessary to dissolve the tablet in a larger amount of solution, such as 2½ ml. Then one-fifth of 2½ ml, or ½ ml, can be administered.

Prepared vials or ampules

Many medications are already in liquid form and ready for use. For example, meperidine hydrochloride (Demerol) is often distributed in large vials and prepared in dilutions of 50 mg per ml. Thus if the order calls for 100 mg, the nurse injects 2 ml, and if it calls for 75 mg, the nurse injects 1½ ml. To calculate the volume of solution that contains a certain milligram dosage, the nurse uses this formula:

$$\frac{\text{D (amount desired)}}{\text{H (amount on hand)}} = \text{Amount (volume) wanted}$$

$$\frac{40\text{ mg}}{50\text{ mg}} = \frac{4}{5}\text{ ml}$$

Example problem Prepare 4 mg of a drug from a vial containing 20 mg in a 5 ml solution. Formula:

$$\frac{\text{Drug available}}{\text{Amount of solution}} = \frac{\text{Dose wanted}}{x\text{ ml}}$$

$$\frac{20\text{ mg}}{5\text{ ml}} = \frac{4\text{ mg}}{x\text{ ml}}$$

Therefore:

$$\frac{20}{5} = \frac{4}{x}$$

Cross multiply:

$$20x = 20$$

$$x = \frac{20}{20}$$

$$x = 1\text{ ml}$$

Assessment

Assessment pertinent to the administration of medications includes:

1. Nursing history
2. Clinical assessment of the patient at the time of and following the drug administration

Nursing Medication History

The nursing history includes information about the drugs that the patient is taking currently or has taken recently. This includes prescription drugs, over-the-counter drugs such as antacids, alcohol and tobacco, and nonsanctioned drugs such as marijuana.

An important part of the history is the patient's knowledge of his or her drug allergies. Some patients can tell a nurse, "I am allergic to penicillin, adhesive tape, and curry." Other patients may not be sure about allergic reactions. An illness occurring after a drug was taken may not be identified as an allergy, but the patient may associate the drug with an illness or unusual reaction. The patient's physician can often give information about allergies. During the history, the nurse tries to elicit information about drug dependencies. The frequency with which drugs are taken and the patient's perceived need for them are measures of dependence.

Clinical Signs

The nurse needs to assess clinical signs when administering drugs. Specifically, the nurse assesses the patient's condition prior to the drug administration, the effect of the drug on the patient, and signs of undesirable side effects and toxicity.

The nature of assessment prior to the administration of the drug depends on the patient's illness, his or her condition, and the route of administration. Patients who breathe with difficulty have their respirations assessed before the administration of any drug. If the patient is acutely ill, the nurse should assess the patient's vital signs, color, and perception of how he or she feels. Depending on the route of administration ordered, the nurse may collect additional data. If the patient is nauseated or vomiting, oral administration may not be desirable. Prior to a subcutaneous injection, the nurse assesses the injection site for tenderness, hardness, swelling, scarring, itching, burning, or localized inflammation. If these are present, another site should be chosen.

After administration, the nurse assesses the effect of the drug and is alert to possible adverse side effects or signs of toxicity. The times of assessment depend to some degree on the time the effect is anticipated. For example, following the administration of furosemide (Lasix) by mouth, the nurse should measure urine output the day the drug is taken. It is important to assess the drug's action in light of knowledge about the intended action and possible adverse reactions. Therefore, it is important that nurses have a thorough knowledge of the drugs they are administering.

Administering Medications

Steps in Administering Medications

When administering any drug, regardless of the route of administration, the nurse follows five steps:

1. Identification of the patient
2. Administration of the drug
3. Provision of adjunctive nursing care as indicated
4. Recording
5. Evaluation of the patient's response to the drug

Identifying the patient

Identifying a patient sounds simple and usually is, but errors can and do occur, usually because a patient gets a drug intended for another. In hospitals, most patients wear some means of identification, such as wristbands with their names and hospital identification numbers. To prevent mistakes, nurses also ask the patient's name or state the name clearly and then listen to the patient's response before administering any medication.

Administering the drug

Equally important is giving the correct drug. Medication orders and cards or lists need to be read carefully and checked against the name on the medication envelope or on the drawer in which the patient's medications are kept if a medication cart is used. The medication is then administered in the dosage and by the route ordered.

Adjunctive nursing intervention

Patients may need help when receiving medications. They may require physical assistance, for instance, in assuming positions for intramuscular injections, or they may need explanations about the medications and guidance about measures to enhance drug effectiveness and prevent complications, e.g., drinking fluids. Some patients convey fear about their medications. The nurse can allay fears by listening carefully to patients' concerns and giving correct information. Patients may give the nurse information regarding their drugs. A patient may say that an analgesic is effective for only 10 or 15 minutes, another patient may feel nauseated about 20 minutes after ingesting a drug, a third patient may feel dizzy each afternoon at about the same time, and a fourth may have pain in the right leg. This type of information needs to be recorded and, when appropriate, relayed to the physician. In some cases, simple nursing measures can relieve the problem, for instance, the nurse can provide milk with a medication to a patient with nausea; in other instances, it may be necessary for the physician to reassess the needs of the patient.

Recording

Once complete, the intervention is recorded on the patient's record. The facts recorded are name of the drug, dosage, method of administration, specific relevant data such as pulse rate (taken in most settings prior to the administration of digitalis), and any other pertinent information. The record should include the exact time of administration and in most agencies the signature of the nurse providing the medication. Often medications that are given regularly are recorded on a special flow record, whereas p.r.n. or stat medications are recorded separately on the nurse's notes.

Evaluating patient response

The response of the patient to a medication can often be detected directly after intravenous administration, 10 to

20 minutes after an intramuscular or subcutaneous injection, and anywhere from immediately to several days after oral administration. For example, the ingestion of aluminum hydroxide gel (Amphojel) often provides almost immediate relief to a patient with epigastric pain; on the other hand, the effects of an antibiotic may not be noticeable for 3 or 4 days.

The kinds of behavior that reflect the action or lack of action of a drug are as variable as the purposes of the drugs themselves. The anxious patient may show the effects of a tranquilizer by behavior that reflects a lowered stress level, for example, slower speech or fewer random movements. The effectiveness of a sedative can often be measured by how well a patient slept; the effectiveness of an antispasmodic, by how much pain the patient feels. In all nursing activities, nurses need to be aware of the medications that a patient is taking and record their effectiveness as assessed by the patient and the nurse on the patient's chart. If appropriate, the nurse may also report the response of the patient to the senior nurse and to the physician directly.

Guidelines for Administering Medications

1. Although medications are prescribed chiefly by physicians, the nurses who administer them are responsible for their own actions and should question orders they consider incorrect. The physician's order should include the name of the medication, the dosage, and the method and frequency of administration. The order may include additional directions, e.g., "withhold dosage if the pulse is below 60."

2. Before administering a medication, the nurse must be knowledgeable about the drug. Most nursing units have a drug reference book, for example, the *United States Pharmacopeia* (*USP*), the *National Formulary*, and the *Homeopathic Pharmacopoeia of the United States.* In Canada, the *British Pharmacopoeia* is frequently used.

3. Federal laws govern the use of narcotics and barbiturates. Narcotics and barbiturates are kept in a drawer or cupboard with a double lock. Special forms are used for recording them. The data usually required are the name of the patient, drug, and physician; date; time of administration; dosage; and signature of the person who prepared and administered the drug.

4. Medication cards are used in some agencies as guides for preparing medications. A card normally includes the patient's name, room and bed number, name of the drug, dosage, and times and method of administration. In some agencies, the date on which the order was prescribed and the date on which it expires are also included.

5. Nurses must concentrate on the task to avoid errors while preparing and giving medications.

6. Five rights guide nurses preparing medications: right drug, right dose, right patient, right time, and right route.

7. The drug preparation must be appropriate to the route prescribed.

8. To prevent an error when preparing medications, the nurse reads the label on the container three times: before taking it off the shelf, while pouring the medication, and after placing it back on the shelf.

9. The nurse who prepares medications must also administer and chart them. He or she is the only person who can confirm the medication.

10. When preparing medications, do not use the following:

- **a.** Medications from unmarked containers or containers with illegible labels
- **b.** Medications that are cloudy or have changed color
- **c.** Medications that have a sediment at the bottom unless the medication requires shaking before use

Return such medications to the pharmacy. Write the reason for their return on the label.

11. Never return medications to a container or transfer medications from one container to another. This practice avoids mixing drugs or placing a drug in the wrong container.

12. Identify the patient correctly and carefully, using the appropriate means of identification, e.g., the identification bracelet.

13. With rare exceptions, patients have the right to know the name and the action of the drug they are taking, and they have the right to refuse a medication. Medications that are refused must be discarded and the reason for refusal recorded.

14. Provide the correct adjunctive nursing measures with the medication, e.g., measure a pulse rate before giving a digitalis preparation or notify the physician before giving the drug if the apical pulse is below 60.

15. Medications should not be left at the bedside, with the exception of antacids, nonnarcotic cough syrups, nitroglycerin, lotions or ointments, certain eye medications, and inhalants. Check agency policies about each of these. When medications are left at the bedside, determine from the patient when she or he takes or applies them.

16. Give medications within 30 minutes of the time ordered, except for preoperative medications, which must be given at the exact time ordered, or medications that are ordered to be given hourly or every 2 hours (e.g., eye medications prior to surgery).

17. If a patient vomits after taking an oral medication, report the fact to the responsible nurse and state the names of all medications given. Withhold the medication(s). Often the physician reorders the same drug by a different route, for example, subcutaneously or intramuscularly.

18. Special precautions must be observed for certain drugs. Most agencies require that two qualified nurses double-check the dosages of anticoagulants, insulin, digitalis preparations, and certain IV medications. Check agency policies.

19. After a medication has been administered, record it on the patient's chart. The recording should include the time, the name of the drug, the dosage, the method of administration, and any related data. Some agencies require that the method of administration be specified if it is other than oral; the oral route is usually not specified in the record.

20. Most agencies have an official list of abbreviations used in medication orders and in recording. See Appendix A for commonly used abbreviations.

21. Evaluate the effectiveness of a medication a suitable time after its administration. For example, the effectiveness of an intramuscularly injected analgesic can be evaluated 10 to 20 minutes after administration.

22. Medications are usually discontinued before surgery, and the physician writes new orders after the surgery. New orders are generally given for drugs a newly admitted patient takes at home or when a patient is transferred to another service within an agency or outside the agency. Check agency policies.

23. When medications are intentionally omitted, e.g., before surgery or a diagnostic test, record the omission and the reason on the patient's chart. It may also be necessary to notify the prescriber.

24. Medication errors sometimes occur. When an error is made, report it immediately to the responsible nurse so that corrective measures can be implemented promptly. Errors are usually documented on an unusual incident form that becomes a part of the agency's file. Check the policies and practices of the agency.

Developmental Considerations in Administering Medications

Knowledge of growth and development is essential for the nurse administering medications to children. The nurse needs to know how to approach a child and what explanations and methods are required. Adolescents, pregnant women, and elderly patients also have special needs.

Infants and Children

Oral medications

Oral medications for children are usually prepared in liquid sweetened forms to make them more palatable. Some drugs are not palatable, and the nurse can mask the taste with honey, jam, juice, or any suitable sweetener. The parents may provide suggestions about what method is best for their child. Necessary foods such as milk or orange juice should not be used to mask the taste of medications because the child may develop unpleasant associations and refuse that food in the future. Artificial sweeteners may be used for diabetic children. Not all children reject unsweetened medicine. Some may be content with a sip of juice or a mint before and after taking a medication. Nurses are encouraged to be aware of the tastes of the medications they are giving, which allows them to answer questions honestly. For example, in response to "Will it taste bad?" the nurse may reply, "It tastes like strawberry to me" or ". . . like sour lemon. Tell me what you think it tastes like." Most children accept this challenge to experiment and learn.

Toddlers who are in the independent "no" stage challenge the nurse's ability to gain the child's cooperation. It is common for toddlers to push medications away or to close their mouths in refusal. This behavior may reflect dislike of medicines, a need to control the situation, or a desire to take the medicine independently. A nurse can offer encouragement by holding the child, acknowledging the child's distaste for the medicine, offering a simple explanation about why it is needed, and expressing faith in the child's ability to manage this situation independently. A spoon, a glass, or a straw may help toddlers take medications. A few words of praise go a long way. The nurse should encourage the child to participate as much as possible, for example, by holding the glass or by choosing between a straw or a spoon. Forcing medications is futile; it communicates hostility and engenders distrust. If the child does not spit out the medication in response to force, the child will no doubt intentionally vomit the medication soon after. It is important, too, that nurses not convey to the child, either verbally or nonverbally, negative attitudes they may have about the medication.

By the age of 4 to 6 years children are generally able to take pills. Some children of 2 years have already learned to swallow pills. To teach children to swallow pills, the nurse tells them to put the pill near the back of the tongue and then to wash it down with water, milk, or juice. Recognition and praise elicits the cooperation of most young children, and seeing other children taking medications will help.

When older children refuse to take medications, the nurse encourages them to discuss their feelings about the drugs and to share suggestions they have. Coaxing and bribing will not get the child to cooperate. It is better to convey an attitude of expectancy and helpful cooperation. For example, it is better to say, "I have your green pill for you, Johnny" than "Johnny, will you please take your green pill?" If given a few choices, such as whether to take a pill or a liquid, most children cooperate more readily. On rare occasions children resist all strategies to get them to take a medication. In that case, the situation needs to be analyzed individually. If all attempts fail, the physician needs to be consulted.

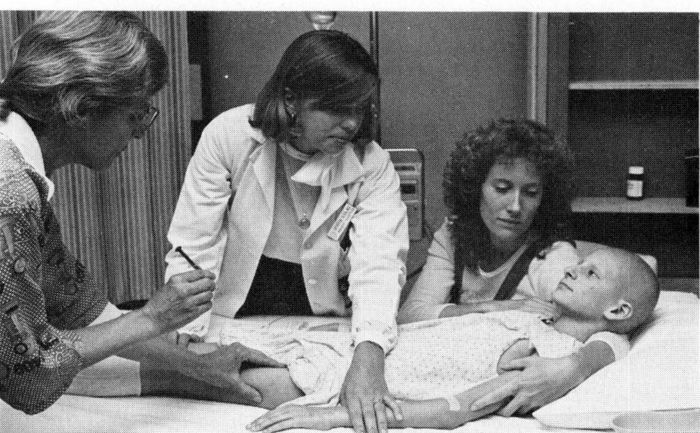

Figure 37–5 Holding a child during an intramuscular injection.

Injectable medications

Children fear any procedure in which a needle is used because they anticipate pain or because the procedure is unfamiliar and threatening. The nurse needs to acknowledge that the child will feel some pain. Denying this fact only deepens the child's distrust. Very young infants may not experience painful stimuli with the same sensitivity as children because infants have delayed reactions to stimuli. They also have limited experiences and thus feel less anticipatory fear or anxiety. By the age of approximately 6 months, infants have memory of past pain and therefore begin to anticipate pain and cry when they see a needle and syringe. By the age of 10 months or a year, the infant may make active attempts to wriggle away or to push the equipment aside. Thus when administering injections to young children, the nurse restrains them to protect them from injury. After the injection, it is important for the nurse (or the parent) to cuddle and speak softly to the infant and give the child a toy to dispel the child's association of the nurse only with pain.

The reasoning ability of toddlers and preschoolers is immature. They often view an injection as punishment for some "bad" behavior, real or imagined, particularly if they are hospitalized. They may believe their parents abandoned them and therefore do not want them or want them punished. Although it is difficult for children of this age to understand why the procedure is necessary even when they receive simple explanations, children who are prepared can and usually do muster coping mechanisms. For example, one child who was to receive an immunization found the situation easier to deal with when he was encouraged to tell the nurse, "You better be quick!" All injections should be given as rapidly as possible, and children must be adequately restrained. Even though a child says, "I'll hold still," another nurse needs to be present for safety. Two nurses may be required to restrain some 4-year-olds. See Figure 37–5 for one method of holding a child during an intramuscular injection.

Children should be told about the injection shortly before it is given. Even if this knowledge increases anxiety, the child should be told the truth. It is also important to find out how the child copes with pain and to support those coping methods. By recognizing the child's developmental level, the nurse can formulate an approach that provides meaningful support. For example a preschooler (5 years old) who is developing a conscience could view an injection as punishment. By telling the child that injections are never used as punishment and giving the child a simple, honest explanation of the injection, the nurse allays guilt and fear.

Children and adolescents should be encouraged to vent their feelings before and after the treatment. Young children may do this in play; adolescents may require support for open discussion.

Participation of parents often can be elicited, although many parents choose not to be involved in restraining their children. If they do participate, they can often console or divert their children during the injection. The nurse may gain children's cooperation by involving them in the procedure, for instance, by asking them on which side they want the injection or by allowing them to swab the site.

Elderly People

Older people can present special problems in relation to medications. Most of their problems are related to physiologic changes, to past experiences, and to established attitudes toward medications.

Physiologic changes in elderly persons usually involve:

1. Altered memory
2. Less acute vision
3. Decrease in kidney function resulting in slower elimination of drugs and higher drug concentrations in the bloodstream for longer periods

4. Less complete and slower absorption from the gastrointestinal tract
5. Increased proportion of fat to lean body mass, which facilitates retention of fat-soluble drugs and increases potential for toxicity.
6. Decreased liver function, which hinders biotransformation of drugs
7. Decreased organ sensitivity, which means that the response to the same drug concentration in the vicinity of the target organ is less in older people than in the young
8. Altered quality of organ responsiveness, resulting in adverse effects becoming pronounced before therapeutic effects are achieved; for example, in older people, digitalis often produces arrhythmia, nausea, or vomiting, before slower and stronger cardiac contractions are achieved.

Many of these changes enhance the possibility of cumulative effects and toxicity. For example, impaired circulation delays the action of medications given intramuscularly or subcutaneously. Digitalis, which is frequently taken by elderly people, can accumulate to toxic levels and be lethal.

It is not uncommon for elderly patients to take several different medications daily. The possibility of error increases with the number of medications taken, whether self-administered at home or administered by nurses in a hospital. The greater number of medications also compounds the problem of drug interactions, because much is yet to be learned about the effects of drugs given in combinations. A general rule to follow is that elderly patients should take as few medications as possible.

Like the very young, elderly persons usually require smaller dosages of drugs, especially of sedatives and other central nervous system depressants, because their effects are greater on older patients. Reactions of the elderly to medications, particularly sedatives, are unpredictable and often bizarre. It is not uncommon to see irritability, confusion, disorientation, restlessness, and incontinence as a result of sedatives. Nurses therefore need to observe patients carefully for untoward reactions. Chloral hydrate is an effective sedative for elderly people. The use of alcohol (e.g., brandy) as a bedtime relaxant and as an appetizer before meals is becoming more common. The moderate use of alcohol by people who are accustomed to it can contribute to a sense of well-being.

Attitudes of elderly people toward medical care and medications vary. Elderly people tend to believe in the wisdom of the physician more readily than younger people. Some older people are bewildered by the prescription of several medications and may passively accept their medications from nurses but not take them. Others may be suspicious of medications and actively refuse them. For this reason, the nurse is advised to stay with patients until they have taken the medications.

Elderly people are mature adults capable of reasoning. Therefore, the nurse needs to explain the reasons for and effects of medications, particularly to ambulatory geriatric patients. This education can prevent the common occurrence of patients taking medications long after there is a need for them, or it can prevent patients from discontinuing a drug too quickly. For example, patients should know that diuretics will cause them to urinate more frequently and may reduce ankle edema. Instructions about medications need to be given to all patients prior to discharge from a hospital. These instructions should include when to take the drugs, what effects to expect, and when to consult a physician.

Because some patients are required to take several medications daily and because visual acuity and memory may be impaired, it is important for the nurse, in consultation with the physician if necessary, to develop simple, realistic plans for patients to follow at home. For example, most people, including elderly people, can have difficulties remembering to take drugs. If they are scheduled to be taken with meals or at bedtime, patients are not as likely to forget. Some patients may take their medications and then an hour later not remember whether they took them. One solution to forgetfulness is to use a special container or glass strictly for medications. If the container or glass is empty, the person knows that he or she took the pills. Loss of visual acuity presents problems that can be overcome by writing out the plan in a print large enough to be read. In some situations the help of a spouse, son, or daughter can be enlisted.

Oral Medications

Oral medications are generally the least expensive and the most easily taken of all drugs. As long as a patient can swallow, they are readily administered. Adjustments may need to be made if the patient is very young or very old or has difficulty swallowing solids. In these cases powders can often be mixed in a small amount of liquid for easier ingestion, scored tablets can be broken, and other tablets can be crushed for easier swallowing.

Enteric coated tablets and capsules should not be broken in this manner, however, because the coating usually serves a purpose, such as protecting the medicine from being inactiviated by gastric juices.

Most oral medications are absorbed in the small intestine, although small amounts can be absorbed through the oral and stomach mucosas. Sublingual medications, for example, are to a large degree absorbed into the capillaries under the tongue. Liquid medications are more readily absorbed in the stomach than tablets or capsules. Some capsules are designed to dissolve in the stomach, whereas others dissolve in intestinal juices. Some oral medicines are particularly irritating to mucous membranes. The unpleasant effects of such a drug can often be prevented by diluting the drug if it is a liquid or by advising the patient to take it after a meal or with milk, unless the latter is contraindicated.

The speed and degree of absorption of drugs from the gastrointestinal tract are somewhat unpredictable. Absorption depends on a number of factors, particularly the presence of food, which may inhibit absorption. There are other disadvantages to oral administration of some medicines; for example, hydrochloric acid is irritating to oral and gastric mucosa and can damage a patient's teeth. This drug is normally well diluted with water and taken with a straw. Other drugs such as elixir of ferrous sulphate can stain a patient's teeth and remove tooth enamel if precautions are not taken. Some medications are inactivated to some degree by gastrointestinal secretions, and therefore the speed of absorption greatly affects the amount of effective drug absorbed.

Oral medications are contraindicated when a patient is vomiting, has gastric or intestinal suction, or is unconscious and unable to swallow. Such patients in a hospital usually are on orders "nothing by mouth" (NPO, nothing per ora, nil per os).

Procedure 37–1 Administering Oral Medications

Equipment

1. A medication tray or cart.
2. Medication cards or list. To save time and avoid retracing steps, arrange the cards in the order in which you will give the medications. Plan to give medications first to patients who do not require assistance, and last to those who do.
3. Disposable medication cups. Small paper cups are needed for tablets and capsules; for liquids waxed or plastic calibrated medication cups are needed.

Preparation

1. Check the date on the medication order and verify its accuracy. It should contain the following:
   a. Patient's name
   b. Name of the drug and dosage
   c. Time for administration
   d. Route of administration, for example, oral (p.o.), subcutaneous or hypodermic (H), intramuscular (IM), or intravenous (IV)

   Records of medication orders include the physician's order, which is usually on the patient's chart, the Kardex record, and the medication card. The surest check is to compare the medication card against the physician's order. In some settings a medication Kardex or computer printout is used instead of medication cards. This Kardex or printout is usually kept in the medications room or in the medication cart. Any discrepancies in the order should be clarified with the responsible nurse or the physician, whichever is appropriate in the agency.
2. Wash hands to remove microorganisms, thus keeping medications and equipment clean and preventing transfer of microorganisms from one patient to another.
3. Read the medication card, and take the appropriate medication from the shelf, drawer, or refrigerator. The medication may be dispensed in a bottle, box, or envelope.
4. Compare the label of the medication container against the order on the medication card. If these are not identical, recheck the patient's chart. If there is still a discrepancy, check with the responsible nurse.
5. Prepare the correct amount of medication for the required dose, without touching the container and contaminating the medication.
   a. If administering tablets or capsules from a bottle, pour the required number into the bottle cap and then transfer the medication to the paper cup. See Figure 37–6. Usually all tablets or capsules to be given to the patient are placed in the same paper cup. Medica-

Procedure 37–1, continued

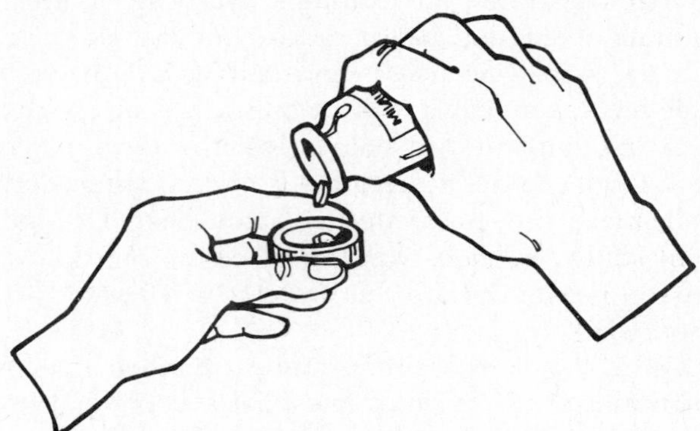

Figure 37–6

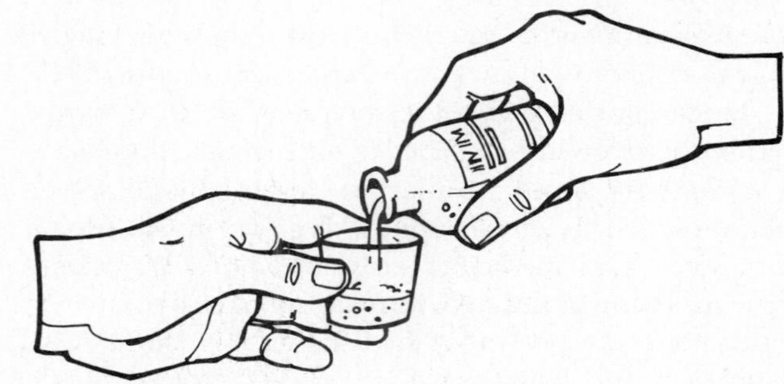

Figure 37–7

tions that require specific assessments, e.g., pulse measurements, respiratory rate or depth, or blood pressure, must be kept separate from the others.

b. If administering a liquid medication, remove the cap, and place it upside down on the countertop to avoid contaminating it. Hold the bottle with the label next to your palm so that if any spills, the label will not become soiled and illegible. See Figure 37–7. Hold the cup at eye level and fill it to the desired level, using the bottom of the *meniscus* (crescent-shaped upper surface of a column of liquid) as the measurement guide.

c. If administering an oral narcotic from a narcotic dispenser, expose the tablet by turning the dial or tearing off the numbered unit dose and drop it into the cup. These containers are sectioned and numbered. Whenever the nurse removes a tablet, the nurse must record the fact on the appropriate narcotic control record and sign it.

d. Open unit dose medications at the patient's bedside.

6. Place the prepared medication(s) and medication card together on the tray or cart.

7. Check the label on the container again, and return the bottle, box, or envelope to its storage place.

Intervention

1. Identify the patient by comparing the name on the medication card with the name on the patient's identification bracelet or by asking the patient to tell you his or her name.

2. Explain to the patient the purpose of the medication and how it will help, using language that he or she can understand. Include relevant information about effects, e.g., tell the patient receiving a diuretic that he or she can expect an increase in urine.

3. Assist the patient to a sitting position or, if not possible, to a lateral position. These positions facilitate swallowing and prevent aspiration.

4. Take the required assessment measures, e.g., pulse and respiratory rates or blood pressure. The pulse rate is taken before administering digitalis preparations and often as an indicator of pain prior to giving analgesics. Blood pressure is taken before giving hypotensive drugs. The respiratory rate is taken prior to administering narcotics, since narcotics depress the respiratory center. If the rate is below 12, the responsible nurse should be consulted.

5. Give the patient sufficient water or juice to swallow the medication if appropriate. Fluids ease swallowing and facilitate absorption from the gastrointestinal tract. Liquid medications are generally diluted with 15 ml (½ oz) of water to facilitate absorption. Some medications, e.g., antacids, cough syrups, and oils, are not diluted. Check agency practices.

6. If the patient is unable to hold the pill cup, use the pill cup to introduce the medication into the patient's mouth. Putting the cup to the patient's

Procedure 37–1, continued

mouth avoids contamination of the medication and of the nurse's hands.

7. If the patient has difficulty swallowing, have him or her place the medication on the back of the tongue before taking the water. Stimulation of the back of the tongue produces the swallowing reflex.
8. If the medication is harmful to tooth enamel or irritating to the oral mucous membrane, e.g., liquid iron preparations, have the patient use a glass straw and drink water following the medication.
9. If the patient says that the medication you are about to give is different from what he or she has been receiving, do not give the medication without checking the original order.
10. If the medication has an objectionable taste, have the patient suck a few ice chips beforehand (ice numbs the taste buds) or give the medication with juice, applesauce, or bread to mask the taste.
11. Stay with the patient until all medications have been swallowed.
12. Wash hands.
13. Record the medication given, dosage, time, any complaints of the patient, and the signature of the nurse. If there are other patients who require medications, give these out before charting.
14. Replace supplies in the appropriate place. Wipe the tray, rinse medication cups if they are to be washed, or dispose of disposable containers.
15. Return the medication card to the slot of next time due.
16. Return to the patient within 30 minutes to evaluate the effects of the medication, e.g., relief of pain.

Parenteral Medications

Parenteral routes commonly used by nurses to administer medications are subcutaneous, intramuscular, and intradermal. In some settings, intravenous medications are also given by nurses, although the type of medication a nurse can administer by this route may be restricted by agency policy. Parenteral medications are absorbed more quickly than oral medications and are irretrievable once injected. Therefore, it is important that they be prepared and administered carefully and accurately. Preparing and administering parenteral medications often involves mixing drugs, preparing powdered drugs, and employing sterile technique.

Equipment

Syringes

Several kinds of syringes are used for injections. Three commonly used types are the standard hypodermic syringe, the insulin syringe, and the tuberculin syringe. See Figure 37–8. Most syringes used today are made of plastic, are individually packaged for sterility, and can be disposed of together with the needles after use. Nondisposable glass syringes may be used in some areas. Once used, they need to be resterilized before further use.

Hypodermic syringes come in 2, 2.5, and 3 ml sizes. These syringes usually have two scales marked upon them, the minim and the milliliter scales. The milliliter

Figure 37–8 Three kinds of syringes: **A,** hypodermic; **B,** insulin; and **C,** tuberculin.

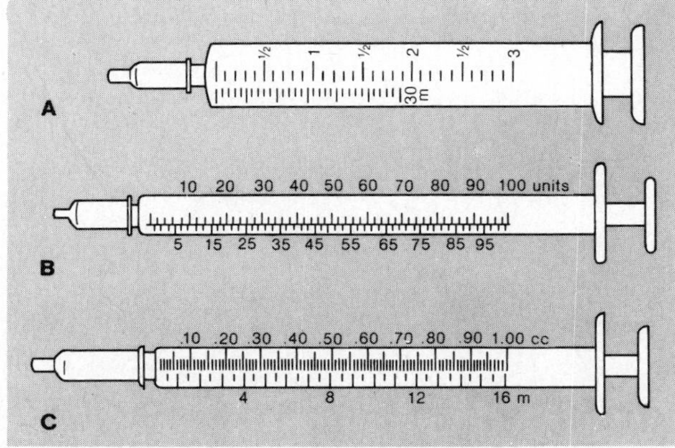

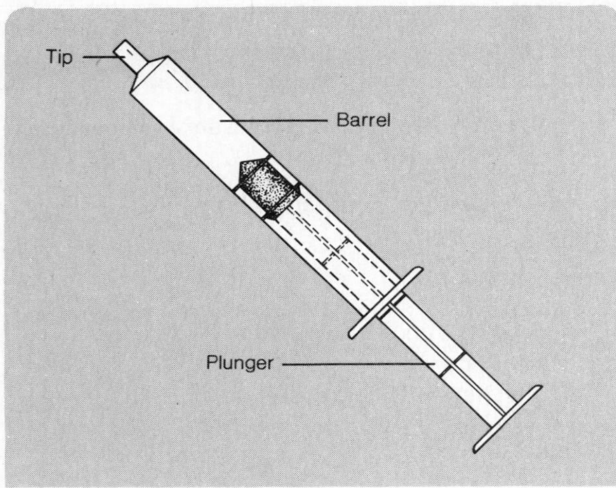

Figure 37–9 Parts of a syringe.

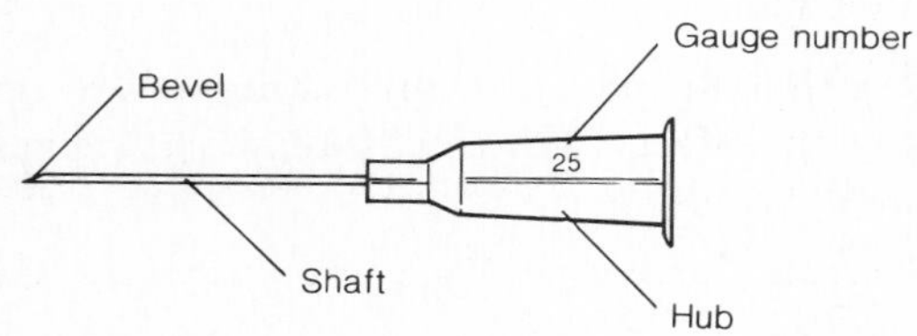

Figure 37–10 Parts of a needle.

Figure 37–11 Sizes of injection needles commonly used.

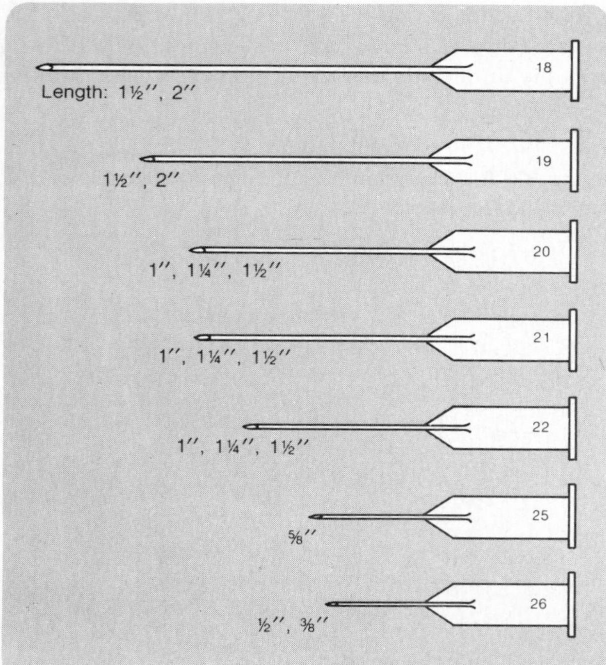

scale is normally used; the minim scale is used for very small dosages, such as epinephrine minims ṫṫṫ H.

Insulin syringes are similar to hypodermic syringes except that they have a scale especially designed for insulin. Insulin syringes have a 100 unit calibrated scale intended for use with U100 insulin. This scale is replacing the U40 and U80 scales used for 40 unit and 80 unit insulin. These syringes are also available in both disposable and nondisposable types.

The tuberculin syringe was designed to administer tuberculin. It is narrow and calibrated in tenths and hundredths of a milliliter (up to 1 ml) on one scale and in sixteenths of a minim (up to 1 minim) on the other scale. This syringe can also be used to administer other drugs, particularly when small or precise measurement is indicated, for example, for an infant dosage.

There are other sizes of syringes, for example, the 5, 10, 20, and 50 ml syringes. These are not generally used to administer drugs directly to patients but often are useful, for example, when adding sterile solutions to intravenous flasks or for irrigating wounds.

All syringes have three parts: the tip of the syringe, which connects with the needle; the barrel or outside part, on which the scales are printed; and the plunger, or part that fits inside the barrel. See Figure 37–9.

Needles

Needles are made of stainless steel or other metals; some are disposable. A needle has three parts: the hub, which fits onto the syringe; the cannula or shaft, which connects to the hub; and the bevel of the needle, which is the slanted part at the tip of the needle. See Figure 37–10. The bevel may be short or long. A long bevel provides a sharp needle, used for subcutaneous and intramuscular injections. Short bevels are used for intravenous injections; a long bevel is not used because it might become occluded if it rests against the side of a blood vessel.

Needles have three variables: the slant of the bevel; the length of the shaft, which varies from ¼ to 5 inches; and the gauge or diameter of the shaft, which varies from 14 to 27 gauge. The larger the gauge, the smaller the diameter of the cannula. For subcutaneous injections, it is usual to use a 24 to 26 gauge needle, ⅜ to ⅝ inch long. Obese patients may require a 1 inch needle. For intramuscular injections, a longer needle with a larger gauge is used, for example, 20 to 22 gauge and 1 to 1½ inches long. See Figure 37–11 for relative sizes of needles.

Syringes and needles can be obtained together or separately. Plastic disposable syringes and needles in individual sterile plastic containers with plastic needle protectors are common today.

Ampules and vials

Ampules and vials are frequently used to package parenteral medications. See Figure 37–12. An *ampule* is a glass container that usually holds a single dose of a drug. The ampule is made of clear glass and has a constricted neck. Some ampule necks have colored marks around them and some are scored. If the neck is not scored, it is filed with a small file before opening. Frequently the drug is in the upper stem of the ampule above the neck as well as in the main portion of the ampule. Before opening the ampule, the nurse needs to flick the upper stem several times with a fingernail to bring all the medication down to the main portion of the ampule. Before opening an ampule, the nurse places a piece of sterile gauze on the far side of the ampule neck and breaks off the top by bending it outward. The sterile gauze protects the nurse's fingers from the glass.

To remove the medication from the bottom of the ampule, the nurse inserts a hypodermic needle and withdraws the amount of drug required. If the ampule contains a single dose, the nurse may need to tip the ampule slightly to obtain all the medication.

A *vial* is a small glass bottle sealed with a rubber cap. Vials may contain only a single dose but often hold multidoses, for example, 50 ml. Vials usually have a metal cap that protects the rubber seal; the cap is readily removed. Before withdrawing medication from a vial, the nurse swabs the rubber cap with a disinfectant, often 70% alcohol. Then the nurse draws into the syringe a volume of air equal to the volume of medication to be withdrawn, inserts the needle into the vial through the rubber cap, and injects the air into the vial. The air allows the medication to be withdrawn easily. The bevel is kept above the medication to avoid creating bubbles. The drug is then withdrawn into the syringe by inverting the vial, holding it upward at eye level, and extracting the plunger.

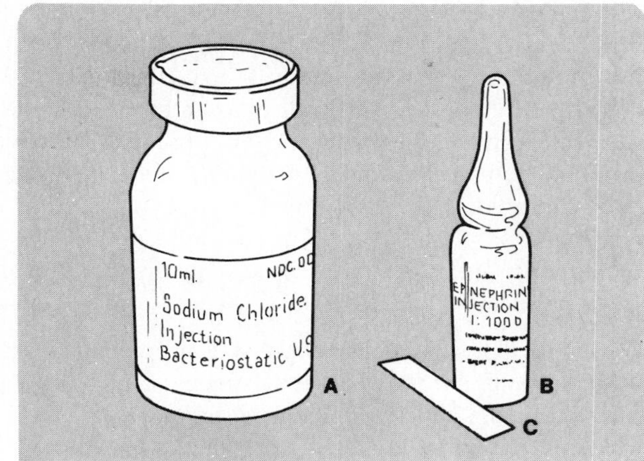

Figure 37–12 **A,** vial; **B,** ampule; and **C,** ampule file.

Mixing Drugs

Frequently patients need more than one drug injected at the same time. To spare the patient the experience of being injected twice, two drugs (if compatible) are often mixed together in one syringe and given as one injection. It is common, for instance, to combine two types of insulin in this manner or to combine injectable preoperative medications such as morphine or meperidine (Demerol) with atropine or scopolamine. Drugs can also be mixed in intravenous solutions. When uncertain about drug compatibilities, the nurse should consult a pharmacist before mixing the drugs.

Mixing drugs from two vials

When withdrawing and mixing medications from two different vials, the nurse takes care not to contaminate the medication remaining in one vial with the other medication. To do this safely, the nurse inserts into vial A a needle attached to a syringe containing the needed volume of air and injects a volume of air equal to the volume of medication to be withdrawn. The tip of the needle must not touch the solution. The nurse withdraws the needle and repeats the procedure with vial B; the nurse again injects a volume of air equal to the volume of medication to be withdrawn. The nurse then withdraws the required amount of medication from vial B. In this way vial B is not contaminated by medication from vial A. The nurse then attaches a new, sterile needle to the syringe, inserts it into vial A, and withdraws the required amount of medication into the syringe. The syringe now contains a mixture of medications from vials A and B and neither vial is contaminated by microorganisms or by medication from the other vial. For information on mixing two types of insulin, see the section on preparing insulin.

Mixing drugs from one vial and one ampule

Because ampules do not require the addition of air prior to withdrawal of the drug, it is recommended that the nurse prepare the medication from the vial first, and then withdraw the medication from the ampule.

Preparing Powdered Drugs

Several drugs, such as penicillin, are dispensed as powders in vials. A liquid (solvent or diluent) must be added to these powders before they can be injected. The technique of adding a solvent to a powdered drug to prepare it for administration is called *reconstitution.*

Powdered drugs usually have printed instructions (enclosed with each packaged vial) that describe the amount and kind of solvent to be added. Commonly used solvents are sterile water or sterile normal saline. Some preparations are supplied in individual-dose vials; others are multidose vials. When multidose vials are reconstituted, the nurse needs to label the vial with the date it was prepared and the amount of drug contained in each milliliter of solution. Once reconstituted, the medication in the vial is usually stored in a refrigerator.

Following are two examples of the preparation of powdered drugs:

1. *Single-dose vial:* Instructions for preparing a single-dose vial direct that 1.5 ml of sterile water be added to the sterile dry powder, thus providing a single dose of 2 ml. The volume of the drug powder was 0.5 ml.
2. *Multidose vial:* A dose of 750 mg of a certain drug is ordered for a patient. On hand is a 10 g multidose vial. The directions for preparation read, "Add 8.5 ml of sterile water, and each milliliter will contain 1.0 g or 1000 mg." Thus after adding the solvent the nurse will give 750/1000 or ¾ ml (0.75 ml) of the medication.

Preparing Insulin

Insulin is prepared in units rather than milligrams or grains. It is available in 40, 80, and 100 units per milliliter of solution. Insulin syringes are described earlier in this chapter. It is essential when preparing insulin that the appropriate calibrations on the syringe be used; for example, the 40 unit scale on the syringe is used only when administering 40 unit insulin and the 80 unit scale only for 80 unit insulin.

Because insulin is watery, the needle gauge used can be as small as possible (26 gauge). Insulin preparations are stored in the refrigerator to prevent deterioration. Preparations that have changed in appearance should never be used, and the solution should be well mixed prior to administration to ensure an accurate concentration and dose. Because shaking the vial can make the medication frothy, a vial of insulin is usually rotated between the palms of the hands and inverted end to end to mix it thoroughly.

Mixing insulin from two vials

There are several types of insulin. They have the same basic action but vary in their time of action. Some act within 2 hours and last for 8 to 10 hours, whereas others act within 6 hours and last for 24 to 36 hours. See Table 37–7 for types of insulin and their actions. Many hospitalized patients are given two types of insulin, short and long acting. These different types vary in content.

Table 37–7 Types of Insulin and Their Actions

Name and classification	Onset of action	Peak action	Duration of action	Time of administration	Time when hypoglycemic reactions can occur
Rapid acting					
Crystalline zinc (CZ)	Within 1 hour	2 to 4 hours	5 to 8 hours	Before meals and when needed	Between meals
Regular	Within 1 hour	2 to 4 hours	5 to 8 hours	↓	Between meals
Semilente	Within 1 hour	6 to 10 hours	12 to 16 hours	Before breakfast	Around lunch
Intermediate acting					
Globin zinc*	Within 2 to 4 hours (faster as dose increases)	6 to 10 hours	18 to 24 hours (longer as dose increases)		Around dinner time or before bedtime
Lente	Within 2 to 4 hours	8 to 12 hours	28 to 32 hours		
Neutral protamine hagedorn (NPH) (Isophane insulin)*	Within 2 to 4	8 to 12 hours	28 to 30 hours		↓
Slow acting					
Protamine zinc (PZ or ZP1)*	4 to 6 hours	16 to 24 hours	24 to 36 hours or more		During night or early morning
Ultralente	8 hours	16 to 24 hours	36 hours or more	↓	↓

*These insulins have a modifying protein added (protamine or globulin).

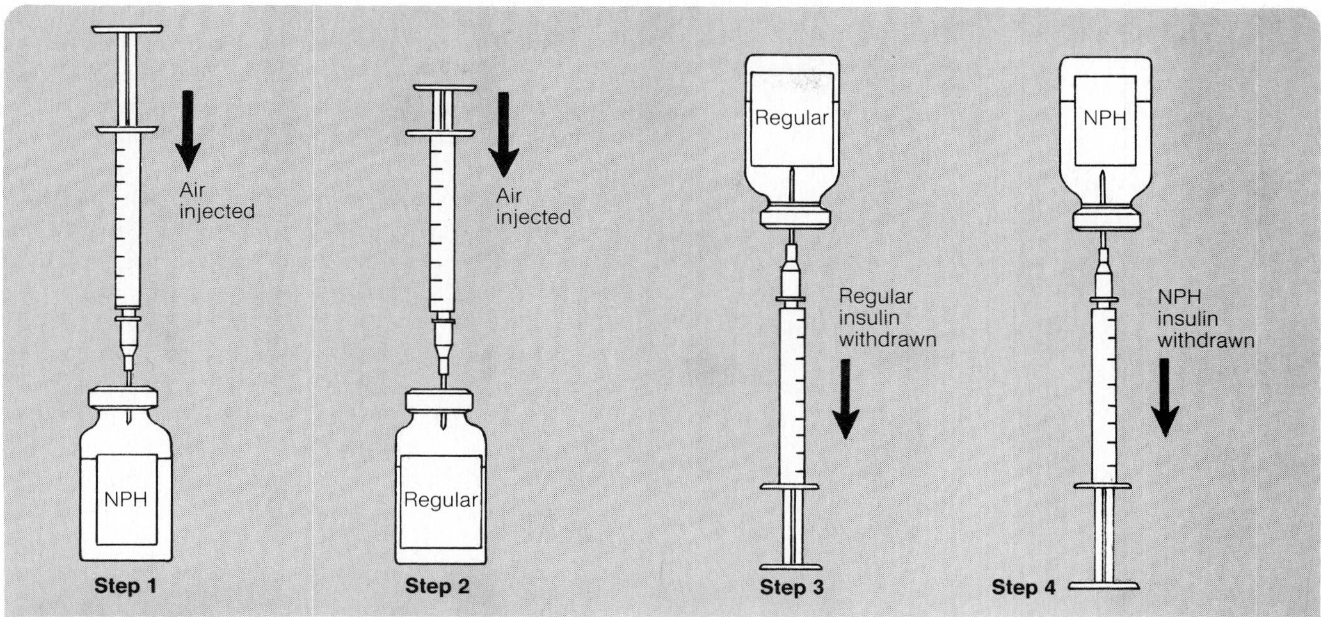

Figure 37–13 Mixing two types of insulin.

Chemically, insulin is a protein that, when hydrolyzed in the body, yields a number of amino acids. Some insulin preparations, in addition, contain a modifying protein, such as globulin or protamine, that slows absorption. This fact is relevant to the mixing of two insulin preparations for injection. Vials of insulins that do *not* have additional protein added should never be contaminated with insulins from vials that contain additional protein. For example, regular insulin (crystalline zinc insulin, CZ) should never be adulterated with other insulin such as protamine zinc, which has added protein.

To prepare two types of insulin in one syringe, the nurse must first inject air into the vial of insulin with protein added, even though this is the insulin drawn into the syringe last.

Example The nurse is to administer 10 units of CZ and 30 units of NPH insulin, which contains protamine, to a patient at 0730 hours.

Step 1. Inject 30 units of air into the NPH vial and withdraw the needle. (There should be no insulin in the needle.) The needle should not touch the insulin.
Step 2. Inject 10 units of air into the CZ vial and immediately withdraw 10 units of CZ insulin.
Step 3. Reinsert the needle into the NPH insulin vial and withdraw 30 units of NPH insulin. (The air was previously injected into the vial.) See Figure 37–13.

By using this method, the nurse does not add NPH insulin to the CZ insulin.

Subcutaneous Injections

Subcutaneous administration is the injection of a drug into the subcutaneous tissue of the body. It is also referred to as hypodermic injection. This method of administration has a number of advantages. The drug is almost completely absorbed from the tissues, provided that blood circulation is normal. Thus the amount of drug absorbed is predictable. The patient's state of consciousness or ability to swallow do not affect subcutaneous injection. The drug administered in this manner generally acts in 30 minutes. The chief disadvantage of this method, as is true of all methods of parenteral administration, is that the skin is broken by the insertion of a needle. Any break in the skin poses the risk of infection, particularly if aseptic technique is not employed.

The sites of the subcutaneous tissue used for a hypodermic injection are usually the outer upper arms or the anterior thighs. These are convenient sites for injections, and they normally offer adequate area and have satisfactory circulation. Patients who administer their own

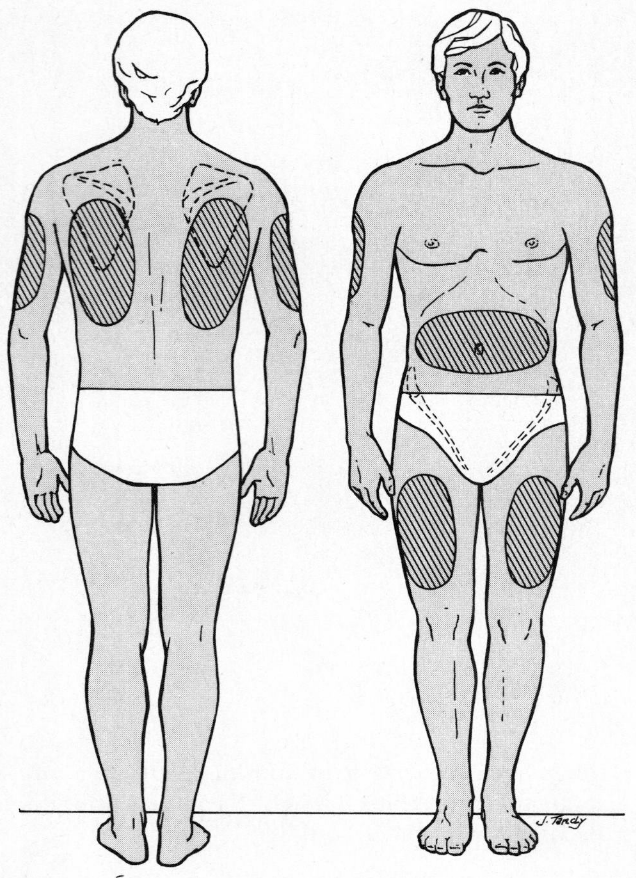

injections, for example, those who have diabetes mellitus, usually use the subcutaneous tissue of the anterior thighs and abdomen. Sites on the upper back below the scapulae are also used by nurses and physicians when administering subcutaneous injections. See Figure 37–14.

It is often advisable to alternate sites if a patient is taking or receiving a number of injections. Patients who administer their own injections must devise a plan for alternative sites. See Figure 37–15.

Figure 37–14 Sites of the body commonly used for subcutaneous injections.

Figure 37–15 A system of alternating injection sites on the body for the administration of insulin. **A,** sites used by the nurse; and **B,** sites used by the patient.

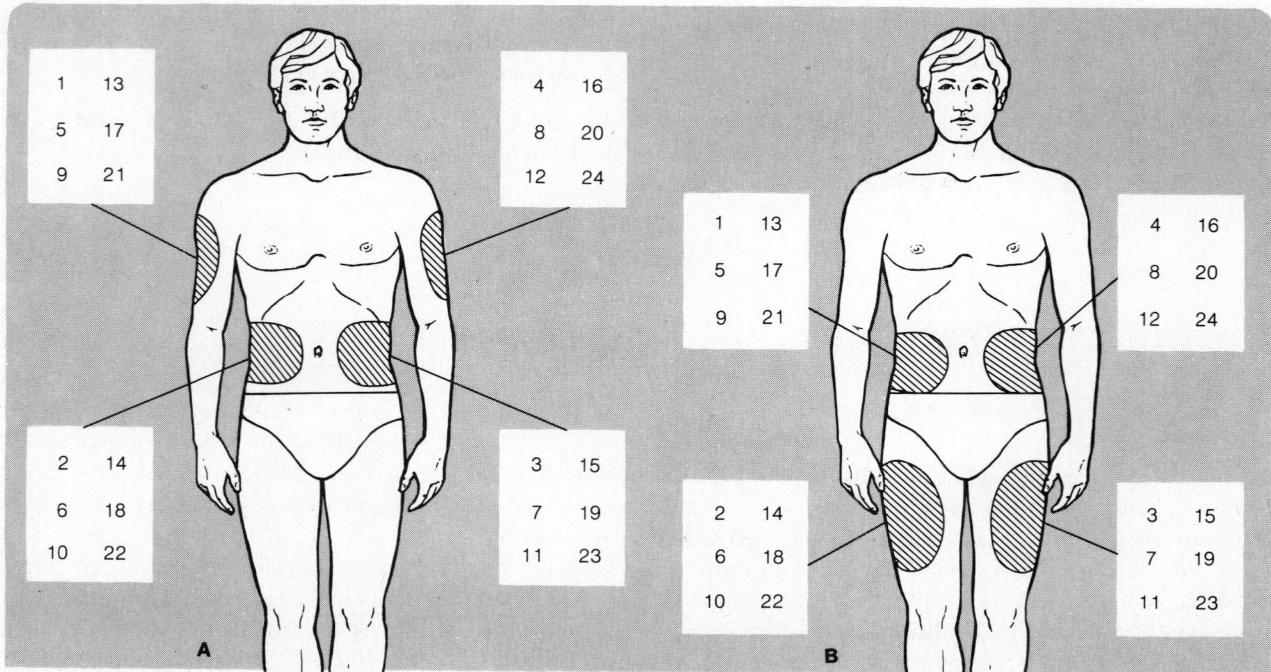

Procedure 37–2 Administering a Subcutaneous Injection

Equipment

Wash hands using a surgical hand wash before assembling the supplies to avoid transmitting microorganisms to the patient or to the sterile equipment.

1. The patient's medication card or list.
2. A vial or ampule of the correct sterile medication.
3. A sterile syringe and needle. Generally a 2 ml syringe and a 25 gauge needle are used for subcutaneous injections. The length of the needle depends on the amount of adipose tissue and the angle used to administer the injection. Generally, a ⅝ inch needle is used for adults when the injection is administered at a 45° angle; a ½ inch needle is used at a 90° angle. Shorter needles, e.g., ⅜ inch, may be used for children, and longer ones, e.g., 1 inch, may be necessary for very obese adults. To determine the appropriate length of the needle for a 90° angle injection, pinch a fold of skin between your thumb and forefinger at the injection site, then measure the width of the skin fold by placing a needle that will not be used for the injection against the skin surface. The appropriate needle length is one-half the width of the skin fold (Pitel 1971). When this method of measuring is used, the needle is inserted without pinching the skin.
4. Sterile disinfectant-soaked swabs to clean the top of a medication vial and the injection site.
5. Dry sterile gauze for opening an ampule.

Preparation

1. Check the medication order. See Procedure 37–1, page 957.
2. Prepare the drug dosage.

From a vial

1. Mix the solution, if necessary, by rotating the vial between the palms of the hands, not by shaking.

   Rationale Some vials contain aqueous suspensions, which settle when they stand. In some instances shaking is contraindicated, because it may cause the mixture to foam. For vials containing only a powder, and requiring the addition of a liquid such as sterile water, the nurse follows the manufacturer's directions. It is important always to withdraw an equivalent volume of air from the vial before adding the fluid.

2. Remove the protective metal cap and clean the rubber seal with a disinfectant, such as 70% alcohol, on sterile gauze. Rub in a rotary motion.

   Rationale The disinfectant cleans the seal so that the needle will not be contaminated when it is inserted.

3. Remove the cap from the needle, taking care to pull the cap straight off to avoid contaminating the needle. See Figure 37–16. Then draw up into the syringe an amount of air equal to the volume of the medication to be withdrawn.
4. Carefully insert the needle into the vial through the center of the rubber cap, maintaining the sterility of the needle.
5. Inject the air into the vial with the bevel of the needle above the surface of the medication.

   Rationale The air creates positive pressure inside the vial, which allows the medication to be drawn out easily. The bevel is kept above the medication to avoid creating bubbles.

6. Invert the vial and hold it at eye level while withdrawing the correct dosage of the drug into the syringe. See Figure 37–17.
7. Withdraw the needle from the vial and replace the cap over the needle, thus maintaining its sterility.

Figure 37–16

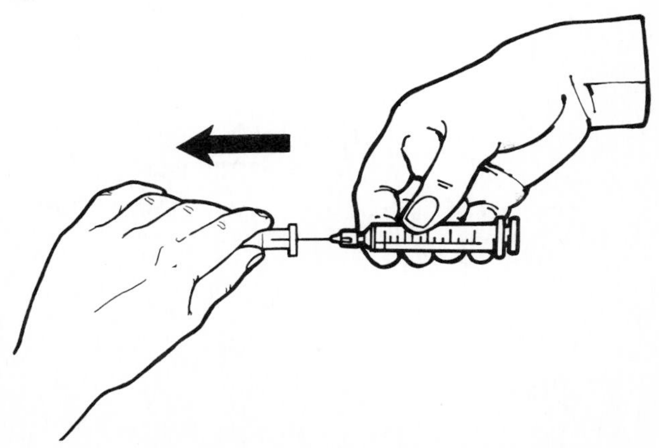

Procedure 37–2, continued

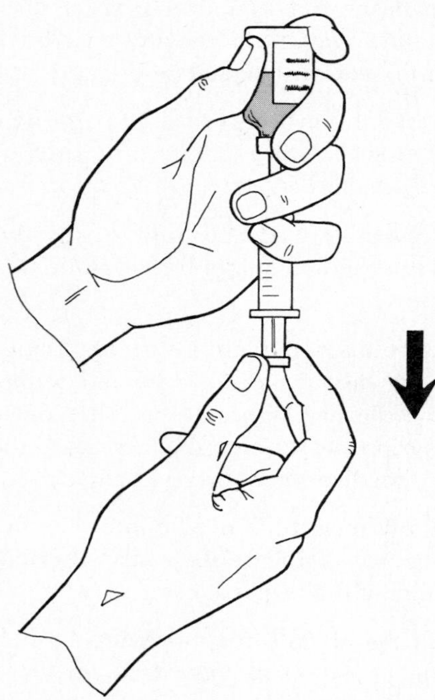

Figure 37–17

8. Place the syringe on the tray or cart.
9. Dispose of the vial or return it to its storage place.

From an ampule

1. Flick the upper stem of the ampule several times with a fingernail.

   Rationale This will bring all the medication down to the main portion of the ampule. Ampules that do not have a very constricted neck may not pose this problem.

Figure 37–18

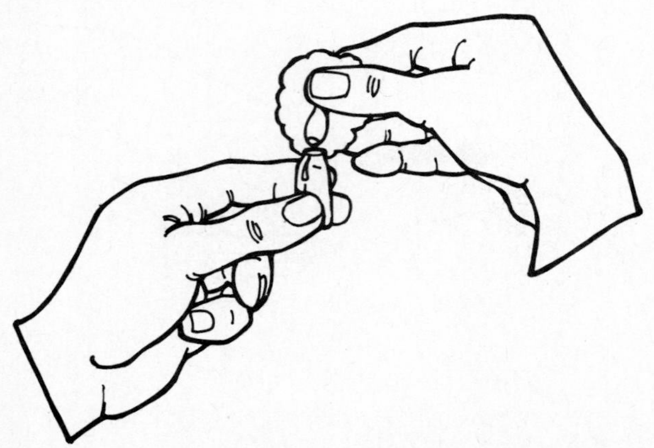

2. File the neck of the ampule if necessary.
3. Place a piece of sterile gauze on the far side of the ampule neck, and break off the top by bending it outward. See Figure 37–18.

   Rationale The sterile gauze protects the nurse's fingers from the glass.

4. Assemble the syringe and needle, if not preassembled. Hold the barrel of the syringe in the middle, and insert the plunger. Maintain sterility except at the uppermost end of the syringe, which is the only part touched by the hand. Attach the needle to the barrel by holding the hub of the needle. Maintain the sterility of the remainder of the needle and the tip of the syringe.
5. Remove the cap from the hypodermic needle, insert the needle in the ampule, and withdraw the amount of drug required for the dosage. If using a single-dose ampule, tip the ampule slightly to obtain all the medication.
6. Cover the needle to maintain its sterility.
7. Place the syringe on the tray or cart.
8. Dispose of the ampule and any unused solution.

Intervention

1. Identify the patient and explain the procedure.
2. Select a site free of tenderness, hardness, swelling, scarring, itching, burning, or localized inflammation. Select a site that has not been used frequently.

   Rationale These conditions could hinder the absorption of the medication. These signs could also increase the likelihood of an infection at the injection site.

3. Provide privacy.

   Rationale The use of some body sites, e.g., the abdomen, necessitates exposure of the patient.

4. As agency policy dictates, clean the site with an antiseptic swab. Start at the center of the site and clean in a widening circle. Allow the area to dry thoroughly. Place the swab between the

Procedure 37–2, continued

third and fourth fingers of the nondominant hand for later use.

Rationale Recommendations differ about the necessity of cleaning the skin prior to injections. Some believe that the antiseptic lessens the number of microorganisms on the skin; others (Dann 1966; Lacey 1968) think that cleaning destroys the normal antibacterial properties of the skin.

5. Remove the needle cap while waiting for the antiseptic to dry. Pull the cap straight off to avoid contaminating the needle.

   Rationale The needle will become contaminated if it touches anything but the inside of the cap, which is sterile.

6. Expel any air bubbles from the syringe by inverting the syringe and gently pushing on the plunger until a drop of solution can be seen in the needle bevel. If air bubbles still remain, flick the side of the syringe barrel.

   or

   When it is important that the entire amount of medication be administered, leave 0.2 ml of air in the syringe (Wong 1982:1237).

   Rationale This small amount of air ensures that only air remains in the needle bore and that all the medication is injected into the patient.

7. Grasp the syringe in your dominant hand by holding it between your thumb and fingers with your palm facing upward for a 45° angle insertion or with the palm downward for a 90° angle insertion. See Figure 37–19.

8. Using the nondominant hand, pinch or spread the skin at the site, and pierce it with the bevel upward for a 45° angle (see Figure 37–20), using a firm steady push.

   Rationale Recommendations vary about whether to pinch or spread the skin. Pinching the skin is thought to desensitize the area somewhat and thus lessen the sensation of needle insertion. Spreading the skin can make it firmer and facilitate needle insertion. Some recommend neither pinching nor spreading the skin (Pitel 1971). The nurse needs to judge which method to use depending on the patient's tissue firmness.

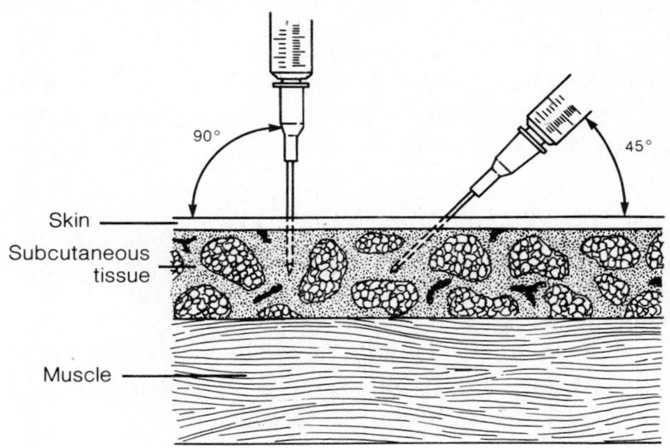

Figure 37–19

9. When the needle is inserted, move your nondominant hand to the barrel of the syringe and your dominant hand to the end of the plunger.

10. Aspirate by pulling back on the plunger. If blood appears in the syringe, withdraw the needle, discard the syringe, and prepare a new injection. If blood does not appear, continue to administer the medication.

Figure 37–20

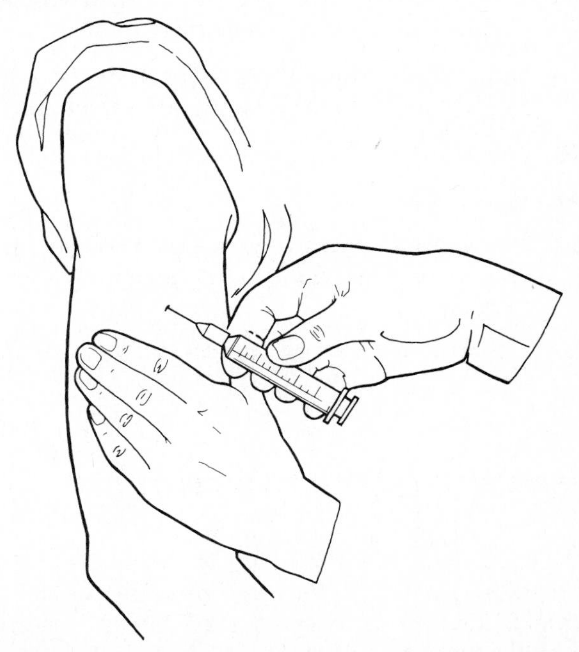

Procedure 37–2, continued

Rationale This step determines whether the needle has entered a blood vessel. Subcutaneous medications may be dangerous if placed directly into the bloodstream; they are intended for the subcutaneous tissues, where they are absorbed more slowly.

11. Inject the medication by holding the syringe steady and depressing the plunger with a slow, even pressure.

    Rationale Holding the syringe steady and injecting the medication at an even pressure minimizes discomfort for the patient.

12. Remove the needle quickly, pulling along the line of insertion and supporting the tissues with your nondominant hand.

    Rationale This step minimizes the patient's discomfort.

13. Massage the site lightly with a sterile disinfectant soaked swab or apply slight pressure.

    Rationale Massage is thought to disperse the medication in the tissues and facilitate its absorption.

14. If bleeding occurs, apply pressure to the site until it stops. Bleeding rarely occurs after subcutaneous injection.

15. Dispose of supplies according to agency procedure. Needle covers should be reapplied.

    Rationale Proper disposal protects the nurse and others from injury and contamination.

16. Assist the patient to a comfortable position.

17. Wash hands.

18. Record the medication given, dosage, time, route, any complaints of the patient, and your signature.

19. Replace supplies as appropriate.

20. Assess the effectiveness of the medication 15 to 30 minutes after the injection or as appropriate, depending on the medication.

Variations for a heparin injection

The subcutaneous administration of heparin requires special precautions because of its anticoagulant properties.

1. Select a site on the abdomen above the level of the iliac crests.

   Rationale These areas are away from major muscles and are not involved in muscular activity, as the arms and legs are; thus, the possibility of hematoma is reduced.

2. Use a ½ inch, 25 or 26 gauge needle, and insert it at a 90° angle. Draw 0.1 ml of air into the syringe when preparing the heparin, and inject it after the heparin.

   Rationale This step fills the needle with air and prevents any leakage of heparin into the intradermal layers when the needle is inserted and when the needle is withdrawn, thus minimizing the possibility of a hematoma.

3. Check agency practices regarding aspiration.

   Rationale Some agencies recommend that the nurse not aspirate to determine whether a blood vessel has been entered, because this causes the needle to move and increases the possibility of hematoma formation. Small blood vessels may rupture, causing bleeding and severe bruising.

4. Do not massage the site after the injection.

5. Alternate sites of subsequent injections.

Intramuscular Injections

The intramuscular injection route is ordered frequently for medications that irritate subcutaneous tissue, for example, penicillin and paraldehyde. Also, the speed of absorption is faster than by the subcutaneous route because of the greater blood supply to the body muscles. Muscles can usually take a larger volume of fluid without discomfort than subcutaneous tissues, although the amount varies among people, chiefly with muscle size and condition.

Only healthy muscles should be used for injections.

A normal, healthy muscle has the following characteristics:

1. It is soft when relaxed and firm when tensed.
2. The relaxed muscle has no palpable hardened masses.
3. Firm palpation is not uncomfortable to the patient.

If a muscle is painful to touch or if there are any hardened areas, using that muscle for an injection is usually contraindicated. Areas with complications such as abscesses, necrotic and sloughing tissue including skin, and damaged nerves and bones are to be avoided. During the injection, damage to a nerve can cause the patient pain and perhaps permanent disability. Damage to bones by a needle can result in an inflammatory reaction such as periostitis (inflammation of the periosteum of the bone), but this is extremely rare even when a bone is struck during an injection. These complications are the chief disadvantages of using intramuscular injections.

The exact amount of medication that any muscle can comfortably absorb at once will vary, but usually 3 ml is considered the maximum for a large muscle. Babies, the elderly, and emaciated patients are usually unable to tolerate this amount; usually 2 ml is the maximum volume for them. Nurses must use their own judgment as to the safe maximum volume, considering (a) size of the muscle, (b) health of the muscle, (c) adequacy of the blood supply, and (d) viscosity or irritant properties of the drug.

Sites

Selecting the appropriate site for an intramuscular injection is critical. Not only should a large, healthy muscle be used, but also the site should have no large nerves or blood vessels and be free of infection and abrasions. When a person is to receive several injections, it is essential to alternate sites to avoid overusing and irritating one muscle. For babies and very young children the quadriceps muscles on the anterior and lateral aspects of the thighs are the sites of choice. The gluteal muscles of babies and children who cannot yet walk are not sufficiently well developed to receive injections. The proximity of the large sciatic nerve and the danger of damaging it usually mitigate against placing injections in the gluteal muscles of children younger than 3 years.

Dorsogluteal

The dorsogluteal site is in the thick muscles of the buttocks. The injection site must be chosen carefully to avoid striking the sciatic nerve, major blood vessels, or bone. There are two methods of establishing the exact site, which is the upper outer aspect of the upper outer quadrant of the buttock, about 5 to 8 cm (2 to 3 in) below the crest of the ilium:

1. Divide the buttock into imaginary quadrants as in Figure 37–21. The vertical line extends from the crest of the ilium to the gluteal fold. The horizontal line extends from the medial fold to the lateral aspect of the buttock. Locate the upper outer aspect of the upper outer quadrant. It is important to palpate the crest of the ilium so that the site chosen is high enough. Visual calculations alone can result in an injection that is too low and injures the patient.
2. Palpate the posterior superior iliac spine, then draw an imaginary line to the greater trochanter of the femur. This line parallels the sciatic nerve. The injection site is lateral and superior to this line. See Figure 37–22.

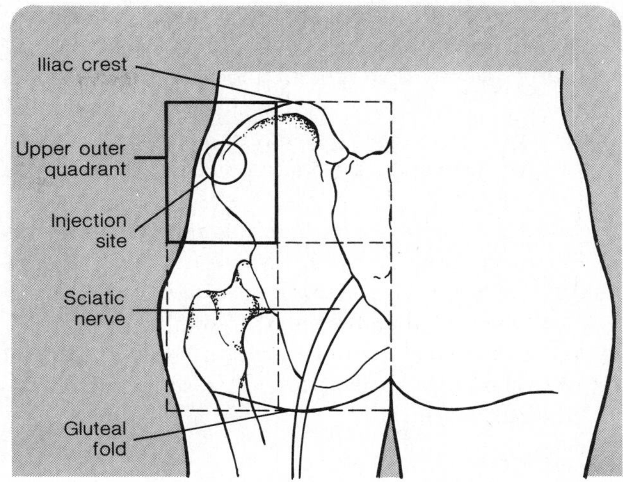

Figure 37–21 One method for establishing the dorsogluteal site for an intramuscular injection.

Figure 37–22 A second method for establishing the dorsogluteal site for an intramuscular injection.

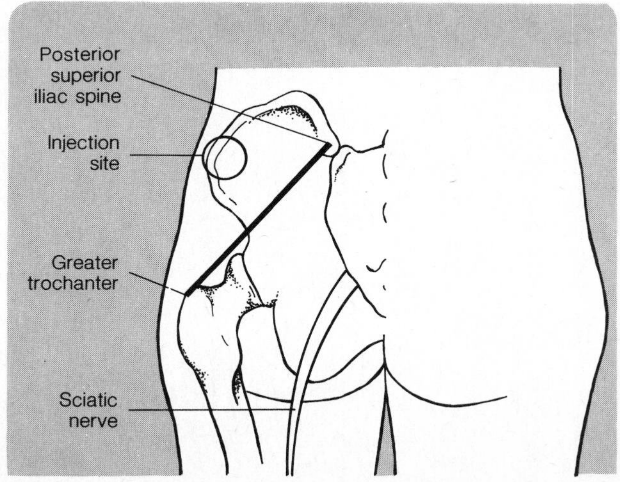

In the past, the dorsogluteal was the site most commonly used for intramuscular injections. However, because some people have difficulty locating it, this site is losing favor. Only those with well-developed gluteal muscles can receive injections in this site. Because these muscles are developed by walking, it is generally not used for children under 3 years.

To administer an injection into this site, the nurse has the patient assume a prone position with the toes pointing medially. A side-lying position can also be used, with the upper leg flexed at the thigh and the knee and placed in front of the lower leg. Both these positions promote relaxation of the gluteal muscles, which reduces the pain of injection.

Ventrogluteal

The ventrogluteal site (von Hochstetter's site) is in the gluteus medius muscle, which lies over the gluteus minimus. This site is gaining favor because the area has no large nerves or blood vessels and less fat than the buttock. It is also farther from the rectal area and tends to be less contaminated, an important factor if the patient is incontinent.

To establish the exact site, the nurse places the palm of the hand on the greater trochanter, with the fingers toward the patient's head. The right hand is used for the left hip, and the left hand for the right hip. The nurse places the index finger on the anterior superior iliac spine and extends the middle finger dorsally, palpating the crest of the ilium and then pressing below it. The injection site is in the center of the triangle formed by the index finger, the third finger, and the crest of the ilium. See Figure 37–23.

This site is suitable for both children and adults. The patient can assume a back- or side-lying position, with the knee and hip flexed to relax the gluteal muscles.

Figure 37–23 The ventrogluteal site for an intramuscular injection.

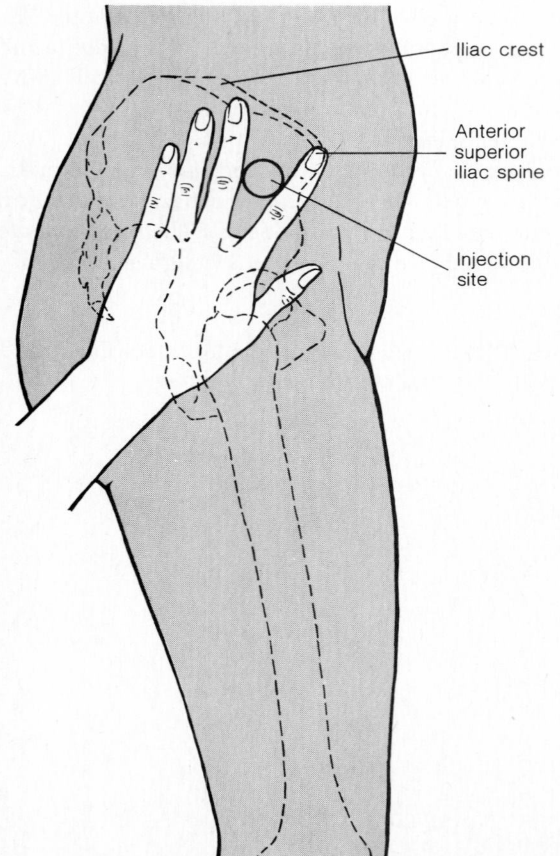

Vastus lateralis

The vastus lateralis muscle is usually thick and well developed in both adults and children. It is increasingly recommended as the site of choice for intramuscular injections because there are no major blood vessels or nerves in the area. It is situated on the anterior lateral aspect of the thigh. The middle third of the muscle is the suggested site. It is established by dividing the area between the greater trochanter of the femur and the lateral femoral condyle into thirds and selecting the middle third. See Figure 37–24.

The patient can assume a back-lying or a sitting position during an injection into this site. For young children, the muscle is bunched before injection.

Rectus femoris

The rectus femoris muscle, in the quadriceps muscle group, can also be used for intramuscular injections. This site is on the anterior aspect of the thigh. See Figure 37–25. It can be used for infants, children, and adults when other sites are contraindicated. Its chief advantage is that the patient who administers his or her own injections can reach this site easily. Its main disadvantage is that an injection here causes some people considerable discomfort if the muscle is not well developed.

The patient assumes a sitting or back-lying position for an injection at this site.

Deltoid and triceps

The deltoid site is on the lateral aspect of the upper arm. It is not used often for intramuscular injections, because it is a relatively small muscle and very close to the radial nerve and radial artery. To locate the densest

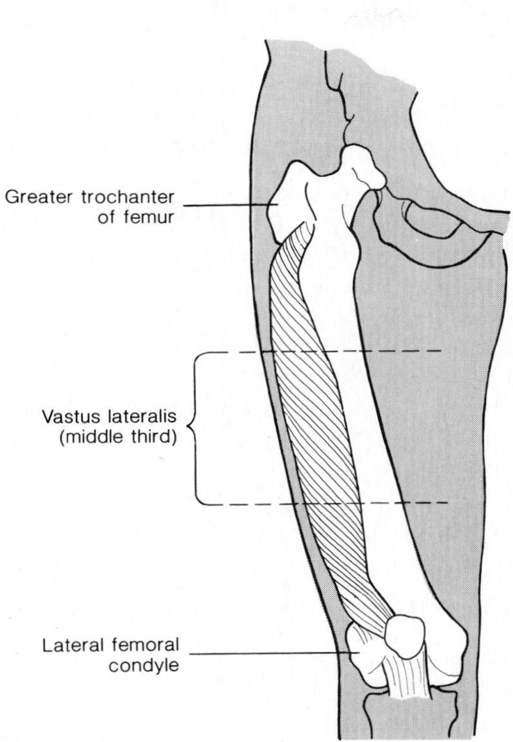

Figure 37–24 The vastus lateralis site for an intramuscular injection.

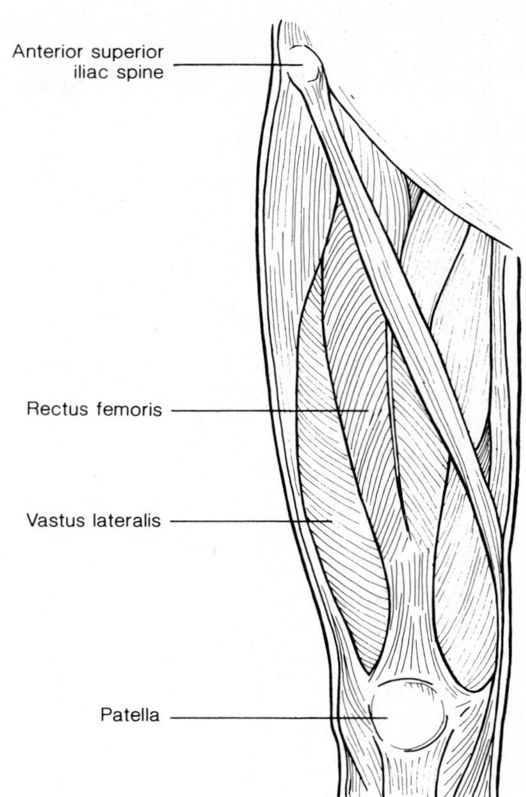

Figure 37–25 The rectus femoris muscle of the upper right thigh, used for intramuscular injections.

part of the muscle, the nurse palpates the lower edge of the acromial process and the midpoint, in line with the axilla, of the lateral aspect of the arm. A triangle within these boundaries approximates the location of the deltoid muscle, about 5 cm (2 in) below the acromial process. See Figure 37–26.

The lateral head of the triceps muscle on the posterior aspect of the upper arm can also be used as an injection site. The site of choice is about midway between the acromial process and the olecranon process of the ulna (the elbow). This site is not often used unless other sites are contraindicated.

Sitting or lying positions can be assumed for injections into deltoid and triceps sites.

Figure 37–26 The deltoid muscle of the upper arm, used for intramuscular injections.

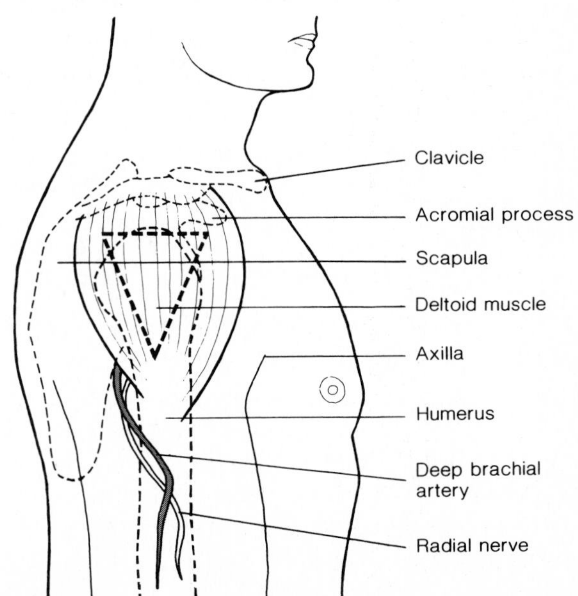

Procedure 37–3 Administering an Intramuscular Injection

Equipment

Wash hands using a surgical hand wash before assembling the supplies to avoid transmitting microorganisms to the patient or to the sterile equipment. The following supplies are needed:

1. The medication card or the patient's chart.
2. The sterile medication. This is usually provided in an ampule or vial. See Procedure 37–2.
3. A sterile syringe and needle. Choose the size of syringe appropriate for the amount of solution to be administered. Usually a 2 to 5 ml syringe is needed. Some medications, such as paraldehyde, require a glass syringe, because the medication interacts with plastic. The size and length of the needle are determined by the muscle to be used, the type of solution, the amount of adipose tissue covering the muscle, and the age of the patient. A large muscle such as the gluteus medius usually requires a 20 to 23 gauge needle, 1½ to 3 inches long, whereas the deltoid muscle requires a smaller, 23 to 25 gauge needle, ⅝ to 1 inch long. Oily solutions such as paraldehyde require a thicker needle, e.g., 21 gauge instead of 23 gauge. Also, the greater the amount of adipose tissue over the muscle, the longer the needle must be to reach the muscle. Therefore, 3 inch needles may be needed for obese patients, whereas 1½ inch needles are used for thinner people. Infants and young children usually require smaller, shorter needles such as 22 to 25 gauge, ⅝ inch to 1 inch long.
4. A swab saturated in an antiseptic solution for cleaning the site.
5. Dry sterile gauze, if an ampule must be opened.

Preparation

1. Check the medication order. See Procedure 37–1.
2. Prepare the correct dosage of the drug from a vial or ampule. See Procedure 37–2.

If the medication is particularly irritating to subcutaneous tissue, the nurse changes the needle on the syringe before the injection. Because the outside of the new needle is free of medication, it does not irritate subcutaneous tissues as it passes into the muscle.

Intervention

1. Identify the patient and explain the procedure. See Procedure 37–1, Intervention steps 1 and 2.
2. Select the intramuscular site for adequate muscle mass. The skin surface over the site should be free of bruises, abrasions, and infection. Determine if the size of the muscle is appropriate to the amount of medication to be injected. An average adult's deltoid muscle can usually absorb 0.5 to 2 ml of medication, whereas the gluteus medius muscle can absorb 1 to 5 ml (Newton and Newton 1979:19), although 5 ml may be very painful. The site should not have been used frequently. If injections are to be frequent, sites should be alternated.
3. Provide privacy if the patient will be exposed.

   Rationale Exposure of the body may embarrass the patient.
4. Establish the exact site for the injection and explain to the patient. See the discussion of sites earlier in this chapter.
5. Clean the site with an antiseptic swab. Using a circular motion, start at the center and move outward about 5 cm (2 in).
6. Remove the needle cover. See Procedure 37–2.
7. Invert the syringe and expel any excess air that has accidentally entered the syringe, leaving only 0.2 to 0.3 ml of air. It may be necessary to flick the syringe to move the bubbles out. The remaining air will rise to the plunger end when the needle is pointed downward.

   Rationale The amount of air should be sufficient to clear medication from the bore of the needle.
8. Use the nondominant hand to spread the skin at the site.

   Rationale Spreading the skin makes it firmer and facilitates needle insertion. Under some circumstances, e.g., when the patient is emaciated or an infant, the muscle may be bunched.
9. Holding the syringe between the thumb and forefinger, pierce the skin quickly at a 90°

Procedure 37–3, continued

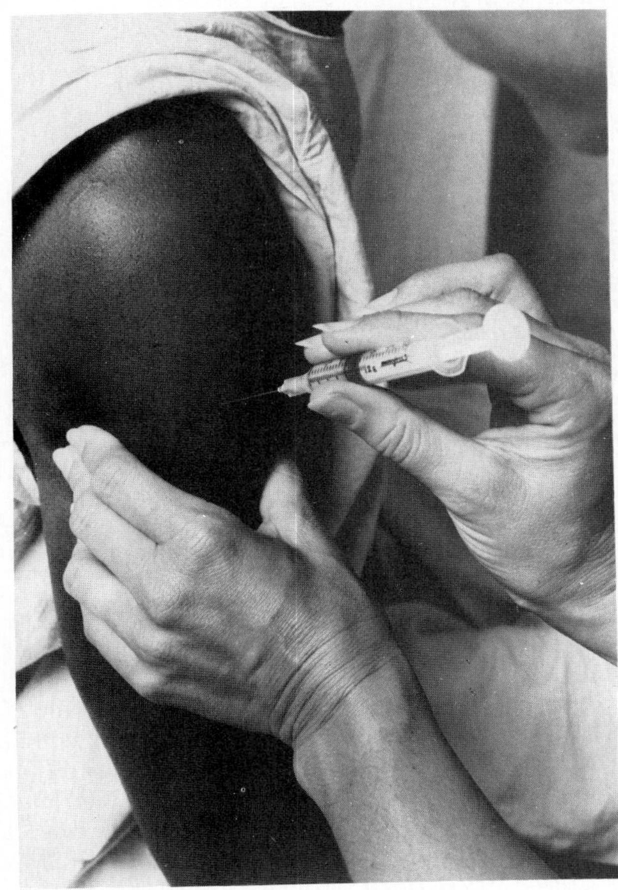

Figure 37–27

angle (see Figure 37–27) and insert the needle into the muscle (see Figure 37–28).

Rationale Using a quick motion lessens the patient's discomfort.

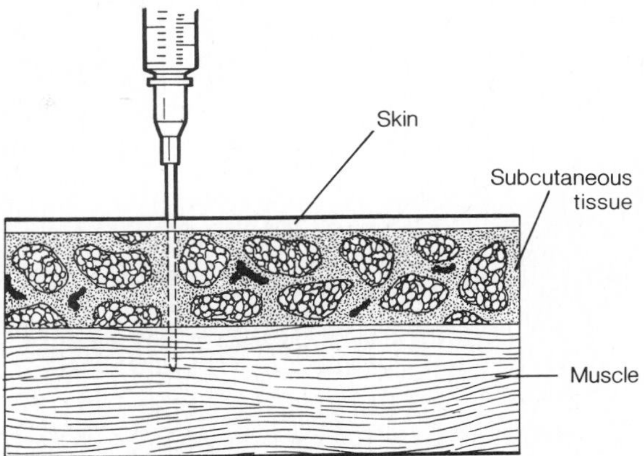

Figure 37–28

10. Aspirate by pulling back on the plunger. If blood appears in the syringe, withdraw the needle, discard the syringe, and prepare a new injection.

Rationale This step determines whether the needle is in a blood vessel.

11. If blood does not appear, inject the medication steadily and slowly, holding the syringe steady.

Rationale Injecting medication slowly permits it to disperse into the muscle tissue, thus decreasing the patient's discomfort. Holding the syringe steady minimizes discomfort.

12. See steps 12 through 20, Procedure 37–2, for withdrawing the needle, massaging the site, disposing of supplies, recording, and conducting follow-up assessment.

Intramuscular Variation (Z-Track)

A Z-track intramuscular injection is a special technique used to administer intramuscular medications that are highly irritating to subcutaneous and skin tissues. The technique is the same as the technique for an intramuscular injection, except that the skin and subcutaneous tissue at the site of the injection are pulled about 2.5 to 3.5 cm (1 to 1½ in) to one side of the site before the needle is inserted. See Figure 37–29, *A*. Traction is maintained for 10 seconds before the needle is removed. During this time, muscle tissues relax and begin to absorb the medication. When the skin returns to its normal position, the needle track is interrupted, and the medication does not seep into the needle track or subcutaneous tissue. See Figure 37–29, *B*. The site is not massaged because massage might cause seepage into delicate tissue.

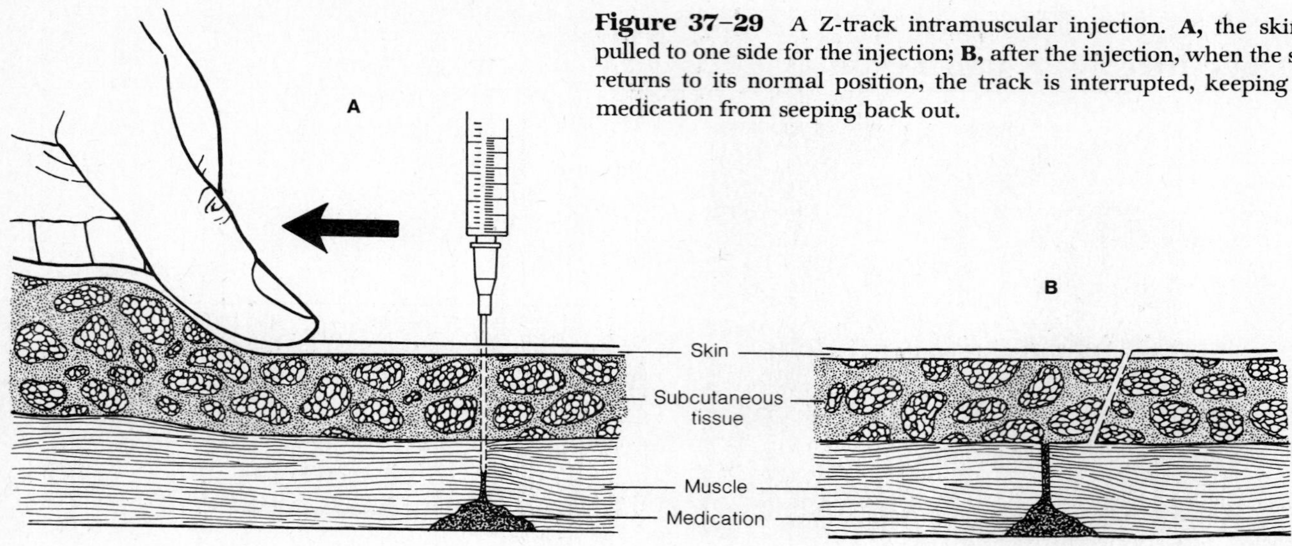

Figure 37–29 A Z-track intramuscular injection. **A,** the skin is pulled to one side for the injection; **B,** after the injection, when the skin returns to its normal position, the track is interrupted, keeping the medication from seeping back out.

Intradermal Injection

An intradermal (intracutaneous) injection is the administration of a drug into the dermal layer of the skin just beneath the epidermis. Usually only a small amount of liquid is used, for example, 0.1 ml. This method of administration is frequently indicated for allergy and tuberculin tests and for vaccinations.

Common sites for intradermal injections are the inner lower arm, the upper chest, and the back beneath the scapulae. See Figure 37–30.

The equipment normally used is a 1 ml syringe calibrated into hundredths of a milliliter. The needle is short and fine, frequently a 25, 26, or 27 gauge, ¼ inch to ⅝ inch long. The preparation is similar to that for a subcutaneous injection.

After the site is cleaned, the skin is held tautly, and the syringe is held at about a 15° angle to the skin, with the bevel of the needle upward. The bevel is thrust through the epidermis into the dermis, and then the fluid is injected. The drug produces a small bleb just under the skin. See Figure 37–31. The needle is then withdrawn quickly, and the site is very lightly wiped with an antiseptic swab. The area is not massaged because the medication may disperse into the tissue or out through the needle insertion site. Intradermal injections are absorbed slowly through blood capillaries in the area.

Figure 37–30 Sites of the body commonly used for intradermal injections.

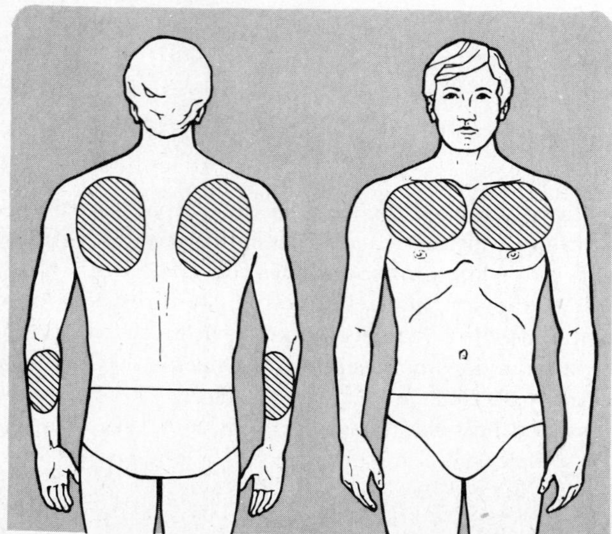

Figure 37–31 For an intradermal injection: **A,** the needle enters the skin at a 15° angle; and **B,** the medication forms a bleb under the epidermis.

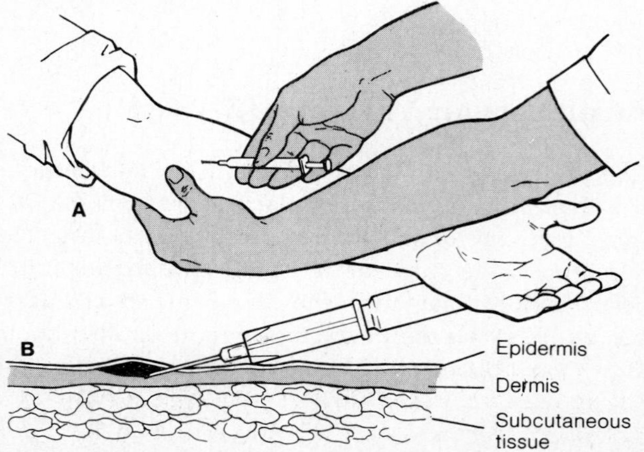

Intravenous Medications

Medications are administered intravenously via:

1. Intravenous bottle or bag
2. Volume-control administration set
3. Additional intravenous container
4. Intravenous push (bolus)

Because IV medications enter the patient's bloodstream directly, they are appropriate when a rapid effect is required (e.g., in a life-threatening situation such as a cardiac arrest). The IV route is appropriate when medications are too irritating to tissues to be given by other routes, e.g., levarterenol bitartrate (Levophed) for acute hypotension. When an IV line is already established, this route is desirable because it avoids the discomfort of other parenteral routes.

There are, however, potential hazards in giving IV medications: infection and rapid, severe reactions to the medication. To prevent infection, sterile technique is used during all aspects of IV medication techniques. To safeguard the patient against severe reactions, the nurse must administer the drug slowly, taking several minutes and following the manufacturer's recommendations. The patient is assessed closely during the administration, and the medication is discontinued immediatelv if an untoward reaction occurs. Common signs of an adverse reaction are: noisy respirations, changes in pulse rate, chills, nausea, and headache. If any adverse signs occur, the nurse notifies the physician or responsible nurse.

The patient is also assessed for signs of problems associated with IV therapy, such as an infection at the IV site or fluid infiltration. For information about techniques for administering IV medications, see Kozier and Erb (1982:1109–23).

Topical Applications

Dermatologic Medications

Dermatologic medications are commonly applied for one of the following reasons:

1. To decrease itching (pruritus)
2. To lubricate and soften the skin
3. To cause local vasoconstriction or vasodilation
4. To increase or decrease secretions from the skin
5. To provide a protective coating to the skin
6. To apply an antibiotic or antiseptic to treat or prevent infection

Inunction is the application of topical drugs meant to be absorbed through the epidermis. Such drugs must be rubbed in. Drugs are not readily absorbed through the epidermis; however, they can be absorbed into the lining of the sebaceous glands and sweat pores. Absorption is facilitated by washing the area well before the application, using a pharmaceutical preparation with a base, such as alcohol, that mixes with fat, and using a drug that is fat soluble.

Dermatologic preparations include lotions, emollients, liniments, ointments, pastes, and powders.

Lotions

Lotions are liquids that often contain an insoluble powder, e.g., calamine lotion, and need to be shaken before use. Lotions may have a soothing effect on the skin or may be mildly acid or alkaline. The lotion is poured onto sterile gauzes or cotton balls and patted onto the affected area. Lotions are not rubbed on because rubbing irritates the rash or pruritus for which the lotion is applied.

Emollients

Emollients also soothe the skin or mucous membranes. Emollients are fatty or oily substances, e.g., olive oil or liquid petrolatum, to which medications are sometimes added. Examples of emollients are lanolin, petroleum jelly, and cold cream; they are applied in the same manner as lotions.

Liniments

Liniments are liquids that usually contain an *anodyne* (pain reliever) or a *rubefacient* (agent that reddens the skin). Liniments are frequently applied to stimulate circulation to an area by vasodilatation of the capillaries. The nurse pours some liniment into the hands and rubs it into the patient's skin with long, firm, smooth strokes. Gloves are normally not indicated for the application of a liniment. Liniment should be at room temperature. A cold liniment causes discomfort and vasoconstriction of the area rather than dilation.

Ointments

Ointments are semisolid preparations of a medication in a base, e.g., petrolatum. Some ointments are soothing, others are antimicrobial or astringent. Ointments are usually applied with a tongue blade or with gloves if the area is large. Sterile technique is essential if there are open wounds, and the nurse wears gloves if the patient has infected skin areas. Gloves protect the nurse and prevent transmission of organisms. The ointment is taken out of the jar with a sterile tongue blade and placed on sterile gauze. Once the ointment is removed from the jar, the cap is replaced. The nurse spreads the ointment with a second tongue blade or sterile gloved hand. The affected area should be well but not overly covered. If the ointment is opaque, no skin should be visible through the medicine. Some ointments, such as cortisone preparations, need to be applied very thinly. Sterile dressings are often applied over the area so that the patient does not inadvertently wipe off the ointment and soil his or her clothes.

Pastes

Pastes are similar to ointments but tend to absorb secretions and penetrate the skin less than ointments. An example is zinc oxide paste, which is used to protect excoriated areas from urine and feces. Pastes are applied in the same manner as ointments.

Powders

Powders are nonabsorbable finely ground medications, usually applied to protect the skin. Examples are talcum powder and cornstarch. The disadvantages of powders are that they do not adhere to dry skin surfaces and tend to cake on moist surfaces. A powder is generally sprinkled on the area, usually after cleaning, and then covered with a dressing so that it will stay on the site.

Figure 37–32 Instilling eye drops onto the lower conjunctival sac.

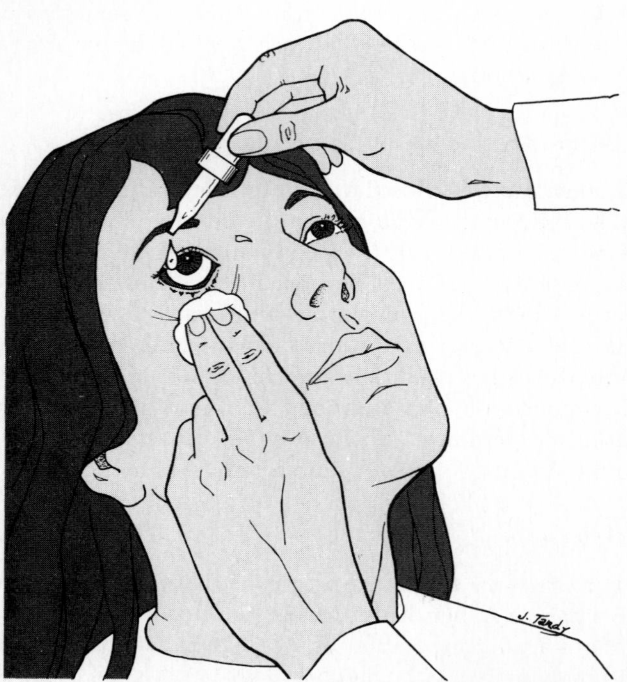

Ophthalmic Instillations

Instillation of eye drops

The patient assumes a sitting position with the head slightly hyperextended and holds a tissue to soak up the excess medication that leaves the eye. The nurse wipes the lids and lashes gently from the inner to the outer canthus with a cotton ball dampened with saline solution.

The nurse instructs the patient to look at the ceiling and exposes the lower conjunctival sac by placing several fingers on the patient's cheek just below the affected eye and drawing the skin downward. Using a side approach, the nurse brings a dropper filled with the eye medication over the conjunctival sac and instills the ordered number of drops in the center or outer part of the lower conjunctival sac. The dropper should be 1 to 2 cm above the sac. See Figure 37–32. The dropper should touch neither the cornea nor the mucous membrane of the conjunctival sac. The skin is permitted to return to its normal position, and the patient asked to close the eye gently, not squeeze it shut. Closing the eye spreads the medication over the eyeball. With a cotton ball or gauze swab, the nurse presses firmly on the nasolacrimal duct for several seconds before the eye is closed, to prevent medication from running out of the eye down the duct. Finally, the nurse wipes the eyelids gently from the inner to the outer canthus to remove excess medication and, if needed, applies an eye pad and secures it with tape.

Instillation of eye ointment

For the insertion of an ointment into the eye, the patient assumes the same position and the nurse draws down the lower lid as described in the section on instillation of eye drops. Holding the ointment tube in the other hand, the nurse approaches the eye from below, and squeezes about 2 cm of ointment from the tube onto the conjunctival sac, moving from the inner aspect to the lateral aspect. See Figure 37–33. The patient closes the eye and moves it to spread the ointment unless this is contraindicated.

Otic Instillations

Some ear instillations treat disease or relieve pain, but many otic instillations are softening agents that aid the removal of ear wax. The prescribed medication, the medicine dropper, and the medicine card are required.

The patient assumes a side-lying position with the ear being treated uppermost. The nurse wipes the external auditory meatus with a cotton-tipped applicator and straightens the ear canal, as follows: If the patient is an adult, or child over 3, the nurse pulls the auricle up and back; if a child under 3 years, downward and backward. The prescribed drops are normally instilled at room temperature. Following the instillation, the tragus of the ear is pressed two or three times to move the drops inward, unless contraindicated. See Figure 37–34. The patient remains in the side-lying position for about 5 minutes. This position prevents the drops from escaping and allows medication to reach all sides of the canal cavity. A small piece of cotton fluff is inserted loosely into the meatus of the auditory canal for 15 to 20 minutes; the cotton should not be pressed into the canal. A piece of cotton at the meatus helps retain the medication in the ear when the patient is up. If pressed tightly into the canal, the cotton interferes with the action of the drug and the outward movement of normal secretions.

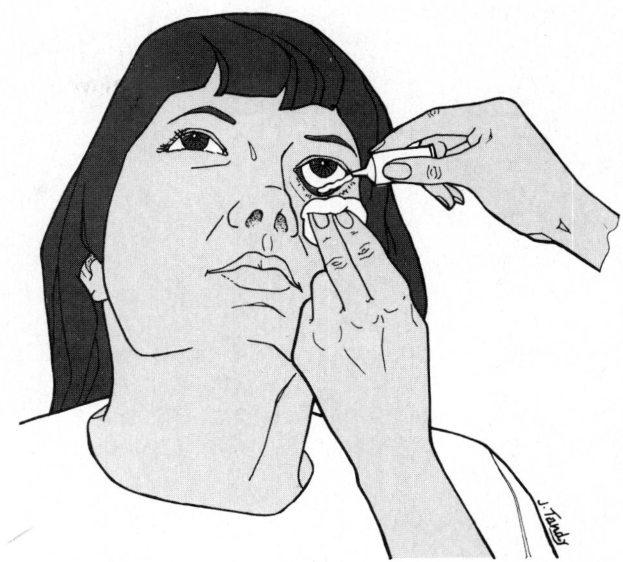

Figure 37–33 Instilling eye ointment onto the lower conjunctival sac.

Nasal Instillations

Usually nose drops are instilled for their astringent effect (to shrink swollen mucous membranes) or to treat infections of the nasal cavity or sinuses. The equipment required is the medication solution, which usually comes in a bottle with an attached dropper, disposable tissues, and a tray for the equipment. Prior to the instillation, the patient blows the nose to clear the nasal passages.

The patient assumes a back-lying position. For treating the opening of the eustachian (auditory) tube, the patient can assume a dorsal recumbent position. The drops flow into the pharynx, where the eustachian tube opens. To treat the ethmoid and sphenoid sinuses, the nurse has the patient assume a back-lying position with the head over the edge of the bed or a pillow under the shoulders so that the head is tipped backward. This is the Proetz position. See Figure 37–35. To treat the maxillary and frontal sinuses, the nurse has the patient assume the same back-lying position, with the head turned toward the side to be treated. This is the Parkinson position. See Figure 37–36. The nurse makes sure that the patient is positioned so that the correct side is accessible if only one side is to be treated. If the patient's head is over the edge of the bed, it must be supported by the nurse's hands so that the neck muscles are not strained.

Once the patient has assumed one of the above positions, the nurse administers the drops. The dropper is held just above the nostril, and the drops are directed toward the midline of the superior concha of the ethmoid bone as the patient breathes through his or her mouth. If the drops are directed toward the base of the nasal cavity, they will run down the eustachian tube. The mucous membranes of the nostrils should not be touched to avoid injury to tissue and contamination of the dropper. The nurse has the patient remain in this position for 5 to 10 minutes so that the solution will flow into the desired area. The nurse discards medication remaining in the dropper before returning the dropper to the bottle.

To administer nose drops to an infant, the nurse places a pillow under the infant's shoulders and allows the child's head to fall back slightly over the edge of the

Figure 37–34 Following an otic instillation, the tragus is pressed two or three times.

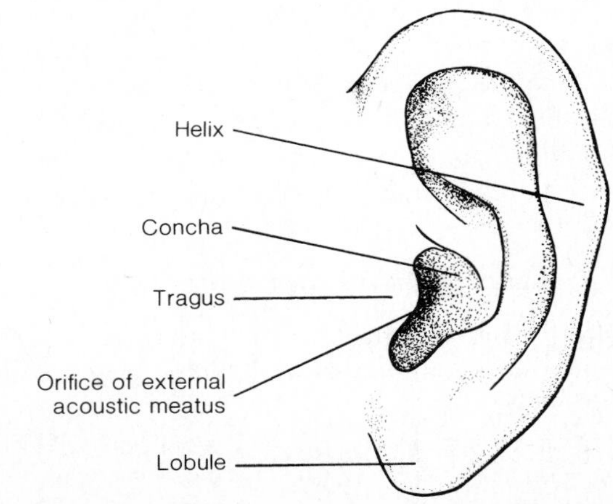

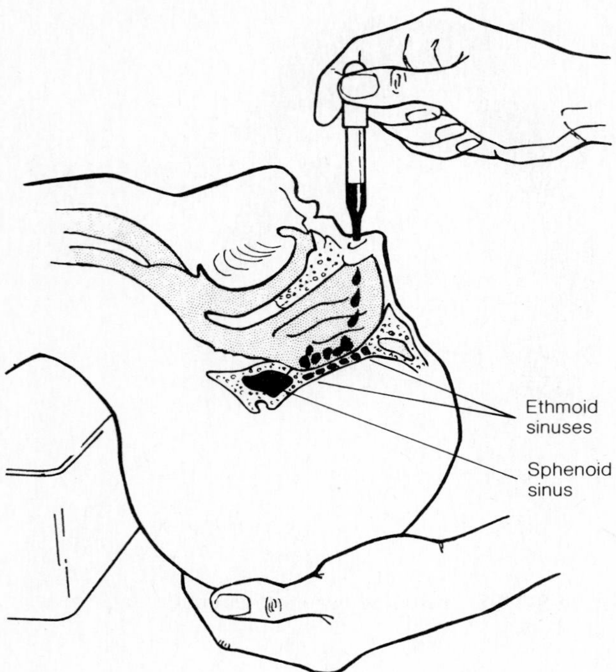

Figure 37–35 Proetz position.

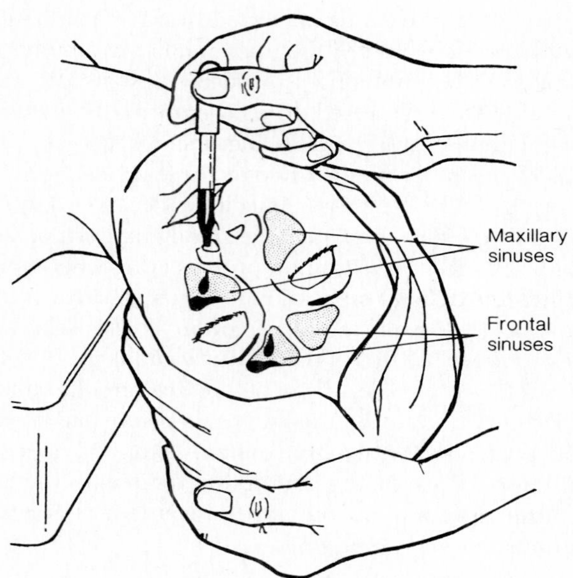

Figure 37–36 Parkinson position.

pillow onto the nurse's arm. This arm can also be used to restrain the infant's arms. The other hand can be used to administer the nose drops.

Vaginal Instillations

Vaginal medications are inserted as creams, jellies, foams, suppositories, or irrigations (douches). Vaginal irrigation is discussed in Chapter 40, page 1044. Medical aseptic technique should be used. Vaginal creams, jellies, and foams are applied with a tubular applicator and plunger. Suppositories are inserted with the index finger of a gloved hand. Vaginal medications are inserted to treat a vaginal infection topically or to relieve vaginal discomfort, e.g., itching or pain.

Prior to the instillation, the nurse asks the patient to urinate since a full bladder can make treatment uncomfortable. Privacy is essential for this procedure. The nurse assists the patient to a back-lying position with the knees flexed and the hips rotated laterally. The patient is draped as for catheterization (see page 723). Adequate lighting on the vaginal orifice is necessary.

Instillation of a vaginal suppository

Suppositories are designed to melt at body temperature, so they are generally stored in the refrigerator to keep them firm for insertion. The nurse unwraps the suppository, puts it on the opened wrapper, and dons gloves to prevent contamination. Next, the nurse lubricates the smooth or rounded end of the suppository to facilitate its insertion. The rounded end is inserted first.

To insert the suppository, the nurse lubricates the gloved index finger and exposes the vaginal orifice by separating the labia with the nondominant hand. The suppository is placed about 8 to 10 cm (3 to 4 in) along the posterior wall of the vagina, or as far as it will go. See Figure 37–37. (The posterior wall of the vagina is about 2.5 cm [1 in] longer than the anterior wall because the cervix protrudes into the uppermost portion of the anterior wall. The anterior wall is usually about 6 to 7.5 cm [2½ to 3 in] long.) The nurse withdraws the finger, removes the gloves by turning them inside out, and places them on a paper towel. Turning the gloves inside out prevents the spread of microorganisms. The patient remains lying in the supine position for 5 to 10 minutes after the insertion. The hips may also be elevated on a pillow. The patient remains lying down to allow the melted medication to flow into the posterior fornix.

Instillation of a vaginal cream

The nurse fills the applicator with the prescribed cream, jelly, or foam. Directions are provided with the manufacturer's applicator. With the gloved nondominant hand, the nurse exposes the vaginal orifice. A second glove may also be worn to protect the nurse's hands from microorganisms. The nurse inserts the applicator gently about 5 cm (2 in) and pushes the plunger until the applicator is empty. See Figure 37–38. The applicator is removed and placed on a paper towel to contain microorganisms and prevent their spread. Next, the nurse removes the glove, turns it inside out, and places it on the paper towel. The patient needs to remain supine for 5 to 10 minutes following the instillation. Finally, the nurse applies a clean perineal pad and a T-binder if there is excessive drainage.

Rectal Instillations

Rectal suppositories are a convenient and safe method of giving certain medications. The advantages of rectal instillation include:

1. It avoids irritation of the upper gastrointestinal tract.
2. Some medications are absorbed well across the mucosal surface of the rectum.
3. Rectal suppositories are thought to provide higher bloodstream levels (titers) of medication, since the venous blood from the rectum is not transported through the liver (Hahn et al. 1982:99).

Rectal medications may have a local effect (e.g., a laxative suppository to soften feces and stimulate defecation) or a systemic effect (e.g., an aminophylline suppository to dilate the patient's bronchi and ease breathing).

Prior to the insertion, the nurse helps the patient to a lateral position with the upper leg acutely flexed. Next, the nurse unwraps the suppository, puts it on the opened wrapper, and dons a glove or fingercot on the hand that will insert the suppository. The glove or fingercot prevents contamination of the nurse's hand by rectal microorganisms and feces. The nurse lubricates the smooth, rounded end of the suppository to prevent anal friction and tissue damage during insertion and lubricates the gloved index finger as well. To relax the patient's anal sphincter, the nurse asks the patient to breathe through the mouth. The suppository is inserted gently into the anus and along the wall of the rectum with the gloved index finger. In adults, suppositories are inserted to a depth of 10 cm (4 in); in children or infants, 5 cm (2 in) or less. See Figure 37–39. To be effective, the suppository needs to be placed along the wall of the rectum rather than embedded in feces. The nurse withdraws the finger, removes the fingercot or glove by turning it inside out, and places it on a paper towel. Turning it inside out contains the rectal microorganisms and prevents their spread. To dispel the patient's urge to expel the suppository, the nurse presses the patient's buttocks together for a few seconds. If a laxative suppository has been given, the nurse asks the patient to retain it for as long as possible (e.g., 15 to 20 minutes). The call signal should be within easy reach so that the patient can summon assistance to use the bedpan or toilet.

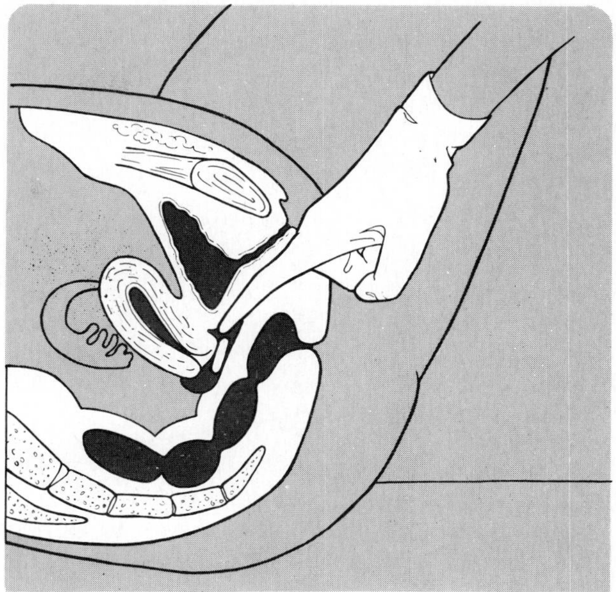

Figure 37–37 Instillation of a vaginal suppository.

Figure 37–38 Instillation of a vaginal cream with an applicator.

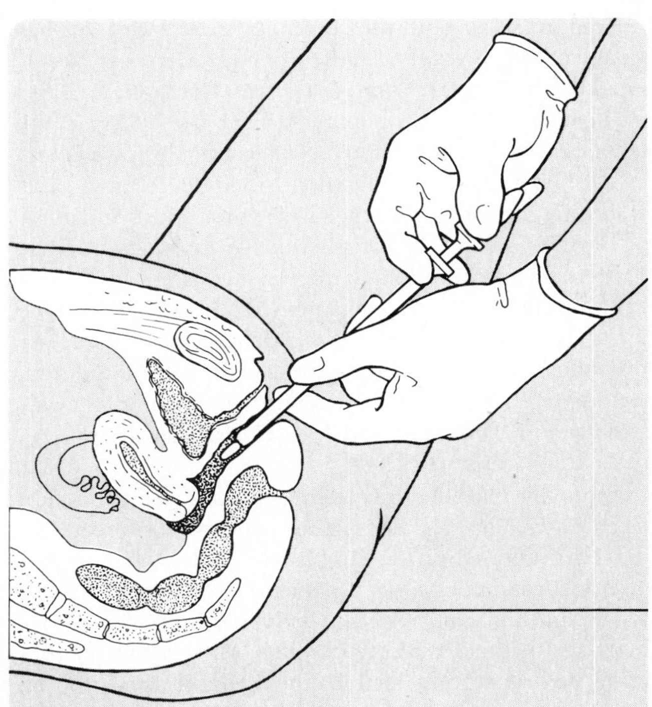

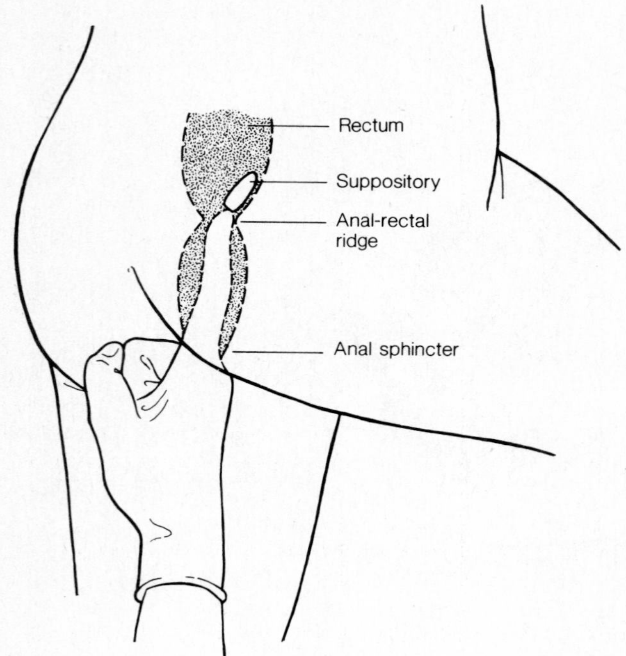

Figure 37–39 A rectal suppository is inserted along the rectal wall beyond the anal-rectal ridge (i.e., beyond the internal sphincter).

Summary

Drugs come from four main sources: plants, minerals, animals, and synthetics. Drugs derived from these sources must be pure and uniform in strength so that dosages are predictable. Official drugs are those designated by the Federal Food, Drug, and Cosmetic Act and are listed in pharmacopoeias such as the *USP* and the *British Pharmacopoeia*. Formularies are also published.

Legal aspects of medications include federal laws governing the control of drugs such as narcotics and nursing legislation in the jurisdiction of nursing practice. Written records itemizing the drug, dosage, date and time of administration, recipient of the drug, and the signature of the nurse giving the drug are essential. For controlled drugs, additional policies are implemented, such as double checks by two nurses prior to the administration of a drug and locked cupboards for narcotics and barbiturates.

Drugs are classified according to their overall action in the body. Primary actions are stimulation or inhibition of tissue or organ functions. Several factors influence these actions: drug concentrations, absorbability, circulation through the body, metabolism of the drug, and excretion of metabolites. Many other factors influence drug action, such as the age and weight of the individual, genetic factors, psychologic factors, specific illness, time of administration, and environment. The effects of drugs are characterized as therapeutic and side effects or unexpected effects are allergies, tolerances, cumulative and idiosyncratic effects, and harmful interactions. Routes of administration of medications are: oral, sublingual, buccal, parenteral (intramuscular, subcutaneous, intravenous, intradermal), and topical (dermatologic preparations, instillations, and inhalations).

Four types of medication orders exist: the standing order, the stat order, the single order, and the p.r.n. order. Essential parts of the medication order are (a) the patient's name, (b) the date and time of administration, (c) the name of the drug, (d) the dosage, (e) the method of administration, and (f) the signature of the person writing the order. The dosage of drugs can be prescribed in three systems: the apothecaries' system, the metric system, and the household system. It is important for the nurse to understand and be able to convert among these three systems.

Nurses often need to calculate fractional dosages. Calculations may be necessary when preparing preoperative medications for adults or when measuring dosages for infants and children. When determining dosages for infants and children, the nurse makes calculations using the child's body weight and body surface area.

Nursing assessment pertinent to medications and their administration includes taking a nursing medication history and evaluating clinical signs related to the patient's condition. When administering drugs nurses follow five steps: (a) identify the patient, (b) administer the correct amount of drug by the appropriate route, (c) provide adjunctive nursing care, (d) record the measure, and (e) evaluate the effectiveness of the drug's action. The nurse must also consider the age and individual needs of the patient. Recommended techniques for administering oral, subcutaneous, intramuscular, intradermal, and topical medications are outlined. In addition, nurses require skills in mixing drugs and preparing injections of powdered drugs and insulin.

Suggested Activities

1. In a laboratory setting, get a classmate to play the role of patient. Determine the following injection sites:

- **a.** Right ventrogluteal (IM)
- **b.** Left dorsogluteal (IM)
- **c.** Left deltoid (IM)
- **d.** Right vastus lateralis (IM)
- **e.** Left arm (subcutaneous)
- **f.** Right back (intradermal)

Mark each site with a piece of adhesive tape. Have your sites checked by an instructor and explain how you chose them.

2. In a clinical setting, list the medications ordered for two patients. Determine which orders are (a) stat, (b) standing, and (c) p.r.n. Identify the agency medication policies that apply to these drug orders.

3. In a clinical setting, identify problems that patients of various age groups may have in taking oral medications. Identify the nursing measures that assist patients to take those oral medications.

4. Determine the different ways medications are administered intravenously in a clinical setting.

5. Interview two elderly patients taking daily medications. Assess their understanding of the medications.

Suggested Readings

Bell, S. K. March 1980. Guidelines for taking a complete drug history. *Nursing 80.* 10:10–11.
A complete drug history tool is organized into three sections: over-the-counter drugs, prescription drugs, and a general health history.

Deberry, P.; Jefferies, L. P.; and Light, M. R. December 1975. Teaching cardiac patients to manage medications. *American Journal of Nursing* 75:2191–93.
A teaching program was planned and implemented for patients who would be taking medications upon leaving the hospital. Teaching techniques and learning difficulties are described. This article offers students ideas for assisting patients.

Drehobl, P. September 1980. Quadriceps contracture. *American Journal of Nursing.* 80:1650–51.
Quadriceps contractures can be caused by repeated intramuscular thigh injections. At greatest risk are premature infants and full-term infants on long-term intramuscular antibiotic therapy. This author outlines measures nurses can take to prevent this problem.

Goldberg, P. B. May-June 1980. Drugs and the elderly: Why do older adults need different dosages? *Geriatric Nursing.* 1:74, 76–77.
Aging affects drug absorption, action, and elimination. Elderly adults need smaller doses.

Kalant, H., and Kalant, O. J. 1972. *Drugs, society, and personal choice.* Don Mills, Ontario: General Publishing Co. Ltd., with the cooperation of the Research Division, Addiction Research Foundation of Ontario.
This small book helps all people, including nurses, be better informed about drugs. Current problems are discussed together with special drugs, the reasons for nonmedical use of drugs, and the physical and psychologic consequences of drug use. Also included is a chapter on evaluating the effects of drug use.

Lambert, M. L. March 1975. Drug and diet interactions. *American Journal of Nursing* 75:402–6.
Included in this article are food malabsorption, drug malabsorption, and the interactions between drugs and food and fluids. A helpful list gives the nurse a guide at a glance as to how and when to administer certain drugs.

Weeks, H. F. January-February 1980. Administering medication to children. *Maternal-Child Nursing* 5:63.
Drug dosage based on body size is explained as well as some of the differences between the adult's and child's metabolic systems. Approaching the child correctly and teaching parents are important.

Willig, S. June 1964. Drugs: Dispensing-administering. *American Journal of Nursing* 64:126–31. Reprinted in Meyers, M. E., editor. 1967. *Nursing fundamentals.* Dubuque, Iowa: William C. Brown Co.
What is the position of the nurse when neither a physician nor a pharmacist is present during part of the 24-hour hospital day? The nurse-physician relationship laws governing labeling and repackaging, drug-related lawsuits, and insurance coverage are discussed.

Wolanin, M. O. November-December 1981. Nursing therapy, drug therapy, or both? *Geriatric Nursing* 2:408–10.
The author discusses the administration of analgesics, comfort measures such as touch, warmth, interaction, relaxation, and rocking. Nursing measures that support the action of laxatives are also included.

Selected References

Bahruth, A. June 1973. Keeping track of injection sites. *Nursing 73* 3:51.

Brandt, P. A.; Smith, M. E.; Ashburn, S. S.; and Graves, J. August 1972. IM injections in children. *American Journal of Nursing* 72:1402–6.

Burke, E. L. December 1972. Insulin injection, the site and the technique. *American Journal of Nursing* 72:2194–96.

Carr, J. J.; McElroy, N. L.; and Carr, B. L. December 1976. How to solve dosage problems in one easy lesson. *American Journal of Nursing* 76:1934–37.

Chezem, J. L. September 1974. Consultation: Aspirating before IM injections. *Nursing 74* 4:87.

Clark, J. B.; Queener, S. F.; and Karb, V. B. 1982. *Pharmacological basis of nursing practice.* St. Louis: C. V. Mosby Co.

Cohen, M. R. April 1981. Medication errors. *Nursing 81.* 11:9.

Dann, T. C. August 1966. Routine skin preparation before injection—is it necessary? *Nursing Times* 62:1121–22.

Evans, M. L., and Hansen, B. D. May-June 1981. Administering injections to different-aged children. *Maternal Child Nursing* 6:194–99.

Foerst, H. November 1979. Drug-prescribing patterns in skilled nursing facilities. *American Journal of Nursing* 79:2002–3.

Gaerlan, M. November 1980. Living and working with drugs. *The Canadian Nurse.* 76:35–42.

Galton, L. August 1976. Drugs and the elderly: What you should know about them. *Nursing 76* 6:39–43.

Geolot, D. H., and McKinney, N. P. May 1975. Administering parenteral drugs. *American Journal of Nursing* 75:788–93.

Gilman, A. G.; Goodman, L. S.; and Gilman, A. 1980. *The pharmacological basis of therapeutics.* 6th ed. New York: Macmillan Publishing Co.

Gotz, B. E., and Gotz, V. P. August 1978. Staying well while growing old: Drugs and the elderly. *American Journal of Nursing* 78:1347–51.

Hahn, A. B.; Barkin, R. L.; and Oestreich, S. J.K. 1982. *Pharmacology in nursing.* 15th ed. St. Louis: C. V. Mosby Co.

Hays, D. June 1974. Do it yourself the Z-track way. *American Journal of Nursing* 74:1070–71.

Hayter, J. November-December 1981. Why response to medication changes with age. *Geriatric Nursing* 2:411–16.

Kennedy, B. March 1981. Self-medication. *Canadian Nurse* 77:36–37.

Kolesar, G. November 1980. It could happen to you—nurses, physicians and pharmacists. Part 1. *The Canadian Nurse.* 76:20–22.

Kozier, B., and Erb, G. 1982. *Techniques in clinical nursing: A comprehensive approach.* Menlo Park, Calif.: Addison-Wesley Publishing Co.

Lacey, R. W. April 1968. Antibacterial action of human skin. *British Journal of Experimental Pathology.* 49:209–15.

Lambert, M. L. March 1975. Drug and diet interactions. *American Journal of Nursing.* 75:402–6.

Lang, S. H.; Zawacki, A. M.; and Johnson, J. E. May 1976. Reducing discomfort from injections. *American Journal of Nursing* 76:800–1.

Mayers, M. H. November-December 1981. Legal guidelines. *Geriatric Nursing* 2:417–21, 441.

The Medical Letter. 24 October 1974. Drugs and alcohol. *The Medical Letter*, New Rochelle, N.Y. Reprinted in *American Journal of Nursing* (January 1976) 76:65.

Newton, D. W., and Newton, M. July 1979. Route, site, and technique: Three key decisions in giving parenteral medication. *Nursing 79* 9:18–21, 23, 25.

Nurse's Reference Library Series. 1982. *Drugs.* Springhouse, Pa.: Intermed Communications, Inc.

Nursing 80 Photobook Series. 1980. *Giving medications.* Horsham, Pa.: Intermed Communications.

Paech, G. November 1980. Drug abuse: A health-oriented approach . . . use? or abuse? *The Canadian Nurse.* 76:18–19.

Pitel, M. January 1971. The subcutaneous injection. *American Journal of Nursing* 71:76–79.

Rodman, M. J., and Smith, D. W. 1979. *Pharmacology and drug therapy in nursing.* 2nd ed. Philadelphia: J. B. Lippincott Co.

Skeist, R., and Carlson, G. November-December 1981. Storing medications safely. *Geriatric Nursing* 2:429–32, 441.

Stewart, D. Y.; Kelly, J.; and Dinel, B. A. August 1976. Unit-dose medication: A nursing perspective. *American Journal of Nursing* 76:1308–10.

Whaley, L. F., and Wong, D. L. 1979. *Nursing care of infants and children.* St. Louis: C. V. Mosby Co.

Wong, D. L. August 1982. Significance of dead space in syringes. *American Journal of Nursing* 82:1237.

Chapter 38

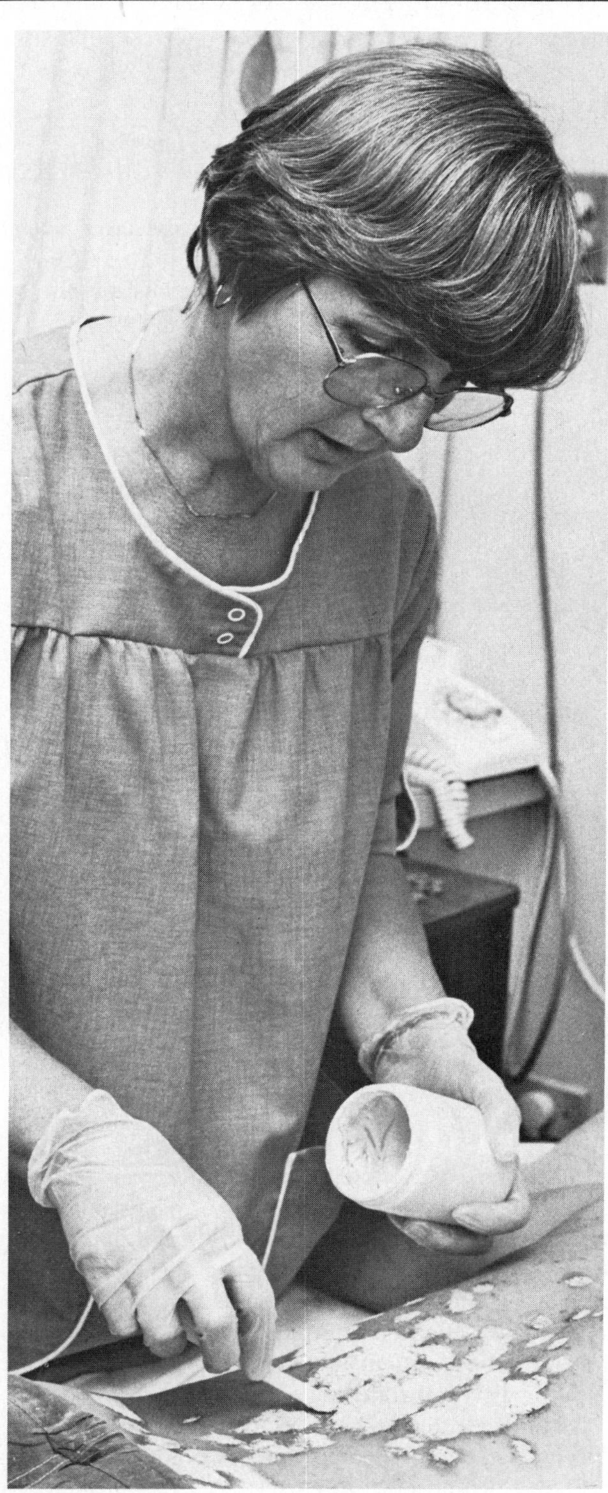

Special Procedures

CONTENTS

(Continued on next page)

Intravenous Cholangiography
Intravenous Pyelography (IVP)
or Urography (IVU)
Angiography
Myelography
Organ Scan

Objectives

1. Know essential terms and facts related to assisting patients undergoing special procedures
   - **1.1** Define selected terms
   - **1.2** Describe various procedures
   - **1.3** Recognize purposes of specific procedures
   - **1.4** Identify assessment data required for specific procedures
   - **1.5** Identify education needs of patients about to have certain tests and treatments
   - **1.6** Outline measures to prepare the patient physically for specific procedures
   - **1.7** Give reasons for essential aspects of specific procedures
   - **1.8** Outline essential follow-up measures for specific procedures

Terms

abdominal paracentesis
angiography
anoscopy
ascites
atrioventricular (AV) node
barium enema
barium swallow
bronchogram
bronchoscopy
cannula
cardiac monitor
cholecystogram (oral cholecystography)
cisternal puncture
colonoscopy
cystoscopy
depolarization (cardiac)
electrocardiogram (ECG, EKG)
electrocardiograph
electroencephalogram
electroencephalograph
electromyogram
electromyograph
endoscope
esophagoscopy
fasciculation
gastroscopy
intravenous cholangiogram
intravenous pyelogram
intravenous pyelography (IVP)
intravenous urography (IVU)
laryngoscopy
lumbar puncture (LP)
myelogram
pneumoventriculogram
polarization (cardiac)
proctoscopy
proctosigmoidoscopy
Purkinje's fibers
repolarization (cardiac)
retrograde pyelogram
scan
sigmoidoscopy
sinoatrial (SA) node
thoracocentesis (thoracentesis)
tomography
trocar
ventriculogram

An important nursing function is assisting with tests and treatments ordered by physicians. Nurses have dual responsibilities: They not only help prepare and reassure patients but also assist during the procedures.

Tests and treatments are frightening to many people. People may fear pain, the results of tests, or their reactions to either the pain or the findings of a test. Fear of the unknown increases these misgivings. It is important for the nurse to be aware of the needs of patients and families and to help them meet these needs.

The nurse is often responsible for certain aspects of tests or treatments. For example, it is frequently a nursing function to assemble the equipment before tests or treatments performed in a clinical nursing unit or a physician's office. The nurse is also responsible for assessing the patient during and after the procedure. Many tests and treatments require special nursing intervention afterward. The nurse is responsible for certain pretest interventions that help assure success. A well-prepared patient is likely to experience the least possible discomfort during tests.

Diagnosis after tests often requires the services of specialists in laboratory tests, radiologic (roentgenographic) techniques, cardiac testing, etc. The nurse helps coordinate the services of these personnel, assists in scheduling, and helps the patient meet schedules.

General Nursing Guidelines

Psychologic Preparation

The patient and possibly the support persons need explanations of why a test or treatment is necessary and what it will entail. This explanation needs to be adjusted to the patient's needs. A small child requires a different explanation than a curious adult. Some persons want to know every detail, but others need only a general explanation. It is important that the nurse be honest with the patient; if the patient will feel sharp pain during the test, it is better to say so than to not mention it.

Often patients want to know where the test will take place, who will do it, how long it will last, and when the results will be available. The last question is often associated with fear. The nurse can base answers on experience and the physician's opinion. If the results are delayed, it is important to explain the delay to the patient and follow up to get the results.

As a general rule, it is wise not to offer information about possible complications and severe reactions. If, however, the patient asks questions about complications and reactions, the nurse should answer honestly, presenting the facts objectively and accurately without exaggeration. When a child is undergoing tests, the family will probably require assistance. The well-informed family, able to anticipate how the child will feel and when they will be able to visit, is better able to offer support.

Physical Preparation

Some tests require special preparation, e.g., a cleaning enema before a barium enema or sedation before a bronchoscopy. In some instances special lighting and drapes are required at the patient's unit. Just before paracentesis and other treatments, the patient needs to assume a special position. When a physician orders sedatives or tranquilizers as needed (p.r.n) before a test, the nurse often decides when or whether to administer them. It is important that the nurse be sensitive to the patient's emotions and aware of excessive anxiety.

Assembling Equipment

It is usually a nursing responsibility to assemble the equipment for tests and treatments carried out at a hospitalized patient's bedside or in an adjacent clinical treatment room. It is also a nursing responsibility to maintain the sterility of sterile equipment. When a patient goes to another unit such as the radiology department, that department assumes responsibility for assembling the equipment.

Many hospitals today use prepackaged disposable sets, which require a minimum of setting up. The set should be checked to see that it contains all required equipment. If the nurse is unsure, it is important to check the agency policy and procedure and make necessary adjustments to the set.

Assisting the Patient

During the treatment or test the nurse needs to observe the patient and provide emotional support. The nurse should be sensitive to signs of distress such as pallor, profuse sweating, accelerated pulse, or signs of nausea or acute pain. Any sign needs to be reported to the person conducting the procedure immediately. The nurse can support the patient by providing information such as, "It will be only 2 minutes more," "The needle is all the way in now," or "You won't feel any additional discomfort." Sometimes the nurse can distract the patient by asking questions; however, some patients do not respond well to this tactic, and the nurse must be sensitive to the patient's wishes.

Assisting with the Procedure

In some instances the nurse hands equipment to the person carrying out the procedure or makes notes on findings made during the procedure, such as the spinal fluid pressure of a patient having a lumbar puncture. Nurses need to know what will be expected of them during tests or procedures and whenever possible anticipate the needs of the person conducting the test.

Assisting after the Procedure

After the procedure the nurse's first responsibility is to assist the patient to a prescribed or comfortable position. For example, after a lumbar puncture, the patient must assume a dorsal recumbent position. Family members need to be told when a procedure is completed and when they can see the patient. It is best to remove equipment before visitors enter because visitors sometimes find long needles and similar equipment disquieting.

Caring for Equipment and Specimens

After the test or treatment the nurse returns the equipment to the appropriate area or disposes of it according to agency policy. Equipment that is not disposed of is washed and rinsed and appropriately distributed for further handling.

Specimens must be appropriately labeled. Hospital specimens usually are marked with the patient's name, identification number, and date. Some specimens require special care if not sent directly to the laboratory. Some urine specimens are refrigerated, and some fecal specimens must be kept warm so microorganisms will not die.

Recording

After the procedure, the nurse is responsible for making appropriate entries on the patient's record. The information recorded includes the treatment or test performed, the time, who carried it out, whether a specimen was taken, specific information such as spinal fluid pressures, and the patient's response.

Nursing Assessment after the Procedure

The nurse assesses the patient's condition after any test or treatment. The interval between assessments depends on the patient's reaction to the test. Even if there have been no adverse reactions, the nurse needs to assess a patient's condition 30 minutes after the test, at which time the nurse makes appropriate adjustments in care. Some patients feel nauseated half an hour after thoracentesis and other procedures, for example.

Examinations Involving Electric Impulses

A number of machines measure and record electric impulses. The *electrocardiograph* receives impulses from the heart, the *electroencephalograph* from the brain, and the *electromyograph* from muscles. All these machines have electrodes that attach to body parts. The electrodes are sensitive to electric activity, which is recorded graphically. The graphic reading can also be shown on an oscilloscope screen.

Figure 38–1 The placement of electrodes on the chest of an adult for electrocardiography.

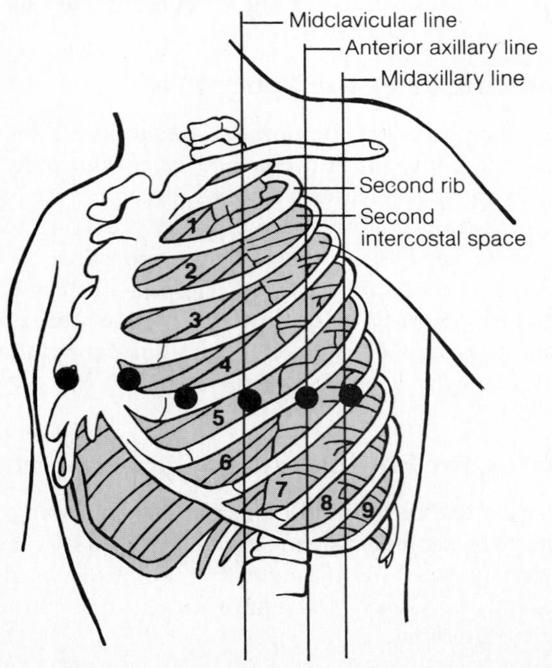

Electrocardiography

An *electrocardiogram* (*ECG* or *EKG*) is a graph of electric impulses from the heart. Electrodes are attached by leads to the electrocardiograph. The electrodes are attached to the patient's body by paste, suction cups, or tape. One electrode is attached to the lower part of each limb, and a fifth electrode is moved to six different positions on the chest. The first position is on the right sternal border; subsequent positions follow the general outline of the heart around to the left sternal border and laterally as far as the midaxillary line. See Figure 38–1.

The heart muscle is said to be *polarized* or charged when it is at rest. When the muscle cells of the ventricles and the atria contract, they *depolarize* or lose their charge. During a resting stage, they regain their electric charge or *repolarize*. Cardiac depolarization and repolarization are recorded on an electrocardiogram.

The heartbeat is normally initiated at the *sinoatrial (SA) node*, which is located in the upper aspect of the right atrium. The SA node is often referred to as the pacemaker of the heart. The impulse radiates over the atria, causing them to contract. It is then picked up by the *atrioventricular (AV) node*, situated at the base of the atrial septum. The impulse then travels from the AV node down two bundle branches throughout the ventricles of the heart. Both the SA and AV nodes as well as the bundle branches have dense networks of *Purkinje's fibers*, modified cardiac tissue that helps conduct the impulse. As the impulse travels throughout this system the ventricles contract or depolarize. Figure 38–2 shows a normal electrocardiogram and indicates intervals of depolarization and repolarization. The P wave arises when the impulse from the SA node causes the atria to contract or depolarize. The QRS wave occurs with con-

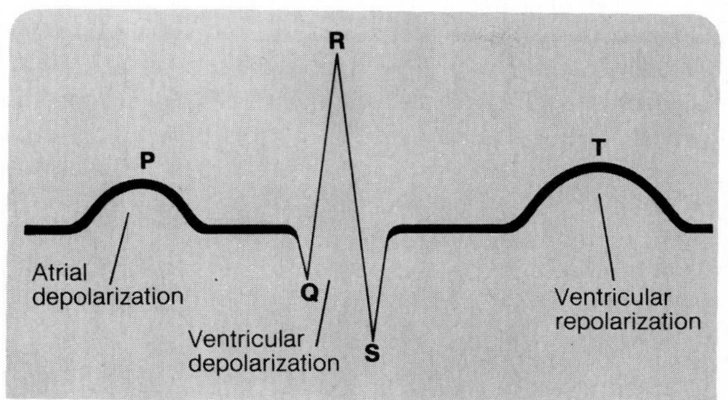

Figure 38–2 Schematic of a normal electrocardiogram.

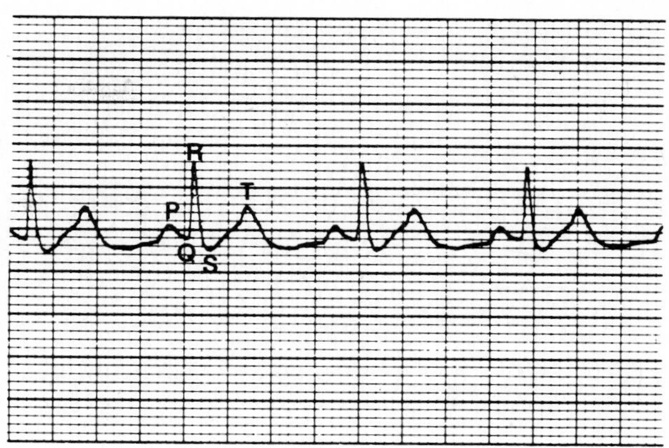

Figure 38–3 A normal electrocardiogram.

traction and depolarization of the ventricles. The T wave represents the resting or repolarization of the ventricles. Repolarization of the atria occurs during the QRS segment of the graph; it is normally not seen on an ECG. The ECG is produced on finely lined paper. The horizontal lines represent the voltage of the electric impulse, and the vertical lines represent time. See Figure 38–3. The graph waves can be abnormal in size, position, and form when cardiac pathology exists.

Patients who require ECGs may go to a special department of a hospital or laboratory. If the patient is very ill, a portable ECG machine can be brought to a bedside in a home or hospital. If the patient is critically ill, the heart may be monitored continually. For such patients, a *cardiac monitor* is used. This machine shows cardiac waves on an oscilloscope.

Electrocardiography is painless and usually takes about 10 minutes. Some physicians order an electrocardiogram as part of routine physical examinations of patients over 40. No special preparation is required before the test.

Electroencephalography

Electroencephalograms (EEGs) are recordings of electric activity in the brain. Electroencephalographs have leads to electrodes that attach to the patient's scalp with paste or small needles. The patient lies in a dorsal recumbent position in a darkened room. The patient may be asked to hyperventilate, and readings may also be taken while the patient sleeps. See Figure 25–1, page 623. If performed on a sleeping patient, the test may take 2 hours; otherwise it lasts no more than 1 hour. The test is normally painless, although the patient may feel occasional pinpricks if needle electrodes are used in the scalp.

Preparation for an EEG VARIES. Some agencies advise that on the day of the test the patient not take stimulants such as coffee or depressants such as alcohol. Usually the patient takes no medications prior to the test, and the nurse shampoos the patient's hair, which should be free of hair spray, hair creams, and the like.

Electromyography

An *electromyogram* is a record of the electric potential created by the contraction of a muscle. Two electrodes are attached with paste or small needles to the skin over the muscle. This test is used to discern muscle abnormalities such as *fasciculation* (abnormal contraction involving the whole motor unit).

Examinations Involving Visual Inspection

Visual inspection or direct visualization techniques involve the use of special instruments called *endoscopes*, which allow visualization of interior parts of the body.

Bronchoscopy and Laryngoscopy

A *bronchoscope* is a lighted instrument, used to visualize the bronchi of the lungs. The examination is referred to as *bronchoscopy*. Prior to the procedure the patient usually fasts for 6 hours and is given a sedative. If a general anesthetic is given, routine preoperative care is given. See Chapter 39. Dentures are removed prior to the examination.

If a general anesthetic is not given, a local anesthetic is sprayed on the patient's pharynx to prevent gagging. The bronchoscope is then inserted to visualize the bronchi. In some instances a section of tissue may be taken for biopsy. After this examination, the patient

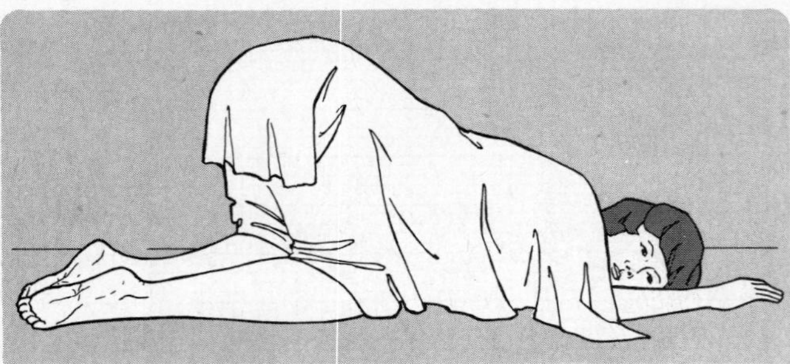

Figure 38–4 The knee-chest position commonly used for examinations of the rectum and colon.

should not take food or fluids until the local anesthetic has worn off and the gag reflex has returned, otherwise the patient could aspirate food and fluid. The possible complications are bleeding due to damaged tissue, laryngospasm, and respiratory distress. A *bronchogram* is a roentgenogram (x-ray film) of the bronchial tree after an iodized oil dye has been instilled. A general anesthetic is usually given before a bronchogram is taken.

A *laryngoscope* is a lighted instrument used to visualize the larynx. The examination is called *laryngoscopy*. The preparation is similar to that for bronchoscopy; local or generalized anesthetic can be used. A biopsy may be taken during the examination.

Precautions afterward include withholding food and fluids until the gag reflex is restored. The nurse needs to observe the patient for laryngospasm and bleeding due to tissue damage.

Gastroscopy and Esophagoscopy

Gastroscopy is the visualization of the interior of the stomach with a lighted instrument called a *gastroscope*. The preparation and care of the patient are the same as for bronchoscopy. *Esophagoscopy* is the examination of the esophagus with a lighted instrument; it is similar to gastroscopy.

Cystoscopy

Cystoscopy is the visualization of the interior of the urinary bladder with a lighted instrument called a *cystoscope*. Usually a general anesthetic is given, and the preparation is similar to that for bronchoscopy. During cystoscopy catheters may be inserted up the ureters into each kidney. Contrast medium is then injected into the kidneys, and x-ray photographs are taken. This procedure is known as *retrograde pyelography*. The x-ray film shows the kidney calyces, the kidney pelvis, the ureters, and the urinary bladder. When a pyelogram is to be taken, the patient is given laxatives and enemas to free the intestines of feces and gas. *Intravenous pyelography* is roentgenography of the kidneys after the injection of dye into the arterial system. An intravenous pyelogram shows the same structures as a retrograde pyelogram. This examination does not require an anesthetic and normally takes about 1 hour.

After cystoscopy, the nurse encourages the patient to drink fluids, which decrease irritation and the possibility of infection.

Proctoscopy, Sigmoidoscopy, and Colonoscopy

Proctoscopy is the examination of the rectum with a lighted instrument *(proctoscope)*. *Sigmoidoscopy* is the examination of the sigmoid colon and the rectum with a lighted instrument *(sigmoidoscope)*. *Proctosigmoidoscopy* is the examination of the sigmoid colon and the rectum with a *proctosigmoidoscope*. *Colonoscopy* is the examination of the entire colon (large bowel) with a lighted instrument *(colonoscope)*. *Anoscopy* is the examination of the anal canal with a lighted instrument called an *anoscope*.

Preparation generally includes laxatives or enemas begun the evening before to clear the bowel of feces. General anesthesia is usually not necessary, although the patient may experience some discomfort. The patient assumes a knee-chest position for the examination. See Figure 38–4. After these examinations, the nurse needs to observe the patient for rectal bleeding because of tissue trauma.

Examinations Involving Removal of Body Fluids and Tissues

Certain body fluids and tissues can help physicians diagnose disease. Table 38–1 lists some common procedures for removing body fluids and tissues. The procedures are normally performed by a physician at the bedside, in an examining room, or sometimes in the emergency department of a hospital. All the procedures described here involve inserting an instrument, often a needle, through the skin and withdrawing some fluid or tissue. The fluid or tissue is usually placed in a special container and sent to the laboratory for examination. Although the procedures for taking specimens are considered safe, each can have complications. Some

Table 38–1 Common Diagnostic or Therapeutic Procedures

Name	Type of specimen	Source	Common tests
Lumbar puncture	Spinal fluid	Subarachnoid space of the spinal canal	Pressure, appearance, sugar, protein, cell count, bacteria, Queckenstedt test
Cisternal puncture	Spinal fluid	Subarachnoid space of the cisterna magna	Ventriculogram, pneumo-ventriculogram
Abdominal paracentesis	Ascitic fluid	Peritoneal cavity	Cell count, cells, specific gravity, protein
Thoracocentesis	Pleural fluid	Pleural cavity	Cell count, protein
Pericardial aspiration	Pericardial fluid	Pericardial sac	Cell count, protein
Bone marrow biopsy	Bone marrow	Iliac crest, posterior superior iliac spine, or sternum	Cells, iron
Liver biopsy	Needle biopsy specimen (liver tissue)	Liver	Carcinoma, cells

agencies require patients to sign consent forms prior to these procedures. In other agencies the general consent form signed by the patient on admission suffices.

Lumbar Puncture

A *lumbar puncture* (LP, spinal tap) is the insertion of a needle into the subarachnoid space of the spinal canal to withdraw cerebrospinal fluid (CSF). An adult normally has about 150 ml of CSF (Guyton 1982:243). The site of a lumbar puncture is usually between the third and fourth or the fourth and fifth lumbar vertebrae. Inserted at this level, the needle does not damage the spinal cord and major nerve roots. See Figure 38–5. The fourth lumbar interspace is the most common lumbar puncture site for adults, but the site is usually lower for infants and small children, whose spinal cord extends almost into the sacral region.

About 800 ml of cerebrospinal fluid (about five times the total volume of fluid in the CSF cavity) is formed daily in adults by the choroid villi in each of the brain's four ventricles. The fluid normally circulates freely through the ventricles, through the subarachnoid space around the brain and spinal cord, and through the central canal of the cord. It is continually reabsorbed into the venous circulation through villi from the arachnoid layer, which extend into the superior sagittal sinus.

Lumbar punctures are carried out for the following diagnostic and therapeutic reasons:

1. To analyze the constituents of CSF
2. To test the pressure of CSF
3. To relieve pressure by removing CSF
4. To inject a spinal anesthetic, dye, or air into the spinal canal

A lumbar puncture is carried out by a physician. The nurse's function is to assist the patient and the physician.

Equipment

A lumbar puncture requires sterile technique. Many hospitals have disposable lumbar puncture kits. The equipment required includes sterile sponges; disinfectant; local anesthetic as well as 21 and 24 gauge needles and syringes for its injection; sterile gloves; mask; lumbar puncture needle 5 to 12.5 cm (2 to 5 in) long, depending on the age and size of the patient (infants require a 5 cm needle); specimen tubes if needed, adapters for needles, manometer to measure spinal fluid pressure, three-way stopcock, and a container for discarded materials.

Preparation

Before the lumbar puncture, the patient arches the back and maintains this position. The nurse can help the patient maintain this position by supporting the back of the patient's neck and knees. See Figure 38–6. Many agencies have sterile fenestrated drapes, which the physician places over the area after scrubbing and gloving.

Technique

The physician applies a disinfectant to the area, injects local anesthetic, and inserts the needle into the intravertebral space. When the flow of CSF is established, the stopcock and manometer are attached to obtain an initial CSF pressure reading. Normal opening pressures

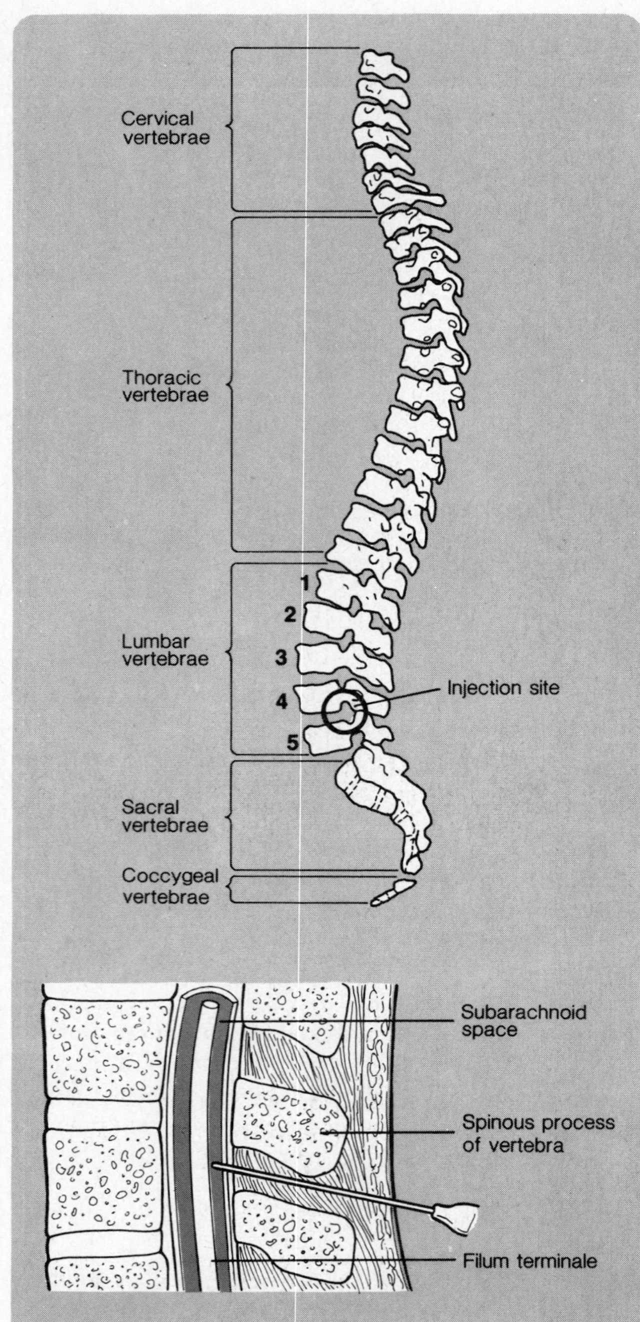

Figure 38–5 A diagram of the vertebral column, indicating a site for insertion of the lumbar puncture needle into the subarachnoid space of the spinal canal.

are 60 to 180 mm of water. Pressures above 200 mm are considered abnormal.

A Queckenstedt test may also be done while the manometer is attached. Someone (often the nurse) exerts digital pressure on one or both of the patient's internal jugular veins. If the patient is normal, digital pressure temporarily increases the manometer reading.

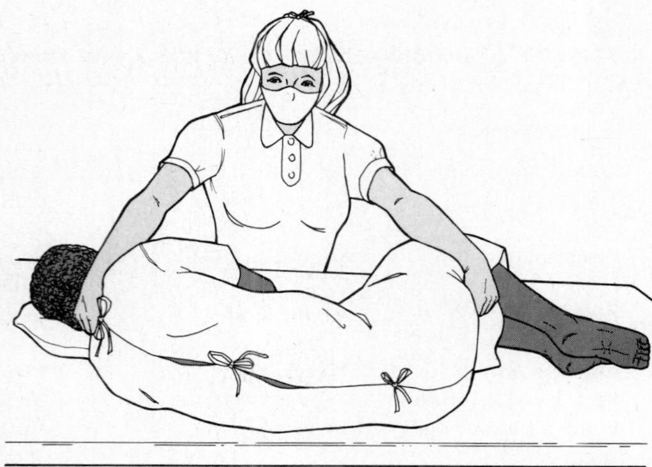

Figure 38–6 Positioning the patient for a lumbar puncture.

If there is a blockage in the spinal canal, digital pressure on the veins affects CSF pressure very little or not at all.

The physician usually takes specimens of CSF and hands the specimen tubes to the nurse, who numbers them in the sequence taken. The physician collects a total of 10 ml of fluid and places 2 to 3 ml of fluid in each specimen tube. Specimens of CSF are often tested in the laboratory for sugar, bacteria, cell count, etc. See Table 38–1. Normal CSF is a clear, colorless fluid. Blood may give the fluid a reddish cast, and infection may make the fluid cloudy.

After collecting the specimens, the physician may take a final (closing) CSF pressure reading before removing the spinal needle.

Follow-up care

After the puncture, the nurse helps the patient assume a dorsal recumbent position, with one pillow under the head. The patient remains in this position for 8 to 24 hours until the body replaces the removed spinal fluid. Some patients get headaches after a lumbar puncture, and the dorsal recumbent position tends to prevent or alleviate it. Analgesics are often ordered and can be given to relieve headaches.

After a lumbar puncture the nurse gathers the equipment; labels specimens and sends them to the laboratory; records data about the lumbar puncture (including the date, time, name of the physician, color and consistency of the fluid, number of specimens, and initial and final pressures); and assesses the response of the patient. The nurse needs to observe and record such signs as pallor, complaints of faintness, changes in pulse rate and other vital signs, changes in degree of consciousness, complaints of headache, and swelling or bleeding at the puncture site. Numbness, tingling, or pain radiating down the legs may indicate nerve irritation and should also be recorded.

Cisternal Puncture

A *cisternal puncture* is similar to a lumbar puncture except that the physician inserts a needle into the subarachnoid space of the cisterna magna. See Figure 38–7. During this procedure, the patient flexes the neck acutely to permit the physician to insert the needle between the first cervical vertebra and the rim of the foramen magnum. Cisternal puncture is necessary for ventriculograms and pneumoventriculograms. A *ventriculogram* is a roentgenogram of the ventricles of the brain after the introduction of an opaque dye. A *pneumoventriculogram* is a roentgenogram of the ventricles of the brain after the introduction of air.

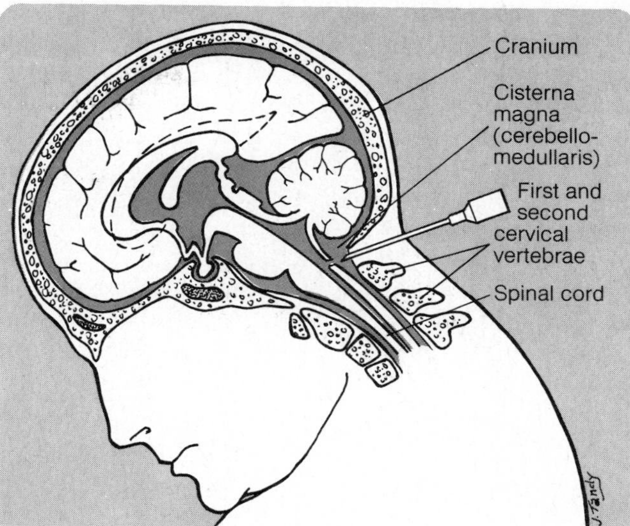

Figure 38–7 During a cisternal puncture, a needle is inserted into the subarachnoid space of the cisterna magna.

Abdominal Paracentesis

Abdominal paracentesis is the removal of fluid from the peritoneal cavity. Normally the peritoneum creates just enough fluid to lubricate the surface of the peritoneum and prevent friction between the peritoneum and the tissues with which it comes in contact; this fluid is absorbed into the lymph circulation through lymph vessels in the peritoneum. However, in patients with cirrhosis of the liver and certain other conditions, large amounts of fluid collect in the cavity; this condition is called *ascites*. Ascites can be treated by restricting fluids and sodium, administering diuretics, and, at times, performing abdominal paracentesis to relieve pressure on the abdominal organs and diaphragm. Paracentesis is also carried out to obtain peritoneal fluid specimens for laboratory study. The fluid is analyzed for types of cells, cell count, specific gravity, and presence of protein.

Equipment

Abdominal paracentesis requires sterile technique. Paracentesis sets are usually available. These contain disinfectant, sponges, local anesthetic, syringe and 24 and 22 gauge needles to administer the anesthetic, sterile gloves, fenestrated drape, small scalpel to make an incision in the abdomen, a needle holder and sutures to sew the incision, dressings, and the aspirating set. The aspirating set generally includes a receptacle for the fluid, tubing, and a trocar and cannula. A *trocar* is a sharp, pointed instrument that fits inside the cannula and pierces, in this case, the peritoneal cavity. A *cannula* is a tube through which plastic tubing can be threaded to drain fluid. The trocar and cannula (and the scalpel, sutures, and needle holder) are needed only if the purpose of paracentesis is to drain fluid. If the purpose is to obtain a specimen, a long aspirating needle attached to a syringe may be used in place of a trocar and cannula. Because the physician makes no incision when simply obtaining a specimen, the scalpel, sutures, and needle holder are not required.

Preparation

Before abdominal paracentesis, the patient should empty the bladder, which if full can be punctured inadvertently when the trocar is inserted. Before starting, the physician needs to know if the patient has been unable to urinate. The sitting position is preferred for abdominal paracentesis because the force of gravity and the pressure of the abdominal organs facilitate the flow of fluid. If the purpose of the procedure is to remove fluid, the nurse needs to measure the abdominal girth at the level of the umbilicus to acquire baseline data for later evaluation. See Figure 38–8. The nurse also records body weight. The patient needs to know that the procedure is usually not painful.

Technique

The physician paints the incision site with disinfectant, anesthetizes the area, and then makes a small incision. A common incision site is midway between the umbilicus and symphysis pubis. The physician inserts the trocar and cannula, removes the trocar, and threads the plastic tubing through the cannula into the abdominal cavity. Fluid in the tubing drains into the container.

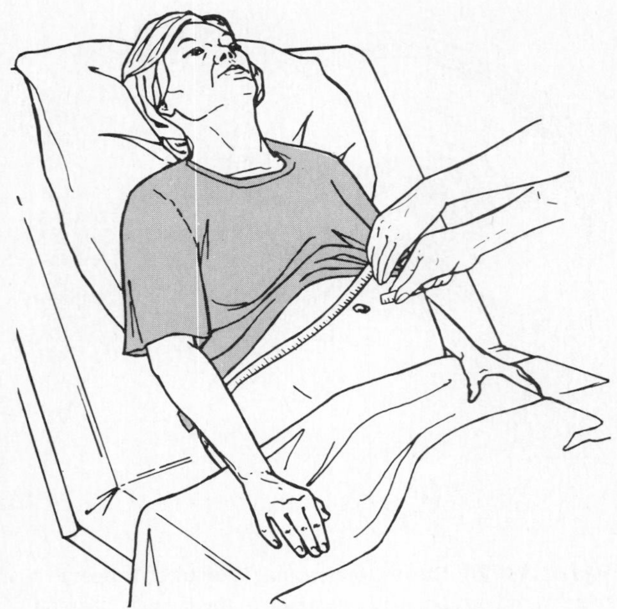

Figure 38–8 Measuring the abdominal girth at the level of the umbilicus before abdominal paracentesis.

The nurse needs to observe the patient carefully during the procedure for signs of shock such as pallor, accelerated pulse rate, sweating, and syncope (fainting). Hypovolemic shock can occur when ascitic fluid is drained too quickly, causing a pressure drop that redirects fluid in the circulatory system to the abdominal area. Ascitic fluid is drained slowly to prevent shock. After paracentesis, the physician removes the cannula and tubing and places a small dressing over the incision. The wound may be sutured. Often patients like the support of an abdominal binder after paracentesis.

Follow-up care

After abdominal paracentesis, the nurse gathers the equipment and labels the specimen, which is sent to the laboratory. Normal ascitic fluid is clear, serous, and light yellow. The protein content is normally low. The nurse records the time, treatment, name of the physician, color and consistency of the fluid, amount of fluid removed, and the response of the patient.

After abdominal paracentesis, the nurse assesses the patient's blood pressure, pulse, and respirations; measures abdominal girth; and weighs the patient. Body weight and abdominal girth, when compared to previous measures, indicate the amount of fluid removed.

Thoracocentesis (Thoracentesis)

Thoracocentesis is the withdrawal of fluid or air from the pleural cavity. Normally there is only enough fluid to lubricate the pleura so that they can move freely. Pleural fluid is removed for both diagnostic and therapeutic purposes. A specimen can be analyzed for the presence of pneumococci, streptococci, and other microorganisms. Aspiration of air or fluid may be indicated to relieve pain, dyspnea, and other symptoms of pleural pressure.

Equipment

The equipment required for thoracocentesis includes local anesthetic, needle and syringe for its administration, disinfectant, gauze swabs, aspirating set, sterile gloves, sterile drapes, mask, container for discarded materials, airtight drainage receptacle, and suction machine or pump to create negative pressure in the drainage receptacle. Because sterile technique must be observed, all supplies and equipment need to be sterile with the exception of the suction machine or pump.

Preparation

The nurse obtains vital signs for baseline data if not readily available and assists the patient to a sitting position with arms stretched upward and forward. See Figure 38–9. This position spreads the ribs, enlarging the intercostal spaces for insertion of the needle. The nurse needs to explain that although the procedure is not normally painful, the patient may experience pressure as the needle is inserted.

Technique

Strict sterile technique is followed. The physician dons sterile gloves, applies antiseptic solution to the patient's skin, administers the local anesthetic, and selects the site of insertion by palpation. This site must be below the level of the fluid if fluid is being removed; a common insertion site is the lower posterior chest. However, the upper anterior chest is often the preferred site if the aim is to remove air. A syringe or stopcock is then attached to the aspirating needle. The stopcock must be in the closed position so that no air enters the pleural space. The physician inserts the needle through the intercostal space to the pleural cavity and in some instances threads a small plastic tube through the needle and then withdraws the needle. (Tubing is less likely to puncture the pleura than a needle.) If using a syringe, the physician pulls on the plunger to draw out the pleural fluid. If using a stopcock, the physician opens it. When a large airtight container is used to receive the fluid, the tubing connects the stopcock to the adapter on the receiving bottle. When the stopcock is opened, the negative pressure in the container, produced by a pump or suction machine, draws the fluid from the pleural cavity. After

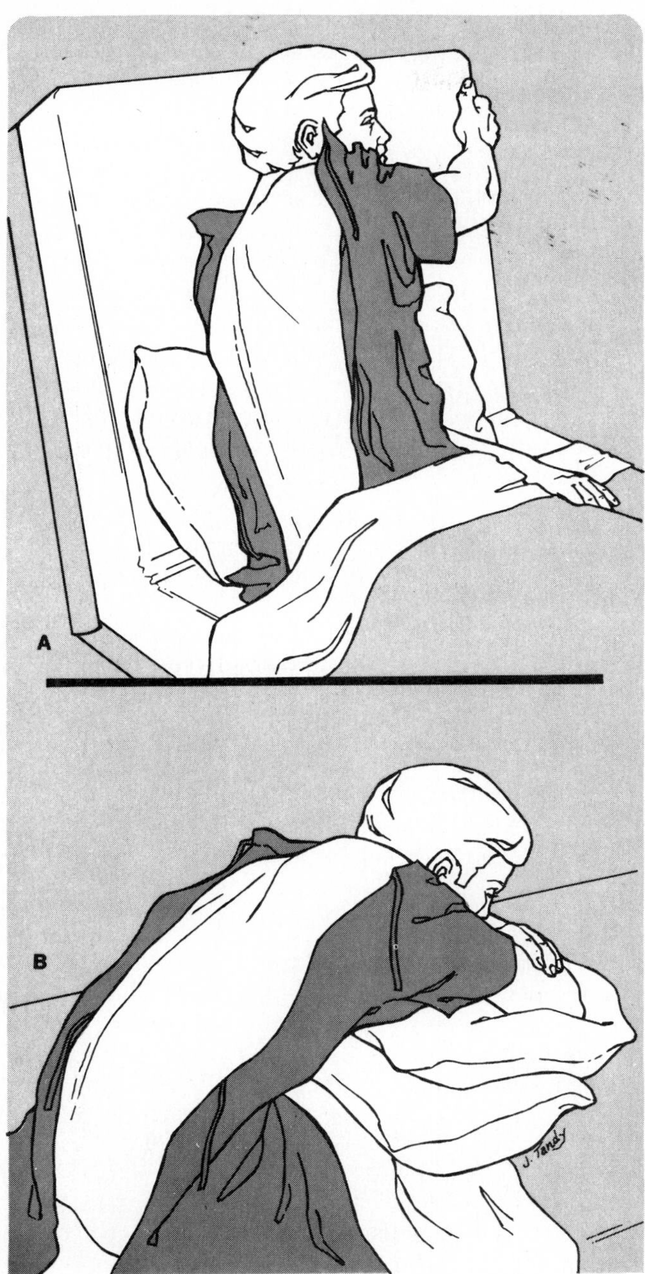

Figure 38–9 Two positions commonly assumed by patients having thoracocentesis: **A,** arm held in front and up; **B,** sitting and leaning forward over pillows.

the fluid is withdrawn, the physician removes the needle or plastic tubing and applies a sterile dressing over the puncture site.

It is important that the patient not cough during this procedure. If the patient has to cough, the physician withdraws the needle slightly so that it does not puncture the pleura. Sometimes a cough suppressant is ordered 30 minutes before thoracocentesis.

Follow-up care

The nurse records the time; treatment; name of the physician; amount, color, and consistency of the fluid; and the response of the patient. Also, the nurse assesses the patient's respirations, particularly noting excessive coughing or blood-tinged sputum (hemoptysis). If thoracocentesis is successful, the patient often feels relief and is able to breathe with less difficulty.

Bone Marrow Biopsy

A bone marrow biopsy is the removal of a specimen of bone marrow for study in a laboratory. The biopsy makes it possible to study a bone marrow specimen for abnormal blood cell development and thus to detect anemia, leukemia, and other diseases of the blood. The sternum and the posterior superior iliac crests are common sites for biopsies. See Figure 38–10.

Equipment

The equipment needed for a bone marrow biopsy includes: skin disinfectant and swabs, local anesthetic as

Figure 38–10 The sternum and iliac crests are common sites for bone marrow biopsies.

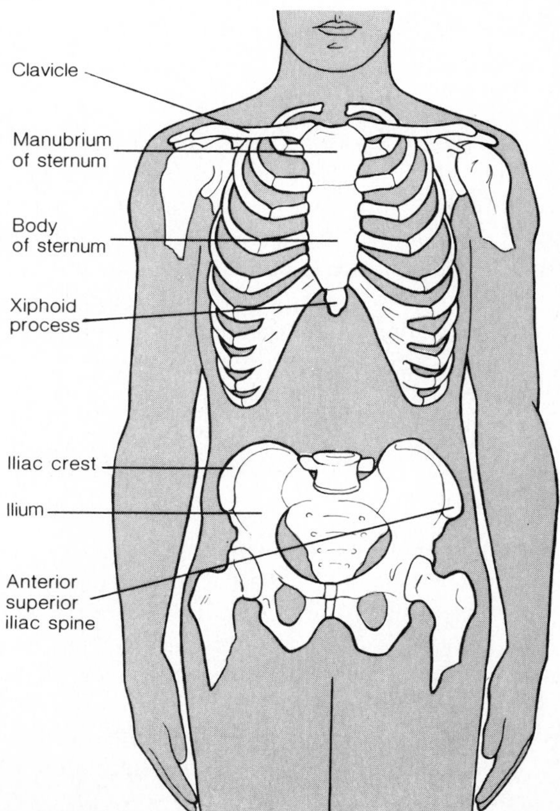

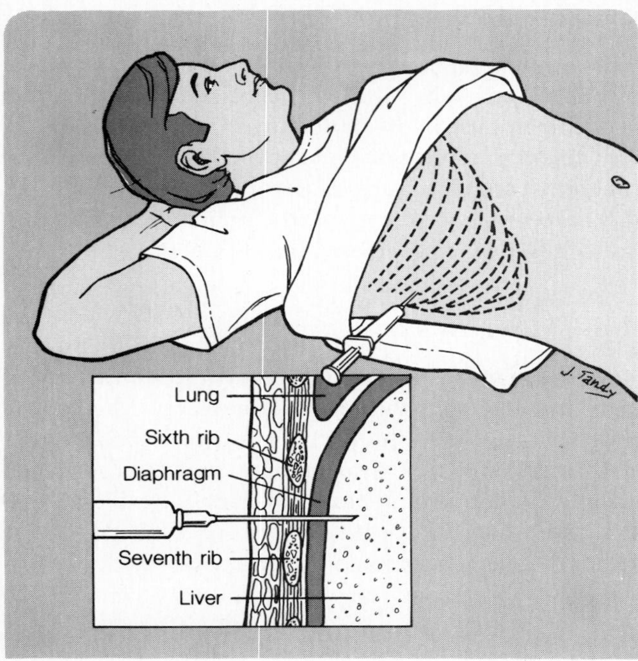

Figure 38–11 A common site for a liver biopsy.

well as a needle and syringe for its administration, bone marrow needle with stylet, aspirating syringe, test tubes (10 ml) or glass specimen slides, small gauze dressing, sterile gloves, sterile drapes, and face masks.

Preparation

Patients need to be informed that the procedure usually takes 15 to 30 minutes, that they may hear a crunching sound and feel pressure as the physician pushes the needle through the cortex of the bone, and that they may feel some pain as the physician aspirates the bone marrow. During a sternal puncture, the patient lies supine with one pillow beneath the head. During a puncture of either iliac crest, the patient commonly lies prone or is positioned according to agency practice. Vital signs are obtained for baseline data if they are not already available.

Technique

The physician dons the sterile gloves, applies the drape, and cleans the skin with disinfectant. The local anesthetic is administered into the skin and into the periosteum of the bone. The physician passes the needle with the stylet through the skin and bone into the red marrow of the spongy bone. Once in the marrow, the stylet is removed and a 10 ml syringe is attached to the needle. The physician pulls on the syringe plunger to withdraw 1 to 2 ml of marrow, replaces the stylet in the needle, and finally removes the needle. The bone marrow specimen is placed in test tubes or on glass slides and a small gauze dressing is applied over the puncture site.

Follow-up care

Following the biopsy, the nurse needs to assess the patient for pain and bleeding from the site; the patient may need an analgesic. The nurse arranges for the specimen with the completed requisition and label to be sent to the laboratory and records the procedure on the patient's chart. The nurse needs to record the procedure, the date and time it was performed, the name of the physician who performed the procedure, the response of the patient, and the fact that specimens were sent to the laboratory.

Liver Biopsy

A liver biopsy is a short procedure, generally performed at the patient's bedside. It requires sterile technique. The physician inserts a needle into the liver to aspirate a sample of liver tissue. The site of insertion is either between two of the right lower ribs (see Figure 38–11) or through the abdomen below the right rib cage. Liver biopsies are usually conducted to facilitate diagnosis of liver disease and to gain information about changes in liver tissue.

Equipment

The equipment needed for biopsy of the liver includes: skin disinfectant and swabs, local anesthetic as well as needle and syringe for its administration, large biopsy syringe and needle, sterile normal saline to clean the biopsy needle after insertion, specimen container with formalin, sterile drapes, sterile gloves, and face mask.

Preparation

Because many patients with liver disease have blood clotting defects and are prone to bleeding, blood tests (e.g., prothrombin time and platelet count) are normally taken well in advance of the test. If the test results are abnormal the biopsy is often contraindicated. Several days before the test, the physician may order an intramuscular injection of vitamin K to reduce the risk of hemorrhage. (Some patients with liver disease may be deficient in vitamin K, necessary for the production of prothrombin, which in turn plays an essential role in blood clotting.)

When explaining the test to the patient, the nurse needs to include:

1. What the physician is going to do; i.e., take a small sample of liver tissue by putting a needle into his or her side or abdomen

2. That the patient will be given a sedative and local anesthetic
3. When and where the procedure will take place
4. Who will be present
5. How long the procedure will take
6. What sensations to expect during the procedure, e.g., mild discomfort as the local anesthetic is injected and slight pressure when the biopsy needle is inserted

It is also vitally important that the patient be told to (and is able to) hold his or her breath for up to 10 seconds when the biopsy needle is inserted and that the patient remain still while the needle is in place.

The patient should fast for at least 2 hours before the procedure and be given a sedative about 30 minutes before. Privacy is provided. The patient lies supine, with the upper right quadrant of the abdomen exposed. Vital signs are obtained for baseline data if they are not already available.

Technique

The physician puts on the sterile gloves, applies an antiseptic to the puncture site, drapes the area with sterile drapes, and injects the local anesthetic. When the area is numb, the patient is instructed to hold his or her breath so the ribs will not move. The physician inserts the biopsy needle and injects a small amount of sterile, normal saline to clear the needle of blood or particles of tissue accumulated during insertion. The physician aspirates some liver tissue by drawing back on the plunger of the syringe, withdraws the needle, and applies pressure to the site to prevent bleeding. A small dressing is then applied to the puncture site.

Follow-up care

The nurse helps the patient to a right side-lying position with a small pillow or folded towel under the puncture site and instructs the patient to remain in this position for several hours. The right lateral position compresses the liver against the chest wall and minimizes the escape of blood or bile through the puncture. The nurse needs to assess the patient's pulse, respirations, and blood pressure every 15 minutes for the first hour following the test or until signs are stable. Complications of the liver biopsy are rare, but a perforated blood vessel can hemorrhage. Also, severe abdominal pain may indicate bile peritonitis (an inflammation of the peritoneal lining of the abdomen), a result of bile leaking from an accidentally perforated bile duct. The nurse checks the biopsy site regularly for localized bleeding. Pressure dressings may be required if bleeding occurs.

The nurse needs to send the labeled specimen and the completed requisition to the laboratory immediately. The nurse then records the procedure on the patient's chart, including the date and time it was performed, the name of the physician, and the response of the patient.

Roentgenographic Examinations

There are several types of roentgenographic examinations. Some body parts, such as bones, are of themselves sufficiently dense to be visible on roentgenograms (x-ray films). Other structures (e.g., the digestive tract, kidney, and blood vessels) must come in contact with contrast media before they are visible on x-ray films. See Figure 38–12.

Contrast media are introduced into the body:

1. Orally or rectally to view the digestive tract (esophagus, stomach, intestines) and gallbladder
2. Intravenously to view the blood vessels, bile ducts, and kidneys
3. Into the subarachnoid space to view the spine and the ventricles of the brain

Scans are x-ray procedures that require a device called a scanner, which includes a scanning device (probe), a computer, a printout machine, and a viewing apparatus. During some scanning procedures (*tomography*), several x-ray beams pass through a body part from different angles. As the x-rays pass through

Figure 38–12 An x-ray film of the small and large intestines filled with a contrast medium.

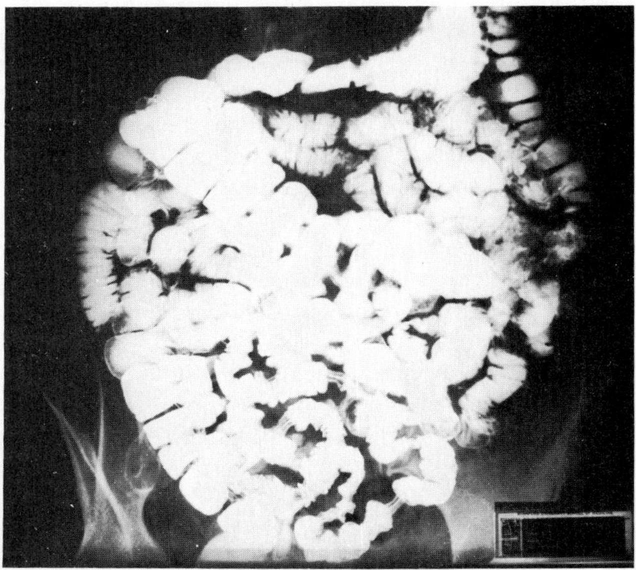

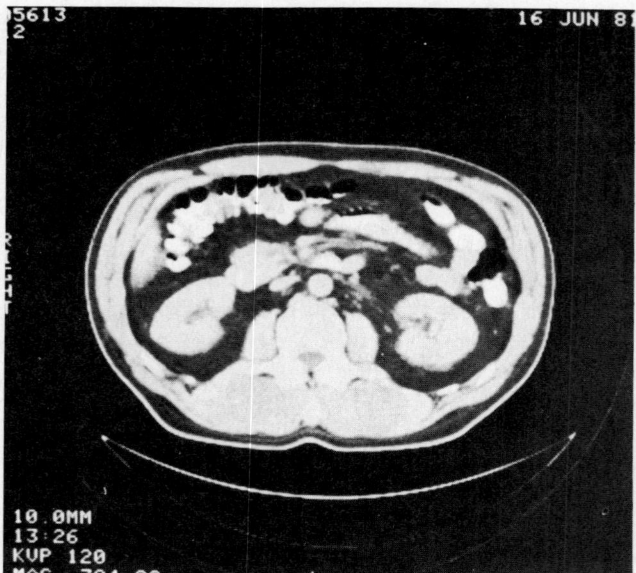

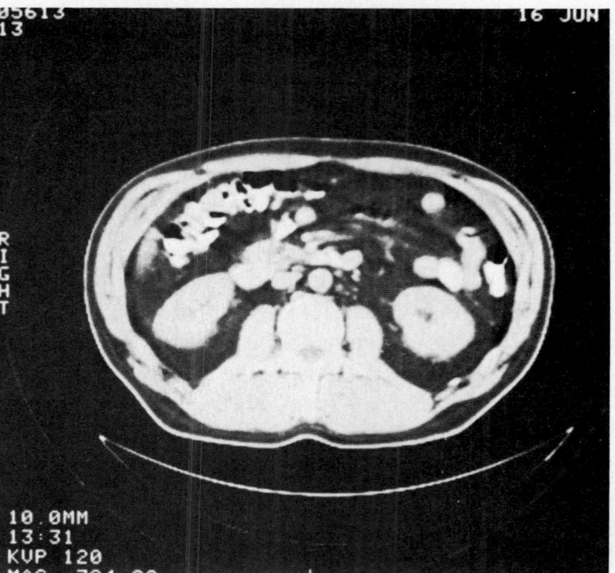

Figure 38–13 A CAT scan showing a cross section of the patient at midabdomen. The spine is at the base; the kidneys are to the left and right of the spine.

different tissues (e.g., fatty tissue, muscle tissue, or a tumor), a movable pen records an image on paper. This image shows variations in the tissues subjected to x-rays. This type of scan is commonly referred to as a CAT scan or CTT scan (computerized transaxial tomogram). See Figure 38–13. The mammogram (x-ray film of the breast) is an example.

In other scanning procedures radioactive materials that have an affinity for specific body tissues are introduced orally or intravenously. For example, radioactive iodine may be given as part of a test to evaluate the function of the thyroid gland, which uses iodine to produce the hormone thyroxin. The thyroid scan lets health personnel see how much of the radioactive iodine the thyroid uses and how the iodine is distributed in the gland. Scans can show the concentration of radioactive particles in any body organ (e.g., brain scan, liver scan, lung scan) and help physicians evaluate the function of an organ or determine the existence of a tumor.

The reasons for roentgenography are:

1. To show abnormalities in the structure or appearance of body organs, e.g., ulcerations in the stomach, tumors, bone fractures, or consolidated infectious material in the lungs
2. To detect impaired function of body organs, e.g., decreased function of the gallbladder or thyroid gland
3. To detect obstructions in body ducts or vessels, e.g., stones in the bile ducts or urinary system, or blood clots in the arteries
4. To determine the extent or spread of malignant tumors

The nurse's role in x-ray procedures is largely to prepare the patient for the examination and provide follow-up care. The nurse must also be alert to complications associated with common x-ray examinations.

Upper Gastrointestinal (GI) Series

The patient swallows barium, and x-ray films are taken of its course through the esophagus, stomach, and duodenum.

Preparation

1. The patient fasts 4 to 6 hours before the test.
2. The nurse explains that:
 a. The patient will feel no discomfort.
 b. The patient will drink a flavored, chalky substance (barium) in the radiology department.
3. The procedure usually takes about 30 minutes.

Follow-up care

1. Administer laxative to eliminate the barium.
2. Observe the regularity of bowel elimination and the passage of barium.

Complications

There may be fecal impaction due to retained barium.

Lower Gastrointestinal Series

The patient is given a barium enema, and x-ray films of the large intestine are taken.

Preparation

1. The patient receives a clear liquid diet 12 to 24 hours before the test to ensure an empty bowel.
2. On the morning of the test, the patient is given enemas until returns are clear and the bowel is free of fecal material.
3. The nurse explains that:
   a. The barium enema will create a feeling of fullness, and the patient may feel the urge to defecate.
   b. The patient may feel slight cramping.
   c. Tubes with balloons may be used to help the patient retain the barium.
   d. The patient will be asked to assume various positions during radiography, e.g., lying on the left side, then lying on the right side.
   e. The patient will expel the barium in the radiology department.
   f. The procedure takes about 30 minutes.

Follow-up care

1. Provide a rest period because the procedure can be tiring.
2. Resume the patient's regular diet; give a light snack as needed.
3. Observe the regularity of bowel elimination and the passage of barium. A cleaning enema may be necessary.

Complications

Fecal impaction due to retained barium may occur.

Cholecystography

The patient swallows a contrast dye, and x-ray films are taken of the gallbladder.

Preparation

1. The patient eats a fat-free supper the evening before the procedure.
2. The patient is checked for allergy to the contrast dye, which contains iodine.
3. In some agencies, a laxative is given the evening before the test. In others, an enema is given the morning of the test.
4. The patient takes six or more contrast pills, e.g., iopanoic acid tablets (Telepaque), at 5-minute intervals the evening before the test. Each tablet is taken with 4 to 6 oz of water.
5. The patient fasts from midnight the night before the test but may drink water.
6. The nurse explains that:
   a. The patient will drink a fatty liquid in the radiology department.
   b. There is usually no discomfort.
   c. The procedure usually lasts about 30 to 45 minutes.

Follow-up care

1. Provide a rest period after the test.
2. Resume the patient's regular diet. Give a light snack if the patient is hungry.

Complications

Some patients are allergic to the contrast dye. Allergic reactions range from mild to severe. Signs of allergic reaction include nausea, vomiting, skin rash, flushing, itching, wheezing, and shock.

Intravenous Cholangiography

X-ray films are taken of the bile ducts after dye is administered intravenously.

Preparation

1. The patient fasts from midnight the night before the test but may drink water.
2. The bowel is cleaned before the test. The patient is either given a laxative the evening before or an enema the morning of the test.
3. The patient is checked for allergy to the contrast dye.
4. The nurse explains that:
   a. Iodine dye will be given intravenously in the radiology department.
   b. Just before the test, the patient may receive an injection of dye in the arm to test for allergic reaction to the dye.
   c. The procedure usually lasts 30 to 45 minutes.

Follow-up care

Resume the patient's regular diet. Provide a light snack if the patient is hungry.

Complications

Some patients are allergic to the contrast dye. Signs of an allergic reaction include itching, hives, wheezing, and shock.

Intravenous Pyelography (IVP) or Urography (IVU)

The patient receives an intravenous injection of radiopaque material, which allows the urinary system (kidney and ureters) to be viewed by roentgenography.

Preparation

1. The patient is given a strong laxative, e.g., castor oil, the afternoon before the test to clear the bowel of fecal material, which can obstruct the view of the urinary system.
2. The patient fasts from midnight the night before the test.
3. The patient is tested for allergy to iodine.
4. The nurse explains that:
   a. The patient will receive an intravenous injection in the radiology department.
   b. The procedure takes about 1 hour.

Follow-up care

1. Encourage the patient to drink fluids and resume the patient's regular diet.
2. Provide for rest. The laxative, together with fasting, can weaken the patient.
3. Observe for adverse reactions to the radiopaque dye.

Complications

Some patients are allergic to the radiopaque dye. Signs of an adverse reaction include itching, hives, wheezing, and shock.

Angiography

Angiography is the roentgenographic visualization of any part of the vascular system. Cerebral angiography is visualization of the vascular system of the brain; coronary arteriography is visualization of the arteries of the heart; renal angiography is visualization of the vascular system of the kidneys; pulmonary angiography is visualization of the vascular system of the lungs; etc. These structures are viewed after a radiopaque material is injected into an artery or vein. The duration of the procedure varies with the part of the vascular system viewed. Some procedures may last up to 3 hours.

Preparation

Preparation varies with the part of the vascular system viewed. Some preparations follow:

1. Before all procedures, the patient is tested for allergy to the radiopaque material.
2. Before some procedures, the patient is sedated.
3. Before some procedures, a catheter is inserted into an artery or vein before the radiopaque material is injected.
4. Before some procedures (e.g., renal angiography) a laxative is administered.
5. The patient usually fasts from midnight the night before any angiography, unless otherwise indicated.
6. The nurse gives appropriate explanations before the test.

Follow-up care

1. Provide bedrest for up to 12 hours.
2. Monitor radial pulse, respirations, and blood pressure every 15 to 30 minutes until vital signs stabilize.
3. Monitor peripheral pulses distal to the puncture site.
4. Observe the injection site for bleeding and swelling.
5. Record discomfort reported by the patient.

Complications

1. Some patients are allergic to the radiopaque material. Signs of allergic reactions include itching, hives, wheezing, and shock.
2. There may be irritation or bleeding at the injection site.
3. Emboli or thrombus formation is a possibility.

Myelography

A contrast material is injected into the subarachnoid space, and x-ray films are taken of the spinal cord, nerve roots, and vertebrae.

Preparation

1. The patient may need to fast from midnight the night before the procedure.
2. If ordered by the physician, sedation is given.
3. The nurse explains that:
   a. In the radiology department, the patient will receive an injection of radiopaque oil via a lumbar or cisternal puncture.
   b. The patient will assume various positions, e.g., side-lying, then prone, then tilted on a table equipped with shoulder and foot supports.
   c. The patient may feel some pain when the oil is removed because it may irritate the nerve roots.
   d. The procedure may take up to 2 hours.

Follow-up care

1. Generally, position the patient flat in bed for 24 hours to minimize headache and nausea. If, however, the dye is not completely removed, elevate the head

above the spine because this position prevents dye from moving to the head and causing meningitis.
2. Monitor vital signs and neurologic status. Be alert to reports by the patient of numbness, pain or tingling in the extremities, muscle weakness, etc.
3. Monitor urinary output.

Complications

1. Postpuncture headache may start a few hours after the test and last for several days up to a week. Generally, the headache occurs when the patient sits up or moves the head suddenly.
2. The contrast media may cause chemical meningitis, characterized by a stiff neck and elevated temperature.
3. Urinary retention is an occasional complication.

Organ Scan

Organ scans are scanning examinations (e.g., brain scan, liver scan, lung scan, etc.) of body organs after oral or intravenous administration of a radioactive substance.

Preparation

1. The patient is given a radioactive substance orally or intravenously.
2. Depending on the radioactive substance used, a blocking agent may be given to prevent uptake of the substance by organs not being studied. For instance, strong iodine solution (Lugol's solution) blocks uptake by the thyroid. The iodine solution is given orally with juice, since its taste is unpleasant. A potassium compound is given for the same purpose if the patient is allergic to iodine. Sodium mercaptomerin, given intramuscularly, blocks the kidney's uptake of the radioactive substance.
3. The patient is checked for allergy to the blocking agent, if used.
4. Sedation is given, if ordered, to children and restless patients.
5. The nurse explains that:

- **a.** There is no need to fear exposure to radiation; exposure is less during a scan than during the usual x-ray examination.
- **b.** The scan is performed in the nuclear medicine department.
- **c.** There is a brief wait while the body distributes the radioactive substance.
- **d.** The patient will feel no discomfort.
- **e.** The patient will be asked to assume various positions and must remain still while the scans are taken.

Follow-up care

Prepare patients for additional scans, performed at varying intervals (e.g., 2 hours, 24 hours, 48 hours, and 72 hours) after the first.

Complications

Some patients are allergic to blocking agents. Allergic reactions range from mild to severe and vary with the blocking agent used.

Summary

When assisting with special procedures, the nurse has these responsibilities:

1. Preparing patients psychologically to alleviate their fear of the unknown and increase their positive participation in the procedure
2. Preparing patients physically, e.g., administering sedatives or cleaning enemas, making sure patients observe fasts if necessary, and positioning patients
3. Assembling equipment for the physician performing the procedure
4. Supporting the patient during the procedure, for example, explaining what is happening
5. Assisting the physician as required, for example, by acquiring specimens
6. Providing follow-up care, including assessing the patient's response, observing for complications, recording the procedure, and handling the specimen appropriately

To fulfill these responsibilities, the nurse must understand the procedure, know what sensations the patient will experience, and be familiar with the complications that can arise.

Suggested Activities

1. In a nursing laboratory, practice preparing for each of the following procedures:
- **a.** Lumbar puncture
- **b.** Paracentesis

c. Thoracocentesis
d. Bone marrow biopsy
e. Liver biopsy

2. In a nursing laboratory, choose a classmate to play the role of the patient. Explain the following procedures:
a. Bronchoscopy
b. ECG
c. Bone marrow biopsy

Reverse roles and have your classmate explain the following procedures to you:
a. Proctoscopy
b. Liver biopsy
c. Cystoscopy

3. In a clinical area, interview four patients who have had one of the above procedures. How did they feel about the procedures? What explanations and preparation were given? What follow-up care was given? Compare your findings with those of other members of your class.

4. Plan nursing interventions to meet the needs of a patient who will be having a test or treatment. Establish criteria by which to assess the patient's response and to evaluate the effectiveness of the test or treatment.

5. In a clinical setting, find opportunities to observe or assist with diagnostic or therapeutic procedures.

Suggested Readings

Blackwell, C. A. February 1975. PEG and angiography: A patient's sensations. *American Journal of Nursing* 75:264–66.
Knowing what a patient feels during a carotid arteriogram and a pneumoencephalogram can help the nurse prepare patients for such procedures.

Hansen, B. D., and Evans, M. L. November-December 1981. Preparing a child for procedures. *The American Journal of Maternal Child Nursing* 6:392–97.
The authors suggest general principles for preparing children before medical procedures. In addition, specific guidelines that outline the child's developmental stage and the nurse's role are provided.

Luciano, K., and Shumsky, C. J. January 1975. Pediatric procedures: The explanation should always come first. *Nursing 75* 5:49–52.
Explanations are important and must be suited to the age of the patient. Infants, toddlers, and their parents need reassurance before pediatric procedures. Ways to communicate with each age group are shown with examples.

Shearer, D.; Collins, B.; and Creel, D. January 1975. Preparing a patient for EEG. *American Journal of Nursing* 75:63–64.
Physical and psychologic preparation of the patient improve the quality of EEG recordings.

Van Meter, M., and Lavine, P. G. April 1975. What every nurse should know about EKGs - Part 1. *Nursing 75* 5:19–27.
Included are the interpretation of EKG readings, the twelve-lead system, and types of rhythms. The electric impulses of the heart's conduction system are explained on pages 26 and 27.

Selected References

Asbury, A. J. 5 July 1973. Electronic equipment in nursing. *Nursing Times* 69:861–63.

Beaumont, E. April 1975. Diagnostic kits. *Nursing 75* 5:28–33.

Byrne, C. J.; Saxton, D. F.; Pelikan, P. K.; and Nugent, P. M. 1981. *Laboratory tests: Implications for nurses and allied health professionals.* Menlo Park, Calif.: Addison-Wesley Publishing Co.

French, R. M. 1975. *Guide to diagnostic procedures.* 4th ed. New York: McGraw-Hill Book Co.

Guyton, A. C. 1982. Human physiology and mechanisms of disease. 3rd ed. Philadelphia: W. B. Saunders Co.

Kozier, B., and Erb, G. 1982. *Techniques in clinical nursing: A comprehensive approach.* Menlo Park, Calif.: Addison-Wesley Publishing Co.

Marici, F. N. October 1973. The flexible fiberoptic bronchoscope. *American Journal of Nursing* 73:1776–78.

Neufeld, A. H. February 1974. Clinical laboratory procedures. *Canadian Nurse* 70:25–44.

Chapter 39

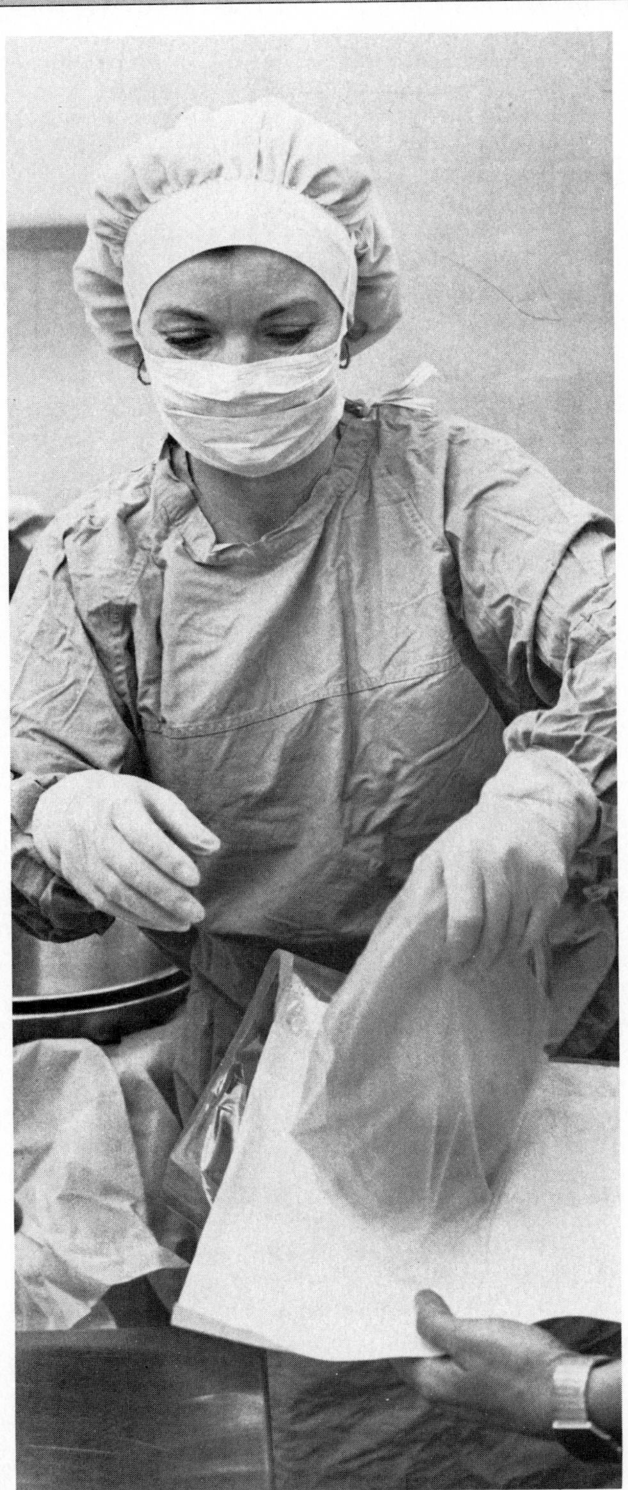

Perioperative Care

CONTENTS

(Continued on next page)

Objectives

1. Know essential terms and facts about surgery, anesthesia, and preoperative planning and care

- **1.1** Define selected terms
- **1.2** Identify the essentials of informed consent
- **1.3** Identify factors that increase surgical risk
- **1.4** Identify common health problems that increase surgical risk
- **1.5** Outline essential information to obtain in the nursing history of a patient having surgery
- **1.6** List common screening tests or examinations performed prior to surgery and the reasons for them
- **1.7** Outline information essential for the nurse to plan preoperative care

2. Understand essential information about preoperative nursing interventions

- **2.1** Identify essentials of teaching patients to move and to carry out leg, coughing, and deep breathing exercises
- **2.2** Identify the nurse's responsibilities for preparing the patient on the day before surgery
- **2.3** Identify essential steps of preoperative skin preparation and the reasons for these steps
- **2.4** Identify the nurse's responsibilities for preparing the patient on the day of surgery
- **2.5** Identify essential steps for inserting a nasogastric tube and the reasons for these steps
- **2.6** Give reasons for routine measures carried out preoperatively

3. Understand essential facts of postoperative nursing assessment and interventions

- **3.1** Identify assessment data required in the initial postoperative period
- **3.2** Identify nursing interventions required in the immediate postoperative period
- **3.3** Identify assessment data required when patients return to the nursing unit from the recovery room
- **3.4** Identify postoperative complications, their causes, and nursing interventions to prevent them
- **3.5** Use essential information from the patient's record to plan postoperative care
- **3.6** Identify general postoperative nursing interventions that relieve discomfort and prevent complications

4. Prepare a patient physically and psychologically for surgery

- **4.1** Provide appropriate preoperative teaching
- **4.2** Prepare the patient adequately on the day before and the day of surgery
- **4.3** Prepare the patient's skin before surgery
- **4.4** Insert a nasogastric tube correctly

5. Provide effective postoperative nursing care to selected patients

- **5.1** Assess patients returning from the recovery room
- **5.2** Gather necessary information from the patient's record to plan postoperative care
- **5.3** With assistance, establish a nursing care plan for the patient
- **5.4** Provide nursing measures to relieve discomfort and prevent complications

Terms

ablative surgery
bronchopneumonia
Cantor tube
caudal anesthetic
constructive surgery
dehiscence
diagnostic surgery
elective surgery
embolus
epidural block
evisceration
exploratory surgery
Harris tube
hypostatic pneumonia
hypovolemic shock
Levin tube
lobar pneumonia
Miller-Abbott tube
nasogastric tube
nerve block
operative (intraoperative)
optional surgery
orogastric tube
palliative surgery
perioperative
postoperative
preoperative
reconstructive surgery
Salem sump tube
singultus
thrombophlebitis
thrombus
tissue perfusion
tympanites
urgent surgery

Operations are traumatic both for patients and their support persons. Today most operations take place in hospitals, which many people associate with pain and death. Many patients equate operations with disfigurement and pain, and the nurse must be sensitive to the psychologic needs of patients having operations.

The *perioperative* period is the time before, during, and after an operation. The *preoperative* period is the time before an operation. The preoperative patient is prepared psychologically and physically for surgery. An important aspect of preoperative nursing is teaching the patient what he or she needs to know. The preoperative period can vary from months to only hours. The *operative* or *intraoperative* period is the time of surgery. It begins with the administration of the anesthetic and terminates when the surgery is completed. The main intraoperative nursing function is to assist the surgical team. The *postoperative* (postsurgical) period is the time following surgery. Major postoperative nursing functions are to help the patient recover from the anesthetic, maintain the patient's body systems, prevent postoperative complications, and prevent undue discomfort. The postoperative period is sometimes divided into the initial postoperative period, during which the patient recovers from the anesthetic, and the continuing postoperative period, after the patient returns to a clinical nursing unit.

The nurse is an essential member of the health team caring for the surgical patient. The nurse prepares patients before operations; often the nurse is responsible for explaining to the patient and family what the operation will entail. After surgery, the nurse helps the patient return to health. Some postoperative patients need to learn certain skills, such as walking with crutches, before they leave the hospital. It is the nurse's responsibility to help patients gain the skills they require. Patients also need skills that help prevent postoperative complications such as pneumonia. Teaching is an important part of the patient's care, and nurses generally are the teachers.

Reasons for Surgery

Surgical procedures can be optional, elective, or urgent. *Optional surgery* is requested by the patient, but it is not necessary for physical health. Usually an operation such as facial plastic surgery is optional and is done for psychologic reasons. *Elective surgery* is surgery the patient chooses to have, such as straightening a bent finger. It is performed for his or her well-being but is not absolutely necessary. *Urgent surgery* is essential for health, such as the removal of an inflamed appendix. Urgent surgery is always essential but not always an emergency. Emergency operations to control internal hemorrhaging are one kind of urgent surgery. Another type of urgent surgery is breast surgery for a malignancy.

The reasons for surgery vary considerably:

1. *Diagnostic surgery* enables the surgeon to confirm a diagnosis. Sometimes a surgeon awaits laboratory analysis of tissue removed during the operation before proceeding with further surgery.

2. *Exploratory surgery* is frequently performed to determine the extent of a pathologic process and sometimes to confirm a diagnosis.

3. *Ablative surgery* is the removal of a diseased organ, such as an inflamed appendix.

4. *Reconstructive surgery* is the restoration of function or normal appearance to damaged tissues, e.g., vaginal repair.

5. *Constructive surgery* is the repair of a congenital malformation, e.g., the repair of a harelip.

6. *Palliative surgery* relieves the symptoms of a disease process, e.g., an intestinal bypass to relieve the symptoms of intestinal obstruction.

Legal Aspects of Surgery

Prior to any surgical procedure patients must sign a surgical consent form. See Figure 39-1. This requirement protects patients from having any surgical procedure they do not want or do not know about. It also protects the hospital and the health personnel from a claim by patients or family that permission was not granted.

Obtaining legal, informed consent to perform surgery is the responsibility of the surgeon. Informed consent is possible only when the patient is told in advance of the character and importance of the surgery, its probable consequences, the chances for success, and alternative measures. Often the responsibility for obtaining consent is delegated to a nurse. For more information about informed consent, see Chapters 3 and 4.

Adults sign their own forms unless they are mentally incompetent or unconscious, in which cases a spouse or next of kin signs for them. Children 19 or younger (18 or younger in some jurisdictions) cannot sign consent forms. A parent or guardian must sign instead. However, some jurisdictions allow teenagers to give consent. In Ontario, a 16-year-old can give consent for surgery. In Quebec, a minor of 14 years can give consent (and be operated on without the parents' knowledge) provided the minor is not hospitalized longer than 12 hours and treatment is not prolonged (Creighton 1981:274). If a minor's parents cannot be found, a court order can be obtained to permit surgery. The consent form becomes a part of the patient's record and goes to the operating room with the patient.

LIONS GATE HOSPITAL

CONSENT FOR EXAMINATION AND TREATMENT

I, the undersigned, do hereby certify that the purpose of this visit or admission of me to Lions Gate Hospital has been explained to me by my physician and I agree that any examination and treatment can be administered which the attending physician or physicians and hospital staff may find necessary for my relief.

Dated this 23 day of August, 1983

(1) Signature of Patient: ____________

(2) Signature of Guardian: James Joffery
(or person authorized
to consent for patient)

Father
(Relationship of above)

Margaret Lane
Signature of Witness

Unconscious
(Reason patient unable to sign)

In situations where it is impossible to obtain a signature on line (1) or (2) above, two physicians shall certify by signing the following:

In the opinion of each of the undersigned physicians the treatment to be carried out is necessary and in the best interest of the continued health and well-being of the patient.

Dated this 23 day of August, 1983

R.W. West, M.D. L.C. Spankie, M.D.

Margaret Lane Margaret Lane
Signature of Witness Signature of Witness

A.456 Rev. 6/78
10M-S-p

Figure 39-1 A sample consent form for surgery and treatment. (Courtesy of Lions Gate Hospital, North Vancouver, British Columbia.)

Preoperative Assessment

Assessing Surgical Risk

The degree of risk involved in a surgical procedure is affected by the patient's (a) age, (b) nutritional status, (c) fluid and electrolyte balance, (d) general health, (e) use of medications, and (f) mental health, including attitude.

Age

Very young and elderly patients are greater surgical risks than children and adults. The neonate's physiologic response to surgery is substantially different from an adult's. Factors that affect the risk are the neonate's circulation, which is largely central, and renal function, which is not fully developed until about 6 months of age. The neonate can respond to an additional need for oxygen only by an increased respiratory rate, and limited blood volume results in a limited fluid reserve. The loss of 30 ml of blood from a neonate is the equivalent of an 850 ml loss from a 200-lb man (Goulding et al. 1965:84–85).

Elderly persons are also at additional risk from surgery. Elderly patients often have impaired circulation due to arteriosclerosis and limited cardiac function. Energy reserves are frequently limited, and hydration and the nutritional status may be poor. In addition, elderly people can be highly sensitive to medications, such as morphine sulfate and barbiturates, frequently used preoperatively and postoperatively.

Nutritional status

Two nutritional problems that can increase surgical risk are obesity and malnutrition due to protein, iron, and vitamin deficiencies. Surgery of obese patients is often deferred except in emergencies. Obese patients have overtaxed hearts and elevated blood pressures. In addition, incisions in overly fatty tissue are difficult to suture and prone to infection. Nutritional deficiencies are seen particularly among elderly and chronically ill patients. Protein and vitamins are needed for wound healing; vitamin K is essential for blood clotting.

Fluid and electrolyte balance

Dehydration and hypovolemia predispose the person to problems during surgery. Electrolyte imbalances often accompany fluid imbalances. Imbalances in calcium, magnesium, potassium, and hydrogen ions are of particular concern during surgery. See Chapter 31.

General health

Operations are least risky when the patient is in general good health. Any infection or pathophysiology increases the risk. Of particular concern are upper respiratory tract infections, which, together with a general anesthetic, can have an adverse effect on respiratory function.

Recent myocardial infarction or any cardiovascular disease can make surgery more dangerous than usual. Renal function is essential for the excretion of body wastes. See Chapter 28. Metabolic and liver function affect healing and the detoxification and elimination of medications. Untreated diabetes mellitus predisposes to infection and impaired tissue healing. When liver function is impaired, the liver cannot detoxify drugs and metabolize carbohydrates, proteins, and fats efficiently. A person whose blood does not coagulate normally may bleed more than is normal or even hemorrhage and go into shock.

Medications

The regular use of certain medications can increase risk of operations. Some of these medications are:

1. Anticoagulants, which increase blood coagulation time
2. Tranquilizers, which can cause hypotension and thus contribute to shock
3. Heroin and other depressants, which decrease central nervous system responses
4. Antibiotics that are incompatible with anesthetic agents, resulting in untoward reactions
5. Diuretics, which can create electrolyte (especially potassium) imbalances

Mental health and attitude

Extreme anxiety can increase the surgical risk. See the discussion of physiologic responses to stress in Chapter 9. The person's anxiety is not always related to the seriousness of the surgical procedure. The surgeon needs to know if a person believes he or she will die during surgery. In some instances professional counseling and a delay in the surgery are indicated.

Patients who have been poorly adjusted for some time may not be able to cope with the additional stress of surgery. People who cope only minimally in a stable, familiar environment can develop full neuroses or psychoses postoperatively.

Physical Examination

If surgery is elective or optional, the physical examination is usually done in the physician's office prior to admission to the agency, but it is done on admission before emergency surgery. In some settings, nurses perform the physical examination. For information about physical examinations, see Chapters 13 and 14. Knowledge of the patient's overall health is essential in preventing complications and reducing surgical risk.

Common health problems that increase surgical risk and may lead to the decision to postpone or cancel surgery include:

1. Cardiac conditions such as angina pectoris, recent myocardial infarction, severe hypertension, or severe congestive heart failure. Well-controlled cardiac problems generally pose little operative risk.
2. Blood coagulation problems that may lead to severe bleeding, hemorrhage, and subsequent shock.
3. Upper respiratory tract infections or chronic obstructive lung diseases such as emphysema. These conditions, especially when exacerbated by the effects of a general anesthetic, adversely affect pulmonary function. They also predispose the patient to postoperative lung infections.
4. Renal disease that impairs adequate excretion of body wastes. Examples are acute nephritis and renal insufficiency.
5. Diabetes mellitus, which predisposes the patient to wound infection and delayed healing.
6. Liver disease such as cirrhosis, which impairs the liver's ability to detoxify medications used during surgery, to produce the prothrombin necessary for blood clotting, and to metabolize nutrients essential for healing.
7. Uncontrolled neurologic disease such as epilepsy.

Nursing History

The nursing history acquired on admission provides patient data that helps the nurse plan preoperative and postoperative care. Although forms vary considerably among agencies, essential preoperative information includes:

1. Physical condition. The patient's general appearance—color, weight, hydration status, and energy level—is noted. Problems such as obesity, malnutrition, dehydration, or marked fatigue may indicate the need for therapy prior to surgery. For instance, the dehydrated patient may need fluids administered intravenously.
2. Mental attitude. Anxiety is a normal response to surgery. However, extreme anxiety can increase the surgical risk and needs to be reported to the physician.
3. Understanding of the surgery. Determining the patient's knowledge about the surgery helps the nurse plan appropriate instruction. A well-informed patient knows what to expect and in general accepts and copes more effectively with surgery and convalescence.
4. Experience with previous surgeries. Some previous experiences may influence the patient's physical and psychologic responses to the planned surgery. For example, a patient who developed a wound infection that caused a gape in a previous incision may demonstrate acute anxiety when a surgical dressing or sutures are removed and may be unwilling to move, believing that movement will cause the wound to gape.
5. Expected outcomes of surgery. Surgery alters patients' body images and life-styles to varying degrees. A middle-aged woman about to have a hysterectomy may feel she will no longer be valued or adequate as a wife and mother; a young man having a hernia repair may worry that he will miss his chance to play in a championship football game. To provide the necessary support for adjustments, nurses need to determine each patient's concerns.
6. Use of medications. Because some medications react with anesthetics or other drugs, the nurse needs to list all medications (birth control pills, diuretics, vitamins, anticonvulsants, insulin, etc.) the patient takes. Certain medications, such as anticonvulsants or insulin, must be continued throughout the operative period to prevent adverse effects. A physician's order to this effect is required, however.
7. Smoking habits. The lung tissue of a person who smokes is chronically irritated, and a general anesthetic irritates it further. When possible, nurses discourage patients from smoking on the day of surgery and are alert for respiratory complications following surgery.
8. Excessive use of alcohol. Moderate use of alcohol does not present a surgical hazard, but heavy, consistent use can lead to problems during anesthesia, surgery, and recovery.
9. Names of family members or friends. Family members or friends provide considerable support to the surgical patient. They need to be recognized and often included in health instruction or follow-up care given to the patient.

Screening Tests

The physician is responsible for ordering all the radiologic and laboratory tests and examinations the patient needs. The nurse's responsibility is to check the orders carefully, to see that they are carried out, and to ensure that the results are obtained prior to surgery.

Some screening tests conducted prior to surgery are:

1. Chest roentgenography to determine the condition of the patient's lungs and in some situations heart size and location. The results may influence both the preoperative sedation ordered and the anesthetic administered.
2. Blood analysis, on the day before surgery when possible. Analysis may include: complete blood count

Table 39–1 Routine Preoperative Screening Tests

Test	Rationale
Urinalysis	To detect urinary tract infections and glucose in the urine
Chest roentgenography	To identify lung pathology and cardiac size
Electrocardiography (usual for patients over 40 years or who have cardiac pathology)	To determine cardiac pathology
Complete blood count (CBC)	To determine hemoglobin and red blood cell count (i.e., the blood's ability to carry oxygen) and white blood cell count, which when elevated signals infection
Blood grouping and crossmatching	To establish blood type in the event a blood transfusion is needed
Serum electrolytes (Na^+, K^+, Mg^{2+}, Ca^{2+}, H^+)	To determine electrolyte imbalances
Fasting blood sugar	To detect metabolic disorders, such as diabetes mellitus
Blood urea nitrogen (BUN)	To assess urinary excretion

(CBC), hemoglobin (Hb or Hgb), and hematocrit (Hct). If substantial blood loss is anticipated during surgery, the physician may order a blood typing and cross-match and sufficient units of blood for a replacement transfusion. When the physician anticipates bleeding problems, an analysis of bleeding or clotting time or prothrombin time may also be ordered. The results of blood tests are important in ruling out many problems that could increase the surgical risk. For example, a high white blood cell count (WBC) may signal an infection; a low red blood cell count (RBC) or low hemoglobin may indicate anemia. Both conditions can delay healing.

3. Urine analysis for all patients before surgery. The results may indicate urinary infection, diabetes, or other abnormalities that warrant treatment prior to surgery. See Table 39–1 for routine preoperative screening tests.

In addition to these routine tests, diagnostic tests directly related to the patient's pathology are usually appropriate (e.g., stomach roentgenography to clarify the pathology before gastric surgery). See Chapter 38.

Preoperative Planning and Nursing Intervention

The overall nursing goal for those caring for preoperative patients is to promote optimal physical and psychologic health, thereby minimizing surgical risk. Nursing subgoals include:

1. Identify and meet the patient's and support persons' learning needs.
2. Promote the patient's peace of mind.
3. Meet fluid and nutritional needs or correct nutritional deficiencies.
4. Promote rest.
5. Reduce number of skin microorganisms and potential for postoperative infection.
6. Prevent bowel or bladder incontinence during anesthesia.
7. Prevent aspiration of vomitus and respiratory obstruction by oral prostheses during anesthesia.
8. Prevent physical trauma to the patient during anesthesia.
9. Protect the patient's personal property during the intraoperative period.
10. Ensure the patient's physical status (e.g., circulation) can be assessed appropriately during the intraoperative period.

Planning also involves the establishment of outcome criteria. For suggested examples, see the section on evaluation, page 1025.

Needs of the Patient and Support Persons

The needs of the patient are often largely learning needs. The surgeon is usually responsible for explaining the surgical procedure to the patient. However, patients often ask nurses questions about the operation after the surgeon has left the hospital unit. If the patient is anxious about the procedure or has questions that the nurse is unable to answer, the nurse notifies the surgeon.

The patient may have specific learning needs about her or his postoperative condition. Learning to attend to a colostomy or the like requires preparation before surgery.

Pain is common postoperatively, and patients are reassured to learn beforehand how to minimize it, e.g., by holding a pillow against the abdomen when moving after abdominal surgery. It is important that patients know they will receive analgesics postoperatively and therefore should experience only minimal discomfort. Most patients who undergo operations also need to learn how to move, breathe deeply, cough, and do leg exercises after surgery. These are discussed later in the chapter.

Patients and their support persons need to know the time and type of surgery. The surgeon usually arranges the date for the surgery and may specify it in the orders. The exact time may not be known until the surgical schedule for the hospital is distributed. The surgeon usually indicates the type of surgery in the preoperative orders on the patient's chart. It is the surgeon's responsibility to explain the surgery; however, often nurses are asked to explain aspects of care.

Duration of the Preoperative Period

The duration of the preoperative period often affects preoperative care and planning. When the preoperative period lasts several days, nurses can draw up a nursing care plan and a teaching plan. See Chapter 17. When the preoperative period is just an hour, only the essentials can be carried out. The learning needs of the patient must be met during the postoperative period.

Availability of Nursing Personnel

Various personnel conduct different aspects of preoperative care. The knowledge and skill required for different interventions vary considerably. The personnel available should carry out those aspects of care for which their education and experience best suit them.

Surgeon's Orders

The surgeon usually indicates the type of surgery in the preoperative orders on the patient's chart. From this information, the nurse determines the kind and extent of skin preparation required, if it is not specified on the order. Agencies usually specify the skin preparation practiced before various kinds of surgery. Special surgeon's orders, such as an enema or the insertion of a catheter or Levin tube, are given before certain surgeries. Some agencies maintain a Kardex file in which the surgeon's preferences are noted (for example, "Saline enema the night before surgery").

Agency Practices

Many agencies outline the nursing responsibilities for preoperative care. Often nurses are responsible for verifying that a consent form has been signed and that the physician has completed the medical history and physical examination. Most hospitals require that these be completed before surgery, except in emergencies.

Preoperative Teaching

Moving, leg exercises, coughing, and deep breathing are important skills for preoperative patients to learn to speed convalescence and help prevent complications.

Figure 39–2 The quadriceps (four muscles of the thigh shown in the anterior view at the top) and gastrocnemius muscles (shown in the posterior view at the bottom) are exercised preoperatively and postoperatively.

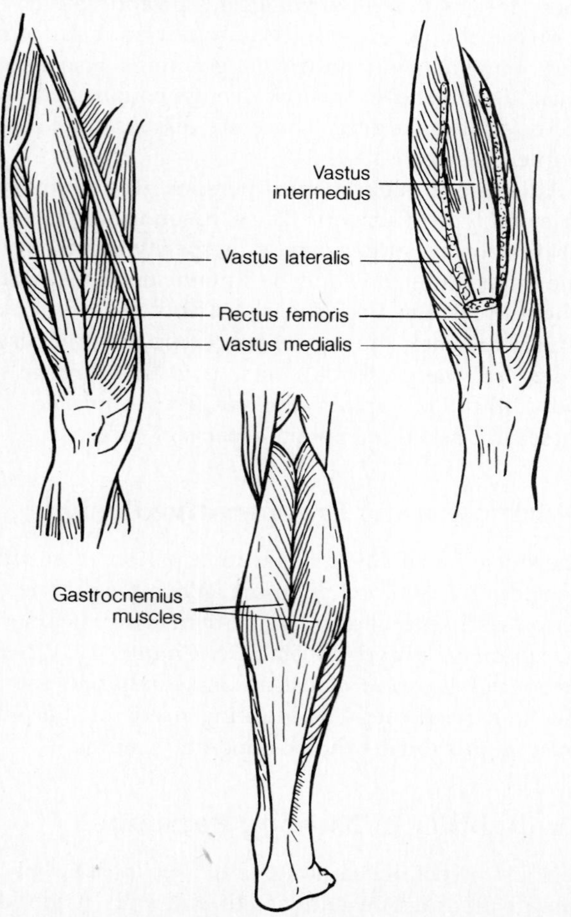

Moving

Turning in bed and early ambulation help patients maintain blood circulation, stimulate respiratory functions, and decrease the stasis of gas in the intestines and resulting discomfort. Patients who practice turning before surgery usually find it easier to do so postoperatively. Some patients require special aids, such as a pillow between the legs, to maintain skeletal alignment. The nursing care plan or the agency procedures specify the kind and duration of movement the patient is to practice.

Leg Exercises

Leg exercises help prevent thrombophlebitis due to slowed venous circulation (venous stasis). The major danger of thrombophlebitis is that thrombi can become emboli and lodge in the arteries of the heart, brain, or lungs, causing serious injury or death.

Leg exercises contract and relax the quadriceps and gastrocnemius muscles. See Figure 39–2. Three exercises that patients need to learn are:

1. Alternate dorsiflexion and plantar flexion of the feet. This exercise is sometimes referred to as calf pumping, since it alternately contracts and relaxes the calf muscles, including the gastrocnemius muscles.
2. Flexion and extension of the knees, along with pressing the backs of the knees into the bed. See Figure 39–3. A patient who cannot raise the legs can do isometric exercises that contract and relax the muscles. See Chapter 24.
3. Raising and lowering the legs alternately from the surface of the bed. The knee of the moving leg is extended. See Figure 39–4. This exercise contracts and relaxes the quadriceps muscles.

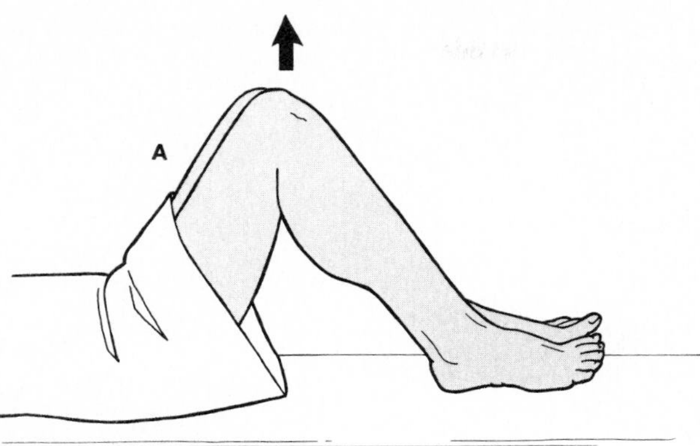

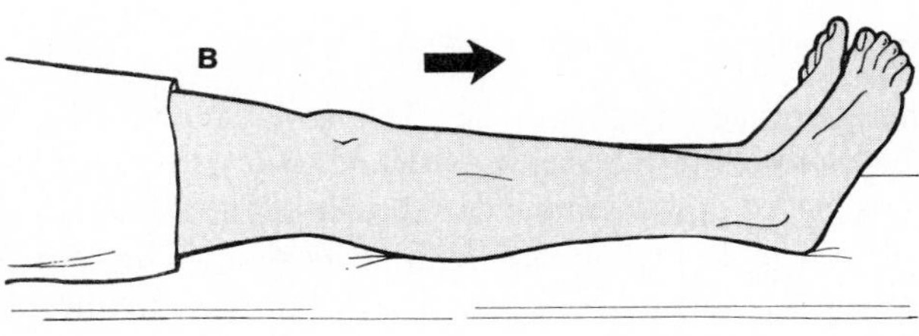

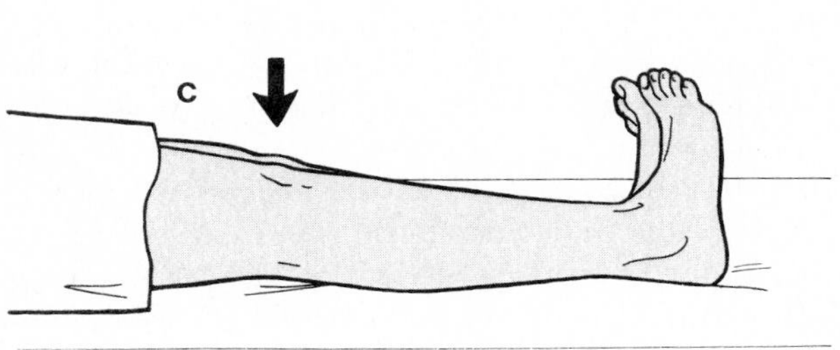

Figure 39–3 Preoperative leg exercises: **A,** flexing the knees; **B,** extending the knees; **C,** pressing the backs of the knees against the bed surface.

The exercises are normally started as soon after surgery as the patient is able. The frequency of exercising depends on the patient's condition and the agency's practices. It is not unusual for patients to do exercises once every waking hour.

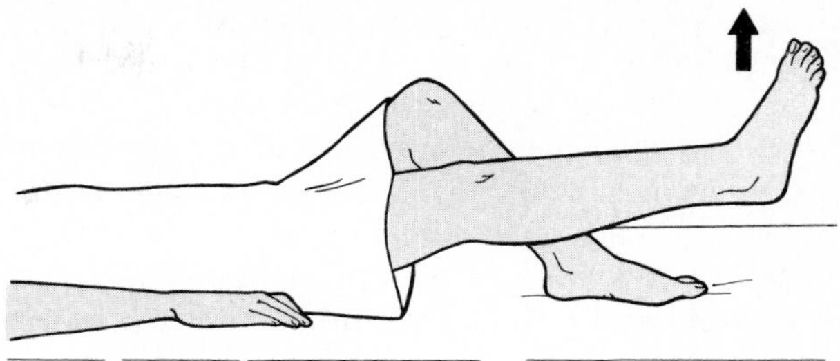

Figure 39–4 Contracting the right quadriceps muscles.

Coughing and Deep Breathing

Coughing and deep breathing exercises help remove mucus, which can form and remain in the lungs due to the effects of a general anesthetic and analgesics. These drugs depress the action of both the cilia of the mucous membranes lining the respiratory tract and the respiratory center in the brain. Deep breathing also aerates lung tissue and thereby helps prevent pneumonia, which may result from stagnation of fluid in the lungs.

While doing deep breathing exercises, the patient inhales and exhales as much air as possible. On inhalation, the diaphragm contracts or flattens, lengthening the chest cavity and pulling the ribcage upward. On exhalation, the diaphragm relaxes or moves upward, and the ribcage is pulled downward. Demonstrating deep breathing to patients is discussed in Chapter 29, page 751.

The number of breaths and the frequency of deep breathing periods vary with the patient's condition. Patients on bedrest and patients recovering from abdominal or chest surgery need to perform deep breathing at least three or four times daily. At each session, the patient should take at least five deep breaths. Patients who are susceptible to pulmonary problems may need deep breathing exercises every hour. Patients with chronic respiratory disease may need special breathing exercises, e.g., pursed-lip breathing and abdominal breathing exercises. See Chapter 29, page 752.

Preoperative Preparation

Psychologic Support

Surgery, and the unknowns patients face during surgery, can produce anxiety in patients and support persons. Some of these unknowns are: What will happen during surgery? How will I feel after the operation? What will the surgeon find?

The nurse needs to find out what specific fears and anxieties patients and support persons have. The patient's self-image may be threatened by disfigurement;

a long hospital stay may mean financial hardship; etc. Once the patient discloses those special concerns, the nurse can offer accurate information and act supportively to help the patient deal with those concerns. Nurses need to listen carefully and not dismiss patients' fears by saying, "Everything will be all right." Often a nurse can relieve anxiety by clarifying patients' misconceptions. By listening carefully, nurses can help patients identify their fears and talk them through.

Children need explanations in language they can understand. The nurse gives information at a rate that keeps their attention and does not overwhelm them. A child may be shown anesthetic equipment and the postanesthesia room ("wakeup room") beforehand. All postoperative care and discomfort should be explained clearly and simply: For example, "You will have a sore tummy." The most important fact to children is when their parents will visit (Luciano 1974:65).

Nutrition and Fluids

Adequate hydration and nutrition promote healing. Nurses need to record any sign of malnutrition. A perioperative record of the patient's weight is one way to assess nutritional status. If the patient is on intravenous fluids or on measured fluid intake, nurses ensure that the fluids are carefully measured. See Chapter 30.

Because anesthetics depress gastrointestinal functioning and because there is a danger the patient may vomit and aspirate vomitus during administration of a general anesthetic, the patient usually fasts at least 6 to 8 hours before surgery. The patient and support persons need to understand the necessity of fasting. Usually, the nurse removes food and fluids from the bedside and places a fasting sign at the bed the evening before surgery. The patient can use a mouthwash if her or his mouth feels dry. If the patient ingests food or fluids during the fasting period, the nurse must notify the surgeon.

Elimination

Depending on the patient's condition, the type of surgery, the physician's order, and agency practice, an enema may be given the evening before surgery. Sometimes a rectal suppository is given instead of an enema, or the enema may be administered the day of surgery. In other instances no special elimination care is given.

Often nurses monitor hydration by measuring fluid intake and output (see Chapter 30) prior to surgery. In some instances, a urinary catheter is inserted the day before or the day of surgery, depending on the surgeon's order and agency practice.

Preoperative Skin Preparation

The purpose of preparing the skin before surgery (preoperative skin preparation) is to destroy microorganisms and thus reduce the chance of an infection.

The skin is shaved the evening before or the day of surgery, as agency policy dictates. In some agencies the patient's skin is "prepped" in a special room just before surgery.

The area prepared is generally larger than the incision area. This practice minimizes the number of microorganisms in the areas adjacent to the incision. Hospital policy dictates how the skin is prepared before various operations.

In some settings, patients are shaved with electric clippers rather than razors. Also, some agencies follow the practice of applying pHisohex, similar germidical soaps, or antiseptic solutions to the shaved areas. Before certain types of surgery, this cleaning is repeated every 4 hours during the patient's waking hours until 2 hours before surgery. Sometimes the shaved area is wrapped in sterile towels between cleanings. Some agencies require that personnel wear sterile gloves and use sterile technique during such cleanings.

Procedure 39–1 Preoperative Skin Preparation

Equipment

1. Adequate lighting that makes the hair on the skin visible
2. A bath blanket to drape the patient

Dry shave

1. Electric clippers with sharp heads and unbroken teeth
2. Scissors for long hair, if needed
3. Antiseptic solution and applicators, if needed

Wet shave

1. Skin preparation set, which contains a disposable razor, compartmentalized basin for solutions, moisture-proof drape to protect the bedding, soap solution, sponges for applying the soap so-

Procedure 39–1, continued

lution, and cotton-tipped applicators for cleaning areas such as the umbilicus

2. Warm water to make the soap solution

Intervention

Before shaving

1. Check the patient's record to verify the surgical site and area to be prepared.
2. Explain to the patient what you plan to do. Adjust the explanation to the patient's needs.
3. Drape the patient. Expose only the area to be shaved at one time. You will shave about 6 inches at a time.

Dry shaving

1. Make sure the area is dry.
2. Shave with clippers; do not apply pressure.

   Rationale Pressure can cause abrasions, particularly over bony prominences.
3. Move the drape and repeat steps 1 and 2 until entire area to be prepared is shaved. If applying antiseptic solution, follow the steps in the section on cleaning and disinfecting, below.

Wet shaving

1. Place the moisture-proof towel under the area to be prepared.
2. Lather the skin well with the soap solution.
3. Stretch the skin taut and hold the razor at about a 45° angle to the skin. Shave in the direction that the hair grows. Use short strokes and rinse the razor frequently.

   Rationale Rinsing removes hairs and lather that can obstruct the blade.
4. Wipe excess hair off the skin with the sponges.
5. Move drape and repeat steps 2–4 until entire area to be prepared is shaved.

Cleaning and disinfecting

1. Clean any body crevices, such as the umbilicus, nails, or ear canals, with applicators and solutions. Dry with swabs.
2. If an antiseptic solution is used, apply it to the area immediately after it is shaved. Leave it the designated time, then dry the area with clean swabs. Agency policy will guide you on whether to use an antiseptic, and if so, which to use and how long to leave it on.
3. Cover the prepared area, if required, with a sterile towel. Hold it in place with adhesive tape.

After shaving

1. After shaving report completion of the skin preparation to the responsible nurse. At some agencies, the skin preparation must be checked by the responsible nurse. Male perineal preparations may be checked by the charge orderly, if the responsible nurse is female. Report to the responsible nurse any abrasions, including those made by the clippers or razor.
2. Remove the waterproof towel and bath blanket carefully so as not to spill the shaved hairs onto the bed.
3. Take the equipment to the service area and dispose of it according to agency practice. Dispose of the bath blanket in the laundry hamper.
4. Record the skin preparation on the patient's chart. Include an assessment of the preparation area (e.g., whether or not abrasions are present) and relevant responses of the patient.

Hygiene

In many settings, patients are bathed with an antimicrobial agent the evening or the morning before surgery. The bath includes a shampoo whenever possible. The patient's nails should be trimmed and free of polish so that the nail beds can be readily assessed for cyanosis and pallor, which are indications of inadequate oxygenation of the blood.

Rest and Medications

Rest restores the body; therefore, patients should rest well prior to surgery. The anesthetist visits the patient preoperatively, discusses with the patient how anesthesia will be achieved, and orders the preoperative medications. Usually a sedative is ordered the night before surgery to ensure the patient sleeps well. Preoperative medications are discussed on page 1012.

Preparation the Day of Surgery

On the day of surgery, the nurse's responsibilities include the following:

1. Vital signs. Take vital signs to obtain comparative baseline data against which to assess the patient's responses during and following surgery. Because any abnormality can cause surgery to be postponed, report promptly abnormalities in any of these signs, e.g., an elevated temperature, to the responsible nurse and to the physician.

2. Fasting and oral care. Ensure that the patient fasts for the prescribed time. The fasting patient may feel thirsty and have a dry mouth. Provide mouthwash and instruct the patient not to swallow water during oral care but just to rinse out the mouth.

3. Hygiene and gowns. Assist the patient with a complete or partial bath, as required. The patient puts on a clean hospital gown, fastened only at the neck or not at all, in accordance with agency policy. An untied gown can be readily removed during the operative and immediate postoperative period. In some agencies, patients wear surgical caps or stockings for added warmth or protection. Also, antiemboli stockings are ordered for patients in some agencies. These stockings compress the peripheral veins and increase the venous return during the inactive period, thus preventing the formation of thrombi or emboli.

4. Hair and cosmetics. Remove or have the patient remove hairpins or clips that may cause pressure or accidental damage to the scalp when the patient is unconscious. Long hair can be braided and fastened with elastic bands to keep it in place. All cosmetics (lipstick, rouge, nail polish, etc.) must be removed, since the color of the skin, lips, and nail beds help nurses and physicians assess circulation during and after surgery. Check agency practice for the removal of nail polish (e.g., with acetone) if the patient does not have nail polish remover.

5. Valuables. Label jewelry, money, and other valuables and place them in safekeeping to avoid their loss or damage and subsequent legal problems. In most agencies valuables are kept in special envelopes and locked in a storage area on the unit. If a patient does not want to remove a wedding band, the nurse can tape it in place. Wedding bands must be removed, however, if there is danger of the fingers swelling following surgery. Some situations warranting removal of a wedding band are surgery of or cast application to an arm and mastectomy that involves removal of the lymph nodes. This surgery may cause edema of the arm and hand.

6. Prostheses. Ensure that all prostheses (artificial body parts, such as partial or complete dentures, contact lenses, artificial eyes, and artificial limbs), as well as eyeglasses, wigs, false eyelashes, and hearing aids, are removed. Partial dentures can become dislodged and choke an unconscious patient. Also check for loose teeth that could become dislodged and aspirated during anesthesia. This is a common problem with 5- or 6-year-old patients having tonsils removed. Agency policy dictates the handling of prostheses. In some agencies they are placed in a locked storage area; in others, they are kept at the patient's bedside.

7. Bowel and bladder. Check that the patient empties the bowel and bladder before surgery. Voiding prevents bowel or bladder incontinence during general anesthesia, prevents constipation postoperatively, prevents obstruction to surgery by a distended bowel or bladder, minimizes risk of injury to the bowel and bladder, and minimizes contamination of the peritoneal cavity if the bladder or bowel is the site of surgery. If an enema is ordered, administer it soon enough on the day of surgery so that the patient has adequate time to expel it. Insert a retention (Foley) catheter if ordered. See Chapter 28. If the patient is unable to void, note this fact on the patient's record.

8. Special orders. Check the physician's orders for special requirements, such as the insertion of a nasogastric tube prior to surgery or the administration of medications, e.g., insulin.

9. Preoperative medications. Check the orders for preoperative medications carefully before administering them. Usually a narcotic (e.g., morphine) and a medication to dry the secretions of the mouth and respiratory tract (e.g., atropine or scopolamine) are given by injection. Sometimes the surgeon orders that oral sedatives (e.g., secobarbital) be administered orally before the injectable medications are given. The narcotic calms the patient before general anesthesia, and the atropine or similar drying drug minimizes the danger that the patient will aspirate secretions into the lungs. Tell the patient that this medication may cause thirst and that he or she may use a mouthwash. After receiving the preoperative medications, the patient remains quietly in bed. Raise the side rails and lower the bed for safety. Place the call light within reach.

10. Recording. In most agencies, personnel use a preoperative checklist to record interventions. See Figure 39–5. Check the agency's forms and follow appropriate recording procedures. It is essential that all pertinent records (laboratory records, x-ray films, consents, etc.) be assembled and completed so that the operating room and recovery room personnel can refer to them.

11. Transfer of the patient to surgery. When the operating room transport person arrives for the patient, carefully check the patient's identification bracelet

Form NS-68

ST. PAUL'S HOSPITAL
Vancouver, B.C.

PRE-OPERATIVE PREPARATION

EVENING PRIOR TO SURGERY—CHECK	Yes	Not Applicable
1. History—completed with signature		
2. Consultation (when necessary) on chart		
3. Treatment and operative consents—signed and witnessed		
4. Telephone no. of next of kin or friend:		
5. Identaband on wrist		
6. Allergy sign on chart and wristband		
7. Operative area prepared		
8. Pre-op bath or shower		
9. Pre-op teaching: a. Attended "Operation Tomorrow"		
b. Demonstrated deep breathing, coughing, and leg exercises		
c. Stated approximate time to OR and return to ward		
d. Stated expectations: • surgery planned		
• incision and dressing area		
• activity progression		
• pain and effect of analgesic		
• NPO, intravenous, diet progression		
• pre-op urine specimen		
e. Verbalized probable discharge plans		
10. H.S. sedation administered or refused—charted on anesthetic record		
11. Fasting sign posted		

DATE ________ SIGNATURE ________

IMMEDIATELY PRIOR TO SURGERY	Yes	Not Applicable
1. Pre-operative urine specimen sent		
2. Reports attached to chart—Lab, X-ray, ECG		
3. Old chart		
4. Addressograph plate attached		
5. Contact lens, wig, jewelry, make-up removed, prosthesis off		
6. Dentures and partial plates removed		
7. Voided ____ Catheterized—time ____ amount ____		
8. Patient in hospital gown		
9. Blood pressure, pulse and respirations taken at least an hour prior to pre-op medication—charted on clinical record		
10. Pre-medication administered and charted on the anesthetic record		
11. Notation made in nurses notes of time to surgery		

DATE ________ SIGNATURE ________

OPERATING ROOM	Yes	Not Applicable
1. Patient identified by circulating nurse		
2. Site of surgery checked by circulating nurse a. Left side ____ Right side ____		
b. Slate ____ Surgeon ____ History ____ Consent ____		

SIGNATURE ________

Figure 39–5 A preoperative checklist (Courtesy of St. Paul's Hospital, Nursing Department, Vancouver, British Columbia.)

against the patient's chart. Generally, one staff member reads the identifying data from the bracelet while another checks it against the patient's record. Do not rely on a drowsy patient to identify himself or herself.

12. Preparation for postoperative care. Prepare the patient's bed and room for the postoperative period. See the instructions for preparing the surgical bed, page 525, in Chapter 21.

Nasogastric Intubation

Gastric intubation is the insertion of a tube into the stomach, through either the nose, the mouth, or a gastrostomy opening. *Nasogastric tubes* can be passed through either the mouth or the nose; however, the nose is preferred because there is less discomfort from the gag reflex. A tube passed through the mouth is often called an *orogastric tube.*

Several types of nasogastric tubes are used for gastric decompression and irrigation. The *Levin tube* is most commonly used for nasogastric intubation. It is a flexible, rubber or plastic, single-lumen tube with holes near the tip. See Figure 39–6, *A.* Inserting a Levin tube is often the nurse's responsibility. The *Salem sump tube* is a nasogastric tube with a double lumen.

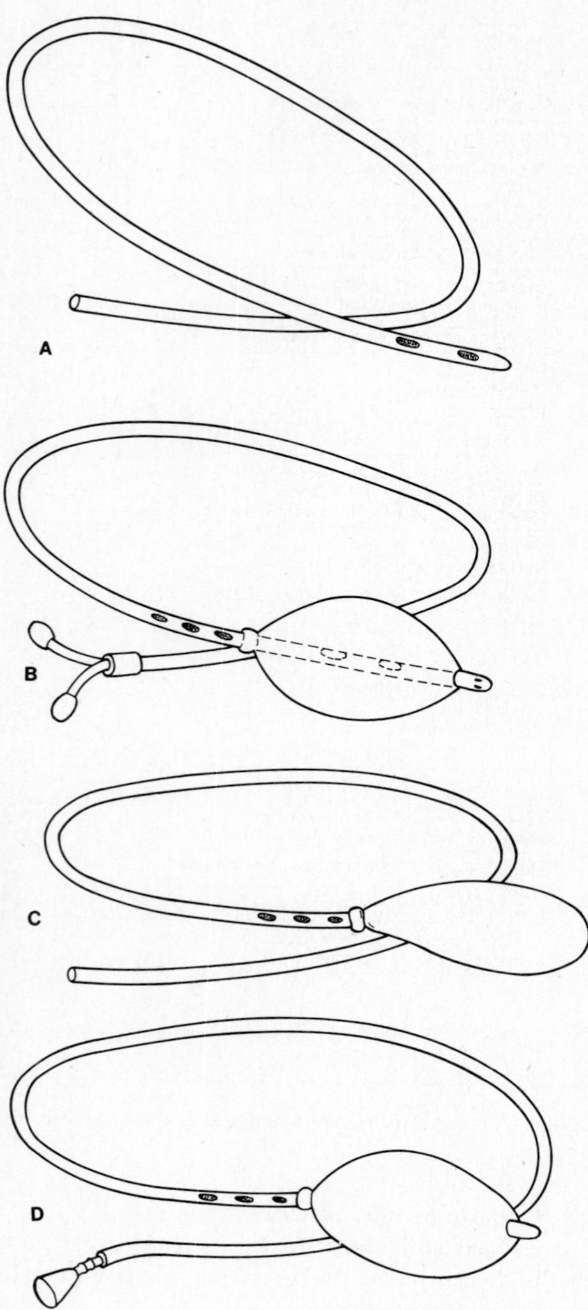

Some tubes pass through the patient's mouth or nose and stomach into the intestines. Physicians and nurse specialists usually insert such tubes. Several types of tubes are inserted this way. The *Miller-Abbott tube* is a double-lumen tube. One lumen leads to a balloon near the tip. See Figure 39–6, *B*. This tube is inserted into the small intestine, usually (a) to obtain secretions for diagnostic study or (b) for irrigation. The external end of the tube has a metal adapter with two openings. One inflates or deflates the balloon; the other drains intestinal secretions. The *Cantor tube* is a single-lumen tube with an inflatable bag at the tip and several holes along the distal end. See Figure 39–6, *C*. The bag is filled with mercury before the tube is inserted. The weight of the mercury causes the tube to move into the intestines. The *Harris tube* is a single-lumen tube with a metal tip. The Harris tube is used for irrigations and suctions. See Figure 39–6, *D*.

Some patients, for instance, those having gastric or duodenal surgery, require the insertion of a Levin (gastric) tube preoperatively. The tube removes fluid and flatus from the stomach, thereby preventing nausea, vomiting, and distention due to reduced peristaltic action after surgery.

Figure 39–6 Four types of tubes used for gastrointestinal suction and irrigation: **A,** Levin; **B,** Miller-Abbott; **C,** Cantor; **D,** Harris.

Procedure 39–2 Inserting and Removing a Nasogastric Tube

Equipment

Although nasogastric tube insertion and removal are not sterile procedures, the nurse washes hands before gathering the equipment to prevent the transfer of microorganisms to the patient. The following items are needed:

1. A gastric tube (plastic or rubber).
2. A solution basin filled with warm water or ice. Rubber tubes are placed on ice to stiffen them for easier insertion. Plastic tubes are placed in warm water to make them more flexible for insertion.

Procedure 39–2, continued

3. A water-soluble lubricant.
4. A 20 to 50 ml syringe with an adapter to attach to the tube. It is used to withdraw stomach contents.
5. A basin in which to collect gastric contents.
6. Nonallergenic adhesive tape, 2.5 cm (1 in) wide, to secure the tube to the face.
7. A clamp (optional) to close the tube after insertion.
8. Suction apparatus, if ordered.
9. A gauze square or a plastic specimen bag and an elastic band to cover the end of the tube, e.g., for preoperative patients.
10. A safety pin and an elastic band to secure the nasogastric tube to the patient's gown.
11. A bib or towel to protect the patient's gown.
12. A glass of water and drinking straw to help the patient swallow the tube.
13. Facial tissues in case the patient's eyes water during the procedure.
14. A stethoscope to assess placement of the tube.

Intervention

Inserting a nasogastric tube

1. Explain to the patient what you plan to do. Adjust the explanation to the patient's needs.

   Rationale A short explanation reassures the patient and allows the nurse to confirm the patient's identity. The passage of a gastric tube is not painful, but it is unpleasant because the gag reflex is activated during insertion.

2. Assist the patient to a high Fowler's position, and support the patient's head on a pillow.

   Rationale It is often easier for the patient to swallow in this position, and gravity helps the passage of the tube.

3. Hyperextend the patient's head to examine the patient's nostrils. Have the patient breathe through each nostril while compressing the other nostril, to select the more patent one.

   Rationale The tube is inserted through the nostril that is more patent.

4. Determine how far to insert the tube in this manner: Use the tube to mark off the distance from the tip of the patient's nose to the tip of the earlobe and then from the tip of the earlobe to the tip of the sternum. Mark this length with adhesive tape if the tube does not have markings.

   Rationale This length approximates the distance from the nares to the stomach. The distance varies among individuals.

5. Lubricate the tip of the tube well with the water-soluble lubricant to ease insertion.

   Rationale A water-soluble lubricant dissolves if the tube accidentally enters the lungs. An oil-based lubricant, such as petroleum jelly, will not dissolve and could cause respiratory complications if it enters the lungs.

6. Insert the tube, with its natural curve toward the patient, into the selected nostril.

7. Have the patient hyperextend the neck, and gently advance the tube toward the nasopharynx. Direct the tube along the floor of the nostril and toward the ear on that side. Provide tissues if the patient's eyes water. If the tube meets resistance, withdraw it, relubricate it, and insert it in the other nostril.

   Rationale Hyperextension reduces the curvature of the nasopharyngeal junction. Directing the tube along the floor avoids the projections (turbinates) along the lateral wall. Slight pressure is sometimes required to pass the tube into the nasopharynx, and some patients' eyes may water at this point. Tears are a natural body response. The tube should never be forced against resistance.

8. Once the tube reaches the oropharynx (throat), have the patient tilt the head forward and encourage him or her to drink and swallow. If the patient gags, stop passing the tube momentarily. Have the patient rest, take a few breaths, and take sips of water to calm the gag reflex.

   Rationale The patient will feel the tube in the throat and may gag and retch. Tilting the head forward facilitates passage of the tube into the posterior pharynx and esophagus rather than into the larynx; swallowing moves the epiglottis over the opening to the larynx.

Procedure 39–2, continued

9. In cooperation with the patient, pass the tube 5 to 10 cm (2 to 4 in) with each swallow, until the indicated length is inserted. If the patient continues to gag and the tube does not advance with each swallow, withdraw it slightly and inspect the patient's throat by looking through the mouth.

Rationale The tube may be coiled. If so, it is withdrawn until it is straight, and the nurse tries again to insert it.

10. Aspirate the stomach contents with a syringe. See Table 26–8 on page 678 for other methods of determining the placement of a nasogastric tube.

Rationale If fluid is removed, the assumption is that the tube is in the stomach. (Stomach contents are clear or yellow with mucus.)

11. If the signs do not indicate placement in the stomach, advance the tube 5 cm (2 in) and repeat the tests.

Figure 39–7

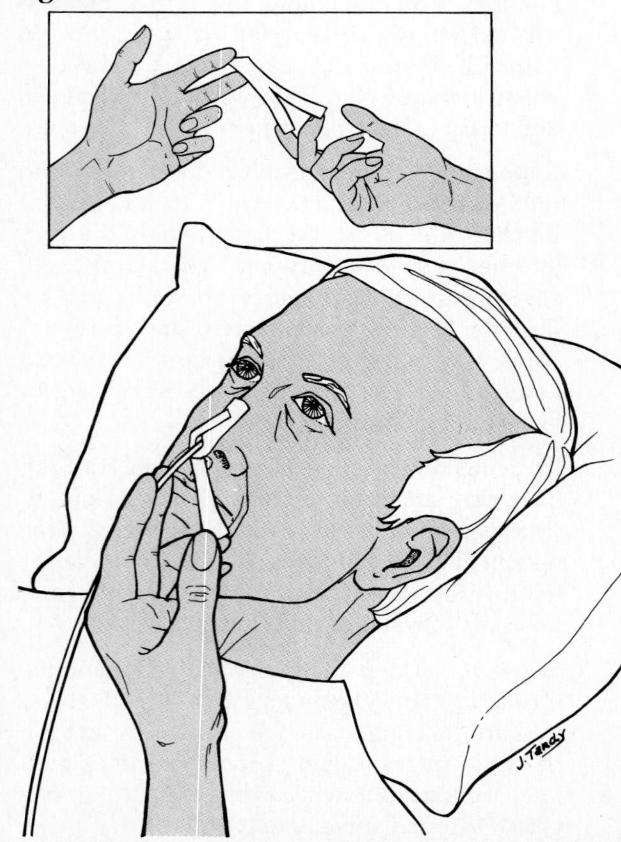

12. Secure the tube by taping it to the bridge of the patient's nose.

a. Cut 7.5 cm (3 in) of tape and split it at one end, leaving a 2.5 cm (1 in) tab at the end.

b. Place the tab over the bridge of the patient's nose, and bring the split ends under the tubing and back up over the nose. See Figure 39–7.

Rationale Taping in this manner prevents the tube from pressing against and irritating the edge of the nostril.

13. Attach the end of the tubing securely to suction, if ordered.

or

Clamp the end of the tubing and cover it with a gauze square or plastic specimen bag and an elastic band. The tube, if inserted preoperatively, is usually clamped.

14. Attach the end of the tube to the patient's gown by one of these two methods:

a. Loop an elastic band around the end of the tubing and attach the elastic band to the gown with a safety pin.

or

b. Attach a piece of adhesive tape to the tube, and pin the tape to the gown.

Rationale The tube is attached to prevent it from dangling and pulling.

15. Record the insertion of the tube and the patient's response (discomfort, etc.) to the insertion.

16. Establish a plan for providing daily nasogastric tube care, including:

a. Inspecting the nostril for discharge and irritation

b. Cleaning the nostril and tube with moistened, cotton-tipped applicators

c. Applying water-soluble lubricant to the nostril if it appears dry or encrusted

d. Changing the adhesive tape as required

e. Giving frequent mouth care, since the patient may breathe through the mouth and cannot drink

17. If suction is applied, ensure that the patency of both the nasogastric and suction tubes is maintained. Irrigations of the tube with 30 ml of normal saline may be required at regular in-

Procedure 39–2, continued

tervals. In some agencies, irrigations must be ordered by the physician.

18. Keep accurate records of the patient's liquid intake and output, and record the amount and characteristics of the drainage.

Removing a nasogastric tube

The removal of a nasogastric tube is ordered by a physician.

1. Turn off the suction, and disconnect the tube from suction apparatus.
2. Remove the adhesive tape securing the tube to the patient's nose. Unpin the tube from the patient's gown.
3. Have the patient take a deep breath and hold it.
4. Steadily and quickly remove the tube while the patient is holding the breath.
5. Dispose of the tube in a bag.
6. Provide tissues for the patient to blow his or her nose, and offer mouthwash if desired.
7. Remove the suction apparatus from the bedside. Measure the amount of fluid drained. Then empty and clean the drainage bottle.
8. Wash hands so as not to transmit microorganisms to others.
9. Record the removal of the tube, the patient's response, and the amount of fluid drained.

Types of Anesthesia

General

General anesthesia is the loss of all sensation and consciousness. A general anesthetic acts by blocking awareness centers in the brain. It can be administered by intravenous infusion, inhalation, or rectal induction.

General anesthetics have certain advantages. Respiration and cardiac function are readily regulated because the patient is unconscious rather than awake and anxious. The anesthesia can be adjusted to the length of the operation and the age and physical status of the patient. Its chief disadvantage is respiratory and circulatory depression. See Table 39–2 for stages of general anesthesia.

Regional

Regional anesthesia is the loss of sensation in one area of the body because sensory impulses to the brain are blocked. A number of methods are employed, such as spinal anesthesia, nerve block, and epidural block. Spinal anesthesia requires a lumbar puncture. See the section on lumbar puncture in Chapter 38. The physician then injects the anesthetic into the spinal canal (subarachnoid space). Commonly used anesthetic agents are procaine hydrochloride (Novocain) and tetracaine hydrochloride (Pontocaine).

A *nerve block* is the injection of an anesthetic agent into a nerve plexus to anesthetize part of the body. For instance, injecting tetracaine into the brachial plexus anesthetizes the arm. An *epidural block* is used commonly in obstetrics. It is the injection of an anesthetic agent between a lumbar interspace but extrathecally. *Caudal anesthesia* is similar to an epidural block except that the needle is inserted through the sacral hiatus into the caudal canal.

Table 39–2 Stages of General Anesthesia

Stage 1	Patient appears drowsy and dizzy.
Stage 2	Patient loses consciousness. Patient can be excited and can move during the initial part of this stage.
Stage 3	This is the stage of relaxation. Reflexes are lost and vital functions are depressed. During this stage surgery is performed.
Stage 4	This is a dangerous stage, when vital functions are too depressed. Patients normally do not enter this stage.

Local

Local anesthesia is the loss of sensation in a small area of tissue. Anesthetic may be sprayed on the skin or mucous membrane or injected into tissue. Cocaine is commonly used in a 4% to 10% solution to anesthetize the eye and mucous membranes. Tetracaine and lidocaine (Xylocaine) are commonly used injectable anesthetic agents. The chief advantage of this method is that the anesthetic acts quickly and has few side effects.

Surgical Procedures

Thousands of surgical procedures are performed in hospitals. Some patients have day surgery: They come to the hospital on the day of the operation and leave the same day after the operation. Other surgical procedures necessitate a longer hospital stay, from a few days to several weeks. The prefixes and suffixes of the names of surgical procedures help the student understand the nature of the operation. See Appendix B.

Initial Postoperative Period: Assessment and Intervention

Nursing intervention immediately after surgery is usually carried out in the hospital recovery room (RR, postanesthetic room, PAR). Recovery room nurses have special skills to care for patients recovering from anesthetics and surgery. Once a patient's condition has stabilized, he or she returns to a clinical nursing area; a day surgery patient returns home.

Postoperative care includes regular, systematic assessment of:

1. Respiratory function
2. Cardiovascular function (circulation)
3. Neurologic status
4. Fluid and electrolyte balance
5. Dressings, tubes, and drains
6. Pain
7. Safety and comfort of the environment

Respiratory Function

The nurse assesses the rate, depth, and quality of respirations as well as the patient's chest movements. See the section on assessing respirations in Chapter 13. Findings need to be compared with the patient's normal respirations recorded on the chart. If respirations appear extremely shallow, the nurse should hold a hand in front of the patient's mouth to feel for exhaled air. If the nurse does not feel exhalations, the nurse auscultates the lungs and notes bilateral air movement.

Respiratory obstruction is the most common recovery room emergency. It may be due to (a) occlusion of the pharynx by the tongue, (b) spasm or edema of the airway, (c) accumulation of secretions in the airway, and (d) aspiration of regurgitated vomitus. Signs of respiratory obstruction include:

1. Restlessness (early sign)
2. Rapid, thready pulse (early sign)
3. Noisy, irregular respirations
4. Use of accessory muscles for breathing, e.g., use of muscles in abdomen or neck and intercostal retractions
5. Apprehension or anxiety
6. Attempts to sit upright
7. Pallor or cyanosis (late sign)

Nursing interventions to maintain adequate respiratory function include:

1. Position unconscious patients on their sides with the face slightly down. Do not place a pillow under the head. This position keeps the tongue forward by gravity, preventing occlusion of the pharynx, and allows drainage of mucus or vomitus out of the mouth rather than down the respiratory tree. To ensure maximum chest expansion, elevate the patient's upper arm on a pillow. If the arm lies against the body, chest expansion is reduced. Once the patient's reflexes return, the patient can assume a back-lying position.
2. Maintain artificial airways in place and apply suction to them until reflexes for controlling coughing and swallowing return. Generally, patients spit out oropharyngeal airways. Endotracheal tubes are not removed until the patient is awake and able to maintain his or her own airway. Before removing airways, first apply suction to the airway and the pharynx. Then help the patient turn, cough, and take deep breaths, provided vital signs are stable.
3. Give oxygen as necessary to hypoventilating patients.
4. Be alert to signs of respiratory complications.

Cardiovascular Function

Cardiovascular function (circulation) is assessed by measuring the blood pressure, taking the pulse, and assessing the color and condition of the skin. If the patient's blood pressure falls more than 20 mm Hg after surgery or falls 5 or 10 mm Hg at each reading, the physician needs to be notified. The pulse is assessed for rate, rhythm, and quality. See Chapter 13, page 308. Apical pulses need to be taken if the radial pulse is thready. Generally, the pulse is slightly faster after surgery, but a pulse above 110 beats per minute or below 60 beats per minute should be reported. Also, a pulse rate markedly above or below the patient's preoperative rate is abnormal. Skin color and condition, particularly that of the lips and nail beds, are indicators of *tissue perfusion* (passage of blood through the vessels). Pale, cyanotic, cool, and moist skin may be a sign of circulatory problems.

Common circulatory problems include hemorrhage and shock, cardiac arrest, and postoperative hypotension. Cardiac arrest is discussed in Chapter 29, page 771. Disruption of sutures and insecure ligation of blood vessels can cause hemorrhage. Shock occurs as a result of massive hemorrhage or cardiac insufficiency. Certain anesthetic agents and muscle relaxants may cause postoperative hypotension. Signs of hemorrhage and shock include:

1. Increase in pulse and respiratory rate
2. Restlessness
3. Lowered blood pressure
4. Cold, clammy skin
5. Thirst
6. Pallor

In addition, bloody drainage on dressings or on bedclothes, often appearing underneath the patient, signals hemorrhage.

Nursing interventions to prevent hemorrhage and shock include:

1. Close observations of vital signs every 15 minutes until signs stabilize and then every 30 minutes
2. Adequate replacement of fluids lost during surgery
3. Application of elastic stockings to prevent pooling of blood in peripheral blood vessels

Neurologic Status

After general anesthesia, patients awaken in the following sequence: responsive to stimuli, i.e., to loud noises or to their names spoken aloud; drowsy; awake but not oriented; alert and oriented (McConnell 1977:34). The return of the patient's reflexes, such as swallowing and gagging, indicates that anesthesia is ending. Time of recovery from anesthesia varies with the kind of anesthetic used, its dosage, and the person's response to it.

To arouse the patient, the nurse calls the patient by name and in a normal tone of voice repeatedly tells the patient that surgery is over and that she or he is in the recovery room.

Fluid and Electrolyte Balance

During surgery, aldosterone production increases, and as a result the body conserves sodium and fluid. Therefore, care must be taken not to overload the body with fluid; however, there must be sufficient fluid to maintain blood pressure. Assessment of fluid and electrolyte balance is discussed in Chapters 30 and 31. All intake and output is monitored. If the patient is receiving blood, the nurse must be alert to signs of adverse reactions.

Dressings, Tubes, and Drains

The nurse regularly inspects dressings and bedclothes beneath the patient for signs of hemorrhage. When recording, the nurse describes the amount of drainage on dressings by the diameter of stains. In addition, the nurse must make certain that all tubes are patent and that tubes and suction equipment are functioning properly. Color, consistency, and amount of drainage is noted.

Pain

As patients emerge from anesthesia, they need analgesics for pain. Analgesics are administered as ordered and when, after assessing the patient's pain, the nurse believes they are needed. Analgesic dosages given in the recovery room (RR) are often reduced by one-quarter to one-third, but their effects are closely evaluated. Sometimes nurses in the RR withhold pain medication from hypotensive patients; however, pain may be the cause of hypotension. Nurses, therefore, need to administer pain medications after assessing the patient's status carefully (McConnell 1977a:36).

Safety and Comfort

A safe environment is one in which patients cannot harm themselves. Nurses need to raise bed side rails and provide warmth. Notifying support persons that the patient is well may comfort both the support persons and the patient.

A safe environment is free of pathogenic microorganisms. Postoperative patients are particularly susceptible to infection because of their weakened condition and because microorganisms can enter the body through the incision.

Continuing Postoperative Period: Initial Assessment

As soon as the patient returns to the nursing unit from the RR, the nurse conducts an initial assessment. The sequence of these activities varies with the situation. For example, the nurse may need to check the physician's stat orders before conducting the initial assessment; in such a case, nursing interventions to implement the orders can be carried out at the same time as assessment. Initial assessment activities include:

1. Determine the time of arrival at the nursing unit.
2. Obtain the vital signs—pulse, respirations, and blood pressure—and compare them with data from the RR.

Figure 39–8 A postoperative initial assessment checklist.

1. **Time of arrival** ____________
2. **Vital signs**
   Pulse ____________
   Respirations ____________
   Blood pressure ____________
3. **Skin**
   Color ____________
   Condition ____________
4. **Level of consciousness**
   Conscious ____________
   Semiconscious ____________
   Unconscious ____________
5. **Dressing**
   Dry ____________
   Drainage present ____________
   Blood ____________
   Intact ____________
6. **Intravenous**
   Type of solution ____________
   Amount in bottle ____________
   Drip rate ____________
   Venipuncture site ____________
7. **Drainage tubes**
   Type ____________
   Attached to suction or drainage container ____________
   Appearance and amount of drainage ____________
8. **Patient position** ____________
9. **Side rails** ____________
10. **Pain**
    Type of analgesic ____________
    Time last given ____________
11. **Other discomforts** ____________
    ____
    ____

3. Note the color and condition (e.g., diaphoresis, coldness) of the patient's skin.
4. Assess the patient's level of consciousness. At this point, most postoperative patients are conscious but drowsy. A fully conscious patient responds verbally, is alert, and is aware of time, place, and person. A semiconscious patient has fluctuating states of awareness. An unconscious patient does not respond verbally, has variable responses to stimuli such as noise or pain, and may be incontinent of urine or feces.
5. Check dressings for moisture or bleeding. Check under the patient for pooled blood. Report blood immediately to the responsible nurse.
6. Note intravenous infusions. Record the type of solution, the amount in the bottle, the drip rate, and the venipuncture site. Obtain additional solutions as ordered. See Chapter 31.
7. Note drainage tubes, such as urinary catheters, and connect them appropriately, e.g., to drainage containers or suction. Verify that fluids are draining and that tubes are not obstructed. Note the amount, color, etc., of the drainage.
8. Determine what position is ordered for the patient. This information is in the patient's chart, in the physician's orders, or in RR records. Patients who have had spinal anesthetics usually lie flat for 8 to 12 hours. Follow agency policy dictating how long the patient lies flat. If the patient is unconscious or semiconscious, place the patient on his or her side, if possible, or in a position that allows fluids to drain from the mouth. Otherwise, follow the patient's preference. Most patients prefer a back-lying position.
9. For the patient's safety, raise the side rails on the bed.
10. Assess the patient's pain or discomfort, and note when the patient last had an analgesic.
11. Record the patient's condition, including your assessment, on the chart. Some agencies provide checklists for this purpose. See Figure 39–8 for a sample checklist. Many hospitals have postoperative routines for regular assessment of patients. In some agencies, assessments are made every 15 minutes until vital signs stabilize, every hour thereafter the same day, and every 4 hours for the next 2 days. It is very important that the assessments be made as frequently as the patient's condition requires.

Nursing Diagnoses

Nursing diagnoses for perioperative patients depend on the condition and needs of the patient. These needs and nursing diagnoses, e.g., fluid and nutritional deficits, are described in other chapters: Nursing diagnoses for most perioperative patients are stated as potential problems.

Most people recover from surgery without incident.

Complications or problems are relatively rare, yet nursing personnel must be aware of the possibility of complications and their clinical signs. Many perioperative nursing measures are meant to prevent complications.

Respiratory Complications

Pneumonia

Pneumonia is often caused by microorganisms such as *Staphylococcus aureus. Lobar pneumonia* involves one or more lobes of the lungs, whereas *bronchopneumonia* is an inflammatory process that originates in the bronchi and involves patches of lung tissue. *Hypostatic pneumonia* is inadequate aeration of the lungs, often due to immobility. The usual clinical signs of pneumonia are elevated temperature, cough, and expectoration of blood-tinged or purulent sputum.

Measures employed to prevent pneumonia include coughing and deep breathing, moving in bed, and early ambulation to aerate the lungs. Nurses notify the physician at the first indication of any clinical signs of pneumonia. Supportive measures usually include bed rest, fluids, oxygen if the patient is in respiratory distress, and medications (e.g., antibiotics) ordered by the physician.

Atelectasis

Atelectasis is often due to mucous plugs blocking the bronchial passageways. The clinical signs include marked dyspnea, cyanosis, pleural pain, prostration, and tachycardia. Coughing, deep breathing, turning, and early ambulation help remove mucus and prevent atelectasis. Sufficient fluid intake helps the sputum remain liquid. If the patient cannot cough out the secretions, suction is used to remove them.

Pulmonary embolism

The clinical signs of pulmonary embolism are sudden chest pain, shortness of breath, and shock. In response, the physician usually initiates anticoagulant therapy to dissolve the embolus. Stasis of blood in the veins, venous injury, increase in blood coagulability, and disease predispose to the formation of emboli. Stasis of blood can occur with prolonged bed rest, obesity, advanced age, burns, and postpartum inactivity. Venous injury can occur during surgery on the legs, pelvis, abdomen, and thorax and from fractures of the pelvis and legs. Increased coagulability can occur with malignancies and may be associated with use of oral contraceptives high in estrogen. Diseases that increase the risk of clot formation include lung and heart disease, infection, and diabetes mellitus (Dossey and Passons 1981:26).

Supportive nursing measures for pulmonary embolism include drug therapy, oxygen if needed to relieve dyspnea, and analgesics for discomfort. Preventive measures include coughing, deep breathing, turning, exercise, and the application of elastic stockings to enhance the venous blood return from the legs. Patients' legs should not be rubbed; rubbing may loosen clots in the veins of the legs.

Circulatory Complications

Hemorrhage

Hemorrhage is a very serious problem that requires early detection and treatment. The escaped blood may appear on the surgical dressing but may remain inside the patient. The clinical signs of hemorrhage are discussed on page 1019. Hemorrhage is usually treated with blood transfusions or intravenous solutions, medications, and oxygen therapy. Extra covers help warm the patient.

Shock

Hypovolemic shock is the result of a markedly reduced volume of circulating fluid due to, for example, hemorrhage. The clinical signs of shock are similar to those of hemorrhage. Nurses need to report such signs immediately to the responsible nurse or physician and be prepared to administer oxygen, medications, intravenous solutions, or blood transfusions.

Thrombophlebitis

Thrombophlebitis is the inflammation of the veins, usually of the legs. The patient often complains of pain, and the affected area is swollen, red, and hot to the touch. Homans's sign (discomfort in the popliteal space upon dorsiflexion of the foot) must be assessed. Bed rest is indicated, together with the application of hot, moist packs, elevation of the legs, and the administration of anticoagulant drugs ordered by the physician. Early ambulation, leg exercises, use of elastic stockings, and ample fluid intake help prevent thrombophlebitis.

Thrombus and embolus formation

A *thrombus* (clot) becomes an *embolus* when it moves from the site where it formed to another area of the body. Thrombi commonly form in the veins where blood flow is slowed (see the discussion of pulmonary embolism earlier in this section). Emboli travel to three major organs: the lungs (pulmonary emboli), the heart (cardiac emboli), and the brain (cerebral emboli). Measures employed to prevent thrombophlebitis also prevent thrombus formation.

Urinary Complications

Urinary retention

Difficulty in voiding following surgery is not an uncommon complication, since anesthetics temporarily depress urinary bladder tone. In addition, urinary retention after surgery involving the rectum, vagina, and lower abdomen is thought to result from spasm of the bladder sphincter.

Urinary retention with overflow can also occur. The patient voids small amounts of urine frequently but retains most of the urine in the bladder. Measuring the patient's fluid intake and output provides data about fluid imbalance and urinary retention. Intake considerably larger than output may indicate retention. The nurse reports urinary retention to the responsible nurse or surgeon if measures to help the patient void are unsuccessful.

Infection

Urinary infection tends to occur with immobilization and limited fluid intake. Clinical signs of urinary infection include a burning sensation during urination, urgency, cloudy urine, and lower abdominal pain. The nurse needs to encourage the patient to take fluids and report the clinical signs to the surgeon. Measures to prevent urinary infections include good perineal hygiene, ample fluid intake, and early ambulation.

Gastrointestinal Complications

Constipation

Constipation can be caused by lack of roughage in the patient's diet and decreased motility of the gastrointestinal tract due to analgesics. Ample fluid intake, a high fiber diet, and early ambulation help prevent constipation.

Singultus

Singultus (hiccups) is produced by intermittent spasms of the diaphragm. The cause may be irritation of the phrenic nerve for a variety of reasons, including abdominal distention. There are many treatments for singultus; a traditional treatment is holding one's breath while drinking a glass of water. Medical treatment varies from carbon dioxide inhalations to intravenous injections of atropine. Hiccups are best prevented by relieving the cause of phrenic nerve irritation.

Distention

Abdominal distention (*tympanites*) can occur as a result of the slowed motility of the intestines. Early ambulation can prevent distention, and such nursing measures as the insertion of a rectal tube may relieve it.

Nausea and vomiting

The patient may report feeling nauseated or "sick to my stomach." Vomiting produces emesis, which needs to be assessed as to appearance and amount. Nursing measures to prevent nausea and vomiting include encouraging the patient to lie still and breathe deeply, keeping the environment free of unpleasant odors, and providing analgesics to prevent severe pain. The physician may order an antiemetic (an agent that prevents nausea and vomiting).

Psychologic Problems

Some patients are depressed after surgery. The patient may learn that the surgeon's findings have serious implications, for example, a malignancy may have been found. Some of the clinical signs of depression are sleep disturbances (excessive sleeping and insomnia), anorexia, tearfulness, loss of ambition, withdrawal, rejection of others, and dejected affect. The loss of health, like other losses, may be grieved.

Nursing interventions include ensuring adequate rest, since sleeping disturbances can aggravate depression; encouraging physical activity, which increases self-esteem and promotes rest; and assisting the patient to express anger and other negative feelings.

Wound Complications

Infection

Some of the clinical signs of wound infection are: purulent exudate, redness, tenderness, elevated body temperature, and odor. Laboratory examination of a specimen of drainage identifies microorganisms causing infection. Nursing intervention includes encouraging fluid intake, keeping the wound clean (see Chapter 40), and preventing the transmission of the microorganisms to others.

Dehiscence

Dehiscence is the opening of a suture line before the incision heals. Small openings are not unusual and may be closed and supported with a sterile butterfly tape. See Chapter 40. The opening always needs to be supported and the wound observed regularly for further opening. For a large dehiscence, the wound is covered with sterile moist towels and the physician is notified.

Evisceration

Evisceration, the extrusion of the internal organs, is a relatively rare but serious complication. A wide opening of an abdominal incision is an emergency. The nurse applies sterile moist dressings over the open area and an abdominal binder (see Chapter 40) to stop the abdominal contents from falling out of the wound. The responsible nurse or surgeon must be notified as soon as the evisceration occurs. Eviscerated patients can go into shock; therefore, the nurse prepares to start an intravenous infusion on the physician's order. The patient is usually taken to surgery immediately for resuturing.

Examples of Nursing Diagnoses

Preoperative period

1. Moderate anxiety related to impending surgery
2. Lack of knowledge related to impending surgery

Postoperative period

1. Potential respiratory complications related to:
  a. Immobility and inadequate lung expansion
  b. Inadequate hydration
2. Potential circulatory complications related to:
  a. Venous stasis
  b. Hemorrhage
3. Potential urinary complications related to:
  a. Site of surgery (specify)
  b. Inadequate fluid intake
  c. Immobility
  d. Anesthesia
4. Potential gastrointestinal complications related to:
  a. Narcotic analgesics
  b. Lack of roughage in diet
  c. Inactivity
  d. Inadequate fluid intake
5. Potential depression or body image disturbance related to surgery (specify)
6. Potential wound complications related to:
  a. Obesity
  b. Lowered resistance

Postoperative Planning and Intervention

The nurse uses assessment data, the surgeon's orders, and the information on the chart to draw up the postoperative nursing care plan. The overall nursing goal is to facilitate the patient's recovery, which includes preventing postoperative problems. See also suggested outcome criteria on page 1025.

From the patient's record check the following:

1. Operation performed
2. Presence of drains, etc., and their location
3. Anesthetic used
4. Postoperative diagnosis
5. Estimated blood loss (EBL)
6. Medications administered in the RR

From the surgeon's postoperative orders check for:

1. Food and fluids permitted by mouth
2. Intravenous solutions and intravenous medications
3. Position in bed
4. Medications ordered, e.g., analgesics, antibiotics
5. Laboratory tests
6. Intake and output, which in some agencies are monitored for all postoperative patients
7. Activity permitted, including ambulation

Note that in some agencies all preoperative orders are automatically canceled with surgery, and new orders are required.

Respiratory Needs

Postoperative nursing intervention to meet respiratory needs is chiefly designed to prevent respiratory complications, such as atelectasis and hypostatic pneumonia. Nursing actions include the following:

1. Encourage the patient to cough and do deep breathing exercises hourly or at least every 2 hours during waking hours for the first few days.
2. Encourage early ambulation, which promotes deep breathing.
3. If the patient cannot ambulate, periodically assist him or her to a sitting position in bed if allowed (this position permits the greatest lung expansion) or turn the patient from side to side every 2 hours. Turning allows alternating maximum expansion of the uppermost lung.
4. Encourage the patient to take fluids as ordered, or maintain IV infusions. Fluids keep the respiratory mucous membranes and secretions moist, thus facilitating the expectoration of mucus during coughing.
5. Use suction if the patient is unable to cough up secretions.
6. Assess the patient's respiratory rate, depth, and rhythm every 4 hours, or whenever the vital signs are taken. Be alert to signs of respiratory problems.

Circulatory Needs

Nursing measures to meet the patient's circulatory needs are provided to prevent thrombophlebitis, shock, and hemorrhage and to assess circulatory status. Nursing interventions include the following:

1. Encourage leg exercises every hour or at least every 2 hours during waking hours. Muscle contractions compress the veins, preventing the stasis of blood in the veins. Contractions also promote arterial blood flow.

2. Encourage early ambulation.

3. Apply tensor bandages up to the knees or antiemboli stockings to support the superficial veins of patients with cardiovascular problems.

4. Encourage adequate fluid intake or maintain IV infusions. Sufficient fluids prevent dehydration and the resulting concentration of the blood that, along with venous stasis, is conducive to thrombus formation.

5. Avoid placing pillows or rolls under the patient's knees. Pressure on the popliteal blood vessels can slow the blood circulation to and from the lower extremities.

6. Assess pulse and blood pressure (see Chapter 13) and assess circulation to the lower extremities. Note the color and temperature of the skin.

Hydration

Postoperative patients often complain of thirst and a dry, sticky mouth. These discomforts are a result of the preoperative fasting period, preoperative medications (such as atropine or scopolamine), and loss of body fluid for a variety of reasons (e.g., blood loss, perspiration, and vomiting). Intravenous infusions are usually given to balance such losses. Nursing measures to meet hydration needs and to relieve thirst or a dry mouth include the following:

1. Maintain IV infusions as ordered.

2. Offer only small sips of water to patients who can have fluids by mouth until they establish tolerance. Large amounts of water can induce vomiting, since anesthetics and narcotic analgesics temporarily inhibit the motility of the stomach.

3. Offer ice chips, if permitted. The patient who cannot take fluids by mouth may be allowed to suck ice chips. Check the physician's orders.

4. Provide mouth care and place a mouthwash at the patient's bedside.

5. Measure the patient's fluid intake and output.

6. Assess the patient for signs of dehydration.

Nutrition

The physician orders the patient's postoperative diet. Depending on the extent of surgery and the organs involved, some patients may be given intravenous fluids and nothing by mouth for a few days. Others may progress from a diet of clear liquids to full fluids, to a light diet, and then to a regular diet within a few days. See Chapter 26.

The nurse supervises nutrition carefully because anesthetics, narcotics, handling of the intestines during abdominal surgery, changes in fluid and food intake, and inactivity all inhibit peristalsis. Nursing care to meet nutritional needs include the following:

1. Maintain IV infusions as ordered.

2. Check the doctor's orders carefully regarding diet.

3. Assess the return of peristalsis by auscultating the abdomen. Gurgling and rumbling sounds indicate peristalsis.

4. Assist the patient to eat as required.

5. Observe the patient's tolerance of the food and fluids ingested.

Comfort and Rest

Pain is usually greatest 12 to 36 hours after surgery and decreases on the 2nd or 3rd day. Analgesics are usually administered every 3 or 4 hours the 1st day, and by the 3rd day most patients require only oral analgesics. Some patients may refuse to take analgesics on a regular schedule because they are not in severe pain. In this situation, inform the patient that analgesics are most effective if given before pain becomes severe. Analgesics also help the patient to do deep breathing exercises, cough, and ambulate. Nursing measures to relieve pain and promote rest include the following:

1. Administer analgesics as ordered and as required.

2. Observe the patient for signs of acute pain, e.g., pallor, perspiration, and tension.

3. Move and position the patient to minimize discomfort.

4. Plan to give analgesics before activities (e.g., ambulation or meals) or rest periods (e.g., at bedtime).

5. Assess the effectiveness of the analgesics.

6. Provide comfort measures that relax the patient, e.g., back rubs, position changes, rest periods, and diverting activities. Tension increases pain perception and responses.

7. Listen attentively to the patient's complaints of pain; note the location, note the type of pain, and determine the cause.

Urinary Elimination

Anesthetics temporarily depress urinary bladder tone, which usually returns within 6 to 8 hours after surgery. Surgery in the pubic area, vagina, or rectum, during which the surgeon may manipulate the bladder, often causes urinary retention. Some postoperative patients have indwelling urinary catheters. Nursing responsibilities in relation to urinary elimination include the following:

1. Measure the liquid intake and output of all patients with intravenous infusions and urinary catheters or other drainage devices. Keep intake/output records for at least 2 days and until the patient reestablishes fluid balance without an IV or catheter in place.

2. Note any difficulties the patient has with voiding, and assess the patient for bladder distention.

3. Report promptly to the responsible nurse if a patient does not void within 8 hours following surgery.
4. Provide measures that promote urinary elimination. For example, help male patients stand at the bedside, ensure that patients are free from pain, ensure that the fluid intake is adequate, and help patients walk.
5. Catheterize a patient if all measures to promote voiding fail. See Chapter 28. In some agencies, catheterization requires a doctor's order.

Fecal Elimination

Abdominal distention due to reduced peristalsis is very common after surgery. Many patients who have had abdominal surgery experience this discomfort about the 3rd day after surgery. Nursing measures to relieve distention include the following:

1. Note and report the passage of flatus.
2. Auscultate the patient's abdomen to confirm the return of peristalsis.
3. Encourage exercises and ambulation, which increase peristalsis.
4. Encourage adequate fluid and food intake when the patient can tolerate these.
5. Administer a rectal tube, enema, or suppository as required and if ordered.

Activity

Ambulation is essential. It prevents respiratory, circulatory, and gastrointestinal problems and also helps prevent general muscle weakness. Generally, patients begin ambulation the evening of the day of surgery or the 1st day after surgery, unless the surgeon orders otherwise. Nursing care in regard to ambulation includes the following:

1. Plan ambulation periods after the patient has taken an analgesic.
2. Make ambulation gradual. Start by having the patient sit on the bed and dangle the feet over the side. Assess his or her tolerance by noting color, respirations, diaphoresis, pulse rate, etc. Take the pulse before moving the patient and again after. Next help the patient stand at the bedside and take a few steps. Increase the distance gradually as the patient's tolerance grows.
3. Provide supportive measures as required. For example, use a pillow to support an abdominal incision, or move the patient's urinary drainage bag or IV pole during ambulation. Give verbal encouragement and reassurance as necessary. See Chapter 15.

Wound Protection

Preventing wound infections and separations is another important nursing function. Nursing responsibilities in regard to wound care include the following:

1. Inspect dressings regularly to ensure they are clean and dry.
2. Ensure that the dressing is fastened securely.
3. Apply abdominal binders as ordered to provide support.
4. Change dressings, using sterile technique as required, when they are soiled with drainage or in accordance with the physician's or nursing orders. See Chapter 40.
5. Inspect the wound for signs of local infection.
6. Assess the patient for signs of generalized infection, e.g., elevated temperature and increased pulse and respiratory rates.
7. Report wound separations promptly.

Evaluation

The outcome criteria for patients who have actual or potential perioperative problems depend on the nursing diagnosis. Some suggested criteria are:

Preoperative period
1. Verbalizes his or her expected outcomes of surgery.
2. Shows no evidence of dehydration, e.g., mucous membranes are moist, skin is not dry, and fluid intake and output are adequate.
3. Skin is intact.
4. Weight is within normal range.
5. Has no upper respiratory infection.
6. Vital signs are normal.
7. Describes planned surgical procedure and its consequences.
8. Demonstrates deep breathing, coughing, and leg exercises to be performed postoperatively.
9. Fasts during the prescribed time.
10. Hemoglobin is normal.
11. Urinalysis is normal.

Postoperative period
1. Carries out leg exercises every 4 hours as instructed.
2. Turns from side to side in bed independently.
3. Coughs and does deep breathing exercises every 2 hours as instructed.
4. Walks to end of hall each morning with assistance.
5. Bilateral air movement in lungs is evident on auscultation.
6. Vital signs are normal.

7. Has no cyanosis or pallor of the skin.
8. Shows no evidence of dehydration.
9. Urine output and fluid intake is adequate.
10. Voiding patterns are normal.
11. Has no signs of infection at site of incision.
12. Dressings are dry.
13. Pain is sufficiently controlled to enable required activity.
14. Bowel activity is satisfactory.
15. Has no abdominal distention.
16. Does not vomit or complain of nausea.

Summary

There are many reasons for surgery and many kinds of operations. Nurses should know why a patient is having an operation. The reason is important in appreciating the patient's point of view and concerns. Before any surgical procedure, the patient must give informed consent by signing a document. If the patient is underage, a parent or guardian must give consent.

Preoperative assessment includes consideration of factors that affect surgical risk, a physical examination, and the taking of a nursing history. A nurse should record observations and report any unusual observation to the surgeon. Preoperative nursing intervention promotes postoperative recovery and helps prevent complications. Teaching deep breathing, coughing, and leg exercises are important aspects of preoperative care. Most patients require preoperative preparation of the skin, and some patients need to have gastric tubes inserted. During surgery the patient is chiefly under the care of the surgeon and the anesthetist.

Patients usually spend the initial postoperative period in the recovery room, where respiratory and cardiovascular functions are monitored closely and neurologic status and fluid and electrolyte balance are closely assessed and controlled. Nurses perform initial assessments when patients return to a clinical nursing unit. Plans for postoperative care are drawn from data from the assessment, the surgeon's orders, and the patient's chart.

Suggested Activities

1. In a laboratory setting, select a partner to play the role of a patient having one of the following operations: (a) appendectomy, (b) left meniscectomy, or (c) surgical correction of an ingrown toenail on the right foot. Plan and conduct the preoperative teaching for the operation selected. Then carry out the appropriate skin preparation for the operation. Have it checked by an experienced nurse.
2. In a laboratory setting, set up a surgical bed unit. Assess another student as you would a returning postoperative patient.
3. In a clinical setting, make a nursing care plan for a preoperative patient. Have the plan checked by the instructor. Implement the plan with appropriate supervision.
4. In a clinical setting, help an experienced nurse "check in" a patient from the recovery room. Observe his or her recording. How did the nurse's assessment compare with yours?
5. In a clinical setting, arrange for supervision while you do an initial assessment of a postoperative patient returning to a nursing unit.
6. In a clinical setting, interview a patient who has had surgery and is recovering well. What does he or she remember about the preoperative care? Was the patient worried? How was he or she assisted during that period? What care would the patient have liked but did not receive?

Suggested Readings

Croushore, T. M. April 1979. Postoperative assessment: The key to avoiding the most common nursing mistakes. *Nursing 79* 9:46–50.

Essential postoperative assessment should include systematic assessment of circulation, respiration, neurologic status, wound, genitourinary function, and gastrointestinal function. Tables for expected wound drainage after abdominal surgery, expected drainage from tube and catheters, common postoperative complications, and a baseline assessment tool for the first critical hours are included.

Goulding, E. J., et al. October 1965. The newborn: His response to surgery. *American Journal of Nursing* 65:84–87.

Excessive blood loss and the danger of aspiration are among the special postoperative concerns when the patient is a newborn.

Luciano, K. November 1974. The who, when, where, what, and how of preparing children for surgery. *Nursing 74* 4:64–65.

Children need special preoperative preparation. Practical guides help the nurse use appropriate vocabulary when providing information to children.

Mezzanotte, E. J. January 1970. Group instruction in preparation for surgery. *American Journal of Nursing* 70:89–91.

Selected patients anticipating abdominal surgery received preoperative instruction as a group. A sample patient instruction sheet is included.

Schumann, D. April 1980. How to help wound healing in your abdominal surgery patient. *Nursing 80* 10:34–40.

Some patients are at high risk of wound complications. Nurses need to learn factors that help or retard healing and nursing interventions appropriate for such patients.

Smith, B. J. October 1978. Safeguarding your patient after anesthesia. *Nursing 78* 8:53–56.

This author outlines guidelines to help nurses deal with the effects of various types of anesthetic agents, drug abuse, and general situations.

Steele, B. G. March 1980. Test your knowledge of postoperative pain management. *Nursing 80* 10:70–72.

A self-test about postoperative pain management includes 26 multiple-choice questions and answers.

Selected References

Blackwell, A. K., and Blackwell, W. January 1975. Relieving gas pains. *American Journal of Nursing* 75:66–67.

Brooks, S. M. 1979. *Fundamentals of operating room nursing.* 2nd ed. St. Louis: C. V. Mosby Co.

Collart, M. E., and Brenneman, J. K. October 1971. Preventing postoperative atelectasis. *American Journal of Nursing* 71:1982–87.

Creighton, H. 1981. *Law every nurse should know.* 4th ed. Philadelphia: W. B. Saunders.

Dossey, B., and Passons, J. M. March 1981. Pulmonary embolism: Preventing it, treating it. *Nursing 81* 11:26–33.

Dziurbejko, M. M., and Larkin, J. C. November 1978. Including the family in preoperative teaching. *American Journal of Nursing* 78:1892–94.

Goulding, E. J., et al. October 1965. The newborn: His response to surgery. *American Journal of Nursing* 65:84–87.

Grubb, R. D. 1979a. *Operating room guidelines: An illustrated manual.* St. Louis: C. V. Mosby Co.

———. 1979b. *Planning ambulatory surgery facilities.* St. Louis: C. V. Mosby Co.

Gruendemann, B. J. 1977. *The surgical patient—behavioral concepts for the operating room nurse.* 2nd ed. St. Louis: C. V. Mosby Co.

Hardgrove, C., and Rutledge, A. May 1975. Parenting during hospitalization. *American Journal of Nursing* 75:836–38.

Healy, K. M. January 1968. Does preoperative instruction make a difference? *American Journal of Nursing* 68:62–67.

Keithley, J. K., and Tasic, P. W. April 1982. A unified approach to assessment of the surgical patient. *American Journal of Nursing* 82:612–14.

King, J., et al. April 1977. The defeated patient. Her worries come first. *Nursing 77* 7:28–33.

Laird, M. August 1975. Techniques for teaching pre- and postoperative patients. *American Journal of Nursing* 75:1338–40.

Libman, R. H., and Keithley, J. April 1975. Relieving airway obstruction in the recovery room. *American Journal of Nursing* 75:603–5.

Luciano, K. November 1974. The who, when, where, what, and how of preparing children for surgery. *Nursing 74* 4:64–65.

McConnell, E. A. September 1975. All about gastrointestinal intubation. *Nursing 75* 5:30–37.

———. March 1977a. After surgery. *Nursing 77* 7:32–39.

———. September 1977b. Ensuring safer stomach suctioning with a Salem sump tube. *Nursing 77* 7:54–57.

———. April 1979. Ten problems with nasogastric tubes . . . and how to solve them. *Nursing 79* 9:78–81.

Marcinek, M. B. November 1977. Stress in the surgical patient. *American Journal of Nursing* 77:1809–11.

Merkatz, R.; Smith, D.; and Seitz, P. June 1974. Preoperative teaching for gynecologic patients. *American Journal of Nursing* 74:1072–74.

Metheny, N. A., and Snively, W. D., Jr. May 1978. Perioperative fluids and electrolytes. *American Journal of Nursing* 78:840–45.

Parsons, M. C., and Stephens, G. J. February 1974. Postoperative complications: Assessment and intervention. *American Journal of Nursing* 74:240–44.

Rau, J., and Rau, M. April 1977. To breathe, or be breathed: Understanding IPPB. *American Journal of Nursing* 77:613–17.

Roberts, M.; Vilinskas, J.; and Owens, G. May 1974. Technicians or nurses in the OR? *American Journal of Nursing* 74:906–7.

Ryan, R. October 1976. Thrombophlebitis: Assessment and prevention. *American Journal of Nursing* 76:1634–36.

Smith, B. J. December 1974. After anesthesia. *Nursing 74* 74:28–32.

Tharp, G. D. December 1974. Shock: The overall mechanisms. *American Journal of Nursing* 74:2208–11.

Walters, J. June 1979. Four practical questions to ask when organizing preoperative classes. *American Journal of Nursing* 79:1090–91.

Wiley, L. April 1974a. Staying ahead of shock. *Nursing 74* 4:19–27.

———. May 1974b. Shock—different kinds, different problems. *Nursing 74* 4:43–52.

———, editor. February 1979. Dealing with depression after radical surgery. *Nursing 79* 9:46–51.

Chapter 40

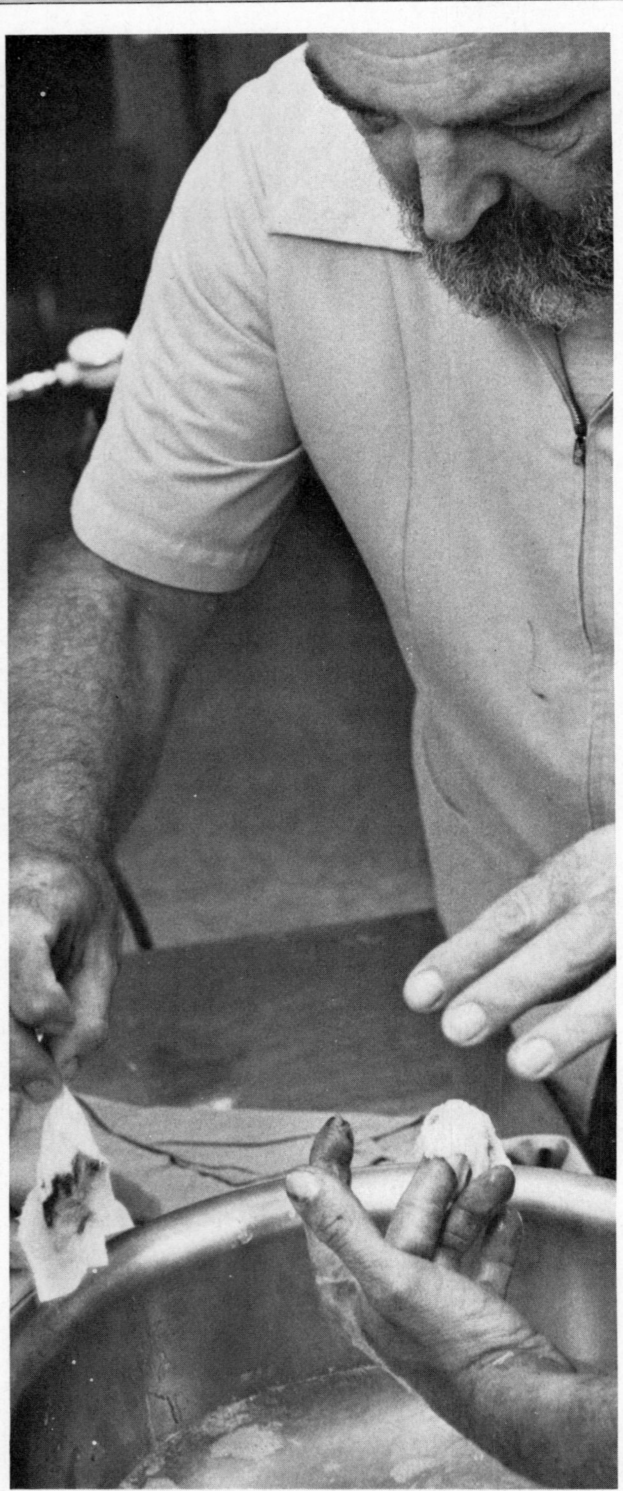

Wound Care

CONTENTS

Objectives

1. Know essential facts about wounds and wound healing

- **1.1** Define terms commonly used to describe wounds
- **1.2** Identify two basic ways in which wounds heal
- **1.3** Identify factors that inhibit wound healing
- **1.4** Identify measures to promote wound healing
- **1.5** Identify assessment factors of a clean, healing wound

2. Understand essential facts about measures for wound care

- **2.1** Identify seven nursing goals of wound care
- **2.2** Compare open and closed methods of wound care
- **2.3** Identify commonly used dressing materials
- **2.4** Identify commonly used types of binders
- **2.5** Identify basic turns used in bandaging
- **2.6** Identify physiologic responses to heat and cold
- **2.7** Identify reasons for implementing selected wound care procedures
- **2.8** Identify essential aspects of wound care procedures outlined in this chapter
- **2.9** Give reasons for selected steps of wound care procedures outlined in this chapter
- **2.10** Identify appropriate assessment and recording data for selected procedures

3. Perform wound care techniques outlined in this chapter safely and effectively

- **3.1** Change a surgical dressing
- **3.2** Clean a Penrose drain site
- **3.3** Shorten a Penrose drain
- **3.4** Remove skin sutures
- **3.5** Irrigate a wound, an eye, an ear, and a vagina
- **3.6** Apply common types of binders
- **3.7** Apply bandages
- **3.8** Apply hot and cold applications

Terms

abrasion
bandage
binder
compress
conduction
contusion
convection
debridement
dehiscence
ecchymotic
edema
exudate
fibrin
fibrous tissue
granulation tissue
hematoma
hot pack
hyperemia
hypothermia
incision
inflammatory process
insulator
irrigation (lavage)
ischemia
laceration
leukocytosis
packing
Penrose drain
primary union (first intention)
pus
pyogenic
radiation
regeneration
retention (stay) suture
secondary union (second intention)
suppuration
suture
trauma

Although the body is remarkably protected from *trauma* (injury) by the skin and by the subcutaneous and adipose tissues, trauma does occur intentionally and unintentionally. Intentional trauma occurs during therapy, such as an operation, venipuncture, or radiation. Although it is therapeutic to remove a tumor, the surgeon must cut into body tissues, thus traumatizing them.

Unintentional wounds are acquired by accident, for example, an arm may be fractured in an automobile accident. If the tissues are traumatized without a break in the skin, the result is a closed wound. A blow from a hard instrument that causes bruising is called a *contusion*, which is considered a closed wound. An open wound occurs when the skin or mucous membrane surface is broken.

Wounds are further described according to the presence or absence of infection. A clean wound is one in which there are no pathogenic organisms. An infected or contaminated wound is one in which pathogens are present. Wounds produced intentionally are generally clean, while unintentional and open wounds are considered contaminated.

One of the functions of the nurse is to promote wound healing, which may involve changing dressings, cleaning and shortening drains, irrigating wound sites, applying heat and cold, and applying bandages and binders. Surgical asepsis is implemented for most of these measures, to prevent the introduction of pathogens into wounds.

Types of Wounds

Wounds are frequently described according to the manner in which the wound is acquired. There are six categories of wounds by this classification: (a) incised, (b) contused, (c) abraded, (d) punctured, (e) lacerated, and (f) penetrating.

An *incised wound* or *incision* is made with a sharp instrument. It can be intentional, such as a cut made with a surgeon's scalpel, or accidental, such as a cut from a sharp knife.

A *contused wound* or *contusion* is a closed wound that occurs as the result of a blow from a blunt instrument. The skin appears bruised (*ecchymotic*) because of the release of blood into the tissues from the damaged blood vessels. Contused wounds are usually unintentional, although contusions of some tissues may occur because of surgical manipulation.

An *abraded wound* or *abrasion* is a type of open wound that occurs as a result of friction, such as a scraped knee from a fall on the road surface. Abraded wounds can also be intentional; for example, in a dermal abrasion the superficial layers of the skin are removed, either by sandpapering or by an abrasive machine, to obliterate scars and pockmarks.

A *punctured wound, stab wound,* or *puncture,* is an open wound made by a sharp instrument that penetrates the skin and underlying tissues. Puncture wounds can be accidental, such as a wound made by stepping on a nail, or intentional, such as a wound made by a surgeon for insertion of a drain. Venipuncture and intramuscular injections are other common puncture wounds induced intentionally.

Lacerated wounds or *lacerations* occur when the tissues are torn apart, producing irregular edges. Lacerations are accidental and often result from accidents involving automobiles or machinery.

A *penetrating wound* is one in which an instrument penetrates deeply into the tissues through the skin or mucous membrane. Usually penetrating wounds are accidental, such as those from bullets or metal fragments. A bullet or other object making a penetrating wound may lodge in an internal organ.

Wound Healing

The body's normal response to injury is the *inflammatory process,* characterized by five cardinal signs: swelling, redness, heat, pain, and impaired function. The process involves a series of events: (a) vascular and cellular changes that create *hyperemia* (excessive blood in the area) and *leukocytosis* (an increase in the number of leukocytes) and are responsible for the five cardinal signs, (b) formation of inflammatory *exudates* (discharges produced by body tissues) of five types—serous, catarrhal, purulent, fibrinous, and sanguineous—and (c) repair of tissues. For detailed information about this process, see Chapter 9, page 187.

Healing can occur in two basic ways: by *regeneration* of tissue (growth of new cells identical to the damaged ones) or by replacement with *fibrous tissue* (scar tissue, which is different from the original cells). If the wound is not large and if cells are not completely destroyed, some tissues of the body can regenerate—that is, new cells are produced and appropriately organized as the specific tissue. Nervous tissue, elastic tissue, and muscle tissue, however, have little, if any, ability to regenerate. Repair of tissues was discussed in detail in Chapter 9, page 188.

Wounds are said to heal by either primary or secondary union (first or second intention). Healing by *primary union (first intention)* usually occurs when the tissue surfaces have been approximated by sutures. Often drains are placed in deep wounds to keep them open until the underlying tissues have healed. Deep wounds need to heal from the inside to the outside surface, so that fluid is not trapped in the wound. Skin regenerates more rapidly than underlying tissues and can seal over before the deeper tissues have healed.

Wound healing by *secondary union (second intention)* requires the formation of considerably more *granulation tissue* (pinkish-white tissue that appears first to fill in an open wound). These wounds are usually large, and the skin edges cannot be approximated; they take much longer to heal, and there is usually extensive scar tissue. Second intention healing also can occur following a wound infection. For information on factors that favor tissue healing, see Chapter 9, page 189.

Factors That Inhibit Wound Healing

1. *Infection.* Infection not only halts the healing process but also damages additional tissue cells, thus increasing the size of a wound, in both width and depth.
2. *Hematomas.* A *hematoma* is a blood clot. Usually blood in a wound is gradually absorbed back into the systemic circulation as debris from the wound. However, a large clot may take weeks to dissolve and be absorbed, thus inhibiting the healing process. Hemato-

mas that inhibit healing for a prolonged period can be removed.

3. *Foreign objects.* Foreign objects, such as a sliver of wood, or microorganisms, can also inhibit healing. The object may cause formation of an abscess before it is removed. This abscess is made up of serum, *fibrin* (a protein found in blood clots), dead tissue cells, and leukocytes (white blood cells), which form a thick liquid called *pus.* This stage in the inflammatory process is known as *suppuration* (pus formation).

If the foreign object is left in the wound, pus will continue to form and will either drain by breaking through the skin surface or be absorbed into the lymphatic system. Microorganisms that cause pus to be formed are called *pyogenic;* not all microorganisms do.

4. *Localized ischemia. Ischemia* is defined as anemia in a body part due to obstruction of the blood flow to the part. Dressings, bandages, and casts that are applied too tightly can cause ischemia. It can also arise from internal obstruction of the blood vessels by a blood clot.

5. *Diabetes.* The presence of diabetes mellitus can also inhibit wound healing. Vascular changes can decrease the blood supply to the area, limiting the nourishment needed for healing.

Measures to Promote Wound Healing

1. Pressure dressings of gauze and elastic adhesive are used initially on incisions or unintentional wounds to prevent hemorrhage and subsequent formation of hematomas that separate wound edges.

2. Sterile technique is used when changing dressings on open wounds or when examining the wound, to prevent infection of the wound.

3. Immunization is confirmed or tetanus antitoxin is given if the tetanus bacillus may be present in a wound.

4. Binders and bandages are used to restrict movement and protect certain wounds from additional injury from stretching and pulling.

5. Patients are assisted to assume positions that encourage the drainage of exudate. For example, if a patient has a wound on the side, a side-lying position on the wound side encourages the flow of drainage.

6. Moist heat (using sterile compresses) may be applied to localize infections and promote healing. Heat brings the tissues additional nourishment and blood components that combat infection.

7. Cold may be applied to closed wounds to reduce swelling and decrease bleeding into the tissues. Cold constricts the arterioles and lessens the flow of blood to the area.

8. Elevation of an injured body part (e.g., a hand) above the level of the heart facilitates the venous return of blood. This reduces swelling and improves circulation within the affected area.

Assessing Wounds

When assessing wounds, the nurse needs to note:

1. The overall appearance of the wound. In a clean, healing wound the area around the wound normally appears reddened due to the inflammatory response. Granulation tissue appears at the skin edges and grows in to fill the wound. By the 7th to 8th day, granulation tissue has covered most wounds. Infected wounds appear excessively reddened and feel hot.

2. The amount, type, and odor of drainage from the wound. The color, consistency, and location of the exudate are assessed. In clean, healing wounds there is normally some serous drainage, and the amount varies with the location of the wound. For example, perineal wounds usually have a large amount of drainage; wounds on the face tend to have little. The serous drainage is clear or slightly brown (because of the presence of some old blood) and watery. New wounds usually have some sanguineous drainage for a few days. Infected wounds have purulent drainage and have an offensive odor.

3. The patient's complaints of discomfort and the location of the discomfort. Generally, incisional pain is severe for up to 3 days postoperatively and is relieved by narcotic analgesics. After that, milder analgesics provide relief. When patients complain of persistent severe pain, an infection or other problem may be the cause.

4. Presence of generalized symptoms of infection such as an elevated body temperature, diaphoresis, or malaise.

5. Presence of *dehiscence* (opening or gaping of the wound edges) and its exact location.

Care of Wounds

Just as there are many types of wounds, there are also many ways of caring for wounds. In general, the care varies with the type of wound, the size of the wound, the amount of exudate present, whether it is an open or closed wound, the location, the personal preference of the physician, and the presence of complicating factors.

Nursing Goals

1. *To prevent infection* from the entrance of microorganisms through the broken protective barriers of the skin and mucous membranes. This is accomplished by using sterile technique when caring for wounds, by using antiseptic on the skin, and, on occasion, by administering antibiotics as prescribed by the physician.

2. *To prevent further tissue damage* of fragile healing wounds from friction or injury. This is done by protecting the wound with dressings and by immobilizing the part with slings or binders.

3. *To promote healing.* This is accomplished by approximating wound edges with sutures (a physician's function), ensuring a good blood supply, supplying essential nutrients, and keeping the area dry.

4. *To clean wounds of foreign debris,* such as pieces of glass or excessive exudates. The former can act as an irritant, and the latter can harbor microorganisms. *Debridement* is the cleaning of an injured area to remove debris, and it is usually performed by the physician. Wounds may be irrigated with water or cleansers such as hydrogen peroxide to clear away organic material prior to cleaning with antiseptics.

5. *To provide means for absorbing inflammatory exudate and to promote drainage.* Rubber or plastic tubes or drains are frequently put into wounds or ducts by the physician during surgery to promote drainage. Some of these drains, commonly referred to as *Penrose drains,* are shortened progressively throughout the healing process. They ensure removal of inflammatory exudates and blood prior to closure of overlying skin. Other drains are placed in ducts, such as the ureter or common bile duct, to ensure patency of the duct and to prevent adhesion or closure of it during healing. Drains or tubes may be attached to suction apparatus to facilitate drainage. A portable vacuum suction (Hemovac) is sometimes used to drain blood and serous exudate from deep surgical wounds, such as those from orthopedic surgery. With this kind of suction, a vacuum is created in an evacuator bag, which gently draws the drainage out of the wound.

6. *To prevent hemorrhage.* Occlusive pressure dressings are commonly applied to surgical incisions for the first few days, until a dressing change is ordered by the physician. In certain body areas, such as the rectum or vagina, long strips of gauze in varying widths are packed into the orifice to apply pressure on blood capillaries and prevent bleeding. This *packing* is usually removed 2 to 3 days after surgery.

7. *To prevent skin excoriation* around draining wounds. This is accomplished by changing saturated dressings as required and by cleaning and drying wounds and surrounding skin areas. When drainage is excessive, as in some bowel surgery (colostomy) or urinary surgery, protective ointments or pastes may be applied to surrounding skin to prevent irritation and excoriation. The frequent removal of adhesive tape can also be irritating to the skin; thus, Montgomery straps or tie tapes are frequently used. See page 1033.

Open and Closed Methods of Care

The closed method of wound care refers to wounds that have a dressing applied, the open method to wounds that do not. Dressings have the following advantages:

1. They help absorb drainage.
2. They protect the wound from microorganisms.
3. They cover unpleasant disfigurements.
4. They can assist in approximating wound edges.
5. They provide emotional reassurance to some people by offering a protective covering.

In some situations, the physician may apply a protective covering such as collodion spray instead of a gauze dressing. This spray hardens like nail polish and can either be peeled from the skin when the wound is healed or be removed with special solutions. A spray covering is often preferred, since the friction of a dressing is eliminated and the wound is always observable through the translucent covering. The wound is kept dry because the spray is moisture-proof. For children, who are active and heal quickly, spray is frequently used. It is not advised for wounds that have drainage.

The open method is used to avoid such disadvantages of dressings as (a) dark, warm, moist environments in which resident and nonresident microorganisms can multiply; and (b) irritation of wounds by friction. Exposing wounds to the air produces drying. This discourages the growth of microorganisms, which need moisture. The open method is frequently employed for burns.

Dressing Materials

Materials to clean wounds

Some nurses prefer cotton balls to clean wounds because of their absorbent qualities, while others prefer gauze squares, claiming that threads of cotton balls can stick to sutures. Cleaning agents vary considerably. Some of the common ones are:

Alcohol 70%

Aqueous and tincture of chlorhexidine gluconate (Hibitane)

Aqueous and tincture of benzalkonium chloride (Zephiran Chloride)

Hydrogen peroxide

Materials to cover wounds

Several sizes of gauze are available to cover wounds. The standard sizes are 10 × 10 cm (4 × 4 in) and 10 × 20 cm (4 × 8 in). The size and the number of pads used

Gussie I 1240
O x2 lg amt

Martin I 240 O 300
Temp 97.9 Ax @ 8 30 pm

Nick I 600 O x3

Della Temp 97.6 Ax

Maude wT 111

Henery 97.5/AX

Henrietta wt. 138

Leela-T. 98.0ax

Joe WT 129

Ida Yoder 97.6/orally

Patsy 98.2/orally

May S. 97.5/AX

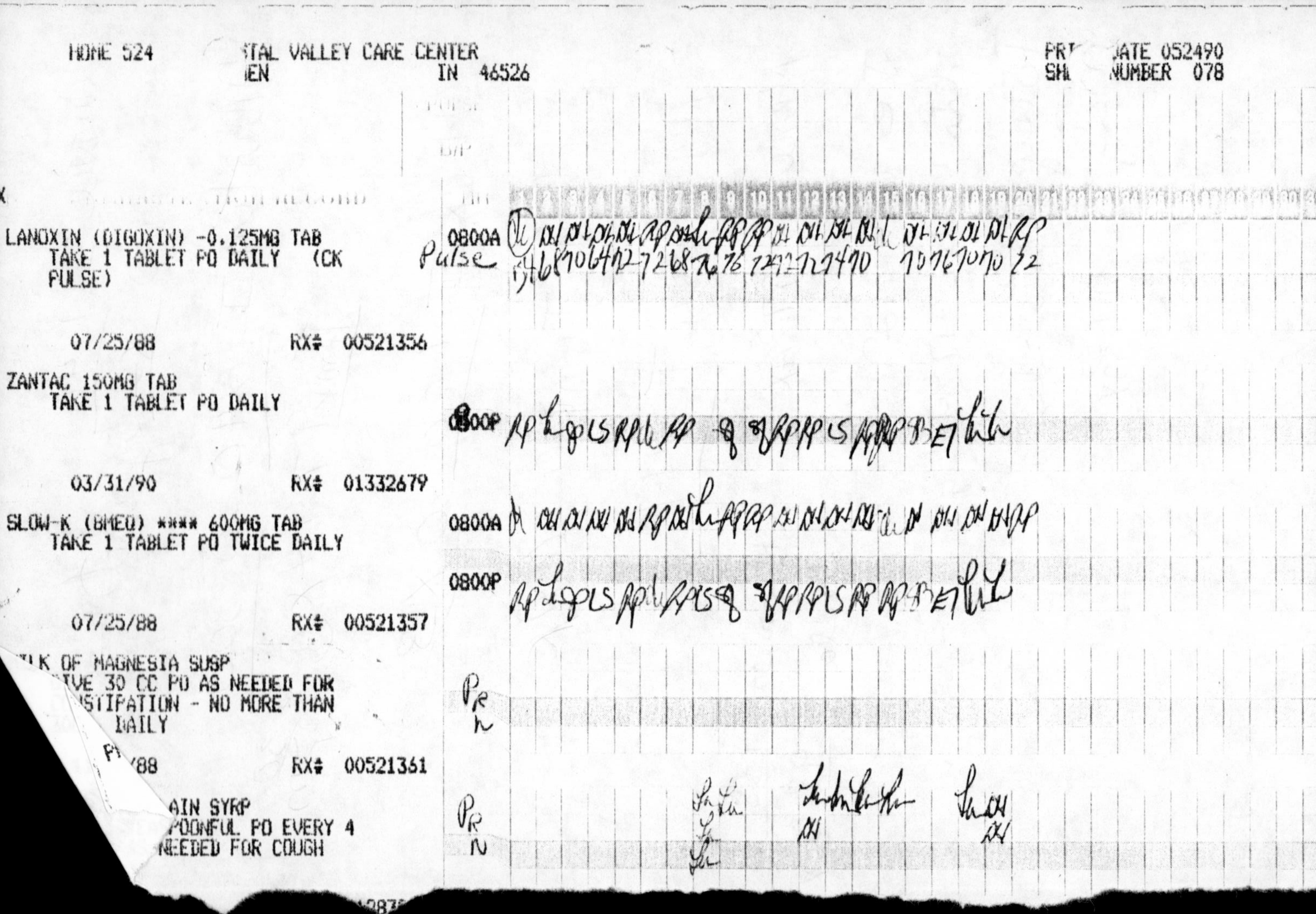

HOME 524

TAL VALLEY CARE CENTER
EN   IN 46526

PRT DATE 052490
SH NUMBER 078

X

LANOXIN (DIGOXIN) -0.125MG TAB
TAKE 1 TABLET PO DAILY (CK
PULSE)

0800A
Pulse

07/25/88 RX# 00521356

ZANTAC 150MG TAB
TAKE 1 TABLET PO DAILY

0800P

03/31/90 RX# 01332679

SLOW-K (8MEQ) **** 600MG TAB
TAKE 1 TABLET PO TWICE DAILY

0800A

0800P

07/25/88 RX# 00521357

LK OF MAGNESIA SUSP
IVE 30 CC PO AS NEEDED FOR
STIPATION - NO MORE THAN
DAILY

PRN

/88 RX# 00521361

AIN SYRP
POONFUL PO EVERY 4
NEEDED FOR COUGH

PRN

Electrolytes: Kozier Tech 683-693

Kozier Funds 777-830

Cardiac: Mason p 267-313

Loebl p 255-290

291-368

depend on the nature of the wound, the amount of exudate, and the location of the wound. These decisions are left to the nurse's judgment. Sometimes the gauze is cut halfway through one side to make it fit around a drain, or it is folded in a special way.

Telfa gauze is a special type of gauze with a shiny, nonadherent surface on one side. It is applied with the shiny surface on the wound. Exudate seeps through this surface and collects on the absorbent side. This kind of dressing is advantageous for wounds with a sticky exudate or newly formed granulation tissue. The dressing does not adhere and therefore does not cause injury to the wound when it is removed.

Larger and thicker gauze dressings, called *surgipads* or *abdominal pads*, are used to cover small gauzes. They not only hold the other gauzes in place but are also absorbent and thus collect excessive drainage. Surgipads are more absorbent on one side, and this side is placed toward the wound; the less absorbent, more protective side is placed outward. The outer side is often indicated with a blue stripe.

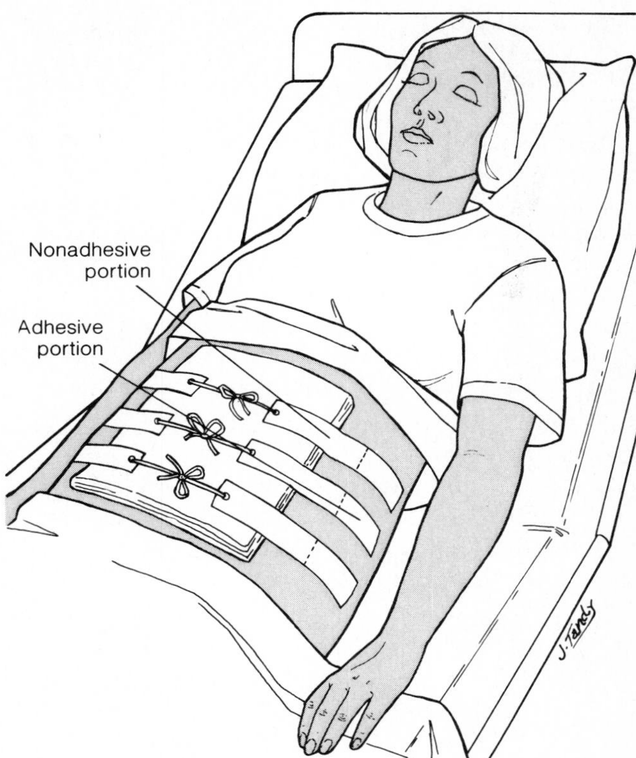

Figure 40–1 Tie tapes are commonly used to secure large dressings that require frequent changing.

Materials to secure dressings

Adhesive tapes After abdominal or other types of surgery, an elastic adhesive tape is commonly applied over wounds because of its ability to compress, thereby controlling hemorrhage. The original tape is removed during the initial dressing change and a lighter dressing applied. Ordinary adhesive tape can be applied in strips across the dressing. It is important to secure the dressing at both ends and across the middle and to use tape of a sufficient width for the dressing and the wound.

Montgomery straps (tie tapes) are commonly used for patients who require frequent dressing changes. See Figure 40-1. These straps prevent skin irritation and discomfort to patients by eliminating the need to remove the adhesive each time the dressing is changed. Nonallergenic tape is used for people who have sensitive skin. If this is not available, tincture of benzoin applied to the skin where the adhesive is to be placed serves as a skin protective.

Bandages and binders There are numerous types of bandages and binders that may be used to secure dressings, as well as to support or immobilize a wound. These are discussed later in this chapter.

Intervention: Changing Dressings

The order for dressings and the frequency of dressing changes are generally prescribed by a physician. Applications of special ointments may also be ordered—for example, "Elase ointment to varicose ulcers and dry dressings twice a day." For a surgical incision, the order may read simply, "Change dressing on the 3rd day postoperatively," and the nurse will then apply skin cleaners and/or antiseptics according to agency policy. Some physicians prefer that nurses reinforce a dressing with surgipads for excessive drainage rather than remove the existing dressing and apply a new one. Others may prescribe a specific solution for cleaning. The nurse reviews the physician's orders and nurses' notes prior to changing a dressing. Notes on the nursing care plan can offer information about the amount of drainage, the quantity of dressing materials required, the patient's allergy to adhesive tape, and scheduled times for dressing changes. It is mandatory that the nurse determine the existence and location of drains before removing dressings, to avoid dislodging a drain. This information can be acquired from the patient's chart and is often on the surgical or anesthetic record or the nursing Kardex.

Some patients are taught to change their own dressings, and the nurse offers assistance as required.

Procedure 40–1 Changing a Dressing

Before assembling the equipment, the nurse dons a face mask, if required, and washes hands using surgical aseptic technique. Many agencies require that a mask be worn for surgical dressing changes to prevent contamination of the wound by droplet spray from the nurse's respiratory tract. The mask is donned before washing the hands because the hands will become contaminated when they touch the hair. A surgical handwash is required before handling sterile equipment.

Equipment

1. A sterile dressing set that includes:
   - **a.** A drape or towel
   - **b.** Cotton balls or gauze squares to clean the wound
   - **c.** A container for the cleaning solution
   - **d.** An antiseptic solution
   - **e.** Two pairs of forceps (thumb or artery)
   - **f.** Gauze dressings and surgipads
   - **g.** Applicators or tongue blades to apply ointments

   If a set is not available, the nurse gathers these items from a central supply cart.
2. Additional supplies required for the particular dressing, e.g., extra gauze dressings and ointment or powder, if ordered.
3. Sterile scissors if needed, e.g., for shaping a dressing. These are added to the sterile set.
4. A waterproof bag for disposal of the old dressings and the used cleaning gauzes.
5. Adhesive tape or tie tapes to secure the dressing.
6. A bath blanket, if necessary, to cover the patient and prevent undue exposure.
7. Acetone or another solution to loosen adhesive, if necessary.

Intervention

Preparing the patient

1. Explain to the patient what you plan to do in terms the patient will understand. Answer specific questions the patient may ask.

   Rationale The patient will be reassured by knowledge of what will happen.
2. Acquire assistance for changing a dressing on an infant or young child.

   Rationale The child might move and contaminate the sterile field or the wound.
3. Provide privacy, and close windows in the room.

   Rationale Privacy enhances the patient's psychologic well-being. Closing the windows, doors, and screens around the bed minimizes air currents, which could transmit microorganisms to the wound.
4. Assist the patient to a comfortable position, in which the wound can be readily exposed. Expose only the wound area, using a bath blanket to drape the patient, if necessary.

   Rationale Undue exposure is physically and psychologically distressing to most patients.
5. Make a cuff on the waterproof bag for disposal of the soiled dressings, and place the bag within reach. It can be taped to the bedclothes or bedside table.

   Rationale Making a cuff on the bag keeps the outside of it free from contamination by the soiled dressings and prevents subsequent contamination of the nurse's hands. Placement of the bag within reach prevents the nurse from reaching across the sterile field and the wound and potentially contaminating these areas.

Removing the soiled dressing

6. Remove binders, if used, and place them aside. Untie Montgomery straps, if used.
7. If adhesive tape was used, remove it by holding down the skin and pulling the tape gently but firmly toward the wound. Use a solvent to loosen the tape, if required.

   Rationale Tape is pulled toward the incision to prevent strain on the sutures or wound. Moistening the tape with acetone or a similar product lessens the discomfort of removal, particularly from hairy surfaces.
8. Remove the outer abdominal dressing or surgipad by hand if the dressing is dry, or using a disposable glove if the dressing is moist. Lift the dressing so that the underside is away from the patient's face.

Procedure 40–1, continued

Rationale The outer surgipad is considered contaminated by the patient's clothing and linen. The appearance and odor of the drainage may be upsetting to the patient.

9. Place the soiled dressing in the waterproof bag without touching the outside of the bag.

Rationale Contamination of the outside of the bag is avoided to prevent the spread of microorganisms to the nurse and subsequently to others.

10. Open the sterile tray. See Chapter 20, page 470.

11. Place the sterile drape beside the wound. See Chapter 20, page 474.

12. Remove the under dressings with tissue forceps, taking care not to dislodge any drains in or near the incision. If the gauze sticks to the drain, use two pairs of forceps, one to remove the gauze and one to hold the drain.

Rationale Forceps are used to remove the under dressings to prevent contamination of the patient's wound by the nurse's hands and contamination of the nurse's hands by wound drainage.

13. Note the type of drainage present, the number of gauzes saturated, and the appearance of the wound.

14. Discard the soiled dressings in the bag. To avoid contaminating the forceps tips on the edge of the paper bag, hold the dressings about 10 to 15 cm (4 to 6 in) above the bag, and drop the dressings into it. After the dressings are removed, discard the forceps or set them aside from the sterile field.

Rationale These forceps are now contaminated by the wound drainage and are discarded before cleaning the wound.

Cleaning and dressing the wound

15. Clean the wound, using artery or tissue forceps and gauze swabs moistened with antiseptic solution. Keep the forceps tips lower than the handles at all times. Use a separate swab for each stroke, cleaning from the incision toward a drain. Discard each swab after use.

Rationale The wound is cleaned from the least to the most contaminated area, i.e., from the drier incision area to a moister drain site, which is considered more contaminated. Forceps tips are always held lower than the handle to prevent their contamination by fluid traveling up to the handle, which is contaminated by the nurse's hand, and back.

a. Clean from the top to the bottom of the incision and from the center to the outside. See Figure 40–2.
or
Clean outward from the incision on one side and then outward on the other side. See Figure 40–3.

b. If a drain is present, clean it after the incision. See page 1036.

c. For irregular wounds, such as a decubitus ulcer, clean from the center of the wound outward, using circular motions.

Figure 40–2

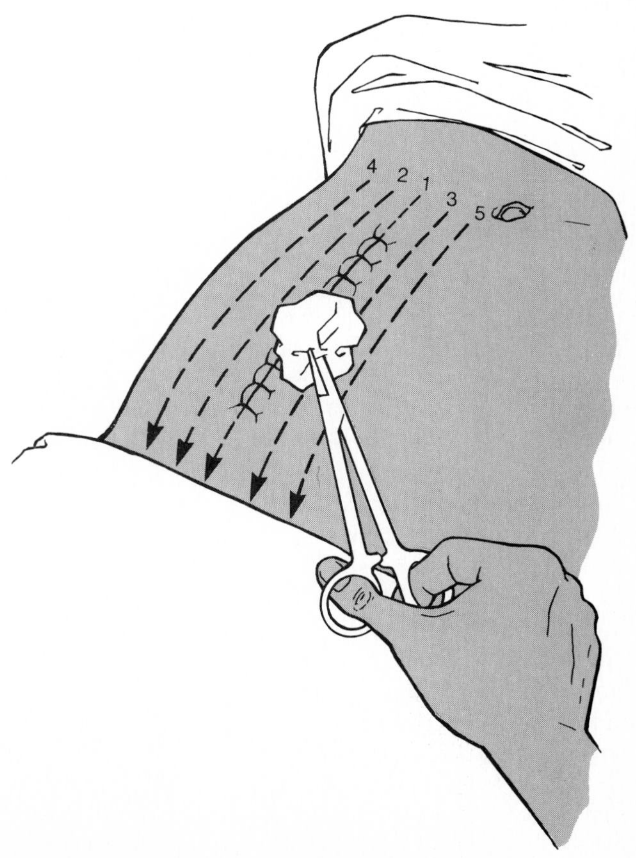

Procedure 40–1, continued

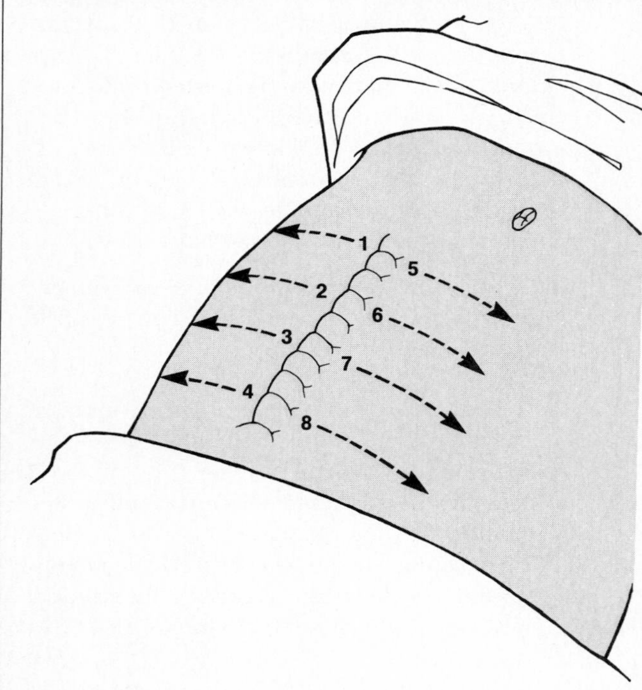

Figure 40–3

16. Repeat the cleaning process until all drainage is removed.

17. Dry the wound in the manner described in step 15, using dry gauze swabs.

18. Apply powder or ointment if required. Shake powder directly onto the wound; use sterile applicators or tongue blades to apply ointment.

    Rationale If drainage is profuse, ointment can protect the skin from irritation. Antibiotic powders or other substances may be ordered by the physician.

19. Apply sterile dressings one at a time over the wound, using sterile forceps. Start at the center of the wound and move progressively outward. Dressings around drain sites may need to be cut (see page 1037). The final surgipad can be picked up by hand, touching only the outside, which is often marked by a blue line down the center.

20. Secure the dressing with tape, Montgomery straps, or a binder.

21. Assist the patient to a comfortable position.

22. Remove the equipment and the bag containing the soiled dressings. Clean the equipment and dispose of the waste bag appropriately.

23. Wash hands.

24. Report changes in the appearance of the wound or drainage to the responsible nurse. Record the dressing change, the wound assessment, and the patient's response.

Intervention: Shortening Penrose Drains

Frequently, flexible rubber drains, called *Penrose drains*, are inserted during abdominal surgery to provide drainage and healing of underlying tissues. These drains may be inserted and sutured through the incision line, but they are most commonly inserted through stab wounds a few centimeters away from the incision line, so that the incision is kept dry. Drains vary in length and width. The length inserted can be 25 to 35 cm (10 to 14 in), and the width, 2.5 to 4 cm (0.5 to 1.5 in). To facilitate drainage and healing of tissues from the inside to the outside, or from the bottom to the top, the physician commonly orders that the drain be pulled out or shortened 2 to 5 cm (1 to 2 in) each day until it falls out. When a drain falls out or is completely removed, the remaining stab wound usually heals within 1 to 2 days. In some agencies this shortening procedure is performed only by physicians; in others, it is performed by nurses.

Shortening of a drain is done in conjunction with a dressing change. Preparation of the patient is the same as for a dressing change. In addition to the dressing change equipment, a sterile safety pin or special drain clamp needs to be added to the dressing tray, to hold the drain end in place above the skin, and straight scissors are needed to cut the drain and to cut gauzes that are placed around the drain site. If the drain is to be shortened for the first time, the suture holding the drain in place needs to be cut and removed. It is essential to confirm the physician's order prior to this procedure.

Cleaning the drain site

The drain site is cleaned after the incision, according to the principle of cleaning from the cleanest to the most contaminated area. Because moist drainage facilitates the growth of resident bacteria, the drain site is

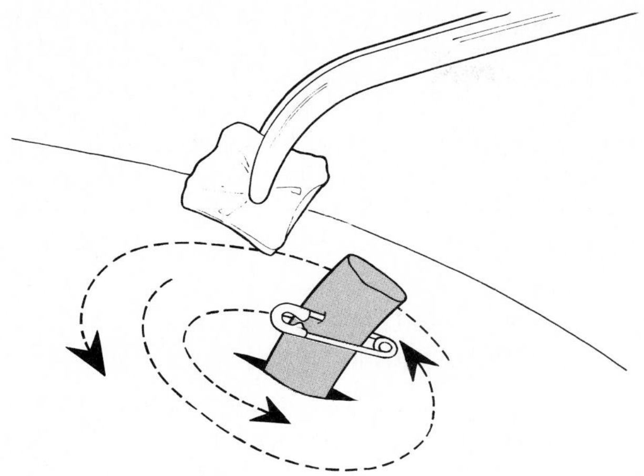

Figure 40–4 Cleaning around a drain site.

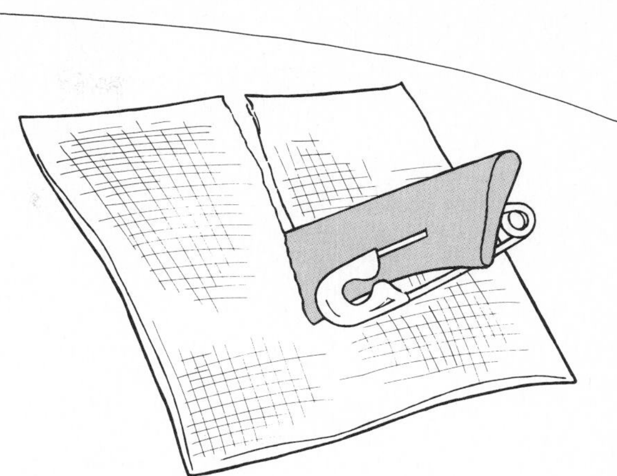

Figure 40–5 Partially split gauze is placed around a Penrose drain.

considered the most contaminated. If the drain is situated in the center of the incision, the incision can be cleaned from the top toward the drain and from the bottom toward the drain, using separate swabs. The skin around the drain is cleaned with an antiseptic swab held with a hemostat. The nurse swabs in half or full circles around the drain site moving outward. See Figure 40–4. Tissue forceps may be used in one hand to hold the drain erect while using the other hand to clean all around it.

Shortening the drain

A Penrose drain shortening proceeds the same as a dressing change up to and including cleaning the incision and the drain site. If the drain is being shortened for the first time the nurse has to cut and remove the suture holding it in place before pulling on the drain to shorten it. See page 1038. If the drain has been shortened previously, a safety pin will be attached to it.

To shorten the drain, firmly grasp it by its full width using a sterile hemostat. Gradually and evenly pull it out the required length. Wearing sterile gloves hold the drain tightly with the fingers against the skin edge and insert the safety pin through the drain over top of the fingers. Fasten the safety pin. This pin keeps the drain from falling back into the incision. Holding the drain securely in place at the skin level and inserting the pin over the fingers prevents the nurse from pulling the drain further out or pricking the patient. Next, cut off the excess drain so that about 2.5 cm (1 in) remains above the skin, and discard the excess in the waste bag. Partially split a 4 × 4 gauze with sterile scissors, and place it snugly around the drain. See Figure 40–5. This dressing prevents the drainage from coming in contact with the skin and causing excoriation. Dress the incision and drain site as described in Technique 40–1, page 1035.

A Penrose drain may also be shortened using two pairs of sterile forceps rather than sterile gloves. See Kozier and Erb (1982:989).

Sutures

Sutures are stitches used to sew body tissues together. A suture can also refer to the material used to sew the stitch. Policies vary about the personnel who may remove skin sutures. In some agencies, only physicians remove sutures; in others, registered nurses and student nurses with appropriate supervision may do so. Various suture materials are used, such as silk, cotton, linen, wire, nylon, and Dacron (polyester fiber) threads. Silver wire clips are also available. The physician prescribes the removal of sutures. Usually skin sutures are removed 7 to 10 days after surgery. Sterile technique and special suture scissors are used. The scissors have a short, curved cutting tip that readily slides under the suture.

Common Methods of Suturing

Sutures can be broadly categorized as either (a) interrupted (each stitch is tied and knotted separately) or (b) continuous (one thread runs in a series of stitches and is tied at only the beginning and the end of the run). Common sutures of the skin include plain interrupted (see Figure 40–6, *A*), mattress interrupted (see Figure 40–6, *B*), plain continuous (see Figure 40–6, *C*), mattress

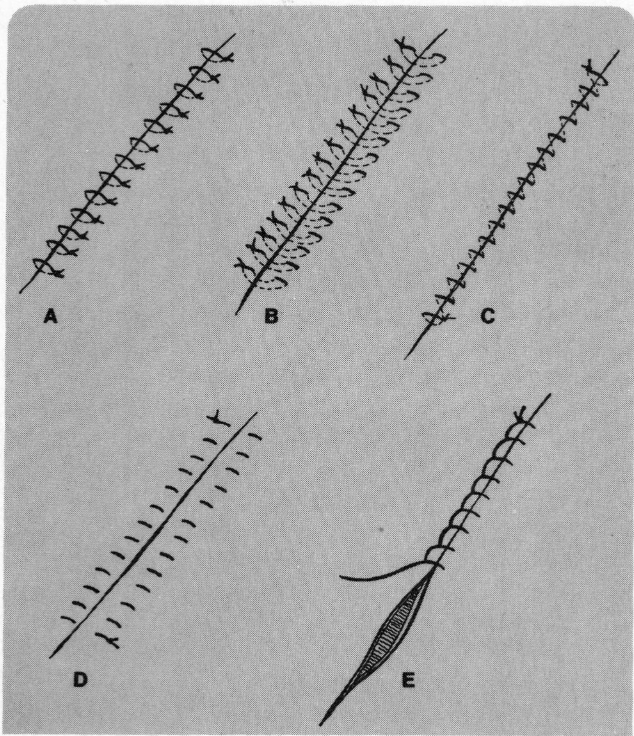

Figure 40–6 Common methods of suturing: **A,** plain interrupted; **B,** mattress interrupted; **C,** plain continuous; **D,** mattress continuous; **E,** blanket continuous.

continuous (see Figure 40–6, *D*), and blanket continuous (see Figure 40–6, *E*).

Guidelines for Removing Sutures

1. The physician's orders must be carefully confirmed. Many times only *alternate* interrupted sutures are removed one day, and the remaining sutures are removed a day or two later.
2. The suture line is usually cleaned with antiseptic solution before and after suture removal as a prophylactic measure to prevent infection.
3. When interrupted sutures were used, alternate ones are removed first. If *dehiscence* (gaping, splitting, or separating) of the wound occurs, the remaining sutures may be left in place.
4. Because suture material that is visible to the eye is in contact with resident bacteria of the skin, this part of the suture is never pulled beneath the skin during removal. Suture material that is beneath the skin is considered free from bacteria. Therefore, for removal, sutures are cut at the skin edge on one side of the visible part. See Figure 40–7. Then the suture is drawn completely out from the other side. Any suture material that is left beneath the skin acts as a foreign body and elicits the inflammatory response.
5. If slight wound dehiscence occurs during the removal of sutures, sterile butterfly tapes are applied to approximate the wound edges as closely as possible.
6. After suture removal, a small dry dressing is applied. The patient is instructed about follow-up wound care. Generally, if the wound is dry and healing well, showers can be taken in a day or two. If wound discharge occurs, the patient is instructed to contact the physician.

Intervention: Removing Skin Sutures

For *plain interrupted* sutures, grasp the suture at the knot with tissue forceps, cut the suture at the skin edge either below the knot or opposite the knot, and pull the thread out in one piece.

Mattress interrupted sutures do not cross the incision line outside the skin and have two threads underlying the skin. Cut the visible part of the suture opposite the knot at either end, when possible, and remove this small visible piece. Then remove the remainder of the suture beneath the skin by pulling the suture out in the direction of the knot. In some sutures, the visible part of the suture opposite the knot is so small that it is possible to cut it only once.

Plain continuous sutures are removed by cutting the thread opposite the knot of the first suture and the thread of the second suture below on the same side. Remove the first stitch and the piece of thread beneath

Figure 40–7 Sutures are cut close to the skin at one side.

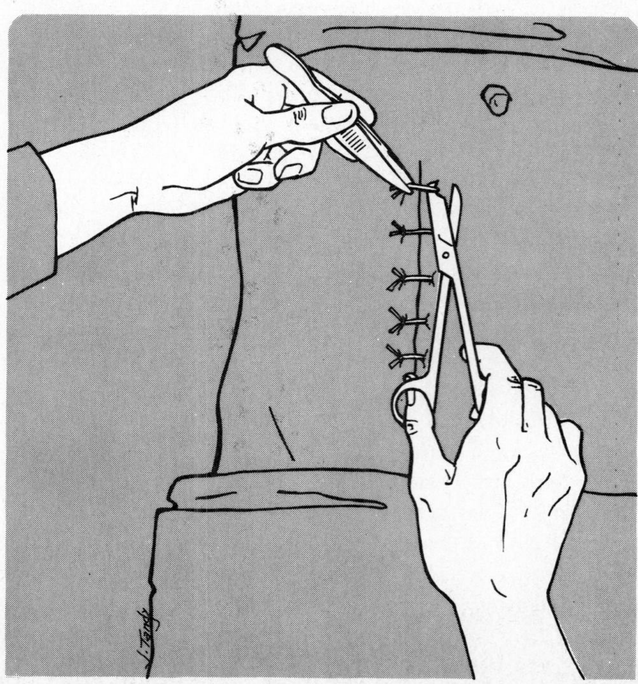

the skin, which is attached to the second stitch, by pulling the knot. Remove the remaining sutures by cutting off the visible part of the thread, pulling the underlying loop up by the next stitch, and again cutting the visible part. Repeat this process until the last knot is reached and removed. After the first stitch is removed, the thread is cut down the same side below the original knot each time.

Blanket continuous sutures are readily removed by cutting the threads that are opposite the looped blanket edge and pulling the stitch out by the looped edge.

Mattress continuous sutures are removed in the manner described for plain continuous sutures. If large pieces of suture material are visible on either side of the incision, cut and remove from side to side of the incision so that visible material is not pulled underneath the skin.

Retention Sutures

Retention sutures, sometimes referred to as *stay sutures*, are very large plain sutures that are seen in some incisions in addition to skin sutures. These large sutures attach underlying tissues of fat and muscle in addition to the skin and are used to support incisions in obese individuals or in situations in which healing may be prolonged. They are frequently left in place longer than skin sutures (14 to 21 days) but may be removed at the same time as the skin sutures. Retention sutures may have rubber tubing over them or may be placed over a roll of gauze extending down the incision line. Both measures prevent these large sutures from irritating the incision. Because there are several forms of retention sutures, the nurse should make inquiries whenever in doubt about their removal.

Irrigations

An *irrigation (lavage)* is the washing or flushing out of an area. It is done for one or more of the following reasons:

1. To clean the area
2. To apply heat and hasten the healing process
3. To apply a medication, such as an antiseptic

Irrigations necessitate the use of sterile technique whenever there is a break in the skin, for example, in a wound irrigation, or whenever a sterile body cavity, such as the bladder, is entered. Some irrigations, however, such as an eye irrigation to remove foreign material, or a vaginal, rectal, or gastric irrigation, are safely conducted using clean technique.

This section discusses procedures for irrigating a wound, eye, ear, or vagina. Urinary catheter or bladder irrigations are discussed in Chapter 28.

Kinds of Irrigators

A number of syringes are used for irrigations. The most common are the Asepto, the rubber bulb, the Toomey, and the Pomeroy. The syringes are often calibrated.

The *Asepto syringe* is a plastic (or glass) syringe with a rubber bulb. See Figure 40–8, *A*. Squeezing the air out of the bulb produces negative pressure, and fluid can be sucked into the syringe. When the bulb is squeezed again, the fluid is ejected from the syringe. Asepto sy-

Figure 40–8 Four types of syringes commonly used for irrigations: **A,** Asepto; **B,** rubber bulb; **C,** Toomey with adapter tip to fit into tubing; **D,** Pomeroy.

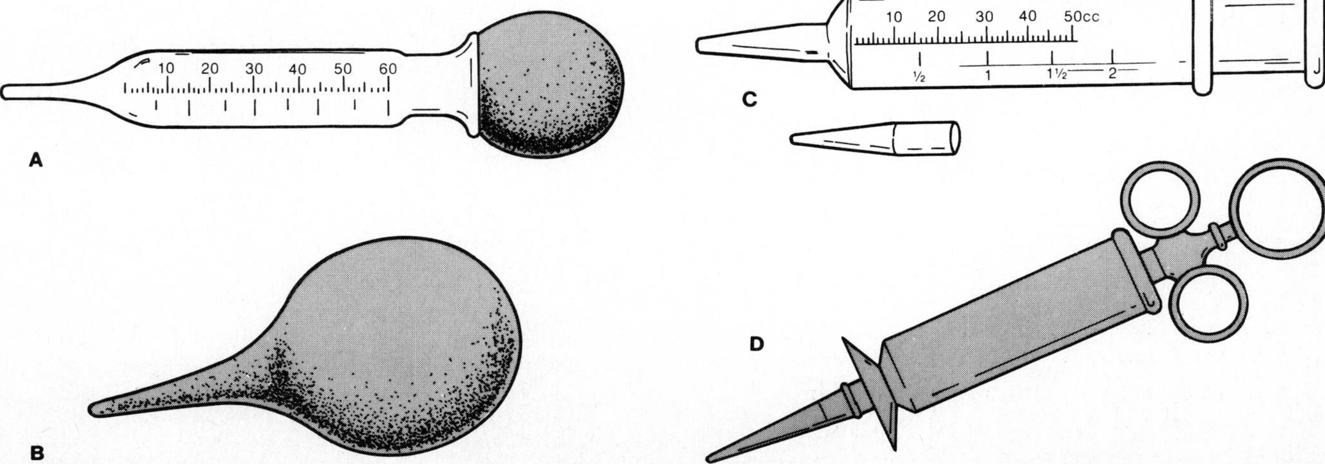

ringes come in several sizes, e.g., 30 ml (1 oz), 60 ml (2 oz), and 120 ml (4 oz).

The *rubber bulb syringe*, also called the *ear syringe*, is often used for irrigating ears. See Figure 40–8, *B*. Like the Asepto syringe, it comes in a range of sizes.

The *Toomey syringe*, which is made of plastic or glass, is also calibrated. See Figure 40–8, *C*. This syringe has a removable tip of metal or plastic that can fit into the end of tubing such as a catheter. Toomey syringes are used for deep wound irrigations that require a catheter and for some types of bladder irrigations.

The *Pomeroy syringe* is sometimes used for an ear irrigation. A shield near the tip end prevents the solution from spraying outward. See Figure 40–8, *D*.

Intervention: Wound Irrigation

Open wounds are frequently irrigated to clean them and to remove excess drainage and sloughing tissue, thereby hastening the healing process. Sometimes the irrigation is designed to apply heat or an antiseptic solution.

Procedure 40–2 Irrigating a Wound

Equipment

1. A dressing set with dressing materials. This is set up as for a dressing change.
2. A sterile irrigating syringe. Bulb syringes are frequently used. For deep wounds with small openings, a sterile straight catheter may also be necessary.
3. A sterile basin for the irrigating solution.
4. A sterile basin to receive the irrigation returns.
5. Irrigating solution, usually 200 ml (6.5 oz) of solution at 32 to 35 C (90 to 95 F), according to the agency's or physician's choice. Dakin's solution and hydrogen peroxide are frequently used.
6. Sterile gloves for the nurse to wear if the wound is to be touched.
7. A waterproof sterile drape to protect the patient and the bed.
8. Sterile petroleum jelly to protect surrounding skin from becoming irritated by certain solutions (e.g., Dakin's solution).
9. A sterile tongue blade to apply the petroleum jelly.

Intervention

1. Explain to the patient what you plan to do, adjusting the explanation to the patient's needs.

   Rationale Knowledge of what the nurse plans to do reassures the patient. The nurse can also identify the patient during the explanation.

2. Assist the patient to a position in which the solution will flow by gravity from the upper end of the wound to the lower end and then into the basin.
3. Wash hands.
4. Proceed as for changing a sterile dressing up through cleaning the wound. See Procedure 40–1, steps 2–15.
5. Place the waterproof drape over the patient and the bed, and position the sterile basin on it below the wound, to catch the irrigating solution.
6. If an irritating solution, such as Dakin's solution, is being used, apply sterile petroleum jelly (using the sterile tongue blade) to the skin around the wound.
7. Using the syringe, run solution over the wound.
8. Continue irrigating until the solution becomes clear (no exudate is present) or until all the solution has been used.

   Rationale The irrigation washes away tissue debris and drainage so that later returns are clearer.

9. Using dressing forceps and sterile gauze, dry the area around the wound.

   Rationale Moisture left on the skin promotes the growth of microorganisms and can cause skin irritation.

10. Apply a sterile dressing to the wound.
11. Assist the patient to a comfortable position.
12. Gather the equipment and dispose of it according to agency practice.
13. Wash hands.
14. Record the irrigation, the solution used, the appearance of the wound, and the appearance of any exudate and sloughing tissue.

Intervention: Eye Irrigation

An eye irrigation is administered to wash out the conjunctival sac of the eye. It is done for any of the following specific reasons:

1. To treat an inflammatory process of the conjunctiva
2. To apply an antiseptic solution
3. To remove a foreign object or an irritating chemical
4. To apply heat or cold to the eye
5. To prepare an eye for surgery

For an eye irrigation in the home, an eye cup is frequently used. The nurse ascertains that the eye cup is clean and that it has no chips along the edge, which could injure the skin.

Procedure 40–3 Irrigating an Eye

Equipment

1. A sterile container for the irrigating solution.
2. Irrigating solution. Usually 60 to 235 ml (2 to 8 oz) of solution at 37 C (100 F) is appropriate.
3. A sterile eye syringe or eye irrigator. An eyedropper can be used if only small amounts of solution are required.
4. A sterile kidney basin to catch the irrigating solution.
5. Sterile cotton balls to dry around the eye after the irrigation.
6. A waterproof drape to protect the patient and the bedclothes.
7. Sterile gloves (optional) to protect the nurse from contamination if the eye is infected.

Intervention

1. Explain to the patient what you plan to do, adjusting the explanation to the patient's needs.

   Rationale The patient is reassured by knowledge of what the nurse plans to do, and the nurse can identify the patient during the explanation.

2. Assist the patient to a comfortable position either sitting or lying. Tilt the patient's head toward the affected eye and ensure that the light source does not shine into the patient's eyes.

   Rationale The patient's head is tilted so that the solution will run from the eye to the basin at the side, not to the other eye. The light source is directed slightly away from the eye particularly if the patient is photophobic.

3. Place the drape to protect the patient, and position the basin against the patient's cheek below the eye on the affected side.

4. Wash hands.

5. Clean the eyelid and lashes with moistened cotton balls, wiping from the inner canthus to the outer canthus.

   Rationale Material on the eyelid and lashes can be washed into the eye if not removed. Cleaning toward the outer canthus prevents contamination of the other eye and the lacrimal duct.

6. Expose the lower conjunctival sac by separating both lids with the thumb and forefinger (see Figure 40–9) or, to irrigate in stages, first hold the lower lid down, then hold the upper lid up. Exert pressure on the bony prominences of the cheekbone and beneath the eyebrow when holding the eyelids.

Figure 40–9

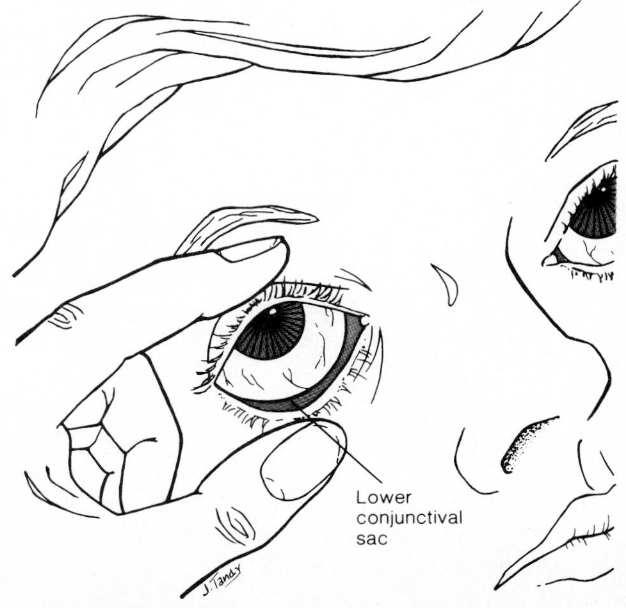

Procedure 40–3, continued

Rationale Separating the lids prevents reflex blinking. Exerting pressure on the bony prominences prevents discomfort from pressure on the eyeball.

7. Hold the eye irrigator about 2.5 cm (1 in) above the eye.

   Rationale At this height the pressure of the solution will not damage the eye tissues and the irrigator will not touch the eye.

8. Irrigate the eye, directing the solution onto the lower conjunctival sac and from the inner canthus to the outer canthus.

   Rationale Directing the solution in this way prevents possible injury to the cornea and prevents fluid and contaminants from flowing down the nasolacrimal duct.

9. Irrigate until the solution leaving the eye is clear (no discharge is present) or until all the solution has been used.

10. Instruct the patient to close and move the eye periodically.

    Rationale Eye closure and movement help to move secretions from the upper to the lower conjunctival sac.

11. Dry around the eye with cotton balls.
12. Gather up the equipment.
13. Assist the patient to a comfortable position.
14. Wash hands.
15. Record the irrigation, solution used, and appearance of the eye, the pupils, and any discharge. Also record whether the returned solution was cloudy, clear, yellow, etc. Report any pain and other mannerisms such as squinting or rubbing the eyes.

Intervention: Ear (External Auditory Canal) Irrigation

Irrigations of the external auditory canal are generally carried out for cleaning purposes, although applications of heat and of antiseptic solutions are sometimes prescribed.

Procedure 40–4 Irrigating the External Auditory Canal

Equipment

1. A container for the irrigating solution.
2. Irrigating solution. About 500 ml (16 oz) of solution is required. Normal saline is frequently used. The temperature is body temperature: for an adult, 37.0 C (98.6 F).
3. A syringe. A rubber bulb or Asepto syringe is frequently used. When large amounts of solution are ordered, a special irrigating nozzle (ear tip) attached to tubing is used, and the solution container is hung from an IV standard.
4. A basin to receive the irrigating solution. A kidney basin is often used because the small curve will fit closely against the head.
5. A moisture-resistant towel to protect the patient (and the bed) from the solution.
6. Applicator swabs for cleaning the external ear.
7. Absorbent cotton balls to dry the pinna of the ear after the irrigation.
8. A thermometer to test the temperature of the solution.

Intervention

1. Explain to the patient what you plan to do. Adjust the explanation to the patient's needs.

   Rationale The patient may experience warmth and occasionally dizziness and discomfort when the fluid comes in contact with the tympanic membrane.

Procedure 40–4, continued

2. Assist the patient to a sitting or lying position with head turned toward the affected ear.

   Rationale The solution can then flow from the ear canal to a basin.

3. Place the moisture-resistant towel around the patient's shoulder under the ear.

4. Place the basin under the ear to be irrigated.

5. Clean the pinna of the ear and the meatus of the ear canal with applicator swabs and solution.

   Rationale Any discharge is removed, so that it will not be washed into the ear canal.

6. Fill the syringe with solution.
   or
   Hang up the irrigating container, and run solution through the tubing and the nozzle.

   Rationale Solution is run through to remove air from the tubing and nozzle.

7. Straighten the patient's auditory canal. For an infant, gently pull the pinna downward. See Figure 40–10, *A*. For an adult, pull the pinna upward and backward. See Figure 40–10, *B*.

   Rationale The auditory canal is straightened so that the solution can flow the entire length of the canal.

8. Insert the tip of the syringe or nozzle into the auditory meatus, and direct the solution gently upward against the top of the canal.

   Rationale The solution will flow around the entire canal and out at the bottom. The solution is instilled gently because strong pressure from the fluid can cause discomfort and damage the tympanic membrane.

9. Continue instilling the fluid until all the solution is used or until the canal is cleaned, depending on the purpose of the irrigation. Take care not to block the outward flow of the solution with the syringe or nozzle.

10. Dry the outside of the ear with absorbent cotton balls.

11. Place a cotton ball in the auditory meatus, to absorb the excess fluid.

12. Assist the patient to a side-lying position on the affected side.

    Rationale Lying with the affected side down helps drain the excess fluid by gravity.

13. Assess the patient's response to the irrigation in terms of discomfort, dizziness, and the appearance and odor of the fluid returns.

14. Remove the equipment from the bedside, and clean or dispose of it appropriately.

15. Wash hands.

16. Record the irrigation; the type, concentration, amount, and temperature of the solution used; the appearance of the returns; and the patient's response in terms of discomfort and dizziness.

17. Return in 15 minutes to assess the drainage on the absorbent cotton ball. Remove the cotton ball if drainage appears complete, and assist the patient to a comfortable position.

Figure 40–10

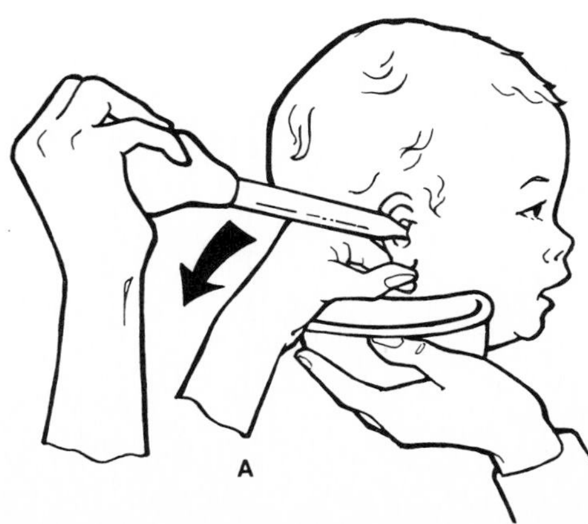

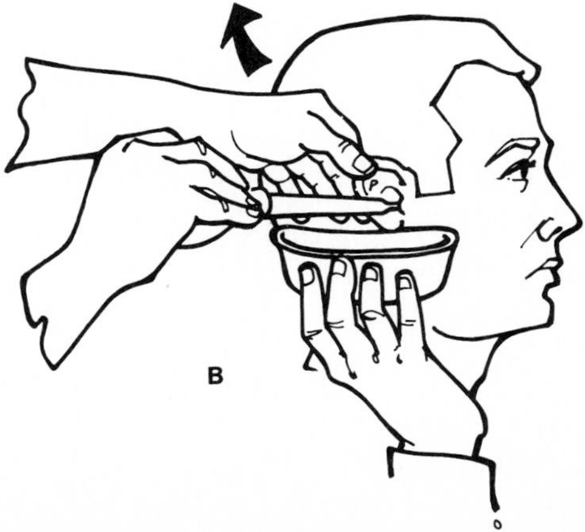

Intervention: Vaginal Irrigation (Douche)

A vaginal irrigation is the washing of the vagina by a liquid at a low pressure. It is similar to the irrigation of the external auditory canal in that the fluid returns immediately after being inserted.

Vaginal irrigations are not usually necessary for female hygiene but are done for the following reasons:

1. To apply an antimicrobial solution that discourages the growth of microorganisms
2. To remove an offensive or irritating discharge
3. To apply heat or cold, for example, in the treatment of inflammation or hemorrhage

Procedure 40–5 Irrigating a Vagina

Equipment

In hospitals, sterile supplies and equipment are used; in a home, sterility is not usually necessary because patients are accustomed to the microorganisms in their environments. Sterile technique is indicated if there is an open wound.

1. A vaginal irrigation set (often disposable) containing:
   a. A nozzle
   b. Tubing and a clamp
   c. A container for the solution
   d. A moisture-resistant drape
2. Irrigating solution. Usually 1000 to 2000 ml at 40.5 C (105 F) is required. Check agency practice. Normal saline, tap water, sodium bicarbonate solution (8 ml of sodium bicarbonate to 1000 ml of water), and vinegar solution (8 ml of vinegar to 1000 ml of water) are commonly used.
3. A thermometer to check the temperature of the solution. This is usually measured before the equipment is taken to the patient.
4. A drape to cover the patient's legs.
5. A bedpan to receive the irrigation returns.
6. Tissues to dry the perineum.
7. Gloves (optional). They may be required to protect the nurse from infection.
8. An IV standard on which to hang the solution container.

Intervention

Preparing the patient

1. Explain the technique to the patient. A vaginal irrigation is normally a painless procedure, and in fact may bring relief from itching and burning if an infection is present. It normally takes about 10 minutes.
2. Provide privacy, and ask the patient to void before the irrigation. If the patient cannot void, check the patient's recent urinary output and percuss or palpate the bladder for urine. See Chapter 28, page 712. If there seems to be urine in the bladder, check with the responsible nurse before starting the procedure.

   Rationale The patient will have less discomfort during the treatment, and the possibility of injuring the vaginal lining is decreased, if the bladder is empty.
3. Assist the patient to a back-lying position with the hips higher than the shoulders so that the solution will flow into the posterior fornix of the vagina. Position the patient on a bedpan, and provide comfortable support for the lumbar region of the back with a roll or pillow. Place the waterproof drape under the bedpan to protect the bedding. Provide a drape for the legs so that only the perineal area is exposed. See Figure 40–11.

Figure 40–11

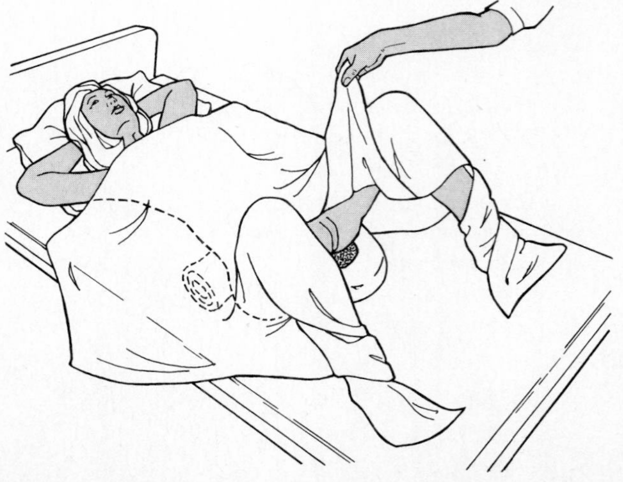

Procedure 40–5, continued

4. Provide perineal care to remove microorganisms.

Rationale This decreases the chance of flushing microorganisms into the vagina.

Irrigating the vagina

5. Clamp the tubing. Hang the irrigating container on the IV standard so that the base is about 30 cm (12 in) above the vagina.

Rationale At this height the pressure of the solution should not be great enough to injure the vaginal lining.

6. Run fluid through the tubing and nozzle into the bedpan.

Rationale Fluid is run through the tubing to remove air and to moisten the nozzle.

7. Run some fluid over the perineal area, then insert the nozzle carefully into the vagina. Direct the nozzle toward the sacrum, following the direction of the vagina.

8. Insert the nozzle about 7 to 10 cm (3 to 4 in), and rotate it several times.

Rationale Rotating the nozzle irrigates all parts of the vagina.

9. Use all the irrigating solution, permitting it to flow out freely into the bedpan.

Rationale Obstructing the flow of the returns could result in injury to the tissues from pressure.

10. Remove the nozzle from the vagina.

11. Assist the patient to a sitting position on the bedpan.

Rationale Sitting on the bedpan will help drain the remaining fluid by gravity.

12. Dry the perineum with tissues.

13. Remove the bedpan.

14. Assess the response of the patient in terms of the color of the fluid returns and the presence of any flecks; discomfort; redness of the vagina; and odor from the vagina.

15. Remove the moisture-resistant towel and the drape.

16. Apply a dressing if indicated.

17. Assist the patient to a comfortable position.

18. Empty the bedpan. Clean the equipment and dispose of it appropriately.

19. Wash hands.

20. On the patient's chart, record the irrigation; the amount, type, strength, and temperature of the irrigating solution; any discomfort etc.; and the response of the patient to the irrigation.

Supporting and Immobilizing Wounds

A *bandage* is a strip of cloth used to wrap the body. Bandages are available in various widths; the most common are 1.5 to 7.5 cm (0.5 to 3 in). They are usually supplied in rolls for easy application to a body part.

A *binder* is a type of bandage. It is a piece of material designed for a specific body part; for example, the triangular binder (sling) fits the arm. Binders are used to support large areas of the body, such as the abdomen, arm, or chest.

Bandages and binders are used for a variety of purposes:

1. To support a wound, e.g., a fractured bone
2. To immobilize a wound, e.g., a strained shoulder
3. To apply pressure, e.g., from elastic bandages to the lower extremities to improve venous blood flow
4. To secure a dressing, e.g., for an extensive abdominal surgical wound
5. To retain splints (this applies chiefly to bandages)
6. To retain warmth, e.g., a flannel bandage on a rheumatoid joint

Support and immobilization are the most common purposes.

Materials

The materials used in bandaging vary widely, according to the purpose of the bandage.

Gauze is one of the most frequently used materials. It is light and porous, and it readily molds to the body. It is also relatively inexpensive and is generally discarded once it becomes soiled. Gauze is used to retain dressings on wounds and to immobilize or support the fingers, hands, toes, and feet. Gauze can be impregnated with petroleum jelly for application to some wounds. Gauze supports dressings well and at the same time permits air to circulate through them.

Flannel is a soft, pliable material that provides warmth to a body part. It is a strong, fairly heavy material, and it can be washed and reused.

Muslin (factory cotton) is another strong material. It is lighter than flannel, but it also supplies good support. Many binders are made of muslin. It can be washed and resued.

Crinoline and Kling are types of woven gauze. Crinoline is loosely woven, yet strong. It is impregnated with plaster of Paris as the base for casts. Kling is woven in such a manner that it will stretch and thus mold to the body.

There are a variety of elasticized bandages, which are generally applied to provide pressure to an area. They may be used as tensor bandages or designed as partial stockings to support the legs and improve the venous circulation. Some elasticized bandages have an adhesive backing and can be secured to the skin. These are most frequently used to retain dressings and at the same time provide some support to a wound.

Plastic adhesive bandages are also used to retain dressings. They are waterproof and thus retain wound drainage or keep an area dry. They have some elastic properties and therefore provide some pressure.

Principles for Use of Bandages and Binders

1. Bandages and binders need to be applied in a way that promotes circulation and does not restrict it. They are applied so that there is even pressure over the area and should be tight enough to serve their purposes without restricting circulation. If possible, the distal end of an extremity should be left uncovered so that the adequacy of the circulation can be readily determined.
2. Symptoms at a distal part of an extremity, such as coldness, bluish discoloration, and a perception of tingling or numbness, usually indicate that circulation is restricted. This fact needs to be reported and the bandage loosened.
3. When a body part is supported, it should be in a position as close to good body alignment as possible. See Chapter 23.
4. Rubbing can cause the skin to become abraded. Therefore skin surfaces should be separated with gauze before bandaging, and bony prominences should be padded.
5. Warmth and moisture facilitate the growth of microorganisms. Therefore binders and bandages need to be changed regularly, unless changing is specifically contraindicated, and the associated skin areas need to be washed and dried. Dirt also promotes the growth of organisms, and its presence indicates that a bandage needs to be changed.

Assessing the Patient

Before applying bandages

1. Observe the affected body surface for any abrasions. Open wounds require a dressing before the bandage is applied.
2. Observe the skin for pallor or cyanosis, which could indicate impaired blood circulation in the area. The color provides baseline data for comparison with observations after the bandage is applied. Any signs of restricted circulation (coldness, cyanosis, swelling, or the patient's complaints of numbness and tingling sensations) should be reported before the bandage is applied.

Before applying binders

1. Assess the affected body area for swelling, discoloration, discomfort, etc.
2. If a dressing is present, determine if it requires changing or reinforcing, depending on the physician's orders.
3. Assess the skin area to be covered by the binder for any abrasions.

Intervention: Bandaging

Guidelines for bandaging

1. Select the material for the bandage according to the purpose of the bandage as well as cost and availability.
2. Select the width of the bandage according to the size of the body part. For example, use a 5 cm (2 in) bandage for an arm, a 2.5 cm (1 in) width for a finger, and a 7.5 to 10 cm (3 to 4 in) width for a leg.
3. Assist the patient to a comfortable position with the part to be bandaged supported in an aligned position, with slight flexion of the joints, unless this is specifically contraindicated.
4. Face the patient to be bandaged unless specifically instructed otherwise (for example, a skull bandage is applied from behind the patient).
5. Hold the roller bandage with the roll facing upward in one hand and the initial part of the bandage in the other hand.
6. Begin by placing the bandage on the limb or part so that the bandage direction will be from distal to proximal and from medial to lateral. Do not begin bandaging over a wound or in an area where pressure is contraindicated, such as the sole of the foot.

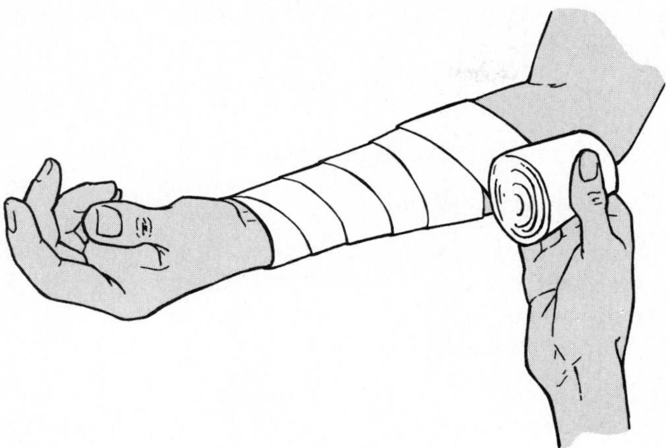

Figure 40–12 A spiral bandage.

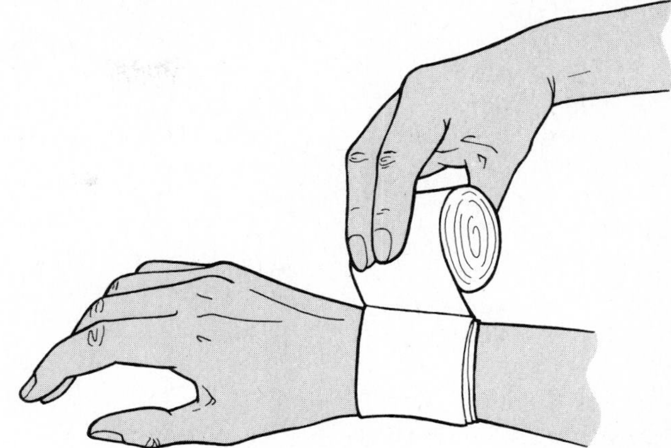

Figure 40–13 A circular bandage.

7. Overlap each bandage turn by two-thirds the width of the bandage and apply the bandage with firm, even pressure.
8. Cover underlying dressings with bandages at least 5 cm (2 in) beyond the edge of the dressing.
9. Pad bony prominences, and separate skin surfaces that would otherwise touch, to prevent friction and subsequent abrasion.
10. Leave the distal aspect of a limb exposed if at all possible, to check the adequacy of the blood circulation.

Basic turns in bandaging

Five basic turns are used in bandaging: spiral, circular, spiral reverse, recurrent, and figure-eight. They are often used in different combinations to bandage different parts of the body.

Spiral turns are used to bandage a part of the body that has about the same circumference throughout, for example, the upper arm or part of the leg. The turns are made at a slight angle, about 30°, and each turn overlaps the preceding one by two-thirds the width of the bandage. See Figure 40–12.

Circular turns are used chiefly to anchor a bandage or to terminate it. They are also used to cover a cylindrical part of the body such as the proximal aspect of the fifth finger. The bandage is wrapped around the body part so that each turn exactly covers the previous turn. See Figure 40–13. Two circular turns are used to anchor and complete a bandage. These are usually not applied directly over a wound because of the discomfort they may cause.

Spiral reverse turns are used to bandage cylindrical body parts that are not of uniform circumference, for example, the lower leg of a muscular person. To make a spiral reverse, bring the bandage upward at a 30° angle, then place the thumb of the free hand on the upper edge of the bandage. Unroll the bandage about 14 cm (6 in), and pronate the hand holding the roll, so that the bandage folds over on itself and continues around the limb. Successive spiral reverses are made at the same point in the turn, each overlapping the previous turn by two-thirds the width of the bandage and at the same angle. See Figure 40–14.

Recurrent turns are used to cover the distal portions of the body such as the hand, the finger, or the stump after an amputation. The bandage is first anchored by two circular turns around the proximal body part, and then the bandage is folded back on itself and brought centrally over the distal end to be covered. Next it is taken to

Figure 40–14 A spiral reverse bandage.

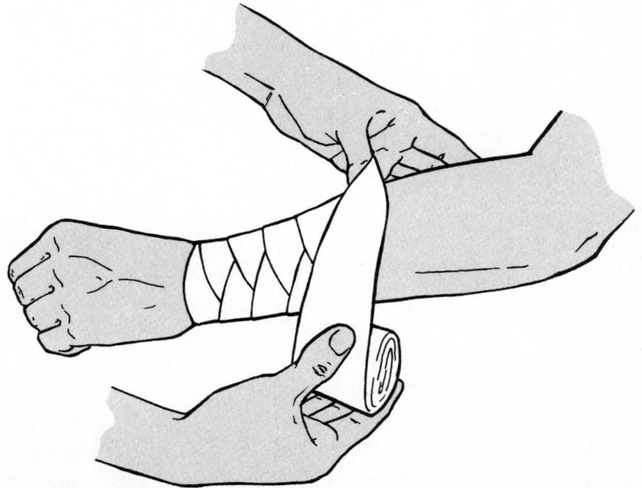

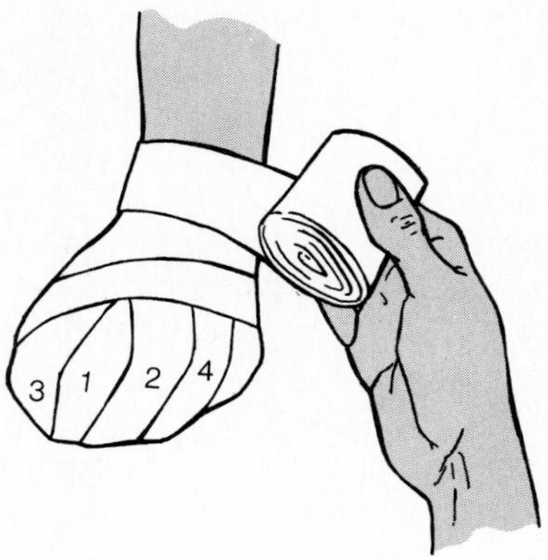

Figure 40–15 A recurrent bandage.

the inferior aspect, where it is held with the other hand and brought back over the end but this time to the right of the center bandage, overlapping one-third the width of the bandage. The roll then is brought back to the left of the center bandage. This pattern of alternate right and left is continued, overlapping all but the first turn by two-thirds the width of the bandage. The bandage is finally secured by two circular turns, which gather in the folded edges of the bandage. See Figure 40–15.

Figure-eight turns are usually used to bandage an elbow, a knee, or an ankle. The bandage is anchored with two circular turns over the center of the joint. Then the bandage is carried above the joint, around it, and below the joint, making figure-eight turns. Each turn works upward and downward from the joint by overlapping the previous turn by two-thirds the width of the bandage. It is anchored by two circular turns above the joint. See Figure 40–16.

In addition to these basic turns, which are used to bandage most areas of the body, there are special bandages for various parts of the body such as skull, ear, and eye bandages.

Intervention: Applying Binders

Common types of binders

There are five commonly used types of binders: the triangular binder (sling), breast binder, scultetus (many-tailed) binder, T-binder (single or double), and abdominal binder.

Triangular binder (sling) The triangular binder is usually made of muslin. It can be applied in a number of ways, but it is usually applied as a full triangle to make a large arm sling that supports the arm, elbow, and forearm. See Figure 40–17.

To make a large arm sling:

1. Place one end of the unfolded triangle over the shoulder of the uninjured side.
2. The binder falls down the front of the patient with the point directed toward the elbow of the injured side.
3. Take the upper corner and carry it around the patient's neck until it hangs over the shoulder on the injured side.
4. Assist the patient to flex the elbow with the thumb upward until the lower arm is at right angles to the upper arm and in front of the binder.
5. Take the lower corner of the binder and bring it up over the arm to the shoulder of the injured side. The tips of the fingers should be visible.
6. Secure this corner to the other end with a reef knot.
7. Bring the point of the bandage at the elbow forward, and secure it neatly with safety pins or adhesive tape if safety pins are contraindicated for any reason.

Figure 40–26 A figure-eight bandage.

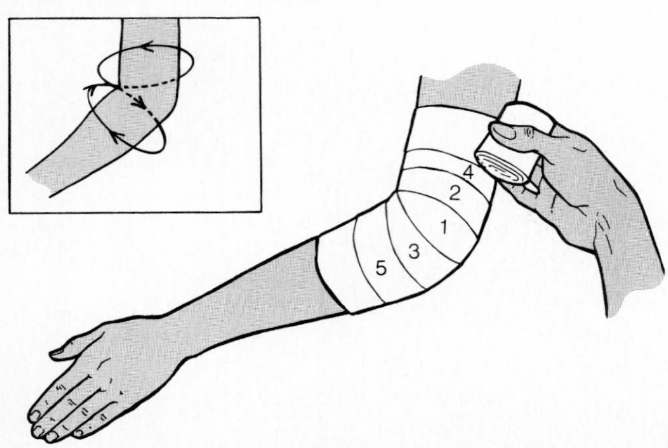

Figure 40–17 A large arm sling.

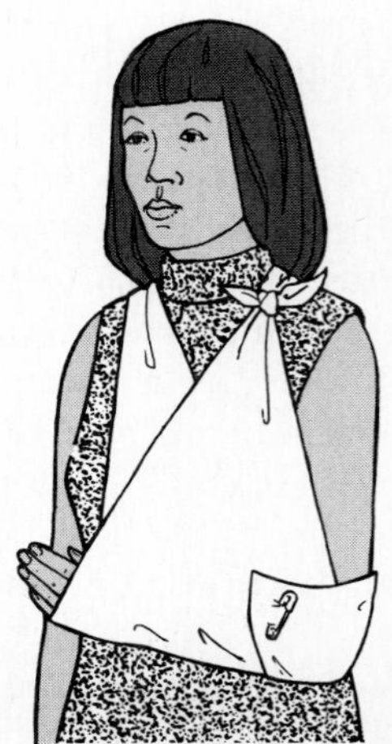

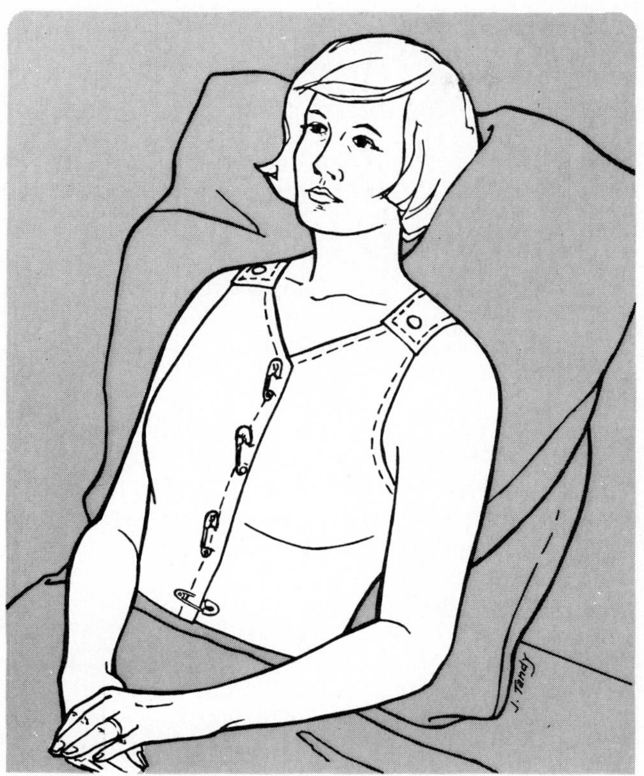

Figure 40–18 A breast binder.

Breast binder Breast binders are used to apply pressure to breasts, for example, when drying up the breasts after childbirth, or to support the breasts, for example, after surgery. In some situations a towel can be used as a breast binder.

The breasts are supported in their normal position, preferably when the patient is sitting. The binder is pinned in front while the patient supports her breasts. The first pin is placed at the nipple line and the next pins are placed alternately above and below the first pin. The lowest pin is placed horizontally so that it will not press into the patient's waist when she bends. The shoulder straps are then fastened. See Figure 40–18.

Scultetus (many-tailed) binder The scultetus binder is used to provide support to the abdomen and, in some instances, to retain dressings. It is usually made of flannel or cotton. The center of the binder is placed under the patient so that the lower edge is at the gluteal fold (over the buttocks). The tails are then brought over to the center of the abdomen from alternate sides, starting at the bottom. See Figure 40–19. Each tail overlaps the preceding one by about half the width of the tail. In thin people the ends of the tails may extend beyond the other side and have to be folded back. The last tail is secured with a safety pin or adhesive tape.

T-binder (single or double) T-binders are usually made of cotton fabric and are used to retain perineal dressings. The bar (top) of the T goes around the patient's waist. The stem of the T passes between the patient's legs, from posterior to anterior. In the *single T-binder*, also referred to as the *female T-binder*, the stem is brought upward and attached to the waistband. The *double T-binder* has two tails, that is, the stem of the T is split into two, for male patients. The two tails are brought up on either side of the penis to the waistband. See Figure 40–20. Double T-binders may be used for female patients if greater support to the perineum is required.

Abdominal binder The abdominal binder is a rectangular piece of cotton that is long enough to encircle a patient's abdomen and overlap about 5 to 7.5 cm (2 to 3 in) for an adult or 2.5 cm (1 in) for an infant. It should be wide enough to reach from the gluteal fold to the patient's waist. It is pinned down the center of the overlap securely and then molded to the patient's body by pinning on the lateral aspects.

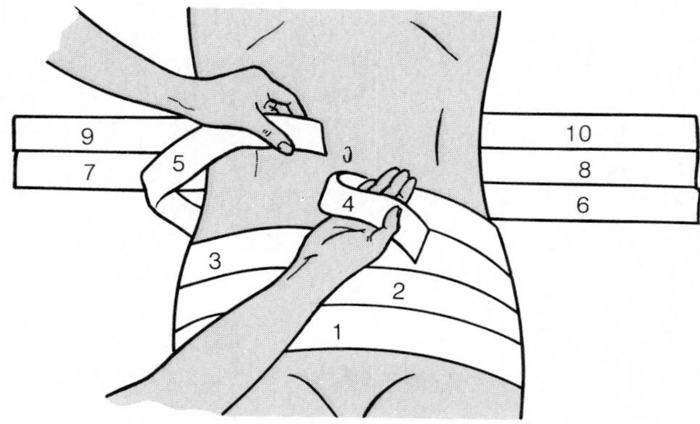

Figure 40–19 A scultetus binder.

Figure 40–20 T-binders: **A,** single; **B,** double.

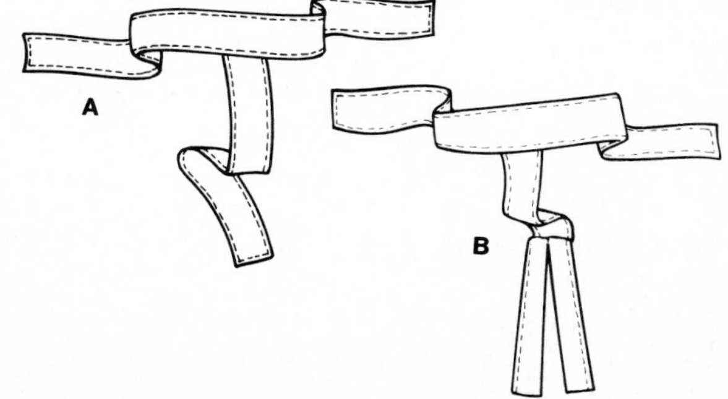

Heat and Cold Therapy

Both heat and cold are applied to the body to support processes involved in the repair and healing of tissues. Hot and cold applications can be applied in either dry or moist forms. The form of choice generally depends upon the exact purpose of the application and the type of wound. For example, an open wound usually indicates the need for sterile, moist compresses or dry heat by radiation to maintain the sterility of the area. Heat to a closed wound is generally applied by a hot pack (hot moist) or an electric pad (hot dry).

A hot application adds heat to a body part; a cold application withdraws heat from the part. Heat is transferred by the processes of conduction, convection, and radiation. *Conduction* means the transfer of heat by molecular interaction; it implies contact between the source of the heat and the body part. An example would be application of a hot water bottle to an abdomen. A substance that inhibits conduction is known as an *insulator*. *Convection* is the transfer of heat by movement of a liquid or gas. An example of transfer by convection is the sitz bath in which the water continues to run. *Radiation* is the transfer of heat in the form of electromagnetic waves through the air. An example of heat applied in this manner is the ultraviolet lamp.

Heat applications are usually classified as radiant, conductive, or conversive. The infrared part of the electromagnetic spectrum produces *radiant heat*; the infrared lamp produces such heat. Penetration of infrared rays is from 1 to 3 mm, depending on whether the wavelengths are near or far. Near wavelengths are 7700–14,000 angstroms (Å), and far wavelengths are 14,000–120,000 Å. (The angstrom is a unit of wavelength of electromagnetic radiation.) Near infrared radiation penetrates about 3 mm and far infrared about 1 mm. Luminous bulbs produce more near infrared radiation and thus have greater penetration than nonluminous filaments, which also produce far infrared radiation.

Conductive heat is provided by the direct application of heat, such as a hot water bag or heated air applied to the body. This heat is relatively superficial; it penetrates 1 to 2 mm and it requires about 20 to 30 minutes to produce the desired effect.

Conversive heat involves the conversion of another form of energy to heat. An example is medical diathermy, where an electric current is used to provide heat to deep tissues. With this method, the resistance of the tissues to the electric current causes the production of heat.

Because heat is often supplied by electrically operated equipment, it is important for nurses to understand some of the properties of electricity and its dangers. For information about electricity, see Chapter 22, page 544.

Physiologic Responses to Heat and Cold

Heat and cold have different effects on the body (see Table 40–1), and their effects vary with the duration of the application.

External heat of short duration

An application of heat of short duration (15 to 30 minutes) has the following effects:

1. Increased temperature of the tissues
2. Vasodilation
3. Increased capillary blood pressure
4. Increased amount of capillary surface available for exchange of fluids and electrolytes, because the capillaries are relaxed
5. Decreased blood viscosity
6. Increased tissue metabolism
7. Sedation with relief of pain and muscle tension

Increasing the temperature of the tissues increases the metabolic activity of the cells involved, and this adds to temperature increase and vasodilation, as more blood flows to the skin. Some of this heat is conducted to underlying tissues. Excessive heat is carried to other body parts by blood flow.

Vasodilation results in a reddening and warming of

Table 40–1 Effects of Hot and Cold Applications

Hot applications	Cold applications
Arteriole vasodilation (reddened skin)	Arteriole vasoconstriction (pale bluish skin)
Decreased stroke volume*	Increased stroke volume*
Increased respiratory rate	Decreased respiratory rate
Increased temperature of local tissues	Decreased temperature of local tissues
Increased amount of capillary surface	Decreased amount of capillary surface
Decreased blood viscosity	Increased blood viscosity
Increased tissue metabolism	Decreased tissue metabolism
Increased capillary blood pressure	Decreased capillary blood pressure
Muscular relaxation	Muscular contraction
Increased number of leukocytes and inflammation	Reduced inflammation

*Stroke volume is the volume of blood ejected from the ventricle of the heart with each contraction.

the skin. The blood flows to the area, which becomes *hyperemic* (has excessive blood). The increase in blood volume facilitates the exchange of nutrients and waste products between the tissues and the blood. The increase in capillary blood pressure also facilitates the movement of nutrients and oxygen from the arterial blood to the tissues. Because the capillaries relax, the surface area of the capillary bed increases, thus increasing the exchange of nutrients and wastes.

When the capillaries of the skin are fully distended, they are capable of holding one-half to two-thirds of the total blood volume. For this reason a person who gets in a hot bath can faint, since dilation of the blood vessels in the skin decreases peripheral resistance, decreases arterial pressure, and thus decreases blood flow to the brain.

The analgesic effects of heat are thought to be due to the equalization of temperature from superficial to deep tissues, but the exact mechanism is not known.

External heat of long duration

Prolonged application of heat to an area decreases the blood flow to the area. This usually occurs after 1 hour of application. Removing the heat for 15 to 30 minutes and then reapplying it reestablishes vasodilation. See page 1053.

Extreme heat

Application of extreme heat has the following effects:

1. Cell metabolism is increased more than the local circulation.
2. Surface arterioles tend to constrict.
3. Muscles tend to remain tense and fail to relax.
4. Cells can be damaged and blisters appear.

External cold of short duration

Application of cold to an area has varying effects, depending on the degree of cold and the length of the application. Cold applications of short duration usually have these effects:

1. Vasoconstriction
2. Increased venous congestion
3. Decreased local tissue metabolism
4. Contraction of the arrector pili muscles
5. Decreasing sensitivity, with a numbing sensation

Vasoconstriction is the first obvious sign after the application of cold. The arterioles of the circulatory system constrict, decreasing the blood supply to the affected part (ischemia). Vasoconstriction results in skin pallor and coolness that can be assessed by touch. The slower circulation and the constriction of the blood vessels result in increased venous congestion, which can be observed from the bluish appearance of the skin. This venous congestion also reduces the amount of fluid entering the tissues, thereby reducing *edema* (accumulation of fluid in the tissues). The decrease in blood flow means that less oxygen and fewer nutrients are available to the tissue cells, which results in decreased tissue metabolism. For this reason, prolonged exposure to cold can result in cell deprivation and subsequent damage.

When cold is applied, particularly over a large area, the body reacts by contracting the arrector pili muscles. This is a normal body response to produce heat by muscle contraction. It can be seen as gooseflesh on the patient.

Another important effect of a cold application is the decreasing sensitivity of the tissues, leading to numbness of the area. This effect is evident when handling snow with the bare hands.

External cold of long duration

It is generally considered unsafe to employ cold applications that would produce skin temperatures below 4.4 C (40 F) for any length of time. The one exception to this general rule is the use of cold in anesthesia.

Cold for a prolonged period can interfere with circulation, healing, cell function, and cell resistance to a point where permanent damage to the tissues results. Prolonged exposure to cold results in vasodilation, as opposed to vasoconstriction. This explains the ruddiness of the skin of a person who has been for a walk in the cold weather.

The symptoms of damaged tissues due to cold are a bluish-purplish mottled appearance of the skin, numbness, stiffness, pallor, and sometimes blisters and pain.

Extreme cold

Extreme cold can damage the cells in the area. The fluid in the tissues can freeze, forming crystals, and the cells can die as a result of the lowered temperature and the lack of oxygen and nourishment.

Perception of Heat and Cold

The skin is well supplied with nerves, blood vessels, and lymph vessels. The temperature receptors in the skin are sensitive to temperatures that are either greater or lesser than that of the skin surface itself, which is 33.9 C (93.0 F). With repeated exposure to either heat or cold, the receptors become less sensitive. Therefore a person can inadvertently damage tissues by not taking adequate precautions during hot and cold applications. For example, a patient who is soaking a hand repeatedly in hot water at home would be wise to take the temperature of the water before putting the hand in it.

Heat and cold are perceived as very cold, cold, cool, tepid, warm, hot, and very hot. The pain receptors are stimulated by extremes in temperature: 45 C (113 F) and above or 15 C (59 F) and below. A person perceives the temperature of hot or cold applications most when the temperature of the skin is changing. That is why a hot water hand soak will feel hottest when the hand is first immersed, not later. Temperatures that are 8.3 C (15.0 F) above the skin temperature and 11.1 C (20.0 F) below the skin temperature stimulate the temperature receptors in the skin. Temperatures around the temperature of the skin—between 33 and 34 C (91.4 and 93.2 F)—are normally undifferentiated. In elderly persons there is decreased sensitivity to localized temperature changes, such as those from hot or cold applications.

Thermal changes are picked up by at least three types of receptors: cold receptors; warmth receptors; and cold pain and warm pain receptors. Both cold and warmth receptors lie close to the surface of the skin. The cold receptors are more plentiful than the warmth receptors, and both vary in density on different parts of the body. For example, there are more cold receptors on the forehead, making it more responsive to cold than to heat. Thermal signals are picked up by the heat or cold receptors and transmitted along the sensory nerves to the central nervous system. The impulses then travel by the lateral spinothalamic tract to the thalamus and to the reticular areas of the brain stem. Some stimuli continue to the somatesthetic cortex and others to the cerebral cortex. As a result of the impulses in the cerebral cortex, the person becomes aware of the sensation of heat or cold.

Tolerance to Heat and Cold

The physiologic tolerance of the body to heat and cold varies according to the following factors:

1. *Part of the body.* The back of the hand is not very sensitive to temperatures, while the inner aspect of the wrist is sensitive.
2. *Size of the part of the body exposed* to the heat or cold. The larger the area exposed, the less the tolerance.
3. *Tolerance of the individual,* which is affected to some degree by age and the condition of the skin, the nervous system, and the circulatory system. The very young and the very old generally have the least tolerance.
4. *Length of exposure* to heat or cold. People feel hot and cold applications most while the skin temperature is changing. After a period of time, tolerance is improved.

See Table 40–2 for recommended temperatures for hot and cold applications.

Heat Applications

Reasons for applying heat

Heat can be applied in a dry form, such as a heating pad, or a moist form, such as a hot compress. Heat is applied for its local effect or its systemic effect. A local effect is one in which the action is confined to a specific area of the body, for example, a finger or a wound. A systemic effect is one in which the body as a whole reacts to the heat; for example, a hot bath warms the entire body. Heat is applied for any of several reasons discussed in the sections that follow.

To relieve muscle spasm Contraction of muscles can be painful, as many people know when they get a "charley horse" in a leg or a wry neck. The application of heat to the area for a short time can relax the muscle that is in spasm and thus dissipate the pain. The underlying mechanism is unknown.

Table 40–2 Recommended Temperatures for Hot and Cold Applications

Description	Centigrade	Fahrenheit	Application
Very cold	Below 15	Below 59	Ice bags
Cold	15–18	59–65	Cold pack
Cool	18–27	65–80	Cold compress
Tepid	27–37	80–98	Alcohol and tepid sponges
Warm	37–40	98–105	Warm bath
Hot	40–46	105–115	Aquathermia, soaks, sitz baths, irrigations, moist sterile compresses, hot water bags for debilitated or young
Very hot	Above 46	Above 115	Hot water bags for adults, heat cradles

To soften exudates When an exudate, produced by the inflammatory response of body tissues, dries, it hardens and can form a crust that adheres to the skin, mucous membrane, or wound. Moist heat in the form of a hot compress softens the exudate, permitting it to be removed.

To hasten the suppuration process When heat is applied to an infected area, the increased circulation brings additional defenders against infection, that is, leukocytes (white blood cells), and takes away toxins that have been produced. The pus that is formed from these elements will consolidate in an area and may subsequently be absorbed into the circulation or drain to the outside of the body. If localization does not occur, the microorganisms may spread to other cells, causing cellulitis; they may be absorbed into the lymphatic system through the tissue fluid and cause an inflammatory process of the lymph vessels (lymphangitis); or they may reach the lymph nodes, where they may either be destroyed or cause a localized inflammation, such as tonsillitis or lymphadenitis.

To hasten healing Heat applied to the body causes vasodilation of the arterioles in the area, which remain dilated. This results in an increased blood supply to the area, bringing additional nutrients for the tissue healing. The arterioles remain dilated for about an hour, after which vasoconstriction takes place. If the heat is removed for 15 to 30 minutes, it can be reapplied and will again cause vasodilation. This is why hot compresses are sometimes alternated with cold compresses.

To warm a part of the body Heat (often dry heat) is applied to warm a particularly cold part of the body. For example, a man with a leg cast may find that his foot is cold because of lack of exercise and the fact that he cannot wear a sock and shoe. A hot water bottle will warm the foot and provide comfort to the patient. The nurse needs to make sure that the coldness of an extremity is not due to impaired circulation. If it is, this is reported immediately for corrective measures.

To reduce congestion in an underlying organ Heat increases blood circulation to the surface on which the heat is applied, redirecting the blood from deeper congested areas. The heat itself penetrates no more than about 2 mm, but a reflex action is set up. The heat acts much like an irritant, stimulating the cutaneous nerve endings, and the stimuli are carried to the spinal cord by the sensory fibers. From there the impulses enter the sympathetic nervous system and go to the internal organs. Thus the blood is redirected away from the organ to the body surface.

To reduce pressure from accumulated fluid The removal of accumulated fluid in a tissue or joint can be facilitated by heat. The heat increases the supply of blood to the area, and the capillaries are available for absorption of fluid. Hence, accumulated fluid is more easily absorbed into the circulation from the tissues.

To increase peristalsis A hot drink or hot food increases the strength of peristaltic waves. This increase in peristalsis can be used to assist patients to establish regular defecation habits. After hot cereal and coffee at breakfast, a patient can learn to use the resulting peristaltic waves for defecation.

To provide comfort and relaxation Heat applied to the body is comforting and relaxing to many people. A warm tub bath relaxes the skeletal muscles and is often used to promote sleep. It is important to remember that very hot applications, that is, those above 46.1 C (115.0 F), produce a reaction similar to cold applications. The superficial blood vessels tend to constrict rather than relax, and the muscles fail to relax.

Factors affecting applications of heat

The following factors affect the use of heat applications to a body area and the degree of heat to be applied:

1. *Size of the body area.* The greater the area of the body, the lower the temperature of the application should be.
2. *Use of moist or dry heat.* Moist heat penetrates better than dry heat. Therefore moist applications of heat do not require as high a temperature as dry applications.
3. *Individual tolerance.* There is wide variation in the degree of tolerance of heat among individuals.
4. *Particular skin area involved.* In any individual, tolerances vary depending on the number of heat receptors present in the body part.
5. *Age and condition of the patient.* Heat is less well tolerated by the very young, the elderly, and people with circulatory problems.

Cold Applications

Reasons for applying cold

Cold can be applied in either moist or dry form. It is used for both systemic and local purposes. Systemically, cold is applied to lower the body's metabolic rate in preparation for certain types of surgery and to lower the body's temperature when it is persistently elevated. Locally, cold is applied for any of the reasons described in the following sections.

To decrease and terminate bleeding Cold constricts the arterioles and increases the viscosity of the blood. It therefore can act to control bleeding and to prevent a hemorrhage.

To anesthetize and reduce pain Cold applications decrease the sensitivity of tissues and create a sensation of numbness. Thus cold can be used as a local anesthetic for a short period of time. This is important to remember when applying cold—because of the numbness, the patient may be unaware that tissues are being damaged.

To reduce inflammation Cold reduces the inflammatory process and slows the suppurative process by causing vasoconstriction and decreasing local tissue metabolism.

To control the accumulation of fluid Because cold constricts the arterioles, fluid accumulation in body tissues is delayed. Therefore cold is applied to prevent swelling due to sprains or tissue trauma.

Factors affecting cold applications

The temperature used for cold applications depends on the purpose of the application, the size of the area to which it is to be applied, and the length of time of the treatment. See Table 40–2. The following factors affect the use of cold applications and the degree of cold to be applied:

1. *Size of the body area.* The greater the area of the body, the higher the temperature of the cold application should be.
2. *Use of moist or dry cold.* Moist cold penetrates better than dry cold; therefore moist applications do not require as low a temperature as dry applications.
3. *Age and condition of the patient.* Elderly patients and people with impaired circulation tolerate cold less well than younger people with good circulation.

Assessing the Patient

Before applying heat

The following clinical signs usually contraindicate the application of heat:

1. *Vasodilation of the area.* Heat will increase the patient's discomfort by increasing the blood circulation (e.g., to a swollen joint) or by increasing the expansion of gases (e.g., in an infected tooth).
2. *Headache.* Vasodilation of the vessels inside the cranium will increase this discomfort.
3. *An inflammatory process such as appendicitis.* The increased blood supply could increase the inflammation and cause the appendix to rupture.
4. *Any possibility of hemorrhage.* Vasodilation will increase bleeding.

Prior to the heat application, the area should be inspected for redness, abrasions, swelling, or bleeding. The nurse also determines whether the patient is experiencing any discomfort.

It is important to assess the patient's capacity to recognize when heat is injurious. Some patients are unable to perceive that heat is damaging the tissues. The nurse also assesses whether the patient is fully conscious or physically debilitated. Patients who are very young, elderly, unconscious, or debilitated often tolerate heat poorly. The body area to which the heat will be applied needs to be assessed for impaired blood circulation. Clinical signs of impairment are numbness or tingling, coolness to the touch, and cyanosis. Areas of poor blood circulation are less tolerant of heat.

If drainage is present, it should be observed for amount, color, and character. The wound and the area around it are assessed for redness, swelling, and discomfort.

Prior to a sitz bath or application of hot compresses to large body areas, the patient's pulse, respirations, and blood pressure are assessed to provide baseline data against which to compare later assessments.

Before applying cold

Nurses need to be aware of symptoms that can contraindicate cold applications. When any of these are observed, they need to be reported:

1. A bluish, purplish appearance to the skin or mucous membrane
2. A cold feeling to the skin or mucous membrane
3. A feeling of numbness
4. Pain due to contracted muscles
5. Shivering and a lowered body temperature

Prior to any cold application, the area is assessed for circulatory deficiencies and decreased sensation. The patient's discomfort is also determined, including any swelling or bleeding.

Prior to a cooling sponge bath, the patient's body temperature, pulse, and respirations are assessed. These provide baseline data against which to compare future assessments. The nurse also watches for signs of a fever, e.g., skin warmth, flushing, complaints of heat or chilling, diaphoresis, irritability, restlessness, general malaise, or delirium.

Before the application of cold moist compresses or packs, any wound is assessed. See the preceding section's discussion of assessing a wound.

Intervention: Applying Heat

Moist heat

Moist applications of heat have the following advantages over dry applications:

1. They soften crusts and exudates.
2. They penetrate more deeply than dry heat.
3. They do not dry the skin.
4. They tend to have a more localized effect, thereby reducing the amount of body fluid that can be lost through diaphoresis.

Sitz baths A sitz bath, or hip bath, is intended to supply moist heat to the patient's pelvic area. The patient is usually immersed from the midthighs to the iliac crests. The temperature of the water should be from 40 to 43 C (105 to 110 F), unless otherwise ordered by the physician, or unless the patient is unable to tolerate the heat. If the purpose of the bath is to assist the patient to relax, the temperature is usually 36.1 to 37.7 C (97 to 100 F). The duration of the bath is generally 15 to 20 minutes, depending on the patient's condition.

Special tubs and chairs, as well as disposable basins, are available for sitz baths. The latter are often used in the home. See Figure 40–21. These tubs are preferable to a regular bathtub, because the patient sitting in a bathtub usually immerses the entire leg in the hot water, and thus the circulation is not directed exclusively to the perineum or pelvic area.

The patient having a sitz bath needs to take care not to place undue pressure on any body part, such as the sacrum or the posterior aspects of the thighs. A stool for the patient's feet can often support the legs, preventing pressure on the thighs. (Some sitz baths are installed at floor level, thus negating the need for a footstool.) Precautions also need to be taken to prevent chilling, burning, or fainting. Often a bath blanket over the patient's shoulders and measures to eliminate drafts during the bath will prevent chilling. Maintaining the temperature of the bath is important. The water should be tested every 10 minutes and hot water added as necessary, taking care to prevent burning the patient. Sometimes patients feel faint and dizzy during a sitz bath. This is particularly true when patients have just had surgery or when the water temperature is above 43 C (109 F). A cold cloth on the back of the patient's neck will often prevent fainting; however, close observation is necessary, and the bath should be terminated if the feeling of faintness persists.

Before taking sitz baths, patients should understand that they are not to touch any wound areas and that they are to signal for a nurse if they feel weak. After rectal surgery, patients need to take a sitz bath after each defecation. Sitz baths may feel uncomfortable initially; however, after 3 to 5 minutes, most patients find them comforting.

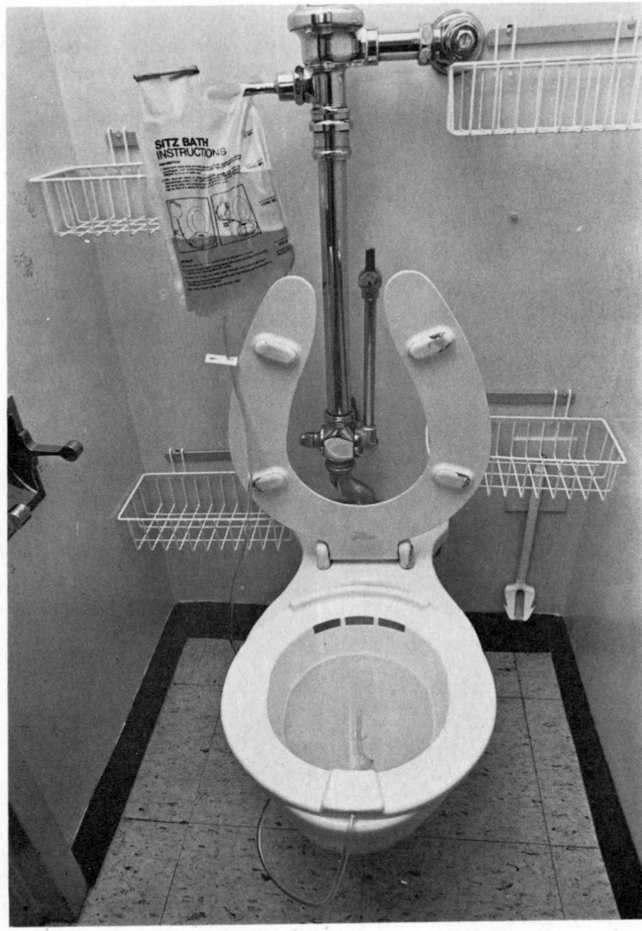

Figure 40–21 A sitz bath used in a hospital.

The nurse makes the following assessments during the bath:

1. Color of the patient's face. Extreme pallor may precede fainting or vomiting.
2. Pulse rate. An accelerated pulse rate may precede fainting.
3. Sensation of faintness, nausea, or extreme pain.
4. Temperature of the water.
5. Appearance of the perineal area.

Hot soaks A soak refers to either immersion of a body part, for example, an arm (see Figure 40–22), in a solution, or the wrapping of a part in gauze dressings that are then saturated with a solution. Soaks may employ either clean technique or sterile technique. The latter is indicated for open wounds, such as a burn or an incision. Dry dressings are usually applied between the soaks.

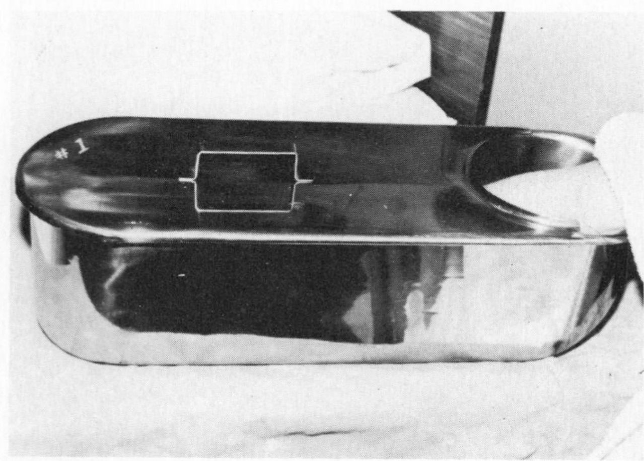

Figure 40–22 An arm soak.

Soaks are usually indicated for the following reasons:

1. To apply heat, thus hastening suppuration and softening exudates
2. To apply medications
3. To clean areas such as wounds in which there is sloughing tissue

The physician's order usually specifies the site for the soak, the type of solution, the temperature of the solution, the length of time for the soak, the frequency, and the purpose. Whether sterile technique is indicated is usually a nursing judgment; if there is a break in the skin, sterile technique is indicated.

The equipment required for a soak is:

1. The specified solution. If a temperature is not ordered, 40.5 to 43.3 C (105 to 110 F) is usually indicated.
2. The container, such as a basin or special arm bath. This should be sterile if there is a break in the skin.
3. A thermometer to test the solution temperature.
4. Towels to support the limb and dry the part after the soak.
5. A sterile drape if sterile technique is used, to cover the part and the solution during the soak.
6. Gauze, if indicated for the soak.

The nurse removes and discards any dressings on the area. After the temperature of the solution has been checked, the part is slowly immersed in the solution. It it is a sterile soak, the affected part is covered with a sterile drape. Ideally the temperature of the solution should be checked every 5 minutes, and solution added or replaced to maintain the appropriate temperature. Normally a soak lasts 15 to 20 minutes. Therefore the patient requires support in a comfortable position to avoid muscle strain. For example, if a hand is to be soaked, the arm can be supported by a pillow.

The nurse makes the following assessments during the soak:

1. Appearance of the area being soaked. Some erythema (redness) is to be expected from the heat of the solution.
2. Pain in the area.
3. Any untoward reactions, such as numbness in the area.

Compresses and moist packs A *compress* is a moist gauze dressing that is applied frequently to an open wound. Sometimes compresses are ordered to be hot, in which case the solution is heated to the temperature ordered by the physician, such as 40.5 C (105 F). Compresses are usually applied using sterile technique when there is a break in the skin; therefore sterile gloves or sterile forceps are needed for their application. A *hot pack (foment)* is a hot moist cloth applied to an area of the body. Frequently wool flannel is used because it holds heat well. Hot packs and hot compresses may be sterile or unsterile and after application are covered with a water resistant material (e.g., Saran Wrap or plastic) to contain the moisture and prevent the transfer of airborne microorganisms to the area.

After a compress or a hot pack has been applied, it is advisable to apply external heat, such as a hot water bottle or heating pad, to help maintain the heat of the application.

The following equipment is required for a moist compress:

1. A container for the solution
2. Solution at the strength and temperature specified by the physician or the agency
3. A thermometer to test the temperature of the solution
4. Gauze squares to soak with the solution and apply to the patient
5. Plastic to insulate the compress, to retain the heat and moisture
6. An insulating towel to help maintain the temperature of the compress
7. A hot water bottle or heating pad (optional) to maintain the heat of the compress
8. Ties, e.g., roller gauze, to fasten the compress in place

For a sterile compress, the container, solution, thermometer, gauze squares, and towel must be sterile. In addition, sterile forceps or sterile gloves are required to maintain the sterility of the gauze when it is wrung out and applied. If a sterile thermometer is not available, the nurse pours a small amount of the solution into a clean basin, measures the temperature with a bath thermometer, and then discards the solution, since it is no longer sterile. The temperature of the rest of the solution is adjusted according to the findings.

The hot compress is prepared by soaking the gauze in the solution. If there is a dressing on the wound, it is removed. The gauze is then wrung out so that it does not drip. For sterile compresses, sterile forceps or sterile gloves are used.

The gauze is then applied to the designated area and molded closely to the body. This improves the transfer of heat because air is a poor conductor of heat or cold. The gauze is then covered with the plastic and the insulating towel to retain the heat and moisture. A hot water bottle or commercial hot pack may be applied over the towel to help retain the heat. It may be necessary to hold the compress in place with ties.

For additional information about hot compresses and moist packs, see Kozier and Erb (1982:967–71).

Dry heat

Dry heat is frequently applied to the body for one or more of the following reasons:

1. To provide comfort
2. To dry the skin or a newly applied plaster of Paris cast
3. To increase blood circulation to an area, such as a decubitus ulcer

Hot water bottles (bags) Hot water bottles, sometimes referred to as *hot water bags*, are frequently used as a source of dry heat in the home. They are being used less often in hospitals because burns can result from their injudicious use. The following temperatures of the water in the bags are considered safe in most situations and provide the desired effect:

Normal adult, 51.6 C (125 F)

Debilitated or unconscious adult, 40.5 to 46.1 C (105 to 115 F)

Child under 2 years, 40.5 to 46.1 C (105 to 115 F)

Agencies that use hot water bags and heating pads may require the patient to sign a release that absolves the agency and its employees from responsibility for any injury incurred in their use.

Hot water bags are usually filled about two-thirds full. The remaining air is expelled and the top secured. The hot water bag is then light and can be readily molded to a body part. Before application, the bag is dried and held upside down to test for leakage. If it is secure, it is then wrapped in a towel or cover and placed on the body site.

Commercial hot packs Dry heat can be supplied by commercially prepared disposable hot packs. See Figure 40–23. Directions on the package tell the nurse how to initiate the heating process. They provide a specified amount of heat for a specified time.

Electric pads Electric pads and blankets have become increasingly popular in recent years. They have the advantage of providing a constant, even heat and of being light and easily molded to a body part. Some electric pads have waterproof covers, and these are highly desirable in situations where moisture is present. Heating pads used in agencies are frequently set to a specific temperature, while those found in homes usually have a more general control to adjust the temperature.

When using electric pads, caution needs to be taken not to insert pins into the pad. A pin can touch a wire inside the pad, damaging the pad and causing a shock to the person holding the pin.

Aquathermia (water-flow) pads The aquathermia or aquamatic pad is a device in which warm distilled water circulates, providing heat to a body part. The pad is attached to a unit run by electricity. The reservoir of the pad is filled two-thirds full, and air bubbles are removed. The desired temperature is set, the pad is covered, and it is placed on the body part. Normal temperature is 40.5 C (105 F), and the treatment is usually continued for 10 to 15 minutes. If unusual redness or pain occurs, the treatment is discontinued and the patient's reaction reported and recorded.

Heat lamps Heat lamps are used to apply dry heat, usually to a small body area with an open wound. They are also used to promote healing of decubitus ulcers.

Figure 40–23 Commercially prepared disposable hot packs.

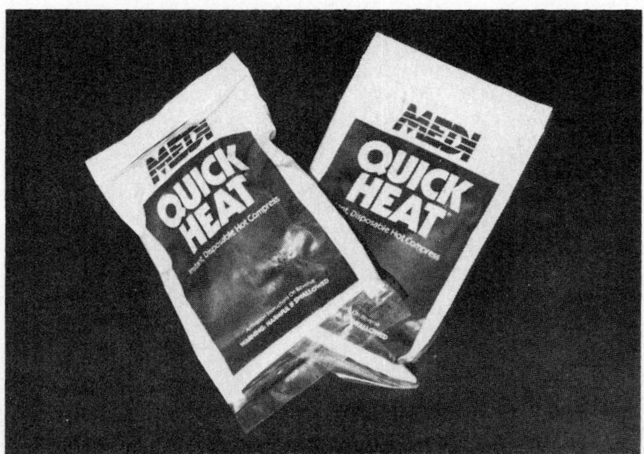

Two types of heat lamps are commonly used: the gooseneck lamp with a 60-watt bulb and the infrared lamp. Two sizes of infrared lamps are commonly available, large and small. Gooseneck and infrared lamps are similar in their use and their action.

Infrared rays penetrate no more than 3 mm of body tissue, and thus they provide heat chiefly to the surface of the skin or mucous membranes. Before a heat lamp is used, the area to be heated should be cleaned and dried. This lessens the likelihood of burning. A heat lamp with a 60-watt bulb or a small infrared lamp is usually placed 45 to 60 cm (18 to 24 in) from the patient. A large infrared lamp is placed 60 to 75 cm (24 to 30 in) away. The treatment usually lasts 15 to 20 minutes, provided the patient is tolerating the heat. The patient should be checked after 5 minutes for discomfort, burning, or any untoward reaction. It is important to caution the patient not to touch the infrared lamp, and the lamp should not be draped or placed under any bedclothes because of the chance of starting a fire. At the first sign of skin redness or discomfort, the treatment should be terminated and the reaction reported and recorded.

Heat cradles Heat cradles are used to provide dry heat to an area, usually to large body areas such as the abdomen, legs, or chest. Heat cradles are made of metal and contain a single bulb or a series of bulbs, often 25 watts each. The cradle is placed over the patient and usually covered with a bath blanket or sheet. The temperature inside the cradle normally should not exceed 51.6 C (125 F), and the treatment normally lasts 10 to 15 minutes. The heat source inside the cradle should be 45 to 60 cm (18 to 24 in) away from the patient.

Intervention: Applying Cold

Moist cold

Moist cold is commonly applied by a cooling sponge bath or by cold moist compresses. The latter are frequently used in a sterile form over open wounds.

Cooling sponge baths The cooling sponge bath uses water or a combination of alcohol and water that is below body temperature. Alcohol evaporates at a low temperature and therefore removes body heat rapidly. However alcohol-and-water sponge baths are less frequently used now than in the past, because alcohol has a drying effect on the skin. The temperatures for cooling sponge baths range from 18 to 32 C (65 to 90 F). A tepid sponge bath generally means one in which the water temperature is 32 C (90 F) throughout the bath. For a cool sponge bath, the water temperature is 32 C (90 F) at the beginning of the bath and is gradually lowered to 18 C (65 F) by adding ice chips during the bath.

The following equipment is needed:

1. A basin for the solution.
2. A bath thermometer to check the temperature of the solution.
3. Solution at the correct temperature. Water or equal portions of 70% alcohol and water are used.
4. Ice chips for a cool sponge bath.
5. Several washcloths and bath towels, or a few washcloths and towels plus several ice bags.
6. A bath blanket.
7. A thermometer to measure the patient's temperature.
8. A fan (optional) to increase air movement around the patient, which lowers the body temperature through convection. If this is used, measures to eliminate drafts during the sponge bath are not taken.

Initially the patient's temperature, pulse, and respirations are assessed and recorded. If the sponge bath is effective, these vital signs should change when taken after the bath (for example, temperature will be reduced).

The nurse provides privacy and covers the patient with the bath blanket. First the patient's face is sponged with plain water and dried. An ice bag may be applied to the patient's head to reduce blood flow. Ice bags or wet washcloths are placed in each axilla and groin, because these areas contain large superficial blood vessels, which help to transfer heat. If washcloths are used, the bed needs to be protected with towels. The washcloths are left in place for about 5 minutes or until they feel warm and then replaced.

The nurse places a bath towel under the patient's arm and sponges the arm slowly and gently for about 5 minutes or as tolerated by the patient. Firm rubbing is avoided because this increases heat production. An alternative method is to place a saturated towel over the extremity and rewet it as necessary. Time is taken for the patient to adjust to the initial reaction of chilliness and for the body to cool. Cool sponges given rapidly for a short period tend to increase the body's heat production mechanism. The patient's arm is then dried, and the procedure is repeated for the other arm and each leg. While sponging the arms and legs, the nurse holds the washcloth briefly over the wrists and ankles where the large blood vessels are close to the skin surface. The patient's vital signs are checked 15 minutes after starting the bath.

While the patient lies on one side, the nurse sponges the back and buttocks for 3 to 5 minutes and then dries them. The washcloths or ice bags are removed from the axillae and groins and those areas dried. The patient's vital signs are rechecked. If the patient's temperature is reduced to slightly above normal, the bath can be terminated. If there is no substantial change, the bath is usually repeated.

If the patient demonstrates any of the following symptoms, the bath should be terminated and the symptoms reported and recorded:

1. Bluish color (cyanosis) of the lips or nails
2. Shivering
3. Accelerated weak pulse

Compresses and moist packs Cold compresses and cold moist packs are applied to patients much as hot compresses and hot moist packs are. See page 1056 and Kozier and Erb (1982:967).

Dry cold

A number of dry cold applications are used for both systemic and local effects. They are often used where there is not an open wound.

Systemic cold: hypothermia *Hypothermia* is an abnormally low body temperature. Measures that produce hypothermia are used to decrease a patient's metabolism and maintain a low body temperature, often for prolonged periods. It is indicated in some instances of cerebral injury and cerebral surgery.

A number of methods are used in therapeutic hypothermia. Nurses are most likely to be involved in hypothermia induced by cooling the body surface. Another method, the extracorporeal method, uses a heart-lung machine (usually during surgery) to cool the blood, thereby reducing the patient's body temperature.

In therapeutic hypothermia by surface cooling, the patient lies between two cooling blankets that are attached to a machine. Coolant circulates within the blankets, cooling the body surface. Surface hypothermia can also be induced by:

1. Covering the patient with a wet sheet over which a fan is directed
2. Covering the patient's body surface with ice bags or plastic bags filled with ice
3. Immersing the patient in a tub of icy water; this is sometimes done for children in the home

The following nursing measures are important in caring for patients who are undergoing hypothermia:

1. Monitor vital signs: temperature, pulse, respirations, and blood pressure.
2. Maintain skin cleanliness and protect the skin with oil as required.
3. Observe the patient for signs of tissue damage and frostbite.
4. Assist the patient to meet basic needs, such as nutrition, elimination, and hygiene.

After a period of hypothermia, a patient's vital signs need to be monitored regularly and frequently until the signs have remained constant for 72 hours.

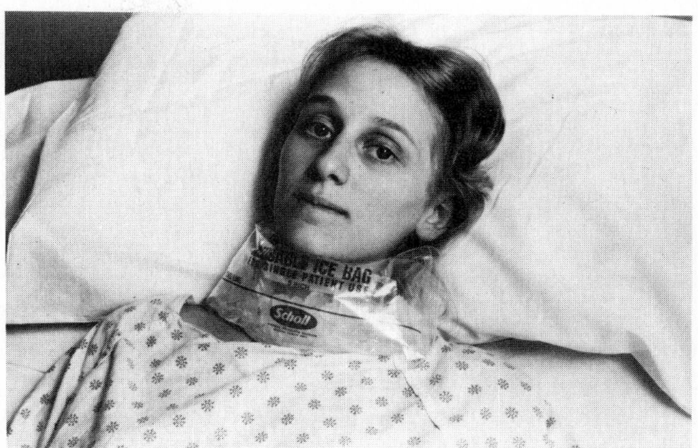

Figure 40–24 A disposable ice collar used to apply cold to the neck area.

Ice bags, ice collars, ice gloves, and disposable ice packs The ice bag, a common device used in many homes and hospitals, is a moderate-sized rubber or plastic bag, with a removable cap, into which pieces of ice can be inserted. Commercially prepared ice bags are available in some agencies. These bags are filled with an alcohol-based solution and sealed; they are kept in freezing units in a central supply area.

An ice collar is similar to an ice bag but is long and narrow. It is designed for use around the neck, though it can be used for other areas.

The ice glove is a rubber or plastic glove that is filled with ice chips and tied at the open end. Gloves are generally used for small body parts, e.g., an eye.

Disposable cold packs are similar to disposable hot packs. They come in a variety of sizes and shapes, and provide a specific degree of coldness for a specific period of time, as indicated on the package. By striking, squeezing, or kneading the package, the nurse activates chemical reactions that release the cold. The manufacturer's instructions must be followed. Most commercially prepared cold packs have soft outer coverings so that they can be applied directly to the body part. See Figure 40–24.

To prepare an ice bag, ice collar, or glove, the nurse places small pieces of ice inside the container until it is two-thirds full, expels excess air, and secures the top to prevent leakage. The container is then covered with a piece of flannel or towel and placed on the patient so that it molds to the body part. The covering absorbs moisture from condensation and needs to be changed when it becomes wet. The bag or other pack should usually be removed 30 to 60 minutes after application and reapplied an hour later for maximum effectiveness, unless the physician's order specifies otherwise.

Summary

A common nursing function is to care for wounds. This may involve changing dressings, shortening and maintaining drains, administering hot and cold applications, applying bandages and binders, and irrigating body parts.

Wounds may be intentional or unintentional. Six categories are classified: incisions, contusions, abrasions, lacerations, punctures, and penetrating wounds. Factors that inhibit wound healing include the presence of foreign objects, hematomas, infections, and localized ischemia. Assessment of wounds includes the overall appearance of the wound, assessment of drainage, the patient's complaints, symptoms of infection, and presence of dehiscence.

The care of wounds varies considerably in accordance with the type of wound, size and location, amount of exudate, presence of complicating factors, and sometimes the personal preference of the physician. Open and closed methods of wound care have advantages and disadvantages that make them appropriate for different circumstances. Various types of dressing materials are indicated for cleaning, covering, and supporting wounds.

Prior to changing dressings the nurse needs to ascertain the physician's orders, the presence of drains, the amount of wound drainage, and the cleaning solutions to be used. The specific techniques involve preparing the equipment, removing soiled dressings, cleaning the wound, and applying clean dressings. Cleaning and shortening a Penrose drain may also be required.

In some agencies registered nurses may be responsible for removing skin sutures. Five common types of sutures are: plain interrupted, mattress interrupted, plain continuous, mattress continuous, and blanket continuous. Each is removed by a specific procedure.

Irrigations are often prescribed to clean wounds, to administer heat, or to apply medications in solution form. The techniques for wound irrigation and for irrigating the eye, the ear, and the vagina have some similarities but each has its own unique steps.

Bandages and binders serve several purposes in the care of wounds, but support and immobilization are the two most common ones. Materials used vary widely and relate to the purpose of the bandage. Examples are flannel, muslin, gauze, and elastic adhesive. The five basic turns required for bandaging specific body parts are: spiral, circular, spiral reverse, recurrent, and figure-eight. Five commonly used types of binders are: the triangular binder, the breast binder, the scultetus (many-tailed) binder, the T-binder, and the abdominal binder.

Heat and cold can be applied in either dry or moist forms. Heat therapy is usually classified as radiant (infrared lamp), conductive (hot water bag), or conversive (medical diathermy). Physiologic responses to heat include an increase in temperature of the tissues, vasodilation, increased capillary blood pressure, decreased blood viscosity, increased tissue metabolism, reduced pain, and muscle relaxation. Responses to cold are generally the opposite, such as decreased temperature of the tissues, vasoconstriction, and muscle contraction. External applications of short duration and of long duration produce different physiologic responses; however the extremes of both hot and cold applications can damage cells. When administering heat or cold applications, the nurse needs to consider: size of the body area, type of application (moist or dry), individual tolerances, specific skin area involved, and age and condition of the patient.

Reasons for heat applications include: relief of muscle spasm, reduction of congestion, provision of comfort and relaxation, and hastening of the suppurative process. Hot moist applications include sitz baths, soaks, compresses, and wet packs. Hot dry applications include hot water bottles, electric pads, heat lamps, and heat cradles.

Cold applications are used to decrease and terminate bleeding, to anesthetize body areas, to reduce inflammation, and to control the accumulation of fluid. Cold moist applications employ tepid or cool sponge baths. Dry cold applications include hypothermia and ice bags. Prior to administering any hot or cold application, the nurse needs to recognize symptoms that contraindicate its use.

Suggested Activities

1. In a clinical area, identify patients who are receiving hot or cold applications. Determine the reasons for these applications and their effects.
2. Observe several surgical incisions or other open wounds, and compare their appearance with the characteristics of clean, healing wounds described in this chapter. Write a sample recording describing the wound, and discuss this with another nurse.
3. Observe several irrigations in a home or agency setting. Describe the irrigation returns in terms of color, clarity, and odor.
4. In a laboratory setting, mark an incision on the abdomen of a classmate, clean the incision, and apply an abdominal dressing using sterile technique.
5. Stitch three different types of sutures into a piece of cloth or tape, and then remove them using sterile technique.

Suggested Readings

Auld, M. E., et al. October 1972. Wound healing. *Nursing 72* 2:36–40.

This article describes how nurses can assist wounds to heal and how nurses may hinder the healing process.

Castle, M. August 1975. Wound care. *Nursing 75* 5:40–44.

Using many photographs, the author describes wound care with particular reference to the practical problems encountered by nurses.

Devney, A. M., and Kingsbury, B. A. August 1972. Hypothermia in fact and fantasy. *American Journal of Nursing* 72:1424–25.

This article provides an overview of the methods of hypothermia and the complications significant to nurses that can ensue.

Rinear, C. E., and Rinear, E. E. January 1975. Emergency bandaging. *Nursing 75* 5:29–35.

Bandaging techniques that are useful in an emergency situation in the community are described. Photographs show some techniques step by step.

Selected References

Gedrose, J. February 1980. Prevention and treatment of hypothermia and frostbite. *Nursing 80* 10:34–36.

Glor, B. A. K., and Estes, Z. E. September-October 1970. Moist soaks: A survey of clinical practices. *Nursing Research* 19:463–65.

Hickey, M. C. January 1965. Hypothermia. *American Journal of Nursing* 65:116–22.

Kozier, B., and Erb, G. 1982. *Techniques in clinical nursing: A comprehensive approach.* Menlo Park, Calif.: Addison-Wesley Publishing Co.

Myers, M. B. September 1971. Sutures and wound healing. *American Journal of Nursing* 71:1725–27.

Nursing 75. October 1975. Wound suction: Better drainage with fewer problems. *Nursing 75* 5:52–55.

O'Dell, A. J. June 1975. Hot packs for morning joint stiffness. *American Journal of Nursing* 75:986–87.

Petrello, J. M. June 1973. Temperature maintenance of hot moist compresses. *American Journal of Nursing* 73:1050–51.

Powell, M. October 1972. An environment for wound healing. *American Journal of Nursing* 72:1862–65.

Waterson, M., consultant. October 1978. Hot and cold therapy. *Nursing 78* 8:44–49.

Weinstock, F. J. October 1971. Emergency treatment of eye injuries. *American Journal of Nursing* 71:1928–31.

Appendices

Appendix A Commonly Used Abbreviations

Abbreviation	Term
abd	abdomen
ABO	the main blood group system
a.c.	before meals *(ante cibum)*
Ac.	acid
A-C	anti-inflammation corticoids
ACTH	adrenocorticotropic hormone
ADH	antidiuretic hormone
ADL	activities of daily living
ad lib	as desired *(ad libitum)*
adm	admitted or admission
AFB	acid-fast bacillus
A/G	albumin-globulin ratio
agit.	shake or stir
$AgNO_3$	silver nitrate
alk	alkaline
AM	morning *(ante meridiem)*
amb	ambulatory
amp	ampule
amt	amount
AP	anteroposterior
A & P	auscultation and percussion; anterior and posterior repair
approx	approximately (about)
aq.	water *(aqua)*
aq. dest.	distilled water *(aqua destillata)*
ARM	artificial rupture of membranes (obstetrics)
ASHD	arteriosclerotic heart disease
A-V	atrioventricular
A & W	alive and well
ax	axillary (armpit)
AZ	Aschheim-Zondek test for pregnancy
Ba	barium
BBB	bundle branch block
BCG	BCG vaccine; ballistocardiograph
BE	barium enema
b.i.d.	twice daily *(bis in die)*
BM (bm)	bowel movement
BMR	basal metabolic rate
BP	blood pressure
BPH	benign prostatic hypertrophy
BRP	bathroom privileges
BS	blood sugar; breath sounds
BSP	bromosulfophthalein (sulfobromophthalein)
BT	bleeding time
BUN	blood urea nitrogen
c̄ (C)	with *(cum)*
C	celsius, centigrade
C-1, C-2, C-3, etc.	cervical vertebrae
Ca	calcium
CA (Ca)	cancer, carcinoma
cap	capsule
CBC	complete blood count
CBD	common bile duct
CBR	complete bed rest
cc	cubic centimeter
CC	chief complaint
CCF	cephalin cholesterol flocculation (liver test)
CCU	coronary care unit
CD	communicable disease
cg	centigram
CHF	congestive heart failure
Cl	chlorine
CNS	central nervous system
c/o	complains of
comp	compound
conc	concentrated
CPD	cephalopelvic disproportion
CPK	creatine phosphokinase
Cr	chromium
CS	cesarean section
C & S	culture and sensitivity
CSF	cerebrospinal fluid
CSR	central supply room
CST	convulsive shock therapy
Cu	copper
CV	cardiovascular; cell volume
CVA	cerebrovascular accident
CVI	cell volume index
CVP	central venous pressure
CVS	cardiovascular system
Cx	cervix
Cysto	cystoscopy examination
CZI	crystalline zinc insulin

Appendix A continued

Abbreviation	Term
DAT	diet as tolerated
dc (disc)	discontinue
D & C	dilation and curettage
DD	differential diagnosis
dg	decigram
Dg	decagram (dekagram)
diff.	differential
dil.	dilute, dissolve
dist	distilled
DOA	dead on arrival
dr	dram; drain; drainage
Dr	doctor
DR	dressing room; delivery room
drsg	dressing
Dx	diagnosis
ECD	expected date of confinement
ECG (EKG)	electrocardiogram
ECT	electroconvulsive therapy
EDD	expected date of delivery
EEG	electroencephalogram
EENT	eye, ear, nose, and throat
e.g.	for example *(exempli gratia)*
elix.	elixir
ENT	ear, nose, and throat
EOM	extraocular movements
eos	eosinophil
ER	emergency room
ESP	extrasensory perception
ESR	erythrocyte sedimentation rate
et al.	and others *(et alii)*
etc.	and the like *(et cetera)*
EUA	examination under anesthetic
exam	examination
F	Fahrenheit
FBS	fasting blood sugar
Fe	iron
FH	family history
FHS	fetal heart sound
fld	fluid
g (Gm, gm)	gram
G	gravida
GA	gastric analysis; general anesthetic
GB	gallbladder
GC (Gc)	gonococcus (gonorrhea)
GI	gastrointestinal
GIT	gastrointestinal tract
GP	general practitioner
gr	grain
gtt	drops *(guttae)*
GU	genitourinary
GUT	genitourinary tract
Gyn	gynecology
h. (hr)	hour *(hora)*
Hb (Hg, Hgb)	hemoglobin
17HC	17-hydroxycorticoids
HCG	human chorionic gonadotropic hormone
HCl	hydrochloric acid
hct (ht)	hematocrit
HCVD	hypertensive cardiovascular disease
hg	hectogram
Hg	mercury
h/o	history of
H_2O	water
HPI	history of present illness
hr	heart rate
h.s.	at bedtime *(hora somni)*
ht	height; hematocrit
Hx	history
ICU	intensive care unit
id.	the same *(idem)*
ID	intradermal
I & D	incision and drainage
i.e.	that is *(id est)*
Ig	immunoglobulin
IM	intramuscular
inf	infusion
inj	injection
invol	involuntary
I & O	intake and output
IOP	intraocular pressure
IPPA	inspection, palpation, percussion, and auscultation
IPPB	intermittent positive pressure breathing
IQ	intelligence quotient
irrig	irrigation
IU	international unit
IV	intravenous
IVP	intravenous pyelogram
JVD	jugular venous distention

Appendix A continued

Abbreviation	Term	Abbreviation	Term
K	potassium	MM	mucous membrane
kg	kilogram	mod	moderate
17KS	17-ketosteroids	mOsm	milliosmole
KUB	kidney, ureter, and bladder	MS	multiple sclerosis; musculoskeletal
L	lumbar; left; liter	MSL	midsternal line
L-1, L-2, L-3, etc.	lumbar vertebrae	MSU	midstream urine
L & A	light and accommodation	myelo.	myelocyte
Lab	laboratory		
Lap	laparotomy	N	nitrogen; normal
LBBB	left bundle branch block	Na	sodium
		NAD	no abnormality detected
LE	lupus erythematosus	NB	note carefully *(nota bene)*; newborn
LH	luteinizing hormone		
liq	liquid	neg	negative
LLE	left lower extremity	neuro	neurology
LLL	left lower lobe	neut.	neutrophil, a variety of white blood cells
LLQ	left lower quadrant		
LMP	last menstrual period	nil (ō)	none
LNMP	last normal menstrual period	no. (#)	number
		noct	at night
LOA	left occiput anterior	non rep.	do not repeat
LP	lumbar puncture	NPN	nonprotein nitrogen
LSK	liver, spleen, kidneys	NPO (NBM)	nothing per ora, by mouth
lt (L)	left		
LUE	left upper extremity	NS (N/S)	normal saline
LUL	left upper lobe	nsq	not sufficient quantity
LUQ	left upper quadrant	NYD	not yet diagnosed
LVH	left ventricular hypertrophy		
		ō	none
lymph.	lymphocyte	O_2	oxygen
		OB (obst)	obstetrics
m	meter; minim; mix	o.d.	daily *(omni die)*
M	thousand; mix	OD	right eye *(oculus dexter)*; overdose
MCH	mean corpuscular hemoglobin		
		o.h.	every hour *(omni hora)*
MCHC	mean corpuscular hemoglobin concentration	OOB	out of bed
		OPD	outpatient department
MCL	midclavicular line	Ophth	ophthalmology
MCU	maximum care unit	OR	operating room
MCV	mean corpuscular volume	Ortho	orthopedics
meds	medications	os	mouth
mEq	milliequivalent	OS	left eye *(oculus sinister)*
mEq/L	milliequivalents per liter	Osm	one osmotically active unit (molecule or ion) per liter
μg	microgram		
mg	milligram	OT	occupational therapy
MH	marital history	OU	both eyes *(oculus uterque)*
MI	myocardial infarction	oz	ounce
mid	middle		
min	minute; minim	p̄	after
mixt	mixture	P	pulse; para
ml	milliliter	PA	posteroanterior; pernicious anemia
mm	millimeter		

Appendix A continued

Abbreviation	Term
Pap	Papanicolaou's smear test
Path	pathology
PBI	protein bound iodine
p.c.	after meals *(post cibum)*
P_{CO_2} (Pa_{CO_2})	partial pressure of carbon dioxide (arterial)
PE (Px)	physical examination
Ped (Peds)	pediatrics
per	by or through
PERLA	pupils equal and reactive to light and accommodation
PET	preeclampsic toxemia
pH	hydrogen ion concentration
P.H.	past history
physio	physiotherapy
PI	present illness
PID	pelvic inflammatory disease
pl. ct.	blood platelet count
PM	afternoon *(post meridiem)*
PMI	point of maximal impulse
p.o.	by mouth *(per os)*
P_{O_2} (Pa_{O_2})	partial pressure of oxygen (arterial)
pop	plaster of Paris
postop	postoperative(ly)
premed	premedication
preop	preoperative(ly)
prep	preparation
p.r.n.	when necessary *(pro re nata)*
Prog	prognosis
pro time	prothrombin time
PSP	phenosulfonphthalein
psych	psychiatry; psychology
pt (Pt)	patient
PT	physical therapy; physical therapist
PUO	pyrexia of unknown origin
PVD	peripheral vascular disease
PZI	protamine zinc insulin
q.	every *(quaque)*
q.a.m. (o.m.)	every morning *(quaque ante meridiem, omni mane)*
q.d.	every day *(quaque die)*
q.h. (q.1h.)	every hour *(quaque hora)*
q.2h., q.3h., etc.	every 2 hours, 3 hours, etc.
q.h.s. (o.n.)	every night at bedtime *(quaque hora somni, omni nocte)*
q.i.d.	four times a day *(quater in die)*
qns	quantity not sufficient
q.o.d.	every other day
qs	sufficient quantity
R	right; respiration; rectal
RBBB	right bundle branch block
RBC (rbc)	red blood cells
rept.	may be repeated
req	requisition
RF	rheumatoid factor
Rh	Rhesus, the Rh factor of blood
Rh Neg	Rhesus factor negative
RISA	radioiodinated serum albumin
R & L	right and left
RLE	right lower extremity
RLL	right lower lobe
RLQ	right lower quadrant
RML	right middle lobe
RR	respiratory rate
Rt (rt, R)	right
RUE	right upper extremity
RUL	right upper lobe
RUQ	right upper quadrant
Rx	take; therapy
$\bar{s}$ (S)	without *(sine)*
sang	sanguineous
SB	sternal border
SC	subcutaneous
SG	specific gravity
SGOT	serum glutamic-oxaloacetic transaminase (aspartate aminotransferase)
SGPT	serum glutamic-pyruvic transaminase (alanine aminotransferase)
SI	seriously ill
Sig. or S.	let it be labeled, write on the label *(signa)*
SMR	submucous resection
SOA	swelling of ankles
SOB (sob)	shortness of breath
soda bicarb	sodium bicarbonate
Sol (sol)	solution
Solv	dissolve
s.o.s.	if necessary *(si opus sit)*
spec	specimen
Sp gr	specific gravity

Appendix A continued

Abbreviation	Term
SR (sed rate)	sedimentation rate
SS (ss)	soap solution, soap suds (enema)
$\overline{SS}$	one-half
staph	staphylococcus
stat.	at once, immediately *(statim)*
st dr	straight drainage
Strep	streptococcus
STS	serologic test for syphilis
subcu	subcutaneous
subling	sublingual (under the tongue)
supp	suppository
susp.	suspension
Sx	symptoms
syr	syrup
T_3	an in vitro test for thyroid function
T_4	a test for thyroxine, the thyroid hormone
T & A	tonsillectomy and adenoidectomy; tonsils and adenoids
tab	tablet
TAB	typhoid, paratyphoid A, and paratyphoid B
TB	tuberculosis
t.i.d.	three times a day *(ter in die)*
TL	team leader
TLC	tender loving care
TNR	tonic neck reflex
To	telephone order
TPI	*Treponema pallidum* immobilization
TPR	temperature, pulse, respirations
Tr.	tincture
TUPR	transurethral prostatic resection
TUR	transurethral resection
U	unit
U/A	urinalysis
ung	ointment
URI	upper respiratory infection
UTI	urinary tract infection
vag	vaginal
VD	venereal disease
VDRL	venereal disease research laboratory (test for syphilis)
viz	namely *(videlicet)*
VO	verbal order
VS (vs)	vital signs
WBC	white blood cells
WF	white female
WM	white male
WNL	within normal limits
wt	weight

Appendix B Root Words, Prefixes, and Suffixes

Word element	Meaning
Root Words	
Circulatory System	
cardio	heart
angio, vaso	vessel
hem, hema, hemato	blood
vena, phlebo	vein
arteria	artery
lympho	lymph
thrombo	clot (of blood)
embolus	moving clot
Digestive System	
bucca	cheek
os, stomato	mouth
gingiva	gum
glossa	tongue
pharyngo	pharynx
esophago	esophagus
gastro	stomach
hepato	liver
cholecyst	gallbladder

Appendix B continued

Word element	Meaning
pancreas	pancreas
entero	intestines
duodeno	duodenum
jejuno	jejunum
ileo	ileum
caeco	cecum
appendeco	appendix
colo	colon
recto	rectum
ano, procto	anus
Skeletal System	
skeleto	skeleton
Respiratory System	
naso, rhino	nose
tonsillo	tonsil
laryngo	larynx
tracheo	trachea
bronchus, broncho	bronchus (plural: bronchi)
pulmo, pneuma, pneum	lung (sac with air)
Nervous System	
neuro	nerve
cerebrum	brain
oculo, ophthalmo	eye
oto	ear
psych, psycho	mind
Urinary System	
urethro	urethra
cysto	bladder
uretero	ureter
reni, reno, nephro	kidney
pyelo	pelvis of kidney
uro	urine
Female Reproductive System	
vulvo	vulva
perineo	perineum
labio	labium (plural: labia)
vagino, colpo	vagina
cervico	cervix
utero	womb; uterus
tubo, salpingo	fallopian tube
ovario, oophoro	ovary
Male Reproductive System	
orchido	testes
Regions of the Body	
crani, cephalo	head
cervico, tracheo	neck
thoraco	chest
abdomino	abdomen
dorsum	back
Tissues	
cutis, dermato	skin
lipo	fat
musculo, myo	muscle
osteo	bone
myelo	marrow
chondro	cartilage
Miscellaneous	
cyto	cell
genetic	formation, origin
gram	tracing or mark
graph	writing, description
kinesis	motion
laparo	flank; through the abdominal wall
meter	measure
oligo	small, few
phobia	fear
photo	light
pyo	pus
roentgen	x-ray
scope	instrument for visual examination
Prefixes	
a, an, ar	without or not
ab	away from
acro	extremities
ad	toward, to
adeno	glandular
aero	air
ambi	around, on both sides
amyl	starch
ante	before, forward
anti	against, counteracting
bi	double
bili	bile
bio	life
bis	two
brachio	arm
brady	slow
broncho	bronchi
cardio	heart
cervico	neck
chole	gall or bile
cholecysto	gallbladder
circum	around
co	together
contra	against, opposite
costo	ribs

Appendix B continued

Word element	Meaning	Word element	Meaning
cysto	bladder	myo	muscle
cyto	cell	neo	new
demi	half	nephro	kidney
derma	skin	neuro	nerve
dis	from	nitro	nitrogen
dorso	back	noct	night
dys	abnormal, difficult	non	not
electro	electric	ob	against, in front of
en	into, in, within	oculo	eye
encephal	brain	odonto	tooth
entero	pertaining to the intestine	ophthalmo	eye
equi	equal	ortho	straight, normal
eryth	red	os	mouth, bone
ex	out, out of, away from	osteo	bone
extra	outside of, in addition to	oto	ear
ferro	iron	pan	all
fibro	fiber	para	beside, accessory to
fore	before, in front of	path	disease
gastro	stomach	ped	child, foot
glosso	tongue	per	by, through
glyco	sugar	peri	around
hemi	half	pharyngo	pharynx
hemo	blood	phlebo	vein
hepa, hepato	liver	photo	light
histo	tissue	phren	diaphragm, mind
homo	same	pneumo	air, lungs
hydro	water	pod	foot
hygro	moisture	poly	many, much
hyper	too much, high	post	after
hypo	under, decreased	pre	before
hyster	uterus	proct	rectum
ileo	ileum	pseudo	false
in	in, within, into	psych	mind
inter	between	pyel	pelvis of the kidney
intra	within	pyo	pus
intro	in, within, into	pyro	fever, heat
juxta	near, close to	quadri	four
lapar	abdomen	radio	radiation
laryngo	larynx	re	back, again
latero	side	reno	kidney
leuk	white	retro	backward
macro	large, big	rhin	nose
mal	bad, poor	sacro	sacrum
mast	breast	salpingo	fallopian tube
medio	middle	sarco	flesh
mega, megalo	large, great	sclero	hard, hardening
meno	menses	semi	half
mono	single	sex	six
multi	many	skeleto	skeleton
myelo	bone marrow, spinal cord	steno	narrowing, constriction
		sub	under

Appendix B continued

Word element	Meaning	Word element	Meaning
super	above, excess	ism	condition
supra	above	itis	inflammation
syn	together	ize	to treat
tachy	fast	lith	stone, calculus
thyro	thyroid, gland	lithiasis	presence of stones
trache	trachea	lysis	disintegration
trans	across, over	megaly	enlargement
tri	three	meter	instrument that measures
ultra	beyond		
un	not, back, reversal	oid	likeness, resemblance
uni	one	oma	tumor
uretero	ureter	opathy	disease of
urethro	urethra	orrhaphy	surgical repair
uro	urine, urinary organs	osis	disease, condition of
vaso	vessel	ostomy	to form an opening or outlet
Suffixes			
able	able to	otomy	to incise
algia	pain	pexy	fixation
cele	tumor, swelling	phage	ingesting
centesis	surgical puncture to remove fluid	phobia	fear
		plasty	plastic surgery
cide	killing, destructive	plegia	paralysis
cule	little	rhage	to burst forth
cyte	cell	rhea	excessive discharge
ectasia	dilating, stretching	rhexis	rupture
ectomy	excision, surgical removal of	scope	lighted instrument for visual examination
emia	blood		
esis	action	scopy	to examine visually
form	shaped like	stomy	to form an opening
genesis, genetic	formation, origin		
gram	tracing, mark	tomy	incision into
graph	writing	uria	urine

Appendix C Commonly Used Symbols

Symbol	Term	Number	Symbol
>	greater than	0	ō
<	less than	½	$\overline{ss}$
=	equal to	1	i
↑	increased	2	ii
↓	decreased	3	iii
♀	female	4	iv
♂	male	5	v
°	degree	6	vi
#	number; fracture	7	vii
ʒ	dram	8	viii
℥	ounce	9	ix
×	times	10	x
@	at		

Appendix D Equivalents

Metric Equivalents

Weights			Volume		
1 picogram	=	10^{-12} gram	1 milliliter	=	1 gram
1 nanogram	=	10^{-9} gram	1 liter	=	1 kilogram = 1000 grams (milliliters)
1 microgram	=	10^{-3} milligram = 10^{-6} gram			
1 milligram	=	1000 micrograms = 10^{-6} gram			
1 centigram	=	10 milligrams = 10^{-1} decigram = 10^{-2} gram			
1 decigram	=	100 milligrams = 10 centigrams = 10^{-1} gram			
1 gram	=	1000 milligrams = 100 centigrams = 10 decigrams			
1 kilogram	=	1000 grams			

Approximate Weight Equivalents: Metric and Apothecaries' Systems

Metric	Apothecaries'	Metric	Apothecaries'
0.1 mg	1/600 grain	30 mg	1/2 grain
1.12 mg	1/500 grain	40 mg	2/3 grain
0.15 mg	1/400 grain	50 mg	3/4 grain
0.2 mg	1/300 grain	60 mg	1 grain
0.25 mg	1/250 grain	100 mg (0.1 gm)	1-1/2 grains
0.3 mg	1/200 grain	150 mg (0.15 gm)	2-1/2 grains
0.4 mg	1/150 grain	200 mg (0.2 gm)	3 grains
0.5 mg	1/120 grain	300 mg (0.3 gm)	5 grains
0.6 mg	1/100 grain	400 mg (0.4 gm)	6 grains
0.8 mg	1/80 grain	500 mg (0.5 gm)	7-1/2 grains
1 mg	1/60 grain	600 mg (0.6 gm)	10 grains
1.2 mg	1/50 grain	1 gram	15 grains
1.5 mg	1/40 grain	1.5 gm	22 grains
2 mg	1/30 grain	2 gm	30 grains
3 mg	1/20 grain	3 gm	45 grains
4 mg	1/15 grain	4 gm	60 grains (1 dram)
5 mg	1/12 grain	5 gm	75 grains
6 mg	1/10 grain	6 gm	90 grains
8 mg	1/8 grain	7.5 gm	120 grains (2 drams)
10 mg	1/6 grain	10 gm	2-1/2 drams
12 mg	1/5 grain	30 gm	1 ounce (8 drams)
15 mg	1/4 grain	500 gm	1.1 pounds
20 mg	1/3 grain	1000 gm	2.2 pounds (1 kilogram)
25 mg	3/8 grain		

Approximate Volume Equivalents: Metric, Apothecaries', and Household Systems

Metric	Apothecaries'	Household
0.06 ml	1 minim (m)	1 drop (gt)
0.3 ml	5 minims	
0.6 ml	10 minims	
1 ml	15 minims	15 drops (gtt)
2 ml	30 minims	
3 ml	45 minims	
4 ml	60 minims (1 fluid dram [fʒ])	60 drops (1 teaspoon [tsp])
8 ml	2 fluid drams	2 teaspoons
15 ml	4 fluid drams	4 teaspoons (1 tablespoon [Tbsp])
30 ml	8 fluid drams (1 fluid ounce [f℥])	2 tablespoons
60 ml	2 fluid ounces	
90 ml	3 fluid ounces	
200 ml	6 fluid ounces	1 teacup
250 ml	8 fluid ounces	1 large glass
500 ml	16 fluid ounces (1 pint)	1 pint
750 ml	1½ pints	
1000 ml (1 liter)	2 pints (1 quart)	1 quart
4000 ml	4 quarts	1 gallon

Glossary

abdominal paracentesis removal of fluid from the peritoneal cavity
abduction movement of a bone away from the midline of the body
abductor muscle a muscle that moves a bone away from the midline of the body
ablative surgery surgery to remove a diseased organ
abrasion wearing away of a structure, such as the skin or teeth
abscess a localized collection of pus and disintegrating body tissues
abstracting forming a summary; isolating or considering separately a particular aspect of an object
acapnia a decreased level of carbon dioxide in the blood
acatalasia a disease characterized by absence of the enzyme catalase, occurring mostly in Japanese people
accommodation (Piaget) the process of change in which a person's cognitive processes are sufficiently matured so that he or she can solve problems that could not be solved previously
accountability being answerable
accreditation a process by which a nongovernmental agency appraises institutions or programs to determine whether they meet established standards for service or training
acetone a flammable, colorless liquid with an ethereal odor, used to remove nail polish
acetylcholine an acetic acid ester of choline, which has an important function in the transmission of nerve impulses at the myoneural junction
aching pain a deep pain of varying degrees of intensity
acholic clay colored and free from bile
acidosis (acidemia) a condition that occurs with increases in blood carbonic acid or with decreases in blood bicarbonate; blood pH below 7.35
acne an inflammatory condition of the sebaceous glands
acromion (acromial process) the lateral projection of the scapula extending over the shoulder joint
active assistive exercise exercise carried out by the patient with some assistance by the nurse
active euthanasia acts performed to shorten a person's life
active exercise exercise carried out by the patient who supplies the energy to move the body parts
active transport movement of substances across cell membranes against the concentration gradient
activity energetic action or being in a state of movement
actual health problem a health problem that currently exists
actual loss a loss identifiable by others
acupuncture a Chinese practice of piercing specific superficial nerves with needles, often to treat pain
acute sharp or severe; describing a severe condition with a sudden onset and short course (as opposed to *chronic*)
adaptation (Piaget) the coping behavior of a person who has the ability to handle the demands of the environment
adaptive mechanisms (coping or defense mechanisms) learned behaviors that assist an individual to adjust to the environment
addiction a term used previously to describe dependence on a drug or habit
adduction movement of a bone toward the midline of the body
adductor muscle a muscle that moves a bone toward the midline of the body
adenohypophysis the anterior part of the pituitary gland
adenosine triphosphate (ATP) a compound that stores energy from glucose oxidation
adherent sticking together, clinging
adhesion a fibrous band or structure by which parts are abnormally held together
adipose fat; of a fatty nature
adolescence a period of life beginning with the appearance of secondary sex characteristics and terminating with somatic growth, usually between ages 11 and 19
adrenal gland an endocrine gland that is located on the superior aspect of the kidney
Adrenalin a trademark name for preparations of epinephrine
adrenocortical arising from the cortex of the adrenal gland
adrenocorticotrophic hormone (ACTH) a hormone produced by the pituitary gland that stimulates the adrenal cortex to produce hormones
adsorbent an agent that attracts other materials or particles to its surface, e.g., charcoal in the stomach and intestines
adventitious breath sounds abnormal breath sounds
advocate one who pleads the cause of another or argues or pleads for a cause or proposal
aeration the process by which the blood exchanges carbon dioxide for oxygen in the lungs
aerobe an organism that requires oxygen to live
aerobic requiring oxygen
affect feelings, emotions
agglutination the process of clumping together
agglutinin a specific antibody formed in blood
agglutinogen a substance that acts as an antigen and stimulates the production of agglutinin
aggression an unprovoked attack or hostile, injurious, or destructive behavior or outlook
agnostic one who believes that the existence of God is unknown
air hunger dyspnea occurring in paroxysms
airway a passageway through which air normally circulates; a device that is inserted through the patient's mouth to maintain the patency of air passages such as the trachea
alarm reaction (Selye) the initial reaction of the body to a stressor
albuminuria the presence of albumin in the urine
aldosterone a hormone produced by the adrenal cortex that regulates the level of sodium in the body
algor mortis the gradual decrease in body temperature after death
alignment (posture) the position of body parts that facilitates body function
alkalosis (alkalemia) a condition that occurs with increases in blood bicarbonate or decreases in blood carbonic acid; blood pH above 7.45
allergy a hypersensitive state
alopecia abnormal loss of hair
alveolus a saclike dilation or cavity in the body (plural: alveoli)
ambulation the act of walking
amino acid one of a group of organic acids containing nitrogen that are considered the components of protein
ammonia dermatitis diaper rash
amphetamine a drug used to stimulate the central nervous system
ampule a small, sealed glass flask, usually designed to hold a single dose of a medication

anabolism a process in which simple substances are converted by the body cells into more complex substances, e.g., building tissue; positive nitrogen balance
anaerobe an organism that does not require oxygen to live
anal canal the terminal aspect of the rectum
analgesic a medication used to alter the perception and interpretation of pain
anal stage (Freud) a stage of human development usually occurring during the 2nd and 3rd years when the child is learning toilet training
anaphylaxis (anaphylactic shock, anaphylactic reaction) a severe allergic reaction
anasarca generalized edema throughout the body
anastomose to join or connect
anatomic position the position of normal body alignment
androgen any substance producing male characteristics
andropause (climacteric) the period of change in men when sexual activity decreases
androsperm sperm bearing a Y chromosome
anemia a condition in which the blood is deficient in red blood cells or hemoglobin
aneroid containing no liquid
anesthesia loss of sensation or feeling; induced loss of the sense of pain
anesthesiologist a physician specializing in the administration of anesthetics
anesthetic bed *see* surgical bed
anesthetist a person such as a nurse who specializes in administering anesthetics
aneurysm dilation of the wall of an artery, a vein, or the heart
anger an emotional state or a subjective feeling of animosity or strong displeasure
angiogram a diagnostic procedure enabling x-ray visualization of the vascular system after injection of a radiopaque dye
angstrom (A) a unit of wavelength of the electromagnetic spectrum
anilingus anal stimulation provided orally
anion an ion carrying a negative charge
ankylosis permanent fixation of a joint; stiffening of a joint
anodyne a medication that relieves pain
anogenital referring to the area around the anus and the genitals
anorexia lack of appetite
anorexia nervosa a psychologic condition in which the person eats little or nothing, leading to emaciation
anoscopy visual examination of the anal canal using a lighted instrument called an anoscope
anoxemia a condition in which the level of oxygen in the blood is below normal
anoxia systemic absence or reduction of oxygen in the body tissues below physiologic levels
answer (legal) a written response to a complaint
antagonist muscle a muscle that acts in the opposite manner to another muscle
antecubital space the area in front of the elbow
anterior of, toward, or at the front
anthelmintic destructive to worms
anthropometric measurement measurement of the size and composition of the body, e.g., height, weight, and skin folds
antibiosis an antagonistic association between organisms
antibiotic a substance produced by microorganisms that has the capacity to inhibit the growth of or kill other microorganisms
antibody a protective substance produced in the body to counteract antigens
anticipatory loss a loss experienced before it actually occurs
antidiuretic hormone (ADH) a hormone that is stored and released by the posterior pituitary gland and that controls water reabsorption from the kidney tubules; also referred to as *vasopressin*
antigen a substance capable of inducing the formation of antibodies
antipyretic a substance that is effective in relieving fever
antiseptic an agent that inhibits the growth of some microorganisms
antiserum (immune serum) a serum that contains antibodies
antrum the portion of the stomach between the fundus and the pylorus
anuria the failure of the kidneys to produce urine, resulting in total lack of urination or output of less than 100 ml per day in an adult
anus the opening of the rectum, the posterior opening of the gastrointestinal tract
anxiety mental uneasiness evidenced by increased level of arousal due to an impending or anticipated threat to self or significant relationships
apathy lack of interest or feeling
Apgar score a system of numerically scoring the condition of a newborn infant
aphasia the inability to communicate by speech, signs, or writing, resulting from an injury or disease
apical beat the heartbeat as heard over the apex of the heart
apical-radial pulse measurement of the apical beat and the radial pulse
apnea cessation of breathing
apocrine gland a large sweat gland whose duct usually opens into a hair follicle
appetite a pleasant sensation in which one desires and anticipates food
appliance (ostomy) a device or bag that is secured to the abdomen to collect either urine or feces
approximate to bring close together (referring to wound or incision edges)
areola the circular area of different color around a central point, such as the circular pigmented area surrounding the nipple of the breast
aromatic having a spicy odor
arrector pili muscle the erector muscle attached to the hair follicle
arrhythmia an irregular pulse rhythm
arteriography x-ray filming of an arterial system after injection of a radiopaque material
arteriosclerosis a condition in which the walls of the arteries become hardened and thickened
artery forceps *see* hemostat
artificial respiration forceful movement of air into and out of the lungs by means external to the person
ascites the accumulation of fluid in the abdominal cavity
asepsis the absence of disease-producing microorganisms
asphyxia a condition resulting from a lack of oxygen in the inspired air
asphyxiation (suffocation) lack of oxygen due to interrupted breathing
aspirate to remove gases or fluids from a cavity by using suction
assault an attempt or threat to touch another person unjustifiably
assertiveness expression of oneself openly and directly without hurting others
assessment in general, an organized collection of data about a patient; in relation to the problem-oriented medical record, the third step of SOAP—that is, analysis and interpretation of the data or diagnosis of a specific problem
assimilation (of a group) the blending of attitudes and beliefs of the members
assimilation (Piaget) the process whereby humans are able to encounter and react to new situations by using the mechanisms they already possess
asthma a disease characterized by spasmodic dyspnea, coughing, and a sense of constriction of the bronchi

astigmatism a refractive error of the eye due to an uneven curvature of the cornea
astringent an agent that causes contraction or shrinkage of tissue; usually applied topically
asymmetric lacking symmetry; showing dissimilarity of corresponding organs on opposite sides of the body
atelectasis collapse of lung tissue
atheist one who denies the existence of God
athetosis involuntary twisting and writhing movements
athlete's foot (tinea pedis) a fungal infection of the foot; ringworm
atony lack of normal muscle tone
atresia absence, closure, or degeneration of a passageway or cavity such as the primordial follicles of the ovaries
atrioventricular (AV) node the neuromuscular tissue of the heart at the base of the atrial septum that conveys impulses to the ventricles
atrioventricular valves cardiac valves between the atria and the ventricles; also referred to as the *tricuspid* and *mitral* valves
atrophy a wasting away or decrease in size of a cell, tissue, body organ, or muscle
attenuate to make thin or to weaken
attitude a feeling tone; a concomitant of behavior
audit a methodical examination and review
auditory related to or experienced through hearing
auricle a chamber of the ear or the heart
auscultation the practice of examining the body by listening to body sounds
authority (in a group) an official or legitimized right to use a given amount or type of power
autoantigen an antigen that originates in the person's own body
autoclave an apparatus that sterilizes, using steam under pressure
autogenous (infection) originating from the patient's own microbial flora
autonomic self-controlling; capable of independent function
autonomy the quality or state of being independent and self-directed without outside control
autopsy (postmortem examination) the examination of a body after death by a physician
axilla the armpit (plural: axillae)
axillary line an imaginary line extending vertically from the anterior fold of the axilla

babbling prelinguistic repetitive sounds produced by infants
Babinski (plantar) reflex in infants up to 1 year, the normal fanning out of the toes and dorsiflexion of the big toe elicited by stroking the sole of the foot (positive Babinski); after 1 year the normal curling of the toes at this stroking (negative Babinski)
bacteriocide an agent capable of destroying some microorganisms
bacteriostatic agent an agent that prevents the growth and reproduction of some microorganisms
balance stability; steadiness; a state of equipoise in which opposing forces counteract each other
Balkan frame a metal frame extending lengthwise over a bed and supported at either end for attaching traction or providing a means of mobility to bedridden patients
bandage a material used to wrap a body part
barbiturate a drug commonly used as a hypnotic and sedative
barium a metallic element commonly used in solution as a contrast medium for x-ray filming of the gastrointestinal tract
barium enema x-ray filming of the large intestine using a contrast medium; also called a *lower gastrointestinal series*
barium swallow x-ray filming of the esophagus, stomach, and duodenum; also referred to as an *upper gastrointestinal series*
barrel chest a chest shape in which the ratio of the anteroposterior diameter to the lateral diameter is 1 to 1
barrier technique *see* reverse protective asepsis
basalis the layer of endometrium of the uterus closest to the myometrium
basal metabolic rate (BMR) the rate at which the body metabolizes food to produce the energy required to maintain body functions at rest
base of support the area on which an object rests
basic human need those things humans require to maintain physiologic and psychologic homeostasis
basilic vein a superficial vein that arises on the ulnar side of the dorsum of the hand, goes up the forearm, and joins the brachial vein to form the axillary vein
battery willful or negligent touching of a person or a person's clothes, which may or may not cause harm
Beau's line a deep line visible across a nail after its growth has been halted and then renewed
bedpan a receptacle used to collect urine and feces from a person confined in bed
behavior modification eliciting and rewarding externally desired behavioral responses to reduce, modify, or eliminate ineffective adaptive coping responses
belief something accepted as true by a judgment of probability rather than actuality
bereavement the state of a person who has experienced the loss of a significant other through death
beriberi a condition due to deficiency of thiamine (vitamin B_1)
bevel a slanting edge
bilateral affecting two sides
bilirubin orange pigment in the bile
bill of rights a summary of fundamental rights and privileges guaranteed to people
binder a type of bandage applied to large body areas, e.g., the abdomen or chest
biologic sex sexual gender genetically determined at conception from the XX or XY chromosomal combination
biopsy the removal and examination of tissue from the living body
biorhythm an inner rhythm that appears to control a variety of biologic processes
biorhythmology study of the biologic rhythms of the body
bisexual experiencing sexual attraction to people of both genders
bleb (wheal) a small, smooth, slightly raised area on the skin, usually filled with fluid
blister a collection of fluid between the epidermis and the dermis
blood pressure the pressure of the blood as it pulsates through the arteries
body image an individual's perception of his or her own physical attributes, body functioning, sexuality, appearance, and state of wellness
body image disturbance negative feelings or perceptions about characteristics, functions, or limits of one's own body or body part
body mechanics the efficient and coordinated use of the body during resting activities and movement
body temperature the internal temperature of the human body
bolus a mass of food or pharmaceutical preparation ready to be swallowed; a mass passing along the gastrointestinal tract; a concentrated mass of pharmaceutical preparation given intravenously
borborygmi abnormally intense and frequent bowel sounds
boundary (systems theory) the line that differentiates the parts of a system from parts external to the system
brachial pulse a pulse located on the inner side of the biceps muscle just below the axilla; usually palpated medially in the antecubital space
bradycardia an abnormally slow heart rate, below 60 beats per minute in an adult
bradypnea abnormally slow respirations; usually fewer than 10 respirations per minute
Braxton Hicks contractions painless, intermittent contractions of the uterus during pregnancy
bronchial sounds normal loud, harsh, hollow blowing sounds heard by auscultation over the trachea and major bronchi

bronchodilator an agent that dilates the bronchi of the lungs
bronchogram an x-ray film of the bronchial tree taken after injection of an iodized oil dye, used as a contrast medium
bronchophony an increase in vocal resonance; an abnormal voice sound heard on auscultation of the chest wall
bronchopneumonia an infection that originates in the bronchi and involves patches of lung tissue
bronchoscope a lighted instrument used to visualize the bronchi of the lungs
bronchoscopy visual examination of the bronchi using a bronchoscope
bronchovesicular sounds combination of bronchial and vesicular sounds heard by auscultation over parts of the chest where a bronchus is near lung tissue
bronchus a large air passageway of the lungs (plural: bronchi)
bruit abnormal blowing, swishing, or rippling sounds heard during auscultation
bubbling gurgling sounds produced as air passes through moist secretions in the respiratory tract
buccal pertaining to the cheek
buffer an agent or system that tends to maintain constancy or that prevents changes in the chemical concentration of a substance
bulimia an uncontrollable compulsion to consume enormous amounts of food and then expel the food by self-induced vomiting
burden of proof (legal) evidence of the defendant's wrongdoing presented by the plaintiff
burning pain pain like the pain of burning skin

cachexia a state of weakness, emaciation, and malnutrition often seen in wasting diseases and terminal malignancies
calcitonin a hormone secreted by the thyroid gland that regulates blood calcium levels
calculus a stone composed of minerals that is formed in the body, e.g., a renal calculus formed in the kidney
calipers an instrument used to measure the thickness of folds of skin
callus hyperplasia or thickening of the horny layer of the epidermis, usually due to pressure
caloric density the number of kilocalories per unit weight of food
caloric value the amount of energy that nutrients or foods supply to the body
calorie (large calorie, kilocalorie, C.) the amount of heat required to raise the temperature of 1 kilogram of water 1 degree centigrade
calorie (small calorie) the unit of heat required to raise the temperature of 1 gram of water 1 degree centigrade
calyx (calix) a cup-shaped organ or cavity
cancellous bone bone of spongy or latticelike structure
cannula a tube with a lumen (channel), which is inserted into a cavity or duct and is often fitted with a trocar during insertion
canthus the angle formed by the upper and lower eyelids; each eye has an inner and an outer canthus
Cantor tube a single-lumen tube inserted through the mouth into the intestines
capillary action the movement of fluid in a tube, caused by the adhesion of the fluid to the wall of the tube
capsule a soft, soluble container for a medication; an anatomic structure enclosing an organ or part of the body; (of a cell) a well-defined, gelatinous layer surrounding a bacterial cell
caput succedaneum edematous swelling of the soft tissues of the part of a newborn's scalp that was encircled by the cervix before it dilated
carbaminohemoglobin the chemical combination of carbon dioxide and hemoglobin
carbohydrate a nutrient composed of carbon, hydrogen, and oxygen, e.g., starches and sugars
carbonic acid the compound formed when carbon dioxide combines with water
cardiac arrest the cessation of heart function
cardiac board a flat board placed under a patient's chest when a patient who requires cardiac massage is lying on a soft surface
cardiac monitor a machine that measures and records the heart function
cardiac output the volume of blood ejected from the heart per minute by ventricular contraction
cardiopulmonary resuscitation (CPR) artificial stimulation of the heart and lungs
caries decay of a tooth or bone
carina the ridge or junction where the main bronchi meet the trachea
carminative an agent that promotes the passage of flatus from the colon
carotid arteries major arteries lying on either side of the trachea and larynx
carotid receptors nerve endings that are found in the carotid bodies and carotid sinuses and that are sensitive to blood pH, changes in blood pressure, and excessive blood CO_2
carrier a person who harbors pathogens but is not ill
cartilage a firm connective tissue found throughout the body
caster a small wheel, often made of rubber or plastic, that permits furniture such as a bed to be moved easily
catabolism a destructive process in which complex substances are broken down into simpler substances, e.g., breakdown of tissue
cataplexy partial or complete muscle paralysis that can occur during narcolepsy
cataract opacity of the lens of the eye or its capsule
catarrh inflammation of the mucous membrane accompanied by a discharge
cathartic a drug that induces evacuation of feces from the large intestine
catheter a tube of plastic, rubber, metal, or other material used to remove or inject fluids into a cavity such as the bladder
cation a positively charged ion
cauda a tail or taillike appendage
caudal anesthetic an anesthetic injected into the caudal canal, below the spinal cord
cavity a hollow space within the body or one of its organs
cecum a dilated pouch that constitutes the first part of the large intestine adjoining the small intestine
cellular fluid *see* intracellular fluid
cellulitis inflammation of cellular tissue
Celsius *see* centigrade
cementum a bonelike connective tissue surrounding the root of a tooth
center of gravity the point at which the mass (weight) of the body is centered
centigrade (Celsius) a thermometer scale used to measure heat; the freezing point of water is 0 C and the boiling point is 100 C
central venous pressure (CVP) a measurement of the pressure of the blood, in millimeters of water, within the vena cava or the right atrium of the heart
cephalhematoma swelling of the scalp due to an effusion of blood between the periosteum and the bone
cephalocaudal proceeding in the direction from head to toe
cerebral death death that occurs when the cerebral cortex is irreversibly destroyed
cerebrospinal fluid fluid contained within the four ventricles of the brain, the subarachnoid space, and the central canal of the spinal cord
certification the practice of determining minimum standards of competence in specialty areas
cerumen waxlike material that protects the auditory canal
cervix the lower end or neck of the uterus, which projects into the vagina
Chadwick's sign a change of the mucous membrane of the vagina to a bluish or violet color during pregnancy

chancre a papular lesion (sore) occurring at the entry of infection in some diseases; the primary sore of syphilis
chart (medical record) a written account of a patient's health history, current health status, treatment, and progress
charting (recording) the process of making written entries about a patient on the medical record
cheilosis cracks or scaling at the corners of the lips
chemical thermogenesis the production of heat by chemical means, e.g., production and circulation of ephinephrine
chemoreceptor a receptor that is sensitive to chemical substances
chemosensitive pain receptors pain receptors stimulated by chemicals
chemotaxis the movement of a cell or an organism in response to a chemical gradient
Cheyne-Stokes respirations rhythmic waxing and waning of respirations from very deep breathing to very shallow breathing with periods of temporary apnea, often associated with cardiac failure, increased intracranial pressure, or brain damage
chill shivering and shaking of the body with involuntary contractions of the voluntary muscles
cholangiogram an x-ray film of the biliary tract taken after the injection of a dye
cholecystogram an x-ray film of the gallbladder after the ingestion of a contrast dye; also called *oral cholecystography*
cholesterol a lipid that does not contain fatty acid but possesses many of the chemical and physical properties of other lipids
chordotomy *see* cordotomy
chorionic gonadotropin (HCG) a hormone produced by the placenta
chorionic somatomammotropin (human placental lactogen) a hormone secreted by the placenta that influences fetal growth
choroid plexus projections of the pia mater into the ventricles of the brain that secrete cerebrospinal fluid
chromosome a structure in the nucleus of a cell that contains DNA and transmits genetic information
chronic persisting over a long time
chyme semifluid material produced by gastric digestion of food in the stomach; it is found in the small and large intestines
cicatrical tissue *see* scar tissue
cicatrix scar
cicatrization formation of a scar
cilia hairlike projections from cells, e.g., of the mucous membrane of the respiratory tract
circadian rhythm rhythmic repetition of certain phenomena each 24 hours
circa dies about a day
circulatory overload a state in which the intravascular fluid compartment contains more fluid than normal
circumcision surgical removal of part or all of the foreskin of the penis; usually performed during infancy
circumduction movement of the distal part of a bone in a circle, with the proximal end remaining flxed
circumference the outer measurement or perimeter, e.g., the distance around the chest
cisterna a space that is enclosed and serves as a reservoir for body fluid
cisternal puncture insertion of a needle into the subarachnoid space of the cisterna magna
citric acid cycle (Krebs cycle) a complex series of chemical reactions by which the acetyl portion of acetyl coenzyme A is broken down to carbon dioxide and hydrogen atoms
civil action a legal action between two or more individuals
civil (private) law rules that regulate or control relationships between people rather than between persons and governments
clavicle the bone commonly known as the collarbone; it articulates with the scapula and the sternum
clean free of pathogenic organisms
clean technique a technique that maintains an area or articles free from pathogens
clergy priests, rabbis, ministers, church elders, deacons, and any other spiritual advisers
client *see* patient
climacteric the point in development when reproduction capacity in the female terminates (menopause) and the sexual activity of the male decreases (andropause)
clinical pharmacist a person who specializes in drugs that are used for treatment, prevention, and diagnosis of disease
clitoris a small round mass of erectile tissue, blood vessels, and nerves located behind the junction of the labia minora; homologous to the penis
closed system a system that does not exchange energy or matter with its environment
closed wound a wound in which there is no break in the skin
clubbing (of nails) an elevation of the proximal aspect of the nail and softening of the nail bed
coagulate to clot
coccidioidomycosis a fungus disease with an acute, benign respiratory infection in the primary stage and a virulent, progressive secondary stage
cochlea a tubular structure in the inner ear that contains the organ for hearing
code of ethics formal guidelines for professional action
cognition the process of knowing, including judgment and awareness
cognitive referring to processes such as remembering, thinking, perceiving, abstracting, and generalizing
cohesive sticking together
cohesiveness (of group) the degree of group unity or oneness
coitus sexual intercourse; from Latin, meaning "a coming together"
coitus interruptus a method of contraception during which the penis is withdrawn prior to ejaculation
colic paroxysmal intestinal cramplike pain
collagen a protein found in connective tissue
colloid substances, such as large plasma protein molecules, that do not readily dissolve in true solutions
colonoscope a lighted instrument used to visualize the interior of the colon
colonoscopy visual examination of the interior of the colon with a colonoscope
colostomy an artificial opening of the colon on the abdomen
colostrum a yellow, milky fluid secreted by the mother's mammary glands a few days before or after childbirth
comatose a state of unconsciousness in which the person shows no response to maximum painful stimuli, absence of reflexes, and absence of muscle tone in the extremities
combustible able to burn; flammable
comedo a mass on the skin consisting of keratin, lipids, fatty acids, and bacteria
commitment (of group) an agreement, pledge, or obligation to do something or follow a course of action
commode a portable, chairlike structure used as a toilet
common law unwritten laws that are binding and upheld by precedent in legal cases rather than statutes
communicable disease (infectious disease) a disease that can spread from one person to another
communication exchange of thoughts, ideas, or feelings between two or more people
compensation an adaptive mechanism in which a person substitutes a certain behavior trait for a characteristic that is perceived to be inadequate
complaint (legal) a document filed by the plaintiff claiming that his or her legal rights have been infringed

compliance in learning, an individual's agreement to learn; in drug therapy, the act of carefully following the prescription
compress a moist gauze dressing that is applied frequently to an open wound; it sometimes is medicated
concave hollowed or rounded inward
concept a complex of ideas that is united to portray a large general idea
conceptual model a basic structure in which a complex of ideas is united to portray a large general idea
concurrent audit an audit relating to present practices
concurrent disinfection measures taken while a patient is infectious to control the spread of the microorganisms
conditioning learning in which a response previously associated with one stimulus becomes associated with another stimulus
condom a sheath or cover, usually made of rubber or plastic, worn over the penis during coitus to prevent conception or infection; it may also be used to catch urine
conduction the transfer of heat from one molecule or object to another by contact
conformity actions in accordance with specified standards
confusion a mental state in which a person appears bewildered and may make inappropriate statements and answers to questions
congenital existing at, and often before, birth
congestion excessive accumulation of blood in a part of the body
congruence (communication) a state in which one's verbal and nonverbal communications convey the same message
conjunctiva the delicate membrane that covers the eyeball and lines the eyelids
conjunctivitis inflammation of the conjunctiva
consciousness a person's normal state of awareness of the environment, self, and others
consensual reaction (eyes) a reaction in which one pupil constricts quickly in response to a bright light and the other pupil constricts also, but more slowly
consent permission given voluntarily by a person in his or her right mind; *informed consent* implies that the individual is knowledgeable about the consent and understands it
constipation passage of small, dry, hard stool or passage of no stool for an abnormally long time
constitutional law law stated in federal, state, or provincial constitutions
constructive surgery surgery to repair a congenitally malformed organ or tissue
consumer a person who uses a service or a product
contact a person who has been near an infected person and thus exposed to pathogenic microorganisms
contact lens a small, plastic corrective lens that fits on the cornea of the eye directly over the pupil
contaminated possessing pathogenic organisms
contour position (of a bed) a position with the head and foot of the bed elevated, creating an angle of about 15°
contraception the prevention of fertilization of the ovum by any method
contract a written or verbal agreement between two or more people to do or not do some lawful act
contraction the normal active shortening or tensing of a muscle
contractual obligation a duty to render service established by a formal or informal contract
contracture permanent shortening of a muscle and subsequent shortening of tendons and ligaments
contusion a closed wound that occurs as a result of a blow from a blunt instrument; a bruise
convection transfer of heat by movement of a liquid or gas, e.g., air currents
conversion an adaptive mechanism of converting a mental conflict into a physical symptom
conversive heat heat that results from the conversion of a primary source of energy
convex curved or rounded like the external surface of a sphere
coping mechanisms *see* adaptive mechanisms
copulation the act of coitus; from Latin, meaning "coupling or joining"
coraje a Chicano term meaning rage in response to a particular situation
cordotomy (chordotomy) surgical severing of the spinothalamic portion of the anterolateral tract of the spinal cord, usually for the purpose of relieving pain
core-gender identity *see* sexual identity
corium *see* dermis
corn a hardening and thickening of the skin forming a conical mass pointing downward into the corium
cornea the transparent covering of the anterior eye that connects with the sclera
corneal reflex irritation of the cornea resulting in a reflex closing of the eyelids
cornification hardening
coronal plane any line or plane dividing the body into anterior (ventral) and posterior (dorsal) portions at right angles to the sagittal plane
coroner a public official who is responsible for investigating any deaths that appear to be unnatural
corpus albicans a mass of white, scarred tissue that replaces the corpus luteum in the ovary when fertilization does not occur
corpus luteum a yellow body formed in the Graafian follicle after the ovum is discharged
cortical bone compact bone
corticoid a term applied to hormones of the adrenal cortex or substances with similar activity
cortisol the most abundant glucocorticoid; also called hydrocortisone
cortisone a hormone produced by the adrenal cortex that has antiinflammatory properties and is involved in the metabolism of glycogen to glucose
costovertebral angle the angle formed by a rib and the spine
cough a sudden expulsion of air from the lungs
counterirritant an agent that produces an irritation with the intent of relieving some other problem
CPR *see* cardiopulmonary resuscitation
cradle cap a yellowish, oily crusting of the scalp of infants
creatinine a nitrogenous waste that is excreted in the urine
credentialing (nursing) the process of determining and maintaining competence in nursing practice
Credé's maneuver manual exertion of pressure on the bladder to force urine out
cremaster the inner layer of striated muscle and connective tissue in the scrotum
crepitus a grating sound caused by bone fragments rubbing together
creps (crepitation) a dry, crackling sound like that of crumpled cellophane, produced by air in the subcutaneous tissue or by air moving through fluid in the alveoli of the lungs
crime an act committed in violation of societal law
criminal action a legal action dealing with disputes between an individual and society as a whole
criminal law law that deals with actions against the safety and welfare of the public
crisis in psychosocial terms, a rapid change or event that disturbs a person's psychologic homeostasis; in fever, the sudden reduction of an elevated body temperature
criterion a standard or model that can be used in judging
crown (of a tooth) the exposed part of the tooth outside the gum, covered by enamel

crutch a device with hand and arm supports used to facilitate walking
crutch palsy weakness of the hand, wrist, and forearm induced by prolonged pressure of a crutch on the axillary nerves
cryptorchidism failure of the testes to descend from the abdominal cavity to the scrotal sacs
crystalline amino acids refined protein used in hyperalimentation
crystalloid salts that dissolve readily in true solutions
culture in microbiology, the cultivation of microorganisms or cells in a special growth medium; in sociology, the beliefs and practices that are shared by people and passed down from generation to generation
culture shock the shock that can occur when an individual changes quickly from one social setting to another where former patterns of behavior are often ineffective
cumulative effect the effect of a drug when the level builds up in the blood
cunnilingus oral stimulation of the clitoris and labia by a partner
cupula a gelatinous dome-shaped structure of the inner ear that contains sensory hair cells
curandero (female: **curandera**) a healer within the Chicano community
curet a spoon-shaped instrument used for removing material from a body cavity
curettage removal of material from the wall of a cavity, e.g., the uterus, with a curet
cuticle the flat, thin rim of skin surrounding the nail
CVP *see* central venous pressure
cyanosis bluish discoloration of the skin, nail beds, and mucous membranes, due to reduced oxygen in the blood
cybernetics the science that deals with the process of communication and automatic control systems
cyst an enclosed cavity or sac lined by epithelium and containing liquid or semisolid material
cystic fibrosis a hereditary condition marked by the accumulation of thick and tenacious mucus in the lungs and the abnormal secretion of saliva and sweat
cystitis inflammation of the urinary bladder
cystocele protrusion of the urinary bladder through the vaginal wall
cystoscope a lighted instrument used to visualize the interior of the urinary bladder
cystoscopy visual examination of the urinary bladder with a cystoscope
cytology the study of the origin, structure, function, and pathology of cells

Dakin's solution a buffered aqueous solution of sodium hypochlorite used as a bactericide
dandruff a dry or greasy, scaly material shed from the scalp
data information
data base (baseline data) all information known about a patient; it includes the physician's history and physical examination, the nurse's assessment and history, and material contributed by other members of the health team
data collection the process of gathering information about a patient or client
deamination the removal of the amino (NH_2) groups by hydrolysis from amino acids
debilitated having lost strength
debride to remove foreign and dying tissue from a wound so that healthy tissue is exposed
deceased dead; a person who is dead
decerebrate posturing a posture indicative of midbrain damage, consisting of extension, adduction, and internal rotation of the arms; extension of the legs with the feet in plantar flexion; and arching of the back
decibel a unit used to measure or describe sound
deciduous teeth temporary teeth that are shed
decision (legal) the outcome of a trial, rendered by a judge
decisional law laws determined by the courts in ruling on cases, rather than by statutes
decoding the process of receiving a communication and converting the message into understandable terms
decortical posturing a posture indicative of damage to the internal capsule and corticospinal tracts above the brain stem; it consists of flexion and adduction of the fingers, wrists, and shoulders; extension and internal rotation of the legs and feet; and rigidity of all extremities
decubitus ulcer an ulcer of the skin and underlying tissues produced by prolonged pressure
decussate to cross over
deductive reasoning making specific observations from a generalization
deep breathing inhaling the maximum amount of air possible, then exhaling
defamation a communication that is injurious to a person
defecation expulsion of feces from the rectum and anus
defendant (legal) person who is claimed to have infringed the rights of another
defense mechanisms *see* adaptive mechanisms
dehiscence a splitting open or rupture
dehydration insufficient fluid in the body
delegate to authorize another as one's representative or to entrust authority to another
delirious experiencing mental confusion, restlessness, and incoherence
demineralization excessive loss of minerals or inorganic salts
demography the study of population statistics
demulcent a drug that coats the intestine, thus protecting the lining
denial an adaptive mechanism in which events, actions, or other matters are unconsciously denied
dental caries tooth decay
dental crown the exposed part of the tooth outside the gum, covered by enamel
dental floss waxed or unwaxed thread used for cleaning between the teeth and the gums
dental plaque deposits on the teeth that serve as a medium for bacterial growth
dental pulp cavity a space in the center of the tooth containing blood vessels and nerves
dental root the part of the tooth that is imbedded in the jaw
dentifrice a paste or powder used to clean or polish the teeth
dentin the internal part of the tooth crown below the enamel
dentures a natural or artificial set of teeth; usually the term designates artificial replacements for natural teeth
deoxyribonucleic acid (DNA) a nucleic acid found in all living cells; it is the carrier of genetic information
dependence reliance
dependent edema edema that collects in the lower parts of the body, where hydrostatic pressure is greatest
dependent nursing function activity by a nurse that is a result of a physician's order
depolarize to reduce toward a nonpolarized state; to cause loss of charge
depression feelings of sadness and dejection, often accompanied by physiologic change; a decrease of functional activity, as in depression of sensorium
dermatologic preparation a medication applied to the skin
dermis (corium) true skin, containing blood vessels, nerves, hair follicles, and glands
detrusor muscle the three layers of smooth muscle that make up the urinary bladder
detumescence the process of returning to a flaccid state, e.g., referring to the penis following ejaculation

development an individual's increasing capacity and skill in functioning, related to growth
developmental crisis a crisis that occurs as a result of stressors impeding development
developmental tasks skills and behavior patterns learned during development
dextrose a sugar; also called *glucose*
diagnosis a statement or conclusion concerning the nature of some phenomenon
diagnostic surgery surgery performed to confirm a diagnosis
dialyzing membrane a membrane that permits water molecules and crystalloids in true solution to move through it but not particles in a colloid dispersion
diapedesis the movement of blood corpuscles through a blood vessel wall
diaphoresis profuse sweating
diaphragm a musculomembranous partition that separates the abdominal and thoracic (chest) cavities
diarrhea defecation of liquid feces and increased frequency of defecation
diastole the period when the ventricles of the heart are relaxed
diastolic pressure the pressure of the blood against the arterial walls when the ventricles of the heart are at rest
diathermy the production of heat in body tissues by high-frequency electric currents
diet the food and fluid regularly consumed by an individual each day
dietitian a person who is skilled in the use of diets in health and disease
diffusion movement of gases or other particles from an area of greater pressure to an area of lower pressure or concentration; the continual intermingling of molecules in liquids, gases, or solids brought about by the random movement of the molecules
diffusion coefficient the rate of solubility of gases in the respiratory membrane
digital performed with the finger
dildo an artificial penis
diploid number the original number of chromosomes in all cells of the body (23 pairs in humans)
diplopia double vision
direct nursing activities activities by a nurse that are carried out in the presence of the patient
disaccharide a sugar consisting of double molecules
discovery (legal) pretrial activities designed to gain all the facts of a situation
disease a morbid (unhealthful) process having definite symptoms
disequilibrium a disturbed state of equilibrium, either mental or physical; an unbalanced condition
disinfectant an agent that destroys pathogens other than spores
disinfection the process by which an article is rendered free of pathogens
disorientation a state of mental confusion; loss of bearings, time, and place
displacement an adaptive mechanism in which an emotional reaction is transferred from one object to another
distal farthest from the point of reference
distention (abdominal) *see* tympanites
distraction a mechanism for relieving pain in which the person's attention is drawn away from the pain
diuresis *see* polyuria
diuretic an agent that increases the production of urine
dorsal of, toward, or at the back
dorsal column stimulator an electrode attached to the dorsal column of the spinal cord for the purpose of relieving pain
dorsal flexion movement of the ankle so that the toes are pointing up
dorsalis pedis pulse a pulse located on the instep of the foot
dorsal recumbent position a back-lying position with the head and shoulders slightly elevated
drain a substance or appliance (usually made of rubber or gauze) to assist in the discharge of drainage from a wound
drainage a discharge from a wound or cavity
dressing a material used to cover and protect a wound
drug (medication) a chemical compound taken for disease prevention, diagnosis, cure, or relief or to affect the structure or function of the body
drug abuse excessive intake of a substance either continually or periodically
drug allergy a hypersensitivity to a drug; the immunologic reaction to a drug
drug dependence inability to keep the intake of a drug or substance under control
drug habituation a mild form of psychologic dependence on a drug
drug interaction the beneficial or harmful interaction of one drug with another drug
drug misuse improper use of common medications in ways that can lead to acute and chronic toxicity
drug tolerance a condition in which successive increases in the dosage of a drug are required to maintain a given therapeutic effect
drug toxicity the quality of a drug that exerts a deleterious effect on an organism or tissue
DT diphtheria and tetanus toxoid
DTP diphtheria toxoid, tetanus toxoid, and pertussis vaccine
dullness (in percussion) decreased resonance or percussion sound that occurs when large amounts of fluid or pus collect in the alveoli
duodenocolic reflex a mass peristaltic movement of the colon stimulated by the presence of chyme in the duodenum
dura (dura mater) the outermost, fibrous membrane covering the brain and spinal cord
dyad a two-person group
dynamic electricity moving electric charges
dysfunction impaired functioning
dyspareunia pain experienced by a woman during intercourse
dyspepsia indigestion
dysphagia difficulty or inability to swallow
dysphasia difficulty speaking
dyspnea difficult and labored breathing in which the patient has a persistent unsatisfied need for air and feels distressed
dysuria painful or difficult urination

ecchymosis a blotchy area or discoloration of the skin; a bruise
ecchymotic appearing like a bruise
eccrine sweat gland a sweat gland that secretes outwardly via a duct
echolalia the repetition by a person of words addressed to him or her
eclampsia convulsions and coma associated with hypertension and proteinuria in pregnant women
ecology the study of the relationship of human beings and the environment
ectoderm the outermost of the three primary germ layers of the embryo
ectopic pregnancy the implantation of the fertilized ovum outside the uterus
ectropion a rolling out of the eyelid
edema excess interstitial fluid
edentulous without teeth
effector organ a muscle or gland that responds to nerve impulses
efferent conveying away from the center
effluent urine or feces discharged through a stoma
ego (Freud) the part of the psyche that maintains its identity; the conscious sense of self
egocentricity concern about oneself

egocentric speech self-centered, noncommunicative speech
ego integrity feeling satisfied with one's life-style and accepting the inevitability of one's life cycle
egophony a type of bronchophony in which the voice has a nasal, bleating quality
ejaculation expulsion of semen from the penis
ejaculatory ducts short tubes that pass through the prostate gland and terminate in the urethra
elective surgery surgery performed for a person's well-being but not absolutely necessary for life
Electra complex (Freud) the female child's attraction to her father; compare with *Oedipus complex*
electrocardiogram (ECG, EKG) a graph of the electric activity of the heart
electrocardiograph a machine that measures and records impulses from the heart on an electrocardiogram
electroencephalogram (EEG) a graph of the electric activity of the brain
electroencephalograph a machine that measures and records impulses from the brain on an electroencephalogram
electrolyte a chemical substance that develops an electric charge and is able to conduct an electric current when placed in water; an ion
electromyogram (EMG) a record of the electric potential created by the contraction of a muscle
electromyograph a machine that measures and records impulses from the muscles on an electromyogram
electron a negatively charged electric particle
emaciation excessive thinness
embalming a process of preserving a body chemically
embolus a blood clot (or a substance, such as air) that has moved from its place of origin and is obstructing the circulation in a blood vessel (plural: emboli)
embryo the derivative of a fertilized ovum that develops into the offspring
embryonic phase the period during which the fertilized ovum develops into an organism; it extends for first 8 or 12 weeks after conception
emesis vomit
emmetropia the normal refraction of the eye, which focuses objects on the retina
emollient an agent that soothes and softens skin or mucous membrane; often an oily substance
empacho a Chicano term for a disease seen primarily in children that includes a swollen abdomen as a result of intestinal blockage
empathy seeing or feeling a situation the way another person sees or feels it
emphysema a chronic obstructive lung disorder in which the terminal bronchioles become distended and plugged with mucus
empirical by observation or experience
emulsification a process by which lipids are broken up and evenly dispersed in an aqueous medium
emulsion a preparation in which one liquid is distributed throughout another
enamel (of a tooth) the hard, inorganic substance that covers the crown of a tooth
encoding the selection of specific signs and symbols to transmit a message
endemic present in a community all the time
endoderm (entoderm) the innermost of the three primary germ layers of the embryo
endogenous developing from within
endometrium the inner mucous membrane lining of the uterus
endorphin a polypeptide found throughout the body that is thought to relieve pain
endosteum the membrane lining a hollow bone
endothelium the layer of endothelial cells lining the blood vessels, cavities of the heart, and serous cavities
enema a solution injected into the rectum and the sigmoid colon
engorgement excessive fullness of an organ or passage
enkephalin a pentapeptide naturally occurring in the brain that has opiatelike effects
enteric referring to the intestines
enteric-coated surrounded with a special coating used for tablets and capsules that prevents release of the drug until it is in the intestines
enteric feeding a feeding administered directly into the small intestine through a tube
enteritis inflammation of the small intestine
enteroclysis the injection of a nutrient or drug into the colon
enterostomal therapist a person who specializes in ostomy care
enterostomy an opening through the abdominal wall into the intestines
entropion an inturned eyelid
enuresis bedwetting
environmental stimulus anything in the environment that arouses or incites action of a receptor (the terminus of a sensory nerve)
enzyme a biologic catalyst that speeds up chemical reactions
epidemic the occurrence of a disease in many people at the same time or in rapid succession in an area
epidemiology study of the occurrence and distribution of disease
epidermis the outermost, nonvascular layer of skin
epididymis a highly coiled duct between the seminiferous tubules of the testes and the vas deferens
epidural outside the dura mater
epidural block injection of an anesthetic between a lumbar interspace into the spinal canal (external to the dura mater)
epinephrine a hormone produced by the medulla of the adrenal glands; it is also manufactured artificially
epistaxis nosebleed
equilibrium a state of balance
erection (penile) lengthening, widening, and hardening of the penis as it becomes congested with blood during sexual arousal
erogenous sexually sensitive
erotic stimuli sensations that cause sexual arousal
eructation ejection of gas from the stomach (belching)
erythema redness that is associated with a variety of rashes
erythematous of the nature of erythema
erythroblastosis fetalis a condition produced in second and subsequent infants borne by Rh negative mothers when the father is Rh positive
erythrocyte red blood cell
erythropoiesis the formation of red blood cells
esophagoscopy visual examination of the interior of the esophagus with a lighted instrument
esophagus the muscular tube that extends from the pharynx to the stomach
espanto a Chicano term for a disease in which the individual is frightened by seeing supernatural spirits or events
ester a compound of alcohol and acid
estrogen a female sex hormone formed by the ovaries, the adrenal cortex, the testes, and the fetoplacental organ
ethics the rules or principles that govern right conduct
ethnic relating to races or to large groups of people with common traits and customs
ethnic group a set of individuals who share a unique cultural and social heritage passed on from one generation to another
ethnicity the condition of belonging to a specific ethnic group
ethnoscience systematic study of the way of life of a designated cultural group to obtain accurate data regarding behavior, perceptions, and interpretations of the universe
etiology cause
Eucharist *see* Holy Communion
eupnea normal respiration that is quiet, rhythmic, and effortless
eustachian (auditory) tube the tube that connects the middle ear with the nasopharynx

euthanasia the act or practice of killing for reasons of mercy
evacuator an instrument for removing fluid or small particles from a body cavity
evaluate to judge or appraise
evaluation the process of identifying the patient's progress toward achievement of established goals, using well-defined outcome criteria; judgment or appraisal
evaporation conversion of liquid into a vapor
eversion turning outward
evisceration extrusion of the internal organs
examine to inspect or investigate
excise to cut off or out
excoriation loss of the superficial layers of the skin
excretion elimination of a waste product produced by the body cells from the body
exhalation (expiration) the act of breathing out; the outflow of air from the lungs to the atmosphere
exophthalmos protruding eyeballs
exotoxin a toxic substance formed by bacteria and found outside the bacterial cell
expected date of confinement (EDC) the projected date of birth of a baby
expectorate to spit up mucus or other materials
expert witness one who by education or experience possesses knowledge that the ordinary layperson does not have
expiration (exhalation) the outflow of air from the lungs to the atmosphere
expiratory reserve volume the volume of air that can be forcefully exhaled after the normal tidal volume
expired dead
exploratory surgery surgery performed to confirm the extent of a pathologic process and sometimes to confirm a diagnosis
extended family the nuclear family plus other relatives such as uncles, aunts, and grandparents
extension increasing the angle of a joint (between two bones); the act of straightening
extensor (muscle) a muscle that acts to straighten a joint thus increasing the angle between two bones
external cardiac massage rhythmic massage of the heart muscle over the sternum
extracellular outside the cells
extracellular fluid (ECF) fluid found outside the body cells
extrathecal outside the sheath, e.g., outside the spinal canal
extravasation the escape of blood from a vessel into the body tissues
extreme unction the sacrament of anointing the sick
exudate material, e.g., fluid and cells, that has escaped from blood vessels and is deposited in tissues or on tissue surfaces during the inflammatory process

fad a practice followed for a time with exaggerated zeal
Fahrenheit a thermometer scale used to measure heat; the freezing point of water is 32 F, and the boiling point is 212 F
fantasy an adaptive mechanism in which wishes and desires are imagined as fulfilled
fasciculation abnormal contraction of a muscle involving the whole motor unit of the muscle
fastigium the highest point
fasting abstinence from eating
fat an organic substance that is greasy and insoluble in water; adipose tissue, a whitish-yellow tissue that forms soft pads between various body organs and serves as an energy reserve; an ester of glycerol with fatty acids
fatty acid the basic structural unit of fat
fear an emotional response to an actual, present danger
febrile pertaining to a fever; feverish
fecal impaction a mass of hardened feces in the folds of the rectum
fecal incontinence inability to control the passage of feces through the anus
feces body wastes and undigested food eliminated from the rectum
feedback a process that enables a system to regulate itself; the response to some of a system's output, which acts as intake for the purpose of exerting influence over a process; in communication, it is the response; in learning, it is the process of relating a person's performance to the desired goal
fellatio the oral stimulation of the male genitals by licking, blowing, or sucking
felony a crime of a serious nature punishable by imprisonment
femoral anteversion the forward tipping or tilting of the femur
femoral pulse the pulse found in the groin at the midpoint of the inguinal ligament
fenestrated perforated to provide a window or opening
fetal heartbeat the heartbeat of the fetus, generally heard through the maternal abdominal wall
fetal phase the stage of development from 8 or 12 weeks after conception until birth
fetus the unborn offspring in the postembryonic state of development
fever elevated body temperature
fiber an indigestible carbohydrate derived from plants
fibrillation involuntary contractions of a muscle; cardiac arrhythmia characterized by extremely rapid, irregular, and ineffective twitchings of the atria or ventricles
fibrin an insoluble protein formed from fibrinogen during the clotting of blood
fibrinous exudate exudate containing large amounts of fibrin
fibroplasia the formation of fibrous tissue
fibrous tissue common connective tissue composed of elastic and collagen fibers
figure-eight bandage a bandage turn usually used for flexed joints in which the bandage makes a figure-eight around and over the joint
first intention healing primary healing of a wound, which occurs when the tissue surfaces have been approximated
fissure a groove or deep fold such as that which separates the lobes of the lung
fistula an abnormal communication or passage usually between two organs or between an organ and the body surface
flaccid weak or lax
flaccid paralysis impaired muscle function with loss of muscle tone
flail chest the ballooning out of the chest wall through injured rib spaces during exhalation and the depression or indrawing of the wall during inhalation
flatness (in percussion) absence of resonance; extreme dullness
flatulence the presence of excessive amounts of gas in the stomach or intestines
flatus gas or air normally present in the stomach or intestines
flexion decreasing the angle of a joint (between two bones); the act of bending
flexor muscle a muscle that acts to bend a joint, decreasing the angle between two bones
flow sheet a record used to chart the progress of specific or specialized data, such as vital signs, fluid balance, or routine medications
flushing transient redness of the skin, often of the face and neck; it may be generalized or restricted to a particular area
follicle (hair) a pouchlike depression in the skin in which a hair is enclosed
follicle stimulating hormone (FSH) a hormone produced by the anterior pituitary gland (adenohypophysis) that stimulates the development of the ovarian follicle
follicular stage *see* preovulatory stage
foment *see* hot pack
fomite an inanimate object other than food that can harbor pathogenic microorganisms and transmit an infection

fontanelle an unossified membranous gap in the bone structure of the skull
footboard a board placed at the foot of a bed against which a patient can brace the feet
foot drop plantar flexion of the foot with permanent contracture of the gastrocnemius (calf) muscle and tendon
forceps an instrument with two blades and a handle used to grasp sterile supplies and to compress or grasp tissues
forensic medicine the application of medical knowledge to the law
foreplay physical stimulation to increase sexual arousal prior to intercourse; also called *precoital stimulation*
foreskin a covering fold of skin over the glans of the penis; also called the *prepuce*
formal operations stage (Piaget) the fourth cognitive developmental stage during 11 to 15 or 16 years
formulary a collection of prescriptions and formulas
Fowler's position a bed sitting position with the head of the bed raised to 45°
fracture a break in the continuity of bone
fracture board a support placed under the mattress of a bed to add rigidity
framework a basic structure supporting a thing
fraud false presentation of some fact or facts with the intention that the information will be acted on by another person
frenulum a fold of mucous membrane that attaches the tongue to the floor of the mouth; a fold on the lower surface of the glans penis that connects it with the prepuce
frequency (of urination) voiding at more frequent intervals than usual
friction rubbing; the force that opposes motion
friction rub *see* pleural rub
frigidity a low or nondetectable sex drive, usually applied to females
frontal plane the plane that divides the body into ventral and dorsal sections
frustration increased emotional tension due to inability to meet goals
fulcrum the fixed point of a lever
functionalis a layer of endometrium that is shed during menstruation
functional residual capacity expiratory reserve volume and the residual volume
funnel chest (pectus excavatum) a congenital defect in which the sternum is depressed and the anteroposterior diameter of the chest is narrowed

gait the way a person walks
gastric pertaining to the stomach
gastrocolic reflex increased peristalsis of the colon after food has entered the stomach
gastroenteritis inflammation of the stomach and the intestines
gastroscope a lighted instrument used to visualize the interior of the stomach
gastroscopy visual examination of the stomach with a gastroscope
gastrostomy a surgical opening that leads through the abdomen directly into the stomach
gauge (of a needle) the diameter of the shaft of a needle
gavage administration of nourishment to the stomach through a nasogastric or orogastric tube; tube feeding
gelatinous like jelly
gender behavior behavior with masculine or feminine connotations
gender identity a person's sense of being masculine or feminine as distinct from being male or female
gender role (sexual role) all that a person says or does to indicate whether the person is male or female
gene the biologic unit of heredity, located on a chromosome
general adaptation syndrome (GAS) a general response of the body to a stressor
generativity (Erikson) concern for establishing and guiding the next generation
genitals the reproductive organs, usually the external ones
genital stage (Freud) the final stage of maturity of an adult
genupectoral position a position in which the weight is borne by the patient's knees and chest and the body is at a 90° angle to the hips
genu valgum a condition in which the medial aspects of the knees touch in the standing position while the feet remain apart; knock-knees
genu varum a condition in which, when the feet are held together, the knees remain apart; bowlegs
geographic poverty the existence of poverty in certain geographic areas of the country
geriatrics the branch of medicine pertaining to elderly people
germicidal possessing the ability to kill microorganisms
germicide an agent that kills some pathogens
gerontology the study of all aspects of the problems of aging
gingiva the gum tissue
gingivitis inflammation of the gums
glans clitoris the exposed part of the clitoris
glans penis the cap-shaped, expansive structure at the end of the penis
glaucoma an eye disease characterized by an increase in intraocular pressure that produces changes in the optic disc and the field of vision
glomerular filtrate fluid formed in the nephron of the kidney that is similar to plasma in composition; the precursor of urine
glossitis inflammation of the tongue
glottis the vocal apparatus of the larynx
glucagon a hormone produced by the alpha cells of the islands of Langerhans in the pancreas; it stimulates the breakdown of liver glycogen
glucocorticoid a hormone produced by the adrenal glands that influences the metabolism of glucose, protein, and fat
gluconeogenesis the process by which the liver converts proteins and fats into glucose
glucose a monosaccharide occurring in food
glycerol the alcohol component of fats
glycogen the chief carbohydrate stored in the body, particularly in the liver and muscles
glycogenesis formation of glycogen
glycogenolysis the breakdown of glycogen to reform glucose
glycolysis the release of energy through the breakdown of glucose
glycosuria the presence of glucose in the urine; glucosuria
goal the end to which a design tends or that a person aims to reach or accomplish; a statement of intent or concern
gonad an ovary or testis
gonorrhea a sexually transmitted (venereal) infection due to *Neisseria gonorrhoeae*
Goodell's sign the softening of the cervix during pregnancy
Good Samaritan act a law that protects physicians and sometimes nurses when rendering aid to a person in an emergency
gout a condition characterized by excessive uric acid in the blood
Graafian follicle a small sac, embedded in the ovary, that encloses an ovum
granulation tissue young connective tissue with new capillaries formed in the wound healing process
granulosa cells a single layer of cells that surrounds the ovum
gravity the force that pulls objects toward the center of the earth
grief emotional suffering often caused by bereavement
grounding process of making an electrical connection between a conductor and the earth or a large body of zero potential
group two or more persons who have shared needs or goals
group dynamics (process) forces that determine the behavior of the group and its members

growth an increase in weight and height; an increase in physical size; the proliferation of cells
guilt the painful emotion associated with transgression of moral-ethical beliefs
gustatory referring to the sense of taste
gynecology the branch of medicine that deals with processes of the female reproductive tract
gynosperm sperm bearing an X chromosome

habitus physique; body build or body type
hair follicle a pouchlike depression in the skin enclosing the root of a hair
hair shaft the visible part of the hair
halitosis bad breath
hallucinate to perceive through the senses something unreal; such as hearing voices or seeing things that do not exist
hallucinogens drugs that cause distortion of the sensory perception
hangnail a shred of epidermal tissue at either side of the nail
haploid number the number of chromosomes (23 single) found in human sperm and egg cells
hapten a substance free of protein that can interact with other substances on antibodies but does not itself cause the formation of antibodies
Harris tube a single-lumen tube with a metal tip that is inserted through the mouth into the intestines
haustrum a saclike formation of a part of the colon, produced by contraction of both the longitudinal and the circular muscles (plural: haustra)
head mirror a mirror worn on the examiner's head that directs light onto an area being examined
health a state of being physically fit, mentally stable, and socially comfortable; it encompasses more than the state of being free of disease
health beliefs concepts about health that an individual believes are true
health-illness continuum a continuum (continuous process) with high-level wellness at one end and death at the other
health maintenance organization (HMO) an organization that provides a wide range of health services on a fixed contract basis, usually geared to preventive medicine
health practice an activity that a person carries out as a result of his or her health beliefs and definition of health
health practitioner a person who provides a health care service
health problem any condition or situation in which a patient requires help to maintain or regain a state of health or to achieve a peaceful death
health state the health of a person at a given time
health team a group of individuals with varying skills whose cooperative efforts are designed to assist people with their health
hectic fever *see* septic fever
Hegar's sign the softening of the lower portion of the uterus during pregnancy
height a vertical measurement extending from the highest point on the head to the surface on which the individual is standing, normally measured in centimeters or inches
hemangioma a large, persistent, bright red or dark purple vascular area of the skin
hematemesis the vomiting of blood
hematocrit the percentage of red blood cell mass in proportion to whole blood
hematoma a collection of blood in a tissue, organ, or body space due to a break in the wall of a blood vessel
hematuria the presence of blood in the urine
hemiplegia the loss of movement on one side of the body
hemoglobin the red pigment in red blood cells that carries oxygen
hemoglobinuria the presence of hemoglobin in the urine
hemolysis rupture of red blood cells
hemopneumothorax a collection of blood and air or gas in the pleural cavity
hemoptysis the presence of blood in the sputum
hemorrhage bleeding; the escape of blood from the blood vessels
hemorrhoids distended veins in the rectum
hemosiderosis deposition of iron in the skin, liver, spleen, and other organs
hemostat (artery forceps) a small pair of forceps used to constrict blood vessels
hemothorax a collection of blood in the pleural cavity
heparin a substance that prevents coagulation of blood
herb a leafy plant that does not have a wood stem and is valued for its medicinal, savory, or aromatic qualities
herbalist an herb doctor; one who prescribes herbs for treating people
Hering-Breuer reflex a reflex that inhibits inspiration
hesitancy (of urination) delay and difficulty initiating voiding
hex a jinx; a spell imposed in witchcraft
high Fowler's position a bed sitting position in which the head of the bed is elevated 90°
hirsutism abnormal hairiness, particularly in women
histology the study of the structure and function of tissues
holism the view that a person is more than the sum of many parts
holophrastic speech a type of speech in which one word expresses a whole sentence
Holy Communion a memorial sacrament practiced by Christians based on the mandate of Jesus Christ at the Last Supper; it is also called the *Eucharist* or the *Lord's Supper*
homeodynamics the continual exchange of energy between human beings and the external environment
homeostasis tendency of the body to maintain a state of balance or equilibrium while continually changing
homogamy mating like with like; inbreeding; reproduction resulting from the union of two identical cells
homogeneity a high degree of likeness of attitudes and beliefs among members of a group
homosexual a person whose primary sexual orientation is to a member of the same sex
hormone a chemical substance that is produced by the body and secreted into the bloodstream and that regulates the activity of certain body organs
hospice a health care facility for the dying
hostility overt antagonism; behavior in which the individual tends to be harmful or destructive
hot pack (foment) a hot moist cloth applied to an area of the body
human chorionic gonadotropin (HCG) a hormone produced by the placenta in the first trimester of pregnancy
humanism concern for human attributes
human placental lactogen *see* chorionic somatomammotropin
humidity the amount of moisture in the air, expressed as a percentage
hunger an unpleasant sensation caused by deprivation of something, especially food
hyaluronidase an enzyme found in tissues; it catalyzes hydrolysis of hyaluronic acid, the cement substance of tissues
hydration the act of combining or being combined with water
hydraulics the branch of physics that deals with the physical actions of liquids
hydrocephalus a disease process resulting in excessive cerebrospinal fluid within the skull
hydrocortisone an adrenocortical steroid produced by the adrenal glands or produced synthetically; also called *cortisol*
hydrolysates hydrolyzed proteins or amino acids
hydrolysis the process of splitting a molecule in the presence of digestive enzymes with the addition of water
hydrometer an instrument used to determine the specific gravity of a fluid

hydrostatic pressure the pressure a liquid exerts on the sides of the container that holds it; also called *filtration force*
hygiene the science of health and its maintenance
hymen a thin fold of mucous membrane separating the vagina from the vestibule
hyperalgesia extreme sensitivity to pain
hyperalimentation administration of hypertonic solutions of carbohydrates, amino acids, and lipids by indwelling intravenous catheters placed into superficial veins or into the superior vena cava via the jugular or subclavian veins; also called *total parenteral nutrition* (TPN)
hypercalcemia excessive calcium in the blood
hypercalciuria excessive calcium in the urine
hyperemia increased blood flow to an area
hyperextension further extension between two bones or stretching out of a joint
hyperextension position a bed position with the head and foot of the bed lowered to form a 15° angle in the bed foundation
hyperglycemia an increased concentration of glucose in the blood
hyperkalemia excessive potassium in the blood
hypernatremia an elevated level of sodium in the blood plasma
hyperopia farsightedness
hyperphosphatemia increased phosphorus levels in the blood
hyperplasia an abnormal increase in the number of cells in a tissue or an organ
hyperpnea an abnormal increase in the rate and depth of respirations
hyperpyrexia an extremely elevated body temperature
hyperreflexia an exaggeration of the reflexes
hyperresonance a lower-pitched sound than resonance
hypersensitivity an exaggerated response of the body to a foreign substance
hypersomnia excessive sleep
hypertension an abnormally high blood pressure
hyperthermia an abnormally high body temperature, sometimes induced as a therapeutic measure
hypertonicity excessive muscle tone or activity
hypertonic solution a fluid possessing a greater concentration of solutes than plasma has
hypertrophy an increase in size of a cell, tissue, or body organ such as a muscle
hyperventilation an increase in the amount of air entering the lungs, characterized by prolonged and deep breaths
hypervolemia an abnormal increase in the body's blood volume
hypnosis an abnormally induced passive state in which an individual responds to suggestions that do not conflict with the person's conscious or unconscious desires
hypnotic (drug) a drug that induces sleep
hypoalbuminemia reduction in the level of albumin in the blood
hypocalcemia decreased calcium in the blood serum
hypochloremia a reduced concentration of chlorides in the blood
hypodermic *see* subcutaneous
hypodermis (subcutaneous tissue) connective tissues beneath the skin
hypodermoclysis the introduction of fluid into the subcutaneous tissues
hypofibrinogenemia an abnormally low level of fibrinogen in the blood
hypoglycemia a reduced amount of glucose in the blood
hypokalemia an abnormally low amount of potassium in the blood
hyponatremia an abnormally low amount of sodium in the blood plasma
hypophosphatemia phosphorus deficiency in the blood
hypophysis *see* pituitary gland
hypostatic pneumonia an infection of lung tissue resulting from poor circulation or stagnation of secretions
hypotension an abnormally low blood pressure
hypothalamus the part of the brain beneath the thalamus that forms the floor and part of the wall of the third ventricle
hypothermia an abnormally low body temperature
hypothesis an assumption made to test its logical or empirical consequences
hypotonicity decreased muscle tone
hypotonic solution a fluid possessing a lesser concentration of solutes than plasma has
hypoventilation a reduction in the amount of air entering the lungs, characterized by shallow respirations
hypovolemia reduction in blood volume
hypovolemic shock a state of shock due to a reduction in the volume of circulating blood
hypoxemia deficient oxygenation of the blood, measured by laboratory means
hypoxia diminished availability of oxygen for the body tissues, due to internal or external causes
hysterectomy surgical removal of the uterus

iatrogenic caused by the physician or medical therapy
id (Freud) the unconscious part of the personality that contains primitive desires and urges and is ruled by the pleasure principle
ideational forming images or objects in the mind
identification an adaptive mechanism by which one feels or thinks as another person does
idiosyncratic effect a different, unexpected, or individual effect from the normal one usually expected from a medication; the occurrence of unpredictable and unexplainable symptoms
ileocecal valve membranous folds between the distal ileum and the entrance to the large intestine (cecum)
ileostomy an artificial opening of the small intestine on the abdomen
ileum the distal portion of the small intestine
illness sickness or deviation from a healthy state or the normal functioning of the total person
illusion a false interpretation of some stimulus
imagination creation by the mind; forming a mental image of something not present to stimulate the senses
imitation copying the behaviors and attitudes of another person
immobility prescribed or unavoidable restriction of movement in any area of a person's life
immunity a specific resistance of the body to infection; it may be natural, endowed resistance or resistance developed after exposure to a disease agent
immunization the process of becoming immune or rendering someone immune
immunoglobulin a part of the body's plasma proteins; also called *immune bodies* or *antibodies*
immunologic reaction production of antibodies in response to an antigen; an allergic reaction
impaction a condition of being firmly wedged or lodged; in reference to feces, a collection of hardened puttylike feces in the folds of the rectum
imperforate abnormally closed; used to describe an opening, such as the anus or the hymen, that is not open
impotence inability to achieve or to maintain an erection sufficiently to perform intercourse
impregnation fertilization of the ovum
incision a cut or wound that is intentionally made, e.g., during surgery
incoherent engaging in actions or speech that lacks cohesion, orderly continuity, relevance, or consistency
incontinence inability to control the elimination of urine (enuresis) or feces (fecal incontinence)
incorporation a process by which people or objects are internalized and become a part of one's understanding

incubation period the time between entrance of a pathogen into the body and the onset of symptoms of the infection
incurvated (ingrown) nail a nail that has grown so that it impinges into surrounding soft tissues
independence self-reliance and self-assertiveness
independent nurse practitioner a nurse who practices independently in the health care system
independent nursing function an activity carried out in the nurse's judgment without the physician's direct order
individual patient supply system (of drugs) medications supplied separately for each patient in specified doses and quantities for a specified period of time
inductive reasoning making generalizations from specific data
induration hardening
infarct a localized area of necrosis (dead cells) usually owing to obstructed arterial blood flow to the part
infection the disease process produced by microorganisms
inference derivation of a conclusion from facts or premises and movement beyond the information to predict or explain
inferential reasoning solving problems by means of inference
inferential statistics statistics that are inferred by generalization from other statistics
inferior situated below
infestation invasion of the body by insects, mites, and/or ticks
infiltration the diffusion or deposition into tissue of substances that are not normal to it
inflammation the tissue response to injury or destruction of cells
influence (in a group) the result of the proper use of power
informed consent *see* consent
infradian rhythm a biorhythm that cycles monthly, such as the human menstrual cycle
infrared heat a radiant type of heat capable of penetrating body tissues to a depth of 10 mm; sources of infrared rays include heat lamps and incandescent light bulbs
infusion the introduction of fluid into a vein or part of the body
ingestion the act of taking in food or medication
ingrown toenail penetration of the edges of the toenail plate into the surrounding tissues
inhalation (inspiration) the act of breathing in; the intake of air or other substances into the lungs
inhalation therapist a respiratory technologist skilled in therapies for patients with respiratory problems
inner canthus the corner of the upper and lower eyelids near the nose
inorganic having no organs; not of organic origin; in chemistry, acids or compounds that do not contain carbon
input information, material, or energy that enters a system
inquest a legal inquiry into the cause or manner of a death
insensible perspiration unnoticeable sweating that evaporates immediately once it reaches the surface of the skin
insertion (of a muscle) the more movable point of attachment of a muscle
insomnia inability to obtain a sufficient quality or quantity of sleep
inspection visual examination to detect features perceptible to the eye
inspiration (inhalation) the act of drawing air into the lungs
inspiratory capacity the tidal volume plus the inspiratory reserve volume
inspiratory reserve volume the volume of air that can be inhaled beyond the normal tidal volume
instillation application of a medication into a body cavity or orifice
insufflator an instrument used to blow air into a part of body, e.g., the rectum
insulator a substance or material that inhibits conduction, e.g., of heat or electricity
insulin a hormone secreted by the beta cells of the islands of Langerhans in the pancreas; also a preparation for administration
integument the skin or covering of the body
integumentary system the skin, hair, and nails
intelligence ability to learn
intensity (in percussion) the loudness or softness of a sound
intercostal between the ribs
intercostal retractions indrawing between the ribs
interdependence a balance between dependence and independence
interdigital between the digits (toes and fingers)
intermittent (quotidian) fever a fever that recurs daily
intermittent positive pressure breathing (IPPB) a breathing pattern in which the lungs are inflated with positive pressure and deflated passively
intern a graduate of a basic health program who is taking planned practical experience, such as nursing or medicine, usually to obtain a license to practice
internal feedback positive or negative responses from oneself about a communication one has given either in writing or verbally
interstitial between the cells of the body's tissues
interstitial cells of Leydig clusters of cells, located between the seminiferous tubules, that secrete male hormones
interstitial fluid fluid found between the body cells
intervention activities performed by the nurse and the patient to change the effect of a problem
intervertebral between the vertebrae
interview a structured consultation used to obtain information or to evaluate the progress of a person
intestinal distention (tympanites) stretching and inflation of the intestines due to the presence of air or gas
intraarterial within or inside an artery
intracardiac within or into the heart muscle
intracellular within a cell or cells
intracellular fluid (cellular fluid, ICF) fluid found within the body cells
intractable pain pain that is resistant to cure or relief
intradermal (intracutaneous) within the skin
Intralipid trademark for an intravenous fat solution that provides concentrated calories during total parenteral nutrition
intramuscular within or inside muscle tissue
intraosseous within or into the bone
intrapleural within the pleural cavity
intrapleural pressure pressure within the pleural cavity
intrapulmonic pressure pressure within the lungs
intraspinal *see* intravertebral
intrathecal within or into the spinal canal
intrauterine inside the uterus
intrauterine device (IUD) a device inserted into the uterus for contraception
intravascular within a blood vessel
intravascular fluid plasma
intravenous within a vein
intravenous cholangiogram an x-ray film of the bile ducts after a contrast dye has been administered intravenously
intravenous pyelogram an x-ray film of the kidneys taken after intravenous injection of a radiopaque dye
intravenous pyelography (IVP) x-ray filming of the kidney and ureters after injection of a radiopaque material intravenously; also called *intravenous urography*
intravenous urography (IVU) *see* intravenous pyelography
intravertebral (intraspinal) within the vertebrae
introjection unconscious acceptance and incorporation of the patterns, attitudes, and ideals of another person as one's own
introversion direction of one's energy and interest toward oneself
intubation insertion of a tube
inunction application of a topical drug to the skin or mucous membrane for absorption
inversion a turning inward

invisible poverty social and cultural deprivation
involution a rolling or turning inward of a particular organ or the entire body, e.g., the uterus after the fetus is expelled
internal rotation a turning toward the midline, e.g., rotation of the hip joint
ion an atom or group of atoms that carry a positive or negative electric charge; an electrolyte
iris the colored, circular membrane of the eye, situated behind the cornea, in the center of which is the pupil
irradiation exposure to penetrating rays, such as x-rays, gamma rays, infrared rays, or ultraviolet rays
irrational confused as to time, place, and/or person
irrigation (lavage) the washing of a body cavity or a wound
irritant a substance that stimulates unpleasant responses, that is, irritates
ischemia lack of blood supply to a body part
islands of Langerhans clusters of endocrine-secreting cells located in the pancreas
isolation *see* protective asepsis
isometric having the same measure or length
isometric muscle contraction tensing of a muscle against an immovable outer resistance, which does not change muscle length or produce joint motion
isometric static exercise exercise in which the patient consciously increases the tension of the muscle without moving the joint
isotonic having the same tonicity as the body fluids; the term is used to compare solutions of the same strength or concentration
isotonic exercise active exercise involving muscle contractions in which there is a marked shortening of muscle length
isotonic muscle contraction shortening of a muscle in the process of doing work that produces joint motion (e.g., range-of-motion exercises or weight lifting)
isthmus a narrow passage connecting two larger parts of an organ

jargon the technical or idiomatic terminology characteristic of a particular group
jaundice a yellowish tinge to the skin and mucous membrane
jejunum the portion of the small intestine that extends from the duodenum to the ileum

Kardex a portable card index file that organizes data about patients in a concise way and often contains nursing care plans
Kelly forceps a type of hemostat
keratin the protein found in epidermis, hair, and nails
keratinized cells dead cells that have been converted to protein
keratotic spots horny growths, such as warts or calluses
ketogenesis the process in which deaminated amino acids are converted into fatty acids, producing ketone bodies (acetone)
ketone any compound containing the carbonyl group, CO, and having hydrocarbon groups attached to the carbonyl group
ketosis a condition in which excessive ketones are formed in the body
kilocalorie (Calorie) the amount of heat required to raise the temperature of 1 kilogram of water 1 degree centigrade
kilogram a unit of weight equal to 1000 grams or approximately 2.2 pounds
kinesiology the study of the motion of the human body
kinesthesia the sense of awareness of the position and the movement of the body parts
kinesthetic referring to awareness of body position and movement
knee-chest position *see* genupectoral position
Korotkoff's sounds sounds of blood produced within the artery with each ventricular contraction
kosher sanctioned by Jewish law
Kussmaul breathing (Kussmaul-Kien respiration) a dyspnea occurring in paroxysms often preceding diabetic coma; air hunger
kwashiorkor a condition occurring in children after weaning as a result of protein and calorie malnutrition; evidenced by growth failure, potbelly, edema, and mental apathy
kyphosis an exaggerated convexity in the thoracic region of the vertebral column, resulting in a stooped posture

labia the fleshy edges of a structure, usually the female genitals
labia majora the two longitudinal folds or lips of skin extending downward and backward from the mons pubis that protect the vaginal and urethral orifices
labia minora small folds of skin lying between the labia majora and the vaginal opening
labored breathing difficult or dyspneic breathing
labyrinth a system of interconnecting canals or cavities
lacerate to tear, rather than cut, a body tissue
lacrimal fluid tears produced by the lacrimal glands that lubricate the eye
lacrimal glands organs that are situated in a depression in the frontal bone at the upper, outer angle of the eye orbit, and that secrete tears
lacrimal sac the opening connecting the tear ducts in the inner canthus of the eye to the nasolacrimal duct, which empties into the nasal cavity
lacrimation the secretion and discharge of tears
lactase an enzyme that acts as a catalyst to convert lactose into glucose and galactose
lactation the secretion of milk; the period of milk secretion
lactiferous conveying or producing milk
lactose a carbohydrate found in milk
lalling repetitive sounds infants make based on what they hear
lanugo fine, woolly hair or down on the shoulders, back, sacrum, and earlobes of the unborn child; it may remain for a few weeks after birth
laryngeal mirror an instrument like a dental mirror used to view the pharynx, larynx, or structures of the mouth
laryngeal stridor a harsh, crowing sound heard during expiration when there is a laryngeal obstruction
laryngoscope a lighted instrument used to visualize the larynx
laryngoscopy visual examination of the larynx with a laryngoscope
laryngospasm spasmodic closure of the larynx
larynx a structure composed of nine cartilages guarding the entrance of the trachea and containing the vocal cords
latency period (Freud) the school-age years (6 to 12 years)
lateral to the side, away from the midline
lateral position a side-lying position
lavage an irrigation or washing of a body organ, such as the stomach
laxative a medication that stimulates bowel activity
learning a permanent change in behavior
learning need a need to change behavior
learning principle an assumption thought to facilitate and maximize learning
legume the fruit or pod of a leguminous plant, such as a pea or bean
lens a transparent, convex body that is the focusing device of the eye
lesion the traumatic or pathologic interruption of a tissue or the loss of function of a body part
lethargy drowsiness; sleeping much of the time when not stimulated
leukocyte a white blood cell
leukocytosis an increase in the number of white blood cells
lever a rigid bar that moves on a fixed axis called a fulcrum
leverage force applied with the use of a lever
Levin tube a single-lumen nasogastric tube
liability the quality or state of being liable
liable legally responsible for one's obligations and actions and obliged to make financial restitution for wrongful acts
libel defamation by means of print, writing, or pictures

libido (Freud) the urge or desire for sexual activity; the energy form or life instinct; also called *sex drive* and *sexual motivation*
license a legal document authorizing an individual to offer knowledge and skills to the public
life expectancy the age to which a person is expected to live
life-style the values and behaviors adopted by a person in daily life
ligament a broad, fibrous band that holds two or more bones together
lightening the descent of the uterus into the pelvic cavity, which usually occurs 2 to 3 weeks before labor begins
line of gravity an imaginary vertical line running through the center of gravity
lingula (of the lung) the superior and inferior segments at the lower half of the long upper lobe of the left lung
liniment a topical liquid applied to the skin frequently to stimulate circulation or to relieve pain
lipid *see* fat
lithotomy position a back-lying position in which the feet are supported in stirrups
living will a statement of a person's wish not to be kept alive by artificial means or "heroic measures"
livor mortis discoloration of the tissues of the body after death
lobar pneumonia an infectious disease of one or more lobes of the lung
lobe a well-defined portion of an organ, e.g., of the lung or brain
local adaptation syndrome (LAS) the reaction of one organ or body part to stress
lochia the vaginal discharge that occurs during the 1st week or 2 after the birth of a baby
lordosis an exaggerated concavity in the lumbar region of the vertebral column
loss an actual or potential situation in which a valued ability, object, person, etc., is inaccessible or changed so that it is perceived as no longer valuable
lotion a liquid that often carries an insoluble powder
louse a parasitic insect that infests mammals (plural: lice)
lumbar puncture (LP, spinal tap) the insertion of a needle into the subarachnoid space at the lumbar region
lumen a channel within a tube, such as the channel of an artery in which blood flows
lung compliance expansibility of the lung
lung recoil the tendency of lungs to collapse away from the chest wall
luteal stage *see* postovulatory stage
lymph a transparent, slightly yellow fluid found within the lymphatic vessels
lymphadenitis inflammation of the lymph nodes
lymphangitis the inflammation of a lymphatic vessel or vessels
lymphatic referring to lymph or lymph vessels
lysis (of a fever) the gradual reduction of an elevated body temperature to normal
lysosome a minute body found in many types of cells; it is involved in intracellular digestion
lysozyme an enzyme in saliva and tears that functions as an antibacterial agent

maceration the wasting away or softening of a solid as if by the action of soaking; often used to describe degenerative changes and eventual disintegration
macrocephaly an abnormally large size of the head
macrophage a large phagocytic cell that destroys microorganisms or harmful cells
malaise a general feeling of being unwell or indisposed
mal de ojo among Chicanos, the belief that disease can result from admiring a part of another person's body, e.g., the hair
malignancy abnormal tissue with a tendency to grow and invade other tissues
malingering the willful feigning of the symptoms of illness to avoid facing something unpleasant
malleolus a rounded prominence on the distal end of the tibia or fibula
malnutrition a disorder of nutrition; insufficient nourishment of the body cells
malpractice professional misconduct or unreasonable lack of professional skill
mammary glands breast tissues that secrete nourishment for the young
mandatory licensure laws that require all persons practicing in a field, such as nursing, to be licensed
manometer an instrument used to measure the pressure of fluids or gases
manslaughter an unlawful killing without previous intent; it is a felony
marasmus a condition of children under 1 year as a result of protein and calorie malnutrition; it is evidenced by wasting, wrinkled skin, thinness, eyes appearing large
margination the aggregating or lining up of substances along a surface or edge, e.g., the lining up of white blood cells against the wall of a blood vessel during the inflammatory process
marijuana an intoxicating agent from the leaves and flowers of the plant *Cannabis sativa*; commonly used in cigarettes and inhaled as smoke
mastectomy surgical removal of the breast
masticate to chew, e.g., food
mastication chewing
masturbation self-stimulation of the genitals or other body parts to derive erotic pleasure
material culture objects, such as eating utensils, and the ways these are used by a society
matriarchy a system of social organization in which the mother is the head of the house or family
matrilineal relating to descent through the female line
maturation the process of becoming mature or fully developed; development of inherited traits
meatus an opening, passage, or channel
mechanosensitive pain receptors pain receptors stimulated by mechanical stimuli
meconium a dark green, mucilaginous material found in the intestines of the newborn
medial toward the middle or midline
medical asepsis practices that limit the number, growth, and spread of microorganisms; clean technique
medical examiner a physician who investigates deaths that appear unnatural and who has advanced education in pathology and forensic medicine
medication (medicine, drug) a chemical or biologic compound administered to humans or animals for disease prevention, cure, or relief, or to affect the structure or function of the body
meiosis a specialized type of cell division that occurs in sperm and egg cells
melanin the dark pigment of the skin
menarche the first menstrual period, occurring sometime between the ages of 9 and 17
meniscus the crescent-shaped structure of the surface of a column of liquid; the crescent-shaped cartilage in the knee joint
menopause cessation of menstruation in the human female, usually occurring between ages 45 and 50
menses menstrual flow
mental defense mechanisms *see* adaptive defense mechanisms
mental well-being a state of contentment, peace of mind, and satisfaction with living and life
mesoderm the middle layer of the three primary developmental germ layers in the ermbryo; it lies between the endoderm and the ectoderm

metabolism the sum of all the physical and chemical processes by which living substance is formed and maintained and by which energy is made available for use by the organism
metacarpal referring to the part of the hand between the wrist and the fingers
metatarsus adductus adduction of the anterior part of the foot with no deformity of the posterior part of the foot
microcephaly an abnormally small size of the head
microglia a type of nerve tissue with migratory cells that act as phagocytes to the waste products of nerve tissues
micronutrient nutrients, such as vitamins and minerals, required in small quantities by the body
microorganism minute living body visible under a microscope
micturate (urinate, void) to pass urine from the body
micturition (urination, voiding) the voluntary expulsion of urine
midclavicular line an imaginary line that runs inferiorly and vertically from the center of the clavicle
midsternal line an imaginary line that runs vertically through the middle of the sternum
milia (whiteheads) small, white nodules usually found over the nose and face of newborns
miliaria rubra a prickly heat rash of the face, neck, trunk, or perineal area of infants
Miller-Abbott tube a double-lumen tube inserted through the nose or mouth into the intestine
milliequivalent (mEq) one-thousandth of an equivalent, which is the chemical combining power of a substance
milliliter (ml) a unit of volume in the metric system approximating 1 cubic centimeter
millimol one-thousandth of a mol
mineralocorticoid a steroid hormone of the adrenal cortex that acts to retain sodium in the body and to excrete potassium
minim the least; the basic unit of volume in the apothecaries' system, equal to 0.0616 ml
misdemeanor a crime less serious than a felony and punishable by a fine or short-term imprisonment or both
mitering a method of folding the bedclothes at the bed corners to maintain them securely
mitosis the process of cell division; the process by which the body replaces cells and grows
MMR combined measles, mumps, and rubella vaccine
mobility ability to move about feely
model a pattern of something to be made
mol a molar solution of a substance
mongolian spots blue or black spots of varying size found largely in the sacral area of Oriental and black infants
monologue a long speech that occurs when there is no listener or responder
monosaccharide a sugar consisting of single molecules
mons pubis a pillow of adipose tissue situated over the symphysis pubis and covered by coarse hair; also called the *mons veneris*
Montgomery's glands sebaceous glands in the areola of the nipple that become enlarged and prominent during pregnancy
Montgomery straps tie tapes used to hold dressings in place
morbidity incidence of disease
mores values of members in a group
morgue a place where dead bodies are temporarily kept before release to a mortician
morning sickness the nausea and vomiting that occur frequently in the mornings during the first trimester of pregnancy
Moro's reflex the startle reflex of infants, in which the arms and legs are extended outward and retracted in response to a sudden stimulus such as a loud noise
morphology form and structure
mortality death; the death rate
mortician a person trained in the care of the dead; also called an *undertaker*
motivation desire
mourning the process through which grief is eventually resolved or altered
mucin the chief constituent of mucus
mucolytic destroying or dissolving mucus
mucous membrane epithelial tissue that forms mucus, concentrates bile, and secretes or excretes enzymes
mucus the lubricating, free slime of the mucous membranes
murmur (cardiac) harsh, rumbling sounds resulting from turbulent blood flow
mydriatic a medication that dilates the pupils of the eyes
myelogram an x-ray film of the spinal cord, nerve roots, and vertebrae after injection of a contrast media into the subarachnoid space
myocardial infarction cardiac tissue necrosis resulting from obstruction of the blood flow to the heart
myocardium the heart muscle; the middle layer of the heart tissue
myometrium the middle, thick, smooth muscle layer of the uterus
myopia nearsightedness

narcolepsy a condition in which an individual experiences an uncontrollable desire for sleep or attacks of sleep at certain intervals
narcotic a strong analgesic
narcotic agonist-antagonist a drug with properties that simulate a narcotic and with properties that act against the effects of a narcotic
narrative notes records of a patient's day-to-day progress which may be keyed to the SOAP format in the POMR or keyed chronologically in traditional patient records
nasogastric tube a plastic or rubber tube inserted through the nose into the stomach
nasopharynx the upper part of the pharynx adjoining the nasal passage
naturopath a nonmedical practitioner who uses such things as light, heat, and water in therapy, but not drugs
nausea the urge to vomit
nebulizer an atomizer or sprayer
necessary cause the one factor that must be present for a specific disease to occur
necrosis nonliving cells or tissue in contact with living cells
necrotic dying
need the lack of something requisite, desirable, or useful
negative feedback (homeostasis) a mechanism in which deviations from normal are sensed and counteracted
negative nitrogen balance a nitrogen output that exceeds nitrogen intake
negligence the omission of something a reasonable person would do or the doing of something a reasonable person would not do; an unintentional tort
neonatal mortality infant death within 28 days of birth
neoplasm any growth that is new and abnormal
nephritis inflammation of a kidney
nephron the functional unit of the kidney
nephrosis a disease of the kidney in which there is malfunctioning kidney tissue without inflammation; also called *nephrotic syndrome*
nerve block chemical interruption of a nerve pathway effected by injecting a local anesthetic
neurectomy interruption of the peripheral or cranial nerves, often to relieve localized pain
neurogenous arising in the nervous system
neurohypophysis the posterior part of the pituitary gland
neurologic pertaining to the nervous system
neuron a nerve cell and its processes; the functional unit of the nervous system
night terrors (pavor nocturnus) nightmares that the person is unable to recall the next morning
nitrogen balance the state of protein nutrition
nocturia (nycturia) increased frequency of urination at night not as the result of increased fluid intake

nocturnal enuresis involuntary urination at night
noncompliance (drug use) failure to follow a prescription
nonmaterial culture the beliefs, customs, languages, and social institutions of a society
nonpathogen a microorganism that does not produce disease under normal conditions
nonproductive cough a dry, harsh cough without secretions
non-rapid-eye-movement sleep *see* NREM sleep
nonverbal communication (body language) communication other than words, including gestures, posture and facial expressions
norm an ideal or fixed standard; an expected standard of behavior of group members
normal saline an isotonic concentration of salt (NaCl) solution
normocephaly normal head circumference
nosocomial referring to or originating in a hospital or similar institution, e.g., a nosocomial disease
NREM sleep (non-rapid-eye-movement sleep) a deep restful sleep state; also called *slow wave sleep*
nuclear family the family unit composed of parents and children
nurse clinician a nurse with advanced skills in a particular area of nursing practice
nursing audit the review of patients' charts to evaluate nursing competence
nursing diagnosis a statement describing a combination of signs or symptoms indicative of an actual or potential health problem that nurses are able, licensed, and accountable to treat
nursing goals goals stated in terms that guide the actions of the nurse
nursing history a record of patient data compiled by nurses using a systematic method
nursing order planned nursing interventions
nursing process a five-step systematic process used in nursing
nursing standards criteria against which nursing care can be evaluated
nutrient an organic or inorganic substance found in food; nutrients are digested and absorbed in the gastrointestinal tract and then used in the body's metabolic processes
nutrition what a person eats and how the body uses it
nutritionist a specialist in food and nutrition
nutritive value the nutrient content of a specified amount of food

obesity weight that is 20% greater than the ideal for height and frame
objective the aim of a maneuver or operation
objective data patient information that can be determined by observation or measurement by laboratory or other means
objective symptom a sign; evidence of a disease or body dysfunction that can be observed and described by others
obligatory heat the heat produced by the body as a result of the metabolism of food
obligatory loss the essential fluid loss required to maintain body functioning
observation the act or power of observing; gathering of information by noting facts or occurrences
obstetrics the branch of medicine dealing with the birth process and related events that precede and follow it
obtunded difficult to arouse from sleep; requiring shaking or a painful stimulus to awaken
obturator a disc or instrument that closes an opening; the obturator of a tracheostomy set fits inside and closes off the end of the outer tube
occult hidden
occupational therapist an individual who helps a patient develop skills necessary for the activities of daily living
Oedipus complex (Freud) the male child's attraction for his mother and accompanying hostile attitudes toward his father; compare with *Electra complex*
ointment a semisolid preparation applied externally to the body
olfactory referring to the sense of smell
oliguria production of abnormally small amounts of urine by the kidneys
opaque not admitting the passage of light
open system a system that exchanges matter, energy, and information with the environment
open wound a wound in which the continuity of the skin or mucous membrane has been interrupted
operative (intraoperative) period the time during surgery
ophthalmoscope an instrument used to examine the interior of the eye
optional surgery surgery requested by the patient but not necessary for health
oral referring to the mouth
oral stage (Freud) the stage of development during the 1st year of life, when the mouth is the principal area of activity
organic referring to an organ or organs; in chemistry, referring to compounds containing carbon; arising from an organism
orgasm the climax of sexual excitement, during which physiologic and psychologic release occurs; orgasm is characterized by rhythmic spasmodic contractions of the genitals
orgasmic dysfunction the inability of females to achieve orgasm
orgasmic platform an increase in size of the outer one-third of the vagina and the labia minora during precoital stimulation
orientation awareness of time, place, and person
orifice an external opening of a body cavity; e.g., the anus is the orifice of the large intestine
origin (of a muscle) the fixed or least movable point of attachment to a bone
orogastric tube a tube inserted through the mouth into the stomach
oropharynx the part of the pharynx that lies between the upper aspect of the epiglottis and the soft palate
orthopnea the ability to breathe only in the upright position, i.e., sitting or standing
orthostatic hypotension low blood pressure in a standing position
orthostatism the erect standing posture of the body
osmol the number of particles in 1 gram molecular weight of a disassociated solute
osmolarity (osmolality) the concentration of solutes in solution; the osmolar concentration of a solution expressed in osmols per liter of solution
osmosis passage of a solvent through a semipermeable membrane from an area of lesser solute concentration to one of greater solute concentration
osmotic pressure pressure exerted by the number of nondiffusable particles in a solution; the amount of pressure needed to stop the flow of water across a membrane
osseous pertaining to bone
ossification the formation of bone or a bony substance
osteoblast a bone-building cell
osteoclast a cell associated with bone resorption and breakdown
osteomalacia the softening of the bones; decalcification of bones in adults
osteomyelitis inflammation of the bone caused by infection and resulting in bone destruction
osteoporosis decrease in bone density; demineralization of bone
-ostomy a suffix denoting the formation of an opening or outlet
otoscope an instrument used to inspect the eardrum and external ear canal
outcome criteria expected alterations in the health status of a patient; standards used to determine the results of nursing interventions for a patient
outer canthus the corner of the upper and lower eyelids away from the nose
output the energy, matter, or information disposed of by a system as a result of its processes
outward rotation a turning away from the midline

oval window an opening between the middle and the inner ear
ovary the female gonad (sexual gland); ova are formed in the two ovaries
overbed cradle a frame placed over a patient in bed to protect the body from contact with the upper bedclothes
overhydration *see* edema
overnutrition the oversupply of calories
overweight weight that is 10% greater than the ideal for height and frame
ovulation the discharge of a mature ovum from the Graafian follicle of the ovary
ovum (egg) the female reproductive cell, which becomes the embryo after fertilization
oxyhemoglobin the compound of oxygen and hemoglobin
oxytocin a hormone secreted by the posterior pituitary gland; oxytocin helps the uterus to contract before, during, and after delivery

pace the distance covered in a step when one walks or the number of steps taken per minute
packing filling an open wound or cavity with a material such as gauze
Paco$_2$ partial pressure of carbon dioxide (arterial blood)
pain a basically unpleasant sensation, localized or general, mild or intense, that represents the suffering induced by stimulation of specialized nerve endings; pain may be threatened or fantasied and may be induced by disease, injury, or mental derangement caused by disease or injury
pain threshold the amount of stimulation required by a person to feel pain
pain tolerance the maximum amount and duration of pain that an individual is willing to endure
palate the roof of the mouth
palliative affording relief but not cure
palliative surgery surgery to relieve the symptoms of a disease process
pallor absence of normal skin color; a whitish-grayish tinge
palmar grasp reflex a reflex, normally present in newborns, that causes the fingers to curl around a small object placed in the palm of the hand
palpation the act of feeling with the hands, usually the fingers
pandemic an epidemic disease that is widespread
panic severe anxiety
Pao$_2$ partial pressure of oxygen (arterial blood)
Papanicolaou (Pap) smear a method of taking sample cervical cells for microscopic examination to detect malignancy
papule a small, superficial, round elevation of the skin
paracentesis the insertion of a needle into a cavity (usually the abdominal cavity) to remove fluid
paradoxical breathing *see* flail chest
paralysis the impairment or loss of motor function of a body part
paramedical having some connection with the practice of medicine
paraphrasing restating a person's message (thoughts and/or feelings) using similar words
paraplegia paralysis of the lower part of the body (including the legs) affecting both motor function and sensation
parasites plants or animals that live on or within another living organism
parasomnia a disorder that interferes with sleep, e.g., somnambulism
parasympathetic (craniosacral) nervous system a branch of the autonomic nervous system
parathyroid hormone (PTH, parathormone) the hormone produced by the parathyroid glands that regulates the calcium and phosphorus levels in the body
parenchyma the functional or essential elements of an organ
parenteral accomplished by a needle; occurring outside the alimentary tract; injected into the body through some route other than the alimentary canal, e.g., intravenously
paresthesia an abnormal sensation of burning or prickling
paronychia inflammation of the tissue surrounding the nail
parotid glands the large salivary glands located below and in front of the ears
parotitis (parotiditis) inflammation of the parotid salivary gland
paroxysm a sudden attack or sharp recurrence; a spasm
partial pressure the pressure exerted by each individual gas in a mixture according to its percentage concentration in the mixture
passive euthanasia allowing a person to die by withholding or withdrawing measures to maintain life
passive exercise exercise during which the muscles do not contract and the nurse, therapist, or patient supplies the energy to move the patient's body part
passivity lethargy; receptivity to outside influence; lack of energy or will
paste a semisolid dermatologic preparation that tends to penetrate the skin less than an ointment
pasteurization application of heat to milk to destroy disease-producing microorganisms
pastoral care an interpersonal relationship that focuses on the spiritual component of another person's life during distress
patent open, unobstructed, not closed
pathogen a microorganism capable of producing disease
pathogenic capable of producing disease
pathology a branch of medicine concerned with the nature of disease
patient (client) a person who seeks help, usually because of illness or injury
patient advocate a person who speaks on behalf of a patient and can intercede on the patient's behalf
patient care standards *see* nursing standards
patient goals goals stated as anticipated patient outcomes, not as nursing activities
patriarchy a social system in which the father is the head of the household or family
patrilineal relating to descent through the male line
pavor nocturnus *see* night terrors
Pco$_2$ partial pressure of carbon dioxide (venous blood)
pectoriloquy exaggerated bronchophony
pediculosis infestation with lice
pediculosis capitis infestation with head lice
peer review review by persons of equal standing
penetrating wound a wound created by an instrument that penetrated the skin or mucous membranes deeply into the tissues
penis the male organ of copulation and urinary excretion
Penrose drain a flexible rubber drain
perceived loss loss experienced by a person that cannot be verified by others
perception the process of understanding something new and then making it part of one's previous experience or knowledge; a person's awareness and identification of a person, thing, or situation
perception checking (consensual validation) verifying the accuracy of listening skills by giving and receiving feedback about what was communicated
percussion the tapping of a body area with short, sharp blows to learn, from the sounds produced, the condition of the body below the tapped area
percussion hammer an instrument shaped like a hammer with a head often made of plastic
pericardial aspiration the removal of fluid from the pericardial sac via an inserted needle
pericardial sac (pericardium) a fibrous sac that surrounds the heart

pericutaneous electric stimulation stimulation of major peripheral nerves by electricity
perimetrium the thin, outer, serous layer of the uterus
perineum the area between the anus and the posterior aspect of the genitals
periodontal disease inflammation of the tissues that surround and support the teeth
perioperative period the time before, during, and after an operation
periorbital around the eye socket
periosteum the connective tissue covering all bones
periostitis inflammation of the periosteum
peripheral at the edge or outward boundary
peripheral nerve implant an electrode implanted in a major sensory nerve for the purpose of relieving pain
peristalsis wavelike movements produced by circular and longitudinal muscle fibers of the intestinal walls; it propels the intestinal contents onward
peristomal referring to the skin area that surrounds a stoma
peritoneal cavity the area between the layers of peritoneum in the abdomen; a potential space
peritoneum the membrane lining the abdominal walls
peritonitis inflammation of the peritoneum
permissive licensure the policy by which practitioners do not have to be licensed to practice but are not protected by the licensing body
personal space the physical distance people prefer to maintain in their interactions with others
perspiration the fluid secreted by the sweat glands for excreting waste products and cooling the body
petechiae pinpoint red spots on the skin
pH a measure of the relative alkalinity or acidity of a solution; a measure of the concentration of hydrogen ions
phagocyte a cell, e.g., a white blood cell, that ingests microorganisms, other cells, and foreign particles
phagocytosis the process by which cells engulf microorganisms, other cells, or foreign particles
phalanx any bone of the fingers or toes (plural: phalanges)
phallic stage (Freud) the stage of development during the 4th and 5th years when sexual and aggressive feelings come into focus associated with the genital organs
phantom pain pain that remains after the perceived location has been removed, such as pain perceived in a foot after the leg has been amputated
pharmacist an individual licensed to prepare and dispense drugs and to make up prescriptions
pharmacology the scientific study of the actions of drugs on living animals and humans
pharmacopoeia a book containing a list of drug products used in medicine, including their descriptions and formulas
pharmacy the skill of preparing, compounding, and dispensing medicines; the place where medicines are prepared and dispensed
pharmacy assistant a member of the health team who in some situations administers drugs to patients
pharynx a musculomembranous sac behind the nose and mouth that connects with the esophagus and bronchi
phimosis an extremely narrowed opening of the foreskin of the penis
phlebitis inflammation of a vein
phlebothrombosis intravascular clotting with marked inflammation of a vein
phlebotomy opening a vein to remove blood
phosphorylation the combining of glucose with phosphate inside a cell
photophobia intolerance to light
photosensitive sensitive to light
phrenic referring to the diaphragm
physiatrist a physician who specializes in rehabilitation medicine; physiatrists use physical aids such as light, heat, and apparatuses
physical pertaining to the body or to physics
physical well-being a state of having one's physical needs met appropriately for homeostasis
physiologic pertaining to body function
physiologic dependence biochemical changes occurring in the body as a result of excessive use of a drug
physiology the science concerned with the functioning of living organisms and their parts
physiotherapist (physical therapist) a member of the health team who provides assistance to patients with musculoskeletal problems
pica a craving for unnatural foods, often during pregnancy, some psychologic conditions, or extreme malnutrition
pigeon chest (pectus carinatum) a chest deformity in which there is a narrow transverse diameter, an increased anteroposterior diameter, and a protruding sternum
pilosebaceous follicle the hair follicle and sebaceous gland complex of the skin
pinna the external part of the ear
pitch (in percussion) the number of vibrations per second or the frequency of vibrations
pitting edema edema in which firm finger pressure on the skin produces an indentation (pit) that remains for several seconds
pituitary gland (hypophysis) an endocrine gland (situated in the brain) that secretes a number of hormones, including adrenocorticotropic hormone and thyrotropic hormone
placebo any form of treatment, e.g., medication, that produces an effect in the patient because of its intent rather than its chemical or physical properties
placenta the tissue attached to the wall of the uterus; the fetus receives nourishment through the placenta, which is expelled as the "afterbirth" after the child is born
placing reflex a reflex of infants demonstrated when the infant is placed vertically with one foot touching the edge of a table; the infant flexes the knee and hip of the same leg and tries to place the foot on the surface of the table
plaintiff the person who files a legal complaint claiming his or her rights have been infringed
plantar flexion movement of the ankle so that the toes point downward
plantar reflex *see* Babinski reflex
plantar wart a wart on the sole of the foot that is sensitive to pressure and caused by the virus papovavirus hominis
plaque a film of mucus and bacteria that forms on the teeth
plasma the fluid portion of the blood in which the blood cells are suspended
pleura the membrane around the lungs; it consists of an outer layer, the parietal pleura, and an inner layer, the visceral pleura
pleural cavity a potential space between the two layers of pleura
pleural rub (friction rub) a coarse, leathery, or grating sound produced by the rubbing together of the pleura
plexus a network, e.g., of nerves or veins
pneumoencephalogram an x-ray film of the cerebrospinal spaces after the introduction of air
pneumonia inflammation of the lung tissue
pneumothorax accumulation of air or gas in the pleural cavity
pneumoventriculogram an x-ray film of the ventricles of the brain after the introduction of air
Po_2 partial pressure of oxygen (venous blood)
polarity the presence of two opposite poles
polarization (of a group) movement by members of a group toward a goal
polarized (cardiac) electrically charged
poliomyelitis an acute viral disease that may cause paralysis

polydipsia excessive thirst
polyneuritis inflammation of many nerves
polypnea an abnormal increase in the respiratory rate
polysaccharide a carbohydrate consisting of dozens of molecules of glucose
polyunsaturated fatty acid a fatty acid that contains two or more double bonds, such as linoleic or arachidonic acid
polyuria (diuresis) the production of abnormally large amounts of urine by the kidneys
POMR (POR) *see* problem-oriented medical record
popliteal referring to the posterior aspect of the knee
population density the number of people per square mile of a given area
port an opening or entrance
portal an entrance
position (in a group) the status or rank one has in a group
positive feedback (homeostasis) a control or regulating mechanism of the body that causes the production of additional hormone
positive nitrogen balance nitrogen input exceeding nitrogen output
positivism the state of being positive; a theory that positive knowledge is based on natural phenomena as verified by empirical sciences
posterior of, toward, or at the back
posterior fornix a vaultlike space at the posterior aspect of the vagina
postmortem examination *see* autopsy
postoperative bed *see* surgical bed
postoperative (postsurgical) period the time following surgery
postovulatory after ovulation
postovulatory stage the part of the female sexual cycle starting immediately after ovulation and lasting about 13 days; also called the *secretory* or *luteal stage*
postpartum occurring after childbirth
postural drainage drainage of secretions from various lung segments by the use of specific positions and gravity
posture the bearing and position of the body; the relative arrangements of the various parts of the body
potency power; the ability of the male to engage in sexual intercourse
potential health problem the presence of risk factors that predispose persons and families to health problems
power ability to influence another person in some way or ability to do something
powerlessness perceived lack of control over events
precedent a prior judicial decision used to justify or confirm a court ruling
precoital stimulation *see* foreplay
precordial thump a sharp blow of the fist to the sternum to restore heart function
precordium the area of the chest over the heart or stomach
preeclampsia an abnormal condition of late pregnancy or the early puerperium characterized by hypertension, albumin in the urine, and generalized edema
prelinguistic pertaining to sounds made by an infant that are not related to language
premature ejaculation the inability to control ejaculation prior to satisfaction of the partner or before 30 to 60 seconds after penetration
preoperational stage (Piaget) the phase of cognitive development that occurs during ages 3 to 7
preoperative period the time before an operation
preoptic center the nerve center anterior to the optic center
preovulatory before ovulation
preovulatory stage the first stage (about 14 days) of the female sexual cycle; also called the *proliferative* or *follicular stage*
prepuberty the period preceding puberty
prepubic urethra the part of the male urethra that is inferior to the pubis
prepuce *see* foreskin
presbycusis loss of hearing due to aging
presbyopia inability of the lens of the eye to accommodate initially to near objects and then to far objects as a result of the aging process
prescription the written direction for the preparation and administration of a remedy
pressoreceptor (baroreceptor) a receptor that is sensitive to changes in pressure, e.g., in the carotid sinus and the arch of the aorta
previable fetus a fetus incapable of extrauterine life
pricking pain pain like the pain of a knife piercing the skin
primary care a type of practice in which the first person to meet the patient, e.g., the nurse, assumes responsibility for care
primary group a small, intimate group in which relations among the members are personal
primary nursing a system of nursing in which the patient is assigned on admission to one nurse, who has primary responsibility for nursing care 24 hours a day
primary union (wound healing) healing that involves the production of minimal scar tissue
primigravida a woman who is pregnant for the first time
primordial follicle the primitive sac or cavity of the ovary that contains the ovum and the granulosa cells
principle a fundamental law or doctrine; assumption
privacy a deserved degree of social retreat that provides a comfortable feeling
privileged communication information given to a professional such as a physician, who is not required to disclose it in a court of law
probate proceedings civil actions relating to wills and estates of deceased persons
probing asking for information chiefly out of curiosity
problem *see* health problem
problem-oriented medical record (POMR, POR) a patient's chart organized according to the patient's problems and recording the reports of several health workers on each problem
process a series of actions directed toward a particular result; in anatomy, a prominence or projection, e.g., of a bone
process recording a word-for-word account of a conversation, including all verbal and nonverbal interactions
proctoclysis a slow instillation of fluid into the rectum
proctoscope a lighted instrument used to visualize the interior of the rectum
proctoscopy visualization of the interior of the rectum with a proctoscope
proctosigmoidoscope a lighted instrument used to visualize the rectum and sigmoid colon
proctosigmoidoscopy visual examination of the rectum and sigmoid colon with a proctosigmoidoscope
prodromal stage the stage of an illness during which there are early manifestations of the disease
productive cough a cough in which secretions are expectorated
progesterone a hormone produced by the ovaries, placenta, and adrenal cortex
prognosis the medical opinion about the outcome of a disease
projection an adaptive mechanism by which a person attributes his or her own characteristics to another
prolactin a hormone produced in the anterior pituitary that stimulates lactation
proliferation rapid reproduction of parts or cells
proliferative (follicular) stage *see* preovulatory stage
pronation turning the palm downward; moving the bones of the forearm so that the palm of the hand turns from anterior to posterior in the anatomic position; also, flat feet
prone (prone position) lying on the abdomen with the face turned to one side
prophylaxis preventive treatment; prevention of disease
proprioceptor a sensory receptor that is sensitive to movement and the position of the body

prostate a gland around the base of the urethra of the male
prostatectomy the removal of the prostate gland
prosthesis an artificial part, e.g., a glass eye, an artificial leg, or dentures
prostration extreme exhaustion
protective asepsis (isolation) setting someone or something apart from others; practices that prevent the spread of infections and communicable diseases
protein an organic substance that is composed of carbon, hydrogen, oxygen, and nitrogen and that yields amino acids upon hydrolysis
proteinuria the presence of protein in the urine
protraction moving a part of the body forward in a plane parallel to the ground
proxemics the study of physical distance between people in their interactions
proximal closest to the point of attachment
proximal fragment the part of a fractured bone nearest the individual's head
prudent diet a diet that is likely to benefit the individual even though it may not prevent disease
pruritus intense itching
psychiatry the branch of medicine that treats behavioral, emotional, or mental disorders
psychogenic (functional) pain pain caused by psychologic factors
psychologic dependence (on a drug) a state of emotional reliance on a drug to maintain one's well-being; a feeling of need or craving for a drug
psychology the study of mental processes and behavior
psychomotor referring to motor actions related to cerebral or psychic activity
psychosomatic concerning the mind and the body; emotional disturbances manifested by physiologic symptoms
ptyalin an enzyme in saliva
ptyalism excessive secretion of saliva
puberty the age during which the reproductive organs become active and secondary sex characteristics develop
public law rules regulating relationships between individuals and government
pudendum *see* vulva
puerperium the period from delivery to about 6 weeks after delivery
pulmonary referring to the lungs
pulmonary capacities the combinations of two or more pulmonary volumes
pulmonary embolus a blood clot that has moved to the lungs
pulmonary resuscitation *see* respiratory ventilation
pulse the wave of blood within an artery that is created by contraction of the left ventricle of the heart
pulse deficit a difference between the apical and the radial pulses
pulse pressure the difference between the systolic and the diastolic pressures
pulse rate the number of pulse beats per minute
pulse rhythm the pattern of pulse beats and of intervals between beats
pulse tension the elasticity of the arteries
pulse volume the force of the blood with each beat produced by contraction of the left ventricle
pulsus regularis equal lapses of time between beats of a normal pulse
puncture (stab) wound a wound made by a sharp instrument penetrating the skin and underlying tissues
pupil the opening at the center of the iris of the eye
Purkinje fibers a network of fibers in the ventricles of the heart that conduct stimuli from the atria to the ventricles
purulent containing pus
purulent exudate an exudate consisting of leukocytes, liquefied dead tissue debris, and dead and living bacteria
pus a thick liquid associated with inflammation and composed of cells, liquid, microorganisms, and tissue debris
pustule a small elevation of the skin or mucous membrane or a clogged pore or follicle containing pus
putrid rotten
pyelogram an x-ray film of the kidney and ureter, showing the pelvis of the kidney
pyemia a generalized, persistent blood poisoning
pyogenic pus-producing
pyorrhea purulent periodontal disease
pyrexia elevated body temperature; fever
pyrogen a substance that produces a fever
pyuria the presence of pus in the urine

quadriplegia the paralysis of all four limbs

rabbi a Jew ordained for professional religious leadership
race classification of humans into subgroups according to specific physical and structural characteristics
radial pulse the pulse point located where the radial artery passes over the radius of the arm
radiation the transfer of heat from a warm object to a cooler object by means of electromagnetic waves, without contact between the two objects; electromagnetic waves used in diagnostic tests and some kinds of therapy
radiation therapy therapy involving x-rays, radium, or other radioactive substances
radiology technologist a member of the health team who takes roentgenograms and assists with other related tests
radiopaque able to block the passage of radiant energy, such as x-rays
rales bubbling or rattling sounds audible on inhalation as air moves through accumulated moist secretions in the lungs
range of motion the degree of movement possible for each joint
rationalization an adaptive mechanism in which one gives socially acceptable reasons for one's behavior
reaction formation an adaptive mechanism in which one behaves exactly opposite to the way one is feeling
readiness the state of being ready; it is used to describe the developmental maturation and growth necessary before one can perform some activities, e.g., walking
receptor (sensor) the terminal of a sensory nerve that is sensitive to specific stimuli
reconstitution the technique of adding a solvent to a powdered drug to prepare it for injection
reconstructive surgery surgery to repair tissues whose function or appearance is damaged
recovery bed *see* surgical bed
recreational therapist a member of the health team who assists patients with activities for recreation
rectocele (proctocele) a protrusion of part of the rectum into the vagina
rectum the distal portion of the large intestine
recumbent length the distance from the soles of the feet to the vertex of the head of a person lying on the back
reduced hemoglobin hemoglobin that has released its oxygen
reduction realignment of fractured bone fragments to their normal position
referred pain pain perceived to be in one area but whose source is another area
reflex an involuntary activity in response to a stimulus
reflexive vocalization nondescriptive sounds infants make in response to various stimuli and environmental conditions
reflexogenic erection an erection of the penis that occurs without apparent sexual stimuli
refractory period the period immediately following orgasm when males cannot respond to sexual stimuli

regeneration the replacement of destroyed tissue cells by cells that are identical or similar in structure and function
regimen a regulated pattern of activity
registration the recording or entering of certain information about individuals
regression reversion to a behavior or state that was acceptable at an earlier age
rehabilitation the restoration of a person who is ill or injured to the highest possible capacity
relapsing fever a fever characterized by periods of normal temperature, lasting 1 or more days, between periods of fever
religion an organized system of worship
remittent fever a fever characterized by a wide range of temperatures, all above normal, over a 24-hour period
REM sleep sleep during which the person experiences rapid eye movement; also called *paradoxical sleep*
renal relating to the kidney
renal dialysis a process in which blood flows from an artery through an artificial membrane that removes impurities; the blood then returns to the patient through a vein
renal pelvis the funnel-shaped upper end of each ureter
rennin a substance secreted by the kidneys when blood sodium levels are low; it controls aldosterone secretion
repolarized (cardiac) requiring an electric charge
repression an adaptive mechanism in which one unconsciously forgets problems or experiences
reservoir a source of pathogens
residual urine the amount of urine remaining in the bladder after a person voids
residual volume (air) the amount of air remaining in the lungs after a person exhales both tidal and expiratory reserve volumes
resistive behaviors behaviors that inhibit involvement, cooperation, or change
resistive exercise exercise in which the patient contracts a muscle against an opposing force, e.g., a weight
resonance a low-pitched, rich sound produced over normal lung tissue when the chest is percussed
respiration the act of breathing; transport of oxygen from the atmosphere to the body cells and transport of carbon dioxide from the cells to the atmosphere
respiratory acidosis (hypercapnia) a state of excess carbon dioxide in the body
respiratory alkalosis a state of excessive loss of carbon dioxide from the body
respiratory arrest the sudden cessation of breathing
respiratory membrane the alveolar walls and the surrounding blood capillaries
respiratory technologist a person who provides diagnostic and therapeutic measures for patients with respiratory problems
respiratory ventilation (pulmonary resuscitation) the inhalation of air into the lungs by artificial means
responsibility reliability and trustworthiness
rest calmness or relaxation without emotional stress
restitution an adaptive mechanism in which one performs restorative acts to relieve guilt
resuscitate to restore life; to revive
resuscitation the application of measures to reestablish breathing
retching the involuntary attempt to vomit without producing emesis
retention (urinary) the accumulation of urine in the bladder and the inability of the bladder to empty itself
retention (stay) suture a large plain suture that attaches to underlying tissues of fat and muscle in addition to the skin; retention sutures are used to support incisions
retina the membrane that lines the back of the eye, receives the image, and is connected to the brain by the optic nerve
retraction moving a part of the body backward in a plane parallel to the ground; the act of drawing back
retrograde pyelogram an x-ray film taken after a contrast medium is injected through ureteral catheters into the kidneys
retroperitoneal behind the peritoneum
retrospective audit an audit of past events
reverse protective asepsis (barrier technique) measures used to prevent certain patients, e.g., those with severe burns, from coming in contact with microorganisms
reverse Trendelenburg's position a position with the head of the bed raised and the foot lowered, while the bed foundation remains unbroken
Rh factor antigens present on the surface of some people's erythrocytes; persons who possess this factor are referred to as *Rh positive,* while those who do not are referred to as *Rh negative*
rhinitis inflammation of the mucous membrane of the nose
rhizotomy interruption of the anterior or posterior nerve root between the ganglion and the spinal cord, often for the purpose of relieving pain
rhonchi coarse, dry, wheezy, or whistling sounds, more audible during exhalation, as the air moves through tenacious mucus or a constricted bronchus
rickets a bone disorder resulting from a deficiency of vitamin D and calcium; decalcification of bone
right a just claim
rigidity stiffness or inflexibility of a muscle
rigor mortis the stiffening of the muscles after death
ritualistic behavior (ritualism) a series of repetitive acts performed compulsively, often to relieve anxiety
roentgen the unit of measurement of gamma rays (γ) or x-radiation
roentgenogram a film produced by photography with x-rays
role the pattern of behavior expected of an individual in a situation or particular group
role conflict a clash between the beliefs, behaviors, etc., imposed by two or more roles fulfilled by one person
rooting reflex a reflex that causes newborns to turn their heads toward the side of a stimulated cheek or lip
rotation turning a bone around its central axis either toward the midline of the body (*internal rotation*) or away from midline of the body (*external rotation*)
round window an opening from the middle ear to the inner ear
rubefacient reddening the skin; a substance that reddens the skin
ruga a ridge or fold in the lining of an organ such as the vagina or the stomach (plural: rugae)

sacrum a triangular bone at the base of the vertebral column
sagittal plane a vertical line or plane dividing the body or its parts into right and left portions
Salem sump tube a double-lumen nasogastric tube
sanction punishment or a measure used to enforce normative behavior of group members
sanguineous bloody
sanguineous exudate an exudate containing large amounts of red blood cells
saphenous vein either of two superficial veins of the leg; the greater one extends from the foot to the inguinal region, while the lesser one extends from the foot up the back of the leg to the knee joint
sarcoidosis a disease in which affected tissues develop epithelioid cell tubercles; commonly affected organs are the lymph nodes, liver, spleen, lungs, skin, eyes, and small bones in the feet and hands
satiety a feeling of fullness as a result of satisfying the desire for food
saturated fat a fat whose molecular structure is saturated with hydrogen, such as fats in meat, butter, and eggs
scab the crust over a superficial wound

scan a specialized type of x-ray procedure involving the use of a scanning device (probe), a computer, a printout machine, and a viewing apparatus
scapula the shoulder blade, a flat, triangular bone at the back of the shoulder
scar (cicatrical) tissue dense fibrous tissue derived from granulation tissue
sclera the white covering of the eye that joins with the cornea
sclerosis a process of hardening that occurs from inflammation and disease of the interstitial substance; the term is used to describe hardening of nervous tissues and arterioles
scoliosis a lateral curvature of a part of the vertebral column
scored marked with a line or groove
scrotum the sac suspended down and behind the penis that contains and protects the testes
scultetus binder an abdominal binder applied in strips that overlap each other
scurvy a condition resulting from vitamin C deficiency
sebaceous gland a gland of the dermis that secretes sebum
seborrheic dermatitis a chronic disease of the skin, characterized by scaling and crusted patches on various body areas, e.g., the scalp
sebum the oily, lubricating secretion of sebaceous glands in the skin
secondary group a group that is generally larger and more impersonal than a primary group
secondary union (second intention) healing that requires the formation of considerable granulation tissue
secretion the product of a gland, e.g., saliva is the secretion of the salivary glands
secretory (luteal) stage *see* postovulatory stage
sedative an agent that tends to calm or tranquilize
segmentation contractions contractions of segments of the intestine in contrast to contractions of large areas of the intestine
self-actualization (Maslow) the highest level of personality development
self-concept the combination of beliefs and feelings one holds about oneself at a given time
self-consistency the aspect of self that strives to maintain a stable self-image
self-esteem self-acceptance; self-worth
self-expectancy what a person wants to become; the power a person perceives he or she has to meet self-expectations
self-ideal *see* self-expectancy
self-image a person's perception of self at a specific time or over a period of time
self-terminating order on a patient's record, an order whose termination time is implicit
semantics the study of the meaning of words
semen seminal plasma combined with sperm
semicircular canals passages shaped like half circles in the inner ear that control the sense of balance by the effect of fluid moving against hairlike nerves
semicomatose pertaining to a state of unconsciousness characterized by reflex movement only when painful stimuli are applied and, in some instances, by decortical or decerebrate posturing
semi-Fowler's position a bed sitting position in which the head of bed is elevated at least 30°, with or without knee flexion
semilunar valves crescent-shaped valves that guard the entrances from the cardiac ventricles into the aorta and pulmonary trunk
seminal plasma substances that are produced by the seminal vesicles, prostate, and Cowper's glands and that energize the sperm and enhance their transport
seminiferous tubules highly coiled tubes that manufacture sperm within each testis
senescence the process of growing old
senility feebleness or loss of mental, emotional, or physical control that occurs in old age
sensitivity quick response, often referring to the response of microorganisms to an antibiotic
sensorimotor stage (Piaget) the initial phase of cognitive development between birth and 2 years
sensoristasis the need for sensory stimulation
sensorium a sensory nerve center
sensory deficit partial or complete impairment of any sensory organ
sensory deprivation (input deficit) insufficient sensory stimulation for a person to function
sensory overload an overabundance of sensory stimulation
septic produced by putrefaction or decomposition
septic (hectic) fever intermittent fever characterized by wide fluctuations and daily periods when body temperature falls to normal or below normal
serosanguineous composed of serum and blood
serous of or like serum
serous exudate a watery exudate composed mainly of serum
serum (blood) blood plasma from which the fibrinogen has been separated during clotting
sex maleness or femaleness; sexual intercourse
sex behavior the behavior associated with sexual intercourse, including physiologic responses and sexual dysfunctions
sex chromosome pair the pair of chromosomes, one from the sperm and one from the ovum, that determine whether gonads develop into testes or ovaries; the sex chromosome pair is designated XX (female) or XY (male)
sex drive *see* libido
sex-typed behavior the action that typically elicits different rewards for one sex or the other
sexual differentiation biologic sex determination of the fetus, during which male genitals or female genitals develop
sexual dimorphism the average differences between males and females in any given species
sexual dysfunction a perceived problem in achieving desired satisfaction of sexuality
sexual identity (core-gender identity) a person's inner feeling or sense of being male or female
sexuality what constitutes male and female; the constitution of an individual in relation to sexual attitudes or activities
sexually transmitted (venereal) disease a disease that can be passed on through intercourse with an infected person
sexual motivation *see* libido
sexual role behavior sexual behavior and gender behavior
shock acute circulatory failure
show expulsion of the mucous plug during labor
shroud a large rectangular or square piece of plastic or cloth used to enclose a body after death
sickle cell anemia a genetic defect of hemoglobin synthesis that accounts for abnormally crescent-shaped erythrocytes; common to Afro-Americans
side effect (of a drug) an outcome that is not intended, such as an unintended action or complication of a drug
sigmoid colon the lower portion of the descending colon of the large intestine; it is shaped like the letter S
sigmoidoscope a lighted instrument used to examine the sigmoid colon
sigmoidoscopy examination of the interior of the sigmoid colon with a sigmoidoscope
Sims's position semiprone position
sings healing ceremonies or rituals carried out by some Native American Indians
singultus hiccups
sinoatrial (SA) node the pacemaker of the heart; the collection of Purkinje's fibers in the right atrium of the heart where the rhythm of contraction is initiated

Skene's glands paraurethral glands that open into the urethra just within the external urinary meatus
slander defamation by spoken words
sleep a state of unconsciousness from which a person can be aroused by appropriate sensory or other stimuli
sleep apnea periodic cessation of breathing during sleep
slipper pan a bedpan with a flattened end to ease placement under the patient; also called a *fracture pan*
smear material spread across a glass slide in preparation for microscopic study
smegma a thick, white, cheeselike secretion that collects between the labia and under the foreskin
SOAP the format used in the POR to record the patient's progress; it has four components: Subjective data, Objective data, Assessment, and Planning
socialization the process by which individuals learn the knowledge, skills, and dispositions of their social group or society
socialized speech the exchange of thoughts between individuals, including questions, answers, commands, and criticisms of others
social worker an individual who assists persons and families with social problems
sociogram a diagram of the flow of verbal communication within a group during a specified period
sociology the study of social relationships and social institutions, such as marriage or education
sociopath a person who is unable to follow society's moral and ethical standards; one who has an antisocial personality
sodium cotransport theory a hypothesis about the mechanism for glucose transport in the presence of sodium
soixante-neuf (69) simultaneous oral-genital stimulation between two persons
solute a substance dissolved in a liquid
solvent the component of a solution that can dissolve a solute
somatic referring to the physical body
somatogenic (organic) pain pain of physical origin
somnambulism sleepwalking
sordes the accumulation of foul matter (food, microorganisms, and epithelial elements) on the teeth and gums
souffle a blowing sound heard by auscultation
source-oriented medical record a traditional patient's chart, organized according to the source of records (i.e., the person or department reporting); it includes separate records for the doctor, the nurse, the social worker, etc.
spasm involuntary contraction of a muscle or muscle group
spastic describing the sudden, prolonged involuntary muscle contractions of patients with damage to the central nervous system
special (therapeutic) diet a diet in which the amount of food, kind of food, or frequency of eating is prescribed
specific gravity the weight or degree of concentration of a substance compared with the weight of an equal amount of another substance used as a standard (e.g., water used as a standard has a specific gravity of 1, while urine in comparison has a specific gravity of 1.010 to 1.025)
speculum a funnel-shaped instrument used to widen and examine canals of the body, e.g., the vagina or nasal canal
sperm the male germ cell (reproductive cell)
spermatogenesis production of sperm
spermicide foam, jelly, or cream inserted in the vagina before intercourse to destroy the sperm chemically
sphincter a ringlike muscle that opens or closes a natural orifice, such as the urethra, when it relaxes or contracts
sphygmomanometer an instrument used to measure the pressure of the blood in the arteries
spinothalamic tract the nerve pathway of the spinal cord in which impulses ascend to the brain
spiral bandage a bandage applied to parts of the body extremities that are of uniform circumference
spiral reverse bandage a bandage applied to extremities of the body that are not of uniform circumference
spiritual belief a belief in a higher power, creative force, divine being, or infinite source of energy; the belief may or may not be associated with an organized religion
spiritual need what a patient needs to maintain, increase, or restore his or her beliefs and faith and to fulfill religious obligations
spirometry the measurement of pulmonary volumes and capacities
splint a rigid bar or appliance used to stabilize a body part
spore a round or oval structure highly resistant to destruction that is formed in some bacterial cells
sprain injury of the ligaments and associated structure of a joint by wrenching or twisting; associated structures include tendons, muscles, nerves, and blood vessels
spreader block (bar) a block of wood or metal that spreads traction tape away from the medial and lateral aspects of the foot in a traction such as a Buck's extension
sputum the mucous secretion from the lungs, bronchi, and trachea that is ejected through the mouth
stability (of a group) the degree of permanence of a group
stab wound *see* puncture wound
stamina staying power or endurance
stammer involuntary repetitions and stops in vocal utterances
standard a measure of quantity, quality, weight, extent, or value that is set up as a rule
standing order on a patient's record, a written order that remains in effect indefinitely
stasis stagnation or stoppage of flow of body fluids, such as intestinal fluids, urine, or blood
static electricity stationary electric charges
station stance; the way a person stands
stature the height of a standing person
statutory law a law passed by a legislature (state, provincial, or federal)
stenosis constriction or narrowing of a body canal or opening
stepping reflex (walking, dancing reflex) a reflex of infants characterized by an up-and-down walking motion of the legs when the infant is held upright with the feet touching a flat surface
stereognosis ability to recognize objects by touching them
stereotype something that conforms to a fixed pattern; an oversimplified judgment or attitude about a person or group
sterile free from microorganisms, including pathogens
sterile field a specified area that is considered free from microorganisms
sterile technique *see* surgical asepsis
sterilization a process that destroys all microorganisms, including spores
sternum the breastbone, a flat elongated bone lying between the ribs and over the heart
stertor snoring or sonorous respiration, usually due to a partial obstruction of the upper airway
stethoscope an instrument used to listen to various sounds inside the body, such as the heartbeats
stimulus anything that arouses or incites action from a receptor
stock supply (of drugs) medications stocked in relatively large quantities in a nursing unit; individual doses are taken from the large supply
stoma an artificial opening in the abdominal wall; it may be permanent or temporary
stomatitis inflammation of the entire mouth
stool (feces) excreted waste products from the large intestine
stopcock a valve that controls the flow of fluid or air through a tube
strabismus squinting or crossing of the eyes; uncoordinated eye movements
strain (of a muscle) overexertion or overstretching of a muscle or part of a muscle

stress a syndrome of signs and symptoms of the body that produces changes in the structure and chemical composition of the body as a response to a stressor; the response may be general or local

stressor any factor that produces stress or alters the body's equilibrium

stretch receptors nerve receptors sensitive to changes in pressure, i.e., in the aorta and carotid sinus; also called *pressoreceptors* or *baroreceptors*

striae gravidarum colorless streaks or lines on the abdomen, breasts, or thighs caused by pregnancy; stretch marks

stricture a narrowing of a passageway or canal

stridor a shrill, harsh, crowing sound made on inhalation due to constriction of the upper airway or layngeal obstruction

stroke volume the amount of blood ejected from the heart with each ventricular contraction

stroma tissue that forms the framework or structure of an organ

stupor a condition of partial or nearly complete unconsciousness; stuporous patients are never fully awakened even when painfully stimulated

stuttering a speech problem evidenced by the repetition of letters or words and prolonged pauses

stylet a metal or plastic probe inserted into a needle or cannula to render it stiff and to prevent occlusion of the lumen by particles of tissue

subarachnoid space the area between the arachnoid membrane and the pia mater

subcostal below the ribs

subcutaneous (hypodermic) beneath the layers of the skin

subcutaneous tissue *see* hypodermis

subjective data patient information that only the patient personally can give, such as thoughts or feelings

sublimation the channeling of unacceptable desires into socially acceptable forms of behavior

sublingual under the tongue

suborbital beneath the cavity or orbit

subscapular below the scapula

substantia gelatinosa gray matter in the dorsal horns of the spinal cord where pain fibers terminate

substernal retractions indrawing beneath the breastbone

substitution replacing one thing with another; an adaptive mechanism in which unattainable or unacceptable goals are replaced with ones that are attainable or acceptable

sucking reflex a reflex sucking action in newborns, initiated by touching their lips

suctioning aspiration of secretions by a catheter connected to a suction machine or outlet

sudden infant death syndrome (SIDS) a condition of some children during the first year, resulting in death during sleep

sudoriferous gland a gland of the dermis that secretes sweat

suicide the taking of one's own life

sulcular technique a dental hygiene technique for removing plaque and cleaning under the gingival margins

superego (Freud) an unconscious part of the psyche that monitors the id and the ego; concerned primarily with ethics, conscience, and social standards

supination turning the palm upward; moving the bones of the forearm so that the palm of the hand turns from posterior to anterior in the anatomic position

supine (supine position) lying on the back with the face upward without support for the head and shoulders; also called *dorsal position*

support system the people and activities that can assist a person at a time of stress

suppository a solid, cone-shaped, medicated substance inserted into the rectum, vagina, or urethra

suppression the willful exclusion of a thought or feeling from consciousness; the sudden stoppage of a secretion or an excretion, e.g., urine

suppuration the formation of pus

supraclavicular retractions indrawing above the clavicles

supraoptic above the eye

supraorbital above the orbit of the eye

suprapubic above the pubic arch

suprasternal retractions indrawing above the breastbone

surfactant a lipoprotein mixture in the alveoli

surgical asepsis measures that render and maintain objects free from microorganisms (sterile)

surgical bed (anesthetic, recovery, or postoperative bed) a bed with the top covers fanfolded to one side or to the end of the bed

susto among Chicanos, a disease of emotional origin; fright caused by natural phenomena such as lightning or loud noises

suture in surgery, a surgical stitch used to close accidental or surgical wounds; in anatomy, a junction line of the skull bones

swallowing reflex a reflex that accompanies the infant's sucking reflex and causes the infant to swallow

symbolization an adaptive mechanism by which objects are used to represent ideas or emotions too painful for a person to express; the creation of a mental image to stand for something

sympathectomy the severing of pathways of the sympathetic nervous system, often to relieve pain of a vascular origin

symphysis pubis the fibrocartilagenous line of union of the bodies of the pubic bones in the median plane

symptom (covert data) *see* subjective data

synapse the junction between two neurons, where nerve impulses are transmitted from one neuron to another

syncope fainting or temporary loss of consciousness

syndrome a group of signs and symptoms resulting from a single cause and constituting a typical clinical picture, such as the shock syndrome

synergist an agent that enhances the action of another so that their combined effect is greater than the effect of either

synovial joint a freely movable joint surrounded by a capsule enclosing a cavity that contains a transparent, viscid fluid

synthesis the process of putting together; assembling the parts of a whole

syphilis a sexually transmitted (venereal) disease caused by the microorganism *Treponema pallidum*

syringe an instrument used to inject or withdraw liquids

system a set of identifiable parts or components

systemic pertaining to the body (or other system) as a whole

systole the period when the ventricles of the heart are contracted

systolic pressure the pressure of the blood against the arterial walls when the ventricles of the heart contract

tablet a medication in solid form that is often compressed and molded

tachycardia an excessively rapid pulse or heart rate, over 100 beats per minute in the adult

tachypnea abnormally fast respirations, usually more than 24 per minute, marked by quick, shallow breaths

tactile pertaining to the sense of touch

tactile (vocal) fremitus vibrations, palpable with the palms of the hands, originating in the larynx and transmitted to the chest wall during speech

talipes equinovarus clubfoot; a foot is malpositioned in plantar flexion at the ankle, with inversion and adduction of the heel and forefoot

Talmud the authoritative written body of Jewish tradition

Taoism Chinese mystical philosophy

tartar the film on teeth, often formed from plaque; dental calculus

T-binder a cloth in the shape of a T often used to retain dressings in the genital region

Td combined tetanus and diphtheria toxoid used for people over 6 years of age; it has less diphtheria toxoid than DT

teaching a system of activities intended to produce learning

technical assault and battery assault and battery without the intent to injure, e.g., when giving a hypodermic injection
temporal pulse a pulse point where the temporal artery passes over the temporal bone of the skull
tenacious sticky, adhesive
tendon a fibrous cord that attaches a muscle to a bone
tenesmus straining; painful, ineffective straining during defecation or urination
terminal hair long, coarse, pigmented body hair
territoriality the pattern of behavior arising from an individual's feeling that certain spaces and objects belong to him or her
testes the male gonads
testosterone a testicular hormone that stimulates the growth of the genitals and the development of male secondary sexual characteristics
tetany a syndrome manifested by muscle twitching, cramps, convulsions, and sharp flexion of the wrist and ankle joints
thalamus the larger and middle portion of the diencephalon of the brain
theory a scientifically acceptable general principle that governs practice or is proposed to explain observed facts
therapeutic healing; supportive of health
therapeutic effect (of a drug) the primary effect desired, or the reason the drug is prescribed
therapy remedial treatment
thermal trauma injury caused by excessive heat or cold
thermosensitive pain receptors pain receptors sensitive to heat and cold
thoracocentesis insertion of a needle into the pleural cavity for diagnostic or therapeutic purposes
thorax the chest cavity
thought disorganization a mental condition evidenced by difficulty remembering what one is saying, confusion about time, inappropriate verbal responses, and sensory distortions
thrombocytopenia an abnormal reduction in the number of platelets in the blood
thrombophlebitis inflammation of a vein followed by formation of a blood clot
thrombosis the development of a blood clot
thrombus a solid mass of blood constituents in the circulatory system; a clot (plural: thrombi)
throughput the process of transforming input so that it is useful to the system
thyroid hormone a hormone produced by the thyroid gland consisting of thyroxine and triiodothyronine
thyroid stimulating hormone (TSH, thyrotropic hormone) a hormone produced by the anterior pituitary gland that stimulates the thyroid gland to produce thyroxine
thyroxine a hormone produced by the thyroid gland
tic a repetitive twitching of the muscles, often of the face or upper trunk
tick a small parasite that bites into tissue and sucks blood
tidal volume the volume of air that is normally inhaled and exhaled
tinea pedis *see* athlete's foot
tinnitus a ringing or buzzing sensation in the ears that is purely subjective
tissue perfusion passage of fluid, e.g., blood, through a specific organ or body part
tolerance the ability to endure without ill effects; the term is often used with reference to taking medications
tomography a scanning procedure during which several x-ray beams pass through the body part from different angles
tone (of a group) the pleasant or unpleasant atmosphere sensed in a group
tonicity the normal condition of tension or tone, e.g., of a muscle
tonic neck reflex a reflex of the newborn, also called the *fencing reflex*, in which, when the head is forcibly turned to one side, the arm and leg on that side are extended while the opposite limbs are flexed
tonometer an instrument used to assess the pressure inside the eye
tonsillectomy the surgical removal of a tonsil or tonsils
tonus the slight, continual contraction of muscles
topical applied externally, e.g., to the skin or mucous membranes
TOPV trivalent oral polio vaccine
torsion twisting
tort a wrong committed by a person against another person or the other person's property
torticollis limited range of motion of the neck, with lateral inclination and rotation of the head away from the midline of the body
tortuous twisted
total lung capacity the maximum volume to which the lungs can be expanded
total parenteral nutrition (TPN) *see* hyperalimentation
tourniquet a device, e.g., a rubber strip, that is wrapped around a body area to compress the blood vessels
toxemia a generalized intoxication due to the absorption of toxins in the body
toxemia of pregnancy a metabolic disturbance during pregnancy; *see* eclampsia, preeclampsia
toxin a poison produced by some microorganisms, animals, and plants
toxoid a modified exotoxin that is no longer toxic but still has the ability to stimulate the production of antibodies
trachea a membranous tube, composed of cartilage, descending from the larynx and branching into the right and left bronchi
tracheal tug an indrawing and downward pulling of the trachea during inhalation
tracheostomy a procedure by which an opening is made in the anterior portion of the trachea and a cannula is introduced into the opening
traction the exertion of a pulling force
transcutaneous electrical stimulation the placement of electrodes on the surface of the skin over a peripheral nerve pathway for the purpose of relieving pain
transfusion (blood) the introduction of whole blood or its components, e.g., serum, erythrocytes, or platelets, into the venous circulation
transudation the passage of serum or other body fluids through a membrane or tissue
transverse plane a horizontal line or plane dividing the body or its parts into superior and inferior portions
trapeze bar a triangular handgrip suspended from an overbed frame
trauma injury
tremor an involuntary muscle contraction, e.g., quivering, twitching, or convulsions
Trendelenburg's position a bed position with the head of the bed lowered and the foot raised, while the bed foundation remains unbroken; in some agencies, the position involves elevation of the knees, with the feet lowered and the head lowered
triage picking, choosing, sorting, and selecting
trial legal proceedings during which all relevant facts are presented to a jury or judge
triglyceride a simple lipid or neutral fat consisting of three fatty acids for each glycerol base
trigone the triangular area at the base of the urinary bladder
trimester a period of 3 months
trocar a sharp, pointed instrument that fits inside a cannula and is used to pierce body cavities
trochanter either of two processes below the neck of the femur
trochanter roll a rolled towel support placed against the hips to prevent external rotation of the legs
troche a lozenge

tubal ligation a surgical tying of the fallopian tubes, rendering the female sterile
tubercle a rounded eminence of bone
tumor an uncontrolled and progressive growth of cells
tunica albuginea a dense, white, fibrous capsule encasing each testis
tunica dartos the middle layer of smooth muscle and tough connective tissue in the scrotum
tuning fork an instrument shaped like a two-pronged fork and make of metal; the prongs vibrate when struck
turgor normal fullness and elasticity
tympanic membrane a membrane separating the external and the middle ear
tympanites (distention) swelling of the abdomen due to the presence of excessive flatus in the intestines or peritoneal cavity
tympany a musical drumming sound produced on percussion over organs that contain gas or air

ulcer a localized sloughing of skin tissue or mucous membrane commonly associated with varicosities or hyperactivity of the gastrointestinal tract
ultradian rhythm a biologic cycle completed in minutes or hours
ultrasound high-frequency, mechanical, radiant energy
ultraviolet referring to radiation having wavelengths shorter than violet rays and longer than x-rays; ultraviolet radiation has powerful chemical properties
umbilicus the navel; the site where the umbilical cord was attached to the fetus
unconscious incapable of responding to sensory stimuli; insensible
unconscious mind (Freud) the mental life of which a person is unaware
undernutrition inadequate caloric intake or nourishment
unilateral affecting one side
unit dose system (of drugs) prepackaged and labeled individual doses of medication for each patient; the amount of medication the patient is to receive at a prescribed hour
universal donor a person with type O blood
universal recipient a person with type AB blood
unpalatable distasteful, unpleasant to the taste
unsterile containing microorganisms; unsterile material may be clean or contaminated
untoward adverse
urban relating to or constituting a city
urea a substance found in urine, blood, and lymph; the main nitrogenous substance in blood
urea frost the appearance of the skin when the salt crystals remain after the evaporation of the sweat in urhidrosis
uremia the retention in the blood of excessive amounts of the byproducts of protein metabolism
ureter the fibrous, muscular tube extending from the kidneys to the urinary bladder
ureterostomy *see* urostomy
urethra the canal extending from the urinary bladder to the outside of the body
urethritis inflammation of the urethra
urgency a feeling that one must urinate
urgent surgery surgery necessary for the patient's health
urhidrosis a condition in which urinous materials, e.g., uric acid and urea, are present in the sweat
urinal a receptacle used to collect urine
urinalysis laboratory analysis of the urine
urinary diversion *see* urostomy
urine the fluid of water and waste products excreted by the kidneys
urobilin the oxidized form of urobilinogen, a compound formed from bilirubin, that is found in feces and occasionally in urine
urostomy (ureterostomy, urinary diversion) an opening through the abdominal wall into the urinary tract that permits the drainage of urine
urticaria an allergic reaction marked by smooth, reddened, slightly elevated patches of skin and intense itching
uterus the womb; the hollow, muscular organ in the female in which the fertilized ovum develops
uvula a small fleshy mass projecting from the soft palate above the base of the tongue

vaccine a suspension of killed, attenuated, or living microorganisms administered to prevent or treat an infectious disease
vagina the canal of the female reproductive tract
vaginal diaphragm a round rubber cup inserted over the cervix of the uterus for contraception
vaginal orifice the external opening of the vagina
vaginal smear vaginal cells placed on a glass slide for laboratory analysis
vaginismus painful, irregular, and involuntary contraction of the muscles around the outer third of the vagina during coitus
Valsalva maneuver forceful exhalation against a closed glottis, which increases intrathoracic pressure and thus interferes with venous return to the heart
value something of worth; a belief held dearly by a person
values clarification a process by which individuals define their own values
vaporization evaporation; conversion of a solid or liquid into a gas (vapor)
varicosity the state of having swollen, distended, and knotted veins, especially in the legs
vas deferens a long tube that extends from the scrotum, curves around the urinary bladder, and empties into the ejaculatory ducts
vasectomy ligation and cutting of the vas deferens, rendering the male sterile
vasoconstriction a decrease in the caliber (lumen) of blood vessels
vasodilation an increase in the caliber (lumen) of blood vessels
vasospasm spasm or constriction of the blood vessels
vector an insect or other animal that transfers pathogens from one host to another
vehicle a transporting agent or medium
vellus fine, nonpigmented body hair
venereal disease *see* sexually transmitted disease
ventilation the movement of air; the act of breathing
ventral of, toward, or at the front; anterior
ventricle a small cavity, such as those located in the brain or the heart
ventriculogram an x-ray film of the ventricles of the brain taken after the introduction of an opaque medium
ventriculography radiologic examination of the ventricles of the brain following the insertion of air or a radiopaque medium
verbal communication communication by the spoken or written word
verdict (legal) the outcome of a trial rendered by a jury
vermin external animal parasites, e.g., ticks, lice, and fleas
vernix caseosa the white, cheesy, greasy, protective material found on the skin of newborns
vertex the top of the head
vertigo dizziness
vesicular sounds normal, quiet, rustling or swishing respiratory sounds heard over the terminal bronchioles and alveoli during auscultation
vestibule a space or cavity at the entrance to a canal; the cleft between the labia containing the vaginal and urethral orifices, hymen, and openings of several ducts
viable fetus a fetus capable of extrauterine life
vial a glass medication container with a sealed rubber cap, for single or multiple doses

vibration a rapid agitation of the hands while pressing on a body area
violence exertion of physical force to injure or abuse
virulence ability to produce disease
virus minute infectious agents smaller than bacteria
viscera large interior organs in body cavities, e.g., the liver and stomach (singular: viscus)
visceral referring to viscera
visceral pain pain originating in the viscera
viscosity the quality of being viscous
viscous thick, sticky
visible poverty lack of money or material resources
visual relating to the sense of sight
vital capacity a lung capacity; the tidal volume plus the inspiratory reserve volume and the expiratory reserve volume
vital (cardinal) signs measurements of physiologic functioning, specifically temperature, pulse, respirations, and blood pressure
vitamins organic chemical substances found in food and essential for normal metabolism and life
vocal resonance vibrations of the larynx transmitted during speech through the respiratory system to the chest wall
void urinate, micturate
volatile evaporating readily
vomitus material vomited; emesis
voodoo the practice of witchcraft or magic
vulva the external female genitals that surround the vaginal orifice and the urethra; also called the *pudendum*

walker a metal, rectangular frame used as an aid to ambulation
weight the heaviness of a body or object, normally measured in kilograms or pounds
wheal *see* bleb
wheeze a whistling sound on exhalation that usually indicates narrowing of the bronchial air passages
will a declaration of how a person wishes to distribute his or her property after death

xiphoid process the lower portion of the sternum
x-rays electromagnetic radiations with extremely short wavelengths

yang in Chinese folk medicine, a positive force that regulates health; it represents the male, warmth, light, and fullness
yin in Chinese folk medicine, a negative force that regulates health; it represents the female, coldness, darkness, and emptiness

zygote the fertilized ovum

Index

weaknesses in nursing education pointed out in the Goldmark Report, recommended graduate instead of student nursing staffs, and called for public support of nursing education.

1939 Graduate School of Midwifery created by the Frontier Nursing Service, Hyden, Kentucky.

1940 Formation of the Nursing Council on National Defense (retitled the National Nursing Council for War Service [NNCWS] in 1941), with representation from major nursing organizations and nursing service agencies, to unify all nursing activities directly or indirectly related to war.

1942 Committee appointed to develop what became the State Board Test Pool Examination (SBTPE). By 1950 all states were using the SBTPE.

—American Association of Industrial Nurses (now the American Association of Occupational Health Nurses) formed.

1943 United States Cadet Nurse Corps established. Through this corps, the federal government subsidized the cost of nursing education, in accelerated programs, for all students agreeing to serve after graduation in civilian or military nursing services for the duration of the war. It was discontinued in 1945.

1946 ANA adopted its economic security (now economic and general welfare) program legitimizing collective bargaining for nurses through their state nurses' associations.

1947 Passage of the Taft-Hartley Act, exempting nonprofit hospitals and other charitable institutions from the obligation to bargain collectively with their employees.

1948 Publication of *Nursing for the future*, report of a far-reaching study of "who would organize, administer, and finance *professional* schools of nursing." Commissioned by the National Nursing Council for War Services and carried out by anthropologist Esther Lucile Brown, the report recommended, among other things, that education for nursing belonged in colleges and universities, not in hospitals.

—NLNE formally established the National Nursing Accrediting Service for nursing educational programs.

—Nationwide movement toward "team nursing" started at Hartford Hospital, Connecticut.

—Metropolitan Demonstration School of Nursing in Windsor, Ontario, operated a 2-year nursing education program (from 1948 to 1952). The Lord Report in 1952 concluded that nurses could be trained at least as satisfactorily in 2 years as in 3 years.

1949 United States Air Force Nurse Corps created.

1950–53 United States nurses served in the Korean war, in Mobile Army Surgical Hospitals (M.A.S.H.).

1951 National Association of Colored Graduate Nurses dissolved itself, to be absorbed into the ANA.

1952 After years of study, the nursing profession in the United States was restructured into two national organizations: the ANA, which remained the membership organization, and the newly formed National League for Nursing (NLN), merging the former NLNE, NOPHN, and ACSN.

—Associate degree education for nursing begun in an experimental project at Teachers College, Columbia University, New York.

—*Nursing Research* launched due to the efforts of the ACSN.

1953 National Student Nurses' Association (NSNA) founded.

—United States Department of Health, Education, and Welfare (DHEW) created. It became the Department of Health and Human Services (DHHS) in 1980.

1954 Association of Operating Room Nurses formed.

1955 American Nurses' Foundation established by the ANA for research purposes.

1956 Federal nurse traineeship program established to aid registered nurses in advanced study.

1960 Publication of *Spotlight on nursing education* by Helen K. Mussallem, report of a pilot project for the evaluation of schools of nursing in Canada.

1963 Publication of *Toward quality in nursing*, report of the Surgeon General's Consultant Group in Nursing, another study of nursing and nursing education that projected the need for more and better prepared nurses.

1964 Ryerson Polytechnical Institute, Toronto, started the first diploma nursing program in Canada within a college institution.

—First Nurse Training Act allocated federal aid for nursing education in the United States.